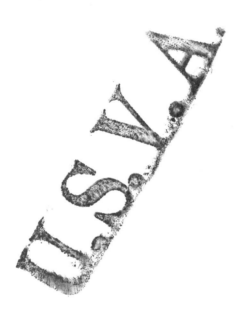

U.S.A.

MW01170340

CURRENT OCULAR THERAPY

CURRENT OCULAR THERAPY 4

FREDERICK T. FRAUNFELDER, M.D.

Professor and Chairman, Department of Ophthalmology,
Oregon Health Sciences University, Casey Eye Institute
Portland, Oregon

F. HAMPTON ROY, M.D., F.A.C.S.

Clinical Associate Professor, Department of Ophthalmology,
University of Arkansas for Medical Sciences;
Baptist Medical Center, Arkansas Children's Hospital;
Doctor's Hospital, St. Vincent Infirmary, Freeway Medical Center,
Little Rock, Arkansas

Associate Editor:

JOAN GROVE
Department of Ophthalmology, Casey Eye Institute
Oregon Health Sciences University,
Portland, Oregon

W. B. SAUNDERS COMPANY
A Division of Harcourt Brace & Company

Philadelphia, London, Toronto, Montreal, Sydney, Tokyo

W. B. SAUNDERS COMPANY
A Division of Harcourt Brace & Company
The Curtis Center
Independence Square West
Philadelphia, PA 19106

NOTICE

The authors and editors of this book have been careful to ensure that drug recommendations are precise and in agreement with standards officially accepted at the time of publication.

It does happen, however, that dosage schedules are changed from time to time in the light of accumulating clinical experience and continuing laboratory studies. This is most likely to occur in the case of recently introduced products.

It is essential that you check the manufacturer's warnings and recommendations for dosage, especially if the drug to be administered or prescribed is one that you use only infrequently or have not used for some time.

THE PUBLISHER

Library of Congress Cataloging in Publication Data

Fraunfelder, FT

Current ocular therapy.

1. Therapeutics Ophthalmological. 2. Ocular
   pharmacology. I. Roy, Frederick Hampton, joint author.
   II. Meyer, S. Martha. III. Title [DNLM: 1. Eye
   diseases—Complications. 2. Eye diseases—Therapy.
   3. Eye manifestations. WW140 F845c]
RE991.F75   617.7'06   79-66715
ISBN   0-7216-4913-0

CURRENT OCULAR THERAPY 4   ISBN   0-7216-4913-0

Copyright © 1995, 1990, 1985, 1980 by W. B. Saunders Company.

Printed in the United States of America.

Last digit is the print number: 9   8   7   6   5   4   3   2   1

CONTRIBUTORS

RICHARD L. ABBOTT, M.D.

Clinical Professor and Director, Corneal and External Disease Service, Department of Ophthalmology, California Pacific Medical Center, San Francisco, California

Erysipelas

ROBERT ABEL, JR., M.D.

Clinical Professor of Opthalmology, Thomas Jefferson University, Senior Staff, Medical Center of Delaware; Senior Staff, St. Francis Hospital; Consulting Staff, Wills Eye Hospital, Philadelphia, Pennsylvania

Allergic Conjunctivitis; Epidemic Keratoconjunctivitis; Keratoconus

IRA A. ABRAHAMSON, M.D.

Associate Professor of Ophthalmology, Assistant Clinical Professor of Family Medicine, University of Cincinnati College of Medicine, Cincinnati, Ohio

Mucocele

WILLIAM A. AGGER, M.D.

Chief, Infectious Disease Section, Gundersen Clinic; Director of Microbiology, Lutheran Hospital, La Crosse, Wisconsin

Sporotrichosis

GARY L. AGUILAR, M.D.

Assistant Clinical Professor of Ophthalmology, University of California, San Francisco, California; Assistant Clinical Professor of Ophthalmology, Stanford University, Stanford, California

Floppy Eyelid Syndrome

AMY AIELLO, M.D.

Active staff of Phoenix Children's Hospital, St. Joseph's Hospital, Phoenix, Arizona

Brown's Syndrome; Marcus Gunn Syndrome

MATHEA R. ALLANSMITH, M.D.

Associate Professor of Ophthalmology, Harvard Medical School, Boston, Massachusetts

Phlyctenulosis

ROY D. ALTMAN, M.D.

Professor of Medicine, University of Miami School of Medicine; Director, Clinical Research, GRECC, and Chief, Arthritis Section, Miami Veteran Affairs Medical Center, Miami, Florida

Angioid Streaks

DUNCAN P. ANDERSON, M.D., F.R.C.S.(C)

Associate Professor of Ophthalmology and Head, Department of Neuro-Ophthalmology, University of British Columbia; Head, Department of Ophthalmology, St. Paul's Hospital, Vancouver, Canada

Meningioma

RICHARD L. ANDERSON, M.D., F.A.C.S.

Professor of Ophthalmology, Chief, Division of Ophthalmic Plastic and Orbital Surgery, University of Utah School of Medicine, Moran Eye Center, Salt Lake City, Utah

Distichiasis; Hypertrichosis

DAVID J. APPLE, M.D.

Professor and Chairman, Department of Ophthalmology; Medical Staff, MUSC Medical Center, Medical University of South Carolina, Charleston, South Carolina

Histiocytosis X

BUDD APPLETON, M.D.

Clinical Professor of Ophthalmology, University of Minnesota School of Medicine; Active staff of St. Paul Ramey Medical Center, and United Hospital, St. Paul, Minnesota

Radiation

LEONARD APT, M.D.

Professor of Ophthalmology; Director Emeritus of the Division of Pediatric Ophthalmology, Jules Stein Eye Institute, University of California School of Medicine, Los Angeles, California

Medulloepithelioma

JAMES V. AQUAVELLA, M.D.

Clinical Professor of Ophthalmology; Director, Cornea Research Laboratory, University of Rochester Medical School, Rochester, New York

Scleromalacia Perforans

ANTHONY C. ARNOLD, M.D.

Associate Professor of Clinical Ophthalmology; Chief, Neuro-Ophthalmology Division, Jules Stein Eye Institute, UCLA School of Medicine, Los Angeles, California

Multiple Sclerosis

KERRY K. ASSIL, M.D.

Assistant Professor of Ophthalmology, Anheuser-Busch Eye Institute, St. Louis, Missouri

Corneal and Conjunctival Calcifications; Herpes Simplex

C. SCOTT ATKINSON, M.D.

Assistant Clinical Professor, University of Pittsburgh, Pittsburgh, Pennsylvania

Congenital and Infantile Cataracts

FELICIA B. AXELROD, M.D.

Professor of Pediatrics and Neurology, New York University School of Medicine, New York, New York

Familial Dysautonomia

PAUL R. BADENOCH, Ph.D.

Senior Hospital Scientist, Department of Ophthalmology, Flinders Medical Centre, Bedford Park, South Australia

Bacterial Conjunctivitis; Bacterial Corneal Ulcers

ANN M. BAJART, M.D., F.A.C.S.

Clinical Instructor in Ophthalmology, Harvard Medical School; Assistant Clinical Professor of Ophthalmology, Tufts New England Medical Center; Surgeon in Ophthalmology, Massachusetts Eye and Ear Infirmary, Boston, Massachusetts

Phlyctenulosis

ANTHONY L. BARBATO, M.D.

Professor of Medicine, Stritch School of Medicine; Executive Vice President for the Medical Center, Loyola University Medical Center, Maywood, Illinois

Hypocalcemia

SUSAN BARKAY, M.D.

Former Head, Department of Ophthalmology, Central Emek Hospital, Afula, Israel

Leptospirosis

SOREN S. BARNER, M.D., M.D.O.S.

Professor of Ophthalmology, Institute for Experimental Research in Surgery, University of Copenhagen; Lecturer in Ophthalmology, Gentofte University Hospital, Copenhagen, Denmark

Astigmatism

JAMES M. BARNETT, M.D.

Consultant, Hackley Hospital and Mercy Hospital, Muskegon, Michigan

Loiasis

GARY P. BARTH, M.D.

Assistant Clinical Professor of Ophthalmology, UCSF; Active Staff, Santa Rosa Memorial Hospital, Santa Rosa, California

Aspergillosis

CHRISTINE E. P- BARTOS, M.D.

Resident, University of Iowa, Iowa City, Iowa; Private Practice, Reed Eye Associates, Pittsford, New York

Central Serous Chorioretinopathy

WILLIAM L. BASUK, M.D.

Active Staff, Pomerado Hospital and North County Ophthalmology, Poway, California

Idiopathic Intracranial Hypertension and Pseudotumor Cerebri

JULES BAUM, M.D.

Research Professor of Ophthalmology, University School of Medicine, Tufts University, Boston Eye Associates, P.C., Chestnut Hill, Massachusetts

Moraxella

ROBERT H. BEDROSSIAN, M.D., M.Sc.

Clinical Associate Professor in Ophthalmology; Oregon Health Sciences University, Portland, Oregon

Myopia

A. ROBERT BELLOWS, M.D.

Assistant Clinical Professor of Ophthalmology, Harvard Medical School; Surgeon, Massachusetts Eye and Ear Infirmary, Boston, Massachusetts

Choroidal Detachment

VITALIANO B. BERNARDINO, JR., M.D.

Professor of Ophthalmology and Associate Professor of Pathology, Jefferson Medical College of Thomas Jefferson University; Attending Surgeon, Wills Eye Hospital, Philadelphia, Pennsylvania; Active Staff, St. Mary's Hospital, Langhorne, Pennsylvania

Melanocytic Lesions of the Eyelids

ROBERT L. BERRY, M.D.

Assistant Clinical Professor of Ophthalmology, University of Arkansas; Medical Advisor, Arkansas Chapter of the Society to Prevent Blindness, Little Rock, Arkansas

Blindness; Echinococcosis; Malaria; Scrub Typhus

JOHN R. BIERLY, M.D.

Assistant Professor of Ophthalmology, University of Kentucky, Lexington, Kentucky

Ligneous Conjunctivitis

ALBERT W. BIGLAN, M.D., F.A.C.S.

Adjunct Associate Professor of Ophthalmology, University of Pittsburgh School of Medicine, Eye and Ear Hospital, Children's Hospital, Pittsburgh, Pennsylvania

Tetanus

ALAN C. BIRD, M.D., F.R.C.S., F.R.C.Ophth.

Professor of Clinical Ophthalmology, Institute of Ophthalmology, London University and Honorary Consultant Moorfields Eye Hospital, London, England

Onchocerciasis

P. D. BLACK, B.Sc., F.R.C.S., F.R.C.Ophth.

Consultant Ophthalmic Surgeon, James Paget Hospital, Gorleston, Great Yarmouth, Norfolk, England

Cerebral Palsy

RAPHAEL S. BLOCH, M.D., F.A.C.S.

Assistant Clinical Professor of Ophthalmology, Albert Einstein College of Medicine, New York, New York; Attending Ophthalmologist, Northern Westchester Hospital Center, Mount Kisco, New York

Homocystinuria

MARK S. BLUMENKRANZ, M.D.

Clinical Professor of Ophthalmology, Stanford University, Co-Director Retinal Service, Menlo Park, California

Acute Retinal Necrosis

MILTON BONIUK, M.D.

Professor of Ophthalmology, Baylor College of Medicine; Active Staff, Methodist Hospital, St. Luke's Episcopal Hospital; Consulting, V.A. Hospital; Consulting, Texas Children's Hospital, Houston, Texas

Cavernous Sinus Thrombosis

VIVIEN BONIUK, M.D.

Associate Professor of Ophthalmology, Albert Einstein College of Medicine, Long Island Jewish Medical Center; Director of Ophthalmology, Queens Hospital Center, New York, New York

Rubella

S. ARTHUR BORUCHOFF, M.D.

Professor of Ophthalmology; Consultant, University Hospital, Boston University School of Medicine, Boston, Massachusetts

Posterior Polymorphous Corneal Dystrophy

WILLIAM M. BOURNE, M.D.

Professor of Ophthalmology, Mayo Medical School; Active Staff, Rochester Methodist Hospital and St. Marys Hospital, Rochester, Minnesota

Fuchs' Corneal Dystrophy

LAURENCE S. BRAUDE, M.D., F.A.C.S., F.R.C.S.(C)

Clinical Assistant Professor, The University of Illinois College of Medicine at Chicago, Chicago, Illinois; Attending Surgeon, Highland Park Hospital, Highland Park, Illinois

Diphtheria

ROBERT J. BROCKHURST, M.D.

Associate Clinical Professor of Ophthalmology, Harvard Medical School; Surgeon in Ophthalmology, Massachusetts Eye and Ear Infirmary, Boston, Massachusetts

Nanophthalmos

MARK A. BRONSTEIN, M.D.

Assistant Clinical Professor of Ophthalmology, College of Medicine, University of California, Irvine, California

Macular Hole

MARION H. BROOKS, M.D.

Professor of Medicine, Loyola University of Chicago Stritch School of Medicine; Chairman, Department of Medicine, Loyola, University Medical Center, Maywood, Illinois

Hypocalcemia

DONNA D. BROWN, M.D.

Virginia Eye Institute, Active staff of St Mary's Hospital, Richmond, Virginia

Staphyloccocal and Mixed Staphylococcal/Seborrheic Blepharoconjunctivitis

STUART I. BROWN, M.D.

Professor and Chairman, Department of Ophthalmology, University of California, San Diego, California

Ocular Rosacea

JOHN D. BULLOCK, M.D., M.S., F.A.C.S.

Professor and Chairman, Department of Ophthalmology; Professor of Plastic Surgery, Wright State University School of Medicine, Dayton, Ohio

Eyelid Coloboma, Choroidal Folds; Nocardia; Oxalosis; Werner's Syndrome

RAYMOND BUNCIC, M.D., F.R.C.S.(C)

Ophthalmologist in Chief, Hospital for Sick Children, University of Toronto, Toronto, Ontario, Canada

Orbital Hypertelorism

RONALD M. BURDE, M.D.

Professor and Chairman, Department of Ophthalmology, Albert Einstein College of Medicine, Bronx, New York

Idiopathic Intracranial Hypertension and Pseudotumor Cerebri

J. DOUGLAS CAMERON, M.D.

Associate Professor of Ophthalmology and Pathology, University of Minnesota, Hennepin County Medical School, Minneapolis, Minnesota

Acrodermatitis Enteropathica

DAVID G. CAMPBELL, M.D.

Professor of Ophthalmology, Dartmouth-Hitchcock Medical Center, Hanover, New Hampshire; Director of Glaucoma Service, Dartmouth-Hitchcock Medical Center, Lebanon, New Hampshire

Ghost Cell Glaucoma; Pigmentary Glaucoma

VICKY CEVALLOS, M.T. (A.S.C.P.)

Ocular Microbiologist, Francis I. Proctor Foundation, University of California, San Francisco, California

Pneumococcus

JOHN W. CHANDLER, M.D.

Professor and Head, Department of Ophthalmology and Visual Sciences, College of Medicine, University of Illinois at Chicago, Chicago, Illinois

Diphtheria

SURESH R. CHANDRA, M.D.

Professor of Ophthalmology, University of Wisconsin Medical School Staff, University Hospital; Consultant, V.A. Hospital and Freeport Hospital, Madison, Wisconsin

Diabetes Mellitus

DEVRON H. CHAR, M.D.

Professor, Departments of Ophthalmology, Radiation Oncology, and the Francis I. Proctor Foundation; Director, Ocular Oncology Unit, University of California School of Medicine, San Francisco, California

Neuroblastoma; Orbital Metastases

STEVE CHARLES, M.D.

Clinical Professor of Ophthalmology, University of Tennessee Center for Health Sciences, Memphis, Tennessee

Proliferative Vitreoretinopathy

RICHARD M. CHAVIS, M.D.

Clinical Assistant Professor of Ophthalmology, Georgetown University Medical Center, Washington, District of Columbia

Liposarcoma

MICHAEL CHERINGTON, M.D.

Clinical Professor of Neurology, University of Colorado School of Medicine; Chairman, Lightning Data Center, St. Anthony Hospital, Denver, Colorado

Botulism

GEORGE N. CHIN, M.D., F.A.C.S.

Active Staff, Northwest Hospital, Seattle, Washington

Typhoid Fever

STEVEN S. T. CHING, M.D.

Associate Professor of Ophthalmology, University of Rochester School of Medicine; Attending Strong Memorial Hospital, University of Rochester, Rochester, New York

Infectious Mononucleosis

LAURIE E. CHRISTENSEN, M.D.

Assistant Professor of Ophthalmology, Department of Ophthalmology, Casey Eye Institute, Portland, Oregon

Ophthalmia Neonatorum

LEONARD CHRISTENSEN, M.D.

Professor of Ophthalmology, Oregon Health Sciences University, Portland, Oregon; Retired

Iris Bombé

STEPHEN P. CHRISTIANSEN, M.D.

Assistant Professor of Ophthalmology, Jones Eye Institute, University of Arkansas for Medical Sciences; Active Staff, Arkansas Children's Hospital, The University Hospital of Arkansas, and John L. McClellan Memorial V.A. Hospital, Little Rock, Arkansas

Robin Sequence; Tyrosinemia II

GEORGE A. CIOFFI, M.D.

Active Staff, Legacy Health Systems, St. Vincent Hospital, and SW Washington Hospitals, Devers Eye Institute, Portland, Oregon

Glaucoma Associated with Intraocular Lenses

GREGORY L. COHEN, B.S.

Medical Student, New York Medical College, Valhalla, New York

Macular Hole

WILLIAM H. COLES, M.D., M.S.

Professor and Chairman, Department of Ophthalmology, State University of New York Health Science Center; Clinical Director, Erie County Medical Center, Buffalo, New York

Cockayne's Syndrome; Indirect Global Ruptures and Sharp Scleral Injuries

DAVID R. CORNBLATH, M.D.

Associate Professor of Neurology, Johns Hopkins University School of Medicine; Active Staff, Johns Hopkins Hospital, Baltimore, Maryland

Myasthenia Gravis

DOUGLAS J. COSTER, F.R.C.S.

Professor of Ophthalmology, Flinders Medical Center, Bedford Park, Adelaide, South Australia

Bacterial Conjunctivitis; Bacterial Corneal Ulcers

DAVID E. COWEN, M.D.

Assistant Professor, Ophthalmic Plastic and Reconstructive Surgery; Director, Orbital and Lacrimal Service, University of Kentucky College of Medicine, Lexington, Kentucky

Alacrima

J. BROOKS CRAWFORD, M.D.

Clinical Professor of Ophthalmology, University of California, San Francisco, California

Keratoacanthoma

R. PITTS CRICK, F.R.C.S.(Eng), F.R.C.Ophth.

Emeritus Lecturer in Ophthalmology, School of Medicine and Dentistry of King's College and Honorary Consultant Ophthalmic Surgeon, King's College Hospital, London, England

Uveoparotid Fever

HAROLD E. CROSS, M.D. Ph.D.

Clinical Assistant Professor of Surgery, University of Arizona Health Sciences Center; Tucson, Arizona

Microspherophakia

LUIZ CARLOS CUCÉ, M.D.

Professor and Chairman, Department of Dermatology, School of Medicine of São Paulo, São Paulo, Brazil

American Mucocutaneous Leishmaniasis

RICHARD D. CUNNINGHAM, M.D., M.S.

Professor, Division of Ophthalmology, Scott and White Clinic, Texas A & M University College of Medicine and Texas A & M University Health Science Center; Senior Consultant, Scott and White Hospital; Consultant, Olin Teague Veterans Administration Hospital, Temple, Texas

Lacrimal Gland Tumors

ROBERT A. D'AMICO, M.D.

Clinical Professor of Ophthalmology, New York University School of Medicine; Chairman of Ophthalmology, St. Vincent's Hospital and Medical Center, Bayley Seton Hospital, and Cabrini Medical Center, New York, New York

Familial Dysautonomia

ROGER A. DAILEY, M.D.

Assistant Professor of Ophthalmology, Casey Eye Institute, Oregon Health Sciences University, Portland, Oregon

Dacryocystitis; Entropion; Epicanthus; Marcus Gunn Syndrome; Optic Foramen Fractures; Sebaceous Gland Carcinoma

LOUIS DAILY, M.D., Ph.D.(Ophth.)

Clinical Associate Professor of Ophthalmology, Baylor College of Medicine; Senior Attending in Ophthalmology, The Methodist Hospital, Houston, Texas

Retinoschisis

STUART R. DANKNER, M.D., F.A.C.S.

Assistant Professor of Ophthalmology, Johns Hopkins School of Medicine; Director, Pediatric Ophthalmology Service, Sinai Hospital; Attending Staff, GBMC, Baltimore, Maryland

Acquired Nonaccommodative Esotropia

S. DAROUGAR, M.D., D.T.M.&H., F.R.C.Path, D.Sc.

Emeritus Professor, University of London; Director, Preventive Medicine Research Unit, I.O. International Ltd., London, England

Trachoma

FREDERICK H. DAVIDORF, M.D.

Professor of Ophthalmology; Director, Vitreo-Retinal Division, The Ohio State University College of Medicine, Columbus, Ohio

Ocular Metastatic Tumors

HOLLY W. DAVIS, M.D.

Associate Professor of Pediatrics, University of Pittsburgh School of Medicine; Director, Pediatric Emergency Medicine, Children's Hospital of Pittsburgh, Pittsburgh, Pennsylvania

Tetanus

CHANDLER R. DAWSON, M.D.

Professor of Ophthalmology, University of California, Director, Francis I. Proctor Foundation for Research in Ophthalmology; Attending Physician, UCSF Hospital, San Francisco, California

Inclusion Conjunctivitis; Pharyngoconjunctival Fever

RONALD E. DEI CAS, M.D.

Fellow, Oculoplastic and Reconstructive Surgery, Children's Hospital of Philadelphia, Philadelphia, Pennsylvania

Liposarcoma

NICK W. H. M. DEKKERS, M.D.

Ophthalmologist, St. Elizabeth Hospital, Tilburg, The Netherlands

Rubeola

ROBERT C. DELLA ROCCA, M.D., F.A.C.S.

Surgeon Director, Ophthalmic Plastic, Reconstructive, and Orbital Service, New York Eye and Ear Infirmary, New York, New York; Clinical Professor of Ophthalmology, New York Medical College, Valhalla, New York

Eyelid Contusions, Lacerations, and Avulsions

BEATRICE M. DIAS, M.D.

Fellow, Dermatology, Memorial Sloan-Kettering Cancer Center, New York, New York

Kaposi's Sarcoma

ANGELO M. DIGEORGE, M.D.

Emeritus Professor of Ophthalmology, Temple University Health Sciences Center, Philadelphia, Pennsylvania

Waardenburg's Syndrome

A. LUISA DILORENZO, M.D., B.S.

Chief Resident, Kresge Eye Institute, Wayne State University, Detroit, Michigan

Tuberculosis

PETER J. DOLMAN, M.D., F.R.C.S.(C)

Clinical Assistant Professor, Department of Ophthalmology, University of British Columbia; Oculoplastic Surgeon, Vancouver General Hospital, Vancouver, British Columbia, Canada

Nonspecific Orbital Inflammatory Syndromes

GEORGE N. DONNELL, M.D.

Emeritus Professor, University of Southern California School of Medicine, Los Angeles, California

Galactosemias

JOHN J. DONNELLY, Ph.D.

Department of Ophthalmology, Scheie Eye Institute, Philadelphia, Pennsylvania

Ascariasis

DONALD J. DOUGHMAN, M.D.

Professor, Department of Ophthalmology, University of Minnesota Health Sciences Center, Minneapolis, Minnesota

Acrodermatitis Enteropathica

STEPHEN M. DRANCE, M.D.

Emeritus Professor of Ophthalmology, Department of Ophthalmology, University of British Columbia; Active Staff, Vancouver Hospital and Health Sciences Center, Vancouver, British Columbia, Canada

Low-Tension Glaucoma

MARK S. DRESNER, M.D., F.A.C.S.

Division Chief, Ophthalmology, Palm Beaches Medical Center; Active Staff, Good Samaritan Medical Center and St. Mary's Hospital, West Palm Beach, Florida

Herpes Simplex; Pellucid Marginal Corneal Degeneration

ROBERT C. DREWS, M.D., F.R.C.Ophth.

Professor of Clinical Ophthalmology, Washington University School of Medicine; Active Staff, Barnes Hospital and Bethesda General Hospital, St. Louis, Missouri

Adult Cataracts

ROBERT M. DRYDEN, M.D., F.A.C.S.

Clinical Professor of Ophthalmology, Department of Ophthalmology, University of Arizona, Tucson, Arizona

Periocular Squamous Cell Carcinoma

STEVEN P. DUNN, M.D.

Assistant Clinical Professor, Oakland University, Rochester, Michigan; Director Corneal and External Disease Service, William Beaumont Hospital, Royal Oak, Michigan

Amyloidosis

HOWARD M. EGGERS, M.D.

Associate Professor of Clinical Ophthalmology, Columbia University; Associate Attending, The Presbyterian Hospital, New York, NY

Oculomotor (Third Nerve) Paralysis

MICHAEL D. EICHLER, M.D.

Fellow, Oregon Health Sciences, University Internal Medicine, Tigard, Oregon

Lymphoid Tumors

MEDHAT M. EL HENNAWI, M.Ch.(Ophth.)

Professor of Ophthalmology, Faculty of Medicine, University of Alexandria, Alexandria, Egypt

Vernal Keratoconjunctivitis

RICHARD ELANDER, M.D.

Clinical Professor of Ophthalmology, Jules Stein Eye Institute, University of California School of Medicine, Los Angeles, California

Myopia

PHILIP P. ELLIS, M.D.

Professor and Chairman, Department of Ophthalmology, University of Colorado Health Sciences Center, Denver, Colorado

Intraocular Foreign Body—Steel or Iron

ROBERT M. ELLSWORTH, M.D.*

Former Emeritus Professor, Department of Ophthalmology, New York Hospital, Cornell Medical College, New York, New York

Retinoblastoma

ROY J. ELLSWORTH, M.D.

Ophthalmologist; Active Staff, St. Alphonsus Hospital; Medical Director, Lions Eye Bank, Boise, Idaho

Rabies

FRANK P. ENGLISH, F.R.A.C.O., F.R.C.S.

Australian Government Consultant Ophthalmologist and Research Associate, Queensland Institute Medical Research, Brisbane, Australia

Demodicosis

DAVID L. EPSTEIN, M.D.

Professor and Chairman of Ophthalmology, Department of Ophthalmology, Duke University Hospital, Durham, North Carolina

Lens-Induced Glaucoma

EDWARD EPSTEIN M.B., Ch.B., D.O.M.S.

Consultant Ophthalmologist, Boksburg Hospital, Johannesburg, South Africa

Coenurosis

WILLIAM L. EPSTEIN, M.D.

Professor of Dermatology, University of California, San Francisco, California

Poison Ivy, Oak, or Sumac Dermatitis

JOSEPH ESHAGIAN, M.D.

Clinical Instructor, Queen of Angels Hollywood Presbyterian Medical Center; Staff Ophthalmologist, St. Vincent's Hospital, Los Angeles, California

Chronic Progressive External Ophthalmoplegia

ROGER A. EWALD, M.D.

Clinical Assistant Professor, University of Illinois College of Medicine; Attending Staff, Carle Clinic, Urbana, Illinois

Solar Retinopathy

FUÁD S. FARAH, M.D.

Professor of Medicine, Chief of the Section of Dermatology, State University of New York Health Science Center, Syracuse, New York

Cutaneous Leishmaniasis

BISHARA M. FARIS, M.D., F.A.C.S.

Clinical Professor of Ophthalmology, Boston University School of Medicine; Lecturer on Ophthalmology, Harvard Faculty of Medicine, Boston, Massachusetts

Scleral Staphyloma and Dehiscences

MARIANNE E. FEITL, M.D.

Assistant Professor of Ophthalmology, University of Chicago; Active Staff, University of Chicago Hospital, Chicago, Illinois

Juvenile Glaucoma

STEPHEN S. FEMAN, M.D.

Professor of Ophthalmology, School of Medicine Vanderbilt University Medical Center, Nashville, Tennessee

Thalassemia

T. J. FFYTCHE, F.R.C.S., F.R.C.Ophth.

Consultant Ophthalmic Surgeon, St. Thomas's Hospital, Moorfields Eye Hospital, and Hospital for Tropical Diseases, London, England

Leprosy

ERIN S. FOGEL, M.D.

Assistant Instructor of Ophthalmology, Medical College of Wisconsin, Milwaukee, Wisconsin

Lattice Corneal Dystrophy

JAMES C. FOLK, M.D.

Professor of Ophthalmology, College of Medicine; Vitreo-Retinal Service, The University of Iowa Hospitals and Clinics, Iowa City, Iowa

Central Serous Chorioretinopathy; The White Dot Syndromes

RICHARD K. FORSTER, M.D.

Professor of Ophthalmology, Bascom Palmer Eye Institute, Department of Ophthalmology, University of Miami School of Medicine, Miami, Florida

Bacterial Endophthalmitis

C. STEPHEN FOSTER, M.D., F.A.C.S.

Professor of Ophthalmology, Harvard Medical School; Director Immunology Service, Massachusetts Eye and Ear Infirmary, Boston, Massachusetts

Candidiasis

ROBERT E. FOSTER, M.D.

Associate Staff, Cleveland Clinic Foundation, Division of Ophthalmology, Cleveland, Ohio

Branch Retinal Vein Occlusion

---

* Deceased

F. T. FRAUNFELDER, M.D.

Professor and Chairman of Ophthalmology, Oregon Health Sciences University; Director, Casey Eye Institute, Portland, Oregon

Conjunctival, Corneal or Scleral Cysts; Conjunctival or Corneal Intraepithelial Neoplasia (CIN) and Squamous Cell Carcinoma; Electrical Injury; Erythema Multiforme Major; Hemophilus Influenzae; Hordeolum; Hypothermal Injury; Lymphoid Tumors; Mycosis Fungoides; Schistosomiasis; Trichiasis; Xanthelasma

F. W. FRAUNFELDER, M.D.

Intern, Providence Medical Center, Portland, Oregon

Erythema Multiforme Major; Hypothermal Injury; Schistosomiasis

JEFFREY FREEDMAN, M.B., B.Ch., Ph.D., F.R.C.S.E.

Professor of Clinical Ophthalmology, State University of New York Health Science Center, Brooklyn, New York

Xeroderma Pigmentosum

H. MACKENZIE FREEMAN, M.D.

Associate Clinical Professor of Ophthalmology, Harvard Medical School; Surgeon, Massachusetts Eye and Ear Infirmary, Boston, Massachusetts

Peripheral Retinal Breaks and Degeneration; Scleral Staphyloma and Dehiscences

MITCHELL H. FRIEDLAENDER, M.D.

Director, Cornea and Refractive Surgery, Division of Ophthalmology, Scripps Clinic and Research Foundation, La Jolla, California

Atopic Dermatitis; Contact Dermatitis; Urticaria and Hereditary Angioedema

ALAN H. FRIEDMAN, M.D.

Clinical Professor of Ophthalmology and Pathology, Department of Ophthalmology, Mount Sinai School of Medicine, New York, New York

Vogt-Koyanagi-Harada Syndrome

JOSEPH FRUCHT-PERY, M.D.

Senior Lecturer, Hadassah University Hospital and Hebrew University; Head, Cornea Service, Department of Ophthalmology, Hadassah University Hospital, Jerusalem, Israel

Ocular Rosacea

WAYNE E. FUNG, M.D.

Clinical Professor of Ophthalmology, Department of Ophthalmology, California Pacific Medical Center, San Francisco, California

Cystoid Macular Edema

DONALD A. GAGLIANO, M.D.

Chief of Ophthalmology, U.S. Army Medical Research Detachment, Division of Ocular Hazards; Assistant Clinical Professor of Surgery, Uniformed Services, University of Health Sciences, Brooks AFB, Texas

Sickle Cell Disease

STEPHEN GANCHER, M.D.

Associate Professor, Department of Neurology, Oregon Health Sciences University; Active Staff, University Hospital and VA Medical Center, Portland, Oregon

Parkinson's Disease

JAMES P. GANLEY, M.D., Dr. P.H.

Professor and Chairman, Department of Ophthalmology, Louisiana State University Medical Center, Shreveport, Louisiana

Coccidioidomycosis

MARK S. GANS, M.D.

Assistant Professor, Department of Ophthalmology, McGill University, Montreal, Quebec, Canada

Idiopathic Intracranial Hypertension and Pseudotumor Cerebri

HERBERT J. GERSHEN, M.D.

Active staff, Kaiser Foundation Hospitals, San Francisco and Hayward, California

Chalazion

GRANT GILLILAND, M.D.

Assistant Clinical Professor of Ophthalmology, University of Texas Southwestern Medical School; Active Staff, Baylor University Medical Center, Parkland Hospital, Children's Medical Center, Dallas, Texas

Sebaceous Gland Carcinoma

WILLIAM B. GLEW, M.D.

Senior Attending Surgeon and Ophthalmology Department Chair, Washington Hospital Center; Associate Professor of Ophthalmology, George Washington University School of Medicine, Washington, District of Columbia

Psoriasis

KENNETH M. GOINS, M.D.

Assistant Professor Cornea and Refractive Diseases, Visual Sciences Center, University of Chicago, Chicago, Illinois

Ichthyosis

DANIEL H. GOLD, M.D.

Clinical Professor of Ophthalmology, Department of Ophthalmology, University of Texas Medical Branch, Galveston, Texas

Sarcoidosis

MICHAEL H. GOLDBAUM, M.D.

Associate Professor of Ophthalmology, Department of Ophthalmology, University of California; Director of Ophthalmology, Servie, V.A. Medical Center, Co-Director, Retina-Vitreous Service, San Diego, California

Central or Branch Retinal Artery Occlusion

STUART H. GOLDBERG, M.D.

Associate Professor of Ophthalmology, Department of Ophthalmology, Penn State University College of Medicine, Hershey, Pennsylvania

Eyelid Coloboma; Nocardia; Werner's Syndrome

JEROME N. GOLDMAN, M.D., F.A.C.S.

Associate Clinical Professor of Ophthalmology, Center for Sight, Georgetown University Medical Center, Washington, District of Columbia

Acquired Syphilis; Congenital Syphilis

GEORGE M. GOMBOS, M.D., F.A.C.S.

Emeritus Professor, State University of New York, Health Science Center at Brooklyn; Chief of Ophthalmology, Veterans Administration Medical Center, Brooklyn, New York

Traumatic Cataract

ERNESTO GONZALEZ, M.D.

Associate Professor of Dermatology, Harvard Medical School; Dermatologist, Massachusetts General Hospital, Boston, Massachusetts

Photosensitivity and Sunburn

BAIRD S. GRIMSON, M.D.

Professor of Ophthalmology and Neuro-Ophthalmology, University of North Carolina School of Medicine, Chapel Hill, North Carolina

Cluster Headache; Trigeminal Neuralgia

LEWIS R. GRODEN, M.D.

Clinical Associate Professor of Ophthalmology, Department of Ophthalmology, University of South Florida School of Medicine; Active Staff; University Community Hospital, Tampa, Florida

Molluscum Contagiosum

STUART A. GROSSMAN, M.D.

Director, Neuro-Oncology; Associate Professor of Oncology, Medicine and Neurosurgery, Johns Hopkins University School of Medicine; Active Staff, Johns Hopkins Hospital, Baltimore, Maryland

Hodgkin's Disease

ARTHUR S. GROVE, JR., M.D.

Assistant Professor of Ophthalmology, Harvard Medical School; Director of Orbital and Plastic Surgery, Massachusetts Eye and Ear Infirmary, Boston, Massachusetts

Dermoid

ROBERTO GUERRA, M.D.

Professor of Ophthalmology; Head, Institute of Clinical Ophthalmology, University of Modena Medical School; Active Staff, University of Modena Medical School Hospital, Eye Clinic, Modena, Italy

Drug-Induced Optic Atrophy

FRONCIE A. GUTMAN, M.D.

Senior Consultant, Division of Ophthalmology, Cleveland Clinic Foundation; Associate Clinical Professor of Ophthalmology, Case Western Reserve University School of Medicine; Active Staff, Cleveland Clinic Foundation, Cleveland, Ohio

Branch Retinal Vein Occlusion

HESKEL M. HADDAD, M.D.

Clinical Professor of Ophthalmology, New York Medical College, Attending, Beth Israel Hospital North, New York, New York

Hypothyroidism

WILLIAM S. HAGLER, M.D.

Associate Professor of Ophthalmology, Emory University School of Medicine, Atlanta, Georgia; Clinical Associate Professor of Ophthalmology, Medical College of Georgia, Augusta, Georgia

Toxocariasis

BARRETT G. HAIK, M.D.

Professor of Ophthalmology; Clinical Professor of Pediatrics, Tulane University School of Medicine; Director of Ophthalmic Oncology and Orbital Disease, Tulane University School of Medicine, New Orleans, Louisiana

Capillary Hemangioma; Cavernous Hemangioma

MICHAEL HALSTED, M.D.

Private Practice, Eye Physicians Omaha, Omaha, Nebraska

Seborrheic Blepharitis

KAY-UWE HAMANN, M.D.

Lecturer for Neuro-ophthalmology, University Eye Hospital (Privatdozent for Neuro-ophthalmology, University Hospital Hamburg), Hamburg, Germany

Acute Idiopathic Polyneuritis

HIRAM H. HARDESTY, M.D.

Emeritus Associate Clinical Professor, Case Western Reserve University School of Medicine; Emeritus Associate Clinical Professor, University Hospitals, Cleveland, Ohio

Intermittent Exotropia

R. D. HARLEY, M.D., Ph.D., F.A.C.S.

Professor Emeritus and Former Chairman, Department of Ophthalmology, Temple University Health Sciences Center; Former Director, Pediatric Ophthalmology, Wills Eye Hospital; Consulting Surgeon; Wills Eye Hospital, Philadelphia, Pennsylvania

Congenital Fibrosis of the Extraocular Muscles

SOHAN SINGH HAYREH, M.D., Ph.D., D.Sc., F.R.C.S.

Professor of Ophthalmology, School of Medicine, University of Iowa; Director of Ocular Vascular Division, Department of Ophthalmology, University of Iowa Hospitals and Clinics, Iowa City, Iowa

Ischemic Optic Neuropathy

THOMAS R. HEDGES, JR., M.D.

Professor of Ophthalmology, University of Pennsylvania and Emeritus Chief of Section in Ophthalmology and Neuro-Ophthalmology, The Elliott Regional Neurologic Center, The Pennsylvania Hospital, Philadelphia, Pennsylvania

Bell's Palsy, Headache

THOMAS R. HEDGES, III, M.D.

Associate Professor of Ophthalmology and Neurology, Tufts University School of Medicine; Director of Neuro-Ophthalmology, New England Eye Center, Boston, Massachusetts

Bell's Palsy

J. TIMOTHY HEFFERNAN, M.D.

Clinical Instructor, University of Washington, Seattle, Washington

Lid Retraction

EUGENE M. HELVESTON, M.D.

Professor of Ophthalmology; Chief Section of Pediatric Ophthalmology, Indiana University School of Medicine; Active Staff, Indiana University Hospitals, Indianapolis, Indiana

Abducens (Sixth Nerve) Paralysis; Congenital Esotropia; Extraocular Muscle Lacerations; Superior Oblique Palsy; Thyroid Extraocular Muscle Disorders

HUGH L. HENNIS, M.D., Ph.D.

Active Staff, Glaucoma Service, Carolina Eye Associates; Attending Staff, Presbyterian Hospital, Charlotte, North Carolina

Histiocytosis X

ROGER L. HIATT, M.D.

Professor and Chairman of Ophthalmology, Department of Ophthalmology, University of Tennessee, Memphis, Tennessee

Corneal Abrasions, Contusions, Lacerations, and Perforations

DAVID A. HILES, M.D.

Clinical Professor of Ophthalmology, Department of Ophthalmology, University of Pittsburgh; Director, Children's Eye Services, Children's Hospital of Pittsburgh, Pittsburgh, Pennsylvania

Congenital and Infantile Cataracts

BARTON L. HODES, M.D.

Professor of Ophthalmology, University of Arizona Health Sciences Center; Active Staff, University Medical Center, Kino Community Hospital, Tucson, Arizona

Phacoanaphylactic Endophthalmitis

HAROLD J. HOFFMAN, M.D., B.Sc.(Med.), F.R.C.S.(C)

Professor of Ophthalmology, University of Toronto; Chief of Neurosurgery, Hospital for Sick Children, Toronto, Ontario, Canada

Craniopharyngioma

JAMES D. HOGAN, M.D.

Department of Dermatology, Gundersen Clinic, La Crosse, Wisconsin

Pruritus

JOHN B. HOLDS, M.D.

Assistant Professor of Ophthalmology and Otolaryngology, St. Louis University School of Medicine; Active Staff, St. Louis University Medical Center, St. Louis, Missouri

Distichiasis

GARY N. HOLLAND, M.D.

Professor of Ophthalmology, UCLA School of Medicine; Director, UCLA Ocular Inflammatory Disease Center, Jules Eye Institute, Los Angeles, California

Acquired Immunodeficiency Syndrome (AIDS)

JACK L. HOLLINS, M.D.

Assistant Clinical Professor, Department of Ophthalmology, University of Kentucky Medical Center, Lexington, Kentucky

Fungal Endophthalmitis

DAVID J. HOPKINS, M.B.Ch.B., F.R.C.S., F.R.C.Ophth.

Consultant Ophthalmic Surgeon, Bradford Hospitals NHS Trust and Airedale Hospital NHS Trust, Bradford, Yorkshire, England

Hallermann-Streiff-Francois Syndrome

RICHARD B. HORNICK, M.D.

Vice President, Medical Education, Orlando Regional Healthcare System, Orlando, Florida

Q Fever

DAVID S. HULL, M.D.

Professor of Ophthalmology, Medical College of Georgia, Augusta, Georgia

Proteus; Pseudoxanthoma Elasticum

JEFFREY J. HURWITZ, M.D., F.R.C.S.(C)

Professor of Ophthalmology; Director Oculoplastics Program, University of Toronto; Ophthalmologist-in-Chief, Mount Sinai Hospital, Toronto, Ontario, Canada

Alacrima

B. THOMAS HUTCHINSON, M.D.

Associate Clinical Professor of Ophthalmology, Harvard Medical School, Boston, Massachusetts

Aphakic and Pseudophakic Pupillary Block

ROBERT A. HYNDIUK, M.D.

Professor of Ophthalmology, The Eye Institute, Medical College of Wisconsin; Senior Attending Staff, John L. Doyne Hospital, Froedtert Memorial Lutheran Hospital, Children's Hospital of Wisconsin, Zablocki Medical Center, Elmbrook Medical Center, Milwaukee, Wisconsin

Bacillus Species Infections; Granular Corneal Dystrophy; Lattice Corneal Dystrophy; Ocular Vaccinia

D. ROGER ILLINGWORTH, M.D., Ph.D.

Professor of Medicine, Division of Endocrine Diabetes and Clinical Nutrition, Department of Medicine, Oregon Health Sciences University, Portland, Oregon

Abetalipoproteinemia and Homozygous Familial Hypobetalipoproteinemia

DOUGLAS A. JABS, M.D.

Professor of Ophthalmology and Medicine; Director, Ocular Immunology Service, The Wilmer Ophthalmological Institute, The Johns Hopkins University School of Medicine, Baltimore, Maryland

Ankylosing Spondylitis; Scleroderma

JERRY C. JACOBS, M.D.

Professor of Clinical Pediatrics; Director of Section of Pediatric Rheumatology, Columbia University College of Physicians and Surgeons, New York, New York

Juvenile Rheumatoid Arthritis

EDWARD A. JAEGER, M.D.

Professor of Ophthalmology, Jefferson Medical College; Attending Surgeon, Wills Eye Hospital; Active Staff, Riddle Memorial Hospital, Media, Pennsylvania

Down's Syndrome

AMY R. JEFFERY, M.D.

Neuro-Ophthalmology Fellow, Wills Eye Hospital, Philadelphia, Pennsylvania

Choroidal Folds; Oxalosis

RICHARD P. JOBE, M.D.

Clinical Professor of Surgery (Plastic), Stanford University; Active Staff, Stanford Medical Center and El Camino Hospital, Stanford, California

Lagophthalmos

THOMAS JOHN, M.D.

Former Director of Cornea and Contact Lens Service, University of Chicago, Chicago, Illinois; Associate Member of Professional Staff, Little Company of Mary Hospital, Evergreen Park, Illinois

Ascariasis

DAVID W. JOHNSON, M.D.

Assistant Professor of Ophthalmology, University of Colorado Health Sciences Center; Director, Vitreo-Retinal Service, University Hospital, Denver, Colorado

Intraocular Foreign Body—Steel or Iron

IRA SNOW JONES, M.D.

Clinical Professor Emeritus of Ophthalmology, Columbia University College of Physicians and Surgeons, New York, New York

Lymphangioma; Rhabdomyosarcoma

IAN H. KADEN, M.D.

Attending Surgeon, Sparrow Hospital, Lansing, Michigan

Mumps

PAUL H. KALINA, M.D.

Assistant Professor of Ophthalmology; Senior Associate Consultant, Mayo Clinic, Scottsdale, Arizona

Choroidal Detachment

ROBERT E. KALINA, M.D.

Professor and Chair of Ophthalmology, Department of Ophthalmology, University of Washington School of Medicine, Seattle, Washington

Choroidal Neovascular Membranes; Retinopathy of Prematurity

SATOSHI KASHII, M.D., Ph.D.

Associate Professor of Ophthalmology, Faculty of Medicine, Kyoto University; Head of Neuro-Ophthalmology and Orbital Surgery; Director of Ophthalmology Outpatient Clinic, Kyoto University Hospital, Kyoto, Japan

Idiopathic Intracranial Hypertension and Pseudotumor Cerebri

PETER R. KASTL, M.D., Ph.D.

Professor of Ophthalmology and Biochemistry, Tulane University School of Medicine; Active Staff, Eye, Ear, Nose and Throat Hospital, Tulane University Hospital, New Orleans, Louisiana

Juvenile Corneal Epithelial Dystrophy; Macular Corneal Dystrophy

MICHAEL KAZIM, M.D.

Assistant Clinical Professor of Ophthalmology and Clinical Surgery, Columbia College of Physicians and Surgeons, Columbia University, New York, New York

Lymphangioma

B. H. KEAN, M.D.*

Clinical Professor Emeritus of Tropical Medicine and Public Health, Cornell University Medical College, New York, New York

Trichinosis

RONALD V. KEECH, M.D.

Associate Professor of Ophthalmology, University of Iowa College of Medicine and University of Iowa Hospitals and Clinics, Iowa City, Iowa

Dissociated Vertical Deviation; Functional Amblyopia

PAUL C. KEENAN, M.D.

Clinical Instructor, Department of Ophthalmology, Georgetown University; Fellow, Cornea and External Disease, University Ophthalmic Consultants of Washington, District of Columbia

Lacrimal Hypersecretion; Lacrimal Hyposecretion; Sjögren's Syndrome

T. E. KELLY, M.D., Ph.D.

Professor, University of Virginia; Director, Division of Medical Genetics, University of Virginia School of Medicine, Charlottesville, Virginia

Mucopolysaccharidosis I-H; Mucopolysaccharidosis I-H/S

NANCY G. KENNAWAY, D. Phil.

Professor of Medical Genetics, Department of Molecular and Medical Genetics; Director of Pediatric Metabolic Laboratory, Oregon Health Sciences University, Portland, Oregon

Gyrate Atrophy of the Choroid and Retina with Hyperornithinemia

JOHN S. KENNERDELL, M.D.

Professor of Ophthalmology, Medical College of Pennsylvania; Adjunct Professor of Ophthalmology, University of Pittsburgh; Chairman, Department of Ophthalmology, Allegheny General Hospital, Pittsburgh, Pennsylvania

Orbital Graves' Disease

MARSHALL P. KEYS, M.D.

Clinical Associate Professor of Ophthalmology, Georgetown University, Washington, District of Columbia

Dyslexia

MARILYN C. KINCAID, M.D.

Clinical Professor of Ophthalmology and Pathology, St. Louis University School of Medicine; Staff, St. Louis University Hospital and Cardinal Glennon Hospital, St. Louis, Missouri

Pediculosis and Phthiriasis

JAMES L. KINYOUN, M.D.

Professor of Ophthalmology, Department of Ophthalmology, University of Washington School of Medicine; Ophthalmologist, University of Washington Medical Center and Retina-Vitreous Specialist, Seattle, Washington

Wegener's Granulomatosis

---

* Deceased

TREVOR H. KIRKHAM, M.D., D.O., F.R.C.S.

Professor of Neurology and Neurosurgery, McGill University; Neuro Ophthalmologist, Montreal Neurological Hospital, Montreal, Quebec, Canada

Mandibulofacial Dysostosis

LEONARD S. KIRSCH, M.D., F.R.C.S.(C)

Clinical Instructor; Fellow of Diseases and Surgery of the Retinal and Vitreous, Department of Ophthalmology, University of California, San Diego, California

Central or Branch Retinal Artery Occlusion

YOSHIAKI KITAZAWA, M.D., Ph.D.

Professor and Chairman, Department of Ophthalmology, Gifu University School of Medicine, Tsukasa-Machi, Gifu, Japan

Primary Angle-Closure Glaucoma

TERO KIVELÄ, M.D.

Senior Lecturer in Experimental Ophthalmology, University of Helsinki, Faculty of Medicine; Ophthalmologist and Ophthalmic Pathologist, Department of Ophthalmology, Helsinki University Central Hospital, Helsinki, Finland

Periocular Merkel Cell Carcinoma

MICHAEL L. KLEIN, M.D.

Professor of Ophthalmology, Oregon Health Sciences University, Casey Eye Institute; Active Staff, Casey Eye Institute and St. Vincent Hospital and Medical Center; Courtesy, Good Samaritan Hospital, Portland, Oregon

Age-Related Macular Degeneration; Eales' Disease

STEPHEN A. KLOTZ, M.D.

Associate Professor of Medicine and Microbiology and Immunology, University of Kansas School of Medicine; Chief of Infectious Disease Section, Veterans Affairs Medical Center, Kansas City, Missouri

Coccidioidomycosis

DAVID L. KNOX, M.D.

Associate Professor of Ophthalmology, Johns Hopkins University School of Medicine; Active Staff, Johns Hopkins Hospital, Baltimore, Maryland

Crohn's Disease and Ulcerative Colitis

FELIX O. KOLB, M.D., F.A.C.P.

Clinical Professor of Medicine, University of California; Consultant, Endocrinology and Metabolism, California-Pacific Medical Center, San Francisco, California

Hypoparathyroidism

J. SCOTT KORTVELESY, M.D.

Assistant Clinical Professor, University of Hawaii School of Medicine; Staff, Department of Ophthalmology, Straub Clinic and Hospital, Honolulu, Hawaii

Orbital Graves' Disease

JAY H. KRACHMER, M.D.

Professor and Chairman of Ophthalmology, Department of Ophthalmology, University of Minnesota Medical School, Minneapolis, Minnesota

Amyloidosis; Infectious Mononucleosis

INGRID KREISSIG, M.D.

Professor and Chairman of Ophthalmology, Retina and Vitreous, University of Tuebingen, Germany; Adjunct Professor of Clinical Ophthalmology, New York Hospital, Cornell Medical Center, New York, New York

Retinal Detachment

GREGORY B. KROHEL, M.D.

Clinical Professor of Ophthalmology and Neurology, Albany Medical College; Attending, Albany Medical Center, Albany, New York; Consultant, Samaritan Hospital, Troy, New York

Orbital Cellulitis and Abscess

THEODORE KRUPIN, M.D.

Professor, Northwestern University Medical School, Department of Ophthalmology; David Shoch Professor of Ophthalmology, Northwestern University, Chicago, Illinois

Juvenile Glaucoma

FRANCOISE LAGOUTTE, M.D.

Honor Professor, University of Bordeaux; Clinique, Rive Droite, Cenon Cedex, France

Fuchs' Dellen

PETER R. LAIBSON, M.D.

Professor of Ophthalmology, Thomas Jefferson School of Medicine; Director, Cornea Service, Wills Eye Hospital, Philadelphia, Pennsylvania

Epithelial Basement Membrane Dystrophy and Recurrent Erosion; Pseudomonas Aeruginosa

BYRON L. LAM, M.D.

Assistant Professor; Director of Neuro-Ophthalmology, Jones Eye Institute, University of Arkansas for Medical Sciences, Little Rock, Arkansas

Hyperparathyroidism; Lid Myokymia; Rocky Mountain Spotted Fever

LAURENT LAMER, M.D., F.R.C.S.(C)

Associate Professor of Ophthalmology, University of Montreal. On active staff, Notre-Dame Hospital, Montreal, Quebec, Canada

Newcastle Disease

ROGER H.S. LANGSTON, M.D., C.M., F.A.C.S.

Residency Program Director, Department of Ophthalmology; Active Staff, Cleveland Clinic Foundation, Cleveland, Ohio

Infectious Crystalline Keratopathy

BAILEY L. LEE, M.D.

Assistant Professor of Ophthalmology, University of Texas Health Center, San Antonio, Texas

Dislocation of the Lens

DAVID A. LEE, M.D., M.S., F.A.C.S.

Associate Professor of Ophthalmology, UCLA School of Medicine; Chief, Glaucoma Division, Jules Stein Eye Institute, Los Angeles, California

Glaucoma Following Bleb Failure

MICHAEL A. LEMP, M.D.

Clinical Professor of Ophthalmology, Georgetown University; Attending, Georgetown University Hospital and Sibley Memorial Hospital; Consultant, Walter Reed Army Medical Center, Washington, District of Columbia

Lacrimal Hypersecretion; Lacrimal Hyposecretion; Sjögren's Syndrome

CHARLES R. LEONE, JR., M.D.

Clinical Professor of Ophthalmology, University of Texas Health Science Center; Chief of Surgery, St. Luke's Hospital, San Antonio, Texas

Oculoauriculovertebral Dysplasia

GLENN J. LESSER, M.D.

Senior Clinical Fellow in Oncology, Johns Hopkins Oncology Center, Baltimore, Maryland

Hodgkin's Disease

ROBERT L. LESSER, M.D.

Associate Clinical Professor of Ophthalmology, Department of Ophthalmology and Visual Science, Yale University School of Medicine, New Haven, Connecticut

Creutzfeldt-Jakob Disease

MARK R. LEVINE, M.D.

Clinical Professor of Ophthalmology, Case Western Reserve University School of Medicine; Chief, Division of Ophthalmology, Mt. Sinai Medical Center; Head, Section of Oculoplastic Surgery, University Hospitals of Cleveland, Cleveland, Ohio

Orbital Implant Extrusion

NORMAN S. LEVY, M.D., Ph.D., F.A.C.S.

Co-Clinical Associate Professor, Department of Community Health and Family Medicine, University of Florida, Gainesville, Florida

Neurilemoma

RICHARD A. LEWIS, M.D., M.S.

Professor of Ophthalmology, Department of Ophthalmology Medicine, Pediatrics, and Molecular and Human Genetics, Baylor College of Medicine, Houston, Texas

Neurofibromatosis-1

JEFFREY M. LIEBMANN, M.D.

Associate Clinical Professor of Ophthalmology, New York Medical College; Active Staff, New York Eye and Ear Infirmary, New York, New York

Ocular Hypertension

THOMAS J. LIESEGANG, M.D.

Professor and Chairman of Ophthalmology, Department of Ophthalmology, Mayo Clinic Jacksonville, Chairman, St. Luke's Hospital, Jacksonville, Florida

Azotobacter; Fuchs' Heterochromic Iridocyclitis

HARVEY LINCOFF, M.D.

Professor of Ophthalmology, Cornell University Medical Center; Attending Surgeon, New York Hospital, New York, New York

Retinal Detachment

RICHARD D. LISMAN, M.D., F.A.C.S.

Clinical Associate Professor of Ophthalmology, New York University School of Medicine; Clinic Chief, Division of Ophthalmic Plastic Surgery, Manhattan Eye and Ear Hospital, New York, New York

Ectropion; External Orbital Fractures; Internal Orbital Fractures

DAVID LITOFF, M.D.

Active Staff, Danbury Hospital, Danbury, Connecticut, and Stamford Hospital, Stamford, Connecticut

Iris Prolapse

HUNTER L. LITTLE, M.D., F.A.C.S.

Clinical Professor of Surgery (Ophthalmology), Stanford University Medical Center, Stanford, California; Palo Alto Retinal Group, Menlo Park, California

Subretinal Neovascular Membranes

LOIS A. LLOYD, M.D., F.R.C.S.(C)

Associate Professor of Ophthalmology, University of Toronto; Senior Consultant of Ophthalmology, Toronto Hospital; Active Staff, The Hospital for Sick Children, Toronto, Ontario, Canada

Orbital Hypertelorism

WILLIAM C. LLOYD III, M.D., F.A.C.S.

Clinical Associate Professor of Surgery, Uniformed Services University of the Health Sciences, Bethesda, Maryland; Staff Ophthalmologist and Director of Ophthalmic Pathology, Brooke Army Medical Center, Fort Sam Houston, Texas

Melanocytic Lesions of the Eyelids

REGAN A. LOGAN, M.D.

Clinical Fellow, Vanderbilt University Medical Center, Nashville, Tennessee

Bacillus Cereus; Blastomycosis

RONALD R. LUBRITZ, M.D.

Clinical Professor of Medicine (Dermatology), Tulane University School of Medicine, New Orleans, Louisiana

Actinic and Seborrheic Keratosis

MALCOLM N. LUXENBERG, M.D.

Professor and Chairman, Department of Ophthalmology, Medical College of Georgia; Active Staff, Medical College of Georgia Hospitals and Clinics, Augusta, Georgia

Crystalline Corneal Dystrophy; Hyperlipoproteinemia; Tularemia

IAN A. MACKIE, F.R.C.S., F.R.C.Ophth

Emeritus Associate Specialist, St. Georges Hospital, Tooting, London, England

Neuroparalytic Keratitis

SCOTT M. MACRAE, M.D.

Associate Professor of Ophthalmology, Cornea and External Disease Services, Oregon Health Sciences University, Casey Eye Institute, Portland, Oregon

Cat-Scratch Disease

LARRY E. MAGARGAL, M.D., F.A.C.S.

Clinical Associate Professor of Ophthalmology, Thomas Jefferson University; Associate Surgeon Retina Service; Co-Director Retina Vascular Unit, Wills Eye Hospital, Philadelphia, Pennsylvania

Retinal Vein Obstruction

STEPHEN K. MAGIE, M.D.

Chief, Department of Ophthalmology, Baptist Medical Center; Active Staff, St. Vincents Medical Center, Little Rock, Arkansas

Ocular Histoplasmosis

SID MANDELBAUM, M.D.

Associate Clinical Professor of Ophthalmology, Albert Einstein College of Medicine; Active Staff, Long Island Jewish Medical Center; Assistant Attending Surgeon, Manhattan Eye, Ear and Throat Hospital, New York, New York

Bacterial Endophthalmitis

GEORGE E. MARAK, JR., M.D.

Clinical Professor of Ophthalmology, Georgetown University Medical Center, Washington, District of Columbia

Sympathetic Ophthalmia

DANIEL MARCHAC, M.D.

Professor College Medicine, Hopitaux de Paris, Paris, France

Anophthalmos

PETER B. MARSH, M.D.

School of Medicine, Oregon Health Sciences University, Portland, Oregon

Optic Foramen Fractures

RONALD J. MARSH, F.R.C.S., F.R.C.Ophth.

Recognized Teacher, Institute of Ophthalmology and Imperial College, St. Mary's Hospital; Consultant Ophthalmologist, Moorfields Eye Hospital, London, England

Herpes Zoster

BRUCE M. MASSARO, M.D., M.P.H.

Associate Professor of Ophthalmology; Ophthalmic Plastic and Reconstructive Surgery, Eye Institute, Department of Ophthalmology, Medical College of Wisconsin, Milwaukee, Wisconsin

Ocular Vaccinia

KANJIRO MASUDA, M.D.

Professor and Chairman of Ophthalmology, University of Tokyo School of Medicine, Tokyo, Japan

Behçet's Disease

IRENE E. H. MAUMENEE, M.D.

Professor of Ophthalmology and Pediatrics, Department of Ophthalmology, Johns Hopkins University School of Medicine, Baltimore, Maryland

Congenital Hereditary Endothelial Dystrophy; Mucopolysaccharidosis I-S

MALCOLM L. MAZOW, M.D.

Walter and Ruth Sterling Professor of Ophthalmology; Director of Pediatric Ophthalmology, University of Texas, Houston, Texas

Convergence Insufficiency

REX M. MCCALLUM, M.D.

Assistant Professor of Medicine, Division of Rheumatology, Allergy, and Immunology, Duke University Medical School, Durham, North Carolina

Cogan's Syndrome

JAMES P. MCCULLEY, M.D.

David Bruton Jr. Professor and Chairman, Department of Ophthalmology, University of Texas Health Science Center, Dallas, Texas

Seborrheic Blepharitis; Staphylococcal and Mixed Staphylococcal/ Seborrheic Blepharoconjunctivitis

JOHN G. MCHENRY, M.D.

Assistant Professor of Ophthalmology, Wayne State University, Detroit, Michigan

Compressive Optic Neuropathies; Inflammatory Optic Neuropathies; Traumatic Optic Neuropathy; Vasculopathic Optic Neuropathies

DAVID J. MCINTYRE, M.D., F.A.C.S.

Honorary Visiting Professor, Shanghai University, Shanghai Ching, China

After-Cataracts

SAUL MERIN, M.D.

Professor of Ophthalmology, Hebrew University of Jerusalem; Head, Unit of Ophthalmology, Mt. Scopus, Hadassah University Hospital, Jerusalem, Israel

Retinitis Pigmentosa

HENRY S. METZ, M.D.

Clinical Professor of Ophthalmology and Former Chairman of the Department of Ophthalmology, University of Rochester School of Medicine, Rochester, New York

A-Patterns; Duane's Retraction Syndrome; V-Patterns

ROGER F. MEYER, M.D.

Professor of Ophthalmology, University of Michigan School of Medicine, Ann Arbor, Michigan

Mumps

BENJAMIN MILDER, M.D.

Professor of Clinical Ophthalmology, Washington University School of Medicine, St. Louis, Missouri

Actinomycosis; Dacryolith; Lacrimal System Contusions and Lacerations

KEVIN N. MILLER, M.D.

Private practice, Ophthalmologist, Las Vegas, Nevada

Histiocytosis X

NEIL R. MILLER, M.D.

Frank B. Walsh Professor of Neuro-Ophthalmology; Professor of Ophthalmology, Neurology, and Neurosurgery, Johns Hopkins Medical Institutions, Baltimore, Maryland

Hodgkin's Disease; Myasthenia Gravis; Temporal Arteritis

JOHN A. MILLS, M.D.

Associate Professor of Medicine, Harvard Medical School, Boston, Massachusetts

Polyarteritis Nodosa

MARY BETH MOORE, M.D.

Active staff of Kaiser Permanente Medical Center, Sacramento, California

Acanthamoebae

WILLIAM R. MORRIS, M.D.

Associate Professor of Ophthalmology, Department of Ophthalmology, University of Tennessee, Memphis, Tennessee

Filamentary Keratitis; Mooren's Ulcer

JOHN C. MORRISON, M.D.

Associate Professor of Ophthalmology, Glaucoma Service, Department of Ophthalmology, Oregon Health Sciences University, Casey Eye Institute, Portland, Oregon

Glaucoma After Ocular Contusion; Malignant Glaucoma; The Glaucoma Suspect

LYNNE H. MORRISON, M.D.

Assistant Professor of Dermatology, Oregon Health Sciences University, Portland, Oregon

Cicatricial Pemphigoid

PETER H. MORSE, M.D., F.A.C.S.

Professor of Ophthalmology, University of South Dakota School of Medicine, Central Plains Clinic, Sioux Falls, South Dakota

Engelmann's Disease

P. K. MUKHERJEE, M.S.

Professor and Head of Department of Ophthalmology; Pt. J.N.M. Medical College, D. K. Hospital, Raipur, India

Congenital Pit of the Optic Nerve; Rhinosporidiosis; Thelaziasis

RALPH MULLER, Ph.D., D.Sc.

International Institute of Parasitology, St. Albans, Herts, United Kingdom

Dracunculosis

GONZALO MURILLO, M.D.

Associate Professor of Ophthalmology, Universidad Mayor de San Andres, La Paz, Bolivia

Sparganosis

AIDAN MURRAY, F.R.C.S.

Lecturer in Ophthalmology, University College; Consultant, Ophthalmic Surgeon, Cork Regional Hospital, Cork, Ireland

Uveoparotid Fever

KHALAD A. NAGY, M.D.

Assistant Lecturer in Ophthalmology, Tanta University, Tanta, Egypt

Allergic Conjunctivitis; Epidemic Keratoconjunctivitis; Keratoconus

MICHAEL A. NAIDOFF, M.D.

Associate Professor of Ophthalmology, Jefferson Medical College of Thomas Jefferson University; Associate Surgeon, Wills Eye Hospital, Philadelphia, Pennsylvania

Melanocytic Lesions of the Eyelids

JOHN M. NASSIF, M.D.

Clinical Instructor, Department of Ophthalmology, University of California, San Diego, California

Eyelid Contusions, Lacerations and Avulsions

KAMAL M. NASSIF, M.D.

Associate Clinical Professor of Ophthalmology, Eye Institute, Medical College of Wisconsin, Milwaukee, Wisconsin

Granular Corneal Dystrophy

HELLMUT F. NEUBAUER, M.D.

Professor Emeritus of Ophthalmology, Department of Ophthalmology, University of Cologne, Cologne, West Germany

Iris Lacerations, Holes, and Iridodialysis

THOMAS P. NIGRA, M.D.

Clinical Professor and Chairman, Department of Dermatology, Washington Hospital Center, Washington, District of Columbia

Psoriasis

MOGENS S. NORN, M.D., Ph.D.

Professor of Ophthalmology, University of Copenhagen. On active staff of Medical Historical University of Copenhagen, Copenhagen, Denmark

Keratoconjunctivitis Sicca

COREY M. NOTIS, M.D.

Clinical Instructor of Ophthalmology, Cornell University Medical College, New York, New York

Retinoblastoma

JULIAN J. NUSSBAUM, M.D.

Chairman, Department of Ophthalmology, Henry Ford Hospital, Detroit, Michigan

Peripheral Retina Breaks and Degeneration

DENIS M. O'DAY, M.D.

Professor and Chairman, Department of Ophthalmology and Visual Sciences, Vanderbilt University School of Medicine, Nashville, Tennessee

Bacillus Cereus; Blastomycosis

EAMON P. O'DONOGHUE, M.B., B.Ch., B.A.O., F.R.C.S.(Ed.)

Ophthalmic Surgeon, Moorfield's Eye Hospital, London, England

Relapsing Polychondritis

JAY JUSTIN OLDER, M.D., F.A.C.S.

Clinical Professor of Ophthalmology; Director, Oculoplastic Service, University of South Florida College of Medicine, Tampa, Florida

Blepharophimosis

H. BRUCE OSTLER, M.D.

Clinical Professor of Ophthalmology, Francis I. Proctor Foundation, University of California, San Francisco, California

Pneumococcus

EARL A. PALMER, M.D.

Professor of Ophthalmology and Pediatrics, Oregon Health Sciences University, Casey Eye Institute; Active Staff, University Hospitals OHSU, Portland, Oregon

Brown's Syndrome

FRANK PARKER, M.D.

Professor and Chairman, Department of Dermatology, Oregon Health Sciences University, Portland, Oregon

Vitiligo

MARSHALL M. PARKS, M.D.

Clinical Professor of Ophthalmology, George Washington University Medical Center; Senior Attending, Children's National Medical Center, Washington, District of Columbia

Lenticonus and Lentiglobus; Monofixation Syndrome

JOHN A. PARRISH, M.D.

Professor, Department of Dermatology, Harvard Medical School; Dermatologist-in-Chief, Massachusetts General Hospital, Boston, Massachusetts

Photosensitivity and Sunburn

GISSUR J. PETURSSON, M.D.

Professor of Ophthalmology; Director, Glaucoma Service, University of Arkansas for Medical Sciences, Little Rock, Arkansas

Filtering Blebs

ROSWELL R. PFISTER, M.D.

Clinical Professor of Ophthalmology, University of Alabama; Director of Eye Research, Brookwood Medical Center, Birmingham, Alabama

Alkaline Injury

DAVID A. PLAGER, M.D.

Associate Professor of Ophthalmology, Section of Pediatric Ophthalmology and Strabismus, Indiana University Medical Center, Indianapolis, Indiana

Slipped Extraocular Muscle

STEVEN M. PODOS, M.D.

Professor and Chairman, Department of Ophthalmology, Mount Sinai School of Medicine, New York, New York

Ocular Hypertension; Plateau Iris

FRANK M. POLACK, M.D., F.A.C.S.

Adjunct Professor, Department of Ophthalmology, College of Medicine, University of Florida, Gainesville, Florida

Reis-Bücklers' Superficial Corneal Dystrophy

J. POLETTI, M.D.

Chief of Ophthalmology, Hospital of Tarbes, Tarbes Cedex, France

Brucellosis

ZANE F. POLLARD, M.D.

Head of Pediatric Ophthalmology Fellowship at the James Hall Eye Center; Active Staff, Scottish Rite Children's Hospital, Atlanta, Georgia

Toxocariasis

TIMOTHY P. POWERS, M.D.

Clinical Instructor of Ophthalmology, Medical University of South Carolina, Storm Eye Institute, Charleston, South Carolina

Histiocytosis X

RONALD C. PRUETT, M.D.

Associate Clinical Professor of Ophthalmology, Harvard Medical School; Surgeon, Massachusetts Eye and Ear Infirmary, Boston, Massachusetts

Persistent Hyperplastic Primary Vitreous

JOSE S. PULIDO, M.D.

Associate Professor, Department of Ophthalmology, Medical College of Wisconsin; Active Staff, The Eye Institute, Medical College of Wisconsin, Milwaukee, Wisconsin

Bacillus Species Infections

ALLEN M. PUTTERMAN, M.D.

Professor of Clinical Ophthalmology; Director, Oculoplastic Service, University of Illinois College of Medicine, Chicago, Illinois

Madarosis; Orbital Fat Herniation

EDWARD L. RAAB, M.D.

Professor of Ophthalmology and Pediatrics; Director of Pediatric Ophthalmology and Strabismus, Mt. Sinai School of Medicine; Attending Ophthalmic Surgeon, Mt. Sinai Hospital, New York, New York

Accommodative Esotropia

MAURICE F. RABB, M.D.

Professor of Ophthalmology, Department of Ophthalmology, University of Illinois at Chicago; Chief, Division of Ophthalmology, Mercy Hospital and Medical Center and Medical Retina Service, Illinois Masonic Medical Center, Chicago, Illinois

Sickle Cell Disease

JOHN M. RAMOCKI, M.D.

Assistant Professor of Ophthalmology, Wayne State Medical School, Kresge Eye Institute; Chief of Ophthalmology, Veteran's Administration Medical School, Allen Park, Michigan; Staff, Hutzel Hospital, Detroit, Michigan

Optic Neuritis

LAWRENCE A. RAYMOND, M.D.

Associate Professor of Ophthalmology; Director, Retina and Vitreous Service, University of Cincinnati Medical Center, Cincinnati, Ohio

Dirofilariasis

AUGUST L. READER, III, M.D., F.A.C.S.

Clinical Associate Professor of Ophthalmology, University of Southern California School of Medicine; Attending Surgeon, Cedars-Sinai Medical Center, Los Angeles, California

Hysteria, Malingering and Anxiety States

MANOLITO R. REYES, M.D.

Visiting Assistant Professor, UCLA Jules Stein Eye Institute, Department of Medicine, Los Angeles, California; Associate Professor, Far Eastern University, Nicanor Reyes Medical Foundation, Manila, Philippines

Glaucoma Following Bleb Failure

L. F. RICH, M.D., M.S.

Associate Professor of Ophthalmology; Director, Cornea and External Disease Service, Casey Eye Institute, Oregon Health Sciences University; Staff, Oregon Health Sciences University Portland, Oregon

Conjunctival Lacerations and Contusions; Pterygium and Pseudopterygium; Relapsing Fever

CLAUDIA U. RICHTER, M.D.

Clinical Assistant of Ophthalmology, Harvard Medical School; Assistant Surgeon of Ophthalmology, Massachusetts Eye and Ear Infirmary, Boston, Massachusetts

Aphakic and Pseudophakic Pupillary Block

ROBERT RITCH, M.D.

Professor of Clinical Ophthalmology, New York Medical College, Valhalla, New York; Chief of Glaucoma Service and Surgeon Director, The New York Eye and Ear Infirmary, New York, New York

Ocular Hypertension; Plateau Iris

MICHAEL C. ROBERSON, M.D.

Associate Clinical Professor of Ophthalmology, University of Arkansas College of Medicine; Active Staff, Baptist Medical Center and University Hospital, Little Rock, Arkansas

Fungal Keratitis; Irritative Conjunctivitis

JOSEPH E. ROBERTSON, JR., M.D.

Associate Professor of Ophthalmology, Retina-Vitreous Service, Department of Ophthalmology, Casey Eye Institute, Oregon Health Sciences University; Active Staff, University Hospital and St. Vincent's Hospital and Medical Center, Portland, Oregon

Diffuse Unilateral Subacute Neuroretinitis; Epimacular Proliferation; Familial Exudative Vitreoretinopathy; Intraocular Foreign Body—Nonmagnetic Chemically Inert

JEFFREY B. ROBIN, M.D.

Associate Professor, Eye Center, Department of Ophthalmology, University of Illinois College of Medicine, Chicago, Illinois

Gonococcal Ocular Disease

STEVEN B. ROBIN, M.D.

Clinical Assistant Professor of Ophthalmology, University of Minnesota Medical School, Minneapolis, Minnesota

Gonococcal Ocular Disease

JOHN H. ROCKEY, M.D., Ph.D.

Professor of Ophthalmology, Scheie Eye Institute, Presbyterian-University of Pennsylvania Medical Center, Philadelphia, Pennsylvania

Ascariasis

SHIYOUNG ROH, M.D.

Ophthalmology Resident, New England Eye Center, Tufts University School of Medicine, Boston, Massachusetts

Angiomatosis Retinae; Polyarteritis Nodosa

JAIME ROIZENBLATT, M.D.

Associate Professor of Ophthalmology, Sao Paolo University School of Medicine, Sao Paulo, Brazil

American Mucocutaneous Leishmaniasis

PAUL E. ROMANO, M.D., M.S.O.

Editor and Publisher, Binocular Vision and Eye Muscle Surgery, Gainesville, Florida

Juvenile Xanthogranuloma; Traumatic Hyphema

HILARY J. RONNER, M.D.

Assistant in Ophthalmology, Harkness Eye Institute; Assistant Attending, Manhattan Eye Ear and Throat Hospital; Adjunct in Ophthalmology, Lenox Hill Hospital, New York, New York

Rhabdomyosarcoma

JACK ROOTMAN, M.D., F.R.C.S.(C)

Professor of Ophthalmology and Pathology, University of British Columbia, Vancouver General Hospital; Active Staff, Vancouver Hospital and Health Sciences Center and British Columbia Children's Hospital; Consulting, British Columbia Cancer Agency, British Columbia, Canada

Nonspecific Orbital Inflammatory Syndromes

ARTHUR L. ROSENBAUM, M.D.

Clinical Faculty, Jules Stein Eye Institute/UCLA; Chief, Division of Pediatric Ophthalmology, Los Angeles, California

Esotropia-High AC/A Ratio

JAMES T. ROSENBAUM, M.D.

Professor of Medicine, Ophthalmology and Cell Biology, Casey Eye Institute; Active Staff, Oregon Health Sciences University, Portland, Oregon

Interstitial Nephritis; Lyme Disease; Rheumatoid Arthritis; Systemic Lupus Erythematosus; Uveitis

F. HAMPTON ROY, M.D., F.A.C.S.

Associate Clinical Professor of Ophthalmology, University of Arkansas Medical Center; Active Staff, Baptist Medical Center, St. Vincent's Hospital, Arkansas Children's Hospital, University of Arkansas Medical Center, and Freeway Medical Center, Little Rock, Arkansas

Fibrosarcoma; Listeriosis; Mikulicz's Syndrome; Spider Bites; Sturge-Weber Syndrome

MELVIN L. RUBIN, M.D.

Professor and Chairman, Department of Ophthalmology, University of Florida School of Medicine, J. Hillis Miller Health Center, Gainesville, Florida

Anisometropia

RICHARD S. RUIZ, M.D.

Professor and Chairman, Department of Ophthalmology, The University of Texas Medical School; President, Medical Staff, Hermann Hospital, Houston, Texas

Vitreous Wick Syndrome

K. MATTI SAARI, M.D.

Professor and Chairman, Department of Ophthalmology, University of Turku; Associate Head, Department of Ophthalmology, Turku University Hospital, Turku, Finland

Reiter's Disease; Yersiniosis

BIJAN SAFAI, M.D., D.S.C.

Attending Physician and Chief, Dermatology Service, Memorial Solan-Kettering Cancer Center; Professor of Medicine (Dermatology), Cornell Medical Center; Adjunct Member, Rockefeller University School of Medicine, New York, New York

Kaposi's Sarcoma

JOHN R. SAMPLES, M.D.

Professor of Ophthalmology, Glaucoma Service, Department of Ophthalmology, Casey Eye Institute, Oregon Health Sciences University, Portland, Oregon

Benign Essential Blepharospasm; Corticosteroid-Induced Glaucoma; Glaucoma Associated with Elevated Venous Pressure; Hemifacial Spasm; Pediatric Aphakic Glaucoma; Rubeosis Iridis; Streptococcus

DAVID J. SCHANZLIN, M.D.

Professor and Chairman, St. Louis University Medical School, St. Louis University Health Science Center; Medical Staff, Anheuser-Busch Eye Institutes, St. Louis University Hospital, Cardinal Glennon Hospital for Children, and St. Mary's Health Center, St. Louis, Missouri

Corneal and Conjunctival Calcifications; Herpes Simplex; Pellucid Marginal Corneal Degeneration

ABRAHAM SCHLOSSMAN, M.D., F.A.C.S.

Clinical Associate Professor of Ophthalmology, State University of New York Health Sciences Center, Brooklyn, New York; Associate Clinical Professor, Department of Ophthalmology, Mt. Sinai School of Medicine; Attending Surgeon, Manhattan Eye Ear and Throat Hospital, New York, New York

Glaucomatocyclitic Crisis

LEE K. SCHWARTZ, M.D.

Associate Clinical Professor, California-Pacific Medical Center, Department of Ophthalmology; Chief, Department of Ophthalmology, University of California and Mt. Zion Medical Center, San Francisco, California

Floppy Eyelid Syndrome

WILLIAM E. SCOTT, M.D.

Professor of Ophthalmology, Department of Ophthalmology, University of Iowa College of Medicine, Iowa City, Iowa

Accommodative Spasm

ERNESTO I. SEGAL, M.D.

Resident, Department of Ophthalmology, University of Texas Medical Branch, Galveston, Texas

Sarcoidosis

JANET B. SERLE, M.D.

Associate Professor of Ophthalmology, Mt. Sinai School of Medicine, Department of Ophthalmology; Active Staff, Mt. Sinai School of Medicine, New York, New York

Ocular Hypertension

DAVID SEVEL, M.D., Ph.D., F.A.C.S.

Head, Division of Ophthalmology; Instructor, Department of Pathology, University of California, Scripps Clinic, La Jolla, California, San Diego, California

Clostridium Perfringens; Leiomyoma

ROBERT N. SHAFFER, M.D., F.A.C.S.

Clinical Professor Emeritus of Ophthalmology, University of Southern California School of Medicine, San Francisco, California

Open-Angle Glaucoma

H. JOHN SHAMMAS, M.D.

Clinical Professor of Ophthalmology, University of Southern California; Active Staff, Children's Hospital, Los Angeles, California; Medical Director, M/S Surgery Center and Staff, St. Francis Hospital, Lynwood, California

Escherichia Coli; Iris Melanoma

CAROL L. SHIELDS, M.D.

Associate Professor, Thomas Jefferson University; Associate Surgeon, Oncology Service, Wills Eye Hospital, Philadelphia, Pennsylvania

Malignant Melanoma of the Posterior Uvea; Glaucoma Associated with Intraocular Tumors

JERRY A. SHIELDS, M.D.

Director, Ocular Oncology Service, Wills Eye Hospital, Thomas Jefferson University; Consultant, Children's Hospital of Philadelphia, Philadelphia, Pennsylvania

Malignant Melanoma of the Posterior Uvea; Glaucoma Associated with Intraocular Tumors

M. BRUCE SHIELDS, M.D.

Professor of Ophthalmology, Duke University Medical Center, Durham, North Carolina

Glaucoma Associated with Anterior Uveitis; Iridocorneal Endothelial Syndrome

WILLIAM T. SHULTS, M.D.

Clinical Associate Professor, Oregon Health Sciences University, Casey Eye Institute; Active Staff, Good Samaritan Hospital and Medical Center, Portland, Oregon

Superior Oblique Myokymia; Tolosa-Hunt Syndrome

JERRY N. SHUSTER, M.D.

Active Staff of Florida Hospital-Orlando, Orlando, Florida

Traumatic Hyphema

GLEN W. SIZEMORE, M.D.

Professor of Medicine, Department of Endocrinology, Loyola University Stritch School of Medicine, Maywood, Illinois

Hypocalcemia

HARVEY H. SLANSKY, M.D.

Instructor of Clinical Ophthalmology, Harvard Medical School; Staff, Emerson Hospital, Lexington, Massachusetts

Acid Burns

WILLIAM S. SLY, M.D.

Alice A. Doisy Professor and Chairman, Edward A. Doisy Department of Biochemistry and Molecular Biology, St. Louis University School of Medicine, Active Staff, Cardinal Glennon Children's Hospital, St. Louis, Missouri

Mucopolysaccharidosis VII

PATRICIA W. SMITH, M.D.

Attending Physician, Wake Medical Center, Rex Hospital, and Raleigh Community Hospital, Raleigh, North Carolina

Epithelial Ingrowth; Intraocular Epithelial Cysts

RONALD E. SMITH, M.D.

Professor and Chairman, University of Southern California School of Medicine and The Doheny Eye Institute; Staff, Doheny Eye Hospital, LAC and USC Medical Center, Los Angeles, California

Propionibacterium Acnes

GILBERT SMOLIN, M.D.

Clinical Professor, University of California, Research Ophthalmologist, Proctor Foundation; Active Staff, Moffitt and Long Hospitals, Peninsula-Mills Hospital, and Seton Hospital, San Francisco, California

Bee Sting of the Cornea

DAVID B. SOLL, M.D., F.A.C.S.

Clinical Professor of Surgery (Ophthalmology), University of Medicine and Dentistry of New Jersey, Robert Wood Johnson Medical School at Camden; Head, Division of Ophthalmology, Cooper Hospital University Medical Center, Camden, New Jersey; Director, Division of Ophthalmology, Frankford Hospital, Philadelphia, Pennsylvania

Enophthalmos

STEPHEN SOLL, M.D.

University of Medicine and Dentistry of New Jersey, Robert Wood Johnson Medical School at Camden, Ocuplastics Service, Camden, New Jersey

Ectropion; Internal Orbital Fractures

STEPHEN E. SOLOMON, D.O.

Assistant Clinical Professor of Pediatrics and Ophthalmology, Michigan State University College of Human Medicine, East Lansing, Michigan; Active Staff, Sinai Hospital, Detroit, Michigan, Hurley Hospital, Flint, Michigan, and St. Joseph/Mercy, Pontiac, Michigan

Mucopolysaccharidosis IV

ALFRED SOMMER, M.D., M.H.Sc.

Professor of Ophthalmology, Epidemiology, and International Health, Johns Hopkins University; Active Staff, Johns Hopkins University, Department of Ophthalmology, Baltimore, Maryland

Hypovitaminosis A

HAROLD F. SPALTER, M.D.

Professor of Clinical Ophthalmology, Columbia University College of Physicians and Surgeons; Attending Ophthalmologist, Columbia Presbyterian Medical Center, New York, New York

Juvenile Rheumatoid Arthritis

ROBERT T. SPECTOR, M.D., F.A.C.S.

Private practice, Sight Foundation, Fort Lauderdale, Florida

Fabry's Disease

DANIEL H. SPITZBERG, M.D., F.A.C.S.

Clinical Associate Professor of Ophthalmology; Staff, Methodist Hospital of Indiana and St. Vincent's Hospital, Indianapolis, Indiana

Influenza; Pars Planitis; Toxoplasmosis

THOMAS C. SPOOR, M.D., M.S., F.A.C.S.

Professor of Ophthalmology and Neurosurgery, Wayne State University; Active Staff, Hutzel Hospital and Harper Hospital, Detroit Medical Center, Detroit, Michigan

Compressive Optic Neuropathies; Inflammatory Optic Neuropathies; Optic Neuritis; Traumatic Optic Neuropathy; Tuberculosis; Vasculopathic Optic Neuropathies

DERECK T. SPRUNGER, M.D.

Clinical Assistant Professor of Ophthalmology, Indiana University School of Medicine; Staff, Methodist Hospital of Indiana, Indianapolis, Indiana

Thyroid Extraocular Muscle Disorders

ROBERT L. STAMPER, M.D.

Professor and Chairman, California Pacific Medical Center, San Francisco, California

Ankyloblepharon; Symblepharon

WALTER J. STARK, M.D.

Professor of Ophthalmology; Director, Corneal Service, Johns Hopkins University, The Wilmer Institute, Baltimore, Maryland

Epithelial Ingrowth; Intraocular Epithelial Cysts

GEORGE O. STASIOR, M.D.

Assistant Clinical Professor, Department of Ophthalmology, Albany Medical College, Albany, New York

Orbital Cellulitis and Abscess

THOMAS L. STEINEMANN, M.D.

Assistant Professor, Corneal and External Disease, Department of Ophthalmology, University of Arkansas for Medical Sciences, Jones Eye Institute; Attending Staff, University of Arkansas Medical Center Hospital and Arkansas Children's Hospital; Consulting Staff, John L. McClellan Veteran's Administration Hospital, Little Rock, Arkansas

Giant Papillary Conjunctivitis; Staphylococcus; Terrien's Marginal Degeneration

ROGER F. STEINERT, M.D.

Assistant Clinical Professor, Harvard Medical School; Associate Surgeon, Massachusetts Eye and Ear Infirmary, Boston, Massachusetts

Posterior Polymorphous Corneal Dystrophy

PAUL STERNBERG, JR., M.D.

Thomas M. Aaberg Professor of Ophthalmology, Emory University School of Medicine, Atlanta, Georgia

Dislocation of the Lens

KARL G. STONECIPHER, M.D., F.A.A.O.

Director, Cornea and Keratorefractive Service, Southeastern Eye Center, Greensboro, North Carolina

Corneal Neovascularization

ALAN SUGAR, M.D.

Professor and Associate Chair of Ophthalmology, W.K. Kellogg Eye Center, University of Michigan Medical School, Ann Arbor, Michigan

Dermatophytosis; Impetigo; Koch-Weeks Bacillus

JOEL SUGAR, M.D.

Professor of Ophthalmology and Director of the Cornea Service, University of Illinois Medical Center, Active Staff, University of Illinois Eye and Ear Infirmary, Chicago, Illinois

Corneal Edema

JOHN H. SULLIVAN, M.D.

Clinical Professor of Ophthalmology, University of California School of Medicine, San Francisco, California

Blepharochalasis; Ptosis

KENNETH C. SWAN, M.D.

Professor of Ophthalmology, Oregon Health Sciences University, Casey Eye Institute; Senior Consultant, Casey Eye Institute, Oregon Health Sciences University Hospitals and Clinics, Portland, Oregon

Cicatricial Pemphigoid; Fibrous Ingrowth; Iris Cysts; Recurrent Late Hyphema from Focal Wound Vascularization

K. NOLEN TANNER, M.D., Ph.D.

Assistant Clinical Professor, Oregon Health Sciences University; Active Staff, St. Vincent Hospital and Good Samaritan Hospital, Portland, Oregon

Accommodative Insufficiency; Low Vision Aids

AHTI TARKKANEN, M.D.

Professor and Director, Helsinki University Eye Hospital, Faculty of Medicine; Head, Department of Ophthalmology, University of Helsinki, Helsinki, Finland

Exfoliation Syndrome

WILLIAM TASMAN, M.D.

Professor and Chairman of Ophthalmology, Department of Ophthalmology, Jefferson Medical College; Ophthalmologist-in-Chief, Wills Eye Hospital; Surgeon, Wills Eye Hospital; Consulting Surgeon, Children's Hospital, and Attending Surgeon, Chestnut Hill Hospital, Philadelphia, Pennsylvania

Coats' Disease

BRUCE C. TAYLOR, M.D.

Clinical Associate Professor of Ophthalmology, University of Texas, Southwestern Medical School, Dallas, Texas

Vitreous Hemorrhage

DANIEL M. TAYLOR, M.D., F.A.C.S.

Solomon Professor of Surgery, University of Connecticut Health Center; Senior Attending Surgeon, New Britain General Hospital; Associate Attending, Dempsey Hospital and Senior Attending, Hospital for Special Care, New Britain, Connecticut

Expulsive Hemorrhage

KLAUS D. TEICHMANN, M.D., F.R.C.S.(C), F.R.A.C.O.

Consultant Ophthalmic Surgeon, King Khaled Eye Specialist Hospital, Riyadh, Saudi Arabia

Orbital Hemorrhages

RICHARD R. TENZEL, M.D.

Clinical Emeritus Professor, University of Miami School of Medicine, North Miami Beach, Florida

Lid Retraction

THOM S. THOMASSEN, M.D.

Assistant Professor, Department of Surgery, Division of Ophthalmology, Uniformed Services University of the Health Sciences, Bethesda, Maryland; Staff Ophthalmologist, Mercy Hospital, Janesville, Wisconsin

Intraocular Foreign Body—Copper

LAWRENCE G. TOMASI, M.D., Ph.D

Associate Professor of Pediatrics, Loma Linda University School of Medicine; Active Staff, Loma Linda University Medical Center, Loma Linda, California

Maple Syrup Urine Disease

ANDREA CIBIS TONGUE, M.D.

Assistant Clinical Professor of Ophthalmology, Oregon Health Sciences University, Portland, Oregon

Basic Exotropia; Oculocerebrorenal Syndrome

HARVEY W. TOPILOW, M.D.

Associate Clinical Professor of Ophthalmology, Albert Einstein College of Medicine; Attending Surgeon Retina Service, Montefiore Hospital and Medical Center, Bronx, New York; Attending Surgeon Retina Service, New York Eye and Ear Infirmary, New York, New York

Cysticercosis

ELIAS I. TRABOULSI, M.D.

Associate Professor of Ophthalmology and Pediatrics, Johns Hopkins School of Medicine; Staff, Johns Hopkins Hospital, Baltimore, Maryland

Mucopolysaccharidosis II; Mucopolysaccharidosis III

RAMESH C. TRIPATHI, M.D., Ph.D., F.A.C.S.

Professor and Chairman of Ophthalmology, Department of Ophthalmology, University of South Carolina School of Medicine, Columbia, South Carolina

Corneal Mucous Plaques

DAVID T. TSE, M.D., F.A.C.S.

Professor of Ophthalmology, Department of Ophthalmology, Bascom Palmer Eye Institute, University of Miami, Miami, Florida

Hypertrichosis

YUKIO UCHIDA, M.D.

Emeritus Professor, Department of Ophthalmology, Tokyo Women's Medical College, Tokyo, Japan

Varicella

E. MICHAEL VAN BUSKIRK, M.D.

Professor of Ophthalmology, Oregon Health Sciences University; Chief of Ophthalmology, Legacy Portland Hospitals, Portland, Oregon

Glaucoma Associated with Intraocular Lenses; Postoperative Flat Anterior Chamber

WOODFORD S. VAN METER, M.D.

Associate Clinical Professor, University of Kentucky School of Medicine, Department of Ophthalmology; Staff, Central Baptist Hospital, St. Joseph Hospital, Humana Hospital, and University of Kentucky Medical Center, Lexington, Kentucky

Fungal Endophthalmitis

DAVID W. VASTINE, M.D.

Chief of Ophthalmology, Highland General Hospital, San Francisco, California; Consultant in Cornea and External Disease, California Pacific Medical Center, San Francisco, California

Ankyloblepharon; Symblepharon

JACLYN VIDGOFF, Ph.D.

Active Staff, Department of Immunology, American Red Cross, Portland, Oregon

Mucopolysaccharidosis VI

N. D. VISWALINGAM, M.B.B.S., D.O.

Associate Specialist, Moorfields Eye Hospital; Research Associate, Institute of Ophthalmology, London, England

Trachoma

MICHAEL D. WAGONER, M.D.

Associate Professor of Ophthalmology, Harvard Medical School; Director, Cornea Service, Massachusetts Eye and Ear Infirmary, Boston, Massachusetts

Phlyctenulosis

JON D. WALKER, M.D.

Assistant Professor, Retina and Uveitis, Department of Ophthalmology, Ohio State University, Columbus, Ohio; Fellow, Vitreoretinal, University of Iowa, Iowa City, Iowa

The White Dot Syndromes

R. BRUCE WALLACE, III, M.D., F.A.C.S.

Assistant Clinical Professor of Ophthalmology, Tulane School of Medicine, New Orleans, Louisiana; Director, Laser and Surgery Center, Alexandria, Louisiana

Detachment of Descemet's Membrane

THOMAS J. WALSH, M.D.

Professor of Ophthalmology and Neurology, Yale Eye Center for Clinical Research, New Haven, Connecticut

Papilledema

DAVID S. WALTON, M.D.

Associate Clinical Professor of Ophthalmology, Harvard Medical School; Board of Surgeons, Massachusetts Eye and Ear Infirmary, Boston, Massachusetts

Aniridia; Infantile Glaucoma; Weill-Marchesani Syndrome

MARTIN WAND, M.D.

Associate Clinical Professor of Ophthalmology, University of Connecticut School of Medicine, Farmington, Connecticut; Senior Surgeon, Hartford Hospital, Hartford, Connecticut

Acinetobacter; Open-Angle Glaucoma

ARDEN H. WANDER, M.D.

Associate Professor of Clinical Ophthalmology, University of Cincinnati Medical Center; Active Staff, University of Cincinnati Hospital and Cincinnati Children's Hospital Medical Center; Attending Staff, Cincinnati Veteran's Administration Hospital, Cincinnati, Ohio

Superior Limbic Keratoconjunctivitis; Thermal Burns

PETER G. WATSON, M.D., F.R.C.S., F.R.C.Ophth.

Head, Department of Ophthalmology, University of Cambridge; Consultant, Addenbrooke's Hospital, Cambridge; Consultant, Moorfields Eye Hospital, Cambridge, London

Episcleritis; Relapsing Polychondritis; Scleritis

ROBERT C. WATZKE, M.D.

Professor of Ophthalmology, Oregon Health Sciences University, Casey Eye Institute; Teaching Faculty Member, University Hospital, Portland, Oregon

Choroidal Ruptures

RICHARD J. WEINBERG, M.D., F.A.C.S.

Clinical Assistant Professor of Ophthalmology, Georgetown University; Active Staff, Fairfax Hospital and Georgetown University Hospital, Washington, District of Columbia

Fusobacterium

MARK H. WEINER, M.D.

Active medical staff, St. Mary's Hospital, J.F.K. Medical Center, Palm Beach Regional Hospital, Palm Beach, Florida

External Orbital Fractures

THOMAS A. WEINGEIST, M.D., Ph.D

Professor and Head, Department of Ophthalmology, University of Iowa Hospitals and Clinics, University Hospitals, Iowa City, Iowa

Fabry's Disease

GEORGE W. WEINSTEIN, M.D.

Professor and Chairman, Department of Ophthalmology, West Virginia University; Active Staff, West Virginia University Hospital, Morgantown, West Virginia

Hyperopia

JOHN J. WEITER, M.D., Ph.D

Associate Clinical Professor of Ophthalmology, Harvard Medical School; Active Staff, Massachusetts Eye and Ear Infirmary, New England Medical Center, Newton-Wellesley Hospital, Salem Hospital, and Holy Family Hospital, Boston, Massachusetts

Angiomatosis Retinae; Polyarteritis Nodosa

RICHARD G. WELEBER, M.D.

Professor of Ophthalmology and Molecular and Medical Genetics, Casey Eye Institute, Oregon Health Sciences University, Portland, Oregon

Abetalipoproteinemia and Homozygous Familial Hypobetalipoproteinemia; Gyrate Atrophy of the Choroid and Retina with Hyperornithinemia; Mucopolysaccharidosis VI; Refsum's Disease

FLEMING D. WERTZ, M.D.

Assistant Professor, Uniformed Services University of the Health Sciences, Bethesda, Maryland; Assistant Chief and Residency Program; Director Walter Reed Army Medical Center, Washington, District of Columbia

Intraocular Foreign Body—Copper

IGOR WESTRA, M.D.

Clinical Instructor, Oregon Health Sciences University, Portland, Oregon; Active Staff, New Hanover Regional Medical Center, Cape Fear Memorial Hospital, Wilmington, North Carolina

Ciliary Body Concussions and Lacerations

JOHN P. WHITCHER, JR., M.D., M.P.H.

Clinical Professor of Ophthalmology, Department of Ophthalmology, University of California School of Medicine; Research Ophthalmologist, Francis I. Proctor Foundation for Research in Ophthalmology, San Francisco, California

Acute Hemorrhagic Conjunctivitis

JOHN H. WILKINS, M.D.

Clinical Instructor of Ophthalmology, Oregon Health Sciences University; Active Staff, Good Samaritan Hospital and Medical Center, Portland, Oregon

Gout

HUGH P. WILLIAMS, F.R.C.S., F.R.C.Ophth.

Consultant Ophthalmic Surgeon, North Middlesex Hospital, Edmonton, London, England

Thygeson's Superficial Punctate Keratopathy

DAVID J. WILSON, M.D.

Associate Professor of Ophthalmology; Director, Christensen Eye Pathology Laboratory, Casey Eye Institute, Oregon Health Sciences University, Portland, Oregon

Chorioretinal Concussions and Lacerations; Conjunctival Melanotic Lesions; Ewing's Sarcoma; Mucormycosis; Ocular Hypotony; Retinal Emboli

FRED M. WILSON II, M.D.

Professor of Ophthalmology; Co-Director of Cornea and External Ocular Disease Service, Department of Ophthalmology, Indiana University School of Medicine, Indianapolis, Indiana

Papilloma

WARREN A. WILSON, M.D.*

Galactosemias

RICHARD L. WINSLOW, M.D.

Clinical Associate Professor of Ophthalmology, University of Texas Southwestern Medical Center, Dallas, Texas

Vitreous Hemorrhage

---

* Deceased

JONATHAN D. WIRTSCHAFTER, M.D., F.A.C.S.

Professor of Ophthalmology, Neurology and Neurosurgery, Frank E. Burch Chair in Ophthalmology, University of Minnesota Medical School; Attending Ophthalmologist, University Hospital, Minneapolis, Minnesota

Osteopetrosis

JOHN L. WOBIG, M.D.

Associate Professor of Ophthalmology; Chief, Oculoplastic Service, Lester T. Jones Chair of Oculoplastics, Oregon Health Sciences University, Department of Ophthalmology, Casey Eye Institute, Portland, Oregon

Basal Cell Carcinoma; Congenital Anomalies of the Lacrimal System; Dacryoadenitis; Epiphora

J. REIMER WOLTER, M.D.

Professor of Ophthalmology, retired, still active in Department of Pathology, University of Michigan, Ann Arbor, Michigan

Arteriovenous Fistula

IRA G. WONG, M.D.

Clinical Professor of Ophthalmology, Department of Ophthalmology, Stanford University Medical Center, Stanford, California; Associate Clinical Professor or Ophthalmology, Proctor Foundation for Research in Ophthalmology, University of California, San Francisco, California

Bee Sting of the Cornea

PETER J. WONG, M.D.

Private practice, Long Island Eye Surgical Center, Long Island, New York

Periocular Squamous Cell Carcinoma

RANDALL V. WONG, M.D.

Active Staff, Part-time, Johns Hopkins University, Baltimore, Maryland

Cystinosis

VERNON G. WONG, M.D.

Emeritus Professor of Ophthalmology, Georgetown University Medical Center, Washington, District of Columbia

Cystinosis

THOMAS O. WOOD, M.D.

Clinical Professor of Ophthalmology, University of Tennessee; Active Staff, Baptist Memorial Hospital, The Regional Medical Center, Memphis, Tennessee

Filamentary Keratitis; Mooren's Ulcer

ROBERT D. YEE, M.D., F.A.C.S.

Professor and Chairman of Ophthalmology, Department of Ophthalmology, Indiana University School of Medicine, Indianapolis, Indiana

Nystagmus

BRIAN R. YOUNGE, M.D.

Consultant, Department of Ophthalmology, Mayo Clinic and Mayo Foundation; Associate Professor of Ophthalmology, Mayo Medical School, Rochester, Minnesota

Carotid Cavernous Fistulas and Cavernous Sinus Arteriovenous Malformations; Optic Gliomas

PREFACE

Current Ocular Therapy has been a highly successful book because its premise is to save clinicians time by providing concise data available at their fingertips. Not infrequently, ophthalmologists photocopy a disease section for the patient's education, again to increase their efficiency. In this edition, major CPT codes have been added to expedite the billing process. The fourth edition deletes a few diseases; however, 15 new topics have been added. The consultants were chosen on the basis of their experience and recent publications. Each has explained his or her method of treatment in a concise format, with an emphasis on recent developments in therapy. In this way, we have made available to the user an authoritative method of management with the most recent clinical advances.

In addition to therapy, drug dosages and methods of administration are included in the text. They have been checked against officially accepted standards. However, clinical experience, new data, differences in opinion among authorities, and individual clinical situations require that the physician exercise his or her own judgment in the choice and use of a drug. In particular, the physician is advised to check the product information included in the drug's package inset before drug administration, especially if the drug is one with which he or she is unfamiliar.

Throughout this book, we have used nonproprietary or generic names. These drugs are listed in alphabetical order, followed by many of their proprietary or trade names, in the Drug Roster at the end of this book. If a particular proprietary drug is not manufactured in the United States, the country of origin is given in parentheses after its name. Combination drugs are seldom included.

The preparations available and usual dosages indicate routes of administration for these drugs. The inclusion of a drug in this list does not indicate approval or disapproval of its use in any category, nor does it imply its efficacy or safety of action. When various indications have dictated different dosage ranges, a broad range from the lowest to highest dosage has been given, regardless of indications.

A few of these drugs have been given special symbols in the book. An asterisk (*) denotes that the particular route of administration is not approved by the FDA. A few drugs are included that are investigational or are presently not approved by the FDA for any indication; these drugs are represented by a dagger (†). If a drug has not been approved by the FDA for the specific indication, the drug is labeled with double dagger (‡). Indicated dosages above the manufacturer's recommended level have been noted with a section mark (§). Some of these drugs may subsequently be released as approved new drugs or with new indications for their use. For the reader's convenience, efforts have been made to include in the Drug Roster those drugs not sanctioned by the FDA for the specific drug dosage, method of use, or indication. Information concerning the preparation or administration of these drugs has been collected from published data or provided by the consultant.

We have had contributions from more than 400 consultants throughout the world. In sincere gratitude for their time and effort, we have acknowledged the contributors in the front of this book.

We wish to express our appreciation and pay special tribute to our Associate Editor, Ms. Joan Grove, who has worked long and hard with devotion and skill to create this book.

F. T. Fraunfelder
F. Hampton Roy

CONTENTS

Part I   GENERALIZED DISORDERS

SECTION 1   INFECTIOUS DISEASES

SECTION 4   NUTRITIONAL DISORDERS

SECTION 5   DISORDERS OF PROTEIN METABOLISM

SECTION 6   DISORDERS OF CARBOHYDRATE METABOLISM

SECTION 7   DISORDERS OF LIPID METABOLISM

SECTION 8   OTHER METABOLIC DISORDERS

SECTION 15   NEOPLASMS

BENIGN

SECTION 16 MECHANICAL AND NONMECHANICAL INJURIES

SECTION 17   UNCLASSIFIED DISEASES OR CONDITIONS

Part II   EYE AND ADNEXA

SECTION 23   EYELIDS

SECTION 24   GLOBE

SECTION 25   INTRAOCULAR PRESSURE

SECTION 26   IRIS AND CILIARY BODY

PART I

GENERALIZED DISORDERS

INFECTIOUS DISEASES

Bacterial Infections

ACINETOBACTER 041.9
(Herellea Vaginicola, Mima Polymorpha)

MARTIN WAND, M.D.

Hartford, Connecticut

The taxonomic saga of *Acinetobacter* continues to unfold at a rapid pace. Since the publication of the last review in 1990, the genus *Acinetobacter* has now been expanded to 17 distinct genospecies, and certainly more genospecies will be identified with more sophisticated techniques. Because this bacterium is ubiquitous and because it does not have many distinctive characteristics, our early inability to specifically identify this organism resulted in taxonomic chaos. Multiple names were given to what is now known to be a single genospecies, and the same name was given to what are now known to be different genospecies. At this writing, the genus *Acinetobacter* is a member of the *Neisseriaceae* family (which includes *Neisseria*, *Moraxella*, and *Kingella*). Of the 17 distinct genospecies so far identified, only 2 have been reported in the ophthalmic literature. *Acinetobacter lwoffi*, last known as *Acinetobacter calcoaceticus* var. lwoffi, and *Acinetobacter baumanii*, last known as *Acinetobacter calcoaceticus* var. anitratus, are probably still better known to ophthalmologists as *Mima polymorpha* and *Herellea vaginicola*, respectively. The true importance of this pathogen in ophthalmology remains uncertain for several reasons: (1) this taxonomic confusion is still evident in current ophthalmic literature, (2) it is an ubiquitous opportunistic organism able to colonize normal and diseased tissue so that a mixed flora is frequently cultured from a specimen, and (3) on gram stain, it is frequently misinterpreted as (or mimics) other Gram-negative coccobacilli (hence, one of its first names, *Mima polymorpha*). For the purposes here, it is sufficient to identify *Acinetobacter* as an aerobic, gram-negative, non-motile coccobacillus that is oxidase negative and non-nitrate reducing and does not ferment glucose.

Recently, studies have shown that *Acinetobacter* strains can be found in virtually 100 per cent of soil and fresh water samples and that it is part of the normal flora of fresh meats. It has been found to be part of the normal bacteria flora of almost every part of the human body, especially the skin, and has also been isolated from many objects in the hospital setting. Some species have been found to be resistant to soaps, disinfectants, and sterilizing irradiation and have been found to be viable for up to 13 days on dry Formica surfaces. In general, it is an avirulent organism that tends to be an opportunist. However, several major changes have occurred since the last review to alter its clinical importance. With the greater prevalence of immunosuppressed patients, either medically or HIV induced, and the more frequent utilization of invasive techniques, the normal host defense mechanisms in patients are compromised more frequently. As a result, *Acinetobacter* and other multiple-drug-resistant, gram-negative opportunistic bacteria have overtaken gram-positive bacteria as the leading cause of nosocomial infections. Although the number of reports of ocular involvement with this organism is still small, there has definitely been an increase over the past 5 years.

The other major change has been the emergence of greater drug resistance in this bacteria. In the early 1970s, *Acinetobacter* infections were often successfully treated with ampicillin, cephalosporins, gentamicin, and carbenicillin. However, rapid and multiple drug resistance has appeared in *Acinetobacter*, with newer antibiotics barely able to keep ahead of developing resistance. *Acinetobacter* strains naturally resistant to cephalosporins have been isolated; multiple-drug antibiotic resistance has been shown to be transposable by plasmids both to and from other *Acinetobacter* and to other gram-negative bacteria; and beta-lactamases, aminoglycoside-inactivating enzymes have been identified as well.

With regard to antibiotic recommendations, several points need emphasis. Because different genospecies have markedly different antibiotic sensitivities, the new taxonomic classifications make most of the previously published antibiotic studies suspect, if not obsolete. Recent studies have shown a synergistic effect with certain antibiotics that by themselves are only moderately effective against this bacteria. At the present time, most strains

3

of *Acinetobacter* are resistant to ampicillin, carbenicillin, cefotaxime, chloramphenicol, and gentamicin; amikacin resistance seems to be developing rapidly. *Acinetobacter lwoffi* is susceptible to most antibiotics, including chloramphenicol, which has been used in the past to differentiate this species from *Acinetobacter baumanii*, which has multiple drug resistance. For *Acinetobacter baumanii*, the most effective antibiotics, in descending order, are co-trimoxazole, polymyxin-B, sulbactam, doxycycline, and imipenem. Although many antibiotics show an additive effect, few show a synergistic effect. The combinations that have a synergistic effect for *Acinetobacter* are carbenicillin with an aminoglycoside antibiotic, imipenem with ciprofloxacin, imipenem with amikacin, and amikacin with ceftazidime. Although clinical experience with the fluroquinolones (e.g., ciprofloxacin, ofloxacin) is limited, they may in time become very useful agents owing to their high tissue penetration characteristics. Interestingly, in pharmacokinetic studies done in normal volunteers, a 500-mg and 400-mg oral dose of ciprofloxacin and ofloxacin, respectively, attained serum concentrations comparable with their 400-mg intravenous formulation. Ciprofloxacin is also available in an ophthalmic solution. Minocycline, a tetracycline, also has a high degree of microbiologic activity against *Acinetobacter* species and has exceptional tissue penetration. However, at the present time, tobramycin and imipenem seem to be the most effective across-the-board antibiotics.

THERAPY

Systemic. Systemic infections require systemic therapy. Intravenous tobramycin and/or imipenenem or some other synergistic combinations are indicated pending results of cultures and sensitivity studies.

Ocular. The topical ophthalmic antibiotic of choice is 0.3 per cent tobramycin solution or ointment, administered every 1 to 6 hours depending on the severity of the ocular involvement. Ciprofloxacin ophthalmic solution 0.3 per cent may prove to be an effective substitute. Tetracycline ointment is another alternative. Unfortunately, some of the newer effective antibiotics have not been formulated for topical use yet. For severe ocular infections, subconjunctival injections of the appropriate antibiotics should be considered. In cases of endophthalmitis, intravitreal antibiotics at the time of vitrectomy have been shown to be sight-saving. Other usual treatment modalities include warm compresses and mydriatic/cycloplegics where appropriate. The above recommendations are only for diagnosed cases of *Acinetobacter* infections. Because these organisms are great mimickers of other gram-negative rods, especially *Neisseria gonorrhoeae*, a severe ocular infection must be treated with broad-spectrum antibiotics until the diagnosis is bacteriologically confirmed and the antibiotic sensitivity known.

Ocular or Periocular Manifestations

Conjunctiva: Follicular conjunctivitis; keratoconjunctivitis resembling keratitis sicca; ophthalmia neonatorum; purulent conjunctivitis.

Cornea: Marginal ulcers; perforations; superficial punctate keratitis.

Eyelids: Blepharitis; edema.

Posterior Pole: Endophthalmitis, post-trauma or vitrectomy.

PRECAUTIONS

There is no clinical or microscopic way to differentiate a hyperacute *Acinetobacter* eye infection from one caused by *Neisseria gonorrhoeae*. On smear, both organisms appear as gram-negative intra- and extracellular diplococci. Since gonococcal conjunctivitis is a systemic disease requiring systemic and topical therapy with penicillin and since *Acinetobacter* is resistant to penicillin, it is critical to keep *Acinetobacter* in mind in the differential diagnosis of a hyperacute conjunctivitis, and treatment should be initiated with broad-spectrum antibiotics until the cause of the infection is known. Because transferable resistance factors to antibiotics have been shown in *Acinetobacter*, antibiotic sensitivity must be determined before starting single-specific therapy.

COMMENTS

With better taxonomy, newer bacteriologic techniques of identifying this organism, more immunocompromised patients, and more invasive intraocular procedures being performed, *Acinetobacter* is becoming a more important infectious organism in ophthalmology. It is important to maintain a high index of suspicion since this ubiquitous opportunistic bacteria can manifest itself in protean ocular infections.

References

Allen DM, Hartman BJ: *Acinetobacter* species. *In* Mandell GL, Douglas RG, Bennett JE (eds): Principle and Practice of Infectious Diseases, 3rd ed. New York: Churchill Livingstone, 1990, pp 1690–1770.

Bouvet PJM, Jeanjean S: Delineation of new proteolytic genomic species in the genus *Acinetobacter*. Res Microbiol *140*:291–299, 1989.

Mark DB, Gaynon MW: Trauma-induced endophthalmitis caused by *Acinetobacter anitratus*. Br J Ophthalmol 67:124–126, 1983.

Melki TS, Sramek SJ: Trauma-induced *Acinetobacter lwoffi* endophthalmitis. Am J Ophthalmol 113:598–599, 1992.

Peyman GA, Raichand M, Bennett TO: Management of endophthalmitis with pars plana vitrectomy. Br J Ophthalmol 64:472–475, 1980.

Traub WH, Spohr M: Antimicrobial drug susceptibility of clinical isolates of *Acinetobacter* species (*A. baumannii, A. haemolyticus,* genospecies 3, and genospecies 6). Antimicrob Agents Chemother 33:1617–1619, 1989.

Wand M, Olive GM Jr, Mangiaracine AB: Corneal perforation and iris prolapse due to *Mima polymorpha.* Arch Ophthalmol 93:239–241, 1975.

ACQUIRED SYPHILIS 095.8

(Acquired Lues, Lues Venera, Malum Venereum)

JEROME N. GOLDMAN, M.D., F.A.C.S.

Washington, District of Columbia

Acquired syphilis is an infectious disease that is usually transmitted sexually by the fastidious spirochete, *Treponema pallidum,* which produces a typical localized lesion, a chancre, in the region of contact about 3 weeks after inoculation. The chancre remains for several weeks and disappears without treatment. It is frequently intravaginal and therefore unrecognized in women. Associated regional lymphadenopathy is typical. Transmission probably takes place during this period of *primary syphilis.*

All syphilis serology tests are nonreactive in the earliest stages of primary syphilis so that diagnosis initially is based on the clinical picture, with confirmation by dark-field examination of chancre scrapings. Later in the early stage, the treponemal tests (FTA-ABS and MHATP) become positive first, followed by nontreponemal reactivity—VDRL, RPR, and Wasserman (cardiolipin) tests.

Secondary syphilis has its onset within weeks to months after infection. During this stage, the organism is disseminated hematogenously, with potential distribution even by way of the smallest blood vessels to every known portion of the human anatomy. Generalized eruptions of the skin and mucous membranes, fever, and diffuse lymphadenopathy characterize this stage. Such episodes may be recurrent.

During the secondary stage, ocular manifestations are common and include iridocyclitis, panuveitis, chorioretinitis, retinitis, papillitis, optic perineuritis, retinal periphlebitis, cystoid macular edema, involvement of the second and seventh cranial nerves, and retinal detachment. The FTA-ABS test is almost always positive in this stage; VDRL testing is significantly positive about 70 per cent of the time, as are the other nontreponemal tests.

Latent syphilis follows the secondary stage. By definition, it is devoid of clinical manifestations; there is no anatomic or cerebrospinal evidence of syphilis. A positive serologic test for syphilis is the only indication of the disease.

Late (tertiary) syphilis may be asymptomatic or may cause symptoms in any part of the body invaded by *T. pallidum* during dissemination. Clinical manifestations of late syphilis occur 20 or more years after the original infection when it is untreated or treated inadequately. Cranial nerve involvement (particular of the second and seventh nerves) and optic atrophy are most frequently seen in tertiary-stage syphilis.

THERAPY

Systemic. *T. pallidum* remains exquisitely sensitive to penicillin in vitro after more than 40 years of clinical use, and no failures of penicillin therapy in clinical or experimental syphilis have been attributed to intrinsic resistance of the organism to penicillin. Penicillin acts upon the cell walls of *T. pallidum* during growth and division, which are thought to occur every 30 hours. After a treponemicidal level of penicillin makes contact with the organism in vitro, increasing the concentration is no longer effective. The large doses of penicillin described in the therapy section are therefore probably necessary only to achieve treponemicidal levels in protected areas, such as the eye or central nervous system. Longer periods of exposure in the spirochete to these levels do have greater efficacy, however.

The recommended* penicillin regimen for primary, secondary, or latent syphilis of less than 1 year's duration is 2.4 million units of benzathine penicillin G administered by intramuscular injection in a single dose. If alternatives to penicillin are desired, doxycycline, 100 mg twice daily, or tetracycline, 500 mg four times daily, is recommended.

The recent literature questions this recommended treatment of syphilis. Ceftriazone, which is currently used to treat gonorrhea, is known to be effective in incubating syphilis and may also prove to be effective in later stages.

For patients who are allergic to penicillin, doxycycline, 100 mg orally twice daily, or 500 mg of oral tetracycline four times daily is recommended for two weeks. Compliance has been shown to be better with the doxycycline regimen. Erythromycin, 500 mg four times daily for 14 days, is a third alternative. Serologic follow-up is essential when these alternative therapies are employed.

Even with penicillin, treatment failures can occur. Whichever regimen is used, patients should be reexamined clinically and serologically at 3 months and at 6 months. If nontreponemal antibody titers have not declined fourfold (two tubes) by 3 months in primary or secondary syphilis or in 6 months in early latent syphilis or if clinical signs or symptoms are present, patients should have a CSF examination and be treated accordingly, provided there has no been reinfection.

In cases of (1) latent syphilis of indeterminant time or more than 1 year's duration, (2) late benign syphilis without complications of neurosyphilis, or (3) cardiovascular syphilis, the recommended therapy regimen is of longer duration than that for primary syphilis. A weekly intramuscular injection of 2.4 million units of benzathine penicillin G is administered for 3 consecutive weeks.

When alternatives to penicillin are chosen, the same daily doses for doxycycline or tetracycline should be used. However, the treatment period is extended from 2 weeks to 4 weeks.

CSF examination is recommended in all patients with syphilis of more than 1 year's duration. Before 1 year, it is clearly indicated when the following conditions are present:

1. Neurologic signs or symptoms
2. Treatment failure
3. Serum nontreponemal antibody = 1.32 or stronger
4. Other suspected evidence of active syphilis (aortitis, iritis, gumma)
5. Nonpenicillin therapy planned
6. Positive HIV antibody test

Treatment of neurosyphilis requires a more rigorous treatment schedule. Aqueous crystalline penicillin G is the preferred penicillin treatment. A daily dosage of 12 to 24 million units daily is required; 2 to 4 million units should be administered intravenously every 4 hours for 10 to 14 days. Another potentially successful regimen is the daily regimen of 2.4 million units of procaine penicillin G intramuscularly plus 500 mg of probenecid orally four times daily for 10 to 14 successive days. If the CSF is consistent with neurosyphilis, patients should be treated for neurosyphilis.

Some authorities recommend additional intramuscular injections of 2.4 million units of benzathine penicillin G weekly for 3 weeks after the intravenous treatment is completed. There is no alternative to penicillin therapy for neurosyphilis, so that skin testing and desensitization should be undertaken.

CSF examination should be repeated every 6 months. If there is neither a reduction of the CSF abnormality in 6 months nor a return to normalcy within 2 years, the neurosyphilis regimen should be repeated.

Ocular. No treatment for ocular syphilis is currently endorsed by the Centers for Disease Control, but the treatment schedule for neurosyphilis is usually followed. In recent clinical practice, intravenous infusion of as much as 24 to 36 million units daily has been reported as curative. The combined use of probenecid not only acts on the renal tubules to raise serum levels but also competitively blocks penicillin reabsorption by the ciliary body from the aqueous humor and maintains higher intraocular levels of the antibiotic. This

is especially important because of the known dissemination of *Treponema pallidum* in the secondary stage and because of the natural course of syphilis, in which ocular, as well as central nervous system manifestations, appear many years later.

Steroids and topical cycloplegics should be used when necessary for anterior segment inflammation. Applications of prednisolone or dexamethasone eyedrops or ointment should be sufficient when administered as for most anterior segment inflammations. Atropine, homatropine, or cyclopentolate may be instilled two to four times daily when there is iris irritation and during more severe attacks of iritis. Glaucoma medications that do not stimulate inflammation, such as epinephrine derivatives or beta blockers, may be used when indicated for elevated intraocular pressure.

In acute, subacute, or chronic anterior ocular inflammation for which local and systemic treatment does not seem to be effective, subconjunctival injections of dexamethasone should be given for 3 to 5 days. The inferior cul-de-sac should be anesthetized with 0.1 per cent proparacaine. The syringe should then be filled with 0.5 ml to 1.0 ml of dexamethasone, followed by 0.5 ml of 1 per cent lidocaine in the same syringe either subconjunctivally or sub-Tenon's using a 27-gauge or 30-gauge needle.

Ocular or Periocular Manifestations

(P) indicates manifestations of primary syphilis; (S) indicates those of secondary syphilis; and (T) indicates signs of tertiary, late, or neurosyphilis.

Conjunctiva: Chancre (P); conjunctivitis (S).
Cornea: Interstitial keratitis (usually monocular) (S).
Extraocular Muscles: Gumma (T); palsy (T); ptosis (T).
Eyelids: Chancre (P); exanthem (S).
Iris: Gumma (T); iritis (S); posterior uveitis (S).
Lacrimal System: Dacryoadenitis (S); dacryocystitis (S).
Optic Nerve: Atrophy (T); gumma (T); optic neuritis (S); papilledema (S); optic perineuritis (S).
Pupil: Abnormalities (T).
Retina: Arteritis (S); gumma (T); pigmentary degeneration (T); retinitis (S); choroiditis (S); macular scars (S, T).
Sclera: Episcleritis (S); gumma (T); scleritis (S).
Vitreous: Vitreitis (S).
Other: Visual field defects (T).
Acknowledgment. The author is grateful to Dr. K. Stone of the Division of STD/HIB Prevention, Centers for Disease Control, for her advice and assistance.

References

Arruga J, et al: Neuroretinitis in acquired syphilis. Ophthalmology 92:262–270, 1985.

Brooks AM, et al: Interstitial keratitis in untreated latent (late) syphilis. Aust NZ J Ophthalmol 14:127–132, 1986.

Deschenes J, Seamone CD, Baines MD: Acquired ocular syphilis, diagnosis and treatment. Ann Ophthalmology 24:134–138, 1992.

Deschenes J, Seamone CD, Baines MD: The ocular manifestations of sexually transmitted diseases. Can J Ophthalmol 25(4):177–185, 1990.

deSouza EC, et al: Unusual central chorioretinitis as the first manifestation of early secondary syphilis. Am J Ophthalmol 105:271–276, 1988.

Folk JC, et al: Syphilitic neuroretinitis. Am J Ophthalmol 95:480–486, 1983.

Gass JD, Braunstein RA, Chenoweth RG: Acute syphilitic posterior placoid chorioretinitis. Ophthalmology 97(10):1281–1297, 1990.

Halperin LS, Berger AS, Grand MG: Syphilitic disc edema and periphlebitis. Retina 10(2):196–203, 1990.

McLeish WM, Pulido JS, Holland S, Culberston WW, Winard K: The ocular manifestations of syphilis in the human immunodeficient virus type I. Ophthalmology 97(2):196–203, 1990.

Mendelsohn AD, Jampol LM: Syphilitic retinitis. A cause of necrotizing retinitis. Retina 4:221–224, 1984.

Poitevin M, et al: Syphilis in 1986. J Clin Neuro-Ophthalmol 7:11–19, 1987.

Spoor TC, et al: Ocular syphilis. J Clin Neuro-Ophthalmol 3:197–202, 1983.

STD Treatment Guidelines. MMWR 38 (number S-8):5–13, 1989.

Syyvers B, Coche F: Syphilitis uveitis: Apropos of 2 cases. Bull Soc Belge Ophthalmol 239:79–86, 1990.

Tamesis RR, Foster CS: Ocular syphilis. Ophthalmology 97(10):1281–1287, 1990.

Veldman E: Neuroretinitis in secondary syphilis. Doc Ophthalmol 1:23–29, 1986.

Wilhelmus KR, Yokoyama CM: Syphilitic episcleritis and scleritis. Am J Ophthalmol 104:595–597, 1987.

AZOTOBACTER 041.9
(Azobacter)

THOMAS J. LIESEGANG, M.D.

Jacksonville, Florida

Azotobacter is a large gram-negative aerobic rod belonging to the family Azotobacteraceae. It is ubiquitous in aerobic soil and water throughout the world in both temperate and tropical zones. The organism has many distinctive features, including large size, pleomorphism, gram stain variability, a distinctive cyst stage, and occasionally extensive production of a slime layer. It can appear as rods, cocci, or yeast-like cells within nature or under certain culture conditions. Even a single pure clone of *Azotobacter* may show varying morphologic characteristics. When grown in a nitrogen-free medium, the organism appears gram negative, but becomes more pleomorphic as the culture ages. The organism does not form spores, but has a characteristic thick-walled spherical, dormant cyst under certain circumstances. The cysts are resistant to ultraviolet radiation and drying and, under suitable conditions, can germinate into the vegetative cells from which they arose. Vegetative cells are mobile by means of flagella, but on induction of encystment, these cells lose motility and become spherical.

The genus comprises four species differentiated by their predominant shape, motility, ratio of amino acids, presence of fluorescent pigment, and various biochemical tests. All four species (*A. beijerinckii, A. chroococcum, A. paspali, A. vinelandii*) grow readily on routine culture media at 35° C. On blood agar, colonies are small, waxy, and slightly opaque. As the culture ages, colonies turn yellow or light tan. On carbohydrate media, extensive capsule or slide layers are produced.

Azotobacter is unique in its high respiratory rate and ability to fix atmospheric nitrogen and synthesize plant hormones. It plays an important role in the terrestrial ecosystem because of its ability to fix substantial amounts of nitrogen, especially in established grasslands and forests. It has been applied as a "bacterial fertilizer" for plants. In the laboratory *Azotobacter* grows best over a free nitrogen media.

A series of ten cases of *Azotobacter* keratitis was reported from Houston over an 8-year period. During the same period, this ocular microbiology laboratory reported the recovery of *Azotobacter* from the conjunctiva on three other occasions, although they were not isolated from the area of pathologic infection. There were no distinctive biomicroscopic signs characteristic of *Azotobacter* keratitis; some of the cases were characterized by a considerable corneal suppuration and subsequent scarring after resolution of the infection. Some patients had predisposing factors and some had foreign body injury, but others had no recognized predisposing factor. All four species have been isolated in association with keratitis. Plentiful large pleomorphic gram-negative rods were detected in the corneal smears, with some smears demonstrating gram-positive rods or the distinctive cysts as well. Two of the ten cases had a mixed bacterial infection. The organism grew on blood and chocolate agar, as well as thyoglycolate and brain heart infusion broth, within a few days of inoculation. Standard disc-diffusion tests have demonstrated uniform sensitivity to gentamicin, neomycin, chloramphenicol, erythromycin, bacitracin, cephalothin, and ampicillin. The clinical response in these cases suggests that gentamicin or another aminoglycoside should be effective against the various species. An animal model and extensive antimicrobial testing have not been done.

On the basis of the similarity of the organisms, some cases of *Azotobacter* have probably been incorrectly identified as *Moraxella*. The large pleomorphic size, the gram-negative forms, and the presence of cysts usually distinguish the *Azotobacter* on corneal smears. The colonial features, motility, biochemical tests, and inducement of the characteristic cyst stage confirm the presence of *Azotobacter*.

THERAPY

Ocular. The organisms seem to be sensitive to most antimicrobial therapy, although this has not been extensively tested. The microbial keratitis has been treated with topical and subconjunctival* gentamicin with subsequent resolution of the infection, although corneal scarring has limited the vision of most patients.

Ocular or Periocular Manifestations

Cornea: Suppurative corneal infection with subsequent scarring.

PRECAUTIONS

Azotobacter is probably misdiagnosed as *Moraxella* keratitis frequently. Careful review of the gram stain should enable differentiation.

COMMENTS

Azotobacter has never been reported as a pathogenic organism in any other organ system in humans. There are distinctive morphologic features of *Azotobacter* keratitis, but it has probably not been recognized in microbiology laboratories. The organisms are usually plentiful on the gram stain, and search of the smear should confirm the variable morphologic appearance, and perhaps the cyst. The organism grows readily on all media. The definitive characterization of the organism requires growth in a nitrogen-free media or the demonstration of the dormant cyst stage. The organism has been sensitive to all antibiotics.

References

Jensen HL: The Azotobacteriaciae. Bacteriol Rev *18*: 195–214, 1954.

Kennedy C, Toukdarian A: Genetics of *Azotobacter*. Application to nitrogen fixation and related aspects of metabolism. Annu Rev Microbiol *41*: 227–258, 1987.

Liesegang TJ, Jones DB, Robinson NM: *Azotobacter* keratitis. Arch Ophthalmol 99:1587–1590, 1981.

Norris JR, Chapman HM: Classification of *Azotobacter*. In Gibbs GM, Shapton DA (eds): Identification Methods For Microbiologists. New York, Academic Press, 1968, pp 19–27.

BACILLUS CEREUS 005.8

REGAN A. LOGAN, M.D.,
and DENIS M. O'DAY, M.D.

Nashville, Tennessee

Bacillus cereus is an aerobic gram-positive bacillus that is now recognized as a highly virulent pathogen. The organism enters the eye either as a result of penetrating trauma with a contaminated metallic foreign body or as a metastatic infection that occurs most frequently in drug addiction. *Bacillus* species rank second only to staphylococci as the most common pathogen isolated in post-traumatic endophthalmitis. In one study, *B. cereus* was noted to be the most common contaminant of injection paraphernalia.

Infection with *B. cereus* results in the development of a fulminating panophthalmitis, accompanied by fever and leukocytosis. The course is extremely rapid. Characteristically, a ring abscess of the cornea develops approximately 48 hours after infection as a manifestation of panophthalmitis caused by *B. cereus*, *Pseudomonas aeruginosa*, or *Proteus* species. However, at this point infection may be well established, and a return to useful vision is unlikely. Retinal periphlebitis is an earlier sign of endophthalmitis and may precede hypopyon formation or corneal changes. In most reported cases, the eye is blind within 72 hours of the onset of infection. These disastrous effects on ocular tissue seem to be related to a specific exotoxin elaborated by the organism, and the virulence of a particular strain may be related to the amount of toxin produced.

THERAPY

Systemic. The mainstay of systemic treatment for *B. cereus* infection is the daily intravenous administration of 40 mg/kg of clindamycin and 4 mg/kg of gentamicin in divided doses. Unlike most gram-positive bacilli, *B. cereus* in resistant to the natural and semisynthetic penicillins, as well as the cephalosporins. However, because there may be difficulty initially with the specific identification of *B. cereus* as opposed to the other gram-positive bacilli, penicillin or a cephalosporin should be administered concurrently with clindamycin and gentamicin to which *B. cereus* is susceptible. A reasonable combination would be 250,000 units/kg of aqueous penicillin G administered intravenously daily. Antibiotic therapy should be continued systemically for at least 7 days.

Ocular. In view of the grave nature of the infection, periocular, intravitreal, and topical ophthalmic antibiotics are recommended in addition to intravenous therapy. Clindamycin may be particularly useful because of the therapeutic levels achievable in the eye after systemic and periocular administration. Separate subconjunctival injections of 34 mg of clindamycin* and 40 mg of gentamicin* are recommended daily. This periocular antibiotic therapy should be continued for several weeks. In addition, fortified gentamicin[§] (13 mg/ml) and clindamycin* (50 mg/ml) eyedrops should be given every 30 minutes. Recently, the combination of 1 mg of vancomycin* with 100 µg of gentamicin* has been suggested for intravitreal use.

Topical and periocular corticosteroids should be administered concurrently with the antibiotics in an attempt to control the host inflammatory response. Subconjunctival injection of 4 mg of dexamethasone* daily is recommended. Topical ocular 1 per cent prednisolone acetate[§] may be used hourly. Corticosteroid and topical antibiotic therapy may be needed for several months.

Surgical. In light of the fulminating course of this disease, an extensive vitrectomy should be performed as soon as infection is suspected. At this time, intravitreal injection of 450 µg of clindamycin* and 250 µg of gentamicin* should be used. Serious consideration should be given to further intravitreal antibiotic therapy in the next 48 hours.

Ocular or Periocular Manifestations

Anterior Chamber: Hypopyon.
Choroid or Retina: Extensive necrosis.
Cornea: Ring abscess.
Globe: Panophthalmitis, progressing to phthisis.
Orbit: Cellulitis with proptosis.
Vitreous: Abscess.

A small but definite risk of pseudomembranous colitis caused by an overgrowth of *Clostridium difficile* in the small bowel is associated with the systemic administration of clindamycin. However, local administration of clindamycin in the doses recommended has not been known to give rise to this adverse side effect.

Systemic gentamicin is potentially nephrotoxic and should be administered with caution in patients with renal impairment. The actual dose should be calculated on the basis of lean body weight, aiming for a peak level of 6 to 8 µg/ml and a trough of 2 µg/ml. Gentamicin blood levels should be checked 24 hours after the initial dose. Once these levels are stabilized, gentamicin levels can be monitored every 4 to 5 days. Serum creatinine levels can be used to check renal function every 2 to 3 days.

The concurrent administration of corticosteroid and antibiotics carries with it the risk of enhancing microbial proliferation. However, this risk seems justified in the face of the speed and destructive nature of this infection.

COMMENTS

The best hope of salvaging eyes infected with *B. cereus* seems to lie with early diagnosis and prompt treatment. Thus, penetrating trauma with a metallic foreign body occurring in a dirty environment or an apparent metastatic infection in a suspected drug addict should always suggest the possibility of an infection by this organism. Fever and leukocytosis in conjunction with panophthalmitis in either setting are especially suggestive of this pathogen, as intraocular infection by most other micro-organisms usually does not produce systemic signs. In such circumstances, an immediate diagnostic and therapeutic vitrectomy is indicated, with antibiotic therapy being initiated before surgery if an undue delay is anticipated. Although the prognosis is extremely poor, several eyes have now been saved with useful vision by following the above approach.

References

Affeldt JC, et al: Microbial endophthalmitis resulting from ocular trauma. Ophthalmology 94:407–413, 1987.
Davey RT Jr, Tauber WB: Post-traumatic endophthalmitis: The emerging role of *Bacillus cereus* infection. Rev Infect Dis 9:110–123, 1987.
Mandelbaum S, Forster RK: Postoperative endophthalmitis. Int Ophthalmol Clin 27:95–106, 1987.
O'Day DM, et al: The problem of *Bacillus* species infection with special emphasis on the virulence of *Bacillus cereus*. Ophthalmology 88:833–838, 1981.
Packer AJ, Weingeist TA, Abrams GW. Retinal periphlebitis as an early sign of bacterial endophthalmitis. Am J Ophthalmol 96:66, 1983.
Shadsuddin D, et al: *Bacillus cereus* panophthalmitis: Source of the organism. Rev Infect Dis 4:97–103, 1982.
Tuazon CU, et al: Serious infections with *Bacillus* sp. JAMA 241:1136–1140, 1979.

BACILLUS SPECIES INFECTIONS 041.8

JOSE S. PULIDO, M.D.,
and ROBERT A. HYNDIUK, M.D.

Milwaukee, Wisconsin

The genera *Bacillus* are ubiquitous bacteria that are gram-positive, aerobic, spore-forming rods. Spore formation allows these species to survive even in very hostile environments, including high temperatures and even ultraviolet radiation. Soil contamination of a wound, foreign body, or puncture site allows tissue inoculation of these organisms.

B. anthracis infections cause anthrax. This

zoonotic disease occurs from exposure to live-stock, especially sheep or goats or their products including wool or hides. Anthrax infection can be cutaneous, inhalational, or gastrointestinal. In the United States this is a rare disease but it still occurs in underdeveloped countries. The anthrax malignant pustule is the most characteristic disease form and produces a papulo-vesicular lesion. Though rare, pustules can develop on the lids, and they can then progress to ulceration followed by gangrene, orbital cellulitis, and septicemia.

B. cereus is the most common and most virulent species of *Bacillus* that causes ocular infection. The most important ocular infection caused by *B. cereus* is an endophthalmitis, usually post-traumatic, which is usually associated with soil-contaminated foreign bodies. In one series of post-traumatic endophthalmitis, there was a 40 per cent incidence of *Bacillus* species. Clinically established *B. cereus* endophthalmitides of longer than 24 hours duration have uniformly resulted in blindness. In a rabbit model, only 100 *B. cereus* organisms were necessary to develop a fulminant endophthalmitis within 24 hours.

Toxins and various proteases, including hemolysins, lecithinases, phospholipases, collagenases, and sphingomyelinases, are probably involved in the devastating inflammation caused by *B. cereus*. Further discussion of *B. cereus* can be found in the preceding article. Because it is a soil contaminant, many infections caused by *B. cereus* as well as other *Bacillus* species are mixed infections in association with other microbial species.

Other *Bacillus* species have been rarely associated with ocular infections, including *B. thurigiensis*, *B. subtilis*, *B. licheniformis*, and *B. alvei*. Of 54 cases of bacillus endophthalmitis reported between 1987 and 1991, 34 were speciated, and of these, 27 (79 per cent) were *B. cereus*, 4 (12 per cent) were *B. licheniformis* and 3 (9 per cent) were *B. subtilis*.

Clinical suspicion should be high in cases of endophthalmitis or keratitis in association with soil contamination or intravenous drug abuse. Treatment should begin immediately after appropriate cultures have been obtained without waiting for culture results. If a foreign body is present, it too should be sent for culture. The organisms grow easily on most media. Speciation is not done in most laboratories, and cultures are often read out as "*Bacillus* species." In certain hospital microbiology laboratories, bacilli are considered contaminants, and the cultures are discarded. Laboratory personnel need to know the ocular significance of these organisms. A gram stain demonstrates straight rod-shaped bacteria with rounded or square ends.

THERAPY

Systemic. For *Bacillus anthrax*, the treatment of choice is penicillin. This is in marked contrast to other bacillus species that produce beta-lactamases and are therefore resistant to penicillin, semi-synthetic penicillins, and cephalosporins. However, in general, bacillus species that are responsible for ocular infections are sensitive to vancomycin and gentamicin. In one series 100 per cent of the organisms were sensitive to either one of these agents. There seems to be synergism between these two antibiotics. Amikacin, in contrast, has not shown this synergism with vancomycin. Clindamycin is an alternative to vancomycin, but there is a higher resistance by *Bacillus* species to this antibiotic though again there is apparent synergism with gentamicin.

Ocular. Treatment of ocular bacillus infections depends on which specific part of the eye or orbit is involved, as well as the route of infection.

Endophthalmitis. Since intraocular *Bacillus* infections tend to do poorly without immediate and aggressive treatment, intravitreal, topical, and subconjunctival antibiotics should be instituted promptly. Intravitreal gentamicin* (100 µg) in combination with vancomycin* (1000 µg) or clindamycin* (500 to 1000 µg) is given. Subconjunctival injections include gentamicin* (20 mg) with either vancomycin* (25 mg) or clindamycin* (25 mg). Topical antibiotics, including vancomycin§ (50 mg/ml) or clindamycin§ (50 mg/ml), along with topical gentamicin§ (13.4 mg/ml) should be administered every 30–60 minutes. In the presence of established severe *Bacillus* endophthalmitis, systemic antibiotics should also be given to avoid panophthalmitis and orbital cellulitis. Vancomycin (15–30 mg/kg/day) or clindamycin (1000 mg/d) can be used.

Corneal Ulcers. After ruling out the possibility that a corneal infection is not part of a panophthalmitis, topical antibiotics alone are the preferred treatment. Either vancomycin§ (50 mg/ml) or clindamycin§ (50 mg/ml) is administered in association with gentamicin§ (13.4 mg/ml) initially every 30 minutes, and then the dosing is titrated depending upon clinical response.

Orbital Cellulitis. Many cases of orbital cellulitis are associated with panophthalmitis. These cases should be treated as in severe *Bacillus* endophthalmitis. If the eye is not involved, then systemic treatment for orbital cellulitis should be vancomycin (500 mg/q6) and gentamicin (1 mg/kg/q8h).

Surgery. With severe necrotizing panophthalmitis, consideration should be given to enucleation to decrease the possibility of systemic seeding or orbital cellulitis. In cases of orbital abscess, drainage should be performed. In cases of endophthalmitis, pars plana vitrectomy should be performed as soon as the possibility of bacillus endophthalmitis is entertained since no vision is reported to have been saved once the characteristic ring ulcer develops. In cases of intraocular foreign bodies with possible soil contamination, vitrectomy in combination with foreign body removal and prophylactic intraocular antibiotics should be considered. At this time the recommended prophylactic intraocular dosages are vancomycin* 500–1000 μg and gentamicin* 100 μg.

Ocular or Periocular Manifestations

Conjunctiva: Purulent or pseudomembranous conjunctivitis.
Cornea: Ring abscess; ulcer.
Globe: Endophthalmitis; panophthalmitis.
Lids: Papulovesicular lesion; preseptal cellulitis.
Orbit: Cellulitis; abscess.

PRECAUTIONS

Intravitreal antibiotics have a high possibility of causing retinal toxicity so it is important to determine that the concentration and dose to be given are exact. This is particularly true with the use of gentamicin for which the toxic doses are still unknown. Usually, 100 μg or less of gentamicin is tolerated even in vitrectomized eyes.

Systemic toxicity of parenterally or orally administered antibiotics needs to be considered. Systemic gentamicin, for instance, can cause nephrotoxicity and ototoxicity. If parenteral gentamicin is to be given, careful attention to renal status as well as peak and trough gentamicin levels should be paid during the course of treatment. However, even careful monitoring of serum levels of aminoglycosides may not prevent ototoxicity, and we rarely recommend its use. Systemic vancomycin may not only cause pseudomembranous colitis but also ototoxicity and nephrotoxicity, especially if given in combination with aminoglycosides. Clindamycin can cause pseudomembranous colitis.

It is important that microbiology laboratory personnel be aware that *Bacillus* species cause severe ocular infections and that growth is not just a laboratory nonpathogenic contaminant.

Acknowledgment. Supported in part by an unrestricted grant from Research to Prevent Blindness, New York.

References

Boldt HC, Mieler WJ: Endophthalmitis. *In* Hyndiuk TK (ed): Infections of the Eye: Diagnosis and Management. Boston, Little, Brown, 1993.
Boldt HC, Pulido JS, Blodi CF, et al: Rural endophthalmitis. Ophthalmology 96:1722–1726, 1989.
Brinton GS, Hyndiuk RA, Abrams G, et al: Posttraumatic endophthalmitis. Arch Ophthalmol 102:547–550, 1984.
Kervick GN, Flynn HW, Alfonso E, et al: Antibiotic therapy for *Bacillus* species infections. Am J Ophthalmol 110:683–687, 1990.
Mieler WF, Ellis MK, Williams DF, et al: Retained intraocular foreign bodies and endophthalmitis. Ophthalmology 97:1532–1538, 1990.
O'Day DM, Smith RS, Gregg CR: The problem of *Bacillus* species infection with special emphasis on the virulence of *Bacillus cereus*. Ophthalmology 88:833–838, 1981.
Vahey JB, Flynn HW: Results in the management of *Bacillus* endophthalmitis. Ophthal Surg 22:681–686, 1991.
Weber DJ, Saviteer SM, Rutala WA, et al: In vitro susceptibility of *Bacillus* spp. to selected antimicrobial agents. Animicrob Agent Chemother 32:642–645, 1988.

BOTULISM 005.1

MICHAEL CHERINGTON, M.D.

Denver, Colorado

Botulism is a paralyzing disease caused by the most toxic substance known to humans. The toxin is produced by the bacterium *Clostridium botulinum*. Eight immunologic distinct toxins have been identified. Human cases are almost always due to type A, B, or E. When contaminated seafood is found to be responsible, the toxin present is often type E.

Botulism toxin is heat labile and thus is often destroyed by the cooking process. By contrast, the spores of *C. Botulinum* are heat resistant. When spores are present in food, actively multiplying bacilli produce the toxin at room temperature under anaerobic conditions at a pH of 4.6 or above. The toxin causes paralysis of skeletal muscles by interfering with the release of acetylcholine.

The clinical symptoms of botulism usually occur within 12 to 36 hours after ingestion of contaminated food. The signs and symptoms begin in the cranial nerve territory (blurred vision, dysarthria, dysphagia) and then descend. This pattern distinguishes botulism from the Guillain-Barré syndrome, which is characterized by ascending paralysis.

In botulism, respiratory paralysis can follow quickly and can be fatal unless treated. Alertness, mentation, and the sensory system remain normal. The pupils are usually normal, particularly early in the disease. Patients with severe botulism almost always have marked extraocular muscle weakness, including ptosis. Weakness of the face, tongue, pharynx, neck, and sometimes the limbus occurs. Weakness progresses until it reaches a plateau at about 4 to 5 days. Although the weakness is bilateral, it is often asymmetric. Severe respiratory paralysis can occur within the first day. Symptoms of parasympathetic dysfunction may include gastrointestinal ileus and dryness of the mouth and eyes. Deep tendon reflexes are reduced in proportion to the degree of muscular weakness. Recovery, if it occurs, is prolonged but nearly total. Laboratory confirmation usually requires the detection of toxin in the contaminated food or in the patient's serum or stool.

THERAPY

Systemic. The role of guanidine‡ in the treatment of botulism remains that of an adjunct to therapy and not that of a cure. It has helped some but not all patients. The initial oral daily dose is 15 mg/kg administered in divided doses.

Supportive. The major treatment of botulism is good medical care, which consists of providing artificial ventilation for the patients with respiratory paralysis. Tracheotomy and positive pressure support are usually required. Mechanical assistance to respiration may be needed for as long as weeks or months. Early administration of antitoxin may be of value in cases of type E botulism. The literature and experience suggest that antitoxin is less effective in types A and B botulism. Corticosteroid treatment has not been beneficial.

Ocular or Periocular Manifestations

Extraocular Muscles: External ophthalmoplegia.
Eyelids: Ptosis.
Pupil: Variable response.

PRECAUTIONS

Increasing the dose of guanidine may result in considerable epigastric distress and nausea. These side effects are problematic because guanidine has not been approved for parenteral administration and must be given orally. Serious side effects of guanidine include bone marrow suppression and renal toxicity.

Recently, another drug, 4-aminopyridine†, has been reported to be effective in reversing the neuromuscular block of botulism. Unfortunately, it has little or no benefit in reversing the paralysis of respiratory muscles. In this respect, it is similar to the action of guanidine. Both guanidine and 4-aminopyridine have serious side effects that may be encountered, particularly with prolonged usage. The most serious side effects seen with guanidine have occurred when its use has been prolonged, usually in illnesses, such as myasthenia syndrome. Therefore, clinicians must weigh risk-benefit ratios. Both of these drugs should be considered experimental at this time.

COMMENTS

In some clinical situations the diagnosis cannot be confirmed by serologic means because of a delay in diagnosis. In these situations particularly, electrophysiologic studies can often provide additional diagnostic information. The most often-noted electrophysiologic abnormality is a reduced amplitude of muscle action potentials.

The treatment of botulism remains good medical and nursing intensive care.

Infant botulism is becoming recognized more frequently. Most cases of infant botulism have an onset before 6 months of age. Patients often have a weak cry, are hypotonic, and develop ptosis and other extraocular palsies. Infant botulism results when ingested spores of *C. botulinum* germinate in the intestinal tract and produce toxin. In some infants, there is a history of being fed honey.

Wound botulism is a rare form of botulism that almost always occurs in adults. Recently, wound botulism has been reported in drug abusers. It results from toxin produced when *C. botulinum* bacteria infect a wound.

A very recent development in the history of this disease has been the use of the neurotoxin as a therapeutic tool. Botulinum toxin A was first reported in 1981 as a treatment for strabismus and has since been used in the treatment of hemifacial spasm, blepharospasm, cervical dystonia, and other dystonias.

References

Cherington M: Botulism. Ten-year experience. Arch Neurol 30:432–437, 1974.
Cherington W: Botulism. Semin Neurol 10:27–31, 1990.
Jankovic J, Brin MF: Therapeutic uses of botulinum toxin. N Engl J Med 324:1186–1194, 1991.
Jenzer G, et al: Autonomic dysfunction in botulism B. A clinical report. Neurology 25:150–152, 1975.
Konig H, Gassman HB, Jenzer G: Ocular involvement in benign botulism B. Am J Ophthalmol 80:430–432, 1975.
Pickett J, et al: Syndrome of botulism in infancy: Clinical and electrophysiologic study. N Engl J Med 295:770–772, 1976.
Scott AB: Botulinum toxin injection into extraocular muscles as an alternative to strabismus surgery. Ophthalmology 87:1044–1049, 1980.
Terranova W, Palumbo JN, Breman JG: Ocular findings in botulism type B. JAMA 241:475–477, 1979.

BRUCELLOSIS 023.9
(Malta Fever, Mediterranean Fever, Melitococcosis, Undulant Fever)

J. POLETTI, M.D.

Tarbes, France

Brucellosis is an infectious disease common to animals and humans. The responsible bacteria are nonmotile, gram-negative aerobic coccobacilli. For humans, the common sources of infection are ingestion of milk products and occupational contact with infected animals.

Brucellosis is very polymorphous. The

acute septicemic phase does not result in many ocular symptoms. During the subacute form of focal brucellosis, osteo-articular, hepatosplenic, glandular, cardiac, respiratory, nephric, and neuromeningeal localizations may occur. Most of the ocular manifestations noticed at this time are related to neuromeningeal involvement. However, during the chronic phase, uveitis and other allergic ocular manifestations are seen more frequently, often isolated from any general context of malaise, pain, neurovegetative disorders, or localized foci. The iridocyclitis is frequently of rapid onset, evanescent, and recurrent. After some relapses, a granulomatous uveitis may develop. Posterior uveitis is often masked by a vitreous opacity; multiple nodular exudates with weak inflammatory or hemorrhagic reactions may also result. At this stage of infection, the Wright's sero-agglutination reaction is often negative, and the skin reaction to *Brucella* antigen is usually positive but contraindicated due to a syndromal reaction risk.

THERAPY

Systemic. In the acute phase, rest and antibiotic therapy for 45 to 60 days are recommended.

In the subacute and chronic phases, antibiotic therapy may be useful to erase quiet foci and persistent bacteria. The usual daily adult dose is 0.2 gm of doxycycline and 0.9 gm of rifampicin, administered for 3 to 6 months. A short course of oral corticosteroid therapy may be necessary prior to this treatment. After remission of chronic brucellosis, specific desensitizing antigen[†] therapy may be administered by intradermal or subcutaneous route. Very small initial doses of the inactivated vaccines should be used, and a slow progression in administration should be made to avoid syndromal reactions.

Ocular. During the uveitis phase, topical ophthalmic atropine and corticosteroids minimize the damage to the eye during an attack and lessen the duration of the ocular disease. Local corticosteroids are also helpful during desensitization to prevent syndromal ocular reaction.

Ocular or Periocular Manifestations

Conjunctiva: Conjunctivitis.
Cornea: Annular keratitis with rounded subepithelial infiltrates; other keratitis; ulcer.
Extraocular Muscles: Paralysis.
Eyelids: Blepharitis.
Lacrimal System: Dacryoadenitis.
Optic Nerve: Papilledema; retrobulbar or optic neuritis.

Retina: Edema; hemorrhages; venous disorders; retinal detachment.
Sclera: Episcleritis; scleritis.
Uvea: Anterior, intermediate, posterior, panuveitis.
Other: Cataract; decreased intraocular pressure (early); secondary glaucoma (late).

PRECAUTIONS

The thrust of treatment must be essentially preventive. Hygiene systemic animal vaccination and human vaccination* (after sensitizing test) of professionally or geographically exposed individuals are effective control measures.

The treatment of chronic brucellosis and of its ocular allergic manifestations is difficult. It is based upon a specific antigen therapy not approved in many countries. It requires a special control and is not usually given to elderly patients or to others with visceral weaknesses. Its efficiency must be checked with repeated dosages, until a normalization of Witmer's relation is achieved.

COMMENTS

The ocular brucellosis diagnosis must be authenticated by the calculation of Witmer's relation between ocular and serous specific antibodies. If this dosage is not available, a presumptive diagnosis will be given by significant values of serologic tests (buffered antigen, indirect immunofluorescence, passive hemagglutination, specific agglutination test; detection of circulating immune complexes) and by the cell immunity test (lymphocyte transformation, inhibition of leukocyte migration), showing a retarded hypersensitivity.

References

Comité mixte FAO-OMS d'experts de la brucellose, 6ème rapport—WHO, Technical report number 740–1986.
Poletti J, Poletti A, Larmande A: Diagnostic and therapeutic problems in brucellosis uveitis. Med Trop 41:523–525, 1981.
Renoux GM, Larmande A, Poletti JA: Le diagnostic biologique de la brucellose oculaire. Arch Ophthalmol 37:767–769, 1977.
Renoux M, et al: Hémagglutination passive, transformation lymphoblastique et migration des leucocytes appliquées au diagnostic des brucelloses. Dev Biol Stand 31:145–156, 1976.
Rolando IM, Carbone AO: Circulating immune complexes in the pathogenesis of human brucellar uveitis. Chibret Intern J Ophthalmol 3:30–38, 1985.

* "Vaccin inactivé brucellique PI" and "Test brucellique PS" Mérieux Institute (France, Portugal, Brazil).

CLOSTRIDIUM PERFRINGENS 000.5

DAVID SEVEL, M.D., Ph.D., F.A.C.S.

La Jolla, California

Clostridium perfringens is a gram-positive, rod-shaped, anaerobic bacillus. It is the most important cause of gas gangrene infection, which occurs predominantly in traumatized, ischemic skeletal muscle but has also been described in the abdominal wall and uterus.

C. perfringens endophthalmitis is rare and occurs as an opportunistic infection. It is associated with a perforating injury, frequently by an intraocular foreign body. *C. perfringens* septicemia may also cause metastatic endophthalmitis. Metastatic endophthalmitis due to *C. perfringens* originating from the biliary tract may occur. In the absence of trauma to the eye, early detection of the primary source of the infection is emphasized. The infection characteristically develops within 24 hours of a penetrating injury. Severe ocular pain, marked edema of the lids, chemosis, and early elevation of the intraocular pressure are the hallmarks of this infection. Bloody or coffee-colored discharge is noted, and hypopyon and air bubbles are characteristically present in the anterior chamber. Intraocular necrosis rapidly ensues, and the patient becomes febrile as a systemic toxicity develops. *C. perfringens* orbital cellulitis may occur as an extension of the eye infection or either primarily in the orbit and is then associated with a retained intraorbital foreign body.

THERAPY

Systemic. The successful treatment of *C. perfringens* is dependent on early diagnosis. A major prerequisite is the correct collection and transportation of the ocular exudate or orbital specimen to the laboratory. The fluid specimen is kept in the syringe and either inoculated without delay into thioglycolate broth or placed in an anaerobic jar (Gaspak). By far, the most satisfactory method of inoculation is in a prereduced anaerobic bottle, which provides a flat agar surface for evaluation of the number and morphologic characteristics of the colonies.

The gram stain determines the initial choice of antibiotic. If large, uniform gram-positive rods are noted, 1 to 3 million units of sodium penicillin G are administered intravenously every 3 to 4 hours. These massive doses of penicillin serve the purpose of prolonging the period during which surgical intervention can be successful. Although systemic antibiotics cannot control the relentless destruction of the eye associated with *C. perfringens* endophthalmitis, they can prevent orbital extension of the condition. If the patient is sensitive to penicillin, 1 gm of cefazolin every 4 hours should be given intravenously. This antibiotic is effective against penicillinase-producing staphylococci, but can cause renal complications.

If gram-positive and gram-negative organisms are observed on gram stain, a combination of 3 million units of sodium penicillin G every 4 hours and 1 gm of chloramphenicol every 6 hours is administered intravenously. Chloramphenicol is a good alternative drug in the highly penicillin-allergic patient. It is preferable to tetracycline or clindamycin in view of the resistance of some clostridia to these agents.

It takes 24 hours or longer to culture the anaerobes. In the interim period, 1 gm of intravenous chloramphenicol is given every 6 to 8 hours so as to cover other anaerobes that may be present.

Once the infection is controlled either by vitrectomy, evisceration, or orbital surgery, 500 mg of ampicillin are given orally every 6 hours. In addition, chloramphenicol is administered orally in a dosage of 500 mg every 8 hours for 1 week and reduced to 250 mg every 6 hours for a second week.

Amoxicillin, 500 mg, may be administered orally every 6 hours instead of the ampicillin, or in the more acute phase, cefotaxime, 2 gm, is given intravenously every 4 hours for 7 days.

The indications for gas gangrene antitoxin are shock and hemolytic anemia. The dosage is 50,000 units intravenously every 6 hours for 1 to 2 days. Gas gangrene antitoxin is of little use in the prophylaxis of gas gangrene and is of questionable value in treatment.

Hyperbaric oxygen treatment does not seem to be efficacious for *C. perfringens* ophthalmitis, but may be of use if there is orbital involvement. Before hyperbaric oxygen is administered, myringotomy tubes are inserted into the eardrums, and the patient is given two 2-hour treatments in a hyperbaric oxygen chamber filled and ventilated with 100 per cent oxygen at a pressure of 3 atmospheres (approximately 30 pounds per square inch).

Ocular. Antibiotic therapy is of prophylactic value and is usually combined with a surgical procedure. Subconjunctival injections of 0.5 to 1.0 million units of sodium penicillin G* or 100 mg of cephaloridine* and 20 mg of gentamicin* are given to cover a mixed infection.

Surgical. A prerequisite for the treatment of *C. perfringens* infection is excision of the necrotic, highly toxic tissue. In the early stages (within 24 hours) of *C. perfringens* endophthalmitis, vitrectomy and instillation of intravitreal antibiotics are indicated. For mixed infection, the dosage of intravitreal infusion fluid is 10 μg of cephaloridine* and 8 μg of gentamicin.*

It seems that once *C. perfringens* endophthalmitis is established treatment will not salvage vision because of the severe toxicity generated by the organism. If the infection is confined to the eye, evisceration is indicated. However, if there is obvious evidence of extension of the reaction beyond the confines of the eye into the orbital tissue, enucleation combined with a partial exenteration of the necrotic and macroscopically involved orbital tissue is indicated. Any intraocular or intraorbital foreign bodies should be removed. These steps are essential to prevent the systemic syndrome of gas gangrene, which is a life-threatening condition.

Ocular or Periocular Manifestations

Anterior Chamber: Gas bubbles; hypopyon.
Cornea: Penetrating wound.
Globe: Endophthalmitis; proptosis.
Other: Acute rise of intraocular pressure; chemosis; coffee-colored discharge; eyelid edema; severe ocular pain.

PRECAUTIONS

Once *C. perfringens* endophthalmitis gains a foothold, the destructive process seems to be irreversible. Rapid necrosis of the intraocular tissue ensues, and neither antibiotics nor gas gangrene antitoxin is of any use. Although hyperbaric oxygen may be of avail if there is orbital involvement, it is unlikely to be efficacious for the intraocular infection.

COMMENTS

Vitrectomy with intravitreal injection of antibiotics could theoretically be of value in gas-gangrene endophthalmitis, as involved toxic and infected tissue are excised.

References

Bristow JH, Kassar B, Sevel D: Gas gangrene panophthalmitis treated with hyperbaric oxygen. Br J Ophthalmol 55:139–142, 1971.
Davis CE, et al: Simple method for culturing anaerobes. Appl Microbiol 25:216–221, 1973.
Frantz JF, et al: Acute endogenous panophthalmitis caused by *Clostridium perfringens.* Am J Ophthalmol 78:295–303, 1974.
Levitt JM, Stam J: *Clostridium perfringens* panophthalmitis. Arch Ophthalmol 84:227–228, 1970.
Nangia V, Hutchinson C: Metastatic endophthalmitis caused by *Clostridium perfringens.* Br J Ophthalmol 76:252–253, 1992.
Obertynski H, Dyson C: *Clostridium perfringens* panophthalmitis. Can J Ophthalmol 9:258–259, 1974.
Sevel D, et al: Gas in the orbit associated with orbital cellulitis and paranasal sinusitis. Br J Ophthalmol 57:133–137, 1973.

CONGENITAL SYPHILIS 090.9

JEROME N. GOLDMAN, M.D., F.A.C.S.

Washington, District of Columbia

Congenital syphilis occurs when *Treponema pallidum* passes across the placenta from a mother whose infection is in the primary, secondary, or early latent stage. The condition may become clinically apparent in utero, at birth, shortly after birth, or between late childhood and middle adolescence (7 to 17 years of age).

Clinical symptoms are apparent at birth only in the most severe cases. The usual signs in the infant under 2 years are hepatosplenomegaly, skin rash, snuffles, nonviral hepatic jaundice, anemia (nephrotic syndrome), or pseudoparalysis.

The older child may have such nonocular stigmata as anterior bowing of the shins ("sabre shins"), frontal bossing, "mulberry molars," "Hutchinson's teeth," "saddle nose," rhagades, or Clutton joints.

Typically, the ophthalmologist is consulted in late childhood because of binocular interstitial keratitis that is invariably associated with anterior uveitis. Before penicillin was available, the ocular inflammation persisted for months. Superficial and deep corneal neovascularization may develop, but it ultimately resolves, leaving the characteristic sheath of translucent scar tissue immediately anterior to Descemet's membrane. A network of relatively clear, branching, linear canals may weave through the opalescent scar as a hallmark of the inflammatory process. After adolescence, the scarred, irregularly thinned corneas with interstitial keratitis typically remain quiescent.

The anterior chamber activity usually damages the chamber angle sufficiently so that secondary glaucoma frequently appears many years later in a quiet eye. The onset of inner ear inflammation, resulting in bilateral deafness, may occur at this time, although it more typically presents later in adolescence or even three decades later.

Also appearing in these late periods are chorioretinitis, retinal periphlebitis, or posterior uveitis, which is sometimes associated with anterior uveitis. The residue seen in the inner eye are the "pepper-and-salt" fundus or the typical "bone corpuscular" pigmented and atrophic areas in the midperiphery with ring scotomata mimicking retinitis pigmentosa. Optic atrophy is also seen in congenital syphilis.

Only very early syphilis (intrauterine through 10 weeks postpartum) is infectious.

Infants

The Centers for Disease Control recently revised its criteria for reporting cases of congenital syphilis and distinguished these new criteria from those for making a diagnosis. Between 70 per cent and 100 per cent of untreated, infected mothers will have infected babies. Therefore, any infant whose mother had untreated, questionably treated, or inadequately treated syphilis is diagnosed *Presumptive,* and should be reported and treated, even if asymptomatic and seronegative. Stillborns of such mothers are also reported. Using the prior, more ambiguous criteria as well as the new criteria, Cohen et al. (1990) found there to be a fivefold increase in reported cases.

Diagnostically, the clinician also considers presumptive any infant with a treponemal test for syphilis, as well as those with the following: (1) evidence of congenital syphilis on physical examination, (2) evidence of congenital syphilis on long bone x-rays, (3) reactive CSF VDRL (although this is occasionally indicative of a high blood titer in the infant, rather than an indication of neurosyphilis), or an otherwise unexplained elevation of the CSF cell count or total protein, or (4) reactive FTA-ABS on antibody absorbed-19S-IgM antibody.

One of the difficulties in making the diagnosis is that the newborn may be seropositive because of the passive transfer of maternal antibodies. Nontreponemal antibodies that are thus acquired, as well as in those infants who are infected and treated adequately, will decrease in titer during the first year.

THERAPY

Infants. Penicillin is the drug of choice because it is effective and incurs no risk to the fetus other than the Jarisch-Herxheimer reaction described below. The CDC recommends that all newborns with congenital syphilis be treated with crystalline penicillin, 50,000 units/kg/dose, intravenously every 8 to 12 hours for 10 to 14 days. Procaine penicillin is not recommended, nor is any alternative drug to penicillin. Benzathine penicillin G is no longer considered an acceptable alternative, although Zenker and Perman (1991) discuss a few instances in which it might be considered.

Nontreponemal tests should be used to evaluate the effectiveness of treatment. If effective, titers will decrease and should disappear within 1 year. Treponemal tests should not be used to evaluate treatment because they usually remain positive. If there is CSF involvement, lumbar punctures should be repeated, and the fluid reexamined until the CSF cell count is normal. If the cell count does not continue a downward trend, if the CSF-VDRL is still reactive at 6 months, or if the cell count is not normal after 2 years, the infant should be retreated.

Older Infants and Children. No distinction is made in the revised CDC criteria or the recent literature between those under 2 years of age and those older than 2. Children older than 2 years of age discovered to have syphilis were previously given a CSF exam to rule out congenital syphilis. If the child was thought to have congenital syphilis (if the CSF was abnormal), he or she was to receive 200,000–300,000 units kg/day of IV aqueous crystalline penicillin G (administered as 50,000 units/kg every 4 to 6 hours for 10 to 14 days). Children thought to have acquired syphilis but who had a normal neurologic examination were to be treated with benzathine penicillin G, 50,000 units/kg IM up to the adult 24 million units/day dose.

Skin testing and oral desensitization are indicated if there is suspected penicillin allergy. These methods are described in the section on Acquired Syphilis. Alternative therapy is not considered to be effective. Children with acute interstitial keratitis secondary to congenital syphilis may require systemic medication, as well as local treatment. The CDC guidelines do not specifically address whether the intramuscular regimen described above or the intravenous treatment described for ocular involvement in the section on Acquired Syphilis should be followed. Since the eye is so protected, penicillin intravenous therapy prorated according to the child's weight along with probenecid would be reasonable. In addition to systemic treatment, topical ophthalmic corticosteroids and cycloplegics may also be useful in relieving the symptomatology of the acute inflammatory interstitial keratitis. Subconjunctival corticosteroids are occasionally administered when there has been no dramatic clinical response within a week.

Surgical. Keratoplasty may be required if the interstitial keratitis results in a severe corneal opacity that impairs vision. Spiral organisms that take on fluorescent antibody markers are sometimes found in aqueous humor. A history of syphilis and/or a positive FTA-ABS (or other treponemal) test is an indication for treatment. When patients with a quiescent, old interstitial keratitis undergo penetrating keratoplasty, the surgeon should anticipate greater postoperative intracameral inflammation than is usual in corneal transplants. More frequent and higher dosages of topical, subconjunctival, and systemic corticosteroids may prove necessary to quiet the inflammation and prevent graft rejection.

PRECAUTIONS

When the syphilis-infected woman is treated with penicillin during pregnancy, the fetus may be lost as the result of the Jarisch-Herxheimer (J-H) reaction in the mother. There is no known way to prevent this reaction. Yet, because of the high risk of the fetus of an untreated mother becoming infected, the possibility of the J-H reaction does not warrant withholding or modifying treatment. Nor is the modification of treatment of the mother warranted for fear that the fetus will be adversely affected by large doses of penicillin. There is no evidence that such an adverse effect can occur. Monthly follow-up is mandatory so that retreatment can be instituted when necessary. The antibody reaction is the same in pregnant and in nonpregnant women.

HIV testing: In cases of congenital syphilis, it is recommended that the mother be treated for HIV serology; if the test is positive, the mother should be counseled and the infant referred appropriately.

COMMENTS

The best treatment for congenital syphilis is its prevention through the adequate treatment of syphilis during pregnancy. Pregnancies should be followed with serologic testing, since syphilis may be subclinical and nonetheless still affect the fetus. Where there is serologic conversion of the mother, treatment of the pregnant mother is indicated and might prevent passage of the infection to the child. Children of such mothers should be treated according to the most recent CDC revisions and closely followed if serologically negative.

Treatment of the ocular manifestations of congenital syphilis in older children and adults should be guided by the knowledge that former regimens for treating syphilis may not be adequate. Even with current recommended levels of penicillin and duration of treatment for congenital syphilis, the neonatal death rate is still about 10 per cent. Prevention at the present time is more desirable than therapy.

Acknowledgment. The author is indebted to Dr. K Stone of the CDC for her assistance and advice.

References

Budell JW: Treatment of congenital syphilis. J Am Vener Dis Assoc 168–171, 1976.

Cohen DA, Boyd D, Pabhudas I, Mascola L: The effects of case definition, maternal screening, and reporting criteria on rates of congenital syphilis. Am J Public Health 80:316–317, 1990.

Collart P, et al: Significance of spiral organisms found, after treatment, in late human and experimental syphilis. Br J Vener Dis 40:81–89, 1964.

Crane MJ: The diagnosis and management of maternal and congenital syphilis. J Nurse Midwifery 37(1):4–16, 1992.

Duke-Elder S (ed): System of Ophthalmology. St Louis, CV Mosby, 1965, Vol. Viii, pp. 815–832.

Fletcher JL Jr, Gorden RC: Perinatal transmission of bacterial sexually transmitted diseases. Part I: Syphilis and gonorrhea. J Fam Prac 30:448–456, 1990.

Goldman JN: Clinical experience with ampicillin and probenecid in the management of treponene-associated uveitis. Trans Am Acad Ophthalmol Otolaryngol 74:509–514, 1970.

Goldman JN, Girard KF: Intraocular treatment in treated congenital syphilis. Arch Ophthalmol 78:47–50, 1967.

Maleville J, Larregue M, Ball M, Geuiaux M: Diverse aspects of congenital syphilis (Fr).

Sanchez PJ: Congenital syphilis. Adv Pediatr Infect Dis. 7:161–180, 1992.

Smith JL, Israel CW: The presence of spirochetes in late seronegative syphilis. JAMA 199:126–130, 1967.

Smith JL, Israel CW: Spirochetes in the aqueous humor is seronegative ocular syphilis. Persistence after penicillin therapy. Arch Ophthalmol 77:474–477, 1967.

STD Treatment Guidelines, 1989. MMWR 38(5–8):9–11, 1989.

Thompson SE III: Treatment of syphilis in pregnancy. J Am Vener Dis Assoc 3:159–167, 1976.

Zenker PN, Perman SM: Congenital syphilis: Trends and recommendations for evaluation and management. Pediatr Infect Dis J 10:516–522, 1991.

DIPHTHERIA 032.9

LAURENCE S. BRAUDE, M.D., F.A.C.S., F.R.C.S.(C),

and JOHN W. CHANDLER, M.D.

Chicago, Illinois

Diphtheria is an acute infectious disease caused by *Corynebacterium diphtheriae*, a gram-positive, club-shaped organism. Only those strains that are latently infected by a bacterial virus, diphtheria phage B, produce exotoxin and are capable of producing diphtheria. The toxin is responsible for the most common systemic complications of diphtheria affecting the heart and nervous system. Cranial nerve involvement can include the third, fourth, and sixth nerves. *C. diphtheriae* is essentially a surface saprophyte, most commonly affecting the nasopharyngeal area. Cutaneous diphtheria seems to be more frequently associated with external ocular involvement. External ocular disease includes tender, red, swollen eyelids; membranous or pseudomembranous conjunctivitis; and corneal ulcers and perforation.

THERAPY

Systemic. In addition to topical therapy, 10,000 to 100,000 units of diphtheria antitoxin are also given systemically after appropriate testing for sensitivity has been done. This total dose should be given at one time, rather than in split doses over a long period. For doses less than 20,000 units, the intramuscular route is convenient. When this method is used, only one-half of the dose should be given intramuscularly and the remainder intravenously. Alternatively, the entire amount of antitoxin may be given intravenously in 100 or 200 ml of isotonic saline over 30 minutes.

Antibiotics are believed to have little effect on the clinical course of diphtheria involving the respiratory tract, but they may be of benefit in terminating the toxin production. Antibiotic therapy is of value because this infection is typically mixed with other bacteria, including staphylococci and pneumococci, and many other organisms. In the very severe cases, streptococci are often present, and there is evidence that tissue damage is due to the mixed infection, rather than to the diphtheria bacillus toxin alone. Additional benefits of antibiotics are hastening clearance of the carrier state and prevention of spread of the organism to others.

Penicillin is the drug of choice. Intramuscular administration of 600,000 units of procaine penicillin G twice daily for 7 to 16 days is usually adequate. Oral penicillin V may be substituted after the third day in patients with uncomplicated infections. Intravenous penicillin G in a daily dose of 4 to 6 million units divided into four doses may be used with intravenous solutions. In patients allergic to penicillin, intravenous erythromycin may be used in a daily dose of 25 to 50 mg/kg for 10 to 14 days. It should be noted that erythromycin resistance has been seen in some recent outbreaks. In addition, *C. diphtheriae* is frequently resistant to cephalexin, colistin, lincomycin, and oxacillin. The organism is usually sensitive to ampicillin, clindamycin, tetracycline, and rifampin. Regardless of the antibiotic, therapy should be continued for at least 7 days.

Steroids have been used to prevent or ameliorate myocarditis, but Harnisch (1980) feels corticosteroids or corticotrophins are not of value in the treatment of diphtheria or any of its complications.

Ocular. If there is clinical suspicion that the disease is due to *C. diphtheriae*, therapy should be instituted immediately and not withheld until laboratory confirmation is obtained, because the severity of the disease is dependent upon the amount of exotoxin absorbed prior to initiation of specific therapy. Treatment of external ocular diphtheria has two goals: neutralization of toxin and eradication of live organisms.

Since the diphtheria toxins irreversibly bind to tissue, antitoxin is effective only against circulatory toxins: once the clinical manifestations of the toxins appear, they cannot be reversed by antitoxin administration. Antitoxin treatment thus blocks only circulating toxins and toxins still to be formed. There are several regimens for the topical and systemic administration of antitoxin, and the amount given is often based on an empiric decision. In general, the more severe the disease or the more extensive the membrane formation, the greater is the amount of antitoxin required.

After giving a test dose to rule out anaphylactic reactions, 10,000 to 100,000 units of diphtheria antitoxin* are topically applied to the involved eye every 4 to 6 hours for 24 to 48 hours. Diphtheria antitoxin* may also be considered for subconjunctival injection as an alternative to topical application.

Commercially available immune and hyperimmune globulin preparations have low diphtheria antitoxin titers and are not useful. However, there is an investigational preparation that may be useful in special circumstances. It consists of a high-titer gamma globulin preparation[‡] made from the blood of persons with high titers of antitoxin. It was intended for use in prophylaxis, but should be considered for treatment of markedly allergic individuals. It may be given solely to persons who are allergic to horse serum. It is obtainable from the Communicable Disease Division, State Department of Public Health, Lansing, Michigan. The treatment dose has not been established. This preparation should never be given intravenously.

Antibiotics are not effective against the toxin, but are indicated for the eradication of the bacilli and superinfections. Repeated instillations of 1000 units/gm of sodium penicillin G or 0.5 per cent erythromycin ointment are administered in addition to systemic antibiotics.

If the disease involves the eyelid skin, cutaneous diphtheria responds well to local application of compresses soaked in penicillin solution (250 to 500 units/ml) and intramuscular injection of 20,000 units of diphtheria antitoxin. A canthotomy should not be done to facilitate opening the lids; since the raw wound invariably becomes infected, the canthotomy actually increases the area of toxin absorption.

The diphtheria membrane usually sloughs away spontaneously during convalescence. Membranes should not be peeled off, as this leaves a raw, bleeding surface and hastens absorption of toxin. With this caveat, a glass rod or cotton-tipped applicator may be used intermittently to break early symblepharon formation in the fornices.

Supportive. Patients with diphtheria should be isolated and hospitalized. Bedrest is important for 3 weeks because of the frequency of myocardial involvement. Aspirin and codeine may be indicated for relief of pain.

Ocular or Periocular Manifestations

Conjunctiva: Catarrhal, membranous, pseudomembranous, or purulent conjunctivitis; hyperemia; petechiae; symblepharon; xerophthalmia.

Cornea: Keratitis; perforation; ulcer.

Extraocular Muscles: Accommodative spasm or paralysis; convergence paralysis; divergence paralysis; paralysis of third, fourth, or sixth nerve.

Eyelids: Blepharitis; cellulitis; cicatrization; edema; entropion; meibomianitis; necrosis; ptosis; trichiasis.

Lacrimal System: Dacryoadenitis; dacryocystitis.

Other: Cataract; central retinal artery occlusion; optic neuritis; preauricular lymphadenopathy.

PRECAUTIONS

Before antitoxin administration, tests for hypersensitivity to horse serum are mandatory. If the patient is allergic to horse serum, antitoxin may be administered following desensitization, or if available, human diphtheria immune globulin may be substituted. Rarely, a patient may exhibit such marked hypersensitivity that antiserum cannot be administered without the risk of death. The heart rate of all patients should be carefully monitored during administration of diphtheria antitoxin because anaphylaxis may occur. In addition, all diphtheria patients should receive careful cardiac monitoring for developing myocarditis. Drugs with depressant effects on the heart must be used with extreme caution in diphtheria patients.

Patients with diphtheria should be quarantined until two successive cultures of the eye, skin, or other infected areas, taken at 24-hour intervals, are negative. If antibiotics have been given, cultural studies should not be initiated until at least 24 hours after cessation of therapy.

COMMENTS

Approximately 200 cases of nonocular diphtheria are reported annually in the United States. The newborn is usually protected by transplacental globulin from the mother, although a few nonocular severe infections in newborns have been reported. Healthy carriers of the organisms, who are themselves not susceptible, are a source of infection to others, but this means of spreading diphtheria has become less important in populations with widespread immunization. However, recent outbreaks of diphtheria in the United States have involved groups of individuals without adequate immunization histories. The disease may be seen in fully immunized persons, in whom it is usually mild and rarely fatal. Death is most frequent in the very young and elderly. As a rule, the longer the delay in the administration of antitoxin, the greater the incidence of complications and death.

References

Chandler JW, Milam DF: Diphtheria corneal ulcers. Arch Ophthalmol 96:53–56, 1978.
Duke-Elder S (ed): System of Ophthalmology. St. Louis, CV Mosby, 1976. Vol. XV, p 46.
Eller JJ: Diphtheria. In Conn HF (ed): Current Therapy. Philadelphia, WB Saunders, 1982, pp 15–19.
Harnisch JP: Diphtheria. In Isselbacher KJ, et al (eds): Harrison's Principles of Internal Medicine, 9th ed. New York, McGraw-Hill, 1980, pp 671–675.
Rogell G: Infectious and inflammatory diseases. In Duane TD (ed): Clinical Ophthalmology. Hagerstown, MD, Harper & Row, 1982, Vol. V, pp 33: 9–10.
Shaw EB: Diphtheria. In Conn HF, Conn RB Jr (eds): Current Diagnosis 6. Philadelphia, WB Saunders, 1980, pp 167–170.
Top FH, Wehrle PF: Diphtheria. In Wehrle PF, Top FH Sr (eds): Communicable and Infectious Diseases, 9th ed. St. Louis, CV Mosby, 1981, pp 197–210.

ERYSIPELAS 035
(St. Anthony's Fire)

RICHARD L. ABBOTT, M.D.

San Francisco, California

Erysipelas is an acute, localized inflammation of the skin and subcutaneous tissue that is characterized by redness, edema, and induration. Although it is a disease affecting primarily adults between 60 and 80 years old, its incidence is increasing in younger age groups. The pathogenic organisms are usually group A beta-hemolytic streptococci, although occasional group B, C, and G strains have been identified. The site of infection is the extremities or face. The primary facial infection is often a nasopharyngitis from which the organism is transferred to the skin through an abrasion or a minute wound.

Erysipelas may begin with an abrupt onset of fever, chills, malaise, and nausea. A definite zone of redness soon appears, with edema, tenderness, and a well-defined, advancing border. In the more severe cases, vesicles may form on the surface. Typically, the infection involves the lymphatic spaces and is spread through these channels to neighboring areas. Constitutional symptoms include high temperature, headache, vomiting, and localized pain. Without treatment, the disease is usually self-limited and runs its course in 4 days to several weeks. As the facial lesions spread, ocular involvement consisting of marked edema and erythema of the lids often occurs. The edema is frequently extensive enough to prevent opening of the eyes. The disease may also progress to gangrene of the eyelids. Although less common, inflammation spreads from the lids to the conjunctiva, producing chemosis and external ophthalmoplegia. Other complications include dacryoadenitis, orbital thrombophlebitis, cellulitis, abscess, and cavernous sinus thrombosis. A late result in chronic infections may be a solid edema or elephantiasis of the eyelids.

Most often it is difficult to identify the inciting organism definitively. The use of blood cultures, needle aspirates, or biopsy specimens has yielded less than 10 per cent positive cultures.

THERAPY

Systemic. Penicillin G is the drug of choice in treating erysipelas. Treatment should be instituted promptly and continued for 10 to 14 days to prevent the possibility of systemic spread. Intravenous penicillin G should be given in a minimum divided daily dosage of 6 million units. Once there is evidence of clinical improvement, the route of administration can be changed to oral medication. Potassium penicillin V should be given daily in four divided doses of 250 mg for the duration of the 10- to 14-day therapy period.

In patients sensitive to penicillin, erythromycin may be substituted. Erythromycin may be given orally in an initial dosage of 500 mg four times daily for several days and then reduced to 250 mg four times daily for 10 days. In severely ill patients, 500 mg of the drug should be given intravenously twice a day for the first 2 or 3 days before oral therapy is begun.

Ocular.   In severe cases resulting in tissue destruction and lid necrosis, meticulous cleaning and debridement of the wounds on a daily basis should be the mainstay of local therapy. The wounds are surgically debrided and cleansed with a 1:1 solution of hydrogen peroxide and sterile saline and repacked daily with iodoform gauze. The use of warm saline compresses and topical broad-spectrum antibiotic ointments helps accelerate the healing process and may prevent secondary bacterial contamination. The application of topical erythromycin ointment within the cul-de-sac helps prevent the occurrence of a secondary bacterial conjunctivitis.

If there is a significant degree of lid contracture in the healing process, exposure keratitis may develop. This condition is best treated initially with tear substitute and lubricating ointments. Surgical repair of a cicatricial ectropion or other lid deformities may be required. It is prudent, however, to wait a minimum of 3 to 6 months before considering surgical intervention to allow the healing process to stabilize and reduce the likelihood of an under- or overcorrection.

Supportive.   Attention should be given to the patient's physical, nutritional, emotional, and recreational activity needs. Hospitalization is usually indicated, with the patient on bedrest. The patient should be isolated until fever subsides, and strict hygienic measures should be employed by all hospital personnel who have contact with an infected patient. Alcohol and tepid sponge baths may be used to reduce high temperature. Vital signs should be monitored regularly.

Ocular or Periocular Manifestations

Conjunctiva: Chemosis; exudative or membranous conjunctivitis.
Cornea: Superficial punctate keratitis secondary to bacterial toxins or exposure with lid ectropion (late); ulcerative keratitis.
Eyelids: Abscess; blepharitis; ectropion; elephantiasis; erythema; gangrene; madarosis; marked edema; necrosis; trichiasis.

Iris: Iridocyclitis.
Lacrimal System: Dacryoadenitis; dacryocystitis.
Orbit: Abscess; cellulitis; thrombophlebitis.
Vitreous or Retina: Chorioretinitis; metastatic vitreous abscess.

PRECAUTIONS

Because erysipelas usually begins abruptly and may progress rapidly, appropriate antimicrobial therapy must be instituted as soon as possible. The diagnosis may be made on the basis of the clinical presentation of the illness, and intravenous penicillin G or its substitute should be started immediately. Regardless of which drug is used, it is essential that treatment in full doses be given over a period of at least 10 days because relapses are relatively common.

Cultures and sensitivities should be obtained for confirmation of the diagnosis only if there is exudate readily available for these studies. Needle aspiration from the lids or orbit is contraindicated in patients with erysipelas because of the possibility of spread of the infection and injury to other structures.

The differential diagnosis must include ophthalmic herpes zoster, allergic contact dermatitis, myosis of collagen disease, trichinosis, and angioneurotic edema.

COMMENTS

Although lower extremity involvement is most common when affecting the face, the erysipelas exanthem most frequently appears in the region of the eye, with the sites of predilection being the eyelid and the inner canthus. The pathophysiology of lid necrosis seems to be related to the release of proteolytic enzymes by the streptococcal organisms, which dissolve connective tissue bridges and allow rapid spread of the bacteria. Because the skin of the lid is so thin, large amounts of fluid can accumulate, thereby raising the tissue pressure and shutting off capillary circulation. Thus, the combination of diffuse bacterial spread and diminished blood supply leads to destruction and necrosis of the lid tissue.

For treatment to be effective, one must make an early diagnosis and institute maximum parenteral antibiotic therapy combined with local debridement and topical antibiotic application. It is recommended that this therapy be continued for a minimum of 10 to 14 days until all evidence of the infection has resolved. Long-term therapy consists of lid plastic surgery after all healing processes have stabilized.

References

Abbott RL, Shekter WB: Necrotizing erysipelas of eyelids. Ann Ophthalmol 11:381–384, 1979.

Bellows J: Ocular complications of erysipelas. Arch Ophthalmol *11*:678–683, 1934.

Bellows JG: Acute bacterial infections. *In* Sorsby A (ed): Modern Ophthalmology, 2nd ed. Philadelphia, JB Lippincott, 1972, Vol. 2, pp 90–91.

Chartier C, Grosshans E: Erysipelas. Intl J Dermatol *29*:459–467, 1990.

Ochs MW, Dolwick MF: Facial erysipelas: Report of a case and review of the literature. J Oral Maxillofac Surg *49*:1116–1120, 1991.

Ronnen M, Suster S, Satewach-Millet M, et al: Erysipelas. Changing Faces. Intl J Dermatol 24:169, 1986.

Scott PM, Bloome MA: Lid necrosis secondary to streptococcal periorbital cellulitis. Ann Ophthalmol *13*:461–465, 1981.

Stewart WD, Danto JL, Maddin S: Dermatology: Diagnosis and Treatment of Cutaneous Disorders, 3rd ed. St. Louis, CV Mosby, 1974, p 218.

ESCHERICHIA COLI 008.0

H. JOHN SHAMMAS, M.D.

Los Angeles, California

Escherichia coli is a gram-negative rod found as a normal commensal in the gastrointestinal tract from which it may spread to infect contiguous structures when normal anatomic barriers are interrupted. This bacillus can also be found in association with other pathogenic organisms in perforated or inflamed conditions. The urinary tract is the usual portal of entry; however, once infection has occurred in a primary focus, further spread to distant organs may occur by means of the bloodstream. Septicemia is the most serious complication of *E. coli* infections. It occurs frequently in immune-deficient patients, in debilitated elderly patients with diabetes mellitus, in patients with urinary tract infection or biliary or intraperitoneal sepsis, and following abortions or pelvic surgery. Enterotoxigenic *E. coli* may cause a gastroenteritis, most commonly in children under 2 years of age.

Ocular involvement is rare and may result in a mucopurulent conjunctivitis. Metastatic endophthalmitis may occur from *E. coli* septicemia, and the usual portal of entry is the central retinal artery. The course of the endophthalmitis is acute; necrosis of the intraocular tissues and loss of vision can occur in less than 24 hours.

THERAPY

Systemic. Choice of an appropriate antimicrobial in *E. coli* infections depends upon the site and type of infection, as well as its severity. A number of antibiotics are effective against the bacillus, but no particular drug is uniformly active against all strains of *E. coli*, so sensitivity testing should guide the choice of antibiotics.

For less severe *E. coli* infections, the initial treatment of choice may be 2 to 4 gm of ampicillin a day administered intramuscularly or intravenously. For more severe infections, the dose could be 6 to 12 gm daily.

Aminoglycosidic antibiotics are the most commonly used against coliform bacillary infections, including *E. coli*. They include kanamycin, gentamycin, amikacin, and tobramycin.

Kanamycin is generally indicated for the initial treatment of serious *E. coli* infections. Severe urinary tract infections that seem to be resistant to other antimicrobials have responded to daily doses of 15 mg/kg of kanamycin intramuscularly in divided doses every 6 to 8 hours.

Alternative treatment may be with 3 to 5 mg/kg of parenteral gentamicin, administered in divided doses every 8 hours. In severe infections that appear to be resistant to kanamycin and gentamicin, amikacin is indicated. Amikacin is given in daily doses of 15 mg/kg in two or three equally divided doses.

In severe cases of sepsis, a combination of antibiotics is given. It usually includes ampicillin and an aminoglycoside, the choice of which is based on knowledge of local susceptibility patterns. Ampicillin and cefatazime (a potent third-generation cephalosporin) is a suitable alternative, especially if an aminoglycoside-resistant nosocomial organism is suspected.

Neomycin appears to be most effective against *E. coli* gastroenteritis. An oral daily dosage of 25 mg/kg is usually indicated for 1 or 2 days.

Ocular. In *E. coli* conjunctivitis, 0.5 per cent chloramphenicol, 0.3 per cent gentamicin, or 0.3 per cent tobramycin solutions are applied topically every 4 hours until the infection appears to be resolved.

Early systemic and local antibiotic therapy is essential for E. coli *endophthalmitis.* Blanket local antibiotic therapy should consist of 20 mg of subconjunctival gentamicin,* 0.3 per cent gentamicin or tobramycin, and 0.5 per cent chloramphenicol solutions every 2 hours. In very severe cases, intravitreal injection of 100 to 300 μg of gentamicin* can be used.

Steroids administered in combination with antibiotics may reduce the massive inflammatory response of the eye, which is often as destructive as the infection. Two mg of dexamethasone* may be injected subconjunctivally and repeated when necessary.

Secondary involvement of the uveal tract may necessitate use of a cycloplegic/mydriatic. One per cent cyclopentolate drops may be applied topically twice daily to aid in the relief of uveitis.

Supportive. Hospitalization is necessary for more severe forms of *E. coli* infection. Infants with *E. coli* gastroenteritis should be isolated and monitored carefully; fluid and electrolyte levels must be maintained, since dehydration can occur rapidly in these patients.

Surgical. Subcutaneous infections are not uncommon in debilitated patients. Drainage of pus and removal of foreign bodies may be necessary.

Ocular or Periocular Manifestations

Anterior Chamber: Cells and flare; gas bubbles; hyphema; hypopyon.
Conjunctiva: Chemosis; hyperemia, pseudomembranous or purulent conjunctivitis.
Cornea: Edema; keratitis; ulcers.
Globe: Panophthalmitis; purulent endophthalmitis.
Other: Increased intraocular pressure; ocular pain; uveitis; visual loss.

PRECAUTIONS

It is advisable to check the serum levels of the aminoglycosides to ensure therapeutic levels and avoid toxicity, since the therapeutic to toxic ratio is very narrow. Monitoring of renal and eighth nerve functions is recommended during therapy with these drugs, particularly for patients with reduced renal function. Concurrent and/or sequential systemic use of potentially neurotoxic or nephrotoxic drugs should be avoided.

Isolation and antimicrobial therapy of contacts are essential to abort epidemic infantile diarrhea. Many *E. coli* infections are hospital acquired, so strict hygienic measures are essential.

COMMENTS

E. coli is rarely found in the normal flora of the conjunctiva. It is most commonly seen as a source of infection in ophthalmia neonatorum. *E. coli* endophthalmitis is a rare complication of *E. coli* septicemia. It has a poor prognosis, and early diagnosis and treatment are essential if useful vision is to be retained.

References

Aronson SB, Elliott JH: Ocular Inflammation. St. Louis, CV Mosby, 1972, pp 103–105, 112–114, 228–230.
Asbell P, Stenson S: Ulcerative keratitis, survey of 30 years laboratory experience. Arch Ophthalmol 100:77–83, 1982.
Baum JL: Initial therapy of suspected microbial corneal ulcers. I. Broad antibiotic therapy based on prevalence of organisms. Surv Ophthalmol 24:97–116, 1979.
Bonadio WA, Smith DS, Madagame E, Machi J, Kini N: *Escherichia coli* bacteremia in children. A review of 91 cases in 10 years. Am J Dis Child 145:671–674, 1991.
Jones DB: Initial therapy of suspected microbial corneal ulcers. II. Specific antibiotic therapy based on corneal smears. Surv Ophthalmol 24:97–116, 1979.
Jones DB: Decision making in the management of microbial keratitis. Ophthalmology 88:814–820, 1981.
Krachmer JH, Purcell JJ Jr: Bacterial corneal ulcers in cosmetic soft contact lens wearers. Arch Ophthalmol 96:57–61, 1978.
Lissner GS, Romano PE: Pneumatosis oculi and spontaneous hyphema in association with pneumatosis intestinalis. Am J Ophthalmol 88:708–713, 1979.
Nelson JD: Pocketbook of Pediatric Antimicrobial Therapy. Baltimore, Williams & Wilkins, 1991, pp 2–5.
Shammas HF: Endogenous *E. coli* endophthalmitis. Surv Ophthalmol 21:429–435, 1977.
Turck M, Schaberg D: Infections due to enterobacteriaceae. *In* Isselbacher KJ, et al. (eds): Harrison's Principles of Internal Medicine, 9th ed. New York, McGraw-Hill, 1980, pp 629–634.

FUSOBACTERIUM 039

RICHARD J. WEINBERG, M.D., F.A.C.S.
Washington, District of Columbia

Fusobacterium is a gram-negative, non-spore-forming, anaerobic bacillus that is a normal inhabitant of the mouth and respiratory, intestinal, and urogenital tracts. Infection is usually secondary to an underlying disease, surgical procedure, or therapy that impairs the normal defense of the host. *Fusobacterium* infection of the skin may also occur following animal or human bites. It is often found in association with spirochetes. The clinical manifestations of *Fusobacterium* infections include tissue necrosis, abscess formation, and septic thrombophlebitis, as well as foul odor and gas in tissue or discharges. *Fusobacterium* infections may cause abscess formation in the brain, lung, liver, or intra-abdominal area; empyema; and necrotizing pneumonia. Ocular manifestations in the more acute cases may include a purulent conjunctivitis, but ulcerative and even gangrenous manifestations may also occur. Acute or chronic infection in the lacrimal system may be present as dacryocystitis or suppurative canaliculitis. Rarely, cellulitis, tenonitis, or metastatic panophthalmitis may also occur in *Fusobacterium* infections. Corneal ulceration is possibly associated with, but is usually secondary to combined infections.

THERAPY

Systemic. Antimicrobial therapy may be indicated in *Fusobacterium* infections involving vital organs or when systemic manifestations are present. Chloramphenicol and clindamycin are the antibiotics of choice; however, chloramphenicol is preferred for patients with infections of the central nervous system because clindamycin does not effectively penetrate the blood-brain barrier. Both antibiotics can be administered orally, but parenteral therapy is advisable for patients with severe infection. Chloramphenicol should be administered parenterally or orally in a daily dose of 50 mg/kg divided into four equal portions, and parenteral clindamycin should be administered in a daily dose of 0.6 to 2.7 gm divided into two to four equal doses. The oral adult dosage for clindamycin is 150 to 450 mg every 6 hours.

Penicillin is also active against most anaerobes other than *Bacteroides fragilis* and occasional strains of *Fusobacterium varium*. The dosage of penicillin G should be at least 6 to 8 million units daily in seriously ill patients or in infections with relatively resistant strains. Ampicillin and cephaloridine are usually comparable to penicillin G, but several other penicillins and cephalosporins are less active. Fusobacteria are generally resistant to the aminoglycosides.

Ocular. Topical antibiotic therapy may be necessary in ocular *Fusobacterium* infections. Topical penicillin G ointment in a concentration of 1000 units/gm may be used every 3 hours. One per cent chlortetracycline ointment or 10 or 15 per cent sulfacetamide drops may also be used several times daily for conjunctivitis or canaliculitis. In canaliculitis, however, a definitive cure may not be effected until all concretions that may be present are removed either by surgery or mechanical expression.

Supportive. In *Fusobacterium* infections, anticoagulant therapy and venous ligation should be considered in patients with thrombophlebitis and multiple septic pulmonary infarctions. If shock or disseminated intravascular coagulation occurs, general supportive measures are important aspects of therapy.

Surgical. Drainage of abscess cavities or local suppurative lesions is of prime importance in the management of patients with *Fusobacterium* infections. The perforation should be closed promptly and devitalized tissues and foreign bodies removed as soon as possible. This is often all that is required for cure in many patients.

Ocular or Periocular Manifestations

Conjunctiva: Chemosis; follicular or purulent conjunctivitis; gangrene.
Lacrimal System: Canaliculitis; dacryocystitis.
Orbit: Abscess; cellulitis; fistula.
Other: Corneal ulcer(?); extraocular muscle tenonitis; eyelid edema; panophthalmitis.

PRECAUTIONS

Since most strains of *Fusobacterium* are highly sensitive to penicillin, chloramphenicol, tetracycline, and clindamycin, susceptibility tests generally serve as a good guide to drug therapy. However, chloramphenicol or clindamycin therapy should be administered with care, since both drugs may cause serious adverse drug-related effects. Chloramphenicol may cause nausea and vomiting, and serious, even fatal blood dyscrasias may occur. Likewise, clindamycin can cause severe colitis, which may end fatally. Precautions to minimize the possibility of aspiration will also be helpful in preventing anaerobic pulmonary infection.

COMMENTS

Therapy with antimicrobial agents in *Fusobacterium* infections must be intensive and prolonged. These infections have a considerable tendency to relapse. If the diagnosis is suspected early and appropriate therapy instituted promptly, the prognosis for recovery is good. The prognosis will vary with the site and extent of lesion; a high mortality may occur in patients with brain abscess, necrotizing pneumonia, liver abscess, endocarditis, or sepsis. Gram-stained specimens may be confused with *Actinomyces* because of similar morphology and variable gram-staining characteristics.

References

Bowers BT, Simmons JR: Surgical management of diverticulum of the canaliculus. Arch Ophthalmol *83*:61–62, 1970.

Burns RP, et al: Unilateral conjunctivitis and canaliculitis due to Fusospirochetal infection. Arch Ophthalmol *59*:235–242, 1958.

Finegold SM: Disease due to non-spore-forming anaerobic bacteria. *In* Wyngaarden JB, Smith LH Jr (eds): Textbook of Medicine, 16th ed. Philadelphia, WB Saunders, 1982, pp 1503–1507.

Lin RG, Arcala AE: Fusobacterium septicemia with otitis media and mastoiditis. Postgrad Med *57*: 159–160, 1975.

Ormerod D, et al: Anaerobic bacterial endophthalmitis in the rabbit. Invest Ophthalmol *27*:115–117, 1986.

Weinberg RJ, et al: Fusobacterium in presumed *Actinomyces* canaliculitis. Am J Ophthalmol *84*:371–374, 1977.

GONOCOCCAL OCULAR DISEASE 098.4

JEFFREY B. ROBIN, M.D.,
and STEVEN B. ROBIN, M.D.

Hoffman Estates, Illinois

Gonorrhea is one of the oldest described infectious diseases affecting humans. Caused by the gram-negative diplococcus, *Neisseria gonorrhoeae*, gonorrhea is a major cause of morbidity throughout the world and is presently the most common reportable disease in the United States (over 800,000 reported cases in 1985). The incidence of gonorrhea, once thought to be on the decline, has been steadily rising since 1984, although rates in some demographic segments, such as male homosexuals, have decreased. Epidemiologic risk factors for gonorrhea include age, sex, sexual preference, race, socioeconomic status, marital status, and accessibility to health care. The spread of gonorrhea is difficult to control because the main vector for the disease is the asymptomatic carrier.

Gonorrhea primarily affects two patient populations: young, sexually active adults and neonates born to infected mothers. In fact, *N. gonorrhoeae* was, until recently, the major cause of ophthalmia neonatorum. Unlike the adult population, the incidence of gonococcal infections in newborns has been markedly decreasing; this is believed to be the result of more widespread antenatal screening and the use of prophylactic antibiotics.

The gonococcal organism, first identified by Neisser in 1879, primarily attacks mucosal epithelium. Gonorrhea is relatively easy to diagnose, given the characteristic appearance of gram-negative diplococci, many of which can be found inside epithelial and leukocytic cells. The introduction of specific culture medium for *Neisseriae*, developed in 1964 by Thayer and Martin, has further facilitated laboratory diagnosis. Differentiation from *N. meningitidis* is accomplished on the basis of sugar fermentation reactions.

Gonorrhea is a potentially multisystem disease, affecting not only the genitourinary tract but also the joints, skin, pharynx, meninges, heart, liver, and eye. Extragenitourinary involvement may occur via hematogenous spread or direct inoculation. Ocular involvement in adults is usually the result of direct hand-eye inoculation; cases have also occurred from laboratory contamination and from the use of urine as a folk-remedy eye wash. Additionally, rare cases of gonococcal conjunctivitis have been associated with direct hematogenous spread from the genitourinary tract. Gonococcal ophthalmia neonatorum is nearly always caused by direct inoculation of the neonate's eyes during passage through an infected birth canal.

Ocular involvement in both adults and neonates is characterized by an acute, copiously purulent conjunctivitis. Involvement may start unilaterally, but may eventually involve both eyes. The *N. gonorrhoeae* organism is one of the few bacteria that is capable of penetrating the intact corneal epithelium. Therefore, corneal ulcerations, abscesses, and perforations commonly occur in untreated gonococcal ocular infections.

The history of gonorrhea therapy has been marked by landmark discoveries and by the ongoing development of antibacterial resistance. Credé, in 1881, introduced silver nitrate for the prophylaxis of gonococcal ophthalmia neonatorum, thereby rapidly reducing the incidence of this neonatal infection. Sulfonamides, introduced in 1939, were the first agents identified to treat established gonococcal infections successfully. Resistance rapidly developed to sulfonamides, however, and penicillin became the drug of choice. Recently, beta-lactamase-producing gonococci, resistant to both penicillin and ampicillin, have become worldwide in distribution. These penicillinase-producing strains of *N. gonorrhoeae* (PPNG) have become predominant in several areas of the world, including several cities in the United States. Additionally, some strains of *N. gonorrhoeae* have chromosomally mediated resistance to penicillin and tetracycline; these chromosomally resistant *N. gonorrhoeae* (CMRNG) strains can be quite difficult to treat. The continued development of antimicrobial resistance by this organism has forced an ongoing evaluation of treatment regimens.

THERAPY

Systemic. The mainstay of systemic therapy for gonorrhea has been the use of parenteral antibiotics, most commonly penicillin. However, because of the continuing development of antimicrobial resistance, the treatment of gonorrhea has periodically been reevaluated. In 1989, for the treatment of gonococcal ophthalmia in adults, the Centers for Disease Control (CDC) recommended a single intramuscular dose of 1 gm ceftriaxone as outpatient therapy. This superseded the prior 1985 recommendation of 10 million units of aqueous penicillin G (given intravenously, with 1.0 gm oral probenecid to decrease renal excretion, daily for 5 days), which proved insufficient in the face of rising PPNG strain incidence. The latter regimen may still be effective, but is more labor intensive, and should only be used on a documented non-PPNG strain.

Other third-generation cephalosporin regimens, namely 500 mg of intravenous cefotaxime or 1 gm of ceftriaxone four times daily for 5 days, have also been found effective. For gonococcal ophthalmia neonatorum the CDC in 1989 recommended either ceftriaxone 25–50 mg/kg per day intravenously or intramuscularly in single daily doses, or cefotaxime 25 mg/kg intravenously or intramuscularly every 12 hours, with either drug given as a 7-day course. If meningitis is present, the regimen should cover 10–14 days. As with adults, effective treatment of uncomplicated gonococcal ophthalmia in neonates has been recently achieved with single-dose ceftriaxone therapy, 50 mg/kg up to 125 mg. Of course, as in adult disease, the prior 1985 therapy of crystalline penicillin G, 100,000 units/kg a day in two intravenous equal doses (four equal doses if infant is more than 1 week old), may be given if the gonococcal isolate is proven susceptible to penicillin.

Recently, gonococcal conjunctivitis without keratitis has been successfully treated with a single-dose regimen of intramuscular antibiotics on an outpatient basis. Of course, an assessment of the patient's capability for follow-up and compliance is an essential component in making the decision for outpatient therapy.

Based on the above recommendations and recent trends, the following systemic treatment regimen is recommended. For uncomplicated gonococcal conjunctivitis, a single dose of 1.0 gm of intramuscular ceftriaxone together with a 7-day oral course of tetracycline (250 mg four times daily) or doxycycline (100 mg twice daily) is an effective combination to treat both gonococcal and chlamydial infections. Alternative therapy for those patients with documented penicillin allergy should involve 2.0 gm of spectinomycin in one intramuscular dose. In more severe cases, particularly with corneal involvement, the patient should be hospitalized and treated with 1.0 gm of ceftriaxone intravenously two times daily for 3 to 5 days; penicillin-allergic patients should receive 2.0 gm of spectinomycin intramuscularly twice daily over a 3- to 5-day course. For neonatal infections, a single intramuscular dose of 125 mg of ceftriaxone is used. If ceftriaxone is contraindicated, gentamicin should be used intravenously in appropriate pediatric doses. Infants born to mothers with untreated gonorrhea are at high risk of infection and therefore should be treated as above.

Recently, the fluoroquinolones have emerged as a new therapeutic choice in the treatment of both gonococcal and chlamydial infection. Ofloxacin, temafloxacin, norfloxacin, and ciprofloxacin have been found effective against both organisms, although no extensive controlled study has yet shown the efficacy of these treatments in ocular gonococcal or chlamydial disease in relation to current modalities.

Ocular, topical antimicrobial agents seem to be ineffective in completely treating gonococcal ophthalmia. They can be used, however, as adjuncts to systemic antibiotics. Topical gentacmicin, erythromycin, or bacitracin can be used four times daily. The final choice should be based upon antibiotic sensitivities.

An essential aspect of topical therapy is copious irrigation of the purulent exudate. The gonococcal exudate may contain toxins of live bacteria. It is produced at such a rate that irrigation with 50 ml of sterile saline may be required as often as every hour. Frequent, copious irrigation is especially important for the treatment of gonococcal ophthalmia neonatorum.

Ocular or Periocular Manifestations

Anterior Chamber: Cellular reaction; hypopyon; endophthalmitis.

Conjunctiva: Chemosis; acute purulent exudate; hemorrhages.

Cornea: Punctate epithelial keratitis; marginal, sterile stromal infiltrates; epithelial defects; infectious stromal infiltrates; stromal ulcerations; descemotocele; perforation, opacification.

Eyelids: Erythema; edema.

PRECAUTIONS

The changing face of microbial sensitivity and resistance has forced continual reevaluation of therapy for gonococcal ophthalmia. Because of the increasing frequency of PPNG infections and also because gonococcal ocular infections can rapidly progress and threaten vision, it is now justifiable to begin appropriate therapy while awaiting the results of antimicrobial sensitivities. It is recommended therefore to avoid agents to which *N. gonorrhoeae* has demonstrated documented resistance, such as penicillin, erythromycin, ampicillin, and tetracycline, and instead use a third-generation cephalosporin as the first-line systemic antibiotic. These agents, such as ceftriaxone, have a broad spectrum of sensitivity, are effective against *N. gonorrhoeae* do not seem to be affected by beta-lactamase, and seem to be relatively safe. When administered intravenously, ceftriaxone rapidly achieves high blood levels; this therapeutic route seems to be ideal for gonococcal ophthalmia with corneal involvement. Because of the excellent results produced by therapy with third-generation cephalosporins, penicillin allergy should be appropriately documented before using potentially less effective agents, such as spectinomycin.

COMMENTS

Appropriate systemic therapy is the mainstay of treatment for gonococcal ocular infections. In all cases, patients must be evaluated on a daily basis. Complete follow-up examinations, with negative cultures, are essential to confirm treatment efficacy. If follow-up is questionable or if there is corneal involvement, patients should be hospitalized. Additionally, treatment regimens should be supplemented with appropriate patient counseling and education, as well as contact tracing.

Gonococcal ophthalmia is frequently accompanied by other venereally transmitted diseases. All patients therefore should have serologic tests for syphilis and, if suspected, HIV exposure. Additionally, because laboratory confirmation of chlamydial infections is difficult, it is reasonable to include anti-chlamydial treatment in the therapeutic regimen, especially in heterosexuals. In most cases, a 7- to 14-day course of oral tetracycline or doxycycline is effective; in tetracycline-allergic patients, neonates, or lactating women, oral erythromycin stearate is an appropriate alternative.

References

Centers for Disease Control: 1985 STD treatment guidelines. MMWR 34:81S–90S, 1985.

Centers for Disease Control: Table 1. Summary—cases specified notable diseases, United States. MMWR 35:810, 1987.

Centers for Disease Control: 1989 Sexually transmitted disease treatment guidelines. MMWR 38(5–8):21–27, 1989.

Centers for Disease Control: Plasmid-mediated antimicrobial resistance in Neisseria gonorrhoeae—United States, 1988 and 1989. MMWR 39(17): 284–287, 293, 1990.

Haase DA, et al: Single-dose therapy of gonococcal ophthalmia neonatorum with ceftriaxone. N Engl J Med 315:1382–1385, 1986.

Judson FN: Treatment of uncomplicated gonorrhea with ceftriaxone: A review. Sex Transm Dis 13: 199–202, 1986.

Kestelyn P, Bogaerts J, Stevens AM, Piot P, Meheus A: Treatment of adult gonococcal keratoconjunctivitis with oral norfloxacin. Am J Ophthalmol 108(5):516–523, 1989.

Lutz FB Jr: Single-dose efficacy of ofloxacin in uncomplicated gonorrhea. Am J Med 87(6C):69S–74S, 1989.

Pareek SS: Conjunctivitis caused by beta-lactamase-producing Neisseria gonorrhoeae. Sex Transm Dis 12:159–160, 1985.

Segreti J: In vitro activity of temafloxacin against pathogens causing sexually transmitted disease. Am J Med 91(6A):24S–26S, 1991.

Ullman S, Roussel RJ, Forster RK: Gonococcal keratoconjunctivitis. Surv Ophthalmol 32:199–208, 1987.

Wan WL, et al: The clinical characteristics and course of adult gonococcal conjunctivitis. Am J Ophthalmol 102:575–583, 1986.

Zajdowicz TR, et al: Laboratory-acquired gonococcal conjunctivitis: Successful treatment with single-dose ceftriaxone. Sex Transm Dis 11:28–29, 1983.

HEMOPHILUS INFLUENZAE 041.5

F. T. FRAUNFELDER, M.D.

Portland, Oregon

Hemophilus influenzae infection is one of the most important and serious bacterial infections in children; in the United States, it is the leading cause of childhood bacterial meningitis. The most common site of infection for most diseases is the upper respiratory tract. Otitis media, sinusitis, epiglottitis, bronchitis, and pneumonia may occur by contiguous spread from the focus. Alcoholism, smoking, chronic lung disease, and HIV infections are important risk factors. Type b (Hib) is the most common strain associated with most *Hemophilus* infections, except in ocular infections when type d is usually identified. The *Hemophilus* species usually associated with conjunctivitis is the Koch-Weeks bacillus, *H. aegyptius*, which often causes a primary conjunctivitis without other foci of *Hemophilus* infections. Although primary ocular infections with *H. influenzae* were thought to usually be involved secondarily to systemic bacterial infection, this is no longer the case (Jacobson et al, 1988). *H. influenzae* is an important ocular pathogen in adults, causing conjunctivitis, orbital cellulitis, corneal ulcers, and endophthalmitis.

THERAPY

Systemic. Systemic therapy will most often be dictated be a physician other than an ophthalmologist since the ocular infection is usually secondary to another source, i.e., meningitis, epiglottitis, septic arthritis, cellulitis, pneumonia, etc. Most cases of Hib disease require hospitalization, especially in children. Drugs of choice are the third-generation cephalosporins—cefotaxime or ceftriaxone—although intravenous ampicillin and chloramphenicol in combination can be used until the sensitivity of the organism is known. For susceptible strains, amoxicillin given orally is preferred. Other agents may be used for ampicillin-resistant strains or for those of unknown susceptibility; for example, combinations of trimethoprim-sulfamethoxazole, a sulfonamide combination with erythromycin, cefaclor, cefiximine, or amoxicillin-clavulanic acid. Oral chloramphenicol, although effective, is rarely used except in children who have already been exposed to it parenterally, since its hematologic risk is real. Therapy is usually continued for at least 2 weeks.

Ocular. Topical ocular antibiotic therapy varies with the severity of the ocular and/or systemic disease. For routine conjunctivitis, application of topical ophthalmic sulfonamides is recommended four times daily. Chloramphenicol eyedrops are probably the treatment of choice only in severe infections, as is true for treatment in other parts of the body. If high doses of systemic chloramphenicol have already been given in the treatment of systemic infection, topical ocular chloramphenicol may also be indicated since hemopoietic exposure will have already occurred.

The conjunctival sac may be irrigated with a saline solution or boric acid eyewash a few times daily to remove conjunctival secretions. Cold compresses applied for 5 minutes three times daily may provide some comfort. The eyelids should otherwise be kept open, and the eyelashes should be coated with an antibiotic ointment at night to prevent the eyelids from sticking together.

Ocular or Periocular Manifestations

Anterior Chamber: Exudates.
Conjunctiva: Chemosis; follicles, hyperemia; mucopurulent conjunctivitis.
Cornea: Infiltration; opacity; pannus.
Other: Cellulitis; dacryoadenitis; extraocular muscle tenonitis; exudative anterior uveitis; eyelid edema; vitreous opacity.

PRECAUTIONS

Topical ocular chloramphenicol is not without risk and should not be used unless specifically indicated. Because of the well-known hemopoietic effects of chloramphenicol, conjunctivitis without other complications rarely requires its use, unless chloramphenicol has already been given systemically.

COMMENTS

Many antibiotics are satisfactory, depending on the severity and site of infection. In vitro sensitivities are indicated and even mandatory for most infections. A significant increase in antibiotic resistance has been noted in *Hemophilus influenzae* infections, especially with ampicillin and chloramphenicol. Purified PRP vaccine for Hib produces greater than 90 per cent protection of infants immunized at 2 years of age and older. Ongoing clinical trials will dictate whether the efficiency of these conjugate vaccines warrants their use for those and older children. However, in children 15 months of age or older, these vaccines may be combined with diphtheria toxoid or other proteins.

Families should be warned that close contact with these patients can result in a greater risk of acquiring this infection. In fact, some family members should be placed on a prophylactic dose of rifampin, 20 mg/kg/day (maximum adult dose 600 mg/day orally for 4 successive days). There is some controversy on using prophylaxis, and consultation with the pediatrician or infectious disease specialist is advised before undertaking this treatment.

References

Al-Hazzaa SAF, Tabbara KF: Bacterial keratitis after penetrating keratoplasty. Ophthalmology *95(11)*:1504–1508, 1988.
Gigliotti F, et al: Efficacy of topical antibiotic therapy in acute conjunctivitis in children. J Pediatr *104*:623–626, 1984.
Granoff DM, Daum RS: Spread of *Haemophilus influenzae* type b: Recent epidemiologic and therapeutic considerations. J Pediatr *97*:854–860, 1980.
Jacobson JA, Call NB, Kasworm EM, et al: Safety and efficacy of topical norfloxacin versus tobramycin in the treatment of external ocular infections. Antimicrob Agents Chemother *32(12)*:1820–1824, 1988.
Millard DD: *Haemophilus influenzae* type b: A rare case of congenital conjunctivitis. Pediatr Infect Dis J 7:363–364, 1988.
Newton NL Jr, Reynolds JD, Wood RC: Cortical blindness following *Hemophilus influenzae* meningitis. Ann Ophthalmol 17:193–194, 1985.
Pach JM: Traumatic *Haemophilus influenzae* endophthalmitis. Am J Ophthalmol *106*:497–498, 1988.
Powell KR, Kaplan SB, Hall CB, et al: Periorbital cellulitis. Clinical and laboratory findings in 146 episodes, including tear countercurrent immunoelectrophoresis in 89 episodes. Am J Dis Child *142*:853–857, 1988.
Walterspiel JN, et al: Ampicillin and chloramphenicol resistance in systemic *Hemophilus influenzae* disease. JAMA *251*:884–885, 1985.

KOCH-WEEKS BACILLUS 041.5
(Hemophilus Influenzae Biogroup Aegyptius, Hemophilus Aegyptius)

ALAN SUGAR, M.D.

Ann Arbor, Michigan

Koch-Weeks bacillus, *Hemophilus influenzae biogroup aegyptius*, is a small gram-negative coccobacillus or slender rod. It was initially recovered as a secondary invader in trachoma and as a cause of epidemic "pink eye." It is now considered to be a subspecies of *H. influenzae*, but it rarely causes systemic illness. It is cultured on blood or chocolate agar, and growth is enhanced around *Staphylococcus* colonies and in a high carbon dioxide atmosphere.

The typical illness is an acute conjunctivitis with a brief incubation period, often less than 24 hours, in children or young adults. The onset is usually in the warmer months; it is most common in the tropical and subtropical climates of the Middle East and North Africa, where it may be spread by ocular secretions and flies. Severe conjunctival injection, frequently with chemosis and bulbar conjunctival hemorrhage, occurs with increasing mucoid or mucopurulent discharge for the first 3 days. Lid edema may be present for about 5 days. Preauricular node swelling and tenderness occur. Without treatment, the conjunctivitis usually clears in 10 to 14 days, but it may relapse or become a chronic papillary conjunctivitis. In infants, the course may be mild and chronic or acute and severe with pseudomembranes. The cornea may be involved, with inferior limbal ulcers beginning on the second or third day; central ulcers with possible perforation may develop rarely. Phlyctenular keratoconjunctivitis with potential corneal scarring may follow healing. It has been postulated that Koch-Weeks infections are often superimposed on trachoma and increase scarring. Although systemic illness is unusual, a fulminant and often fatal bacteremia with purpuric skin lesions, following resolution of the conjunctivitis, has recently been recognized and is known as Brazilian purpuric fever. This disease is caused by a specific clone of the organism.

THERAPY

Systemic. Intravenous antibiotic therapy is indicated for orbital cellulitis and Brazilian purpuric fever.

Ocular. *H. aegyptius* conjunctivitis responds rapidly to treatment with most ophthalmic antibiotics, including sulfacetamide, chloramphenicol, polymyxin B, gentamicin, tobramycin, and tetracycline. The administration of hourly drops during the day with ointment used at bedtime leads to resolution in 3 days.

Ocular or Periocular Manifestations

Conjunctiva: Acute or chronic conjunctivitis; chemosis; injection; mucoid, mucopurulent, or purulent discharge; pseudomembrane; subconjunctival hemorrhage; phlyctenules.
Cornea: Infiltrates; marginal ulcer, phlyctenule; scarring; perforation.
Eyelids: Edema; cellulitis.
Other: Orbital or periorbital cellulitis; tearing; photophobia; iritis.

PRECAUTIONS

Adequate therapy is necessary to prevent recurrence or development of chronic conjunctivitis. Repeated reinfection is common in endemic regions, and antibiotic resistance may develop. Culture and sensitivity testing should be performed in severe or prolonged cases.

COMMENTS

The relationship between *H. aegyptius* infection and trachoma infection is unclear, but the two may coexist. Systemic illness—Brazilian purpuric fever—although rare, is cause for future concern.

References

Brazilian Purpuric Fever Study Group. Brazilian purpuric fever, identified in a new region of Brazil. J Infect Dis 165(suppl):16–19, 1992.
Dawson CF: Epidemic Koch-Weeks conjunctivitis and trachoma in the Coachilla Valley of California. Am J Ophthalmol 49:801–808, 1960.
Fedukowicz HB, Stetson S: External Infections of the Eye. 3rd ed. New York, Appleton-Century-Crofts, 1985, pp 66–69.
Taylor HR, Kolarczyk RA, Johnson SL, Schachter J, Prendergast RA: Effect of bacterial secondary infection in an animal model of trachoma. Infect Immun 44:614–616, 1984.

LEPROSY 030.9
(Hansen's Disease)

T. J. FFYTCHE, F.R.C.S., F.R.C.Ophth.

London, England

Leprosy is a disease caused by the acid-fast bacillus *Mycobacterium leprae*; it is communicable and probably transmitted by droplets, although the exact method of its spread remains uncertain.

The skin, peripheral nerves, mucous membranes, testes, and eyes are primarily involved because the organisms have an affinity for neural tissues in those parts of the body where the temperature is relatively low. The disease results in disfigurement and loss of mobility, and in a significant number of patients the deformities may be accompanied by visual impairment. In many countries leprosy still carries the social stigma that has persisted through ignorance for centuries.

The clinical picture of the disease is influenced by the immunity of the host, which is highest in the paucibacillary form (PB) and lowest in the multibacillary form (MB). Ocular involvement may occur indirectly in both types of leprosy through the combined effects of damage to the superficial branches of the trigeminal and facial nerves, with consequent corneal hypesthesia and exposure keratopathy. Direct invasion of the anterior part of the globe, which is susceptible because of its relatively low temperature, occurs in multibacillary disease and can produce chronic changes in the cornea, iris, and ciliary body with few early symptoms. An acute and often severe inflammatory reaction may occur in MB disease as part of a response to circulating immune complexes, known as erythema nodosum leprosum (ENL), and can cause iridocyclitis, episcleritis, or scleritis. ENL may develop spontaneously or as a result of changes in therapy, an intercurrent infection, or stress.

THERAPY

Systemic. The development of resistant organisms to standard anti-leprosy drugs, together with noncompliance, has led to a radical reappraisal of the therapy for the disease over the last decade and the introduction of multidrug therapy (MDT) in most centers. In paucibacillary disease the regime recommended by the WHO consists of 100 mg of dapsone daily as self-medication and 600 mg of rifampin once a month under surveillance, with treatment continued for at least 6 months. In multibacillary disease the WHO recommends 100 mg of dapsone and 50 mg of clofazimine daily as self-medication and once-monthly supervised doses of 600 mg of rifampin and 300 mg of clofazimine. Treatment in MB cases should be continued for at least 2 years and preferably until negative skin smears are obtained. Doses are reduced proportionally for children.

To avoid permanent neural and ocular damage, acute reactions in leprosy require energetic therapy. Treatment includes the use of analgesics and systemic corticosteroid preparations. In addition, control of the reaction can be facilitated by giving clofazimine, chloroquine, and thalidomide (if available).

More traditional therapies, such as chaulmoogra oil and herbal remedies, persist in many parts of the world. Attempts to improve cell-mediated immunity by means of a vaccine derived from the nine-banded armadillo are still undergoing clinical trials, and prophylactic BCG vaccination has been found to give some protection in several areas where the disease is endemic.

Ocular. The ocular manifestations of leprosy are influenced by many factors and may vary according to ethnic groups. Four main causes of blindness can occur on their own or in combination: lagophthalmos leading to exposure keratopathy, corneal hypesthesia predisposing to corneal ulceration, acute or chronic iridocyclitis, and secondary cataract.

Exposure keratopathy resulting from facial nerve involvement combined with corneal hypesthesia may result in corneal ulceration and secondary infection. A facial nerve paralysis can occur after an acute neuritis in all forms of leprosy as part of a sudden change in cellular immunity, known as a reversal reaction. It should be treated by energetic measures: protection of the cornea with lubricating eyedrops and broad-spectrum antibiotic drops and ointment. The neuritis may respond to systemic steroid therapy. Lid surgery may be necessary in the later stages.

The acute iridocyclitis that occurs in ENL responds to conventional anti-inflammatory treatment with local mydriatic and steroid drops. During an attack, 1 per cent atropine should be used three times daily together with 2 hourly dexamethasone; the dosage can be reduced as the inflammation subsides. In severe cases, subconjunctival injections* of steroids and mydriatics may be necessary. If secondary glaucoma develops, oral hypotensive agents, such as 250 mg of acetazolamide four times daily, should be added to this regime.

In multibacillary disease, a chronic iridocyclitis resulting in iris atrophy and profound miosis may occur and cause considerable visual loss. Because this condition does not respond to local mydriatic or steroid therapy in the late stage, attempts should be made to dilate the pupils with daily instillations of 5 per cent phenylephrine or 1 per cent atropine before the atrophy becomes too advanced.

Surgical. Lid surgery is designed to prevent corneal damage from exposure caused by facial nerve paralysis: procedures range from simple lateral tarsorrhaphy to more elaborate operations, such as temporalis transfer. Malpositions of the lids also require

surgical correction in order to avoid secondary corneal disease, and an infected lacrimal sac, which can provide a reservoir of infection, should be removed. The leprous eye tolerates intraocular surgery reasonably well, provided that there is no active inflammation, and such procedures as optical iridectomy, cataract surgery, and keratoplasty may be performed safely. There is no contraindication to intraocular lens implantation in paucibacillary cases, but in multibacillary disease, when chronic iridocyclitis is present, it should be avoided.

Ocular or Periocular Manifestations

Cornea: Corneal hypesthesia; corneal ulcer; exposure keratopathy; leproma; pannus; superficial stromal keratitis; thickened corneal nerves.

Episclera and Sclera: Episcleritis; scleritis; staphyloma.

Eyebrows: Madarosis; nodules; thickening of the skin.

Eyelids: Blepharochalasis; distichiasis; ectropion; entropion; lagophthalmos; madarosis; nodules; trichiasis.

Iris: Iridocyclitis, acute or chronic; iris atrophy; iris pearls; nodular leproma; synechiae.

Lacrimal System: Dacryocystitis, acute or chronic; epiphora; nasolacrimal duct obstruction.

Pupil: Anisocoria; corectopia; diminished or absent response to light; miosis; occlusio pupillae; polycoria; seclusio pupillae.

Others: Decreased intraocular pressure; paralysis of seventh nerve; phthisis bulbi; secondary cataract; secondary glaucoma.

PRECAUTIONS

The institution of multidrug therapy has been a significant factor in the control of eye complications, and compliance with treatment is very important for its success. Patients on dapsone should be watched closely for signs of toxicity, which may include anorexia, nausea and vomiting, neuropathy, anemia and agranulocytosis, and the drug should not be given to patients with glucose-6-phosphate dehydrogenase (G6PD) deficiency. Clofazimine can provoke diarrhea and causes a red-black discoloration of the skin and urine that may be disturbing to the patient. Rifampin may give rise to gastrointestinal and respiratory symptoms, acute renal failure, thrombocytopenic purpura, hepatic reactions, and skin rashes. The use of topical and systemic steroids should be monitored carefully to avoid steroid-induced glaucoma and secondary cataract.

COMMENTS

Visual impairment in leprosy is caused mainly by damage to the cornea through paralysis of the facial and trigeminal nerves, by cataract, and by the complications of acute and chronic iridocyclitis. Because patients are often unaware of ocular involvement, it may go undetected at a stage when preventive measures would be most effective. Therefore, education for leprosy workers to screen for eye disease, and for patients on self-care and drug compliance, therefore becomes fundamentally important. The aim of therapy should be the prevention of ocular changes by attention to eye protection and hygiene and to the early diagnosis of intraocular disease. Once the eye is affected, continuous supervision should be the goal, even after the patient has completed MDT and is classified as "cured." Whenever late complications develop, attempts should be made to preserve useful vision by medical and surgical measures. This may often mean that long-standing prejudices and the stigma of the disease have to be overcome in order to avoid blindness, which is especially tragic in these already disabled and disadvantaged individuals.

References

Brand M, ffytche TJ: Eye complications of leprosy. *In* Hastings R (ed): Leprosy. New York, Churchill Livingstone, 1985.
Brand MB: The Care of the Eye in Hansen's Disease, 2nd ed. Carville LA, Gillis W Long Hansen's Disease Centre, 1987.
Courtright P, Johnson GJ: Prevention of Blindness in Leprosy, rev ed. London, International Centre for Eye Health, 1991.
Ffytche TJ: Ocular leprosy. Trop Doct 15:118–127, 1985.
Tharangaraj RH, Yawalkar SJ: Leprosy. Basel, Ciba Geigy, 1986.

LEPTOSPIROSIS 100.9

SUSAN BARKAY, M.D.

Afula, Israel

Leptospirosis is an acute systemic disease with endemic or epidemic occurrence. It is caused by the smallest pathogenic spirochete, the *Leptospira interrogans*, which comprises some 170 serovars (serotypes). These serovars have been differentiated on the basis of distinct agglutinogenic properties, but they are indistinguishable by morphologic, cultural, and physiologic properties. These 170 serovars fall into about 20 serogroups on the basis of common, overlapping antigenic components.

Leptospiras are harbored by animal hosts, including lower mammalians, such as rats, mice, and raccoons, as well as domestic animals, cattle, swine, and dogs. Infected animals seldom show overt illness, although in some countries they cause a problem for veterinarians. Most carrier animals have asymptomatic infection of the renal tubules with long-lasting leptospiruria, which serves as the source of the disease in humans. In warm seasons *Leptospira* can survive for weeks in moist soil or alkaline water, and most cases of infection occur during the summer and autumn months.

Humans can acquire the disease through contact with urine or tissues of infected animals via abraded skin or mucous membranes. Direct transmission from person to person is possible, but rare.

Leptospiras penetrate tissues mechanically. After peritoneal inoculation in animal experiments, there is a rapid invasion of the leptospiras into the bloodstream. After 24 hours, they are present in virtually all organs and can be recovered from the blood, CSF, the brain, and also the anterior chamber of the eyes. Similar observations have been made in several cases of human disease. The tissue damage caused by *Leptospira* is probably of a toxic nature, and its virulence seems to depend on toxin production.

Systemic Manifestations

Leptospirosis is a biphasic illness. After an incubation period of 3 to 26 days, leptospiras invade the bloodstream and CSF, causing an acute febrile illness, occasionally in very severe form, with high temperatures, chills, muscular pains, pulmonary manifestations, gastrointestinal disturbance, and a skin rash, either petechial or purpuric. In this stage, jaundice is not a usual finding. A characteristic sign is an almost asymptomatic conjunctival effusion.

At this "leptospiremic" phase, *Leptospira* can be cultured with semisolid (Fletcher's or Stuart's) media from the blood or CSF. After the tenth day, they disappear from the blood and CSF and are excreted with the urine (sometimes until the eleventh month). The leptospiremic phase ceases.

An almost asymptomatic interval of some days follows, after which the immune phase sets in. In this phase, there is a high degree of individual variability, with some patients being almost asymptomatic and others becoming severely ill. About 50 per cent of the patients have a high fever state with meningismus, and 25 per cent have meningitis with elevated protein values and pleocytosis in the CSF. Encephalitis; Guillain-Barré syndrome; optic, abducens, facial, and auditory nerve defects; radiculitis; peripheral nerve lesions; and myocarditis are other complications. The second phase may last from a few days to as long as several weeks.

In some cases, in Weil's syndrome the course is extremely serious. Jaundice appears after the first days with hepatic enlargement, and fever is high and persistent. Pyuria, hematuria, and peak elevations of blood urea nitrogen occur as signs of acute tubular necrosis. A diffuse vasculitis may occur with general hemorrhagic manifestations, such as epistaxis, hemoptysis, gastrointestinal bleedings, and subarachnoidal hemorrhage.

The clinical signs of the immune phase parallel the appearance of *Leptospira* antibodies in the blood at the end of the first week, reaching their peak in the third or fourth week. During this period of the disease, serologic tests should be done. They are complicated owing to the large number of antigenically distinct leptospiral serotypes, but very often it is sufficient to test only for the organism known to be present in the endemic area. The microscopic agglutination-lysis test against living *Leptospira* has the highest sensitivity. The simple agglutination test, using killed *Leptospira*, is a good diagnostic aid, but is less accurate since nonspecific reactions may occur. After the tenth day of illness and until the third month when complement-fixing antibodies are present in the serum, the complement fixation test is also an excellent diagnostic aid.

Blood for serologic tests should be examined during the acute illness and also during the convalescent period. A fourfold titer rise is considered diagnostic. If only one specimen is available, a titer of 1:1600 gives strong presumptive evidence of the diagnosis.

Ocular Manifestations

Ocular findings have been reported in 3 per cent to 92 per cent of cases of leptospirosis. This wide range is probably due to the varying enthusiasm and knowledge of clinical observers.

In the first days of the disease is found a conjunctival infection involving the anterior part of the globe and the conjunctiva of the lower lid. There is a characteristic clinical picture: the conjunctiva is pink in color (except in jaundiced patients in which it is yellow), and the engorged conjunctival and episcleral vessels anastomose with dilated pericorneal vessels, thus giving the impression of a reticulum. Usually there are no subjective complaints, no lacrimation, and no discharge. However, discharge, if present, contains *Leptospira* and may be the source of further infection. This picture tends to disappear during convalescence.

In the immune phase, as part of the central nervous system involvement, palpebral herpes and optic neuritis may develop with or without iridocyclitis. This condition is usually self-limited and of short duration.

Most important, however, are the late uveitis cases which occur long after the general features of the disease have subsided in apparently healthy persons. Indeed, cases have been reported after 5 years. There is usually an acute, moderate, bilateral iridocyclitis with hyperemia of the iris. Yet, severe exudative inflammation with mutton fat precipitates, dense posterior synechiae between the iris and lens, and even hypopyon and secondary glaucoma are quite common. Choroiditis, retinal hemorrhages and exudates, and peculiar vitreous membranes running from the optic disc toward the anterior segment have been described, with a course of absorption lasting for years. Blindness as a final outcome has been reported.

The pathogenesis of the uveitis as a late complication is not clear. *Leptospira* organisms have been isolated from the anterior chamber, but antibodies have been also found in other, similar uveitis cases. It has been suggested that the *Leptospira* can survive a long time in the eye, as they do in the pelvis of the kidney, in spite of high levels of antibodies in the general circulation. It is possible that those organisms that survive can excite an inflammation in the form of late uveitis only after systemic immunity has faded.

THERAPY

Systemic. There is no specific treatment for leptospirosis, but there is general agreement that treatment with high doses of antimicrobials reduces complications. They must be administered in the first 2 to 4 days of the illness during the leptospiremia. Initiating antimicrobial treatment after the fifth day of the disease is not considered worthwhile.

Penicillin G, 2.4 million units IV/day, or tetracycline, 0.5 gm orally every 6 hours, is recommended for a period of 7 days. Within a few hours of the initial dose of penicillin, a Jarisch-Herxheimer type of reaction may occur, indicating that the drug possesses some in vivo antileptospiral activity. Doxycycline, 0.1 gm orally twice a day for 7 days, may favorably affect the course of leptospirosis.

Careful management of fluid and electrolyte balance is required in cases of renal failure. In severe cases of tubular necrosis, hemodialysis or peritoneal dialysis is indicated.

Ocular. In cases of iridocyclitis, 1% atropine should be administered three times daily, with 0.5% ophthalmic prednisolone drops three to six times daily. If this treatment fails, subconjunctival betamethasone* injections, 1–1.5 mg, may be given. In severe cases, oral prednisone, 40 mg to 80 mg daily, is indicated.

Ocular or Periocular Manifestations

Anterior Chamber: Cells; flare; hypopyon.
Conjunctiva: Conjunctivitis; hemorrhages.

Cornea: Keratic precipitates.
Extraocular muscles: Muscle palsies.
Eyelids: Herpes.
Iris: Posterior synechiae.
Lens: Cataract.
Optic nerve: Neuritis.
Pupil: Seclusion.
Retina: Hemorrhages; exudates.
Vitreous: Peculiar vitreous strands.
Other: Secondary glaucoma; visual loss.

PRECAUTIONS

From the etiologic point of view, diagnosis of *Leptospira* uveitis is not simple. In endemic areas and in cases where there is a short interval between the systemic disease and uveitis, it is not difficult to find the connection. However, in many cases of severe uveitis, the forerunner was an uncomplicated febrile disease of short duration that occurred months or sometimes years before. In those cases, diagnosis is difficult and often presumptive. It must rest on the history of systemic illness with characteristic anamnestic data and clinical signs of leptospirosis sometimes experienced much earlier, on exclusion of other causes, and on positive serologic tests.

The prognosis of the disease in an icteric form is mostly good. Recovery is complete, except for the rare cases with residual renal tubular dysfunction. Still, it should be kept in mind that there is a case-fatality rate of 3 to 6 per cent. In jaundiced patients with Weil's syndrome, mortality ranges from 25 per cent to 40 per cent in untreated cases.

Most uveitis cases respond well to treatment, and even in the severe forms there is mostly a complete recovery. However, there are cases with long-lasting courses, causing cataract formation or secondary glaucoma and thus severe visual impairment.

COMMENTS

Leptospirosis was once regarded primarily as an occupational disease among farmers, dairy workers, veterinarians, rice and sugar cane field workers, and the like. However, it has become more and more a recreational hazard to hunters, fishermen, and swimmers in endemic areas. In the past decade, infection from contact with dogs has become more frequent, particularly among children.

Leptospirosis is a preventable disease that can be avoided with adequate prophylactic methods. Recently progress has been made in developing useful vaccines against leptospiral infections. Until safe polyvalent vaccines are developed, hygienic precautions should be taken in cooperation with veterinary services and health care authorities.

References

Barkay B, Garzozi H: Leptospirosis and uveitis. Ann Ophthalmol 16:164–168, 1984.

Braude AI: Medical Microbiology and Infectious Disease. Philadelphia. WB Saunders, 1980, pp 437–441, 1143–1146, 1839–1847.

Duke-Elder S (ed): System of Ophthalmology. London, Henry Kimpton, 1965, Vol VIII, pp 201–203.

Duke-Elder S (ed): System of Ophthalmology. London, Henry Kimpton, 1966, Vol IX, pp 322–325.

Jawetz E, Melnick JL, Adelberg EA: Review of Medical Microbiology, 14th ed. Los Altos, CA: Lange Medical Publications, 1979, pp 259–260.

Masuzawa T, Suzuki R, Yanagihara Y: Microbiology. Immunology 35(3):199–208, 1991.

Sanford JP: In Braunwald, et al (eds): Harrison's Principles of Internal Medicine, 11th ed. New York, McGraw-Hill, 1987, pp 652–655.

Walsh TJ, Hoyt C: Clinical Neuro-Ophthalmology, 3rd ed, Vol II. Baltimore: Williams & Wilkins, 1969, pp 1548–1551.

LISTERIOSIS 027.0
(Listerellosis)

F. HAMPTON ROY, M.D., F.A.C.S.

Little Rock, Arkansas

Listeria monocytogenes is found in soil and plants. It is a non-spore-forming, gram-positive, non-acid-fast, diphtheroid-like rod. Listeriosis septicemia commonly causes abortion in pregnant women and neonatal death.

Listeriosis, which causes a general infection or meningitis, is more likely to infect the eye. The conjunctivitis caused by this organism may be purulent or nonpurulent. Contaminated amniotic fluid causes a purulent conjunctivitis more commonly seen in newborn infants. The nonpurulent conjunctivitis is usually associated with meningitis or encephalitis caused by listeriosis.

Corneal involvement is rare, having been reported in only two cases. Both started with a keratitis caused by listeriosis with a central corneal ulcer. In one case, pupillary block glaucoma occurred after a heavy fibrinous reaction in the anterior chamber. Laser iridotomy was unsuccessful in treating the glaucoma. Cephalosporins and gentamicin used both subconjunctivally and as fortified drops helped heal the corneal ulcers. The diagnosis was made in both cases by a corneal smear and culture.

Endophthalmitis caused by listeriosis is rare. In the English literature from 1967 to 1990, only three cases were reported. Listeriosis is more common in immunosuppressed individuals. The manifestations include severe uveitis with an elevated intraocular pressure. Large pigmented precipitates can be present over the posterior surface of the cornea. A hypopyon is brown to black in color and is fibrinous. A severe fibrinous alteration of the aqueous may occur with a secondary glaucoma.

THERAPY

Systemic. Ampicillin and gentamicin have a synergistic effect against *L. monocytogenes*. Intravenous administration of 2 gm of ampicillin every 4 hours and 100 mg of gentamicin every 8 hours may be given for 5 days. After this treatment, the patient may be maintained on oral tetracycline and ampicillin with topical ophthalmic gentamicin. Oral tetracycline, of course, should only be used for adults.

Ocular. When there is a hypopyon, an anterior chamber tap should be done. This procedure helps ensure early diagnosis and treatment. Intravitreal injections of 200 to 400 mg of gentamicin* can be administered at the time of paracentesis.

The endophthalmitis may be treated with a combination systemic antibiotic and ocular therapy; 100 mg of ampicillin* may be administered for 7 days sub-tenon. Usually after the intraocular treatment, little is gained by further ocular therapy. Hourly gentamicin drops for the first 3 days and then every 2 hours while the patient is hospitalized is a reasonable dosage level, with gentamicin ointment being applied at night. Atropine, of course, can be instilled for cycloplegia.

PRECAUTIONS

Listeriosis may be enhanced by the use of steroids, which should be used cautiously.

Listeriosis is an opportunistic infection that occurs in immunosuppressed individuals. If a tan to brown hypopyon is present in an immunocompromised individual, *L. monocytogenes* must be considered along with a possible endogenous endophthalmitis. The fibrinous reaction may remain for a long period of time in the anterior chamber, reducing visual acuity. With paracentesis the laboratory may mistake *L. monocytogenes* for a nonpathologic diphtheroid with this polymorphonuclear response.

COMMENTS

A general listeria infection should be treated early with antibiotics. A delay in therapy may result in death. Early treatment of endophthalmitis is important to reduce the long-term effect on vision.

References

Abbott RL, Forster RK, Rebell G: *Listeria monocytogenes* endophthalmitis with a black hypopyon. Am J Ophthalmol 86:715–719, 1978.

Azimi PH, Koranyi K, Lindsey KD: *Listeria monocytogenes*. Synergistic effects of ampicillin and gentamicin. Am J Clin Pathol 72:974–977, 1979.

Bagnarello AG, et al. *Listeria monocytogenes* endophthalmitis. Arch Ophthalmol 95:1004–1005, 1977.

Ballen PH, Loffredo FR, Painter B: *Listeria* endophthalmitis. Arch Ophthalmol 97:101–102, 1979.

Boisivon A, Guiomar C, Carbon C: In vitro bactericidal activity of amoxicillin, gentamicin, rifampicin, ciprofloxacin and trimethoprim-sulfamethoxazole alone or in combination against *Listeria monocytogenes*. Eur J Clin Microbiol Infect Dis 9:206–209, 1990.

Decker CF, Simon GL, DiGioia RA, Tuazon CU: *Listeria monocytogenes* infections in patients with AIDS: Report of five cases and review. Rev Infect Dis 13:413–417, 1991.

Forster RK, et al: Further observations on the diagnosis, etiology, and treatment of endophthalmitis. Trans Am Ophthalmol Soc 73:221–230, 1975.

Goodner EK, Okumoto M: Intraocular listeriosis. Am J Ophthalmol 64:682–686, 1967.

Holland S, Alfonso E, Gelender H, Heidemann D, Mendelsohn A, Ullman S, Miller D: Corneal ulcer due to *Listeria monocytogenes*. Cornea 6:144–146, 1987.

Skogberg K, et al: Clinical presentation and outcome of listeriosis in patients with and without immunosuppressive therapy. Clin Infect Dis 14:815–821, 1992.

Zimianski MC, Dawson CR, Togni B: Epithelial cell phagocytosis of *Listeria monocytogenes* in the conjunctiva. Ophthalmology 13:623–626, 1974.

LYME DISEASE 104.8

JAMES T. ROSENBAUM, M.D.

Portland, Oregon

Lyme disease is a spirochetal disease caused by infection from the tick-borne organism, *Borrelia burgdorferi*. The disease is endemic in geographic areas that support the appropriate life cycle of the tick. Deer, mice, lizards, and birds are commonly involved in this life cycle. In the United States, the disease is most common along the Northeastern seaboard. Other foci of disease include the northern portions of the Midwest and areas along the Pacific coast. The disease has been reported worldwide, including in portions of Europe and Japan.

As in another spirochetal disease, syphilis, many clinicians describe three stages of Lyme disease. Stage I is exemplified by a characteristic expanding skin lesion, erythema chronicum migrans, that begins at the site of the tick bite. This rash is sufficiently characteristic as to be virtually diagnostic, but its presence is not inevitable. Meningeal and flu-like symptoms are also common in stage I disease. Weeks to months after this initial stage of the disease, cardiac, neurologic, or joint disease may dominate the clinical illness (stage II disease). Finally, after months of latency, stage III disease is characterized by chronic neuropsychiatric or joint manifestations.

Serologic tests to demonstrate antibodies to *B. burgdorferi* are the mainstay of diagnosis. However, these tests are fraught with difficulty. First, during the initial stages of disease antibodies may not have yet developed. Second, the tests available suffer from many problems, including standardization, reproducibility, sensitivity, and specificity. The detection of antibodies is not sufficient by itself to establish a diagnosis of Lyme disease.

The most common ocular manifestation of Lyme disease is conjunctivitis during stage I. Cranial nerve palsies that affect ocular motility, especially Bell's palsy, are also relatively common. Papilledema, optic neuritis, keratitis, exudative choroiditis, iritis, posterior uveitis, and retinal vasculitis have also been described.

THERAPY

Systemic. The treatment of Lyme disease depends on the stage of disease, the organ affected, and of course, the age of the patient. All stages of Lyme disease should be treated with antibiotics, but the efficacy of antibiotics for late disease, which may in part be immune-mediated, is less consistent.

Options for early Lyme disease include doxycycline, 100 mg twice a day for 10 to 21 days; amoxicillin, 500 mg three times per day for 10 to 21 days; or azithromycin, a 500-mg loading dose followed by 250 mg per day for a total of 5 days of therapy. Probenecid, 500 mg three times per day, can be added to potentiate the amoxicillin. Options for cardiac, neurologic, or joint disease include prolonged courses of doxycycline; penicillin G, 20 million units intravenously per day in divided doses for up to 21 days; or ceftriaxone, 2 gm intravenously for 14 to 21 days. Children younger than age 9 should not receive tetracyclines, such as doxycycline. Penicillin and amoxicillin are the drugs of choice if the patient is pregnant.

Ocular. For ophthalmic disease, treatment is usually dictated by the other manifestations of the disease and its stage. Conjunctivitis should respond to regimens that are effective for early Lyme disease. Optic neuritis or Bell's palsy should be treated as for other neurologic manifestations. Some observations suggest that oral corticosteroids or intra-articular steroids may reduce the efficacy of antibiotic regimens. By analogy, then, the use of oral or periocular corticosteroid injections without antibiotic coverage may be contraindicated for such a problem as uveitis. Topical corticosteroids are a reasonable adjunct for therapy for conjunctivitis, keratitis, or anterior uveitis.

Ocular or Periocular Manifestations

Choroid: Diffuse choroiditis.
Conjunctiva: Conjunctivitis.
Cornea: Keratitis (involving epithelial basement membrane, superficial and deep stroma).
Extraocular Muscles: Bell's palsy; paresis of third, fourth, or sixth nerve.
Iris: Iridocyclitis.
Optic Nerve: Papilledema; pseudotumor cerebri, optic atrophy.
Retina: Detachment; vasculitis.
Other: Decreased vision; diplopia; periorbital edema; endophthalmitis.

COMMENTS

Antibiotic therapy may be complicated by a Jarisch-Herxheimer-like reaction. Newer diagnostic tests, such as the polymerase chain reaction for *B. burgdorferi*-specific nucleic acids, may improve diagnostic accuracy. Even in endemic areas, the risk of infection is low enough so that prophylactic antibiotics after a tick bite are not warranted. Additional antibiotics, such as oral cefuroxime, are being studied.

References

Aaberg TM: The expanding ophthalmologic spectrum of Lyme disease. Am J Ophthalmol 107:77, 1989.

Kauffmann DJH, Wormser GP: Ocular Lyme disease: Case report and review of the literature. Br J Ophthalmol 74:325, 1990.

Luger SW, Krauss E: Serologic tests for Lyme disease. Arch Intern Med 150:761, 1990.

Massarotti EM, Rahn DW, Messner RP, Wong JB, Johnson RC, Steere AC: Treatment of early Lyme disease. Am J Med 92:396, 1992.

Rahn DW: Lyme disease: Clinical manifestations, diagnosis, and treatment. Arth Rheum 20:201, 1991.

Rahn DW, Malawista SE: Lyme disease: Recommendations for diagnosis and treatment. Ann Int Med 114:472, 1991.

Rosenbaum JT, Rahn DW: Prevalence of Lyme disease among patients with uveitis. Am J Ophthalmol 112:462, 1991.

Rothova A, Kuiper H, Spanjaard L, Dankert J, Breebaart AC: Spiderweb vitritis in Lyme borreliosis. Lancet 337:490, 1991.

Winterkorn JMS: Lyme disease: Neurologic and ophthalmic manifestations. Surv Ophthalmol 35:191, 1990.

MORAXELLA 372.02

JULES BAUM, M.D.

Boston, Massachusetts

Formerly called the diplobacillus of Morax-Axenfeld, *Moraxella lacunata* induces either an angular blepharoconjunctivitis or an infectious corneal ulcer. It is a gram-negative aerobic rod-shaped or coccoid diplobacillus. Organisms formerly called *M. liquefaciens* are indistinguishable from *M. lacunata* and have been incorporated into the latter species.

At the turn of the century, many investigators found the *Moraxella* diplobacillus to be the most commonly diagnosed cause of conjunctivitis. More recently, the reported incidence of *Moraxella* conjunctivitis and blepharoconjunctivitis has decreased dramatically and has ranged from 0.1 to 1.0 per cent of all forms of conjunctivitis in the Western world. *Moraxella* characteristically induces a chronic angular (outer angle) blepharoconjunctivitis with follicles and a typical erythematous eczematoid appearance of the skin at the lateral canthus. *Moraxella* ocular infection is rarely seen in young children. Without treatment, the disease may persist for months or even years. This is also true of staphylococcal blepharoconjunctivitis, now the most frequent cause of angular blepharoconjunctivitis. Rarely, *Moraxella* produces an acute severe conjunctivitis.

M. lacunata may also induce a severe corneal ulcer that is usually associated with a hypopyon. The ulcer may be superficial or deep, central or peripheral. Similar ulcers produced by *M. nonliquefaciens* cannot be distinguished clinically from ulcers induced by *M. lacunata* (or *M. lacunata* subsp *liquefaciens*).

THERAPY

Ocular. *Moraxella* is sensitive to most antibiotics, including penicillin, and treatment of the blepharoconjunctivitis is relatively simple. Proteases produced by the organism cause the maceration of the skin at the canthus, and 0.25 to 0.5 per cent zinc sulfate eyedrops or ointment counteracts the effect of the proteases. After cultures have been obtained, both topical antibiotic and zinc sulfate therapy should be given three to four times daily until the disease process has resolved. The choice of antibiotic may be modified on the basis of in vitro susceptibility results. Treatment of a *Moraxella* corneal ulcer should conform to the initial treatment of any suspected corneal ulcer (see Bacterial Corneal Ulcers p. 478).

Ocular or Periocular Manifestations

Conjunctiva: Chronic catarrhal angular conjunctivitis; follicles; mucopurulent discharge.
Cornea: Central or peripheral ulcer with or without hypopyon.
Eyelids: Chronic blepharitis; eczema and maceration; lateral canthal skin erythema.
Other: Iridocyclitis secondary to corneal ulcer.

PRECAUTIONS

Since *Moraxella* ocular disease usually occurs in a poor and alcoholic population, compliance is often a problem; every effort should be made to impress on the patient the importance of compliance.

COMMENTS

Moraxella ocular infections tend to occur most frequently, but not exclusively, in a derelict, malnourished, alcoholic population. Nasal and conjunctival cultures for *Moraxella* were positive in 12.9 per cent and 0.3 per cent, respectively, of normal subjects in a recent series, whereas similar cultures taken from a derelict alcoholic population yielded positive cultures in 35 per cent and 5.5 per cent, respectively. Although *Moraxella* is part of the normal flora of the respiratory tract, its incidence may be higher in a derelict population. It is curious that, whereas *M. liquefaciens* is the species most often part of the normal nasal flora, the more frequent ocular pathogen is *M. lacunata*.

References

Baum J, Fedukowicz HB, Jordan A: A survey of *Moraxella* corneal ulcers in a derelict population. Am J Ophthalmol 90:476–480, 1980.

Baum JL, Jones DB: Initial therapy of suspected microbial corneal ulcers. Surv Ophthalmol 24:97–116, 1979.

Chandler RL, Bird RG, Smith MD, Anger HS, Turfrey BA: Scanning electron microscope studies on preparations of bovine cornea exposed to *Moraxella bovis*. J Comp Pathol 93:1–8, 1983.

Fedukowicz HB: External Infections of the Eye: Bacterial, Viral and Mycotic, 2nd ed. New York, Appleton-Century-Crofts, 1978.

Jackman SH, Rosenbusch RF: In vitro adherence of *Moraxella bovis* to intact corneal epithelium. Curr Eye Res 3:1107–1112, 1984.

Lennette EH, et al (eds): Manual of Clinical Microbiology, 3rd ed. Washington, DC, American Society for Microbiology, 1980.

Ringvold A, Vik E, Bevanger LS: *Moraxella lacunata* isolated from epidemic conjunctivitis among teenaged females. Acta Ophthalmol (Copenh) 63:427–431, 1985.

van Bijsterveld OP: Acute conjunctivitis and *Moraxella*. Am J Ophthalmol 63:1702–1705, 1968.

van Bijsterveld OP: The incidence of *Moraxella* on mucous membranes and the skin. Am J Ophthalmol 74:72–76, 1972.

van Bijsterveld OP: Host-parasite relationship and taxonomic position of *Moraxella* and morphologically related organisms. Am J Ophthalmol 77:545–554, 1973.

NOCARDIA 039

JOHN D. BULLOCK, M.D., M.S., F.A.C.S.,
Dayton, Ohio
and STUART H. GOLDBERG, M.D.
Hershey, Pennsylvania

Nocardiosis is typically caused by *Nocardia asteroides*, which is named for the starlike appearance of the colonies on agar plate. Once thought to be a fungus, it is now classified in the bacterial family Nocardiaceae, which includes aerobic *Actinomycetes* having a complex cell wall. The organism reproduces by fragmentation of its hyphae into bacillary and coccoid elements. It is distinguished by a propensity for filamentous growth with true branching. A natural soil saprophyte, it is often found in decaying organic matter. The organisms are gram-positive and often show an intermittent or beaded staining pattern with gram stain. Gomori methenamine silver stain also demonstrates the organisms well. In culture, they tend to grow slowly, but will grow within a wide temperature range on virtually any bacterial, fungal, or mycobacterial medium that lacks antibiotics.

Systemic nocardiosis is a chronic, progressive, localized, or disseminated infection that usually invades the body via the respiratory tract. When the lung is involved the clinical picture can resemble bronchitis or pneumonia similar to that seen with tuberculosis or other bacterial or fungal infections. Nocardial organisms can also cause mycetoma (maduromycosis or Madura foot), a chronic, deep subcutaneous tissue and bone infection usually of the lower extremity. Between 20 to 50 per cent of cases of nocardiosis are in otherwise healthy patients, but it is much more common in debilitated, immunosuppressed patients. The patient presents with cough and low-grade fever. Malaise, weight loss, and night sweats may occur. The radiologic appearance is that of a rapidly developing lobar or segmental infiltrate. Central nervous system dissemination occurs in 25 to 40 per cent of cases. Other sites of dissemination include the skin and subcutaneous tissues, kidney, liver, and lymph nodes. Ocular involvement has been reported in 3 per cent of cases of systemic nocardiosis. Diagnosis can be made by blood culture, sputum culture, or direct aspiration of material.

Ophthalmic *N. asteroides* infection occurs either exogenously or endogenously. Exogenous ocular disease arises as a superficial infection, usually following trauma, with or without intraocular extension. In endogenous ocular nocardiosis, the organisms reach the eye hematogenously in an immunologically normal, immunosuppressed, or immunocompromised patient. Endogenous ocular nocardiosis occurs at a mean age of 46 years, with a male-to-female ratio of 4:1, and is bilateral in 30 per cent of patients.

THERAPY

Systemic. Most strains of *N. asteroides* are sensitive to sulfonamides. The treatment of choice is 6 to 10 gm/day of sulfadiazine or sulfisoxazole. Treatment must be prolonged. Immunologically intact patients require a minimum of 6 weeks of therapy, whereas immunosuppressed patients are treated for a year.

Ocular. Nocardial keratitis and scleritis may be treated with hourly 15 to 30 per cent sulfacetamide eyedrops with or without hourly topical ampicillin (40 to 100 mg/ml), or topical trimethoprim (16 mg/ml)/sulfamethoxazole (80 mg/ml) given every half hour[§] initially. Oral administration of trimethoprim/sulfamethoxazole in a dosage of 320 mg of trimethoprim and 1.6 gm of sulfamethoxazole should be given twice a day. The use of steroids in the treatment of nocardial keratitis is controversial. Subconjunctival injection of trimethoprim/sulfamethoxazole,[*] scleral débridement, and scleral grafting have been employed to treat nocardial scleritis. Therapy of nocardial endophthalmitis with a variety of systemic and topical antibiotics is frequently unsuccessful. Many of these eyes go on to blindness, evisceration, and enucleation. A reported case of exogenous endophthalmitis in an immunocompetent patient was successfully treated with vitrectomy, penetrating keratoplasty, and intraocular, topical, and systemic antibiotics.

Ocular or Periocular Manifestations

Anterior Chamber: Hypopyon.
Cornea: Keratoconjunctivitis; ulcerative keratitis.
Globe: Endophthalmitis.
Iris: Anterior uveitis.
Lacrimal System: Dacryocystitis.
Orbit: Chronic cellulitis.
Sclera: Scleritis.
Vitreous or Retina: Chorioretinitis; subretinal abscess.

PRECAUTIONS

Immunosuppressive medications should be reduced in patients with nocardiosis. In primary isolation from clinical material, the colonies of *N. asteroides* can take as long as 2 to 4 weeks to appear. Because of this long time interval, a high index of suspicion is necessary to make the diagnosis microbiologically. Culture plates tend to be overgrown by contaminants and may be discarded before *Nocardia* colonies grow.

COMMENTS

Healthy individuals have only a 15 per cent mortality from nocardiosis. Nonimmunosuppressed patients with an underlying disease have a mortality of approximately 20 per cent from nocardiosis, whereas patients who are taking immunosuppressive medications and have nocardiosis have a mortality of 80 to 100 per cent. The probability of surviving nocardiosis is increased by rapid diagnosis, discontinuation or marked reduction of immunosuppressive medication, and prolonged, aggressive, and accurate antimicrobial therapy. Eight of fourteen reported immunocompromised patients with endogenous nocardial endophthalmitis died. The diagnosis of nocardial endophthalmitis was established antemortem in only two of these patients.

N. asteroides is a facultative, intracellular parasite that can persist and grow within macrophages. The basis of nocardial pathogenicity is its cell wall, which is composed of complex lipids, peptides, and polysaccharides.

Common histopathologic features of nocardial endophthalmitis include a suppurative and necrotizing inflammatory response in the choroid and retina along with subretinal abscesses.

References

Brooks JG, Mills RAD, Coster DJ: Nocardial scleritis. Am J Ophthalmol 114:371–372, 1992.

Bullock JD: Endogenous ocular nocardiosis: A clinical and experimental study. Trans Am Ophthalmol Soc 81:451–531, 1983.

Chen CJ: *Nocardia asteroides* endophalmitis. Ophthalmic Surg 14:502–505, 1983.

Climenhaga DB, Tokarewicz AC, Willis NR: *Nocardia* keratitis. Can J Ophthalmol 9:284–286, 1984.

Donnenfeld ED, Cohen EJ, Barza M, Baum J: Treatment of *Nocardia* keratitis with topical trimethoprim-sulfamethoxazole. Am J Ophthalmol 99:601–602, 1985.

Ferry AP, Font R, Weinberg RS, Boniuk M, Schaffer CL: Nocardial endophthalmitis: Report of two cases studied histopathologically. Br J Ophthalmol 72:55–61, 1988.

Gregor RJ, Chong CA, Augsburger JJ, Eagle RC, Carlson KM, Jessup M, Wong S, Naids R: Endogenous *Nocardia asteroides* subretinal abscess diagnosed by transvitreal fine-needle aspiration biopsy. Retina 9:118–121, 1989.

Katten HM, Pflugfelder SC: *Nocardia* scleritis. Am J Ophthalmol 110:446–447, 1990.

King LP, Furlong WB, Gilbert WS, Levy C: *Nocardia asteroides* infection following scleral buckling. Ophthalmic Surg 22:150–152, 1991.

Srinivason M, Shaarma: *Nocardia asteroides* as a cause of corneal ulcer. Arch Ophthalmol 105:464, 1987.

PNEUMOCOCCUS 041.2
(Streptococcus Pneumoniae)

H. BRUCE OSTLER, M.D.,
and VICKY CEVALLOS, M.T. (A.S.C.P.)

San Francisco, California

Commonly known as pneumococcus, *Streptococcus pneumoniae* is a gram-positive lancet-shaped coccus characteristically appearing as diplococcus but occasionally singly or in short chains. The normal habitat of the pneumococcus is the upper respiratory tract of humans. It is also present in the eyes of a small percentage of healthy individuals.

The pneumococcus is the primary etiologic agent in all types of pneumonias in the United States and the most frequent cause of otitis media in children. Pneumococcus has also been implicated in meningitis and septicemia. Infections with pneumococcus occur through droplets released from infected patients.

Pneumonia is often preceded by an upper respiratory infection. The infection is usually sudden, with a shaking chill, sharp pain in the involved hemithorax, cough with early sputum production, fever, and headache. Gastrointestinal symptoms are often present.

Ocular disease occurs from direct invasion by the organism. In newborns, the pneumococcus may cause ophthalmia neonatorum. In the adult, the organism is a common cause of dacryocystitis. *S. pneumoniae* is a true corneal pathogen. It also frequently causes an acute catarrhal conjunctivitis.

THERAPY

Systemic. With few exceptions *S. pneumoniae* is susceptible to penicillin, the cephalosporins, vancomycin, erythromycin, clindamycin, chloramphenicol, trimethoprim, and bacitracin. The quinolone ciprofloxacin is somewhat less active than the B-lactam agents against *S. pneumoniae*.

Treatment of choice is procaine penicillin (300,000 to 600,000 units at 12-hour intervals) for pneumococcal pneumonia. It is inadvisable to rely on oral therapy for acutely ill patients. Patients with mild infection who are otherwise healthy, however, can be treated safely with an initial intramuscular injection of procaine penicillin G (300,000 to 600,000 units) followed by oral penicillin V (250 mg every 6 hours) for 10 days. Aqueous potassium penicillin G, 40,000 to 50,000 units/kg divided in four equal portions every 6 hours, should be given to patients with overwhelming disease with the potential for cardiovascular collapse. Alternate drugs that may be used for the patient allergic to penicillin include erythromycin (250 mg every 6 hours) and vancomycin (500 mg every 12 hours). Cefazolin (1 gm every 8 hours) and other cephalosporins are effective. However, clinical cross sensitivity reactions to penicillin occur in about 8 to 15 per cent of patients.

In the United States, 5 to 10 per cent of *S. pneumoniae* strains are resistant to penicillin. Bacteremia and meningitis caused by highly resistant strains and meningitis due to intermediately resistant strains should be treated with agents other than penicillin. Therapy of these infections may include chloramphenicol (if susceptible) or cefotaxime, ceftriaxone, or vancomycin, possibly with the addition of rifampin, depending on the patient's response and such factors as the serum bactericidal activity. Pneumoniae caused by intermediately resistant strains may be treated in most cases with high-dose penicillin alone.

Ocular. Topical ophthalmic antibiotics normally suffice for the treatment of a conjunctivitis due to pneumococcus. Bacitracin[§] (10,000 units/ml) should be given every hour during the first day and then four times daily for 1 week. Erythromycin ophthalmic ointment (0.5 per cent) may be substituted for the bacitracin.

For suppurative keratitis, central corneal ulcers due to *S. pneumoniae*, one should give topical fortified aqueous penicillin G* (100,000 units/ml) every half hour during the day and every hour during the night. Bacitracin[§] (10,000 units/ml) or cefazolin* (50 mg/ml) topically may be substituted for the penicillin. Subconjunctival cefazolin* (50 to 100 mg) or penicillin* (0.5 to 1.0 million units) should also be given every 12 to 24 hours for the first few days. If perforation seems imminent, systemic antibiotics as outlined under endophthalmitis should be started.

A gram stain can be of great value in identifying *S. pneumoniae* in corneal scrapings. With this stain, the organisms are seen as gram-positive cocci in pairs with the unattached ends of each cocci slightly pointed outward, giving the organisms their lancet shape morphology. A capsule surrounding each pair of cocci can often be seen as well.

For treatment of endophthalmitis caused by pneumococcus, intravitreal cefazolin* (2.25 mg) should be administered immediately after aspiration of vitreous or vitrectomy. A daily dosage of 20 to 40 million units of aqueous penicillin G divided into four equal portions should be administered intravenously. In patients with a history of hypersensitivity to penicillin, cefazolin (15 mg/kg/day divided into three equal doses) intravenously, erythromycin (15 to 20 mg/kg/day divided into four equal doses) intravenously, or lincomycin (600 mg three times daily) may be substituted for the penicillin. Subconjunctival injections, as outlined above for treatment of corneal ulcers, should also be given.

Cycloplegics are indicated in order to prevent posterior synechiae and reduce pain in patients with suppurative keratitis or endophthalmitis. One or two drops of 1 per cent atropine or 1 per cent cyclopentolate may be instilled one to three times daily.

Orbital cellulitis caused by pneumococcal infection should be treated with aqueous penicillin G intravenously as outlined above. An otolaryngologist should evaluate and treat the paranasal sinuses, if indicated.

Acute dacryocystitis caused by pneumococcus requires adequate and prompt drainage of the lacrimal sac. When the dacryocystitis is no longer acute, the patency of the nasolacrimal system should be reestablished. If periodacryocystitis has occurred, either 250 mg of oral penicillin V every 6 hours or 600,000 units of intramuscular aqueous procaine penicillin G daily may be used. In ad-

dition, drainage of the nasolacrimal sac should be reestablished. In instances of hypersensitivity to penicillin, 250 to 500 mg of oral erythromycin four times daily may be substituted.

Secondary glaucoma, which can occur in central corneal ulcers or endophthalmitis, may require the use of a systemic carbonic anhydrase inhibitor or a topical beta blocker. The usual oral adult dosage is 250 mg of acetazolamide four times daily.

Supportive. A new pneumococcal capsular polysaccharide vaccine is recommended for the prevention of pneumococcal infection in high-risk patients. Such high-risk patients include the elderly, patients with an underlying disease that adversely affects pulmonary function, and immunosuppressed patients. The vaccine is not indicated for more widespread use at this time, but may be indicated in the future if penicillin-resistant pneumococci become more common.

Ocular or Periocular Manifestations

Anterior Chamber: Hypopyon.
Conjunctiva: Acute catarrhal conjunctivitis; chemosis; hyperemia; membranous, pseudomembranous, purulent, or ulcerative conjunctivitis; petechial subconjunctival hemorrhages (superiorly).
Cornea: Anterior staphyloma; epithelial keratitis; leukoma; perforation; serpiginous ulcer.
Globe: Endophthalmitis; panophthalmitis.
Other: Dacryocystitis; exudative anterior uveitis; orbital cellulitis; palpebral edema; preauricular lymphadenopathy; secondary glaucoma.

PRECAUTIONS

Systemic therapy for ocular pneumococcal infection, except for endophthalmitis and orbital cellulitis, offers little or no advantage over topical and subconjunctival therapy. In addition to a risk of toxicity, systemic therapy yields comparatively low levels of the appropriate drug in the affected ocular tissues. The organism is usually resistant to neomycin, gentamicin, and polymyxin B. Thus, Neosporin, the principal constituents of which are neomycin and polymyxin B, is a poor choice in the treatment of pneumococcal infections. Strict guidelines for the use of corticosteroids in the treatment of pneumococcal infections are not currently available, and one is cautioned in the use of this drug.

References

Applebaum PC: World-wide development of antibiotic resistance in Pneumococci. Eur J Clin Microbiol 6:367–373, 1987.
Conte JE, Barriere SL: Manual of Antibiotics and

Infectious Diseases, 5th ed. Philadelphia, Lea and Febiger, 1984 pp 25–26.

Hoeprich PD: Bacterial pneumonias. *In* Hoeprich PD (ed): Infectious Diseases, 3rd ed. Hagerstown, MD, Harper & Row, 1983, pp 347–360.

Jones DB: Early diagnosis and therapy of bacterial corneal ulcers. Int Ophthalmol Clin 13:1–29, 1973.

Klugman KP: Pneumococcal resistance to antibiotics. Clin Microbiol Rev 3:171–196, 1989.

Lauer BA, Reller LB: Serotypes and penicillin susceptibility of pneumococci isolated from blood. J Clin Microbiol 11:242–244, 1980.

Lentnek A, LeFrock JL, Molavi A: *Streptococcus pneumoniae. In* Levison, ME (ed): The Pneumonias: Clinical Approaches to Infectious Diseases of the Lower Respiratory Tract. Littleton, MA, John Wright, 1984, pp 261–271.

Mandell GL, Sande MA: Antimicrobial agents: Penicillins and cephalosporins. *In* Gilman AG, Goodman LS, Gilman A (eds): The Pharmacological Basis of Therapeutics, 7th ed. New York, Macmillan, 1985, pp 1115–1145.

Okumoto M, Smolin G: Pneumococcal infections of the eye. Am J Ophthalmol 77:346–352, 1974.

Robins-Brown RM, et al: Resistance mechanisms of multiply resistant pneumococci: Antibiotic degradation studies. Antimicrob Agents Chemother 15:470–474, 1979.

Sande MA, Mandell GL: Antimicrobial agents: Tetracyclines, chloramphenicol, erythromycin, and miscellaneous antibacterial agents. *In* Gilman AG, Goodman LS, Gilman A (eds): The Pharmacological Basis of Therapeutics, 7th ed. New York, Macmillan, 1985, pp 1170–1198.

PROPIONIBACTERIUM ACNES 040

RONALD E. SMITH, M.D.

Los Angeles, California

Propionibacterium acnes is a fastidious gram-positive non-spore-forming, pleomorphic, anaerobic bacterium that has been associated with a wide variety of ocular infections. Infectious corneal ulcers, conjunctivitis, dacryocystitis, and frank bacterial endophthalmitis have been reported. More recently, a new syndrome possibly related to *P. acnes* has emerged. This postcataract extraction syndrome includes chronic recurrent postoperative uveitis with large keratic precipitates. Infiltrates occur in the capsular bag with recurrent hypopyon. There may be gradual progression to more typical signs of infectious endophthalmitis. It is possible that *P. acnes*, in addition to producing disease as a replication infectious agent, may act as an immunopotentiater in the presence of residual lens material and an intraocular lens in such cases.

THERAPY

Systemic. Cases of corneal ulceration and frank infectious endophthalmitis due to *P. acnes* require appropriate intensive antibiotic therapy as in any such case. Culturing the organism may be difficult, and culture techniques that take into consideration the anaerobic culture requirements of the organism are necessary. Penicillin derivatives are usually effective.

Ocular. Therapy of the postcataract extraction/intraocular lens (IOL) "*P. acnes* syndrome" is less well established. There is usually a favorable response to high-dose topical steroids in early phases, with resolution of keratic precipitates and hypopyon and return of good vision. However, this form of postoperative inflammation often returns or remains chronic and may gradually progress to more frank endophthalmitis in the vitreous cavity. At this stage, vitreous aspiration and culture with antimicrobial therapy by systemic, intravitreal,* and subconjunctival* routes are probably indicated.

Surgical. If frank infectious endophthalmitis is present due to *P. acnes*, intravitreal* antibiotics and vitrectomy are indicated. The usual criteria for vitrectomy in microbial endophthalmitis may be employed. The role of capsulectomy and removal of residual lens material and the removal of the intraocular lens itself are controversial at this time. In some instances, recurrence of inflammation is a clinical problem because residual lens material in the presence of the intraocular lens may encourage further inflammation related to immunopotentiation by the *P. acnes* organism itself.

Ocular or Periocular Manifestations

Anterior Chamber: Recurrent hypopyon; precipitates in the capsular bag and on the intraocular lens.

Cornea: Corneal edema with large keratic precipitates.

Vitreous Cavity (advanced cases): Cells in the vitreous; other evidence of bacterial endophthalmitis.

PRECAUTIONS

It is very difficult to culture *P. acnes*. Consultation with a microbiology laboratory may be necessary to ensure proper identification of this organism.

The therapy of the newly described "*P. acnes* syndrome" remains controversial. It is not clear what role the removal of the intraocular lens or the posterior capsule may play in the management of this entity. The rationale for removal of the capsule relates to the possible role of residual lens material that remains after extracapsular cataract extraction. Also, removal of at least part of the posterior capsule permits better penetration of antibiotics and eliminates the sequestered location of bacteria.

In the treatment of the postcataract extraction/IOL "*P. acnes* syndrome," some authorities have recommended immediate removal of the posterior capsule and residual lens material and the intraocular lens. Others favor a staged approach consisting of posterior vitrectomy and partial capsulectomy. The importance of intravitreal antibiotics that are effective against the organism is generally accepted, along with a vitrectomy if the infectious inflammatory condition has progressed. Topical and systemic corticosteroids are also helpful to reduce the phacoantigenic component of this ocular inflammatory condition.

References

Beatty RF, Robin JB, Trousdale MD, Smith RE: Anaerobic endophthalmitis caused by *Propionibacterium acnes*. Am J Ophthalmol 101:114–116, 1986.

Jones DB, Robinson NM: Anaerobic ocular infections. Trans Am Acad Ophthalmol Otolaryngol 83:309–331, 1977.

Meisler DM, Palestine AG, Vastine DW, Demartini DR, Murphy BF, Reinhart WJ, Zakov N, McMahon JT, Cliffel TP: Chronic *Propionibacterium* endophthalmitis after extracapsular cataract extraction and intraocular lens implantation. Am J Ophthalmol 102:733–739, 1986.

Meisler DM, Zakov ZN, Bruner WE, Hall GS, McMahon JT, Zachary AA, Barna BP. Endophthalmitis associated with sequestered intraocular *Propionibacterium acnes*. Am J Ophthalmol 104:428–429, 1987.

Smith RE: Inflammation after cataract surgery. Am J Ophthalmol 102:788–790, 1986.

PROTEUS 041.9

DAVID S. HULL, M.D.

Augusta, Georgia

Proteus organisms are gram-negative bacilli found as free-living saprophytes in water, soil, and dead or decaying organic substances. They are enterobacteria and a component of the normal flora of the mammalian intestine; they may cause an opportunistic infection in a weakened host. The pathogenic species in humans include *P. mirabilis, P. vulgaris,* and *P. penneri*; of these *P. mirabilis* is implicated most frequently in human infections. A former *Proteus* species, *P. morganii*, has been reclassified as *Morganella morganii*. A third genus is called *Providencia* and includes the former *Proteus rettgeri*, which is now classified as *Providencia rettgeri*.

Parts of the body that may be affected by *Proteus* infection include the skin, ears, mastoid, sinuses, eyes, peritoneal cavity, bone, urinary tract, meninges, lungs, and bloodstream. The majority of *Proteus* infections are hospital acquired, and patients with long-term indwelling urinary tract catheters are particularly at risk. Cutaneous infections occur most often in surgical wounds, particularly after antimicrobial therapy. *Proteus* species have been recovered from 2.6 per cent of normal eyes, with *P. mirabilis* being the most common. Ocular infection by *Proteus* organisms is uncommon, but when it occurs it is usually severe and carries a relatively poor prognosis. Most *Proteus* infections of the eye occur following trauma to the eye; however, *Proteus* bacteremia may result in secondary ocular involvement. Postoperative *Proteus* infection can be particularly troublesome, since the *Proteus* bacilli replace the more susceptible flora eradicated by post-operative antibiotics. Ocular infections in which *Proteus* organisms have been implicated include scleritis, keratitis, corneal ulcers, necrotic inflammation of the eyelid, endophthalmitis, and panophthalmitis. As in other types of bacterial endophthalmitis, panophthalmitis often results in loss of the eye.

THERAPY

Systemic. For *Proteus* infections, ampicillin, gentamicin, and tobramycin are frequently effective. However, because of the emergence of multiple drug-resistant strains of *Proteus*, a complete microbiologic evaluation with drug testing is necessary to rationally formulate effective chemotherapy. *Proteus mirabilis* is usually responsive to ampicillin or amoxicillin. Second choices include a cephalosporin or aminoglycoside. Other *Proteus* species may respond to an aminoglycoside (gentamicin, tobramycin, amikacin, netilmicin) or third-generation cephalosporin. Second choices include broad-spectrum penicillins (ticarcillin, piperacillin, mezlocillin, azlocillin). Third choices include aztreonam and imipenem.

Ocular. Ciprofloxacin 0.3 per cent ophthalmic solution may be effective for treatment of *Proteus* infections of the external eye. For severe *Proteus* infections of the external eye, suggested treatment includes subconjunctival injections of 20 mg of gentamicin* or 20 mg of tobramycin* daily. In addition, topical fortified 14 mg/ml gentamicin§ ophthalmic drops or fortified 14 mg/ml tobramycin§ ophthalmic drops may also be applied two or three times hourly.

Ocular or Periocular Manifestations

Conjunctiva: conjunctivitis; edema; exudates.
Cornea: Abscess; descemetocele; edema, exudates; folds in Descemet's membrane; keratitis; perforation; ulcer.

Eyelids: Edema; infiltration; gangrene; necrosis.
Globe: Endophthalmitis; panophthalmitis.
Sclera: Scleritis.
Other: Anterior uveitis; dacryocystitis; hypopyon; paralysis of seventh nerve.

PRECAUTIONS

Proteus organisms, as may other enteric species, may carry resistant factors, and antibiotic susceptibility tests should be done on clinical isolates. *Proteus* corneal ulceration may rapidly lead to perforation and require surgical intervention.

Because the aminoglycosides are potentially nephrotoxic, the renal function of all patients must be monitored carefully during administration of aminoglycoside antibiotics. Aminoglycosides have been implicated in severe vestibular and auditory dysfunction, particularly in patients with impaired kidney function. Patients should be carefully observed for signs of damage to the eighth nerve.

Because of the similarity of structure of penicillins and cephalosporins, patients may manifest cross-reactive allergic reactions.

COMMENTS

Proteus organisms have a tendency to produce infection in locations previously infected by other bacilli. These organisms are frequently cultured from superficial wounds, draining ears, and sputum. *Proteus* infection, especially *P. vulgaris*, may occur as a sequela to previous antibiotic treatment.

References

Leibowitz HM: Antibacterial effectiveness of ciprofloxacin 0.3% ophthalmic solution in the treatment of bacterial conjunctivitis. Am J Ophthalmol 112:29S–33S, 1991.

Neu HC: Pathophysiologic basis for the use of third generation cephalosporins. Am J Med 88(4A):3S–11S, 1990.

Okumoto M, et al: *Proteus* species isolated from human eyes. Am J Ophthalmol 81:495–501, 1976.

Parunovic A: *Proteus mirabilis* causing necrotic inflammation of the eyelid. Am J Ophthalmol 76:543–544, 1973.

Sande MA, et al: Antimicrobial agents. *In* Gilman AG, Rall TW, Nies AS, Taylor P (eds): Goodman and Gilman's—The Pharmacological Basis of Therapeutics. New York, Pergamon Press, 1990, pp 1018–1046.

Schein OD, et al: Microbial keratitis associated with contaminated ocular medications. Am J Ophthalmol 105:361–365, 1988.

Smolin G: *Proteus* endophthalmitis. Arch Ophthalmol 91:419–420, 1974.

Weber DJ, et al: Endophthalmitis following intraocular lens implantation: Report of 30 cases and review of the literature. Rev Infect Dis 8:12–20, 1986.

PSEUDOMONAS AERUGINOSA 041.7

PETER R. LAIBSON, M.D.

Philadelphia, Pennsylvania

Pseudomonas aeruginosa, an opportunistic gram-negative, motile rod is a bacterial organism that can cause one of the most serious infections of the cornea. *Pseudomonas* infections of the cornea cause severe damage because of their ability to produce proteases, which rapidly cause stromal necrosis with resultant corneal thinning and perforation. *Pseudomonas* corneal ulcers can cause corneal perforation in 24 hours, whereas infections due to staphylococcal, streptococcal, or *Haemophilus* organisms may take days to weeks to cause severe corneal thinning and perforation, although this is uncommon with these organisms.

The *Pseudomonas* infection characteristically starts in a small central or paracentral area and spreads rapidly. However, it can also start peripherally, and when the infection occurs near the limbus and extends into the sclera, the prognosis for ocular recovery is poor.

In recent years, the incidence of corneal ulcers caused by *Pseudomonas* has significantly increased. This increase in directly linked to the use of contact lenses, particularly extended-wear soft contact lenses used overnight. Even disposable contact lenses used for 1 week and then discarded have caused corneal ulceration due to *Pseudomonas* infection.

Pseudomonas is the most common gram-negative bacterial organism isolated from infections related to soft and hard contact lens use. In some studies, it is even more commonly cultured from contact lens-related ulcers than are gram-positive organisms. These ulcerations may be the result of the patient's failure to follow the manufacturer's advice concerning sterilization and appropriate changes of solution. Even with proper care, however, the use of soft contact lenses overnight presents a significantly increased risk for developing microbial keratitis. In addition to obtaining positive cultures from the corneal ulcer, the organisms are often recovered from the contact lens solutions, the contact lens containers, and the contact lens itself.

THERAPY

Systemic: Usually systemic therapy is not necessary for bacterial corneal ulcers, including *Pseudomonas* ulcers. However, with extensive involvement of the cornea, particularly when *Pseudomonas aeruginosa* involves the limbus and sclera, systemic medication is indicated. In those cases, daily injections of tobramycin, 4 mg/kg, and/or ciprofloxacin 500 mg twice daily are used. Mezlocillin, ticarcillin, and piperacillin have also been used for intravenous therapy with severe limbal and scleral involvement of *Pseudomonas*.

Ocular A corneal ulcer caused by *P. aeruginosa* must be diagnosed and treated as soon as possible because of the rapid destruction of stromal collagen by enzymes produced with this infection. In the past, subconjunctival injections* of fortified aminoglycosides were commonly used, but today, the frequent application of fortified topical medication§ is preferred. These fortified medications are now readily available from most pharmacies that dispense ophthalmic drugs, particularly at eye centers, because most pharmacists know how to change regular-strength aminoglycoside to fortified concentrations. The drug of choice for known *Pseudomonas* infection is fortified tobramycin,§ rather than gentamicin.§ In studies performed on *Pseudomonas* corneal ulcers at Wills Eye Hospital almost 30 per cent of the *Pseudomonas* isolates were intermediately affected by gentamicin, whereas they were strongly inhibited by tobramycin. In our experience at Wills Eye Hospital, all *Pseudomonas* isolates were sensitive to tobramycin.

Since fortified medications are readily available, use of topical drops every 15 minutes for the first several hours and then every 30 minutes for the next 24 hours is indicated, rather than subconjunctival medications. Other topical medications that have been effective in treating *Pseudomonas* ulcers are Ciloxan 0.3 per cent and fortified topical drops, such as mezlocillin, ticarcillin, and piperacillin.

Corneal ulcerations with or without hypopyon should be scraped first before instituting antibiotics. These scrapings should be looked at with gram stain for bacterial organisms and with Giemsa stain for cell type. After the scrapings and cultures are performed, topical antibiotics are applied. The antibiotic of choice is fortified tobramycin§ (15 mg/ml) every 15 minutes if the ulcer is severe or every 30 minutes for the first day or two. This medication should be given around the clock. If it is unclear whether this is a gram-positive or gram-negative organism, the use of fortified cefazolin* (100 mg/ml) is also recommended either every 30 minutes, 1 hour, or 2 hours around the clock between applications of the fortified tobramycin. In addition to the antibiotics, atropine should be applied for cycloplegia and antiglaucoma medications instituted if the pressure is elevated. Under no circumstances should steroids be used in the early stages of any *Pseudomonas* infection. Once the ulcer shows signs of response, the topical drops can be tapered slowly.

If one is sure that *P. aeruginosa* alone is responsible for the corneal ulcer, then tobramycin is usually sufficient for appropriate therapy. Topical antibiotics may be tapered according to the response of the bacterial ulcer, but should be continued for at least 1 to 2 months after the epithelial ulceration has healed. Once the epithelial ulceration has healed, the judicious use of topical steroids may be employed to limit the stromal inflammation and eventual scarring. Although steroids have been used following epithelial healing, tobramycin drops should also be used as a prophylactic medication to prevent recurrence of *Pseudomonas* infection. Recurrent *Pseudomonas* infection is common if the antibiotic is tapered too quickly while steroids are being used even in very low doses.

The use of a collagenase inhibitor is still controversial, and very few ophthalmologists use these medications today in conjunction with stromal melting caused by *Pseudomonas* infections. In the past, 10 or 20 per cent solutions of acetylcysteine* have been employed four or five times a day.

Surgical. When endophthalmitis occurs secondary to cataract extraction, filtering blebs, or corneal or retinal surgery and this infection is caused by *P. aeruginosa*, the visual outcome is very poor. Immediate vitrectomy is indicated along with intravitreal injection* of antibiotics and corticosteroids, depending upon the severity of the infection. Early vitrectomy with intravitreal antibiotics is essential if there is any hope of salvaging vision in these severe postoperative infections caused by *Pseudomonas*.

PRECAUTIONS

Although one must carefully monitor the systemic levels of tobramycin when systemic therapy is being used, treatment with topical fortified drops to the cornea does not require this monitoring. For this reason, most bacterial corneal ulcers alone are treated with topical medication, which is highly effective in reaching the site of bacterial growth rapidly. The use of frequent topical drops every 15 or 30 minutes is more effective in treating a corneal ulcer caused by *Pseudomonas* than is systemic medication. If systemic medication is needed for endophthalmitis or scleral involvement, one must obtain peak and trough antibiotic levels 30 minutes before and 30 minutes after antibiotic infusion. If the systemic levels are satisfactory every other day, serum creatinine levels should be obtained because systemic aminoglycosides, such as tobramycin, can cause kidney failure. The patient on long-term systemic antibiotics should also be followed by an internist.

The use of corticosteroids in bacterial corneal ulcers or endophthalmitis is very controversial. Once the *Pseudomonas* corneal ulcer seems to be brought under control with appropriate local therapy, steroids may be used judiciously. The rule is that steroids are to be used very cautiously in any patient with corneal ulcer caused by *Pseudomonas* because of the problem of recurrent infections, as mentioned previously. Corticosteroids should be used in the lowest effective dosage and accompanied by antibiotics.

COMMENTS

Serious infections caused by *Pseudomonas* have become a problem because of their increasing frequency, particularly in soft daily-wear and extended-wear contact lens users. The chief characteristics of this organism are its antibiotic resistance and rapid and deep spread with resulting corneal thinning and perforation. Corneal perforation has been seen within 24 hours of the onset of a *Pseudomonas* corneal ulcer. All suspicious corneal ulcers should be treated with fortified preparations of tobramycin until the culture definitely shows the absence of a gram-negative organism.

The prognosis is very grave for scleral involvement and *P. aeruginosa* endophthalmitis.

References

Clemmons CS, et al: Pseudomonas ulcers following patching of corneal abrasions associated with contact lens wear. CLAO J 13:3, 1987.

Cohen EJ, et al: Corneal ulcers associated with contact lenses including experience with disposable lenses. CLAO J 17(3):173–176, 1991.

Donnenfeld ER, et al: Changing trends in contact lens associated corneal ulcers: An overview of 116 cases. CLAO J 12:145–149, 1986.

Poggio EC, et al: The incidence of ulcerative keratitis among users of daily wear and extended wear soft contact lenses. N Engl J Med 321:779–783, 1989.

RELAPSING FEVER 087.9
(Recurrent Fever)

L.F. RICH, M.D., M.S.

Portland, Oregon

Relapsing fever is an infectious spirochetal disease caused by either *Borrelia recurrentis* or *Borrelia novyi*. Another spirochetal infection, Lyme disease, is caused by *Borrelia burgdorferi*. The spirochetes of the genus *Borrelia* that cause relapsing fever are transmitted by the human body louse (causing an edemic form of the disease) or members of the *Ornithodoros* tick family. The clinical course of infection transmitted by either vector tends to be similar. It is characterized by toxemia and recurring febrile paroxysms separated by afebrile periods. Relapses duplicating the original attack recur at intervals of 1 to 2 weeks and become progressively less severe. Recovery usually occurs after two to ten relapses. Ocular involvement in relapsing fever is not uncommon, particularly in the tick-borne form of the disease. The ocular symptoms usually occur during periods of relapse, rather than in the initial febrile attack. Common ocular manifestations may include extraocular muscle paralysis, uveitis, conjunctivitis, a transient interstitial keratitis, palpebral edema, and visual impairment. Retrobulbar neuritis and optic atrophy may be produced if there has been meningeal involvement.

Diagnosis can be made during the febrile phase of the illness by demonstration of the organisms in the peripheral blood with Giemsa or Wright stain.

THERAPY

Systemic. The medication of choice is tetracycline, given orally in an adult dosage of 0.5 gm every 6 hours for 7 days and followed by 1 gm daily for another 5 days. This treatment usually clears all infection and prevents the occurrence of relapses. Alternative treatment may be with aqueous procaine penicillin G, which is given in a dosage of 600,000 units daily by intramuscular injection for 10 days.

Recent information suggests that combination therapy with both tetracycline and aqueous procaine penicillin G may be even more effective than use of either drug singly. Such combination treatment avoids the severe reaction that invariably follows tetracycline treatment and clears any residual brain infection. In this therapy, 400,000 units of aqueous procaine penicillin G are given by intramuscular injection on the first day. This treatment is followed the next 7 days by 500 mg of oral tetracycline, given every 6 hours.

Ocular. For uveitis, 2 per cent homatropine or 0.25 per cent scopolamine eyedrops may be applied twice daily to keep the pupil dilated and produce cycloplegia. Topical corticosteroid eyedrops may be used during waking hours to reduce inflammation, and an ointment containing 0.05 per cent dexamethasone may be applied at night before retiring.

Supportive. The patient with relapsing fever is extremely ill; therefore, careful nursing is essential. Bedrest is indicated for all patients with this infection. Liberal fluids and proper nutrition are necessary. Since relapse may lead to the false assumption that the infection has run its course, the patient should not be allowed to undertake strenuous work until complete recovery is certain.

Ocular or Periocular Manifestations

Anterior Chamber: Hypopyon.

Conjunctiva: Conjunctivitis; discharge; hemorrhages.

Cornea: Band-shaped keratopathy; dendritic keratitis; interstitial keratitis.

Optic Nerve: Atrophy (secondary to meningeal involvement); retrobulbar neuritis (secondary or meningeal involvement).

Retina: Exudates; hemorrhages; venous engorgement.

Vitreous: Exudates; opacity.

Other: Decreased visual acuity; icterus; ocular pain; paralysis of sixth or seventh cranial nerve; photophobia; ptosis, uveitis; visual loss.

PRECAUTIONS

A Jarisch-Herxheimer reaction occurs quite commonly after administration of high doses of tetracycline or penicillin. Recent evidence indicates that the Jarisch-Herxheimer reaction with tetracycline may be greatly diminished if penicillin is given prior to administration of the tetracycline. Therefore, combination therapy may produce better results than use of either drug by itself. Complete bedrest for at least 48 hours after treatment with tetracycline or penicillin is recommended.

COMMENTS

Louse-borne relapsing fever has been reported from all continents, occurring most frequently in overcrowded areas where unhygienic conditions prevail. This disease is still a serious problem in the Near East, the Mediterranean Basin, and tropical America.

The prognosis is serious in both forms of the disease if no treatment is given. Tick-borne relapsing fever is an especially grave disease, since neurologic and ophthalmologic involvement often occurs in this type of relapsing fever. Death has occurred from hyperpyrexia with convulsions, myocardial failure, or hepatic coma; however, treatment of relapsing fever has greatly reduced mortality from the disease.

References

Bryceson ADM, et al: Louse-borne relapsing fever. A clinical and laboratory study of 62 cases in Ethiopia and a reconsideration of the literature. Q J Med 39:129–170, 1970.

Burgdorfer W: The relapsing fevers. In Hunter GW III, Swartzwelder JC, Clyde DF: Tropical Medicine, 5th ed. Philadelphia. WB Saunders, 1976, pp 137–146.

Duke-Elder S (ed): System of Ophthalmology. St. Louis, CV Mosby, 1976, Vol XV, p 138.

Ginsberg SP: Corneal problems in systemic disease. In Duane T (ed): Clinical Ophthalmology. Hagerstown, MD, Harper & Row, 1982, Vol V, pp 43: 1–23.

Magnarelli LA: Serologic diagnosis of Lyme disease. Ann NY Acad Sci 539:154–161, 1988.

Rogell G: Infectious and inflammatory diseases. In Duane TD (ed): Clinical Ophthalmology. Hagerstown, MD, Harper & Row, 1982, Vol V, pp 33: 14–15.

Salih SY, Mustafa D: Louse-borne relapsing fever. II. Combined penicillin and tetracycline therapy in 160 Sudanese patients. Trans R Soc Trop Med Hyg 71:49–51, 1977.

Southern PM Jr, Sanford JP: Relapsing fever. A clinical and microbiological review. Medicine 48: 129–149, 1969.

Warrell DA, et al: Pathophysiology and immunology of the Jarisch-Herxheimer-like reaction in louse-borne relapsing fever: Comparison of tetracycline and slow-release penicillin. J Infect Dis 147:898–909, 1983.

STAPHYLOCOCCUS 041.1

THOMAS L. STEINEMANN, M.D.

Little Rock, Arkansas

Staphylococci are gram-positive bacteria of the family Micrococcaceae. They are aerobic (facultatively anaerobic) and nonmotile and tend to grow in grapelike clusters. The Micrococcaceae family can be further divided into two groups based upon coagulase production. Coagulase, an enzyme that causes plasma to coagulate, has been regarded as a marker for virulence. Although most severe staphylococcal infections are caused by coagulase-positive organisms and many researchers believe that coagulase production indicates the likelihood that a strain is potentially pathogenic, there is no evidence that coagulase itself is directly responsible for disease signs and symptoms.

Whereas coagulase-positive organisms comprise one species (S. aureus), coagulase-negative staphylococci are further divided into 11 species. In the past most coagulase-negative staphylococci were collectively referred to as *Staphylococcus albus* because of the white colony growth pattern on agar plates, in contrast to S. aureus, which elaborates a golden pigment. More recently S. albus has been referred to as Staphylococcus epidermidis. The term Staphylococcus epidermidis is still used by some to include all coagulase-negative staphylococci in a generic sense. Strictly speaking, however, coagulase-negative staphylococci have been further speciated by biotyping, a scheme based on specific biochemical properties.

Components of the cell wall of S. aureus include peptidoglycan, protein A, and teichoic acid polymers, all of which may contribute to pathogenicity. S. aureus also produces several enzymes and toxins that have been implicated as important pathogenic factors. These secreted extracellular enzymes include hyaluronidase and lipase, which may help the organism survive in tissues. Many strains also produce toxins that damage membranes and exert a cytotoxic effect on a variety of cells, including leukocytes, fibroblasts, and epithelial cells of the cornea and conjunctiva. Most of the staphylococci isolated from skin infections are S. aureus. S. aureus gains access to underlying tissues, often after surgery or trauma, creating a characteristic local abscess lesion. Colonization of the nose, skin, and scalp may begin early in childhood and continue throughout life. These sites probably serve as a source of ocular infection.

Coagulase-negative staphylococci have historically been regarded as contaminants when recovered in culture media, probably because they are the predominant normal skin flora and are often present on mucous membranes. Rarely do they cause skin infections. However, they are now clearly recognized as opportunistic pathogens of increasing importance, especially in hospital-acquired infections. They are most commonly associated with infections involving prosthetic devices, such as intraocular lenses, and intravenous lines. It has been shown that many strains produce an exopolysaccharide ("slime" or "biofilm" substance) that facilitates bacterial adherence to prosthetic surfaces and may be a factor in resistance to host defenses and antimicrobial therapy.

Staphylococci may infect any portion of the eye or orbital structures. Lid infections are common and may be chronic. They often reflect lowered host resistance; the infection is often directly spread from the conjunctiva or nasolacrimal system. Atopy is a common predisposing condition. Staphylococci remain a common cause of acute and chronic conjunctivitis, suppurative keratitis, marginal corneal (catarrhal) infiltrates, phlyctenulosis, and hordeola. Orbital infections can occur, either from staphylococcal septicemia or via direct spread from contiguous structures, such as lid abscesses or infected teeth). Staphylococci are the most common cause of acute or delayed endophthalmitis in postoperative cataract patients.

THERAPY

Systemic. Specific antimicrobial therapy is chosen based upon the site and severity of the infection and the antimicrobial sensitivities of the organism involved. The increasing prevalence of staphylococcal infections reflects the frequency with which the organism has developed antimicrobial resistance. In fact, fewer than 20 per cent of staphylococci strains are still sensitive to penicillin. However, most community-acquired staphylococcal infections are still sensitive to synthetic penicillinase-resistant penicillins. Methicillin and nafcillin are equally effective parenteral agents. Both may be given in daily doses of 150 to 200 mg/kg. Doses should be administered at 4- to 6-hour intervals. Oral or intramuscular dicloxacillin (500 mg) four times daily can also be used to treat penicillinase-producing staphylococci.

Cephalosporins are an acceptable alternative to semisynthetic penicillinase-resistant penicillin in patients who have had prior reactions to penicillin. Cefazolin can be given intramuscularly or intravenously in a maximum dose of 1 gm every 6 hours. Oral preparations, such as cephalexin, can be given for less serious infections. The usual oral dosage is 250 to 500 mg every 6 hours.

For those infections caused by methicillin-resistant staphylococci, vancomycin remains the drug of choice for parenteral treatment. Dosages of 500 mg are given over a 1-hour period every 6 hours. Vancomycin levels greater than 30 μg/ml should be avoided because of potential renal damage and ototoxicity. Oral rifampin may be particularly useful as an adjunctive treatment to either parenteral or local therapy. Emergence of resistance,

however, is rapid, and this drug should never be used as a single antistaphylococcal agent. Oral dosages of 300 to 600 mg are usually given every 12 hours. Rifampin may also be useful in combination with other antimicrobials for the elimination of the staphylococcal carrier state.

Fluoroquinolones, such as ciprofloxacin, are newer agents that show great promise in the treatment of resistant infections. They are highly active in vitro and in vivo against methicillin-resistant and methicillin-susceptible staphylococci. The usual dosage is 200 to 400 mg intravenously or orally every 12 hours. However, resistance has been increasingly documented, especially in nosocomial infections. Therefore, fluoroquinolones should not be used as a single agent in the treatment of methicillin-resistant staphylococcal infections. Fluoroquinolone therapy in combination with other antibiotics is potentially promising, but requires further study.

Ocular. Staphylococcal infections of the lid may be treated with a variety of antimicrobial ointments, including sulfacetamide (10 per cent), erythromycin (0.5 per cent), or bacitracin (5,000 units/gm). Frequency and duration of treatment should be based on the severity of the infection and the clinical response. Less severe forms of conjunctivitis also usually respond to sulfacetamide 10 per cent ophthalmic drops every 6 hours. A recently introduced antimicrobial eyedrop (Polytrim) combines trimethoprim sulfate (0.1 per cent) and polymyxin B sulfate (10,000 unit/ml). Trimethoprim is effective against many aerobic gram-positive bacteria, including many strains of staphylococci.

Chronic staphylococcal blepharitis and meibomian keratoconjunctivitis can be treated effectively with oral tetracycline. Treatment is initiated at 1–2 gm/day until signs and symptoms are controlled. After control is attained, low-dose (250 mg/day) maintenance therapy is continued for months or years to prevent recurrences. The mechanism of action seems to be mediated by reducing staphylococcal lipase production, not eliminating the bacteria.

Conjunctivitis caused by methicillin-resistant staphylococci has been increasingly recognized, especially in patients in long-term care facilities. In these cases, topical vancomycin is effective and can be prepared by dissolving injectable vancomycin hydrochloride in phosphate-buffered artificial tears at a concentration of 25 to 50 mg/ml.

Keratitis is typically treated with topical antibiotic drops as primary therapy based upon corneal scrapings obtained for culture and sensitivity. The empiric use of fortified antibiotic concentrations to obtain higher corneal drug levels is widely accepted. Fortified aminoglycosides (gentamicin, 14 mg/ml) and cephalosporins (cefazolin, 50 mg/ml) are usually effective in treating staphylococcal keratitis. Methicillin-resistant staphylococcal keratitis has, however, recently been reported. For these infections aminoglycosides and cephalosporins are probably inadequate treatment. Two separate case reports have described the effective use of vancomycin (50 mg/ml) and commercially available ciprofloxacin (3 mg/ml) drops.

Other common corneal diseases caused by staphylococci include marginal (catarrhal) infiltrates and phlyctenulosis. Both are caused by chronic staphylococcal colonization of the external ocular surface and lids and are thought to represent an immune reaction to staphylococcal exotoxins deposited in the cornea or conjunctiva. Treatment is directed at eliminating the antigen load by frequent lid scrubs with mild shampoo and antibiotic drops or ointment. This therapy is sometimes used in conjunction with topical steroids to diminish immunologically mediated inflammation.

A complete discussion of the management of endophthalmitis is beyond the scope of this chapter. Please see the section, Endophthalmitis, for details.

Supportive: Inspissated secretions of lid glandular structures may occur both externally (glands of Zeiss) or internally (meibomian glands). These secretions often contribute to chronic staphylococcal surface disease, such as blepharitis or hordeolum, and may be treated by applying moist warm lid compresses. Excessive oil secretion may also be treated by gently expressing the material with fingertip pressure or by using cotton-tipped applicators. Daily lid hygiene to remove oil, lid debris, and scaling is accomplished with a mild baby shampoo or commercially available lid hygiene packs. Localized abscesses that do not spontaneously drain with moist heat may require incision and drainage.

Ocular or Periocular Manifestations

Anterior Chamber: Cells and flare; hypopyon.

Conjunctiva: Hyperemia; papillary response; purulent conjunctivitis; chemosis, phlyctenulosis.

Cornea: Punctate epithelial keratopathy; suppurative keratitis; perforation; marginal (catarrhal) infiltrates; phlyctenulosis; crystalline keratopathy.

Eyelids: Collarettes; lid margin vascularization; tylosis; meibomianitis; lash follicle folliculitis; lid margin ulceration; eczematoid dermatitis; angular blepharitis; trichiasis; madarosis; poliosis; hordeolum; chalazion; ectropion; entropion; edema, abscess; cellulitis; pseudoptosis.

Globe: Endophthalmitis; panophthalmitis; intraocular lens contamination; scleral ulceration.

Iris: Nongranulomatous anterior uveitis; posterior synechiae.

Orbit: Cellulitis; osteomyelitis; periosteitis.

Other: Dacryocystitis; increased intraocular pressure; dacryoadenitis.

PRECAUTIONS

Emergence of methicillin-resistant *S. aureus* and penicillin- and methicillin-resistant *S. epidermidis* is a concern in nosocomial infections. Every attempt should be made to isolate the organism and perform sensitivities to a wide range of antimicrobials. Sensitivity patterns may differ from hospital to hospital.

The physician must keep in mind the potentially hazardous side effects of systemic antimicrobial therapy. BUN, creatinine, and electrolyte levels must be measured before antibiotic administration and at 3-day intervals thereafter. Peak and trough antibiotic serum concentrations should be measured to determine the safety and adequacy of intravenous antibiotic therapy.

COMMENTS

Staphylococci are common worldwide causes of blepharitis, conjunctivitis, and keratitis. In the past, *S. aureus* was implicated as the single most responsible organism for endophthalmitis. Recent reports indicate that *S. epidermidis* is now the most commonly cultured intraocular pathogen, accounting for 40 per cent of postoperative and posttraumatic endophthalmitis. This is consistent with the finding of *S. epidermidis* as the most common isolate from conjunctival cultures. Since these organisms can be resistant to penicillinase-resistant penicillins, treatment should be guided by culture and sensitivity results.

References

Archer GL: Staphylococcus epidermidis and other coagulase-negative staphylococci. *In* Mandell GL, Douglas RG Jr, Bennett JE (eds): Principles and Practice of Infectious Diseases, 3rd ed. New York, Churchill Livingstone, 1990, pp 1511–1518.

Davis JL, et al: Coagulase-negative staphylococcal endophthalmitis. Ophthalmology 95:1404–1410, 1988.

Dougherty JM, et al: The role of tetracycline in chronic blepharitis. Invest Ophthalmol Vis Sci 32: 2910–2875, 1991.

Goodman DF, Gottsch JS: Methicillin-resistant *S. epidermidis* keratitis treated with vancomycin. Arch Ophthalmol 106:1570–1571, 1988.

Insler MS, et al: Successful treatment of methicillin-resistant *S. aureus* keratitis with topical ciprofloxacin. Ophthalmology 98:1690–1692, 1991.

Leibowitz HM: Clinical evaluation of ciprofloxacin 0.3% ophthalmic solution for treatment of bacterial keratitis. Am J Ophthalmol 112:34S–47S, 1991.

Limberg MB: A review of bacterial keratitis and bacterial conjunctivitis. Am J Ophthalmol 112: 2S–9S, 1991.

Ostler HB: Bacterial infections. *In* Ostler HB: Diseases of the External Eye and Adnexa, 1st ed. Baltimore, Williams & Wilkins, 1993, pp 369–377.

Steinart R: Current therapy for bacterial keratitis

and bacterial conjunctivitis. Am J Ophthalmol 112:10S–14S, 1991.

Waldvogel FA: Staphylococcus aureus (including toxic shock syndrome). *In* Mandell GL, Douglas RG Jr, Bennett JE (eds): Principles and Practice of Infectious Diseases, 3rd ed. New York, Churchill Livingstone, 1990, pp 1489–1510.

STREPTOCOCCUS 041.0

JOHN R. SAMPLES, M.D.

Portland, Oregon

Streptococci and aerococci are gram-positive, catalase-negative cocci that may appear singly, in pairs, in short chains, or in long chains. These organisms are facultative anaerobes, although some strains can grow poorly under aerobic conditions. *Streptococcus* is a ubiquitous organism and is part of the normal flora of the mouth, pharynx, and the intestinal tract of humans.

Streptococci may be classified according to a serologic system based upon antigenic carbohydrate extracted from the cell wall. Based on both the chemical composition and immunologic reactivity of this carbohydrate, streptococci can be divided into 18 groups (A through H and K through T). The organisms within each of these groups are similar.

Some streptococci are not grouped on the basis of carbohydrate antigenicity, including the anaerobes, but according to their ability to produce hemolysis. Alpha-hemolysis is denoted by a greenish color of the sheep red blood cells that surround the colony, which indicates the incomplete or partial lysis of red blood cells. Beta-hemolysis is denoted by a clear zone surrounding the colony, which indicates the complete lysis of blood cells. Gamma-hemolysis indicates that there is no lysis of erythrocytes surrounding the colony. Two compounds, termed hemolysins, cause beta-hemolysis. One is streptolysin-O, which is antigenic and oxygen-sensitive. The other is streptolysin-S, which is nonantigenic and resistant to oxygen. If only aerobic incubation is used when streptococci are identified, oxygen will neutralize the activity of streptolysin-O and cause beta-hemolytic colonies to be overlooked.

The alpha-hemolytic *Streptococcus* that is the most common and important human pathogen is *Streptococcus pneumonia*. Although there is only one species of this organism, frequently termed pneumococcus, there are 83 distinct serotypes. On gram stain, this organism appears as oval or spherical gram-positive diplococci with distal ends that are pointed or lancet shaped. This organism is responsible for conjunctivitis, endophthalmitis, and dacryocystitis and is becoming increasingly resistant to pen-

icillin. As a result, when the organism is isolated, antimicrobial susceptibility testing may be helpful. Alpha-hemolytic streptococci are found as part of the normal flora of the mouth and pharynx. Nonetheless, they may be pathologic agents as in acute or subacute bacterial endocarditis.

Beta-hemolytic streptococci are probably the most common streptococcus to cause human disease. *S. pyrogenese*, a group A organism, has been isolated from the eyelids in conjunctivitis, in periorbital cellulitis, in endophthalmitis, and keratitis. Its normal habitat is the nasopharynx, skin, and rectum. These organisms are harmful in three ways: through direct invasion, through the elaboration of erythogenic toxin that is an exotoxin responsible for scarlet fever, and by provoking immunoresponses resulting in delayed postinfectious syndromes, such as acute rheumatic fever and acute glomerulonephritis. *S. agalactiae* (Group B) has been isolated in neonatal conjunctivitis, endophthalmitis accompanying meningitis, and adult endophthalmitis. *S. equisimilis* (Group C) has been identified as a cause of endophthalmitis and conjunctivitis.

Aerococci are alpha-hemolytic gram-positive cocci that have been identified in subacute bacterial endocarditis and urinary tract infections. They are not known to be pathogens in the eye.

THERAPY

Systemic. Traditionally, penicillin has been regarded as the drug of choice for streptococcal infections. However, with the emergence of penicillin resistance, therapy needs to be tailored to the antibiotic sensitivity of the infecting organism. Generally, the alpha-streptococci, including pneumococcus, are resistant to aminoglycosides and polymyxin B, but are susceptible to cephalosporins, erythromycin, clindamycin, bacitracin, vancomycin, and chloramphenicol. The beta-streptococci, excluding enterococci, are susceptible to penicillin, cephalosporins, erythromycin, bacitracin, vancomycin, clindamycin, and chloramphenicol. Enterococci usually respond to a combined therapy that includes both penicillin or vancomycin, as well as an aminoglycoside.

Penicillin is the drug of choice for pneumococcal pneumonia. Unless complications are present, the presently advocated high-dose regimes provide little advantage over the standard daily dose of 1.2 to 2.4 million units. The many alternative drugs available for the treatment of pneumococcal infections include erythromycin, clindamycin, cephaloridine, and other cephalosporins. Although cephalosporins have excellent bactericidal activity against pneumococci, they must be used with caution in a penicillin-allergic patient. It should be kept in mind that first- and second-generation cephalosporins are ineffective in the treatment of meningitis. Clindamycin is also ineffective against meningitis, but chloramphenicol is an acceptable alternative for pneumococcal meningitis. A mutation pneumococcal gene that includes penicillin-binding proteins groups I and II decreases the affinity of these proteins for penicillin and leads to the increase in penicillin resistance. A type 57 pneumococcus has been identified in Durbin, South Africa, which is completely resistant to penicillin, ampicillin, cephaloridine, erythromycin, chloramphenicol, and clindamycin. The strain has remained sensitive to vancomycin, rifampin, and bacitracin. This organism has produced at least 15 cases of pneumonia and meningitis. A multiple resistant Type 6-B pneumococcus was identified in Colorado in 1980. This organism was resistant to penicillin G, chloramphenicol, and tetracycline and was isolated from the cerebrospinal fluid of an infant who had meningitis. The organism was sensitive to rifampin, ampicillin, and chloramphenicol. Penicillin-resistant pneumococci have also been isolated in cases from Brooklyn, New York.

Pneumococcal vaccines are excellent, safe immunogens that produce long-lasting antibody titers. However, children younger than 2 years of age respond poorly to the vaccine. There have been few side effects reported, except for mild erythema and pain at the injection site. The efficacy of the vaccine remains controversial largely because of an ongoing failure to demonstrate its effectiveness. For this reason, it has not been well accepted for clinical use, with less than 25 per cent of vaccine candidates being immunized. The vaccine is generally recommended in healthy adults older than 65 years and in adults with chronic respiratory disease, immunosuppression, cirrhosis, alcoholism, renal failure, Hodgkin's disease, myeloma, and those who are asplenic or have a splenic dysfunction.

Group A streptococci continue to be uniformly sensitive to penicillin, which remains the drug of choice. The dosage and duration vary enormously, ranging from 10 days of low-dose therapy for pharyngitis to prolonged high-dose intravenous therapy for osteomyelitis. Cephalosporins are effective substitutes in penicillin-allergic patients, but they must be used with caution because of the risk of an allergic cross-reactivity. As mentioned above, other alternatives include erythromycin, vancomycin, and clindamycin. Group B streptococci are sensitive to clinically achievable levels of penicillin, but the minimum inhibitory concentrations are somewhat higher than those for group A streptococci. Other streptococci, including anaerobes, are almost uniformly penicillin sensitive.

Ocular. Patients with conjunctivitis or eyelid involvement by *Streptococcus* should be treated systemically, as well as locally. Topical treatment may consist of the use of bacitracin or erythromycin ointment. Hot compresses and the removal of any impetiginous crust may be helpful.

Streptococcal conjunctivitis can usually be successfully treated with erythromycin or bacitracin alone.

When a streptococcal ulcer is evident, both topical and systemic therapy are indicated. Topical ophthalmic antibiotics, including erythromycin, bacitracin, or cefazolin,* should be given every hour while awake and every 2 hours at night. Subconjunctival injection of sodium penicillin G,* 0.5 to 1.0 million units, or 50 to 100 mg of methicillin* should be considered. Since this type of injection is painful, analgesia is advocated.

Streptococcal endophthalmitis requires prompt initiation of vigorous treatment with systemic, local, intraocular, and subconjunctival injections of antibiotics and steroids. At the time of vitrectomy or vitreous tap for culture, intracameral instillation of 250 µg of cephaloridine* or 1 mg of methicillin* with 0.1 mg of subconjunctival dexamethasone* is initiated. This is supplemented with topical application of 250 to 1,000 units/ml of bacitracin§ or 100,000 units/ml of sodium penicillin G.§ Orbital cellulitis secondary to *Streptococcus* should be treated with systemic antibiotics.

Supportive. Treatment of symptoms is important in patients with streptococcal sore throat. Analgesia for relief of headache, adequate hydration, and treatment of other symptoms are all necessary.

Ocular or Periocular Manifestations

Conjunctiva: Chemosis; mucopurulent or purulent conjunctivitis; hyperemia.
Cornea: Hyperesthesia infiltration; ring ulcer; central ulcer.
Eyelids: Blepharitis; dermatitis; impetigo; madarosis; scarletina rash.
Globe: Endophthalmitis; proptosis; lacrimal system dacroadenitis; dacrocystitis.
Optic Nerve: Optic neuritis.
Orbit: Abscess; cellulitis; thrombophlebitis.

PRECAUTIONS

Penicillin must always be used with caution in patients who have a history of allergy or asthma. Cephalosporins must be used with the understanding that they may be cross-reactive with penicillin.

COMMENTS

Streptococci are common bacterial pathogens in humans that produce infections in many tissues of the body. Because transmission may occur, vigorous hygiene is well advised in caring for these patients.

References

Abbott RL, Shekter WB: Necrotizing erysipelas of the eyelids. Ann Ophthalmol 11:381–384, 1979.

Brinser JH: Ocular bacteriology. *In* Tabbara KF, Hyndiuk RA (eds): Infections of the Eye. Boston, Little Brown, 1986.

Jacobs MR, Kornahof HJ, Robbins-Browne et al: Emergence of multiply resistant pneumococci. N Engl J Med 299:735, 1978.

Leveille AS, McMullan FD, Cavanaugh HD: Endophthalmitis following penetrating keratoplasty. Ophthalmology 83:38–39, 1977.

Liesegang TJ, Samples JR, Waller RR: Suppurative interstitial ring keratitis due to streptococcus. Ann Ophthalmol 16:392–396, 1984.

Multiply resistant pneumococcus—Colorado. MMWR 30:197, 1981.

Okumoto M, Smolin G: Pneumococcal infections of the eye. Am J Ophthalmol 77:345–352, 1974.

Scott PM, Bloome MA: Lid necrosis secondary to streptococcal periorbital cellulitis. Ann Ophthalmol 13:461–465, 1981.

Wannamaker LW, Ferrieri P: Streptococcal infections—updated. DM; Disease–A–Month. Oct:1–40, 1975.

TETANUS 037
(Lockjaw)

ALBERT W. BIGLAN, M.D., F.A.C.S., and HOLLY W. DAVIS, M.D.

Pittsburgh, Pennsylvania

Tetanus is an acute neuromuscular disease characterized by rigidity and spasm. This condition results from intoxication by the neurotoxin tetanospasmin, which is produced by autolysis of the anaerobic spore-forming bacteria, *Clostridium tetani*. Symptoms may be local or systemic and are characterized by uncontrolled reflex spasms of voluntary muscles. There are four clinical forms reflecting variations in the predominant site of action of the toxin: local, generalized, cephalic, and neonatal.

Local tetanus causes rigidity of the muscles in close proximity to the site of infection. In many cases it is a precursor of generalized disease.

The first symptoms of generalized tetanus are stiffness of the jaw, neck, and possibly the tongue. This stiffness is followed by masseter rigidity resulting in trismus, risus sardonicus, dysphagia, and back and shoulder stiffness. Subsequently, a generalized increase in muscle tone and irritability supervenes, punctuated by intensely painful tetanic spasms in response to stimulation. These spasms are characterized by opisthotonos, flexion and adduction of the upper extremities with fists clenched, and extension of the lower extremities. In severe cases autonomic dysfunction manifested by hypertension, tachycardia, and diaphoresis may occur. Major complications include acute upper airway obstruction and vocal cord and diaphragmatic paralysis.

Upon recovery, complete muscle function usually returns.

Cephalic tetanus is a rare form of tetanus occurring in 1.1 per cent of the patients with generalized tetanus. Cephalic tetanus refers to a paradoxic cranial nerve palsy especially involving the lower cranial nerves in a person with generalized tetanus. After recovery, patients with cephalic tetanus may have residual weakness of the muscles innervated by the affected nerve.

Neonatal tetanus occurs in infants whose umbilical stumps are contaminated by soil or feces and who are born to nonimmunized mothers. It is extremely rare in the United States.

The organism, *C. tetani*, is an anaerobic, spore-forming rod found in soil and animal feces. Tetanus occurs in nonimmune patients with damaged tissue contaminated with *C. Tetani* spores. Even minor wounds can serve as portals of entry, although burns, surgical wounds, compound fractures, septic abortions, contaminated umbilical stumps, and puncture wounds are at highest risk. The spores produce exotoxins, of which the most important is tetanospasmin. The toxin disseminates locally and hematogenously and binds to presynaptic membranes at the neuromuscular junction of motor neurons. It then enters the neurons where it inhibits the release of neurotransmitters. Once inside the neuron, it is protected from the action of antitoxin. The toxin also travels by retrograde axonal transport to the neuronal cell bodies in the spinal cord and brainstem where it is released into the extracellular space. From there it moves into the synapses of inhibitory cells and prevents the release of the inhibitory neurotransmitters, glycine and gamma-aminobutyric acid (GABA), from the presynaptic terminal. This inhibition results in an increase in the resting firing rate of motor neurons, which produces muscular rigidity. The motor system then responds to afferent stimulation with intense, painful sustained contraction of both agonist and antagonist muscles, termed *tetanic spasm*. The incubation period is from 3 to 21 days. Symptoms occur in the head and neck first and the limbs last.

The incidence of tetanus in the United States is approximately 90 cases per year and has been constant over the past decade. Seventy-two per cent of cases occur after an acute injury, either a puncture or laceration. Most cases are acquired from injury outdoors. About 8 per cent of cases are the result of major trauma or are animal related.

Tetanus is a preventable condition. Approximately 60 per cent of reported cases occur in patients 50 years of age or older due to failure to maintain immunity by receiving booster doses of vaccine on a regular basis. Random serologic tests demonstrate a lack of protective levels of antibody in 50 per cent of persons 60 years of age or older.

TABLE 1. Tetanus Prophylaxis Immunization

Infants: primary vaccination
Intramuscular 0.5 cc DTP: at 2, 4, and 6 months of age and a booster at 15 to 18 months
> Children under 7 years old, not previously immunized in the first year of life

Intramuscular 0.5 cc DTP: 3 doses, 2 months apart followed by a fourth dose 6 to 12 months later
> Children over 7 years old: not previously immunized

Intramuscular 0.5 cc Td (contains a smaller dose of diphtheria toxoid) two doses, 1 to 2 months apart and third dose 6 to 12 months later
> Children over 7 years old and adults previously mmunized

Intramuscular Td every 10 years

DTP: Diphtheria and tetanus toxoids and pertussis vaccine.
Td: Tetanus and diphtheria toxoids.

THERAPY

Prophylactic. Tetanus is preventable. Every person should receive a vaccination series to produce active immunity to tetanus neurotoxin. The type of material used for vaccination and the schedule of administration depend on the age of the patient and his or her exposure to trauma (Tables 1 and 2).

The requirement for additional immunization will depend on the immunization status and on the condition of the wound. Complete primary immunization with tetanus toxoid (DTP or Td) will provide lasting protection for non-tetanus-prone wounds for 10 years or longer. If a fresh wound is tetanus prone (deep or severe puncture), a booster is appropriate if the patient has not received tetanus toxoid within the preceding 5 years (Table 2).

Patients who have not completed a full immunization series may require tetanus toxoid and passive immunization with 250 units of intramuscular human tetanus immune globulin (TIG). When TIG is used with tetanus toxoid (DTP or Td), separate syringes and injection sites should be used.

Systemic. The goals of treatment of tetanus are to stop the production of toxin by surgical debridement and antibiotics, to neutralize circulating toxin by administering antitoxin, and to provide supportive measures.

First, antitoxin, available as human tetanus immune globulin (TIG), is given intramuscularly. The currently recommended dose is 3000 to 6000 units, although recent evidence suggests that 500 IU may be adequate. This is followed by wound debridement if surgically indicated. Metronidazole, 500 mg every 6 hours for 10 days, is the antimicrobial treatment of choice. Penicillin is best avoided as it has GABA-A antagonist activity.

In mild cases of generalized tetanus or cases with dysphagia or respiratory difficulties, supportive care consists of management in a quiet dark room with minimal handling and administration of benzodiazapines (GABA-A agonists) for control of spasms and sedation. Diazepam is titrated in doses of 5 to 10 mg every 3 to 4 hours, or lorazepam, is given in 2-mg doses two to three times daily.

Moderate cases—those with pronounced spasticity, dysphagia, and respiratory problems—require endotracheal intubation or tracheostomy in addition to sedation.

Severe cases with gross spasticity and major spasms require paralysis with vecuronium†, 6 to 8 mg/hr and artificial ventilation. Very severe cases with sympathetic overactivity require management of tachyarrhythmias and blood pressure with labetalol, 0.25–1.0 mg/minute, and require sedation with morphine or general anesthesia.

Simultaneous with management of the acute episode, active immunization should be started using 0.5 ml of tetanus toxoid (Td) intramuscularly, with subsequent doses to complete the active immunization series. This is important because the levels of toxin produced even in severe cases are not enough to stimulate adequate production of protective antibody.

TABLE 2. Summary Guide to Tetanus Prophylaxis in Routine Wound Management

HISTORY OF ABSORBED TETANUS TOXOID (DOSES)	CLEAN, MINOR WOUNDS		ALL OTHER WOUNDS*	
	Td(+)	TIG 250 U IM	Td(+)	TIG
Unknown or < three	Yes	No	Yes	Yes
≥ Three (‡)	No(§)	No	No(‖)	No

*Such as, but not limited to, wounds contaminated with dirt, feces, soil, and saliva; puncture wounds; avulsions; and wounds resulting from missiles, crushing, burns, and frostbite.
+For children over 7 years old, DTP (DT, if pertussis vaccine is contraindicated) is preferred to tetanus toxoid alone. For persons ≥ 7 years of age, Td is preferred to tetanus toxoid alone.
‡If only three doses of fluid toxoid have been received, then a fourth dose of toxoid, preferably an absorbed toxoid, should be given.
§Yes, if more than 10 years since last dose.
‖Yes, if more than 5 years since first dose. (More frequent boosters are not needed and can accentuate side effects.)

Ocular. Tetracycline ointment should be applied to the eye every 2 to 6 hours. Cycloplegia with atropine may be used to manage uveitis after trauma. In patients receiving prolonged respiratory therapy, care for the globe with frequent lubrication and protection of the cornea is essential. Temporary tarsorrhaphy may be necessary in patients with accompanying seventh cranial nerve palsy.

Surgical. Careful debridement and removal of foreign material, both intraocular and periocular, in any tetanus-prone wound should be accomplished. Primary closure of the wound or wounds is recommended.

Ocular or Periocular Manifestations

Conjunctiva: Chemosis; hyperemia; necrosis.
Cornea: Exposure keratitis and ulcer (secondary to seventh cranial nerve palsy or prolonged respirator care).
Extraocular Muscles: Nystagmus; palsy of the sixth, third, and fourth cranial nerves (in decreasing frequency); spasm.
Eyelids: Lagophthalmos; blepharospasm; ptosis (may be associated with a third nerve palsy); tonic spasm (pseudoptosis).
Orbit: Abscess; panophthalmitis; trauma changes.

PRECAUTIONS

The extent of injury is not related to the susceptibility for tetanus. A trivial wound or an insect bite can produce tetanus, although most cases arise from severe globe or orbital trauma. Time from the injury to the onset of symptoms may be as long as 2 to 3 weeks. Patients without prior immunization should be observed closely during this period. Local reactions to DTP are common and do not indicate sensitization; however, severe and fatal reactions can occur.

Immunosuppressive therapy may suppress the immune response, and routine vaccinations should be deferred if possible during such therapy. Mild febrile illness is not a reason to defer routine vaccinations.

COMMENTS

Tetanus cases occur in unimmunized or inadequately immunized patients. Mortality is high for patients with generalized tetanus and ranges from 15 to 46 per cent. The coexistence of cephalic tetanus does not adversely affect mortality. Spores of *C. tetani* are ubiquitous, and there is no natural immunity to tetanus toxin. Therefore, all patients with penetrating injuries should be given appropriate prophylaxis. If a severe case of clinical tetanus develops, intensive medical care is required, and referral to a tertiary care center is indicated.

References

Ahmadsyam Salom, Treatment of Tetanus, British Medical Journal *291*:648, 1985.
Biglan AW, Ellis FD, Wade TA: Supranuclear oculomotor palsy and exotropia after tetanus. Am J Ophthalmol *86*:666–668, 1978.
Bleck TP: Pharmacology of tetanus. Clin Neuropharmacol *9*:103–120, 1986.
Diphtheria, tetanus, and pertussis. Guidelines for vaccine prophylaxis and other preventive measures. Ann Intern Med *95*:723–728, 1981.
Edmondson RS, Flowers MW: Intensive care in tetanus: Management, complications, and mortality in 100 cases. Br Med J *1*:1401–1404, 1979.
Immunization Practices Advisory Committee: Diphtheria, Tetanus and Pertussis: Recommendations for vaccine use and other preventative measures. Recommendations of the immunization practices advisory committee (ACIP). MMWR *40*:1–28, 1991.
Roos, KL: Tetanus Seminars in Neurology. *11*:206–214, 1991.
Rothstein RJ, Baker FJ II: Tetanus. Prevention and treatment. JAMA *240*:675–676, 1978.
Wetzel JO: Tetanus following eye injury. Report of case: Review of literature. Am J Ophthalmol *25*: 933–944, 1942.

TUBERCULOSIS 010.0

THOMAS C. SPOOR, M.D., M.S., F.A.C.S., *and* A. LUISA DILORENZO, M.D., B.S.

Detroit, Michigan

Tuberculosis (TB) is a communicable disease caused by the acid-fast bacillus, *Mycobacterium tuberculosis*. It occurs primarily as a pulmonary infection, being almost exclusively spread by air-borne transmission through tiny droplet nuclei that remain suspended in the air for prolonged periods of time. However, the bacillus may also be widely disseminated hematogenously. Tuberculosis infection of the eye is rare and may occur as either a primary or secondary infection. Primary ocular infection is often a conjunctivitis, probably introduced into the eye by contaminated hands, fomites, or exposure to dust or sputum particles containing tubercle bacilli. In secondary infection (hematogenously spread), tubercles may be present in or on any part of the eye. Tuberculous allergic manifestations (phlyctenular keratitis and conjunctivitis) are more common than ocular infection. Ocular symptoms may also result from infection of adjacent structures (sinuses and orbit) or from intracranial involvement of the optic pathways.

There has been a dramatic change in the incidence of tuberculosis in the United States. Until 1984, there was a steady decline in the number of cases from over 84,000 cases in 1953 to a nadir of 22,000 cases in 1984. In 1984 the longstanding annual decline abruptly ended, and from 1984 to 1991, 39,000 more cases were reported than would have been expected had the previous downward trend continued (There were 26,000 cases reported in 1990 alone.) Much of the recent increase in cases is attributed to the development of tuberculosis in HIV-infected persons. In these individuals, there is a higher disease attack rate and shorter incubation period associated with newly acquired tuberculosis and a higher mortality rate associated with the disease. Other susceptible individuals include the elderly, the urban poor, and those individuals who come from countries where TB is endemic; for example, Hispanic, Haitian, and southeast Asian immigrants. Recently the emergence of multidrug-resistant tuberculosis (MDR TB) has become a serious nationwide concern.

The overall increasing incidence of tuberculosis has brought more persons with active tuberculosis into institutional settings, many of which serve populations of HIV-infected persons. As a result, persons in hospitals, hospices, homeless shelters, and prisons are at increased risk.

THERAPY

Systemic. To prevent the emergence of drug-resistant mutants, two effective drugs are always needed to treat tuberculosis. Owing to the slow generation time of the mycobacteria and the long periods of metabolic inactivity, prolonged courses of drug treatment are also necessary. Presently, curative short-course therapy lasting for 6 months is available. It consists of isoniazid 300 mg, rifampin 600 mg, and pyrazinamide 2 gm daily for 2 months and then continuing with isoniazid and rifampin for an additional 4 months. More prolonged treatment is recommended in patients with HIV infection because the efficacy of standard therapy in such patients is uncertain. When there is isoniazid resistance or intolerance, ethambutol in a dosage of 15 mg/kg may be substituted and treatment duration increased to 12 months in HIV-negative individuals and to 18 months in HIV-positive individuals. In cases of rifampin intolerance, ethambutol is also used in addition to isoniazid and pyrazinamide. Treatment lasts for 18 to 24 months in HIV-negative individuals or for 12 months after cultures are negative, whichever is longer in HIV-positive individuals.

When the mycobacteria are resistant to two or more drugs, (MDR TB), the course of treatment increases from 6 months to 18 to 24 months, and the cure rate drops from nearly 100 per cent to less than 60 per cent.

Ocular. Systemic treatment is necessary for metastatic ocular tuberculosis and may also be necessary for primary ocular tuberculosis. Topical ophthalmic corticosteroids and cycloplegics may be necessary to control inflammation and prevent scarring due to keratitis and iritis. Secondary infection should be treated vigorously with topical antibiotics as sensitivities warrant. Localized lid lesions may be excised surgically.

Supportive. Rest, good diet, and improved general hygiene may be used as supportive measures to increase the patient's resistance.

Ocular or Periocular Manifestations

Choroid: Disseminated choroiditis; isolated tubercles.

Conjunctiva: Follicular, hypertropic granulomatous, papillary, or purulent conjunctivitis; hyperemia; miliary ulcer, phlyctenules; polypoid "fibroma"; subconjunctival nodules (tuberculomas).

Cornea: Interstitial or sclerosing keratitis; mutton-fat keratic precipitates; pannus; phlyctenules; ulcer.

Eyelids: Blepharitis, cellulitis, edema; hyperemia; lupus tuberculosis; meibomianitis.

Iris: Granulomatous anterior uveitis; nodules.

Lacrimal System: Chronic dacryoadenitis; dacryocystitis; tuberculous pericystitis.

Motility: Internuclear ophthalmoplegia; gaze palsies.

Optic Nerve: Atrophy, optic neuritis (associated with tuberculous meningitis); optochiasmic arachnoiditis.

Orbit: Chronic cellulitis, fistula formation; periosteitis; primary abscess (extension from lacrimal gland or sinuses).

Retina: Exudative retinitis; periphlebitis.

Sclera: Perforation; scleritis, ulcer.

Other: Hypopyon, preauricular, submaxillary or cervical lymphadenopathy; tuberculous panophthalmitis; vitreous hemorrhages.

PRECAUTIONS

The major problem in tuberculosis treatment programs is patient default, which can be as high as 40 to 60 per cent. This rate is highest in countries with limited resources. Therefore, the new shortened courses of treatment have helped improve patient compliance.

There are many alternative effective drug regimens, and toxicity is a factor in the choice of therapy. Hepatitis, which is of great concern, occurs in persons taking isoniazid with either rifampin or ethambutol and in more of those taking pyrazinamide. Alcohol and barbiturates predispose patients to isoniazid hepatotoxicity. Isoniazid is also known to deplete pyridoxine and may induce a peripheral or optic neuropathy. Persons with such predisposing factors as old age, diabetes, alcoholism, and malnutrition should be given pyridoxine concomitantly with isoniazid; the usual dose is 50 mg daily. Ethambutol may induce a dose-related optic neuritis that has been shown to be irreversible on discontinuation of the drug. It is excreted by the kidney in the active form, and therefore, patients with renal failure should have their visual acuity and color vision monitored frequently. Disadvantages of streptomycin include fetal ototoxicity if given during pregnancy, as well as eighth nerve dysfunction, which is particularly troublesome in patients over 50 years of age who may be unable to compensate for the loss of vestibular function.

Early reports have suggested that patients with HIV infection and tuberculosis tolerate antituberculosis medications well. Recently, however, there have been reports of increased adverse effects to rifampin. Limited data suggest that the combination of zidovudine (AZT) and antituberculosis medications is well tolerated. Antifungals used in AIDS-related infections have a complex interaction with isoniazid and rifampin, limiting their efficacy. Ketoconazole inhibits the absorption of rifampin, which can result in the failure of tuberculosis treatment.

COMMENTS

Phlyctenular keratoconjunctivitis is the most common form of external ocular tuberculosis. Conjunctival lesions are more commonly found on the palpebral than the bulbar conjunctiva and may be diagnosed by biopsy with appropriate stains and cultures. Orbital and sinus involvement are also reported infrequently.

The diagnosis of tuberculosis by the ophthalmologist is often indirect and is based upon the clinical picture, a positive purified protein derivative, and response to therapy. The ophthalmologist must consider tuberculosis as a possible etiology for any chronic anterior uveitis or disseminated choroiditis. One must also be aware that ophthalmic complications can occur secondary to the treatment of systemic tuberculosis.

References

Barnes PF, Bloch AB, Davidson PT, Snider DE: Tuberculosis in patients with human immunodeficiency virus infection. N Engl J Med 324:1644–1650, 1991.

Cangemi FE, Friedman AH, Josephberg R: Tuberculoma of the choroid. Ophthalmology 87:252–258, 1980.

Daniel Thomas M: Tuberculosis. *In* Harrison's Principles of Internal Medicine, 12th ed. New York, McGraw-Hill, 1991, pp 637-645.

DeVita EG, Maio M, Sadun A: Optic neuropathy in ethambutol-treated renal tuberculosis. J Clin Neuro-Ophthalmol 7:77–83, 1987.

DeVoe AG, Locatcher-Khorazo D: The external manifestations of ocular tuberculosis. Trans Am Ophthalmol Soc 62:203–212, 1964.

Fedukowicz HB: External Infections of the Eye: Bacterial, Viral, and Mycotic, 2nd ed. New York, Appleton-Century-Crofts, 1978, pp 136-141.

Inocencio FP, Ballecer R: Tuberculosis granuloma in the midbrain causing wall-eyed bilateral inter-nuclear ophthalmoplegia. J Clin Neuro-ophthalmol 5:31–35, 1985.

Locatcher-Khorazo D, Seegal BC: Microbiology of the Eye. St. Louis, CV Mosby, 1972, pp 119–130.

Management of persons exposed to multidrug-resistant tuberculosis—United States. MMWR 41:1–70, 1992.

Pearson ML, Jereb JA, et al: Nosocomial transmission of multidrug-resistant *Mycobacterium tuberculosis*. Ann Intern Med 117:191–196, 1992.

Prevention and control of tuberculosis in US communities with at-risk minority populations—United States. MMWR 41:1–23, 1992.

Prichard JG, Raleigh J: Tuberculosis and other mycobacterial diseases. *In* Conn's Current Therapy. Philadelphia, WB Saunders, 1986, pp 167-174.

Schlaegel TF Jr, O'Connor GR: Tuberculosis and syphilis. Arch Ophthalmol 99:2206–2207, 1981.

Smith JL: Should ethambutol be barred? (Editorial). J Clin Neuro-Ophthalmol 7:84–86, 1987.

Spoor TC, Harding SA: Orbital tuberculosis. Am J Ophthalmol 91:644–647, 1981.

TULAREMIA 021.9
(Deerfly Tularemia, Pahvant Valley Plague, Rabbit Fever)

MALCOLM N. LUXENBERG, M.D.

Augusta, Georgia

Tularemia is an acute infectious disease caused by *Francisella tularensis*, a gram-negative coccobacillus. The disease occurs throughout the United States, but is most common in the Southeast. The organism has been recovered from many wild mammals, some domestic animals (such as the cat), and many insects. The most important reservoir hosts in the United States are wild game, primarily rabbits, ticks, and other blood-sucking arthropods, with wild game being the most important vectors east of the Mississippi River and ticks being the overall most important vectors, especially west of the Mississippi River. The route of entry is through the skin or mucous membranes, with human infection most frequently occurring after contact with tissues or body fluids of an infected animal or from the bite of an infected insect. Less frequently, infection can be acquired by inhalation of infectious aerosols, by ingestion of contaminated water, or by eating inadequately cooked meat from an affected animal. Two cases were recently reported in which infection was apparently acquired by contact with rabbit feet, which were given as good luck charms, from an infected animal. Infection can occur at any time of the year, involves all age groups, and is seen most frequently in adult men who are outdoorsmen or hunters.

The incubation period is approximately 3 to 5 days, after which a nodular ulcerated lesion develops at the site of entry. Most patients then have a rapid onset of fever, chills, malaise, and headache. This condition usually evolves into a clinical syndrome of which there are several types, with the ulceroglandular form being most common and the oculoglandular type least common. The portal of entry in the latter type is usually via the conjunctiva. The oculoglandular form is most frequently unilateral and is characterized by purulent conjunctivitis, nodular-ulcerative lesions of the conjunctiva, chemosis, periorbital edema, pain, and lymphadenopathy. Less commonly seen are corneal infiltrates, ulceration, scarring, and vascularization. Dacryocystitis occasionally occurs. In rare instances, there may be perforation of the cornea and endophthalmitis with loss of the eye. Laboratory diagnosis is difficult as gram stains of exudate are usually negative, the organism does not grow on routine media, and biopsies of lesions rarely reveal the organism with standard stains. Most cases are diagnosed by serologic testing, with a fourfold rise in the tularemia agglutination titer considered to be diagnostic. Unfortunately, the agglutination titers are usually negative for the first 2 weeks after the initial infection and do not reach their maximum for 2 to 3 months. However, a recent report suggests that a microagglutination test may demonstrate higher titers and detect infection earlier than other tests.

THERAPY

Systemic. Streptomycin, which is bactericidal for the organism, is the drug of choice for the treatment of tularemia, and a rapid response to treatment, often within 48 hours, is seen in most cases. A daily dose of 15 to 20 mg/kg is given intramuscularly in divided doses for up to 14 days. In selected cases, gentamicin, which is also bactericidal, may be used in a daily dose of 5 mg/kg as a therapeutic alternative to streptomycin. Relapses are uncommon with these agents. Tetracycline may be used, but is bacteriostatic for *F. tularensis*, and relapses occur more frequently with this drug, especially if it is used for less than 14 days. A loading dose of 30 mg/kg of tetracycline is given orally, followed by 30 mg/kg in divided doses for 14 days. There has been limited clinical experience with tobramycin. A recent case report suggests that imipenem/cilastatin (Primoxin) may be useful in treating tularemia patients who have renal disease when streptomycin or gentamicin cannot be used.

Ocular. Topical gentamicin or tetracycline eyedrops should be used along with the systemic therapy. Initially they should be administered every 2 to 3 hours for 1 to 2 days and can then be decreased to four times a day for 7 to 10 days if the infection is responding adequately. Cycloplegic drops should be used as needed. Cool compresses may provide symptomatic relief, especially in the acute phases.

Supportive. Because tularemia is a serious systemic illness, medical consultation, preferably from a specialist in infectious diseases, should be obtained to help with the overall management, including the selection and dosage of antibiotics.

Ocular or Periocular Manifestations

Conjunctiva: Chemosis; marked hyperemia; nodular ulcerative granuloma; purulent conjunctivitis.
Cornea: Infiltrates; opacity; perforation, ulcer; vascularization.
Eyelids: Edema; nodular ulcerative lesions.
Globe: Endophthalmitis.
Lacrimal System: Dacryocystitis.
Other: Ocular pain; periorbital edema; preauricular or cervical lymphadenopathy.

PRECAUTIONS

The dosage of streptomycin and gentamicin must be carefully adjusted depending on the patient's age and renal function. The patient should be properly monitored for the possible development of toxicity from medications, such as streptomycin, which can damage the labyrinthine system.

COMMENTS

The diagnosis of tularemia infection of the eye can be difficult as the condition is uncommon and routine laboratory tests are usually negative, especially in the earlier stages. Therefore, a high index of suspicion is important, and a careful history for exposure to known vectors must be obtained. Once the diagnosis is made or strongly suspected, treatment should be started as quickly as possible, preferably with streptomycin, as the response to treatment is better and relapses less frequent if therapy is initiated within the first 2 weeks of illness.

References

Bloom ME, Shearer WT, Barton LL: Oculoglandular tularemia in an inner city child. Pediatrics 51: 564–566, 1973.
Boyce JM: *Francisella tularensis* (tularemia). In Mandell GL, Douglas RG Jr, Bennett JE: Principles and Practice of Infectious Diseases. New York, John Wiley & Sons, 1979, pp 1784-1788.
Evans ME, et al: Tularemia and the tomcat. JAMA 246: 1343, 1981.
Evans ME, et al: Tularemia: A 30-year experience with 88 cases. Medicine 64:251–269, 1985.
Francis E: Oculoglandular tularemia. Arch Ophthalmol 28:711–741, 1942.
Guerrant RL, et al: Tickborne oculoglandular tularemia. Arch Intern Med 136:811–813, 1976.
Hanna C, Lyford JH: Tularemia infection of the eye. Ann Ophthalmol 3:1321–1325, 1971.
Lee HC, Harowitz E, Linder W: Treatment of tularemia with imipenem/cilastatin sodium. South Med J 84:1277–1278, 1991.

Mason WL, et al: Treatment of tularemia, including pulmonary tularemia, with gentamicin. Am Rev Respir Dis *121*:39–45, 1980.

Ryan-Porvuer K, Whitehead PY, Leggiadro RJ: An unlucky rabbit's foot. Pediatrics *85*:598–600, 1990.

Sato T, Frijita H, Ohara Y, & Homma M: Microagglutination test for early and specific serodiagnosis of tularemia. J Clin Microbiol *28*:2372–2374, 1990.

TYPHOID FEVER 002.0

GEORGE N. CHIN, M.D., F.A.C.S.

Seattle, Washington

Typhoid fever is an acute febrile illness caused by the ingestion of and the intestinal invasion by *Salmonella typhi*, a gram-negative bacillus found only in humans. Prevalent in those regions of the world lacking sanitary water and sewage systems, its transmission can occur through ingestion of contaminated food or water, contact with an acute case of typhoid fever, or contact with a chronic asymptomatic carrier. Transmission through direct fecal-oral contact is more common among children.

Typhoid fever is characterized by sustained fever, headache, chills, sore throat, coughing, nausea, vomiting, diarrhea, constipation, abdominal pain, anorexia, muscle pain, weakness, dizziness, and, occasionally, seizures. The onset is usually gradual, and the illness achieves maximum severity during the second or third week, with marked weakness, abdominal discomfort and distention, "rose spots" rash, cervical adenopathy, hepatomegaly, splenomegaly, rales, and occasional neurologic manifestations, such as mental dullness. Recovery, characterized by declining fever, begins by the end of the third or fourth week. The most prominent major complications are intestinal hemorrhage and perforation, which can occur during the third week, often heralded by a sudden drop in temperature and increased pulse.

Ocular manifestations of typhoid fever are rare and may include lid abscesses, corneal ulcers, uveitis, vitreous hemorrhage, retinal hemorrhage and detachment, panophthalmitis, optic neuritis, extraocular muscle palsies, orbital thrombosis, and orbital abscesses. Ocular complications of this nature are probably a result of direct invasion by the organism into the ocular tissues, but some, such as vitreous hemorrhage after typhoid vaccination, may be hypersensitivity phenomena.

THERAPY

Systemic. Diagnosis of typhoid fever is made through isolation of *Salmonella* organisms from cultures of blood, urine, stool, bone marrow aspirates, or skin biopsies of "rose spots." Once the illness is confirmed, prompt antimicrobial therapy should begin. Chloramphenicol is the preferred antibiotic, given orally or intravenously in daily dosages of 50 mg/kg divided into four doses for at least 14 days. A general sense of improvement and well-being can be expected within 48 hours. The febrile episode may continue for 5 to 7 days and should not be interpreted as treatment failure.

Numerous reports over the last 15 years have documented the presence of chloramphenicol-resistant strains of typhoid fever. When these are present, ampicillin should be administered orally or intravenously in dosages of 100 mg/kg per day in four divided doses for at least 14 days. Most of the *S. typhi* chloramphenicol-resistant strains have been found in Mexico, India, and southeast Asia.

When isolates are shown to be resistant to both chloramphenicol and ampicillin, a trimethoprim-sulfamethoxazole‡ combination has proven to be a reasonably effective alternative. This combination of 320 to 640 mg of trimethoprim with 1.6 to 3.2 gm of sulfamethoxazole may be given orally or intravenously in two divided doses for 2 weeks. Slow intravenous infusion of 160 mg of trimethoprim and 800 mg of sulfamethoxazole diluted in 250 ml of 5 per cent dextrose in water may be administered every 12 hours. Rapid infusion or bolus injection should be avoided.

Severely toxemic patients may benefit from a short course of systemic corticosteroids, such as 60 mg of intravenous prednisolone. Corticosteroid therapy should be rapidly tapered and discontinued after the third day.

Treatment of chronic carriers of *S. typhi* consists of oral ampicillin in daily doses of 3 to 6 gm for 4 to 6 weeks. Chloramphenicol has no influence on the chronic typhoid fever carrier state. Radiographic examination of the biliary tract is essential during the initial assessment, since the gallbladder is the nidus of the chronic carrier state in the majority of such patients. If gallbladder disease is not evident, prolonged administration of ampicillin may end the carrier state. All chronic carriers should be discouraged from handling food and must be carefully instructed in the importance of hand washing. The appropriate public health officials should be notified.

Ocular. In addition to systemic antibiotics, ocular infection with salmonellosis should be treated with frequent topical chloramphenicol and/or periocular injection of ampicillin* when indicated. Lid abscesses should be drained and specimens carefully handled for culture. Topical application of a chloramphenicol ointment may be applied to the wound. All purulent conjunctival discharges should be irrigated with saline. Conjunctivitis and corneal ulcers should be treated with an hourly application of 0.5 per cent chloramphenicol ophthalmic solution, with appropriate smears and cultures taken to rule out secondary invaders. If corneal perforation occurs, the general method of treatment includes pressure bandage, tissue adhesives, or blowout patch.

Uveitis can be treated with 1 per cent atropine ophthalmic solution three times a day to keep the pupil dilated and prevent synechiae. Prednisolone, 1 per cent ophthalmic suspension, should also be instilled hourly to control the inflammation and should be tapered according to its response.

Orbital infection and vitreous, retinal, optic nerve, and intraocular muscle involvement are much more difficult to treat. Since their pathogenesis is unknown, no effective treatment has been found. Exudative nonrhegmatogenous retinal detachment has been shown to respond to oral administration of 40 to 60 mg of prednisone for 3 days, which controls the exudative fluid. When endophthalmitis or panophthalmitis is present, the prognosis for visual recovery is poor. To relieve ocular pain, hot packs or compresses 10 to 15 minutes three times a day may be effective.

Supportive. Supportive care with particular attention given to nutritional requirements, adequate hydration, and correction of electrolyte disorders is of utmost importance during the initial phase of managing typhoid fever patients. All patients should be hospitalized under enteric isolation precaution in order to prevent spreading the disease to other patients and hospital personnel. Vital signs and white blood cell count must be carefully monitored. Bedrest during the initial phase is essential; ambulation should be gradual. Tepid sponge baths or cooling blankets can reduce the temperature of individuals with severe hyperpyrexia. Codeine rather than aspirin should be used in treating headache, since salicylates can produce wide swings in temperature with very uncomfortable chills and sweats, in addition to their effects on blood platelets and irritating action on the bowels. Hypothermia and hypotension occur in some patients after administration of salicylates. A high caloric liquid diet should be provided to those capable of oral intake. Those who cannot eat should be given intravenous infusion supplemented with vitamins.

Transfusion is indicated if significant intestinal hemorrhaging occurs. Typing and crossmatching should be done at the time of initial diagnosis of typhoid fever. If perforation is suspected, emphasis should be placed on efforts to combat shock and decompression of the bowels. Additional antimicrobials may be added to control peritonitis. Small perforations may localize and can be managed without surgical intervention. Typhoid patients are considered poor surgical risks.

Ocular or Periocular Manifestations

Conjunctiva: Chemosis; conjunctivitis; subconjunctival hemorrhages.

Cornea: Ulcer.
Extraocular Muscles: Conjugate gaze paralysis; paralysis; tenonitis.
Eyelids: Abscess; hemorrhages.
Globe: Endophthalmitis; panophthalmitis.
Iris: Iritis; uveitis.
Optic Nerve: Disc edema; optic neuritis.
Orbit: Abscess; cellulitis; orbital vein thrombosis.
Retina: Central retinal artery emboli; edema; exudative detachment; hemorrhages; venous engorgement.
Vitreous: Hemorrhages.
Other: Central scotoma; choroiditis; dacryoadenitis; hypopyon; ocular pain; paralysis of accommodation; visual loss.

PRECAUTIONS

Because salicylates can produce severe hypothermia and vascular collapse, they should be avoided in patients with typhoid fever. Laxatives and enemas should be avoided despite constipation, since they may precipitate intestinal hemorrhage and ulcer perforation.

All patients receiving chloramphenicol should be monitored for bone marrow toxicity, and a complete blood count should be obtained. Chloramphenicol-induced granulocytopenia may occur and is reversible with discontinuation of the antibiotic. Aplastic anemia is rare, but may follow the use of chloramphenicol.

Renal function should be monitored in patients receiving trimethoprim and sulfamethoxazole, and a creatinine clearance should be done. The most frequent clinical side effects seen with these drugs are rash, nausea, and vomiting; megaloblastic anemia may also occur. In any event, the drugs should be reduced or discontinued if these adverse reactions occur. Patients receiving trimethoprim, sulfamethoxazole, or ampicillin should be monitored for hypersensitivity reactions.

Although immunization with typhoid vaccine provides significant immunity against typhoid infection, protection is not complete and can be readily overcome by a large dose of organisms. Nevertheless, immunization is recommended for those individuals living or traveling in areas where the disease is endemic and for persons working with the organism in the laboratory. Family members of a chronic carrier should also be vaccinated. Immunization of a person living within the United States is not necessary. Because of the extremely low prevalence of the disease and of carriers in the United States, mass vaccination against typhoid, even in such disasters as floods, is rarely needed. Adults should receive 0.5 ml of vaccine on two separate occasions 1 to 2 weeks apart. The vaccine causes a transient titer elevation of agglutinins against typhoid O antigens for several months and a persistent elevated titer for H antigens. The yearly booster is required to maintain immunity.

Local health authorities should be made aware of all typhoid fever patients so that appropriate field investigation can begin to determine the source of infection. Precautions should be observed to prevent the spread of infection from persons with active cases or from carriers. Stool specimens should be cultured during convalescence at weekly intervals. Three consecutive negative stool cultures usually indicate that a carrier state does not exist. On the other hand, a positive culture 4 months after treatment indicates that a carrier state may have developed. Chronic or convalescing carriers should not be allowed to prepare food until clear documentation shows that at least three or more stool cultures are negative for typhoid bacilli. Carriers should be cautioned regarding routine sanitary techniques.

COMMENTS

As many as 20 per cent of all patients with typhoid fever who are successfully treated with chloramphenicol may relapse. In most cases, relapse appears as a brief febrile illness 2 to 4 weeks after the completion of antimicrobial therapy. Relapses usually do not require treatment due to the self-limiting nature of the illness, but retreatment with antibiotics for 1 week may be necessary if symptoms persist longer than 36 to 48 hours. Therapy is identical to that of the initial episode.

The mortality rate of typhoid fever before the introduction of chloramphenicol was about 12 per cent. Mortality presently stands at 2 to 3 per cent in patients treated with proper antibiotic therapy and 10 per cent in untreated patients. Causes of death include toxemia, inanition, pneumonia, and intestinal perforation and hemorrhage. Death is primarily observed in infants, the aged, or individuals with malnutrition or other underlying diseases.

References

Bajpai PC, Dikshit SK: Bilateral optic neuritis and encephalitis complicating typhoid fever. J Indian Med Assoc 30:54–57, 1958.

Calhoun FP: Ocular complications due to typhoid inoculations. Arch Ophthalmol 48:553–558, 1919.

Dhir SP, et al: Salmonella lid abscess. Indian J Ophthalmol 24:27–28, 1977.

Doughman DJ: Treatment of corneal thinning and perforation. JCE Ophthalmol, January, 1978, pp 15–23.

Foote SC, Hook EW: Salmonella species (including typhoid fever). In Mandell GL, Douglas RG Jr, Bennett JE: Principles and Practice of Infectious Diseases. New York, John Wiley & Sons, 1979, pp 1730–1750.

Herzog C: Chemotherapy of typhoid fever: A review of literature. Infection 4:166–173, 1976.

Hook EW, Guerrant RL. Salmonella infections. In Isselbacher KJ, et al (eds): Harrison's Principles of Internal Medicine, 9th ed. New York, McGraw-Hill, 1980, pp 641-648.

Lewis PJ, Jones BL: Vitreous haemorrhage after typhoid cholera inoculation. Med J Aust 2:914, 1974.

Mathur JS, et al: Post typhoid retinal detachment. J All-India Ophthalmol Soc 18:135–137, 1970.

Prélat: Un cas d'iridocyclite bilatérale au cours de la vaccination antityphoidique (T.A.B.). Arch Ophthalmol 35:742–746, 1916-1917.

Warren JW, Hornick RB: Immunization against typhoid fever. Annu Rev Med 30:457–472, 1979.

YERSINIOSIS 020.9

K. MATTI SAARI, M.D.

Turku, Finland

Yersiniosis is a disease caused by infection with the gram-negative bacilli *Yersinia enterocolitica* or *Y. pseudotuberculosis*. Plague bacterium has been reclassified as *Y. pestis*. A wide range of clinical manifestations have been attributed to these bacilli, and they vary according to the age and condition of the patient. In the infant, gastroenteritis with high fever is common. Older children often experience acute abdominal symptoms, which may include acute terminal ileitis or mesenteric adenitis. Adults may present with enteritis, including diarrhea, nonspecific abdominal pain, nausea, vomiting, and fever. Nonpurulent reactive arthritis, often with myalgia, is more common in young and middle-aged adults, and erythema nodosum is more usual in women in late middle age. Less common symptoms include carditis, septicemia, glomerulonephritis, hepatitis, and hemolytic anemia.

Pyogenic ocular involvement (microbial invasion of the eye) is very rare in patients with yersiniosis; however, Parinaud's oculoglandular syndrome with ensuing corneal perforation and panophthalmitis leading to visual loss has been reported. Reactive ocular inflammation (the causative agent cannot be isolated from the eye), including acute anterior uveitis, conjunctivitis, and Reiter's syndrome, is occasionally associated with *Yersinia* infection in patients with HLA-B27 antigen.

THERAPY

Systemic. Most *Y. enterocolitica* strains are resistant in vitro to ampicillin, amoxicillin, carbenicillin, and penicillin and are sensitive to gentamicin, kanamycin, tobramycin, tetracycline, chloramphenicol, and to the combination of sulfamethoxazole and trimethoprim. However, success with these drugs is not uniform. Drug therapy must be started promptly when the diagnosis of yersiniosis is suspected. Usually, 250 to 500 mg of tetracycline are given orally every 6 hours for 10 days. If chloramphenicol is given, the dosage should be 250 to 500 mg orally every 4 to 6 hours or 500 mg every 6 hours by intravenous injection. Alternatively, 160 mg of trimethoprim and 800 mg of sulfamethoxazole may be given orally two to three times daily. Gentamicin is given by intramuscular injection in an initial dosage of 0.8 mg/kg, followed by 0.4 mg/kg every 6 hours. Therapy should be continued for at least 24 to 48 hours after symptoms and fever have subsided.

Ocular. With conjunctival *infections*, fortified gentamicin§ (14 mg/ml) eyedrops should be given hourly for 8 days, and then one drop should be given every 6 hours until the infection seems to be resolved. With corneal involvement, subtenon injection of 20 to 40 mg of gentamicin* daily for 4 to 5 days, followed by two more injections on alternate days, may be indicated. If corneal perforation occurs, a corneal patch graft may be indicated to seal the perforation.

Topical 1 per cent atropine solution may be used for uveitis, and one drop may be given every 6 hours. If the patient is sensitive to atropine, 0.25 per cent scopolamine may be substituted.

Reactive conjunctivitis associated with *Yersinia* infection usually resolves in 1 week without treatment. Reactive iritis should be treated with topically administered corticosteroids (0.1 per cent dexamethasone or 0.5 to 1 per cent prednisolone) every hour daily, corticosteroid ointment for the night, and 0.25 per cent scopolamine three times a day. In cases with fulminant onset of intraocular inflammation, systemic corticosteroids, beginning with 40 to 60 mg of oral prednisolone daily and followed by reduction of the dosage, may be used. In patients with reactive ocular inflammation after *Yersinia* infection, antibiotic therapy should be applied only in cases where high levels of IgM antibodies indicate recent infection, when *Yersinia* can be cultured from the stools, or when diarrhea or abdominal pains are still present or closely connected with the illness. Associated *Yersinia* infection should be treated with 250 mg of tetracycline orally every 6 hours for 10 days.

Surgical. The management of *Y. enterocolitica* endophthalmitis and panophthalmitis is extremely difficult, and most eyes are lost at this stage of the disease. Emergency pars plana vitrectomy may be indicated to remove the infectious organisms, to confirm their antibiotic sensitivity by vitreous culture, and to enable intravitreal injection of 0.1 mg of gentamicin.* The postoperative therapeutic regimen should include systemic antibiotics, daily subtenon injections of 20 to 40 mg of gentamicin* or 20 to 40 mg of tobramycin,* and topical instillation of fortified gentamicin§ (14 mg/ml) or tobramycin§ (11 mg/ml) eyedrops every 30 minutes for the first few days and then tapered.

Supportive. Supportive care may consist of intravenous fluid, pressor drugs, and oxygen, when required.

Ocular or Periocular Manifestations

(P) indicates pyogenic manifestations; (R) indicates reactive manifestations.

Anterior Chamber: Cells and flare (P,R); fibrinous exudates (R).

Conjunctiva: Chemosis (R); edema (P); follicles (R); granulomatous conjunctivitis (Parinaud's) (P); hyperemia (P,R); mucopurulent conjunctivitis (P,R); necrosis (P); ulcer (P).

Cornea: Clouding (P); perforation (P); ulcer (P).

Globe: Endophthalmitis (P); panophthalmitis (P).

Iris: Acute anterior uveitis (P,R), posterior synechiae (P,R); vasodilation of iris vessels (R).

Retina: Disc edema (R); hemorrhages (P); macular edema (R); vascular constriction (P).

Vitreous: Cells (R).

Other: Cataract (P); hypopyon (P); ocular pain (P,R); photophobia (P,R); visual loss (P).

PRECAUTIONS

Since yersiniosis may present with such a wide spectrum of symptoms, diagnosis may easily be missed. This infection should always be considered in patients with fever of unknown origin. This fact is underlined by the possibility of fatal complications from the disease, especially in malnourished patients and those who develop sepsis. When a diagnosis of yersiniosis is suspected, stool and conjunctival discharges should be cultured. Serologic diagnosis is available at reference laboratories. An elevated erythrocyte sedimentation rate is characteristic for yersiniosis in patients of all ages.

Adverse effects caused by tetracyclines include nausea, enterocolitis, superinfections, and photosensitivity. Patients taking tetracyclines should not sunbathe. Products containing aluminum, magnesium, or calcium ions (antacids, milk, and milk products) decrease the absorption and should not be taken during the hour before or 2 hours after an oral dose of tetracycline. Tetracyclines should be avoided during pregnancy and in children below 8 years because of irreversible deposition of the substance in growing teeth and bones.

Gentamicin should be used with caution in patients who have renal impairment. Both nephrotoxicity and neurotoxicity with involvement of the eighth cranial nerve have been reported with the use of gentamicin.

Chloramphenicol may have severe side effects, although these are rather uncommon. Adverse effects reported with this drug include skin rashes, fever, gastrointestinal disturbance, bone marrow depression, and the gray-baby syndrome.

COMMENTS

The mode of transmission of *Yersinia* bacilli is not fully understood. The bacilli have been isolated from a wide number of wild and domestic animals, and transmission to humans by contact with infected animals may occur in some instances. However, the primary mode of transmission seems to be fecally contaminated food and water. It also seems likely that the disease may be spread by contact with infected persons.

Although serious complications may occur in debilitated and older patients, the prognosis in *Yersinia* infections is generally good, especially if diagnosis can be made and treatment started relatively early. In children, *Y. enterocolitica* diarrhea is often self-limiting, and the role of antibiotic therapy is unclear. Subacute localizing forms of infection sometimes appear in patients with *Y. pseudotuberculosis* infection, particularly those with concurrent underlying disease.

References

Bottone EJ (ed): Yersinia enterocolitica. Boca Raton, FL, CRC Press, 1981.
Butler T: Plague and Other Yersinia Infections. New York, Plenum Medical Book Co., 1983.
Chin GN, Noble RC: Ocular involvement in *Yersinia enterocolitica* infection presenting as Parinaud's oculoglandular syndrome. Am J Ophthalmol *83*:19–23, 1977.
Mäki M et al: Yersiniosis in children. Arch Dis Child *55*:861–865, 1980.
Mattila L et al: Acute anterior uveitis after yersinia infection. Br J Ophthalmol *66*:209–212, 1982.
Saari KM, et al: Ocular inflammation associated with *Yersinia* infection. Am J Ophthalmol 89:84–95, 1980.
Saari, KM, et al: Acute anterior uveitis and conjunctivitis following yersinia infection in children. Int Ophthalmol 9:237–241, 1986.
Saari KM: The eye and reactive arthritis. *In* Toivanen A and Toivanen P (eds): Reactive Arthritis. Boca Raton, FL, CRC Press, Inc, 1988, pp 113–124.

Chlamydial Infections

INCLUSION CONJUNCTIVITIS 077.0
(Paratrachoma, *Chlamydia*)

CHANDLER R. DAWSON, M.D.

San Francisco, California

The chlamydiae are obligate intracellular organisms derived from bacteria that now comprise three species: *Chlamydia trachomatis*, *Chlamydia psittaci*, and *Chlamydia pneumoniae*. *C. trachomatis*, almost exclusively a human pathogen, includes the agents of classic trachoma (always associated with serotypes A, B, Ba, and C) and of inclusion conjunctivitis or paratrachoma (serotypes D, E, F, G, H, I, J, and K); these organisms infect the epithelium of mucoid surfaces and were once identified as the TRIC (trachoma-inclusion conjunctivitis) agents. The *C. trachomatis* agents also include the agents of lymphogranuloma venereum (serotypes L1, L2, and L3) that infect deeper tissues but not epithelial surfaces and are more pathogenic in animal systems.

Like lymphogranuloma venereum, serotypes D through K are sexually transmitted, and the secondary eye involvement in adults occurs in about 1 in 300 genital cases. Exposure of the infant in the birth canal yields a rate of ocular infection of 35 to 50 per cent of exposed newborns, resulting in chlamydial ophthalmia neonatorum. Infection of the eyes of adults occurs from sexual partners or from autoinoculation of infective genital discharges into the eye. Genitally transmitted chlamydial infections are the major cause of nongonococcal urethritis in men and of cervicitis and salpingitis in women and cause a number of other diseases.

Infants exposed to chlamydial infection from the mother's cervix during birth develop ophthalmia neonatorum at 5 to 12 days of age. Of infants exposed during delivery, 10 to 20 per cent also develop chlamydial respiratory disease with pneumonia as late as 6 months postpartum; the infection involves the gastrointestinal tract as well. Neonatal ophthalmia presents as tearing with moderate discharge and swelling of the lids. The eyes are usually red and inflamed, and there is infiltration and swelling of the conjunctiva. If untreated, chlamydial conjunctivitis in newborns may resolve spontaneously in 5 to 9 months, but has been known to persist for years with development of chronic follicular conjunctivitis, corneal neovascularization (vascular pannus), and conjunctival scarring. Infants with chlamydial respiratory disease may present from 2 to 6 months of age with rhinitis, cough, and a pertussis-like inspiratory whoop, and they frequently have eosinophilia.

In adults, ocular chlamydial infection produces chronic follicular conjunctivitis with keratitis. Because this adult disease is difficult to distinguish from the clinical findings in early trachoma, the term "paratrachoma" is used to describe the whole spectrum of eye disease with genitally transmitted chlamydial infection. Ocular chlamydial disease occurs most frequently in adults between the ages of 18 and 30. The eye disease usually has an acute onset in one eye with watering and mucoid discharge, sticking of lids in the morning, foreign body sensation, hyperemia of the conjunctiva, and sometimes swelling of the lids. On examination, there is a swollen preauricular node, follicular conjunctivitis with easily visible conjunctival lymphoid follicles, and a diffuse inflammatory response with fine tarsal papillae and diffuse infiltration. Superficial keratitis includes fine and larger macropunctate epithelial erosions, subepithelial infiltrates similar to those of epidemic keratoconjunctivitis, limbal infiltration, and superficial neovascularization.

Laboratory procedures to identify chlamydial infections include Giemsa staining of smears; isolation in cell culture; direct fluorescent monoclonal antibodies (DFA) staining (Microtrak, Syva Co.) of smears; enzyme immunoassay (EIA) test (Chlamydiazyme, Abbott Laboratories; Pharmacia EIA; Microtrak, Syva Co.); nucleic acid hybridization assay (Gen. Probe, Pace 2 Chlamydia kit, Gen. probe, San Diego); the Kodak Sure-cel chlamydia test kit (Eastman-Kodak, Rochester, NY), which is particularly useful for occasional cases and does not require special training or equipment; polymerase chain reaction diagnostic tests for chlamydia, which are still under development; and serum antibody levels measured by complement fixation (CF) or microimmunofluorescent (MIF) tests. Microscopic examination of Giemsa-stained conjunctival smears is still very effective in detecting neonatal chlamydial infections because the inclusions are so numerous, but this procedure is less sensitive in adult inclusion conjunctivitis. The DFA and ELISA tests are now widely available in hospital and other laboratories and are highly sensitive for identifying chlamydial infection in the conjunctiva of both adults and neonates. Cell culture techniques are less available, but are highly sensitive and highly specific. The presence of serum IgM antibody against chlamydia in newborns suggests a systemic infection, particularly pneumonia.

THERAPY

Systemic. Because infection is not limited to the eye in either neonatal infants or adults, it is necessary to use systemic antimicrobial treatment. Moreover, the sexual consorts of adults or parents of infants must also receive a full course of therapy. For infants, effective therapy is provided by oral erythromycin, 40 mg/kg daily in four divided doses for a minimum of 2 weeks. Adults with chlamydial eye infections should receive tetracycline or erythromycin. Effective treatment includes daily administration of 1 to 2 gm of tetracycline in four divided doses for 2 to 3 weeks; doxycycline, 100 mg twice daily; and erythromycin in doses of 1 to 1.5 gm daily in four divided doses for 2 to 3 weeks. The use of erythromycin estolate or ethylsuccinate is known to carry a high risk of toxic hepatitis, and erythromycin is also generally less well tolerated than oral tetracyclines. Azithromycin, an analogue of erythromycin, is very long acting and, treatment with a single 1-gm dose is now recommended for adults with genital infections, but a higher dose may be needed for chlamydial conjunctivitis. One gram daily for 5 days should be effective in adults, however. Because oral sulfonamides must be given for at least 3 weeks to be effective, they have a high risk of producing systemic sensitivity.

Ocular. Local antimicrobial treatment with tetracycline or erythromycin ointment to the eye is not necessary for patients on full oral therapeutic doses of antibiotics. It has been shown that the topical treatment alone is extremely slow and only partially effective in treating adult or neonatal inclusion conjunctivitis, and relapses are frequent. Topical sulfonamide alone is even less effective than topical tetracyclines or erythromycin. Moreover, because the infection is systemic, local therapy alone should be discouraged. For the occasional adult patient who develops an anterior iritis with inclusion conjunctivitis, the use of topical corticosteroids carries no more risk than to any other patient, as long as the patient is under systemic treatment with antimicrobials or has received a full course of systemic treatment. When used without systemic antichlamydials, topical corticosteroids are definitely not indicated for the treatment of the conjunctivitis or keratitis even when combined with topical antimicrobial therapy, because that regimen simply results in prolongation of the disease.

Topical rifampin* ointment has been used in the treatment of ocular chlamydial infections but, as with all topical antimicrobials, is of limited use. Moreover, rifampin and its derivatives are available only for investigational use in the eye in the United States.

Ocular or Periocular Manifestations

Conjunctiva: Cicatrization (rare); follicular conjunctivitis, hyperemia; marked papillary infiltration.
Cornea: Anterior stromal opacities; diffuse, fine punctate, or macropunctate keratitis; marginal infiltration; pannus ulcer (rare); vascularization.
Eyelids: Edema.
Other: Anterior uveitis; irritation.

PRECAUTIONS

Anterior uveitis that is nongranulomatous and self-limited may develop in patients with HLA B27 positive lymphocytes, apparently as a response to chlamydial infection. The uveitis does not respond to antimicrobial treatment for the conjunctival disease, but can be readily suppressed with adequate doses of topical corticosteroids. Recurrent episodes of uveitis occur with this syndrome, but they are unrelated to chlamydial infection.

Conjunctival scar formation may result in patients who receive prolonged courses of topical corticosteroids without appropriate antimicrobial therapy.

COMMENTS

For the prophylaxis of chlamydial ophthalmia in newborns, tetracycline or erythromycin ointment is not significantly more effective than Credé prophylaxis with 1 per cent silver nitrate.

References

Beem MO, Saxon EM: Respiratory-tract colonization and a distinctive pneumonia syndrome in infants infected with *Chlamydia trachomatis*. N Engl J Med 296:306–310, 1977.

Dawson CR, et al: Inclusion conjunctivitis and Reiter's syndrome in a married couple. *Chlamydial* infections in series of both diseases. Arch Ophthalmol 83:300–306, 1970.

Grossman M, et al: Prospective studies in chlamydia in newborns. *In* Mardh P (ed): Chlamydial Infections. Amsterdam, Elsevier Biomedical, 1982.

Mordhorst CH, Dawson C: Sequelae of neonatal inclusion conjunctivitis and associated disease in parents. Am J Ophthalmol 71:861–867, 1971.

Schachter J, Dawson CR: Human Chlamydial Infections. Littleton, MA, Publishing Sciences Group, 1978.

Schachter J, Moncada J, Dawson CR, Sheppard J, Courtright P, Said ME, Zaki S, Hafez F, Lorincz A: Nonculture methods for diagnosing chlamydial infection in patients with trachoma: A clue to the pathogenesis of the disease? J Infect Dis 158(6):1347–1352, 1988.

Sexually transmitted diseases. Treatment guidelines 1985. MMWR 34(4S):75S–108S, 1985.

Warren R, Dwyer B, Plackett M, et al: Comparative evaluation of detection assays for *Chlamydia trachomatis*. J Clin Microbiol 31:1663–1666, 1993.

TRACHOMA 076

N. D. VISWALINGAM, M.B.B.S., D.O., *and* S. DAROUGAR, M.D., D.T.M.&H., F.R.C.Path., D.Sc.

London, England

Trachoma, a chronic keratoconjunctivitis, is the most common cause of ocular morbidity and preventable blindness in the world. It is a major public health problem in the rural population of developing countries, particularly in Africa and Asia. The World Health Organization has estimated that 500 million people have trachoma and that approximately five million are blind because of its complications. Recent data suggest that, in most countries of the Middle East, trachoma is no longer a major public health problem because of improvements in the economy, standards of living, hygiene, and health care and the introduction of trachoma control and prevention of blindness programs.

Trachoma is generally caused by *Chlamydia trachomatis* serovars A,B,Ba, and C. *Chlamydia trachomatis*, a member of the Chlamydiaceae family, are gram-negative, obligate intracellular bacteria. Other important members of the *C. trachomatis* species are *C. trachomatis* serovars D to K, which cause genital infections and sexually associated ocular infections. *C. trachomatis* D to K serovars can occasionally cause signs similar to trachoma, i.e., follicular conjunctivitis with pannus and/or conjunctival scarring.

In rural populations, trachoma is generally asymptomatic or causes mild symptoms that patients accept without complaint. In more sophisticated urban populations, patients with active trachoma may complain of watering, mucopurulent discharge, redness, swelling of the lids, ptosis, irritation, foreign body sensation, and itching in one or both eyes. In advanced cases of trachoma with severe conjunctival scarring and keratitis, patients may complain of having thick lids, dry eyes, moderate to severe foreign body sensation, and blurred vision.

Clinical signs develop in lids, the bulbar and palpebral conjunctiva, the limbus, and the cornea. The lids may become mildly swollen and erythematous. The bulbar conjunctiva may show a mild redness, edema (chemosis), and vascular congestion. Occasionally follicles may develop in the upper and lower fornices.

Signs in the palpebral conjunctiva include hyperemia, diffuse infiltration, papillae, follicles, and scars. Papillary response is more severe in the upper and lower tarsal conjunctiva. During the early stage, papillae may present as small red dots. In the advanced stage, the papillae may become much larger, each consisting of a dense collection of inflammatory cells around congested vessels.

Follicles that present as round, elevated, and avascular lesions may occur in the whole conjunctiva. Follicle size varies between 0.2 and 3 mm in diameter. In the upper and lower tarsus, they appear as small yellowish-to-gray white spots against a red background. In the upper and lower fornices, the follicular response is more severe and follicles are larger. The follicles are made up of a dense collection of lymphocytes and monocytes and, to a lesser degree, plasma cells and macrophages. In fully developed follicles (mature), the inflammatory cells are organized around a germinal center.

Conjunctival scars commonly occur in advanced cases of trachoma. In mild cases, scars present as a fine focal area or are stellate or linear. In more severe cases, diffuse or synechial scars may develop. Patients with severe scarring are likely to develop trichiasis and entropion.

At the limbus, vascular congestion, edema, follicles, and Herbert's pits may develop. Follicles are generally small and transient, but occasionally large follicles occur in a row over the corneal-scleral border. After their rupture, a unique depression called Herbert's pits develops.

Corneal signs in trachoma include epithelial and subepithelial punctate keratitis, diffuse infiltration, pannus, and scars. Epithelial punctate keratitis (EPK) is generally small and commonly occurs in the upper half of the cornea in association with pannus. Subepithelial punctate keratitis (SEPK) is coarse and sometimes visible to the naked eye. The SEPK is similar to that seen in chlamydial ocular infection that is sexually transmitted and in adenovirus SEPK.

The pannus consists of epithelial vascularization and associated diffuse infiltration and EPK. The size of the pannus varies in relation to the severity and course of trachoma. In the early stage it is small and only detectable by slit-lamp examination, although in florid cases its size may be about 2 to 3 mm and it is generally associated with cloudiness. The pannus is more prominent in the upper half of the cornea, but it can occur in the lower half of the cornea.

The potentially blinding complications of trachoma are severe scarring of the tarsal conjunctiva, severe subconjunctival and peritarsal fibrosis, trichiasis, entropion, and dry eye. Trichiasis and entropion may cause corneal erosion resulting in ulceration, corneal scarring, and an eventual loss of vision. These complications generally occur in the older age group, particularly in mothers with several young children suffering from active trachoma.

Trachoma may present in different clinical forms. In infants it presents as moderate to severe papillary conjunctivitis similar to bacterial conjunctivitis. In older babies (over 6 months old) some follicles may develop in the upper or lower fornix. In areas with a high prevalence of moderate or severe trachoma, classical trachoma—follicular conjunctivitis with pannus and/or scarring—develops in children. In older, school-aged children and adolescents, follicular conjunctivitis is commonly associated with advanced pannus and conjunctival scarring.

Clinical diagnosis of classical forms of trachoma is based on the presence of follicles on the upper tarsal conjunctiva with either pannus, conjunctival scarring, or Herbert's pits. In atypical trachoma—that is, papillary or follicular conjunctivitis without pannus or conjunctival scarring—other conditions considered in the differential diagnosis include bacterial conjunctivitis; other forms of chlamydial conjunctivitis; viral conjunctivitis, particularly adenovirus and herpes simplex virus conjunctivitis; allergic conjunctivitis; follicu-

losis, which is common in young children; and toxic follicular conjunctivitis caused by topically applied drugs and eye cosmetics.

Laboratory tests are not required for the diagnosis of classical trachoma. However, they are useful for the diagnosis of atypical forms of the disease in individual cases, for epidemiologic studies, and for assessing the efficacy of treatment or control measures. Useful laboratory techniques include the following:

Cell culture for isolation of *Chlamydia trachomatis*, which is considered to be the gold standard test

Direct detection of chlamydial inclusions or elementary bodies in conjunctival smears (DFA) using fluorescein-labeled monoclonal antibody

Direct detection of *Chlamydia* in clinical specimens using enzyme immunoassays (EIA); the sensitivity of DFA and EIA for the diagnosis of chlamydial infection is slightly lower than the culture tests

DNA hybridization test and polymerase chain reaction test, which are highly sensitive for detecting chlamydial antigens; they are considered to be more useful for epidemiologic and immunopathologic studies of trachoma than for diagnosis because of their complexity and cost

Serologic tests: The presence of specific antibodies to *C. trachomatis* A to C in blood or local discharges (tears) indicates exposure to trachoma agents and may assist in the diagnosis of atypical trachoma. The micro-immunofluorescence test using pools of *C. trachomatis* A,B,C; *C. trachomatis* D to K; and representatives of *C. pneumoniae* and *C. psittacci* is the method of choice. This test detects type- or subspecies-specific antibodies and can differentiate between antibodies to *C. trachomatis* A to C (causing trachoma) and *C. trachomatis* D to K (causing genital infection and associated ocular infection) and *C. pneumoniae*. It is shown that up to 50 per cent of the population of developed and developing countries may have antibodies to *C. pneumoniae*.

THERAPY

C. trachomatis is highly sensitive to tetracyclines, erythromycin and related macrolides, and rifampin and, to a lesser degree, to sulfonamides.

Topical. Continuous topical therapy with tetracyclines (chlortetracycline, oxytetracycline, or tetracycline), rifampin, or erythromycin eye ointment, three times daily for 6 weeks, is effective. The ophthalmic solution may require five daily applications for 8 weeks. In the rural areas, patient compliance is poor due to their inability to apply ointment and the ointment's adverse reactions.

Systemic. Trachoma is effectively treated with oral antibiotics. A 3-week course of 15 mg/kg of body weight of tetracycline or erythromycin (divided into four doses) or 1.5 mg/kg of doxycycline (one dose daily) or 30 mg/kg of sulfamethoxazole (divided in four doses) is recommended. In babies and preschool children, a 3-week course of systemic erythromycin, 50 mg/kg of body weight daily (divided in four doses), in syrup should be used.

Chemotherapy when applied properly and diligently will cure most cases of trachoma in an urban setting. However, in rural settings, it is advisable to treat other family members simultaneously to prevent reinfection.

New macrolides, such as azythromycin, have been shown to be highly effective against chlamydial genital infections. Studies are in progress to evaluate their efficacy in chlamydial ocular infections.

Surgical. Trichiasis and entropion are the major blinding complications of trachoma. Several lid operations are available to correct these lid deformities. However, the effectiveness of these lid operations in rural settings is not very high.

PRECAUTIONS

Topical tetracycline or rifampin eye ointment may cause irritation, allergic responses, or temporary blurring of vision. The concurrent topical application of corticosteroids is not recommended because of hazards associated with the topical use of steroids. Corticosteroids may mask signs and symptoms of trachoma, and rebound of the disease may occur when they are discontinued.

Oral tetracycline should not be given to babies, preschool children, and pregnant women.

COMMENTS

In rural communities with a high prevalence of blinding trachoma, continuous topical or systemic treatment of all individuals is not feasible. The World Health Organization recommends an intermittent topical treatment in which tetracycline eye ointment is applied twice daily for 5 consecutive days for each of 6 months. This method of therapy is designed to reduce the severity of the disease and the shedding of infectious agents, hence interrupting the transmission of trachoma. However, in recent studies on the prevention and control of trachoma, the failure rate of intermittent topical therapy of mass populations

was found to be very high. This may have been due to the inability or unwillingness of parents to use the eye ointment properly and regularly in their own eyes and in the eyes of their children, lack of supervision in most villages, spoilage of ointment because of excessive heat and melting of the base, and exchange of ointment with other families. For moderate to severe trachoma, the results of pilot projects using an oral dosage of 5 mg/kg of doxycycline or 35 mg/kg of sulfalene[+] once monthly for 6 to 8 months or once weekly for 3 weeks were as effective as the intermittent therapy using tetracycline eye ointment. These drugs were administered by health workers who treated considerable numbers of patients daily. Although the initial cost of the drug was rather high, the reduction of trachoma and the very low failure rate make this regimen cost effective. In these studies, there were no serious side effects, but minor side effects, such as nausea, vomiting, and skin rashes, were observed in about 5 per cent of patients. Parenteral vaccination gives partial or temporary protection from trachoma, but may cause hypersensitivity of the eye and exacerbation of clinical signs.

References

Al-Rifai KM: Trachoma through history. Int Ophthalmol 12:9–14, 1988.

Darougar S, Jones BR: Trachoma. Br Med Bull 39: 117–122, 1983.

Darougar S, et al: Family-based suppressive intermittent therapy of hyperendemic trachoma with topical oxytetracycline or oral doxycycline. Br J Ophthalmol 64:291–295, 1980.

Darougar S, et al: Topical therapy of hyperendemic trachoma using rifampicin, oxytetracycline, or spiramycin eye ointments. Br J Ophthalmology 64:37–42, 1980.

Darougar S, et al: A double-blind comparison of topical therapy of chlamydial ocular infection (TRIC infection) with rifampicin or chlortetracycline. Br J Ophthalmol 65:549–552, 1981.

Dawson CR, Jones BR, Tarizzo ML: Guide to Trachoma Control. Geneva, World Health Organization, 1981.

Jones BR: The prevention of blindness from trachoma. Trans Ophthalmol Soc UK 95:16–33, 1975.

Olson CM: In herpes or chlamydial infections, immune response may be key factor in lost vision [news]. JAMA 261:819–820, 1989.

Schachter J, Moncada J, Dawson CR, Sheppard J, Courtright P, Said ME, Zaki S, Hafiz SF, Lorincz A: Non-culture methods for diagnosing chlamydial infection in patients with trachoma: A clue to the pathogenesis of the disease? J Infect Dis 158:1347–1352, 1988.

Tabbara KF, Cooper H: Minocycline levels in tears of patients with active trachoma. Arch Ophthalmol 107:93–95, 1989.

Treharne JD: The microbial epidemiology of trachoma. Int Ophthalmol 12:25–29, 1988.

Mycotic Infections

ACTINOMYCOSIS 039.9

BENJAMIN MILDER, M.D.

St. Louis, Missouri

Actinomycosis is a noncontagious infection caused by a group of organisms, the *Actinomyces*. The disease is often described as a mycotic infection, although this anaerobic organism is not a true fungus. The species most often identified in ocular disease is the *Actinomyces israelii*.

Actinomycosis is usually acquired by chewing on or otherwise making contact with contaminated straw or hay. Thus, it is a disease of rural settings and is transmitted to the orbit and ocular structures by way of the mouth or nasal passages.

The principal sites of actinomycosis are cutaneous, cervicofacial, thoracic, and abdominal. In the facial area, the buccal cavity, teeth, and mandible are most commonly involved. Invasion of the lacrimal system is usually unaccompanied by other concurrent clinical manifestations of actinomycosis.

THERAPY

Systemic. Significant improvement in actinomycosis patients may be expected when either penicillin or tetracycline antibiotics are administered in high doses over long periods of time. The tetracyclines are the drugs of choice for oral administration, administered in dosages of 500 mg every 6 hours. Minocycline dosage is 100 mg every 12 hours. A suitable alternative is penicillin G, which may be administered topically*, subconjunctivally*, or systemically. In severe infections, adequate therapeutic levels require intramuscular or intravenous administration. Daily recommended dosages are 25,000 to 50,000 units/kg in divided doses every 4 hours. The treatment should be continued for several weeks after clinical cure.

Ocular. For corneal ulcers, therapeutic concentrations can be obtained rapidly by the subconjunctival route. The recommended dosage is 0.5 to 1 million units of penicillin G*.

Natamycin has been used for the topical treatment of blepharitis, conjunctivitis, and keratitis of mycotic origin, particularly if the fungus has not been identified. However, if *Actinomyces* is known to be the causative agent, the drug of choice is sodium penicillin G, used as eye drops* in a concentration of 500,000 units/ml.

Surgical. Aspiration or surgical drainage is a valuable adjunct to the chemotherapy of actinomycotic lesions of the lids and orbit. Since the larger orbital lesions tend to be "honeycombed," care must be taken to ensure that the incision is adequate and pockets of abscess are opened.

In *Actinomyces* canaliculitis, small concretions can be expressed through the punctum by massaging the canaliculus. However, since this form of canaliculitis tends to be resistant to therapy, the definitive cure may require slitting the canaliculus to remove the concretions and the infected mucosal lining. It is essential that the slitting be limited to the horizontal limb of the canaliculus as far as the ampulla and that this be performed on the conjunctival aspect of the lid, not on the lid margin. The punctum should never be included in such an incision. The canaliculus, thus opened, is curetted to remove infected mucosa. It is not necessary to close the canaliculotomy wound with sutures. Surgical excision of firm nodules in the subconjunctival tissues may also be indicated.

Ocular or Periocular Manifestations

Anterior Chamber: Hypopyon.

Conjunctiva: Angular, catarrhal, or pseudomembranous conjunctivitis; mucopurulent discharge; ulcer; yellow nodules.

Eyelids: Abscess; fibrosis; yellow nodules.

Iris: Anterior uveitis secondary to keratitis and corneal ulceration.

Lacrimal System: Canaliculitis with fullness in the region of the canaliculus, pouting of the punctum and creamy pus exuding from the punctum, often with "sulfur granules"; dacryocystitis (rare).

Orbit: Abscess; infiltration; proptosis.

PRECAUTIONS

Older methods, such as irradiation and sulfonamides, have not been shown to be effective in the treatment of actinomycosis. Amphotericin B also is of no value. When the canaliculus has been opened and curetted, one "old-fashioned" remedy that may still be of value is the application of tincture of iodine to destroy the remaining canalicular mucosa.

COMMENTS

Actinomycosis is disappearing because of the wide use of modern therapeutic agents. Such drugs as the penicillins and tetracyclines are now used prophylactically after dental extraction and in other conditions that might evolve into actinomycosis. However, the disease still exists, especially in the rural Midwest.

Actinomycosis tends to run an extremely chronic course, but spontaneous resolution has been reported even after many months. Favorable prognosis in the cervicofacial forms is directly related to early diagnosis and specific therapy based on microscopic confirmation of the organism.

REFERENCES

Bennett JE: Actinomycosis. In Isselbacher KJ, et al (eds): Harrison's Principles of Internal Medicine, 9th ed. New York, McGraw-Hill, 1980, pp 734–735.

Blanksma LJ, Slijper J: Actinomycotic dacryocystitis. Ophthalmologica 176:145–149, 1978.

Bohigian GM: Handbook of External Diseases of the Eye. Fort Worth, Alcon, 1980, p 163.

Korting GW: The Skin and Eye: A Dermatologic Correlation of Diseases of the Periorbital Region. Philadelphia, WB Saunders, 1973, pp 52–54.

Leigh RJ, Good EF, Rudy RP: Ophthalmoplegia due to actinomycosis. J Clin Neuro-Ophthalmol 6:157–159, 1986.

Seal DV, et al: Lacrimal canaliculitis due to Arachnia (Actinomyces) propionica. Br J Ophthalmol 65:10–13, 1981.

ASPERGILLOSIS 117.3

GARY P. BARTH, M.D.

Santa Rosa, California

Aspergillosis is a systemic infection caused by the ubiquitous saprophytic, *Aspergillus* fungi. In most cases, the respiratory system serves as the portal of entry.

The disease is prevalent in the southern United States, India, and Africa. Its frequency is highest among grain farmers and feeders or breeders of poultry or pigeons. Ocular and orbital involvement is rare and may be associated with complications of infected sinuses, trauma, surgery, intravenous drug abuse, or immunosuppression. Occasionally, it has no known cause. Infection reaches the orbit by direct extension and is characterized by chronic nonnecrotizing, granulomatous inflammation and fibrosis. Orbital aspergillosis is characterized by slowly progressive unilateral proptosis, ocular pain, and decreased vision. Keratomycosis due to *Aspergillus* accounts for nearly 50 per cent of all reported cases of oculomycosis.

THERAPY

Systemic. Amphotericin B is the most reliable drug for the treatment of aspergillosis. However, because of its toxicity, an intravenous test dose of 1.0 mg dissolved in 50 to 150 ml of 5 per cent dextrose in water should be given. The dose can then be progressively increased in 5- to 10-mg increments to a daily maximum of 0.5 to 0.6 mg/kg. Fulminant infections can be treated with daily doses as high as 0.8 to 1.0 mg/kg during the first 2 weeks.

Rifampin[‡] has shown activity against *Aspergillus* when used in combination with the detergent effects of amphotericin B. The antimetabolite flucytosine also acts synergistically with amphotericin B. An oral dose of 37.5 mg/kg of flucytosine[‡] every 6 hours may be used in combination with 0.3 mg/kg of intravenous amphotericin B daily.

Synthetic imidazoles have been found to be variably effective against many *Aspergillus* infections. A single daily dose of 0.4 to 1.0 gm of ketoconazole[‡] may be administered orally. Miconazole[‡] may be given intravenously in doses of 10 to 15 mg/kg every 8 hours.

Systemic steroids may be necessary in visual loss and proptosis caused by allergic *Aspergillus* sinusitis.

Ocular. Five per cent natamycin ophthalmic suspension is available for the treatment of *Aspergillus* corneal infection. Natamycin is similar to amphotericin B in its activity against *Aspergillus*, but is more stable in suspension and much less irritating to the conjunctiva. Amphotericin B* in a 0.1 to 0.3 per cent suspension can be used until natamycin can be obtained. In severe cases, either drug can be used hourly for the first 48 hours.

In cases refractory to natamycin therapy, 1 or 2 per cent miconazole* can be substituted. Four per cent thiabendazole* or 1 per cent clotrimazole* has also been reported to be effective against *Aspergillus* infections.

Subconjunctival injection of 1 mg of amphotericin B and intravitreal doses of 5-10 μg of amphotericin B have been used in *Aspergillus* endophthalmitis, but the risk of retinal toxicity has not been established.

Surgical. Orbital involvement with *Aspergillus* is a life-threatening problem. Prompt medical therapy should be combined with surgical drainage. In a corneal ulcer caused by *Aspergillus*, débridement of the fungal growth may allow better penetration of antifungal drops. A penetrating keratoplasty may be required in cases that are refractory to medical therapy. In cases with intraocular *Aspergillus* a vitrectomy may be necessary.

Ocular or Periocular Manifestations

Anterior chamber: White mass.
Cornea: Abscess; keratitis; keratoconjunctivitis.
Globe: Endophthalmitis; choroidal infarct; retinal detachment; posterior ischemic neuropathy; central retinal artery occlusion.
Lacrimal system: Canaliculitis; dacryocystitis.
Orbit: Proptosis, abscess.

PRECAUTIONS

Proper diagnostic procedures are essential for establishing the diagnosis of *Aspergillus* infection. In suspected *Aspergillus* keratitis, at least six to eight scrapings with a Kimura spatula from the bed of the infection are needed. Intravitreal and anterior chamber aspirates should be concentrated by the use of a filter or by centrifugation. Orbital biopsy material should be plated soon after collection, since *Aspergillus* is a ubiquitous organism and false-positive results could occur if the specimen were to remain unnecessarily exposed. If the organism can be cultured, either Sabouraud's media (Emmon's modification) or blood agar will usually be positive within 48 hours. Blood cultures are routinely negative even in fulminant cases. Gram, Giemsa, and Grocett's methanemine-silver stains are better than potassium hydroxide for detecting the branching septated hyphae. Specific antifungal treatment should be withheld until a diagnosis of a fungal infection can be established. Once antifungal therapy has been initiated, negative scrapings do not indicate elimination of the infection.

Medical therapy of aspergillosis is made more difficult by the poor ocular penetration of most drugs, the toxicity associated with their use, the length of time that therapy must be continued, and the lack of published studies documenting their effectiveness. The poor ocular penetration and toxicity preclude systemic use of drugs in *Aspergillus* keratitis. Side effects may include a dose-related febrile reaction, anorexia, nausea, decreased weight, hypokalemia, thrombophlebitis, bone marrow depression, and nephrotoxicity. Natamycin in drop form is well tolerated, but may produce necrosis and granulomas following subconjunctival injection. Flucytosine can cause rash, gastrointestinal intolerance, hepatic dysfunction, and leukopenia. Ketoconazole has been known to cause nausea, rash, pruritus, and severe hepatitis. Patients treated with ketoconazole should have their liver enzymes and liver function tests monitored regularly. Miconazole can cause pruritus, phlebitis, thrombocytosis, hyperlipidemia, and hyponatremia. Since cardiorespiratory arrest has been associated with the first intravenous dose of miconazole, the initial dose is best administered by the physician.

COMMENTS

Therapy of *Aspergillus* infections is often complicated by a delay in diagnosis, the previous use of corticosteroids, and the long-term use of the antifungal medications. In vitro sensitivity tests are not completely reliable and should serve only as a guide to the clinical response. When a penetrating keratoplasty is performed, the subsequent use of corticosteroids should be delayed as long as possible to prevent reactivation of the fungus.

References

Denning DW, Stevens DA: Antifungal and surgical treatment of invasive aspergillosis. Rev Infect Dis 12:1147–1169, 1990.

Dunlop IS, Billson FA: Visual failure in allergic *Aspergillus* sinusitis: Case report. Br J Ophthalmol 72:127–130, 1988.
Jampol LM, et al: Retinal and choroidal infarction from *Aspergillus*: Clinical diagnosis and clinicopathologic correlations. Trans Am Ophthalmol Soc. 86:442–435, 1988.
Harris GJ, Will BR: Orbital *Aspergillosis*. Ophthalmol Plast Reconstr Surg,5:207–211, 1989.
O'Day DM, et al: The evaluation of therapeutic responses in experimental keratomycosis. Curr Eye Res 11:35–44, 1992.
Roney P, et al: Endogenous *Aspergillus* endophthalmitis. Rev Infect Dis 8:955–958, 1986.
Sihota R, et al: *Aspergillus* endophthalmitis. Br J Ophthalmol 71: 611–613, 1987.
Vitale AT, et al: Orbital *Aspergillosis* in an immunocompromised hosts Am J Ophthalmol 113: 725–726, 1992.
Weinstein JM, et al: Posterior ischemic optic neuropathy due to *Aspergillus fumigatus*. Clin Neuro-Ophthalmol 9:7–13, 1989.

BLASTOMYCOSIS 116.0

REGAN A. LOGAN, M.D., and DENIS M. O'DAY, M.D.

Nashville, Tennessee

Blastomycosis, a chronic fungal disease caused by *Blastomyces dermatitidis*, produces granulomatous lesions that may involve any part of the body, with a predilection for the skin, lung, and bones. Ocular involvement can occur by direct extension from lesions involving the face and eyelids or by hematogenous dissemination from a primary pulmonary lesion. The lids seem to be the ocular structure that is most commonly involved in blastomycosis. Intraocular involvement is rare, with only nine cases being reported in the world literature.

THERAPY

Systemic. All forms of extrapulmonary blastomycosis should be treated systemically. Severely ill patients are treated with amphotericin B. Before the intravenous administration of amphotericin B, an initial test injection should be given over a period of 2 to 4 hours in a dosage of 1 mg in 250 ml of 5 per cent dextrose in water. This dose is then gradually increased in 2- to 5-mg increments every 24 hours until a daily dose of 30 to 40 mg is reached. This dosage is then administered until a total dose of 2 gm is achieved.

In an attempt to avoid the toxic effects of amphotericin B, oral antimycotic agents have been investigated. Non-life-threatening blastomycosis can be treated with oral ketoconazole 400 mg/day for six months. Itraconazole has shown promise in the treatment of blastomycosis and may soon be another alternative to amphotericin B. The efficacy of fluconazole in blastomycosis has not been studied sufficiently to make recommendations and comparative studies are needed.

Ocular. Amphotericin B can be administered topically using an intravenous preparation diluted to a concentration of 0.15 per cent. Optimal dosing frequency is not known. Subconjunctival injection of amphotericin B has been poorly tolerated.

Miconazole is tolerated by subconjunctival injection at a daily dose of 5 mg of undiluted intravenous preparation.* It may be administered topically as a 1 per cent solution* prepared from the intravenous form of the drug and given hourly.

Ketoconazole can also be administered as a topical preparation at 1 to 5 per cent concentrations. The optimal dosing frequency is not known.

Surgical. Surgical drainage of lid or orbit abscesses may be indicated with antifungal therapy given before and after surgery.

Ocular or Periocular Manifestations

Anterior Chamber. Hypopyon.
Choroid: Focal choroiditis.
Cornea: Descemetocele; perforation; stromal keratitis; ulcer.
Eyelids: Abscess leading to cicatrization; entropion; papules; pustules.
Iris: Anterior uveitis; nodules.
Orbit: Abscess; cellulitis.

PRECAUTIONS

Intravenous usage of amphotericin B may result in two types of reactions: idiosyncratic and dose related. Idiosyncratic reactions occur rarely, but can be lethal and include grand mal seizures, vertigo, flushing and anaphylaxis, thrombocytopenia, acute liver failure, generalized pain, ventricular fibrillation, and cardiac arrest. Dose-related side effects, which are more common, include anemia, hypokalemia, fever, and chills. Less commonly, leukopenia, thrombocytopenia, renal failure, thrombophlebitis, nausea and vomiting, anorexia, and headaches may occur. Topical application of amphotericin B may result in burning, chemosis, epithelial clouding, and punctate epithelial erosions.

The toxic effects of intravenous ketoconazole are less severe, with nausea and vomiting being the most common. Rarely, ketoconazole may cause hepatocellular damage, and liver transaminase levels should be monitored during therapy. When administered topically, ketoconazole is well tolerated.

Miconazole administered topically or by subconjunctival injection has shown minimal toxicity. Because the adverse reactions to intravenous miconazole are frequent and severe, this drug is rarely administered intravenously.

COMMENTS

Ocular infection with blastomycosis is so rare that the most appropriate therapy remains an unsettled question. In those instances where corneal involvement occurs, consideration should be given to the topical administration of miconazole in combination with systemic therapy. Experience with infection in other tissues indicates that treatment should be for a prolonged period. There is some evidence that an impaired cell-mediated immunity facilitates infections with *B. dermatitidis*. This has been observed especially in children. In such circumstances, attention to appropriate parenteral alimentations is an important prerequisite for a return to normal immunologic function.

References

Barr CC, Gamel JW: Blastomycosis of the eyelid. Arch Ophthalmol *104*:96–97, 1986.
Bradsher RW: Blastomycosis. Clin Infect Dis *14*: S82–90, 1992.
Chesney JC, et al: Pulmonary blastomycosis in children. Amphotericin B therapy and a review. Am J Dis Child *133*:1134–1139, 1979.
Fitzsimmons RB, Ferguson AC: Cellular immunity and nutrition in refractory disseminated blastomycosis. Can Med Assoc J *119*:343–346, 1978.
Johns KJ, O'Day DM: Pharmacologic management of keratomycosis. Surv Ophthalmol *33*:178–188, 1988.
Lewis H, et al: Latent disseminated blastomycosis with choroidal involvement. Arch Ophthalmol *106*:527–530, 1988.
Rodrigues MM, Laibson P, Kaplan W: Exogenous mycotic keratitis caused by *Blastomyces dermatitidis*. Am J Ophthalmol *75*:782–789, 1973.
Safnek JR, Hogg GR, Napier LB: Endophthalmitis due to *Blastomyces dermatitidis*: Case report and review of the literature. Ophthalmology *97*:212–216, 1990.
Vida L, Moel SA: Systemic North American blastomycosis with orbital involvement. Am J Ophthalmol *77*:240–242, 1974.

CANDIDIASIS 112.9

C. STEPHEN FOSTER, M.D., F.A.C.S.

Boston, Massachusetts

Candidiasis, an infection caused by the yeast fungus family of *Candida*, may occur as a result of local or generalized infection by any member of this family; *Candida albicans* is by far the most common species identified in cases of human candidiasis. When the infection is local in such sites as the vagina, mouth, or skin, the clinical problem is not usually life threatening and frequently responds rapidly to local, appropriate antifungal therapy. However, local candidiasis in vital structures and in the eye or systemic infections caused by *Candida* are frequently considerably more devastating.

Generalized candidiasis is uncommon, but may occur in two settings: (1) systemic dissemination in drug addicts, in the debilitated patient, or in the immunosuppressed patient and (2) chronic mucocutaneous candidiasis (CMCC), a distinct clinical entity involving immune and/or immunoregulatory dysfunctions. Four groups of CMCC have been described: early CMCC, late-onset CMCC, familial CMCC, and juvenile familial polyendocrinopathy with candidiasis. Early CMCC is the most severe form; in addition to the persistent *Candida* colonization of the skin, hair, nails, and mucous membranes, *Candida* granulomata form and produce substantial disfiguring of the patient. Approximately half of the patients with early CMCC also have some form of endocrinopathy, such as hypoparathyroidism, diabetes mellitus, Addison's disease, or hypothyroidism. Late-onset CMCC is the mildest form of chronic mucocutaneous candidiasis, with clinical involvement usually only of the oral cavity and occasionally the nails. As the name implies, this form of the disease typically is seen in elderly individuals. Familial CMCC is transmitted as an autosomal recessive trait and is usually not associated with endocrinopathy. The disease is mild to moderate in severity. Juvenile familial polyendocrinopathy with candidiasis is characterized by mild to moderate candidiasis and endocrinopathy, usually in the form of hypoparathyroidism or Addison's disease. Other disorders not infrequently seen in patients with CMCC are pernicious anemia, iron-deficiency anemia, chronic active hepatitis, ovarian dysfunction, and keratoconjunctivitis.

The immunologic defects most commonly found in patients with CMCC include anergy to *Candida* antigen, impaired in vitro lymphocyte responsiveness to stimulation with *Candida* antigens (impaired blastogenic transformation and impaired lymphokine production), and occasional elaboration of serum factors (usually antibodies) that inhibit lymphocyte responsiveness to *Candida* antigens in vitro, even from normal donors.

Ocular involvement with *Candida* infestation may occur as a result of local inoculation or from endogenous colonization. Any part of the eye may be affected. Local inoculation most typically results in *Candida* keratitis, although *Candida* conjunctivitis, blepharitis, canaliculitis, or dacryocystitis may occur. Endogenous spread usually results in retinitis, uveitis, and/or endophthalmitis.

THERAPY

Systemic. Ketoconazole is the current therapy of choice for chronic mucocutaneous candidiasis, is probably also a useful component in the therapeutic management of patients with disseminated systemic candidiasis, and is a useful adjunct in the treatment of patients with keratomycosis. Oral administration of 200 to 400 mg of ketoconazole daily results in relatively high levels of penetration into the cornea and aqueous humor.

Flucytosine likewise penetrates the ocular structures relatively well after oral administration. The usual oral daily dose of flucytosine is 150 mg/kg in divided doses. Most *Candida* isolates are usually quite sensitive to flucytosine, but resistance can develop relatively rapidly, particularly if the administered dose is suboptimal.

Amphotericin B is an additional agent that may be used systemically in candidiasis therapy. Amphotericin B may be given by slow intravenous infusion under specific guidelines, primarily for patients with progressive and potentially fatal infections.

Fluconazole, a newer antifungal agent (see below), has been used unsuccessfully in the care of patients with systemic candidiasis, and it seems to penetrate the eye after systemic administration.

Ocular. A 5 per cent suspension of natamycin may be administered every 1 to 2 hours for the treatment of a *Candida* corneal ulcer. However, two major problems confront the ophthalmologist who must rely on natamycin. Many *Candida* isolates are not highly sensitive to this drug, and none of the polyene antibiotics, including natamycin, penetrates the ocular structures well. Although these drugs may be effective in curing very superficial ocular surface infections with *Candida*, deeper corneal ulcers frequently do not respond to this therapy.

Two other classes of antifungal agents are considerably more effective in treating infections caused by *Candida*: the imidazoles and flucytosine.

The imidazole agents are usually highly effective against ophthalmic *Candida* infections. Clotrimazole has been successfully used to treat patients with *Candida* corneal ulcers, without evidence of significant ocular toxicity; clotrimazole* cream may be applied eight to twelve times a day for 6 weeks. Miconazole penetrates well into the cornea and anterior chamber after topical or subconjunctival administration. Undiluted 1 per cent intravenous miconazole* solution may be applied topically every hour for the treatment of *Candida* keratitis. In addition, subconjunctival injection of 10 mg of miconazole* every 48 hours may also be used for deep *Candida* keratitis. Although intense conjunctival inflammation has been reported after subconjunctival injection of this drug, significant evidence of toxicity was not present.

Fluconazole is marketed as Diflucan tablets (50, 100, and 200 mg) and as intravenous aqueous solution (2 mg/ml). It is a selective inhibitor of fungal cytochrome P-450 sterol

C-14 alpha-demethylation and hence has a re-markable safety record thus far in systemic therapy, primarily of *Candida* or *Cryptococcus* infections.

Topical administration of a 1 per cent so-lution in sterile water and oral administration of 200 to 400 mg per day have been used re-cently in the care of selected patients with ker-atomycosis. Penetration of fluconazole into the cornea is excellent, and this drug, the first of a new class of synthetic bis-triazole com-pounds, is one of the few advances made re-cently in the antifungal field.

None of the antifungal agents penetrates into the vitreous cavity well after systemic ad-ministration, and the intravenous administra-tion of amphotericin B can be associated with substantial undersirable side effects. Side ef-fects can be alleviated with saline loading and every other day therapy. Intravitreal admin-istration of antifungal agents is controversial, but limited data suggest that up to 5 μg of amphotericin B* or 40 μg of miconazole* ad-ministered intravitreally may be a reasonable therapeutic choice for management of *Candida* endophthalmitis with vitreal involvement.

The preferred regimen for the management of *Candida* includes 1 per cent flucytosine* ad-ministered every hour on the hour, alternat-ing with 0.15 per cent amphotericin B every hour on the half hour.

Management of intraocular *Candida* infec-tions may include 150 mg/kg of oral flucy-tosine and intravenous therapy of amphoter-icin B combined with surgical therapy and intraocular antifungal administration.

Surgical. The surgical management of oc-ular *Candida* infections may range from a pro-cedure as mild as periodic expression of the meibomian glands for *Candida* meibomianitis, periodic curettage of the canaliculus for *Can-dida* canaliculitis, and daily scraping débride-ment of *Candida* corneal ulcer to therapeutic penetrating keratoplasty or therapeutic vitrec-tomy. Each of these surgical modalities is im-portant in the adequate care of patients with *Candida* infections of the eye. Curettage of an infected canaliculus, irrigation of an infected lacrimal sac, and frequent expression of in-fected meibomian glands are essential to the successful eradication of *Candida* infections in these regions. Daily débridement of a *Candida* corneal ulcer not only removes necrotic and in-fected material but also enhances the penetra-tion of topically applied antifungal agents.

The decision about the need for and tech-nique of therapeutic penetrating keratoplasty in a case of advanced or progressing *Candida* keratitis is complex. Most ophthalmologists probably delay too long in the face of a wors-ening case of *Candida* corneal ulcer before pro-ceeding with therapeutic penetrating kerato-plasty. The decision to proceed with this therapeutic modality should be made before the process progresses into the anterior cham-ber and extends to the corneal periphery, where total excision of the affected area

would be extremely difficult. Intraocular ex-tensions or the development of "malignant fungal glaucoma" or both are absolute indi-cations for surgical intervention.

The safety and efficacy of therapeutic vit-rectomy for infectious endophthalmitis have not been proven, but there are some obvious theoretical attractions to this therapeutic mo-dality. Some surgeons feel that it is important to remove as much of the "abscess" of in-fected material in the vitreous cavity as pos-sible and to instill antifungal agents locally into the vitreous cavity when *Candida* endoph-thalmitis with vitreous involvement is present.

Ocular or Periocular Manifestations

Anterior Chamber: Cells and flare; hypo-pyon.

Conjunctiva: Cicatrization; follicular, pseu-domembranous, or purulent conjunctivitis; necrotic ulcer; phlyctenulosis.

Cornea: Dendritic, epithelial, or superficial punctate keratitis; opacity; stromal infiltrate, with or without feathery edges and "satellite" lesions; stromal vascularization.

Eyelids: Blepharitis; cheesy material ex-pressible from meibomian glands; eczema; edema; granuloma; hyperemia; pustules.

Globe: Atrophy; endophthalmitis; panoph-thalmitis.

Lacrimal System: Calcareous cast; dacryo-cystitis; epiphora; occlusion of lacrimal canaliculi.

Optic Nerve: Granulation; hyperemia; in-filtration; papillitis; perivasculitis.

Retina: Atrophy; embolism; exudative de-tachment; perivasculitis; Roth's spot; vascular engorgement.

Vitreous: Abscess, cellular reaction; con-densation; fluffy, white exudates.

Other: Decreased visual acuity; hemor-rhages, retrobulbar abscess.

PRECAUTIONS

Although fungi rank behind bacteria and viruses in overall incidence as causes of ocu-lar infections, they often produce greater structural and functional damage to the eye. This is partly due to the fact that fungal in-fections often develop slower and the diag-nosis may be delayed. Also, their propensity to mimic other infections or neoplastic dis-eases is often a problem to the ophthalmolo-gist, and effective treatment may be missed or delayed thereby. Deficiencies of current ocular antifungal agents also limit the opportunity for specific treatment of these micro-organ-isms. Amphotericin B is not a good ocular an-tifungal agent. It is highly irritating and does not reach the anterior chamber in effective levels after parenteral, subconjunctival, or topical administration. There is no evidence to indicate that nystatin is more effective than amphotericin B against *Candida*. Natamycin penetrates the eye so poorly that it is useful only for superficial infections, and it is not the most effective antifungal agent against *Candida*.

It is usually unwise to initiate broad-spectrum antifungal therapy for a suspected fungal ulcer or suspected fungal endophthalmitis. The best defense against eventual confusion in the face of a deteriorating clinical picture in a patient with infectious keratitis or endophthalmitis is an adequate initial diagnostic effort that guarantees the successful isolation of the caustic organism, so that ultimate identification and selection of specific therapy are possible. Therefore, for a corneal ulcer, adequate corneal scrapings for smears and for cultures on multiple media are essential. In suspected endophthalmitis, aqueous or vitreous samples are similarly essential; in any case of aphakic endophthalmitis or vitreal involvement in endophthalmitis, a vitreous tap should be considered mandatory.

COMMENTS

The use of systemic and/or topical corticosteroids in the management of patients with infectious keratitis or endophthalmitis, including those cases caused by *Candida* is controversial. It is clear that corticosteroids can inhibit the host response to the infecting organism and can thereby promote undesirable progression of the infectious process. It also seems clear, however, that excessive inflammatory host responses can be highly destructive and can produce undesirable permanent structural alterations to the eye. Some clinicians believe that it is possible and desirable to modify such excessive host responses with corticosteroids while simultaneously not over-depressing the host immune response, so that adequate eradication of the organism occurs without excessive inflammatory-response-induced tissue destruction. In an animal model of *Candida* keratitis, dosages of topical corticosteroids considerably less than those commercially available were required to achieve such balance. Decisions regarding the appropriate use of corticosteroids in these settings are complex and extremely tricky. At the very least, it should be strongly emphasized that steroid therapy has no place in the management of an ocular infection, unless the causative organism has been isolated and definitively identified and specific therapy to which the organism is sensitive has been instituted. Commercially available topical steroid preparations should probably not be used in the care of patients with keratomycosis.

References

Foster CS: Miconazole therapy for keratomycosis. Am J Ophthalmol 91:622–629, 1981.

Foster CS, et al: Ocular toxicity of topical antifungal agents. Arch Ophthalmol 99:1081–1084, 1981.

Heinenmann MH, Bloom AF, Horowitz J: *Candida*

albicans endophthalmitis in a patient with AIDS. Case report. Arch Ophthalmol 105:1172–1173, 1987.

Insler MS, Urso LF: *Candida albicans* endophthalmitis after penetrating keratoplasty. Am J Ophthalmol 104:57–60, 1987.

Malecaze F, Bessieres MH, Bec P, Fleutiaux S, Mathis A, Sequela JP: Immunologic analysis of the aqueous humour in *Candida* endophthalmitis. I: Experimental study. Br J Ophthalmol 72: 309–312, 1988.

Mathis A, Malecaze F, Bessieres MH, Arne JL, Seguela JP, Bec P: Immunologic analysis of the aqueous humour in *Candida* endophthalmitis II: Clinical study. Br J Ophthalmol 72:313–316, 1988.

Parrish CM, O'Day DM, Hoyle TC: Spontaneous fungal corneal ulcer as an ocular manifestation of AIDS. Am J Ophthalmol 104:302–303, 1987.

Tolentino F, et al: Retinal and lens toxicity studies of intravitreal miconazole. Invest Ophthalmol Vis Sci 19(Suppl):114, 1980.

COCCIDIOIDOMYCOSIS 114.9

JAMES P. GANLEY, M.D., Dr. P.H.,

Shreveport, Louisiana

and STEPHEN A. KLOTZ, M.D.

Kansas City, Kansas

Coccidioidomycosis is an infectious disease caused by *Coccidioides immitis*, a dimorphic fungus whose free-living or saprobic state is restricted to the semi-arid Lower Sonoran life zone. Hence, in the United States, it is endemic to southeast California, southern Arizona and New Mexico, and southwestern Texas. Elsewhere in the Western hemisphere, *C. immitis* can be found in Mexico, Central America, and parts of South America. Primary infection occurs after the inhalation of airborne arthroconidia that transform into spherules, thus beginning the parasitic phase of the fungal life cycle. Primary infection is almost always contained by the host and is often asymptomatic. White women, however, are particularly prone to develop a characteristic syndrome known as "valley fever" or "desert rheumatism." Conjunctivitis or episcleritis, along with erythema nodosum or erythema multiforme and arthritis, is prominent in this syndrome. Individuals with valley fever develop a positive skin test reaction to coccidioidin and simultaneously develop measurable tube precipitin antibodies in the serum. Uncommonly, primary infection is not contained by the host, and progressive cavitary pulmonary disease (typically in men with pre-existing lung disease) or extrapulmonary dissemination of the fungus may occur (in pregnant women, in persons with diabetes mellitus, or in men of dark-skinned races). Patients with impaired cell-mediated immunity caused by such drugs as corticosteroids or concurrent infection with the human immunodeficiency virus are at particular risk for relapsing infection and/or extrapulmonary dissemination. Disseminated disease with *C. immitis* is occasionally the defining opportunistic infection for the diagnosis of AIDS in patients infected with a human immunodeficiency virus. Furthermore, with the advent of the AIDS epidemic, patients with disseminated disease are being treated the world over, far outside the endemic area of *C. immitis*.

Chorioretinal lesions occur in up to 9 per cent of individuals with documented disease; the majority of these lesions are asymptomatic and resolve spontaneously without therapy. No relationship has been associated between the presence of these asymptomatic lesions and the severity of systemic disease. Most documented cases of symptomatic intraocular involvement cause significant visual loss and ocular morbidity; these cases tend to be associated with progressive systemic coccidioidomycosis. The major symptomatic intraocular manifestations are chronic granulomatous iridocyclitis, choroiditis, and retinitis; endophthalmitis has also been described. Posterior ocular involvement is usually focal, but may be diffuse; overlying vitreous reaction varies from only mild involvement to marked turbidity.

Granulomatous lesions of eyebrow, lids, and palpebral conjunctiva have been reported. Anterior segment manifestations, including phlyctenular conjunctivitis, episcleritis, and scleritis, usually occur with primary pulmonary infection and are often associated with erythema nodosum. These manifestations are considered to be hypersensitivity responses to the coccidioidal antigen and usually subside along with the primary infection without treatment. Rarer ocular manifestations of *C. immitis* infection include orbital and optic nerve granulomas and extraocular nerve palsies secondary to intracerebral infection.

THERAPY

Systemic. Amphotericin B remains the drug of choice in the initial treatment of life-threatening disease. Intravenous therapy is indicated in disseminated disease, including progressive periocular and intraocular involvement. Lid granulomata are often associated with other granulomata of the skin and often resolve with amphotericin B therapy. The penetration of amphotericin B into the cerebral spinal fluid occurs at levels below the minimal inhibitory concentration of the drug, but unlike cryptococcal meningitis, which responds to intravenous therapy alone, coccidioidal meningitis requires intrathecal*, intracisternal*, or intraventricular* therapy as well. Amphotericin B binds to ergosterol contained within fungal plasma membranes and in doing so induces membrane defects. It possesses considerable immunoadjuvant effects, as well as antifungal properties. Amphotericin B is administered intravenously in dextrose and water; it precipitates in saline. Premedication with aspirin or acetaminophen and diphenhydramine (or meperidine, if reactions are severe) reduces or eliminates uncomfortable reactions that commonly occur during administration. It is customary to administer a 1 mg test dose in 100 to 200 ml of 5 per cent dextrose in water over 1 to 2 hours; this test dose should be followed with therapeutic doses (up to 0.6 mg/kg) administered over 4 to 6 hours. If nausea, headache, or fever is particularly troublesome, extending the time of infusion to 8 hours is often helpful. After stabilization of the patient's condition, a double dose may then be given on alternate days, thus allowing outpatient treatment. A total dose of 2 to 2.5 gm or frequently more is required. Total doses of 9 gm or more, lifelong intrathecal injections, or permanent oral azole therapy may be required in patients in whom remission is slow, those with meningitis, or those with AIDS. The duration of therapy depends on the patient's extent of disease, response to therapy, and reduction in the complement-fixation antibody titers, not by the total amount of amphotericin B administered.

The efficacy and safety of a new formulation of amphotericin B administered intravenously in liposomes have been demonstrated with other fungi. Liposomes are cleared by the reticuloendothelial system, thus sparing amphotericin B-induced toxicity to such target organs as the kidney. This is a particularly attractive strategy in treating such diseases as histoplasmosis in which the reticuloendothelial system is characteristically parasitized by the fungus. However, the short shelf-life of the liposome preparation limits its current usefulness, and its efficacy in coccidioidomycosis is unknown.

Azoles are now the preferred therapy for non-life-threatening disease. Although strict comparison has been difficult to achieve, the newer azoles, itraconazole and fluconazole, seem superior to amphotericin B in the treatment of disease that is not fulminant. Their mode of action is by inhibition of the cytochrome P-450 enzyme system, resulting in a reduction of ergosterol in fungal cell membranes.

Ketoconazole, the first oral azole, has shown promise in the treatment of non-life-threatening coccidioidomycosis. In daily doses of 400 mg orally it was successful in the treatment of disseminated disease without meningitis. Using extremely stringent criteria, a cure was established in 30 to 40 per cent of patients treated with ketoconazole. It has been used concurrently with amphotericin B for the treatment of coccidioidomycosis in AIDS patients. It is useful in limited pulmonary disease caused by *C. immitis*, as well as in the treatment of such deep-seated infections as arthritis or osteomyelitis. Toxicity from high-dose ketoconazole limits its usefulness for the treatment of meningitis.

Ketoconazole, however, has been surpassed in clinical efficacy by itraconazole and fluconazole. Itraconazole at 300-400 mg orally per day showed impressive activity in the treatment of chronic coccidioidal meningitis (80 per cent response rate). The drug was also effective in the treatment of nonmeningeal coccidioidomycosis. Itraconazole at these doses has few side effects. Fluconazole at 50-400 mg orally per day has also been used as sole therapy for the treatment of coccidioidal meningitis. The drug is available for intravenous use as well. It has demonstrated effectiveness similar to itraconazole, but preliminary impressions are that patients treated with fluconazole may have a higher relapse rate than those treated with itraconazole.

Ocular. Amphotericin B has poor intraocular (aqueous humor and vitreous) penetration when administered intravenously, unless large doses are used, which increases the risk of renal toxicity. Subconjunctival injection of amphotericin B* is sometimes used for severe fungal endophthalmitis in a dosage of 0.75 to 5.0 μg in 1.0 ml aqueous suspension, but its efficacy in coccidioidal endophthalmitis is unknown. Subconjunctival injections likewise result in poor penetration into the vitreous of experimentally inflamed eyes. Intracameral injection* has been used in severe anterior uveitis along with intravenous therapy without any clear benefit, and experimentally this procedure produces a severe vitritis with scarring.

Ocular or Periocular Manifestations

Anterior Chamber: Cells; flare; hypopyon.
Choroid: Atrophic scars; diffuse chorioretinitis; focal choroiditis; granulomas.
Conjunctiva: Conjunctivitis (bulbar); granulomas (palpebral); phlyctenules (bulbar); ulcer (palpebral).
Cornea: Mutton-fat keratic precipitates; necrotic inflammatory foci; perforation; superficial infiltrate.
Extraocular Muscles: Abducens paralysis; diplopia.
Eyelids: Edema; granuloma.
Globe: Endophthalmitis.
Iris or Ciliary Body: Granulomatous iridocyclitis; peripheral anterior synechia; posterior synechia.
Optic Nerve: Atrophy; juxtapapillary granuloma; neuritis; optic nerve granuloma; papilledema.
Orbit: Granuloma.
Retina: Edema; exudates; focal retinitis; hemorrhages; perivascular sheathing.
Scleral and Episcleral: Episcleritis; scleritis.
Vitreous: Exudates; vitritis.

PRECAUTIONS

Immunosuppressive therapy, especially using corticosteroids, is a primary factor in increasing the risk of dissemination and should be reduced or discontinued where possible. An initial improvement in the ocular lesions may be seen with topical and systemic corticosteroids, but an exacerbation of ocular inflammation usually follows their continued use and results in progressive destruction of the eye.

Treatment with amphotericin B results in significant but predictable toxicity that can be managed with modest dose reduction if necessary. Nephrotoxicity causes a reduction in the glomerular filtration rate and therefore an elevation of blood urea nitrogen. To avoid uremic symptoms, a reduction in dose and interval is recommended in patients with a serum creatinine greater than 3.0 mg/dl. Both reversible and permanent nephrotoxicity occur, but the latter is rarely clinically apparent. Hypokalemia develops as a consequence of renal tubular acidosis and can be treated with oral potassium supplements. A reversible normocytic, normochromic anemia is an expected complication, but usually does not require transfusion. Amphotericin B should be infused slowly. Rapid administration (in less than 60 minutes) is associated with potentially lethal hyperkalemia that is presumably caused by cell death associated with binding of amphotericin B to cholesterol in host plasma membranes.

Both ketoconazole and itraconazole require an acid pH in the stomach for absorption. Therefore, patients with achlorhydria or those who are receiving antacids or histamine H_2 blockers are not suitable candidates for treatment with these drugs. Ketoconazole also interferes with steroidogenesis in humans. Testicular and adrenal dysfunction occur, manifesting clinically as gynecomastia and oligospermia; minor elevations in liver function tests may occur. Idiosyncratic hepatic failure is a rare but fatal reaction. Patients who experience prohibitive side effects with the azoles or who are simultaneously taking rifampin, phenytoin, or carbamazepine should receive amphotericin B.

Miconazole, a first generation azole, because of its Cremaphor carrier induces intense pruritus in half of the patients receiving it, as well as occasional anaphylactoid reactions. Because of these and other adverse reactions and the fact that it is available only as an intravenous drug, miconazole has fallen into disfavor.

COMMENTS

Measurement of serum tube precipitin and complement-fixation antibody titers, radiographs, and geographic exposure are important in diagnosing coccidioidomycosis. Coccidioidin and spherulin skin testing are valuable epidemiologic tools; the former is important in judging response to therapy. Therapy is best supervised by clinicians experienced in the vagaries of this disease. A full and complete ophthalmic examination is indicated in anyone with ocular symptoms or signs. Confirmation of the diagnosis should be sought by culture or, if possible, by tissue diagnosis. Anterior chamber or vitreous paracentesis may be indicated in some cases.

The detection of acute peripheral chorioretinal lesions associated with coccidioidomycosis does not necessarily imply the presence of active disseminated disease requiring treatment. Frequently, these lesions are self-limiting, leaving asymptomatic, atrophic chorioretinal scars. They should be followed periodically, and the decision regarding treatment should depend on ocular disease progression, as well as the overall coccidioidal disease status.

References

Blumendranz MS, Stevens DA: Endogenous coccidioidal endophthalmitis. Ophthalmology *87*: 974–984, 1980.

Blumendranz MS, Stevens DA: Therapy of endogenous fungal endophthalmitis. Miconazole or amphotericin B for coccidioidal and candidal infection. Arch Ophthalmol *98*:1216–1220, 1980.

Danetta A, et al: Coccidioidomycosis in the acquired immunodeficiency syndrome. Ann Intern Med *106*:372–379, 1987.

Drutz DJ: Amphotericin B in the treatment of coccidioidomycosis. Drugs *26*:337–346, 1983.

Drutz DJ, Catanzaro A: Coccidioidomycosis. Am Rev Resp Dis *117*:559–585, 727-771, 1978.

Galgiani JN, et al: Ketoconazole therapy of progressive coccidioidomycosis. Comparison of 400- and 800-mg doses and observations at higher doses. Am J Med *85*:603–610, 1988.

Glasgow BJ, et al: Miliary retinitis in coccidioidomycosis. Am J Ophthalmol *104*:24–27, 1987.

Graybill JR: Future directions of antifungal therapy. Clin Infect Dis *14*:S170–S181, 1992.

Rodenbiker HT, Ganley JP: Ocular coccidioidomycosis. Surv Ophthalmol *24*:263–290, 1980.

Rodenbiker HT, et al: Prevalence of chorioretinal scars associated with coccidioidomycosis. Arch Ophthalmol *99*:71–75, 1981.

Tucker RM, et al: Itraconazole therapy for chronic coccidioidal meningitis. Ann Intern Med *112*: 108–112, 1990.

Tucker RM, et al: Treatment of coccidioidal meningitis with fluconazole. Rev Infect Dis *12*:S380–S389, 1990.

Tucker RM, et al: Interaction of azoles with rifampin, phenytoin, and carbamazepine: In vitro and clinical observations. Clin Infect Dis *14*:165–174, 1992.

DERMATOPHYTOSIS 110.9
(Epidermophytosis, Epidermomycosis, Ringworm, Rubrophytia, Tinea, Trichophytosis)

ALAN SUGAR, M.D.

Ann Arbor, Michigan

Dermatophytosis refers to superficial infection of the skin by the ringworm fungi; *Trichophyton, Epidermophyton,* and *Microsporum* are among the common species causing cutaneous infection. Clinically, dermatophytoses are classified by the involved skin area, such as tinea capitis (ringworm of the scalp), tinea corporis (of body skin), and tinea pedis (athlete's foot). Ocular or periocular involvement is rare and is usually a result of facial infection. This group of fungi affects only keratinized tissue and is therefore usually limited to superficial infection. Lesions begin as red papules that become red, circular, scaly patches. As the lesions enlarge centrifugally, the center may clear, leaving a typical ringworm pattern. There is usually very little underlying inflammation. Marginal blepharitis, lid ulcers, and loss of lashes or brow hair may occur secondary to facial or scalp involvement. Allergy to fungi-dermatophytid reactions can occur causing noninfected vesicular lesions on the hands and rarely allergic conjunctivitis. The diagnosis can be confirmed by examination of skin scrapings under the microscope after adding a drop of 10 per cent potassium hydroxide. Cultures on Sabouraud's medium, kept at room temperature, grow in 2 to 3 weeks.

THERAPY

Systemic. Extensive involvement or lesions unresponsive to topical treatment may be treated with oral griseofulvin. A dosage of 125 to 250 mg for children or 500 mg for adults of the microsize crystalline form is given in a single dose after a meal. The ultramicrosize crystalline form requires half of the above dosage, 3.3 mg/lb in children. Because the drug is incorporated into keratin slowly and is fungistatic, at least 4 to 6 weeks of treatment are required. For severe infections or in patients allergic to griseofulvin, daily administration of ketoconazole in a dosage of 50 to 200 mg for children or 200 to 400 mg for adults may be used. Fluconazole may also be given as 150 mg once weekly for 1 to 4 weeks. Itraconazole, terbinafine, and other new agents are being studied.

Topical. Antifungal creams can be successful in treating milder lesions of the face, scalp, and lids. The available agents include 1 per cent clotrimazole, 2 per cent miconazole, 1 per cent tolnaftate, 1 per cent econazole, and 1 per cent haloprogin. The medication should be applied twice daily after the involved skin is gently cleansed, and treatment should be continued for 1 week after the lesion clears. Care should be taken in the application of these antifungal agents because they are irritating if applied to the eye. Involved lashes should be epilated.

Ocular or Periocular Manifestations

Conjunctiva: Infectious or allergic conjunctivitis.
Cornea: Fungal ulcer (very rare).
Eyebrows: Folliculitis; madarosis; scaly rash.
Eyelids: Blepharitis; dermatitis; edema; madarosis; ulcer.

PRECAUTIONS

As in other fungal infections, corticosteroids may mask the nature of the dermatophytosis, may increase its severity, and may prolong its course. Premature discontinuation of topical or systemic antifungals may be followed by relapse of the infection.

COMMENTS

Ocular and periocular involvement with dermatophytosis is rare and usually is an extension from involved scalp or facial skin. Tinea capitis—scalp ringworm—occurs most frequently in children in hot humid weather. Other forms occur in adult men. As in other fungal infections, such systemic disease as malignancy or diabetes and systemic steroids may be predisposing factors.

References

Duke-Elder S: System of Ophthalmology. St. Louis, CV Mosby, 1974, Vol XIII, pp 175–179.
Fedukowicz HB, Stetson S: External Infections of the Eye. Bacterial, Viral, and Mycotic, 3rd ed. East Norwalk, CT, Appleton-Century-Crofts, 1985, pp 194–196.
Francois J, Rysselaerre M: Oculomycoses. Springfield, IL, Charles Thomas, 1972, pp 229–245.
Korting GW: The Skin and Eye. A Dermatologic Correlation of Disease of the Periorbital Region. Philadelphia, WB Saunders, 1973, pp 50–54.
Lachapelle JM, De Doncker P, Tennstedt D, et al: Itraconazole compared with griseofulvin in the treatment of tinea corporis/cruris and tinea pedis/manus. Dermatology 184:45–50, 1992.
Montero-Gei F, Perera A: Therapy with fluconazole for tinea corporis, tinea cruris, and tinea pedia. Clin Infect Dis 15(Suppl):77–81, 1992.
Ostler HB, Okumoto M, Halde C: Dermatophytosis affecting the periorbital region. Am J Ophthalmol 72:934–938, 1971.

MUCORMYCOSIS 117.7
(Phycomycosis)

DAVID J. WILSON, M.D.

Portland, Oregon

Mucormycosis is an acute, severe infection caused by fungi of the order Mucorales and the class Phycomycetes. Some authors prefer the term *phycomycosis* to describe this disease because fungi of orders other than Mucorales are pathogenic to humans. Several terms have been used in the ophthalmic literature to describe this entity, including rhino-orbitocerebral, rhinocerebral, craniofacial, spheno-orbital, and orbital mucormycosis or phycomycosis.

Mucormycosis represents an opportunistic infection in which a ubiquitous organism (normally found in soil, air, and as a common bread mold) becomes a pathogen in humans under a variety of metabolic situations. Diabetes, particularly when ketoacidosis is present, is by far the most common predisposing condition; it is present in 40 to 80 per cent of patients. Other predisposing conditions include chronic renal failure, leukemia, lymphoma, metabolic acidosis, and cirrhosis. Mucormycosis with no underlying disease has been reported, but these cases are quite rare.

The classic presentation of mucormycosis is a diabetic patient who initially complains of rhinitis, sinusitis, and facial pain with rapid progression to signs and symptoms of orbital cellulitis and orbital apex syndrome. With cerebral involvement, severe headache, altered mental status, and signs of cavernous sinus or internal carotid artery thrombosis become manifest. The diagnosis of mucormycosis requires the demonstration of the characteristic broad, nonseptate, branching hyphae in tissue, as well as culture of the fungi. These fungi have a marked predilection for invading arteries, which characteristically produces thrombosis with extensive coagulative necrosis and gangrene.

THERAPY

Early diagnosis is critical and has been credited with the tremendous reduction in mortality seen in this disease since 1979. A combination of surgical débridement of necrotic tissue, systemic and local antifungal (amphotericin B) administration, and correction of the underlying metabolic defect is essential for successful management of this disease.

Systemic. Amphotericin B is the antifungal agent of choice. Because of the numerous systemic side effects of this medication, it should be administered under the direction of a physician familiar with its use. After administration of a test dose, a regimen of 0.3 mg/ kg dissolved in 500 ml of 5 per cent dextrose in water has been recommended for intravenous administration over a 1- to 3-hour period each day. This should be advanced to a daily dose of 0.5 to 0.6 mg/kg. Amphotericin B is continued as indicated by the patient's clinical course, and total doses of over 4 gm are often required.

Ocular. Histologic evaluation of debrided tissue may give some indication of adequacy of therapy. Local irrigation and packing of the orbit with gauze containing 1 mg/ml of amphotericin B have been advocated as measures to limit the amount of disfiguring debridement that must be done.

Surgical. Complete debridement of all necrotic tissue must be performed. Since mucormycosis begins as an infection of the sinuses and may spread to the orbit and brain, debridement may require the combined efforts of an ophthalmologist, otolaryngologist, and neurosurgeon.

Supportive. Standard medical techniques are employed to correct the basic metabolic defect. It is usually advisable to admit the patient to a medical service where the metabolic defect can be managed and the patient can be monitored for toxicity from amphotericin B.

Ocular or Periocular Manifestations

Conjunctiva: Chemosis; hyperemia; suppuration.
Cornea: Clouding; ulcer; anesthesia.
Eyelids: Ptosis; edema; discoloration; necrosis.
Globe: Proptosis.
Pupil: Dilation; absent reaction to light.
Other: Decreased visual acuity; orbital and facial pain; diplopia; paralysis of extraocular muscles; nasal or palatal eschar or ulcer; headache; altered mental status; orbital apex syndrome; cavernous sinus thrombosis; internal carotid artery occlusion.

PRECAUTIONS

Mucormycosis is a life-threatening disease, and early diagnosis is essential in its successful management. Mucormycosis can be mistaken for bacterial orbital cellulitis or sinusitis with cavernous sinus thrombosis. Awareness of the epidemiology is helpful in alerting the clinician to the possibility of mucormycosis. Corticosteroids do not have a role in the management of mucormycosis and may exacerbate the condition. Amphotericin B is an extremely toxic drug and should be administered under the guidance of a physician skilled in its use.

COMMENTS

Three principles should guide the treatment of patients with mucormycosis: correction of predisposing metabolic abnormalities, surgical debridement of nonviable tissues, and use of systemic amphotericin B.

References

Castelli JB, Pallin JL: Lethal rhinocerebral phycomycosis in a healthy adult: A case report and review of the literature. Ophthalmology 86:696–703, 1978.
Kohn R, Hepler R: Management of limited rhino-orbital mucormycosis without exenteration. Ophthalmology 92:1440–1444, 1985.
Lie K-J, et al: Phycomycosis of the central nervous system associated with diabetes mellitus in Indonesia. Am J Clin Pathol 32:62–70, 1959.
Parfrey NA: Improved diagnosis and prognosis of mucormycosis: A clinicopathologic study of 33 cases. Medicine 65:113–123, 1986.
Schwartz JN, Donnelly EH, Klintworth GK: Ocular and orbital phycomycosis. Surv Ophthalmol 22:3–28, 1977.

OCULAR HISTOPLASMOSIS 115
(Presumed Ocular Histoplasmosis Syndrome)

STEPHEN K. MAGIE, M.D.

Little Rock, Arkansas

Originally described in 1951, the ocular histoplasmosis syndrome or the presumed ocular histoplasmosis syndrome affects an estimated population of 2000 young and middle-aged adults per year. The classical triad consists of peripapillary chorioretinal scarring, punched-out "inactive" chorioretinal scars, and hemorrhagic or neurosensory macular lesions or disciform macular scars. The histoplasmic capsulatum organism has been implicated as the cause of the chorioretinal scars with secondary subretinal neovascular membranes (SRN). The loss of central vision generally occurs many years after the initial acute phase.

Endemic to the Ohio and Mississippi River valleys, *Histoplasma capsulatum* initially causes a generally mild upper respiratory type infection. Acute asymptomatic multifocal chorioiditis probably occurs at this early stage. The condition in the active stage may be indistinguishable from the clinical entity of multifocal choroiditis with panuveitis. The paramount feature in multifocal choroiditis is intraocular inflammation, although the course may vary with relatively quiet periods. Acute inflammatory findings alone help differentiate ocular histoplasmosis from multifocal chorioiditis. Experimental evidence suggests that the chronic lesion—chorioretinal scars or "histo spots"—may not indeed represent inactive lesions. The lesions are often associated with chronic inflammatory cell infiltrates. Loss of central vision is associated with the development of SRN. The presenting symptoms in most patients are blurred central vision, metamorphopsia, micropsia, and central scotomas. If the symptoms are in the nondominant eye, the patient may inadvertently discover the visual loss when the dominant eye is covered. In addition to the classic triad, patients with AIDS can develop disseminated histoplasmosis. The histoplasmic capsulatum organism has been observed pathologically in lesions of retinitis, optic neuritis, and uveitis in AIDS patients. Endogenous and exogenous endophthalmitis have been reported.

THERAPY

Systemic. Pharmacologic therapy in the past has been limited to the systemic use of high-dose steroids. Currently, the use of high-dose steroids in the management of SRN is unwarranted. The use of systemic chemotherapy, such as interferon-alpha, is currently investigational, but may hold promise for the future.

Ocular. The Macular Photocoagulation Study (MPS) has demonstrated that laser treatment is effective for extrafoveal SRN (200–2500 mm from the center of the foveal avascular zone) and juxtafoveal SRN (1–199 mm from the center of the foveal avascular zone). Although the MPS has shown a long-term benefit in patients with age-related macular degeneration, the central acuity results are poor. Treatment of subfoveal SRN with laser is still far from perfect. Laser photocoagulation for subfoveal SRN in ocular histoplasmosis patients has not been shown to yield a long-term benefit. It is well known that some patients maintain relatively good central vision even in the presence of subfoveal SRN. Both argon and krypton laser photocoagulation have shown beneficial results. Yet, even in experienced hands, the rate of persistent vessels or recurrent vessels as defined by the MPS is significant. Persistent vessels are associated with a much poorer visual outcome. Systemic hypertension is the only patient-related factor that has been associated with persistent vessels.

Timely clinical evaluation of the patient with fluorescein angiography is essential in the management of patients with suspected SRN. Dilated fundus examination with contact lens evaluation and comparison to the angiographic findings are essential.

Surgical. Surgical management with subretinal dissection of the neovascular complex has been reported.

Ocular or Periocular Manifestations

Choroid, Retina, Vitreous: Atrophic posterior segment scars; "histo spots"; peripapillary atrophy; subretinal neovascularization; choroiditis; endophthalmitis.

Macula: Neurosensory detachment; subretinal hemorrhage; subretinal exudate.

PRECAUTIONS

Systemic treatment with antifungal agents, such as amphotericin B, is not indicated in the absence of actively replicating organisms. Patients with subretinal neovascularization should not be treated with corticosteroids. Histoplasmic choroiditis should be included in the differential diagnosis of any patient with AIDS and active choroiditis, retinitis, or optic neuritis.

Patients need to be educated about their disease and its guarded prognosis. They need proper instruction in monitoring it closely, such as using Amsler grid testing to detect acute visual changes. Close follow-up observation with repeated fluorescein studies to detect persistent or recurrent vessels is essential. Typically, patients are followed at intervals of 2 to 3 weeks for the first few months after laser treatment.

COMMENTS

Ocular histoplasmosis with subretinal neovascularization is a frustrating disease both to the patient and the physician. Patients are generally at a time in their lives where visual loss can adversely affect their occupation and can keep them from reaching their fullest potential. These patients need education about their disease, tremendous compassion, and encouragement.

In addition to the advances made by the ongoing laser treatment trials, the future holds promise for improvement in visual outcomes with both surgical and pharmacologic treatment modalities.

References

Anderson A, Taylor C, Azen S, et al: Immunopathology of acute experimental histoplasmic choroiditis in the primate. Invest Ophthalmol Vis Sci 28:1195–1199, 1987.

Anderson A, et al: Immunopathology of chronic experimental histoplasmic choroiditis in the primate. Invest Ophthalmol Vis Sci 33:1637–1641, 1992.

Fung WE: Interferon alpha$_{2a}$ for treatment of age-related macular degeneration. Am J Ophthalmol 112:349–350, 1991.

Krause AC, Hopkins WG: Ocular manifestation of histoplasmosis. Am J Ophthalmol 34:564–566, 1951.

Macular Photocoagulation Study Group. Argon laser photocoagulation for ocular histoplasmosis: Results of a randomized clinical trial. Arch Ophthalmol 101:1347–1357, 1983.

Macular Photocoagulation Study Group. Argon laser photocoagulation for neovascular maculopathy: Three year results from randomized clinical trials. Arch Ophthalmol 104:694–701, 1986.

Macular Photocoagulation Study Group. Persistent and recurrent neovascularization after krypton laser photocoagulation for neovascular lesion of ocular histoplasmosis. Arch Ophthalmol *107:* 344–352, 1989.

Macular Photocoagulation Study Group. Laser photocoagulation of subfoveal neovascular lesions in age-related macular degeneration: Results of a randomized clinical trial. Arch Ophthalmol. *109:*1220–1231, 1991.

Pulido JS, Folberg R, et al: *Histoplasma capsulatum* endophthalmitis after cataract extraction. Ophthalmology 97:217–220, 1990.

Specht CS, Mitchell KT, et al: Ocular histoplasmosis with retinitis in a patient with acquired immune deficiency syndrome. Ophthalmology 98: 1356–1359, 1991.

Thomas MA, Grand MG, Williams DF, et al: Surgical management of subfoveal choroidal neovascularization. Ophthalmology 99:952–968, 1992.

RHINOSPORIDIOSIS 117.0

(Oculosporidiosis)

P. K. MUKHERJEE, M.S.

Raipur, India

Rhinosporidiosis is a chronic infective granuloma most commonly affecting nasal mucosa. Because the nose is frequently involved and the first reported case was a chronic granuloma of the nostril, the name rhinosporidiosis was given to this condition. It may also involve the nasopharynx, lacrimal sac, conjunctiva, and the postnasal space by direct continuity. It may be seen in the larynx, palate trachea, bronchus, and maxillary sinus as well. Rhinosporidiosis can infect other parts of the body far from the nose, such as the urethra, vulva, vagina, and rectum. Lesions of skin and bone have also been reported. It seems that only few organs, such as the brain and heart, are immune to the disease. The disease occurs naturally both in humans and animals independently or may spread from one to the other.

The organism, once believed to be a sporozoan, is now considered to be a fungus belonging to class Phycomycetes. The organism starts its life cycle as a parasite measuring 8 μ, but grows by nuclear division until it reaches a size about 200 to 300 μ and contains 40,000 nuclei that form 16,000 spores. The spores appear round or oval and measure 2-10 μ in size. After implantation in mucosa or a mucocutaneous area, the infective spores enter deeper and lead a parasitic life. They increase in size by asexual multiplication and, in time, develop into a sporangium.

The sporangium measures about 300 to 500 μ in diameter and has a double-walled envelope; the outer one is chitinous and the inner one consists of cellulose. The mature sporangium may contain as many as 16,000 spores. It bursts at a weak spot in its wall, and spores are discharged into the tissue to begin the cycle again.

The disease has a wide distribution, mostly in the tropics. Cases reported from nontropical countries are sporadic and have a history of migration from the tropics. It is seen more commonly in tropical countries in part because of their moderate to heavy annual rainfall, which results in a humid climate. The countries most affected are India, Ceylon, Indonesia, and the Phillipines. The greatest number of cases are found in India and Ceylon. In India, the distribution is not uniform; it is seen mostly in the South Central and Southern states. Surprisingly, no case has been reported from Australia or New Zealand.

The mode of infection is not well understood. Males are more frequently affected, with 75 per cent of cases seen in males under 20 years of age. Almost all infected patients have a habit of bathing in common village pools along with cattle. The cattle in the endemic area show frequent involvement. Yet, the fungus has neither been cultured under artificial conditions nor have experiment lesions been produced in animals. The possible mode of infection could be water borne or air borne. One hypothesis is that the spore reaches the person's mucous membrane while bathing in an infected pond and becomes lodged in natural recesses in the mucosal fold (conjunctival fornices) or pathologic strictures (nasolacrimal duct stenosis) where it proliferates to produce a typical lesion. Wide systemic dissemination may be blood borne or by continuity of the mucous membrane (from the nasal mucosa down to the trachea, bronchus, and lungs or spread from the oropharynx to gastrointestinal tract). Genitourinary tract involvement is most probably retrograde from the external genitals to the bladder or pelvic organs.

The typical lesion is a pedunculated fleshy mass ranging from few millimeters to few inches in size; occasionally, it is sessile. The mass is red in color due to the abundance of vascularity, and the surface is rough and shows fine capillaries on it. On the surface are multiple brown or white dots representing old and immature sporangia, respectively. The tissue is friable, and the slightest trauma causes bleeding, resulting in epistaxis, hemoptysis, hematuria, or bleeding from conjunctiva.

The diagnosis in endemic areas is not difficult, but in nonendemic areas it may be confused with chronic granuloma-like tuberculosis, syphilis, burst chalazia, or a new growth, either a hemangioma, papilloma, or malignancy. However, the reverse is also true, as the above-mentioned conditions are often confused with rhinosporidiosis in endemic areas.

The diagnosis is best confirmed by histopathology of the excised tissue. Under high power of the microscope, sporangia in wet preparation of small tissue removed from the growth have been demonstrated in most of the ocular cases. Free spores can be isolated in the tears of an affected person as well.

The ocular lesion has two modes of presentation, one being spread from the nose and the other being involvement of the ocular structure without nasal or systemic involvement. The latter type of lesion is designated as primary rhinosporidiosis of the eye or oculosporidiosis, which accounts for 10 per cent of all cases.

Patients with conjunctival involvement seek medical help earlier than those with an affected lacrimal sac, because the fleshy red growth attracts attention earlier. A conjunctival growth overhanging the cornea may cause foreign body sensation and lacrimation. The conjunctival growth is a solitary chronic granuloma that can be sessile or pedunculated. Growth arising from fornices are more likely to develop long pedicles than those arising from tarsal conjunctiva or the limbus. The pedunculated growth is a flat, leaf-like, red mass with crenated edges. The surface is rough and has multiple white dots that represent sporangia; it bleeds on manipulation.

The sclera is very rarely involved, although a scleral staphyloma may result. Generally, a conjunctival growth overlies the staphyloma.

The lacrimal sac is most commonly affected in the form of chronic dacryocystitis. The sac presents a typical appearance. The skin over the swelling has an orange peel appearance; the swelling is soft, nontender, and compressible. There is no regurgitation, and complete block of the nasolacrimal duct is rare. Erosion of the surrounding bone is common. The sac may be secondarily infected, presenting as cellulitis. Bilateral involvement is rare.

THERAPY

Ocular. Ocular involvement does not require any specific drug therapy. No known drug is effective against rhinosporidiosis. However, associated conjunctivitis may be treated with appropriate broad-spectrum antibiotics.

Surgical. The most satisfactory results are obtained by complete surgical removal of the growth. Surgery can be undertaken under topical anesthesia, but children may require general anesthesia. The conjunctival growth is grasped with blunt and flat forceps without trauma to the growth and is pulled away from the conjunctiva. The pedicle is cut by sharp scissors, and the cut distal stump retracts immediately. Because of profuse hemorrhage, it may be necessary to tie the stump or use thermal cautery. In most cases, using a firm-pressure bandage is sufficient. For small conjunctival growths, cryoapplication is sufficient to convert the whole mass into an ice ball, resulting in shrinkage of the growth.

In scleral staphyloma, best results are obtained by applying cryo all around the staphyloma. The overlying conjunctiva is dissected clear from the staphyloma, and the scleral bulges are indented with silicone or a Silastic sponge of a suitable size. The buckle must overlap the staphyloma by about 1 mm on each side. A posteriorly placed scleral staphyloma is clearly visible with an indirect ophthalmoscope. The conjunctiva is replaced over the buckle. The eye may be made soft by use of intravenous mannitol during manipulation. Diathermy is contraindicated as this may perforate the staphyloma and cause intractable bleeding.

Management of chronic dacryocystitis due to rhinosporidiosis is less satisfactory than that of conjunctival growth. Unless meticulous care is taken to remove the growth in one sitting, recurrence is frequent, especially if nasal growth is not taken care of simultaneously. The procedure consists of dissection of the friable growth, mostly by blunt dissection from the surrounding structure without rupture. If the mass is ruptured, there is profuse hemorrhage that obscures the field and promotes recurrence, which is more difficult to manage.

Ocular or Periocular Manifestation

Conjunctiva: Sessile or pedunculated granuloma bleeding from the growth.
Lacrimal System: Chronic dacryocystitis.
Sclera: Scleral staphyloma.
Other: Lacrimation due to growth rubbing over the cornea.

PRECAUTIONS

Care should be taken not to rupture the sac while removing it. Doing so leads to intractable bleeding.

COMMENTS

Involvement of ocular adnexa is very common. In endemic areas, rhinosporidiosis may be confused with other chronic granuloma or malignancy.

References

Acharya PV, Gupta RL, Darbari BS: Cutaneous rhinosporidiosis. Indian Dermatol Vener 39:22–23, 1973.

Darbari BS, Gupta RL, Shukla IM, Arora MM: Rhinosporidiosis in Raipur. A clinicopathological study of 348 cases. Indian J Pathol Bact 15:105–107, 1972.

De Doncker, RML, deKeize RJ, Oosterhuis JA, Maes, A: Scleral melting in a patient with conjunctival rhinosporidiosis. Br J Ophthalmol 74:635–637, 1990.

Gupta RL, Darbari BS, Dwevedi MP, Billore OP, Arora MM: An epidemiological study of rhinosporidiosis in and around Raipur. Indian J Med Res 64:1293–1299, 1976.

Krishnan MM, Kawatra VK, Rao VA, Ratnakar C: Diverticulum of the lacrimal sac associated with rhinosporidiosis. Br J Ophthalmol 70:867–868, 1986.

Lamba PA, Shukla IM Ganapathy M: Rhinosporidium granuloma of conjunctiva with scleral ectasia. Br J Ophthalmol 54:565–568, 1970.

Mukherjee PK, Shukla IM, Despande M, Pravenna K: Rhinosporidiosis of the lacrimal sac. Indian J Ophthalmol 30:513–514, 1982.

Naik RS, Siddiqui RA, Naik V: Urethronasal rhinosporidiosis. J Indian Med Assoc 72:238–239, 1979.

Savino DF, Margo CE: Conjunctival Rhinosporidiosis. Light and electron microscopic study. Ophthalmology 90:1482–1489, 1983.

Shukla IM, Darbari BS, Arora MM, Gupta RL, Arora NP: Ocular rhinosporidiosis. Proc All-India Ophthalmol 21:133–137, 1970.

SPOROTRICHOSIS 117.1

WILLIAM A. AGGER, M.D.

La Crosse, Wisconsin

Sporotrichosis is a chronic fungal infection caused by *Sporothrix schenckii*. Infection usually occurs when the spores are traumatically inoculated into the skin, often on the extremities and occasionally in or about the eyes. The most common type of the disease is the localized subcutaneous variety. This lesion usually occurs on exposed skin and is characterized by nodules or pustules that may develop into small ulcers. If the condition is not treated, similar nodules may develop along the lymphatics draining the area. The disease often becomes chronic, resulting in enlargement of the regional lymph nodes.

An uncommon skin manifestation of sporotrichosis is the fixed cutaneous type, which appears as a verrucous patch in individuals with good host defenses.

Rarely, systemic disease may develop in compromised hosts, such as alcoholics, or patients with HIV infection. After inhalation of spores, an initial pulmonary lesion is followed by hematogenous spread. In this type of disease, the pathogen may metastasize widely, causing granulomas in the joints, genitourinary system, skin, or eyes.

Ocular involvement in sporotrichosis is uncommon. It usually occurs as a result of a primary infection, often on the eyelids, and rarely as a result of a disseminated infection. When the eyelid is the site of disease, a fixed verrucous lesion or, more commonly, one or more subcutaneous nodules appear, often producing a secondary purulent and ulcerative blepharitis. Secondary to the palpebral infection, preauricular adenopathy, dacryocystitis, and orbital abscesses may develop.

Other rare manifestations of ocular sporotrichosis include conjunctivitis, scleritis, and keratitis. Intraocular sporotrichosis may occur after perforation of a corneal ulcer, trauma to the eye, or metastasis. The usual intraocular form of the disease is uveitis, which may be either granulomatous, with mutton-fat keratic precipitates or nongranulomatous.

THERAPY

Systemic. The drug of choice in cutaneous sporotrichosis is potassium iodide. Ten drops of a saturated solution of potassium iodide are given orally three times daily. Doses are increased, as tolerated, to a total daily dose of 120 drops. This regimen should be continued for 1 month after the skin lesions have cleared.

In disseminated sporotrichosis, an initial intravenous dose of 0.25 mg/kg of amphotericin B is indicated. Daily dosage may then be increased to 0.4 mg/kg and continued to a total dose of between 1.5 and 2.5 gm. Only if unusual circumstances occur, such as renal insufficiency, should the dose be reduced.

Flucytosine[‡] and ketoconazole[‡] give inconsistent results, whereas itraconazole[†] therapy has been successful in nonocular disease in a moderate number of patients.

Ocular. The primary treatment of eyelid disease usually consists of systemic potassium iodide, in addition to ophthalmic administration of amphotericin B. Depending on the severity of the disease, amphotericin B[*] (1.5 mg/ml in D5W) eyedrops may be sufficient to treat sporotrichotic conjunctivitis. In patients with sporotrichosis of the lacrimal canaliculi or sac, local irrigation and topical administration of amphotericin B may be effective.

For patients with sporotrichotic corneal ulcers, systemic treatment should be supplemented with topical amphotericin B ophthalmic solution, administered hourly during the day and every other hour at nighttime. Adjunctive therapy includes subconjunctival injection of amphotericin B[*] and cycloplegics.

In sporotrichotic endophthalmitis, vitrectomy is probably the treatment of choice. Intravitreal injection of 5 to 10 ug of amphotericin B has been recommended, along with systemic therapy, by some clinicians.

Ocular or Periocular Manifestations

Conjunctiva: Granulomatous or purulent conjunctivitis; ulcerative oculoglandular conjunctivitis.

Cornea: Keratitis; perforation; ulcer.

Eyelids: Verrucous patch; purulent or ulcerative blepharitis; subcutaneous abscess.

Globe: Endophthalmitis; panophthalmitis.

Iris: Atrophy; uveitis, granulomatous or nongranulomatous, hypopyon.

Lacrimal System: Dacryocanaliculitis; dacryocystitis; fistula.

Orbit: Abscess; erosion of bony wall; fistula; osteitis; periosteitis.

Sclera: Abscess; scleritis.
Other: Preauricular lymphadenopathy.

PRECAUTIONS

Simple aspiration of secondary nodules can be useful for diagnosis, but except for intra-vitreal infection, surgery is usually contraindicated in patients with sporotrichosis.

The patient receiving potassium iodide treatment should be observed for evidence of iodism; if it appears, the dosage should be reduced or discontinued. Reactions may include acneiform rashes, coryza, bronchitis, stomatitis, gastritis, parotid swelling, conjunctivitis, and eyelid edema. Mild iodide sensitivity may lessen or disappear despite continued therapy.

Saline solution should not be used to dilute amphotericin B because it may cause amphotericin B to precipitate. Because of the well-known toxicity of amphotericin B, dosage with this drug must be individualized. Fever, nausea, nephrotoxic reactions, and electrolyte disturbances are common side effects of this drug. Topical ophthalmic concentrations greater than 5 per cent are irritating and can cause corneal erosions. The ophthalmologist should note that intraocular penetration of topical and subconjunctival amphotericin B is poor.

COMMENTS

If left untreated, sporotrichosis will develop into a chronic condition. If endophthalmitis or anterior uveitis fails to respond to steroid therapy, the ophthalmologist should consider paracentesis of the anterior chamber or vitreous aspiration to confirm infection. Appropriate microscopy and cultures for bacteria, mycobacteria, and fungi should be done. Once intraocular sporotrichosis has developed, the prognosis for useful vision is very grave, even with treatment. Although iodide treatment is successful in the subcutaneous forms of sporotrichosis, it is unfortunately not effective in the treatment of deep tissue disease. In these cases, amphotericin B is required.

References

Agger WA, Caplan RH, Maki DG: Ocular sporotrichosis mimicking mucormycosis in a diabetic. Ann Ophthalmol 10:767–771, 1978.
Allen HF: Amphotericin B and exogenous mycotic endophthalmitis after cataract extraction. Arch Ophthalmol 88:640–644, 1972.
Axelrod AJ, Peymon GA, Aplle DJ: Toxicity of intravitreal injection of amphotericin B. Am J Ophthalmol 76:578–583, 1973.
Brunette I, Stulting RD: *Sporothrix schenckii* scleritis. Am J Ophthalmol 114:370–371, 1992.
Clarkson JG, Green WR: Endogenous fungal endophthalmitis. *In* Duane TD (ed): Clinical Ophthalmology. Hagerstown, MD, Harper & Row, 1982, Vol III, pp 11:23–27.
Francois J, Rysselaere M: Oculomycoses. Springfield, IL, Charles C Thomas, 1972, pp 370–386.
Kurosawa A, et al: *Sporothrix schenckii* endophthalmitis in a patient with human immunodeficiency virus infection. Arch Ophthalmol 88:376–380, 1988.
Restrepo A, Robledo J, Gomez I, Tabares AM, Gutierrez R: Itraconazole therapy in lymphangitic and cutaneous sporotrichosis. Arch Dermatol 122:413–417, 1986.
Stern GA, Fetkenhour CL, O'Grady RB: Intravitreal amphotericin B treatment of *Candida* endophthalmitis. Arch Ophthalmol 98:89–93, 1977.
Witherspoon CD, Kuhn F, Owens SD, White MF, Kimble JA: Endophthalmitis due to *Sporothrix schenckii* after penetrating ocular injury. Ann Ophthalmol 22(10):385–387, 1990.

Rickettsial Infections

Q FEVER 083.0
(Query Fever)

RICHARD B. HORNICK, M.D.

Orlando, Florida

Q fever is the name attached to the infections produced by *Coxiella burnetii*. The name comes from the frustration that Derrick encountered when he was unable to isolate a bacterial pathogen from workers in an abattoir who were part of an outbreak of a febrile illness. Thus, he called this Q (for query) fever. Even though the organism continues to be classified as a *Rickettsia*, its intracellular growth characteristics are different from those of the other *Rickettsia*. It is a highly infectious agent; probably infection with only one organism may cause disease in humans. Diagnosis is confirmed by serologic tests because attempts at isolation of the organism are dangerous due to its high infectivity. Reported infections are rare, about 15 to 20 per year. Infections are usually asymptomatic. Serologic surveys indicate as high as 40 per cent of a population exposed to cattle, sheep, and goats may have demonstrable circulating antibodies. Persons who are ill have a mild, self-limiting, febrile illness that is characterized by fever, severe intractable headache, and myalgia. About half of such patients can be shown to have pneumonitis. Ten per cent may develop hepatitis; however, as many as 85 per cent of patients may have abnormal liver function tests. Rarely, chronic infection of the heart valves occurs. Rash is not a manifestation of this infection.

Ocular involvement in Q fever is unusual, and ocular manifestations as the only evidence of the disease are very rare. Lesions involving the eye are probably a consequence of the vasculitis that is the hallmark of rickettsial infections. The organisms multiply in the endothelial cells of small blood vessels. Most patients have a severe headache with associated photophobia, and the pain is frequently retro-orbital in location. The pathogenesis of this pain is probably related to the vasculitis. Conjunctivae are injected, but no exudate occurs. Uveitis occurs very rarely; however, thorough evaluation of *C. burnetii* as a cause of uveitis has not been carried out. Lesions in the retina are also unusual, but evidence of the vasculitis may occur as hemorrhages, edema, and engorgement of veins. As a consequence of immune reactions, episcleritis can conceivably occur. Two recent case reports indicate that involvement of the extrinsic and intrinsic ocular muscles can occur. One patient had Miller Fisher syndrome with bilateral ptosis, sixth nerve paralysis bilaterally, and upgaze paralysis. Residual symptoms persisted for 7 months. Another patient had Q fever meningoencephalitis with bilateral abducens nerve paralysis, optic neuritis, and abnormal CSF findings. These findings were reversible.

THERAPY

Systemic. No antibiotic has demonstrated equal in vivo therapeutic effectiveness to tetracycline and chloramphenicol, which remain the drugs of choice for treatment of rickettsial infections. Either tetracycline or chloramphenicol in a dosage of 0.5 gm every 6 hours can produce good therapeutic responses. Antibiotic therapy should be continued for 7 to 10 days for the patient with pneumonitis. Duration of antibiotic therapy for such ocular manifestations as uveitis seen secondary to Q fever is unknown. Steroid therapy for symptoms related to Q fever has not been evaluated; however, in other rickettsial infections, steroids have been used with some success for patients in shock.

Ocular. In those rare patients who develop episcleritis, topical corticosteroid drops can be used to reduce the erythema. These patients must also receive concurrent systemic antibiotic therapy. The steroids will interfere with the host's attempts to contain the *C. burnetii* and thus the need for the antibiotic.

PRECAUTIONS

Adverse effects of antibiotic and steroid treatment need to be kept in mind. Gastrointestinal disturbances, such as nausea, vomiting, and diarrhea, can be associated with tetracycline therapy. The occurrence of diarrhea requires that the drug be stopped immediately and the patient evaluated for the possibility of antibiotic colitis. Chloramphenicol is less likely to cause these same problems, but antibiotic colitis has been reported in patients receiving chloramphenicol. The risk of bone marrow depression after chloramphenicol administration is about 1 in 20,000 to 40,000. Steroid therapy may interfere with immune mechanisms necessary to suppress the infectious processes.

COMMENTS

Q fever is acquired primarily by inhalation of infected aerosols. Large domestic animals are the usual sources of contamination. To date, these animals have not been demonstrated to be compromised by *C. burnetii* infection, although huge numbers of organisms are shed with the placentas of these animals and the area around some slaughterhouses can be shown to be contaminated with these rickettsiae. *C. burnetii* bacteria are very resistant to environmental decremental forces and will persist for years on surfaces where they have been deposited. After drying, they can be readily transmitted by windborne dust. Ingestion of milk from infected cows may be a source of inapparent infection, as well as overt disease. Infected ticks may be responsible for transmitting the disease among animals, but this mode of transmission has not been proven in humans. Person-to-person spread of the disease is unlikely, but pathologists have acquired such while performing autopsies on infected patients.

References

D'Angelo LJ, Baker EF, Schlosser W: Q fever in the United States. 1948–1977. J Infect Dis *139*:613–615, 1979.

Derrick EH: "Q" fever, A new fever entity: Clinical features, diagnosis and laboratory investigation. Med J Aust 2:281–299, 1937.

Diaz OA, et al: Miller Fisher syndrome Associated with Q fever. J Neurol Neurosurg Psychiatr 53: 615–616, 1990.

Duke-Elder S (ed): System of Ophthalmology. St. Louis, CV Mosby, 1976, Vol XV, p 135.

Dupont IIL, et al: Q fever hepatitis. Ann Intern Med 74:198–206, 1971.

Shaked Y, Samra Y: Q fever meningoencephalitis associated with bilateral abducens nerve paralysis, bilateral optic neuritis and abnormal cerebrospinal fluid findings. Infection *17*:394–395, 1989.

ROCKY MOUNTAIN SPOTTED FEVER 082.0

BYRON L. LAM, M.D.

Little Rock, Arkansas

Rocky Mountain spotted fever is a severe acute infectious disease caused by the obligate, intracellular bacteria *Rickettsia rickettsii* and transmitted through the skin by the bite and excretions of infected ticks. The two major vectors in the United States are the wood tick, *Dermacentor andersoni*, in the Rocky Mountain states and the dog tick, *Dermacentor variabilis*, in the eastern and southern states. Dogs have been shown to harbor the organism, and young adults and children are most often infected. Approximately 700 cases with a mortality of 3 to 6 per cent are reported annually in the United States, with the majority occurring during the spring and summer months in the West, South Central, and South Atlantic regions. The organism invades the endothelial and smooth muscle cells of blood vessels, producing a systemic vasculitis with increased vascular permeability. Loss of serum proteins, decreased blood volume, and thrombi over damaged endothelial cells result in hypoperfusion and circulatory failure.

After a prodrome of fever and malaise, approximately 90 per cent of patients develop a maculopapular rash between the third and fifth day of the illness. The rash gradually becomes petechial and first involves the distal extremities, including the palms and soles. The rash subsequently spreads toward the trunk. Symptoms include high fever, lethargy, headache, myalgia, abdominal pain, and nausea and vomiting. Dehydration and edema often ensue, and splenomegaly, hepatomegaly, interstitial pneumonitis, and encephalitis may occur.

Ocular manifestations of Rocky Mountain spotted fever and scrub typhus are similar. These manifestations are usually limited to petechial lesions on the bulbar conjunctiva as part of the systemic vasculitis. Anterior nongranulomatous uveitis has been reported. Fundus changes are caused by vasculitis with retinal hemorrhages, cotton-wool spots, retinal edema, and increased vascular engorgement and tortuosity. Optic disc edema may occur, presumably from ischemia, and periorbital edema may be present in severe cases. Ocular histopathology from a case clinically consistent with Rocky Mountain spotted fever showed retinal and choroidal vasculitis, arteriolar occlusions, and focal infiltrates of chronic inflammatory cells.

THERAPY

Systemic.   The specific antibiotics are doxycycline, tetracycline, and chloramphenicol. Seriously ill patients require intravenous administration. Oral doses of doxycycline 100 mg twice a day or tetracycline 500 mg four times a day are recommended for adults who are not acutely ill. Likewise, oral doses of doxycycline, 2.2 mg/kg/day with an initial dose of 2.2 mg/kg twice a day for 1 day, or tetracycline 50 mg/kg/day in four divided doses are recommended for children over the age of 8 who are not acutely ill. In more seriously ill patients, intravenous doses of tetracycline 500 mg four times a day are given for adults and 30 mg/kg/day in four divided doses are given for children over the age of 8. Chloramphenicol is an alternative in adults in whom tetracycline is contraindicated (e.g., because of allergy, or pregnancy) and in children younger than 8 years of age. In children, chloramphenicol is given as 100 mg/kg/day intravenously in four divided doses and then 50 mg/kg/day orally in four divided doses. For adults, chloramphenicol is given as 500 mg to 750 mg four times a day intravenously or orally. These antibiotics are rickettsiostatic, and final elimination of the organism is achieved by host immune mechanisms. Therapy is continued for 7 to 10 days or until the patient is afebrile for 2 to 3 days.

Ocular.   After proper systemic antibiotic therapy is instituted, ocular signs and symptoms resolve rapidly. Moderately severe iridocyclitis should be treated with topical cycloplegics along with topical corticosteroids, although no specific information is available. Similarly, no data are available regarding enhanced resolution of conjunctivitis by topical antibiotics.

Supportive.   Intravenous fluids and electrolyte management are crucial to overcome dehydration and to support blood pressure. Anticonvulsants, analgesics, antipyretics, oxygen, mechanical ventilation, and other modalities may be necessary depending on the involvement of various organ systems.

Ocular or Periocular Manifestations

Conjunctiva: Petechiae; conjunctivitis.
Cornea: Keratic precipitates.
Eyelids: Edema.
Iris: Anterior nongranulomatous uveitis; iris nodules.
Optic Nerve: Disc edema.
Orbit: Edema.
Retina: Vasculitis; arteriolar occlusions; cotton-wool spots; edema; exudates; hemorrhages; vascular engorgement and tortuosity.

PRECAUTIONS

Rocky Mountain spotted fever is a potentially fatal disease, and early treatment with appropriate antibiotics is the key prognostic factor. Therapy should be instituted as soon as the disease is suspected since serologic tests will not become reliably positive for 7 to 10 days after onset of symptoms. The Weil-

Felix test has poor sensitivity and specificity and should not be used to diagnose the disease during the acute phase. Other commonly used serum tests include latex agglutination, indirect hemagglutination assay, and indirect immunofluorescent antibody assay. Recently, the polymerase chain reaction has successfully demonstrated *R. rickettsii* in patients with severe disease, but it is not widely available and its clinical utility is not yet proven. Biopsied skin lesions may be tested with direct immunofluorescence and immunoperoxidase, but these tests are also not widely available.

Bronchopneumonia is a common complication, resulting in accumulation of pulmonary fluid and impaired gas exchange. In these patients, fluids must be administered with caution because of susceptibility to vascular overload and acute pulmonary edema. Thus, orbital edema is an important sign of increased extravascular volume.

Intravascular coagulation accompanies the disease process, and thrombocytopenia should not be regarded arbitrarily as an indication of drug toxicity. The onset of encephalitis carries a grave prognosis, and a significant fatality rate of 3 to 6 per cent persists, which is usually attributable to delay in diagnosis and institution of specific antibiotic therapy.

COMMENTS

Ophthalmologists rarely participate in the management of patients with Rocky Mountain spotted fever in whom fulminant systemic symptoms overwhelm mild ocular manifestations. The ocular changes are probably underestimated and usually resolve within 3 weeks of therapy. Early recognition prompting timely treatment with appropriate antibiotics is crucial to reduce mortality and morbidity.

References

Cherubini TD, Spaeth GL: Anterior nongranulomatous uveitis associated with Rocky Mountain spotted fever. Arch Ophthalmol *81*:363–365, 1969.

Duffey RJ, Hammer E: The ocular manifestations of Rocky Mountain spotted fever. Ann Ophthalmol *19*:301–306, 1987.

Kamper C: Treatment of Rocky Mountain spotted fever. J Pediatr Health Care *5*:216–222, 1991.

Kirk JL, Fine DP, Sexton DJ, Muchmore HG: Rocky Mountain spotted fever. A clinical review based on 48 confirmed cases, 1943-1986. Medicine *69*: 35–45, 1990.

Presley GD: Fundus changes in Rocky Mountain spotted fever. Am J Ophthalmol *67*:263–267, 1969.

Raab EL, Leopold IH, Hodes HL: Retinopathy in Rocky Mountain spotted fever. Am J Ophthalmol *68*:42–46, 1969.

Smith TW, Burton TC: The retinal manifestations of Rocky Mountain spotted fever. Am J Ophthalmol *84*:259–262, 1977.

Sulewski ME, Green WR: Ocular histopathologic features of a presumed case of Rocky Mountain spotted fever. Retina *6*:125–130, 1986.

Weber DJ, Walker DH: Rocky Mountain spotted fever. Infect Dis Clin N Am *5*:19–35, 1991.

SCRUB TYPHUS 081.2
(Japanese River Fever, Mite-Borne Typhus, Rural Typhus, Tropical Typhus, Tsutsugamushi Disease)

ROBERT L. BERRY, M.D.

Little Rock, Arkansas

Scrub typhus is an acute febrile illness caused by *Rickettsia tsutsugamushi* or *R. orientalis*. This organism is endemic to a large area of the Far East bounded by Japan, Pakistan, and Australia. It is transmitted to humans by the larva (chiggers) of several mite (*Leptotrombidium*) species. The name derives from the "scrub" or wasteland favored by the rodent hosts carrying the mites. Tsutsugamushi, the Japanese name, was used much earlier than scrub typhus, but the latter name was widely used by the soldiers of World War II in whom many thousands of cases developed.

The classic presentation, seen in 60 per cent or more of cases, is an initial papule progressing to an ulcer or eschar at the site of the chigger bite. Invariably, there is moderate to high-grade continuous fever, very often accompanied by frontal headache and significant regional lymphadenopathy. Chest pain, blurred vision, conjunctivitis, and maculopapular rash are common. The spectrum of the disease is wide, however, and often the characteristic signs are not present. Mild disease is difficult to diagnose, and the disease is much more common than originally thought. A definite clinical diagnosis of scrub typhus is often difficult to achieve, and specific laboratory confirmation (by immunofluorescent technique) is expensive and rarely available early enough to influence patient management. Some studies of tropical workers show it to be the most common cause of febrile illness requiring hospitalization.

The acute phase of the untreated disease lasts 2 to 3 weeks, followed by a prolonged convalescence. Serious or fatal respiratory, neurologic, cardiovascular, or hematologic complications may develop during the second week of untreated illness. Prompt diagnosis and the use of appropriate antibiotics rapidly alter the clinical course of the disease.

Ocular findings in scrub typhus are particularly striking and may be of diagnostic aid in the early stages of the disease. Although the marked flush, conjunctival hyperemia, conjunctivitis, and periorbital edema are seen with other infectious diseases, a distinguishing feature of scrub typhus is the marked retinal vein engorgement. This retinopathy usually occurs in the second or third week of the disease and persists for many weeks and well into the period of convalescence.

THERAPY

Systemic. Broad-spectrum antibiotics are effective in the treatment of this disease and should be initiated early in the illness. Tetracycline is probably the drug of choice because it eliminates symptoms of scrub typhus more rapidly than chloramphenicol, and relapses are uncommon unless an incomplete course of therapy is administered. A daily adult dosage of 2 gm of tetracycline should be administered in four equal doses. The recommended daily dosage of tetracycline for children is calculated on the basis of 25 to 50 mg/kg.

A single oral dose of a long-acting tetracycline, such as 200 mg of doxycycline, may be as effective as a 7-day course of tetracycline in the treatment of scrub typhus. Doxycycline should not be given on an empty stomach.

Chloramphenicol may also be effective for the treatment of scrub typhus. The daily chloramphenicol dosage should be calculated on the basis of 39 mg/kg.

Antibiotics should be continued for at least 7 to 10 days. Doing so allows time for the patient's immunologic defense to develop appropriate antibodies and to prevent relapses.

Ocular. Cycloplegics are used to put the ciliary body at rest and control the anterior uveitis and photophobia. One drop of 1 per cent atropine, 5 per cent homatropine, or 0.25 per cent scopolamine may be used in the involved eye two to four times daily. Local corticosteroid eyedrops are also effective for control of inflammation. One drop of 0.1 per cent dexamethasone, 0.12 per cent prednisolone acetate, or 1 per cent prednisolone phosphate may be used two to four times daily.

Supportive. Adjunctive therapy includes bedrest, fluid and electrolyte replacement, and adequate protein intake. The patient should be hospitalized and observed for potential complications secondary to inadequate or delayed therapy, such as circulatory collapse, renal failure, anemia, or hypoproteinemia. These patients should also be carefully observed for disseminated intravascular coagulation.

Ocular or Periocular Manifestations

Conjunctiva: Hemorrhages; hyperemia.
Cornea: Keratic precipitates; ulcers.
Eyelids: Cicatrization; ecchymosis; edema; madarosis.
Iris: Anterior uveitis; synechiae.

Retina: Edema; exudates, hemorrhages, venous engorgement.
Vitreous: Haze.
Other: Decreased visual acuity; enlarged blind spot; fixation nystagmus; irritation; lacrimation; paracentral scotoma; photophobia.

PRECAUTIONS

In addition to its greater potential for bone marrow toxicity, chloramphenicol is somewhat slower than tetracycline in reducing the fever and other clinical manifestations of scrub typhus. Therefore, chloramphenicol should be restricted to only those patients in whom there is a contraindication to tetracycline administration.

All tetracyclines have relatively low toxicity at usual dosage levels. However, tetracycline use in children under 8 years of age is contraindicated because of possible temporary depression of bone growth and permanent changes in teeth. Gastrointestinal disturbances occur in about 10 per cent of patients receiving 2 gm or more of tetracycline daily. Gastric irritation and vomiting following single-dose administration of doxycycline may necessitate that some doses be repeated. Strict adherence to the instructions that the drug should be taken after a meal usually eliminates gastric irritation and vomiting. Intolerance to doxycycline may be more marked than to tetracycline.

COMMENTS

Single-dose therapy for scrub typhus would shorten the time that patients spend in the hospital and might allow treatment to be given on an outpatient basis because consumption of the antibiotic could be assured.

References

Brown GW: Recent studies in scrub typhus: A review. J Roy Soc Med 71:507–510, 1978.
Brown GW, et al: Scrub typhus: A common cause of illness in indigenous populations. Trans Roy Soc Trop Med Hyg 70:444–448, 1977.
Brown GW, et al: Single-dose doxycycline therapy for scrub typhus. Trans Roy Soc Trop Med Hyg 72:412–416, 1978.
Chamberlain WP Jr: Ocular findings in scrub typhus. Arch Ophthalmol 48:313–321, 1952.
Kitagawa M: A rare case of acute neuroretinitis due to tsutsugamushi disease. Jpn J Clin Ophthalmol 33:1047–1052, 1979.
Paul SR, Karanth S, Dickson D: Scrub typhus along the Thai-Kampuchean border; new treatment regimen. Trop Doc 17:104–107, 1987.
Pogge RC: Tsutsugamushi fever in Arizona. Ariz Med 31:832–833, 1974.
Ramanathan M, Abidin M, Balachand V: The diagnosis of scrub typhus: An evaluation. Med J Malaysia 42:61–64, 1987.
Scheie HG: Ocular changes associated with scrub typhus: Study of 451 patients. Arch Ophthalmol 40:245–267, 1948.

Sheehy TW, Hazlett D, Turk RE: Scrub typhus. A comparison of chloramphenicol and tetracycline in its treatment. Arch Intern Med 132:77–80, 1973.

Twartz JC, et al: Doxycycline prophylaxis for human scrub typhus. J Infect Dis 146:811–818, 1982.
Wang CL, et al: Neonatal scrub typhus: A case report. Pediatrics 89:965–968, 1992.

Viral Infections

ACQUIRED IMMUNODEFICIENCY SYNDROME (AIDS) 042.9

GARY N. HOLLAND, M.D.

Los Angeles, California

AIDS is the most severe condition in a spectrum of clinical disorders caused by human immunodeficiency virus, type 1 (HIV-1). HIV-1 can infect a variety of cells, but its most serious effects are due to infection of CD4+ ("helper") T-lymphocytes. The resulting immunologic abnormalities make patients susceptible to life-threatening opportunistic infections and lead to the development of unusual neoplasms through unknown mechanisms. HIV-2 is a related retrovirus that also causes AIDS. It is found more commonly in African patients.

The term "AIDS" was created by the Centers for Disease Control for epidemiologic purposes to describe the most serious cases of HIV infection; individuals are given a diagnosis of AIDS if they have one or more specific "indicator diseases" that result from HIV infection, including serious opportunistic infections such as *Pneumocystis carinii* pneumonia, unusual neoplasms such as Kaposi sarcoma, and HIV encephalopathy. The spectrum of HIV-associated conditions also includes the acute, transient mononucleosis-like syndrome that can follow initial infection; a syndrome of persistent generalized lymphadenopathy, chronic fever, weight loss, and diarrhea (commonly referred to as AIDS-related complex [ARC]); and asymptomatic infections. It is not known how many HIV-infected individuals will eventually develop AIDS, but it is estimated that at least 50 per cent will do so within 10 years after being infected with HIV.

Infection with HIV occurs through sexual intercourse, receipt of contaminated blood products, or congenital transmission from an infected mother to her unborn child. Groups at high risk for HIV infection include homosexual and bisexual men, intravenous drug abusers, and heterosexual partners of HIV-infected individuals. Male-to-female transmission occurs more readily than female-to-male transmission during heterosexual intercourse. Routine testing of blood donors for HIV antibodies has reduced the risk of infection for hemophiliacs and recipients of whole blood transfusions.

Ocular disorders are among the common manifestations of AIDS. The majority of patients develop one or more ophthalmic disorders during the course of their illness. Most disorders fall into four categories: lesions related to microvascular disease (cotton-wool spots, retinal hemorrhages, conjunctival microvasculopathy); opportunistic ocular infections; neoplasms of the ocular surface, adnexa, and orbit; and neuro-ophthalmic abnormalities related to intracranial infections and neoplasms. CMV retinopathy is the most common sight-threatening disease associated with AIDS.

THERAPY

Systemic. Three drugs have been approved by the Food and Drug Administration (FDA) for specific treatment of HIV infection: zidovudine (500–600 mg/day), didanosine (200–600 mg/day), and zalcitabine (1.125–2.25 mg/day, approved only for use in combination with zidovudine). Zidovudine has been shown to increase patient survival and ameliorate the severity of secondary opportunistic infections. The effect of these drugs on the incidence and severity of ophthalmic disease has not been studied specifically.

There have been several anecdotal reports that zidovudine alters the course of CMV retinopathy or halts its progression, presumably through its immunopotentiating effect since it has no in vitro activity against CMV. It is doubtful that zidovudine therapy alone will be effective treatment for CMV retinopathy in the vast majority of patients, however. The role of zidovudine as an adjunct to specific anti-CMV therapy remains to be determined.

It has been hypothesized that HIV infection of ocular tissues can cause uveitis in the absence of secondary opportunistic infections. Zidovudine therapy has been reported anecdotally to cause resolution of anterior chamber and vitreous inflammatory reactions. Zidovudine should never be used as initial therapy, however, until a thorough examination and laboratory investigation rule out a secondary infectious cause.

Despite the availability of antiretroviral drugs, the mainstay of AIDS therapy remains the treatment of secondary opportunistic infections and neoplasms. Patients are best treated by a team of physicians that may include infectious disease specialists, immunologists, oncologists, neurologists, radiation oncologists, pediatricians, and ophthalmologists. The evaluation and systemic treatment of ocular infections should be conducted with the assistance of infectious disease specialists, since autopsy studies indicate that intraocular infections are usually associated with widely disseminated disease.

Two drugs have been approved by the FDA for the treatment of CMV retinopathy: ganciclovir and foscarnet. Both can halt or slow the progression of CMV retinopathy in immunocompromised patients. However, they do not eradicate virus from the eye; virus can be recovered from the retina after treatment, and reactivation of the retinopathy occurs after cessation of drug therapy. Patients therefore must receive chronic low-dose therapy to prevent disease recurrence. Even with continued treatment, eventual reactivation or slow spread of infection is common.

Based on clinical experience with these drugs, dosing regimens have been established empirically that consist of an induction phase (ganciclovir: 5 mg/kg intravenously every 12 hours for 14 days; foscarnet: 60 mg/kg every 8 hours for 14 days) followed by a maintenance phase (ganciclovir: 5 mg/kg intravenously daily or 6 mg/kg every 24 hours for 5 days out of 7; foscarnet: 90 mg/kg daily). A foscarnet maintenance dose of 120 mg/kg/day has been used by some investigators; this higher dose may provide better control of CMV retinopathy and increased survival without an appreciable increase in toxicity. The drugs are available only in intravenous preparations. A permanent indwelling catheter is usually placed in patients receiving maintenance therapy.

An oral formulation of ganciclovir is being investigated. However, because of its low bioavailability it will probably be useful only for maintenance therapy, and induction therapy for the initial control of infection and reinduction therapy for disease reactivation will still require intravenous medication.

Ganciclovir has bone marrow toxicity; many AIDS patients receiving the drug become neutropenic. Neutropenia can be treated with leukocyte growth factors (sargramostim [granulocyte-monocyte colony stimulating factor, GM-CSF]; filgrastim [granulocyte colony stimulating factor, G-CSF]). Concurrent use of one agent can allow continued use of ganciclovir at full doses in many patients with a history of neutropenia.

Foscarnet has renal toxicity, which is the most common reason that its use must be discontinued. It can also cause anemia and abnormalities in calcium metabolism.

The efficacies and toxicities of ganciclovir and foscarnet have been compared in a large multicenter study. There was no difference between treatment groups for major ophthalmic end-points, including final visual acuity or time to disease reactivation and progression. There was a difference in survival; median survival for patients treated with foscarnet was 12.6 months, whereas median survival for patients treated only with ganciclovir was 8.5 months. The cause of the differential survival was not determined, but may be related to the fact that foscarnet has antiretroviral activity as well. In addition, patients treated with ganciclovir were less able to tolerate zidovudine, because it is also a bone marrow suppressant. In the future, survival patterns may change; didanosine, dideoxycytosine (which can be used with ganciclovir), and leukocyte growth factors (which allow the concurrent use of full-dose ganciclovir and zidovudine) were not widely available at the time of the trial. There was also a difference in morbidity between treatment groups. Patients receiving foscarnet were more likely to switch to ganciclovir because of drug side effects than vice versa. The choice between ganciclovir and foscarnet for initial therapy of CMV retinopathy should be individualized for each patient on the basis of these various factors.

Reactivation of CMV retinopathy can usually be brought back under control by a repeat 2-week course of higher-dose, induction-level therapy ("reinduction") with the same drug being used for maintenance therapy. Most patients will continue to have reactivations, and they may come at increasingly short intervals. Several treatment strategies have been used for late reactivations; they include alternating ganciclovir and foscarnet, combining ganciclovir and foscarnet, and continuously administering induction-level ganciclovir with concurrent use of a leukocyte growth factor. Which is most effective of these regimens has not been determined.

Patients who cannot tolerate any systemic administration of drug may benefit from the intravitreal administration of ganciclovir (see the section on Ocular Therapy below).

Successful treatment will preserve vision, but cannot restore vision already lost because of retinal necrosis. Patients should be informed of the symptoms of infection, which include floaters, visual field changes, and blurring, and should seek medical attention immediately if they occur. Ganciclovir or foscarnet therapy is usually begun immediately in patients with vision-threatening lesions in one or both eyes: those adjacent to or inside the major temporal vascular arcades and those adjacent to the optic nerve head. Because of the toxic effects of drug therapy and the slow rate with which lesions enlarge, it may be appropriate to delay treatment of more anterior lesions in some patients until progression is documented.

Retinal destruction in CMV retinopathy is caused by the productive viral infection of retinal cells. It is not a secondary effect of inflammation. Steroids therefore should play no role in the treatment of CMV retinopathy.

Varicella-zoster virus (VZV) retinopathy is treated with intravenous acyclovir (10–20 mg/kg every 8 hours for at least 10 days), although results have generally been poor because of its rapidly progressive nature. After the initial course of therapy, patients probably should receive maintenance therapy with acyclovir, but the amount of drug required to prevent reactivation has not been determined.

Toxoplasmic retinochoroiditis responds to treatment with antiparasitic drugs, but the best therapy has not been established. The most commonly used drugs are pyrimethamine in combination with one of the following antibiotics: sulfadiazine, clindamycin, tetracycline (if other drugs cannot be tolerated), or spiramycin (not available in the United States). With treatment, lesions involute and scar, and inflammation resolves. Reactivation of lesions is common unless at least one drug is continued on a chronic basis. The majority of retinal destruction in immunocompromised patients with toxoplasmosis results from the proliferation of parasites, rather than from inflammation. Therefore, steroid therapy is probably of little value in these patients.

All patients suspected of having ocular syphilis should be referred for evaluation of the cerebrospinal fluid to rule out neurosyphilis. Drug regimens appropriate for the treatment of neurosyphilis should be used in all patients with ocular disease: at least 10 days of aqueous crystalline penicillin G (2-4 million units intravenously every 4 hours) or aqueous procaine penicillin G (2.4 million units intramuscularly each day) with probenecid (500 mg orally 4 times daily). The efficacy of penicillin therapy may be altered in HIV-infected patients; it is believed that the rate of treatment failures is increased. Patients should be observed closely after treatment for evidence of disease recurrence.

Systemic corticosteroids should be used with caution in patients with HIV infection. Although commonly used in the treatment of zoster ophthalmicus, ocular toxoplasmosis, and other uveitic disorders in immunocompetent individuals, their use in patients with AIDS may result in additional, unacceptable immunosuppression. Furthermore, they probably contribute little to the management of most sight-threatening lesions. As stated above, retinal necrosis in CMV retinopathy and ocular toxoplasmosis results primarily from cellular destruction by the proliferating pathogens, rather than from the associated inflammatory response.

Chemotherapy is the first line of defense against multifocal Kaposi sarcoma and should be administered under the direction of an oncologist. Drugs used successfully to induce regression of tumors (including ophthalmic lesions) are doxorubicin, bleomycin, and vinblastine. An appropriate indication for treatment of conjunctival tumors is the presence of large bulky lesions that are cosmetically disturbing, interfere with eyelid function (rare), or produce discomfort because of mass effect (the tumors themselves are not painful). Appropriate indications for treatment of eyelid tumors are entropion formation and trichiasis resulting from large indurated tumors, ulceration of tumor-involved eyelid margins, and enlarging tumors that may eventually result in these complications. Local therapy for ophthalmic lesions is necessary only if systemic therapy is unsuccessful, or cannot be tolerated, in cases where an immediate response is needed to prevent complications (trichiasis, ulceration of the eyelid margin), or if the patient has isolated ophthalmic lesions.

Ocular. Intravitreal injections of ganciclovir* have been used in patients with CMV retinopathy who are neutropenic and therefore cannot receive intravenous ganciclovir. A dose of 200 μg in 0.1 cc is delivered via the pars plana to the midvitreous. Doses as high as 400 μg in 0.1 ml have been used in refractory cases. Injections are given twice weekly until the disease is brought under control; maintenance of quiescent lesions with one injection per week then can be considered. Experience with this treatment is limited, and issues regarding drug toxicity after repeated injections have not been resolved. An implantable device that slowly releases ganciclovir into the vitreous is under investigation. Intravitreal ganciclovir therapy probably should be reserved only for those cases with progressive, sight-threatening infections in patients who cannot tolerate systemic administration of adequate doses of either ganciclovir or foscarnet.

Laser therapy of CMV retinopathy has been attempted, but it does not seem to be capable of preventing the spread of CMV retinopathy.

Cryotherapy can be used to treat conjunctival or eyelid Kaposi sarcoma. Eyelid lesions treated with a circulating liquid nitrogen probe at −30°C using a freeze-thaw-freeze-thaw technique have resolved without recurrence over many months of follow-up. Cryotherapy can also be used to treat molluscum contagiosum lesions on the eyelids. Lesions do shrink, but frequently they do not resolve completely, even with repeated treatments.

Surgical. Repair of retinal detachments in patients with CMV retinopathy is the most commonly performed ophthalmic surgical procedure in patients with AIDS. Detachments occur in at 25 per cent of patients, and the risk increases with the duration of infection. Because of extensive hole formation in areas of necrotic retina, vitrectomy and the use of silicone oil for retinal tamponade are the most commonly used procedures. Recurrent detachments are frequent.

As in immunocompetent hosts, vitrectomy may be necessary for treatment of those rare cases of fungal endophthalmitis that occur in patients with AIDS.

Large molluscum contagiosum lesions of the eyelids may require complete surgical excision. Curettage is less effective for treatment of lesions than in immunocompetent hosts.

Surgical excision of Kaposi sarcoma lesions

of the conjunctiva or eyelids is rarely necessary because of their good response to systemic chemotherapy, irradiation, or cryotherapy. If surgery is necessary for diagnostic examination or to debulk large tumors, they can be excised easily without excessive bleeding despite their vascular nature. Even total excision of isolated tumors is not curative because of the multifocal nature of this neoplasm.

Topical. Herpes simplex virus epithelial keratitis associated with AIDS tends to be more severe and to recur more frequently than when it occurs in immunocompetent patients. Lesions seem to respond to topical antiviral therapy (trifluridine 1 per cent, administered every 2 hours up to nine times daily), but resolution of lesions even with treatment may take 3 weeks or longer. Lesions should be treated until the dendriform or geographic lesions have have completely resolved. Continued use of topical antiviral medication to prevent recurrences is not indicated.

Persistent dendriform keratitis resembling herpes simplex virus epithelial keratitis but caused by a productive varicella-zoster virus infection can occur in patients without severe zoster lesions of the skin. This infection seems to respond to treatment with topical acyclovir ointment* (a formulation not available in the United States), but not to topical trifluridine.

Vigorous topical antibiotic therapy for secondary bacterial infections of the cornea, based on culture results and sensitivity testing, may be curative in selected cases despite the severe immunosuppression of AIDS.

Topical steroid therapy for the mild iridocyclitis that accompanies necrotizing viral infections of the retina is not necessary.

Irradiation: Local irradiation may be effective palliative treatment for Kaposi sarcoma lesions that involve the conjunctiva and/or eyelids in lieu of systemic chemotherapy. Administration of 2000 to 3000 centigrays (cGy) in 200 to 300 cGy fractions over a 3-week period by means of a 6-MeV linear accelerator (while shielding the eye) or a 100-kvp superficial radiation unit has been reported to cause total or near-total resolution of lesions with minimal side effects for 4 months or longer. Recurrences after 6 months are common. It has not been determined whether cryotherapy or irradiation is more effective for local therapy of Kaposi sarcoma.

Radiation therapy to decrease tumor mass also may be a useful adjunct to chemotherapy of Burkitt lymphoma involving the orbit.

Ocular or Periocular Manifestations

Anterior Segment: Iridocyclitis (syphilitic, secondary to retinal infections, idiopathic).

Choroid: Infections (pathogens that affect primarily the choroid but may have retinal involvement include *Mycobacterium avium* complex, *Mycobacterium tuberculosis*, *Cryptococcus neoformans, Candida albicans, Histoplasma capsulatum, Pneumocystis carinii, Sporotrichum schenckii*); choroidal effusion of unknown cause with forward displacement of ciliary body and angle-closure glaucoma.

Conjunctiva: Microvascular changes (dilated capillaries, isolated vascular fragments, vessel segments of irregular caliber, microaneurysms, sludging of blood flow); conjunctivitis (*Chalmydia trachomatis*, serotype L2 [lymphogranuloma venereum], molluscum contagiosum, idiopathic).

Cornea: Dendriform keratitis (herpes simplex virus, varicella-zoster virus); fungal ulcers (*Candida species*, unrelated to trauma); secondary bacterial ulcers.

Eyelids and Periocular Skin: Molluscum contagiosum; zoster ophthalmicus; Kaposi sarcoma.

Optic Nerve: Ischemic optic neuropathy; infection (CMV); papilledema (frequently associated with cryptococcal meningitis); optic atrophy.

Orbit: Neoplasms (Kaposi sarcoma, Burkitt lymphoma); pseudotumor.

Retina: Lesions attributable to retinal microvasculopathy (cotton-wool spots, retinal hemorrhages, microaneurysms, ischemic maculopathy); infections (pathogens that affect primarily the retina include CMV, *Toxoplasma gondii*, herpes simplex virus, *Nocardia sp.*, *Treponema pallidum*, varicella-zoster virus, endogenous bacteria); isolated retinal vasculitis of unknown cause.

Other: Neuro-ophthalmic signs of intracranial disease (cranial nerve palsies, visual field defects, pupillary abnormalities); sudden, severe, bilateral visual loss associated with cryptococcal meningitis (mechanism unknown); vitritis of unknown cause.

PRECAUTIONS

Physicians administering treatment must be aware of the risks associated with some antimicrobial therapies. Allergic reactions to sulfonamides occur commonly in patients with AIDS. Patients given sulfadiazine for treatment of toxoplasmosis should be observed closely for the development of rashes. Neutropenia occurs in many patients who receive ganciclovir. Absolute neutrophil counts usually rise with cessation of treatment, but irreversible neutropenia and death have been associated rarely with ganciclovir use. Ganciclovir-resistant strains of CMV have been isolated from patients receiving long-term treatment. Foscarnet may cause severe renal toxicity with azotemia, anemia, and abnormalities in calcium metabolism.

Care should be taken to minimize factors predisposing to opportunistic infections. Maintenance of nonspecific natural defenses, such as normal eyelid function and an intact corneal epithelium, are the most important means of decreasing serious infections of the ocular surface. Careful attention should be directed to the eyelid margins, looking for development or progression of Kaposi sarcoma lesions, which can cause entropion formation and trichiasis. Patients whose corneas have been compromised by previous disease should be observed carefully; neurotrophic keratitis following herpetic infections, for example, may be more susceptible to secondary bacterial ulcers. HIV-infected patients who develop contact lens-associated infections may be less able to combat these infections than their immunocompetent counterparts.

Iatrogenic factors can increase the risk of certain infections. Intraocular fungal infections are rare unless patients develop candidemia, which can be caused by contaminated indwelling catheters.

Patient care activities put health care workers at very low risk for HIV infection, although infection has occurred after needlestick accidents or prolonged exposure of open skin lesions to contaminated blood. The risk of such infection seems to be approximately 0.3 per cent. Nevertheless, all physicians, including ophthalmologists, should take great care to avoid such exposures. Caution should be taken with sharp instruments during ocular surgery. Needles should be placed in puncture-resistant containers immediately after use; resheathing of needles before disposal is not necessary and may result in needlestick injuries.

HIV has been identified in tears and ocular fluids, but there is no evidence that virus transmission has ever occurred by exposure to tears or contaminated instruments. Nevertheless, our understanding of HIV transmission remains incomplete, and precautions therefore are warranted to prevent virus transmission during ophthalmic examinations and procedures. Precautions should be employed with all patients since HIV infection may not be apparent.

Gowns, masks, and eye goggles are recommended if there is a possibility of contact with splashed blood or infected body fluids during examinations, invasive procedures, or laboratory studies. They are not necessary for routine ophthalmic examinations. Gloves may be worn if excessive lacrimation is expected or if the examiner has open lesions on the hands. Gloves should be worn in touching mucous membranes, open skin lesions, or body fluids. Although gloves will not prevent needlestick injuries, their use during fluorescein and retrobulbar anesthesia injections will prevent exposure to blood from the injection site or dripping from the needle. Coughing patients may be asked to wear masks to prevent the air borne spread of secondary pathogens.

Disposable items contaminated by blood or body fluids should be placed in watertight containers. Reusable instruments should be sterilized by standard techniques. Other contaminated devices should be wiped clean after direct contact with the ocular surface and then soaked in one of the following solutions for 10 minutes or longer: a *fresh* solution of 3 per cent hydrogen peroxide, 0.525 per cent sodium hypochlorite (1:10 dilution of household bleach), 70 per cent ethyl alcohol, or 70 per cent isopropyl alcohol. Instruments then should be thoroughly rinsed with water and dried before reuse. It is believed that applanation tonometer tips can be disinfected by wiping with a pledget soaked with 70 per cent isopropyl alcohol followed by air drying. Surfaces contaminated with blood or body fluids may be cleaned with a 2 per cent phenolic solution, e.g. Amphyl.

Contact lenses from trial fitting sets should be disinfected after every patient use by either of the following methods: commercially available hydrogen peroxide contact lens disinfecting solution or heat disinfection (78-80°C, 172-176°F) for at least 10 minutes. Some contact lenses will not tolerate heat disinfection. Specific recommendations for a given lens can be obtained from its manufacturer. Various commercially available chemical sterilizing solutions for contact lenses have not been fully evaluated for their ability to inactivate HIV in clinical situations.

HIV also has been identified in corneal tissue. Currently all cornea donors are screened for the presence of HIV antibodies, and tissue is not accepted from individuals known to be members of high-risk groups, regardless of their antibody status. There is no evidence, however, that HIV transmission by penetrating keratoplasty occurs, despite the fact that tissue has been used from donors discovered in retrospect to be HIV-infected.

COMMENTS

Accurate diagnosis of HIV-related ophthalmic disorders may have important implications for the overall care of patients. Disseminated infections, for example, may be apparent first in the eye. Early referral to specialists in other fields will allow more successful treatment of nonocular disorders.

AIDS is a uniformly fatal disease. Treatment of its secondary ophthalmic disorders is generally palliative since neoplasms are rarely cured and infections are rarely eliminated after they develop. Instead, therapy is aimed at controlling existing disease. Prolonged therapy may be required to prevent recurrences, but chronic prophylactic treatment to prevent ophthalmic infections is currently not practical. Prophylaxis against CMV retinopathy will be a potential use for oral ganciclovir or other oral agents if a better understanding of risk factors allows for the identification of patients at highest risk for this infection. Chronic topical antibiotic prophylaxis against ocular surface infections might be selectively used for antibiotic-resistant organisms or fungi.

The goal of therapy is to improve or maintain the quality of life for patients before they die. Clinicians must weigh the morbidity of various medications or operations against their potential benefits before beginning treatment. Factors to consider include visual potential, life expectancy for a given patient, and the need for other medications that may interfere with treatment. Some patients may decide against certain treatments, such as prolonged intravenous therapy for extensive unilateral retinal infections or repair of a unilateral total retinal detachment, because of the associated cost, inconvenience, side effects, and poor visual potential.

The understanding of AIDS and its treatment is evolving rapidly. The findings and recommendations contained herein are based on experience with the syndrome through mid-1992. Additional ocular disorders will undoubtedly be identified, and knowledge about disease pathophysiology will improve as the epidemic spreads. Existing therapies will be refined, and new drugs will become available. To provide appropriate care for patients, practicing ophthalmologists need to remain abreast of these developments.

References

Centers for Disease Control: Recommendations for preventing possible transmission of human T-lymphotropic virus type III/lymphadenopathy-associated virus from tears. MMWR 34:533–534, 1985.

Dugel PU, et al: Treatment of ocular adnexal Kaposi's sarcoma in the acquired immune deficiency syndrome. Ophthalmology 99:1127–1132, 1992.

Heinemann MH: Long-term intravitreal ganciclovir therapy for cytomegalovirus retinopathy. Arch Ophthalmol 107:1767–1772, 1989.

Holland GN, et al: Treatment of cytomegalovirus retinopathy with ganciclovir. Ophthalmology 94: 815–823, 1987.

Holland GN, et al: Ocular toxoplasmosis in patients with the acquired immunodeficiency syndrome. Am J Ophthalmol 106:653–667, 1988.

Irvine AR: Treatment of retinal detachment due to cytomegalovirus retinitis in patients with AIDS. Trans Am Ophthalmol Soc 89:349–363, 1991.

Margolis TP, et al: Varicella-zoster virus retinitis in patients with the acquired immunodeficiency syndrome. Am J Ophthalmol 112:119–131, 1991.

Palestine AG, et al: A randomized, controlled trial of foscarnet in the treatment of cytomegalovirus retinitis in patients with AIDS. Ann Intern Med 115:665–673, 1991.

Pepose JS, et al: Acquired immunodeficiency syndrome: Pathogenic mechanisms of ocular disease. Ophthalmology 92:472–484, 1985.

Schuman JS, Orellana J, Friedman AH, Teich SA: Acquired immunodeficiency syndrome (AIDS). Surv Ophthalmol 31:384–410, 1987.

Shuler JD, et al: Kaposi sarcoma of the conjunctiva and eyelids associated with the acquired immunodeficiency syndrome. Arch Ophthalmol 107: 858–862, 1989.

Studies of Ocular Complications of AIDS Research Group, in Collaboration with the AIDS Clinical Trials Group: Mortality in patients with the acquired immunodeficiency syndrome treated with either foscarnet or ganciclovir for cytomegalovirus retinitis. N Engl J Med 326:213–220, 1992.

ACUTE HEMORRHAGIC CONJUNCTIVITIS 077.4
(AHC, Epidemic Hemorrhagic Keratoconjunctivitis)

JOHN P. WHITCHER, Jr., M.D., M.P.H.

San Francisco, California

Acute hemorrhagic conjunctivitis, a new disease entity first reported in 1969 in Ghana, has since become pandemic, with the first epidemic in the United States occurring September, 1981, in Key West, Florida. The etiologic agent, which has been isolated from patients worldwide including one patient in Florida, has been designated as enterovirus type 70, a new member of the enterovirus group.

Interestingly, another viral agent, coxsackievirus 24 variant (CA24v), has also been isolated in several epidemics since its first appearance as a cause of AHC in Taiwan in 1985. Evolutionary analysis of enterovirus 70 and CA24v, using the nucleotide sequence, indicates that the two viruses branched off from the prototype strain in 1984 approximately 18 months before the first epidemic of AHC due to CA24v occurred in Taiwan. The epidemiologic importance of this observation is profound because exposure to one strain does not convey immunity to the other.

After a short incubation period of 24 to 48 hours, patients experience an explosive onset of irritation, foreign body sensation, and periorbital pain. In several hours, a full-blown conjunctivitis develops with lid edema, chemosis, seromucous discharge, and complaints of photophobia and tearing. Both eyes are usually involved, and preauricular lymphoadenopathy with variable tenderness is present. Subconjunctival hemorrhages are invariably present, beginning as small petechiae on the bulbar conjunctiva and quickly spreading to cover both the bulbar and palpebral conjunctiva. Moderate follicular hypertrophy is present, as well as a fine, diffuse, epithelial keratitis. In the majority of patients, the acute conjunctivitis subsides spontaneously in 3 or 4 days, with residual conjunctival hemorrhages and corneal epithelial staining remaining as long as 7 to 14 days. Systemic symptoms are rare, although several cases of lumbosacral radiculomyelitis have been reported late in the course of the disease, at a rate of 1 in 10,000 cases.

THERAPY

Ocular. Topical broad-spectrum antibiotics, such as 10 per cent sulfacetamide eyedrops, may be used to prevent secondary bacterial infection. One drop instilled into both eyes four times daily is sufficient.

Topical corticosteroids are not usually indicated. The rapid course of the infection leads to quick resolution without complications in most cases.

Supportive. Because acute hemorrhagic conjunctivitis is extremely contagious, strict hygiene should be observed. Family members are especially at high risk of infection.

Ocular or Periocular Manifestations

Conjunctiva: Chemosis; follicular conjunctivitis; petechial bulbar hemorrhages (which rapidly coalesce on the palpebral conjunctiva also); seromucous discharge.

Cornea: Fine, diffuse, epithelial keratitis present centrally or superiorly.

Other: Lacrimation; lid edema; periorbital pain; photophobia; preauricular lymphadenopathy with variable tenderness; a transient low-grade iritis.

PRECAUTIONS

As in the case of epidemic keratoconjunctivitis, transmission of acute hemorrhagic conjunctivitis seems to be mainly by eye-to-hand-to-eye contact. Contaminated instruments or medications may also be implicated, and great care should be taken by the physician examining patients with the disease not to unwittingly transmit it to other individuals. Careful handwashing and cleansing of instruments are essential.

It is likely that acute hemorrhagic conjunctivitis is now endemic in many populations where there were previous epidemics. The presence of continuing sporadic infections has been demonstrated by significant titers of virus neutralizing antibody to enterovirus type 70 in many young children in Ghana, even though a major epidemic has not occurred there in over 15 years.

COMMENTS

Even though acute hemorrhagic conjunctivitis is an extremely symptomatic and highly visible ocular disease occurring in epidemic proportions, complications are fortunately rare. Prolonged visual disability does not occur as in some cases of epidemic keratoconjunctivitis, and patients recover with remarkably few sequelae. Because of the relatively benign course of the disease, overtreatment with topical antibiotics and corticosteroids should be avoided.

References

Acute hemorrhagic conjunctivitis caused by coxsackievirus A24-Caribbean. MMWR *36*:245–251, 1987.

Acute hemorrhagic conjunctivitis—Key West, Florida. MMWR *30*:463–464, 1981

Asbell PA, de la Pena W, Harms D, et al: Acute hemorrhagic conjunctivitis in central America: First enterovirus epidemic in the western hemisphere. Ann Ophthalmol *17*:205–209, 1985.

Babalola OE, Amone SS, Samaila E, et al: An outbreak of acute hemorrhagic conjunctivitis in Ka-

duna, Nigeria. Br J Ophthalmol *74(2)*:89–92, 1990.

Chatterjee S, Quarcoopome CO, Apenteng A: Unusual type of epidemic conjunctivitis in Ghana. Br J Ophthalmol *54*:628–630, 1970.

Isolation of enterovirus 70 from a patient with acute hemorrhagic conjunctivitis—Key West, Florida. MMWR *30*:497, 1981

Kuritsky JN, Weaver JH, Bernard KW, et al: An outbreak of acute hemorrhagic conjunctivitis in central Minnesota. Am J Ophthalmol *96*:449–452, 1983.

Lin KH, Takeda N, Miyamura K, et al: The nucleotide sequence of 3c proteinase region of the coxsackievirus A24 variant: Comparison of the isolates in Taiwan in 1985-1988. Virus Genes *5(2)*: 121–131, 1991.

Minami K, et al: Seroepidemiologic studies of acute hemorrhagic conjunctivitis virus (enterovirus type 70) in West Africa. I. Studies with human sera from Ghana collected eight years after the first outbreak. Am J Epidemiol *114*:267–273, 1981.

Sklar VE, Patriarca PA, Onorato IM, et al: Clinical findings and results of treatment in an outbreak of acute hemorrhagic conjunctivitis in Southern Florida. Am J Ophthalmol *95*:45–54, 1983.

Whitcher JP, et al: Acute hemorrhagic conjunctivitis in Tunisia. Report of viral isolations. Arch Ophthalmol *94*:51–55, 1976.

Wright PW, Stauss GH, Langford MP: Acute hemorrhagic conjunctivitis. Am Fam Physician *45(1)*: 173–178, 1992.

Wulff H, Anderson LJ, Pallansch MA, et al: Diagnosis of enterovirus 70 infection by demonstration of IgM antibodies. J Med Virol *21*:321–327, 1987.

CAT-SCRATCH DISEASE 372.02

SCOTT M. MacRAE, M.D.

Portland, Oregon

Cat-scratch disease is a self-limited disease most often seen in children and characterized by local lymphadenopathy. The disease is usually preceded by a history of a cat scratch, bite, or lick. Less commonly, the disease may result from exposure to another animal, such as a rabbit or monkey. Typically, from 1 to 4 weeks after exposure, a red papule or rash or both occur at the inoculation site with subsequent lymphadenopathy. Low-grade fever, malaise, and lymph node discomfort may be present. Although complications are rare, hepatosplenomegaly, mediastinal masses, thrombocytopenic purpura, encephalitis, and osteolytic lesions have been documented. A skin test in which cat-scratch (Hanger Rose) antigen is injected intradermally into the volar surface of the forearm confirms the diagnosis, although false-negative results may occur early in the course of the disease. Other causes of regional lymphadenopathy, such as tularemia, sporotrichosis, tuberculosis, syphilis, and coccidioidomycosis, should be considered. Parinaud's oculoglandular syndrome occurs in 5 per cent of all cases. Rarely, a neuroretinitis may occur. This syndrome is characterized by unilateral palpebral conjunctival involvement with granulomatous nodules surrounded by follicles, chemosis, and injection, as well as preauricular lymph node enlargement. The conjunctival nodules may occasionally ulcerate. Recently, a gram-negative intracellular rod similar to lepothrix has been noted in conjunctiva, skin, and lymph nodes using a Warthin-Starry silver impregnation stain.

THERAPY

Supportive. The treatment of cat-scratch disease is palliative. If discomfort or fever occurs, analgesics, warm compresses, and antipyretics are warranted. A conjunctival biopsy of the granuloma may shorten the course of the disease and provides a specimen to rule out the infectious agents noted earlier. Excisional biopsy of the lymph node usually is not indicated, since it may lead to a persistent draining sinus. Lymph node needle aspiration may be necessary if there is marked suppuration and painful adenopathy. Systemic and topical antibiotics and steroids do not seem to affect the course of the disease and are of dubious value. If patients develop systemic symptoms, treatment with TMP-SMX may be useful.

Ocular or Periocular Manifestations

Conjunctiva: Acute and chronic conjunctivitis; granuloma or nodules; serous (nonpurulent) discharge.
Retina: Neuroretinitis.
Other: Tender or nontender preauricular or cervical lymphadenopathy.

PRECAUTIONS

Familial outbreaks of cat-scratch disease have been reported, but are unusual. The cats seem to be infectious only for several weeks. Transmission of the disease between humans has never been documented.

COMMENTS

Cat-scratch disease is a diagnosis of exclusion in which other more debilitating diseases should be ruled out. The diagnosis is based on a history of exposure to cats, the identification of the inoculum site, lymphadenopathy, and a positive cat-scratch skin test. Patients usually experience only mild discomfort, and the lymphadenopathy usually resolves in 30 to 90 days without sequelae.

References

Carithers HA: Oculoglandular disease of Parinaud. A manifestation of cat-scratch disease. Am J Dis Child 132:1195–1200, 1978.

Carithers HA, Carithers CM, Edwards RO Jr: Cat-scratch disease: Its natural history. JAMA 207: 312–316, 1969.

Chin GN, Hyndink RA: Parinaud oculoglandular conjunctivitis. In Duane TD (ed): Clinical Ophthalmology. Hagerstown, MD, Harper & Row, 1982, Vol IV, pp 4:1-8.

Collip PJ: Cat-scratch disease therapy (Letter). Am J Dis Child 143:1261, 1989.

Marcy SM, Kibrick S: Cat-scratch disease. In Top FH Sr, Wehrle PF (eds): Communicable and Infectious Disease, 8th ed. St. Louis, CV Mosby, 1976, pp 154-160.

Margileth AM: Cat scratch disease. In Wyngaarden JB, Smith LH Jr (eds): Textbook of Medicine, 16th ed. Philadelphia, WB Saunders, 1982, pp 1695-1697.

Ulrich, GG, et al: Cat scratch associated with neuroretinitis in a 6-year-old girl. Ophthalmology 99:246–249, 1992.

Wear DJ, et al: Cat-scratch disease: A bacterial infection. Science 221:1403–1405, 1983.

Wear DJ, et al: Cat-scratch disease bacilli in the conjunctiva of patients with Parinaud's oculoglandular syndrome. Ophthalmology 92:1282–1287, 1985.

EPIDEMIC KERATOCONJUNCTIVITIS 077.1
(EKC)

ROBERT ABEL, JR., M.D., and KHALAD A. NAGY, M.D.

Wilmington, Delaware

Epidemic keratoconjunctivitis (EKC) is a highly communicable, acute, external ocular inflammatory disease. The most frequent cause of "pink eye" is adenovirus types 8 and 19, although other serotypes can be responsible. After a 5- to 12-day incubation period, the disease is characterized by acute onset of a unilateral, then bilateral papillary or follicular conjunctival reaction, with focal corneal epithelial lesions and regional lymphadenopathy. A frequent symptom is the lids being stuck together in the morning; marked inflammation and serous discharge may also be present. Approximately 2 weeks after the onset, the conjunctivitis subsides and discrete subepithelial opacities slowly appear, presumably at the site of previous epithelial lesions. When these opacities are located centrally, vision may be impaired. If uveitis develops, these opacities may be associated with photophobia and rarely pain. These typical opacities spontaneously regress over a period of months; however, they may rarely persist for as long as several years.

Giemsa staining of conjunctival scrapings demonstrates degenerated epithelial cells with many lymphocytes and few polymorphonuclear cells (PMNs). Cell cultures are frequently positive in the acute phase, whereas a fourfold antibody rise may provide retrospective confirmation. More laboratories are making direct and indirect immunofluorescent techniques and the new immunoperoxidase staining available. Cambridge Biosciences, Inc., makes an office-based ELISA test called Adeno Clone, which gives a positive result in 1 hour.

Adenovirus can cause EKC (serotypes 2–4, 7–11, 14, 16, 19, and 29), pharyngoconjunctival fever, hemorrhagic conjunctivitis, chronic papillary conjunctivitis, and recurrent keratitis.

THERAPY

Systemic. Analgesics may be employed for patient comfort, although their use is generally not emphasized. In a double-blind trial in England, oral amantadine was found to be an effective prophylactic agent. Topical 1 per cent silver nitrate has been useful in a number of cases and remains our treatment of choice.

Ocular. Artificial tears applied four times daily or even hourly provide symptomatic relief and dilute the desquamative debris. Topical decongestants may decrease conjunctival congestion, but often do not provide as much relief of discomfort as do cold packs applied to the eyes. Topical corticosteroids and cycloplegics are useful in anterior uveitis. Corticosteroids are generally reserved for patients with significant iritis or with corneal opacities in the visual axis. If corticosteroids are used, they should be tapered very gradually. Pretreatment of rabbits with 0.1 per cent 5-HPMPC demonstrated ocular titers of the virus.

Supportive. Since spread occurs readily by hand-to-eye transmission, patients must be instructed to avoid touching their eyes and then touching others. Frequent washing of the hands and use of separate linen are very important to quarantine the infection.

Ocular or Periocular Manifestations

Conjunctiva: Diffuse papillary or follicular conjunctivitis; hyperemia; marked chemosis; pseudomembrane or true membrane formation; subconjunctival hemorrhages.

Cornea: Discrete subepithelial central opacity (late); punctate epithelial keratitis; scattered epithelial erosions.

Eyelids: Blepharospasm; edema; serous discharge with slight crusting.

Other: Anterior uveitis (rare); epiphora; periocular, submaxillary, or cervical lymphadenopathy; photophobia.

PRECAUTIONS

Although treatment of adenovirus infection has been long awaited, there is still no effective therapy available for this worldwide epidemic disease. Antiviral agents and topical interferon have not been proven to be clinically effective. Topical and systemic antibiotics have been used to eliminate bacterial or chlamydial etiology. Topical corticosteroids are rarely employed, except for iritis, because of the delayed resolution of the corneal opacities; early administration of these agents does not prevent the development of the subepithelial opacity.

Numerous hospital and community outbreaks have been documented in the literature. Spread occurs both by direct hand-to-eye transmission and by contact with tonometers and other eye instruments. It is vital that physicians, patients, and personnel in medical facilities wash their hands frequently to avoid transmission of this potentially epidemic disease. Patients should likewise be instructed in good hygienic techniques.

COMMENTS

Epidemic keratoconjunctivitis and other serotypes of adenovirus are usually limited to ocular disease in adults. With children, there is a greater chance of systemic findings associated with the conjunctivitis. Rarely, epidemic keratoconjunctivitis may be seen in conjunction with a bacterial infection (such as Koch-Weeks bacillus), in which case copious exudate and dissemination of the virus can occur more readily.

References

Abel R. Jr: Adenovirus keratoconjunctivitis and new approaches to prophylaxis. Ann Ophthalmol 9:13, 1997.

Dawson C, Darrell R: Infections due to adenovirus type 8 in the United States. I. An outbreak of epidemic keratoconjunctivitis originating in a physician's office. N Engl J Med 268:1031–1034, 1963.

Dawson CR, Hanna L, Togni B: Adenovirus type 8 infections in the United States. IV. Observations on the pathogenesis of lesions in severe eye disease. Arch Ophthalmol 87:258–268, 1972.

Dawson CR, et al: Adenovirus type 8 keratoconjunctivitis in the United States. III. Epidemiologic, clinical, and microbiologic features. Am J Ophthalmol 69:473–480, 1970.

Gordon Y, Romanowski J, Araullo-Cruz T: Antiviral efficacy of S-HPMPC against adenovirus in NZ-rabbit ocular model ocular microbiology and immunology group. Presented at the 25th Annual Meeting, American Academy of Ophthalmology, October, 1991, Anaheim, CA.

Liesegang TJ: Biology and molecular aspects of herpes simplex and varicella zoster, viral infection. Ophthalmology 99(5):781–785, 1992.

Sprague JB, et al: Epidemic keratoconjunctivitis. A severe industrial outbreak due to adenovirus type 8, N Engl J Med 289:1341–1346, 1973.

Vastine DW: Viral disease: Adenovirus and mis-

cellaneous viral infections. In Smolin G, Thoft RA (eds): Viral Diseases in the Cornea, 2nd ed. Boston, Little Brown, 1987, p 216.
Vastine DW, Wilmer BI, Anicetti VR: Detection of adenovirus, herpes simplex virus, and chlamydia by an immunoperoxidase staining technique. Presented to the Annual Meeting of ARVO, May, 1981, Sarasota, FL.

HERPES SIMPLEX 054.9

KERRY K. ASSIL, M.D.,
MARK S. DRESNER, M.D., F.A.C.S.,
and DAVID J. SCHANZLIN, M.D.

St. Louis, Missouri

Herpes simplex virus, a large complex DNA virus, commonly infects the skin and mucous membranes in the regions of the mouth, genitalia, and eye. The initial attack is generally self-limited and is often subclinical. However, herpetic disease is recurrent, and a wide range of clinical manifestations can result from infection with this agent.

Primary herpes infection of the eye is characterized by vesicles on the skin of the lids, follicular conjunctivitis, and, sometimes, punctate keratitis. After primary infection, recurrent disease is usually in the form of dendritic ulceration of the cornea; however, epithelial ulceration can occasionally assume an amoebic or geographic form. This more severe form of epithelial herpetic keratitis frequently occurs in patients using topical corticosteroid preparations. Between 10 and 20 per cent of patients with herpetic ulceration of the cornea subsequently develop underlying stromal inflammation. The stromal involvement may be associated with deep vascular ingrowth (interstitial keratitis) or may be disciform in configuration, due to severe endothelial disease, with stromal edema. The stromal patterns of involvement are usually associated with uveitis. Indolent (metaherpetic) ulceration occurs when healing of the epithelium is compromised by the underlying stromal inflammation or can be secondary to medication toxicity.

THERAPY

Ocular. Therapy for *primary herpes infection* of the eye is directed at removal of virus from the cornea and adjacent skin. Cultures of the cornea may be made for virus, but should also be made for bacteria if secondary infection is suspected. Presence of viral antigens or viral DNA may also be confirmed by immunohistochemical stains or by the polymerase chain reaction (PCR). The diagnosis is, however, generally based on a typical history and presence of a characteristic epithelial dendrite.

To inhibit virus replication and prevent corneal infection, topical idoxuridine, vidarabine, or trifluridine may be used; ointments should be instilled five times a day and eye drops instilled every hour while the patient is awake. Oral acyclovir is a more current, preferred treatment. However, patients with renal dysfunction may not be able to tolerate oral acyclovir. A cycloplegic may also be prescribed to relieve photophobia and ciliary spasm, and frequent follow-up is advised. No topical antiviral medication is effective in the treatment of herpes simplex skin lesions.

Recurrent herpetic epithelial keratitis has historically been treated by débridement combined with trifluridine or vidarabine. Débridement, which when used alone is considered suboptimal therapy, is performed after instillation of topical anesthetic (4 per cent cocaine or 0.5 per cent proparacaine) into the conjunctival sac. Cocaine has the advantage of loosening the corneal epithelium. The loose epithelium at the edge of the dendritic figure is wiped away with a sterile cotton-tipped applicator or with the edge of a knife blade or platinum spatula. After débridement, a cycloplegic drug is instilled into the conjunctival sac, and a semipressure patch is applied. The patient is asked to return in 48 hours. If the epithelial defect has an irregular appearance on reexamination or has the branching appearance of a dendritic or geographic ulcer at any point, débridement and patching are repeated or antiviral drug therapy is started.

Triflurothymide, a pyrimidine analogue, is the drug of choice in the United States for topical ophthalmic antiviral therapy. Although similar in structure to idoxuridine, it is twice as potent, and because of its biphasic solubility, it is tenfold more soluble and can achieve therapeutic intraocular concentrations. It is considered more efficacious than idoxuridine in the treatment of dendritic and geographic ulcers and superior to vidarabine for geographic ulcers. Trifluridine is the least vulnerable of the three antiviral agents to resistant viral strains. There is no cross-allergenicity between trifluridine, idoxuridine, and vidarabine.

One per cent trifluridine is administered nine times daily for 10 days and is tapered thereafter; 1 per cent idoxuridine can be administered every waking hour and every 2 hours at night. Three per cent vidarabine ointment, a purine analogue, is prescribed five times daily.

The most recent ophthalmic drug available in the treatment of herpes simplex is acyclovir.* It is a prodrug: thymidine kinase, specified by the herpes virus, activates acyclovir by phosphorylation. Host cells have a different phosphorylating enzyme that only minimally activates acyclovir. This gives the drug a 3000 times greater effect against herpes simplex virus than against the host. Its toxicity compares favorably to trifluridine, vidarabine, or idoxuridine. Acyclovir and trifluridine heal approximately the same percentage of ulcers, but acyclovir heals dendritic ulcers more rapidly. It is not yet available in the United States for topical ophthalmic use.

Many ophthalmologists now consider oral acyclovir to be the treatment of choice for ocular herpetic disease. This is particularly true for patients with recurrent disease in whom chronic suppression is desired. Recommended therapy for active disease is 200 mg oral dose, five times per day. For chronic suppression, as little as one tablet every other day may be sufficient. The attempt to augment or modify the host's immunologic milieu has led some investigators to study the role of cimetidine as an adjunct to standard antiviral therapy. The efficacy of this modality has not been fully established.

Stromal herpetic keratitis usually occurs in patients who have had previous attacks of epithelial herpes. In the presence of an epithelial defect, no corticosteroids should be used; rather, the patients should be treated with antiviral therapy and a short-acting cycloplegic agent to keep the pupil moving. If no epithelial defect is present and topical corticosteroid therapy is felt to be indicated, therapy should begin with the minimal prescriptive dosage. The dose is then gradually increased until the desired effect is obtained. The least amount of corticosteroid necessary to achieve the desired effect should be used and therapy tapered as soon as clinically feasible. As with all corticosteroid therapy, the patient should be followed closely. The concerns of steroid use in patients with severe stromal keratitis center on the possibilities of immunosuppression and delayed wound healing with the potential for corneal perforation. With the availability of systemic acyclovir, clinicians no longer believe that stromal keratitis is simply an immune-mediated response to inactive viral antigens. Acyclovir alone is often sufficient to quiet eyes with prior severe chronic keratitis. Antiviral medication should be continued as long as corticosteroids are utilized. Elevation of intraocular pressure may be treated with timolol and systemic acetazolamide if necessary.

Disciform herpetic disease presents as a pattern of local stromal corneal edema with underlying folds in Descemet's membrane and keratic precipitates. It is almost always accompanied by a moderate-to-severe anterior chamber reaction. The treatment of disciform keratitis is generally similar to that of stromal herpes. If the lesion is paracentral and does not cause significant visual impairment, the patient can be managed with cycloplegic agents and the lesion will resolve with time. If there is a significant decrease in visual acuity, topical corticosteroids can be used in combination with an antiviral cover and cycloplegics. Recurrent disciform keratitis is often responsive to chronic suppressive doses of acyclovir. Glaucoma should be treated with timolol and systemic acetazolamide as necessary.

Indolent stromal ulceration is managed with antiviral and corticosteroid therapy along with a soft contact lens to prevent corneal drying. When there is melting of the cornea, care must be taken not to stop corticosteroid therapy abruptly, as doing so may lead to rebound inflammation and increase the melting process, thereby resulting in perforation. The anticollagenolytic activity of tetracycline may help retard corneal melting when applied as a topical ointment. One should also consider the possibility of medication-induced toxicity when faced with chronic nonhealing epithelial defects.

Supportive. Epithelial disease usually runs a short course of several days, and an initial dose of a short-acting cycloplegic, such as 5 per cent homatropine, is usually sufficient. With stromal keratitis and uveitis, the long-acting effect of atropine is preferred.

The presence of bacterial infection complicating herpetic keratitis is sufficiently uncommon to make the routine administration of antibiotics unnecessary. However, any rapid change in the nature of the corneal lesion should arouse suspicion of a bacterial infection, and one should instigate appropriate investigations and treatment.

Surgical. Keratoplasty should be considered when descemetocele formation and perforation are imminent. If the cornea perforates, the best management is keratoplasty, performed as expediently as possible. Sealing of a perforated descemetocele with a tissue adhesive and fitting with a soft contact lens often result in reformation of the anterior chamber in preparation for definitive corneal transplantation.

Keratoplasty for corneal scarring, secondary to stromal herpes simplex virus, should be done with caution. Most corneal transplant surgeons wish to have the patient remain without recurrent disease for 6 to 12 months before considering the procedure. With the availability of acyclovir, the prognosis of patients with corneal scarring has improved.

Ocular or Periocular Manifestations

Conjunctiva: Follicular conjunctivitis; hyperemia.

Cornea: Dendritic, geographic, or metaherpetic ulcer; disciform keratitis; hypesthesia; irregular (nondisciform) keratitis; lipid keratopathy; stromal scarring; vascularization.

Iris: Anterior uveitis, atrophy.

Other: Cataract; hypopyon; increased intraocular pressure; occlusion of nasolacrimal canaliculi; preauricular lymphadenopathy; scleritis; vesicular blepharitis.

PRECAUTIONS

The major problem related to therapy is the difficulty in achieving a precise débridement that does not damage Bowman's layer. There is also the fine balance between the beneficial antiinflammatory action of steroids on the balance of virus and host and the toxicity of the antiviral compounds.

Some forms of débridement are particularly injurious. The use of sharp instruments, cryotherapy, or strong chemicals, such as phenol or iodine, should be avoided as unnecessarily damaging. Adequate débridement can usually be achieved by brushing the epithelial lesions with a cotton-tipped applicator, a technique that is not only convenient but effective in that epithelial healing is rapid (usually within 24 hours) with resultant early disappearance of pain and discomfort. Any tendency for recurrent lesions to form in the early period after healing can be overcome by using a topical antiviral for 7 to 10 days after débridement.

Topical corticosteroids are effective in suppressing the inflammatory response of herpetic keratitis. However, their inappropriate use may result in severe epithelial disease or stromal necrosis, increased tendency toward recurrence, elevation of the intraocular pressure, and lens changes. Patients requiring topical corticosteroids for suppression of the inflammatory response usually require the drug for a period of months, and withdrawal is often complicated by recurrence of inflammation. The immunosuppressive complications of steroid administration can largely be avoided by the concurrent administration of antiviral therapy. Patient cooperation is a prerequisite for the safe administration of corticosteroids in herpetic keratitis. The availability of oral acyclovir has decreased the dependence on steroids for the management of HSV keratitis.

All topical antiviral medications currently available for clinical use in the United States are toxic, with signs of toxicity being similar for all such drugs. Punctate epithelial keratopathy, limbal follicles, a follicular conjunctival response, ptosis, punctal stenosis, and contact dermatitis can occur at any time after 10 to 14 days of therapy. In mild cases of antiviral toxicity, epithelial changes may be the only manifestation. Idoxuridine is the most toxic topical antiviral agent in clinical use, whereas vidarabine and trifluridine seem to be less toxic. Topical acyclovir is not yet available in the United States. Oral acyclovir should be used with caution in patients who have renal disease.

COMMENTS

The major difficulties in treating herpetic keratitis are related to the tendency for recurrence and the management of stromal disease. Several mechanisms seem responsible for the recurrences. In latent form, herpes simplex virus can be present in the cells of the cornea and in the central connections of the trigeminal nerve, particularly in the trigeminal ganglion. Disturbance of the nerve results in activation of the virus and the passage of particles centrifugally along the nerve, with shedding from the nerve endings. Lesions tend to occur when the balance between latency and host defenses is disturbed, such as during febrile illnesses, during menses, or on exposure to sunlight.

The toxic potential of antiviral agents should always be considered in patients who heal poorly, as these agents are inhibitors of cell division. Although continuous ocular drug delivery systems are currently under investigation, the limitations of such systems in preventing recurrences are related to the unacceptable toxicity from the chronic use of currently available topical medications.

References

Colin J, Malet F, Chastel C: Acyclovir in herpetic anterior uveitis. Ann Ophthalmol 23:28–30, 1991.

Coster DJ, Jones BR, Falcon MG: Role of debridement in the treatment of herpetic keratitis. Trans Ophthalmol Soc UK 97:314–317, 1977.

Falcon MG: Rational acyclovir therapy in herpetic eye disease. Br J Ophthalmol 71:102–106, 1987.

Falcon MG, et al: Management of herpetic eye disease. Trans Ophthalmol Soc UK 97:345–349, 1977.

Herbort CP, Buechi ER, Matter M: Blunt spatula debridement and trifluorothymidine in epithelial herpetic keratitis. Curr Eye Res 6:225–228, 1987.

McGill J, Fraunfelder FT, Jones BR: Current and proposed management of ocular herpes simplex. Surv Ophthalmol 20:358–365, 1976.

Ohashi Y, et al: Demonstration of herpes simplex virus DNA in idiopathic corneal endotheliopathy. Am J Ophthalmol 112:419–423, 1991.

Parlato CJ, et al: Role of debridement and trifluridine (trifluorothymidine) in herpes simplex dendritic keratitis. Arch Ophthalmol 103:673–675, 1985.

Pavan-Langston D: Diagnosis and management of herpes simplex ocular infection. Int Ophthalmol Clin 15:19–35, 1975.

Rong BL, et al: Detection of herpes simplex virus thymidine kinase and latency-associated transcript gene sequences in human herpetic corneas by polymerase chain reaction amplification. Invest Ophthalmol Vis Sci 32:1808–1815, 1991.

Williams HP, Falcon MG, Jones BR: Corticosteroids in the management of herpetic eye disease. Trans Ophthalmol Soc UK 97:341–344, 1977.

HERPES ZOSTER 053.9

RONALD J. MARSH, F.R.C.S., F.R.C.Ophth.

London, England

Herpes zoster is an acute vesicular eruption caused by varicella-zoster virus, which is morphologically identical to the virus that causes chickenpox. It may be activated by a local lesion involving the posterior root ganglia, by systemic disease (particularly Hodgkin's disease), recently by early HIV infection, or by immunosuppressive therapy. The disease may occur at any age, but it is more common after 50 years of age. Ophthalmic herpes zoster is a variable disease ranging from trivial to devastating. Inadequate management may lead to disastrous eyelid scarring, neuralgia, loss of the eye, and even suicide. In about 50 per cent of ophthalmic zoster cases, ocular complications occur. They fall primarily into those associated with inflammatory changes, those resulting from nerve damage, and those secondary to tissue scarring.

THERAPY

Systemic. Acyclovir has been used extensively in herpes zoster infection. There is good evidence that intravenous administration is effective in preventing the severe dissemination of disease in immunosuppressed patients. The role or oral acyclovir in otherwise healthy patients is uncertain. It was first claimed that a dose of 400 mg daily for 5 days reduced the incidence and severity of ocular complications. More recently, it has been suggested that, if the dose is doubled to 800 mg daily for 7 days and administered within 2 days of the rash, better results are achieved. However, there seems to be no effect on postherpetic neuralgia, although there is brief early analgesia.

Although some authorities believe that the use of routine systemic steroids results in fewer zoster complications, the increased risk of systemic spread of the disease should be considered. Systemic corticosteroids are indicated only in progressive proptosis with total ophthalmoplegia hemorrhagic bullae of the skin and at the onset of optic neuritis or contralateral hemiplegia. These conditions are most probably due to occlusive vasculitis that threatens sight and are therefore a logical indication for this means of therapy. An initial oral daily dosage of 60 mg of prednisone may be given, which may be rapidly reduced to a maintenance dose. Oral administration of 50 to 100 mg of flurbiprofen* three times daily is useful in cases of severe scleritis, episcleritis, and sclerokeratitis that have not responded fully to the strongest of doses of topical ophthalmic steroids. Indeed, mild and moderate cases of episcleritis may be treated with flurbiprofen alone.

Pain is notoriously difficult to treat and is generally the most severe within the first 2 weeks. During this acute phase, patients should be given sufficient drugs to suppress their pain. Mild analgesics, such as acetaminophen or propoxyphene, should be tried initially before stronger analgesics, such as pentazocine or meperidine, are used. The anti-inflammatory content of these drugs is also useful. In addition, the pain and paresthesia of postherpetic neuralgia generally tend to be worse at night and are aggravated by heat and wind. Extra analgesia may be needed at these times. Sublingual buprenophrine* may be particularly useful in cases of refractory intermittent neuralgia. Severe irritational neuralgia may be treated with piriton 4 mg or chlorpromazine 25 mg twice a day.

Depression frequently occurs during the acute phase of herpes zoster and may also be an important component of postherpetic neuralgia. It is important to treat this depression, and amitriptyline is particularly useful.

Ocular. The mainstay of therapy for ocular complications of herpes zoster is steroids. During the acute stage when lid vesicles are discharging and forming crusts or a mucopurulent conjunctivitis is present, antibiotic-steroid solutions may be applied to the eye and continued for at least 3 weeks after the onset of the rash. Tetracycline ointment should be applied twice daily to chronically scarred or inflamed lid margins since they become a focus for staphylococcal secondary infection if left untreated.

Steroids should be used for all moderate or severe inflammatory lesions and are essential for those linked with vasculitis. At the first evidence of severe episcleritis, scleritis, sclerokeratitis, or iritis, 0.1 per cent dexamethasone suspension should be instilled every 4 hours and ointment applied at night. Prompt treatment at the start of vasculitis reduces the ischemic and fibrotic scarring that usually develops. Once control is achieved, the potency and frequency of administration can be reduced. The iritis of herpes zoster frequently causes elevation of intraocular pressure; this is true even with low-grade anterior uveitis. Fortunately, steroid therapy alone usually controls this pressure elevation within a few days. Although this complication generally occurs at the onset of the disease, it may appear as a late relapsing phenomenon years after the acute attack.

The inflammatory keratitis of herpes zoster responds well to steroid therapy and does not require such high doses as the above. In fact, very mild keratitis often resolves without any treatment over 2 to 3 months. The dose of topical steroids should be titrated against the degree of disease activity in the eye. This is a slow, cautious process and may extend over a period of years. As well as reducing the frequency of administration of the drug, serial logarithmic dilutions or a change to another weaker steroid (from dexamethasone to a betamethasone or prednisolone) may be made. Many patients can titrate their own dose, which may be reduced to as little as 0.03 per cent prednisolone once a day to maintain control.

Fairly common ocular complications in herpes zoster are the loss of corneal sensitivity and damage to the mechanisms that produce a stable precorneal tear film. A combination of artificial tears and mucolytics helps stabilize the tear film and improves the health of the corneal epithelium. Bandage lenses are best avoided in all cases of keratitis where there is loss of corneal sensation because of the risk of hypopyon ulcer formation. Acute melting neuroparalytic ulcers have been successfully treated by botulinum toxin-induced ptosis.

Topical ophthalmic antiviral treatment, including acyclovir,* seems to have no significant value in ocular zoster, and in fact, idoxuridine seems to have an adverse effect on an already compromised corneal epithelium.

Surgical. A lateral half-tarsorrhaphy should be carried out immediately in all cases of neurotrophic ulceration and may be necessary in cases of chronic exposure and neuroparalytic keratitis. It can be difficult to persuade patients to accept this treatment, but it provides rapid healing and security and dramatically reduces outpatient visits. Emergency grafting may have to be done in cases of neurotrophic ulceration with perforation. The prognosis is not as good in these situations as considerable difficulty may be encountered in establishing a stable corneal epithelium over the graft.

Corrective lid surgery may need to be considered for lid margin deformities, such as ectropion and trichiasis. It is urgently required when there is full thickness loss of the lid margin.

Neglected disciform keratitis or sclerokeratitis frequently gives rise to dense scarring and lipid deposits in the central cornea. These patients tend to do well with perforating corneal grafts, provided that the cornea is not too vascularized.

Topical. Routinely, in the crusting phase, an antibiotic-steroid ointment, such as neomycin and hydrocortisone, is applied to the eyelids and skin two or three times daily. Topical antiviral agents in the form of idoxuridine dissolved in dimethyl sulfoxide have been used for treating the acute lesions of ophthalmic zoster. Although the rash tends to heal faster with this treatment, there is some doubt of its effectiveness in preventing postherpetic neuralgia. Topical treatment for postherpetic neuralgia includes stellate ganglion block given in the early stage of the disease; TENS is given in the later stages along with skin massage using a lubricant, such as lanolin, or an active agent, such as capsaicin.

Supportive. Patients with acute ophthalmic herpes zoster are often very ill, aged, and infirm. It is very difficult for them to take their treatment, feed themselves, and rest at home, and the kindest course is to admit them for 1 week to the hospital. The patient should be in partial isolation until the vesicles have dried (usually within 5 days). It is preferable that personnel in contact with the patient at this stage have had chickenpox, since they possibly could acquire varicella from the patient. The converse, however, is not true. Patients should be reassured that the duration of the rash is short and that the neuralgia is usually short-lived.

Ocular or Periocular Manifestations

Conjunctiva: Fatty granuloma; nonspecific conjunctivitis.

Cornea: Dendrites; disciform, neuroparalytic, neurotrophic, punctate, or stromal nummularis keratitis; lipid deposits; mucous plaques; recurrent ulcer; stromal cicatrization; stromal loss; vascularization.

Eyelids: Cicatricial entropion; neuralgia; paralysis; trichiasis; zoster rash.

Iris: Anterior uveitis; atrophy; distortion.

Sclera: Atrophy; episcleritis; scleritis.

Other: Cataract; optic neuritis; paralysis of third, fourth, or sixth nerve; proptosis; secondary glaucoma.

PRECAUTIONS

The important essentials of steroid management are careful follow-up and examination to detect toxic side effects. A significant number of patients on topical steroids develop glaucoma and cataract after long-term use. Secondary infection may occur when using steroids in patients with neurotrophic keratitis. It may be difficult differentiating steroid glaucoma from hypertensive iritis, particularly in mucous plaque keratitis; a helpful measure is to increase the dose of steroid and review in 2 days. When the steroid is confirmed as the culprit, fluromethalone drops should be substituted. The dose of steroids should be reduced as soon as possible to avoid lens opacities, although in some cases it is impossible to know whether to attribute the cataracts to the chronic iritis. Regular slit-lamp examination and applanation are therefore essential.

It should be emphasized that the acute edema that occurs shortly after the onset of the rash is not due to bacterial cellulitis and will resolve without antibiotics within a few days.

COMMENTS

One of the most important features of the ocular complications in herpes zoster is their tendency to recur, even years after the rash. It should be remembered that some relapses may occur when the original attack of herpes zoster has either been forgotten or was so mild as to pass unnoticed. The stimulus for the relapse is often unknown, although the precipitous withdrawal of topical steroids is a potent cause. Therefore, follow-up must be long and thorough in those with ocular involvement, and topical steroids must be slowly and cautiously withdrawn (over years, if necessary). Adequate analgesia must be administered. Those patients referred to an ophthalmologist from their family physicians have a much lower incidence of dermatologic nonmetastatic tumors than those referred from a hospital internist.

References

Adams CGW, Kirkness CM, Lee JP: Botulinum toxin A-induced protective ptosis. Eye 1:603–608, 1987.
Bucci FA, Gabriels CF, Krohel GB. Successful treatment of postherpetic neuralgia with capsaicin. Am J Ophthalmol 106:758–759, 1988.
Cobo LM, et al: Oral acyclovir in the therapy of acute herpes zoster ophthalmas: An interim report. Ophthalmology 92:1574–1583, 1985.
Dawber R: Idoxuridine in herpes zoster: Further evaluation of intermittent topical therapy. Br Med J 2:521–526, 1974.
Jeul-Jenson BE, MacCallum PO: Herpes Simplex, Varicella and Zoster. Philadelphia, JB Lippincott, 1972, pp 163–171.
Marsh RJ: Herpes zoster keratitis. Trans Ophthalmol Soc UK 93:181–192, 1973.
Marsh RJ: Current management of ophthalmic herpes zoster. Trans Ophthalmol Soc UK 96:334–337, 1976.
Marsh RJ: Idoxuridine (IDU) in dimethyl sulfoxide (DMSO) in the treatment of ophthalmic zoster. Ophthal Digest 39:17–19, 1977.
Marsh RJ, Fraunfelder FT, McGill JI: Herpetic corneal epithelial disease. Arch Ophthalmol 94:1899–1902, 1976.
McKendrick HW, et al: Oral acyclovir in acute herpes zoster. Br Med J 293:1529–1532, 1986.
Peterslund NA, et al: Acyclovir in herpes zoster. Lancet 2:827–830, 1981.
Stevens DA, Merigan TC: Interferon, antibody, and other host factors in herpes zoster. J Clin Invest 51:1170–1178, 1972.

INFECTIOUS MONONUCLEOSIS 075

JAY H. KRACHMER, M.D.,

Minneapolis, Minnesota

and STEVEN S.T. CHING, M.D.

Rochester, New York

Infectious mononucleosis is a clinical syndrome of adolescents and young adults which is characterized by malaise, fever, sore throat, and generalized lymphadenopathy. Other systemic involvement may include splenomegaly (50 per cent), hepatomegaly (20 per cent), headache, vomiting, jaundice, palatal petechiae, and skin rash. Complications can be seen in any organ system. The etiologic agent of infectious mononucleosis is usually the Epstein-Barr virus (EBV). Mononucleosis syndromes can also be produced by cytomegalovirus (CMV), acute human immunodeficiency virus (HIV) infection, hepatitis, and *Toxoplasma gondii*. The primary infection with the EBV may present clinically with less than the full syndrome; in children, the infection may be indistinguishable from other upper respiratory infections.

The ocular system may be involved directly by the virus or indirectly via the central nervous system. The most common ocular involvement is a follicular conjunctivitis.

Laboratory findings indicative of EBV infection are atypical lymphocytosis and heterophile antibodies to ox or sheep erythrocytes. Because of the possibility of false-negative heterophile antibodies (5 to 10 per cent), specific serologic testing for EBV infection can be performed. Early infection generates early antigen (EA) antibodies and gamma M antibodies to viral capsid antigens (VCA). After several months, anti-EA and gamma M anti-VCA become negative. Evidence of past infection is indicated by the presence of antibodies to Epstein-Barr nuclear antigens (EBNA) and gamma G antibodies to VCA. These latter antibodies may be present for life.

THERAPY

Systemic. The disease is self-limited and usually only supportive therapy is necessary. Rest during the acute illness and gradual resumption of normal activity are recommended. Acetaminophen or aspirin may be used to decrease fever and sore throat. Systemic corticosteroids have been used to shrink obstructing tonsils. Acyclovir and its congeners inhibit in vitro EBV replication. In immunocompetent hosts, acyclovir decreases virus shedding from the oropharynx; however, the clinical course of the disease does not seem to be altered. In immunocompromised individuals, high doses of systemic acyclovir have been effective in selected cases of EBV-related lymphoproliferative disorders.

Ocular. The conjunctivitis may be treated with cool compresses. Topical steroids have been used to treat the stromal keratitis and iritis. One case of epithelial dendritic keratitis seemed to respond to topical ophthalmic acyclovir.* Systemic corticosteroids have been used in cases of extensive neurologic involvement, but their efficacy is uncertain.

Ocular or Periocular Manifestations

Conjunctiva. Follicular, granulomatous, or membranous conjunctivitis; subconjunctival hemorrhages; hyperemia.

Cornea. Punctate epithelial keratitis; dendritic keratitis; stromal keratitis as nummular opacities, subepithelial infiltrates, or ring shaped opacities.

Lacrimal System. Dacryoadenitis; dacryocystitis; Sjögren's syndrome.

Neuro-ophthalmologic. Accommodation

paresis; convergence deficiency; hemianopsia; nystagmus; ophthalmoplegia; optic neuritis; papilledema.

Sclera. Episleritis; scleritis.

Uvea. Iritis; vitritis; multifocal choroiditis with retinal pigment epithelial disturbance; punctate outer retinitis.

PRECAUTIONS

In childhood and adolescence, the disease may present symptoms similar to other upper respiratory illnesses. Aspirin should not be used in this age group because of the association of aspirin, influenza, and Reye's syndrome.

COMMENTS

There is evidence of EBV chronic infection in salivary and lacrimal glands in normal individuals. This phenomenon occurs in a greater frequency in patients with Sjögren's syndrome. Whether this is a consequence of Sjögren's syndrome or it is causally involved in the pathogenesis of this disease remains to be elucidated.

Almost 100 per cent of individuals over 30 years of age demonstrate evidence of past EBV infection, but few have had the clinical syndrome of infectious mononucleosis. With the availability of specific EBV antibody testing, the practitioner should keep this infection in mind when searching for etiologies of puzzling ocular disease.

References

Aaberg TM, O'Brien WJ: Expanding ophthalmologic recognition of Epstein-Barr virus infections. Am J Ophthalmol 104:420, 1987.

Darrel RW (ed): Viral Diseases of the Eye. Philadelphia, Lea & Febiger, 1985, pp 112–117.

Feigin RD, Cherry JD: Textbook of Pediatric Infectious Disease, 3rd ed., Philadelphia, WB Saunders, 1992, pp 1547–1557.

Matoba AY: Ocular disease associated with Epstein-Barr virus infection. Surv Ophthalmol 35: 145–150, 1990.

Pflugfelder SC, et al: Amplification of Epstein-Barr virus genomic sequences in blood cells, lacrimal glands, and tears from primary Sjogren's syndrome patients. Ophthalmology 97:976–984, 1990.

Raymond LA, et al: Punctate outer retinitis in acute Epstein-Barr virus infection. Am J Ophthalmol 104:424, 1987.

Tiedeman JS: Epstein-Barr viral antibodies in multifocal choroiditis and panuveitis. Am J Ophthalmol 103:659, 1987.

Wong KW, et al: Ocular involvement associated with chronic Epstein-Barr virus disease. Arch Ophthalmol 105:788, 1987.

Wyngaarden WB, Smith JC: Cecil Textbook of Medicine, 19th ed. Philadelphia, WB Saunders, 1992, pp 1838–1840.

INFLUENZA 487.1

DANIEL H. SPITZBERG, M.D., F.A.C.S.

Indianapolis, Indiana

Influenza is an acute respiratory infection of specific viral etiology. There are three distinct antigenic types of influenza virus, designated A, B, and C. Although type C usually produces only a minor illness, antigenic types A and B can cause major epidemics. This disease often occurs sporadically or in localized outbreaks, particularly in schools or military camps and usually in the fall or winter season. The characteristics of influenza include the sudden onset of headache, fever, malaise, muscular aching, substernal soreness, nasal stuffiness, and nausea. In this condition, the temperature rises abruptly and usually subsides over 2 to 3 days. Coryza, nonproductive cough, sore throat, mild pharyngeal infection, flushed face, and conjunctival redness are common symptoms. Influenza may cause necrosis of the respiratory epithelium, which predisposes the body to secondary bacterial infections. Influenza early in pregnancy has been said to result in multiple congenital deformities in the fetus, including the occurrence of anencephaly and congenital cataract. Ocular complications may include acute catarrhal conjunctivitis, superficial punctate or interstitial keratitis, palpebral edema, and secondary bacterial infections. A usually bilateral, self-limited nongranulomatous anterior uveitis may occur during convalescence. It can become chronic with exacerbation and remission.

THERAPY

Systemic. Prophylactically, amantadine protects 50 to 70 per cent of recipients exposed to influenza A viruses and is indicated for patients over 1 year of age during influenza A outbreaks, especially individuals for whom influenza would entail a grave risk (such as the elderly). It may be most effective in individuals who already have antibodies against influenza A virus strains; therefore, previous vaccination does not interfere with and may augment its effect. Amantadine also may have therapeutic value if given promptly after the first symptoms of infection appear. Administration of 100 mg of amantadine twice daily should be continued for at least 10 days.

Ocular. In cases of mild uveitis, 5 per cent homatropine solution should be applied topically four times daily to decrease pain. Influenzal uveitis can become chronic, with exacerbations and remissions. Patients with this type of uveitis respond well to topical ocular corticosteroid therapy for short periods of time. Topical ophthalmic 0.12 per cent prednisolone can be added two or three times a day to the regimen for a week to control low-grade uveitis.

Catarrhal marginal ulcers are an immunologic response and should be treated with 0.12 per cent prednisolone solution four times daily.

Supportive. Bedrest and gradual return to full activity are advisable to reduce complications. Codeine in an adult oral dosage of 15 to 60 mg may be used to depress the cough reflex and is more effective than salicylates for the treatment of headache and myalgia. Salicylates often increase discomfort by causing sweats and chills. Antibiotics should be reserved for treatment of bacterial complications.

Ocular or Periocular Manifestations

Conjunctiva: Catarrhal conjunctivitis; hyperemia; subconjunctival hemorrhages.

Cornea: Dendritic ulcer due to herpes simplex; erosion; interstitial or superficial punctate keratitis; marginal ulcer.

Extraocular Muscles: Myalgia; paralysis of third or fourth nerve; tenonitis.

Lacrimal System: Dacryoadenitis; dacryocystitis.

Orbit: Cellulitis; panophthalmitis.

Retina: Angiospasm; edema; exudates; hemorrhages; stellate retinopathy; venous thrombosis.

Other: Accommodative spasm; cataract (congenital); episcleritis; mydriasis; myopia; optic neuritis (associated with encephalitis); uveitis.

PRECAUTIONS

If the fever persists for more than 4 days, if cough becomes productive or if the white count rises about 12,000/cubic millimeter, secondary bacterial infection should be ruled out or verified and treated.

Routine yearly immunization with polyvalent influenza virus vaccine for high-risk groups is strongly recommended. Persons of all ages who suffer from chronic rheumatic heart diseases, other cardiovascular diseases, chronic bronchopulmonary diseases, diabetes mellitus, or Addison's disease should be considered for prophylactic treatment. Pregnant women and persons 65 years or older should also be considered, regardless of their previous state of health.

COMMENTS

The duration of uncomplicated influenza is 1 to 7 days, and complete recovery is the rule. However, pre-existing respiratory disease and secondary bacterial pneumonia can lead to a fatal outcome. Most fatalities are due to bacterial pneumonia. Pneumococcal pneumonia is most common, but staphylococcal pneumonia is most serious.

In general, serious ophthalmic complications are rare; however, secondary bacterial infections must be watched closely. The cornea is usually the site of most serious ocular complications. This area, along with the anterior chamber, is where the main follow-up examinations should be centered.

References

Grossman M, Jawetz E: Infectious diseases: Viral and rickettsial. *In* Krupp MA, Chatton MJ (eds): Current Medical Diagnosis and Treatment. Los Altos, Lange, 1982, pp 821–822.

Knight V: Influenza. *In* Isselbacher KJ et al (eds): Harrison's Principles of Internal Medicine, 9th ed. New York, McGraw-Hill, 1980, pp 785–789.

Rabon RJ, Louis GJ, Zegarra H, Gutman FA: Acute bilateral posterior angiopathy with influenza A viral infection. Am J Ophthalmol 103:289–293, 1987.

Schlaegel TF Jr: Uveitis associated with viral infections. *In* Duane TD (ed): Clinical Ophthalmology. Hagerstown, MD, Harper & Row, 1982, Vol IV, pp 46:1–13.

MOLLUSCUM CONTAGIOSUM 078.0

LEWIS R. GRODEN, M.D.

Tampa, Florida

Molluscum contagiosum is a self-limited, mildly contagious skin disease caused by a pox-virus. Typical lesions are small dome-shaped, umbilicated, shiny skin-colored papules. The lesions are usually not inflamed and are most often asymptomatic. Lesions on the eyelid or lid margin can be inconspicuous and hidden by the lashes; less commonly, lesions are found on the conjunctiva and rarely on the cornea. The corneal findings usually involve the superior third of the eye and can progress to a trachoma-like picture. The follicular conjunctivitis and keratitis associated with molluscum contagiosum are toxic reactions to the virus, not infectious processes.

THERAPY

Surgical. Molluscum contagiosum is best managed by simple excision of the lesion. This can be done under local infiltration anesthesia, using scissors or a scalpel blade. Eradication of the lesion can also be achieved using electrocautery.

Incision and curettage effectively remove the viruses that pack the core of the molluscum contagiosum lesion. Curettage can be done with either a curette, needle, or comedo extractor.

Cryosurgery is also effective treatment. Light freezing followed by the curettage decreases the risks of cryosurgery and effectively removes the lesion.

The application of chemical caustics, such as liquefied phenol, silver nitrate, or trichloroacetic acid, may also effect a cure.

Ocular or Periocular Manifestations

Conjunctiva: Molluscum contagiosum lesions; scarring; subacute or chronic follicular conjunctivitis.

Cornea: Fine epithelial keratitis; keratinization; molluscum contagiosum lesions; pannus; pseudodendrite; subepithelial infiltration; ulcer.

Lacrimal System: Epiphora; punctal occlusion.

Other: Foreign body sensation; photophobia; visual loss.

PRECAUTIONS

Although cryosurgery is effective in the treatment of molluscum contagiosum, it must be used with caution as it can lead to depigmentation of dark skin. Both cryosurgery and chemical caustics can also cause excess scarring. Although such drugs as cantharidin are valuable for skin lesions, they should not be used around the eyes, as scleral erosion can occur.

At one time, systemic sulfonamides were suggested as adjunctive therapy to surgery. However, such use is no longer recommended.

COMMENTS

The ocular findings clear rapidly after eradication of the molluscum contagiosum lesion. If the lesions are untreated, however, the ocular disease can lead to a trachoma-like picture and visual loss. The ocular and periocular lesions of molluscum contagiosum are often associated with lesions elsewhere, particularly in the genital areas. Venereal contact is a common means of transmission, and contaminated cosmetics can also spread the virus. Although usually a self-limiting disease, molluscum contagiosum can be progressive in an immunosuppressed individual.

References

Charles NC, Friedberg DN: Epibulbar molluscum contagiosum in acquired immunodeficiency syndrome. Ophthalmology 99:1123, 1992.

Cobbold RJC, MacDonald A: Molluscum contagiosum as a sexually transmitted disease. Practitioner 204:416–419, 1970.

Duke-Elder S (ed): System of Ophthalmology. St. Louis, CV Mosby, 1965, Vol VIII, pp 376–379.

Grayson M: Diseases of the Cornea. St. Louis, CV Mosby, 1979, pp 116–118.

Kohn SR: Molluscum contagiosum in patients with acquired immunodeficiency syndrome (Letter). Arch Ophthalmol 105:458, 1987.

Rodrigues MR, et al: Methods for rapid detection of human ocular viral infections. Ophthalmology 86:452–464, 1979.

MUMPS 072.9

IAN H. KADEN, M.D.,
and ROGER F. MEYER, M.D.

Ann Arbor, Michigan

Mumps is a acute contagious disease caused by the mumps virus, which is transmitted by droplet on direct contact. The ports of entry are the nose, mouth, and possibly conjunctiva. The incubation period averages 18 days. One attack usually produces lifelong immunity. A generalized viremia carries the virus to the susceptible tissues. The parotid and other salivary glands are usually affected, but their involvement is only one aspect of a widely disseminated disease. The testicles and ovaries may also be affected. The major systemic complications are those that affect the central nervous system, including mumps meningitis, encephalitis, myelitis, polyradiculitis, and cranial neuritis. They may be present individually or in combination. Deafness can occur after mumps and may be profound. The ocular manifestations of mumps, in approximate order of frequency, include dacryoadenitis, optic neuritis, conjunctivitis, scleritis, keratitis, uveitis, retinitis, and ocular muscle palsies. Mumps in the mother during the early months of pregnancy may result in congenital abnormalities. Diagnosis of mumps infection can be confirmed by acute and convalescent serologic studies.

THERAPY

Ocular. There is no specific treatment for mumps infection. Warm moist compresses are generally sufficient to improve patient comfort and reduce ocular swelling.

If iritis is present, atropine may be used to put the ciliary body at rest. In normal adults, one or two topical ocular instillations of 1 per cent atropine produce cycloplegia, which begins within 25 minutes and persists for 3 to 5 days.

The course of scleritis, keratitis, and uveitis may be shortened by the use of topical corticosteroids. One or two drops of 1 per cent prednisolone two to four times daily may control the inflammation. Oral or intravenous steroids may be indicated for more severe cases of uveitis and for optic neuritis or neuroretinitis.

Supportive. The mumps virus has been

shown to be present in the saliva as long as 7 days before and 9 days after the appearance of parotid swelling; until the parotid swelling subsides, the patient should be isolated. Bed-rest is recommended during the febrile period. Analgesics, such as 300 to 600 mg of aspirin every 6 to 8 hours, may be used for relief of headache and fever. If additional sedation is necessary, codeine in a dosage of 15 to 60 mg every 3 to 4 hours should prove adequate.

Ocular or Periocular Manifestations

Conjunctiva: Chemosis; follicular or papillary conjunctivitis; hyperemia; subconjunctival hemorrhages.
Cornea: Interstitial keratitis with stromal infiltration and edema; opacity (congenital); punctate epithelial keratitis; ulcer.
Extraocular Muscles: Paralysis; tenonitis.
Eyelids: Edema; hyperemia.
Globe: Exophthalmos, microphthalmos (congenital).
Lacrimal System: Dacryoadenitis, epiphora.
Optic Nerve: Atrophy; disc hyperemia; optic neuritis, papillitis, neuroretinitis.
Sclera: Episcleritis; scleritis.
Other: Anterior uveitis; central retinal vein occlusion; cortical blindness; posterior subcapsular lens opacity (congenital); posterior uveitis (congenital); transient glaucoma; vitreous hemorrhages.

PRECAUTIONS

Since there is no specific treatment for mumps infection, therapy should be directed toward relief of symptoms and prevention of complications. Because of the potential hazard of corticosteroid therapy, its use in mild cases is not recommended. Antimicrobial drugs are of no value, except when secondary bacterial infections are present.

COMMENTS

A live, attenuated mump virus vaccine was licensed in the United States in 1968. It is safe and highly effective. Adverse reactions are rare except for the occasional case of parotitis. It is provided as a combined vaccine with measles and rubella vaccines and is recommended for routine immunizations of children over 1 year of age.
A resurgence of mumps infection in recent years has revitalized interest in mandatory universal immunization. The resurgence has occurred among teens and young adults, many of whom belong to what is thought to be a relatively underimmunized cohort of children born between 1967 and 1977. Seronegativity for mumps may be as high as 15 per cent of the 15- to 24-year-old population. Demonstration of mumps vaccination is recommended before college attendance or employment in medical care settings, where the consequences of disease spread may be severe.

References

Centers for Disease Control: Mumps—United States, 1985–1988. MMWR 3:101–105, 1989.
Foster RE, et al: Mumps neuroretinitis in an adolescent. Am J Ophthalmol 110:91–93, 1990.
Hayden GF, et al: Current status of mumps and mumps vaccine in the United States. Pediatrics 62:965–969, 1978.
Kelly PW, et al: The susceptibility of young adult Americans to vaccine-preventable infections. JAMA 266:2724–2729, 1991.
Krishna N, Lyda W: Acute suppurative dacryoadenitis as a sequel to mumps. Arch Ophthalmol 59:350–351, 1958.
Love A, Malm G, Rydbeck R, Norrby E, Kristensson K: Developmental disturbances in the hamster retina caused by a mutant of mumps virus. Dev Neurosci 7:65–72, 1985.
Meyer RF, Sullivan JH, Oh JO: Mumps conjunctivitis. Am J Ophthalmol 78:1022–1024, 1974.
Polland W, Thorburn W: Transient glaucoma as a manifestation of mumps. A case report. Acta Ophthalmol 54:779–782, 1976.
Riffenburgh RS: Ocular manifestations of mumps. Arch Ophthalmol 66:739–743, 1961.
Strong LE, Henderson JW, Gangitano JL: Bilateral retrobulbar neuritis secondary to mumps. Am J Ophthalmol 78:331–332, 1974.
Swan JW, Penn RF: Scleritis following mumps. Report of a case. Am J Ophthalmol 53:366–368, 1962.

NEWCASTLE DISEASE 077.8

LAURENT LAMER, M.D., F.R.C.S.(C)

Montreal, Quebec

Newcastle disease, caused by a paramyxovirus, is primarily a serious epizootic pneumoencephalitic infection of fowls. In humans, the disease is usually transmitted by contact with infected poultry. It produces an acute follicular conjunctivitis with slight serous discharge and enlarged preauricular lymph nodes. Characteristic ocular symptoms include burning, foreign body sensation, pain, redness, tearing, and photophobia. The infection usually has an abrupt onset; the bulbar conjunctivae become injected and chemotic, follicles appear on the tarsus of the caruncle, and the lid may become edematous. The conjunctivitis is usually unilateral. Corneal involvement is rare; however, a fine epithelial keratitis or round subepithelial opacities may develop. In patients who experience systemic involvement, there may be fatigue, a slight elevation of temperature, headaches, and mild arthralgia.

THERAPY

Ocular. There is no specific treatment for Newcastle disease. Therapy should be directed toward preventing complications, reducing secondary bacterial infection, and relieving symptoms. The use of topical ocular broad-spectrum antibiotics, such as a mixture of neomycin, polymyxin B, and bacitracin, may be of some value, although this has not been definitively demonstrated. The application of hot compresses gives some systemic relief.

Systemic. Bedrest may be indicated in more severe cases. The patient should be instructed to avoid eyestrain or any activity that might increase the severity of the ocular affections.

Ocular or Periocular Manifestations

Conjunctiva: Chemosis; exudates; follicular conjunctivitis; hemorrhages; hyperemia; mucopurulent discharge.
Cornea: Fine keratic precipitates; round central subepithelial opacity.
Eyelids: Edema; follicles.
Other: Decreased accommodation; decreased visual acuity; irritation; lacrimation; ocular pain; photophobia; preauricular lymphadenopathy.

PRECAUTIONS

Newcastle disease is a benign, self-limited disease that normally runs its course in 7 to 10 days. In rare instances, some blurring of vision or difficulty of accommodation may persist for a short period of time.

COMMENTS

Newcastle disease occurs as a disease of poultry throughout the world. Human infection usually occurs through conjunctival contact, primarily in poultry workers and laboratory personnel. Although human-to-human transmission of the disease has not been documented, it seems likely that it may occur.

There is some concern that the Newcastle disease virus may develop into a more serious human pathogen. The virus, a parainfluenza type, has demonstrated its genetic plasticity by assuming four pathologic forms.

References

Charan S, Mahajan VM, Rai A, Balaya S: Ocular pathogenesis of Newcastle disease virus in rabbits and monkeys. J Comp Pathol 94:159–163, 1984.
Duke-Elder S (ed): System of Ophthalmology. St. Louis, CV Mosby, 1965, Vol VIII, pp 369–372; 1976, Vol XV, p 110.
Hanson RP: Paramyxovirus infections. In Hubbert WT, McCulloch WF, Schnurrenberger PR (eds): Diseases Transmitted from Animals to Man, 16th ed. Springfield, IL, Charles C Thomas, 1975, pp 851–858.
Lamer L: Sur un cas de conjonctivite de la maladie de Newcastle. Can J Ophthalmol 4:390–393, 1969.
Schemera B, Toro H, Herbst W, et al: Conjunctivitis and disorders of general health status in humans caused by infection with Newcastle disease virus. DTW 94:383–384, 1987.
Zehetbauer G, Kunz C, Thaler A: Cases of pseudo fowl plague (Newcastle disease) in man in lower Austria. Wien Klin Wochenschr 83:878–880, 1971.

OCULAR VACCINIA 999.0

BRUCE M. MASSARO, M.D., M.P.H.,
and ROBERT A. HYNDIUK, M.D.

Milwaukee, Wisconsin

Vaccinia is an infection caused by the DNA-containing laboratory virus used for smallpox prophylaxis. Vaccination with this live virus can result in infection of ocular tissues as a result of hand or fomite transfer from a primary vaccination site (76 per cent) or from the site of another individual (20 per cent). An incubation period of 7 to 10 days precedes development of a severe, typically unilateral blepharoconjunctivitis. Nonimmune patients are generally more severely affected than previously vaccinated patients. The overall incidence of accidental vaccinial infection is 18.8 per million vaccinations.

The eyelid skin is most commonly affected. Single or multiple lesions, initially papulovesicular, become pustular or ulcerated or both. Severe lid edema and erythema, regional lymphadenopathy, and an acute febrile illness with myalgias occur. Scarring is more severe in nonimmune patients and those with eczema. Vaccinial conjunctivitis may occur with or without blepharitis and is often purulent with possible membrane formation or frank ulceration. Orbital cellulitis may develop. Vaccinial infections of the lids and conjunctiva generally last about 10 days and resolve without sequelae. As is the case in herpetic canalicular obstruction, vaccinial infection of the upper lacrimal drainage system mucosal epithelium can produce scarring with canalicular and punctal stenosis or occlusion. Epiphora may develop acutely or shortly after the blepharoconjunctivitis.

Corneal infection usually occurs in association with eyelid or conjunctival infection or both. It may range in intensity from a mild superficial punctate keratitis to a disciform necrotizing stromal keratitis with possible corneal perforations. Nonimmune patients with ocular vaccinia develop significant keratitis in 20 to 50 per cent of cases, whereas only 10 per cent of those previously vaccinated suffer this complication. Stromal keratitis may occur as late as 2 to 3 months after the original infection and is felt to be immune in origin, unlike corneal epithelial disease, which presents acutely and reflects replicating virus. Giemsa-stained scrapings of infected tissues display diagnostic eosinophilic intracytoplasmic inclusion bodies (Guarnieri's bodies).

THERAPY

Systemic. Vaccinia immune globulin (VIG) is gamma globulin fractionated from serum in patients vaccinated a few months before blood donation. VIG is effective in modifying the complications of systemic and ocular vaccinia and is especially helpful in cases with orbital cellulitis. It is available from the American Red Cross Regional Blood Centers and the Centers for Disease Control. VIG is given intramuscularly in a dosage of 0.6 ml/kg. No more than 5 ml should be injected at one site, and no more than 20 ml should be given at one time. The dose may be repeated in 48 hours if no improvement occurs.

Ocular. For vaccinial infection of the lids or conjunctiva without corneal involvement, investigational use of topical antiviral medications may help prevent the development of keratitis. A combination of 3 per cent vidarabine[+] ophthalmic ointment five times daily and 1 per cent trifluridine[+] solution every 2 hours during waking hours is probably more effective than idoxuridine. Idoxuridine[+] can be administered as 0.5 per cent ophthalmic solution every hour during the day and every 2 hours at night.

If corneal involvement has occurred, investigational use of vidarabine, trifluridine, or idoxuridine in the dosages outlined above will probably be effective in the resolution of the epithelial stage of the keratitis (due to multiplying virus). Both vidarabine and trifluridine have been shown to be significantly more effective than idoxuridine for the treatment of vaccinial keratitis. The antivirals should be continued topically for one week after there is an absence of macropunctate epithelial fluorescein staining. Whether acyclovir* or other newer antiviral agents are effective in treating ocular vaccinia is not known. Topically applied interferon-alpha* has been shown to be effective in treating the punctate epithelial and ulcerative keratitis of ocular vaccinia.

Good hygiene should be maintained, with warm, moist compresses applied to the eye as needed. Topical antibiotics should be given twice daily to prevent bacterial superinfection. Topical corticosteroids may be used for significant active stromal keratitis if the epithelium has healed and topical antiviral coverage is maintained. Cycloplegics should be used as needed for iritis.

Surgical. In cases of progressive necrotizing keratitis, lamellar or penetrating keratoplasty may be indicated.

Ocular or Periocular Manifestations

Conjunctiva: Chemosis; hyperemia; non-follicular, catarrhal, or purulent conjunctivitis; ulceration of palpebral or bulbar conjunctiva.

Cornea: Epithelial ulceration; fine or coarse punctate epithelial keratitis; interstitial, disciform, or necrotizing stromal keratitis; stromal scarring; vascularization.

Eyelids: Edema; erythema; pustules; ulcers; vesicles.

Lacrimal: Canaliculitis with canalicular and/or punctal stenosis and epiphora.

Other: Anterior uveitis, choroiditis; extraocular muscle palsies secondary to postvaccinial encephalitis; optic neuritis; orbital cellulitis; preauricular lymphadenopathy.

PRECAUTIONS

Although useful in the presence of vaccinial blepharitis or orbital cellulitis, VIG should not be used if keratitis is present. Experimental results show that the use of VIG in the presence of established keratitis may actually result in prolonged, more extensive stromal inflammation and subsequent stromal scarring. Topical corticosteroids may aggravate the acute stage of the disease. However, once the corneal epithelium has healed and significant stromal inflammation or anterior uveitis is present, topical corticosteroids may be used cautiously, along with topical antiviral coverage. Systemic steroids should be avoided.

COMMENTS

Ocular vaccinia is now rarely seen because routine childhood smallpox vaccination ended in the early 1970s. The World Health Organization declared the world free of smallpox in May 1980, and vaccination of civilians is indicated only for laboratory workers directly involved with smallpox-related viruses. Vaccination is no longer recommended for international travel. However, all active military personnel are vaccinated for strategic defensive reasons. As more men and women born after 1970 enter military service, the percentage of those undergoing primary vaccination continues to increase with an attendant increased risk for systemic dissemination. Patients at risk include those with atopic or other forms of dermatitis, those undergoing immunosuppressive therapy, and those with a systemic disease that compromises the immune status, such as AIDS.

Acknowledgment. Supported in part by an unrestricted grant from Research to Prevent Blindness, Inc. and supported in part by Ophthalmic Research Core Grant EY-01931.

References

deLuise VP: Viral conjunctivitis. *In* Tabbara KF, Hyndiuk RA (eds): Infections of the Eye: Diagnosis and Management. Boston, Little Brown, 1986, pp 437–460.

Duke-Elder S (ed): System of Ophthalmology. St. Louis, CV Mosby, 1965, Vol VIII, pp. 360–367.

Fulginiti VA, et al: Therapy of experimental vaccinial keratitis. Effect of idoxuridine and VIG. Arch Ophthalmol 74:539–544, 1965.

Harley RD, Stefanyszyn MA, et al: Herpetic canalicular obstruction. Ophthal Surg 18:367–370, 1987.

Hyndiuk RA, et al: Treatment of vaccinial keratitis with vidarabine. Arch Ophthalmol 94:1363–1364, 1976.

Hyndiuk RA, et al: Treatment of vaccinial keratitis with trifluorothymidine. Arch Ophthalmol 94: 1785–1786, 1976.

O'Brien WJ: Antiviral agents. In Tabbara KF, Hyndiuk RA (eds): Infections of the Eye: Diagnosis and Management. Boston, Little Brown, 1986, pp 257–274.

Pavan-Langston D: Ocular antiviral therapy. Int Ophthalmol Clin 20:149–161, 1980.

Redfield RR, et al: Disseminated vaccinia in a military recruit with human immunodeficiency virus (HIV) disease. N Engl J Med 316:673–676, 1987.

Ruben FL, Land JM: Ocular vaccinia: An epidemiologic analysis of 348 cases. Arch Ophthalmol 84:45–48, 1970.

virus may persist longer in the conjunctiva, although the conjunctivitis is milder. Epidemics of PCF occur in the summer and in association with poorly chlorinated swimming pools.

There are several reports of chronic adenovirus ocular infections. Boniuk et al. (1965) isolated Ad type 2 from the eye of a patient with chronic keratitis. Darougar and his associates (1977) reported a case of recurrent papillary conjunctivitis that persisted for 16 months and from which Ad type 19 was isolated 12 months after its onset. Pettit and his group (1979) described three cases of chronic keratoconjunctivitis associated with Ad types 3, 4, and 5. In two of these three patients, there was active epithelial keratitis, and the third patient had purulent conjunctivitis and subepithelial opacities. All three patients received topical corticosteroids early in the course of their diseases. Our group at the Proctor Foundation isolated Ad type 5 from a patient with longstanding superficial punctate keratitis of Thygeson and folliculosis.

Although the role of adenovirus infection was not clear, in these patients with longstanding disease the adenoviruses could well cause chronic disease of the external eye. Unusual forms of Ad infection have been reported in patients with immunosuppression.

PHARYNGOCONJUNCTIVAL FEVER 372.02
(Acute Follicular Conjunctivitis, Adenovirus Conjunctivitis, PCF, Syndrome of Beal)

CHANDLER R. DAWSON, M.D.

San Francisco, California

Pharyngoconjunctival fever (PCF) and acute follicular conjunctivitis are the most common manifestations of ocular adenovirus (Ad) infection. Adenovirus follicular conjunctivitis can occur without other signs or as PCF in association with pharyngitis and fever. In either form, the conjunctivitis usually has an acute onset. It is usually unilateral at onset with involvement of the second eye within a week and preauricular lymphadenopathy on the side of the affected eye. The virus probably is transmitted by finger-to-eye spread or by respiratory droplets directly onto the conjunctival surface. After an incubation period of 5 to 12 days, the disease starts with hyperemia, watery discharge, and follicle formation. In PCF, the conjunctivitis is accompanied by pharyngitis and fever and occasionally by gastrointestinal symptoms. Systemic signs occur in about one-third of patients with Ad type 4 conjunctivitis and are less common with Ad type 3. The conjunctivitis subsides gradually in 7 to 15 days during which time virus can regularly be found in the conjunctiva and upper respiratory tract; Ad type 3

THERAPY

Ocular. Antiviral drops and topical interferon have not been generally useful for treating adenovirus conjunctivitis. Astringent drops may diminish hyperemia and relieve symptoms. Topical antibiotics may be used to prevent secondary bacterial infections. If the keratitis is particularly severe, mydriatic drops (cyclopentolate, homatropine) may be used to alleviate discomfort. Topical corticosteroids[‡] have not been shown to be effective and carry a certain risk because follicular conjunctivitis due to herpes simplex virus can be accompanied by corneal ulceration, which is made worse by steroids.

Supportive. Management is primarily supportive. Patients should be reassured that the condition is self-limited (less than 15 days) and rarely results in serious complications. Other general supportive measures include antipyretics to control fever and iced compresses to the eyes if there is swelling and pain.

Ocular or Periocular Manifestations

Conjunctiva: Acute follicular conjunctivitis; chemosis; hyperemia; punctate hemorrhages; serofibrinous exudates.

Cornea: Marginal infiltration; superficial punctate keratitis; occasional residual subepithelial opacities.

Eyelids: Blepharospasm; edema, pseudoptosis.

Other: Lacrimation; periorbital pain; photophobia; preauricular and submandibular lymphadenopathy.

PRECAUTIONS

Patients and their families need to be told how to prevent the spread of adenovirus on towels, pillows, and hands.

COMMENTS

There are 41 currently known serotypes of adenovirus subdivided into six groups (A, B, C, D, E, and F) based on DNA restriction enzyme analysis genome typing. The causes of PCF and adenovirus conjunctivitis include Ad types 3 and 7, which belong to group B, and Ad 4, the only type in group E. All of the types associated with epidemic keratoconjunctivitis are in group D, which has 29 serotypes, including Ad types 8, 19, and 37.

Worldwide, Ad types 1, 2, 3, 5, and 7 are isolated most frequently, whereas types 4, 6, and 8 are found much less often. After the initial infection, the Ad group C (Ad 1, 2, 5, and 6) may persist as a latent infection in the lymphoid tissues of the nasopharynx and gastrointestinal tract. Children are usually infected with the endemic types before the age of 2 years. Types 3 and 7 are associated with "swimming pool conjunctivitis," as well as with lower respiratory disease in children younger than 6 years of age. Types 4, 7, and 21 are the major cause of epidemics of acute respiratory disease in military recruits and cause sporadic pneumonia in children. Types 40 and 41 are associated with diarrheal disease in hospitalized pediatric patients. Adenoviruses, as can other latent viruses, can present as chronic infections in immunosuppressed patients.

References

Aoki K, et al: Clinical and aetiological study of adenoviral conjunctivitis with special reference to adenovirus types 4 and 19 infections. Br J Ophthalmol 66:776–780, 1982.

Boniuk M, Phillips CA, Friedman JB: Clinic adenovirus type 2 keratitis in man. N Engl J Med 273:924–925, 1965.

Bryden AS, Chesworth C: An assessment of Adenoclone EIA: A monoclonal based, group specific enzyme assay for adenovirus diagnosis. Serodiagn Immunotherap Infect Dis 2:341–347, 1988.

Darougar S, Quinlan MP, Gibson JA, Jones BR: Epidemic keratoconjunctivitis and chronic papillary conjunctivitis in London due to adenovirus type 19. Br J Ophthalmol 61:76–85, 1977.

Dawson CR: Follicular conjunctivitis. *In* Wilson LA (ed): External Diseases of the Eye. Hagerstown, MD, Harper & Row, 1979, pp 57–75.

Hierholzer JC: Adenoviruses in the immunocompromised host. Clin Microbiol Rev 5(3):262–274, 1992.

Horvath J, Palkonyay L, Weber J: Group C adenovirus DNA sequences in lymphoid cells. J Virol 59:189–192, 1986.

Ishii K, et al: Comparative studies on aetiology and epidemiology of viral conjunctivitis in three countries of East Asia—Japan, Taiwan and South Korea. Int J Epidemiol 16:98–103, 1987.

Pettit TH, Holland GM: Chronic keratoconjunctivitis associated with ocular adenovirus infection. Am J Ophthalmol 88:748–751, 1979.

Tullo AB: Adenovirus infections. *In* Easty DL (ed): Virus Disease of the Eye. Chicago, Year Book Medical Publishers, 1985, pp 257–270.

RABIES 071

ROY J. ELLSWORTH, M.D.

Boise, Idaho

Rabies is an acute viral infection of the central nervous system (CNS). The virus is almost always transmitted to humans from the bite of an infected wild animal. Raccoons, foxes, bats, skunks, wolves, llamas, and unvaccinated cats and dogs frequently carry the rabies virus. Bites inflicted during an unprovoked attack from an animal displaying inappropriate behavior are the most likely to result in the transmission of rabies.

Transmission of rabies from human-to-human was first reported by Houff et al. in 1979 as the result of a corneal transplant from a patient who was suspected of having died from Guillain-Barré syndrome. Since then, five other cases have been reported following human corneal transplantation.

The virus is transmitted from the animal's infected salivary glands and incubates in the victim's muscle cells for 10 days to 8 months before moving along the peripheral nerve to the CNS. This prolonged incubation period allows adequate time for prophylactic treatment to be effective.

Pain around the wound site is usually present along with a prodrome of flulike symptoms. Rabies is a systemic illness affecting many organ systems. It can be classified into two types: furious and paralytic. Patients with furious rabies show signs of rage and hyperactivity. Paralytic symptoms are those of progressive flaccid paralysis and are often mistakenly diagnosed as Guillain-Barré syndrome. Difficulty swallowing fluids and excess secretions require close monitoring during the acute neurologic phase, which usually lasts 1 week before coma and respiratory arrest. A few documented cases of rabies have recovered with aggressive treatment and supportive care.

Serum antibodies can usually be detected between 6 and 13 days after exposure.

If a domestic animal is suspected of having

rabies, it should be confined and observed for 10 days for abnormal behavior. If a wild animal is suspected of carrying the rabies virus, it should be killed and examined for CNS Negri bodies or the virus itself by an appropriate laboratory.

THERAPY

Systemic. Treatment should begin before the diagnosis is confirmed by study of the suspected animal or serum antibodies. Vigorous wound care to the area should begin with soap and water and should be followed by cleaning the bite with 1 per cent povidone-iodine or 1 to 2 per cent benzalkonium chloride. Tetanus prophylaxis should also be given along with antibiotic therapy for both aerobic and anaerobic bacteria. Rabies vaccination should be started as soon as possible using human diploid-cell vaccine or rabies vaccine absorbed, in conjunction with human rabies immunoglobulin. These methods are nearly 100 per cent effective in providing and inducing protective antibodies. They must be given before the virus has invaded the central nervous system, after which time it is almost always fatal. Rabies vaccine absorbed and human diploid-cell are given concomitantly with human rabies immunoglobulin.

Rabies vaccine absorbed is available from the Michigan Department of Health. Human diploid-cell vaccine (IMOVAX Rabies, Merieux) is available commercially. Both vaccines are best given intramuscularly. Human rabies immunoglobulin (Hyperab, cutter; Imogan Rabies, Meriux) is given to provide passive immunity until the victim's natural immunity response is mounted by the vaccines.

Ocular or Periocular Manifestations

Neurologic Stage: Paralysis of extraocular muscles, third, fourth, or seventh nerve; eyelid-retraction; retinal edema and hemorrhages; lacrimation; photophobia; aerophobia; hydrophobia; and difficulty swallowing.

Prodromal Stage: Headache; pain and itching around the wound site.

COMMENTS

Six cases of human-to-human rabies infections have been documented following corneal transplantation from donors with no history of being bitten by an animal. Rabies symptoms are nonspecific and can mimic other diseases. These cases, along with the transmission of the Creutzfeldt-Jakob virus by corneal transplantation, make it important to exclude donors who die from postinfectious polyneuritis or unexplained encephalopathy.

Rabies infections in humans are fatal if not treated. Postexposure treatment with human diploid-cell vaccine or rabies vaccine absorbed along with human rabies immunoglobulin is almost always successful if initiated early in the incubation period.

References

Centers for Disease Control: Human-to-human transmission of rabies by a corneal transplant—Idaho. MMWR 28:109–111, 1979.

Centers for Disease Control: Human-to-human transmission of rabies via corneal transplant—Thailand. MMWR 30:475, 1981.

Centers for Disease Control: Human-to-human transmission of rabies via a corneal transplant—France. MMWR 29:25–26, 1989.

Duffy P, et al: Possible person-to-person transmission of Creutzfeldt-Jacob disease. N Engl J Med 290:692–693, 1974.

Frenia ML, Lafin SM, Barone JA: Features and treatment of rabies. Clin Pharmacol 2, 1992.

Gode GR, Bhide NK: Two rabies deaths after corneal grafts from one donor (Letter). Lancet 2 (8614):791, 1988.

Groleau G: Rabies. Emergency Med Clin N Am. 10, 1992.

Haltia M, Tarkkanen A, Kivelia T: Rabies: Ocular pathology. Br J Ophthalmol 73:61–67, 1989.

Houff SA, et al: Human-to-human transmission of rabies virus by corneal transplant. N Engl J Med 300:603–604, 1979.

RUBELLA 056.9
(German Measles)
VIVIEN BONIUK, M.D.
New York, New York

Rubella has been known as a clinical entity for almost 200 years. It is viral in origin, caused by a member of the toga-virus group with one antigenic type. In 1941, Gregg made the astute clinical observation that a peculiar type of congenital cataract was associated with the occurrence of a rubella epidemic 9 to 10 months earlier. This observation led to the description of the congenital rubella syndrome (CRS), which is a well-defined and well-described group of ocular, cardiac, and other organ system abnormalities resulting from exposure to the rubella virus during embryonic life. The rubella epidemic of 1964 to 1965 afforded an opportunity for multidisciplinary study of the effects of the rubella virus and led to development of a vaccine, resulting in a 98 to 99 per cent reduction in the incidence of rubella and congenital rubella syndrome (CRS) since 1969.

Since rubella infrequently causes significant ocular and systemic complications in the postnatal period, attention here is directed only to CRS. Although several cases of acute rubella retinal pigment epitheliitis have been reported in adults, they have not led to serious sequelae. The effects in utero are explainable by the observation that chronic infection by the rubella virus causes cells to have a prolonged doubling time and shortened survival; therefore, organ systems infected with virus during their active growing period will be underdeveloped and abnormal.

Depending on the stage of gestation during which rubella is acquired, there is a wide spectrum of systemic features ranging from stillbirths to the most minimally detectable damage to the retinal pigment epithelium and the pigmented epithelium in the organ of Corti. Other systemic abnormalities are prematurity by weight and mental and physical developmental retardation that persists into childhood. Also included are thrombocytopenic purpura, pancytopenia, large skull with bulging anterior fontanel, encephalitis, various neurologic anomalies, hepatosplenomegaly, radiologically observable bone changes, pancreatic insufficiency, esophageal atresia, and cleft palate. Various types of cardiac anomalies may be present and are frequently associated with ocular defects.

The most common ocular findings in congenital rubella syndrome are retinopathy; a peculiar central, often eccentric, dense nuclear cataract; and microphthalmos. Less frequent findings are iris hypoplasia with pigment epithelial defect, nystagmus and strabismus, congenital glaucoma, and corneal haze due to transient keratitis, which may leave a permanent scar. The pigmentary changes of the retina may show progression in early childhood, and there have been ten reported cases of subretinal neovascularization and disciform macular detachment as late complications. CRS must be considered in the differential diagnosis of subretinal neovascular membranes in the pediatric age group.

THERAPY

Surgical. As soon as the child's condition permits, the congenital rubella cataract should be completely aspirated. Postoperative treatment with mydriatics should be intensive and continued for at least 3 months; parents should be cautioned about the importance of punctal occlusion after eyedrop administration. Early optical correction of aphakia is essential.

The glaucoma secondary to the congenital rubella syndrome behaves as a phenotypic congenital glaucoma. Other ocular abnormalities, such as strabismus, are treated in a manner consistent with basic therapeutic principles.

PRECAUTIONS

A multidisciplinary approach to treatment of these children is essential because of the presence of multiple anomalies associated with physical and mental developmental delay. It is essential that they be followed in centers familiar with coordination of therapy in order to maximize their development.

COMMENTS

The incidence of rubella in pregnancy is directly related to the pool of susceptible women in that age group and their exposure to those recently infected with rubella virus. Recent epidemiologic data indicate that most cases reported now occur in young adults (those over 15 years of age), which include women of childbearing age who are at high risk; prior prevalence predominated in the under 14 years of age group. Therefore, the incidence of reported congenital rubella syndrome has not decreased substantially in recent years.

In the United States, laws require vaccination against rubella for school entry, which should ultimately reduce the adult pool; however, particularly susceptible at this time are those individuals in health care facilities providing care for women of childbearing age. Special attention (state-mandated) is paid to the immunization status of health care workers. The risk of severe congenital malformation after rubella vaccination is low, even should it be given to a pregnant women; however, to avoid this risk, women known to be pregnant should not be vaccinated and conception should be avoided for 3 months after vaccination. CRS has been reported in the offspring of previously vaccinated women. Rubella immunity should be tested before each pregnancy.

References

Boniuk V: Rubella. Int Ophthalmol Clin *15*:229–241, 1975.

Collis WJ, Cohen DN: Rubella retinopathy: A progressive disorder. Arch Ophthalmol *84*:33, 1970.

Condon R, Bower C: Congenital rubella after previous maternal vaccination (Letter). Med J Aust *156*(12): 882, 1992.

Deutman AF, Grizzand WS: Rubella retinopathy and subretinal neovascularization. Am J Ophthalmol *85*:22, 1978.

Gerber SL, Helveston EM: Subretinal neovascularization in a 10-year-old child. J Pediatr Ophthalmol Strabismus *29*:250–251, 1992.

Gerstle C, Zinn KM: Rubella-associated retinitis in an adult: Report of a case. Mt Sinai J Med NY *43*:303–308, 1976.

Greaves WL, et al: Prevention of rubella transmission in medical facilities. JAMA *248*:861–864, 1982.

Hayashi M, Yoshimura N, Kondo T: Acute rubella retinal pigment epitheliitis in an adult. Am J Ophthalmol *93*:285–288, 1982.

Preblud SR, et al: Fetal risk associated with rubella vaccine. JAMA *246*:1413–1418, 1981.

RUBEOLA 055.9
(Measles, Morbilli)

NICK W.H.M. DEKKERS, M.D.

Tilburg, The Netherlands

Rubeola is an acute, extremely communicable febrile disease, which primarily used to affect young school-aged children. In the developed world, the rapidly increasing rate of immunization has caused a shift toward the older age groups, whereas in developing countries, mainly the very young (6 months to 2 years) are affected. Rubeola is caused by a paramyxovirus and is characterized by a catarrhal inflammation of the respiratory tract and subepithelial conjunctivitis in the prodromal phase of the disease, followed by a maculopapular rash. The viral epithelial keratoconjunctivitis, late in the prodromal phase and in the exanthematous stage, starts in the exposed parts of the conjunctiva and progresses toward the central cornea. Separate lesions can coalesce into large corneal erosions. Corneal ulcers and perforations, which are rare complications in well-nourished patients, can result from bacterial or viral (herpetic) superinfections and are usually associated with protein-energy malnutrition. Infection with the virus in utero has been associated with cataracts, dacryostenosis, pigmentary retinopathy, and cardiopathy.

THERAPY

Systemic. Mild antipyretics and analgesics, such as aspirin, may be indicated for relief of fever, myalgias, and headache. Systemic antibiotics are not indicated, except in cases of secondary bacterial infections.
Ocular. The conjunctivitis and keratitis are usually of a mild and self-limiting nature. Eye care can be restricted to normal cleansing of the eyelids to remove crusts and secretions caused by conjunctivitis. In debilitated children, the application of eye ointment three or four times daily prevents the development of exposure keratitis and the progression of the keratitis into large corneal erosions.
Supportive. Low illumination reduces photophobia.

Ocular or Periocular Manifestations

Rare, apart from conjunctival and corneal signs.
Anterior Chamber: Hypopyon (associated with corneal ulcers and perforations).
Choroid: Posterior uveitis.

Conjunctiva: Kopliks' spots; subepithelial conjunctivitis, sometimes with follicles and hemorrhages (prodromal stage).
Cornea: Viral epithelial keratoconjunctivitis (exanthematous stage) as a common sign; rarely erosion, ulcer, adherent leukoma.
Eyelids: Blepharospasm; cellulitis; edema.
Iris: Prolapse; synechiae.
Lacrimal System: Dacryoadenitis; dacryocystitis; dacryostenosis (congenital).
Optic Nerve: Atrophy; retrobulbar or optic neuritis (associated with visual hallucinations, homonymous hemianopsia, and sixth nerve palsy).
Retina: Edema; pigmentary retinopathy (congenital); vascular construction (may simulate central retinal artery occlusion).
Other: Accommodative spasm; hemianopsia; mydriasis; orbital cellulitis; paralysis of sixth nerve; secondary glaucoma, strabismus.

PRECAUTIONS

Routine immunization with live, attenuated measles vaccine has considerably changed the epidemiology of measles. This makes the clinical diagnosis a more difficult one than it used to be. In severe immunosuppression as in protein-energy malnutrition, the characteristic rash is lacking and the measles infection is clinically not diagnosed.

COMMENTS

In the United States and Europe, measles is a relatively mild disease. On the contrary, measles is associated with high mortality and considerable morbidity in developing countries.
The incidence of blindness after measles can be as high as 1 per cent. This corneal blindness is caused by a combination of factors: measles, malnutrition, vitamin A deficiency, traditional treatment, and secondary bacterial or viral infection.

References

Dekkers NWHM: The cornea in measles. Doc Ophthalmol 52:1–120, 1981.
Dekkers NWHM: The cornea in measles. *In* Darrell RW (ed): Viral Infections of the Eye. Philadelphia, Lea & Febiger, pp 239–250, 1985.
Frederique G, Howard RO, Boniuk V: Corneal ulcers in rubeola. Am J Ophthalmol 68:996–1003, 1969.
Morley DC, Martin WJ, Allen I: Measles in East and Central Africa. E Afr Med J 44:497–508, 1967.
Sanford-Smith JH, Whittle HC: Corneal ulceration following measles in Nigerian children. Br J Ophthalmol 63:720–724, 1979.

VARICELLA 052.9
(Chickenpox)

YUKIO UCHIDA, M.D.

Tokyo, Japan

Varicella is a mild, highly contagious exanthem of childhood characterized by fever and vesicular eruptions in successive crops on the skin and mucous membranes. It is transmitted by droplet infection and caused by the varicella-zoster virus, a member of the herpes virus group. Although the majority of children and nonimmune adults recover promptly without sequela, rare but severe complications, such as pneumonia and encephalitis, have been known to occur. Ophthalmic involvement consists primarily of unilateral small, papular, phlyctenular eruptions along the lid margin, on the semilunar fold of the conjunctiva, and, most commonly, at the limbus.

THERAPY

Systemic. Systemic antibiotics may be administered when secondary infections occur. Zoster immunoglobulins can be used to prevent the development of the disease in children who are immunologically compromised and have been exposed to varicella. Zoster immunoglobulins work favorably when given within 3 days after the exposure. Immunization by a live attenuated virus vaccine seems to be effective in high-risk children. Intravenous acyclovir[‡] may be used successfully for severe varicella pneumonitis.

Ocular. There is no specific therapy for varicella. Cool compresses may be used to relieve the pruritus. For photophobia and discomfort caused by keratitis and uveitis, mydriatic-cycloplegics may be used. One drop of 1 per cent atropine solution may be instilled into the conjunctival sac once to twice daily. Vesicles or ulcers of the outer eye may become secondarily infected. Therefore, topical antibiotics, such as erythromycin, gentamicin, or tobramycin, should be used prophylactically to prevent infection. Antibiotic ointment may be applied on the skin three times daily and solution be instilled into the conjunctival sac four to six times daily. Antiviral agents, such as vidaradine,[‡] trifluridine,[‡] or acyclovir,[*] have not proved to be of value clinically against stromal keratitis and uveitis; however, they seem to have some therapeutic effect on epithelial lesions. Vidarabine or acyclovir ointment may be administered into the conjunctival sac five times daily, and trifluridine ophthalmic solution may be instilled five to nine times daily.

The use of topical corticosteroid should be avoided, except for severe nonuclerative stromal keratitis with uveitis. In this situation, a small amount of corticosteroids (one drop of 0.1 per cent dexamethasone three times daily at most) should be used in combination with cycloplegia, and the medication must be tapered gradually as a response is attained.

Supportive. Patients should rest in bed while they are febrile and remain at home until cutaneous eruptions become crusted. An antipyretic may be administered while patients are febrile, but the use of salicylates, such as aspirin, should be avoided in children. Because secondary infection of the cutaneous lesion with *Staphylococcus* or *Streptococcus* is common, the patient's skin should be kept clean. The fingernails of the patient should be trimmed to prevent secondary skin infections caused by scratching.

Ocular or Periocular Manifestations

Conjunctiva: Hyperemia; phlyctenular lesion at limbus; ulcer; vesicles.

Cornea: Descemetocele; opacity; pseudodendritic epithelial lesion; punctate epithelial keratitis; stromal disciform or interstitial keratitis; ulcer; vesicles.

Eyelids: Cicatrization of lid margin; distortion of cilia; ulcer; vesicles.

Optic Nerve: Optic Neuritis; papilledema.

Retina: Diffuse retinitis; exudative retinitis; acute retinal necrosis; hemorrhagic retinopathy; periphlebitis.

Sclera: Scleritis.

Other: Anterior uveitis, cataract; external ophthalmoplegia; internal ophthalmoplegia; phthisis bulbi.

PRECAUTIONS

Treatment of varicella is essentially symptomatic. Systemic corticosteroids are contraindicated because these drugs are known to cause dissemination of the disease. Once stromal keratitis has been treated with topical corticosteroids, it is difficult to withdraw these drugs without recurrence of the disease, even if the medication is tapered. Therefore, initiation of this therapy should be withheld if possible, and it must be restricted to severe cases.

COMMENTS

The ocular vesicles or ulcers of varicella resolve spontaneously with minimal scarring. Unilateral serous iridocyclitis occasionally occurs as a separate entity, but is self-limited. Rare intraocular involvement, such as retinitis or optic neuritis, may cause transient loss of vision; however, recovery of vision is the usual outcome. Stromal keratitis of the disciform type may occur at different periods after the onset, from several weeks or months. When it is treated with topical corticosteroids, pseudodendritic lesions that harbor the virus occasionally appear in the corneal epithelium. These lesions, however, do not seem to develop into large ulcers.

References

Duke-Elder S (ed): System of Ophthalmology. St. Louis, CV Mosby, Vol VIII, 1965, pp 337–339.

McGill J, Chapman C: A comparison of topical acyclovir with steroids in the treatment of herpes zoster keratouveitis. Br J Ophthalmol 67:746–750, 1983.

Uchida Y, Kaneko M, Hayashi K: Varicella dendritic keratitis. Am J Ophthalmol 89:259–262, 1980.

Wilhelmus KR, Hamil MB, Jones DB: Varicella disciform stromal keratitis. Am J Ophthalmol 111: 575–580, 1991.

Wilson FM II: Varicella and herpes zoster ophthalmicus. In Tabbara KF, Hyndiuk RA (eds): Infections of the Eye. Boston, Little Brown, 1986, pp. 369–386.

SECTION 2

PARASITIC DISEASES

ACANTHAMOEBAE 136.9

MARY BETH MOORE, M.D.

Dallas, Texas

Two genera of small free-living amoebae can cause infections in humans. Amoebae of the *Naegleria* species are flagellated and gain access to the central nervous system by penetration of the nasal mucosa and direct invasion of the cribiform plate following a swim in contaminated water. The acute, necrotizing encephalitis that follows is rapidly fatal and may last 5 to 7 days. In contrast, amoebae of the *Acanthamoeba* species are nonflagellated and relatively less aggressive. They cause a slowly progressive, usually fatal granulomatous encephalitis that may last weeks or months. The route of infection is thought to be hematogenous.

Corneal infections are also caused by direct contact either with a foreign body contaminated with *Acanthamoeba* or with a contaminated soft or hard contact lens. Contact lenses become contaminated when rinsed or stored in homemade saline solution, distilled water, tap water, or well water. Contamination may also occur when a patient wears contact lenses while swimming in contaminated water or immersing in a contaminated hot tub. Commercially prepared preserved and nonpreserved saline solution can become contaminated once opened, and currently available disinfection methods may not eradicate the organism. Repeated inoculation onto the cornea via a contaminated contact lens results in a chronic, smoldering, painful keratitis.

Species responsible for corneal infections include *A. castellanii, A. polyphaga, A. culbertsoni, A. hatchetti,* and *A. rhysodes.* The organism exists in two forms: the motile, replicating trophozoite and the sessile, dormant cyst. It inhabits soil and water, and the cysts can become air-borne. The trophozoite feeds on bacteria and releases enzymes that may facilitate tissue invasion.

The number of reported cases of *Acanthamoeba* keratitis has increased significantly over the past 5 years. Initially, patients underwent multiple failed grafts or enucleation because of delayed diagnosis, and in some cases, the diagnosis was not made until tissue specimens were examined retrospectively. However, recently, early recognition and appropriate treatment have resulted in medical and surgical eradication of the infection and preservation of good vision. The most common misdiagnosis is herpes simplex keratitis because of the similar ocular pain, pseudodendrites, nonsuppurative keratitis, and initial positive response to topical steroids. The clinical course of *Acanthamoeba* keratitis is characterized by infection in young, healthy individuals, intense ocular pain, waxing and waning keratitis, pseudodendrites, recurrent epithelial defects, anterior stromal ring infiltrate, radial neuritis, and disciform keratitis. Diffuse anterior and posterior scleritis, scleral nodules, and uveitis have also been reported to be caused by *Acanthamoeba.* Organisms have been recovered from an anterior chamber paracentesis and have been seen on the iris surface histopathologically, thus raising the possibility of intraocular invasion. Fundus involvement is rare and thought to be due to hematogenous spread.

THERAPY

Systemic. A single, daily dose of 200 to 600 mg of ketoconazole[‡] or itraconazole,[‡] 100 to 200 mg daily, with meals, may be used for severe infections; however, it is not known if therapeutic levels of these drugs are achieved in the cornea. Sulindac, 200 mg or less, four times a day, may be used to relieve ocular pain. Oral narcotics may be required to alleviate severe ocular pain, which may last several weeks or months. However, long-term use of narcotics should be avoided.

Ocular. Medical therapy is evolving as more drugs are tested, found to be effective in vitro, and applied to the clinical situation. Currently, the accepted approach is topical ophthalmic treatment with one or more of the following: 0.1 per cent propamidine,[†] 0.15 per cent dibromopropamidine,[†] 0.1 per cent pentamidine,[‡] 1 per cent miconazole[‡] and 1 per cent clotrimazole, in combination with neomycin/polymyxin B/gramicidin[‡] or paromomycin[‡] solution. Both propamidine and pentamidine are members of the aromatic amines, which have well-documented antiparasitic properties. The antifungal imidazoles and antibacterial aminoglycosides inhibit growth of amoebae in vitro.

Polyhexamethylene biguanide (PHMB), a polymeric biguanide disinfectant, is reported to be effective in patients with uncontrolled refractory keratitis. In vitro, dimethyl sulfoxide (DMSO) 30 per cent was cysticidal when

113

combined with propamidine isethionate. DMSO presumably acts as a carrier for the amoebicidal drug, enabling its penetration into the normally drug-resistant cyst.

Initial treatment is intensive. A typical regimen includes propamidine and neomycin/polymyxin B/gramicidin solutions; each drop is given every hour or more frequently and then tapered over 1 month to four times a day. This maintenance therapy is continued for 1 year in an attempt to eradicate cysts that might persist in the cornea. Reactivations during maintenance therapy are treated as vigorously as initial infections. Because these drops are toxic, some patients develop medicamentosal conjunctivitis. This condition is reversible once the dose is reduced. Therefore, therapy with these drops should not be reduced because of toxicity.

The use of topical steroids[‡] is controversial. Cellular host defense mechanisms against amoebae consist of macrophages and neutrophils. Steroids inhibit that arm of defense and, as with fungal and mycobacterial infections for which drugs alone may be only partially effective, may potentiate or prolong the infection. Unfortunately, patients are usually started on steroids before the correct diagnosis is made, and they then become dependent on them for control of pain and inflammation. It is important to try to wean them off steroids as quickly as possible. A topical mydriatic-cycloplegic may be used to dilate the pupil and prevent ciliary spasm.

Surgical. The timing and role of penetrating keratoplasty are also controversial. Some clinicians advocate medical treatment for 1 year to eradicate the organism before surgery, thus avoiding grafting into an infected host bed. There are several reports of successful medical cures that resulted not only in saving the eye but also in preserving good vision. Others advocate early surgery to remove all organisms before they spread to the periphery. However, the extent of the infection is not always apparent on slit-lamp examination, and recurrences in the graft can lead to repeated graft failures, uncontrolled glaucoma, cataract, wound melt and dehiscence, and phthisis.

Other. One method used to prevent recurrences after penetrating keratoplasty is to freeze the recipient bed at the time of surgery. Cryotherapy may kill trophozoites, but it does not eradicate cysts, which survive freezing temperatures and can potentially excyst to reinfect the graft. Cryotherapy may also cause increased intraocular inflammation and retrocorneal fibrous membrane formation, resulting in graft failure. Conjunctival flaps were tried in the first reported cases. However, they failed because of progression of the infection under the flap, which resulted in necrosis and melting of the flap. For therapy of extreme ocular pain that is unresponsive to the treatment described earlier, an absolute alcohol, retrobulbar block (0.3 to 0.6 ml of absolute al-

cohol, or 1 to 2 ml of 50 per cent alcohol, mixed with 1 to 2 ml of .75 per cent marcaine) may be given. This block is painful; therefore, intravenous sedation before its administration is recommended.

Ocular or Periocular Manifestations

Anterior Chamber: Cells and flare; fibrin strands; hypopyon.

Conjunctiva: Chemosis; ciliary flush; hyperemia.

Cornea: Pseudodendrite; persistent or recurrent epithelial defects; subepithelial infiltrates; elevated corneal epithelial lines; punctate anterior stromal infiltrates; diffuse patchy anterior stromal infiltrates; full or partial anterior stromal ring infiltrate; disciform keratitis; radial neuritis; double-ring infiltrate; stromal cysts; stromal necrosis; descemetocele; perforation; graft rejection.

Eyelids: Reactive ptosis; hyperemia; edema.

Iris: Nongranulomatous anterior uveitis; posterior synechiae.

Sclera: Nodular scleritis; diffuse anterior and posterior scleritis.

Other: Decreased visual acuity; *severe* ocular pain (out of proportion to the clinical findings); photophobia; epiphora; secondary glaucoma; vitritis; retinal perivasculitis; papillitis; chorioretinitis.

PRECAUTIONS

Topical ophthalmic miconazole is acidic and poorly tolerated by patients. Clotrimazole is currently used for infections that do not respond to propamidine, dibromopropamidine, or neomycin/polymyxin B/gramicidin combination.

Liver functions must be monitored in patients administered ketoconazole or sulindac, and neither drug should be used in pregnant women or women of childbearing age.

COMMENTS

The diagnosis of infection by *Acanthamoebae* is difficult. It requires a high index of suspicion, persistence, and an experienced observer and laboratory personnel. In a patient wearing contact lenses, a painful keratitis and a culture that is negative and unresponsive to antibacterial and antiviral therapy should alert the practitioner to the possibility of an amoebic infection. Using calcofluor white and immunofluorescent antibody staining of corneal scrapings and tissue biopsy specimens, and cultures on nonnutrient agar plates precoated with *E. coli* can improve the chances of a positive diagnosis. Positive cultures of contact lenses, contact lens paraphernalia, and saline solutions may lend support for the diagnosis of amoebic keratitis when appropriate laboratory tests are repeatedly negative. Because this can be a devastating infection that is unresponsive to current medical and surgical therapy, prevention is extremely important. Practitioners who fit contact lenses must ensure that patients do not use nonsterile fluids to rinse, store, or disinfect their lenses.

References

Berget ST, Monodino BJ, Hoft RH, et al: Successful medical management of *Acanthamoeba* keratitis. Am J Ophthalmol *110*:395, 1990.
Driebe WT Jr, Stern GA, Epstein RJ, et al: *Acanthamoeba* keratitis: Potential role for topical clotrimazode in combination chemotherapy. Arch Ophthalmol *106*:1196, 1988.
Ishibashi Y, Matsumoto Y, Kabata T, et al: Oral braconazole and topical miconogole with debridement for *Acanthamoeba* keratitis. Am J Ophthalmol *109*:121, 1990.
Larkin DFP, Kilvington S, Dart JKG: Treatment of *Acanthamoeba* keratitis with polyhexamethylene biguanide. Ophthalmology *99*:185, 1992.
Moore MB, McCulley JP: *Acanthamoeba* keratitis associated with contact lenses: Six cases of successful medical treatment. Invest Ophthalmol Vis Sci *28*(Suppl):371, 1987.
Saunders PPR, Proctor EM, Rollings DF, et al: Enhanced killing of *Acanthamoeba* cysts in vitro using dimethylsulfoxide. Ophthalmology *99*:1197, 1992.
Wright P, Warhurst D, Jones BR: *Acanthamoeba* keratitis successfully treated medically. Br J Ophthalmol *69*:778, 1985.

AMERICAN MUCOCUTANEOUS LEISHMANIASIS 085.5

JAIME ROIZENBLATT, M.D.,
and LUIZ CARLOS CUCÉ, M.D.

São Paulo, Brazil

American mucocutaneous leishmaniasis is a zoonosis that occurs endemically in certain areas in Latin America; it is caused by the flagellate protozoa *Leishmania braziliensis braziliensis* and more rarely by *L. braziliensis panamensis*. The American form of leishmaniasis resembles the Oriental cutaneous type in that it is characterized by specific ulcerating granulomas of the skin; however, American leishmaniasis is distinguished from *L. tropica* by the frequent presence of mucocutaneous lesions. Like all types of leishmaniasis, American mucocutaneous leishmaniasis is transmitted to humans by the bite of the infected female *Phlebotomus* sandfly. The initial lesion normally occurs in exposed parts of the body, and those who work in forests are most frequently affected. Reservoirs other than humans include wild rodents, such as rats, mice,

agoutis, and pacas, that are common in the neotropics. The human being is only an accidental member in the biologic cycle of this zoonosis. The incubation period varies from 2 to 8 weeks, after which an erythematous papule develops at the site of inoculation and gradually increases in size by peripheral extension. The papule may vesiculate, ulcerate, or take a mulberry appearance. Regional adenopathy may be noted in the initial stages.

Generally, the lesions are secondarily infected. The disease may follow an apparently benign and self-limiting course; the ulcer usually heals within a year, leaving a typical scar at the site of the lesion. After 1 or 2 years, mucocutaneous lesions may develop in the nasal mucosa; the nasal cartilage usually is invaded and destroyed, resulting in a deformity known as "tapir's nose." The involvement of the nasal fossae, pharynx, soft palate, floor of the mouth, and tonsils, as well as the upper respiratory tract and larynx, may cause difficulty in breathing, feeding, and deglutition. In its preference for cartilages, the ear may also be invaded and destroyed. The mucocutaneous involvement occurs as a result of direct spread to the original lesion or hematogenous and even lymphatic dissemination. In addition to the previously discussed forms, a disseminated anergic form may occur in which there is widespread involvement of the skin by infiltrative lesions.

Ocular findings associated with American mucocutaneous leishmaniasis involve the eyelids and conjunctiva. Eyelid edema, scarring, or even destruction of the tarsus and nodular granulomas of the tarsal or bulbar conjunctiva may develop. Ulceration of the conjunctiva and cornea, and interstitial keratitis, have also been described. Rare cases of iridocyclitis have been reported, and in one instance *Leishmania sp.* was isolated from the aqueous humor. The eye may be involved by contiguous spread from the eyelid and conjunctiva, by hematogenous spread, or by inoculation of the conjunctiva by the patient's own fingers.

THERAPY

Systemic. Only sporadic forms of American mucocutaneous leishmaniasis are self-limiting. If the initial lesion is present or if there are already signs of systemic spread, particularly of mucocutaneous involvement, systemic treatment should be instituted immediately.

The drug of choice is antimony meglumine.[†] It is the most often used antimonate at present due to its low toxicity and good therapeutic results. The daily dose of antimony meglumine is 10 to 20 mg/kg for adults, with a maximum daily dosage of 850 mg and 4 to 6 mg/kg for children. The drug can be administered intramuscularly in children and intravenously in adults, by slow infusion, for

15 to 25 days. This course can be repeated two or more times after 15- to 20-day intervals.

Equally efficient is stibogluconate sodium, given intramuscularly or intravenously in daily doses of 10 to 20 mg/kg for 6 to 10 days. In the United States, antimony meglumine and stibogluconate sodium are available from the Centers for Disease Control in Atlanta.

In resistant cases and particularly when there is extensive mucocutaneous involvement, the drug of choice is amphotericin B. Slow infusion of 0.5 to 1.0 mg/kg diluted in 500 ml of a 5 per cent dextrose in water solution may be administered over a 6- to 8-hour period every 1 to 2 days. Fresh solutions should be prepared for each injection. The drug should be protected from light during administration. For cutaneous forms, a total dose of 1.5 to 2.0 gm is given; it may be increased up to 3 gm until the patient is clinically cured.

Cycloguanil pamoate[+] has not shown more significant results than the previously discussed drugs. Therefore, its use is not indicated.

Ocular. Topical ocular antibiotics are indicated to prevent secondary bacterial infection of conjunctival or corneal defects. Topical steroids and atropine alleviate iridocyclitis. Cool compresses may give symptomatic relief. Sunglasses will aid in photophobia.

Supportive. Secondary infection in mucocutaneous leishmaniasis should be controlled by use of appropriate antimicrobial drugs. Cauterization of the verrucose lesions and plastic surgery for facial disfigurement may sometimes be necessary. Surgery should only be considered after a long interval has passed after the patient is clinically cured; otherwise, it may have disastrous effects.

Ocular or Periocular Manifestations

Conjunctiva: Papulonecrotic and ulcerative lesions; phlyctenulas; symblepharon.

Cornea: Abscess; diffuse keratitis; granulomatous and ulcerative lesions; interstitial keratitis.

Eyelids: Cicatrization and destruction of the tarsus; "hard" edema; nodular or ulcerating granuloma.

Iris: Iritis, iridocyclitis.

PRECAUTIONS

American mucocutaneous leishmaniasis is a form of human leishmaniasis that is sometimes very resistant to therapy and has a high relapse rate. The duration of the disease and the patient's immune status are in part responsible for these different responses to medication. Treatment should be continued until an apparent cure is obtained, and the patient should be observed for an extended period. If the drug of choice seems to be ineffective, it is advisable to try a second course

of therapy with this same drug before using alternative drugs. Complement-fixing antibody should not be detectable 6 to 12 months after the apparent clinical cure. In chronic leishmaniasis, it is very uncommon to find the parasite. However, the diagnosis can be confirmed with the Montenegro skin test, which is positive in more than 90 per cent of patients with this disease. In recent cases, impression smears, aspirates, and punch biopsy specimens should be taken from the edge of suspicious skin lesions when possible. If a biopsy is not possible because of location, scrapings from a slit made in involved skin can be cultured or stained for organisms in fresh ulcers. The characteristic amastigotes appear and are more easily recognized in smears than in tissue sections. Recent techniques that may permit direct and rapid diagnosis in tissue samples are either blotting with radiolabeled DNA probes or the immunoperoxidase method using species-specific monoclonal antibodies.

Adverse effects with the use of antimony meglumine and stibogluconate sodium are not common. However, their toxicity and use should be monitored carefully. The most frequent adverse effects include chills, fever, coughing, vomiting, muscle and joint stiffness, arthralgia, bradycardia, and anaphylactoid reactions. The intravenous administration of amphotericin B usually produces chills, fever, vomiting, headache, and hypersensitivity reactions. Phlebitis is also often a problem with the intravenous administration of amphotericin B, and 100 to 150 mg of hydrocortisone may be added to the infusion to prevent this complication. Intravenous infusion by means of a pediatric scalp vein minimizes the risk of thrombophlebitis. Tolerance may be enhanced by temporarily lowering the dose or administering aspirin, diphenhydramine, or phenothiazines. Therapeutically active amounts of amphotericin B may impair kidney and liver function and produce anemia (impaired iron utilization by bone marrow). Electrolyte disturbances (hypokalemia, distal tubular acidosis), shock, and a variety of neurologic symptoms also may occur.

COMMENTS

American leishmaniasis occurs most frequently in rural areas among forest workers. The disease occurs more often in men than in women, probably because of the greater number of men in these occupations. Prophylactic measures include the use of repellents and nets and continuous surveillance in endemic areas. Eradication of the *Phlebotomus* with insecticides may have disastrous ecologic consequences and should be used only as a last resort or in endemic situations.

The patient may also be an incidental source of infection, and prompt treatment will render him or her noninfective to sandflies. A vaccine has been tested, but it offered only 50 per cent efficacy, and the immunity it provides is only transitory.

The prognosis in mucocutaneous leishmaniasis is much more serious than in cutaneous leishmaniasis because of the destructiveness of mucocutaneous lesions and the resistance sometimes found to therapy. The prognosis is good if treatment is begun early, preferably before mucocutaneous lesions develop.

References

Chu FC, Rodrigues MM, Cogan DG, Neva FA: Leishmaniasis affecting the eyelids. Arch Ophthal 101:84–91, 1983.

Duke-Elder S (ed): System of Ophthalmology. St. Louis, CV Mosby, 1976, Vol XV, pp 85–86.

Falqueto A, Sessa PA: Leishmaniose tegumentar americana. In Veronesi R (ed): Doenças Infecciosas e Parasitárias, 8th ed. Rio de Janeiro, Guanabara Koogan, 1991, pp 750–762.

Ferrari TCA, Guedes ACM, Oréfice F, Genaro O, Pinheiro SRA, Marra MA, Silveira ILN, Miranda MO: Isolation of Leishmania sp. from aqueous humor of a patient with cutaneous disseminated leishmaniasis and bilateral iridocyclitis (preliminary report). Rev Inst Med Trop São Paulo 34(4): 296–298, 1990.

Livni N, Abramovitz A, Londner M, Okon E, Morag A: Immunoperoxidase method of identification of Leishmania in routinely prepared histological sections. Virchows Arch (Pathol Anat) 401:147–51, 1983.

Mayrink W, Williamns P, Costa CA, Magalhães PA, Melo MN, Dias M, Lima AO, Michalick MSM, Carvalho EF, Barros GC, Sessa PA, Alencar JTA: An experimental vaccine against American dermal leishmaniasis: Experience in the State of Espírito Santo, Brazil. Ann Trop Med Parasitol 79(3):259–269, 1985.

Neva FA: Diagnosis and treatment of cutaneous leishmaniasis. In Remington JS, Swartz MN (eds): Current Clinical Topics in Infectious Diseases. New York, McGraw-Hill, 1982, Vol 3, p 364.

Pearson RD, Sousa AQ: Leishmania species: Visceral (kala-azar), cutaneous, and mucosal leishmaniasis. In Mandell GL, Douglas RG Jr, Bennett JE (eds): Principles and Practice of Infectious Diseases, 3th ed. New York, Churchill Livingstone, 1990, pp 2066–2077.

Roizenblatt J: Interstitial keratitis caused by American (mucocutaneous) leishmaniasis. Am J Ophthalmol 87:175–179, 1979.

Webster LT: Drugs used in the chemotherapy of protozoal infections. In Gilman AG, Goodman LS, Gilman A (eds): The Pharmacological Basis of Therapeutics, 8th ed. New York, Macmillan, 1990, pp 1008–1017.

Wirth DF, Rogers WO, Barker R Jr: Leishmaniasis and malaria: New tools for epidemiologic analysis. Science 234:975–979, 1986.

ASCARIASIS 127.0

THOMAS JOHN, M.D.,
JOHN J. DONNELLY, Ph.D.,
and JOHN H. ROCKEY, M.D., Ph.D.

Philadelphia, Pennsylvania

Ascariasis results from the ingestion of infective eggs of the roundworm, *Ascaris lumbricoides* (or rarely, *A. suum*). Larvae hatch from the ova in the small intestines, penetrate the intestinal wall, and are carried via the portal venous system and lymphatics through the liver to the lungs. There they penetrate into and migrate up the respiratory passages and are swallowed; the adult worms mature in the small intestines. In severe infections, larvae may pass through the lungs into the general circulation and may reach such structures as the eye and periocular tissues. Ascariasis may be asymptomatic, or pulmonary disease (Loeffler's eosinophilic pneumonitis, asthma), abdominal disease (small intestine, biliary duct or pancreatic duct obstruction, intussusception, volvulus, appendicitis, diverticulitis, perforation, hepatic abscess), or type I hypersensitivity reactions (urticaria, acute conjunctivitis, acute laryngeal obstruction, wheal-and-flare dermal reactions) to ascarid antigens mediated by high titer IgE antibody may develop. Intraocular or periocular (within nasolacrimal system) localization of an ascarid larva is rare, being an accident of aberrant larval migration.

THERAPY

Systemic. The drug of choice is mebendazole, which blocks glucose uptake by the parasite. It has a wide antiparasitic spectrum and gives a cure rate of 95 to 100 per cent for *Ascaris necator*, and *Enterobius*; hence, it is useful in mixed infections. Mebendazole is administered orally in a dosage of 100 mg twice daily for 3 consecutive days. Pyrantel is an alternative drug of choice for treating ascariasis. A single oral dose of 11 mg/kg (maximum 1 gm) is given for adults and children. Pyrantel paralyzes the worms, which then are expelled intact, and a laxative is usually not required. Piperazine is also very effective and less expensive but more toxic than the previous two agents. It blocks neuromuscular junctions and produces paralysis of the ascarid, leading to expulsion of the worm. For adults, a single daily oral dose of 3.5 gm given on 2 consecutive days is recommended; for children, 75 mg/kg (daily maximum, 3.5 gm) may be administered in the same fashion. Oral thiabendazole in a dose of 25 mg/kg (daily maximum, 3 gm) taken twice daily after meals is also effective in the treatment of ascariasis. Likewise, levamisole,[†] which seems to act by inhibiting succinate dehydrogenase in the muscles of the worm, results in paralysis and expulsion of the worm.

Ocular. Most of the ocular allergic manifestations of ascariasis may be resolved with systemic antiparasitic therapy. Anterior uveitis may be treated with topical corticosteroids and mydriatic/cycloplegics. Depending on the severity of the uveitis, the frequency of steroid drops may range from hourly application to once every other day. Subconjunctival injections* of corticosteroids may be used if necessary. The strongest and longest-acting cycloplegic is atropine. It may be used topically one to four times daily, depending on the degree of inflammation. For milder uveitis, 0.5 per cent scopolamine or 2 to 5 per cent homatropine may be used. Systemic corticosteroids are indicated when other forms of corticosteroids have failed or posterior inflammatory reaction of chorioretinitis is present. Photocoagulation has been used to kill intraocular parasites, but may cause an increased allergic reaction because of the release of parasite antigens.

Supportive. Hospitalization is usually limited to patients with severe infections and complications. Such patients may require correction of fluid and electrolytes, transfusions, and high caloric intake. Saline enemas may be useful to remove worms that may be present in the large bowel. Intestinal obstruction, if present, is initially treated conservatively with nasogastric suction and intravenous fluids. After vomiting is controlled, piperazine may be given through the nasogastric tube in a dosage of 65 mg/kg (maximum, 1.0 gm) every 12 to 24 hours for six doses. If there is no improvement, it may be possible to manipulate the bolus of worms into the large bowel during laparotomy. Only if this procedure is unsuccessful should enterotomy and removal of the worms be attempted.

Ocular or Periocular Manifestations

Conjunctiva: Conjunctivitis; subconjunctival parasite; xerosis.
Eyelids: Edema; urticaria.
Iris: Uveitis.
Lacrimal System: Egress of larva via lacrimal punctum.
Lens: Subluxation.
Optic Nerve: Papilledema.
Orbit: Pseudotumor.
Retina: Edema: hemorrhagic macular chorioretinitis, periphlebitis.
Vitreous: Recurrent hemorrhages.
Other: Scotoma; secondary glaucoma; visual loss.

PRECAUTIONS

In multiple intestinal helminthic infections, ascariasis should be treated first in order to prevent migration of ascarids. Before elective surgery, patients should be dewormed because worms can penetrate the intestinal wall, especially in the region of surgical anastomosis.

Pyrantel should be used with caution in patients with preexisting liver dysfunction. Its safe usage in pregnancy and in children under 2 years of age has not been established. Likewise, mebendazole is contraindicated during pregnancy and has not been investigated extensively in children below the age of 2. Piperazine is contraindicated in renal or hepatic insufficiency and in epileptic patients. Its accumulation in the presence of renal insufficiency may produce neurotoxic signs.

During examination of the feces, fertilized ova are easy to recognize, whereas unfertilized ova assume bizarre shapes and may be mistaken for debris. Rarely, infections may be due only to male worms.

COMMENTS

Ascariasis, a worldwide helminthic infection, is the most common helminthiasis that affects humans. One quarter of the world's population is infected with *A. lubricoides*. Although cosmopolitan, ascariasis is most common in the tropics where sanitation is poor and is endemic in the rural southwestern United States. Susceptibility to infection and serious complications are greatest in childhood. Ascariasis is usually accompanied by minor symptoms, although severe complications can develop. Elevated blood eosinophil levels usually are present only during the tissue migratory phase. Eggs appear in the feces 60 to 75 days after the ingestion of infective eggs. Examination of feces may help establish the diagnosis. Visceral larva migrans due to the related ascarid *Toxocara canis* may be differentiated by the ELISA (enzyme-linked immunosorbent assay) immunoassay. Other ascarids, such as *Baylisascaris procyonis*, also may cause ocular larva migrans. In the United States, the worm load is usually modest. Cure rate is high with adequate therapy. The case-fatality rate of intestinal obstruction in the United States is 3 per cent. Treatment of ascariasis may be nutritionally advantageous for children with heavy worm burdens and marginal protein availability.

References

Beck JW, Davies JE: Medical Parasitology, 3rd ed. St. Louis, CV Mosby, 1981, pp 136–140.
Blumenthal DS: Ascariasis. *In* Wyngaarden JB, Smith LH Jr (eds): Textbook of Medicine, 16th ed. Philadelphia, WB Saunders, 1982, pp 1768–1769.
Cook GC: The clinical significance of gastrointestinal helminths: A review. Trans Roy Soc Trop Med Hyg *80*:675–685, 1986.
Duke-Elder S (ed): System of Ophthalmology. St. Louis, CV Mosby, 1976, Vol XV, pp 15–16.
Gass JDM, Braunstein RA: Further observations concerning the diffuse unilateral subacute neuroretinitis syndrome. Arch Ophthalmol *101*:1689, 1983.
Glickman LT, Schantz PM: Epidemiology and pathogenesis of zoonotic toxocariasis. Epidemiol Rev *3*:230–250, 1981.

Most H: Treatment of common parasitic infections of man encountered in the United States. (First of two parts). N Engl J Med 287:495–498, 1972.

Schlaegel TF Jr, Knox DL: Uveitis and parasitoses. In Duane TD (ed): Clinical Ophthalmology. Hagerstown, MD, Harper & Row, 1982, Vol IV, pp 52:1–16.

Sharma S: Advances in the treatment and control of tissue-dwelling helminth parasites. Prog Drug Res 30:473–547, 1986.

Turner JA: Drug therapy of gastrointestinal parasitic infections. The ACG Committee of FDA-related matters. Am J Gastroenterol 81:1125–1137, 1986.

COENUROSIS 123.8

EDWARD EPSTEIN, M.B., Ch.B., D.O.M.S.

Johannesburg, South Africa

Coenurosis is an infestation in an intermediate host with the cystic larval stage of the dog tape worm. Previously classified as genus *Multiceps sp.*, modern taxonomy prefers genus *Taenia*—*T. multiceps*, *T. serialis*, and *T. glomeratus*. Unlike a cysticercus, the coenurus is a thin-walled cyst containing many scoleces, and it has no daughter cysts as do hyatids. The cysts can be up to 20 mm in diameter and may occur in grapelike clusters. Carnivores, dogs, foxes, and wolves harbor the adult worm, whereas the intermediate hosts are a variety of herbivorous or omnivorous domestic and wild animals, such as sheep, goats, cattle, deer, and cats; rarely humans serve as intermediate hosts.

In humans, the coenurus develops in muscles, subcutaneous tissue, nervous system, and the eye. The brain is often involved, and the clinical manifestations are those of a space-occupying lesion or lesions—headache, loss of weight, somnolence, ataxia, visual disturbance, and neck and shoulder stiffness. The coenurus may involve any part of the globe and its muscles, and subconjunctival infestation is found in young children, mainly toddlers. It is thought that this infestation might be due to direct contamination of the conjunctival sac with the voided ova—oncospheres—from the ground, vegetation, or the fur of dogs. In adults, the spread is via the blood after ingestion.

Diagnosis is easy when the cyst is subconjunctival, in the anterior chamber or the vitreous. Other sites present difficulty, and ultrasound, computed tomography, and magnetic resonance imaging scans are useful. A false-positive Casoni's and hydatid complement-fixation test may occur. The eosinophil count may be only 3 per cent. Price et al. (1989) have reported data that point to a possible serodiagnostic test.

THERAPY

Ocular. Uveitis in these cases is treated just as are other uveitis conditions, depending on the severity. Topical cycloplegics and steroids and, in certain instances when the disease is quite severe, subtenon and systemic steroids are of value.

Specific drug therapy for the coenurus has not as yet been established. Price et al. (1989) have reported a seemingly successful use of praziquantel in posterior abdominal wall cysts in a primate, the spectacled langur. The diagnosis was established in an excised subcutaneous cyst. Dosage was 50 mg/kg/day for 14 days as used in human cysticercosis. Repeat CT scans showed a reduction in the size and calcification of previously active cysts. However, a pretreatment scan also showed calcified cysts, which indicates a natural defense process.

Ibechukwa and Onwukene (1991) gave praziquantel 25 mg/kg/daily for 3 days to a patient with the coenurus in the vitreous, whom they had watched for 3 months. Ten days later the cyst burst with severe inflammatory sequelae. A repeat course (not detailed) was given, and eventually the eye settled and cleared showing a total retinal detachment with pre- and subretinal scarring. It might thus be worthwhile trying a 2-week course of praziquantel, 50 mgm/kg/day, and observing the case for a further week. If no obvious improvement follows, one should then proceed surgically.

Surgical. Surgery is the treatment of choice at present. Its success depends upon the accessibility of the cyst. However, as the outcome if the cyst is left is devastating, even leading to enucleation, an attempt at removal should always be made.

First, measures to soften the eye as much as possible are used. For subretinal or intrachoroidal cysts, a suitably sized and located scleral "trapdoor" flap is raised. The rectus muscle involved need not be detached. The position of the anterior and posterior ciliary arteries and the vena vorticosa must be kept in mind and treated if necessary to avoid hemorrhage. A longitudinal line of light diathermy is applied along the proposed line of incision in the meridian of the greatest bulge and repeated as the incision is deepened. The longitudinal direction permits extension posteriorly should the cyst prove too large to be eased through the initial incision, although a fairly large cyst can mold and be expressed through a 3 to 5 mm opening.

Cysticerci in the vitreous have been successfully removed by pars plana vitrectomy. Probably a coenurus can be dealt with in the same way. There have not been any recorded cases of that procedure, however. Vitrectomy apparatus, if not available, is not absolutely necessary as cysticerci have been removed successfully by other surgical methods from the vitreous. A Flieringa ring is placed near the equator. An intravitreous drip is fitted as for vitrectomy for use if required. A suitably sized and located scleral flap is raised over the pars plana. A latitudinal 4 to 5 mm incision is made through the pars plana using the diathermy knife technique described above. A 3-mm diameter canula connected by suitable silicone tubing to a 5-ml syringe is used to suck the cyst from the eye. The procedures can be done under direct vision with a monocular or binocular headband ophthalmoscope. Should the cyst break, the intravitreous drip is started and the cyst removed piecemeal. A vitreous cryoprobe or a pair of nontoothed long-shanked fine forceps can also be used to grip the cyst.

The intact cyst is easily seen by direct vision through the pupil, but if it ruptures a highminus contact lens might be required to remove the fragments of the cyst.

Equipment must be on hand to treat and plomb retinal breaks should they occur.

Ocular or Periocular Manifestations

Anterior Chamber: Cells; flare; hypopyon.
Choroid and Retina: Detachment; edema; granuloma.
Conjunctiva: Coenurus cysts; conjunctivitis.
Cornea: Infiltration; keratic precipitates.
Globe: Pain; proptosis; scleritis.
Iris: Anterior uveitis; posterior synechiae; coenurus.
Other: Increased intraocular pressure; miosis; visual loss; vitreal haze.

COMMENTS

Intraocular helminthic infestations occur rarely. When the parasite has invaded the vitreous or anterior chamber, the diagnosis is simple. However, when the cyst is subretinal and especially within the uvea, diagnosis becomes more difficult. Parasitic cysts usually produce signs of iritis, inflammation, and localized swelling and have been misdiagnosed as scleritis. A careful peripheral fundoscopy should always be done.

References

Boase AJ: Coenurus cyst in eye. Br J Ophthalmol 40:183–185, 1956.
Epstein E: Intraocular cysticercus. Case report, surgical removal. S Afr Med J 22:625, 1948.
Epstein E, Proctor NSF, Heinz J: Intraocular coenurosis infestation. S Afr Med J 33:602–604, 1959.
Ibechukwu BI, Onwukene KE: Intraocular coenurus. Br J Ophthalmol 75:430–431, 1991.
Johnstone HG, Jones OW Jr: Cerebral coenurosis in an infant. Am J Trop Med 30:431–441, 1950.
Price C, et al: Coenuriasis in a spectacled langur. Am J Trop Med Hyg 34:27–30, 1989.
Wainright J: Coenurosis. J Pathol Bacteriol 73:347–354, 1957.
Williams PH, Templeton AC: Infection of the eye by tapeworm Coenurus. Br J Ophthalmol 55:766–769, 1971.

CUTANEOUS LEISHMANIASIS 085.4
(Old World Leishmaniasis, Oriental Sore, Tropical Sore)

FUÁD S. FARAH, M.D.

Syracuse, New York

The leishmaniases represent a group of clinical diseases caused by various species of *Leishmania*. The systemic form of the disease (visceral leishmaniasis, kala azar), is common in the Mediterranean basin, India, Sudan, and Kenya. It is caused by *L. donovani* and *L. infantum*. The cutaneous form of the disease (CL) seen in the Near East, Mediterranean basin, Ethiopia, and Kenya and some parts of the former Soviet Union (Old World leishmaniasis) is caused by *L. tropica* (major and minor), *L. ethiopica*, and *L. infantum*. Mucucutaneous leishmaniasis (MCL) that occurs in Central America, Mexico, and Brazil (New World leishmaniasis) is caused by *L. mexicana, L. braziliensis,* and *L. amazonensis.* Thus, the skin is involved in both Old World and New World leishmaniases.

The clinical manifestations of CL can generally be divided into localized and disseminated involvement. Acute CL appears on an exposed area accessible to sandfly bites (the responsible vector). The initial lesion is a small papule resembling an insect bite that persists, enlarges, and becomes firm and adherent. It is asymptomatic except for mild pruritus. With time, central ulceration develops and is followed by healing, with a characteristic scar within a year of onset. Although numerous cutaneous lesions resulting from multiple sandfly inoculations may be seen, CL is usually localized to a single lesion. Chronic CL is rare and is usually seen in elderly patients. It is expected that those with immune deficiency may develop chronic disease. The face is most commonly affected. Ulceration does not occur, and the lesions are persistent and do not heal. *Leishmania* recidiva follows the same course as acute CL in the early stages and is indistinguishable from it. However, after the lesions have healed, usually within 1 year, there is reactivation of the parasite, and new lesions appear months or years later at the original scar. Disseminated cutaneous leishmaniasis is characterized by multiple lesions rich in parasites and is associated with a specific cell-mediated immune response defect against the *Leishmania*.

The mucocutaneous (MCL) form of the disease is more serious and may be life threatening. Both the skin and the upper respiratory passages are involved. It begins as a small papule similar to CL, but in contrast to CL the initial lesion does not heal but rather extends to involve the mucosa and cartilage of the nose and the pharynx. The larynx is rarely involved. There is marked disfigurement, malnutrition, infection, and respiratory failure.

Ocular manifestations are limited to the eyelids and occur in 2 to 5 per cent of patients.

THERAPY

CL is self-limited, and the treatment depends on the extent of the disease and the expected deformity if untreated. Cryotherapy with liquid nitrogen or carbon dioxide is very effective in treating localized lesions and results in cosmetically acceptable scars. Surgical excision is not recommended for routine use, but may be effective for the small early single lesion.

Systemic. CL lesions respond to pentavalent antimonials and antimalarials. Stibogluconate sodium and antimony meglumine are effective in patients with multiple lesions. Antimony meglumine[†] is administered intramuscularly in daily doses of 60 to 100 mg/kg for 10 to 12 days. The course may be repeated after 1 to 2 weeks until the lesions are cured, usually in about 30 to 40 days. For acute leishmaniasis, cycloguanil pamoate administered as an intramuscular injection of 5 to 6 mg/kg is preferred. Intralesional injections of chloroquine* and pentamidine* isethionate may benefit some patients. Amphotericin B is of limited use in CL, but is more appropriate in MCL. Ketoconazole[‡] has been tried in CL and MCL. Experimentally, it eliminates 80 to 95 per cent of the parasites in *L. tropica*-infected macrophages. Pyrazolopyridines (alluputinol and allopurinol ribonucleosides) also show promise.

COMMENTS

Although there is greater understanding of the pathophysiology and immunology of leishmanial infections, more investigation is still needed for treatment to achieve a high degree of success. Uncomplicated acute CL should be managed by using the treatments with the least side effects. Aggressive therapy may be required in refractory cases and where cosmetic considerations are of particular importance. Secondary bacterial infection should be treated if present.

References

Berman JD: Activity of imidazole against *Leishmania tropica* in human macrophages cultures. Am J Trop Med Hyg 30:566–569, 1981.

Chu FC, Rodrigues MM, Cogan DG, Neva FA: Leishmaniasis affecting the eyelids. Arch Ophthalmol 101:84–91, 1983.

Duke-Elder S (ed): System of Ophthalmology. St. Louis, CV Mosby, Vol. XV, 1976, pp 85–86.

Farah FS: Protozoan and helminth infections. *In* Fitzpatrick TB, et al (eds): Dermatology in General Medicine. Textbook and Atlas, 3rd ed. New York, McGraw-Hill, 1987, pp 2477–2495.

Farah FS: Leishmaniasis. *In* Demis, et al (eds): Clinical Dermatology. Hagerstown, MD, Harper & Row, 1988, pp 1–21.

Francois J, et al: Ocular manifestations of Leishmaniasis. Ann Oculist 206:295–305, 1973.

Guerra R, Tosi P, Molinelli G: Leishmaniasis of the lid in Tuscany. Ophthalmologica 168:193–196, 1974.

Neal RA, Croft SL, Nelson DJ: Antileishmanial effect of allopurinol ribonucleoside and related compounds allopurinol, thiopurinol, thiopurinol ribonucleoside and of formycin B sinefungin and lipidine WR 6026. Trans Roy Soc Trop Med Hyg 19:122–128, 1985.

Weinrauch L, Livshin R, El-On J: Cutaneous leishmaniasis treated with ketoconazole. Curtis 32: 288–289, 1983.

CYSTICERCOSIS 123.1

HARVEY W. TOPILOW, M.D.

New York, New York

Humans may serve as either the definitive host of the adult pork tapeworm (Cestoda), *Taenia solium*, or the intermediate host, harboring the larval form, *Cysticercus cellulosae*. T. is endemic in India, South America, Africa, and Asia.

Gravid proglottid segments of the adult worm release eggs in the stool, which are then ingested by the usual intermediate host, the hog. In the hog's intestine, the cestode embryo is released from the egg, penetrates into vascular channels, and is carried to all parts of the body, predominantly to striated muscle. Once the embryo lodges in a small vessel, it transforms into the encysted cysticercus or larval stage. Humans become infected by eating undercooked pork containing viable cysticerci, which mature in the human intestine to the adult worm.

Humans may also ingest the ova either via reverse peristalsis if the adult worm inhabits the intestine or, more commonly, by eating food or water contaminated with cestode ova, thus becoming an intermediate host. Just as in the hog model, the embryo released from the ingested ova penetrates the bowel wall vasculature to embolize throughout the human host, encyst, and develop as cysticerci or "bladder worms." This systemic infestation with the larval organism constitutes cysticercosis.

Cysticerci are commonly found in the brain, muscle, skin, and the eye. They may cause muscular pain and fever and may mimic meningoencephalitis or brain tumor.

Ocular involvement occurs in half of affected patients. Bilateral ocular involvement and multifocal uniocular involvement are extremely rare. The most common intraocular locations for cysticerci are the subretinal space or the vitreous. There are numerous reports of cysticerci invading the anterior chamber, subconjunctival space, orbit, and the eyelids.

Optic atrophy due to prolonged papilledema from central nervous system cysticercosis has also been reported.

The embryo reaches the choroid via the posterior ciliary arteries, alterating the overlying pigment epithelium as the cyst develops. Formation of a large cyst in the subretinal space often produces an exudative retinal detachment. Perforation of the retina by the cysticercus results in a free-floating intravitreous cyst. If the inflammatory response in the retinal pigment epithelium is adequate, the small retinal tear created by the entrance of the cyst into the vitreous is sealed, and an atrophic chorioretinal scar results. If the retinal break is larger and remains open, a rhegmatogenous retinal detachment can then occur.

THERAPY

Surgical. The most effective recognized means for preserving function in an eye with subretinal or intravitreous cysticerci is surgical removal of the larva. Severe inflammation caused by toxic products from the dead larva destroys the eye in 80 per cent of cases in which the cyst is not removed. Therefore, every attempt should be made to remove a subretinal or intravitreous cysticercus.

Intravitreous cysticercosis is best treated by removing the parasite using a vitrectomy instrument via the pars plana. This technique provides excellent visualization of the larva by using a precorneal contact lens, operating microscope, and endoillumination. It makes lens extraction, which is required in open-sky vitrectomy, unnecessary. The cyst is soft and pliable and is readily sucked into the cutting port. The specific instrumentation used is not critical as any of the currently available vitrectomy units are adequate. In some designs the suction-cutter and endoillumination and irrigation capabilities are on the same probe, thereby requiring only a single sclerotomy. Others require three separate sclerotomies to accommodate separate probes for suction-cutting, endoillumination, and an infusion cannula. The only advantage of the latter design relates to the fact that the cysticercus is often "photophobic," scurrying away from such sources of bright light as the endoillumination probe. If the endoilluminator and suction-cutter are contained on the same probe, it is often necessary to chase the parasite through the vitreous as it flees from the endoilluminator light. If the light and suction-cutter are separate, it may be easier to guide the parasite toward the suction-cutter for removal.

A subtotal vitrectomy is performed to remove any toxic products released from the cyst, and a periocular corticosteroid injection is given at the conclusion of surgery. Postoperatively, the mild vitreous inflammation often seen is usually well controlled by topical corticosteroids and mydriatics.

Subretinal cysticercosis is best managed by first carefully localizing the parasite with indirect ophthalmoscopy and scleral depression. A transilluminating diathermy probe is useful in localization. The exact position of the parasite is outlined on the sclera with a marking pen. A lamellar scleral dissection is performed over the cyst, and the scleral bed is treated with diathermy to produce a firm retinal-retinal pigment epithelial adhesion once the retinal is reattached. A radial sclerotomy is performed over the center of the cyst. The exposed choroid is treated with diathermy using confluent applications of low intensity and long duration to coagulate small blood vessels and minimize bleeding.

Transillumination of the sclerotomy site is used to identify patent choroidal vessels that require additional diathermy. It is also used to verify that the cysticercus has not moved. The knuckle of exposed choroid is incised, and the cyst is extruded from the eye by maintaining gentle pressure on the globe. A solid silicone implant is placed within the scleral bed beneath scleral flaps with an encircling band to create a permanent buckling effect and to close any retinal breaks created by the parasite or surgical manipulation.

In certain cases, a posteriorly located subretinal cyst containing a dead parasite may be collapsed and fibrosed to such a degree that it cannot be removed. In such cases, vitreous traction on the retina overlying the cyst can be successfully relieved by a localized buckling procedure. Systemic, periocular*, and topical corticosteroids may be required to control the intraocular inflammation resulting from the dead retained parasite.

Ocular or Periocular Manifestations

Optic Nerve: Atrophy; papilledema.
Retina: Break; chorioretinal scar; exudative or rhegmatogenous retinal detachment.
Other: Cysticerci present almost anywhere in or around the eye; ocular pain; uveitis.

PRECAUTIONS

The gravity of cysticercosis is reflected by the 40 per cent mortality of patients with central nervous system involvement and the fact that in certain underdeveloped nations 2 to 4 per cent of all autopsies reveal cysticercosis as the cause of death. Therefore, once the infection is diagnosed, it is of utmost importance to begin an exhaustive search for the organisms in the central nervous system. In addition, careful fecal examination of the patient and the family members should be undertaken to determine whether the patient harbors the adult cestode or has been infected by a family member.

COMMENTS

Intraocular cysticercosis usually results in blindness unless the parasite is surgically removed from the eye. While the cysticercus is alive, it induces a mild-to-moderate inflammatory response. A violent inflammatory reaction ensues when the parasites dies, often resulting in destruction of the globe.

References

Bartholomew RS: Subretinal cysticercosis. Am J Ophthalmol 79:670–673, 1975.

Hutton WL, Vaiser A, Snyder WB: Pars plana vitrectomy for removal of intravitreous cysticercus. Am J Ophthalmol 81:571–573, 1976.

Kapoor S, Kapoor MS: Ocular cysticercosis. J Pediatr Ophthalmol Strabismus 15:170–172, 1978.

Messner KH, Kammerer WS: Intraocular cysticercosis. Arch Ophthalmol 97:1103–1105, 1979.

Perry HD, Font RL: Cysticercosis of the eyelid. Arch Ophthalmol 96:1255–1257, 1978.

Santos R, et al: Management of subretinal and vitreous cysticercosis: Role of photocoagulation and surgery. Ophthalmology 86:1501–1504, 1979.

Shea M, et al: Intraocular *Taenia crassiceps* (Cestoda). Trans Am Acad Ophthalmol Otolaryngol 77:778–783, 1973.

Topilow HW, et al: Bilateral multifocal intraocular cysticercosis. Ophthalmology 88:1166–1172, 1981.

Wood TR, Binder PS: Intravitreal and intracameral cysticercosis. Ann Ophthalmol 11:1033–1036, 1979.

Zinn KM, Guillory SL, Friedman AH: Removal of intravitreous cysticerci from the surface of the optic nervehead. A pars plana approach. Arch Ophthalmol 98:714–716, 1980.

DEMODICOSIS 133.8

FRANK P. ENGLISH, F.R.A.C.O., F.R.C.S

Brisbane, Australia

Demodectic infestation of humans is characterized by the presence of two congeric species on the same host: *Demodex folliculorum*, which is found in the hair and eyelash follicles, and *Demodex brevis*, which infests the meibomian and sebaceous glands and the gland component of the pilosebaceous unit. These metazoans are virtually ubiquitous in the adult population and are predominantly located in the facial area involving the eyelids, eyebrows, forehead, and nasal region. They are also found in the oral, mammary, axillary, and pubic regions. All phases of their development can be seen, including the immature and mature stages.

D. folliculorum lies in the hair follicle with its head downward and feet facing the epithelial surface. Its sharp chelicerae puncture epithelial cells, allowing evacuation of cytoplasm by the parasite. Later, its trifid claws shred these damaged cells as they move upward, which contributes to the bulk of diagnostic cuffing seen in infestation.

D. brevis consumes glandular cells in its particular locus. In heavy infestation, it may affect the lipid layer of the tear film coacervate.

Patients complain of itching and burning of the eyelids, with crusting and loss of lashes. The pruritis is episodic and may parallel oviposition activity. Normally, the parasite's existence is torpid; however, in egg laying there is a bout of frenetic activity lasting several hours. This mite causes granulomata of the skin characterized by pain and swelling of tissue. Histopathologic studies of a chalazion have revealed giant and chronic inflammatory cellular reaction around the site of the acarid.

Many crumpled dead parasites are observed often unwittingly by the ophthalmologist in the daily office routine for they are located in debris on the lid margin and sometimes straddle the cilia. The observer is actually scanning a graveyard of mites. The parasites are seen when the lid is scrubbed with a moist cotton-wool applicator that is placed in a droplet of saline on a slide and examined with light microscopy.

Demodectic mites undergo two molting periods in development, and the cast exoskeletons of immature specimens are also seen with high magnification. The observer is rewarded with an exquisite view of the exoskeleton of the acarid and is able to identify with clarity the body contours and even ruptures in the integument at the time of ecdysis.

THERAPY

Ocular. Assessment of the degree of infestation is mandatory. With high magnification on the slit lamp, experienced observers can often identify mites lying in the mouths of follicles. They are only seen in profile with the patient gazing downward. Where there is cellular detritus build-up on the margin, their presence can be camouflaged, and they are only highlighted by carefully removing this material with jeweler's forceps. Generally, however, diagnosis is established by examination of epilated lashes with light microscopy.

In heavy infestation, mite nests occur. These conglomerates resemble cuffing, but contain many eggs and parasites in all stages of development. It is important to recognize and remove these colonies that act as a reservoir of infestation.

Although it has been traditional practice to treat the eyelid margin with an ether scrub, doing so only results in partial evacuation from the follicles, and the application needs to be repeated. Ether cleanses the eyelid, but has little effect on this acarid. A suitable substitute for ether is saline. After a drop of anesthetic has been applied to the eye, a saturated cotton-wool applicator is used to cleanse the eyelashes and dislodge nests. This maneuver is less dangerous than ether therapy. After this procedure, a course of sulfa-cetamide or neomycin/polymyxin B/bacitracin ophthalmic ointment is applied at nighttime for a few weeks. This treatment reduces concomitant bacterial infection and slows down the migration of parasites. The life cycle is believed to be longer than previously estimated, and it may be necessary to prolong therapy in recalcitrant cases.

Patients are prone to recurrence as it is impossible to eradicate the mite completely. Cryotherapy on isolated mites offers promise, but the real answer will be found in the development of an effective acaricide. An effective agent against the house dust mite has been developed in Australia by Allersearch. The formula contains an alcohol-based benzyltannate complex that apparently has a neurotoxic effect. I have found that this substance also destroys demodectic mites resulting in vacuole formation within the acarid, and clinical trial studies are warranted. Tarsal massage is valuable in reducing the population of *D. brevis*, especially when there has been a history of recurrent meibomianitis.

Ocular or Periocular Manifestations

Conjunctiva: Erythema.
Eyebrows or Eyelids: Blepharitis; cuffing; follicular distension and hyperplasia; hyperemia; hyperkeratinization; madarosis; meibomian gland destruction; mite colonies; granuloma; exoskeleton of dead parasites; acarid exuviae; eyelid tumor; rarely active movement of mite; deposition of broken mite egg shells on the lid margin.
Other: Pruritis.

PRECAUTIONS

Extreme care is necessary in ether application to the lid margin to avoid spillage onto the cornea. The amount of ether necessary to kill an isolated mite is staggering, and realistically, there cannot be a clinical parallel.

In the general management of demodicosis, it is important not to induce the state of symbiophobia. This condition is causing increasing concern among dermatologists.

COMMENTS

Demodecosis is associated with specific pathology of the eyelids. There is also a potential bacterial vector role allowing passage of bacteria from the depths of the follicle to the integumentary surface. *D. brevis* has the ability to penetrate the dermis with resultant inflammation, producing a granuloma.

A study of the feeding habits of these mites raises the suspicion of a viral vector role. This role could be particularly significant, especially for the smaller acarid.

Scanning electron microscopy of human eyelid specimens obtained by surgery reveals the tails of parasites protruding alongside eyelashes and cilia of the eyelid and more recently occurring freely on the skin surface.

Fissures occur in the extruded tip, which eventually breaks off causing spillage of its contents onto the eyelid. Demodectic mites have been noted to carry *Mycobacterium leprae* bacilli and fungi, and this feature causes concern.

Electron microscopy also has revealed the presence of discarded cracked mite eggshells on the intermarginal strip. Few people have observed the emergence of the larva from the egg, but the late Dr. Tullos Coston viewed this process and photographically recorded the eggshell breaking apart. Like the discarded opisthosoma, they are chitinous in nature and would account for those hard gritty objects felt on rubbing the eyelids, which have the vernacular title of "sleep" in the English language and the more colorful annotation "eye faeces" in Mandarin. It is not known whether these chitinous objects are those highly reflectile particles that are sometimes observed in the precorneal tear film and if so in time could lodge in the nasolacrimal passages in increasing numbers to interfere with their patency. I have noted however that in an idle moment on the slit lamp one can dislodge a mite from a lash and cause it to be swilled around in the lacrimal lake to lodge easily in the orifice of the inferior lacrimal punctum.

The discovery of free-living parasites on the skin surface raises the question of what happens in the microgravity milieu experienced by astronauts. If free floating and inhaled, they may pose a pulmonary hazard, as some years ago the eminent North American parasitologist, Dr. Harold Brown, noted that demodectic mites can produce pneumonitis.

References

Ayres S Jr, Ayres S III: Demodectic eruptions (demodicidosis) in the human. Arch Dermatol 83: 816–827, 1961.

Borrel A: Lepre et Demodex. Acarienes et Lepre. Ann Inst Pasteur, Paris. 23:125–128, 1909.

Coston TO: *Demodex folliculorum* blepharitis. Trans Am Ophthalmol Soc 65:361–392, 1967.

Duke-Elder S (ed): System of Ophthalmology. St. Louis, CV Mosby, 1974, Vol XIII, p 228.

English FP, Cohn D: Demodex infestation of the sebaceous gland. Am J Ophthalmol 95:843–844, 1983.

English FP, Iwamoto T, Darrell RW, DeVoe AG: The vector potential of *Demodex folliculorum*. Arch Ophthalmol 84:83–85, 1970.

English FP, Nutting WB: Demodicosis of ophthalmic concern. Am J Ophthalmol 91:362–372, 1981.

English FP, Nutting WB: Feeding characteristics in demodectic mites of the eyelid. Aust J Ophthalmol 9:311–313, 1981.

English FP, Nutting WB: Eyelid mite nests. Aust J Ophthalmol 10:187–189, 1982.

English FP, Nutting WB, Cohn D: Demodectic infestation of the meibomian glands. Am J Ophthalmol 95:261–262, 1983.

English FP, Nutting WB, Cohn D: Demodectic oviposition in the eyelid. Aust NZ J Ophthamol *13*: 71–73, 1985.

English FP, Cohn D, Groeneveld ER: Demodectic mites and chalazion. Am J Ophthalmol *100*:482–483, 1985.

English FP, Zhang GW, McManus DP, Campbell P: Electron microscopic evidence of acarine infestation of the eyelid margin. Am J Ophthalmol *109*:239–240, 1990.

English FP, Zhang GW, McNanus DP, Horne FA: The presence of the parasite *Demodex folliculorum* on the skin surface of the eyelid. Aust NZ J Ophthalmol *19*:229–234, 1991.

Norn MS: *Demodex folliculorum*. Incidence, regional distribution, pathogenicity. Dan Med Bull *18*:14–17, 1971.

Wolf R, Ophir J, Avigad J, Lengy J, Krakowski A: The hair follicle mites (*Demodex sp.*). Acta Dermatol Venereol (Stockholm) *68*:535–536, 1988.

DIROFILARIASIS 027.8

LAWRENCE A. RAYMOND, M.D.

Cincinnati, Ohio

Dirofilariasis is a zoonotic infection caused by several species of *Dirofilaria*, nematodes that naturally parasitize animals. Their life cycles are complicated. The adults produce microfilariae that circulate in blood. The microfilariae are ingested by mosquitoes wherein they progress to an infective stage. Infective larvae gain access to the new host through the skin, and development starts. There are at least three *Dirofilaria* species known to occur in the human eye or periocular tissues, but many other filaroids of humans and animals can be found in these locations. Most *Dirofilaria* infections are in the subcutaneous tissues, usually presenting as painless nodules. When the parasite dies, there is an inflammatory reaction with marked polymorphonuclear cell infiltrate, mostly eosinophils. At this stage, the nodule becomes painful, and the patient may consult the physician.

The incidence of *Dirofilaria* infections in humans is low; a disproportionate number of cases affecting the eye or periorbital tissues are reported, but the location in the eye or near the eye may cause patients to consult a physician more often. When the parasite is in the conjunctiva or anterior chamber, the patient may see it and seek consultation. If it is in the vitreous or retina, the patient may note a moving shadow. In either case, *Dirofilaria* and other filarial parasites should be considered in the differential diagnosis. When the parasite is in a nodule, the diagnosis is made by the pathologist examining the specimen removed from the patient.

Species of *Dirofilaria* found in ocular and periocular tissues are *D. repens*, *D. tenuis*, and *D. immitis*. *D. repens*, occurring naturally in

the subcutaneous tissues of dogs, foxes, and cats in Europe, Africa, the former Soviet Union, and Asia, has been referred to as *D. conjunctivae* when present in humans. *D. tenuis*, a parasite of the subcutaneous tissues of the raccoon in the southeastern United States, also was referred to as *D. conjunctivae* until 1965 when its true nature was demonstrated. Both *D. repens* and *D. tenuis* are responsible for infections in the conjunctiva, the eyelid, and rarely the lacrimal canal. These parasitic infections usually present as a nodule, or rarely, the nematode is detected before it encapsulates. *D. immitis*, a cosmopolitan parasite of the right ventricle and pulmonary arteries of dogs, has an early developmental phase in the subcutaneous tissues. Most infections with *D. immitis* in humans occur in the lungs where they produce small infarct-like lesions, but the parasite has been recovered from the anterior chamber of the eye on at least two occasions in Australia and from the posterior chamber once in Malaysia. In the United States, a parasite that was morphologically indistinguishable from *D. immitis* and *D. lutrae* has been recovered from the orbit at least twice.

In endemic areas of human filarial infections other than from *Dirofilaria*, such as *Brugia malayi* and *Wuchereria bancrofti*, the parasites have been found often in the eye. In the United States, a *Dipetalonema arbuta*-like worm in pleural and peritoneal cavities of the porcupine has been removed from the anterior chamber of a human eye.

THERAPY

Surgical. If the nematode is migrating in the retina area outside of the macular area, photocoagulation may be used. The purposes of photocoagulation are to prevent damage of the retinal pigment epithelium by *Dirofilaria* and to avoid migration of the parasite into the optic nerve, macula, or vitreous with resultant uveitis.

Surgical excision of the inflammatory nodule containing the parasite in the eyelid, periorbital region, or subconjunctival area is the treatment of choice. Surgical removal of the living intraocular *Dirofilaria* from the anterior chamber or vitreous preserves eyesight and decreases the associated uveitis.

Ocular or Periocular Manifestations

Anterior Chamber: Cells and flare; free nematode present.

Conjunctiva: Chemosis; hyperemia; nodules; nonencapsulated parasite beneath bulbar conjunctiva.

Extraocular Muscles: Tenonitis.

Eyelids or Eyebrows: Nodules.

Orbit: Inflammatory pseudotumor; pain; proptosis.

Retina: Macular degeneration; migrating nematode; unilateral pseudoretinitis pigmentosa.

Sclera: Nodules.

Vitreous: Free nematode present.

Other: Diplopia; irritation; itching; lacrimation; lowered amplitudes on electroretinogram; uveitis; visual loss.

PRECAUTIONS

Because the patient is infected with only a single nematode, systemic treatment with diethylcarbamazine is usually not indicated. If diethylcarbamazine is administered to these patients with intraocular location of a living parasite, allergic responses may occur after the death of the nematode. These reactions may include urticaria, fever, gastrointestinal disturbance, and lymphadenitis. Corticosteroids need to be given with caution in patients with secondary bacterial infection.

COMMENTS

Dirofilaria can incite inflammatory reactions in ocular tissues. When the parasite is located within the conjunctiva, eyelid, anterior chamber, or vitreous and can be removed, symptomatic inflammation is relieved. Also, retrieval of the parasite allows for identification of the species. When a filarial worm is migrating in the retina away from the macula, photocoagulation is the treatment of choice.

References

Beaver PC: Intraocular filariasis: A brief review. Am J Trop Med Hyg 40:40–45, 1989.

Font RL, Neafie RC, Perry HD: Subcutaneous dirofilariasis of the eyelid and ocular adnexa. Report of six cases. Arch Ophthalmol 98:1079–1082, 1980.

Guterbock WM, Vestre WA, Tood KS Jr: Ocular dirofilariasis in the dog. Mod Vet Pract 62:45–47, 1981.

Moorhouse DE: *Dirofilaria immitis*: A cause of human intra-ocular infection. Infection 6:192–193, 1978.

Orsoni JG, Coggiola G, Minazzi P: Filaria conjunctivae. Ophthalmologica 190:243–246, 1985.

Raymond LA, et al: Living retinal nematode (filarial-like) destroyed with photocoagulation. Ophthalmology 85:944–949, 1978.

Skrjabin KL: Invasions a filariides chez l'homme en l'URSS. Med Parasitol Parasite Dis 9:119–127, 1940.

Thomas D, et al: The *Dirofilaria* parasite in the orbit. Am J Ophthalmol 82:931–933, 1976.

Vodovozov AM, Jarulin GR, Djakonowa SW: *Dirofilaria* im Glaskörper des Menschen. Ophthalmologica 166:88–93, 1973.

DRACUNCULIASIS 125.7
(Dracontiasis, Dracunculosis, Guinea Worm Infection)

RALPH MULLER, Ph.D., D.Sc.

St. Albans, England

Dracunculiasis is an infection of connective and subcutaneous tissues by the nematode, *Dracunculus medinensis*. Clinical effects are produced primarily by the gravid female when she discharges her larvae near the skin surface, usually on the extremities. There are symptoms of local itching, urticaria, and burning pain at the site of a small blister. As the blister bursts, the anterior end of the nematode gradually appears through the ulcerated skin. Secondary infection is common, and invasion of the deeper tissues is a rare complication. These complications may include tetanus, septicemia, arthritis, paraplegia, constrictive pericarditis, or urogenital involvement. Ocular manifestations in dracunculiasis are uncommon, but can include allergic reactions, such as intense eyelid edema and conjunctival hyperemia. The parasite may also be found in the tissues of the eyelid or subconjunctiva, or very rarely, it may localize behind the globe.

THERAPY

Systemic. Several drugs have recently been found to be effective in facilitating expulsion or removal of worms, rapid resolution of symptoms, and healing of ulcers. These drugs include niridazole, thiabendazole, and metronidazole. Niridazole is given orally in a dosage of 25 mg/kg daily for 7 days, and the dosage is normally divided. Thiabendazole should be given orally in a dosage of 25 mg/kg twice daily for 2 days. Metronidazole may be used as an alternative drug and is administered orally in a dosage of 250 mg three times daily for 10 days. Although it is unlikely that any of these drugs will have direct antiparasitic activity, they do reduce tissue reaction.

Supportive. Bedrest is indicated, with the affected part being elevated. Strict hygienic measures should be observed; the ulcer should be kept clean, and secondary infection should be controlled with antibiotics. Guinea worms that have emerged through an ulcer may be wound gradually around a small stick and thus removed over a period of about 1 month. Sterile dressings and acriflavine cream should be applied daily during this procedure in order to prevent secondary infection.

Surgical. Surgical extraction of the worm is recommended only when the worm can be palpated subcutaneously, but has not yet emerged through the skin. Worms should be carefully removed intact; otherwise, sever cellulitis may result.

Abscesses caused by worms bursting in the tissues or secondary infection may be incised and aspirated, if necessary. True guinea worm abscesses caused by the gravid female's expulsion of larvae may require incision, evacuation, and primary closure of the abscess under antibiotic cover. Guinea worm cysts or calcified worms may be extracted by surgery, if necessary.

Ocular or Periocular Manifestations

Conjunctiva: Abscess; conjunctivitis; erythema; hyperemia; nematode present.
Eyelids: Abscess; edema; erythema; nematode present; cystic mass; urticaria.
Globe: Nematode present; proptosis; cystic mass.
Orbit: Nematode present; abscess.

PRECAUTIONS

Niridazole should be taken after meals to minimize gastric irritation. Metronidazole may cause abdominal discomfort and breathlessness. Some patients object to the bitter taste of the drug, so care should be taken to see that patients actually take it. Simultaneous administration of an antihistamine often blocks uncomfortable side effects.

Surgical extraction of the guinea worm may be very difficult, since the worm may lie very tortuously. Great care should be taken to see that the entire worm is removed intact because sepsis almost always results if the worm is broken and may lead to cellulitis, abscess formation, or septicemia.

COMMENTS

Dracunculiasis is primarily a disease of poverty, particularly in remote rural communities without safe drinking water. Infection occurs through the ingestion of water from ponds containing infected cyclops, the intermediate host of the parasite. It is most common in the countries of sub-Saharan Africa. Although usually not a serious disease, provided that complications do not ensue, it is incapacitating and can be economically important to poor rural communities. An international effort to eradicate the disease worldwide by 1995 has already been successful in Pakistan and India. Measures include provision of safe drinking water, filters, health education, and treatment of ponds.

References

Burnier M Jr, Hidayat AA, Neafie R: Dracunculiasis of the orbit and eyelid: Light and electron microscopic observations of two cases. Ophthalmology 98:919–924, 1991.
Diallo JS: Manifestations Opthalmologiques des Parasitoses. Paris, Masson, 1985, pp 248–250.
Duke-Elder S (ed): System of Ophthalmology. St Louis, CV Mosby, 1976, Vol XV, p 47.
Hopkins DR, Ruiz-Tiben E: Dracunculiasis eradi-
cation: Target 1995. Am J Trop Med Hyg 43:296–300, 1990.
Kale OO, Elemile T, Enahoro F: Controlled comparative trial of thiabendazole and metronidazole in the treatment of draconculiasis. Ann Trop Med Parasitol 77:151–157, 1983.
Muller R: Guineaworm eradication: Four more years to go. Parasitol Tod 8:352–357, 1992.

ECHINOCOCCOSIS 122.9
(Echinococciasis, Hydatid Cyst, Hydatidosis)

ROBERT L. BERRY, M.D.

Little Rock, Arkansas

Echinococcosis is an infection caused by larval forms (hydatid cysts) of *Echinococcus multilocularis, E. granulosus, E. vogeli,* or *E. orligarthrus.* The most common host for *E. granulosus* is the intestine of a dog, although it can be found in other domestic animals. The human is an intermediate host who is infected by ingestion of food containing the eggs of the organism. The ovum hatches in the intestinal tract, and the embryo penetrates the intestinal wall to enter the portal circulation. The infection is usually due to eating unboiled vegetables contaminated by the feces of dogs or cats. The eggs may also be carried directly from the dog or cat to the mouth of the child or adult. The disease is more prevalent in rural areas of the world, such as East Africa, the Middle East, and South America.

The most common sites of hydatid cyst are the liver (60 to 70 per cent) and lungs. Factors that determine the final location of the cysts are not well defined, but include anatomic and physiologic factors of the host.

Although subretinal, vitreous, and anterior chamber hydatid cysts have been reported, the orbit is the primary ophthalmologic location. One to 2 per cent of the cases of human echinococcosis have an orbital location. Inside the orbit, hydatid cysts tend to be located superiorly, and some may erode the orbital roof and become intracranial. Hydatid cysts of the orbit tend to occur most often in persons under 30 years of age. Although there is evidence that infected individuals may not manifest systemic symptoms for long periods of time, this is not usually the case in orbital hydatidosis, where even small cysts can cause serious complications. The ocular history is relatively short, from 1 to 12 months, and is characterized by firm, unilateral, progressive, nonpulsating exophthalmos. Chemosis, lid edema, and orbital cellulitis may develop as a consequence of rupture or secondary infection. Other findings may include mechanical restriction of ocular motion (which may reach total ophthalmoplegia), visual impairment, papilledema or papillitis, retinal striae, and exposure keratitis due to extensive proptosis.

THERAPY

Systemic. Medical treatment of echinococcosis has centered on the broad-spectrum antihelminthic agent mebendazole.[‡] Mebendazole has a demonstrated ability to sterilize hydatid cyst cavities. A recently completed 10-year clinical trial of continuous therapy demonstrated increased life expectancy, subjective improvement, substantial radiologic decrease in the size of the liver lesions, and lack of progression of distant metastases.

Mebendazole is given in daily oral doses of 20 mg for the first 3 or 4 days. If no idiosyncratic reactions are encountered, the daily dosage may be increased to 3 or 4 gm for a period of at least 30 days. BCG vaccine[‡] administration has been shown effective in suppressing the growth and metastasis of experimental *E. multilocularis* infections, raising the possibility that effective immunotherapeutic modalities may be available in the future.

Surgical. The major treatment of this lesion is surgical excision of the cyst. The cyst is surgically exposed through a transconjunctival or transpalpebral approach for the anterior cysts and a lateral orbitotomy after frontal craniotomy for the most frequently encountered cases involving a superior or medial position. Except for the small cysts that can be removed entirely, the usual technique is to puncture the cyst and aspirate the hydatid fluid. Subsequently, the fluid of the cyst is replaced with either 1 per cent formaldehyde in saline or 70 per cent alcohol and left in place for 5 minutes before surgical excision of the membrane.

Ocular or Periocular Manifestations

Conjunctiva: Chemosis; conjunctivitis; granuloma; hydatid cysts.
Cornea: Abscess; keratitis.
Eyelids: Edema; granuloma; hydatid cysts; ptosis; widening or asymmetry of palpebral fissure.
Globe: Exophthalmos; pain; phthisis bulbi; proptosis.
Lacrimal System: Hydatid cysts in the lacrimal gland.
Optic Nerve: Atrophy; optic neuritis; papilledema.
Orbit: Abscess; hydatid cysts; erosion of bony walls.
Retina: Hydatid cysts; detachment; hemorrhages.
Vitreous: Hydatid cysts; opacity.
Other: Cataract; disturbances of conjugate movement; hypopyon; ocular pain; secondary glaucoma; visual loss.

PRECAUTIONS

Surgical removal of the cysts must be done with great care so that multiple scoleces ("hydatid sand") are not scattered into adjacent tissue. Sterilization of the cyst with formaldehyde or alcohol may prevent additional seeding in the event of accidental rupture of the cyst. Accidental rupture of the cyst may produce a severe inflammatory reaction that is responsive to systemic corticosteroid treatment.

COMMENTS

Environmental control measures have been shown to reduce the incidence of echinococcosis. Contact with infected dogs, particularly fecal contamination of hands and feet, should be avoided. Infected carcasses should be burned or buried to prevent access by animals to material containing scoleces. Dogs should also be treated if found to be infected with this organism.

Hydatid cyst should be included in the differential diagnosis of unilateral proptosis in patients from countries where echinococcosis is endemic.

References

Cook BR: *Echinococcus multilocularis* infestation acquired in U.K. Lancet *337*:560–561, 1991.
Lerner SF, et al: Hydatid cyst of the orbit. Arch Ophthalmol *109*:285, 1991.
Morales AG, et al: Hydatid cysts of the orbit: A review of 35 cases. Ophthalmology *95*:1027–1032, 1988.
Musio CF, Linos D: Echinococcal disease in an extended family and review of the literature. Arch Surg *124*:741–744, 1989.
Rausch RL, et al: Consequences of continuous mebendazole therapy in alveolar hydatid disease with a summary of a 10-year clinical trial. Ann Trop Med Parasitol *80*:403–419, 1986.

LOIASIS 125.2
(African *Loa Loa* Eye-Worm Disease)
JAMES M. BARNETT, M.D.

Muskegon, Michigan

Loiasis is a chronic parasitic infection caused by the filariae *Loa loa*. The larva stage of the *L. loa* worm is transferred to humans by bites of the female deer fly of the genus *Chrysops*. The larvae migrate to the human subcutaneous tissue and mature to adults. The male and female adults copulate, and thereafter microfilariae are released. These microfilariae migrate into the bloodstream via the lymphatics. The microfilariae can be picked up in the bite of another deer fly, and thus, the circle is complete. Infection may be asymptomatic for as long as 15 years. The most common clinical manifestations are "calabar swellings." These transient swellings are areas of localized subcutaneous edema. They may occur anywhere, but are especially common around medium-sized joints and areas exposed to trauma, such as legs, hands, and orbits. The onset of the lesion is often heralded by local pain and itching. An edematous, nonerythematous swelling 10 to 20 cm in diameter then develops, lasts for several days, and subsides slowly. These swellings recur irregularly either at the same site or in various locations.

The adult worm occasionally migrates under the skin, producing a prickly, crawling sensation. Periocular skin and subconjunctiva are common sites. When the worm passes under the conjunctiva, it may be visualized directly. Often, males will follow a female on her subcutaneous or subconjunctival path. The worms produce an edematous conjunctivitis that may last for several days.

THERAPY

Systemic. Diethylcarbamazine is the drug of choice and is effective against the parasite in all stages of development. The oral dosage in adults and children is 2 mg/kg three times a day after meals for 14 to 21 days. A small dose should be given initially to determine if there are any adverse effects to diethylcarbamazine.

Surgical. Surgical extraction of the worm is advised when it appears superficially in the periocular skin or conjunctiva. Worms typically move directly under the bulbar conjunctiva where they can be seen. A drop of 0.59 per cent proparacaine hydrochloride is used to anesthetize the conjunctiva. The worm is grasped through the conjunctiva with a forcep and held firmly while a suture is placed through the conjunctiva and around the worm and tied in place. Finally, the conjunctiva is buttonholed, and the worm is extracted. Female adult worms measure about 60 mm, whereas males are 30 mm in length.

Ocular or Periocular Manifestations

Conjunctiva: Conjunctivitis; parasites present.
Eyelids: Edema.
Other: Lacrimation.

PRECAUTIONS

Adverse reactions can occur with the administration of diethylcarbamazine in loiasis. These reactions may include headache, dizziness, nausea, and fever. Destruction of the microfilariae may cause serious allergic reactions manifested by severe pedal edema, intense itching, dermatitis, fever, colic, and lymphad-

enitis. Rarely, a fatal allergic encephalitis or anaphylactic reaction has occurred in patients treated with this drug for loiasis. Endocardial fibrosis developed in a Peace Corps worker in east Africa treated with diethylcarbamazine for *Loa loa*. The concomitant administration of antihistamines or corticosteroids is advisable to minimize allergic reactions. Patients with known longstanding exposure to *Loa loa* and high microfilariae blood levels should be started on very small doses of diethylcarbamazine, which can be increased in the absence of allergic reactions. If reactions are severe, the dosage of diethylcarbamazine should be reduced or treatment interrupted.

COMMENTS

Loiasis is endemic in western and central Africa. Most cases diagnosed in the United States are in people who have resided in these endemic areas. The infections can last in certain individuals for as long as 30 years. It is necessary that ophthalmologists be aware of loiasis, particularly in this age of global travel. It has been shown that loiasis can be prevented with the use of 5 mg/kg of diethylcarbamazine for 3 days each month while exposure lasts. One should use caution in giving prophylaxis to patients who have resided in west or central Africa as diethylcarbamazine can cause a fatal reaction due to the death of microfilariae.

The American deer fly, *C. atlanticus* (which is endemic in the Mississippi Gulf Coast), has been shown experimentally to maintain the *Loa loa* parasite in an infective state. Large numbers of infective larvae were commonly recovered from experimentally infected flies. Therefore, *C. atlanticus* could theoretically transmit *Loa loa* from human to human within the United States.

The prognosis of loiasis is good with treatment. Without treatment, loiasis is annoying and uncomfortable, but is rarely life threatening. Penetration of the worms into the eye is rare, and generally there are no serious sequelae to the subconjunctival parasite.

References

AMA Drug Evaluations, 6th ed. New York, John Wiley & Sons, 1986, pp 1606.
Barnett JM, Wolter JR: *Loa loa*: The African eye worm observed in Michigan. J Pediatr Ophthalmol 8:23–25, 1971.
Duke-Elder S (ed): System of Ophthalmology. St. Louis, CV Mosby, 1965, Vol VIII, pp 402–405.
Farrer WE, Wittner M, Tanowitz HB: African eye worm (*Loa loa*) in a tourist. Ann Ophthalmol 13:1177–1179, 1981.
Gibbs RD: Loiasis: Reports of three cases and literature review. J Natl Med Assoc 71:853–854, 1979
Jaccard A, Lortholary O, Visser H: Diethylcarbamazine and human loiasis (Letter). N Engl J Med 5:320, 1989.
Loa loa: A pathogenic parasite (Editorial). Lancet 6:554, 1986.

Nutman TB, Miller KO, Mulligan M, Reinhardt GN, Currie BJ, Steel C, Ottese EA: Diethylcarbamazine prophylaxis for human loiasis. Results of a double-blind study. N Engl J Med *319*:752–756, 1988.

Oberg MS, McGowen BA, Kleiman DA: Loiasis 15 years after exposure. Tex Med *83(2)*:36–37, 1987.

Olness K, Franciosi RA, Johnson MM, Freedman DO: Loiasis in an expatriate American child: Diagnostic and treatment difficulties. Pediatrics *80*: 943–946, 1987.

Webster LT: Drugs used in the chemotherapy of helminthiasis. *In* Goodman LS, Gilman AG (eds): The Pharmacological Basis of Therapeutics, 7th ed. New York, Macmillan, 1985, pp 1010–1011.

MALARIA 084.6

ROBERT L. BERRY, M.D.

Little Rock, Arkansas

Malaria is an infectious febrile disease that is sometimes a severe and chronic protozoan infection. It is still a major cause of illness and death worldwide; in 1984 over ten million cases were reported. Mortality is principally in children younger than age 5 and in nonimmune adults, e.g., tourists. The number of malaria cases reported in the United States has increased over the past decade. In 1988 1,023 cases of malaria were reported to the Centers for Disease Control. The overall U.S. mortality rate from malaria is estimated to be 4.2 per cent.

Malaria is most commonly transmitted to humans through the bite of an infected *Anopheles* mosquito (primary host). Transmission also occurs from mother to fetus or with use of a common syringe by drug addicts (secondary host). The causative organism is one or more of the *Plasmodium* species: *P. falciparum, P. vivax, P. malariae,* and *P. ovale.*

Symptoms of malaria develop as early as 8 days or as late as several months after exposure. Malaria often begins with nonspecific malaise, which is followed shortly by a characteristic shaking chill and rapidly rising temperature that is usually accompanied by headache and nausea; the initial episode ends with profuse sweating. After a fever-free interval, the cycle of chills, fever, and sweating is repeated either daily (*P. falciparum,* 36 to 48 hours), every other day (*P. vivax* and *P. ovale,* 48 hours), or every third day (*P. malariae,* 72 hours). Duration of an untreated primary attack varies from a week to a month or longer. Relapses are common in all forms, except *P. falciparum* malaria, and may occur at irregular intervals for several years. *P. falciparum* malaria is also known as pernicious subtertian, malignant, and estivoautumnal malaria and is the most severe form.

THERAPY

Systemic. Malaria is treated by chemotherapeutic agents given systemically to suppress the disease, to manage an acute attack, or as curative therapy. Chloroquine is still the drug of choice, but in some areas chloroquine-resistant malaria has emerged. Suppressive therapy consists of 500 mg (300 mg base) of oral chloroquine administered once or twice weekly. This therapy protects travelers to malarious areas by suppressing the erythrocytic infection and thus the clinical manifestations of malaria. It is started 1 week before arrival in an endemic area and should be continued for 4 to 6 weeks after leaving the area, since its continued use results in parasitic eradication of sensitive strains of *P. falciparum.* In *P. vivax, P. ovale,* and *P. malariae,* 26.3 mg (15 mg base) of primaquine must be given daily for 14 days in conjunction with or after the discontinuation of chloroquine.

An acute attack of any type of malaria, except drug-resistant *P. falciparum* malaria, can be treated by chloroquine. The dose is 1 gm (600 mg base) of oral chloroquine, followed by 500 mg (300 mg base) in 6 hours and then 500 mg (300 mg base) daily for 2 days. The total dose is 2.5 gm (1.5 gm base). Comatose or vomiting patients may be given 250 to 375 mg (200 to 300 mg base) of intramuscular chloroquine every 6 hours. Oral therapy with chloroquine should be resumed as soon as possible.

Chemoprophylaxis of chloroquine resistant strains of *P. falciparum* consists of 250 mg per week of mefloquine. This therapy should also be started 1 week before arrival in an endemic area and continued for 4 to 6 weeks after leaving the area.

An acute attack of chloroquine-resistant *P. falciparum* malaria can be treated orally with pyrimethamine-sulfadoxine, three tablets as a single dose, and doxycycline, 100 mg twice daily for 3 days. If this treatment fails, quinine sulfate, 650 mg three times daily for 3 days, may be given or halofantrine 500 mg every 6 hours for six doses plus doxycycline 100 mg twice daily for 3 days.

Parenteral therapy for all malaria consists of quinine dihydrochloride 600 mg in 300 ml normal saline over 2 to 4 hours; it is repeated every 8 hours until oral therapy can be started. An alternate parenteral therapy consists of quinidine gluconate 10 mg per kg loading dose (maximum dose, 600 mg) in normal saline slowly over 1 hour, followed by continuous infusion of 0.002 mg per kg per minute for a maximum of 3 days.

Ocular. The most frequent ocular complication associated with malaria is herpes simplex keratitis, and appropriate topical management should be instituted. Iritis may also accompany an attack of malaria and is treated routinely with topical steroids and cycloplegics. Other ophthalmic abnormalities that occur with malaria generally resolve as the disease process subsides, with the exception of ischemic optic nerve lesions and large macular hemorrhages that may result in permanent sequelae.

Ocular or Periocular Manifestations

Choroid or Retina: Hemorrhages with or without edema (small peripheral, large central); vaso-occlusion.

Conjunctiva: Enlarged horizontally oriented conjunctival vessels in the intrapalpebral zones; icterus; pallor; petechiae; subconjunctival hemorrhages.

Cornea: Herpes simplex keratitis; herpes zoster keratitis; interstitial keratitis; nonherpetic keratitis; stromal opacification.

Extraocular Muscles: Paresis of third, fourth, or sixth nerve (transient).

Eyelids: Blepharitis; edema; herpes zoster involvement; neuralgia and hyperalgesia or various ocular sensory nerves (particularly the supraorbital and infraorbital nerves); ptosis.

Iris: Iridocyclitis; iritis.

Lens: Cataracts (rare).

Optic Nerve: Atrophy: hyperemia; papillary hemorrhages; papilledema; retrobulbar or optic neuritis.

Pupil: Anisocoria; reflex disturbances.

Vitreous: Hemorrhages; opacity.

PRECAUTIONS

Chloroquine is the drug of choice in all types of malaria, except drug-resistant *P. falciparum* malaria. Side effects secondary to chloroquine may include corneal deposits (epithelial whorls) and retinopathy. Retinopathy is best detected by serial visual fields, color testing, and direct macular exam. Infants and children are particularly susceptible to parenteral chloroquine overdosage, and severe reactions and deaths have been reported.

COMMENTS

Persons traveling to areas where malaria is endemic should take protective measures to reduce contact with the mosquito vector. Travelers should attempt to remain in a well-screened area between dusk and dawn. When going out in the evening, they should wear protective clothing and use insect repellent that contains N, N-diethyl-m-toluamide. Travelers taking malaria chemoprophylaxis should continue the therapy for 4 to 6 weeks after leaving an endemic area.

Currently, a malaria vaccine is being developed, but general use is several years away.

References

Bell RW: Ophthalmologic findings in malaria. Ann Ophthalmol 7:1439–1442, 1975.

Johnson LW: Preventive therapy for malaria. Am Fam Physician 44:471–478, 1991.

Nussenzweig V, Nussenzweig RS: Progress toward malaria vaccine. Hosp Pract 25:45–57, 1990.

Playfair JM, et al: Modern vaccines. Lancet 335: 1263–1266, 1990.

Ross JVM: Ocular complications associated with malaria. Eye Ear Nose Throat Monthly 32:707–711, 1953.

ONCHOCERCIASIS 125.3

ALAN C. BIRD, M.D., F.R.C.S., F.R.C.Ophth.

London, England

Onchocerciasis results from infection with the nematode, *Onchocerca volvulus*. The human is the definitive host. The transmission of *O. volvulus* requires the intervention of a vector, the blood-sucking black fly of the genus *Simulium*. The fly becomes infected by the intake of microlariae from humans, and infection occurs by insertion of immature adult worms. Adult worms can be found in fibrous nodules that are characteristically subcutaneous and are most easily identified over bony prominences, such as the rib cage, pelvis, and head. The offspring of the adults—microfilariae—are mobile and migrate in subcutaneous tissue, but can also be found in the blood. In the eye, they can be seen in the cornea, aqueous humor, and vitreous. There are some reports of microfilariae within the neuroretina, and they have also been located by histopathology in the optic nerve. In patients infected within the first year of life, viable microfilariae cause little or no tissue reaction; however, dead microfilariae produce considerable focal inflammation with subsequent tissue destruction. In these patients, microfilariae can be found in large numbers in the skin and eye. In patients infected in later life, the live microfilariae seem to evoke an inflammatory response, and the identifiable population of microfilariae is low.

Dead microfilariae cause localized corneal stromal disease around the dead worm that resolves spontaneously. A continued high population of microfilariae causes progressive sclerosis of the corneal stroma, which usually begins in the lower part of the cornea and spreads upward. Anterior uveitis is accompanied by downward movement of the pupil. In the fundus, the chorioretinal scarring characteristically is seen temporal to the fovea; it progresses to a ring of change in the peripheral macula. In advanced disease, there is confluent atrophy of the entire macular region. Optic nerve disease is manifest as swelling of the optic nerve that, within months, causes arcuate scotomata. As the disease develops, total loss of peripheral field may occur so that the patient may remain with a small central field but normal acuity.

Apart from ocular disease, the major impact of onchocerciasis is on the skin. Chronic generalized dermatitis gives rise to itching and hyperpigmentation. It is also believed that progressive fibrosis may give rise to elephantiasis. There is little good information concerning involvement of other systems. The microfilariae seem to have widespread distribution in the body, although their effects on various internal organs are unknown. There seems to be significant variation in the expression of the disease in different parts of the world, which may be related to differences in *Onchocerca*, host response, or biting habits of the vector.

Diagnosis can be made on the basis of a known history of contact with the disorder and identification of microfilariae in tissues in the eye or in skin snips. A small dose of diethylcarbamazine causes microfilariae death and a consequent inflammatory response that is manifest as fever, esosinophilia, and skin rash; this is known as the Mazotti test.

THERAPY

Systemic. Two drugs have been used in the past for the treatment of onchocerciasis. Diethylcarbamazine is very effective in causing microfilarial death, but has little effect on the adult worm. Massive microfilarial death generates secondary inflammation resulting in visual loss and considerable dermatitis, lymphadenopathy, and arthralgia. Attempts have been made to modify the inflammatory response with systemic corticosteroids, although doing so seems to reduce the microfilaricidal effect of the drug. The severe consequences of diethylcarbamazine treatment have caused this form of treatment to be abandoned. Likewise, suramin causes death of adult worms and is also microfilaricidal. However, this form of treatment is associated with severe systemic diseases and, in particular, may induce renal failure.

Over the last few years, a new microfilaricidal drug, ivermectin,[†] has been introduced. It seems to be effective in causing reduction of microfilariae within the body over a period of 3 months. It is believed that this drug kills microfilariae, although their disappearance is much slower than with diethylcarbamazine and little inflammatory response is seen. There is also some evidence that ivermectin affects the germinal epithelium of the adult worm, as manifested by large numbers of dysmorphic microfilariae around the adult worms. Phase 3 studies have failed to show any major complications of this form of treatment, although its widespread use must await the completion of phase 4 studies. The form of treatment seems to be eminently practical, since a single oral dose of 12 mg seems to cause disappearance of microfilariae for up to a year. Although this treatment does not eradicate onchocerciasis from the individual, there are high hopes that annual dosing within a population may control the disorder.

Ocular. Local anti-inflammatory agents are effective in controlling ocular inflammation.

Surgical. Excision of subcutaneous nodules containing adult worms has been practiced for some time. It is evident that the load of microfilariae in the eye bears some relationship to the number of subcutaneous nodules in the head. Removal of these subcutaneous nodules reduces the microfilarial load. Although this reduction has some effect, it does not eradicate the infection, and the use of this treatment in a large population is relatively impractical.

Supportive. Vector control has been used in widespread areas of Africa by the World Health Organization. It has proved to be effective, although it requires repeated spraying of the area and is expensive. It is unlikely that vector control represents a practical long-term solution to the problem.

PRECAUTIONS

In the eye, punctate inflammatory disease at the level of the pigmented epithelium may result secondary to diethylcarbamazine treatment. A more important complication is the onset or aggravation of optic neuritis. There are reports of patients suffering visual loss as a result of treatment.

References

Anderson J, Fugslang H: Further studies on the treatment of ocular onchocerciasis with diethylcarbamazine and suramin. Br J Ophthalmol 62:450–457, 1978.

Anderson J, Fugslang H, Marshall TF deC: Effects of suramin on ocular onchocerciasis. Trop Med Parasitol 27:279–296, 1976.

Bird AC, Anderson J, Fugslang H: Morphology of posterior segment lesions of the eye in patients with onchocerciasis. Br J Ophthalmol 60:2–20, 1976.

Dadzie KY, et al: Ocular findings in a double-blind study of ivermectin versus diethylcarbamazine versus placebo in the treatment of onchocerciasis. Br J Ophthalmol 71:78–85, 1987.

De Sole G, et al: Adverse reactions after large-scale treatment of onchocerciasis with ivermectin: Combined results from eight community trials. Bull WHO 67:707–19, 1989.

Green BM, et al: Comparison of ivermectin and diethylcarbamazine in the treatment of onchocerciasis. N Engl J Med 313:133–138, 1985.

Newland HS, et al: Effect of single-dose ivermectin therapy on human *Onchocerca volvulus* infection with onchocercal ocular involvement. Br J Ophthalmol 72:561–569, 1988.

Taylor HR, et al: Treatment of onchocerciasis. The ocular effects of ivermectin and diethylcarbamazine. Arch Ophthalmol 104:863–870, 1986.

PEDICULOSIS AND PHTHIRIASIS 132.9

MARILYN C. KINCAID, M.D.

St. Louis, Missouri

Pediculosis refers to infestation by *Pediculus humanus* var. *corporis* and *Pediculus humanus* var. *capitis*, body and head lice, respectively. These lice are similar to each other in appearance and interbreed freely. Infestation by *Phthirus pubis*, the pubic louse, is called phthiriasis and is by far the most common type of louse infestation of the ocular region. Both types of lice lay eggs on the hair shafts; the eggs, or nits, are firmly adherent, resisting both mechanical and chemical removal.

Pediculus organisms are 2 to 4 mm long and have long slender legs that allow them to move about freely to feed. These lice are typically passed from person to person by close contact either with another infested person or with contaminated clothing or bedding. Infestation of the cilia is very rare and occurs only when there is massive infestation of the adjacent scalp hair.

Phthirus pubis is also called the crab louse because of its shape. At 2 mm, it is smaller than *Pediculus* and has a broad, shield-like body. This louse is much less mobile than *Pediculus*. Its legs are thicker with claw-like feet, and it prefers sites where the distance between adjacent hairs is similar to its grasping span, particularly the pubic hair but also axillary, chest, and beard hair, as well as the eyelashes. Thus, phthiriasis is primarily a sexually transmitted disease of adults. However, *Phthirus* also causes 1 per cent of all lice infestations of scalp hair and can occur in infants.

Both types of lice are associated with conditions of crowding or poor personal hygiene, but may occur in all socioeconomic groups.

THERAPY

Topical. In cooperative adults and older children, when the infestation is mild, physical removal of the involved lashes under direct visualization may be sufficient. Cryotherapy has been found effective in killing both adult lice and nits and is likewise feasible in older children and adults.

Topical white petrolatum smothers the adult lice and should be applied twice daily for 10 days to eradicate the emerging nits. Some authors have found this treatment to be only partially effective, however.

Lindane (gamma benzene hexachloride) 1 per cent shampoo is an effective pediculocide that is available by prescription. It is used as a single application to the head and body and can be repeated after 7 days if necessary, since it is less effective against the nits. Central nervous system toxicity has been reported

from absorption through the skin, particularly in infants. This preparation is also irritating to the eye, and its use on the lashes is not recommended. However, some authors have used it successfully after applying an antibiotic ointment to the eye to act as a mechanical barrier.

A recently available agent, 1 per cent permethrin creme rinse, has been shown to be effective against both *Pediculus* and *Phthirus*. It is not specifically recommended for use around the eye, but is apparently nonirritating to the eye according to the manufacturer (Burroughs-Wellcome).

A-200 Pyrinate (Norcliff Thayer) is a solution of pyrethrins, piperonyl butoxide, kerosene, and other ingredients and is available without a prescription. This agent is effective, but is toxic to the corneal epithelium, causing erosions with secondary ulceration and necrosis. The toxic agent may in fact be one of the "inert" ingredients.

Recently, 20 per cent fluorescein[‡] was observed to be effective in killing *Phthirus*, but to date there has been no larger therapeutic trial of this apparently nontoxic agent. No information is available regarding whether it kills the nits.

One per cent yellow mercuric oxide[‡] and 3 per cent ammoniated mercury[‡] ophthalmic ointments have been recommended as effective when used twice daily for a week.

Cholinesterase inhibitors, including physostigmine ointment,[‡] kill the adult lice but not the nits. These agents cause cholinergic side effects—both local, such as ciliary spasm, and systemic, such as trembling and ataxia. An aqueous solution of the organophosphate insecticide malathion[†] has been described in the British literature as nontoxic and effective against both adult lice and nits, but it is not yet available in the United States.

Supportive. In adult patients, phthiriasis is usually acquired from sexual contacts, so the patient may also have other sexually transmitted diseases. Reinfestation may occur if sex partners are not examined and treated. Phthiriasis is less common in children than in adults, and although it may be contracted from an adult caregiver, the possibility of sexual abuse must be considered when a child has phthiriasis. In all cases, family members should be examined and treated, if necessary. The patient may also have other sites of infestation, so the entire body should be examined. Clothing, bedding, hair brushes, and combs should be sterilized by heating to 50° C, achieved by using the highest available washer and dryer temperature settings. Any cosmetics used around the eyes should be discarded.

Reexamination 7 to 10 days after treatment is important in order to detect inadequate treatment, newly emerging adult lice, or reinfestation.

Ocular or Periocular Manifestations

Conjunctiva: Follicular conjunctivitis (may cause more symptoms than the actual lid infestation, so a high index of suspicion is required for prompt diagnosis).

Cornea: Marginal keratitis (rare).

Eyelids: Infestation (manifest by direct visualization of lice and nits, reddish-brown louse feces, and maculae ceruleae, the blue spots on the skin indicative of louse bites); pruritus; blepharitis; secondary infection with preauricular lymphadenopathy.

PRECAUTIONS

Because most of the pediculocides are much less effective against nits than against adult lice, re-examination at 7 to 10 days is necessary, with retreatment as indicated.

Several of the agents noted above are irritating or toxic to the eye, and should be used cautiously. Agents requiring a prescription should be nonrefillable. Pruritus that persists after the lice are eradicated may indicate hypersensitivity to the pediculocide.

COMMENTS

Pediculosis of the ocular region is extremely rare and is generally an extension of heavy scalp infestation. Phthiriasis is more common and in many circumstances can be considered a venereal disease. Adequate treatment and follow-up are necessary to prevent ongoing or recurrent infestation.

References

Awan KJ: Cryotherapy in phthiriasis palpebrarum. Am J Ophthalmol 83:906–907, 1977.

Burns DA: The treatment of *Pthirus [sic] pubis* infestation of the eyelashes. Br J Dermatol 117:741–743, 1987.

Couch JM, Green WR, Hirst LW, de la Cruz ZC: Diagnosing and treating *Phthirus pubis* palpebrarum. Surv Ophthalmol 26:219–225, 1982.

Kalter DC, Sperber J, Rosen T, Matarasso S: Treatment of pediculosis pubis: Clinical comparison of efficacy and tolerance of 1% lindane shampoo vs. 1% permethrin creme rinse. Arch Dermatol 123:1315–1319, 1987.

Kirschner MH: *Phthirus pubis* infestation of the eyelashes. JAMA 248:428, 1982.

Mathew M, D'Souza P, Mehta DK: A new treatment of Pthiriasis [sic] palpebrarum. Ann Ophthalmol 14:439–441, 1982.

Pe'er J, BenEzra D: Corneal damage following the use of the pediculocide A-200 Pyrinate. Arch Ophthalmol 106:16–17, 1988.

Silburt BS, Parsons WL: Scalp infestation by *Phthirus pubis* in a 6-week-old infant. Pediatr Dermatol 7:205–207, 1990.

Singh S, et al: *Phthirus pubis* infestation of the scalp: Report of three cases. Rev Infect Dis 12:560, 1990.

SCHISTOSOMIASIS 120.9
(Bilharziasis)

F. W. FRAUNFELDER, M.D.,
and F. T. FRAUNFELDER, M.D.

Portland, Oregon

Schistosomiasis affects more than 200 million people worldwide (approximately 400,000 infected individuals in the Americas currently); several hundred million more reside in endemic areas which puts them at risk of exposure to the parasites. Consequently, schistosomiasis with its associated morbidity is a major public health problem of subtropical and tropical areas. Five main species infect the human host: *Schistosoma haematobium, S. mansoni, S. japonicum, S. intercalatum,* and *S. mekongi.* Each species is endemic in certain geographic areas of the world with *S. haematobium* widespread in Africa and the Arabian peninsula, and *S. japonicum* infection found in the Far East, parts of mainland China, Japan, Taiwan, the Philippines, Indonesia, Thailand, Laos, Cambodia and Malaysia. *S. mansoni* infection used to be limited to Africa but now commonly occurs in Brazil, Venezuela and certain Caribbean islands. *S. intercalatum* are found in Central and West Africa and *S. mekongi,* the most recently identified schistosome species, are endemic in some parts of Southeast Asia.

Adult schistosomes live in the veins of the host's viscera, and each species infects certain areas. Eggs of the adult female flukes penetrate the wall of the adjacent viscus and are released into the urine or feces. If the eggs in the human excreta reach water, they hatch with each egg releasing a free-swimming miracidium. Miracidia enter species of fresh water snails which are the intermediate hosts of these parasites. Inside the snail, each miracidium develops into a sporocyst which, in turn, gives rise to daughter sporocysts. These daughter sporocysts produce many thousand cercariae which leave the snail and are released into the water. Cercarial rapidly penetrate the skin of man and make their way to the peripheral circulation becoming schistosomula. Cercarial penetration of the skin may be asymptomatic, however, transient pruritic dermatosis is common ("swimmer's itch") along with the characteristic features of fever, arthralgia, cephalgia, and pulmonary symptoms.

Complications of infection stem from eggs encysting in viscera or migrating in the bloodstream. Superinfection, liver fibrous degenerations, splenic fibrous degeneration with portal hypertension (*S. mansoni* and *S. japonicum*), renal insufficiency (*S. haematobium*), and genital lesions (*S. haematobium*) are the consequences.

Ocular manifestations are the result of *S. haematobium* mainly and *S. japonicum* secondarily. Allergic ocular manifestations occurring at the same time as infestation are the most common sequelae, however, aberrant schistosoma eggs or adults may develop ocular features. These include hyperplasia of the lacrimal glands or inflammatory nodules in the conjunctiva or lids. Aberrant adults may result in parasites located in the orbital veins or in the eye. During infestation, "cercarian" conjunctivitis and palpebral or orbital edema may develop. Uveitis, chorioretinitis, retinal venous thrombosis, chorioretinal artery occlusion, and optic neuritis have been reported during egg implantation. Recently, inflammation of the retinal pigment epithelium caused by *S. mansoni* has been reported with lesions resembling those of acute multifocal placoid pigment epitheliopathy.

THERAPY

Systemic. There are a variety of antischistosomals effective against parasites of this nature with the most effective agent being praziquantel[†] with a buried subconjunctival mattress stitch. Praziquantel has several advantages over other agents including single daily oral administration, low incidence of toxicity and side effects, and marked antiparasitic activity. The recommended dose for infection with *S. haematobium, S. intercalatum,* or *S. mansoni* is 40 mg/kg of body weight administered once. For *S. japonicum* infection, it is recommended to administer 30 mg/kg twice in one day, and for *S. mekongi,* 20 mg/kg three times in one day. Side effects include abdominal pain, headache, dizziness, and skin rashes. Amoscanate[†] has recently been reported to be a highly effective agent against most species of schistosomes which infect humans, however reversible hepatotoxicity is a noted side effect. Oxamniquine[†] is an alternate drug for *S. mansoni.*

Ocular. Treatment as above suffices for ocular therapy unless complications develop. "Cercarian" conjunctivitis and other allergic reactions may need to be treated with topical corticosteroids. Arterial occlusions may require systemic and topical ophthalmic corticosteroids.

Surgical. Excision of nodules or granulomas on the eyelids or anterior segment are rarely necessary. The parasite may occasionally need to be removed from the globe or from an orbital vein.

Ocular or Periocular Manifestations

Anterior Chamber: Hyphema; presence of parasite.
Choroid or Retina: Arterial occlusion; edema; nongranulomatous posterior uveitis; phlebitis; inflammation of retinal pigment epithelium.
Conjunctiva: Granuloma; hyperemia; proliferation of papillae, xerosis.
Cornea: Pigmentation.

Eyelids: Edema; granuloma; urticaria.
Iris: Iridocyclitis.
Lacrimal System: Adenitis.
Optic Nerve: Optic neuritis.
Orbit: Edema; presence of parasite in veins; pseudomotor.

PRECAUTIONS

Diagnosis of schistosomiasis must be based on the clinical presentation, travel history and finding parasite eggs in excreta. Quantification of infection and assessment of viability of the eggs are important procedures for planning therapy and evaluation of prognosis. Antischistosomal therapy, if given early, may lead to reversal of pathologic lesions. In more advanced cases, disease spread can be halted and further damage prevented from chemotherapeutic agents.

COMMENTS

Eradication of schistosomiasis is not a realistic goal with the currently available tools and the economic and social structure of the endemic areas. A more realistic approach would be control of disease and reduction of transmission by targeted chemotherapy combined with focal mollusciciding if required. Continued health education, raising socioeconomic standards and abandoning obsolete agricultural practices offer means for progress in containing this infection.

References

Ashton N, Cook C: Allergic granulomatous nodules of the eyelids and conjunctiva. Am J Ophthalmol 87:1–28, 1979.
Dickinson AJ, Rosenthal AR, Nicholson KG: Inflammation of the retinal pigment epithelium: A unique presentation of ocular schistosomiasis. Br J Ophthalmol 74(7):440–442, 1990.
Milligan A, Burns DA: Ectopic cutaneous schistosomiasis and schistosomal ocular inflammatory disease. Brit J Dermatol 19(6):793–798, 1988.
Shapiro TA, Were JB, Talalay P, Bueding E, Rocco L, Danso K, Massof R, Green R, Mellits ED, Lietman PS: Clinical evaluation of amoscanate in healthy male volunteers. Am J Trop Med Hyg 35(5):945–953, 1986.

SPARGANOSIS 123.5

GONZALO MURILLO, M.D.

La Paz, Bolivia

Sparganosis is an infestation in humans caused by the sparganum or plerocercoid larvae of *Diphyllobotrium*-related tapeworms belonging to the genus *Spirometra* after ingestion (usually in drinking water) of a cyclops bearing the plerocercoid larvae; ingestion of infected uncooked frog, snake, fish, or more infrequently pork meat containing plerocercoid larvae; and the application of infected fresh frog or snake flesh as a poultice. The frog and snake tissues contain the *Sparganum* that is capable of invading human tissues. The definite hosts for *Spirometra* are dogs and cats. The infection often presents as a tumoral-type lesion in any part of the body, mainly as a painful subcutaneous swelling as these tissues become invaded by the *Sparganum*.

A marked eosinophilia is usually present. Although the disease is rare, it predominates in Asia, is less frequent in Africa, and is found sporadically in North and South America. The eye, orbital, and periorbital tissues may be involved, with intense pain, irritation, and inflammation; subconjunctival, orbital, and palpebral edema; profuse lacrimation; and sometimes destruction of the globe. The onset of subconjunctival infestation occurs with an intensely itchy conjunctivitis, photophobia, or blepharospasm. This causes toxemia and the formation of nodules around the parasites. The retrobulbar infestation produces lagophthalmos and corneal ulceration, upper eyelid chemosis, and ptosis. Elephantiasis of the eyelids may develop when the *Sparganum* is localized in the lymphatic vessels.

THERAPY

Surgical. The preferred method of treatment is to kill the worms by injection of 2 to 4 ml of 40 per cent ethyl alcohol with epinephrine-free procaine in the lesion and then the surgical excision of the nodules. Also the parasites may be killed by the intravenous injection of novarsenobenzol[†] (adults 300 to 450 mg, children 70 to 150 mg) administered every 4 to 5 days given two to six times daily. Alternatively, neoarsphenamine[†] in intravenous injection could be given in a dosage usually ranging from 150 to 600 mg. There is no established medical therapy.

Ocular or Periocular Manifestations

Conjunctiva: Chemosis; conjunctivitis; nodules.
Cornea: Corneal ulcer.
Eyelids: Blepharospasm; edema; nodules; ptosis; lagophthalmos; elephantiasis.
Orbit: Cellulitis; edema; granuloma.
Other: Lacrimation; ocular pain; photophobia; acneiform pustules in affected skin.

PRECAUTIONS

Some adverse reactions following the injection of ethyl alcohol, procaine, neoarsphenamine, or novarsenobenzol could appear, including local skin irritation, eczematoid skin,

or allergic contact dermatitis with ethyl alcohol. With procaine the known side effects are arterial hypotension, and cardiac and respiratory failure. With neoarsphenamine, flushing of the face, edema of the lids, profuse diaphoresis, and hypotension could occur immediately after the intravenous injection.

COMMENTS

In most of the cases after the intravenous injection of neoarsphenamine or novarsenobenzol, it is mandatory to surgically excise the nodules containing the parasites. Tarsorrhaphy has been used also to preserve the cornea until the parasite is excised or rejected.

References

Faust EC, Rusell PF, Jung RC: Craig and Faust's Clinical Parasitology, 8th ed. Philadelphia, Lea & Febiger, 1974, pp 516–519.
Leon LA, Almeida R, Mueller JF: A case of ocular sparganosis in Ecuador. J Parasitol 58:184–185, 1972.
Plore JJ: Cestode (tapeworm) infections. In Isselbacher KJ, et al (eds): Harrison's Principles of Internal Medicine, 9th ed. New York, McGraw-Hill, 1980, p 917.

THELAZIASIS 128.9

P. K. MUKHERJEE, M.S.

Raipur, India

Thelaziasis is a nematode infection of ocular tissue caused by *Thelazia callipaeda* and is commonly found in Japan, China, Burma, Bangladesh, India, and some parts of North and Central America. About ten species of *Thelazia* have been identified in the conjunctival sac, lacrimal gland, and lacrimal canal of dogs, cats, horses, sheep, black bears, and deer; a similar number of species has been identified in birds.

The involvement of the human eye is less common than in animals or birds. In humans, the ocular adnexa, including the conjunctiva, lid, and lacrimal passages, are involved more frequently. Intraocular involvement is least common. Although the complete life cycle of *Thelazia* has not yet been worked out, transmission to humans probably occurs by an arthropod host, such as the fly. It is speculated that the eggs are laid in the conjunctival sac or lacrimal duct, and the complete life cycle may take place there. Intraocular penetration may occur either through an abraded cornea or through the sclera after subconjunctival involvement.

THERAPY

Systemic. Diethylcarbamazine[‡] may be used to destroy the microfilariae if surgical methods are not desirable. An oral dose of 50 mg diethylcarbamazine three times daily for 14 days may prove effective.

Ocular. Therapy depends on the part of the ocular tissue that is involved. If the cornea or anterior chamber is involved, one drop of 1 per cent atropine daily with 0.5 or 1.0 per cent prednisolone or 0.1 per cent dexamethasone several times a day may control the inflammation.

Surgical. Surgical therapy is the method of choice in the ocular management of thelaziasis. The adult worm is removed from the anterior chamber by paracentesis under subdued light to prevent it from migrating to the posterior chamber. If the worm is attached to the iris or has formed an iris nodule, a sector iridectomy may be necessary. Removal of the worm from the conjunctiva or lacrimal passage should be performed with forceps or cotton-tipped applicator, and the conjunctival nodules may need to be excised.

Ocular or Periocular Manifestations

Anterior Chamber: Cells and flare; worm present.
Conjunctiva: Nodules; worm present.
Eyelids: Ectropion; edema; nodules.
Iris: Nodules; worm attached to the iris stroma.
Lacrimal System: Increased tear secretion; worm present.
Other: Irritation; ocular pain; photophobia.

PRECAUTIONS

Frequent instillation of atropine may kill the worm, which is not desired, since necrosis of the worm would further stimulate an intraocular inflammation. The systemic administration of diethylcarbamazine may cause a serious allergic reaction due to destruction of the microfilariae, which is manifested by intense pruritus, dermatitis, and fever. The concomitant administration of antihistamines or corticosteroids is advisable to minimize allergic reactions.

COMMENTS

Involvement of the human eye by this parasite is relatively uncommon and is usually confined to the conjunctiva and the lids. Intraocular involvement is most uncommon, although it has been reported.

References

Duke-Elder S (ed): System of Ophthalmology. St. Louis, CV Mosby, 1974, Vol XIII, p 193.

Joseph A: Ocular thelaziasis. A case report. Ind J Ophthalmol 33:113–114, 1985.
Mukherjee PK, Verma S, Agrawal S: Intraocular thelazia. A case report. Ind J Ophthalmol 25:41–42, 1978.
Schultz GR: Intraocular nematode in man. Am J Ophthalmol 70:826–829, 1970.

TOXOCARIASIS 128.0

ZANE F. POLLARD, M.D.,
and WILLIAM S. HAGLER, M.D.

Atlanta, Georgia

Toxocariasis is an infection caused mainly by the dog roundworm, *Toxocara canis*. There are a few reported cases in the literature of human intestinal infection with *Toxocara cati*, the common ascarid of the cat, but there has been no documented proof of visceral larval migrans or ocular toxocariasis caused by this larvae. The ovum of *T. canis* is ingested orally, and the larvae hatch in the intestine and penetrate the mucosa to spread throughout the body. "Visceral larva migrans" is the term used when there is liver and/or lung involvement. The brain, heart, eye and orbit can also be involved. Eye involvement is termed "ocular toxocariasis." Before the late 1970s, the diagnosis was made by demonstrating larvae in a liver biopsy or in studying enucleated eyes for the presence of larvae or an eosinophilic abscess. At the present time, the clinical diagnosis of visceral larva migrans and ocular toxocariasis is confirmed by the ELISA (enzyme-linked immunosorbent assay) test. This test has a high sensitivity and specificity because the antigen used is the *Toxocara*-embryonated egg. Occasionally in patients with ocular toxocariasis the serum titers are normal, but titers performed on the aqueous are elevated. The diagnostic titer for ocular toxocariasis is felt to be 1:8, whereas the titer needed to confirm the diagnosis of visceral larva migrans is 1:32. However, a titer lower than 1:8 should not deter one from making the diagnosis of ocular toxocariasis in the face of strong clinical evidence because 85 per cent of cases show a decrease in titers over a period of 6 months to 6 years from the time of the initial examination, 10 per cent show a rise in the titer, and 5 per cent show stable titers in the 5 to 6 years after the initial diagnosis. Some patients presenting with low titers may have had high titers in the past.

Visceral larva migrans usually presents around 2 years of age, whereas the average presentation of ocular toxocariasis is 7.5 years. Elevated white blood cell count and eosinophilia as high as 30 per cent are often seen with visceral larva migrans, but only occasionally with ocular toxocariasis. Hepatosplenomegaly is usually seen with visceral larva migrans, but only rarely with ocular toxocariasis. The immunology of this disease, which produces only rare involvement of the eye in visceral larva migrans and likewise presents only rarely with visceral involvement in cases of ocular toxocariasis, is not yet understood. It was thought that a positive titer for *Toxocara* would exclude the diagnosis of retinoblastoma, which might clinically be confused with ocular toxocariasis in some cases. However, cases of retinoblastoma with positive titers for *Toxocara* have been seen. Although the eye of these patients contained only retinoblastoma, the positive titer for *Toxocara* pointed to a prior infection with *Toxocara*.

A 27-gauge needle can be used to aspirate the aqueous to check for titers to *Toxocara*, as well as to look for eosinophils in cases in which the diagnosis is in doubt. In children this procedure is done under general anesthesia.

Several cases of ocular toxocariasis have also had high titers for toxoplasmosis. This is quite understandable as the contamination of the soil with *Toxocara* eggs by the dog can easily be matched by contamination of the soil with the *Toxoplasma* oocyst by the cat.

The prognosis for ocular toxocariasis is quite poor with 80 per cent of untreated eyes becoming legally blind (20/200 or less). The greatest number of cases have been reported in the United States followed by England and Australia. A few cases have been reported in France, Belgium, Germany, Ireland, Israel, Greece, Japan, Poland, Italy, Hungary, Mexico, Netherlands, Argentina, and Venezuela.

THERAPY

Systemic. Fifteen years ago, 15 mg/kg of diethylcarbamazine[‡] on a daily basis was used for 3 weeks to treat toxocariasis. Today, thiabendazole has replaced diethylcarbamazine as the leading anthelminthic for toxocariasis. Thiabendazole[‡] is administered (25 to 50 mg/kg/day) in two divided doses each day for 7 to 10 days. Occasionally, the course is repeated for a second or third time. This anthelminthic is used in combination with systemic steroids because it is felt that the reaction to the dead nematode is very devastating to the eye. Prednisone in the dosage of 2 mg/kg/day is used for 3 weeks to control the vitritis. In some cases the steroids alone have been able to clear the vitreous. Topical steroids are useful if iritis is present. The ocular absorption of thiabendazole is unknown. A recent report on the use of oral thiabendazole in patients with the diagnosis of diffuse unilateral subacute neuroretinitis, who had moderately intense vitritis, was most encouraging. It is felt that this entity is due to a nematode infection of the retina. The most frequent side effects of thiabendazole are anorexia, nausea,

vomiting, and dizzyness. Elevation of SGOT and hyperglycemia with leukopenia and hematuria have been reported, as well as Stevens-Johnson syndrome. Blurring of vision, hypotension, enuresis, and perianal rash have rarely been reported.

Surgical. There are many cases in which various types of surgical treatment are helpful. Peripheral retinal detachment is common, which may develop because of contraction of the vitreous base that can produce a peripheral dialysis. A standard scleral buckling procedure alone may be effective; in a few cases that procedure was all that was necessary for a successful result.

In the majority of patients requiring surgery, there is also a significant detachment of the posterior retina that either involves or threatens the macula. The detachment is usually caused by prominent vitreous bands that can only be removed by vitrectomy techniques. A lensectomy is necessary in many of these patients, either because of cataract formation or in order to completely remove the extreme anterior attachments of the vitreous bands. In addition to the vitrectomy and lensectomy, a scleral buckling procedure may be required.

In some instances a vitrectomy alone can be used to remove opaque vitreous. Of course, adequate time should be given for medical treatment to work before performing a vitrectomy.

With the exception of lesions at the fovea, laser photocoagulation of the nematode larvae can be performed if the media is clear enough. Extensive application of burns must be given to destroy the larvae because a partially destroyed larva may cause a severe inflammatory reaction.

The use of various combinations of these surgical procedures can result in stability or improvement in visual acuity, although reactivation of the uveitis has rarely been seen after surgery. Because the natural history and the rate of progression of ocular toxocariasis are not well documented, ophthalmologists should follow these patients very closely and perform surgery whenever a macular detachment occurs or seems eminent or whenever a progressive peripheral detachment occurs.

Some outstanding visual results with surgical treatment have been obtained. Several cases improved from 20/400 or less to 20/40 and 20/30. Of course, if the macula has already been destroyed by a posterior detachment or granuloma, central visual acuity cannot be improved, but stability of peripheral vision can be expected in most cases.

Ocular or Periocular Manifestations

Cornea: Larvae; nummular keratitis.
Globe: Diffuse nematode endophthalmitis.
Iris: Granuloma (may be associated with hypopyon).

Lens: Cataract; larvae.

Optic nerve: Granuloma (growing from the surface of the optic nerve into the vitreous); optic neuritis; papillitis.

Retina: Detachment (often confused with retinoblastoma); focal posterior granuloma; peripheral inflammatory granuloma (appearing as a unilateral pars planitis but sometimes also associated with a retinal detachment); retinal fold or vitreous band from the peripheral mass to the optic nerve or posterior pole.

Other: Strabismus.

PRECAUTIONS

Children's sandboxes can be decontaminated by replacing the sand or by steam sterilization. It is estimated that there are between 60 and 80 million dogs in the United States and 30 million cats. Treatment of these animals with piperazine or pyrantel pamoate has been quite effective in managing toxocariasis. Infections in puppies are more common than in the adult dog. A public health awareness of this problem plus a concerted effort to have all dogs and cats dewormed will reduce the incidence of this disease.

COMMENTS

Epidemiologic surveys are being performed to determine the exact incidence and distribution of this disease in the United States. In some areas of Georgia, ELISA titers have been positive in 10 per cent of control groups. In one county in Georgia, 3 per cent of controls tested had positive titers for *Toxocara*. The percentage of dogs with intestinal toxocariasis has been reported to vary from 20 to 86 per cent.

References

Brown DH: Ocular *Toxocara canis*. J Pediatr Ophthalmol 7:182–191, 1970.

Felberg NT, Shields JA, Federman JL: Antibody to *Toxocara canis* in the aqueous humor. Arch Ophthalmol 99:1563–1564, 1981.

Gass JD, Callanan DG, Bowman B: Oral therapy in diffuse unilateral subacute neuroretinitis. Arch Ophthalmol 110:675–680, 1992.

Hagler WS, et al: Results of surgery for ocular *Toxocara canis*. Ophthalmology 88:1081–1086, 1981.

Liesegang TJ: Atypical ocular toxocariasis. J Pediatr Ophthalmol 14:349–353, 1977.

Pollard ZF: Long-term follow-up in patients with ocular toxocariasis as measured by ELISA titers. Ann Ophthalmol 19:167–169, 1987.

Pollard ZF, et al: ELISA for diagnosis of ocular toxocariasis. Ophthalmology 86:743–749, 1979.

Rhones JAA, Pratt CB, Johnson WW: Thiabendazole in visceral larva migrans. Am J Dis Child 121:226–229, 1971.

TOXOPLASMOSIS 130.9
(Ocular Toxoplasmosis, Toxoplasmic Iridocyclitis, Toxoplasmic Retinochoroiditis)

DANIEL H. SPITZBERG, M.D., F.A.C.S.

Indianapolis, Indiana

This infection is caused by the protozoal parasite, *Toxoplasma gondii*, which invades and multiplies asexually within the cytoplasm of nucleated host cells. As host immunity develops, multiplication slows, and the parasite develops cysts within cells. These cysts have a predilection for the brain, eye, and muscle. As a result, various symptoms, such as recurrent retinochoroiditis, hydrocephalus, intracerebral calcification, and central nervous system manifestations, may develop. Although ocular toxoplasmosis may not make its first appearance until adulthood, most infections with *T. gondii* are congenital in origin and have a predilection for the nerve fiber layer. Microphthalmos, posterior uveitis, optic atrophy, iritis, strabismus, and nystagmus are the ocular signs most often associated with severe congenital toxoplasmosis and may be well developed at birth. Ophthalmoplegia and nystagmus are usually due to central nervous system involvement. Before toxic systemic medications are prescribed, the ophthalmologist should document the possibility of toxoplasmosis (by a toxoplasmosis titer positive at any level) and should rule out tuberculosis (by performing the tuberculin skin test down to PPD#2) and syphilis (by obtaining a negative FTA-ABS test).

THERAPY

Systemic. *Corticosteroids should not be used without specific antimicrobials.* At one time, it was popular to treat toxoplasmic retinochoroiditis with corticosteroids alone, but occasionally the patients' immunity is not strong enough to prevent the rampant multiplication of the parasite, resulting in serious damage.

Depending on the severity and the location of the retinochoroiditis, one should use up to four drugs: trisulfapyrimidines (sulfadiazine, sulfamethazine, and sulfamerazine), pyrimethamine, clindamycin, and corticosteroids. Since these drugs work in different ways, they may be synergistic; however, synergism has only been demonstrated for pyrimethamine and triple sulfa. Although small peripheral retinal lesions do not demand any medication, patients with large severe ones near the macula or optic disc probably should receive all four drugs (quad therapy). The major defense against *T. gondii* is a cellular response in which immune competent lymphocytes and macrophages participate. In the future, treatment may be directed more toward enhancing the body's immunity than toward the use of antiparasitic drugs.

If only one drug is chosen, trisulfapyrimidines should be the first choice because of their minimal expense, good tolerance, lack of spoilage, and simplicity of use; however, this drug is difficult to find. One must avoid most of the newer sulfonamides because they are less effective. The usual dosage of trisulfapyrimidines as 1 to 1.5 gm given orally four times daily.

The alternate first or second choice would be clindamycin,[‡] usually in a dosage of 300 mg every 6 hours. This is an expensive drug and has not yet been approved by the FDA for toxoplasmosis and probably never will be because of the infrequency of toxoplasmosis and the expense of obtaining such approval. A less expensive but less effective alternative to clindamycin is 500 mg of tetracycline[‡] four times daily.

The major problem with pyrimethamine is that it is nauseating and requires two additional steps. One needs to prescribe at least 3 mg of leucovorin a week and obtain a platelet count for depression of the bone marrow at least once a week. A loading dose of 50 mg of pyrimethamine four times a day the first day is followed by 25 mg twice a day thereafter.

Corticosteroids should not be used without the cover of at least one antitoxoplasmic agent, and one must be careful not to use them in an immunosuppressive dosage. Either 100 mg of prednisone every other day after breakfast or periocular injections* every 2 to 3 weeks are recommended.

Ocular. Subtenon injection of steroids* may produce immediate dramatic improvement in patients with ocular toxoplasmosis. In addition, topical local anesthetics should be applied at least five times over the area to be injected. The head should be tilted so that gravity will pull the anesthetic into the cul-de-sac. An injectable anesthetic is not necessary nor advisable. A 2-ml syringe is used to inject 0.5 ml of the 80 mg/ml concentration of methylprednisolone. The easiest place to make the injection is inferotemporally. The point of the needle should be placed 3 to 4 mm in front of the cul-de-sac and between blood vessels and pushed into the hilt *following the curve* of the sclera. One is helped to follow the curve of the sclera by the use of lateral motion of the needle over an area of 5 mm. This is a most valuable maneuver, since it allows one to hug the sclera as the needle goes in. The barrel of the syringe must be moved a large distance as one goes around the eyeball in order to keep the needle point near the eye. Keeping the needle near the eye with the aperture facing the sclera cuts down on the patient's discomfort and increases the penetration of the steroid because the medication will be closer to the sclera and not out in the orbital tissues. This lateral motion also avoids impaling the eyeball, since the ophthalmologist will immediately be aware that the sclera has been engaged if such a movement is used. By putting the injection far back, the side effects of chemosis and ptosis are decreased and the white material is not visible. If repeated injections are necessary, the superotemporal quadrant is usually varied with the inferotemporal. If a patient develops an allergy to methylprednisolone, the diagnosis should be confirmed by intradermal injection of 0.01 ml and read at 2 days, and the patient should be switched to triamcinolone (40 mg/ml).

Surgical. Freezing the active lesion has been employed in an attempt to kill resistant *T. gondii* and thus to quiet the lesion. This technique should be reserved for unusual cases. The entire lesion may be frozen and thawed three times in one sitting.

Although photocoagulation does kill cysts of *T. gondii*, it also damages normal retina and cannot be relied upon to eradicate all the cysts. Photocoagulation of an active lesion may occasionally be of value in those that have failed to heal after several months of medical treatment or in those patients who cannot tolerate the medication.

Vitrectomy is indicated only for patients with dense membranes and greatly reduced vision. This treatment is not indicated for punctate opacities.

Ocular or Periocular Manifestations

Cornea: Keratic precipitates.
Extraocular Muscles: Esotropia; nystagmus.
Iris: Iritis; synechiae.
Optic Nerve: Atrophy; disc edema; papillitis.
Pupil: Anisocoria; persistent membrane.
Retina: Macular edema; retinitis.
Sclera: Scleritis; thickening.
Vitreous: Cells; exudates; haze; posterior vitreous detachment.
Other: Cataracts; lymphadenopathy; microphthalmos.

PRECAUTIONS

Pseudomembranous colitis may develop with the use of clindamycin; however, this danger is greatly reduced if trisulfapyrimidines are used. If clindamycin is prescribed, patients should be warned to discontinue use of the drug if they have four or more bowel movements a day than is normal for them. In addition, the prescription for clindamycin should be limited to a 1-week supply with three refills.

Sometimes a blood picture resembling macrocytic anemia result from administration of pyrimethamine. Platelet counts should be monitored weekly in these patients. This bone marrow depression can be prevented in most patients by the oral dosage of leucovorin in any drink without alcohol. This regimen is superior to waiting for thrombocytopenia to develop and then using leucovorin. The use of folic acid, which inactivates the pyrimethamine, should be avoided.

COMMENTS

No method of preventing attacks has been designed at the present time. Patients should be advised to take good care of their general health and to have some medication, such as triple sulfonamides, on hand to take immediately with the first symptoms of a recurrence. It is crucial to start therapy as early as possible, especially before the onset of retinal necrosis if the lesion is near the disc or macula.

Many infants survive acute infection and have no complications or sequelae; however, some have healed scars in the fundus and may develop retinochoroiditis later in life.

References

Dobbie JG: *Toxoplasma* retinochoroiditis. Successful isolation of *Toxoplasma gondii* from the subretinal fluid of the living human eye. Ann Ophthalmol 2:509–513, 1970.

Eyles DE, Coleman N: Synergistic effect of sulfadiazine and Daraprim against experimental toxoplasmosis in mouse. Antibiotics Chemother 3: 483–490, 1953.

Fitzgerald CR: Pars plana vitrectomy for vitreous opacity secondary to presumed toxoplasmosis. Arch Ophthalmol 98:321–323, 1980.

Frenkel JK, Hitchings GH: Relative reversal by vitamins (p-aminobenzoic, folic, and folinic acids) of the effects of sulfadiazine and pyrimethamine on *Toxoplasma*, mouse and man. Antibiotics Chemother 7:630–638, 1957.

Ghartey KN, Brockhurst RJ: Photocoagulation of active toxoplasmic retinochoroiditis. Am J Ophthalmol 89:858–864, 1980.

Tabbara KF, O'Connor GR: Treatment of ocular toxoplasmosis with clindamycin and sulfadiazine. Ophthalmology 87:129–134, 1980.

Tessler HH: Quadruple therapy offers rapid, effective results in ocular toxoplasmosis. Ophthalmology Times 5:27, 1979.

TRICHINOSIS 124
(Trichinellosis)

B. H. KEAN, M.D.

New York, New York

Almost 30 million people throughout the world are infected with *Trichinella spiralis*; most of the cases of trichinosis occur in the United States, but only a few hundred are reported each year because the disease is unrecognized or so mild as to produce few symptoms. The disease is acquired by the ingestion of poorly cooked meat, especially pork, or ground beef contaminated by pork in the grinder. Less frequently, the meat of other mammals, such as bear, fox, and walrus, is involved. An epidemic in which 325 persons became ill due to the consumption of poorly cooked horse meat imported from Connecticut was reported in France.

After meat containing encysted larvae is ingested, the gastric juices release the parasites that develop in the upper portion of the small intestine. The adult females measure 3 to 4 mm by 60 um, and males are one-third of that size. After 4 days of maturation, the adults produce larvae at the rate of 1000 daily for several weeks while embedded in the mucosa. The larvae disseminate throughout the entire body, but have a predilection for striated muscle, which is invaded and where encystment eventually takes place.

It is customary to divide the stages of trichinosis into the intestinal, the visceral (muscular), and convalescent phases, but there is considerable overlap among them. Systemic symptoms of trichinosis may include gastrointestinal disturbances, especially diarrhea; fever; generalized muscle pains, sometimes severe; and eosinophilia, often pronounced.

The ophthalmologist is often the first to see the patient and has a unique opportunity to suspect the diagnosis. Bilateral edema of the eyelids, barely recognizable or severe enough to shut the eyes, presents as the first symptom of the disease in most patients. There is no consensus regarding the exact mechanism of the edema that may occur from the 6th to the 22nd day of infection, but it certainly is associated with the invasion of the eye muscles and the resulting myositis. Such mistaken diagnoses as kidney disease, mumps, angioneurotic edema, and erysipelas have been made.

Other ophthalmic signs of trichinosis may include pain on motion of the eye muscles, pain in one or both eyes, headaches associated with fever, chemosis, and subconjunctival and retinal petechial hemorrhages. Rarer are disturbances in vision, including blurring, strabismus, exophthalmos, nystagmus, photophobia, diplopia, and visual hallucinations. Tiny striated hemorrhages close to the inferior temporal vein have also been reported.

The symptoms and the inevitable eosinophilia make a clinical diagnosis relatively easy. Definitive diagnosis is made by the use of several different serologic tests; the bentonite flocculation test is the most widely used, with a rising titer considered convincing. Muscle biopsy, if positive, is conclusive.

THERAPY

Systemic. If the diagnosis is made early (in the first week) 200 mg of mebandazole[‡] twice a day for 3 to 5 days may be helpful in reducing the intestinal worm load and hence the number of larvae released. This stage is rarely recognized except in epidemics.

In the muscular stage of severe infection, mebendazole,[‡] 200 to 300 mg three times a day for 5–10 days is recommended. Thiabendazole[‡] may be used instead; the usual oral dose is 25 mg/kg, given in divided doses for 3 days and repeated after an interval of 24 to 48 hours. The drug should be taken after meals. Recently, mebendazole has been replacing thiabendazole because it is better tolerated. Both drugs may produce a hypersensitivity reaction, and both are contraindicated in pregnancy. In severe cases, 60 mg of prednisone daily should be used in conjunction with one of these anthelminthics.

Some advocate the use of mebendazole and thiabendazole in grater doses and for longer duration than we have recommended. Albendazole and flubendazole are under study as substitutes for mebendazole, but are not available in the United States.

Ocular. Ocular therapy is directed primarily to relief of the severe ocular pain that results from larval invasion of ocular musculature. Topical corticosteroids usually provide significant relief and help reduce swelling. A solution of 0.2 per cent hydrocortisone drops may be used four times daily until symptoms subside. In severe cases, topical corticosteroids may be accompanied by subconjunctival corticosteroid injections; 5 mg/ml of hydrocortisone* is the recommended dosage. Cycloplegics are indicated if anterior uveitis is evident.

Supportive. If the infection is mild and there is no evidence of encephalitis or myocarditis, symptomatic treatment may be sufficient. These patients should be confined to bed and fed high-calorie, protein-rich diets. Ice packs to the eyes, used intermittently, are often welcome. Pain relievers should be used freely, but aspirin should be avoided because it may increase the number and extent of the hemorrhages. Hospitalization is recommended for patients with severe trichinosis.

Consultation with an infectious disease expert is desirable.

Ocular or Periocular Manifestations

Conjunctiva: Chemosis; conjunctivitis; diffuse hemorrhages (splinter); petechiae.
Extraocular Muscles: Encysted parasites; paresis or paralysis of the sixth nerve.
Eyelids: Edema; erythema.
Globe: Exophthalmos; immobility; proptosis.
Iris: Anterior uveitis.
Optic Nerve: Disc hyperemia; optic neuritis; papilledema.
Pupil: Loss of rapid adaptation to light changes.
Retina: Edema; exudates; hemorrhages.
Other: Decreased accommodation; diplopia; dyschromatopsia; ocular pain; orbital edema; photophobia; scotoma; secondary glaucoma; visual field defects; visual loss.

References

Campbell WC, Denham DA: Chemotherapy. In Campbell WC (ed): Trichinella and Trichinosis. New York, Plenum Press, 1983, pp 335–366.
Drugs for parasitic infections. Med Lett 34:17–26, 1992.
Duke-Elder S (ed): System of Ophthalmology. St. Louis, CV Mosby, 1976, Vol XV, pp 159–160.
Horse-meat associated trichinosis in France. MMWR 35:291–298, 1986.
Hoskins DW: Trichinellosis (trichinosis). In Wyngaarden JB, Smith LH Jr (eds): Textbook of Medicine, 18th ed. Philadelphia, WB Saunders, 1988, pp 1911–1912.
Michelson MK, Schantz PM: Trichinosis. In Gorbach SL, Bartlett JG, Blacklow NR (eds): Infectious Diseases. Philadelphia, WB Saunders, 1992, pp 1314–1328.

SECTION 3

ENDOCRINE DISORDERS

HYPERPARATHYROIDISM
252.0

BYRON L. LAM, M.D.

Little Rock, Arkansas

Hyperparathyroidism is a group of disorders in which there is excessive secretion of parathyroid hormone, which may be caused by a primary disorder of the parathyroid gland or be secondary to diseases that produce low serum calcium. Primary hyperparathyroidism may be due to a parathyroid adenoma (80 per cent of cases), parathyroid hyperplasia (15 to 20 per cent), or parathyroid carcinoma (2 to 4 per cent). Primary hyperparathyroidism is more common in women, and the incidence increases after age 50. In addition, primary hyperparathyroidism is the most consistent feature of multiple endocrine neoplasia type 1, occurring in over 90 per cent of clinical cases.

Secondary hyperparathyroidism is often caused by chronic renal failure, rickets, Fanconi's syndrome, renal tubular acidosis, and intestinal malabsorption syndromes. Unlike other forms of hyperparathyroidism in which serum calcium is elevated and serum phosphate is low or normal, the serum calcium in secondary hyperparathyroidism is low or normal and the serum phosphate is elevated. The term "tertiary hyperparathyroidism" is used when hyperparathyroidism persist after the cause of secondary hyperparathyroidism is corrected. Some of these patients have a parathyroid adenoma, which presumably results from prolonged stimulation. Increased production of parathyroid hormone can also be caused by drugs, such as lithium.

The symptoms of hyperparathyroidism are nonspecific and include muscle weakness, bone pain, abdominal pain, nausea and vomiting, and mental changes. These symptoms are encompassed by the phrase, "stones, bones, abdominal groans, and psychic moans." Complications of the disorder include pancreatitis, peptic ulcer, renal calculi, bone demineralization (osteitis fibrosa cystica and osteopenia), and muscular atrophy from neuromuscular dysfunction. In addition, hyperreflexia, depression, emotional liability, and slow mentation are prominent features. Diagnosis is established by abnormal levels of serum calcium, serum parathyroid hormone, and urine cAMP (a product of renal tubular cells).

Most ocular manifestations of hyperparathyroidism result from calcium deposition in ocular tissues. However, such calcification can occur in other conditions of hypercalcemia without hyperparathyroidism, such as in some cases of chronic renal failure. Calcium deposits on the conjunctiva, cornea, and sclera are attributed to hypercalcemia and local alkalosis, presumably from diffusion of carbon dioxide into air. Calcium deposits may also be found on the iris epithelium, ciliary processes, and ciliary muscles. Both hyperparathyroidism and hypoparathyroidism can rarely cause papilledema.

THERAPY

Systemic. Although asymptomatic patients may not require treatment, they should be monitored periodically for renal, skeletal, and gastrointestinal abnormalities. Treatment is required in symptomatic patients and in patients with evidence of complications. In primary hyperparathyroidism, surgical removal of the abnormal gland(s) is usually curative. Acute severe hypercalcemia (>15 mg/dl) is treated by hydration with saline solutions up to 1 L/hr and diuresis with such agents as intravenous furosemide 20 to 80 mg every 1 to 2 hours or intravenous ethacrynic acid 10 to 40 mg every 1 to 2 hours. The goal is to maintain urine output and to promote calcium excretion. Occasionally, intravenously mithramycin, an antibiotic that retards bone absorption, at 25 to 50 µg/kg on alternate days and intravenous disodium etidronate, a bisphosphonate, at two to four doses of 10 to 15 µg/kg on alternate days may be required. Oral phosphate at a daily dose of 1 to 2 gm will temporarily lower serum calcium, but it should not be continued on a long-term basis because of the risk of additional tissue calcification. After serum calcium has decreased to a safe level (<13 mg/dl), therapy is continued with at least 3 liters of fluid daily, sodium chloride tablets 400 to 600 meq daily, and oral furosemide 40 to 160 mg or ethacrynic acid 50 to 200 mg daily. Although the production of parathyroid hormone has been shown to be decreased by histamine and beta-adrenergic agents, there have been no convincing responses in hyperparathyroidism to either beta blockade with propranolol or histamine blockade with cimetidine. Lithium-induced

143

hyperparathyroidism responds to the cessation of lithium.

Surgical. If a parathyroid tumor is found, surgical removal is indicated. In hyperplasia of all glands, three and a half glands are removed. If the glands in the neck are normal, exploration extending to the mediastinum may be necessary. Postoperative hypoparathyroidism requires oral calcium and oral vitamin D or its analogue. Patients with severe bone disease may recalcify the skeleton rapidly in the postoperative period ("hungry bone syndrome"). This condition can result in severe and sustained hypocalcemia, which may require intravenous calcium solutions.

Ocular. In patients with symptomatic band keratopathy, removal of the calcium deposits may be attempted. After mechanical denuding of the corneal epithelium, a diluted solution of 0.5 per cent ethylenediamine tetraacetic acid (EDTA) is applied to the area with a Weck-Cel sponge for 5 to 30 minutes. In refractory cases, more concentrated EDTA (1 to 2 per cent) may be used, and gentle scraping is necessary.

Ocular or Periocular Manifestations

Conjunctiva: Calcification; glass-like crystals.
Cornea: Band keratopathy; bleb; opacity.
Optic Nerve: Papilledema; atrophy.
Retina: Vascular engorgement.
Other: Scleral calcification; orbital rim mass.

PRECAUTIONS

If serum calcium rises to dangerous levels, the patient may complain of metallic taste, thirst, headache, and drowsiness; stupor and death may follow if serum calcium reaches 20 mg/dl. Red gritty eyes with band keratopathy may be the presenting sign of hyperparathyroidism. Patients on digitalis preparations may show digitalis toxicity when serum calcium rises.

COMMENTS

Primary hyperparathyroidism should be suspected in patients with recurring renal calculi, bone disease, pancreatitis, peptic ulceration, and other evidence of multiple endocrine neoplasia, particularly if there is a family history. Parathyroid hormone has been shown to exaggerate both hypertension and anemia. Since the advent of automated biochemical screening, most cases of primary hyperparathyroidism have been found in asymptomatic patients. The diagnosis is confirmed by the finding of hypercalcemia with a raised level of serum parathyroid hormone. Normally, a raised serum calcium from other causes should suppress parathyroid function. The one exception is the syndrome of hypercalcemia and peptide production by some nonparathyroid malignancies; such peptides react in the same way as parathyroid hormones on the assay. Secondary hyperparathyroidism occurs in many clinical situations and is apparent in most patients with renal failure from the time they begin to show phosphate retention.

The management of hyperparathyroidism is usually within the realm of internists and specialized surgeons. Ophthalmic evaluation is prompted in symptomatic patients with corneal and conjunctival calcifications or in rare patients with optic disc edema. The calcium salts are deposited extracellularly in the corneal layers and tend to persist long after the serum calcium have normalized.

References

Aurbach GD, Marx SJ, Spiegel AM: Hyperparathyroidism. *In* Wilson JD, Foster DW (eds): Williams Textbook of Endocrinology, 8th ed. Philadelphia, WB Saunders, 1992, pp. 1429–1445.

Cogan DG, Albright F, Bartter FC: Hypercalcemia and band keratopathy. Report of nineteen cases. Arch Ophthalmol 40:624–638, 1948.

Golan A, et al: Band keratopathy due to hyperparathyroidism. Ophthalmologica 171:119–122, 1975.

Naiman J, Green RW, D'Heurle D, et al: Brown tumor of the orbit associated with primary hyperthyroidism. Am J Ophthalmol 90:565–571, 1980.

Sampson MJ, van't Hoff W, Bicknell EJ: The conservative treatment for mild hyperparathyroidism. Br Med J (Clin Res) 296:1016–1017, 1988.

Scholz DA, Purnell DC. Asymptomatic primary hyperparathyroidism. 10-year prospective study. Mayo Clin Proc 56:473–478, 1981.

HYPOCALCEMIA 275.4

MARION H. BROOKS, M.D.,
ANTHONY L. BARBATO, M.D.,
and GLEN W. SIZEMORE, M.D.

Maywood, Illinois

Hypocalcemia may be found in patients with hypoproteinemia, hypoparathyroidism, chronic renal failure, hypomagnesemia, malabsorption syndrome, acute pancreatitis, osteoblastic metastases and other malignant disorders, rickets or osteomalacia, sepsis, and after the administration of such drugs as anticonvulsants, bisphosphonates, and plicamycin and the transfusion of large quantities of citrated blood. A decrease in serum calcium does not always indicate a disturbance of calcium homeostasis. Patients with hypoproteinemia often have a low total but normal ionized calcium level. Under these circumstances, there are no symptoms attributable to hypocalcemia, and calcium replacement is unnecessary. By contrast, low ionized calcium concentrations cause neuromuscular and ectodermal cell dysfunction, and treatment is needed to relieve and reverse the symptoms, signs, and complications of hypocalcemia. Neuromuscular irritability may manifest as fatigue, anxiety or depression, muscle spasms, perioral and distal limb paresthesias, gait disturbances, cardiac arrhythmias, and frank tetany with carpal-pedal spasm, laryngeal spasm, and seizures. Ectodermal abnormalities may include dry skin; the loss of scalp, eyelid, or eyebrow hair; brittle nails; hypoplastic dentition; and cataracts. Bedside maneuvers that suggest hypocalcemia include positive Chvostek's or Trousseau's signs.

Cataracts are the best-known ocular complication of hypocalcemia, but the loss of eyebrows or eyelashes and papilledema also occur.

THERAPY

Systemic. The major therapeutic objective in all forms of hypocalcemia is restoration and maintenance of serum calcium concentrations in the vicinity of 8.5 to 9.5 mg/dl without the development of hypercalciuria or hypercalcemia. The therapeutic regimen used to achieve this goal depends on the cause of hypocalcemia and the response of the individual patient to therapy.

In chronic hypoparathyroidism, low parathyroid hormone is associated with the diminished conversion of vitamin D to its active metabolite, calcitriol, by the kidney. As a consequence, the intestinal absorption of calcium and the mobilization of calcium from bone are impaired, resulting in hypocalcemia. Adequate serum calcium can often be maintained in mild hypoparathyroidism with calcium supplements alone, but administration of both vitamin D and calcium are usually required to increase serum calcium significantly in patients with hypoparathyroidism. Vitamin D may be administered in the form of ergocalciferol, dihydrotachysterol, or calcitriol (1,25-dihydroxyvitamin D_3). The daily dose of ergocalciferol varies from 25,000 to 200,000 IU, depending upon the patient's response. Some authorities prefer to use dihydrotachysterol in a dose of 0.125 to 5.0 mg per day since this preparation has a shorter half-life, is three times as potent as ergocalciferol on a weight basis, and does not require 1 alpha hydroxylation by the kidney to exert its metabolic effects. Despite these theoretical advantages, dihydrotachysterol is more expensive than ergocalciferol and has not been demonstrated to be unequivocally superior to the latter in the treatment of hypoparathyroidism. Treatment with calcitriol is advantageous because this form of vitamin D is fully active in increasing intestinal calcium absorption and, when compared to ergocalciferol, has a more rapid onset of action (hours) and a faster metabolic clearance (days). In view of the markedly enhanced potency of calcitriol relative to other preparations of vitamin D, the daily dose is usually in the range of 0.25 to 2.0 μg per day. The dose of any vitamin D preparation must be individualized for each patient. Since the full effect of a given dose may not be apparent for a long period of time, increments in dosage should not be made more often than every 2 to 3 weeks.

In addition to vitamin D, calcium supplements are generally needed to restore serum calcium levels to normal. Several caveats are important. First, the failure to appreciate that replacement doses of calcium are expressed in terms of *elemental* calcium, rather than the calcium salt, is a common therapeutic error. Elemental calcium constitutes only 9.3 per cent of the weight of calcium gluconate, 18.4 per cent of the weight of calcium lactate, and 40 per cent of the weight of calcium carbonate. Because of the relatively low *elemental* calcium content of calcium gluconate and lactate tablets compared to calcium carbonate, it is often necessary to prescribe a large number of these tablets each day to provide the 1 to 3 gm of elemental calcium required by patients with hypoparathyroidism. For example, to achieve a daily calcium intake of 2 gm would require 43 500-mg tablets of calcium gluconate or 16 650-mg tablets of calcium in comparison to 8 650 mg tablets of calcium carbonate. Second, all calcium salt preparations are not equal. The bioavailability of calcium in various preparations may differ markedly because of different disintegration and dissolution characteristics of the tablets. Therefore, pharmacists and physicians must ensure adequate calcium bioavailability in the preparations that they provide. Third, calcium carbonate tablets should not be taken during fasting when gastric acid secretion is minimal. Optimal absorption occurs when calcium carbonate tablets are taken in equal portions four times daily with meals. Finally, some patients absorb a particular calcium preparation more efficiently than another or prefer a particular preparation because it has fewer side effects. These patients may require or prefer calcium citrate tablets, calcium glubionate syrup, or calcium lactate or carbonate powder "dissolved" in water or juice.

Hypocalcemia develops in chronic renal failure because there is inadequate renal parenchyma to convert 25-hydroxyvitamin D to calcitriol despite high parathyroid hormone levels. Administration of calcitriol in a dose of 0.25 to 1.0 μg per day to patients undergoing chronic dialysis often restores serum calcium and parathyroid hormone levels to normal and prevents the development of renal osteodystrophy. In some patients with renal failure, calcium supplements and oral phosphate binding agents are required to reduce serum phosphate levels by interfering with intestinal phosphorus absorption.

Hypocalcemia due to hypomagnesemia is most often encountered in patients with alcoholism. In this situation, the secretion of parathyroid hormone and its biologic activity are impaired as a consequence of magnesium depletion. The restoration of total body magnesium stores to normal by the administration of magnesium salts is usually associated with an increase in the serum calcium concentration.

The hypocalcemia associated with malabsorption syndromes, rickets, osteomalacia, osteoblastic metastases and other malignant disorders, and the administration of anticonvulsants usually responds to treatment of the underlying disease, together with administration of vitamin D and calcium supplements in doses similar to those used in the treatment of hypoparathyroidism.

Hypocalcemia that develops in response to parathyroidectomy, acute pancreatitis, or the transfusion of large quantities of citrated blood may be associated with the acute onset of tetany and may require intravenous calcium administration for relief of symptoms. Administration of 10 ml of 10 per cent calcium chloride or calcium gluconate solutions may be used. However, since extravasation of calcium solutions into soft tissues elicits a marked inflammatory response, it is preferable to prepare a solution containing 200 mg of elemental calcium in 100 ml of 5 per cent dextrose in water and to administer this solution over a 10-minute period through an indwelling catheter in a large peripheral vein. If symptoms recur, the infusion may be repeated at 6 to 8-hour intervals, or calcium may be administered at a slower rate by constant intravenous infusion.

Dairy products contain calcium, but are also rich in phosphate, which can interfere with the absorption of calcium from the intestine and can increase serum phosphate levels. For this reason, the excessive intake of dairy products should be discouraged. Administration of parathyroid hormone has no role in the therapy of chronic hypocalcemia at this time.

Surgical. Because the neuromuscular and metabolic abnormalities associated with hypocalcemia increase the risk of anesthesia and surgery, elective procedures should be postponed until normocalcemia is restored. In addition, cataract extraction in hypocalcemic patients may be associated with an increased risk of postoperative hemorrhage.

If the oral intake of calcium and vitamin D is limited as a consequence of surgery, serum calcium levels must be monitored carefully. If hypocalcemia develops, replacement therapy should be instituted intravenously.

Ocular or Periocular Manifestations

Conjunctiva: Conjunctivitis.
Eyebrows or Eyelids: Blepharitis; blepharospasm; madarosis; pigmentation; ptosis.

Lens: Flake-like, crystalline, punctate, or zonular cataracts.
Optice Nerve: Papilledema.
Other: Decreased visual acuity; diplopia; photophobia; strabismus.

PRECAUTIONS

Hypervitaminosis D with hypercalcemia and hypercalciuria leading to renal damage from nephrocalcinosis or nephrolithiasis are potentially serious complications of therapy with calcium and vitamin D. Vitamin D intoxication often develops unexpectedly in patients who have had stable serum calcium levels for prolonged periods. In general, the smallest dose of vitamin D that will provide the desired effects should be used, and patients should be taught to recognize the symptoms of hypercalcemia and to alert their physician if they occur. The physician should measure serum and urinary calcium levels at weekly intervals during the initiation of therapy, at monthly intervals for 6 months, and every 3 to 6 months thereafter when serum calcium levels seem to have stabilized. If hypercalcemia or hypercalciuria develops, supplemental calcium and vitamin D must be discontinued immediately, and adequate hydration must be ensured with oral or parenteral fluids. When the hypercalcemia is severe, administration of 60 to 80 mg of prednisone daily will usually restore serum calcium to normal within days. Hypercalcemia associated with the use of ergocalciferol may persist for several months because of the large stores of this agent in adipose tissue and skeletal muscle. By contrast, hypercalcemia produced by calcitriol lasts for only a few days. This fact, plus the similar cost for therapeutically comparable daily doses, causes many physicians to prefer calcitriol to ergocalciferol for the treatment of chronic hypocalcemia.

The dose of calcium and vitamin D may need to be increased during pregnancy, lactation, or the administration of phenytoin or phenobarbital. Conversely, the requirement for calcium and vitamin D may decrease in patients receiving thiazide diuretics. Care must also be exercised when calcium and vitamin D are administered to patients receiving digitalis preparations, since hypercalcemia can lead to the development of digitalis intoxication and cardiac arrhythmias.

Laboratory evaluation of patients suspected of having hypocalcemia should always include measurement of total serum protein, albumin, urea nitrogen, creatinine, calcium, phosphate, magnesium, electrolytes, and pH. If the total calcium level is low, the ionized calcium should be measured; additional studies, including serum parathyroid hormone, will be necessary to define the cause of the hypocalcemia.

COMMENTS

Chronic renal failure with an inability to synthesize calcitriol is the most common cause of hypocalcemia. Malabsorption that limits the availability of both calcium and vitamin D is the next leading cause, followed by hypoparathyroidism. Although hypoparathyroidism is usually an iatrogenic disease that develops after thyroid or parathyroid surgery, it may also occur spontaneously in an idiopathic form or as pseudohypoparathyroidism.

Because hypocalcemia cataracts are not reversible, attempts should be made to prevent their development or progression. Careful monitoring of serum calcium and phosphate in all patients initially for 3 days and subsequently at 3 and 6 months after thyroidectomy, parathyroidectomy, or radical neck dissection is mandatory because the patient may remain asymptomatic despite significant hypocalcemia. The progression of hypocalcemia cataracts is variable in that they may be found as early as 10 days or as late as 22 years after thyroidectomy. The lenticular changes resulting from hypocalcemia are suggestive but not pathognomonic of this disorder and vary from minute, white, punctate opacities to complete opacification of the lens. Despite these variations, there is general agreement that early recognition and vigorous therapy will often prevent the development or halt the progression of cataracts in hypocalcemic patients.

References

Bronsky D, et al: Idiopathic hypoparathyroidism and pseudohypoparathyroidism: Case reports and review of the literature. Medicine 37:317–352, 1958.

Brooks MH: Lenticular abnormalities in endocrine dysfunction. In Bellows JG (ed): Cataract and Abnormalities of the Lens. New York, Grune & Stratton, 1975, pp 291–294.

Buckwalter JA, et al: Postoperative hypoparathyroidism. Surg Gynecol Obstet 101:657–666, 1955.

Carr CJ, Shangraw RF: Nutritional and pharmaceutical aspects of calcium supplementation. Am Pharmacy NS27:49/149-57/157, 1987.

Morris DA: Cataracts and systemic disease. In Duane TD (ed): Clinical Ophthalmology. Hagerstown MD, Harper & Row, 1982, Vol. V, pp 41:1–2.

Okamo K, et al: Comparative efficacy of various vitamin D metabolites in the treatment of various types of hypoparathyroidism. J Clin Endocrinol Metab 55:238–243, 1982.

Schneider AB, Sherwood LM: Pathogenesis and management of hypoparathyroidism and other hypocalcemic disorders. Metabolism 24:871–898, 1975.

Zaloga GP, Chermow B: Hypocalcemia in critical illness. JAMA 256:1924–1929, 1986.

HYPOPARATHYROIDISM 252.1

FELIX O. KOLB, M.D., F.A.C.P.

San Francisco, California

Hypoparathyroidism is caused by a deficient secretion of parathyroid hormone or, more rarely, resistance to its action due to a receptor defect "pseudohypoparathyroidism." This disorder usually occurs after thyroidectomy, surgery for parathyroid tumor, x-ray irradiation, massive radioactive iodine administration for cancer, or idiopathic conditions. Transient hypoparathyroidism in newborns may result from magnesium deficiency, maternal hypercalcemia, or intake of cow's milk containing large amounts of phosphate. Hypoparathyroidism is characterized by decreased blood calcium and increased serum phosphate in the absence of renal failure. Parathormone levels are low or absent in hypoparathyroidism and elevated in pseudohypoparathyroidism. This disorder may cause tetany, muscle cramps, stridor, carpopedal spasms, and convulsions. Lethargy, personality changes, and mental retardation are evident in chronic cases. Some patients show basal ganglia calcifications best seen on CT scan. The signs of Trousseau and Chvostek may also be present. Idiopathic hypoparathyroidism may be associated with candidiasis, Addison's disease, and thyroiditis due to an autoimmune disorder. The incidence of hypoparathyroidism occurs equally in both sexes and rarely is familial.

The major ocular manifestation in chronic hypoparathyroidism is cataract, characterized by numerous bilateral discrete polychromatic opacities, usually in the cortices and subcapsular zones of the lens. Other ocular complications may include keratoconjunctivitis, blepharospasm, photophobia and diplopia, papilledema, increased intracranial pressure (pseudotumor cerebri), and loss of eyebrows.

THERAPY

Systemic. Acute hypoparathyroidism usually occurs after thyroid surgery and requires immediate treatment. Intravenous infusion of 5 to 10 ml of 10 per cent calcium chloride or 10 to 20 ml of 10 per cent calcium gluconate (preferably dissolved in 500 to 1000 ml of 5 per cent dextrose in water) may be given until tetany ceases. Oral calcium salts and ergocalciferol or its more active analogues should be started as soon as possible to maintain the serum calcium level. Calcium carbonate is the oral calcium salt of choice, and 1 to 2 gm of calcium carbonate two to three times daily are sufficient. Alternatively, 8 gm of calcium gluconate[§] or 4 to 8 gm of calcium lactate[§] powder may be administered orally three times daily. Calcium citrate, 3 to 6 gm/day, is better absorbed in most patients. Ergocalciferol may be administered in a daily dosage of 40,000 to 200,000 units (1 to 5 mg). In some patients, up to 7 or 8 mg of ergocalciferol may be needed daily. When a more rapid action is required to control severe hypocalcemia, crystalline dihydrotachysterol (DHT) in a dosage of 0.8 to 2.4 mg may be indicated. After several days, a daily dosage of 0.2 to 1.0 mg will usually maintain blood calcium at a normal level. In addition, daily administration of 10 to 20 ml of oral aluminum hydroxide may be given 1 hour after meals to help lower the serum phosphate level in the initial stage of treatment. In cases refractory to ergocalciferol or DHT, 50 to 100 μg of calcifediol[§] two times daily or preferably 0.25 μg of calcitriol[§] three to four times daily may be needed. Once calcium is normalized, lower doses of calcium, ergocalciferol, or DHT will maintain a normal calcium level. Chlorthalidone[‡] given in a dosage of 50 mg with a low-sodium diet can control mild hypoparathyroidism without the use of ergocalciferol. Magnesium supplementation may be needed.

Ocular. For ocular keratitis and keratoconjunctivitis, 0.5 or 1 per cent methylcellulose solution may be applied four times daily in combination with 1.5 per cent cortisone ointment every 4 hours to lubricate the eye artificially and to control inflammation.

Supportive. A high-calcium, low-phosphorus diet is important in the treatment of hypoparathyroidism. Patients should omit such foods as milk and cheese during acute hypoparathyroidism, because of their high phosphate content.

Surgical. Cataracts may remain stable if hypocalcemia is corrected. If a cataract matures, lens extraction may be performed. There is no apparent increase in postoperative complications compared with other surgery.

Ocular or Periocular Manifestations

Conjunctiva: Conjunctivitis.
Cornea: Epithelial defects; keratitis; nodules; pannus.
Eyebrows: Madarosis.
Eyelids: Blepharospasm; madarosis; ptosis.
Lens: Punctate opacities; subcapsular cataracts.
Optic Nerve: Edema; optic neuritis; papilledema.
Other: Diplopia; myopia; photophobia.

PRECAUTIONS

Although the treatment of hypoparathyroidism with vitamin D is effective, it is hazardous because the patient's condition may so easily slip over into serious hypercalcemic toxicity. Hypervitaminosis D is a frequent complication of the treatment of hypoparathyroidism, and serum calcium must be monitored frequently and the dosage adjusted accordingly. The serum calcium level should be maintained in the low normal range. In severe vitamin D intoxication, corticosteroids may be effective antidotes. Intravenous calcium chloride or calcium gluconate should not be overused to treat tetany or irreversible tissue calcification will occur. Phenothiazine drugs should be administered with caution in hypoparathyroid patients, since they may precipitate dystonic reactions.

COMMENTS

In the prognosis of hypoparathyroidism, some changes may be reversible, but the dental changes, cataracts, and brain calcifications are permanent. Papilledema and increased intracranial pressure disappear with therapy.

The ease of misdiagnosing hypoparathyroidism with convulsion and papilledema as a brain tumor is apparent. The possibility of hypoparathyroidism should be borne in mind when cataracts develop in young children who may have few symptoms, except some mental changes.

References

Along U, Chau JC: Hypocalcemia from deficiency of and resistance to parathyroid hormones. Adv Pediatr 32:439, 1985.

Avioli LV: The therapeutic approach to hypoparathyroidism. Am J Med 57:34–42, 1974.

Bajandas FJ, Smith JL: Optic neuritis in hypoparathyroidism. Neurology 26:451–454, 1976.

Breslau NA, Pak CYC: Hypoparathyroidism. Metabolism 28:1261–1276, 1979.

Cheek JC, Riggs JE, Lilly RL: Extensive brain calcification and progressive dysarthria and dysphagia associated with chronic hypoparathyroidism. Arch Neurol 90:1038–1039, 1990.

Hanno HA, Weiss DI: Hypoparathyroidism, pseudohypoparathyroidism, and pseudo-pseudohypoparathyroidism. Arch Ophthalmol 65:238–242, 1961.

Haussler MR, Cordy PE: Metabolites and analogues of vitamin D. Which for what? JAMA 247:841–844, 1982.

Illum F, Dupont E: Prevalences of CT-detected calcifications in the basal ganglia in idiopathic hypoparathyroidism and pseudohypoparathyroidism. Neuroradiology 27:32–37, 1985.

Okano K, et al: Comparative efficacy of various vitamin D metabolites in the treatment of various types of hypoparathyroidism. J Clin Endocrinol Metab 55:238, 1982.

Parfitt AM: Surgical, idiopathic, and other varieties of parathyroid hormone-deficient hypoparathyroidism. *In* DeGroot LJ (ed): Endocrinology, 2nd ed. Philadelphia, WB Saunders, 1989, Vol 2, pp 1049–1064.

Phillipson B, Angelin B, Christensson T, Einarsson K, Leijd B: Hypocalcemia with zonular cataract due to idiopathic hypoparathyroidism with a note on the prevalence of severe hypocalcemia in a health screening. Acta Med Scand 203:223–229, 1978.

Rao SD, Kleerskoper M, Tolia K, Matkovic V, Parfitt AM: Hypoparathyroidism and biochemical screening. Ann Intern Med 95:655, 1981.

HYPOTHYROIDISM 244.9
(Cretinism, Hypothyroid Goiter, Juvenile Hypothyroidism, Myxedema)

HESKEL M. HADDAD, M.D.

New York, New York

Hypothyroidism is a disease caused by the lack of or decrease in systemic thyroid hormones, which results from a deficiency of the thyroid gland or its function. Hypothyroidism may have different specific causes: (1) primary damage of the thyroid gland (loss of thyroid tissue), which may be congenital, as in cretinism, due to surgery (Thyroidectomy), or after treatment with radioactive iodine after thyroiditis or infectious diseases of the thyroid glands, such as mumps; (2) tumor infiltration of the thyroid gland, either primary or metastatic thyroid carcinoma; or (3) deficiency of iodine in the diet, as in endemic goiter. Hypothyroidism could also be secondary to reduced stimulation of the thyroid gland by the pituitary, as in Simmonds' disease, or after hypophysectomy or may be associated with feedback inhibition of TSH (thyroid-stimulating hormone) secretion by the pituitary gland due to the use of exogenous thyroid hormone. This mechanism is often used in the treatment of hypothyroid goiter and occasionally in the management of thyroid nodules.

In infancy and childhood, hypothyroidism results in generalized suppression of the body systems and growth, primarily bone formation. Hypophyseal dysgenesis, as recognized radiologically in the newborn, is the first clinical sign of cretinism, even before the full-blown picture of the disease develops in the infant. Whereas the retardation of growth reduces weight gain in children, myxedema and swelling of the skin induce a weight gain in adults.

In hypothyroidism, the skin becomes dry and scaly, with yellowish discoloration due to increased carotene in the circulation (carotenemia). The skin is usually pale and cold. In myxedema, the skin appears edematous and thick. The edema may occasionally be localized on the tibia and other bony protuberances. Hair growth may be slowed, and there is a retardation in cuticular growth, especially of the nails and the hair of the armpits and face. This retardation is also manifested by thin brittle hair and alopecia. The mental processes may become dulled and cerebration slow. Mental retardation ensues in infants if the condition is not corrected promptly. The cardiovascular system displays bradycardia, hypotension, enlargement of the heart by myxedema, and decreased electrocardiographic parameters with poor circulation, which may further enhance the edema.

Ocular manifestations may include loss of the hair of the eyebrows, especially their temporal third or half. The lids become edematous, but in contrast to endocrine exophthalmos edema, the periorbital myxedema is intradermal with almost bullous formations of the skin. Occasionally hypothyroidism may induce increased tear flow. The conjunctiva becomes pale and appears gelatinous, in contrast to the chemosis and hyperemia noted in hyperthyroidism and Graves' disease, and the sclera has a very grayish-white appearance. Occasionally superficial punctate keratopathy is associated with hypothyroidism, especially when it is related to neoplastic destruction of the thyroid gland. There is marked sluggishness of the circulation by funduscopic examination with venostasis. In very rare conditions, an exophthalmos may develop, especially after thyroiditis or Hashimoto's struma. The intraocular pressure tends to be low, but with tonography, there is an association of reduction in the outflow facility, as well as in intraocular pressure, which is directly related to the changes in the coefficient of scleral rigidity. There is also a decreased tear secretion resembling keratoconjunctivitis sicca.

THERAPY

Systemic. Management of hypothyroidism is established with thyroid replacement therapy. Although the optimal dosage is determined by the patient's clinical response, replacement therapy in an adult can usually be satisfied with 195 mg of thyroglobulin (thyroid extract) daily. Alternatively, levothyroxine may be administered orally in a daily dosage of 0.1 to 0.3 mg or liothyronine in a dosage of 25 to 75 μg. Synthetic thyroid hormone derivatives are not recommended as initial therapy nor for use in children.

Ocular. Most of the ocular symptoms clear after the systemic disease is treated. Topical ophthalmic lubricants containing methylcellulose or petrolatum may be useful for conjunctival irritation and blepharitis aggravated by lid edema. Carbonic anhydrase inhibitors, such as 125 to 250 mg of acetazolamide or 25 to 50 mg of methazolamide one to four times daily, may be useful to alleviate edema, as the treatment for hypothyroidism is advanced.

PRECAUTIONS

It is imperative that patients treated for myxedema or cretinism be given initial small doses of thyroglobulin to prevent induced cardiac stress and to alleviate the edema of the heart gradually and thus promote better circulation. Otherwise, such patients may develop sudden cardiac failure. Combinations of thyroid products are not recommended because of their higher biologic activity.

In those cases of hypothyroidism caused by failure of the pituitary, attention should be paid to treating the other hormonal deficiencies, particularly adrenal insufficiency. Treatment of the thyroid alone may precipitate severe Addison's disease and may be fatal.

COMMENTS

Usually, the prognosis of hypothyroidism is excellent if recognized and treated early. If not recognized and treated promptly in infancy, however, hypothyroidism can cause permanent mental retardation (cretinism). The association of diabetes with hypothyroidism may create another hazard to the health of the patient, especially if the thyroid is treated without the proper adjustment of diabetic control. The alleged increased incidence of cataract or glaucoma with hypothyroidism does not seem to be corroborated by current statistics.

References

Arffa RC: Diseases of the Cornea. Chicago, Yearbook Publishers, 1991.

Brownlie BEW, Newton OAG, Singh SP: Ophthalmopathy associated with primary hypothyroidism. Acta Endocrinol 79:691–699, 1975.

Haddad HM: Tonography and visual fields in endocrine exophthalmos: Report on 29 patients. Am J Ophthalmol 64:63–67, 1967.

Mahto RS: Ocular features of hypothyroidism. Br J Ophthalmol 56:546–549, 1972.

McDougall IR: Treatment of hyper- and hypothyroidism. J Clin Pharmacol 21:365–384, 1981.

Swanson JW, Kelly JJ Jr, McConahey WM: Neurological aspects of thyroid dysfunction. Mayo Clin Proc 56:504–512, 1981.

Wortsman J, Wavak P: Palpebral redundancy from hypothyroidism. Plast Reconstr Surg 65:1–3, 1980.

SECTION 4

NUTRITIONAL DISORDERS

CROHN'S DISEASE AND ULCERATIVE COLITIS
555.9
(Granulomatous Ileocolitis, Regional Enteritis, Terminal Ileitis)

DAVID L. KNOX, M.D.

Baltimore, Maryland

Crohn's disease and ulcerative colitis are the two most common inflammatory bowel diseases. Regional enteritis, terminal ileitis, and granulomatous ileocolitis are synonyms that emphasize different features of Crohn's disease. The spotty or regional nature of the disorder affects the enteric canal anywhere from the esophagus to the rectum. It is felt by some that large aphthous ulcers of the tongue and buccal mucosa are also a manifestation.

Deep focal ulceration of the mucosa, visualized either by proctosigmoidoscopy or on the surface of excised ileum, is a major feature. Some ulcers form fistulas from bowel to bowel, bowel to skin, or bowel to bladder or vagina. Histopathologically, ulcers and thickened gut wall contain acute and chronic inflammatory cells, and, most characteristically, epithelioid and giant cells.

In contrast, ulcerative colitis is characterized by widespread surface ulceration that may at times become fulminant and lead to perforation. Epithelioid and giant cells are not seen in tissue from patients with ulcerative colitis.

Etiologies have not been proven for either disease. Certain facts have been observed by the author. Crohn's disease often occurs in siblings or in several generations of family members, who, along with the patient, also have multiple allergies. Many of the patients were not breast fed or had colic and other troubles with feeding of cow's milk formula.

The initial symptoms are often quite mild, depending on the segment of intestine that is involved. Multiple symptoms of intestinal discomfort, excessive gas, and intermittent diarrhea, mistakenly classified as "irritable bowel syndrome," may precede for months or years an insidious or explosive onset of severe diarrhea, rectal bleeding, fever, malaise, and weight loss in the patient with Crohn's disease. Adolescents may have had an enigmatic failure to grow. The disease can begin at any age, but most patients present in their twenties and thirties, males a little earlier than fe-

males. In total, the number of cases in males equals those in females. The disease is protean, highly variable, unpredictable, and of different duration and recurrence patterns. There are some patients whose courses leave the clinician with the thought that the disease has "burned itself out."

Diagnosis depends primarily on histopathology, but clinical features determined by history, proctocolonoscopy, and radiologic features, such as the "string sign" in the terminal ileum, are the bases of the diagnosis of Crohn's disease. Ulcerative colitis is diagnosed primarily by colonoscopy and biopsy, but radiologic features include the loss of haustral markings and frequently polyps.

THERAPY

Systemic. Treatment is difficult, primarily because etiologic mechanisms have not been defined. Family physicians, internists, gastroenterologists, and general surgeons, all with slightly different educations, experiences, and psychologic natures, are the primary and secondary managers of these patients. In their desperation, patients often seek the care of many different physicians. An ophthalmologist should never try to manage these patients alone, but should work closely with other experienced practitioners.

Systemic complications of Crohn's disease include arthritis, erythema nodosum, pyoderma gangrenosum, anemia, and amyloidosis. Malnutrition and weight loss are so obviously a result of bowel disease that they are not emphasized, although they are important. Often, complications of ulcerative colitis are the same as those of Crohn's disease with the exception of hepatitis, which can progress to cirrhosis and death.

Complications may occur without obvious activity of the Crohn's disease, concurrent with obvious activity, or as indicators of subclinical activity. Ocular complications occur in about 10 per cent of patients with Crohn's disease and, in the author's experience, less frequently in patients with ulcerative colitis.

The following treatments are those used by other physicians treating patients observed by the author in Baltimore, Maryland. Systemic corticosteroids are the most commonly used agents, because of their standardization, availability, familiarity, and, most importantly, their effectiveness. Initial high doses

151

rapidly reduce abdominal pain, nausea, fever, and diarrhea. Gradual tapering over weeks or months to maintenance doses brings stability to the patient.

Azulfidine (sulfasalazine) or other sulfa-containing drugs are used so frequently that they must have some value. Cytotoxic agents, such as Immuran* (azothiaprin), are used for patients whose disease does not respond to the above agents. General supportive measures, such as a liquid or low-roughage diet, pain medication, and antispasmodic drugs, give relief.

Surgical. Surgical intervention is required for intestinal obstruction, abscess from rupture or fistula, large mass of inflamed ileum and adjacent tissue, severe pain, intractable rectal disease, or fistula alone. Some surgeons, activists by nature, advise excision of the involved ileum in a patient whom other practitioners might elect to follow medically. For severe ulcerative colitis with multiple polyps or associated liver disease, total colectomy is advised.

Many patients do very well after surgery. Gut symptoms cease, extraintestinal complications, such as arthritis, subside, and the patients return to relatively normal lives unless they have ileostomies or colostomies. Other patients have intermittent disease that needs continuing medical or surgical management. A few patients have relentless, progressive disease.

Ocular. Ocular complications can be divided into three groups. Primary complications, which are associated with the activity of the Crohn's disease, occur with high frequency and respond to systemic therapy, such as systemic corticosteroids or surgical excision. Secondary complications result from another complication of Crohn's disease, and coincidental complications occur so frequently in normal people that they are considered not related.

Primary complications of Crohn's disease are a specific epithelial and anterior stromal keratopathy, limbal corneal infiltrates, subconjunctival hemorrhage, episcleritis, scleritis, acute iritis, chronic iridocyclitis, macular edema, retinal vasculitis, and papillitis. Orbital inflammation can produce proptosis, pain, and limited movement from either myositis or general inflammation. Optic neuritis can cause the loss of vision in one or both eyes or by chiasmal involvement. Episcleritis has been, in the author's experience, the most common ocular complication of Crohn's disease so that it is both a diagnostic point in the differentiation of Crohn's from ulcerative colitis and an indicator of activity of the basic disease.

Secondary complications of Crohn's disease are night blindness and dry eyes from vitamin A deficiency induced by the patient's reduced intake of vegetables that irritate the gut and because either an absent or diseased ileum prevents the normal absorption of vitamins. Refraction changes occur when patients start or stop taking systemic corticosteroids. Cataracts occur after the prolonged use of corticosteroids or because of chronic iridocyclitis. Exudative retinal detachment has been seen in two patients. Only after drainage of a psoas abscess did one patient improve. The other patient had posterior scleritis that improved with systemic corticosteroids. Optic disc edema occurred in two patients, presumably from posterior scleritis. Scleromalacia from scleritis occurred in one patient and *Candida* endophthalmitis from intravenous nutrition in another.

Coincidental complications of Crohn's disease include conjunctivitis, recurrent corneal erosion, glaucoma, and generalized retinal artery narrowing. Ulcerative colitis is complicated in the eyes by iritis and iridocyclitis.

Treatment of ocular complications begins with identification of the type of complication. Primary complications require attention to the intestinal disease and clarification of its status. More aggressive treatment either medically or surgically may be indicated. The ophthalmologist must work closely with other practitioners. Acute iritis requires topical corticosteroids, cycloplegics, and at times systemic corticosteroids. Limbal corneal infiltrates and episcleritis frequently respond to topical steroids.

Chronic iridocyclitis in patients with Crohn's disease or ulcerative colitis is a difficult problem. It is closely associated with active gut disease and has responded to excision of involved intestinal tissue. Systemic corticosteroids given for both conditions help, but are not curative. The characteristic keratopathy of Crohn's disease does not impair vision and is not painful; therefore, it requires no therapy. Macular edema syndromes usually respond to systemic corticosteroids.

Secondary complications require first the recognition that an intervening process be identified and treated. Dry eyes and night blindness are managed by giving the patient vitamin A, either parenterally or by a liquid preparation for oral ingestion and easy absorption. Exudative retinal detachment requires clarification as to whether it is secondary to scleritis or a remote abscess. Cataract is managed according to its nature. Early posterior subcapsular opacities have, in the author's experience, stopped progressing when systemic corticosteroids were stopped. However, activity of the intestinal disease may require continuation of corticosteroids. In young people, visually disabling cataract is well managed by extracapsular, irrigation-aspiration techniques through a small limbal incision.

Papillitis from posterior scleritis usually responds to systemic corticosteroids. Endophthalmitis from either bacteria or fungi can be aggressively managed by diagnostic and therapeutic vitrectomy, which provides an organism for culture and removes the mass of infected vitreous. Appropriate antimicrobial therapy depends upon identification and sensitivity studies.

Coincidental ocular disease requires only that the ophthalmologist recognize that it is not related to the intestinal disorder. Management is the same as would be given to any patient.

Management of a patient with an ocular complication of Crohn's disease or ulcerative colitis is difficult and time consuming. Efforts must be expended to clarify the status of the intestinal disease and to communicate with the other physicians involved.

References

Blase WP, Knox DL, Green WR: Granulomatous conjunctivitis in 2 patients with Crohn's disease. Br J Ophthalmol 68:901–903, 1984.

Ellis PP, Gentry JH: Ocular complications of ulcerative colitis. Am J Ophthalmol 58:779–784, 1964.

Hopkins DJ, et al: Ocular disorders in a series of 332 patients with Crohn's disease. Br J Ophthalmol 58:732–737, 1974.

Kirshner JB, Shorter RG: Recent developments in "nonspecific" inflammatory bowel disease, Parts 1 and 2. N Engl J Med 306:775–785 and 306:837–848, 1982.

Knox DL, Bayless TM: Gastrointestinal and ocular disease. In Mausolf FA (ed): The Eye and Systemic Disease. St. Louis, CV Mosby, 1975, pp 333–348.

Knox DL, Schachat AP, Mustonen E: Primary, secondary and coincidental ocular complications of Crohn's disease. Ophthalmology 91:163–173, 1984.

Knox DL, Snip RC, Stark WJ: The keratopathy of Crohn's Disease. Am J Ophthalmol 90:862–865, 1980.

Korelitz BI, Coles RS: Uveitis (iritis) associated with ulcerative and granulomatous colitis. Gastroenterology 52:78–82, 1967.

Macoul KL: Ocular changes in granulomatous ileocolitis. Arch Ophthalmol 84:95–97, 1970.

Ruby AJ, Jampol LM: Crohn's disease and retinal vascular disease. Am J Ophthalmol 110:349–353, 1990.

Salmon JF, Wright JP, Bowen RM, Murray AD: Granulomatous uveitis in Crohn's disease: A clinicopathologic case report. Arch Ophthalmol 107:718–719, 1989.

Schulman MF, Sugar A: Peripheral corneal infiltrates in inflammatory bowel disease. Ann Ophthalmol 13:109–111, 1981.

HYPOVITAMINOSIS A
264.9
(Xerophthalmia)

ALFRED SOMMER, M.D., M.H.Sc.

Baltimore, Maryland

Hypovitaminosis A is the presence of depleted tissue stores, usually reflected in low serum levels, of vitamin A. Most often, inadequate dietary intake is the cause. Interference with absorptive, storage, or transport capacities, such as in liver disease, sprue, cystic fibrosis, regional enteritis, and chronic gastroenteritis, can have the same effect. The primary ocular changes indicating vitamin A deficiency are night blindness and xerophthalmia. As a rule, these eye lesions tend to be most serious in the younger age groups, although night blindness is often difficult to substantiate in a small child. Even mild vitamin A deficiency, unaccompanied by clinical xerophthalmia, can increase a child's risk of severe infectious disease and death. High-dose vitamin A supplementation is now recommended for all children with measles who may be at risk of vitamin A deficiency and all children with moderate to severe measles, even in the absence of specific clinical signs of xerophthalmia. Acute decompensation of vitamin A status is thought to account for half of all measles-associated corneal destruction and the exacerbation of measles complications that accounts for half or more of all measles-associated mortality.

THERAPY

Systemic. The primary treatment for hypovitaminosis A is rapid replenishment of vitamin A stores. In patients with normal absorptive and storage capacities, oral administration of 200,000 IU of vitamin A[§] in oil for 2 successive days, followed by an additional dose 1 to 2 weeks later, is adequate. In patients with severe gastroenteritis, the initial dose might preferably be intramuscular injections of 100,000 IU of vitamin A in water. Patients with severe protein-energy malnutrition require additional large oral doses every 2 to 4 weeks until their protein status improves. Patients with persistent, underlying malabsorption might be handled by repeated high dosages of oral therapy, with the adequacy determined by periodic serum vitamin A determinations. When this oral therapy is ineffective, periodic parenteral administration of water-miscible vitamin A may be necessary. Children with measles, with or without ocular lesions, should be treated in the same way as children with clinical xerophthalmia: 200,000 IU vitamin A orally on 2 successive days.

Ocular. Corneal lesions frequently fail to respond to systemic therapy for 2 to 4 days. Although tretinoin is not licensed for use as a topical ophthalmic drug, 0.1 per cent tretinoin* in arachis oil applied three times daily will hasten corneal healing during the first critical days of therapy.

Corneal ulcers should be carefully observed and cultured to rule out secondary bacterial infections. Topical broad-spectrum antibiotic ointments may be applied several times daily as prophylaxis until healing is complete. Artificial tears may be used as needed. In children especially, a firm shield should protect ulcerated eyes.

Surgical. Classical vitamin-A-responsive lesions usually improve within 1 week of therapy, and most heal within 2 to 4 weeks. However, Bitot's spots that are not responsive to vitamin A may require simple excision. Most localized corneal ulcers are peripheral and tend to become plugged with iris; they do not require tectonic grafts. Limbal to limbal necrosis (keratomalacia) rapidly obliterates the anterior chamber and is rarely if ever helped by surgery.

Supportive. Adequate food intake, with particular reference to the amount and quality of dietary protein and calories, is important.

Ocular or Periocular Manifestations

Conjunctiva: Bitot's spot; xerosis.
Cornea: Edema; erosion; haziness; keratomalacia; opacity; perforation; punctate keratitis; ulcer; xerosis.
Lacrimal System: Loss of tear film wetting action.
Retina: Degeneration; depigmentation; opacity.
Other: Night blindness; scotoma; visual loss.

PRECAUTIONS

Care is required in the diagnosis of vitamin-A specific conjunctival epithelial changes. Not every slight degree of dryness or thickening of the conjunctiva should be ascribed to vitamin A depletion. Severe corneal changes, especially ulceration and keratomalacia, often occur in the absence of milder signs of vitamin A deficiency (night blindness, conjunctival xerosis, Bitot's spots). Many patients with corneal involvement have severe generalized malnutrition or systemic diseases (gastroenteritis, tuberculosis) that interfere with vitamin A metabolism and wound healing and require immediate attention.

Under no circumstances should oil-miscible vitamin A be used for parenteral therapy. The vitamin is released slowly, if at all, from the injection site.

Use of topical ophthalmic tretinoin can lead to increased scarring and should be reserved for eyes with corneal xerosis, nonaxial ulcers, or for one eye of patients with axial ulcers in both.

COMMENTS

The most sensitive clinical test for vitamin A deficiency is measurement of dark adaptation. Determination of vitamin A concentration in the serum is less reliable, since the serum level may not fall below 0.2 µg/ml until the body's reserves are extensively depleted. The relative dose-response test is a useful index of liver vitamin A stores, without the need for a biopsy. It is thus the most practical, sensitive indicator of substandard vitamin A status available for the management of chronic, marginal deficiency. A therapeutic trial with vitamin A is safe and invariably simpler, less expensive, and more definitive in potential cases of clinical disease than are the various criteria for assessing vitamin A status.

Many of these patients have inadequate aqueous tears, as well as a deficiency of goblet cells and mucus. Tears may be unable to spread over the epithelial surface and maintain a moist protective tear film. The corneal epithelium may be damaged by evaporation and can become susceptible to secondary bacterial infection.

Vitamin A deficiency is a systemic disease that ophthalmologists are often in the position to detect first. Adequate attention must be paid to potential systemic effects and the need for supportive therapy.

References

Barclay AJG, Foster A, Sommer A: Vitamin A supplements and mortality related to measles: A randomised clinical trial. Br Med J 294:294–296, 1987.

Foster A, Sommer A: Corneal ulceration, measles, and childhood blindness in Tanzania. Br J Ophthalmol 71:331–343, 1987.

Hussey GD, Klein M: A randomized, controlled trial of vitamin A in children with severe measles. N Engl J Med 323:160–164, 1990.

Sommer A: Nutritional Blindness: Xerophthalmia and Keratomalacia. New York, Oxford University Press, 1982.

Sommer A, Emran N: Topical retinoic acid in the treatment of corneal xerophthalmia. Am J Ophthalmol 86:615–617, 1978.

Sommer A, et al: Vitamin-A-responsive panocular xerophthalmia in a healthy adult. Arch Ophthalmol 96:1630–1634, 1978.

Sommer A, Emran N, Tamba T: Vitamin A responsive punctate keratopathy in xerophthalmia. Am J Ophthalmol 87:330–333, 1979.

Sommer A, et al: History of nightblindness: A simple tool for xerophthalmia screening. Am J Clin Nutr 33:887–891, 1980.

Sommer A, et al: Oral versus intramuscular vitamin A in the treatment of xerophthalmia. Lancet 1:557–559, 1980.

Sommer A, et al: Protein deficiency and treatment of xerophthalmia. Arch Ophthalmol 100:785–787, 1982.

Sommer A, et al: Impact of vitamin A supplementation on childhood mortality: A randomised controlled community trial. Lancet 1:1169–1173, 1986.

SECTION 5

DISORDERS OF PROTEIN METABOLISM

CYSTINOSIS 270.0

RANDALL V. WONG, M.D.,
and VERNON G. WONG, M.D.

Washington, District of Columbia

Cystinosis is a rare, recessively inherited error of metabolism characterized by increased intracellular (nonprotein) levels of free cystine that appear to be localized within lysosomes. Cystine accumulates within the bone marrow, reticuloendothelial cells, kidneys, cornea, and conjunctiva. Three forms of cystinosis—nephropathic, intermediate, and benign (also known as infantile, adolescent, and adult)—have been described, and in all three forms crystal deposits develop in the cornea and conjunctiva.

The most severe form, nephropathic, becomes symptomatic in the first few years of life and is characterized by polyuria, polydipsia, progressive renal failure (Fanconi's syndrome), rickets, and growth retardation. Late in the course of nephropathic cystinosis, severe hypothyroidism, splenomegaly, and hepatomegaly may be seen at times. The intermediate form has variable renal failure and presents later in life. Death is common within the first decade in nephropathic cystinosis, whereas patients with benign cystinosis, true to its name, seem to have a normal life expectancy.

Ocular symptoms include photophobia and crystal deposits (tinsel-like and glistening) located in the cornea and conjunctiva. An early ocular finding is a peripheral pigmentary retinopathy that will progress to visual impairment.

THERAPY

Systemic. Therapeutic attempts to remove or reduce the cystine load in the cells, thereby reversing or retarding further damage, have been made with penicillamine[†] and ascorbic acid,[†] but have been found to be ineffective. Oral mercaptamine[†] at daily doses of 30 to 90 mg/kg seems to be of benefit when instituted early in the disease.

Mercaptamine has been shown to lower cystine levels in vitro and in vivo, and growth can be improved and renal deterioration delayed or prevented.

Ocular. Treatment of the photophobia associated with all forms of this disease is symptomatic. Dark glasses and avoidance of bright light are partially effective. Mercaptamine 0.1 per cent eyedrops have been shown to clear corneal crystals in a limited number of children.

Surgical. Treatment of renal failure associated with the nephropathic and intermediate forms has been achieved with renal transplant. The success of this method is sufficient to recommend it when renal failure supervenes.

Successful corneal transplantation has been achieved in one reported case, but recurrent crystal deposition may occur later.

Supportive. Adequate fluid intake, vitamin D supplements, and control of chronic acidosis and hypophosphatemia are important in the nephropathic and later in the intermediate forms of cystinosis. Dietary restriction of cystine and methionine is not effective.

Ocular or Periocular Manifestations

Choroid: Crystal deposits.
Conjunctiva: Crystal deposits.
Cornea: Crystal deposits (initially confined to anterior stroma, but progress to full thickness).
Iris: Crystal deposits.
Retina: Pigment epithelial degeneration (nephropathic form).
Other: Lacrimation; photophobia.

PRECAUTIONS

Mercaptamine therapy has been reported to cause reversible seizures in the higher dosage range of 90 mg/kg.

Long-term follow-up in renal transplant patients demonstrated progression of corneal crystal deposition, as well as progressive retinal pigment degeneration involving the posterior pole and occasionally the macula. Decrease in visual acuity has also been documented. It would seem that, although renal transplant prolongs life, it does not halt progression of the disease.

155

COMMENTS

The ophthalmologist commonly makes the diagnosis of cystinosis by noting the deposition of crystals in the cornea and conjunctiva, but multiple myeloma may also present a similar appearance. The diagnosis of cystinosis can be confirmed by an assay of cystine content of a conjunctival biopsy specimen, cultured skin fibroblasts, or polymorphonuclear leukocytes. A pulse-label technique can be used with amniotic cells to provide an in utero diagnosis of the homozygote state. The heterozygote state can also be detected, but cystine values may overlap normal values.

References

Gahl WA, et al: Cystinosis: Progress in a prototypic disease. Ann Intern Med 109:557–569, 1988.

Kaiser-Kupfer MI, et al: Removal of corneal crystals by topical cysteamine in nephropathic cystinosis. N Engl J Med 316:775–779, 1987.

Kaiser-Kupfer MI, et al: Clear graft two years later after keratopathy in nephropathic cystinosis. Am J Ophthalmol 105:318–319, 1988.

Katz B, et al: Recurrent crystal deposition after keratopathy in nephropathic cystinosis. Am J Ophthalmol 104:190–191, 1987.

Sanderson PO, et al: Cystinosis: A clinical, histopathologic, and ultrastructural study. Arch Ophthalmol 91:270–274, 1974.

Schneider JA, Schulman JD, Seegmiller JE: Cystinosis and the Fanconi sydrome. In Stanbury JB, Wyngaarden JB, Frederickson DS (eds): The Metabolic Basis of Inherited Disease, 4th ed. New York, McGraw-Hill, 1978, pp 1660–1682.

Wong VG: Ocular manifestations in cystinosis. Birth Defects 12:181–186, 1976.

Wong VG, Lietman PS, Seegmiller JE: Alterations of pigment epithelium in cystinosis. Arch Ophthalmol 77:361–369, 1967.

Yamamoto GK, et al: Long-term ocular changes in cystinosis: Observations in renal transplant recipients. J Pediatr Ophthalmol Strabismus 16:21–25, 1979.

HOMOCYSTINURIA 270.4

RAPHAEL S. BLOCH, M.D., F.A.C.S.

Mount Kisco, New York

Homocystinuria is a genetically determined error of the metabolism of methionine, one of the essential amino acids. Its incidence has been estimated to vary from 1 in 50,000 to 1 in 200,000 live births. The disorder is most commonly caused by the absence or deficiency of cystathionine beta-synthase, an enzyme that is active in one step of the catabolic pathway through which methionine is ultimately degraded to cysteine. As a consequence of this biochemical defect, there are increased concentrations of methionine and homocyst(e)ine in body fluids and diminished concentrations of cysteine. Elevated tissue levels of homocyst(e)ine are postulated to be responsible for the extensive connective tissue abnormalities observed in this disease. Homocystinuria is inherited by the autosomal recessive mode, but there is considerable heterogeneity in both its biochemical and clinical expressivity. Nearly half of the patients retain a small but measurable amount of beta-synthase activity; this group is less severely affected and more responsive to therapy than those with total absence of the enzyme.

The clinical signs of homocystinuria are not apparent at birth. Beginning in early childhood, however, there is progressive involvement of the eye and nervous, skeletal, and vascular systems. Developmental delays may be detected in the first year, e.g., failure to sit or crawl in the appropriate age range. Mental retardation is evident by mid-childhood in about half of all patients. Subluxation of the lens occurs by the age of 10 in most cases, is usually bilateral, and is often the diagnostic feature of the disease. In later childhood the patients are typically tall and thin, blond and blue-eyed, with elongated digits, knockknees, and diffuse osteoporosis on x-ray. The most ominous complication of homocystinuria is the propensity to thromboembolism. This may occur at any age, can involve both the arterial and venous vasculature of any organ, and results in a mortality rate of approximately 25 per cent before age 30.

It is of interest that heterozygosity for homocystinuria, estimated to occur in 1 to 2 per cent of the population and previously viewed as an asymptomatic carrier state, has recently been implicated as a significant risk factor for atherosclerotic vascular disease.

THERAPY

Systemic. Initially, the only therapy for homocystinuria was nutritional—restriction of dietary intake of methionine and supplementation with oral cysteine. Several low-methionine "medical foods," formulated from both natural and synthetic sources, are commercially available. Such a regimen has been effective in preventing or ameliorating some of the complications of homocystinuria, including the rate of lens dislocation.

At present, pharmacologic doses of pyridoxine (vitamin B_6),* ranging up to 1.2 gm daily, are tried in all cases. Pyridoxine is a cofactor for the deficient enzyme, and its administration results in marked biochemical improvement within several weeks in a significant percentage of patients. Responsiveness to pyridoxine is strongly correlated with detectable residual cystathionine beta-synthase activity. Current studies suggest that, in responsive patients, pyridoxine is effective in reducing the incidence of thromboembolic events, as well as lens dislocation.

Pyridoxine therapy may be supplemented with oral folic acid, another member of the vitamin B complex, that enhances the re-methylation of homocysteine back to methionine.

For those individuals not responsive to pyridoxine, an alternative approach to management is the use of chemical agents that reverse the catabolic degradation of methionine, thereby preventing the build-up of homocysteine to toxic levels. Betaine,* in doses of 6 gm daily, has been successfully employed for this purpose, with substantial biochemical and clinical improvement. More recently, betaine has also been used as supplemental treatment in pyridoxine responders, effectively normalizing plasma homocysteine levels after the ingestion of methionine.

Ocular. Refractive errors should be treated with conventional optical correction for as long as possible. Acute glaucoma caused by incarceration of the ectopic lens in the pupil is an emergency condition and is preferably managed with mydriasis and pressure on the cornea, with the patient supine in order to reposition the lens in the posterior chamber. This treatment should be followed by miotic therapy to help retain the lens behind the pupil and a peripheral iridotomy (laser or surgical) to prevent subsequent episodes of pupillary block. In the event that the lens cannot be dislodged, it is advisable to perform the iridotomy and then repeat the repositioning procedure.

Surgical extraction of the dislocated lens is usually a procedure of last resort for impaired vision or pupillary block, as it carries a high risk of vitreous loss and hemorrhage.

Ocular or Periocular Manifestations

Globe: Buphthalmos; posterior staphyloma.
Lens: Subluxation; dislocation; spherophakia; cataract.
Optic Nerve: Atrophy.
Retina: Peripheral cystoid degeneration; peripheral pigmentary degeneration; retinal detachment; retinal artery occlusion.
Uvea: Pigment atrophy of iris and choroid.
Other: Myopia; glaucoma with or without pupillary block; strabismus.

PRECAUTIONS

There is significant morbidity and mortality from thromboembolism following all surgery in homocystinuria, including ophthalmic procedures. The risk is greatest with general anesthesia, which is usually mandatory for young or retarded patients; local anesthesia is also dangerous when it is injected in proximity to important blood vessels. Optimal perioperative management includes adequate hydration, reduction of blood viscosity and platelet adhesiveness with the infusion of

dextran, and early postoperative ambulation. Conventional anticoagulant therapy is not advisable, but a regimen of dipyridamole or aspirin to inhibit platelet aggregation may be helpful in the postoperative period.

COMMENTS

Early diagnosis and treatment are the keys to effective prevention of the complications of homocystinuria. Mass neonatal screening programs have successfully detected this and several other treatable metabolic diseases. Because of the relatively early appearance of ocular abnormalities, particularly lens subluxation, the ophthalmologist can play a critical role in the diagnosis and management of this sight-threatening and life-threatening disorder.

References

Burke J, et al: Ocular complications in homocystinuria—early and late treated. Br J Ophthalmol 73: 427–431, 1989.
Clarke, R, et al: Hyperhomocysteinemia: An independent risk factor for vascular disease. N Engl J Med 324:1149–1155, 1991.
Cross H, Jensen A: Ocular manifestations in the Marfan syndrome and homocystinuria. Am J Ophthalmol 75:405–420, 1973.
Elsas L, Acosta P: Nutrition support of inherited metabolic diseases. In Shils M, Young V (eds): Modern Nutrition in Health and Disease, 7th ed. Philadelphia, Lea & Febiger, 1988, pp 1363–1367.
Mudd S, Levy H, Skovby F: Disorders of transsulfuration. In Scriver C, et al (eds): The Metabolic Basis of Inherited Disease, 6th ed. New York, McGraw-Hill, 1989, pp 693–734.
Mudd S, et al: The natural history of homocystinuria due to cystathionine beta-synthase deficiency. Am J Hum Genet 37:1–31, 1985.
Parris W, Quimby C: Anesthetic considerations for the patient with homocystinuria. Anesth Analg 61:708–710, 1982.
Wilcken D, et al: Homocystinuria—The effects of betaine in the treatment of patients not responsive to pyridoxine. N Engl J Med 309:448–453, 1983.
Wilcken D, et al: Homocystinuria due to cystathionine beta-synthase deficiency—The effects of betaine treatment in pyridoxine-responsive patients. Metabolism 34:1115–1121, 1985.

MAPLE SYRUP URINE DISEASE 270.3
(Branched-Chain Ketoaciduria, MSUD)

LAWRENCE G. TOMASI, M.D., Ph.D.
Loma Linda, California

Maple syrup urine disease (MSUD) is an autosomal recessive disorder characterized by a marked elevation in branched-chain amino acids (leucine, isoleucine, and valine) and their respective ketoacids in the serum. The disease derives its name from the odor similar to maple sugar (burned sugar) in the urine. The enzymatic defect is in the oxidative decarboxylation of these ketoacids by a high-molecular-weight multienzyme complex that involves five closely linked enzymatic reactions and multiple co-factors, including thiamine and lipoic acid. The variability in the symptomatology of the disorder has been correlated with the level of residual enzymatic activity. Currently, the enzymatic abnormalities in MSUD are grouped as follows: (1) classical, (2) intermittent, (3) intermediate, (4) thiamine-responsive, and (5) E_3-deficient phenotypes. These variant groups represent mutations that involve different reactions in the multienzyme complex or, alternatively, may be multiple alleles for a single genetic locus.

The more classical presentations include initial symptoms of poor weight gain, vomiting, lethargy, and seizures that are related to the elevated blood levels of the branched-chain amino acids and their metabolites, particularly leucine. Although leucine-induced hypoglycemia commonly accompanies the metabolic derangement, the mechanisms by which central nervous system injury occurs remain uncertain. Postulated mechanisms include an inhibition of protein synthesis secondary to the disturbed free amino acid pool and/or an inhibition of glutamic acid decarboxylation by the elevated branched-chain ketoacids, leading to altered levels of the putative neurotransmitter gamma-aminobutyric acid (GABA).

Late signs of central nervous system injury include generalized increased muscle tone, opisthotonus, coma, microcephaly, and severe psychomotor delay, with death occurring in untreated patients secondary to an intercurrent infection. In those with classical MSUD, death may occur in the first week of life and almost certainly within the first year.

Neuropathologic studies on patients succumbing during the first month of life demonstrate only a sponginess of the white matter attributed to edema. In those patients who survive well into the first year, a deficiency in myelin and an astrocytosis are noted that are similar to that described in patients with other aminoacidopathies, such as phenylketonuria. These nonspecific alterations within the central nervous system reflect a delay in myelinogenesis, rather than defective synthesis or increased destruction of the myelin. More recently, these neuropathologic findings can be demonstrated antemortem by CT scan or magnetic resonance imaging (MRI). Mild to moderate atrophy with a marked diffuse, low-density attenuation of the white matter has been described in both the cerebellum and the cerebral hemispheres. In addition, abnormalities of the gray matter within the globus pallidus as well as the thalamus are de-

scribed, a finding that may be unique to MSUD. A reversibility of these abnormalities within the gray matter has been reported after dietary treatment. Status spongiosus, together with dysmyelination, is the pathologic counterpart of the CT and MRI abnormalities.

Increasingly, variants of MSUD have been reported in which intermittent central nervous system dysfunction occurs, rather than the overwhelming illness of the classical disease. Age of onset in these patients is usually in the first decade of life, but has been reported at 40 years of age, with intermittent episodes of lethargy, nystagmus, ataxia, and seizures usually in association with an intercurrent infectious illness. Two recent reports reflect this variability. The mother of a child with intermittent MSUD, and thus an obligatory carrier of the trait, demonstrated neurologic symptoms at 40 years of age that were responsive to dietary therapy. A 15-year follow-up of an infant with thiamine-responsive MSUD reported that the adolescent had a normal social life and attended a regular high school. She exhibited neither epilepsy nor behavioral abnormalities, and her current IQ was 85 on the WISC-R. She had experienced five episodes of metabolic decompensation over this 15-year period with clinical symptomatology of seizures and coma, one of which was of sufficient severity to require peritoneal dialysis.

In such patients, the characteristic elevation in serum and urine branched-chain amino acids and ketoacids is present, although these abnormalities may not be discernible during symptom-free intervals. Confirmation of the diagnosis by direct assay of the branched-chain oxidative decarboxylase activity in either white cells or cultured fibroblasts of patients is possible either during an acute attack or during symptom-free intervals. In general, age of onset and severity of symptoms are related to residual enzymatic activity; classical MSUD patients demonstrate less than 2 per cent of normal activity, whereas those with the mildest symptoms have enzymatic activity levels of between 8 and 15 per cent of normal values. Recent studies have precluded a defect in either the transcription of DNA or the processing of RNA in selected cultures of MSUD fibroblasts.

Ocular manifestations have been reported in both classical MSUD and its variants. Their incidence and prevalence, however, are markedly increased in the variant forms perhaps because such signs in classical MSUD are masked by a severe encephalopathy. In contrast to other inborn errors of metabolism in which complex sphingolipids accumulate from conception within the lysosome (i.e., Tay-Sachs disease), these branched-chain amino acids are readily removed from the fetus via the placenta during gestation. Thus, symptoms of MSUD are absent at birth, may become apparent within the first week of life, and fluctuate with both the infant's protein intake and general metabolic status. The commonly noted decreased visual attentiveness on initial presentation is almost certainly due to cerebral cortical rather than ocular dysfunction, with its severity related to the infant's level of consciousness. The optic atrophy described in the older untreated patients has a gray rather than a white hue, reflecting the generalized defect in myelination described throughout the central nervous system, as demonstrated neuropathologically by Franke and co-workers. Disturbances in ocular movements include gaze paresis either upward, combined vertical and horizontal, or adductor. Ptosis and sluggish pupillary light reaction also are commonly reported signs. Nystagmus is a frequently reported finding with the initial clinical symptomatology and also during the recovery phase with treatment. As an initial finding in these patients, it may represent the subtle seizures that are described with the encephalopathy. During recovery, it should not be confused with the progression of the neurologic symptoms. The localization of the dysfunction within the neuro-ophthalmologic pathways is unclear, but diffuse cerebral edema, subtle seizures, and a thiamine-dependent variant should have a greater consideration in the differential diagnosis.

THERAPY

Systemic. Since the branched-chain amino acids cannot be synthesized in animals, therapy of MSUD, as in other aminoacidopathies, is based on dietary control of these essential amino acids. Unlike phenylketonuria, however, such dietary control must be lifelong. In classical MSUD, an amino acid mixture tailored to the patient's weight and growth potential is utilized, whereas patients with the variant form require less stringent dietary control. Frequently, at the time that the diagnosis is initially made, the levels of the branched-chain amino acids and ketoacids are extremely elevated, which produces severe neurologic symptoms and signs that may be life threatening. A similar picture occurs episodically in patients on a prescribed diet or in those with a variant form, usually during an intercurrent illness. As a rule, parenterally administered fluids containing glucose and electrolytes, followed by an amino acid diet in which the branched-chain amino acids are omitted, will reverse these findings. Occasionally, this standard regimen is unsatisfactory, and an exchange transfusion or peritoneal dialysis may be lifesaving.

Ocular. Strabismus therapy may require glasses, patching, or surgery. Ptosis surgery may be indicated if warranted by the cosmetic or functional deficit.

Ocular or Periocular Manifestations

Extraocular Muscles: Nystagmus; ophthalmoplegia.
Eyebrows or Eyelids: Elevation; epicanthal folds; ptosis.
Optic Nerve: Atrophy.
Pupil: Decreased or absent reaction to light.
Other: Convergent strabismus; cortical visual inattentiveness.

PRECAUTIONS

Early diagnosis and dietary treatment are imperative to prevent mental retardation and death. In classical MSUD, generalized systemic symptoms are more prominent than the ocular manifestations. On the other hand, ophthalmoplegia is a relatively uncommon sign in the newborn nursery and has been the initial feature in many infants who become symptomatic during the neonatal period and early infancy. An easily obtainable and rapid screening test for urinary ketoacids utilizing 2,4-dinitrophenylhydrazine is available in most hospitals. Although more specific assays are necessary to establish the diagnosis, this screening test remains useful because of its widespread availability and infrequent false-negative results.

The ophthalmologist is more likely to be confronted with one of the variant forms of MSUD or the patient whose classical MSUD is under treatment but has decompensated with the metabolic stress of an infectious illness. In either case, both the ocular manifestations and biochemical abnormalities will only be present during the period of decompensation. Thus, the screening test for urinary ketoacids will be a useful addition to the diagnostic studies utilized in the evaluation of these ocular manifestations.

COMMENTS

The mean incidence of MSUD from various studies is 1:250,000. Although dietary treatment prolongs life and prevents mental retardation, such patients are exceedingly difficult to manage in comparison to those with the more commonly encountered phenylketonuria, which has a disease incidence of 1:13,000. In the United States, all 50 states screen for phenylketonuria, whereas 20 states presently are screening for MSUD. Difficulties in management include the necessity to balance three amino acids in the diet, their ubiquitous presence in food from which they cannot be removed, frequent life-threatening decompensations that occur in patients while on treatment, and the apparent need to continue dietary management throughout the life span. Computerized dietary management plans have been reported for both infants and adults.

Although screening the population for heterozygotes has not proven feasible because of the rarity of this condition, antepartum diagnosis is available to families who are at risk because of an affected child. The enzyme is normally present in fibroblasts grown from amniotic fluid cells, and affected fetuses have been identified in utero.

References

Chabria S, Tomasi LG, Wong PWK: Ophthalmoplegia and bulbar palsy in variant form of maple syrup urine disease. Ann Neurol 6:71–72, 1979.

Ellingsen LI, Haugstad TS, Holm H: Tailoring of the diet for the individual in maple syrup urine disease: Long-term home dietary treatment of an adult patient with MSUD by monitoring of daily intake with a personal computer. A case report. Hum Nutr Appl Nutr 39A:130–136, 1985.

Franke G, et al: Ophthalmologische und histopathologische befunde bei Ahornsirup-Krankheit. Ophthalmology 80:457–459, 1983.

Holmgren G, et al: Intermittent neurological symptoms in a girl with a maple syrup urine disease (MSUD) variant. Neuropediatrics 11:377–383, 1980.

Hu CW, et al: Isolation and sequencing of a cDNA encoding the decarboxylase (E1) alpha precursor of bovine branched-chain alpha-keto acid dehydrogenase complex. Expression of E1 alpha mRNA and subunit in maple-syrup-urine-disease and 3T3-L1 cells. J Biol Chem 263:9007–9014, 1988.

Mantovani JF, et al: MSUD: Presentation with pseudotumor cerebri and CT abnormalities. J Pediatr 96:279–281, 1980.

Naughten ER, et al: Early diagnosis and dietetic management in newborn with maple syrup urine disease. Birth to six weeks. J Inherited Metab Dis 8(Suppl 2):131–132, 1985.

Paul TD, Naylor EW, Guthrie R: Urine screening for metabolic disease in newborn infants. J Pediatr 96:653–656, 1980.

Schriver CR, et al: So-called thiamine-responsive maple syrup urine disease: 15-year follow-up of the original patient. J Pediatr 107:763–765, 1985.

Suzuki S, et al: Cranial computed tomography in a patient with a variant form of maple syrup urine disease. Neuropediatrics 14:102–103, 1983.

Tanaka K, Rosenberg LE: Disorders of branched chain amino acid metabolism. In Stanbury JB, et al (ed): The Metabolic Basis of Inherited Disease, 5th ed. New York, McGraw-Hill, 1983, pp 440–473.

Taylor D: Ophthalmological features of some human hereditary disorders with demyelination. Bull Soc Belge Ophthalmol 208:405–413, 1983.

Uziel G, Savoiardo M, Nardocci N: CT and MRI in maple syrup urine disease. Neurology 38:486–488, 1988.

OCULOCEREBRORENAL SYNDROME 270.8
(Lowe's Syndrome)

ANDREA CIBIS TONGUE, M.D.

Lake Oswego, Oregon

Oculocerebrorenal (OCRL) or Lowe's syndrome is an X-linked recessive metabolic disorder characterized by congenital cataracts, glaucoma, hypotonic facies with frontal bossing and deep-set eyes, mental and motor retardation, muscular hypotonia, areflexia, hyperexcitability, and renal tubular dysfunction (Fanconi's syndrome) with proteinuria, aminoaciduria, metabolic acidosis, inability to acidify urine, rickets, and osteomalacia. Ocular abnormalities and proteinuria may be the only stigmata present during early infancy and the first stage of the disease. Aminoaciduria may not be present until 1 year of age or later. Neurologic abnormalities likewise are often not striking during the first year, but are noted in all affected infants over 1 year of age. Metabolic abnormalities appear during the second stage and can be ameliorated by supportive systemic therapy. During the third stage, metabolic abnormalities may disappear, and systemic therapy may no longer be necessary. Joint dislocation and scoliosis can develop secondary to hypotonia and joint hypermobility. Mental retardation is usually profound, but some patients with IQs of 70 and 80 have been reported. Behavioral changes with aggressive behavior have been reported in 20 to 40 per cent of patients, usually after age 5, and improving in one-third during the teens. Patients with supportive metabolic therapy may live to be 30 or 40 years old, succumbing generally from infections or renal failure due to glomerular involvement.

A primary biochemical defect has not been identified, and there is no biochemical assay that confirms the diagnosis of OCRL. The incidence of OCRL is estimated to be 1 in 200,000 live births. The disorder is X-linked recessive and has been mapped to the Xq24-26 region.

THERAPY

Systemic. Supportive treatment is aimed at correcting the metabolic abnormalities caused by the proximal renal tubular malfunction. Fluid replacement, alkali therapy, correction of electrolyte imbalance, and supplements of vitamin D ameliorate the metabolic acidosis, rickets, and osteomalacia.

Surgical. Removal of dense cataracts is indicated in the hope of preventing marked visual impairment. However, visual acuity is not expected to be better than 20/100, even with optimal treatment results. The surgeon should be prepared to perform a posterior capsulotomy and anterior vitrectomy, since the flat discoid lenses are strongly adherent to the anterior vitreous in many patients.

Management of glaucoma is essentially the same as for other types of congenital or infantile glaucomas. The etiology of glaucoma is not clear, but in some patients, it may be secondary to angle anomalies or to pupillary block.

Corneal keloid formation in older children may cause significant visual impairment, initiating an attempt at corneal surgery. Keloids, however, recur and are a most difficult management problem. Exposure and trauma to the epithelium may be contributing factors to the keloid formation, since they are typically in the lower half to two-thirds of the cornea. Rarely, they may be seen in the superior cornea, which is covered by the upper lid. Several months after cataract surgery, one patient was observed to develop keloid formation at the entry site of the irrigation canula in the inferior temporal cornea adjacent to the limbus. Another patient developed keloids after persistent punctate epithelial keratitis of the inferior cornea, secondary possibly to exposure and recurrent staphylococcal keratitis. This raises the question whether corneal incisions should be avoided in these patients. Other patients have been reported to have keloids without a history of preceding trauma.

To minimize corneal epithelial trauma, spectacle correction of the aphakia may be preferable to contact lens correction. Likewise, efforts should be made to minimize corneal exposure; partial tarsorrhaphy may be helpful.

Of interest is the formation of fibroids, desmoids, and noninflammatory swelling of joints and extremities in a number of OCRL patients. The pathophysiology may be similar to corneal keloids.

Ocular or Periocular Manifestations

Anterior Chamber: Embryonic angle.
Cornea: Edema; keloid formation; megalocornea; microcornea (rare); opacity; pannus; thickened Descemet's membrane.
Globe: Buphthalmos; microphthalmos.
Iris and Ciliary Body: Atrophy, hypoplasia and segmental aplasia of dilator pupillae muscle; poorly developed ciliary muscle; posterior synechia; rudimentary ciliary processes.
Lens: Cataracts; microphakia; posterior lenticonus.
Orbit: Deep-set eyes; orbital fat atrophy.
Retina: Lange's folds; sclerosis and hyalinization of retinal vessels.
Other: Glaucoma; miosis; nystagmus; strabismus.

PRECAUTIONS

Any male infant with congenital cataracts should be suspected of having OCRL. It is important to remember that proteinuria may be the only other early manifestation of the disorder. Typically, the cataracts are flat, discoid, and central. Often, the pupil is miotic and resistant to mydriatics. Glaucoma is not a necessary accompaniment of the disease, but occurs in about 50 per cent of the patients. In older children, degenerative changes of the cornea with vascularization and keloid formation are significant factors in causing further visual impairment.

COMMENTS

Prompt recognition of the disease is necessary for the institution of appropriate systemic therapy and amelioration of the metabolic abnormalities. Genetic counseling with identification of possible carrier females is important. The ophthalmologist is in the position of identifying OCRL heterozygotes because of the lens abnormalities that they demonstrate. Lens abnormalities include punctate opacities usually greater than 15 to 25 per quadrant (usually more than 100 per lens), subcapsular plaques, linear opacities, and posterior polar cataracts. If appropriate genetic counseling is to be carried out, careful slit-lamp examination with the pupil dilated is therefore mandatory in all females who are at risk for being a carrier of the OCRL gene. Gene mapping has located the abnormality to the Xq24-26 region.

The recurrence risk for having an affected male for a woman who is a heterozygote is 25 per cent for each pregnancy, and 50 per cent if the fetus is a male. Each female offspring of a heterozygous female has a 50 per cent chance of inheriting the abnormal gene. If a female is not identified by slit-lamp examination to be a heterozygote but there is a family history of OCRL, the risk is estimated to be 6 per cent that she is a nonpenetrant carrier, and the risk for her having an affected son is estimated to be 1.5 per cent. Examination of chromosomes by RFLP analysis is useful in establishing the carrier state in females with negative slit-lamp examinations in families with OCRL. Unaffected male offspring of heterozygous females do not carry the gene and do not produce affected offspring.

References

Abassi V, Lowe C, Calcagno PL: Oculo-cerebrorenal syndrome. A review. Am J Dis Child *115*: 145–168, 1968.
Cibis G, et al: Corneal keloid in Lowe's syndrome. Arch Ophthalmol *100*:1795–1799, 1982.
Cibis G, et al. Lenticular opacities in carriers of Lowe's syndrome. Ophthalmology *93*:1041–1045, 1986.
Charnas LR, Gahl WA: Oculocerebrorenal syndrome of Lowe. Adv Pediatr *38*:75–107, 1991.

TYROSINEMIA II 270.2
(Pseudodendritic Keratitis, Recessive Keratosis Palmoplantaris, Richner-Hanhart Syndrome)

STEPHEN P. CHRISTIANSEN, M.D.

Little Rock, Arkansas

Tyrosinemia II is an autosomal recessive metabolic disorder caused by deficiency of hepatic cytoplasmic tyrosine aminotransferase (cTAT). The gene for this enzyme has been mapped to chromosome 16q 22.1. Hepatic mitochondrial TAT levels are normal. Cytoplasmic TAT catalyzes the conversion of tyrosine to p-hydroxyphenylpyruvic acid (p-HPPA). Deficiency of cTAT results in elevated plasma tyrosine concentration, tyrosinuria, and tyrosyluria. In affected patients, plasma tyrosine ranges from 16 to 62 mg/dl (normal, 0.6 to 2.1 mg/dl).

Patients with this disorder have characteristic ocular and skin lesions. It is thought that tyrosine crystallizes within cells, initiating an inflammatory cascade. Most patients develop bilateral pseudodendritic keratitis early within the first year of life. Onset is variable, however, and ranges from 2 weeks of age to late in the second decade. Some patients never develop ocular findings. Ocular involvement is usually heralded by pain, photophobia, tearing, and conjunctival injection.

The keratitis has been described as stellate or branching and is initially restricted to the epithelium. It is often confused with herpes simplex keratitis. However, the bilateral presentation, minimal staining with fluorescein or rose bengal, negative viral studies, normal corneal sensation, and lack of response to topical antiviral therapy allow one to rule out a herpetic etiology.

As the disease progresses, corneal ulceration, subepithelial and stromal scarring, and corneal neovascularization may occur with resultant visual loss. Cataracts and glaucoma have also been described in untreated patients. Nystagmus and exotropia have been noted in some patients with tyrosinemia II; these may be a consequence of visual loss, rather than a primary effect of the disease.

Cutaneous lesions typically occur with or after the eye lesions. They begin as blisters or erosions on the palms and soles, particularly on the tips of the digits and the thenar and hypothenar eminences. The blisters crust and eventually become hyperkeratotic. The lesions are painful but not pruritic and often present in a linear distribution. The severity of cutaneous involvement may wax and wane independently of systemic or topical therapy. Some authors have described symptomatic improvement in ocular and cutaneous symptoms during the summer months.

Mental retardation, learning disability, behavioral anomalies, microcephaly, growth retardation, and seizures have been noted in some patients with tyrosinemia II, but are, at best, inconsistent findings. One patient has been described with multiple congenital anomalies.

THERAPY

Systemic. The mainstay of therapy in tyrosinemia II is dietary restriction of tyrosine and phenylalanine intake. This diet may be initiated with a prepared formula, such as the Mead Johnson 3200 AB diet. As plasma tyrosine levels decrease, the diet may be liberalized, with the goal of therapy to maintain plasma tyrosine in the range of 10 mg/dl. Reduction of plasma tyrosine results in fairly rapid resolution of both ocular and cutaneous lesions, both of which will recur if an unrestricted diet is resumed. The effect of dietary control on the occurrence of mental retardation in tyrosinemia II is unknown. Oral retinoids have been used to control cutaneous lesions even when dietary compliance is poor. No other systemic or topical treatments have proven effective to date, including steroids.

Ocular. The early ocular manifestations of tyrosinemia II respond rapidly to dietary therapy. Therefore, initial ocular therapy is usually symptomatic. Topical corticosteroid, antiviral, and antibiotic therapy have all been shown to be ineffective. If corneal scarring or neovascularization has affected the visual axis, lamellar or penetrating keratoplasty may be necessary. Keratitis may recur in the graft if plasma tyrosine is not controlled. One author has suggested that topical corticosteroids after penetrating keratoplasty may promote recurrence of keratitis in the graft. Excimer laser photokeratectomy may be useful in this disorder if corneal scarring and neovascularization are superficial.

Ocular or Periocular Manifestations

Conjunctiva: Discrete plaques; hyperemia; mucous discharge; papillary hypertrophy.

Cornea: Stellate or pseudodendritic keratitis; erosion; ulceration; haze; scarring; neovascularization.

Lens: Subcapsular cataract.

Other: Glaucoma; nystagmus; strabismus; ocular pain; photophobia; visual loss.

PRECAUTIONS

Patients with tyrosinemia II may first present with ocular symptoms and signs. Thus, it is imperative that the ophthalmologist consider this metabolic cause of keratitis during the initial evaluation. Clinical suspicion of this disorder can be easily confirmed with amino acid studies. Early diagnosis and dietary intervention may ultimately prevent visual loss.

COMMENTS

Tyrosinemia II is distinct from tyrosinemia I, another recessive disorder caused by a deficiency of fumarylacetoacetate hydrolase. Patients with tyrosinemia I also have elevated levels of tyrosine and its metabolites. However, these patients do not have the characteristic cutaneous or ocular findings of patients with tyrosinemia II. Rather, they characteristically have hepatic and renal dysfunction or failure.

References

Balato N, Cusano F, Lembo G, Santoianni P: Tyrosinemia type II in the two cases previously reported as Richner-Hanhart syndrome. Dermatologica 173:66–74, 1986.

Goldsmith LA, LaBerge C: Tyrosinemia and related disorders. *In* Scriver CR, Beaudet AL, Sly WS, Valle D (eds): The Metabolic Basis of Inherited Disease. New York, McGraw-Hill, 1989, vol 1, pp 547–562.

Heidemann DG, Dunn SP, Bawle EV, Shepherd DM: Early diagnosis of tyrosinemia type II. Am J Ophthalmol 107:559–560, 1989.

Lohr KM, Hyndiuk RA, Hatchell DL, Kurth CE: Corneal organ cultures in tyrosinemia release chemotactic factors. J Lab Clin Med 105:573–580, 1985.

Ney D, Bay C, Schneider JA, Kelts D, Nyhan WL: Dietary management of oculocutaneous tyrosinemia in an 11-year-old child. Am J Dis Child 137:995–1000, 1983.

Sayar RB, von Domarus D, Schafer HJ, Beckenkamp G: Clinical picture and problems of keratoplasty in Richner-Hanhart syndrome (tyrosinemia type II). Ophthalmologica 197:1–6, 1988.

Shear CS, Nyhan WL: Tyrosinemia II, Oregon Type. *In* Buyse ML (ed): Birth Defects Encyclopedia. Dover, MA, Center for Birth Defects Information Services, 1990, pp 1724–1725.

SECTION 6

DISORDERS OF CARBOHYDRATE METABOLISM

DIABETES MELLITUS 250.

SURESH R. CHANDRA, M.D.

Madison, Wisconsin

Diabetes mellitus is a complex disorder of carbohydrate, lipid, and protein metabolism characterized clinically by hyperglycemia and the relative or absolute lack of insulin. It is a common disorder that is prevalent world-wide. In the United States, the prevalence of diabetes is 2 per cent of the population. These figures are based on known diabetic patients and do not include the large reservoir of un-diagnosed diabetics. The development of diabetes is influenced by multiple factors, both genetic and environmental. The disease may develop in the first and second decades of life (type I) or in middle and late life (type II); more than half of the diabetic individuals above the age of 40 years are overweight. It occurs more commonly in females than males (3:2), and a family history of diabetes is positive in 25 per cent of patients. The disease is generally transmitted as a recessive trait without sex linkage.

Although the discovery of insulin has led to increased longevity of diabetics, the longer duration of the disease is associated with an increased incidence of secondary complications, consisting of accelerated atherosclerosis and a triad of retinopathy, nephropathy, and neuropathy.

Diabetic retinopathy is the second leading cause of new blindness and the leading cause of blindness in adults under the age of 65 in the United States. The prevalence of diabetic retinopathy is strongly related to the duration of diabetes. The prevalence of clinically detectable diabetic retinopathy is less than 25 per cent in patients with less than 5 years duration of diabetes, about 50 per cent when diabetes has been present for 5 to 15 years, and exceeds 75 per cent in patients who have had diabetes for more than 15 years. There is evidence to suggest a strong relationship between hyperglycemia and the incidence and progression of diabetic retinopathy.

THERAPY

Systemic. Adult-onset diabetic patients whose diabetes cannot be controlled with diet alone or those who are unwilling or unable to adhere to a restrictive diet can be controlled with oral hypoglycemic agents or insulin. Oral hypoglycemic agents are useful only in adult-onset diabetics (type II). Tolbutamide (1.5 gm twice a day), acetohexamide (750 mg twice a day), and chlorpropamide (175 mg twice a day) are some of the commonly used oral hypoglycemic agents.

Most juvenile-onset diabetic patients (type I) and some maturity-onset diabetics (type II) who are uncontrolled with diet and oral hypoglycemic agents require insulin. Single or multiple injections of one or more of various long- and short-acting insulins may be used in combination to control the hyperglycemia. The majority of insulin-dependent diabetics require between 1 and 4 units of insulin per hour or 10 to 20 units for each main meal.

Ocular. Various pharmacologic agents have been tried to treat diabetic retinopathy. Clofibrate‡ has been used in an attempt to reduce the amount of hard exudates, and calcium dobesilate† has been tried to decrease the capillary fragility and abnormal permeability. However, neither of these drugs is of practical use for diabetic retinopathy in the United States.

It has been suggested that the increased platelet aggregation in diabetic retinopathy may be responsible for its development and progression, perhaps by promoting small vessel obstruction. Aspirin, a potent inhibitor of platelet aggregation, is not beneficial in retarding diabetic retinopathy as shown by the randomized National Eye Institute-sponsored Early Treatment Diabetic Retinopathy Study (ETDRS).

Surgical. At the present time, photocoagulation is the treatment of choice for proliferative diabetic retinopathy. The beneficial effect of photocoagulation has been demonstrated by the ETDRS. In this study, the beneficial effect of the treatment was observed in both proliferative and severe nonproliferative retinopathy, but was of greater clinical importance in those eyes with the following high-risk characteristics: (1) moderate to severe disc neovascularization, defined as new vessels greater than one-fourth to one-third the area of the disc and (2) mild disc neovascularization or retinal neovascularization elsewhere, if preretinal or vitreous hemorrhage was present. Although both argon laser and xenon arc photocoagulation were shown to be beneficial, the argon technique was preferred because side effects (decreases in visual acuity and peripheral visual fields) were less frequent.

The treatment technique most commonly used is called "panretinal" or "scatter" treatment. It consists of the application of several hundred 500-micron diameter burns to the midperipheral and peripheral portions of the retina. Treatment extends posteriorly to two disc diameters from the center of the macula in the temporal quadrants and one-half disc diameter nasal to the optic disc. In addition, focal treatment using moderate-intensity confluent burns may be applied to new vessels on the surface of the retina. The total number of burns is usually 1200 to 1600, each with a duration of 0.1 to 0.2 seconds. Power is adjusted to achieve a moderately white burn. The treatment is applied on an outpatient basis under topical or retrobulbar anesthesia. Focal treatment to new vessels on the optic disc is not necessary.

Regression of disc neovascularization is usually apparent very soon (days to weeks) after treatment, but is not always complete or permanent. When substantial regression of disc neovascularization is not obtained (and maintained), one or more additional scatter treatments over previously untreated retina are often followed by satisfactory regression.

The risk-benefit ratio of photocoagulation in patients with mild to moderate nonproliferative retinopathy is being evaluated by the ETDRS. The ETDRS demonstrated that photocoagulation treatment is beneficial in diabetic macular edema.

Before photocoagulation was widely accepted, pituitary ablation was advocated for patients with rapidly progressive "florid" retinopathy. Because of its attendant mortality and morbidity and because of the effectiveness and safety of photocoagulation, this procedure is rarely used today.

In some cases of traction retinal detachment with or without retinal break, scleral buckling or scleral resection may be useful. In most cases, a pars plana vitrectomy procedure is necessary.

Vitrectomy surgery is used to treat eyes with severe vitreous hemorrhage, tractional retinal detachment, and extensive preretinal membrane formation. In vitrectomy, long-standing vitreous hemorrhage is removed from the eye, and the traction caused by fibrous scar tissue is relieved. The vitreous is replaced with physiologic solution to restore transparency. The National Eye Institute's Diabetic Retinopathy Vitrectomy Study (DRVS) demonstrated that, in patients with nonresolving diabetic vitreous hemorrhage, early vitrectomy is beneficial in type I diabetics but did not provide any advantage in type II diabetics. The study also showed that vitrectomy is beneficial in advanced proliferative diabetic retinopathy.

In patients with neovascular glaucoma, panretinal photocoagulation is often followed by regression of rubeosis iridis and neovascularization in the anterior chamber angle. In some early cases, photocoagulation plus conventional antiglaucoma medical therapy may be sufficient to control intraocular pressure. Direct photocoagulation of new vessels extending across the chamber angle has also been advocated. When peripheral anterior synechiae are extensive, filtering surgery is required, but the results are often unsatisfactory.

Supportive. The goal of diabetic management should be to educate the patient about diabetes and its complications and to help the patient lead as normal a life as possible. This can be achieved by teaching the patient and family about diabetes and the importance of self-care through regular habits, avoidance of dietary and other excesses and deficiencies, maintenance of normal weight, and finally applied common sense.

Dietary management remains the most important factor in the practical management of diabetes mellitus. The diabetic diet should maintain the prescribed balance between carbohydrates, protein, fat, vitamins, and minerals in order to maintain the patient's ideal body weight.

Ocular or Periocular Manifestations

Ciliary Body: Glycogen deposits in pigment epithelium; thickening of basement membrane.

Cornea: Endothelial pigment deposits; hypesthesia; poor epithelial healing.

Extraocular Muscles: Paralysis of third or sixth nerve.

Iris: Ectropion uveae; glycogen deposits in pigment epithelium; pupillary abnormality; rubeosis iridis.

Lens: Cataracts; pigment deposits on epithelium; premature presbyopia.

Macula: Edema; heterotopia.

Optic Nerve: Atrophy; papillopathy.

Retina: Cotton-wool spots (soft exudates); detachment; dilation and beading of retinal veins; hard exudates; hemorrhages (superficial, deep, and preretinal); intraretinal microvascular abnormalities; microaneurysms; neovascularization and fibrous proliferation; sclerosis of retinal arterioles.

Vitreous: Asteroid hyalosis; detachment; hemorrhages.

PRECAUTIONS

A good control of diabetes may be beneficial in the prevention of diabetic retinopathy. There is some evidence that coexistent hypertension may have an adverse effect on the progression of diabetic retinopathy. Pregnancy carries a high risk of deterioration of retinopathy and significant visual loss in patients with proliferative or severe nonproliferative retinopathy. There is controversy regarding the possible increased risk of cardiovascular complications associated with the prolonged use of oral hypoglycemic agents.

The most common side effects of panretinal photocoagulation observed in the ETDRS are a mild to moderate decrease in visual acuity and constriction of peripheral visual fields. These harmful side effects were more commonly observed with xenon arc than with argon photocoagulation.

Until the results of the DRVS are available, vitrectomy is indicated in long-standing vitreous hemorrhage and retinal traction involving the macula.

COMMENTS

Diabetic retinopathy poses a major threat of blindness in patients with diabetes mellitus. Treatment with photocoagulation reduces this threat significantly. Careful periodic ophthalmoscopic examinations, preferably through dilated pupils, should be performed on all patients. If the patient develops diabetic retinopathy, its progression should be monitored by an ophthalmologist who can seek specialized care, such as photocoagulation or vitrectomy, at an appropriate time.

References

Blankenship GW, Skyler JS: Diabetic retinopathy: A general survey. Diabetes Care 1:127–137, 1978.

Bresnick GH: Diabetic retinopathy. In Peyman GA, Sanders DR, Goldberg MF (eds): Principles and Practice of Ophthalmology. Philadelphia, WB Saunders, 1980, pp 1205–1276.

Diabetic Retinopathy Study Research Group: Photocoagulation treatment of proliferative diabetic retinopathy. Clinical application of (Diabetic Retinopathy Study) findings: DRS Report Number 8. Ophthalmology 88:583–600, 1981.

Diabetic Retinopathy Vitrectomy Study Research Group: Early vitrectomy for severe vitreous hemorrhage in diabetic retinopathy. Two year results of a randomized trial; Diabetic Retinopathy Vitrectomy Study Report Number 2. Arch Ophthalmol 103:1644–1652, 1985.

Early Treatment Diabetic Retinopathy Study Research Group: Photocoagulation for diabetic macular edema. Early Treatment Diabetic Retinopathy Study Report Number 1. Arch Ophthalmol 103:1796–1806, 1985.

Kahn HA, Bradley RF: Prevalence of diabetic retinopathy. Age, sex, and duration of diabetes. Br J Ophthalmol 59:345–349, 1975.

Kahn HA, Moorhead HB: Statistics on Blindness in a Model Reporting Area, 1969–1970 (DHEW Publication No. NIH 73–427). Washington, DC, Government Printing Office, 1973.

Klein R, Klein B, Davis MD: Wisconsin epidemiologic study of diabetic retinopathy. Prevalence and severity of diabetic retinopathy and its association with risk factors in participants diagnosed to have diabetes mellitus after age 29 years. Preliminary report. Invest Ophthalmol Vis Sci 22(Suppl):68, 1982.

GALACTOSEMIAS 271.1

WARREN A. WILSON, M.D.,
and GEORGE N. DONNELL, M.D.

Los Angeles, California

Galactosemia can result from more than one inborn error of galactose metabolism. The most important source of the sugar is milk, where it is found in the form of the disaccharide lactose. Lactose is hydrolyzed in the intestine to its monosaccharides, glucose and galactose. These are absorbed and used for energy and the synthesis of several galactose-containing cell components.

Three major enzymatic reactions are involved in the metabolism of galactose. In the first step of galactose metabolism, galactokinase catalyzes the phosphorylation of galactose. In the second step, which is mediated by the enzyme galactose-1-phosphate uridyltransferase, the galactose-1-phosphate formed is exchanged with glucose-1-phosphate of uridine diphosphoglucose to form uridine diphosphate galactose. The third reaction catalyzed by uridine diphosphogalactose 6 epimerase transforms uridine diphosphogalactose to uridine diphosphoglucose.

Defects in each of the three major steps have been described. All of the disorders are inherited as autosomal recessive traits; both parents are obligatory heterozygotes and exhibit about one-half of normal erythrocyte enzyme activity.

In galactokinase deficiency, galactose accumulates in the blood and overflows into the urine. Galactitol is formed in tissues from galactose. Cataracts and pseudotumor cerebri are the important clinical findings, and they are thought to result in part from galactitol accumulation in the target organs.

Transferase deficiency has a frequency of approximately 1 in 60,000 births. The gene coding for the enzyme resides on chromosome number 9 and recently has been cloned using oligonucleotide probes.

The presenting symptoms of galactosemia associated with transferase deficiency usually manifest a few days after feedings containing lactose have been started and include vomiting, jaundice, hepatomegaly and severe infections. If untreated the mortality rate is high.

In survivors, mental retardation and cataracts become evident.

It has been recently recognized that even those patients diagnosed and treated early have significant long-term sequelae. Abnormalities of neuropsychologic functioning are common and are manifested by below-average intelligence, psycholinguistic abnormalities, and poor academic performance. Defects in expressive language word retrieval have been reported in more than half of the patients. Ataxia, tremors, and incoordination have been described in about 20 per cent of these patients. Hypergonadotrophic hypogonadism occurs in more than 90 per cent of the galactosemic females and is characterized by failure of secondary sexual development and menstrual abnormalities.

Lenticular cataracts have been observed in about one-half of the patients due to transferase deficiency. Cataracts involve the embryonal and fetal nuclei and have been described as zonular and lamellar. Lens changes have been documented as early as 20 weeks of gestation. Although the central clouding may be dense, these cataracts rarely, if ever, become mature, even in patients undiagnosed at 6 months or more. Originally, it was thought that significant regression of the opacities occurred when infants were placed on the proper diet; however, this has not been the case. Some residual opacities are observed in most patients.

Two types of epimerase deficiency have been described. In one type, the enzyme deficiency is limited to blood cells and is clinically benign. The other type, which has a very low frequency, has been associated with clinical manifestations similar to those described for patients with transferase deficiency.

THERAPY

Systemic. The management of kinase and transferase deficiencies is essentially the same and involves the withdrawal of lactose-containing foods (milk and its products). It is important that the diet be maintained throughout life. Clearly, compliance requires the cooperation of patients, their parents, and the assistance of a nutritionist. The acute systemic manifestations of galactosemia usually resolve after the initiation of a lactose-free diet.

Ocular. Dietary compliance will prevent the progression of cataract formation, but does not result in the complete regression of lens changes. The management of the lenticular changes in galactosemia are the same as for congenital cataracts resulting from other causes.

References

Donnell GN, Bergren WR: The galactosemias. *In* Raine DN (ed): Treatment of Inherited Metabolic Diseases. New York, American Elsevier, 1974, pp 91–144.

Kaufman FR, et al: Hypergonadotrophic hypogonadism in female patients with galactosemia. N Engl J Med 304:994–998, 1981.

Juergen Reichardt, et al: Cloning and characterization of CDNA encoding human galactose-1-phosphate uridyltransferase. Mol Biol Med 5: 107–115, 1988.

Oberman AE, et al: Galactokinase deficiency cataracts in identical twins. Am J Ophthalmol 74: 887–892, 1972.

Vannas, et al: Lens changes in a galactosemic fetus. Am J Ophthalmol 80:726, 1975.

Wilson WA: Cataracts and galactose metabolism. Trans Am Ophthalmol Soc 65:661–704, 1967.

Wilson WA: Surgery of congenital and childhood cataracts. Trans Pac Coast Otoophthalmol Soc 59: 207–219, 1978.

Wilson WA, Donnell GN: Cataracts in galactosemia. Arch Ophthalmol 690:215–222, 1958.

Wilson WA, Donnell GN, Koch R: Galactosemia, a twenty-five-year follow-up. *In* XXII Concilium Ophthalmologicum Paris 1974, Acta Paris, Masson, 1976, Vol I, pp 740–744.

MUCOPOLYSAC-CHARIDOSIS I-H 277.5

(Dysostosis Multiplex, Hurler Syndrome, MPS I-H, Pfaundler-Hurler Syndrome)

T. E. KELLY, M.D., Ph.D.

Charlottesville, Virginia

Mucopolysaccharidosis I-H is an autosomal recessive syndrome characterized by deficiency of lysosomal enzyme α-L-iduronidase, which allows the mucopolysaccharides, dermatan sulfate and heparan sulfate, to accumulate in cells throughout the body. The primary manifestations include skeletal abnormalities, enlargement of the spleen and liver, corneal clouding, and mental retardation. Although the child may develop normally for the first few months, typical Hurler manifestations usually begin to appear in the first or second year of life. Clouding of the cornea is present in all patients with this disease. Buphthalmos and megalocornea may also be present. Retinal degeneration occurs in many cases, and optic atrophy is also common. The eyebrows are typically bushy and coarse, and the eyelids are thickened and coarse.

THERAPY

Systemic. Considerable enthusiasm has been generated in England for the use of bone marrow transplantation in the management of inborn errors of metabolism. There have been several reports of successful transplantation in patients with MPS I-H with evidence of enhanced mucopolysaccharide degradation and clinical improvement. This approach is still highly experimental, and there are several major problems: the onset of lysosomal storage diseases is prenatal; the morbidity and mortality of bone marrow transplantation are high; and there is doubt that the changes in viscera observed after a successful transplant will extend to the skeleton and central nervous system, the major organs involved in the mucopolysaccharidoses.

Supportive. The physician should offer the parents sympathetic guidance in dealing with the gross deformities and mental retardation that may develop in these patients. Genetic counseling is also indicated for parents because of the 25 per cent recurrence risk and the availability of prenatal diagnosis.

Surgical. Surgical treatment is supportive; it may include repair of hernias and hydroceles, orthopedic surgery for skeletal deformities, or adenoidectomy to provide relief from the persistent upper airway obstruction present in Hurler patients. Penetrating keratoplasty or lamellar corneal graft may be used for corneal clouding. Hydrocephalus and associated papilledema may require shunting of cerebrospinal fluid.

Ocular or Periocular Manifestations

Cornea: Interstitial clouding; megalocornea.
Eyebrows: Bushy; coarse.
Eyelids: Coarse eyelashes; edema; ptosis; tylosis.
Iris: Acid mucopolysaccharide deposits.
Lens: Acid mucopolysaccharide deposits; congenital anterior polar cataract.
Optic Nerve: Atrophy; cupping; disc edema; disc hyperemia.
Orbit: Enlarged optic foramen; hypertelorism; small.
Retina: Detachment; macular edema; pigmentary degeneration.
Sclera: Acid mucopolysaccharide deposits.
Other: Anisocoria; buphthalmos; convergent strabismus; decreased visual acuity; nystagmus.

PRECAUTIONS

Administration of general anesthesia is complicated by excessive pharyngeal secretions, laryngospasm, cardiac abnormalities, increased frequency of cardiac arrest, hypoxia, and hypotension. Postoperative obstruction or infection may occur in the respiratory tract and require tracheotomy. Many of these complications may be avoided if large doses of atropine are given in the preinduction period and postoperative narcotics are withheld as much as possible.

Plasma infusion is not a practicable means of therapy. Improvement is temporary, if present at all. There are dangers of fluid overload in those patients whose cardiovascular status is compromised.

COMMENTS

The prognosis for the Hurler patient is not encouraging. Mental retardation is invariably present and is especially severe and progressive after the first year, usually reaching a plateau after several years. Deformities of the respiratory tract in this syndrome may cause choking on solid foods or the nasal regurgitation of liquids. Some patients may have unexplained spells of cyanosis or even apnea. Death usually occurs in the first decade of life either from cardiac involvement or increased susceptibility to pneumonia and bronchitis.

In 1992, the structural gene coding for the enzyme, alpha-L-iduronidase, was cloned and sequenced from the distal short arm of chromosome number 4. It is to be expected that analysis of mutations in patients representing the various clinical phenotypes of MPS-I will improve our understanding of the variability of this disease. Further, this knowledge holds the promise of the eventual development of gene therapy as a means of treating the otherwise inevitable progressive course of this disease.

References

Bloch RS, Henkind P: Ocular manifestations of endocrine and metabolic diseases. *In* Duane TD (ed): Clinical Ophthalmology. Hagerstown, MD, Harper & Row, 1982, Vol V, pp 21:10–12.
Francois J: Ocular manifestations of the mucopolysaccharidoses. Ophthalmologica *169*:345–361, 1974.
Hobbs JR: Bone marrow transplantation for inborn errors. Lancet 2:735–739, 1981.
Hobbs JR, et al: Reversal of clinical features of Hurler's disease and biochemical improvement after treatment by bone-marrow transplantation. Lancet 2:709–712, 1981.
Nowaczyk MJ, Clarke JT, Morin JD: Glaucoma as an early complication of Hurler's disease. Arch Dis Child 63:1091–1093, 1988.
McKusick VA: Heritable Disorders of Connective Tissue, 4th ed. St. Louis, CV Mosby, 1972, pp 528–548.

MUCOPOLYSAC-CHARIDOSIS I-H/S 277.5
(Hurler/Scheie Syndrome, MPS I-H/S)

T. E. KELLY, M.D., Ph.D.

Charlottesville, Virginia

Mucopolysaccharidosis I-H/S is an autosomal recessive syndrome characterized by deficiency of lysosomal enzyme α-L-iduronidase, which allows the mucopolysaccharides, dermatan sulfate and heparan sulfate, to accumulate in cells throughout the body. The primary manifestations include corneal opacities, cardiac enlargement, umbilical and inguinal hernias, and multiple skeletal changes. Mild mental retardation may be present. Micrognathia and severe acne are features peculiar to this form of mucopolysaccharidosis. Ocular findings also include both diffuse corneal clouding and pigmentary retinopathy. Buphthalmos and megalocornea may also be present. The eyebrows are typically bushy and coarse, and the eyelids are thickened and coarse.

THERAPY

Systemic. Considerable enthusiasm has been generated in England for the use of bone marrow transplantation in the management of inborn errors of metabolism. There have been several reports of successful transplantation in patients with MPS I-H with evidence of enhanced mucopolysaccharide degradation and clinical improvement. This approach is still highly experimental, and there are several major problems: the onset of lysosomal storage diseases is prenatal; the morbidity and mortality of bone marrow transplantation are high; and there is doubt that the changes in viscera observed after a successful transplant will extend to the skeleton and central nervous system, the major organs involved in the mucopolysaccharidoses.

Supportive. The physician should offer the parents guidance in dealing with the gross deformities and mental retardation that may arise in these patients. Life expectancy of these patients is into the twenties, and surgical and medical management of individual problems is appropriate.

Genetic counseling is indicated for parents as a 25 per cent recurrence risk exists. Carrier detection should also be available for other relatives.

Surgical. Surgical treatment is supportive. It may include repair of hernias and hydroceles, orthopedic surgery for skeletal deformities, or adenoidectomy to provide relief from the persistent upper airway obstruction present in these patients. Tympanoplasty and hearing aids may be required to preserve hearing. Penetrating keratoplasty or lamellar corneal graft is the treatment of choice for corneal clouding. Hydrocephalus and associated papilledema may be relieved by shunting of cerebrospinal fluid.

Ocular or Periocular Manifestations

Cornea: Bullous keratopathy; clouding; megalocornea; punctate opacity; thickening.
Eyebrows: Bushy; coarse.

Eyelids: Coarse eyelashes; edema; ptosis; tylosis.
Globe: Buphthalmos; proptosis.
Iris: Acid mucopolysaccharide deposits; distortion; folding, thickening.
Lens: Acid mucopolysaccharide deposits; congenital anterior polar cataract.
Optic Nerve: Atrophy; cupping; disc edema; disc hyperemia.
Orbit: Enlarged optic foramen; hypertelorism; small.
Retina: Detachment; macular edema; pigmentary degeneration; tapetoretinal degeneration.
Sclera: Acid mucopolysaccharide deposits; thickening.
Other: Anisocoria; constriction of visual fields; convergent strabismus; decreased visual acuity; night blindness; secondary glaucoma.

PRECAUTIONS

Plasma infusion is not a practicable means of therapy. Improvement is temporary, if present at all. However, the danger of fluid overload is present in those patients whose cardiovascular status is compromised. Such patients manifest heart disease as cardiomyopathy, conduction defects, and valvular heart disease. Several have died during induction of anesthesia for minor procedures. General anesthesia should be approached with caution.

COMMENTS

The Hurler syndrome and the Scheie syndrome share a common metabolic defect; in both, the enzymatic deficiency is α-L-iduronidase. The mutation in both is presumed to be allelic, and thus it is felt that the inheritance of a Hurler gene and a Scheie gene results in a genetic compound with an intermediate phenotype, the Hurler/Scheie syndrome. This phenotype is distinct, although intermediate in severity between the Hurler and Scheie syndromes. Patients with mucopolysaccharidosis I-H/S usually succumb after protracted cardiac failure. Mental deficiency and dwarfism are less severe than in the Hurler syndrome, although the pattern of radiographic changes is similar. Additional atypical mucopolysaccharidosis patients with the same specific biochemical defect and similar features of Hurler syndrome suggest that several genetically distinct forms of α-L-iduronidase deficiency exist.

References

Chijiiwa T, Inomata H, Yamana Y, Kaibara N: Ocular manifestations of Hurler/Scheie phenotype in two sibs. Jpn J Ophthalmol 27:54–62, 1983.

Hobbs JR: Bone marrow transplantation for inborn errors. Lancet 2:735–739, 1981.

Hobbs JR, et al: Reversal of clinical features of Hurler's disease and biochemical improvement after treatment by bone-marrow transplantation. Lancet 2:709–712, 1981.

Kajii T, et al: Hurler/Scheie genetic compound (mucopolysaccharidosis IH/IS) in Japanese brothers. Clin Genet 6:394–400, 1974.

Kelly TE: The mucopolysaccharidoses and mucolipidoses. Clin Orthop 114:116–136, 1976.

Lavery MA, Green WR, Jabs EW, Luckenbach MW, Cox JL: Ocular histopathology and ultrastructure of Sanfilippo's syndrome, type III-B. Arch Ophthalmol 101:1263–1274, 1983.

MUCOPOLYSAC-CHARIDOSIS I-S 277.5

(MPS I-S, Scheie Syndrome)

IRENE E.H. MAUMENEE, M.D.

Baltimore, Maryland

Mucopolysaccharidosis I-S is an autosomal recessive syndrome characterized by deficiency of the lysosomal enzyme α-L-iduronidase, which allows the mucopolysaccharides, dermatan sulfate and heparan sulfate, to accumulate intracellularly throughout the body. The primary manifestations include severe progressive corneal clouding and retinal degeneration, joint contractures, facial coarseness, hammer toes, and carpal tunnel syndrome. Glaucoma is a late complication. Aortic regurgitation occurs, but cardiac decompensation at an early age is usually not a major problem. The onset of symptoms in this relatively mild disease usually is after the age of 5 years, although corneal clouding, stiff fingers, and umbilical or inguinal hernias may be detected sooner.

THERAPY

Systemic. Several therapeutic approaches are currently being tried to restore the ability to degrade or clear storage material. Such therapy requires either induction of enzyme synthesis, enhancement of any residual enzyme activity, or replacement therapy through bone marrow transplantation.

Surgical. Surgical treatment may include repair of hernias and hydroceles or orthopedic surgery for skeletal deformities. Penetrating keratoplasty is the treatment of choice for corneal clouding. Hydrocephalus and associated papilledema may be relieved by shunting of cerebrospinal fluid in others, papilledema is probably due to scleral thickening secondary to MPS deposits.

Supportive. Genetic counseling is indicated for the parents, who have a 25 per cent risk of having another similarly affected child. There is no mental involvement, life expec-

tancy is close to normal, and patients may lead fruitful normal lives. The resulting facial coarseness is only mildly debilitating. Chronic care is not needed until very late in the disease, when blindness, cardiac insufficiency, or marked joint stiffness may have occurred.

Ocular or Periocular Manifestations

Cornea: Clouding (more striking in the peripheral than central cornea); punctate opacities; thickening.

Eyebrows: Bushy; coarse.

Eyelids: Coarse eyelashes; edema; tylosis.

Iris: Acid mucopolysaccharide deposits; distortion; folding; thickening.

Optic Nerve: Disc edema; atrophy.

Retinal: Macular edema; tapetoretinal degeneration.

Sclera: Acid mucopolysaccharide deposits; thickening.

Other: Anisocoria; cataracts; constriction of visual fields; decreased visual acuity; glaucoma (secondary to mucopolysaccharide deposits in trabecular meshwork, also angle-closure attacks); proptosis.

PRECAUTIONS

Administration of general anesthesia is complicated by excessive pharyngeal secretions, laryngospasm, cardiac abnormalities, increased frequency of cardiac arrest, hypoxia, and hypotension. Postoperative obstruction or infection in the respiratory tract may require tracheostomy. Many of these complications may be avoided if large doses of atropine are given in the preinduction period and postoperative narcotics are withheld as much as possible.

COMMENTS

Originally classified as MPS V because of the distinctive phenotype, the Scheie syndrome is currently designated as MPS I-S. Clinically, the patients with MPS I-H and MPS I-S have many similarities (corneal clouding, hepatosplenomegaly, cardiovascular abnormalities, and certain skeletal deformities), but they differ in three important respects. In contrast to patients with MPS I-H, patients with MPS I-S are not dwarfed, are free of neurological and mental deficits (except for the signs of the carpal tunnel syndrome), and have normal life expectancy.

References

Collins MZ: Optic nerve head swelling and optic atrophy in the systemic mucopolysaccharidoses. Ophthalmology 97:1445–1449, 1990.

Crocker AC: Present status of treatment of the mucopolysaccharidoses. Birth Defects 10:113–124, 1974.

François J: Ocular manifestations of the mucopolysaccharidoses. Ophthalmologica *169*:345–381, 1974.

Hussels IE, et al: Treatment of mucopolysaccharidoses. Birth Defects *10*:212–238, 1974.

Kelly TE: The mucopolysaccharidoses and mucolipidoses. Clin Orthop *114*:116–136, 1978.

Legum CP, Schorr S, Barman ER: The genetic mucopolysaccharidoses and mucolipidoses. Review and comment. Adv Pediatr *22*:305–347, 1976.

MUCOPOLYSACCHARIDOSIS II 277.5

(Hunter Syndrome , MPS II)

ELIAS I. TRABOULSI, M.D.

Baltimore, Maryland

Mucopolysaccharidosis II is the only known X-linked disorder of mucopolysaccharide metabolism. One in 132,000 male newborns is affected in the United Kingdom, as opposed to 1 in 34,000 in Israel; this discrepancy is thought to be due to genetic drift. MPS II is caused by a deficiency of iduronate sulfatase that results in the intracellular accumulation and excessive urinary excretion of two mucopolysaccharides, chondroitin sulfate B and heparitin sulfate. Several researchers, including Bunge et al. (1992), have reported the molecular characterization of the mutations associated with MPS II. Mucopolysaccharidosis II is thought to exist in two clinically and genetically distinct forms. In the severe form (MPS IIA), mental retardation and neurologic changes are almost indistinguishable from those found in mucopolysaccharidosis I-H. Other clinical signs of MPS IIA include gargoyle-like facies, dwarfism, hepatosplenomegaly, deafness, and early death by age 15. In the mild type (MPS IIB), intelligence is not impaired, and survival into adulthood and even procreation have been observed. The corneas remain clear until the fourth decade of life. Collins and co-workers (1990) reported papilledema in about 20 per cent of patients with MPS II and optic atrophy in another 10 per cent. Retinal degeneration is another important ocular feature of this disorder.

THERAPY

Systemic. Several experimental approaches have been used in an attempt to enhance the degradation of the stored material. Such therapy is based on induction of enzyme, activation of any residual enzyme activity, or replacement therapy with exogenous enzyme. Perfusions of fresh plasma from a normal donor are administered at regular intervals in order to provide a supply of the particular deficient enzyme. There is no evidence to date that plasma infusion has caused any improvement by either reversing the severe skeletal changes or contributing to the catabolism of the stored mucopolysaccharides. Fibroblast and bone marrow transplantation therapy is also being investigated and may be of some usefulness in the future.

Supportive. The physician should offer the parents sympathetic guidance in dealing with the deformities and resultant complications that characterize both forms of Hunter syndrome. Genetic counseling and prenatal diagnosis are offered to families with an affected child.

Surgical. Surgical treatment is supportive; repair of hernias and hydroceles or orthopedic surgery for skeletal deformities may be necessary. Hydrocephalus and associated papilledema, if severe enough to warrant surgical intervention, may be relieved by shunting of cerebrospinal fluid.

Ocular or Periocular Manifestations

Cornea: Acid mucopolysaccharide deposits; stromal haze (late).

Eyebrows or Eyelashes: Bushy; coarse, proptosis.

Eyelids: Edema; ptosis; tylosis.

Iris or Ciliary Body: Acid mucopolysaccharide deposits.

Optic Nerve: Atrophy; cupping; disc hyperemia; papilledema.

Retina: Diminished electroretinogram; pigmentary degeneration.

Sclera: Acid mucopolysaccharide deposits; thickened.

PRECAUTIONS

Administration of a general anesthetic may be complicated by excessive pharyngeal secretions, laryngospasm, cardiac abnormalities, increased frequency of cardiac arrest, hypoxia, or hypotension. Postoperative obstruction or infection may occur in the respiratory tract and may require tracheotomy. Many of these complications may be avoided if large doses of atropine are given in the preinduction period and if postoperative narcotics are withheld as much as possible.

COMMENTS

Mucopolysaccharidosis II is an X-linked disorder. Hence, the disease is only transmissible from mother to son. Parents at risk should be informed that there is a 50 per cent chance that their son will be affected and a 50 per cent chance that their daughter will be a carrier. Carrier females do not manifest any signs of the disease.

Prenatal diagnosis is possible and is at the present time the most effective way to deal with MPS II. Amniocentesis or chorionic villus biopsy is performed in pregnancies where the mother has previously given birth to an affected son. Amniotic cells are cultured and examined for a deficiency of iduronate sulfatase. If such is found, the pregnancy can be interrupted early. It is also possible to measure the levels of iduronate sulfatase in the mother's serum; these levels rise between the 6th and 12th week if the fetus is normal, but do not increase if the fetus is affected.

References

Beck M, Cole G: Disc oedema in association with Hunter's syndrome: Ocular histopathological findings. Br J Ophthalmol 68:590–594, 1984.

Bunge S, Steglith C, Beck M, Rosenkranz W, Schwinger E, Hopwood JJ, Gal A: Mutation analysis of the iduronate-2-sulfatase in patients with mucopolysaccharidosis type II (Hunter syndrome). Hum Molec Genet 1:335–339, 1992.

Collins MLZ, Traboulsi EI, Maumenee IH: Optic nerve head swelling and optic atrophy in the systemic mucopolysaccharidoses. Ophthalmology 97:1445–1449, 1990.

Di Natale P, Neufeld EF: Biochemical diagnosis of mucopolysaccharidoses, mucolipidoses and related disorders. Perspect Inherit Metab Dis 2: 113–123, 1979.

Frangieh GT, Traboulsi EI, Kenyon KR: The mucopolysaccharidoses. In Gold DH, Weingeist TA (eds): The Eye in Systemic Disease. Philadelphia, JB Lippincott, 1990, pp 372–377.

Gibbs DA, et al: The treatment of lysosomal storage diseases by fibroblast transplantation: Some preliminary observations. Birth Defects 16:457–474, 1980.

Jolly RD, Desnick RJ: Inborn errors of lysosomal catabolism—Principles of heterozygote detection. Am J Med Genet 4:293–307, 1979.

Legum CP, Schorr S, Berman ER: The genetic mucopolysaccharidoses and mucolipidoses: Review and comment. Adv Pediatr 22:305–347, 1976.

McDonnell JM, Green WR, Maumenee IH: Ocular histopathology of systemic mucopolysaccharidosis, type II-A (Hunter syndrome, severe). Ophthalmology 92:1772–1779, 1985.

Neufeld EF, Muenzer J: The mucopolysaccharidoses. In Scriver CR, Beaudet AL, Sly WS, Valle D (eds): The Metabolic Basis of Inherited Disease, 6th ed. New York, McGraw-Hill, 1989, Vol II, pp 1565–1587.

MUCOPOLYSAC-CHARIDOSIS III 277.5

(MPS III, Sanfilippo Syndrome)

ELIAS I. TRABOULSI, M.D.

Baltimore, Maryland

Mucopolysaccharidosis III is inherited as an autosomal recessive trait and is characterized by excessive tissue storage and urinary excretion of heparitin sulfate. There are four subtypes, designated A, B, C, and D, which are indistinguishable clinically. The A form is caused by a deficiency of heparan sulfate sulfatase, the B form by a deficiency of N-acetylglucosaminidase, the C form by a defect in acetyl CoA: alpha-glucosaminide N-acetyl transferase, and the D form by a defect in N-acetylglucosamine-6-sulfate sulfatase. The various forms of MPS III are nonallelic (the mutations occur at separate genetic loci).

Severe mental retardation and neurologic deterioration are the most prominent clinical signs. Mental and neurologic deficiencies progress to extreme degrees within a few years, and death usually occurs by 10 to 15 years of age. Seizures and aggressive behavior have been noted in most patients. Growth and physical development are within normal limits, and skeletal abnormalities are minimal. The corneas remain clear, but retinal pigmentary degeneration is common. Collins and coworkers (1990) reported a 5 per cent prevalence of papilledema and a 14 per cent prevalence of optic atrophy in MPS III.

THERAPY

Systemic. Several experimental approaches have been used in an attempt to enhance the degradation of the stored material. Such therapy is based on induction of enzyme synthesis, activation of any residual enzyme activity, or replacement therapy with exogenous enzyme. A major modality is plasma therapy, in which perfusions of fresh plasma from a normal donor are administered at regular intervals in order to provide a supply of corrective factor (the particular deficient enzyme). There is no evidence to date that plasma perfusion causes any improvement by either reversing the severe mental and neurologic changes or contributing to the catabolism of the stored heparan sulfate (apart from a transient effect). Enzyme replacement therapy using HLA-compatible fibroblasts is a promising hope for the future.

Supportive. Genetic counseling is indicated for parents who already have an affected child. They should be informed of the 25 per cent statistical probability of producing affected children in future pregnancies. There is no surgical or medical treatment available that would contribute to the well-being of the patient.

Ocular or Periocular Manifestations

Cornea: Acid mucopolysaccharide deposits.
Eyebrows: Bushy; coarse.
Iris or Ciliary Body: Acid mucopolysaccharide deposits.
Lens: Acid mucopolysaccharide deposits.
Optic Nerve: Rarely papilledema; optic atrophy.

Retina: Pigmentary degeneration.
Sclera: Acid mucopolysaccharide deposits.

PRECAUTIONS

As the physical features of mucopolysaccharidosis III are usually minimal, this disorder may not be included in the differential diagnosis of a child with progressive central nervous system disorder. The urine of patients suspected of having this disorder should be tested for excess mucopolysaccharides, and skin fibroblasts should be cultured and examined for the enzymatic defect. Unless these examinations are undertaken in children who undergo progressive mental deterioration after normal early development, the diagnosis of MPS III may be overlooked.

COMMENTS

Prenatal diagnosis is possible. Amniocentesis or chorionic villus biopsy is performed in pregnancies where the mother has previously given birth to an affected child. Amniotic cells are cultured and assays are performed for all of the enzymes involved in MPS III. If one of the enzymes is found to be deficient, pregnancy can be interrupted early.

References

Berman ER: Diagnosis of metabolic eye disease by chemical analysis of serum, leukocytes and skin fibroblast tissue culture. Birth Defects 12:15–51, 1976.

Collins MLZ, Traboulsi EI, Maumenee IH: Optic nerve head swelling and optic atrophy in the systemic mucopolysaccharidoses. Ophthalmology 97:1445–1449, 1990.

Dean MF, et al: Enzyme replacement therapy by transplantation of HLA-compatible fibroblasts in Sanfilippo A syndrome. Pediatr Res 15:959–963, 1981.

Del Monte MA, Maumenee IH, Green WR, Kenyon KR: Histopathology of Sanfilippo's syndrome. Arch Ophthalmol 101:1255–1262, 1983.

Frangieh GT, Traboulsi EI, Kenyon KR: The mucopolysaccharidoses. *In* Gold DH, Weingeist TA (eds): The Eye in Systemic Disease. Philadelphia, JB Lippincott, 1990, pp 372–377.

Lavery MA, et al: Ocular histopathology and ultrastructure of Sanfilippo's syndrome, type III-B. Arch Ophthalmol 101:1255–1262, 1983.

Legum CP, Schorr S, Berman ER: The genetic mucopolysaccharidoses and mucolipidoses: Review and comment. Adv Pediatr 22:305–347, 1976.

Neufeld EF, Muenzer J: The mucopolysaccharidoses. *In* Scriver CR, Beaudet AL, Sly WS, Valle D (eds): The Metabolic Basis of Inherited Disease, 6th ed. New York, McGraw-Hill, 1989, Vol. II, pp 1565–1587.

MUCOPOLYSAC-CHARIDOSIS IV 277.5
(Chondro-Osteodystrophy, Keratosulfaturia, Morquio-Brailsford Syndrome, Morquio Syndrome, MPS IV)

STEPHEN E. SOLOMON, D.O.

East Lansing, Michigan

Mucopolysaccharidosis IV is a progressive autosomal recessive disorder characterized by an enzyme deficiency of N-acetylgalactosamine-6-sulfate sulfatase (type A) and B-galactosidase (type B), resulting in an abnormal accumulation of keratan sulfate in tissues and excretion in the urine. Severe skeletal deformity is the hallmark of the disease. Although the classical clinical and radiographic features of Morquio's syndrome are present at birth, they become distinctive at 2 years of age. Joint laxity and shortness of stature prompt medical attention, with radiographic confirmation by demonstration of flat vertebrae (platyspondyly universalis) and odontoid hypoplasia. Advancing age brings exaggeration of the multiple skeletal abnormalities, with deficient linear growth beyond age 5. Midface hypoplasia coupled with a depressed nasal bridge and protrusion of the mandible results in the classic mucopolysaccharidosis facies. Cardiac manifestations occur secondary to respiratory failure caused by kyphoscoliosis and restricted chest movements, although aortic regurgitation may occur primarily. Teeth are severely affected and have very thin enamel (type A). Subtle corneal changes may appear at an early age, but are not grossly apparent until approximately 8 years of age. Glaucoma and retinal pigmentary changes have recently been reported. Optic atrophy is rare.

THERAPY

Systemic. Methods to regulate the synthesis or to enhance the metabolism or excretion of mucopolysaccharides are not available. Direct gene replacement is futuristic. Several clinical trials involving enzyme replacement therapy and tissue organ transplantation have been carried out. To date, infusion of plasma and purified enzymes and the implantation of cultured fibroblasts and amnion cells (HLA negative) have failed to produce quantitative clinical effects.

Supportive. The intelligence of patients with MPS IV is usually normal. With sympathetic guidance, these individuals can achieve age-appropriate levels of education. A hearing aid may be of some value in patients with hearing loss from recurrent otitis media.

Parents of affected children have a 25 per cent risk of having another affected child. Prenatal diagnosis is available by enzyme assay from cultured amniotic fluid cells or by analysis of amniotic fluid MPS derived from fetal tissue.

Surgical. Some surgeons have advocated prophylactic posterior spinal fusion of the upper cervical spine to prevent atlantoaxial subluxation or translocation with resultant spinal cord compression and cervical myelopathy. Myringotomy tubes may be necessary for alleviation of chronic otitis media.

There is generally no need to resort to penetrating keratoplasty in children with MPS IV since visual deficit is usually mild.

Ocular or Periocular Manifestations

Conjunctiva: Acid mucopolysaccharide deposits.
Cornea: Clouding.
Optic Nerve: Atrophy.
Retina: Pigmentary degeneration.
Trabecular Meshwork: Glaucoma.

PRECAUTIONS

At the present time, there is no specific treatment for MPS IV. The risks of complications associated with anesthesia and postoperative respiratory obstruction need to be appreciated before even simple procedures are undertaken. Hyperextension of the neck should be avoided.

COMMENTS

Patients with MPS IV usually die in their third or fourth decade of life from cor pulmonale caused by the severe abnormalities of the chest and spine. Variation in the clinical manifestations are common, and very mild cases can be encountered. Patients with mild forms of MPS IV may survive into their sixties. Interestingly, recent findings of retinal involvement in MPS IV were demonstrated in a patient of advanced age. It was proposed that the retinal involvement in this disease is mild but progressive and therefore is not seen in younger patients, but becomes apparent in older persons with Morquio's syndrome. In addition, those patients with MPS IV who reach advanced age display characteristic CT findings in spite of having normal intelligence, suggesting mucopolysaccharide deposition in cortical matter.

References

Cahane M, Treister G, Abraham FA, Melamed S: Glaucoma in siblings with Morquio syndrome. Br J Ophthalmol 74:382–383, 1990.

Dangel ME, Tsou BH: Retinal involvement in Morquio's syndrome. Ann Ophthalmol 17:349–354, 1985.

Iwamoto M, Nawa Y, Maumenee IH, Young-Ramsaran J, Matalon R, Green WR: Ocular histopathology and ultrastructure of Morquio syndrome. Graefes Arch Clin Exp Ophthalmol 228:342–349, 1990.

Matalon R: Mucopolysaccharidoses. *In* Gershwin ME, Robbins DL (eds): Musculoskeletal Diseases of Children. New York, Grune & Stratton, 1983, pp 277–284.

McKusick VA, Neufeld EF: The mucopolysaccharide storage diseases. *In* Stanbury JB, Wyngaarder JB, Fredrickson DS, et al (eds): The Metabolic Basis of Inherited Disease, 5th ed. New York, McGraw-Hill, 1983, pp 512–520.

Nelson J, Grebbell FS: The value of computed tomography in patients with mucopolysaccharidosis. Neuroradiology 29:544–549, 1987.

Yuen M, Fensonn AH: Diagnosis of classical Morquio's disease: N-acetyl-galactosamine-6-sulfate sulfatase activity in cultured fibroblasts, leukocytes, amniotic cells and chorionic villi. J Inher Metab Dis 8:80–86, 1985.

MUCOPOLYSAC-CHARIDOSIS VI 277.5
(Maroteaux-Lamy Syndrome)

RICHARD G. WELEBER, M.D.,
and JACLYN VIDGOFF, Ph.D.

Portland, Oregon

Mucopolysaccharidosis VI is an autosomal recessive trait with an enzyme deficiency of sulfogalactosamine sulfatase (N-acetyl-galactosamine-4-sulfatase or arylsulfatase B), which causes dermatan sulfate to accumulate within the body. Excessive amounts of dermatan sulfate or chondroitin sulfate B are also present in the urine. There seem to be both mild and severe phenotypes, which may represent different allelic genes. Patients with an intermediate degree of severity have recently been described. The physical findings resemble those of mucopolysaccharidosis I-H with respect to growth retardation, skeletal deformities, and coarse facial features; however, intellectual development is normal. A prominent forehead and sternal protrusion are frequently noted soon after birth. Restriction of joint motion may begin by the first year. Growth retardation is first noted at the age of 2 or 3 years, and skeletal growth may cease entirely after 8 years. By the sixth year, all patients have hepatomegaly, and about half have enlarged spleens. Deafness and inguinal hernias are common. Cardiac involvement (aortic and mitral valvular stenosis) is frequent and, with respiratory complications, is the most serious threat to patients. Generally, the life span is longer than in patients with mucopolysaccharidosis I-H, although, with the severe phenotype, survival past the mid-twenties is rare. The significant ocular manifestations of mucopolysaccharidosis VI are corneal clouding, which is moderate in degree and develops early, glaucoma, and optic atrophy. Papilledema has been reported and is thought to be associated with hydrocephalus.

THERAPY

Systemic. Several experimental approaches are currently being tried to restore the ability to degrade or clear the storage material. These include induction of enzyme synthesis, enhancement of any residual enzyme activity, and replacement therapy with exogenous enzyme. Plasma therapy, in which perfusions of fresh plasma are administered in order to provide a corrective factor for the particular enzymatic deficiency, may provide short-term biochemical improvement, but significant difficulties with long-term plasma therapy limit this approach. Another experimental approach is transfusion of lymphocytes. However, at present, neither of these forms of therapy has been of lasting benefit. Bone marrow transplantation has been tried in patients with several forms of MPS, including MPS VI, with subsequent normalization of glycosaminoglycan excretion and ultrastructural appearance of the liver, decrease in hepatosplenomegaly, and increase in joint mobility. However, clearing of corneal cloudiness, which has occurred with bone marrow transplantation in other forms of MPS, has not been seen in MPS VI. Bone marrow transplantation is a major procedure with high morbidity and mortality (30 per cent mortality when HLA-identical sibs were used as donors). Considering the risks, high expense, and questionable outcome, bone marrow transplantation should be considered experimental and restricted to carefully selected and monitored patients.

Supportive. The physician should offer sympathetic guidance in helping the parent deal with the skeletal deformities that arise in these patients. Parents should be informed of available inpatient chronic care facilities. Genetic counseling should be provided to parents and other potential carriers, as well as to patients who reach childbearing age. Both parents of an affected child are carriers of the deficient gene; however, since the gene defect is detectable in amniotic cell cultures, prenatal diagnosis is possible.

Surgical. Surgical treatment is supportive, with repair of hernias and hydroceles, orthopedic surgery for skeletal deformities, or adenoidectomy to provide relief from the persistent nasal discharge, as indicated. Penetrating keratoplasty or lamellar corneal graft has been performed for significant corneal clouding. Hydrocephalus and associated papilledema may be relieved by shunting of cerebrospinal fluid.

Ocular or Periocular Manifestations

Choroid: Thinning.
Ciliary Body: Acid mucopolysaccharide deposits.
Cornea: Acid mucopolysaccharide deposits; clouding; opacity; thickening.
Eyebrows: Bushy; coarse.
Optic Nerve: Atrophy; cupping; papilledema.
Retina: Detachment; macular edema; vascular tortuosity.
Sclera: Acid mucopolysaccharide deposits; thickening.
Other: Coarse eyelashes; decreased visual acuity.

PRECAUTIONS

Atlantoaxial subluxation can occur as a result of hypoplasia of the odontoid process. In addition, neurologic deterioration from myelopathy due to thickening of the dura of the cervical spinal cord and consequent cord compression has been reported. Early surgical decompression seems to be beneficial.

COMMENTS

One of the most outstanding features of mucopolysaccharidosis VI is the normal intellectual capacity of the patients. They usually attend regular schools and pass their examinations without difficulties, although visual and physical handicaps eventually impede their psychomotor performance.

References

Cantor LB, Disseler JA, Wilson FM: Glaucoma in the Maroteaux-Lamy syndrome. Am J Ophthalmol 108:426–430, 1989.

Goldberg MF, Scott CI, McKusick VA: Hydrocephalus and papilledema in the Maroteaux-Lamy syndrome (mucopolysaccharidosis type VI). Am J Ophthalmol 69:969–975, 1970.

Kenyon KR, et al: Ocular pathology of the Maroteaux-Lamy syndrome (systemic mucopolysaccharidosis type VI). Histologic and ultrastructural report of two cases. Am J Ophthalmol 73:718–741, 1972.

Krivit W, Pierpont ME, Ayaz K, Tsai M, Ramsay NKC, Kersey JH, Weisdorf S, Sibley R, Snover D, McGovern MM, Schwartz MF, Desnick RJ: Bone marrow transplantation in the Maroteaux-Lamy syndrome (mucopolysaccharidosis type VI): Biochemical and clinical status 24 months after transplantation. N Engl J Med 311:1606–1611, 1984.

McGovern MM, Lundman MD, Short MP, Steinfeld L, Kattan M, Raab EL, Krivit W, Desnick RJ: Status of bone marrow transplantation in Maroteaux-Lamy syndrome (MPS type 6): Status 40 months after BMT. Birth Defects 22:42–53, 1986.

McKusick VA: Heritable Disorders of Connective Tissue, 4th ed. St. Louis, CV Mosby, 1972, pp 611–627.

Neufeld EF, Muenzer J: The mucopolysaccharidoses. In Scriver CR, Beaudet AL, Sly WS, Valle D (eds): The Metabolic Basis of Inherited Disease, 6th ed. New York, McGraw-Hill, 1989, Vol 2, pp 1565–1587.

Spranger JW, et al: Mucopolysaccharidosis VI (Maroteaux-Lamy's disease). Helv Paediat Acta 25:337–362, 1970.

Stumpf DA, et al: Mucopolysaccharidosis type VI. (Maroteaux-Lamy syndrome). I. Sulfatase B deficiency in tissues. Am J Dis Child *126:*747–755, 1973.

Tamaki N, et al: Myelopathy due to diffuse thickening of the cervical dura mater in Maroteaux-Lamy syndrome: Report of a case. Neurosurgery *21:*416–419, 1987.

MUCOPOLYSAC-CHARIDOSIS VII 277.5
(β-Glucuronidase Deficiency, MPS VII)

WILLIAM S. SLY, M.D.

St. Louis, Missouri

Mucopolysaccharidosis VII is a rarely encountered autosomal recessive disorder caused by a deficiency of β-glucuronidase. The enzyme deficiency causes heparan sulfate, dermatan sulfate and chondroitin-4 or -6-sulfate to accumulate within the body. The disorder is characterized by dwarfism, hepatosplenomegaly, skeletal deformities, mild to moderate mental retardation, hernias, unusual facies, delayed psychomotor development, and frequent symptomatic pulmonary infections. Variable corneal clouding may be present. Phenotypic variation in different pedigrees has been remarkable.

THERAPY

Systemic. Several experimental approaches are currently being tried to restore the ability to degrade or clear the storage material. Such therapy would require induction of enzyme synthesis, enhancement of any residual enzyme activity, or replacement therapy with exogenous enzyme. Other experimental approaches include bone marrow transplantation.

Supportive. The physician should offer the parents sympathetic guidance in dealing with the gross deformities and mental retardation that may arise in these patients. The parents should be informed of any inpatient chronic care facilities that may be available. Genetic counseling is indicated for parents, as the risk of recurrence is 25 per cent in subsequent pregnancies. Prenatal diagnosis is possible from enzyme assays on cells cultured from amniocentesis specimens.

Surgical. Surgical treatment is supportive and might include repair of hernias or orthopedic surgery for skeletal deformities. Penetrating keratoplasty or lamellar corneal graft is the treatment of choice for corneal clouding.

Ocular or Periocular Manifestations

Cornea: Clouding.

PRECAUTIONS

There is no specific treatment for any of the mucopolysaccharidoses. Plasma infusion has occasionally provided temporary improvement, but it is still not a practical means of therapy.

COMMENTS

The phenotypic variability of β-glucuronidase deficiency is quite remarkable and suggests genetic heterogeneity. Recently, several unrelated β-glucuronidase-deficient patients have presented in the newborn period with nonimmune hydrops and have died within the first 12 months. This is the most severe clinical form of the disease; the milder forms resemble the Hunter syndrome phenotype in severity, though symptoms are less progressive in late childhood. Despite considerable variability of β-glucuronidase activity in the plasma and serum of normal individuals, the homozygous-affected patient can readily be diagnosed from serum. For carrier detection, the enzyme should preferably be measured in fibroblast cultures or leukocytes. The relatively simple enzymatic assay on white blood cell lysates provides a means for making or excluding this diagnosis, as well as for determining carrier states. Its application to other patients with mucopolysaccharidoses will help delineate this entity further.

References

Beaudet AL, et al: Variation in the phenotypic expression of β-glucuronidase deficiency. J Pediatr *86:*388–394, 1975.

Gitzelmann R, et al: Unusually mild course of β-glucuronidase deficiency in two brothers (mucopolysaccharidosis VII). Helv Paediatr Acta *33:*413–428, 1978.

Guibaud P, et al: Mucopolysaccharidosis type VII par deficit en beta-glucuronidase: Etude d'une famille. J Genet Hum *27:*29–43, 1979.

Lee JES, Falk RE, Ng WG, Donnell GN: Beta-glucuronidase deficiency; a heterogeneous mucopolysaccharidosis. Am J Dis Child *139:*57–59, 1985.

Nelson A, et al: Mucopolysaccharidosis VII (β-glucuronidase deficiency) presenting as nonimmune hydrops fetalis. J Pediatr *101:*574–576, 1982.

Sewell AC, Gehler J, Mittermaier G, Mayer E: Mucopolysaccharidosis type VII (beta-glucuronidase deficiency): A report of a new case and a survey of those in the literature. Clin Genet *21:*366–373, 1982.

Sly WS, et al: Beta glucuronidase deficiency: Report of clinical, radiologic, and biochemical features of a new mucopolysaccharidosis. J Pediatr *82:*249–257, 1973.

OXALOSIS 271.8

JOHN D. BULLOCK, M.D., M.S., F.A.C.S.

Dayton, Ohio

and AMY R. JEFFERY, M.D.

Philadelphia, Pennsylvania

Oxalosis is a systemic condition characterized by elevated serum and urinary oxalic acid levels. Oxalic acid combines with calcium in the body to produce an overall increase in calcium oxalate. The subsequent deposition of the calcium oxalate in various tissues is histopathologically termed "oxalosis."

Primary oxalosis is a rare autosomal recessive inborn error of carbohydrate metabolism involving an enzymatic defect in the glyoxylate pathway. Both type I (with a deficient peroxisomal alanine: glyoxylate aminotransferase) and type II (which lacks D-glyceric dehydrogenase) are characterized by a chronic excess of serum and urinary oxalic acid.

Secondary oxalosis results from increased serum and urinary levels of oxalic acid from exogenous causes. Pyridoxine or thiamine deficiency, ingestion of oxalate or oxalate precursors (prolonged methyoxyflurane anesthesia, ethylene glycol, xylitol), increased ascorbic acid levels, impaired renal excretion, fat malabsorption syndromes, or chronic dialysis can increase oxalic acid levels.

The diagnosis of oxalosis is made by measuring an increased level of urinary oxalate and, if tissue is available, a pizzolato stain for calcium oxalate. Primary oxalosis is diagnosed after all other sources of oxalic acid are excluded. If any of the previously mentioned sources are present in the face of systemic oxalosis, the diagnosis is presumably secondary oxalosis.

Postmortem studies of patients with oxalosis have noted that calcium oxalate is deposited intracellularly in many organs as fine yellow crystalline particles. Crystalline deposits can cause nephrolithiasis with kidney failure, complete heart block, peripheral vasospasm, and crystalline retinopathy. Retinal crystals are in a widespread distribution similar to a "flecked retina" appearance. All the vascularized tissues of the eye may contain deposits, but the retinal pigment epithelium (RPE) is involved primarily. Eye involvement in oxalosis is uncommon, but when it occurs it is usually in those patients with primary hereditary oxalosis type I or, in the past, in patients given methoxyflurane anesthesia. Eye involvement has been reported in approximately one-third of all patients with primary oxalosis type I.

THERAPY

Primary: There is no satisfactory treatment for primary oxalosis. High fluid intake and phosphate and pyridoxine levels can reduce urinary oxalate and kidney damage. The majority of patients develop renal failure by age 20, and even their transplanted kidneys fail secondary to oxalosis.

Secondary: To treat secondary oxalosis, one should attempt to remove the offending agent, correct a deficiency, or discontinue an oxalate precursor. Hemodialysis or peritoneal dialysis does not remove oxalate with the same efficiency as does the kidney so that patients with chronic renal failure are persistently hyperoxaluric.

For patients with fat malabsorption, cholestyramine can bind oxalate to minimize the oxalosis; a low-fat diet is also helpful.

Ocular or Periocular Manifestations

Eyelids: Stippled with subepidermal oxalate deposits.

Optic Nerve: Optic atrophy.

Retina: Crystalline retinopathy (yellowish-white punctate lesions) in posterior pole extending to equator; subretinal ringlet; large black geographic lesions; macular edema; tractional retinal detachment.

Vessels: Artery, arteriole, and capillary occlusions.

Vitreous: Vitreous hemorrhage.

Other: Neovascular glaucoma.

PRECAUTIONS

When a crystalline retinopathy or flecked retina is found on examination, a clinical history for causes of secondary oxalosis must be conducted. Retinal oxalosis can result in a central or branch arteriolar occlusion and optic atrophy so it must be part of the differential diagnosis for those presentations. The visual prognosis in patients with oxalosis is usually excellent, but it depends on the degree of the oxalate deposition. Oxalosis leading to a maculopathy can cause mild impairment, whereas optic atrophy results in severe visual loss. Retinopathy in oxalosis suggests a more severe form of the disease.

COMMENTS

Histopathologically, patients with hyperoxalosis have an abundance of oxalate crystals scattered in the RPE and uveal structures, but the majority of these crystals are not observed on clinical examination. The posterior pole of the pigment epithelium seems predisposed to oxalate disposition. This may be due to its close relation to the high-flowing choriocapillaris. These crystals may then irritate the RPE, resulting in the hypertrophic black lesions seen on clinical examination. Since calcium oxalate is a blood-borne product, the retinopathy may reflect the high vascularity of the eye.

References

Albert DM, Bullock JD, Lahav M, Caine R: Flecked retina secondary to oxalate crystals from methoxyflurane anesthesia: Clinical and experimental studies. Trans Am Acad Ophthalmol Otolaryngol 79:817–826, 1975.

Bullock JD, Albert DM: Generalized oxalosis with retinal involvement following methoxyflurane anesthesia. Anesthesiology 41:296–302, 1974.

Bullock JD, Albert DM: Flecked retina appearance secondary to oxalate crystals from methoxyflurane anesthesia. Arch Ophthalmol 93:26–31, 1975.

Bullock JD, Albert DM, Skinner HCW, Miller WH, Galla J: Calcium oxalate retinopathy associated with generalized oxalosis, x-ray diffraction and electron microscopic studies of crystal deposits. Invest Ophthalmol 13:256–265, 1974.

Caine RA, Albert DM, Lahav M, Bullock JD: Oxalate retinopathy: An experimental model of a flecked retina. Invest Ophthalmol 14:359–364, 1975.

Garner A: Retinal oxalosis. Br J Ophthalmol 58:613–619, 1974.

Goodkin DA: Ethylene glycol poisoning. Am J Med 88:201, 1990.

Meredith TA, et al: Ocular involvement in primary hyperoxaluria. Arch Ophthalmol 102:584–587, 1984.

Small KW, Letson R, Scheinman J: Ocular findings in primary hyperoxaluria. Arch Ophthalmol 108:89–93, 1990.

Small KW, Scheinman J, Klintworth GK: A clinicopathological study of ocular involvement in primary hyperoxaluria type I. Br J Ophthalmol 76:54–57, 1992.

Wells CG, et al: Retinal oxalosis. Arch Ophthalmol 107:1638–1643, 1989.

SECTION 7

DISORDERS OF LIPID METABOLISM

FABRY'S DISEASE 272.7
**(Angiokeratoma Corporis Diffusum
Universale, Anderson-Fabry Disease,
Glycolipid Lipidosis)**

ROBERT T. SPECTOR, M.D., F.A.C.S.,

Fort Lauderdale, Florida

and THOMAS A. WEINGEIST, M.D.,
Ph.D.

Iowa City, Iowa

Fabry's disease, formerly called angiokeratoma corporis diffusum universale, is a rare glycolipid thesaurosis that results from an X-linked recessive inborn error of metabolism; it is the only lipid metabolism and storage disorder to have this mode of inheritance. Deficiency of the enzyme alpha-galactosidase results in accumulation of ceramide trihexoside and dihexosyl ceramide. Recent studies have implicated additional enzymes.

Cutaneous angiokeratomas and whorl-like corneal dystrophy are the most distinctive physical findings in Fabry's disease. Accumulation of neutral glycosphingolipids in endothelial, perithelial, and smooth muscle cells of the cardiovascular, renal, and cerebrovascular systems results in progressive impairment and premature death. The complete clinical manifestations of Fabry's disease occur only in males (hemizygotes). Fabry's disease is not a symptomatic disease of early childhood, but may be diagnosed before 10 years of age. Children may complain of pain in extremities, and there may be a lack of sweating, giving rise to fevers. With progression, there are complaints of easy fatigability (due to storage in skeletal muscle), poor vision (corneal opacities and cataracts), and psychologic disturbances due to decreased blood flow from thrombus formation in the brain. Early in life, affected males have a reduced alphagalactosidase level in plasma, serum, leukocytes, tears, and skin fibroblasts. An elevated trihexosyl ceramide level in urine, plasma, and skin fibroblasts can also be demonstrated. Multiple wine-red angiokeratomas involve the trunk, fingers, penis, lips, and tongue. Skin lesions may be distributed in the bathing trunk region in hemizygous adults. Death usually occurs before the fourth or fifth decade from renal or cardiac failure or from cerebrovascular disease. Female carriers (heterozygotes) are involved to a lesser extent and usually develop symptoms at a later age. In heterozygous females, Fabry's disease is usually limited to the eyes; life expectancy is nearly normal, since renal and cerebrovascular involvement is uncommon.

Ocular findings in Fabry's disease are often subtle and seldom interfere with vision, but are important when confirming the diagnosis. The most characteristic ocular sign is a fine, whorl-like, superficial corneal opacity that occurs in both affected male subjects and female carriers. On slit-lamp examination, golden-brown pigmentation is visible in the corneal epithelium. This vortex corneal pattern resembles the corneal changes found after chronic ingestion of chloroquine, amiodarone, and other agents that cause a drug-induced lipidosis. The familial corneal dystrophy of Fleischer-Gruber (cornea verticillata), which was once considered a separate entity, has been found to be a manifestation of Fabry's disease. Dilated sausage-shaped conjunctival blood vessels and tortuosity of retinal vessels are common. Two specific types of cataracts occur in Fabry's disease. One type is characterized by granular anterior subcapsular deposits. The other type is an unusual spoke-like posterior subcapsular opacity that is best seen by retroillumination.

In Fabry's disease, decreased visual acuity results primarily from occlusive retinal vascular disease and complications of hypertensive retinopathy. Profound loss of vision from central retinal artery occlusion is sometimes the initial presenting symptom.

Abnormal accumulation of intracytoplasmic lipid occurs throughout endothelial, perithelial, and smooth muscle cells of the eye. Intracellular deposits of lipid also are found in epithelial cells of the conjunctiva, cornea, and lens. Ultrastructural examination of these inclusions reveals that they consist of a single membrane, surrounding concentrically arranged membranous lamellae. The myelin-like structures are not pathognomonic of Fabry's disease.

The histopathologic basis for the whorl-like pattern in the cornea has been the subject of debate. Increasing evidence indicates that it is due to a combination of accumulation of lysosomal granules in the epithelium that have been detected even in the fetus and duplication of the basal lamina of the corneal epithelium.

THERAPY

Systemic. Intravenous administration of purified enzyme (placental alphagalactosidase)† has been investigated, but offers little promise. Phlebotomy does not alter plasma or urinary levels of ceramide trihexoside, and plasmapheresis is ineffective in treating the acroparesthesia of Fabry's disease. Treatment of pain is symptomatic; diphenylhydantoin (20 mg/24 hr) or carbamazepine (200 mg/hr) has been used with variable success.

Surgical. No satisfactory treatment is currently available. Renal transplantation has been performed for amelioration of chronic uremia. Unfortunately, recurrence of the storage disease is common in the renal allograft. The disproportionately high incidence of sepsis in some patients may be due to the deficient immunologic function of lipid-laden leukocytes. Hemodialysis remains an alternative mode of therapy for uremia, but does not alter the accompanying cerebrovascular disease or renal failure.

Ocular or Periocular Manifestations

Conjunctiva: Telangiectasia.
Cornea: Cornea verticillata; whorl-like or spoke like opacity.
Extraocular Muscles: Internuclear ophthalmoplegia.
Eyelids: Edema.
Lens: Anterior and posterior, spoke-like, subcapsular opacity ("Fabry cataract").
Optic Nerve: Disc edema.
Orbit: Periorbital edema.
Retina: Central or branch retinal artery occlusion; hypertensive retinopathy; vascular occlusive disease; vascular tortuosity.

PRECAUTIONS

Genetic counseling and recognition of female carriers are important. The pattern of inheritance is like that of all X-linked recessive disorders. There is an absence of father-to-son transmission. All daughters of an affected male will be carriers (heterozygotes). Half the sons of affected daughters will also have Fabry's disease. Identification of all female carriers is difficult, since 25 to 40 per cent of suspected heterozygotes may have normal alpha-galactosidase levels. Recent studies have shown that, with the use of multiple biochemical tests, carriers can now be identified in more than 90 per cent of cases.

COMMENTS

The diagnosis of Fabry's disease is easily missed, especially in female carriers. The ophthalmologist is in an excellent position to make the diagnosis since corneal changes are the earliest and the most consistent ocular abnormality. Corneal changes occur in about 90 per cent of affected male subjects and may be the only ocular sign in female carriers. The posterior spoke-like cataracts may be pathognomonic. The whorl-like corneal opacities are highly indicative of Fabry's disease, especially if there has been no history of consumption of drugs, such as chloroquine.

References

Beutler E, Westwood B, Dale GL: The effect of phlebotomy as a treatment of Fabry disease. Biochem Med 30:363–368, 1983.

Braine HG, et al: A prospective double-blind study of plasma exchange therapy for the acroparesthesia of Fabry's disease. Transfusion 21:686–689, 1981.

Desnick RJ, Frabowski GA: Advances in the treatment of inherited metabolic disease. Adv Hum Genet 11:281–369, 1981.

Desnick RT, et al: Fabry disease: Molecular diagnosis of hemizygotes and heterozygotes. Enzyme 38:54–64, 1987.

Franceschetti AT: Fabry's disease: Ocular manifestations. Birth Defects 12:195, 1976.

Francois J, Hanssens, M, Teuchy H: Corneal ultrastructural changes in Fabry's disease. Ophthalmologica 176:313, 1978.

Kleijer WJ, et al: Prenatal diagnosis of Fabry's disease by direct analysis of chorionic villi. Prenat Diagn 7:283–287, 1987.

Mathew TH: Recurrence of disease following renal transplantation. Am J Kidney Dis 12:85–96, 1988.

Riegel EM, et al: Ocular pathology of Fabry's disease in a hemizygous male following renal transplantation. Surv Ophthalmol 26:247–252, 1982.

Rodriguez FH, Hoffmann EO, Ordinario AT: Fabry's disease in a hemizygous male following renal transplantation. Surv Ophthalmol 26:247–252, 1982.

Rodriguez FH, Hoffmann EO, Ordinario AT: Fabry's disease in a heterozygous woman. Arch Pathol Lab Med 109:89–91, 1985.

Sakuraba H, et al: Effects of vitamin E and ticlopidine on platelet aggregation in Fabry's disease. Clin Genet 31:349–354, 1987.

Tsutsumi A, et al: Corneal findings in a foetus with Fabry's disease. Acta Ophthalmol 62:923–931, 1984.

Weingeist TA, Blodi FC: Fabry's disease: Ocular findings in a female carrier. A light and electron microscopic study. Arch Ophthalmol 85:169, 1971.

HYPERLIPOPROTEINEMIA 272.4

MALCOLM N. LUXENBERG, M.D.

Augusta, Georgia

Hyperlipoproteinemia is a metabolic disorder characterized by abnormally elevated concentrations of specific lipoprotein particles in the plasma. Hyperlipidemia, which refers to an elevation of the plasma cholesterol and/or triglycerides above the normal range, is present in all these disorders. The hyperlipoproteinemias can be separated into primary and secondary forms, with the secondary form being caused by other diseases, such as diabetes mellitus, pancreatitis, renal disease, or hypothyroidism. They can also be divided into distinct groups that are determined by the pattern of elevation of the plasma lipoproteins. However, these groups are not specific diseases, but may represent the final result of various metabolic disorders. Certain ones can be defined as genetically determined, and their mechanisms and modes of inheritance have been determined. The primary groups include chylomicronemia (exogenous or endogenous hyperlipemia), hypercholesterolemia, dysbetalipoproteinemia (hyperlipoproteinemia type 3), hypertriglyceridemia, mixed hyperlipoproteinemia, and combined hyperlipoproteinemia. Clinical manifestations of the hyperlipoproteinemias are caused by deposition of lipids at various sites throughout the body, such as the skin, tendons, vascular system, and eye. Corneal arcus, lipemia retinalis, and xanthelasma are the most common ocular abnormalities.

THERAPY

Systemic. Various drugs, especially those that lower cholesterol and/or triglycerides, may be beneficial in the management of these disorders. Some of the medications used include clofibrate, gemfibrozil, niacin, cholestyramine resin, colestipol, dextrothyroxine, sitosterols, probucol, and some progestational agents. Gemfibrozil is chemically related to clofibrate and lowers both cholesterol and triglycerides. Because of the possibility of significant side effects and the question whether triglycerides are independent risk factors for atherosclerosis, many physicians use drugs to reduce triglyceride levels only when they exceed 500 mg/100 ml. Cholesterol can be significantly lowered by a group of drugs known as HMG Co-A reductase inhibitors. These include lovastatin (Mevacor) and two newer agents, pravastatin and simvastatin. It has been recommended that patients taking lovastatin have an annual eye examination as lens opacities may develop. However, this possible side effect does not seem to occur with pravastatin and simvastatin.

Supportive. Diet remains the cornerstone of therapy for hyperlipidemia. Weight reduction is desirable, and saturated fat and cholesterol intake may need to be restricted. In addition, alcohol and estrogens should be avoided in certain types of hyperlipoproteinemias.

Surgical. Ileal bypass surgery and plasmapheresis may be used to lower elevated serum lipids in very selected cases of familial hypercholesterolemia. These forms of therapy should only be used by physicians with experience in this field.

Xanthelasma may be surgically excised. Small defects can be primarily closed, whereas large defects may require skin grafting or other plastic surgical repair. Care must be taken to avoid postoperative ectropion in the lower eyelid and lid lag and/or lagophthalmos in the upper eyelid. Xanthelasma may also be removed by photocoagulation.

Ocular or Periocular Manifestations

Choroid: Xanthoma (hypercholesterolemia).

Conjunctiva: Lipemia of limbal vessels (dysbetalipoproteinemia); xanthoma (hypercholesterolemia).

Cornea: Arcus (hypercholesterolemia and dysbetalipoproteinemia); lipid keratopathy (chylomicronemia and hypercholesterolemia).

Eyelids: Eruptive xanthoma (chylomicronemia, dysbetalipoproteinemia, and mixed hypertriglyceridemia); xanthelasma (hypercholesterolemia and dysbetalipoproteinemia).

Iris: Xanthoma (chylomicronemia).

Retina: Lipemia retinalis (chylomicronemia and mixed hypertriglyceridemia); xanthoma (chylomicronemia and hypercholesterolemia).

PRECAUTIONS

Hyperlipoproteinemia may be present in children and young adults, and persons with these disorders can develop abnormalities of the vascular system, including ischemic cardiac disease. Therefore, it is important to obtain appropriate medical evaluation, especially in patients younger than 40 to 45 years of age who have a prominent arcus of the cornea, or xanthelasma, or in any patient with lipemia retinalis, in order to establish a diagnosis and initiate therapy when appropriate. Corneal arcus is commonly seen in normal people, especially in males over the age of 45 years, without associated hyperlipidemia. Although xanthelasma may be present without elevation of the serum lipids, about half of the patients have elevated cholesterol levels. Studies have demonstrated apolipoprotein abnormalities in patients with xanthelasma, including those with normal cholesterol levels. There may also be an increased prevalence of hyperlipidemia in patients with retinal vein occlusion. In many cases, it is difficult or impossible to determine which patients with these findings have hyperlipidemia, especially when there are no other signs of hyperlipoproteinemia. Therefore, one should consider obtaining serum cholesterol and triglyceride studies in any patient with premature arcus or xanthelasma.

COMMENTS

Measurements of plasma lipid and lipoprotein levels should be performed while the patient is on a regular diet after an overnight fast of 12 to 16 hours. Identification of abnormal lipoprotein patterns can often be made after determining serum cholesterol and triglyceride levels and visual inspection of the plasma sample, which has been stored at 4°C. In some cases, it may be necessary to perform electrophoresis and ultracentrifugation of whole plasma specimens to make a diagnosis.

Lipemia retinalis is caused primarily by elevation of the serum triglycerides, which impart a milky color to the blood. The changes are usually not seen until the triglyceride level reaches at least 2000 mg per cent and are best observed, in the early stages, in the peripheral fundus. The vessels initially appear salmon pink, but when the triglyceride level rises further, they assume a whitish appearance. These changes, which begin in the periphery, progress toward the posterior pole as the triglyceride level rises. In severe cases, the vessels are creamy white in color, and it becomes difficult to differentiate arteries from veins. The findings can fluctuate widely from day to day, depending on the triglyceride level. The fundus abnormalities, which improve as the triglycerides return to normal, provide a means of following the patient's course and response to therapy.

Patients suspected or known to have hyperlipoproteinemia should be referred to a physician familiar with these disorders for evaluation and management, as treatment can be difficult, especially regarding the selection and use of specific drugs.

References

Bron AJ: Corneal changes in the dislipoproteinaemias. Cornea 8:135–140, 1989.
Bron AJ, Williams HP: Lipaemia of the limbal vessels. Br J Ophthalmol 56:343–346, 1972.
Brunzel JD, Bierman EL: Chylomicronemia syndrome. Interaction of genetic and acquired hypertriglyceridemia. Med Clin North Am 66:455–468, 1982.
Dodson PM, et al: Retinal vein occlusion and the prevalence of lipoprotein abnormalities. Br J Ophthalmol 66:161–164, 1982.
Feldman EB: Nutrition and diet in relation to hyperlipidemia and atherosclorisis. In Shields M, Olson JA, Shike M (eds): Modern Nutrition in Health & Disease, 8th ed. Philadelphia, Lea & Febiger, 1992.
Fredrickson DS, Goldstein JS, Brown MS: The familial hyperlipoproteinemias. In Stanbury JB, Wyngaarden JB, Fredrickson DS (eds): The Metabolic Basis of Inherited Disease, 5th ed. New York, McGraw-Hill, 1982, pp 655–671.
Havel RJ, Goldstein JL, Brown MS: Lipoproteins and lipid transport. In Bondy PK, Rosenberg LE (eds): Metabolic Control and Disease, 8th ed. Philadelphia, WB Saunders, 1980, pp 393–494.
Havel RJ, Kane JP: Therapy of hyperlipidemic states. Annu Rev Med 33:417–433, 1982.
Kuske TT, Feldman EB: Hyperlipoproteinemia, atherosclerosis risk, and dietary management. Arch Intern Med 147:357–360, 1987.
Margolis S: Treatment of hyperlipemia. JAMA 239:2696–2698, 1978.
Rifkind BM: Corneal arcus and hyperlipoproteinemia. Surv Ophthalmol 16:295–304, 1972.
Spaeth GL: Ocular manifestations of the lipodoses. In Tasman W (ed): Retinal Diseases in Children. New York, Harper & Row, 1971, pp 127–137.
Vinger PF, Sachs BA: Ocular manifestations of hyperlipoproteinemia. Am J Ophthalmol 70:563–573, 1970.

SECTION 8

OTHER METABOLIC DISORDERS

GOUT 274.7
(Hyperuricemia)

JOHN H. WILKINS, M.D.

Portland, Oregon

Hyperuricemia occurs in a group of diseases with an abnormality of purine metabolism(~15 per cent) and/or uric acid excretion(~85 per cent). Gout is the term used to describe the condition in which hyperuricemia and associated urate deposition in joint (tophi), interstitial renal disease, uric acid nephrolithiasis, or characteristic mono- or pauciarticular arthritis occur. Primary gout is due to an inborn error of metabolism resulting in the excess production of urate or in the diminished excretion of uric acid. Secondary gout is caused by an increased breakdown of nucleic acids due to a variety of acquired diseases (e.g., lymphoproliferative diseases) or to decreased renal excretion of uric acid (e.g., renal insufficiency, thiazide diuretics). Hyperuricemia occurs equally in males and females. True gouty arthritis, however, occurs in males much more frequently than in females (20:1) and is usually found in those of middle age. The lifetime prevalence is 3 per 1000 population in the United States, with a peak incidence at age 60 years. Gouty arthritis is much more common in the obese, in heavy ethanol users, and in those who eat foods rich in purines (fish, meat, poultry, especially the solid organs), which may account for its historical association with the upper socioeconomic classes.

The systemic symptoms of gout are caused by the deposition of urate crystals in and about joints, the kidneys, and other tissues. Tissue trauma, cellular destruction, and inflammation ensue. The symptoms of this inflammation include acute pain accompanied by redness, tenderness, and swelling of the affected area. Although the metatarsophalangeal joint of the great toe is the most commonly affected joint followed by the feet, ankles, and knees, urate crystal deposition (tophi formation) can occur in any joint, bursa, or subcutaneous region. Most common severe complications are in the kidney due to nephrolithiasis-associated hydronephrosis or pyelonephritis and renal insufficiency from urate nephropathy.

The most common ocular involvement is chronic bilateral conjunctival redness. Other features are uncommon and include episcleritis, scleritis, conjunctivitis, keratopathy, and keratitis. Although historically uveitis was a frequent finding, more recent series have failed to detect any association.

THERAPY

Systemic. The goals of therapy are to stop the acute attack, prevent recurrent attacks, and avoid systemic complications.

ACUTE. The initial acute inflammatory attack of gout may be treated by either oral nonsteroidal anti-inflammatory drugs (NSAIDs) or colchicine. Indomethacin or naproxen sodium are the most commonly employed NSAIDs to treat the acute episodes; indomethacin 50 mg every 8 hours, or naproxen sodium, 750 mg initially followed by 250 mg every 8 hours for 3 to 7 days. Individuals show response within 24 to 36 hours, and the drug should begin to be tapered by 3 days and stopped by 1 week. Colchicine is an alternative to NSAIDs for an acute attack and should be considered when NSAIDs are contraindicated, as in peptic ulcer disease. Although the exact method of action is not known, colchicine seems to act by inhibiting the migration of granulocytic cells to the inflamed area and by decreasing lactic acid production, which is commonly associated with phagocytosis. Colchicine is also known to prevent cell mitosis, which may explain its ability to prevent the mobilization of leukocytes during inflammation. It also inhibits histamine release from mast cells. If colchicine is given within the first few hours of onset of an acute gouty arthritis attack, it provides dramatic relief in greater than 90 per cent of individuals. Colchicine can be given as an intravenous injection of a single dose of 2 mg diluted in 20 ml of 0.9 per cent sodium chloride solution with excellent results. The major complications from the intravenous form are extravasation and focal necrosis. Alternatively, an oral dose of 1 mg can be given initially, followed by 0.5 mg every 1 to 2 hours; the therapy is stopped as soon as the pain eases or nausea, vomiting, or diarrhea occur. The maximum total dose should be less than 6 mg. However, 50 to 80 per cent of pa-

183

tients treated with oral colchicine will develop dose-limiting gastrointestinal side effects. It is important not to repeat a regimen of oral colchicine within 7 days due to cumulative toxicity. A third alternative is systemic corticosteroids or local injection to the affected joint. Prednisone, 40 to 80 mg given orally, will often resolve an attack within 48 hours. Corticosteroids are usually employed for those individuals who cannot tolerate either NSAIDs or colchicine.

PREVENTIVE. Once the initial attack has resolved, the patient should be evaluated to determine the cause of the attack. A diet low in purines should be prescribed. Both serum uric acid and 24-hour urinary uric acid levels should be determined. If normal or low urinary uric acid levels are found, then a trial of uricosuric agents is indicated. The most commonly employed agents in the United States are probenecid and sulfinpyrazone. Probenecid is begun at a dose of 250 mg twice daily for 1 week and is then increased to 500 mg twice daily and continued. The maximum recommended dose is 2 gm twice daily. Sulfinpyrazone is started at 100 mg twice daily and increased until an adequate serum urate (<6.5mg/dl) level is achieved to a maximum of 400 mg twice daily. The dose of either drug may then be tapered slowly as long as adequate serum urate levels are suppressed and no attacks have occurred in the prior 6 months. If an acute attack of gout occurs while on chronic suppressive therapy, these drugs should be continued and the acute therapeutics added. Allopurinol or other xanthine oxidase inhibitors are indicated for those individuals with hyperuricemia in the presence of an elevated urinary excretion of uric acid (>800 mg/24 hr). They may also be employed in the presence of renal insufficiency, intolerance to uricosuric agents, or for prophylaxis before cytotoxic therapy. Allopurinol is started at 100 mg daily and increased by 100 mg/day at weekly intervals until serum urate is at acceptable levels. The usual dose is 300 mg daily as a single dose. The maximum recommended dose is 800 mg per day. Whether employing uricosuric or xanthine oxidase inhibitors to lower serum uric acid, prophylaxis of acute exacerbations may be also accomplished by the concurrent use of colchicine, 0.5 to 1.5 mg/day, or indomethacin, 25 to 50 mg per day (or another NSAID). It is important to note that all drug doses must be titrated in the presence of renal insufficiency.

Ocular. The therapy of the ocular complications of gout ranges from proper lid hygiene and artificial tears for the conjunctival injection to systemic NSAIDs for the scleritis. Topical steroids (e.g., fluoromethalone 1 per cent one to four times daily) may also be employed to control the conjunctivitis, episcleritis, or scleritis associated with gout. The crystalline- or band-like keratopathy may be treated by superficial keratectomy.

Supportive. The importance of lifestyle changes should also be emphasized. A diet low in purines and in alcohol should be instituted. The obese patient should also be instructed in a weight loss program.

Ocular or Periocular Manifestations

Conjunctiva: Conjunctivitis with scant discharge; tophi; intraepithelial monosodium urate crystals; hyperemia.
Cornea: Crystalline keratopathy in epithelium and anterior stroma; band-like keratopathy.
Extraocular Muscles: Tenonitis.
Lens: Allopurinol-associated cataracts
Sclera: Scleritis; episcleritis.
Uvea: Acute anterior iritis (very rare).
Vitreous: Vitreous opacities.

PRECAUTIONS

NSAIDs are contraindicated in those patients with a history of recent gastrointestinal bleeding or of active peptic ulcer disease. In addition, asthma attacks may be precipitated by NSAIDs. Allopurinol is contraindicated in patients with a history of adverse reaction to this form of therapy(~20 per cent of individuals will have an adverse reaction). Most common adverse reactions are hypersensitivity reactions involving the blood and skin. As these reactions can be so severe as to be life threatening, the medication should be stopped at the first sign of rash or abnormal CBC. Colchicine may potentiate the action of several medications, including most NSAIDs, methotrexate, and aspirin. As with all medications, the risks and benefits should be discussed before initiating therapy.

COMMENTS

Gout is a chronic disease for which there is no cure. The goals of management of individuals with gout are to stop the acute attack, prevent future attacks, eliminate hyperuricemia to avoid the accumulation of urate crystals in tissues, and to identify underlying disorders associated with hyperuricemia.

References

Ferry AP: Ocular abnormalities in patients with gout. Ann Ophthalmol 17:632–635, 1985.
Fishman R, Sunderman F: Band keratopathy in gout. Arch Ophthalmol 75:367–369, 1966.
Fraunfelder FT, et al: Cataracts associated with allopurinol therapy. Am J Ophthalmol 94:137–140, 1982.
Hutchinson J: The relation of certain diseases of the eye to gout. Br Med J 2:995–1000, 1989.
Kelley WN, Schumacher HR: Gout. In Kelley WN, Harris ED, Ruddy S, et al (eds): *Textbook of Rheumatology*, 4th ed. Philadelphia, WB Saunders, 1993, pp 1291–1325.
Lerman S, Megaw JM, Gardner K: Allopurinol therapy and cataractogenesis in humans. Am J Ophthalmol 94:141–146, 1982.

McWilliams JR: Ocular findings in gout. Am J Ophthalmol *35*:1778, 1952.

Slansky HH, Kuwabara T: Intranuclear urate crystals in corneal epithelium. Arch Ophthalmol *80*: 338–344, 1968.

XERODERMA PIGMENTOSUM 757.33

JEFFREY FREEDMAN, M.B., B.Ch., Ph.D., F.R.C.S.E.

Brooklyn, New York

Xeroderma pigmentosum is a rare, autosomal recessive disorder characterized by extreme cutaneous photosensitivity to ultraviolet light, early development of cutaneous malignancies of ectodermal and mesodermal origin on ultraviolet light-exposed areas, severe ophthalmologic abnormalities, and, often, early death from malignancy. Neurologic abnormalities are also sometimes present. The range of harmful ultraviolet light extends to a wavelength of at least 320 nm and possibly even up to and higher than 340 nm. Consequently, such harmful ultraviolet light from sunlight, germicidal lamps, sunlamps, and even some commonly employed fluorescent light tubes must be avoided.

Symptoms of the disease are usually noted by 3 years of age, but may first become apparent in adult life. Photosensitivity is one of the earliest recognized cutaneous signs, characterized by erythema occurring on exposed areas, especially the face, neck, V area of the chest, forearms, and dorsa of hands. The skin lesions can be divided into six stages: stage 1—acute sun sensitivity in infancy, inflammation erythema and bullae; stage 2—pigmented macules and achromic spots in exposed areas; stage 3—telangiectasia of exposed areas; stage 4—atrophy of lids, dryness of conjunctiva, and corneal opacification; stage 5—benign growths, conjunctival inflammatory masses, symblepharon, and papillomas of lids; and stage 6—neoplasms: epithelioma, basal cell carcinoma, and malignant melanoma.

Corneal involvement may be the most common ocular change occurring with xeroderma pigmentosum. Beginning before 2 years of age, vascularization of the inferior half of the cornea may be followed by vascularization of the upper half of the cornea. The vessels regress, leaving a nonvascularized opaque area so that at 2 years of age the entire cornea is opaque. During the active stage of vascularization, the patient may experience intensive photophobia and lacrimation. Presumably, the lower half of the cornea is involved early because of its more direct exposure to the sun,

the upper half being protected by the lid. Histologically, all layers of the cornea appear to be abnormal, with the most prominent change being a degenerative pannus and irregularity of its superficial corneal stroma. Band-shaped nodular dystrophy, also known as climatic droplet keratopathy, has been noted in a patient with xeroderma pigmentosum. Other ocular lesions may include conjunctival pterygia and pinguecula; benign papillomas and fibromas of the iris occur less frequently. Keratoconus may occur in association with xeroderma pigmentosum; it may be the result of disturbances in the cell differentiation and the function of epithelial cells and keratocytes caused by ultraviolet-light-induced deficient DNA synthesis. The fundus of the eye is not affected in xeroderma pigmentosum.

In a survey of 830 patients with xeroderma pigmentosum, ocular abnormalities were reported in 40 per cent of the patients described and were restricted to tissues exposed to ultraviolet radiation (lid, conjunctiva, and cornea). The abnormalities included ectropion, corneal opacity leading to blindness, and neoplasms. Malignant neoplasms develop in many patients with xeroderma pigmentosa and involve the lids, conjunctiva, or corneoscleral limbus. Conjunctival neoplasms include intraepithelial epithelioma, squamous cell carcinomas, and sarcomas. Corneal tumors may be primary or secondary to invasion from the corneoscleral limbus. Corneal neoplasms include epitheliomas, sarcomas, squamous cell carcinomas, and melanomas. In some patients, the malignancies may invade the orbit.

THERAPY

Systemic. Systemic chemotherapy is used only for patients with known metastasis.

Ocular. Methylcellulose drops or soft contact lenses may be used to keep the cornea moist and to protect against mechanical trauma in patients whose lids are severely deformed. Corneal transplantation can be used to treat patients with corneal opacification due to pannus. If corneal transplantation is undertaken, an anti-rejection regimen must be used. The regimen that has been utilized with some success is a combination of steroids and azathioprine. Prednisolone in a dosage of 200 mg daily is given for 5 days. This is reduced by 10 mg per day to 100 mg. When this level is reached, the dosage is dropped by 10 mg per week to a standing dose of 60 mg daily. Azathioprine is given in a dose of 150 mg daily for 1 month and then dropped to 100 mg daily for a minimum period of 6 months. Weekly blood counts and platelet levels must be performed. Azathioprine is stopped if platelets drop below 150,000 or the white cell count below 3000.

Supportive. Since exposure to sunlight results in the skin changes typical of xeroderma pigmentosum, patients must be educated to constantly protect all body surfaces from ultraviolet radiation. In addition to sunlight, ultraviolet exposure may come from germicidal lamps, artificial sunlamps, and to a small extent, the common, unfiltered, cool, white, fluorescent lamps. However, long wavelength ultraviolet radiation from incandescent lamps or sunlight passing through window glass is not known to be harmful. Ultraviolet radiation protection should consist of adopting a lifestyle to minimize the possibility of ultraviolet radiation exposure; wearing protective clothing, glasses, and hairstyles; and using sunscreens. When outdoors, patients should wear long-sleeved clothing, long pants, and wide-brimmed hats. Sunglasses or eyeglasses that are completely opaque to ultraviolet radiation should be worn. The glasses should incorporate side shields to protect the eyelids and periorbital skin, as well as the cornea and conjunctiva. Exposed skin should be covered with physical ultraviolet radiation blocking agents, such as zinc oxide ointment, titanium dioxide compounds, or thick makeup. Chemical sunscreens with the highest sun protection factor ratings should be used; these usually contain para-aminobenzoic acid or its derivatives.

Fibroblasts from patients with xeroderma pigmentosum exhibit an abnormally sensitive response to chemical carcinogens, such as benzapyrene derivatives and others. Exposure to such common environmental carcinogens as cigarette smoke should be minimized.

Early detection of cutaneous and ocular lesions is important to permit treatment with minimal morbidity. Patients should be examined weekly by a family member who has been instructed in the recognition of cutaneous neoplasms. This examination should include the eyes, scalp, ears, mouth, as well as covered skin areas.

Surgical. Premalignant lesions, such as multiple actinic keratoses, may be treated with superficial freezing with liquid nitrogen or with topical application of fluorouracil. Larger areas have been treated with therapeutic dermatome shaving or dermabrasion. These modalities remove the outer, more damaged epidermal layers. The epidermis is then repopulated by cells from follicles or glands, which by virtue of their deeper location have received less ultraviolet radiation exposure. Each melanoma should be treated as if it were the sole primary melanoma, with the surgical procedure dictated by the histology and location of the lesion. Malignant lesions not amenable to the above modalities can be treated with x-ray.

Neoplasms of the lids, conjunctiva, and cornea are usually treated surgically. All conjunctival surfaces must be examined for malignancies as these can occur in the fornices and may be missed unless looked for.

Ocular or Periocular Manifestations

Conjunctiva: Conjunctivitis; inflammatory nodules; malignancies; pigmentation; symblepharon.
Cornea: Exposure keratitis; malignancies; pannus; perforation; ulcer.
Eyelids: Blepharitis; blepharospasm; ectropion; keratoses; malignancies; pigmentation.
Iris: Anterior uveitis; malignancies.
Other: Photophobia; visual loss.

PRECAUTIONS

Psoralens followed by long wavelength ultraviolet radiation should not be used in xeroderma pigmentosum patients. This treatment results in DNA damage, which is not repaired normally in xeroderma pigmentosum cells, and has been reported to result in an increase in skin cancer in patients with xeroderma pigmentosum and psoriasis. Actinic keratoses have been treated with topical fluorouracil, but patients may eventually become refractory to this treatment.

COMMENTS

In patients in whom systemic chemotherapy must be used, care should be exercised to avoid untoward reactions that might result from the use of a chemotherapeutic drug to which the patient might be abnormally sensitive by virtue of defective DNA repair. The dermatologic changes that occur in patients with xeroderma pigmentosum are due to an inherited deficiency in the repair of DNA damage produced by irradiation with ultraviolet light. DNA damage produced by certain chemicals is also not repaired normally by xeroderma pigmentosum cells. The ocular abnormalities in this disorder probably result both from the intrinsic DNA repair defect in those cells of the eye that are irradiated with sunlight and from impairment of the mechanical protection of the ocular accessory organs.

There is no known prevention for the progressive neurologic abnormalities of xeroderma pigmentosum. However, with early diagnosis, appropriate avoidance of harmful ultraviolet light, and prompt treatment of neoplasms, most xeroderma pigmentosum patients without neurologic abnormalities can now survive well into adulthood and lead productive lives.

References

Blanksma LJ, Donders PC, van Voorst Vader PC: Xeroderma pigmentosum and keratoconus. Doc Ophthalmol 64:97–103, 1986.

Freedman J: Xeroderma pigmentosum and band-shaped nodular corneal dystrophy. Br J Ophthalmol 61:96–100, 1977.

Freedman J: Corneal transplantation with associated histopathologic description in xeroderma pigmentosum occurring in a black family. Ann Ophthalmol 11:445–448, 1979.

Kraemer KH: Xeroderma pigmentosum. *In* Dennis DJ, Dobson R, McGuire J (eds): Clinical Dermatology. Hagerstown, MD, Harper & Row, 1980.

Kraemer KH, Lee MM, Scotto J: Xeroderma pigmentosum. Cutaneous, ocular and neurologic abnormalities in 830 published cases. Arch Dermatol *123*:241–250, 1987.

Newsome DA, Kraemer KH, Robbins JH: Repair of DNA in xeroderma pigmentosum conjunctiva. Arch Ophthalmol *93*:660–662, 1975.

Regan JD, et al: Repair of DNA damaged by mutagenic metabolites of benzo(a)pyrene in human cells. Chem Biol Interact *20*:279–287, 1978.

Robbins JH: Significance of repair of human DNA: Evidence from studies of xeroderma pigmentosum. J Natl Cancer Inst *61*:645–656, 1978.

Robbins, JH, et al: Xeroderma pigmentosum. An inherited disease with sun sensitivity, multiple cutaneous neoplasms, and abnormal DNA repair. Ann Intern Med *80*:221–248, 1974.

HEMATOLOGIC AND CARDIOVASCULAR DISORDERS

ARTERIOVENOUS FISTULA 447.0

(Arteriovenous Aneurysm, Arteriovenous Angioma, Arteriovenous Malformation, Cirsoid Aneurysm, Racemose Hemangioma, Varicose Aneurysm)

J. REIMER WOLTER, M.D.

Ann Arbor, Michigan

Arteriovenous (A-V) fistulas are abnormal communications, single or multiple, between arteries and veins by which arterial blood enters the veins directly without traversing a capillary network. These fistulas can be developmental or acquired. Most acquired fistulae occur secondary to penetrating injuries, bone fractures, or blunt trauma. Malignancy, infection, or rupture of arterial aneurysms can also be the cause of A-V communications. Congenital A-V fistulas usually are complex formations of many separate or interconnected lesions, most commonly seen in the head and neck region. Clinical manifestations of A-V aneurysms include formation of a space-taking mass, swelling, edema, hemorrhage, pain, glaucoma, exophthalmus, diplopia, or other disturbances of ocular function. The tissues adjacent to superficial A-V fistulas may be tender, appear either red or cyanotic, and may exhibit hemorrhages and locally increased skin temperatures.

All vascular parts of the eye and its adnexa can be involved with A-V fistulas. They may be part of a more extensive malformation in the eye region, such as the Sturge-Weber syndrome. The major outflow of periocular arteriovenous fistulas is the superior ophthalmic veins, which may expand tremendously and be associated with engorged orbital and conjunctival veins. These veins give the signs and symptoms of venous congestion, and they become arterialized in time. Corneal edema, flare and cells in the anterior chamber, rubeosis iridis, glaucoma, cataract, retinal venous congestion, and intraocular hemorrhages are common manifestations.

THERAPY

Surgical. Resection or x-ray therapy—high-precision proton beam radiotherapy spe-

cifically—is recommended. Ligation or balloon embolization of the feeding artery is not usually applicable for intraocular A-V aneurysms. Yet, photocoagulation and laser coagulation for local obliteration and in panretinal application are used. Before operating on extraocular A-V fistulas, it is important to obtain complete angiographic studies, as well as a thorough clinical examination, Doppler sonography, and other x-ray studies including laminography.

A single fistula can be repaired surgically by reestablishing the continuity of the involved artery by arterrioraphy, end-to-end anastomosis, or grafting. Embolization of feeding arteries using detachable balloons, isobutylcyanoacrylate, or polyvinyl particles has been reported, but can lead to complications. Mild cases may be relatively stationary and should be managed conservatively. Multiple fistulae mainly present as a space-taking problem and can be excised or otherwise obliterated completely.

Eighty-five to 90 per cent of all A-V aneurysms in the eye region are primarily supplied by the carotid circulation. Carotid ligation in the neck and/or intracranial or extracranial ligation, with possible additional ligation of the external carotid and opthalmic arteries, are among the recommended treatments. The superior ophthalmic veins may also be ligated in the orbit through a superior marginal approach or after resection of the outer orbital wall.

Ocular or Periocular Manifestations

Anterior Chamber: Cells and flare; hemorrhage; shallowing; iris involvement; angle closure and acute glaucoma in ciliochoroidal detachment.

Choroid: Choroidal detachment; vascular tumor; hemorrhage; atrophy or scarring.

Conjunctiva: Chemosis; neovascularization; vascular congestion; vascular tumor; hemorrhage; necrosis.

Cornea: Bullous keratopathy; clouding; neovascularization.

Eyelids: Edema; vascular tumor; protrusion; ptosis.

Globe: Exophthalmus; diplopia; glaucoma; blindness in extremes.

Iris: Atrophy; iris tumor; rubeosis; ectropion uveae.

Optic nerve: Congestion; vascular tumor; papilledema; atrophy.

Retina: Vascular tumor; congestion; hemorrhage; degeneration; detachment; macrovessels; twin vessels; vein thrombosis.

Other: Cataract; vitreous hemorrhage; loss of vision; pareses of third or sixth nerves; vascular tumor; and congestion of orbit.

PRECAUTIONS

Even in the absence of operative or postoperative complications, surgical therapy may be complicated by late cerebral signs, such as slowly progressive hemiplegia due to spreading thrombosis. Associated cerebral edema or deterioration of the ocular blood supply may cause late problems; for example, sloughing of the cornea.

COMMENTS

The most common traumatic A-V fistula is caused by rupture of the carotid on its course through the cavernous sinus in fractures at the base of the skull. Others develop in the sphenoid bone, where the artery and veins are intimately apposed. A majority of spontaneous A-V fistulas occur in women, and 25 per cent occur during pregnancy. The prognosis in this condition is not good, and sudden death can occur due to rupture of the cavernous sinus and massive cerebral hemorrhage.

References

Brown GC, Shields JA: Tumors of the optic nerve head. Surv Ophthalmol 29:239–264, 1985.

Chronister CL, Nyman NN, Meccariello AF: Congenital retinal macrovessel. Optometry Vis Sci 68:747–749, 1991.

Coffman JD: Peripheral vascular diseases due to abnormal communications between arteries and veins. Arteriovenous fistula. *In* Beeson PB, McDermot W (eds): Textbook of Medicine, 14th ed. Philadelphia, WB Saunders, 1975, pp 1082–1083.

De Jong PT: Neovascular glaucoma and occurrence of twin vessels in congenital arteriovenous communications of retina. Document Ophthalmolog 68:3–4, 1988.

Flaherty PM, Lieb WE, Sergott RC, Bosley TM, Savino PJC: Color Doppler imaging. A new noninvasive technique to diagnose and monitor carotid cavernous sinus fistulas. Arch Ophthalmol 109:522–526, 1991.

Fourman S: Angle closure glaucoma complicating ciliochoroidal detachment. Ophthalmology 96:646–643, 1989.

Fritz W, Klein HJ, Schmidt K: Arteriovenous malformation of the posterior ethmoidal artery as unusual cause of amaurosis fugax. The ophthalmic steal syndrome. J Clinical Neuro-Ophthal 9:165–168, 1989.

Hanneken AM, Miller NR, Debrun GM, Nauta HJ: Treatment of carotid-cavernous sinus fistulas using a detachable balloon catheter through the superior ophthalmic vein. Arch Ophthalmol 107:87–92, 1989.

Katzen LB, Katzen BT, Katzen MJ: Treatment of carotid-cavernous fistulas with detachable balloon catheter occlusion. Adv Ophthalmol Plast Reconstr Surg 7:157–165, 1987.

Kupersmith MJ, Berenstein A, Choi IS, Warren F, Flamm E: Management of non-traumatic vascular shunts involving the cavernous sinus. Ophthalmology 95:121–130, 1988.

Lucas BC, Eckardt C: Venous vascular anomalies in myelinated retinal nerve fiber layer area. Klin Mbl Augenheilkd 199:454–456, 1991.

Mansour AM, Wells CG, Jampol LM, Kalina RE: Ocular complications of arterio-venous communications of the retina. Arch Ophthalmol 107:232–236, 1989.

Munzenrider JE, Austin-Seymour M, Blitzen PJ, Gentry R, Goitein M, Gragoudas ES, Johnson K, Koehler AM, McNulty P, Moulton G, et al: Proton therapy at Harvard. Strahlentherapie 161:756–763, 1985.

Pauleikhoff D, Wessing A: Arteriovenous communications of the retina during a 17-year followup. Retina 11:433–436, 1991.

Suit H, Urie M: Proton beams in radiation therapy. J Natl Cancer Inst 84:155–156, 1992.

Troost BT, Glaser JS: Aneurysms, arteriovenous communications, and related vascular malformations. *In* Duane TD (ed): Clinical Ophthalmology, Hagerstown, MD, Harper & Row, 1981, Vol II, 17:1–30.

Walsh FB, Hoyt WF: Clinical Neurophthalmology, 3rd ed. Baltimore, Williams & Wilkins, 1969, pp 1714–1735.

Weber J: Techniques and results of therapeutic catheter embolisation. Int Angiol 9:214–223, 1990.

Wolter JR: Arteriovenous fistulas of the eye region. Trans Am Ophthalmol Soc 72:253–281, 1974.

Wolter JR: Arteriovenous fistulas involving the eye region. J Pediatr Ophthalmol 12:22–39, 1975.

Wolter JR: Arteriovenous fistula of the eyelid: Secondary to chalazion. J Pediatr Ophthalmol 14:225–227, 1977.

CAROTID CAVERNOUS FISTULAS AND CAVERNOUS SINUS ARTERIOVENOUS MALFORMATIONS 853.0

BRIAN R. YOUNGE, M.D.

Rochester, Minnesota

Carotid cavernous fistulas (CCFs) are abnormal connections of the carotid arteries directly into the veins of the cavernous sinus; depending on the rate and amount of this shunt, they may produce neuro-ophthalmic manifestations. CCFs are most frequently caused by trauma, although spontaneous fistulas may also occur, particularly in postmenopausal women. A dural sinus arteriovenous fistula (DSAVF) to the cavernous sinus, in contrast, is an acquired spontaneous shunt, usually of the low-flow type, and of complex origin, with feeding vessels from external and internal carotid dural vessels, but it may produce similar ophthalmic manifestations, particularly if the rate of flow is significant. Other predisposing factors include infection, malignancy, aneurysms, carotid dissection, fibromuscular dysplasia, pregnancy, and the Ehlers-Danlos syndrome.

Ocular manifestations (unilateral, bilateral, or even contralateral) include arterialized vessels of the conjunctiva and orbit, proptosis, edema and hyperemia of periorbital structures, papilledema, retinal hemorrhages and macular edema, iritis, iris atrophy, secondary glaucoma, and anterior segment ischemia. Visual loss may supervene from optic nerve compromise or corneal complications, retinal ischemic, or secondary glaucoma and may be accompanied by various extraocular muscle palsies, most commonly third nerve and sixth nerve palsies; aberrant regeneration of the third nerve is common. Bruit audible to the patient is a very annoying symptom and is usually detected by the examiner. Pulsating exophthalmos may also occur in very high-flow shunts. Neither bruit nor exophthalmos is common in clinical DSAVF. Death from rupture of the cavernous sinus is very rare and occurs most often during pregnancy.

THERAPY

Ocular. Although the treatment may be neurosurgical or interventional by the neuroradiologist, these lesions produce almost exclusively ocular complications, and the ophthalmologist needs to be centrally involved in decisions about diagnosis and management. Many of the low-flow shunts spontaneously occlude in time. Sometimes, even the investigational procedure of angiography will precipitate a cure. Many patients can coexist well with a low-flow shunt and have minimal or no symptoms. Previous carotid occlusive "trapping" procedures rendered the eye even more ischemic and were associated with a significant rate of visual loss and risk of cerebral complications. The one-eyed patient with CCF seldom, if ever, needs surgical treatment because the risk of total blindness is not to be taken lightly in a nonlethal disease. Of two such patients described in the literature, one refused treatment of any kind and did well, and the other was subjected to a series of embolization and trapping procedures that resulted in total permanent blindness and a lawsuit against the surgeon. The ophthalmologist must clearly demonstrate to the patient and his or her colleagues the threat to vision, the risks of doing nothing, and the risks of intervention.

In patients with intolerable symptoms or visual compromise, there are now several suitable forms of therapy.

Surgical. CCFs are of two main types: high flow and low flow. The high-flow CCFs are usually direct communications between a rent in the internal carotid artery and the cavernous sinus, and they are most often traumatic in origin. Low-flow CCFs are spontaneous DSAVFs, although some traumatic CCFs are low flow as well. When treatment is indicated for threatened visual loss or other neuro-ophthalmic complications, the high-flow fistulas are best managed by detachable balloon embolization or metallic coil embolization. Low-flow shunts are often managed by observation alone, with expected spontaneous resolution, or with either detachable balloon obliteration or embolization of the external carotid artery, depending on the type of shunt. Other approaches to both types have their advocates and have various degrees of success; platinum wire or other materials have been used via percutaneous catheterization of the dilated superior ophthalmic vein, and radiation therapy has been reported to be successful in low-flow shunts. Rarely, they may require direct attack or other arterial occlusion procedures. The role of the gamma knife or LIWAC is as yet uncertain, but appears promising.

PRECAUTIONS

Complications can ensue, such as cerebral infarction intracranial or subarachnoid hemorrage, or death, transient neurologic defects, ophthalmoplegias, pain, and visual loss; late complications can also occur, including recurrence of the fistula and premature deflation of the balloon. Sometimes, late effects of treatment improve the situation by progressive obliteration of the sites of leakage. Abrupt closure of a fistula may in itself produce neurologic deficits, especially in patients with CCFs of long duration, presumably on the basis of the so-called luxury perfusion phenomenon.

References

Barrow DL, et al: Classification and treatment of spontaneous carotid-cavernous sinus fistulas. J Neurosurg 62:248–256, 1985.

Bitoh S, et al: Irradiation of spontaneous carotid-cavernous fistulas. Surg Neurol 17:282–286, 1982.

Debrun GM, et al: Indications for treatment and classification of 132 carotid-cavernous fistulas. Neurosurgery 22:285–289, 1988.

Halbach VV, et al: Normal perfusion pressure breakthrough occurring during treatment of carotid and vertebral fistulas. AJNR 8:751–756, 1987.

Palestine AG, Younge BR, Piepgras DG: Visual prognosis in carotid-cavernous fistula. Arch Ophthalmol 99:1600–1603, 1981.

Sanders MD, Hoyt WF: Hypoxic ocular sequelae of carotid-cavernous fistulae: Study of the causes of visual failure before and after neurosurgical treatment in a series of 25 cases. Br J Ophthalmol 53:82–97, 1969.

Teng MMH, et al: Occlusion of arteriovenous malformations of the cavernous sinus via the superior ophthalmic vein. AJNR 9:539–546, 1988.

CAVERNOUS SINUS THROMBOSIS 325

MILTON BONIUK, M.D.

Houston, Texas

To many physicians, the term "cavernous sinus thrombosis" implies a severe infectious process of acute onset. The process primarily involves the central nervous system with generalized symptoms and signs of a septic process. The source of infection may be the face, mouth, throat, paranasal sinuses, ear, or teeth. The frequency of this disorder has decreased considerably since the introduction of antibiotics.

In addition to the septic variety, an aseptic form of cavernous sinus thrombosis may be seen with crushing fractures through the sphenoid, after surgical treatment of carotid cavernous fistula and tic douloureux, and in association with phlebothrombosis of the orbital veins.

Diagnosis of aseptic thrombosis is difficult, and the condition is most frequently confused with carotid cavernous fistula. The absence of widening of the pulse pressure with tonometry or tonography, the absence of a bruit, and a negative carotid angiogram should make one suspect this diagnosis; the use of orbital venography, high resolution CT scanning, or MRI with gadolinium (which show irregular filling defects within the dilated sinus) may also be helpful in confirming a suspected diagnosis. Early recognition of this disorder is obviously important, and perhaps neurosurgeons should institute some prophylactic measures that would help prevent this complication. Suspected cases associated with phlebothrombosis of the orbital veins should have a medical workup to rule out underlying causes or systemic diseases, such as a history of oral contraceptives or evidence of dysproteinemia. If inflammation is present, the possibility of cranial arteritis or some collagen vascular disease should be considered in the differential diagnosis.

The most obvious ocular sign of cavernous sinus thrombosis is protosis associated with dilation of the episcleral veins. There may be a variable degree of lid and conjunctival edema. If lagophthalmos and exposure keratitis are present, there may be secondary changes, such as staining and ulceration of the cornea. An afferent pupillary defect or dilation of the pupil secondary to an internal ophthalmoplegia may also be seen. The retina may show dilation of the retinal veins with hemorrhages, and in some cases, there may be retinal ischemia and infarction. The optic disc may be swollen or may show signs of an ischemic optic neuritis. Glaucomatous cupping may be seen in some patients with severe secondary open-angle glaucoma. Motility may be restricted as a result of changes in the extraocular muscles or secondary to involvement of the third, fourth, and sixth cranial nerves.

THERAPY

Systemic. Although most cases of *septic cavernous sinus thrombosis* are of bacterial origin, some cases have been reported in association with mucormycosis and *Aspergillus* organisms. It is important therefore to make a precise diagnosis as soon as possible. Doing so requires immediate blood cultures, as well as skull and sinus x-rays and CT or MRI scanning of the head. In some cases, biopsy and cultures from the paranasal sinuses might be necessary to make a diagnosis.

Once the etiologic agent has been identified, treatment with appropriate antibiotics is indicated. Until the specific organism has been isolated, broad-spectrum coverage should include 2 gm of intravenous methicillin every 4 hours or 2 gm of intravenous cephalothin every 4 hours plus up to 5 to 8 mg/kg of gentamicin injected in three equally divided doses.

If a diagnosis of *aseptic cavernous sinus thrombosis* is established in the acute phase, systemic anticoagulants (heparin and/or warfarin) or the combination of 600 mg of aspirin and 150 mg of dipyridamole might be indicated. One recent study suggests that anticoagulants in combination with antibiotics is indicated early in the treatment to reduce morbidity among survivors. If there is evidence of inflammation, systemic steroids or other anti-inflammatory agents, such as indomethacin or ibuprofen, might be indicated.

Ocular. In the septic variety, there may be tremendous proptosis, conjunctival chemosis, lagophthalmos, and exposure keratitis. These conditions may require the use of artificial tears, lubricating ointment, taping of the lids, intermarginal sutures, or some type of moisture chamber.

The secondary open-angle glaucoma in both septic and aseptic patients is probably secondary to increased episcleral venous pressure. The glaucoma responds poorly to miotics and other forms of medical therapy. If surgery becomes necessary, a trabeculectomy might be indicated, although the dilated episcleral, iris, and angle vessels might lead to serious operative and postoperative hemorrhage. Cryocyclotherapy, or the use of transcleral YAG laser might be good alternatives to trabeculectomy.

Supportive. The septic patient may require antipyretic and analgesic agents. Intravenous fluids and electrolyte therapy may be required in the nauseated or comatosed patient. Patients with aseptic thrombosis may benefit from elevation of the head, which promotes venous drainage and may relieve some of the symptoms.

Ocular or Periocular Manifestations

Conjunctiva: Chemosis; dilation of episcleral veins.
Cornea: Punctate staining; ulcer.
Extraocular Muscles: Third, fourth, or sixth nerve paralysis.
Eyelids: Edema; ptosis.
Globe: Proptosis.
Optic Nerve: Glaucomatous cupping; ischemic neuritis; papilledema.
Pupil: Afferent defect; dilation.
Retina: Hemorrhages; ischemic infarction; venous dilation.
Other: Glaucoma; orbital cellulitis; visual loss.

PRECAUTIONS

With the septic variety of cavernous sinus thrombosis, prompt diagnosis and early institution of appropriate antibiotic treatment are essential for survival of the patient. It is important to continue systemic antibiotics for several weeks after the acute septic phase has subsided in order to prevent a relapse.

The aseptic variety of cavernous sinus thrombosis is less of an emergency and more difficult to diagnose. If the diagnosis is not established in the acute phase, the use of anticoagulants might be of questionable value.

COMMENTS

In the septic variety of cavernous sinus thrombosis, the mortality rate has dropped dramatically since the introduction of antibiotics. Early aggressive treatment with intravenous antibiotics is necessary in the acute phase, and it must be followed by several weeks of oral antibiotics in order to prevent relapses. Late ocular complications, including glaucoma and corneal or motility problems, require periodic ophthalmologic evaluation and treatment.

In the aseptic variety of cavernous sinus thrombosis, the clinical picture and course of the disease are different. It is difficult to make a diagnosis, and carotid angiography is usually necessary to rule out the possibility of a low-flow carotid cavernous fistula. New techniques that may help in diagnosis include CT scanning and MRI with gadolinium. Although anticoagulants and other drugs, such as aspirin and dipyridamole, may be indicated in the acute phases of the disease, treatment in the later stages is mainly directed toward the secondary glaucoma, which is often difficult to control.

References

Ahmadi J, et al: CT observations pertinent to septic cavernous sinus thrombosis. AJNR *6*:755–758, 1985.

Ben-uri R, Palma L, Kaveh Z: Case report: Septic thrombosis of the cavernous sinus: Diagnosis with the aid of computed tomography. Clin Radiol *40*:520–522, 1989.

Boniuk M: The ocular manifestations of ophthalmic vein and aseptic cavernous sinus thrombosis. Trans Am Acad Ophthalmol Otolaryngol *76*: 1519–1534, 1972.

Levine SR, Twyman RE, Gilman S: The role of anticoagulation in cavernous sinus thrombosis. Neurology *38*:517–522, 1988.

Ogundiya DA, Keith DA, Mirowski J: Cavernous sinus thrombosis and blindness as complications of an odontogenic infection: Report of a case and review of literature. J Oral Maxillofac Surg *47*: 1317–1321, 1989.

Sekhar LN, Dujovny M, Rao GR: Carotid-cavernous sinus thrombosis caused by *Aspergillus fumigatus.* J Neurosurg *52*:120–125, 1980.

Van Johnson E, Line LB, Julian BA, Garcia JH: Bilateral cavernous sinus thrombosis due to mycormycosis. Arch Ophthalmol *106*:1089–1092, 1988.

SICKLE CELL DISEASE 282.60

DONALD A. GAGLIANO, M.D.,
San Antonio, Texas
and MAURICE F. RABB, M.D.
Chicago, Illinois

The clinical findings of a patient with sickle cell anemia were first described in 1910, but it was not until 1949 that it was discovered that the disease was due to the presence of an abnormal hemoglobin, which was named hemoglobin S (Hb S). Hemoglobin S is formed by a single amino acid substitution of valine for glutamic acid in the sixth position from the N-terminal end of the beta chain of the hemoglobin molecule. Intracellular polymerization of deoxyhemoglobin S results in distortion of the erythrocyte membrane and the characteristic sickle shape. Sickled erythrocytes can cause rheologic impairment from poor erythrocyte deformability and from the increased adhesion of sickled erythrocytes to vascular endothelium. Very small changes in arterial oxygen tension, even with oxygen saturation above 90 per cent, can result in sickling. The term "sickle cell (SC) disease" is used to refer to the group of conditions in which the presence of Hb S causes significant morbidity. It includes the homozygous state (Hb SS, sickle cell anemia) and the heterozygous states, sickle C disease (Hb SC) and sickle/B thalassemia. Hemoglobin C is formed by a single amino acid substitution of lysine for glutamic acid at the same location on the beta chain of the hemoglobin molecule as the substitution found in Hb S.

Although SC trait (Hb AS) is prevalent in 8 to 10 per cent of African-Americans, patients with (Hb AS) have entirely normal growth, development, and exercise tolerance. In general, no special liability status should be given to individuals with SC trait. However, establishing the diagnosis may be beneficial to individuals who are planning families and in some clinical situations. About 70,000 African-Americans (0.5 per cent) are homozygous for Hb S, and about 16,000 have Hb SC. Although homozygous SC disease may have a multitude of presentations depending on the amount of fetal-hemoglobin (Hb F) present and the presence of other point mutations in the hemoglobin gene, in general, homozygous SC disease is associated with the more severe systemic findings, whereas heterozygous SC disease (Hb SC and Hb S/B thalassemia) is associated with the more severe ophthalmic findings.

THERAPY

Systemic. Patients with SC disease may experience crises that present with vaso-occlusions and are characterized by organ infarction and/or pain; acute hemolysis; sudden enlargement of the liver and/or spleen, caused by the trapping of erythrocytes; and/or the sudden cessation of marrow function. The most common definable cause of crises is infection, most often of the respiratory and urinary tract. Cool, damp, or rainy weather is also associated with increased sickle crises. Patients in crisis should receive treatment for an underlying infection, hypoxia, dehydration, and pain. Preliminary results indicate that pentoxifylline, a hemorrheologic agent, may be beneficial in vaso-occlusive crises. Long-term organ system damage from multiple vaso-occlusive events and chronic hemolytic anemia may result in impairment of multiple organ systems including renal, ocular, cardiopulmonary, cerebrovascular, gastrointestinal, and skeletal. Close medical supervision, genetic counseling, and periodic ophthalmologic evaluations are essential in the management of patients with SC disease.

Based on the pathophysiology of the disease, several treatment strategies have evolved. These approaches include the inhibition of intracellular Hb S polymerization and the polymer effects on the RBC membrane, vasodilation, and the modification of the interaction between the RBC and the blood vessels. Since Hb F (gamma-globin chains) inhibits the tendency of Hb S red cells to polymerize, increasing Hb F levels by activating the gene for fetal-hemoglobin may reduce the hemolytic and vaso-occlusive complications of SC disease. This technique has been successfully accomplished with the administration of 5-azacytidine, hydroxyurea, and, most recently, arginine butyrate.

Ocular. The term "proliferative sickle retinopathy (PSR)" implies the presence of neovascular tissue, and this condition is associated with the most severe vision-threatening sequelae of SC disease. Neovascularization of the retina, in the shape of a sea fan, develops on the venular side of an A-V anastomosis. Fluorescein angiography is currently the best method to identify the presence of neovascularization. The incidence of central visual loss occurs in approximately 12 per cent of eyes with PSR. Traction on the retina by the contracting vitreous results in the development of vitreous hemorrhage, tractional retinal detachment, retinal tears, and rhegmatogenous retinal detachments. Vitreous hemorrhage, which occurs in approximately 5 per cent of eyes with PSR, is more common in SC disease and when there are more than 60 degrees of perfused neovascular tissue. Autoinfarction, or the spontaneous nonperfusion of neovascular membranes, occurs in 20 to 60 per cent of eyes with PSR, with a peak incidence 2 years after the peak incidence of the development of PSR.

Treatment of proliferative sickle retinopathy is directed toward preventing vision loss from vitreous hemorrhage, retinal detachment, and epiretinal membranes. Photocoagulation, applied by various techniques including feeder vessel, focal scatter, and peripheral circumferential scatter, is effective for treating PSR and reducing the risk of vision loss. Because of the potential complications from photocoagulation and the tendency for regression, treatment of PSR in SC patients over age 40 is probably unnecessary. Reported complications from photocoagulation include choroidal neovascularization, retinal breaks, and peripheral choroidal ischemia. In a long-term evaluation, complications from the feeder vessel technique occurred in up to 35 per cent of patients; however, no significant incidence of visual loss due to complications was found.

Surgical. Vitreoretinal surgery in SC patients may be indicated for the treatment of retinal detachments, nonclearing vitreous hemorrhages, or epiretinal membranes. Based on a 71 per cent incidence of anterior segment ischemia in PSR patients undergoing scleral buckling surgery for retinal detachments, the use of prophylactic preoperative exchange transfusions or erythrophoresis has been recommended. However, the risks associated with exchange transfusions, as well as the improvements in vitreoretinal surgical techniques, warrant a careful reevaluation of the use of routine preoperative exchange transfusions, particularly in patients with SC disease. Perioperative measures to reduce the incidence of anterior segment ischemia include (1) using nonsympathomimetic local anesthesia; (2) minimizing the use of topical sympathomimetics; (3) using supplemental oxygen for 48 hours postoperatively; (4) avoiding the manipulation of extraocular muscles; (5) minimizing the use of transcleral diathermy or cryotherapy; (6) avoiding the use of wide encircling scleral buckling elements, expansile concentrations of intraocular gases, carbonic anhydrase inhibitors; (7) using internal drainage of subretinal fluid; (8) closely monitoring and treating elevated intraocular pressure. Anterior segment ischemia following surgery is an emergency with a notoriously poor prognosis, and all attempts should be made to oxygenate the anterior segment. Options include hyperbaric oxygen therapy, continuous supplemental oxygen, and transcorneal oxygen with the use of goggles.

Ocular or Periocular Manifestations

Ocular manifestations of sickle cell disease result from vasoocclusions and may be seen in the conjunctiva, iris, retina, and choroid.

Choroid: Choroidal vascular occlusion; subretinal neovascularization; angioid streaks.

Conjunctiva: Vascular abnormalities, referred to as the conjunctival sickle sign.

Iris: Iris atrophy presenting as asymptomatic segmental white patches on the iris; pupillary irregularity; iris neovascularization.

Optic Nerve: Atrophy; transient, tiny, dark red isolated vascular segments on the surface of the optic disc; disc neovascularization.

Retina: Peripheral retinal vascular occlusions resulting in a nonperfused infarcted area of retina; central retinal artery and macular arteriolar occlusions; epiretinal membranes; retinal, subretinal, and preretinal hemorrhages (salmon-patch hemorrhages); black sunbursts; iridescent granular deposits; proliferative sickle retinopathy (PSR).

PRECAUTIONS

Blood in the anterior chamber (hyphema) in SC patients, including patients with SC trait, is considered a medical emergency, and a sickle screen is warranted on every African-American patient with hyphema. The environment of the anterior chamber promotes sickle hemoglobin polymerization, which can result in an elevated intraocular pressure (IOP) from blockage of the trabecular meshwork. Since SC patients are particularly prone to developing central retinal artery occlusion and optic atrophy even with mildly elevated intraocular pressures, the IOP should be monitored closely and not allowed to be greater than 25 mm Hg for more than 24 hours. Med-

ical management may include topical beta blockers; however, carbonic anhydrase inhibitors should be avoided since they may cause further sickling and a worsening of the outflow obstruction. If after a judicious trial of medical therapy the intraocular pressure remains elevated, surgical intervention with an anterior chamber lavage is indicated.

References

Asdourian G, Nagpal KC, Busse B, Goldbaum M, Patrianakos D, Rabb MF, Goldberg MF: Macular and perimacular vascular remodeling in sickling haemoglobinopathies. Br J Ophthalmol 60:431–453, 1976.

Condon P, Jampol LM, Farber MD, Rabb M, Serjeant G: A randomized clinical trial of feeder vessel photocoagulation of proliferative sickle cell retinopathy: II. Update and analysis of risk factors. Ophthalmology 91:1496–1498, 1984.

Deutsch TA, Weinreb RN, Goldberg MF: Indications for surgical management of hyphema in patients with sickle cell trait. Arch Ophthalmol 102:566–599, 1984.

Farber MD, Jampol MD, Fox P, Moriarty BJ, Acheson RW, Rabb MF, Serjeant GR: A randomized clinical trial of scatter photocoagulation of proliferative sickle cell retinopathy. Arch Ophthalmol 109:363–367, 1991.

Fox PD, Acheson RW, Serjeant GR: Outcome of iatrogenic choroidal neovascularization in sickle cell disease. Br J Ophthalmol 74:17–20, 1990.

Fox PD, Vessey SJ, Forshaw ML, Serjeant GR: Influence of genotype on the natural history of untreated proliferative sickle retinopathy—an angiographic study. Br J Ophthalmol 75:29–31, 1991.

Gagliano DA, Goldberg MF: The evolution of salmon-patch hemorrhages in sickle cell retinopathy. Arch Ophthalmol 107:1814–1815, 1989.

Goldbaum MH, Galinos SO, Apple D, Asdourian GK, Nagpal K, Jampol L, Woolf MB, Busse B: Acute choroidal ischemia as a complication of photocoagulation. Arch Ophthalmol 94:1025–1035, 1976.

Goldberg MF: Classification and pathogenesis of proliferative sickle retinopathy. Am J Ophthalmol 71:649–665, 1971.

Goldberg MF: Retinal vaso-occlusion in sickling hemoglobinopathies. Birth Defects 12:474–515, 1976.

Goldberg MF, et al: Sickled erythrocytes, hyphema, and secondary glaucoma: I. The diagnosis and treatment of sickled erythrocytes in human hyphemas. Ophthalmic Surg 10:17–123, 1979.

Jacobson MS, Gagliano DA, Cohen SB, Rabb MF, Jampol LM, Farber MD, Goldberg MF: A randomized clinical trial of feeder vessel photocoagulation of sickle cell retinopathy. A long term follow-up. Ophthalmology 98:581–585, 1991.

Jampol LM, Green JL, Goldberg MF, Peyman GA: An update on vitrectomy surgery and retinal detachment repair in sickle cell disease. Arch Ophthalmol 100:591–593, 1982.

Jampol LM, Orlin C, Cohen SB, Zanetti C, Lehman E, Goldberg MF: Hyperbaric and transcorneal delivery of oxygen to the rabbit and monkey anterior segment. Arch Ophthalmol 106:825–829, 1988.

Kimmel AS, Margargal LE, Stephens RF, Cruess AF: Peripheral circumferential retinal scatter photocoagulation for the treatment of proliferative sickle retinopathy: An update. Ophthalmology 93:1429–1434, 1986.

Moriarty BJ, Acheson RW, Serjeant GR: Epiretinal membranes in sickle cell disease. Br J Ophthalmol 71:466–469, 1987.

Peachey NS, Gagliano DA, Jacobson MS, Derlacki DJ, Fishman GA, Cohen SB: Correlation of electroretinographic findings and peripheral retinal nonperfusion in patients with sickle cell retinopathy. Arch Ophthalmol 108:1106–1109, 1990.

Perrine SP, Ginder GD, Faller DV, Dover GH, Ikuta T, Witkowska HE, Cai SP, Vichinsky EP, Olivieri NF: A short-term trial of butyrate to stimulate fetal-globin-gene expression in the beta-globin disorders. N Engl J Med 328:81–86, 1993.

Pulido JS, Flynn HW Jr, Clarkson JG, Blankenship GW: Pars plana vitrectomy in the management of complications of proliferative sickle retinopathy. Arch Ophthalmol 106:1553–1557, 1988.

Ryan SJ Jr, Goldberg MF: Anterior segment ischemia following scleral buckling in sickle cell hemoglobinopathy. Am J Ophthalmol 72:35–50, 1971.

Ward A, Clissold SP: Pentoxifylline. A review of its pharmacodynamic and pharmacokinetic properties and its therapeutic efficacy. Drugs 34:50–97, 1987.

Wilhelm JL, Zakov ZN, Holtge GA: Erythrophoresis in treating retinal detachment secondary to sickle-cell retinopathy. Am J Ophthalmol 92:582–583, 1981.

TEMPORAL ARTERITIS
446.5
(Giant Cell Arteritis)

NEIL R. MILLER, M.D.

Baltimore, Maryland

Temporal arteritis is a systemic disease characterized by chronic granulomatous inflammation of the wall of large and medium-sized arteries. Affected arteries show fragmentation of the elastic lamina, necrosis of smooth muscle cells, and infiltration with lymphocytes, epithelial cells, and giant cells. The process has a predilection for the extradural cranial arteries, including the ophthalmic and posterior ciliary arteries, but it may affect the large arteries of the head and neck and the coronary, renal, and peripheral arteries. The cause of temporal arteritis is unknown, but studies demonstrating immunoglobulin deposition in affected vessels suggest that there may be an underlying immunologic defect.

Temporal arteritis occurs almost exclusively in patients over 50 years of age. Its prevalence increases with advancing age, such that 1 per cent of patients 80 years of age or older will develop the disease. Men and women are affected equally.

Most patients with temporal arteritis have constitutional symptoms and signs, including intermittent fever, malaise, anorexia, migratory arthralgia (polymyalgia rheumatica), and weight loss. They may complain of severe temple pain, scalp tenderness, jaw pain or claudication, or ear pain. They often have exquisite tenderness in the region of the superficial temporal artery on one or both sides. One or both arteries may be prominent, but nonpulsatile.

Many patients with temporal arteritis develop visual symptoms as the initial manifestation of the disease. In others, visual symptoms predominate, but a careful history will elicit the constitutional symptoms described above.

Systemic sequelae of temporal arteritis include stroke, heart attack, kidney failure, and arterial insufficiency of the upper and lower extremities. Ocular complications occur in about 50 per cent of patients. The most common ocular disturbance is visual loss, which may affect one or both eyes and which may be partial or complete. The visual loss may result from retinal or choroidal ischemia, central retinal artery occlusion, anterior or posterior (retrobulbar) ischemic optic neuropathy, or cerebral ischemia. Homonymous visual field defects may result from occlusion of one of the posterior cerebral arteries or its branches, with bilateral involvement causing cortical blindness. Diplopia may also occur in patients with temporal arteritis. It results from ocular motor nerve paresis, usually abducens nerve paresis or pupil-sparing oculomotor nerve paresis, and from extraocular muscle ischemia. Some patients develop complete ocular ischemia from occlusion of the ipsilateral internal carotid or ophthalmic arteries.

The diagnosis of temporal arteritis is a *clinical* one. Temporal arteritis should be considered in any elderly patient with acute visual loss, and a careful history should be obtained with respect to the various constitutional symptoms described above. Once the diagnosis is suspected, an emergency erythrocyte sedimentation rate (ESR) should be obtained. The most popular procedure used to perform an ESR is the Westergren method, which is extremely accurate for high ESRs; however, other procedures, such as the Wintrobe and Zeta methods, are also used in some laboratories. If the ESR is elevated or if the ESR is normal but the patient is thought to have a clinical picture compatible with temporal arteritis, therapy should be initiated immediately, and a temporal artery biopsy should be performed within 8 days. The biopsy initially may be performed on one side only. The specimen obtained should be at least 2 cm long. It should be fixed in formalin, imbedded on end, and serially sectioned until the tissue is exhausted. The slides should be examined by a pathologist acquainted with the pathologic appearance of temporal arteritis. If the biopsy specimen is negative, but it is thought that temporal arteritis is a likely diagnosis, the opposite temporal artery should be biopsied. If this biopsy specimen is also negative, the physician should search for another cause of the patient's symptoms, such as an occult malignancy. It is important to obtain a temporal artery biopsy in all patients with suspected temporal arteritis even if the clinical picture is thought to be pathognomonic of the disease because of the potential side effects of systemic corticosteroid therapy.

THERAPY

Systemic. Corticosteroid therapy is the only effective treatment for temporal arteritis. It should therefore be instituted as soon as the diagnosis of temporal arteritis is suspected and blood has been drawn for an ESR. The usual dose is 1.5 to 2.0 mg/kg/day of prednisone or prednisolone in single or divided doses taken orally. Some authors have advocated intravenous corticosteroid therapy for those patients with acute vision loss from anterior or retrobulbar ischemic optic neuropathy. Such patients are given 500 to 1000 mg of methylprednisolone intravenously every 12 hours for 3 to 5 days, after which time they are switched to oral corticosteroids in the dose described above.

Most patients experience relief of systemic symptoms within 24 hours after starting corticosteroid therapy, although vision, once lost, almost never returns and the ESR may take 2 to 14 days to decrease. Even if symptoms abate immediately and the ESR becomes normal, patients should be maintained on a stable dose of corticosteroid for about 2 to 3 weeks. The dose should then be reduced at the rate of no more than 5 to 10 mg/week, and the patient's symptoms and ESR should be monitored on a weekly basis. As long as the patient remains free of symptoms and the ESR remains normal, the corticosteroid dose may be lowered. If symptoms return, the ESR begins to increase, or both, the steroid dose should be increased and kept stable until symptoms once again abate and the ESR normalizes. Alternate-day corticosteroid therapy does not suppress the inflammatory response on the day on which no steroids are taken. It is therefore thought that there is a risk of visual loss in patients placed on this regimen.

It must be remembered that temporal arteritis is often a *chronic* disease that may last for 6 to 18 months and often longer. Patients may therefore require corticosteroid therapy for many months, and attempts to wean them from therapy too fast may result in catastrophic visual or systemic complications from the persistent disease. The anti-inflammation drug, dapsone, may be used *in conjunction with systemic corticosteroids* to reduce the amount of steroids needed to control the disease and to increase the speed at which the steroids can be tapered.

Ocular or Periocular Manifestations

Choroid: Delayed perfusion; ischemia; infarction.

Extraocular Muscles: Diplopia, ophthalmoplegia; abducens nerve paresis; pupil-sparing oculomotor nerve paresis; trochlear nerve paresis.

Eye: Ocular ischemic syndrome.

Eyelid: Ptosis.

Optic Nerve: Ischemic optic neuropathy (anterior and retrobulbar).

Pupil: Relative afferent defect; tonic pupil.

Retina: Central retinal artery occlusion; ischemic retinopathy; cotton-wool spots; hemorrhage.

Other: Cortical blindness; homonymous visual field defects; internuclear ophthalmoplegia.

PRECAUTIONS

Systemic corticosteroid therapy is associated with well-described systemic side effects, especially an increased incidence of bacterial and fungal infections. All patients taking systemic corticosteroids for temporal arteritis should be monitored carefully by an internist, general practitioner, or gerontologist familiar with temporal arteritis and with the systemic side effects of corticosteroid therapy.

References

Caselli RJ, Hunder GG, Whisnant JP: Neurologic disease in biopsy-proven giant cell (temporal) arteritis. Neurology 38:352–359, 1988.

Chambers WA, Bernardino VB: Specimen length in temporal artery biopsies. J Clin Neuro-Ophthalmol 8:121–125, 1988.

Cullen JF, Coleiro JA: Ophthalmic complications of giant cell arteritis. Surv Ophthalmol 20:247–260, 1976.

Eshaghian J: Controversies regarding giant cell (temporal, cranial) arteritis. Doc Ophthalmol 47:43–67, 1979.

Hunder GG, Sheps GG, Allen GL, Joyce JW: Daily and alternate-day corticosteroid regimens in treatment of giant cell arteritis. Ann Intern Med 82:613–618, 1975.

Kyle V, Hazelman BL: Treatment of polymyalgia rheumatica and giant cell arteritis. I. Steroid regimens in the first two months. Ann Rheumat Dis 48:658–661, 1989.

Kyle V, Hazelman BL: Stopping steroids in polymyalgia rheumatica and giant cell arteritis: Treatment usually lasts for two to five years. Br Med J 300:244–245, 1990.

Machado EBV, Michet CJ, Hunder GG, O'Fallon WM, Ballard DJ, Kurland L, Cruz ME: Temporal arteritis: Clinical and epidemiological features from a community-based study, 1950 to 1985. Ann Neurol 22:148, 1987.

Matzkin DC, Slamovits TL, Sachs R, Burde RM: Visual recovery in two patients after intravenous methylprednisolone treatment of central retinal artery occlusion secondary to giant-cell arteritis. Ophthalmology 99:68–71, 1992.

McDonnell PJ: Ocular manifestations of temporal arteritis. Curr Opinion Ophthalmol 1:158–160, 1990.

McDonnell PJ, Moore GW, Miller NR, Hutchins GM, Green WR: Temporal arteritis. Ophthalmology 93:518–530, 1986.

Mehler MF, Rabinowich L: The neuroophthalmological spectrum of temporal arteritis. Ann Neurol 22:147–148, 1987.

Miller NR: Walsh and Hoyt's Clinical Neuro-Ophthalmology, 4th ed. Baltimore, Williams & Wilkins, 1991, Vol. 4, pp 2601–2627.

Nevyas JY, Nevyas HJ: Giant cell arteritis with normal erythrocyte sedimentation rate: A management dilemma. Metab Pediatr System Ophthalmol 10:18–21, 1987.

Paice EW: Giant cell arteritis: Difficult decisions in diagnosis, investigation and treatment. Postgrad Med J 65:743–747, 1989.

Reinitz E, Aversa A: Long-term treatment of temporal arteritis with dapsone. Am J Med 85:456–457, 1988.

Rosenfeld SI, Kosmorsky GS, Klingele TG, Burde RM, Cohn EM: Treatment of temporal arteritis with ocular involvement. Am J Med 80:143–145, 1986.

Slavin ML, Margolis AJ: Progressive anterior ischemic optic neuropathy due to giant cell arteritis despite high-dose intravenous corticosteroids. Arch Ophthalmol 106:1167, 1988.

Wong RL, Korn JH: Temporal arteritis without an elevated erythrocyte sedimentation rate. Am J Med 80:959–964, 1986.

THALASSEMIA 282.4

STEPHEN S. FEMAN, M.D.

Nashville, Tennessee

Thalassemia is a group of hereditary disorders characterized by decreased rates of synthesis of hemoglobin polypeptide chains. In the past, these disorders had a variety of names (Cooley's anemia, thalassemia major, thalassemia minor, etc.); now a more inclusive nomenclature based on the involved polypeptide chain is in common use—alpha-thalassemia, beta-thalassemia, etc. The most common clinical feature of thalassemia is the development of a hypochromic microcystic anemia. In some varieties, however, the thalassemic change represents such a small fraction of total globin synthesis that this feature is difficult to measure with standard techniques.

In general, when a patient has one thalassemia gene and one normal gene, the disorder is thalassemia trait (thalassemia minor in the older literature), and relatively mild anemia is present. When two similar genes are present, there is a severe impairment of hemoglobin synthesis (or thalassemia major). However, thalassemia can be subdivided just as well by identifying the rate of synthesis of polypeptide chains. On that basis, one can describe various degrees of hemoglobin synthesis impairment; doing so results in the more clinically relevant descriptions of severe, mild, and silent forms of thalassemia.

The most common type of thalassemia, which was described by Cooley and Lee in 1925, is a defect in the rate of synthesis of the beta-polypeptide chain of hemoglobin A. This defect causes a relative increase in the levels of hemoglobin A2 and hemoglobin F, along with microcystic hypochromic anemia. In addition, splenomegaly, hepatomegaly, and discoloration of the skin and sclera occur. At one time, it was thought that this disorder had a specific geographic distribution that extended from the Mediterranean through the Middle East, India, and Southeast Asia; it is now found worldwide.

THERAPY

Systemic. Transfusions to prevent the anemia symptoms have been the standard of treatment for many years. In time, such therapy results in an iron overload and hemosiderosis; this complication has been a common cause of death in these patients. However, with the use of iron chelators, such as deferoxamine, this danger is lessened. Splenomegaly becomes a major problem for such patients and can be resolved with splenectomy when needed.

Ocular. The most serious threats to vision occur in patients with thalassemia and sickle cell trait. This hemoglobinopathy is associated with abnormally shaped red blood cells that have difficulty passing through the retinal microcirculation. Retinal microvascular occlusions and foci of ischemic infarctions accompany these changes. Such patients develop peripheral retinal neovascularizations that result in vitreous hemorrhages. The vessels feeding and draining the neovascular growth can be identified by fluorescein angiography. Photocoagulation to occlude the feeding and draining vessels can close the neovascular growth and prevent such hemorrhages. The surrounding area of ischemic retina can be treated with a scatter photocoagulation pattern to reduce the stimulus for recurrent neovascularization and prevent recurring problems in that retinal region.

Ocular or Periocular Manifestations

Conjunctiva: Focal regions of dilated and tortuous vessels.

Lens: Cortical punctate opacities.

Retina: Vascular tortuosity; pigmented chorioretinal scars (black sunburst pattern); iridescent intrarctinal deposits; focal arterial occlusions; neovascularization; hemorrhages; angioid streaks; retinal pigment epithelial degenerations.

Vitreous: Hemorrhages.

PRECAUTIONS

Ocular complications usually indicate that the patient has a combination of thalassemia and some other hemoglobin abnormality. The treatment of the ocular manifestations of the other hemoglobin abnormality offers the greatest visual benefit to the patient.

COMMENTS

Intraocular hemorrhages without neovascularization and visual field defects have been reported in thalassemia patients; treatment of the underlying systemic disorder can prevent additional changes of this type. When retinal neovascular changes are identified, one must search for additional hemoglobin abnormalities. If such features are found, the treatment should be directed to the ocular and systemic manifestations of the coexisting hemoglobinopathy in order to prevent additional visual loss.

References

Condon PI, Serjeant GR: Ocular findings in sickle cell thalassemia in Jamaica. Am J Ophthalmol 74:1105–1109, 1972.

Cooley TB, Lee P: A series of cases of splenomegaly in children with anemia and peculiar bone changes. Trans Am Pediatr Soc 37:29–35, 1925.

Feman SS, Westrich DJ: Macular arteriole occlusions in sickle cell beta-thalassemia. Am J Ophthalmol 101:739–740, 1986.

Gartaganis S, Ismiridis K, Papageogiou O, Beratis NG, Papanastasiou D: Ocular abnormalities in patients with beta-thalassemia. Am J Ophthalmol 108:699–703, 1989.

Goldberg MF, Charache S, Acacio I: Ophthalmologic manifestations of sickle cell thalassemia. Arch Intern Med 128:33–39, 1971.

Magli A, Fusco R, Mettivier V, Pisapia R: Ocular manifestations in thalassemia minor. Ophthalmologica 184:139–146, 1982.

WEGENER'S GRANULOMATOSIS 446.4

JAMES L. KINYOUN, M.D.

Seattle, Washington

Wegener's granulomatosis is a necrotizing, granulomatous vasculitis of the sinuses (upper respiratory tract), lungs (lower respiratory tract), and kidneys. A limited form of the disease exists in which renal lesions are not present. All age groups can be affected, and symptoms include rhinorrhea, sinus pain, cough, malaise, and weight loss. There is no sexual or racial predilection. Although the etiology remains unknown, available evidence (deposition of immune-complexes) indicates that immunopathogenic mechanisms are responsible. Histopathology shows a necrotizing granulomatous vasculitis with infiltrate of neutrophils, lymphocytes, plasma cells, histiocytes, and giant cells. The most common ophthalmic manifestation of this disease is proptosis due to orbital involvement via extension from adjacent sinuses.

THERAPY

Systemic. Cytotoxic drugs have greatly improved the prognosis for patients with Wegener's granulomatosis. Cyclophosphamide[‡] in a daily oral dosage of 2 mg/kg is a successful treatment for most patients, whereas the 2-year mortality rate before this drug was over 90 per cent. Treatment should be continued for 1 year after all signs of active disease have subsided. The erythrocyte sedimentation rate is a useful laboratory test to monitor disease activity.

Systemic corticosteroids (e.g., oral prednisone 60 to 80 mg daily) are recommended to control inflammation during the first 2 weeks of induction therapy with cyclophosphamide. After 2 weeks, the steroids can usually be tapered and discontinued.

Ocular. Specific ocular therapy is not usually necessary because appropriate systemic treatment also alleviates the associated ocular disease.

Surgical. Orbital decompression procedures should be considered in patients with optic nerve compression that is unresponsive to medical treatment. Grafts may be necessary to treat severe corneal and scleral ulceration.

Topical. Surface lubricants, such as petrolatum ointment every 30 minutes to 4 hours, may be necessary for corneal drying caused by proptosis. Topical antibiotic solution or ointment (e.g., tobramycin every 3 to 4 hours) is recommended for patients with corneal ulceration to prevent and treat superinfections. Topical ophthalmic corticosteroid drops, such as 1 per cent prednisolone every 3 to 4 hours, are useful in controlling superficial ocular inflammation (e.g., conjunctivitis, episcleritis, and scleritis) and anterior uveitis. Ciliary spasm associated with uveitis can be treated with topical 1 per cent cyclopentolate every 4 hours.

Supportive. Affected patients will require a minimum of 1 year of drug treatment in addition to possible hospitalizations and surgical procedures, such as biopsies of lung or sinuses. Therefore, considerable health care expenditures are required. Financial assistance for those patients in need will be necessary.

Affected patients need to know the chronicity of this disease, its unknown etiology, the relatively optimistic outlook for most cases, and possible treatment complications. Of primary concern to patients considering parenthood or more offspring is that treatment can cause sterility. Sperm banking may be desired before beginning treatment in male patients. Females should use safe contraceptive methods during treatment because cytotoxic drugs are known to be teratogenic. Normal reproductive functions resume in some, but not all, patients after cytotoxic drug treatment is discontinued.

Irradiation. Irradiation of affected tissues has been attempted to control disease, but is of questionable efficacy and is no longer recommended.

Ocular or Periocular Manifestations

Conjunctiva: Conjunctivitis.
Cornea: Peripheral and central ulcers.
Eyelids: Edema.
Lacrimal System: Obstruction of nasolacrimal duct.
Optic Nerve: Optic neuritis; papilledema.
Orbit: Proptosis.
Retina: Central retinal artery occlusion; vasculitis.
Sclera: Episcleritis; scleritis.
Uvea: Choriocapillaritis; uveitis.

PRECAUTIONS

Complications of treatment with cyclophosphamide include bone marrow suppression, hemorrhagic cystitis, azoospermia, bladder carcinoma, nausea, vomiting, and hair loss. The leukocyte count should be followed closely during therapy (initially every other day and weekly during maintenance therapy) and should not decrease below 3000 cells/ mm^3. Granulocyte count below 1500 cells/ mm^3 increases the risk of infection. Dosages must be decreased at the first signs of bone marrow suppression because the full effect of the present dosage will not be manifest in the white count until 1 week later. Hemorrhagic cystitis can be minimized by adequate hydration, which prevents concentrated urine. Fortunately, hair regrows in most patients who experience hair loss while taking cyclophosphamide.

Complications of systemic corticosteroids include fluid retention, weight gain, "moon" facies, hyperglycemia, osteoporosis, bone fractures, psychologic disturbances, peptic ulcer, and infection. Side effects can be minimized by switching to every other day treatment and discontinuing steroids as soon as inflammation is controlled.

Accurate diagnosis depends on clinical findings (sinus and lung involvement with or without renal disease) and histopathology (granulomatous inflammation with necrotizing vasculitis). Antineutrophil cytoplasmic antibodies (ANCAs) reportedly are useful in the diagnosis and estimation of disease activity. A closely related disease with a poorer prognosis is lymphomatoid granulomatosis, which can be differentiated histopathologically by demonstrating the angiocentric infiltration of atypical lymphoid cells. Other similar diseases include the Churg-Strauss syndrome and necrotizing sarcoid granulomatosis.

COMMENTS

Because ophthalmic symptoms can be the initial manifestation of Wegener's granulomatosis, ophthalmologists should be aware of this disorder. Prompt referral to an internist and early treatment with cytotoxic and immunosuppressive drugs may not only save life but also preserve useful vision. Affected patients will need to be followed by internists and ophthalmologists to monitor treatment effectiveness and the side effects of cytotoxic and immunosuppressive drugs. Depending on disease activity, follow-up examinations daily or at several month intervals are appropriate.

References

Biglan AW, et al: Corneal perforation in Wegener's granulomatosis treated with corneal transplantation: Case report. Ann Ophthalmol 9:799–801, 1977.

Bullen CL, et al: Ocular complications of Wegener's granulomatosis. Ophthalmology 90:279–290, 1983.

Cupps TR, Fauci AS: The vasculitides. In Smith LH Jr: Major Problems in Internal Medicine. Philadelphia, WB Saunders, 1981, Vol. XXI, pp 155–173.

Fauci AS, Wolff SM: Wegener's granulomatosis: Studies in eighteen patients and a review of the literature. Medicine 52:535–561, 1973.

Fauci AS, Haynes BF, Katz P: The spectrum of vasculitis: Clinical, pathologic, immunologic, and therapeutic considerations. Ann Intern Med 89:660–671, 1978.

Haynes BF, et al: The ocular manifestations of Wegener's granulomatosis. Am J Med 63:131–141, 1977.

Kalina PH, et al: Diagnostic value and limitations of orbital biopsy in Wegener's granulomatosis. Ophthalmology 99:120–124, 1992.

Kinyoun JL, Kalina RE, Klein ML: Choroidal involvement in systemic necrotizing vasculitis. Arch Ophthalmol 105:939–942, 1987.

Leavitt RY, Fauci AS: Pulmonary vasculitis. Am Rev Respir Dis 134:149–166, 1986.

Robin JB, et al: Ocular involvement in the respiratory vasculitides. Surv Ophthalmol 30:127–140, 1985.

Soukiasian SH, et al: Diagnostic value of antineutrophil cytoplasmic antibodies in scleritis associated with Wegener's granulomatosis. Ophthalmology 99:125–132, 1992.

Valeriano-Marcet J, Spiera H: Treatment of Wegener's granulomatosis with sulfamethoxazole-trimethoprim. Arch Intern Med 151:1649–1652, 1991.

van der Woude FJ, et al: Autoantibodies against neutrophils and monocytes: Tool for diagnosis and marker of disease activity in Wegener's granulomatosis. Lancet I:425–429, 1985.

DERMATOLOGIC DISORDERS

ACRODERMATITIS ENTEROPATHICA 686.8

J. DOUGLAS CAMERON, M.D.,
and DONALD J. DOUGHMAN, M.D.,

Minneapolis, Minnesota

Acrodermatitis enteropathica is a rare hereditary disease characterized by skin lesions, alopecia, failure to thrive, diarrhea, and impaired immune function with frequent infections. A variety of ocular lesions also may occur. Involvement in siblings, but not in parents, and a history of familial occurrence in 65 per cent of patients suggest an autosomal recessive mode of inheritance. The disease usually manifests itself early in infancy, often just after weaning from human breast milk. Children with this disorder tend to be listless, apathetic, and anorectic and develop psychomotor retardation. Acrodermatitis enteropathica is characterized by a fluctuating course with severe exacerbations. If untreated, the disease is fatal; however, mild cases may improve at puberty and require no further therapy.

The dermatitis consists of vesiculobullous cutaneous eruptions distributed symmetrically, periorificially, and acrally. The areas about the eyes, occiput, elbows, hands, knees, feet, and especially the paronychial areas of the fingers and toes are involved. The skin lesions crust quickly and become psoriasiform; secondary infections, especially with *Candida*, are common. Alopecia involving the scalp, eyebrows, and eyelashes usually follows the dermatitis. Nonspecific conjunctivitis associated with photophobia frequently accompanies the dermatitis. Linear subepithelial corneal opacities are occasionally found during exacerbations of the dermatitis. Punctal stenosis, cataracts, and optic atrophy have also been reported in patients with acrodermatitis enteropathica.

THERAPY

Systemic. Oral zinc therapy (10 to 50 mg of zinc base as zinc sulfate or zinc gluconate per day) produces complete remission in acrodermatitis enteropathica, allowing normal growth with cessation of diarrhea, correction of immune deficiency, and disappearance of skin lesions. In most cases, zinc supplementation must be continued throughout the life span.

Ocular. The development of ocular lesions is generally prevented by oral zinc supplementation. Occasionally, supportive measures, such as artificial tears or dark glasses, may be necessary. Punctal dilation may be required in those cases with punctal stenosis.

Ocular or Periocular Manifestations

Cornea: Anterior corneal scarring; epithelial thinning; linear subepithelial opacities.

Eyebrows or Eyelids: Madarosis; nonspecific blepharitis; vesiculobullous eruptions.

Other: Abnormalities of dark adaptation; lacrimal punctal stenosis; nonspecific conjunctivitis; photophobia.

PRECAUTIONS

There are no recognized untoward effects of supplemental zinc therapy. Some patients have now lived long enough to complete normal pregnancies without teratologic complications. Occasionally, a single dose may cause transient emesis. Iodoquinol is no longer used in the treatment of acrodermatitis enteropathica.

COMMENTS

It was noted initially that feeding with human breast milk would improve the complications of acrodermatitis enteropathica. In the early 1950s, it was found that treatment with the antifungal agent, iodoquinol, improved the signs of acrodermatitis. In 1973, Barnes and Moynahan made the fortuitous discovery that oral zinc therapy produces dramatic improvements in this disease process. Indeed, the beneficial results from iodoquinol therapy were subsequently found to be due to increased zinc absorption caused by this drug. It is now generally accepted that the signs and symptoms of acrodermatitis enteropathica are caused by zinc deficiency and are identical to those seen in animals made zinc deficient by dietary means or with hereditary zinc malabsorption. The mechanism for this disease currently is thought to be depressed intestinal zinc absorption, probably through a failure in the production of a low molecular weight zinc-binding ligand that facilitates zinc absorption.

Severe zinc deficiency is found in a variety of more common processes, such as chronic alcoholism, sickle cell anemia, regional enteritis, short bowel syndrome, and total parenteral nutrition, to name only a few. Ocular abnormalities may complicate these states of acquired zinc deficiency just as in the hereditary disease of abnormal zinc metabolism, acrodermatitis enteropathica. Studies in zinc-deficient animals have recently confirmed the essential role of zinc in normal ocular function.

References

Barnes PM, Moynahan EJ: Zinc deficiency in acrodermatitis enteropathica: Multiple dietary intolerance treated with synthetic diet. Proc Roy Soc Med 66:327–329, 1973.

Cameron JD, McClain CJ: Ocular histopathology of acrodermatitis enteropathica. Br J Ophthalmol 70:662–667, 1986.

Leure-duPree AE: Electron-opaque inclusions in the rat retinal pigment epithelium after treatment with chelators of zinc. Invest Ophthalmol Vis Sci 21:1–9, 1981.

Matta CS, Felker GV, Ide CH: Eye manifestations in acrodermatitis enteropathica. Arch Ophthalmol 93:140–142, 1975.

Racz P, et al: Bilateral cataract in acrodermatitis enteropathica. J Pediatr Ophthalmol Strabismus 16:180–182, 1979.

Sunderman FW Jr: Current status of zinc deficiency in the pathogenesis of neurological dermatological and musculoskeletal disorders. Ann Clin Lab Sci 5:132–145, 1975.

Warshawsky RS, et al: Acrodermatitis enteropathica. Corneal involvement with histochemical and electron micrographic studies. Arch Ophthalmol 93:194–197, 1975.

Wirsching L Jr: Eye symptoms in acrodermatitis enteropathica. A description of a brother and sister, with corneal changes. Acta Ophthalmol 40:567–574, 1962.

ATOPIC DERMATITIS 691.8

(Atopic Eczema, Besnier's Prurigo)

MITCHELL H. FRIEDLAENDER, M.D.

La Jolla, California

Atopic dermatitis is one of the eczematous skin eruptions. It often occurs in childhood, but may be seen in adolescents and adults as well. The incidence in children under 5 years of age is estimated at 3 per cent. Frequently, patients with atopic dermatitis have a history of respiratory allergy or allergic reactions to certain foods. Although immunologic abnormalities have been noted in atopic dermatitis, this condition also seems to represent an abnormal reactivity of the skin to various stimuli. This abnormal skin reactivity may be genetically determined, and it is considered by some to represent a metabolic or biochemical defect. Although patients with atopic dermatitis undergo extensive allergic testing, it is frequently impossible to find a relationship between this condition and a known allergy.

Serum IgE concentrations are generally elevated in patients with atopic dermatitis. Recent evidence indicates that a deficiency of cellular immunity may also exist. Cutaneous delayed hypersensitivity responses to ubiquitous antigens, such as *Candida* and streptokinase-streptodornase, may be poor. A deficiency of T-suppressor cells may be responsible for the failure to terminate IgE antibody responses to certain antigens in atopic dermatitis. IgE binds to mast cells in the skin, initiating the release of histamine and chemical mediators during antigenic stimulation. The overly reactive skin of atopic patients may respond excessively to the effects of histamine and other chemical mediators.

THERAPY

Topical. Topical steroids may be used for the skin lesions. A fluorinated corticosteroid in a water-soluble base, such as triamcinolone or betamethasone, may be applied three times a day to localized skin lesions. For exudative lesions, wet saline dressings may be applied several times a day. For thick and lichenified lesions, 1 per cent crude coal tar in Lassar's paste or cold cream may be effective. Coal tar derivatives, however, can sensitize the skin to strong sunlight.

Systemic. If the skin lesions are widespread and not controlled by topical therapy, oral corticosteroids may be added. As little as 5 to 10 mg of prednisone a day combined with a full regimen of topical treatment may keep a patient relatively free of dermatitis. For acute involvement of large areas of skin, a high dose of prednisone may be given and tapered slowly until skin lesions improve. Long-term use of corticosteroids should be avoided, especially in children, because of the tendency of these drugs to suppress growth.

Antihistamines, such as hydroxyzine, may be given in doses of 5 to 25 mg as often as four times a day to help control itching.

Ocular. If an inciting antigen can be identified in atopic keratoconjunctivitis, it should be eliminated. Topical corticosteroids may be used for short periods of time; however, their long-term usage should be avoided. In general, the lowest dose of corticosteroid required to control the patient's symptoms should be administered as infrequently as possible. Cold compresses and topical vasoconstrictor/antihistamine eyedrops may be all that are necessary to maintain comfort. Some recent success has been obtained with the use of 2 to 4 per cent cromolyn eyedrops. This medication stabilizes mast cells and prevents the release of their mediators.

Surgical. Surgery of atopic cataracts should not be undertaken lightly. Several investigators have reported such complications as severe hemorrhage, retinal detachment, iridocyclitis, and corneal edema. A relatively high incidence of pre- and postoperative retinal detachment has been reported. In patients with keratoconus associated with atopic eczema, penetrating keratoplasty may be carried out with a high degree of success.

Supportive. The skin of atopic dermatitis patients is easily irritated. Therefore, these patients should take care to avoid these factors—bathing too frequently, excessive sweating, chapping in cold weather, scratching, emotional stress, such irritating fabrics as wool and nylon, and nonspecific irritants, such as harsh soaps and detergents.

Ocular or Periocular Manifestations

Conjunctiva: Chemosis; filamentary discharge; giant papillary hypertrophy; hyperemia; linear or stellate scarring; shrinkage of the fornices; Trantas' dots.

Cornea: Cicatrization; keratoconus; punctate staining; vascularization.

Eyelids: Erythema; exudates; scaling and crusting; secondary staphylococcal blepharitis.

Lens: Cataracts.

Retina: Detachment.

PRECAUTIONS

Patients with active atopic dermatitis should not be vaccinated for smallpox because of the danger of developing a disseminated vaccinia infection. Corticosteroids should be used with restraint for ocular and skin manifestations. Cataracts, glaucoma, and secondary infections are known to develop in atopic patients treated excessively with corticosteroids. Surgery of atopic cataracts has been associated with complications, including hemorrhage, retinal detachment, iridocyclitis, and corneal edema.

COMMENTS

Atopic dermatitis is a chronic disease, and manifestations vary depending on the patient's age. A dermatologist should manage the patient's dermatitis. Ocular findings occur in a small percentage of atopic dermatitis patients; however, they can be the most severe aspect of the condition. Supportive treatment with cold compresses and topical vasoconstrictor/antihistamine eyedrops may be all that is required. Topical corticosteroids may be necessary, but should be used with restraint because they may eventually induce cataract formation and other problems. Cromolyn shows great promise in the treatment of this condition, and other antiallergic drugs are also being developed. Since atopic patients are prone to secondary infections, these should be looked for and treated appropriately.

References

Amemiya T, Matsuda H, Uehara M: Ocular findings in atopic dermatitis with special reference to the clinical features of atopic cataract. Ophthalmologica *180*:129–132, 1980.

Christiansen SC: Evaluation and treatment of the allergic patient. Int Ophthalmol Clin *28*:282–293, 1988.

Donshik PC: Allergic conjunctivitis. Int Ophthalmol Clin *28*:294–302, 1988.

Friedlaender MH: Allergy and Immunology of the Eye. New York, Raven, 1993, pp 75–79.

Hanifin JM, Lobitz WC Jr: Newer concepts of atopic dermatitis. Arch Dermatol *113*:663–670, 1977.

Hogan MJ: Atopic keratoconjunctivitis. Am J Ophthalmol *36*:937–947, 1953.

McGeady SJ, Buckley RH: Depression of cell-mediated immunity in atopic eczema. J Allergy Clin Immunol *56*:393–406, 1975.

Tuft SJ, Kemeny DM, Dart JK, Buckley RJ: Clinical features of atopic keratoconjunctivitis. Ophthalmology *98*:150–158, 1991.

Uehara M, Ofuji S: Atopic dermatitis: A discussion of theories concerning its pathogenesis. J Dermatol *7*:231–238, 1980.

CONTACT DERMATITIS 692.9
(Dermatitis Venenata)

MITCHELL H. FRIEDLAENDER, M.D.

La Jolla, California

Contact dermatitis is probably the most common immunologic disease encountered by dermatologists. It results from the exposure of the skin to a wide variety of substances commonly found in the environment, including drugs, dyes, plant resins, preservatives, cosmetics, and metals. There are two varieties of contact dermatitis: (1) irritant, the more common form, and (2) allergic. Irritant contact dermatitis is caused by excessive moisture or by acids, alkalis, resins, or chemicals capable of injuring any person's skin if persistent contact is allowed. Allergy or hypersensitivity plays no role in irritant contact dermatitis. Allergic contact dermatitis, unlike the irritant variety, only occurs in sensitized individuals and involves the mechanism of cell-mediated immunity. In allergic contact dermatitis, an individual becomes sensitized to a given chemical or other sensitizing substance, and on re-exposure to the same chemical, an erythematous delayed skin reaction is elicited.

Irritant dermatitis is provoked by substances with primary irritant properties or by frequent defatting of the skin caused by excessive moisture. With repeated exposure, edema, erythema, vesiculation, and scaling of the skin develop. In allergic contact dermatitis, the sensitizing substances are generally haptens of small molecular weight, which bind to dermal proteins forming complete antigens. Initial exposure to the hapten results in sensitization of T lymphocytes. A second application elicits an inflammatory response.

THERAPY

Systemic. The only form of contact dermatitis that may require systemic corticosteroids is widespread, severe poison ivy dermatitis. A 10- to 14-day course of prednisone may be used in this situation, since it may lessen the intensity of the disease, as well as the loss of time from work or school. Desensitization treatment by the oral and parenteral routes has been tried with poison ivy; however, the efficacy of this mode of therapy is still in dispute.

Ocular. The eye is a frequent site of involvement in contact dermatitis. Such drugs as neomycin, atropine and its derivatives, chloramphenicol, and penicillin and its related compounds may all act as sensitizers. The basis of treatment in contact dermatitis is the removal of the allergen or irritant from the patient's environment. When the allergen is identified, use of the compound containing it should be discontinued and avoided in the future. For conjunctivitis or keratoconjunctivitis associated with drugs that are primary irritant substances or contact allergens, the best treatment is withdrawal of the drug and substitution of an appropriate, nonirritating medication.

Topical. In acute skin lesions, cool saline compresses should be applied. Topical fluorinated corticosteroid lotions, such as triamcinolone or betamethasone, may be used. In chronic lesions, steroid lotions or ointments are also of use.

Supportive. It may be difficult or impractical to remove the allergen or irritant from the patient's environment due to economic or occupational factors. If continued exposure to an allergen is necessary, well-designed clothing may offer suitable protection.

Ocular or Periocular Manifestations

Conjunctiva: Chemosis; papillary reaction; vasodilation; watery discharge.
Cornea: Fine, epithelial, punctate, keratitis; small, yellow, necrotic limbal opacity.
Eyelids: Crusting; eczema; edema; erythematous blepharitis; exudates; lichenification; scaling; vesicles.

PRECAUTIONS

Rubbing the eyes after handling soaps, detergents, or chemicals may provoke a contact dermatitis reaction. Allergic reactions to cosmetics affect primarily the eyebrows and upper lids because of the method of application. Mascara, eyebrow pencil, and face creams may also act as allergens. Nail polish and nail polish hardeners can cause sensitization around the eye by accidental touching of the area. Lip gloss and eye gloss cosmetics contain lanolin fractions that may also act as sensitizers.

Parabens are used in a great many lotions, creams, and cosmetics because they are excellent antimicrobial agents that prevent spoilage from bacterial and fungal growth. Paraben allergy is one of the leading causes of contact dermatitis at the present time. Nickel sulfate is a common sensitizer found in jewelry and undergarments. Chromates used in costume jewelry, leather products, bleaches, and fabrics are also common offenders.

Many ocular medications are excellent contact sensitizers. Neomycin is perhaps the most common. Other antibiotics, anesthetics, and dilating agents, as well as preservatives, can cause similar problems. Development of a red eye while on chronic eyedrops should alert the ophthalmologist to the possibility of contact sensitivity. Patch testing by the dermatologist or simply discontinuation of the medication will generally make the diagnosis apparent.

COMMENTS

Contact sensitivity is a common problem in ophthalmology because of the everyday exposure to chemicals. The best form of treatment is discontinuation of the offending substance. Steroid therapy can reduce symptoms, but is not recommended on a long-term basis. Patch testing can be very helpful in determining the cause of contact dermatitis and in selecting alternative drugs to which the patient is not sensitive.

References

Claman HN, et al: Control of experimental contact sensitivity. Adv Immunol 30:121–157, 1980.
Friedlaender MH: Contact allergy and toxicity in the eye. Int Ophthalmol Clin 28:317–320, 1988.
Friedlaender MH: Allergy and Immunology of the Eye. New York, Raven, 1993, pp 79–82.
Friedlaender MH, Cyr R: Contact sensitivity in the guinea pig eye. Curr Eye Res 1:403–407, 1981.
Mathias CGT, et al: Delayed hypersensitivity to retrobulbar injections of methylprednisolone acetate. Am J Ophthalmol 86:816–819, 1978.
Mathias CGT, et al: Allergic contact dermatitis to echothiophate iodide and phenylephrine. Arch Ophthalmol 97:286–287, 1979.
Nethercott JR, Nield G, Holness DL: A review of 79 cases of eyelid dermatitis. J Am Acad Dermatol 21:223–230, 1989.

ERYTHEMA MULTIFORME MAJOR 695.1

(Erythema Multiforme Exudativum, Stevens-Johnson Syndrome, Toxic Epidermal Necrosis)

F. T. FRAUNFELDER, M.D.,
and F. W. FRAUNFELDER, M.D.

Portland, Oregon

Erythema multiforme is a mucocutaneous inflammatory disorder that is episodic and usually self-limiting. Clinically, the disease presents as a spectrum ranging from the mild form without mucosal involvement, erythema multiforme minor, which is a benign condition with no marked complications, to erythema multiforme major or Stevens-Johnson syndrome, which implies ocular involvement, often with severe bullous-erosive mucocutaneous reactions. Toxic epidermal necrosis (TEN) is the most severe form of this entity, with loss of "sheets" of skin and the threat of recurrence, severe disability, or even death.

Although there are many precipitating causes for erythema multiforme, the most well documented for erythema multiforme minor are recurrent infections with herpes simplex, type I and II. The more common causes of erythema multiforme major are respiratory infections, often with *Mycoplasma pneumoniae*, and drug reactions (caused by sulfonamides, phenytoin, penicillins, phenylbutazone, barbiturates, salicylates, mercurials, and arsenicals).

Erythema multiforme major is a disease of children and young adults, and its pathogenesis is thought to be related to immune complexes, cell-mediated immunity, or both. The prodromal period can consist of fever, malaise, sore throat, and arthralgias. Subsequently, skin eruptions develop and most frequently involve the dorsal hands and feet and extensor surfaces of the forearms and legs. The lesions are erythematous macules that rapidly become papular and frequently enlarge and form the characteristic iris or "bullseye" target lesions. Skin lesions have a cycle of approximately 2 weeks, and recurrent cycles of lesions are not uncommon. Ocular manifestations vary markedly and include severe sicca, total conjunctival and corneal scarring, keratinization of all ocular mucous membranes and lid margins, corneal vascularization, entropion, trichiasis, symblepharon, perforation, and blindness.

THERAPY

Systemic. At the onset of this disease, one cannot predict its eventual ocular course or outcome. Therefore, close observation and consultation with physicians experienced with this potentially devastating entity are imperative. The systemic management is seldom administered by an ophthalmologist, but it is significantly influenced by the ocular course of the disease. Therefore, decisions regarding steroid, antibiotic, and immunosuppressive therapy and hospital management should be made jointly.

Ocular. Not infrequently, the most serious long-term sequelae are ocular, so that close ophthalmic observation once or twice daily is indicated during acute periods. Nursing and care by family members during the acute and chronic phases of this disease are critical to prevent complications. Even with this attention, some patients may become progressively worse regardless of management. The key areas of care include lid hygiene, lubrication, control of secondary infections, attempts to control the inflammatory process, and prevention of secondary scarring. The physician must be aware that preservative-free solutions are recommended and that overzealous topical ocular medications may be toxic to these fragile epithelial surfaces.

It must be emphasized that the most important aspect of ocular care is lid hygiene and lid position. During the acute phase, gentle swabbing of lid discharge is ideal. Ensuring that the lids are not stuck to the globe and preventing lid closure with the resultant exposure to corneal problems require close monitoring. Taking time to explain these concerns to the family and caregivers may prevent many complications.

Preservative-free solutions of various viscosities given by the nursing staff or more likely by a family member may be necessary as often as every 15 minutes. Preservative-free ointments may also be used. However, to be effective, a heavy coating is necessary since all ointments are hydrophobic. This heavy coating causes marked visual impairment in a patient who is often already sensory incapacitated. Therefore, these ointments are best reserved for use during the night.

Periodic ocular cultures are ideal because systemic pathogens from head and body skin lesions can easily be transferred to the eye. The type and frequency of topical ocular antibiotics are debatable. Antibiotics effective against the patient's skin pathogens are preferred. *Pseudomonas* is not uncommon, although *Staphylococcus* is most common. Prophylactically, solutions or ointments applied once or twice daily or close observation is preferred, with more aggressive topical ocular therapy added when a secondary infection occurs. Determining the frequency of antibiotics is based on the clinical picture, i.e., whether an infection is present, the amount of discharge, and how well the ocular tissue is tolerating the topical ocular therapy. Distinguishing toxic responses to topical ocular medication from an exacerbation of the disease may be difficult.

It is important to control the inflammatory process, but how best to do so is controversial. Emphasis should be placed on preventing scarring of the eyelids from the cascade of secondary effects and protecting the integrity of the corneal epithelium. The latter objective is achieved by paying close attention to the eyelids and lashes, as well as limiting conjunctival and episcleral reactions by limiting toxic medications, meticulous hygiene, and the judicious use of steroids. Since the initial ocular inflammatory response is similar to the systemic picture, consultation with the internist about the use of oral steroids is important. If oral steroids are administered, topical ocular steroids may not be necessary or their frequency may be decreased, thereby causing less toxicity to the epithelium. Ocular steroids should seldom be given more than four times daily if they contain preservatives. Systemic immunosuppressive drugs may be indicated, and more often than not, the ocular sequelae are the instigating factors. Again, the drugs will most often be the ones with which the internist is most comfortable.

Daily examination of the fornices, especially the inferior fornex (it is too traumatic to view the upper eyelids, except superficially) for symblepharon formation is imperative in the acute phase. No anesthesia should be used except if absolutely necessary because topical ocular anesthetics are among the most toxic agents to the epithelium. A saline-moistened cotton swab or ointment-coated glass rod may be used. Gentleness in swabbing is the key, along with early intervention. Iatrogenic symblepharon secondary to vigorous swabbing may be a factor in extensive symblepharon formation.

Tretinoin, a topical retinoid (all-trans retinoic acid, a vitamin A analogue) has been shown to reverse conjunctival keratinization. This is a method to treat ocular surface disorders by reversing diseased epithelium; however, the benefit of this drug in treating this disease is unproven.

Surgical. The management of symblepharon formation is controversial and is often based on the ophthalmologist's previous experience. Preventing contact between bulbar and palpebral conjunctiva can be accomplished with a symblepharon ring, scleral shell, or plastic wrap. A piece of plastic wrap can be cut to the width of the palpebral fissure, and three 5-0 nylon mattress sutures placed near the end of the wrap can be passed from the fornix out through the skin. The wrap is subsequently folded over the skin surface, and sutures are passed through the wrap and tied. Use of these devices must be monitored closely because erosion of the conjunctiva can aggravate the problem. These devices are recommended during the acute and postacute phase of the disease. They are seldom of value during the late chronic phase if subconjunctival scarring and contracture occur.

Aberrant eyelashes are significant causes of epithelial disturbance. Simple removal of stray eyelashes may be insufficient because the regrowing stub may be more detrimental than the original eyelash. Permanent eyelash epilation is the goal of long-term control. Cryoepilation or selected electrolysis may be necessary.

In selected cases, punctal occlusion (collagen, silicone, or permanent) may be an effective method for correcting tear deficiency syndromes. In some cases, a tarsorrhaphy, either surgical or with mattress sutures, may be indicated.

Patients suffering from localized conjunctival epidermalization have been treated by tarsal polishing or with grafting from the buccal mucous membrane.

Ocular or Periocular Manifestations

Conjunctiva: Adhesions; catarrhal, pseudomembranous, or purulent conjunctivitis; chemosis; collagen degeneration; cysts; hyperemia; subconjunctival hemorrhages; symblepharon; vesicles; widespread fibrinoid necrosis of arterioles and venules.

Cornea: Cicatrization; dense opacity; infiltration; keratoconjunctivitis sicca; neovascularization; pannus; perforation; punctate keratitis; ulcer.

Eyelids: Blepharitis; blepharospasm; cicatrization; edema; entropion; trichiasis; ulcer.

Globe: Endophthalmitis; immobility; panophthalmitis; phthisis bulbi, rupture.

Lacrimal System: Decreased tear secretion; occlusion of the lacrimal puncta.

Other: Anterior uveitis; cataract; episcleral nodules; miosis; optic neuritis.

PRECAUTIONS

In general, patients with this disease are best followed by an ophthalmologist with prior experience with erythema multiforme major. It is imperative that the ophthalmologist inform the internist of the ocular sequelae, since not infrequently, the internist's knowledge in this area is marginal. Because topical corticosteroids are of questionable value in the treatment of ocular inflammation, they are often indicated in small doses and for short periods of time. Close monitoring of patients on topical corticosteroids is important because of the potential for secondary corneal melt and infection. Contact lenses may be used, but in general have a limited role other than preventing exposure and problems from trichiasis. Long-term contact lens use is to be avoided, if possible, since it seems to stimulate corneal vascularization.

The treatment of erythema multiforme major is not well delineated; however, the above outline provides the greatest opportunity for success. Yet, some patients still do poorly, and even months into the disease after other systemic sequelae have resolved, the ocular complications, including perforation, exacerbate. The ophthalmologist often has the opportunity to get to know these patients better than any other in his or her practice!

References

Arffa RC: Grayson's Diseases of the Cornea. Erythema Multiforme. Chicago, Mosby-Year Book, 1991, pp 563–567.

Foster CS: Cicatricial pemphigoid. Trans Am Ophthalmol Soc 84:527, 1986.

Kozarsky AM, Knight SH, Waring GO III: Clinical results with a ceramic keratoprosthesis placed through the eyelid. Ophthalmology 94:904–911, 1987.

McCord CD, Chen WP: Tarsal polishing and mucous membrane grafting for cicatricial entropion, trichiasis and epidermalization. Ophthalmol Surg 14:1021–1025, 1983.

Mondino BJ: Cicatricial pemphigoid and erythema multiforme. Ophthalmology 7:939–952, 1990.

Ormerod DL, Fong LP, Foster SC: Corneal infection in mucosal scarring disorders and Sjogren's syndrome. Am J Ophthalmol 105:512–518, 1988.

Rakel RE: Erythema multiforme. In Coopman SA, Arndt KA (eds): Conn's Current Therapy. Philadelphia, WB Saunders, 1992, pp 633–635.

Soong HK, Martin NF, Wagoner MD, Alfonso E, Mandelbaum SH, Laibson PR, Smith RE, Udell I: Topical retinoid therapy for squamous metaplasia of various ocular surface disorders. A multicenter, placebo-controlled double-masked study. Ophthalmology 95(10):1442–1446, 1988.

Wright P, Collin JRO: The ocular complications of erythema multiforme (Stevens-Johnson syndrome) and their management. Trans Ophthalmol Soc UK 103:338–341, 1983.

HYPERTRICHOSIS 704.1
(Hirsutism)

DAVID T. TSE, M.D., F.A.C.S.,

Miami, Florida

and RICHARD L. ANDERSON, M.D., F.A.C.S.

Salt Lake City, Utah

There is some overlap between the terms "hirsutism" and "hypertrichosis." Hirsutism is conventionally defined as a disease of women and children in which there is excessive growth of body hair in response to androgens, resulting in a male distribution of hair growth. Hypertrichosis refers to the congenital or acquired presence of excessive hair growth of vellus or lanugo hair in areas that are not usually hairy. Lanugo is a fine, short hair covering the entire body of the developing fetus; it usually completes its growth cycle before birth. Vellus hair is similar to the fetal lanugo hair, but makes its appearance in postnatal life; it is generally unpigmented. Excessive accumulation of vellus hair may give a "peach fuzz" appearance, particularly when localized in the facial region.

Generalized hypertrichosis may affect any part of the body, with the exceptions of the palms and soles. It has been reported in association with the following: congenital hypertrichosis lanuginosa, acquired hypertrichosis lanuginosa, anorexia nervosa and malnutrition, central nervous system disorders, porphyria, dermatomyositis, pretibial myxedema, hypothyroidism, acrodynia, pregnancy, and drug-induced hypertrichosis. In congenital hypertrichosis lanuginosa, the lanugo hair follicles of the fetus persist as lanugo hair follicles into adult life; often these patients exhibit a covering of fine hair over the lids, with the eyebrows similarly affected by the abundant hair growth. Likewise, the hair follicles in acquired hypertrichosis lanuginosa revert to production of the fetal lanugo hair. In these patients, the disorder is often related to an underlying malignancy. In some, hypertrichosis may precede the presentation of the neoplasm by up to 2 years, but in the majority, disseminated malignancy has been present when the increased hair is first noted. Drug-induced hypertrichosis has been associated with cyclosporine, minoxidil, diazoxide, phenytoin, leukocyte A interferon, psoralens, streptomycin, penicillamine, benoxaprofen, tamoxifen, and phenothiazines. In most cases the drug-induced hair growth is not associated with any rise in androgen levels.

Localized hypertrichosis sometimes results from chronic low-grade physical or chemical trauma or hormonal stimulation. It may also be associated with nevi, particularly congenital nevi, and is often seen with porphyria. Topical corticosteroids that are used in patients for the therapy of chronic diseases, such as eczema, psoriasis, and disseminated lupus erythematus, sometimes stimulate hair growth. This has been seen primarily in adults who have used potent fluorinated corticosteroids.

Acquired trichomegaly (an increase in the length of eyelashes) has recently been reported in patients infected with HIV type I. These patients had advanced infection with severe T-helper cell depletion, high levels of p-24 antigenemia, and an inability to tolerate zidovudine therapy. Control of infection with other antiretroviral agents can induce regression of trichomegaly. These reports suggest that acquired trichomegaly of the eyelashes may be a useful cutaneous marker of AIDS. Interferon and cyclosporine can also produce trichomegaly, suggesting that immune dysregulation may be responsible for this unusual clinical finding. In patients presenting with acquired trichomegaly without known precipitating systemic or pharmacologic causes, a search for possible immune system alteration may be indicated.

Hirsutism may be due to physiologic states (precocious puberty, menopause) or endocrinologic states (Cushing's syndrome, malignancies). Congenital ocular hypertrichosis may manifest itself as an increase in the length or the number of eyelashes or brow-lashes. Synophrys (the fusion of eyebrows across the midline), trichomegaly (an increase in the length of cilia), and polytrichia (an increase in number) are common in this condition. Ectopic cilia, reduplication of the ciliary follicles, and cilium inversum are rare hypertrichotic anomalies. Duplication supercilia, in which two rows of eyebrows are present, has also been described.

THERAPY

Supportive. Attempts should be made to determine the cause of the hypertrichosis or hirsutism. If the cause is not physiologic, therapy should be directed at correction of the underlying condition. In the great majority of cases, the hirsutism represents a genetically based normal variation, and the patient can be reassured that the excess hair has no pathologic significance. However, many patients will insist on treatment for cosmetic reasons. In these cases, the least irritating methods should be applied. Cutting or shaving the hair is not likely to irritate the skin. However, there is often a resistance to shaving because of the myth that it stimulates hair to grow faster or more coarsely. One method is to bleach the hair with hydrogen peroxide, thus rendering it less conspicuous. Alternatively, application of a depilatory cream or removal with tweezers may also be beneficial. However, depilatory cream is generally too irritating to use around the eye, and the method does not permanently remove the overgrowth of hair.

Systemic. In patients whose hirsutism presents a problem beyond which can be handled by local physical means, various drug regimens have been used on an empirical basis. New growth of unwanted hair associated with primary adrenal androgenic hyperfunction can often be inhibited by long-term low-dose corticosteroids; a dosage of 5 to 10 mg of oral prednisone daily may be effective. Measurement of plasma and/or urinary parameters after several weeks of glucocorticoids may be of some predictive value. If androgen parameters are lowered by the corticosteroids, the physician is encouraged to pursue long-term management with this agent, providing that secondary side effects are kept at a minimum. Excessive hair growth associated with primary ovarian hyperfunction sometimes may be controlled by a combined progestogen-estrogen combination, usually in the form of oral contraceptives. Again, measurement of androgen parameters after one or more cycles of suppression may encourage the continuation of this therapy.

Recently, the finding that androgenic receptors are present in the hair follicles combined with the availability of several compounds with antiandrogenic properties has afforded new approaches to the treatment of hirsutism. Spironolactone, an aldosterone antagonist, seems to be remarkably effective for the treatment of hirsutism. In one small series, spironolactone at a dose of 200 mg a day was administered to two groups of patients with hirsutism: (1) those with polycystic ovary disease with excessive ovarian androgen production and (2) those with normal androgen levels and idiopathic hirsutism. Treatment with spironolactone resulted in improvement of hirsutism in 19 of 20 patients, with regression in terms of diameter, density, and the rate of facial hair growth within 2 months. Although these results are encouraging, spironolactone is not an entirely benign medication. Until additional data are available from a large number of patients, spironolactone cannot be recommended as an entirely benign and effective treatment for hirsutism.

The oral administration of the powerful antiandrogen, cyproterone acetate,† alone or in combination with ethinyl estradiol,‡ has been found to be successful in several European trials. These progestin-like agents may have several sites of action, including suppression of testosterone production and direct antiandrogen action at one or more target organ sites. This treatment is presently at the investigational stage. Cimetidine‡ has recently been found to have antiandrogenic activity, and preliminary clinical results suggest that this drug may be a safe, effective treatment of androgen-dependent hirsutism.

Surgical. Electrolysis is usually a successful method for permanent hair removal, particularly if there are relatively few hairs; it can also be an effective adjunct along with a medication regimen in more severe cases. Properly performed, electrolysis can be a safe and effective method of hair removal. However, it is a time-consuming, expensive, and moderately uncomfortable procedure. It is generally suitable for only small areas, such as the face and eyelids. Minimal scarring and depigmentation may result. Expertise in this field can be quite variable, since commercial electrolysis is an unlicensed field in many areas. Care should thus be exercised in selecting an electrolysist.

The management of polytrichosis of the eyelids is discussed in the section on distichiasis.

Ocular or Periocular Manifestations

Cornea: Irritative keratitis.
Eyebrows: Excessive cilia; synophrys.
Eyelids: Ectopic cilia; monilethrix; pili torti; polytrichosis; reduplication of ciliary follicles; trichomegaly.

PRECAUTIONS

If there is a diffuse coarsening of hairs, especially in the area of the upper lid, electrolysis may produce poor results. Electrolysis is a tedious procedure that usually requires multiple treatment sessions. A history of keloid formation is an important medical contraindication to electrolysis. Too vigorous electrolysis treatment can produce perceptible cutaneous scarring.

Under no circumstances should radiotherapy be employed in the treatment of hypertrichosis. Permanent depilation can be achieved only at the expense of eventual radiodermatitis, which is both disfiguring and dangerous.

The topical application of depilation waxes or lotions containing barium sulfide or thioglycollates is capable of producing contact dermatitis. Troublesome folliculitis is a frequent complication unless the procedure is carried out under skilled supervision. For this reason, such applications are generally not recommended in the periocular area.

COMMENTS

In at least 90 per cent of women who consider themselves hirsute, the hirsutism is genetically determined and must be considered physiologic. In the small percentage of patients in whom hirsutism is a manifestation of a defined and reversible medical disorder, it is important that an accurate diagnosis be made at an early stage.

Most cases of acquired hypertrichosis are reversible, assuming that the underlying cause is recognized and can be treated. Careful planned investigation by an endocrinologist to identify the etiology is advisable for all such patients, particularly if hormonal abnormalities are suggested.

References

Anderson JAR: An assessment of (1) cyproterone acetate and (2) ethinyl oestradiol and lynoestrenol (Minilyn) in the treatment of idiopathic hirsutism. Br J Dermatol 99:545–552, 1978.

Casanova JM, Puig T, Rubio M: Hypertrichosis of the eyelashes in acquired immunodeficiency syndrome (letter to the editor). Arch Dermatol 123:1599, 1987.

Cumming DC, et al: Treatment of hirsutism with spironolactone. JAMA 247:1295–1298, 1982.

Duke-Elder S (ed): System of Ophthalmology. St. Louis, CV Mosby, 1963, Vol III, pp 873–881.

Kaplan MH, Sadick NS, Talmor M: Acquired trichomegaly of the eyelashes: A cutaneous marker of acquired immunodeficiency syndrome. J Am Acad Dermatol 25:801–804, 1991.

Maguire HC: Diseases of the hair. In Moschella SL, Pillsbury DM, Hurley HJ Jr (eds): Dermatology. Philadelphia, WB Saunders, 1975, pp 1215–1221.

Muller SA: Hirsutism. Am J Med 46:803–817, 1969.

Vigersky RA, et al: Treatment of hirsute women with cimetidine. A preliminary report. N Engl J Med 303:1042, 1980.

ICHTHYOSIS 757.1
(Acquired Ichthyosis, Epidermolytic Hyperkeratosis, Ichthyosis Vulgaris, Lamellar Ichthyosis, X-Linked Ichthyosis)

KENNETH M. GOINS, M.D.

Chicago, Illinois

Ichthyosis refers to a relatively uncommon group of skin disorders characterized by the presence of excessive amounts of dry surface scales. The ichthyosiform dermatoses may be classified according to clinical manifestations, genetic presentation, and histologic findings. Inherited and acquired forms of ichthyosis have been described, and ocular alterations may occur in specific subtypes.

There are four distinct types of inherited ichthyosis: ichthyosis vulgaris, lamellar ichthyosis, epidermolytic hyperkeratosis, and X-linked ichthyosis. Ichthyosis vulgaris is the most common and is inherited as an autosomal dominant trait with an incidence of 1 in 300. In this disorder, dry skin and follicular accentuation (keratosis pilaris) usually appear at puberty. Scaling is most prominent over the trunk, abdomen, buttocks, and legs. The flexural areas, such as the antecubital fossa, are spared.

Epidermolytic hyperkeratosis is an autosomal dominant disorder with an incidence of 1 in 300,000 in the general population. At birth, the skin is moist, red, and tender. Thick verrucous scaling occurs within a few days.

Lamellar ichthyosis, a more severe form of dermatosis, is an autosomal recessive trait with an incidence of 1 in 300,000. Children who are born with lamellar ichthyosis are called "collodion babies" and are covered at birth by a thickened membrane that is subsequently shed. The scaling of the skin involves the whole body with no sparing of the flexural creases. Approximately one-third of children affected with this disorder will develop bilateral ectropion of the cicatricial type that seems to result from excessive dryness of the skin and subsequent contracture. Secondary corneal ulceration may occur secondary to chronic exposure.

X-linked ichthyosis is another severe disorder with an incidence of 1 in 100,000 in male patients. Generalized scaling is present at or shortly after birth. This scaling is most prominent over the extremities, neck, trunk, and buttocks. The flexural creases, palms, and soles are spared. Irregular stromal corneal opacities that are located anterior to Descemet's membrane are found in 16 to 50 per cent of male patients, and this finding may be used to distinguish this form of ichthyosis from all others. Approximately 25 per cent of female carriers have minor corneal opacities, which are not known to affect visual acuity. Previous studies have shown a deficiency of steroid-sulfatase in skin fibroblasts and a marked elevation of plasma cholesterol sulfate in patients with X-linked ichthyosis.

Acquired ichthyosis usually occurs in adults and is manifested as small, white, fish-like scales that are frequently concentrated on the extremities, but may be seen in a generalized distribution. This form of ichthyosis may be associated with internal neoplasia (Hodgkin's lymphoma), systemic illness (sarcoidosis), or the intake of certain medications that interfere with sterol synthesis in epidermal cells (nicotinic acid).

THERAPY

Systemic. Oral retinoids display an impressive antikeratinizing action in ichthyosiform dermatoses. Etretinate (1 mg/kg/day) and isotretinoin (2 mg/kg/day) have been shown to reduce scaling, discomfort, and disfigurement. However, when these drugs are discontinued, the ichthyotic skin recurs, thereby necessitating chronic use. Patients with epidermolytic hyperkeratosis may develop chronic bacterial infections of the skin, necessitating chronic antibiotic therapy. In these cases, benzathine penicillin G, 1.2 million units intramuscularly, is given every 2 to 3 weeks until the skin infection subsides. Oral erythromycin ethyl succinate, 800 mg four times daily, may be substituted in penicillin-allergic patients.

Ocular. In chronic ocular surface disorders associated with ichthyosis, nonpreserved artificial tears (carboxymethylcellulose sodium 0.5 to 1.0 per cent) and ointment (white petrolatum 56.8 per cent, mineral oil 41.5 per cent) are preferred to prevent complications from dryness and exposure. Preservative-free lubricants may be used as often as needed while decreasing the incidence of preservative-related allergies. In cases where poor corneal epithelial adhesion is present, bandage contact lenses and temporary collagen shields may decrease symptoms and promote surface healing.

Topical. To prevent cicatricial ectropion in lamellar ichthyosis, a humidified atmosphere combined with the use of topical moisturizing agents is beneficial. Petrolatum ointment and 10 per cent urea cream applied to the eyelid skin several times daily will help prevent skin contracture. Salicylic acid 2 per cent and retinoic acid 0.1 per cent ointments are also effective, but local irritation may limit their frequency of usage.

Surgical. When cicatricial ectropion develops, despite room humidification and vigorous skin lubrication, there is the danger of corneal breakdown and perforation. Full thickness skin grafts from the forearm, post-auricular, and groin areas may be used to repair the abnormalities successfully. A concomitant medial and/or lateral lid adhesion is recommended in severe cases. The incidence of ectropion recurrence may be decreased if surgery can be postponed until suitable non-scaly patches of skin can be clearly identified to serve as graft donor sites.

Supportive. The mainstays of ichthyosis therapy are frequent bathing with tar soap, removal of surface scales, and application of a water barrier. In disabling cases, oral retinoids may reduce cosmetic disfigurement, depression, and social isolation.

Ocular or Periocular Manifestations

Conjunctiva: Keratinization and thickening secondary to ectropion.
Cornea: Exposure keratitis secondary to ectropion; unilateral megalocornea (lamellar ichthyosis); pre-Descemet's opacities (X-linked ichthyosis); recurrent corneal erosion; band keratopathy; Salzmann's nodules (ichthyosis vulgaris); microphthalmos (rare).
Eyelids: Ectropion (lamellar ichthyosis); blepharitis; meibomian gland absence (rare).

PRECAUTIONS

Because skeletal hyperostosis and arthralgia may occur with chronic oral etretinate and isotretinoin use, this form of treatment is reserved only for those with very severe scaling and cosmetic deformity. Topical dermatologic retinoid preparations are irritating to the conjunctival fornices and therefore should not be directly applied to the eye.

COMMENTS

Since ichthyosis is primarily a skin disorder, periodic evaluation by a dermatologist is recommended. The ophthalmologist may be helpful in the treatment of ocular manifestations and identifying the specific type of ichthyosis, particularly the lamellar and X-linked forms.

References

Baden HP, Imber M: Ichthyosis with an unusual constellation of ectodermal dysplasias. Clin Genet 35:455–461, 1989.

Banse-Kupin L, Pelachyk JM: Ichthyosiform sarcoidosis. J Am Acad Dermatol 17:616–620, 1987.

Costagliola C, Fabbrocini G, Illiano GMP, Scibelli G, Delfino M: Ocular findings in X-linked ichthyosis: A survey on 38 cases. Ophthalmologica 202:152–155, 1991.

Leung PC, Ma GFY: Ectropion of all four eyelids associated with severe ichthyosis congenita: A case report. Br J Plast Surg 34:302–304, 1981.

Mansour AM, Traboulsi EI, Frangieh GT, Jarudi N: Unilateral megalocornea in lamellar ichthyosis. Ann Opththalmol 17:466–470, 1985.

Marano RPC, Ortiz Stradtmann MA, Uxo M, Iglesias E: Ocular findings associated with congenital X-linked ichthyosis. Ann Ophthalmol 23:167–172, 1991.

Orth DH, Fretzin DF, Abramson V: Collodion baby with transient bilateral upper lid ectropion. Review of ocular manifestations in ichthyosis. Arch Ophthalmol 91:206–207, 1974.

Peled I, Bar-Lev A, Wexler MR: Surgical correction of ectropion in lamellar ichthyosis. Ann Plast Surg 8:429–431, 1982.

Sever RJ, Frost P, Weinstein G: Eye changes in ichthyosis. JAMA 206:2283–2286, 1968.

Shelley WB, Shelley ED: Advanced Dermatologic Therapy. Philadelphia, WB Saunders, 1987, pp 1056–1084.

IMPETIGO 684

ALAN SUGAR, M.D.

Ann Arbor, Michigan

Impetigo is a superficial infection of the skin caused by group A *Streptococcus* or *Staphylococcus aureus* or both. It occurs primarily in newborns and young children. Although thought in the past to be mostly streptococcal, recent studies have shown *S. aureus* to be the primary organism in most cases. Impetigo contagiosa is easily transmitted and is the most common skin infection of children. The initial lesions are tiny vesicles in the superficial epidermis that develop into larger pustules. Initially, there is very little underlying erythema. The lesions become covered by a thin crust that thickens to a honey-colored purulent crust and appears to be "tacked on" to the skin. An erythematous base and regional lymphadenopathy may develop, although there are no systemic symptoms. Deeper skin ulceration (ecthyma) may follow. The lesions occur in exposed areas, particularly the face and arms, and are especially common in late summer and after minor skin trauma. An important systemic sequela is the development of glomerulonephritis when nephrogenic streptococcal strains are involved with a 2 to 5 per cent incidence, mostly in children under 6 years old. Bullous impetigo is caused by staphylococci and begins with the development of large bullae, which rupture leaving a thin clear crust. Ocular involvement in impetigo is secondary to periocular skin involvement.

THERAPY

Systemic. Untreated impetigo may become a chronic skin disease and lead to acute glomerulonephritis. Systemic antibiotic therapy is effective treatment, either alone or in combination with topical therapy. Penicillins are rapidly effective for most streptococci, but staphylococci are increasingly resistant. A 10-day course of 250,000 to 500,000 units of oral penicillin V three to four times daily is an adequate regimen. Intramuscular benzathine penicillin G in a single 0.6 to 1.2 million unit injection is effective when compliance is a problem. A 10-day course of 20 to 40 mg/kg of erythromycin may be given in four divided doses. Penicillin-resistant staphylococci in bullous impetigo may be treated with 25 to 50 mg/kg of cloxacillin§ or dicloxacillin§ four times a day for 7 to 10 days. Oral cephalosporins are also effective.

Topical. Traditionally, impetigo has been treated with cleansing of the crusts and scrubbing with bacteriostatic soaps, followed by the application of bacitracin or neomycin ointment. Recent studies, however, have shown that scrubbing may delay healing. Topical 2 per cent mupirocin ointment is as effective as oral erythromycin. It may be used alone and is as effective as systemic antibiotics in preventing glomerulonephritis.

Ocular or Periocular Manifestations

Conjunctiva: Acute bacterial conjunctivitis.
Cornea: Bacterial ulcer (rare).
Eyelids: Blepharitis: cicatricial ankyloblepharon (rare); local skin lesions.

PRECAUTIONS

Isolation and skin wound precautions should be observed to prevent the spread of infection to family members or to other patients. Prophylactic treatment of family members, especially young children, can be effective.

COMMENTS

Topical treatment with mupirocin has gained favor because of its effectiveness against increasingly prevalent erythromycin-resistant staphylococci.

References

Dagan R, Bar-David Y: Double-blind study comparing erythromycin and mupirocin for treatment of impetigo in children: Implications of a high prevalence of erythromycin-resistant *Staphylococcus aureus* strains. Antimicrob Agents Chemother 36:287–290, 1992.

Ferrieri P, Dajani AS, Wannamaker LW: A controlled study of penicillin prophylaxis against streptococcal impetigo. J Infect Dis 129:429–438, 1974.

Margolis HS, et al: Acute glomerulonephritis and streptococcal skin lesions in Eskimo children. Am J Dis Child 134:681–685, 1980.

Mertz PM, Marshall DA, Eaglstein WH, et al: Topical mupirocin treatment of impetigo is equal to oral erythromycin therapy. Arch Dermatol 125:1069–1073, 1989.

Peter G, Smith AL: Group A streptococcal infections of the skin and pharynx. (First of two parts). N Engl J Med 297:311–317, 1977.

Rice TD, Duggan AK, DeAngelis C: Cost effectiveness of erythromycin versus mupirocin for the treatment of impetigo in children. Pediatrics 89:210–214, 1992.

OCULAR ROSACEA 695.3

JOSEPH FRUCHT-PERY, M.D.,
and STUART I. BROWN, M.D.

San Diego, California

Rosacea is a common chronic skin disorder of unknown etiology. It is more prevalent in females and is usually manifested between the ages of 30 to 50 years. Characteristically, the facial flush areas (forehead, nose, and cheeks) and the V of the neck are involved. The presence of telangiectasia pustules and rhinophyma is diagnostic of rosacea, and supporting findings include erythema, hypertrophic sebaceous glands, and papules. Intermittent exacerbation and remissions are common.

Ocular manifestations of rosacea mainly involve the lids, conjunctiva, and cornea. Diffusely hyperemic conjunctiva, blepharitis, meibomianitis or styes are common, and episcleritis may also occur. Corneal involvement includes punctate epithelial erosions, peripheral vascularization, and subepithelial infiltrates with thinning central to vascularization. Corneal perforation may ensue secondary to the infiltrate and thinning. Patients usually complain of burning and tearing and general irritation.

THERAPY

Systemic. Treatment with oral tetracyclines[‡] is necessary to alleviate the symptoms and signs of ocular rosacea. Recent experience shows that doxycycline, a semisynthetic tetracycline, can alleviate ocular symptoms. Although its maximal effect is slower, doxycycline is as efficient as tetracycline and is better tolerated. The dose of 100 mg of doxycycline is given once a day for 6 weeks. If the patient's symptoms have responded, the dose is tapered to 50 mg daily for one month, then 50 mg every other day, and finally stopped. However, if the symptoms remain unchanged, the doxycycline is discontinued, 250 mg of tetracycline is given four times a day, and the dose is slowly tapered according to the patient's symptoms and response.

Improvement is expected within the first 3 weeks; irritation is usually diminished before the signs resolve. Most of the treated patients require some daily medication indefinitely. Abrupt tapering may cause recurrence of the disease, which may be very difficult to treat with full doses of tetracycline, and some of these cases become unresponsive to these drugs.

Ocular. Topical antibiotics are ineffective in ocular rosacea. Topical steroids may be useful to treat subepithelial corneal infiltrates or episcleritis; however, these drugs should always be applied in addition to oral tetracyclines. Associated blepharitis will respond to systemic doxycycline or tetracycline.

Surgical. Small corneal perforations, especially peripheral, may be treated with application of cyanoacrylate adhesive and a bandage soft contact lens or by lamellar patch graft. In patients with large central perforations or with visual disability from scarred and vascularized corneas, a penetrating keratoplasty may be done. Concurrent treatment with tetracycline or doxycycline is crucial during these surgical maneuvers.

Topical. Facial lesions respond to treatment with tetracycline. Patients rarely require topical corticosteroid preparations to decrease signs of the disorder.

Ocular or Periocular Manifestations

Conjunctiva: Hyperemia.
Cornea: Pannus; perforation; punctate erosion (recurrent); subepithelial infiltration; superficial or deep wedge-shaped neovascularization; thinning.
Eyelids: Chalazion; chronic blepharoconjunctivitis; erythema of lid margins; hordeolum; increased meibomian secretions; thickening.
Sclera: Nodular episcleritis.
Other: Burning; decreased visual acuity; foreign body sensation; irritation; pain.

PRECAUTIONS

Tetracycline or doxycycline should not be used in children under the age of 8 years or until enamel deposition on the maturing teeth is completed. Likewise, it should not be given to pregnant or lactating women. Vaginal yeast superinfection may occur and can be treated by gradual tapering of the tetracycline doses or with local antifungal agents. Tetracycline should be administered on an empty stomach, and concurrent administration of antacids, dairy products, or iron preparations is not recommended because gastrointestinal absorption of the drug is diminished by these agents. Doxycycline can be used at any time. Although milk products insignificantly affect the absorption of doxycycline, concurrent antacids or milk products are not recommended with its use.

COMMENTS

The diagnosis of ocular rosacea is often missed. All examinations for external eye disorders should be performed with good illumination and removal of facial makeup if present to enable the discovery of subtle signs. Ocular signs and symptoms may be unilateral, and rosacea patients may present with a unilateral red eye. It is important to counsel patients, since this disease may be chronic and some signs of meibomianitis or blepharitis may persist after most symptoms are relieved.

References

Brown SI, Shahinian L Jr: Diagnosis and treatment of ocular rosacea. Ophthalmology 85:779–786, 1978.

Frucht-Pery J, et al: The effect of doxycycline on ocular rosacea. Am J Ophthalmol 107:434–436, 1989.

Jenkins MS, et al: Ocular rosacea. Am J Ophthalmol 88:618–622, 1979.

Lempert SL, Jenkins MS, Brown SI: Chalazia and rosacea. Arch Ophthalmol 97:1652–1653, 1979.

Marmion VJ: Tetracyclines in the treatment of ocular rosacea. Proc Roy Soc Med 62:11–12, 1969.

Sneddon IB: A clinical trial of tetracycline in rosacea. Br J Dermatol 78:649–652, 1966.

Tolman EL: Acne and acneiform dermatoses. In Moschella SL, Pillsbury DM, Harley HJ Jr (eds): Dermatology. Philadelphia, WB Saunders, 1975, pp 1139–1142.

PHOTOSENSITIVITY AND SUNBURN 692.79

ERNESTO GONZALEZ, M.D.,
and JOHN A. PARRISH, M.D.

Boston, Massachusetts

For obvious reasons, the skin and the eye are the primary targets for the effects of ultraviolet radiation. The enhanced response of these organs to the natural or artificial, nonionizing, electromagnetic radiation is referred to as photosensitivity. On the skin, this phenomenon has variable manifestations depending on such factors as the wavelength, exposure dose and duration, the presence of chemical photoenhancers, and the host's innate defenses (constitutive pigmentation, thickness of the stratum corneum) and immunologic response. The response we are most familiar with is the sunburn reaction, an acute photosensitivity reaction induced by absorption on the skin of ultraviolet radiation in the range of 290 to 320 nm (UVB) after exposure beyond the threshold of redness (erythema) for that skin type. The phenomenon is referred to as acute phototoxicity and is manifested as tender erythema with edema and, in severe cases, vesiculation. Constitutional complaints, such as fever, nausea, chills, and delirium, can be seen in severe cases. Chronic phototoxic reactions have been reported in subjects receiving long-term phototherapy treatment with longer wavelength ultraviolet light (UVA—320 to 400 nm) when used in combination with chemical photosensitizers, such as psoralen (PUVA). The manifestation of this reaction is more insidious, with tender erythema and scaling but minimal edema and no vesiculation. It can be frequently confused with skin disorders, such as psoriasis and eczema, for which the phototherapy treatment

was originally prescribed. Frequent or chronic exposure to ultraviolet radiation will eventually produce a silent, cumulative damage that will have more significant consequences than the symptomatic, acute, or chronic phototoxic reactions. Atrophy of the skin with or without dilated blood vessels (telangiectasia), pigmentary disturbances and, the promotion of such skin tumors as basal cell epithelioma, squamous cell carcinoma, and malignant melanoma are inexorable complications in subjects with no natural or artificial skin photoprotection.

Photosensitivity reactions on the skin can also develop when an altered immunologic state is present in the host and a delayed hypersensitivity reaction is initiated when the skin is exposed to chemical and ultraviolet radiation, primarily UVA. This is called photoallergic reaction and is primarily manifested as an eczematous dermatitis. Endogenously produced abnormal metabolites, such as porphyrins, can also produce photosensitive disorders called porphyrias with vesicles, skin fragility and atrophy, and scarring. Finally, a group of idiopathic photodermatoses that can be genetically determined or acquired can have protean manifestations, such as papules, plaques, or urticarial lesions in which the biochemical alteration has not been elucidated yet. Polymorphous light eruption, referred to commonly as "sun poisoning," is a common pruritic acquired idiopathic photodermatosis that occurs most often in women exposed to strong sunlight; it accounts for approximately 30 per cent of all photosensitive disorders of the skin. Solar urticaria and chronic actinic dermatosis are other forms of idiopathic symptomatic photodermatoses.

The eye is the other organ in the body that is particularly sensitive to the nonionizing wavelengths of optical radiation (280 to 1400 nm) normally present in our environment. Since the normal cornea, aqueous humor, ocular lens, and vitreous humor are almost completely transparent to visible light, visible radiation normally does not cause photic damage to these tissues. These transparent tissues, however, can absorb ultraviolet radiation, and the photic damage will be primarily produced by the high-energy, short wavelength UVB rays absorbed selectively by these tissues.

The most common ocular abnormality caused directly by ultraviolet radiation is photokeratoconjunctivitis, which results from the absorption of short (UVC, 200 to 290 nm) and middle (UVB, 290 to 320 nm) wavelength ultraviolet radiation by the outer viable cell layers of the cornea and conjunctiva. The clinical picture of photokeratitis has a characteristic course. After exposure, a period of latency varies somewhat inversely with the exposure dose, being as short as 30 minutes to as long as 24 hours. Conjunctivitis, often accompanied by erythema of the periorbital skin, is associated with a foreign body sensation, varying degrees of photophobia, lacrimation, and blepharospasm. Corneal pain can be very severe. The individual is usually incapacitated for 6 to 24 hours, but all discomfort usually disappears within 48 hours. Very rarely does exposure result in permanent damage. Unlike the skin, the ocular system does not develop tolerance to repeated exposure.

The "snow blindness" that occurs with prolonged exposure among polar explorers is another example of acute corneal photodamage by UVB radiation where snow serves to reflect 80 per cent of the ultraviolet radiation (compared to 5 per cent from grass). Photokeratitis can also be induced by accidental exposure to high-intensity, artificial ultraviolet light, such as arc welding, or to moderate intensity ones, such as germicidal lamps ("welder's flash"). The use of high-intensity UVB and UVA radiation in the commercial tanning industry has been responsible for photokeratitis among workers in that industry, whereas roofers have been reported to develop photokeratitis from airborne exposure to volatilized coal-tar pitch, a photosensitizer that can be absorbed on the surface of the eye. Laser sources that emit high-intensity, shortwave (UVB—290 to 300 nm) ultraviolet radiation can also produce damage to the cornea. Finally, ultraviolet exposure has been implicated in the development of pterygium and pingueculum as a chronic damage to the conjunctiva.

The normal human cornea and aqueous humor transmit almost all light at wavelengths longer than 300 nm. The ocular lens absorbs almost all UVB radiation while it transmits some ultraviolet A and all visible light, which is primarily absorbed in the retina. This absorption of high-energy, short-wavelength ultraviolet radiation by photochemically generated chromophores in the lens induces photochemical damage during a lifetime of exposure to ambient ultraviolet radiation. For example, 75 per cent of UV light, 300 to 400 nm, is transmitted by lenses in children under 10 years of age, whereas none is transmitted in subjects over 25 years old. The absorption of ultraviolet light by the aging lens is responsible for some forms of cataract formation, but it serves as a filter to protect the retina from photodamage. Of the three major anatomic and morphologic types of senile cataracts (nuclear, cortical, and posterior subcapsular), a recent epidemiologic study revealed that high cumulative levels of UVB environmental exposure increased significantly the risk of cortical cataracts, whereas UVB radiation had a negligible effect on the formation of nuclear cataracts. The study did not find any causal relationship between cataracts and UVA exposure. Case-control studies have also found a similar relation for both cortical and posterior subcapsular opacities. The progressive destruction of the ozone layer in the atmosphere by chlorinated fluorocarbons and other pollutants and the concomitant increased UVB radiation on the surface of the earth further increase the potential for lenticular opacities and photodamage to other UVB ocular absorbers.

Ocular photodamage by intraocular photosensitizers, either endogenously produced, such as tryptophan and porphyrins, or exogenously introduced, such as phenothiazines, nalidixic acid, psoralens used in medicine, or chemical compounds with a benzene or tricyclic rings used in industry, can occur in the lens, choroid, and retina. The widespread use of photochemotherapy with oral 8-methoxypsoralen and high-intensity UVA light sources (PUVA) for multiple dermatologic diseases and the injudicious exposure to UVA with or without chemical photosensitizers for tanning purposes (tanning salons) pose significant threats. The high-intensity, artificial light sources used in these instances are far beyond the normal environmental exposures to UVA. More importantly, a chemical photosensitivity is produced by psoralen as the intraocular chromophore, when it absorbs UVA radiation, produces photoproducts with proteins and DNA cross-links that interfere with DNA replication and cellular proliferation. It has been shown that 8-methoxypsoralen (8-MOP) enters the lens and can be found in the cortex, nucleus, and epithelial cells and diffuses out of the lens in 12 hours if no exposure to UVA radiation occurs during that period. If exposed to UVA (which is abundantly present in sunlight), however, the 8-MOP binds to the lens proteins and DNA and can produce potential cumulative damage with repeated exposures since the lens is completely encapsulated and never sheds any cells. In young children whose lenses transmit UVA and in aphakic patients, PUVA may potentially result in damage to the retina.

The advent of lasers has created a new source of ocular damage. Laser-emitting UV radiation can photochemically induce permanent cataracts within 24 hours, and near-instantaneous cataract formation can be induced thermally by UV laser exposure at the lens absorption band of 365 nm.

The retina in adults is relatively spared from photodamage by UV radiation since it does not receive energy of wavelengths shorter than 390 nm due to the transmittance restriction of the lens. As mentioned before, children under 10 are at higher risk of retinal photodamage from UV light since the ocular lens at that age allows transmission of this radiation to the retina. A small window of UVB and UVA transmittance (less than 10 per cent), centered about 320 nm, is present even during adolescence, which may account for the increasing prevalence of choroidal malignant melanoma due to UV exposure during that age period. Retinal photodamage has been reported by solar exposure in sungazers. Some investigators believe that solar retinopathy can be explained almost entirely by the photochemical effects of shorter wavelengths of visible light (blue region) and the ultraviolet radiation components of the sun's spectrum. On the other hand, no association has been found between long-term exposure to UV radiation and an increased risk for macular degeneration. As mentioned above, retinal damage can occur when chemical photosensitivity is enhanced by deposits of intraocular photosensitizers and exposure to UV light, particularly UVA.

THERAPY

Preventive. Therapeutic intervention, first and foremost, should stress prevention as both sunburn and photosensitivity are preventable conditions. Clothing and avoidance of sun exposure are the simplest measures. For subjects with light complexion, sunscreens with sun protection factor (SPF) of at least 15 should be applied 45 minutes before wetting the skin with sweat or water to allow absorption into the skin. Sunblocks are also effective, but need to be reapplied more frequently since they are not absorbed. Wearing a hat with a wide brim can offer partial protection of facial skin and can reduce ocular exposure to UVB by 50 per cent.

Protection of the eyes from the effects of high-intensity UV radiation requires the isolation of high-intensity UV sources and the use of goggles and other shields with proper filters. Most safety glasses with lenses and side shields made of polycarbonate plastic afford adequate protection against arc welding and snow-laden environment while allowing visible light transmission. Although spectacle sunglasses can block the full spectrum of UV radiation, side shields or wraparounds are important since UV exposure of the angles of the eye can reach as high as 6.6 per cent. Ordinary eyeglasses do not appreciably absorb radiation between 300 to 400 nm. Commercial sunglasses are not necessarily effective absorbers of the longer wavelength of UV light. Darkly tinted sunglasses, for example, can decrease visible light significantly, but may allow the transmission of UV light into ocular tissue. Yellow-tinted or amber-tinted sunglasses may also have similar drawbacks.

Systemic. Acute phototoxic reaction (sunburn) may require cool water soaks or baths when erythema is present or astringent and drying products (Aveeno, Burow's solution) when vesicles/bullae are present. Severe generalized acute phototoxicity (more than 30 per cent body surface) may require systemic corticosteroids in oral doses of 40 to 60 mg of prednisone daily tapered down over 12 to 14 days. This approach offers symptomatic relief, but does not necessarily reduce the duration or intensity of the erythema. Topical steroids provide an intermediate symptomatic improvement between the other topical agents and oral prednisone. Although acute chemical

phototoxic reactions will respond to the above regimen, it is imperative to identify and remove the chemical photosensitizers to prevent further exacerbations or recurrences. Chronic phototoxic reaction produced by high, sustained doses of phototherapy requires discontinuation and eventual adjusting of the phototherapy dose according to the skin type of the subject, as well as the use of topical agents to lubricate and cool the skin or topical steroids to reduce inflammation. Photoallergic reactions require identification of the topical photosensitizers with appropriate photopatch testing since it is essential to remove the culprit for improvement. The use of topical or systemic steroids is indicated, depending on the severity, as there is a predictable response both symptomatically and by suppressing the eczematous dermatitis.

The idiopathic dermatoses require establishing the causative wavelength with phototesting and determining the minimal erythema dose (MED). Response to topical therapy is usually poor, except for the important role that sunscreens or sunblocks play in filtering the incriminating UV radiation. Patients with more symptomatic or extensive disease require systemic therapy with antimalarials, such as hydroxychloroquine (200 mg twice a day) or quinacrine (100 mg twice a day), or preventive therapy with oral prednisone 3 days before exposure to sunlight. Carefully monitored exposures to UV light from artificial sources for 10 to 15 treatments (PUVA or UVB) can induce temporary tolerance in patients with PMLE, solar urticaria, or chronic actinic dermatosis. The treatment of porphyrias may require phlebotomy or low-dose oral chloroquine and should usually be referred to an expert in the field.

Ocular. Symptomatic relief of photosensitivity of the eyelids may be obtained with cold compresses of isotonic saline, Burow's solution 1:40, or plain tap water. Cold compresses reduce the blepharospasm and the accompanying paroxysmal pain. Topical corticosteroids may be applied judiciously for a short time to reduce erythema, pruritus, and edema.

Acute solar conjunctivitis can be improved symptomatically by bandaging the eyes, and broad-spectrum antibiotics may be applied topically to prevent intercurrent infections. In severe cases, homatropine eyedrops may help relieve the ciliary spasm and extreme miosis.

PRECAUTIONS

The use of hydroxychloroquine to treat patients with idiopathic photosensitive disorders, such as PMLE, is not listed in the manufacturer's official directive. Although not as retinotoxic as chloroquine, baseline and periodic eye examinations are indicated when this drug is used since irreversible retinopathy can develop. Atabrine, an antimalarial with a chemical structure not derived from chloroquine, does not produce retinal toxicity, but can cause hematologic disorders.

The risk of inducing glaucoma and cataracts when using topical or systemic steroids needs to be considered. Short courses of fluorinated steroids and even longer courses of hydrocortisone 1 per cent applied topically on eyelids have been incriminated in the production of glaucoma.

All patients receiving PUVA therapy should wear protective sunglasses for at least 12 hours after ingestion of methoxsalen. The sunglasses must be opaque to UVA, should have side shields, and should be worn when driving or when indoors next to a window since UVA is transmitted through window and windshield glass. Suntanning with natural sunlight and especially with high-intensity, artificial UV light (UVA) should be discouraged to avoid both acute and chronic phototoxicity to cutaneous and ocular tissues.

Eye protection with the appropriate goggles for the high-intensity, monochromatic radiation emitted by different laser sources is essential for both the patient and the healthcare worker. Yearly eye examinations are recommended for healthcare workers using laser sources routinely.

References

Barker FM: The effects of UV-A upon the eye. *In* Urbach F (ed): Biological Responses to Ultraviolet A Radiation. Kansas, Valdenmar Publishing, 1992, pp 273–280.

Barker FM, Brainard GC, Dayhawk-Barker P: Transmittance of the human lens as a function of age. Invest Ophthalmol Vis Sci *32S*:1083, 1991.

Hu H: Effects of ultraviolet radiation. Med Clin North Am *74*:509–514, 1990.

Lerman S: Radiant Energy and the Eye. New York, Macmillan, 1980.

Lerman S: Ocular phototoxicity (Editorial). N Engl J Med *319*:1475–1476, 1988.

Taylor HR, West SK, Rosentah FS, et al: Effect of ultraviolet radiation on cataract formation. N Engl J Med *319*:1429–1433, 1988.

POISON IVY, OAK, OR SUMAC DERMATITIS 692.6
(Rhus Dermatitis)

WILLIAM L. EPSTEIN, M.D.

San Francisco, California

Several plants in the *Rhus* genus are capable of producing contact dermatitis. Poison ivy (*Rhus radicans*) dermatitis is by far the most common, but poison oak (*R. toxicodendron*) and poison sumac (*R. vernix*) dermatitis may also occur. The most characteristic lesion is a linear one, appearing on an extremity that has brushed past an offending plant. The rash is initially red and very itchy; it rapidly becomes vesicular and may spread from the patient's extremities to face or genitals. In severe cases, the patient is acutely uncomfortable, due to the oozing, crusting, itching, and smarting that occur during the active stages of infection. Resolution of *Rhus* dermatitis usually occurs in 2 to 3 weeks. Ocular involvement almost always results from transmission of the irritant to the ocular adnexae by the hands. The lids become edematous and hyperemic, vesiculation occurs, and a secondary pyoderma may lead to pustulation. In severe cases, a chemotic conjunctival reaction may be present. The cornea may be involved, causing pain, photophobia, and blepharospasm.

THERAPY

Systemic. If edema becomes noticeable or the dermatitis is severe, systemic corticosteroids may be employed. A repository corticotropin injection of 80 units may be given intramuscularly on the patient's first visit. Repeat injections given on the third and fifth days often provide sufficient relief. However, the dose and frequency of injection depend upon the patient's response. The same degree of control requires an initial dose of 400 to 600 mg of hydrocortisone or its equivalent (80 to 100 mg of triamcinolone or methylprednisolone).

Ocular. Ocular therapy is symptomatic. Cool compresses may provide relief for itching and burning. In the earliest stages before marked vesiculation has occurred, topical corticosteroids, such as 0.2 per cent betamethasone cream, may be applied three times daily to the eyelids for a few days. If conjunctival or corneal involvement occurs, topical ophthalmic corticosteroids, such as 0.05 per cent dexamethasone ointment, may be used four times daily. If an anterior uveitis is present, 5 per cent homatropine one to four times daily may be used.

Supportive. Before vesiculation occurs and during the healing stage, topical corticosteroids may be applied to the affected area. High-potency corticosteroids in a gel base or an optimized vehicle are preferred for skin lesions, whereas topical ophthalmic ointments are necessary for use around the eye. Topical 0.05 to 0.5 per cent fluocinolone, fluocinonide, or betamethasone may be used three times daily.

After vesiculation occurs, conventional therapy relies on the use of cold soaks (Burow's solution 1:40), tepid baths (starch and soda, Aveeno oatmeal), and lotions (calamine without additives). However, drying and cracking of the skin from overzealous bathing should be avoided, as it tends to increase pruritus. Care must be taken not to allow these materials to touch the eye.

Sedatives or antihistamines may help alleviate pruritus. Aspirin may be given in a dosage of 0.6 gm every 3 to 4 hours. Occasionally, 0.5 to 2.0 gm of chloral hydrate at bedtime may be necessary.

Ocular or Periocular Manifestations

Conjunctiva: Chemosis.
Cornea: Infiltration; keratitis.
Eyelids: Blepharospasm; edema; hyperemia; pustules; vesicles.
Other: Ocular pain; photophobia.

PRECAUTIONS

The effectiveness of topical corticosteroids is greatly reduced after vesiculation has begun. Because of the high potency of recommended topical corticosteroids, they should not be used for long periods of time or over large areas of the body. Prolonged use of topical corticosteroids near the periocular area should be avoided because of the potential danger of glaucoma. If systemic corticosteroids are used, the value of a very large initial dose cannot be overemphasized; most failures in this form of therapy are caused by hesitation to use a therapeutic dose of corticosteroid. Flare-ups may occur if the dosage of corticosteroids is reduced too rapidly. Local subcutaneous injections of corticosteroids can cause atrophic changes.

Administration of poison ivy extract is contraindicated in the management of acute cases. It usually produces no effect, and occasionally the dermatitis is aggravated by this therapeutic measure.

COMMENTS

The *Rhus* plants produce a dermatitis by means of a group of antigens common to all three plants. The same group of antigens may also be found in the shell of the cashew nut, the mango rind, Japanese lacquer, Indian marking nut, the ginkgo tree, and several other exotic plants and trees from South America and Southeast Asia. The dermatitis caused by these antigens is more likely to be vesicular and bullous than many other common forms of contact dermatitis.

Rhus dermatitis occurs most commonly in children during spring and summer and in those whose occupations bring them into contact with the species. Poison ivy dermatitis is very common and constitutes a significant source of disability.

References

Duke-Elder S (ed): System of Ophthalmology. St. Louis, CV Mosby, 1974, Vol XIII, p 60.
Epstein WL: Allergic contact dermatitis. *In* Fitzpatrick TB et al (eds): Dermatology in General Medicine, 3rd ed. New York, McGraw-Hill, 1987, pp 1373–1383.
Epstein WL: The poison ivy picker of pennypack park. J Invest Dermatol *88*:7s–11s, 1987.
Grant WM: Toxicology of the Eye, 3rd ed. Springfield, IL, Charles C Thomas, 1986, pp 749–750.

PRURITUS 698.9

JAMES D. HOGAN, M.D.

La Crosse, Wisconsin

Pruritus is an unpleasant sensation perceived in the skin that elicits the response of scratching. It reflects a sensation of generalized itch, whereas itch implies a visible morphologic skin finding usually localized and accompanied by scratching. Pruritus may be sharp and well localized (epicritic), diffuse (protopathic), scattered with multiple distant foci of itching after primary focal itch, or referred itch within the same dermatome of primary focal itch. It may result from physiologic or pathologic causes; as a generalized hyperresponsiveness of itchy skin, such as in urticaria with dermatographism; and, more recently, central neural itch as mediated by the central nervous system without primary cutaneous changes.

Itch receptors' free nerve endings and networks pass through a rich milieu in the dermis of blood vessels, mast cells, and connective tissue, forming a plexus of receptor sites at the dermal-epidermal junction. Itch and pain are separate sensations, though increasing itch stimulus can result in pain. Removal of the epidermis and upper dermis abolishes itch but not pain sensation. Both pain and itch are transmitted to the spinal cord by small diameter fibers and are probably integrated at a common site in the dorsal horn of each spinal segment. Impulse conduction is then transmitted to the contralateral anterolateral spinothalamic tracts of the spinal cord to secondary neuronal relay centers in the thalamus. However, evidence of tertiary cortical itch receptors in the sensory cortex is inferential.

The best-known mediator of itch is histamine. Histamine is known to be present in mast cells surrounding dermal vessels. Serotonin is present in activated platelets; however, serotonin is not found primarily in skin. Epidermal proteases or peptidases obtained from inflamed skin will provoke itch, leading to the conclusion that products obtained from keratinocytes or leukocytes during inflammation may directly activate itch receptors. Additionally, kinin peptides, vasoactive intestinal polypeptides, enkephalin, substance P, and neurotensin all can either modulate itch directly or the sensation of itch. These peptides seem to modulate itch through the release of histamine, as well as having a direct effect on the itch receptor. Prostaglandin E_1 potentiates histamine-induced itching and may have a direct pruritogenic action on nerve endings. Histamine may provoke itch by a direct action in H_1 receptors and perhaps an indirect action due to the secondary release of other mediators. H_2 receptors do not seem to be involved in histamine-induced itch, although H_2 blockers, such as cimetidine, may be beneficial in idiopathic chronic urticaria. Central itch may be mediated by the neuropeptides and endorphins, as naloxone may either inhibit or potentiate the central perception of itch depending on the direction of placebo response, i.e., it may abolish the placebo response or stimulate the placebo response. Direct pathologic itch may be mediated by pruritogenic dihydroxy bile salts as in primary biliary cirrhosis; however, a poor correlation is observed between depletion of the suspected mediator and symptomatic benefit. Additionally, the mediator in uremic pruritus is unknown, although systemic benefit is provided by phototherapy with ultraviolet B (290 to 320 nm) treatment.

Pruritus may be subdivided into the generalized sensation of pruritus without skin changes; pruritus with primary skin lesions, such as macular erythema, papules, vesicles, urticaria, and eczematization; and pruritus with secondary skin lesions of excoriations, secondary infection, or lichenification.

Systemic diseases with focal or generalized itching include the following: *CNS disease* (senile pruritus, multiple sclerosis, psychosis with delusions of parasitosis), *liver disease* (hepatitis, primary biliary cirrhosis, extrahepatic biliary obstruction, drug-induced intrahepatic cholestasis, pruritus gravidarum), *renal disease* (uremic pruritus, secondary hyperparathyroidism), *metabolic disease* (hyperthyroidism; hypothyroidism; hypoglycemia; diabetes; cutaneous paresthesias as numbness, tingling, crawling sensations accompanying peripheral neuropathy; pruritus ani), *hematopoietic disorder* (iron-deficiency anemia, polycythemia vera, paraproteinemia, hypereosinophilic syndrome), and *malignancy* (Hodgkin's disease, carcinoid syndrome, myeloid metaplasia, mycosis fungoides, adenocarcinomas including adenocarcinoma colon with iron-deficiency anemia or hepatic metastases, nasal pruritus with brain tumor, lymphoma, multiple myeloma). Subclinical *drug reactions* (angiotensin-converting enzyme inhibitors; beta blockers; thiazide diuretics; antiarrhythmics, such as quinidine, procainamide, tocainide, encainide, and amiodarone; warfarin; phenothiazines; antidepressants; cocaine; morphine; codeine; aspirin; nonsteroidal anti-inflammatory agents; vitamin B complex) as well as *miscellaneous causes* (excessive bathing, harsh soaps usually advertised as antibacterial that leave no soapy films) may also be responsible for pruritus. Other factors that may induce pruritus include *contact urticaria* to enzymes or fragrances in liquid detergents, fragrance in fabric softeners, optical brighteners in powdered detergents, or fiberglass and *solar exposure*, which causes a type of polymorphous light eruption. Rarely, brachial-radial pruritus, dermatomal pruritus from nerve compression, hereditary pruritus localized to the midback or scapular tip, caffeine-induced pruritus, premenstrual pruritus, aspartame-induced pruritus or frank urticaria, nasal pruritus of atypical angina, autoimmune progesterone dermatitis, mastocytosis, and aquagenic pruritus may occur.

Pruritus may present with the primary cutaneous lesion of urticaria. If present less than 4 weeks, urticaria is classified as *acute* and most often is the result of (1) drug exposure; (2) preceding or intercurrent viral, bacterial, or parasitic infection; (3) immediate, intermediate, or delayed phase food reaction; (4) inhalation allergy, as an intrinsic or extrinsic seasonal or nonseasonal activation of the atopic state; (5) local or systematized *Hymenoptera* or insect venom reaction; or (6) local or systematized contact urticaria to chemicals, cosmetics, etc. *Chronic* urticaria is diagnosed when hives have been present for 4 to 6 weeks or more. Generally, if the individual hive persists for greater than 24 hours, a skin biopsy is indicated to rule out urticarial vasculitis of an idiopathic nature, either associated with hypocomplementemia with or without nephritis or presenting as systemic lupus erythematosus. Pruritus may accompany individual lesions of Henoch-Schönlein purpura and ordinary leukocytoblastic vasculitis. Physical urticaria, such as solar, pressure, aquagenic, vibratory, dermographism, and cholinergic (induced by exercise, heat, stress, or cold) urticaria, should be excluded by history and appropriate testing. Cholinergic urticaria, a common chronic physical urticarial problem, can be diagnosed by observing typical 1- to 3-mm wheals with a surrounding 0.5- to 3-cm zone of erythema. A rare variety of diffuse erythema can also signify cholinergic urticaria. Exercise- or cold-induced cholinergic urticaria may trigger systemic anaphylaxis, and testing must be performed under controlled conditions. Other rare forms of urticaria include adrenergic urticaria, hereditary or acquired angioneurotic edema caused by Cl-esterase inhibitor deficiency, functional protein abnormality, or atypical serum protein as in the acquired form. Life-threatening airway swelling may occur with angioneurotic edema. The acquired form requires a search for associated malignancy. Generally, most chronic urticaria does not have an identifiable etiology and seems to reflect feedback instability in the mast cell population itself.

Ocular pruritus has both exogenous and endogenous etiologies. Examples of exogenous causes that frequently induce bilateral and symmetric identical morphologic eruptions include upper eyelid dermatitis syndrome as elaborated by Howard Maibach. Etiologies may include irritant reactions from mascara and makeup remover, facial soaps, shampoos, or cleansing regimens; accumulative relaxation dermatitis from moisturizers (so-called cosmetic addiction); irritant reactions from airborne particles, such as smog, tobacco smoke, dust, pollen, animal dander, and molds; topical sensitivity to globe lubricants or over-the-counter artificial tears, Murine, Visine, contact lens solution, prescription ophthalmologicals such as timolol, glaucoma drops, or antibacterials; contact or photocontact dermatitis to topical sulfa medicaments. Itching may arise from the development of papillary conjunctivitis in contact lens wearers. Distant site allergic contact dermatitis may occur from nail polish, artificial acrylic nails, sprayed perfume, fragrance or preservatives and stabilizers, detergents and emulsifiers in lubricants and lotions. Frequently, allergic contact dermatitis can arise after exposure to toxic plants, such as poison ivy, oak, and sumac; airborne ragweed; as well as inadvertent exposure to certain sunscreen agents, especially PABA and PABA derivatives. Diagnosis rests on removal of the offending agent with supportive patch testing, provided that a relevant exposure and clinically evident allergic contact dermatitis exist. Patch testing should follow after complete clearing of the eyelid dermatitis, which may take up to 3 months. Since there is a regional variation in the activity between eyelid tissue and back skin, we would recommend traditional patch tests arranged on the upper back from the North American Contact Dermatitis group tray along with fragrances, preservatives, and other materials indicated. Application of the patient's eyelid products can also be patch tested in traditional 48 to 72-hour closed patch tests on the upper back. Alternatively, open use patch tests can be conducted applying the material to the forearm daily for 3 days, then closed patch tests on the antecubital fossa for 3 days, then applied to the neck for 3 days, and then reapplied to one lid only. If redness appears at any stage of the patch testing process, the material should be incriminated as reactive and causal. If redness or irritation develops, one then has the answer, especially if it develops immediately (contact urticaria) or within 24 to 48 hours (allergic contact dermatitis). However, in most cases accumulative irritant dermatitis is responsible for the outbreak and more time must elapse before the process recurs. Often there is an interactive process of cleansing, hydrocarbon irritation from mascara, makeup remover, detergents or emulsifiers that induces a skin loading process that must coexist before dermatitis recurs. In health care workers, spina bifida patients, or atopic eczema patients, orbital and eyelid redness, urticaria and pruritus may be sentinel findings in latex contact urticaria syndrome. This diagnosis and management require a high index of suspicion, careful history and workup, latex allergy testing when appropriate, and environmental engineering to avoid further latex exposure and risk for anaphylaxis.

Intrinsic or endogenous causes of ocular pruritus most frequently accompany the atopic state with a tendency for eyelid and periorbital pruritus with or without visible evidence of eczema. Ocular pruritus frequently accompanies allergic and nonallergic rhinoconjunctivitis as part of the atopic diathesis. In children, chronic eye rubbing may signify seasonal allergies and may heighten eyelid skin sensitivity to seasonal changes, environmental antigens, or airborne contact allergens. Other endogenous skin disorders inducing pruritus include inflammatory psoriasis, ocular rosacea, seborrheic dermatitis especially in infancy, chronic blepharoconjunctivitis, meibomianitis, bacterial infections with *Staphylococcus aureus* and *Pneumococcus*, viral molluscum conjunctivitis, eyelash pediculosis, chronic dacrocystitis, cannaliculitis, and vernal conjunctivitis. Immunobullous diseases, such as cicatricial pemphigoid, adult and childhood linear IgA disease, paraneoplastic pemphigus, Stevens-Johnson syndrome, and drug-induced ocular pseudopemphigoid all may induce itching, pain, and late ocular involvement in such diseases as pemphigus vulgaris, pemphigus foliaceus, and epidermolysis bullosa acquisita. Conjunctival inflammation and pruritus accompany acrodermatitis enterohepatica and necrolytic migratory erythema as well. Ocular inflammation and pruritus often confined to one eyelid margin with accompanying pain or irritation upon digital contact are often presenting symptoms of localized basal cell carcinoma, squamous cell carcinoma, precancerous lesions of actinic keratoses, or sebaceous gland carcinoma of the eyelid or conjunctival surface.

THERAPY

Supportive. An attempt should be made to determine if pruritus is a manifestation of internal disease, a reaction to drugs, associated with primary skin disease elsewhere, or a contact urticarial, irritant, or contact allergic reaction limited to the periorbital region. Therapy should be directed to correcting or avoiding the underlying cause where possible. If all such determinable causes can be excluded, then symptomatic treatment may be directed to the pruritus.

The patient should be advised to avoid scratching the area as doing so lowers the itch threshold and reinforces the itch-scratch cycle. Nails should be trimmed to avoid excoriations. Cultures for bacteria should be obtained as indicated, since altered skin integrity may allow pathogenic staphylococcal or streptococcal colonization that can contribute to pruritogenic stimulus by release of keratinocyte peptidases and cytotoxic antibody production. The patient should avoid fatigue, strain, alcohol, and caffeine as these may lower the itch threshold. A constant climate and avoidance of excessive moisture or dryness are preferable.

Topical. In the active, wet, vesiculated, or exudative phase with secondary infected areas, open compresses with cool tap water or Burow's solution should be applied for 10 to 20 minutes three or four times daily. The compresses should then be removed and the skin allowed to air dry. Calamine lotion may also be applied to enhance drying, if desired. This routine should be repeated until this phase has been converted into a drier state, usually in 3 to 5 days.

If the skin is fissured with eczematization, the skin should again be hydrated with tap water compresses, but then immediately covered with a bland soothing moisturizing lotion, such as Vaseline brand Dermatology Formula Lotion. If redness and itching persist after rehydration, the skin may be covered with a weak steroid cream or ointment, such as 0.025 per cent triamcinolone. If more moisture needs to be retained without promoting maceration, an ointment rather than a cream base should be used. The steroid cream or ointment should be given until symptoms have abated, usually in 5 to 7 days.

In the dry state with lichenification with thickening, hydration compresses with tap water should be applied three to four times daily. Direct application of a weak 1 per cent hydrocortisone ointment may be used until redness and pruritus abate, followed by the daily application of plain USP white petrolatum.

Acceptable topical corticosteroids for the initial control of inflammation include 2.5 per cent hydrocortisone, 0.025 per cent triamcinolone cream or ointment, or 0.2 per cent hydrocortisone valerate cream. After the initial period necessary to control the inflammation, which is usually 5 to 7 days, 1 per cent hydrocortisone should be used to maintain the symptom-free skin until a bland emollient base, such as plain USP white petrolatum, Theraplex Emollient cream or Vaseline Dermatology Formula Lotion, can be applied. The importance of not using stronger steroids in the periocular region cannot be overemphasized because of the need to avoid topical steroid side effects to the thin skin in this area and as not to potentiate the ocular absorption of steroid which, can lead to elevated ocular pressure and precipitate acute angle-closure glaucoma.

Systemic. If systemic therapy is needed to augment topical anti-inflammatory measures, antihistamines may be useful. Initial side effects can be minimized by beginning treatment at night before bedtime and then increasing the dose as the body develops tolerance to the drug. Often, significant antipruritic effect is not established because the full 24-hour dose of the antihistamine is not employed. In children, it is important to establish the full 24-hour dose on a mg/kg scale and then employ the medication in appropriate divided doses. Hydroxyzine has been shown to be a superior antipruritic agent in several studies; however, many comparison trials have not been conducted on an equivalent potency basis, and therefore, a clear choice of the best antihistamine for the individual patient rests on the patient's response to a full dose of what is often an empiric choice. If antipruritic effects are not beneficial, one should then choose another antihistamine H_1 blocker from a different class of parent compound. Ethanolamine derivatives (diphenhydramine), alkylamine derivatives chlorpheniramine ethylenediamine derivatives (tripelennamine), piperazine derivatives (hydroxyzine), phenothiazine derivatives (trimeprazine), or cyproheptadine are examples of other antihistamines from which to choose. Treatment might begin in adults with hydroxyzine at bedtime and an increase to 25 mg five times daily. If this fails to relieve symptoms, the oral dose may be increased to a maximum of 100 mg four times daily. In children, the elixir is useful with a maximum daily dose of 2 mg/kg in divided doses. Tranquilizers, such as 2 to 5 mg of diazepam or 5 to 10 mg of chloridiazepoxide three to four times per day, may be beneficial in allaying anxiety associated with pruritus in some patients. In senile pruritus, doxepin may be useful in the absence of organic causes for itch.

Newer third-generation nonsedating H_1 blockers of the piperidine class include Seldane (terfenadine) 60 mg twice daily, Hismanal (astemizole) 10 mg once daily, and Claritin (loratadine) 10 mg once daily. Double-blind crossover trials show that astemizole is effective as a single agent compared to placebo. Belaich (1990), comparing loratadine 10 mg daily to terfenadine 60 mg twice daily or placebo showed 68 per cent, 55 per cent, and 31 per cent of the loratadine, terfenadine, and placebo groups improved at day 7 and 28 over baseline. Sixty-four per cent of the loratadine, 52 per cent of the terfenadine, and 25 per cent of the placebo groups had a larger complete response in this chronic urticaria group. Monroe (1992) found loratadine comparable to Hydroxyzine and superior to placebo in chronic urticaria and atopic dermatitis groups. Mild sedation can occur; in this study 1 of 20 patients with loratadine experienced this side effect. Other side effects have included weight gain and increased appetite. Rare cardiac toxicity with ventricular arrhythmia and torsades de pointes has been reported with Seldane and Hismanal in specific clinical settings. Patients with known prolongation of QT intervals; patients receiving class 1A antiarrhythmic drugs (quinidine, procainamide, disopyramide) and some class III antiarrhythmic drugs (Sotalol, amiodarone) that prolong QT intervals; patients with underlying hypomagnesemia, hypokalemia, digoxin toxicity, or other conditions predisposing to prolonged QT intervals; or patients with underlying liver disease where metabolism of the drug can be impaired, patients receiving the concomitant administration of macrolide antibiotics, such as erythromycin, clarithromycin, possibly azithromycin, ketoconazole, and itracanazole; patients with severe bradyarrhythmias, and ventricular tachycardias; and patients with a history of drug overdose should not be prescribed these agents. It is expected that loratadine will also be included in this warning. The antihistamine consensus conference found overall that the relative risk of such cardiac events is extremely small and that these medications are very effective and safe when used appropriately and in the recommended dose range.

If necessary, a minimally sedating adjunct regimen would include either 1 mg of azatadine twice daily or 4 mg of chlorpheniramine two or three times daily. For early morning break-through, the addition of 25 mg of hydroxyzine every night has been helpful. For cold-induced urticaria, 10 mg of doxepin three times daily seems to be superior to cyproheptadine. In the elderly, doxepin and other sedating antihistamines should be used with caution, especially at full doses, because of the increased risk of unsteadiness, falls, and injury. Doxepin and other antihistamines with anticholinergic activity are contraindicated in narrow-angle glaucoma and in patients with a tendency toward urinary retention.

Severe allergic contact dermatitis may necessitate systemic steroids. Prednisone beginning at 40 to 60 mg initially, then tapered over 10 to 14 days, will control the immunologically mediated reaction and prevent flare break-through. Other methods that may help include the H_2 blocker cimetidine,[‡] especially in some cases of chronic urticaria. Administration of 300 mg of cimetidine may be given twice daily and titrated to threshold suppression, with special concern for its side effects and problems with long-term usage.

PRECAUTIONS

When more potent steroid creams or ointments are applied, they should be used for as brief a period as possible and in as low a potency as is efficacious. It is now known that repeated applications of topical steroids enhance their potency, and what has little effect initially will become more potent with continued usage. Another factor that enhances potency is frequent application, and twice-daily application is sufficient initially, with subsequent daily application to begin after the symptomatic period has ended. Additionally, absorption through dermatitic skin where the stratum corneum barrier has been broken will increase steroid absorption. This factor along with the extreme thinness of the eyelid skin can dramatically increase potency over one hundred times. It is also known that the absence of fluorinated steroid application is not a guarantee of long-term safety and that steroid-induced toxicity can occur with 1 per cent hydrocortisone alone.

COMMENTS

Other medications in mastocytosis that have proven useful include oral cromolyn sodium[‡] for gastrointestinal mastocytosis. Newer agents include ketotifen,[T] which can inhibit mast cell release of mediators without needing blocking action as do the classic H_1 blockers. Except for some cases of mastocytosis, prostaglandin inhibitors have not been studied for their antipruritic effect, and aspirin[T] may increase or decrease the itch threshold in different patients. Topical cromolyn* has not been shown to have antipruritic action over placebo. Newer studies have shown topical doxepin* to have histamine-induced pruritus blocking effect, although large-scale studies have not been done. Naloxone[‡] has been tested for central itch block, but results are not conclusive to recommend its use for regular antipruritic therapy. For pruritus associated with cholestasis, removal of any cholestatic drug is indicated where possible, and the use of activated charcoal plasma exchange or oral charcoal is helpful. For uremic pruritus, phototherapy with UVB is also helpful in many patients.

Additionally, erythropoietin has been reported successful in severe uremic pruritus in one recent study. PUVA has been reported helpful in pruritus associated with polycythemia vera and myelofibrosis.

References

Belaich S: Comparative effects of loratadine and terfenadine in the treatment of chronic idiopathic urticaria. Ann Allergy 64:191–194, 1990.
Bernard JD: Clinical aspects of pruritus. In Fitzpatrick TB, et al (eds): Dermatology in General Medicine. New York, McGraw-Hill, 1987. pp 78–90.
Bircher AJ: Aquagenic pruritus. Arch Dermatol 124:84–89, 1988.
Bleehan SS, et al: Cimetidine and chlorpheniramine in the treatment of chronic idiopathic urticaria: A multi-centre randomized double blind-study. Br J Dermatol 117:81–88, 1987.
Bubak ME: Allergic reactions to latex among health care workers. Mayo Clin Proc 67:1075–1079, 1992.
DeMarchi S: Relief of pruritus and decrease in plasma histamine concentrations during erythropoietin therapy in patients with uremia. N Engl J Med 326:969–974, 1992.
Denman ST: A review of pruritus. J Am Acad Dermatol 14:375–392, 1986.
Fox RW, et al: The treatment of mild to severe chronic idiopathic urticaria with astemazole: Double blind and open trials. J Allergy Clin Immunol 78:1159–1166, 1986.
Goldsobel AB, et al: Efficacy of doxepin in the treatment of chronic idiopathic urticaria. J Allergy Clin Immunol 78:867–873, 1986.

Grant-Kels JM: Oculocutaneous disease, Part I and II. Dermatol Clin *10*, October 1992.

Hirschmann JV, et al: Cholinergic urticaria: A clinical and histologic study. Arch Dermatol *123*: 462–467, 1987.

Meltzer EO: Comparative safety of H1 antihistamines. Ann Allergy *67*:625–632, 1991.

Monroe EW: Chronic urticaria: Review of nonsedating H₁ antihistamines in treatment. J Am Acad Dermatol *19*:842–846, 1988.

Monroe EW: Relative efficacy and safety of loratadine, hydroxyzine, and placebo in chronic idiopathic urticaria and atopic dermatitis. Clin Ther *14*:17–21, 1992.

Papadopoulas NM: Electrophoretic differentiation of acquired angioedema from hereditary angioedema. Clin Chim Acta *163*:231–234, 1987.

Pola J, et al: Urticaria caused by caffeine. Ann Allergy *60*:207–208, 1988.

Procacci P: Central pruritus case report. Pain *47*: 307–308, 1991.

Shelley WB, Shelley ED: Adrenergic urticaria: A new form of stress induced hives. Lancet *2*:1031–1033, 1985.

Wanderer AA: Clinical characteristics of cold-induced systemic reactions in acquired cold urticaria syndromes. J Allergy Clin Immunol *78*:417–429, 1986.

PSORIASIS 696.1

WILLIAM B. GLEW, M.D.,
and THOMAS P. NIGRA, M.D.

Washington, District of Columbia

Psoriasis vulgaris is a chronic skin disease of unknown etiology affecting 1 to 4 per cent of the population. It is characterized by sharply circumscribed, elevated, thick red plaques of skin covered with coarse, dry, silvery scales. The epidermal cells in patches of psoriasis have lost regulatory control and turn over several times more rapidly than normal epidermal cells. Most patients have minimal amounts of psoriasis limited to such areas as the elbows, knees, scalp, and gluteal cleft; approximately 15 per cent of the psoriatic population have severe generalized psoriasis.

Removal of the silvery scale produces minute bleeding points (Auspitz sign). In an active case of psoriasis, stroking of normal skin with a blunt instrument will result in the development of typical papules a few weeks later in the area of trauma (Köbner phenomenon). This probably accounts for the frequency of psoriasis seen on elbows and knees, since there is constant trauma to these areas.

Psoriasis infrequently affects the skin of the eyelids, but plaques may extend to the conjunctiva where they can cause irritation. Marginal keratitis and uveitis are also uncommon, but may occur more frequently in psoriatics than in the general population. Psoriasis is a capricious disease that can appear at any age.

It is characterized by flares sometimes associated with streptococcal infection and stress, and there can be spontaneous remission of the lesions.

THERAPY

Systemic. Chemotherapy for psoriasis is based on drugs that interfere with the reproduction of epidermal cells. Methotrexate is the only systemic drug approved for use in severe psoriasis. The usual dosage range of methotrexate is 2.5 to 5.0 mg at 12-hour intervals for three doses each week. Monitoring of renal, liver, and bone marrow functions is essential. Other drugs, such as hydroxyurea[†] and aminopterin,[†] have been used to treat psoriasis. In addition, the use of aromatic retinoid etretinate has been shown to be very effective, particularly in association with ultraviolet therapy. For unresponsive cases, cyclosporine[†] has been helpful in doses of 5 mg/kg.

Perhaps the greatest advances in the treatment of psoriasis have come in the areas of phototherapy. Since the 1920s when patients were hospitalized on an average of 21 days and treated intensively (Goeckerman regimen), tar and ultraviolet light therapy have been used to clear psoriasis. This modality has proven safe and effective for psoriasis, although it is time consuming and costly and does not prevent recurrences.

In 1974, a new form of photochemotherapy known as PUVA was developed. This therapy employs the systemic use of psoralen, methoxsalen, which sensitizes the skin to longwave ultraviolet light in the 320 to 400 nm range (UVA). The skin is irradiated with UVA in a carefully monitored chamber 2 hours after ingestion of methoxsalen, resulting in a controlled phototoxic response that is therapeutic. On the average, 90 per cent of patients treated with this modality at intervals of two to three times weekly clear in 21 treatments. They are then maintained in a clearing phase with follow-up treatments every 1 to 4 weeks. After a clearing and short maintenance phase, approximately 60 per cent remain clear for greater than 1 year. This modality has recently been approved by the FDA and must be done under strict protocol only on severe disabling psoriasis. It has a long-term risk of skin carcinogenesis and cataracts.

Since the development of PUVA, there has been a resurgence of ultraviolet light therapy in general for psoriasis. Today, intense sunburn spectrum 280 to 320 nm (UVA) light therapy given in association with the topical application of tar or anthralin derivatives is very effective on an outpatient basis for treating generalized psoriasis. Maintenance and slow tapering of the therapy subsequent to clearing (average 30 treatments) result in a longer remission than the Goeckerman regimen. If patients respond to this therapy and maintain a good remission, PUVA is not necessarily indicated.

Ocular. Keratoconjunctivitis, which may be associated with psorasis even in the absence of facial lesions, responds to ocular steroid drops four times daily and ointment during the night. Uveitis usually responds to 30 mg of oral prednisone daily. Keratitis sicca, trichiasis, cicatrization, symblepharon, and ectropion are rare secondary findings for which a variety of tear replacements and ocular lubricants can be helpful.

Topical. Topical therapy is indicated for minimal psoriasis. The potent fluorinated steroids, such as halcinonide, fluocinonide, betamethasone, and triamcinolone, as well as hydrocortisone, are the most commonly used preparations. Topical pulse therapy with super potent steroids, such as clobetasol, can be done for 2 weeks. Success is problematic when used for longer periods. In the past, occlusive dressings were needed to potentiate the corticosteroid effectiveness. Currently, application of halcinonide two times a day is very effective in most cases. Other modalities of delivering corticosteroids to the skin include the use of impregnated tape or direct injection of 5 mg/ml of triamcinolone in saline into the dermal area of a lesion by raising a wheal.

It is important also to treat the normal skin of psoriatics, since dry skin serves as a locus for the Köbner phenomenon that may result in more extensive psoriasis. Patients should use various preparations of bath oils and topical emollients, such as lotions and creams, to keep their skin healthy and well lubricated.

Finally, coal tar has been effective in treatment and can be used in association with fluorinated steroids in derivative form or by itself in a 5 per cent concentration in white petrolatum in association with ultraviolet light. For the scalp, coal tar shampoos containing sulfur and salicyclic acid or in association with fluorinated steroid solutions are very effective.

PRECAUTIONS

Systemic corticosteroids should not be used in the treatment of psoriasis because of the high doses necessary and the severe exacerbations that often occur after the steroids are stopped.

Methotrexate should be used very carefully. It has the potential risk of hepatic cirrhosis when high cumulative doses have been used or in association with alcohol ingestion. Hematologic function also needs to be monitored for suppression of marrow components.

Phototherapy has been reported to produce skin cancer, as does sunlight. To prevent the development of cataracts associated with phototherapy, adequate ocular photoprotection can be achieved by wearing goggles and spectacles that are tested and confirmed as *opaque to ultraviolet light*. Goggles must be worn during irradiation; wraparound spectacles should be worn after ingestion of photosensitizers and for the 24-hour period of potential photosensitization after each drug dose. Ordinary sunglasses are not adequate.

Phototherapy using UVA and UVB alone has been successful in clearing eyelid psoriasis associated with recurrent blepharitis. Eyelids are nearly opaque to these shorter wavelengths. Patients must keep their eyelids closed during treatment; in cases where eyelid closure is incomplete, UV-impermeable contact lenses must be worn.

COMMENTS

The combination of psoralens and UVA in the treatment of psoriasis is now established as a successful mode of therapy for severe generalized psoriasis, but the increased incidence of skin carcinomas and potential for cataractogenesis mandate continued caution in the administration of this innovative therapy.

References

Current status of oral PUVA therapy for psoriasis: Eye protection revisions. J Am Acad Dermatol 6: 851–855, 1982.

Eustace P, Pierse D: Ocular psoriasis. Br J Ophthalmol 54:810–813, 1970.

Fritsch PO, et al: Augmentation of oral methoxsalen photochemotherapy with an oral retinoic acid derivative. J Invest Dermatol 70:178–182, 1978.

Glew WB, Nigra TP: PUVA and the eye. In Abel AE (ed): Photochemotherapy in Dermatology. New York/Tokyo, Igaku-Shoin, 1992, pp 241–253.

Knox DL: Psoriasis and intraocular inflammation. Trans Am Ophthalmol Soc 77:210–224, 1979.

Lerman S, Megaw J, Willis I: Potential ocular complications from PUVA therapy and their prevention. Invest Dermatol 74:197–199, 1980.

Melski JW, et al: Oral methoxsalen photochemotherapy for the treatment of psoriasis: A cooperative clinical trial. J Invest Dermatol 68:328–335, 1977.

Parrish JA, et al: Photochemotherapy of psoriasis with oral methoxsalen and longwave ultraviolet light. N Engl J Med 291:1207–1211, 1974.

Prystowsky JH, et al: Present status of eyelid phototherapy: Clinical efficacy and transmittance of ultraviolet and visible radiation through human eyelids. J Am Acad Dermatol 26:607–613, 1992.

Roenigk HH Jr, et al: Methotrexate guidelines—revised. J Am Acad Dermatol 6:145–155, 1982.

Sandvig K, Westerberg P: Ocular findings in psoriatics. Acta Ophthalmol 33:463–467, 1955.

URTICARIA AND HEREDITARY ANGIOEDEMA 708.9

(Angioneurotic Edema, Giant Edema, Giant Urticaria, Hives, Nettle Rash, Quincke's Disease)

MITCHELL H. FRIEDLAENDER, M.D.

La Jolla, California

Urticaria is a cutaneous eruption with multiple pathogenic mechanisms that may be immunologic or nonimmunologic. Its prevalence in the general population is high and is estimated to be between 10 and 25 per cent. No specific cause can be found in 70 per cent of patients with chronic urticaria; in others, psychogenic, allergic, and physical factors may play a role.

The skin lesions of urticaria are sharply circumscribed, elevated areas of edema. If the swelling is extensive and involves the subcutaneous tissues, the term "angioedema" is used. Urticaria may be divided into acute and chronic forms. Acute urticaria is often associated with immunologic mechanisms. Chronic urticaria, which lasts more than 8 weeks, frequently has no identifiable cause. At times, emotional or allergic factors may be implicated.

The immunologic mechanisms involved in urticaria are not well understood. The clinical signs of urticaria may be simulated by injection of histamine into the skin. Presumably, histamine and other vasoactive mediators are released from mast cells by immunologic or nonimmunologic means in urticaria.

Hereditary angioedema is characterized by repeated attacks of epithelial edema involving the skin, respiratory tract, and gastrointestinal tract. Urticaria does not occur in this condition, although the skin may be well demarcated. Although hereditary angioedema was first recognized by Osler in 1888, it was only recently discovered that a biochemical abnormality in the complement system exists in this entity. Patients with hereditary angioedema have an inherited deficiency of C1-esterase inhibitor, a protein that inhibits activation of the first component of complement. The deficiency leads to uncontrolled activation of the complement pathway and generation of a kinin-like substance. Repeated episodes of angioedema involving the skin and respiratory tract may lead to death from pharyngeal edema and asphyxiation. About 85 per cent of patients' kindreds have markedly deficient or absent C1-esterase inhibitor. In the remaining 15 per cent, the inhibitor is present in normal amounts, but is functionally inactive.

THERAPY

Systemic. Antihistamines are frequently effective in the control of urticaria and may be effective for angioedema, particularly if administered soon after the onset of symptoms. Daily administration of 30 to 100 mg of hydroxyzine in divided doses has become increasingly popular for the treatment of urticaria, regardless of cause. Beta-adrenergic drugs, such as ephedrine and terbutaline, are now being used as adjuncts to antihistamines for the therapy of urticaria. These drugs elevate intracellular cyclic AMP levels and, in turn, suppress mediator release from mast cells. Systemic corticosteroids may be required for control of severe cases of acute urticaria or angioedema, but in general, they have no place in the regular therapy of chronic urticaria. Aqueous epinephrine may be given subcutaneously for the temporary relief of acute urticaria.

In patients with hereditary angioedema, three groups of medications are useful: antifibrinolytic agents, anabolic steroids and impeded androgens, and fresh-frozen plasma. The antifibrinolytic agent aminocaproic acid[‡] has been used successfully to prevent attacks of hereditary angioedema. The effective dose in adults is 18 gm daily in divided doses. Tranexamic acid[‡] is a newer, more potent antifibrinolytic agent that markedly reduces the frequency of attacks of hereditary angioedema at a dose of 3 gm daily. Methyltestosterone[‡] (an anabolic steroid) and danazol or oxymetholone[‡] (impeded androgens) have been shown to prevent attacks of hereditary angioedema. These drugs induce synthesis of C1 inhibitor. In acute attacks, administration of fresh-frozen plasma as the source of C1 inhibitor provides a rapid method to terminate attacks.

Ocular. Systemic therapy will generally control ocular as well as other systemic manifestations of these two diseases. However, subcutaneous injection or application of cotton pads soaked in 1:1000 epinephrine[‡] may be used for treatment of severe conjunctival edema.

Surgical. If orbital edema develops to such an extent that the globe or optic nerve is threatened, relief from pressure should be provided. The most effective method to remove pressure seems to be an osteoplastic decompression of the lateral orbital wall. This should rarely be necessary.

Supportive. A specific etiologic agent may sometimes be identified in urticaria. In food allergy, the suspected food may be eliminated from the diet for several weeks and subsequently tried again to determine its relation to the urticaria. Drug allergy requires a careful history and elimination of the suspected drug.

In hereditary angioedema, prevention of airway obstruction is essential.

Counseling. Cholinergic urticaria may be associated with exercise, emotional stress, and overheating. Sunlight, trauma, and sudden changes of temperature may also precipitate urticaria due to physical allergy. Sunscreen lotions or topical antipruritic medications, such as calamine lotion, may also be of value in prophylaxis.

Hereditary angioedema may be precipitated by trauma, dental extractions, wearing of tight garments, physical exertion, infections, heat or cold, emotional stress, and menstruation.

Ocular or Periocular Manifestations

Conjunctiva: Chemosis.
Eyelids: Edema; hyperemia.
Optic Nerve: Optic neuritis; papilledema.
Other: Central serous retinopathy; exophthalmos; nystagmus; orbital edema; secondary glaucoma; uveitis; visual field defects.

PRECAUTIONS

Pharyngeal edema is a life-threatening situation that must be treated immediately. Some patients present with abdominal attacks that mimic intra-abdominal crises, and not infrequently patients are subjected to laparotomies. Approximately 50 per cent of cases present before the age of 6 years.

If the eye is not threatened, overenthusiastic treatment is not encouraged, since the edema will usually resolve in a few days. Corticosteroids should not be considered a substitute for epinephrine in the emergency treatment of severe cases.

Antihistamines may cause drowsiness, and patients taking them should be warned not to drive or operate machinery.

COMMENTS

Urticaria has numerous causes, and its pathogenesis is poorly understood. Basically, it is associated with uncontrolled mast cell degranulation and release of mediators. Therapy is designed to prevent mast cell release or inhibit the mediators of inflammation.

Hereditary angioedema is an inherited deficiency of C1-esterase inhibitor and represents a chronic condition that is life threatening. Patients must be counseled intensively, and emergency therapy must be available to them.

References

Ballogh Z, Whaley K: Hereditary angio-oedema: Its pathogenesis and management. Scott Med J 25: 187–195, 1980.
Bielory L, Noble KG, Frohman LP: Urticarial vasculitis and visual loss. J Allergy Clin Immunol 88:819–821, 1991.
Casale TB, Sampson HA, Hanifin J, et al: Guide to physical urticarias. J Allergy Clin Immunol 82: 758–763, 1988.
Christiansen SC: Evaluation and treatment of the allergic patient. Int Ophthalmol Clin 28:282–293, 1988.
Friedlaender MH: Allergy and Immunology of the Eye. New York, Raven, 1993, pp 85–86.
Kaplan AP: The pathogenic basis of urticaria and angioedema: Recent advances. Am J Med 70: 755–758, 1981.
Mathews KP: Management of urticaria and angioedema. J Allergy Clin Immunol 66:347–357, 1980.
Mathews KP: Urticaria and allergic conjunctivitis. Curr Opinion Immunol 2:535–541, 1990.

VITILIGO 709.0

FRANK PARKER, M.D.

Portland, Oregon

Vitiligo is a patchy depigmentary disorder of the skin that is generally progressive over many years and occurs in 1 to 2 per cent of the general population. The depigmentation is due to a destruction of melanocytes in the involved skin. Nearly 40 per cent of patients have a positive family history, with an autosomal dominant inheritance pattern. The depigmentation may appear anywhere on the skin surface, although the lesions most often are symmetrically distributed bilaterally on the backs of the hands, on the forearms, face and neck, around body orifices, and over bony prominences. In over 50 per cent of patients, vitiligo first develops before the age of 20 years. Early lesions may show only patchy loss of melanin pigment; however, total loss of pigment in the involved area is almost invariable as time passes. The borders of the enlarging depigmented areas are sharply delineated and may display mild inflammation, as well as hyperpigmentation. The extent of the disease varies from a few small patches to universal loss of pigment. Hairs in the patches usually lose their pigment. The lesions of vitiligo are benign and asymptomatic. However, the areas are subject to painful sunburn.

Vitiligo frequently begins with the rapid loss of pigment, which may be followed by a lengthy period when the skin color does not change. Later, pigment loss may begin anew. The loss of color may continue until, for unknown reasons, the process stops. Cycles of pigment loss, followed by periods of stability, may continue indefinitely. It is rare for any patient with vitiligo to repigment or regain significant skin color spontaneously.

Vitiligo can take several other forms, such as halo nevi, segmental vitiligo (involving a region supplied by peripheral nerves), veloce vitiligo (rapid graying hair and sudden appearance of extensive vitiligo after an episode of acute emotional or physical trauma), or chemical vitiligo (depigmentation seen on the hands of people working with germicidal detergents or rubber containing monobenzone). Once the process of chemical vitiligo is set in motion locally, loss of pigment cells can occur in parts of the body remote from sites of actual contact.

No matter how extensive vitiligo is, the color of the eyes under ordinary examination does not change. However, 3 of 51 patients with vitiligo studied with a slit-lamp biomicroscope were found to have a focal loss of pigment in the irides. Most common are lesions in the ocular fundus suggestive of chorioretinitis or atrophy of the pigment layers of the eyes. It is likely that destruction of melanocytes in the eye may be an important factor in the pathogenesis of certain types of uveitis. This process could also play an initiating role in sympathetic ophthalmia.

Vitiligo may occur in association with hyper- or hypothyroidism, thyroiditis, alopecia areata, pernicious anemia, juvenile and adult diabetes, and Addison's disease. In addition, vitiligo may be associated with ocular syndromes, such as Vogt-Koyanagi syndrome and sympathetic ophthalmia. Vitiligo may precede the clinical appearance of these conditions by several years and occurs in 8 to 20 per cent of people with these disorders.

The presence of thyroid, adrenal, and gastric parietal cell antibodies in many patients with both vitiligo and endocrine disease suggests a common, perhaps autoimmune origin. The autoimmune theory of vitiligo is further strengthened by the increased prevalence of organ-specific autoantibodies in several, but not all large series of patients with vitiligo. Recently, the presence of a circulating complement-fixing antibody that binds melanocytes of human skin and nevus cells in two patients with vitiligo and multiple endocrine insufficiencies has provided further evidence regarding the autoimmune nature of vitiligo. Presumably, such IgG antibodies play some role in the destruction of the melanocytes in the vitiliginous skin. Other theories regarding the etiology of vitiligo are that (1) abnormal functioning nerve cells may injure nearby pigment cells and (2) the melanocytic cells may be self-destructive (autotoxic).

THERAPY

Supportive. Complete spontaneous cure is unusual. Some temporary and partial repigmentation is detectable in about 50 per cent of patients during the summer months. The treatment of vitiligo is usually unsatisfactory, and in most cases, it is best to advise patients to seek effective cosmetic camouflage.

Topical. Especially in darker-skinned persons, treatment of vitiligo often consists of the application of cosmetic cover creams to the involved areas. Opaque formulations containing zinc oxide are the most favorable camouflaging agents as they combine a broad-spectrum sunscreen agent with a water-resistant opaque base. These preparations come in various shades, imparting a natural look.

The depigmented patches may also be painted with dihydroxyacetone. Cosmetic cover-up lotions containing dihydroxyacetone and certain analine dyes impart fairly natural color to amelanotic areas. Reapplication is required after washing as these compounds are water soluble. Protection from the sun by a benzophene or an aminobenzoic acid sunscreen cream is advisable. Patients with skin types I or II (light skin with little melanin pigmentation who sunburn readily) benefit from artificial suntan formulations containing 5 per cent dihydroxyacetone, which often gives satisfactory skin color. Care should be taken with these preparations as they impart a greenish color to the skin after the formulation is 6 to 9 months old.

In patients whose vitiliginous lesions are limited to a small area, topical application of psoralens followed by ultraviolet light (PUVA therapy) is indicated. Methoxsalen lotion or 0.1 per cent methoxsalen in hydrophilic ointment may be applied to the affected area. After 45 minutes to an hour, the area is exposed to long wavelength ultraviolet light. The first exposure should last 15 seconds; subsequent exposures, every other day, are increased by 15-second increments until a visible erythema has appeared in the affected area. Subsequent exposures are given or slightly increased at this time level until pigment fills in from the normally pigmented skin borders and the perifollicular melanocytes. The distance of the light source to the skin should be kept constant for each exposure.

Steroid preparations may promote repigmentation in vitiligo lesions. Topical betamethasone[†] and clobetasol[†] have been used with variable results. Local injections of corticosteroids[†] have also been used, with 60 per cent of patients' vitiligo responding to a variable degree in one series. Care must be used with such injections, as skin atrophy is a common and unwelcome complication.

Tattooing ferrous oxide[†] pigment into the dermis of vitiliginous areas, if they are of limited extent, may also be of some benefit.

A small group of patients with widespread vitiligo who have not responded to psoralens and UV light or who do not want to commit to 100 to 300 sessions of photochemotherapy and who desire complete depigmentation can be given a trial of 20 per cent monobenzone. This medication is applied to the normal pigmented areas twice daily and decreases pigment in the normal areas within 2 to 3 months. Full depigmentation is achieved in 4 to 12 months in 50 to 60 per cent of patients. Complications from the monobenzone include burning, itching, erythema, dryness, and contact dermatitis.

Systemic. Occasionally, oral psoralens treatment is worth trying, especially when the vitiligo is widespread and the patient highly motivated. Two hours before exposure to natural sunlight or long wavelength ultraviolet light (UVA 320 to 380 nm), a psoralen preparation is given (trioxsalen or methoxsalen). Oral trioxsalen is the preferred drug when sunlight is used because it is less phototoxic than methoxsalen. The patient using trioxsalen should begin with a 1-minute exposure to sunlight, and the times are gradually increased every other day 2 hours after taking the trioxsalen, until visible erythema occurs in the affected areas. If artificial UVA light booths are used, 20 to 40 mg of methoxsalen is given 1 to 2 hours before light exposure. The treatment continues every other day at the time or energy exposure that gives erythema, until repigmentation occurs. This treatment often takes months, and if repigmentation is not seen, increasing the methoxsalen dosage to 60 mg has been advocated. Perifollicular macules of repigmentation in the depigmented areas first appear after 15 to 30 treatments. Complete repigmentation usually requires 200 to 300 treatments. Some repigmentation may be achieved in 15 to 20 per cent of patients. Certain areas of the body are more responsive than others. The face, especially the periorbital area, responds quite well, followed by the neck and trunk. Vitiliginous areas over bony prominences, hands, feet, and mucosa are the most resistant. Young patients often respond more rapidly than older individuals.

Phenylalanine[‡] and UVA light have also been used for treating generalized vitiligo. A success rate of 95 per cent repigmentation has been reported with this method, as well as less sun sensitivity of affected areas after therapy.

Ocular. There is no treatment for uveal or retinal depigmentation.

Ocular or Periocular Manifestations

Choroid: Posterior uveitis.
Eyebrows or Eyelids: Depigmentation of skin and lashes.
Iris: Depigmentation.
Retina: Atrophy; depigmentation.

PRECAUTIONS

In laboratory studies liver toxicity has developed in animals following the use of oral psoralens. However, there seems to be no evidence that such an effect occurs in humans receiving oral psoralens. Patients sometimes experience nausea after receiving oral methoxsalen; however, taking the drug after a glass of milk or a sandwich usually allays the sensation of nausea. Presently, there is some concern that long-term therapy with high-dose oral psoralens plus UVA therapy may result in ocular damage and skin cancers. It is advisable to have the patient undergo a baseline ophthalmologic examination before instituting oral psoralens therapy and have periodic subsequent examinations.

While on PUVA treatments, special protective glasses are recommended on the days the psoralens are taken. After a patient has used either topical or oral psoralens, the skin is also sensitive to ultraviolet light for at least 24 hours. Sunscreens or cover-ups should be used if the patient must be exposed to sunlight for longer periods of time than the therapeutic exposure period. Care should also be taken with topical psoralens, as they may cause intense dermatitis reactions with vesiculation and blistering.

COMMENTS

The etiology of vitiligo remains obscure. Among the various hypotheses that have been proposed to explain the pathogenesis of the disease, autoimmune mechanisms have been prominent. Recent research suggests that a nondermatomal vitiligo may be due to an autoimmune mechanism, whereas a dermatomally distributed vitiligo derives from a disturbance in the sympathetic nerves of the affected area.

References

Albert DM, Nordlund JJ, Lerner AB: Ocular abnormalities occurring with vitiligo. Ophthalmology 86:1145–1158, 1979.

Benmaman O, Sanchez SL: Treatment and camouflaging of pigmentary disorders. Clin Dermatol 6:50–61, 1988.

Cormane RH, et al: Phenylalanine and UVA light for the treatment of vitiligo. Arch Dermatol Res 277:126–130, 1985.

Duke-Elder S (ed): System of Ophthalmology. St. Louis, CV Mosby, 1974, Vol XIII, pp 369–371.

Koga M: Vitiligo: A new classification and therapy. Br J Dermatol 97:255–261, 1977.

Lerner AB, Nordlund JJ: Vitiligo. What is it? Is it important? JAMA 239:1183–1187, 1978.

Lorincz AL: Disturbances of melanin pigmentation. *In* Moschella SL, Pillsbury DM, Hurley JJ Jr (eds): Dermatology. Philadelphia, WB Saunders, 1975, pp 1096–1128.

Lowe D: Pigmentary disturbances. *In* Conn HF (ed): Current Therapy. Philadelphia, WB Saunders, 1982, pp 673–677.

SECTION 11

CONNECTIVE TISSUE DISORDERS

JUVENILE RHEUMATOID ARTHRITIS 714.30
(JA, JRA, Juvenile Arthritis, Still's Disease)

JERRY C. JACOBS, M.D.,
and HAROLD F. SPALTER, M.D.

New York, New York

Juvenile rheumatoid arthritis has been the diagnostic label applied to all forms of persistent arthritis of childhood onset. During the past decade, it has become apparent that currently accepted diagnostic criteria identify a consortium of different disorders with different genetic susceptibility determinants, environmental offsets, pathology, prognoses, and clinical patterns. It has also become apparent that all forms of both "childhood" and "adult" arthritis may begin at any age.

The eyes are frequently affected in two different forms of childhood arthritis: pauciarticular arthritis and spondyloarthritis. Subacute or chronic iridocyclitis occurs primarily in association with pauciarticular arthritis (four or fewer affected joints). Girls are predominantly afflicted (9:1), and the median age of onset is 2 years of age. In 50 per cent of cases, arthritis is limited to the knee at the time of onset, and 74 per cent of cases are nonarticular; 40 per cent of girls in this subset develop uveitis, and half of these patients have a positive test for antinuclear antibody (ANA). The eye inflammation is usually silent and only discovered by routine slit-lamp screening examination, which should be performed every 3 months in this subset. In one series, 92 per cent of these patients possessed human leukocyte antigen (HLA)-DRw5. Those who develop iridocyclitis most frequently do so within the first year after the onset of arthritis, but uveitis may first occur at any time and may recur many years later. Both eyes are ultimately affected in 70 per cent of cases; in 21 per cent of cases the duration of eye disease exceeds 10 years.

Acute iridocyclitis occurs primarily in patients with spondyloarthritis, a form of arthritis related pathologically and genetically to the prototypic disorders—ankylosing spondylitis and Reiter's syndrome. Most patients present with pauciarticular arthritis of the lower extremities. Boys are more frequently afflicted, and the median age of onset is 10 years of age. In one series, 8 per cent of children with this form of arthritis developed uveitis during childhood, but the lifetime risk is probably about 25 per cent. The ANA test is usually negative, but occasionally may be transiently positive at the onset of arthritis. Most patients possess HLA-B27, and a family history of similar arthritis and/or uveitis may frequently be established in these patients. Subacute or chronic iritis is less frequent in this subset, but does occur. Chronic blepharitis and conjunctivitis are also associated with spondyloarthritis.

Iridocyclitis is not known to occur in childhood-onset rheumatoid-factor positive adult rheumatoid arthritis and is rare in polyarticular and systemic-onset (Still's disease) forms of childhood arthritis. However, all forms of arthritis lack precise definition and tend to be confused with each other. Therefore, all children with arthritis require regular slit-lamp examinations for the detection of silent uveitis. In the past, 2 per cent of all children with arthritis lost all vision, the risk of total blindness was much higher in the highly susceptible subsets (6 per cent), and in one recent study, 12 per cent of affected eyes followed longer than 9 years were blind.

THERAPY

Systemic. Nonsteroidal antiinflammatory agents are the drugs of choice in all forms of childhood arthritis. "Slow-acting" agents, such as sulfasalazine, gold salts, penicillamine, and hydroxychloroquine, may be required by some patients. Methotrexate[†] is used in severe cases. All patients and their parents are taught a physical medicine regimen to maintain the functional range of motion of the affected joints.

Ocular. Unless the inflammation is so severe that vision is threatened, all patients are initially treated with mydriatics and topical steroid drops administered at frequent intervals. If vision is threatened or a prompt response is not obtained, 1 to 2 mg/kg of oral prednisone daily in divided doses may be used until the inflammation is completely controlled (usually a few weeks). The dosage should then be changed to an alternate-day regimen (2 to 5 mg/kg, with a daily maximum of 150 mg). Provided the inflammation remains controlled, the dose is gradually reduced with careful monitoring of the eyes. Methotrexate is now being used as an alternative to steroids in some cases. Chlorambucil[‡] is effective, but dangerous.

Surgical. If bilateral complicated cataracts occur at any age and residual vision is unacceptable or if there is no vision in a single eye at an age where amblyopia ex anopsia may result, surgical removal of the cataract may be required. Experience suggests that the optimal surgical technique is phacoemulsification with preservation of the posterior capsule. To control inflammation completely, corticosteroid coverage should be provided beginning the day before surgery, with a sufficient daily dose provided on the day of surgery and throughout the postoperative period. Intraocular steroids are administered by subtenon injection* during the surgery and again, if necessary, during the postoperative period. As soon as the surgical result is assured, the steroids are changed to an alternate-day regimen as detailed earlier. In appropriate cases, such as when the lens is also dislocated or severe vitritis is present, lensectomy with vitrectomy is an alternative procedure. Conventional surgical techniques for complicated cataracts have historically yielded extraordinarily poor results and should no longer be used in these children with chronic uveitis.

Secondary glaucoma must be controlled both before and after surgery; this can usually be accomplished with appropriate drug therapy, but special surgical techniques may also be used if required. Successful restoration of vision after surgery for complicated cataract is dependent upon restoring vision to an eye that is not also blinded by inadequately treated glaucoma or amblyopia ex anopsia.

Band keratopathy may be treated with curettage and chelating agents, such as edetate disodium.* Laser treatment may be effective in resistant cases.

Ocular or Periocular Manifestations

Anterior Chamber: Cells; protein flare.
Cornea: Keratitic precipitates; band keratopathy.
Iris or Ciliary Body: Ciliary flush (rare); iris bombé, synechiae.
Other: Decreased visual acuity; glaucoma; ocular pain (rare); papillitis; photophobia; macular edema; vitreous cells.

PRECAUTIONS

Topical ocular steroids can induce cataract and glaucoma; systemic steroids can also cause these and many other adverse effects, including avascular necrosis of bone, but these risks are acceptable to most patients in an effort to prevent blindness. Aspirin toxicity may produce gastrointestinal, auditory, and metabolic disturbances and increases the risk of Reye's syndrome. Nonsteroidal anti-inflammatory agents are not known to increase the risk of Reye's syndrome, but otherwise have similar risks as aspirin and greater risks of renal complications. A high incidence of serious side effects, including changes in macular retinal pigment epithelium, has discouraged the long-term use of hydroxychloroquine in the treatment of juvenile rheumatoid arthritis. Gold and penicillamine are high-risk agents of uncertain efficacy. Methotrexate increases the risk of infection and may cause liver cirrhosis. Chlorambucil induces leukemia.

COMMENTS

Obsessive screening with early diagnosis and aggressive corticosteroid treatment of uveitis in arthritic children are imperative in preventing visual disability in most children. Recognition of ANA, HLA-DRw5, HLA-B27, and pauciarticular disease as risk factors warranting even more frequent screening and vigilance has also improved the visual prognosis. For children whose vision is compromised as a result of complicated cataracts, newer surgical techniques and improved management have transformed what was an essentially hopeless situation into practically 100 per cent restoration of adequate vision. These newer surgical techniques, including phacoemulsification, lensectomy, and vitrectomy, are supported by dynamic corticosteroid control of postoperative inflammation and by careful attention to glaucoma and the potential for amblyopia ex anopsia. These goals have been primarily achieved in large clinics specializing in the care of eye complications of arthritic children, but may now be extended to other settings where both pediatric rheumatologic support and informed ophthalmologic medical and surgical care are available.

References

Breitgart A, Schwarz-Eywill M, Bauer H, et al: Uveitis: Associations with rheumatic diseases and immunosuppressive therapy with methotrexate. Arthritis Rheum 35:S162, 1992.

Fernandez-Vina MA, Fink CW, Stastny P: HLA antigens in juvenile arthritis. Arthritis Rheum 33: 1777–1784, 1990.

Flynn HW, Davis JL, Culbertson WW: Pars plana lensectomy and vitrectomy for complicated cataracts in juvenile rheumatoid arthritis. Ophthalmology 95:1114–1119, 1988.

Jacobs JC: Pediatric Rheumatology for the Practitioner, 2nd ed. New York, Springer-Verlag, 1993.

Jacobs JC, Berdon WE, Johnston AD: HLA-B27-associated spondyloarthritis and enthesopathy in childhood: Clinical, pathologic, and radiologic observations in 58 patients. J Pediatr 100:521–528, 1982.

Kanski JJ: Uveitis in juvenile chronic arthritis: Incidence, clinical features and prognosis. Eye 2: 641–645, 1988.

Kanski JJ: Screening for uveitis in juvenile chronic arthritis. Br J Ophthalmol 73:225–228, 1989.

Kanski JJ: Juvenile arthritis and uveitis. Surv Ophthalmol 34:253–267, 1990.

Kanski JJ, Shun-Shin GA: Systemic uveitis syndromes in childhood: An analysis of 340 cases. J Ophthalmol 91:1247–1252, 1984.

Merriam JC, Chylack LT, Albert DM: Early-onset pauciarticular juvenile rheumatoid arthritis: A histopathologic study. Arch Ophthalmol 101: 1085–1092, 1983.

Palmer RG, Kanski JJ, Ansell BM: Chlorambucil in the treatment of intractable uveitis associated with juvenile chronic arthritis. J Rheumatol 12: 967–970, 1985.

Petty RE: Current knowledge of the etiology and pathogenesis of chronic uveitis accompanying juvenile rheumatoid arthritis. Rheum Dis Clin North Am 13:19–36, 1987.

Praeger DL, et al: Kelman procedure in the treatment of complicated cataract of the uveitis of Still's disease. Trans Ophthalmol Soc UK 96:168–172, 1976.

Spalter HF: The visual prognosis in juvenile rheumatoid arthritis. Trans Am Ophthalmol Soc 73: 554–570, 1975.

Vawter RL, Macsai M, Fakadej A, et al: Methotrexate for inflammatory eye disease. Arthritis Rheum 35(5S):R12, 1992.

Wolf MD, Lichter PR, Ragsdale CG: Prognostic factors in the uveitis of juvenile rheumatoid arthritis. Ophthalmology 94:1242–1248, 1987.

POLYARTERITIS NODOSA 446.0

(Necrotizing Angiitis, PAN, Periarteritis Nodosa)

JOHN J. WEITER, M.D., Ph.D.,
SHIYOUNG ROH, M.D.,
and JOHN A. MILLS, M.D.

Boston, Massachusetts

Polyarteritis nodosa is a widespread inflammatory and necrotizing vasculitis that usually affects small- and medium-sized muscular arteries, although venous involvement may occur. The lesions are typically focal or segmental, are often in different stages of development, and have a predilection for branch points and bifurcations of vessels. The pathologic hallmark of the disease is acute necrotizing inflammation of the arterial media, with fibrinoid necrosis and extensive inflammatory cell infiltration of all vessel coats and surrounding tissue. Aneurysmal dilations and rupture may occur, and thrombosis and fibrosis may lead to occlusion of the lumen. Such vascular lesions may involve virtually every organ of the body, with characteristic involvement of renal and visceral arteries and sparing of the pulmonary circulation.

The cause of polyarteritis is unknown. It is usually grouped with the so-called collagen diseases and may be mediated by the deposition of immune complexes. The presence of hepatitis B antigen in 30 per cent of patients with polyarteritis nodosa together with the isolation of circulating immune complexes composed of hepatitis B antigen and immunoglobulin, as well as the demonstration by immunofluorescence of hepatitis B antigen, Ig M, and complement in the blood vessel walls, strongly implicates the immune system in the pathogenesis of this disease. Circulating antineutrophil cytoplasmic antibodies (ANCA) have been noted to be associated with small vessel vasculitis. The perinuclear staining pattern (pANCA) has been found to be useful in both diagnosing and monitoring disease activity in patients with active microscopic polyarteritis.

Polyarteritis nodosa has been reported to occur in patients of all ages, although the usual age of onset is between 20 and 50 years. Males are affected more commonly in a ratio of 2.5:1. In a variant of this entity called cutaneous polyarteritis nodosa, the lesions are restricted to the small muscular arteries of the subcutaneous tissue. This localized disease spares visceral arteries and is therefore not a true systemic vasculitis syndrome. The relationship between this disorder and true peri arteritis seems analogous to the relationship between discoid and systemic lupus erythematosus.

Clinical manifestations of polyarteritis nodosa are protean and variable, reflecting the widespread vascular involvement, the degree of ischemia, and the resulting necrosis. The clinical onset may be abrupt, with chills, fever, and tachycardia, or insidious, with low-grade fever, myalgia, arthralgia, anorexia, weight loss, and nonspecific weakness and fatigue. Hypertension occurs in 50 per cent of patients and renal involvement in 75 per cent. Mucous membrane lesions and a wide variety of cutaneous abnormalities develop, including purpura, petechiae, urticaria, subcutaneous nodules, and skin ulceration. Involvement of the gastrointestinal and both central and peri pheral nervous systems is common. Ocular involvement may result as lesions in the cerebral vasculature affect the visual or oculomotor pathways. The retinal and choroidal vasculatures may be affected directly by local lesions or through secondary changes resulting from nephrogenic hypertension. The external eye and anterior segment of the eye rarely may have inflammatory and ischemic lesions. Ocular involvement is relatively uncommon, occurring in 10 to 20 per cent of patients.

THERAPY

Systemic. The 5-year survival rate for untreated patients with polyarteritis nodosa is approximately 10 per cent. This high mortality justifies an aggressive therapeutic approach. The use of corticosteroids has improved the 5-year survival to approximately 50 per cent. Prednisone should be used at a level of 1 to 2 mg/kg and adjusted upward if necessary. Efficacy of therapy should be assessed on the basis of symptom control and degree of organ involvement while the erythrocyte sedimentation rate and white blood cell count are followed. The episodic course of periarteritis nodosa makes the effects of therapy difficult to follow. When the disease seems to be controlled, a slow, cautious, stepwise reduction of corticosteroid dosage may be undertaken at 1- to 2-week intervals. If long-term therapy is required, an alternate-day regimen may be attempted. Although a remission may occur during therapy with corticosteroids, these drugs frequently mask inflammatory activity while the disease progresses.

Cytotoxic agents are gaining greater acceptance in the therapy for polyarteritis nodosa. The combination of corticosteroids and immunosuppressive agents has resulted in an increased survival rate of up to 90 per cent. The most commonly used immunosuppressive agents are azathioprine[‡] and cyclophosphamide.[‡] Cyclophosphamide has induced clinical remission in patients with severe necrotizing vasculitis that had been refractory to other therapeutic modalities. Oral administration of 2 mg/kg of cyclophosphamide daily should be started together with 1 to 2 mg/kg of prednisone daily. If symptoms are controlled after 2 weeks, the prednisone dosage is slowly tapered to an alternate-day regimen, and the cyclophosphamide dosage is adjusted to maintain a white blood cell count of $3000/m^3$.

Ocular. Ocular treatment is generally symptomatic. Early systemic control of the disease with corticosteroids and immunosuppressive agents tends to lessen the ocular symptoms. Inflammation of the anterior segment should be treated with topical corticosteroids and mydriatics. Control of systemic hypertension decreases retinal vascular disease. Retrobulbar injection* of vasodilators may be tried for their antispasmodic effects, but they are often found to be ineffective.

Supportive. Management of complications consists largely of support in the event of organ failure or intervention in the event of hemorrhage or organ infarction. Systemic hypertension should be carefully controlled, since sustained hypertension will add further insult to kidneys already damaged by vasculitis or glomerulonephritis. Furthermore, systemic hypertension is a major contributor to late complications, such as stroke and myocardial infarction. Physical therapy may be employed to sustain muscular tone and arterial function in patients with musculoskeletal involvement, and splints are useful to prevent contractures. Analgesics, such as aspirin, are useful adjuncts for treating myalgias and arthralgias.

Ocular or Periocular Manifestations

Conjunctiva: Edema; hyperemia; subconjunctival hemorrhages; ulcer.

Cornea: Keratoconjunctivitis sicca; marginal ulcer; necrotizing sclerokeratitis.

Extraocular Muscles: Nystagmus; paralysis; tenonitis.

Eyelids: Edema; ptosis.

Globe: Proptosis or pseudotumor (rarely, in contradistinction to Wegener's granulomatosis).

Optic Nerve: Atrophy; disc edema.

Retina or Choroid: Central retinal artery occlusion; cotton-wool spots; edema; exudates; hemorrhages; hypertensive retinopathy; nonrhegmatogenous (exudative) retinal detachment; vasculitis of specific retinal and choroidal arteries.

Sclera: Necrotizing nodular scleritis; nodular episcleritis; sclero-uveitis.

Other: Anterior uveitis; Argyll Robertson pupil; cataracts; cortical blindness; hemianopsia; internuclear ophthalmoplegia.

PRECAUTIONS

Both of the therapeutic agents recommended earlier, corticosteroids and cytotoxic drugs, have significant adverse side effects of which the physician should be aware. The multitude of side effects related to corticosteroid therapy have been reviewed in detail; they include suppression of the hypothalamic-pituitary axis, cataracts, and osteonecrosis. These adverse effects are predictable and related directly to the dosage and duration of therapy; the dosage should therefore be tapered, when possible, to an alternate-day regimen, and the minimal efficacious dose should be determined.

Immediate and long-term complications have been reported with the use of cyclophosphamide. Cyclophosphamide directly suppresses the bone marrow, and this effect should be monitored through peripheral leukocyte counts. Other complications include lower urinary tract problems, such as hemorrhagic cystitis and bladder fibrosis. Finally, any patient undergoing immunosuppressive therapy should be carefully observed for signs of infection, particularly by such opportunistic organisms as cytomegalovirus, *Candida*, and *Toxoplasma gondii*.

COMMENTS

The treatment strategy described earlier is designed to modulate or suppress the immune mechanisms underlying the vasculitis. Other modalities less commonly employed to alter the host immune response are antilymphocyte serum and lymphoplasmapheresis. Plasmapheresis has been used in an attempt to remove immune complexes. This approach is based upon the yet unproven supposition that periarteritis nodosa is an immune complex disease.

Even with treatment, the prognosis is poor. Renal failure, ruptured aneurysms, strokes, and cardiovascular disease are the major causes of death. The cutaneous variant, cutaneous polyarteritis nodosa, runs a chronic course with a good long-term prognosis.

References

Axelrod L: Glucocorticoid therapy. Medicine 55:39–65, 1976.

Conn DL: Polyarteritis. Rheum Dis Clin North Am 16:341–362, 1990.

Cupps TR, Fauci AS: The vasculitides. Major Prob Intern Med 21:1–211, 1981.

Diaz-Perez JL, Winkelmann RK: Cutaneous periarteritis nodosa. Arch Dermatol 110:407–414, 1974.

Frohnert PP, Sheps SG: Long-term follow-up study of periarteritis nodosa. Am J Med 43:8–14, 1967.

Kirkali P, Topaloglu R, Kansu T, Bakkaloglu A: Third nerve palsy and internuclear ophthalmoplegia in periarteritis nodosa. J Pediatr Ophthalmol Strabismus 28:45–46, 1991.

Leib ES, Restivo C, Paulus HE: Immunosuppressive and corticosteroid therapy of polyarteritis nodosa. Am J Med 67:941–947, 1979.

Morgan CM, Foster CS, D'Amico DJ, Gragoudas ES: Retinal vasculitis in polyarteritis nodosa. Retina 6:205–209, 1986.

Schein PS, Winokur SH: Immunosuppressive and cytotoxic chemotherapy: Long-term complications. Ann Intern Med 82:84–95, 1975.

Steinberg AD, et al: Cytotoxic drugs in treatment of nonmalignant diseases. Ann Intern Med 76:619–642, 1972.

Venning MC, Quinn A, Broomhead V, Bird AG: Antibodies directed against neutrophils (C-ANCA and P-ANCA) are of distinct value in systemic vasculitis. Q J Med 77(284):1287–1296, 1990.

PSEUDOXANTHOMA ELASTICUM 757.39
(Grönblad-Strandberg Syndrome, PXE)

DAVID S. HULL, M.D.

Augusta, Georgia

Pseudoxanthoma elasticum is an inherited connective tissue disorder characterized by redundant folds of soft, wrinkled, and lax skin typically located on the neck, lower abdomen, or perineum and in the flexures of the arms, popliteal fossae, axillary, and groin areas. There are two autosomal dominant and two recessive forms of the disease. It usually appears by age 30, although it may appear in childhood or in old age. Although it may affect the elastic tissue of the skin, eyes, or cardiovascular system, the primary defect seems to be premature degeneration and calcium deposition in the dermal elastic fibers. The xanthomatous eruptions are perfectly symmetric, small (1 to 3 mm in diameter), yellow nodules that have a plucked-chicken appearance. The skin is loose, but not hyperelastic. Cardiovascular complications may accompany the disorder. Patients may exhibit hypertension, premature atherosclerosis, coronary insufficiency, angina pectoris, mitral valve prolapse, arterial insufficiency in the extremities, dilation of the aorta, vascular aneurysms, and gastrointestinal or cerebral hemorrhages.

Similar changes occur in the elastic lamina of Bruch's membrane, resulting in the formation of angioid streaks in the fundi of approximately 85 per cent of patients. The combination of characteristic skin changes and angioid streaks is pathognomonic of the Grönblad-Strandberg syndrome. A serous hemorrhagic maculopathy with subretinal neovascular membrane occurs in about 70 per cent of cases. This results in the loss of central vision and visual acuity. Angioid streaks usually occur bilaterally, develop in the second or third decades, and gradually increase over several years. They may not be visible ophthalmoscopically; however, they can be clearly seen on fluorescein angiography. The angioid streaks that occur in the fundus have been well described as resembling cracks in old oil paintings. They tend to radiate from the disc and lie deep to the retinal vessels. They are gray or brown, and there may be small white borders on either side of the stria. They are not connected with the retinal vessels.

Diffuse mottling or peau d'orange, often associated with widespread drusen-like spots, may be the earliest fundus changes in this disease. These disturbances may be present with or without angioid streaks.

THERAPY

Systemic. Treatment is conservative and symptomatic. Hypertension may occur frequently in patients with pseudoxanthoma elasticum and may require treatment. Patients with ischemic symptoms may require arteriography. The cosmetic appearance of the skin may be improved by plastic surgery.

Ocular. Patients with angioid streaks of the fundus and neovascular membranes should be considered for fluorescein angiography. Argon or krypton laser photocoagulation can be used to destroy choroidal neovascularization associated with angioid streaks with good visual results.

Supportive. Genetic counseling is especially important in view of the newly detected autosomal dominant variants of pseudoxanthoma elasticum in which the risk of transmission is increased to 50 per cent.

Ocular or Periocular Manifestations

Choroid or Retina: Angioid streaks; choroidal neovascular membranes; detachment;

macular hemorrhages; mottling; prominent choroidal vessels; scarring.

Cornea: Peripheral opacity.

Other: Exophthalmos (orbital hematoma); optic atrophy; paralysis of extraocular muscles (secondary to vascular lesions of central nervous system); visual field defects; visual loss; vitreal hemorrhages.

PRECAUTIONS

Patients with pseudoxanthoma elasticum may be at increased risk during anesthesia. Coronary artery insufficiency may predispose the patient to arrhythmias and sudden death. Accurate blood pressure readings and electrocardiogram monitoring are essential. A nasogastric tube should be avoided because of the tendency for gastric bleeding. Since even minor trauma can cause retinal hemorrhage, contact sports should be avoided. Prophylactic photocoagulation of angioid streaks in the absence of choroidal neovascularization may cause that condition.

COMMENTS

The underlying defect in pseudoxanthoma elasticum is the abnormal presence of stainable polyanion in the dermal elastic fibers. These polyanions play a role in the subsequent calcification of the affected fibers. The calcium content of skin lesions increases with the severity of the lesions, and the lesions do not occur without deposited calcium. The changes of Bruch's membrane are caused by tears, which later result in angioid streaks. These streaks may subsequently be followed by pigment epithelial degeneration and the formation of choroidal neovascular membranes. Focal retinal degeneration and visual loss seem more related to repeated hemorrhages in the region of reaction to the angioid streaks than to the angioid streaks themselves. The retinal vessels appear normal, and hemorrhages originate from choroidal neovascular membranes.

References

Brancato R, et al: Laser treatment of macular subretinal neovascularization in angioid streaks. Ophthalmologica 195:84–87, 1987.

Eddy DD, Farber EM: Pseudoxanthoma elasticum. Internal manifestations: A report of cases and a statistical review of the literature. Arch Dermatol 86:729–740, 1962.

Francois J, et al: Neovascularization after argon laser photocoagulation of macular lesions. Am J Ophthalmol 79:206–210, 1975.

Gelisken Ö: A long term follow-up study of laser coagulation of neovascular membranes in angioid streaks. Am J Ophthalmol 105:299–303, 1988.

Hull DS, Aaberg TM: Fluorescein study of a family with angioid streaks and pseudoxanthoma elasticum. Br J Ophthalmol 58:738–745, 1974.

Kaplan EN, Henjyoji EY: Pseudoxanthoma elasti-

cum: A dermal elastosis with surgical implications. Plast Reconstr Surg 58:595–600, 1976.

Krechel SLW, Ramirez-Inawat RC, Fabian LW: Anesthetic considerations in pseudoxanthoma elasticum. Anesth Analg 60:344–347, 1981.

Meislik J, et al: Laser treatment in maculopathy of pseudoxanthoma elasticum. Can J Ophthalmol 13:210–212, 1978.

Pope FM: Autosomal dominant pseudoxanthoma elasticum. J Med Genet 11:152–157, 1974.

Pope FM: Two types of autosomal recessive pseudoxanthoma elasticum. Arch Dermatol 110:209–212, 1974.

Wilkinson CP: Stimulation of subretinal neovascularization. Am J Ophthalmol 81:104–106, 1976.

RELAPSING POLYCHONDRITIS 733.99

PETER G. WATSON, M.D., F.R.C.S., F.R.C.Ophth.

Cambridge, England

and EAMON P. O'DONOGHUE, M.B., B.Ch., B.A.O., F.R.C.S. (Ed.)

London, England

Relapsing polychondritis causes inflammation of cartilaginous structures throughout the body, but most commonly affects the nasal, tracheal, and auricular cartilage. The characteristic features of the disease are destruction of cartilage and its eventual replacement with connective tissue. Migratory oligo- or polyarthritis is frequently the earliest sign and is generally progressive. The chondritis typically is of sudden onset and very painful. If the costal, tracheal, and laryngeal cartilage also become involved, the trachea may collapse and death may result from acute bronchial obstruction.

Diagnostic criteria were described by McAdam in 1976 and consist of three or more of the following: (1) recurrent chondritis of both auricles, (2) nonerosive inflammatory polyarthritis, (3) chondritis of nasal cartilage, (4) inflammation of ocular structures, (5) laryngotracheal chondritis, or (6) vestibular or cochlear inflammation. These criteria were modified further by Damiani in 1979 to include histopathologic evidence for the disease. The 5- and 10-year survival rates are 74 per cent and 55 per cent respectively, with death due mainly to infection, vasculitis, and malignancy. Anemia at diagnosis is a poor prognostic indicator at any age, as well as saddle nose deformity and systemic vasculitis in patients under 51 years. Myocardial, aortic, and cardiac valvular involvement in addition to renal and liver dysfunction have also been observed. Ocular involvement occurs in 50 to 65 per cent of patients. The most frequent ocular signs are episcleritis and scleritis.

THERAPY

Systemic. Relapsing polychondritis is a notoriously difficult disease to treat. Treatment is by suppression of the inflammation in the sclera, cartilage, and connective tissue by corticosteroids that are also especially effective against laryngotracheobronchial and external ear manifestations. Prednisone is usually started in a dosage of 60 mg daily, or an equivalent dose of another corticosteroid preparation may be used. In exceptionally severe acute disease, it is sometimes necessary to suppress the inflammation by the use of 500 mg of methylprednisolone, given intravenously in an infusion over a period of at least 1 hour. This may need to be repeated after 2 days. (Perioperative pulsed intravenous methylprednisolone should also be considered when planning surgery to vulnerable tissues.) If this fails to control the condition or there is evidence of raised circulating immune complexes, 500 mg of cyclophosphamide[‡] given intravenously will probably induce a remission of the disease. A second dose may need to be given intravenously after a week, and all therapy may need to be continued. Patients on cyclophosphamide must be well hydrated so that if the drug is given by intravenous infusion it should be followed for 24 hours with intravenous fluids. Most patients can be maintained on low doses of oral steroids, alone, although some will require addition of the immunosuppressive drugs, such as cyclophosphamide[‡] or azathioprine.[‡]

Ocular. Topical ophthalmic corticosteroids are occasionally helpful for recurrent ocular problems. Prednisolone eyedrops or ointment may be applied on an hourly basis for acute episodes and then tapered. One per cent atropine applied one to three times daily may be of value in controlling the uveitis.

Supportive. Any sign of respiratory distress with tracheal inflammation should be observed closely and treated early by intubation. If perichondrial inflammatory masses narrow the airway, surgical removal of the masses and reconstruction of the airway may be indicated.

Since collapse of the nasal cartilage or development of nasal tip deformity usually worsens after surgery, cosmetic surgery is not recommended. In extreme cases of cardiac vascular involvement, valvular replacement with prosthetic valves or aortic aneurysm resection may become necessary symptomatic treatment.

Ocular or Periocular Manifestations

Conjunctiva: Chemosis; conjunctivitis; infiltration.
Cornea: Edema; opacity; perforation; stromal infiltration; thinning; ulcer.
Globe: Phthisis bulbi.

Sclera: Blue coloration; episcleritis; scleritis; thinning.

PRECAUTIONS

Relapsing polychondritis should be considered not only in patients presenting with scleral disease but also in those who develop diffuse joint disease. When the diagnosis has been established, corticosteroid therapy should be started as early as possible. However, it must be remembered that corticosteroids neither stop the disease progression in the more aggressive cases nor the development of potential lethal organ system involvement. There is some evidence that cyclophosphamide may induce a prolonged remission. The use of subconjunctival corticosteroids should be avoided, as diseased sclera may be lost at the site of the injection.

Though there are no specific serologic markers for relapsing polychondritis, antinuclear cytoplasmic auto-antibody (CANCA), which is highly specific for Wegener's granulomatosis, will help discriminate these two conditions in equivocal cases.

Careful radiologic evaluation of major airways and joints is of paramount importance for diagnostic, prognostic and management purposes. Computed tomography is useful in assessing the extent of disease.

The major airways are affected in over 50 per cent of cases. Michet et al. (1986) has reported that the fatality rate due to respiratory problems is closer to 10 per cent.

If elective surgical procedures are considered, they should be undertaken only during periods of remission and with immunosuppression. These patients tolerate anesthesia poorly, especially if tracheobronchial involvement is present and active and expert anesthesia care is required.

COMMENTS

Although relapsing polychondritis is more commonly a chronic, low-grade, episodic disease, it may be a fulminant disease with a rapid downhill course. The critical organ system involved in relapsing polychondritis is the respiratory tract. However, death from ruptured abdominal aneurysms or progressive heart failure secondary to aortic regurgitation has also occurred. Because of the variation in severity and the episodic nature of the disease, careful prolonged follow-up and individualized therapy are the keys to optimal treatment. Aggressive therapy may be necessary during an acute attack.

References

Arkin CR, Masi AT: Relapsing polychondritis: Review of current status and case report. Sem Ar thritis Rheum 5:41–62, 1975.
Booth A, Dieppe PA, Goddard PL, Watt I: The ra-

diological manifestations of relapsing polychondritis. Clin Radiol 40:147–149, 1989.

Damian JM, Levine HL: Relapsing polychondritis—Report of ten cases. Laryngoscope 89:929–944, 1979.

Hayward AW, Al-Shaikh B: Relapsing polychondritis and the anaesthetist. Anaesthesia 43:573–577, 1988.

Isaak BL, Liesgang TJ, Michet CJ: Ocular and systemic findings in relapsing polychondritis. Ophthalmology 93:681–689, 1986.

McAdam LP, et al: Relapsing polychondritis: Prospective study of 23 patients and a review of the literature. Medicine 55:193–215, 1976.

McKay DAR, Watson PG, Lyne AJ: Relapsing polychondritis and eye disease. Br J Ophthalmol 58:600–605, 1974.

Mendelson DS, et al: Relapsing polychondritis studied by computerized tomography. Radiology 157:489–490, 1985.

Michet CJ, et al: Relapsing polychondritis: Survival and predictive role of early disease manifestations. Ann Intern Med 104:74–78, 1986.

Specks U, et al: Anticytoplasmic autoantibodies in diagnosis and follow-up of Wegener's granulomatosis. Mayo Clin Proc 64:28–36, 1989.

RHEUMATOID ARTHRITIS 714.0

JAMES T. ROSENBAUM, M.D.

Portland, Oregon

Rheumatoid arthritis is a systemic, immune-mediated disease that primarily affects females with an onset during middle age. Approximately 80 per cent of patients with rheumatoid arthritis have a positive test for rheumatoid factor, which indicates an IgM type immunoglobulin that binds to an IgG. In general, the arthritis characteristic of rheumatoid arthritis is symmetric. Joints most likely to be affected include the proximal interphalangeal joints of the hands and feet, the metacarpal-phalangeal joints, the metatarsal-phalangeal joints, wrists, ankles, knees, hips, shoulders, and temporomandibular joints. The extra-articular manifestations of rheumatoid arthritis include subcutaneous nodules, vasculitis, pleuropericarditis, leukopenia and anemia as in Felty's syndrome, and interstitial lung disease. The arthritis characteristic of rheumatoid arthritis is generally clinically and radiographically distinct from such other causes of arthritis as systemic-onset juvenile rheumatoid arthritis, ankylosing spondylitis, Reiter's syndrome, and gout.

Keratoconjunctivitis sicca is an extremely common complication of rheumatoid arthritis. In autopsy studies, nearly all patients with rheumatoid arthritis have a lymphocytic infiltration of salivary glands, as is characteristic of Sjögren's syndrome. Patients with rheumatoid arthritis frequently have abnormal Schirmer's tests, abnormal rose bengal staining of the conjunctiva, and complaints related to ocular dryness. Treatment of rheumatoid arthritis does not generally alter the keratoconjunctivitis. Symptomatic therapy for Sjögren's syndrome secondary to rheumatoid arthritis should therefore not differ from treatment for Sjögren's syndrome that is primary, i.e., unassociated with another connective tissue syndrome.

Other ocular manifestations of rheumatoid arthritis include scleritis, episcleritis, peripheral corneal infiltrates (Wessely rings), and marginal corneal thinning (corneal melts). In rheumatoid arthritis, rarely a tendonitis of the sheath of the superior oblique muscle can impair the function of that muscle, resulting in Brown's syndrome. Complications from anterior scleritis include glaucoma and iritis. Although posterior scleritis is a less frequent manifestation of rheumatoid arthritis, it does occur and may be associated with such complications as retinal detachment and disc edema. In contrast to ankylosing spondylitis and some subsets of juvenile rheumatoid arthritis, iritis is not a manifestation of rheumatoid arthritis, unless it occurs secondarily to scleritis or vasculitis.

Scleritis develops most commonly in patients with rheumatoid arthritis who have other extraarticular manifestations of the disease, such as vasculitis and nodules. These patients ordinarily have strongly positive tests for rheumatoid factor. Rheumatoid arthritis is the most common systemic disease associated with scleritis. A painful, necrotizing scleritis should be distinguished from the more indolent condition, scleromalacia perforans. Approximately 50 per cent of all patients with scleromalacia perforans have rheumatoid arthritis, usually in association with subcutaneous nodules. The therapy for either a scleritis or a corneal melt in the setting of rheumatoid arthritis is optimized if the underlying joint disease is well controlled.

THERAPY

Systemic. The therapy for rheumatoid arthritis includes nonsteroidal anti-inflammatory drugs (NSAIDs), more potent medications that are generally considered to be disease-modifying agents, and adjunctive measures, such as physical therapy, rest, and joint protection. The NSAIDs include aspirin, indomethacin, ibuprofen, phenylbutazone, naproxen, piroxicam, ketorolac, nabumetone, diclofenac, etodolac, and tolmetin, among others. These medications work in part by inhibiting the synthesis of prostaglandins. If tolerated, one of these agents should always be included in the therapy for scleritis. Most published reports on scleritis discuss experience with either 25 to 50 mg of indomethacin administered orally three to four times daily or 100 mg of phenylbutazone administered orally three to four times daily. The author's preference is to begin with indomethacin and to consider phenylbutazone if an adequate therapeutic response is not achieved in 2 weeks.

Disease-modifying drugs for rheumatoid arthritis include antimalarials, injectable and oral gold salts, sulfasalazine, penicillamine, and immunosuppressants, including methotrexate,[‡] azathioprine, and cyclophosphamide.[‡] The antimalarials (200 mg of oral hydroxychloroquine two times daily or 250 mg of oral chloroquine once daily) are the least toxic disease-modifying agents. Unfortunately, only about 40 per cent of patients respond to this class of medication, and the onset of benefit is frequently as long as 12 weeks after initiating therapy.

Intramuscular gold injection is the first choice of many rheumatologists when selecting a disease-modifying drug. Either aurothioglucose or gold sodium thiomalate is given by injection as frequently as every week up to a dose of 50 mg. After a total dose of 1 gm, the frequency of injections is generally reduced. The complete blood count and urinalysis must be monitored frequently while either of these drugs is given. About 70 per cent of patients with rheumatoid arthritis will have sustained improvement from gold injections. However, the onset of benefit may be delayed as long as 3 months after the initiation of treatment. Gold may also be taken orally as auranofin, usually at a dose of 3 mg two times daily. Although efficacious, most rheumatologists do not consider oral gold to be as potent as intramuscular gold. The mechanism of action of the orally administered drug may differ from that of the intramuscular drug.

Penicillamine is an alternative to intramuscular gold as a disease-modifying drug. Penicillamine is given orally at daily doses as high as 0.75 to 1.5 gm. The drug is usually begun at a daily dose of 125 mg, and the dosage is increased by 125 mg/day every 2 weeks. As with gold, the complete blood count and urinalysis must be monitored carefully, and 3 months or more may be required before therapeutic benefit is achieved. Toxicity may include loss of taste, thrombocytopenia, nephrotic syndrome, and a variety of presumably immune-mediated side effects.

Sulfasalazine[‡] (2 to 3 gm daily in divided doses) seems to be effective for rheumatoid arthritis, especially if the disease is of recent onset. Its role in severe disease or in the arrest of the progression of erosive bone changes has not been established.

Immunosuppressant drugs are also effective for rheumatoid arthritis. Azathioprine at an oral dose of 1 to 2 mg/kg daily has been approved by the FDA for rheumatoid arthritis. Oral or intramuscular methotrexate,[‡] usually at a dose from 5 to 15 mg weekly, has become extremely popular as a treatment for rheumatoid arthritis. Its unique virtues include a low likelihood of leukopenia at the recommended dose (if the baseline renal function is normal) and a rapid onset of action, such that patients generally benefit within 2 to 3 weeks after initiating therapy. Although methotrexate is an excellent drug for the articular manifestations of rheumatoid arthritis, its role in treating rheumatoid nodules or vasculitis is less established. Since scleritis and corneal melts tend to correlate with these aspects of rheumatoid disease, the role of methotrexate for ocular complications of rheumatoid arthritis has not been established. Cyclophosphamide[‡] (usually 1 to 2 mg/kg daily) is one of the most potent cytotoxic drugs available. It is an excellent choice for a complication of rheumatoid arthritis, such as a corneal melt, if other less toxic modalities of therapy have failed.

Corticosteroids, either orally or injected locally, can provide prompt, but transient improvement in rheumatoid arthritis. In general, a corticosteroid dose greater than what is comparable to 10 mg of prednisone should be used only as a temporary measure in rheumatoid arthritis. An acute ocular complication, such as a scleritis or a corneal melt, might be an indication for a limited course of oral corticosteroids. The long-term safety of prednisone at a daily dose of less than 10 mg is still debated.

The role of cyclosporine,[‡] drug combinations, pulse methylprednisolone, total lymphoid irradiation, and lymphoplasmapheresis is less well established in rheumatoid disease. Recent reports suggest benefit from oral cyclosporine in the treatment of corneal melt.

Ocular or Periocular Manifestations

Cornea: Keratoconjunctivitis sicca; marginal corneal thinning or keratolysis; peripheral corneal infiltrates.

Extraocular: Tendonitis affecting the superior oblique muscle sheath.

Sclera: Anterior or posterior scleritis; episcleritis; scleromalacia perforans.

Other: Complications of scleritis including iritis, glaucoma, exudative choroiditis, disc edema; complications from medications including chrysiasis from gold, retinal pigment changes or corneal opacities from antimalarials, blurry vision from NSAIDs, posterior subcapsular cataracts and glaucoma from corticosteroids.

PRECAUTIONS

Potential toxicities from NSAIDs include gastrointestinal bleeding, such central nervous system effects as mood swings or headache, reduction in glomerular filtration rate and fluid retention, and reduced platelet function. Reversible blurring of vision can also occur with NSAIDs. Optic neuritis may be a rare complication from this class of medications. Phenylbutazone has rarely been associated with a fatal aplastic anemia.

Retinal toxicity should be monitored closely on antimalarial therapy, although it occurs rarely if the recommended doses are not exceeded. Reversible corneal deposits can also induce visual halos in patients receiving antimalarial therapy.

Potential toxicities of gold salts include anemia, leukopenia, thrombocytopenia, rash, stomatitis, flushing, and renal disease. The deposition of gold in the cornea or chrysiasis occurs in 75 per cent of patients who receive a cumulative intramuscular dose greater than 1.5 gm; however, this accumulation is rarely clinically significant.

The long-term use of corticosteroids may be associated with numerous toxicities. Some of these adverse effects, such as osteopenia and a reduced response to infection, are especially troublesome in patients with rheumatoid arthritis.

COMMENTS

Rheumatoid arthritis should be distinguished from other causes of joint inflammation, such as osteoarthritis and Reiter's syndrome. Most patients with rheumatoid arthritis have positive tests for rheumatoid factor and a polyarticular, symmetric arthritis. Only a minority of patients with juvenile rheumatoid arthritis have a disease that resembles that seen in adults.

Keratoconjunctivitis is a frequent manifestation of rheumatoid arthritis. Scleritis affects only a small percentage of patients with rheumatoid arthritis, but rheumatoid arthritis is the systemic disease most commonly associated with scleritis. Patients with scleritis often have other extra-articular manifestations of rheumatoid disease. Optimal treatment for scleritis associated with rheumatoid arthritis includes therapy for the systemic disease, but therapy of the arthritis does not alter ocular dryness.

Many of the medications used to treat rheumatoid arthritis have potential ocular toxicities.

References

Brown SI, Grayson M: Marginal furrows: A characteristic corneal lesion of rheumatoid arthritis. Arch Ophthalmol 79:563–567, 1968.

Felson DT, Anderson JJ, Meenan RF: Use of short-term efficacy/toxicity tradeoffs to select second-line drugs in rheumatoid arthritis. Arthritis Rheum 35:1117–1125, 1992.

Foster CS, Forstot SL, Wilson LA: Mortality rate in rheumatoid arthritis patients developing necrotizing scleritis or peripheral ulcerative keratitis. Effects of systemic immunosuppression. Ophthalmology 91:1253–1262, 1984.

Jayson MIV, Jones DEP: Scleritis and rheumatoid arthritis. Ann Rheum Dis 30:343–347, 1971.

Lyne AJ, Pitkeathley DA: Episcleritis and scleritis.

Association with connective tissue disease. Arch Ophthalmol 80:171–176, 1968.

McGavin DD, et al: Episcleritis and scleritis: A study of their clinical manifestations and association with rheumatoid arthritis. Br J Ophthalmol 60:192–226, 1976.

Watson PG, Hayreh SS: Scleritis and episcleritis. Br J Ophthalmol 60:163–191, 1976.

SCLERODERMA 710.1
(Systemic Sclerosis)

DOUGLAS A. JABS, M.D.

Baltimore, Maryland

Scleroderma is a disorder of connective tissue of unknown etiology characterized by fibrous degenerative changes in the skin and viscera, vascular insufficiency, and vasospasm. It usually affects patients between the ages of 30 and 50 years, and females are affected four times more frequently than males. The skin changes consist of thickening, tightening, and induration, leading to the loss of normal mobility and to contracture (scleroderma). These changes are usually preceded by an edematous phase lasting weeks to months. The fingers (sclerodactyly), arms, and face are usually affected early, but the process may spread to involve the entire body. Raynaud's phenomenon occurs in approximately 90 per cent of patients with scleroderma.

Visceral involvement includes esophageal dysfunction with gastroesophageal reflux, pulmonary fibrosis, cardiac abnormalities (such as pulmonary hypertension and arrhythmias), gastrointestinal hypomotility, and renal disease (scleroderma kidney). Renal failure is a cause of mortality in systemic sclerosis, and it is often associated with the onset of malignant hypertension. Other manifestations include digital ulcers, telangiectasia, polyarthralgias, polyarticular arthritis (occasionally), and myositis.

Scleroderma encompasses a spectrum of clinical diseases ranging from the relatively benign, more slowly progressive CREST syndrome (*c*alcinosis, *R*aynaud's phenomenon, *e*sophageal dysfunction, *s*clerodactyly, and *t*elangiectasia) to more severe disease (systemic sclerosis) with extensive skin disease and visceral involvement. "Overlap" syndromes occur with other connective tissue diseases, such as sclerodermatomyositis and mixed connective tissue disease. The latter is characterized by high titers of antibody to ribonucleoprotein and a combination of features of systemic lupus erythematosus, systemic sclerosis, and polymyositis. Localized benign forms of scleroderma without vascular or visceral disease also occur.

Ocular complications of systemic sclerosis

usually result from involvement of the facial skin and lacrimal glands. Involvement of the eyelids results in tightness of the lids, lagophthalmos, blepharophimosis, and ptosis. Telangiectasia may be present on the lids, and the conjunctival fornices are shortened. Exposure keratitis may occur, but it is not common. Tear secretion is often decreased, which may lead to keratoconjunctivitis sicca. Abnormalities of the conjunctival vessels, including venous dilation, varicosities, vascular sludging, and telangiectasia, are common. Grade IV hypertensive retinopathy with hemorrhages, cotton-wool spots, and papilledema is often present during scleroderma-renal crises.

THERAPY

Systemic. No specific agent or agents have been found that clearly halt the progression of scleroderma. The drug used most often is D-penicillamine,‡ a compound that interferes with the intermolecular cross-linking of collagen. Although retrospective studies suggest benefit, results of penicillamine therapy have thus far been equivocal. Although trials of immunosuppressive agents have been disappointing, one trial of 5-fluorouracil showed a modest benefit in skin scores, Raynaud's phenomenon, and patients' global assessment. Therefore, therapy is often directed toward management of the various complications of the disease.

Ocular. When keratoconjunctivitis sicca or exposure keratitis problems are present, tear substitutes should be used at frequent intervals, and bland lubricating ointments should be used at night.

Supportive. Skin care is essential. Special soaps, creams, and lotions are used to relieve dryness and increase pliability. Ulcerations should be kept clean to avoid secondary infections. Articular complaints may be helped by aspirin or nonsteroidal antiinflammatory drugs. Avoiding cold exposure and the use of warm protective clothing help protect against Raynaud's phenomenon. Calcium channel blockers, such as nifedipine, diltiazem, and verapamil, are used as vasodilator therapy to treat Raynaud's phenomenon and are subjectively efficacious, although their physiologic effect is less certain. Although systemic corticosteroids are used to treat an associated myositis, corticosteroids have no effect on the scleroderma. In several cases, aggressive antihypertensive therapy has been shown to reverse renal failure in the scleroderma-renal crisis.

Ocular or Periocular Manifestations

Choroid: Patchy choroidal nonperfusion.
Conjunctiva: Chemosis, shortened fornices; telangiectasia; varicosities; vascular sludging; venous dilation.

Cornea: Exposure keratitis; keratoconjunctivitis sicca.
Eyelids: Blepharophimosis; lagophthalmos; ptosis; tightness.
Orbit: Periorbital edema.
Retina: Cotton-wool spots; hemorrhages; papilledema; venous thrombosis.
Other: Decreased tear secretion; ocular myositis; paralysis of extraocular muscles; Sjögren's syndrome.

PRECAUTIONS

Because of the high frequency of abnormalities of tear secretion in these patients, tear production should be evaluated. If tear replacement therapy is necessary, it should be started.

COMMENTS

The main ocular manifestations of progressive systemic sclerosis are eyelid involvement (about 65 per cent of cases), decreased tear production (40 to 50 per cent), keratoconjunctivitis sicca (30 per cent), shallow conjunctival fornices (20 per cent), and conjunctival vascular abnormalities (70 per cent). Visual impairment is seldom a problem unless severe corneal damage occurs as a result of dry eyes.

The retinal lesions in progressive systemic sclerosis are clinically and histopathologically indistinguishable from those of malignant hypertension. However, they have been described in one normotensive scleroderma patient and in scleroderma patients with blood pressures lower than expected compared to the severity of fundus changes. This finding suggests an underlying abnormality of the retinal vasculature. Studies using fluorescein angiography have demonstrated patchy choroidal nonperfusion in patients. This change was unrelated to hypertension and seemed to have no effect on retinal function. Results of minor salivary gland biopsies have suggested that lacrimal and salivary gland involvement may be due to either inflammatory lesions (Sjögren's syndrome) or to glandular fibrosis.

References

Casas JA, Saway PA, Villarreal I, Nolte C, Menajovsky BL, Escudero EE, Blackburn WD, Alarcon S, Subauste CP: 5-Fluorouracil in the treatment of scleroderma: A randomized, double-blind, placebo-controlled international collaborative study. Ann Rheum Dis 49:926–928, 1990.

Grennan DM, Forrester J: Involvement of the eye in SLE and scleroderma. A study using fluorescein angiography in addition to clinical ophthalmic assessment. Ann Rheum Dis 36:152–156, 1977.

Horan EC: Ophthalmic manifestations of progressive systemic sclerosis. Br J Ophthalmol 53:388–392, 1969.

Jabs DA: The rheumatic diseases. *In* Tasman W, Jaeger EA (eds): Duane's Clinical Ophthalmology. Philadelphia, JB Lippincott, 1992, Vol 5, pp 1–39.

MacLean H, Guthrie W: Retinopathy in scleroderma. Trans Ophthalmol Soc UK 89:209–220,
1969.

Osial TA Jr, Whiteside TL, Buckingham RB, Singh
G, Barnes EL, Pierce JM, Rodnan GP: Clinical
and serologic study of Sjögren's syndrome in patients with progressive systemic sclerosis. Arthritis Rheum 26:500–508, 1983.

Seibold JR: Scleroderma. In Kelley WN, Harris ED
Jr, Ruddy S, Sledge CB (eds): Textbook of Rheumatology, 3rd ed. Philadelphia, WB Saunders,
1989, pp 1215–1244.

Steen VD, Medsger TA Jr, Rodnan GP: D-Penicillamine therapy in progressive systemic sclerosis
(scleroderma). Ann Intern Med 97:652–659, 1982.

West RH, Barnett AJ: Ocular involvement in scleroderma. Br J Ophthalmol 63:845–847, 1979.

SJÖGREN'S SYNDROME 710.2

(Gougerot-Sjögren's Syndrome)

MICHAEL A. LEMP, M.D.,
and PAUL C. KEENAN, M.D.

Washington, District of Columbia

Sjögren's syndrome is a chronic autoimmune disease characterized by the triad of dry eyes (keratoconjunctivitis sicca), dry mouth (xerostomia), and a connective tissue disease, most commonly rheumatoid arthritis. The majority of patients presenting with keratoconjunctivitis sicca do not have overt evidence of systemic disease. However, those patients with collagen vascular disease, particularly rheumatoid arthritis, have an unusually high incidence of keratoconjunctivitis sicca. Sjögren's syndrome is currently divided into two forms: primary, dry eyes and dry mouth, and secondary, dry eyes and dry mouth in association with systemic autoimmune disease. The disease is characterized by mononuclear infiltration of the main and accessory lacrimal and salivary glands, which leads to the destruction of the lacrimal and salivary glands, resulting in a deficiency of tears and saliva. The evidence supporting an autoimmunue pathogenesis is strong. Sjögren's syndrome has been associated with rheumatoid arthritis, systemic lupus erythematosus (SLE), Wegener's granulomatosis, lymphoproliferative diseases, paraproteinemias, and even drug reactions.

Eighty-five per cent of patients with rheumatoid arthritis and secondary Sjögren's syndrome have an association with HLA DW 4. In contrast, patients with primary Sjögren's syndrome have an increased frequency of HLA DW-2, HLA DW-3, or both. Autoantibodies vary in their expression in different subgroups of Sjögren's syndrome. Autoantibodies to Ro (SSA) and La (SSB) are commonly found in primary Sjögren's syndrome and in Sjögren's syndrome associated with SLE, but not in Sjögren's syndrome associated with RA. Patients with a connective tissue disorder and SSA and SSB antibodies are more likely to develop sicca.

Women are more frequently affected by Sjögren's syndrome than men, in a sex ratio of 9:1. The onset of this condition is gradual, and the true prevalence of Sjögren's syndrome is unknown. The onset of the disease is frequently between the ages of 40 to 60, but it has been reported to occur during childhood and adolescence. Other diseases associated with Sjögren's syndrome include scleroderma, polymyositis, Hashimoto's thyroiditis, panarteritis, interstitial pulmonary fibrosis, and primary biliary cirrhosis. In patients presenting with signs and symptoms of keratoconjunctivitis sicca, questioning might reveal the presence of dry mouth, arthritic complaints, and/or other symptoms.

THERAPY

Systemic. Attention to inflammatory diseases of an autoimmune nature accompanying Sjögren's syndrome is of paramount importance. Systemic corticosteroids play a major role in the management of these conditions. Systemic antimetabolites are useful and occasionally life saving in the management of these conditions.

Ocular. The use of artificial tear supplements remains the mainstay of treatment of keratoconjunctivitis sicca. In the past 15 years, tear substitutes have been improved by the addition of adsorptive polymers for their formulations. The frequent instillation of artificial tears of low viscosity with an adsorptive polymer will manage most cases. A major advance in the use of tear substitutes is the introduction of formulatives without preservatives. Preservatives are toxic to the ocular surface, and frequent applications can lead to a worsening of surface disease. Unit-dose package solutions without preservatives, although costly, can be useful for many patients. Lacrisert, a small pellet of hydroxy propylmethyl cellulose, which dissolves slowly over a 6- to 12-hour period, has been useful in some patients. In the most severe cases, the use of moisture chambers or punctal occlusion or both can be quite helpful. The placing of a small lateral tarsorrhophy has been of benefit in selected patients.

In a subgroup of patients with keratoconjunctivitis sicca, the irritative symptoms are secondary to a marked increase in viscosity of the ocular mucin. The use of acetylcysteine* in 10 to 20 per cent concentrations can decrease the viscosity of the mucin and result in an alleviation of symptoms.

Soft bandage contact lenses have been used to treat corneal surface disease in the dry eye. Their use is discouraged, although they tend to be dramatically effective in the treatment of filamentary keratitis. They carry with them a high risk of infection and other problems, such as lens deposits, and they must be used in conjunction with frequent tear substitutes. The bandage lenses should be limited to those cases that cannot be managed adequately otherwise.

Ocular or Periocular Manifestations

Conjunctiva: Chemosis; hyperemia; lusterless appearance.
Cornea: Mucous plaques; perforation; superficial punctate erosions; thinning; ulcer.
Eyelids: Blepharitis; chalazion; hordeolum; meibomianitis.
Lacrimal System: Decreased tear film stability (rapid break-up time); increased debris in the tear film; increased tear film viscosity.

PRECAUTIONS

Patients with Sjögren's syndrome have decreased ocular surface defense mechanisms associated with keratoconjunctivitis sicca, thereby making them more prone to infections. Moreover, because of the autoimmune nature of their disease, they are more likely to sustain sterile necrotic ulcerations secondary to vasculitis. This combination of susceptibilities makes marginal corneal ulceration and even perforation a possibility. Corticosteroids therefore should be used with great care in the management of these conditions. The management of the systemic manifestations of Sjögren's syndrome should be coordinated with an internist because of the frequent monitoring necessary in anticipation of the side effects of drug therapy.

COMMENTS

One point should be emphasized. The majority of people presenting with keratoconjunctivitis sicca do not have and will not develop discernible systemic disease. Those people, however, who do have evidence of systemic disease conforming to the criteria for Sjögren's syndrome can be reassured that the majority of patients can be managed successfully throughout life without the loss of vision.

References

Coll J, Rives A, et al: Prevalence of Sjögren's syndrome in autoimmune disease. Ann Rheum Dis 46(4):286–289, 1987 Apr.

Farris L: Sjögren's syndrome. *In* Gold D, Weingest T (eds): The Eye and Systemic Disease. Philadelphia, JB Lippincott, 1990, pp 249–263.

Holly FJ, Lemp MA: Tear physiology and dry eyes. Surv Ophthalmol 22:68–87, 1977.

Lemp MA: General measures in management of the dry eye. Int Ophthalmol Clin 27(1):36–43, 1987.

Lemp MA: Recent developments in dry eye management. Ophthalmology 94(10):1299–1304, 1987.

Lemp MA: Dry eye. *In* Spaeth GL, Katz LJ, Parker KW (eds): Current Therapy in Ophthalmic Surgery. Toronto, BC Decker, 1989, pp 96–99.

Manthorpe R, et al: Sjögren's syndrome: A review with emphasis on immunological features. Allergy 36:139, 1981.

Tabbara KF, et al: Sjögren's syndrome: A correlation between ocular findings and salivary gland histology. Trans Am Acad Ophthalmol Otolaryngol 78:467, 1974.

SYSTEMIC LUPUS ERYTHEMATOSUS 710.0

JAMES T. ROSENBAUM, M.D.
Portland, Oregon

Systemic lupus erythematosus (SLE) is an immunologically mediated disease of uncertain etiology that has the potential to affect virtually any organ system. The American College of Rheumatology has suggested 11 diagnostic criteria for SLE. Patients are considered to have lupus if they meet four of the following criteria and have no alternate diagnostic explanation for the abnormalities: (1) malar rash; (2) discoid rash; (3) photosensitive rash; (4) oral ulcers; (5) nonerosive arthritis in two or more joints; (6) pleuritis or pericarditis; (7) glomerulonephritis or proteinuria; (8) seizures or psychosis; (9) hemolytic anemia, leukopenia, lymphopenia, or thrombocytopenia; (10) immunologic laboratory abnormality, such as antibodies to double-stranded DNA or the SM antigen, or a false-positive serologic test for syphilis; and (11) a positive antinuclear antibody test that is not caused by a medication. SLE is much more common in females than males. The prognosis depends largely on the organ system involved.

Keratoconjunctivitis sicca is the most common ocular manifestation of SLE. Cotton-wool spots are seen in as many as 28 per cent of patients with SLE. Some authorities believe that the presence of cotton-wool spots correlates with the likelihood of central nervous system disease. Other potential ocular manifestations of SLE include conjunctivitis, retinal vasculitis or retinal vascular occlusion, optic neuritis, scleritis, episcleritis, marginal corneal ulcer, eyelid rash, central nervous system disease affecting vision or extraocular muscles, and iritis. Papilledema may be present in association with pseudotumor cerebri.

As many as 50 or 60 per cent of patients with SLE have antibodies to a phospholipid known as cardiolipin. These antibodies may prolong the partial thromboplastin time. Because of this laboratory property, antibodies to cardiolipin are sometimes referred to as the lupus anticoagulant, although they are rarely associated with clinical bleeding. In fact, paradoxically, antiphospholipid antibodies are frequently associated with thrombosis. Antibodies to phospholipid may be responsible for false-positive serologic tests for syphilis. Antibodies to cardiolipin may be present without any manifestation of either systemic lupus or other autoimmune disease.

Antibodies to cardiolipin are strongly associated with thrombosis, including deep venous thrombosis, pulmonary embolism, nonbacterial thrombotic endocarditis, and central nervous system infarction. These antibodies may be causally related to spontaneous abortion. Antibodies to cardiolipin have been detected in association with an occlusive retinal vasculitis.

THERAPY

The treatment for SLE depends largely on the organ system that is involved and the severity of that involvement.

Systemic. Arthritis and pleuropericarditis are generally improved by nonsteroidal anti-inflammatory drugs, such as aspirin or indomethacin (75 to 200 mg daily). Antimalarials, including hydroxychloroquine[‡] (200 mg twice daily) and chloroquine[‡] (250 mg once daily), are particularly effective for discoid rash and the serositis. Anticoagulation may be indicated for thrombosis secondary to antiphospholipid antibodies.

Immunosuppressive therapy is indicated for SLE when the disease involves a critical organ, such as the kidney. For active lupus nephritis, monthly boluses of intravenous cyclophosphamide[‡] reduce the risk of end-stage renal failure. Intravenous cyclophosphamide is generally begun at 500 mg/m^2. The dose may be increased, depending largely on hematologic toxicity. Oral corticosteroids or intravenous methylprednisolone may be used to supplement cyclophosphamide. Corticosteroids alone, however, are not as effective as cyclophosphamide for lupus-related renal disease. Other approaches with cytotoxic drugs, such as daily oral azathioprine (1 to 2 mg/kg/day), daily oral cyclophosphamide (1 to 2 mg/kg/day), or weekly methotrexate (7.5 to 15 mg/wk), can be tried for patients who fail or who do not tolerate intravenous cyclophosphamide therapy. Pulse therapy with intravenous methylprednisolone, plasmapheresis, and total lymphoid irradiation are additional forms of immunosuppression that have been tried when more conventional therapy is not efficacious.

The section on rheumatoid arthritis (see page 234) contains additional discussion of therapy with nonsteroidal anti-inflammatory drugs, antimalarials, and cytotoxics.

Ocular. The treatment for sicca is described in the section of Sjögren's syndrome (see page 238). No form of immunosuppressive therapy has been found to increase tear formation.

Topical. Dermatologic manifestations of lupus are usually treated by topical corticosteroid preparations.

Ocular or Periocular Manifestations

Conjunctiva: Conjunctivitis.
Cornea: Keratoconjunctivitis sicca; peripheral corneal infiltrates; marginal corneal ulcer or keratolysis.
Eyelids: Erythematous, hyperkeratotic rash; telangiectasia.
Retina: Cotton-wool spots or cytoid bodies; retinal vasculitis; retinal vaso-occlusive disease including central or branch retinal artery or vein occlusions; secondary hypertensive retinopathy.
Sclera: Scleritis; episcleritis.
Other: Iritis; changes secondary to central nervous system infarction, including cranial nerve palsies, homonymous hemianopsia, nystagmus, and intranuclear ophthalmoplegia.

PRECAUTIONS

The section on uveitis (see page 681) contains a more complete discussion of the adverse effects of corticosteroids.

COMMENTS

Systemic lupus erythematosus is a multi system disease that may involve the eye. Although antinuclear antibodies are characteristic of this disease, a positive test for antinuclear antibodies does not establish a diagnosis in the absence of clinical findings.

The two most common ocular manifestations of systemic lupus are dry eyes and cotton-wool spots.

Patients with lupus who have retinal ischemic events have a greater likelihood of having central nervous system disease. The lupus anticoagulant or antiphospholipid antibodies, such as those to cardiolipin, may be causally related to some instances of retinal vascular occlusion. The treatment for retinal vasculitis may differ from the treatment of anticardiolipin-mediated retinal occlusive disease.

References

Austin HA, et al: Therapy of lupus nephritis. Controlled trial of prednisone and cytotoxic drugs. N Engl J Med 314:614–619, 1986.

Boey ML, et al: Thrombosis in systemic lupus erythematosus: Striking association with the presence of circulating lupus anticoagulant. Br Med J 287:1021–1023, 1983.

Boumpas DT, Austin HA III, Vaughn EM, Klippel JH, Steinberg AD, Yarboro CH, Balow JE: Controlled trial of pulse methylprednisolone versus two regimens of pulse cyclophosphamide in severe lupus nephritis. Lancet 340:741, 1992.

Gold DM, Morris DA, Henkind P: Ocular findings in systemic lupus erythematosus. Br J Ophthalmol 56:800–804, 1972.

Jabs DA, et al: Severe retinal vaso-occlusive disease in systemic lupus erythematosus. Arch Ophthalmol 104:558–563, 1986.

Levine SR, et al: Visual symptoms associated with the presence of a lupus anticoagulant. Ophthalmology 95:686–692, 1988.

Tan EM, et al: The 1982 revised criteria for the classification of systemic lupus erythematosus (SLE). Arthritis Rheum 25:1271–1277, 1982.

Stafford-Brady FJ, Urowitz MB, Gladman DD, Easterbrook M: Lupus retinopathy. Patterns, associations, and prognosis. Arthritis Rheum 31:1105, 1988.

WEILL-MARCHESANI SYNDROME 759.8

DAVID S. WALTON, M.D.

Boston, Massachusetts

The Weill-Marchesani syndrome is an hereditary cause of ectopia lentis and secondary glaucoma. The usual mode of inheritance is autosomal recessive but may be autosomal dominant, and affected persons demonstrate microspherophakia, short stature, stubby hands and feet, and brachycephaly. The affected lenses possess an abnormally small equatorial diameter, can be thickened in the anterior-posterior diameter, and become subluxated. The lens capsule and zonules are abnormal when viewed microscopically. Lens movement usually occurs inferiorly or anteriorly. The abnormal shape of the lens and anterior displacement predispose the eye to the development of glaucoma, which may be acute or chronic and may begin in childhood. The mechanism of the glaucoma is usually secondary to trabecular obstruction caused by pupillary blockage, but the possibility of obstruction by the iris, without pupillary block, due to appositional crowding of the iris against the angle face also must be considered.

THERAPY

Ocular. Lenticular myopia is a constant finding in this syndrome and often is progressive. Appropriate spectacle or contact lens correction is indicated. Astigmatism secondary to subluxation in the coronal plane cannot be corrected by contact lenses and requires spectacle correction.

The loss of vision may occur at a young age secondary to glaucoma. Regular anterior segment examinations are indicated to recognize early the presence of anterior chamber shallowing, increased iris convexity, and narrowing of the filtration angle, which predispose to pupillary block glaucoma. The additional finding of peripheral anterior synechia is an important sign of progressive angle closure.

Medical therapy to prevent angle closure may be helpful in the short term, but must be monitored very carefully. Miotics given to open the angle may increase pupillary block. An alpha-adrenergic antagonist may be the safest choice to accomplish this goal. Mydriasis may also have a beneficial effect on the angle width by lessening pupillary block, but may cause crowding of the angle and secondary glaucoma and also may allow displacement of the lens into the anterior chamber.

Acute glaucoma in this syndrome should be initially managed medically through the use of osmotic agents, carbonic anhydrase agents, and beta-adrenergic blocking agents. Simultaneous medications should also be administered to move the pupil to relieve pupillary block. I would favor the initial use of a weak, short-acting mydriatic followed by careful observation of the pupil size, lens position, and change in iris configuration and angle depth.

When first seen in their adolescence or adult years, patients with this syndrome may have chronic glaucoma secondary to permanent angle-closure glaucoma. Iridectomy, of course, does not reverse this condition, but only prevents further blockage of the trabecular meshwork associated with the continued occurrence of angle closure in the untreated eye. Medical treatment is indicated for the chronic glaucoma.

Surgical. When an eye is at risk for pupillary-block glaucoma in this syndrome, as indicated by the angle iris-lens configuration on gonioscopy, or when there is evidence of past or present pupillary-block glaucoma, laser iridotomy is indicated to relieve or prevent the development of permanent angle closure. It should be remembered that this development is a frequent and early complication in this syndrome, and prophylactic surgery must also be considered for the fellow eye. The more affected eye will often possess a shallower anterior chamber. The opening should be placed as peripherally as possible to prevent blockage of the opening by the lens. Argon laser peripheral iridoplasty may be considered for persistent appositional angle closure following the relief of pupillary block. Laser iridotomy is preferable to surgical iridectomy for the treatment of acute glaucoma secondary to pupillary block in this syndrome. It is to be expected, however, that because of the young age of many patients with this problem and the need to perform any procedure done with general anesthesia, the opportunity to choose laser iridotomy may not be available. If medical treatment has been unsuccessful in correcting the pupillary block in preparation for a surgical iridectomy, surgical relief of the block using a rounded spatula within the anterior chamber should be considered to allow a later surgical iridectomy to be done under more favorable circumstances. Miotics may be safely used in this syndrome after iridectomy or iridotomy to induce miosis and hold the lens behind the iris.

When there is inadequate control of medical treatment for chronic glaucoma, external filtration surgery will be necessary. The considerations relevant to such procedures performed with aphakia must be considered, especially in respect to the potential for vitreous entry into the anterior chamber and filter site.

Supportive. Careful screening of the relatives of patients with this syndrome is indicated. Children with threatening anterior segment findings may be asymptomatic and require prophylactic treatment. Other relatives may possess normal eyes and only the systemic features of this syndrome. Appropriate genetic counseling is indicated for all family members.

Ocular or Periocular Manifestations

Anterior Chamber: Abnormally shallow.
Ciliary Body: Prominence of the uveal meshwork in the ciliary body band region (infrequent).
Cornea: Megalocornea; microcornea; opacities related to lenticulocorneal contact.
Lens: Anterior displacement; inferior displacement; microspherophakia; punctate cortical opacities; increased thickness.
Optic Nerve: Glaucomatous cupping.
Other: Convex iris; lenticular myopia; pupillary block glaucoma; decreased ocular diameter.

PRECAUTIONS

Miotics often increase the severity of the pupillary block mechanism in this syndrome; increased iris-lens contact may develop secondary to the miosis and relaxation of the lens zonules. Angle-closure glaucoma also may be initiated by cycloplegia and pupillary dilation. Surgical iridectomy may be complicated by vitreous loss more readily in the presence of compromised zonules. Subluxation of the lens into the anterior chamber may occur and is not prevented by iridectomy.

COMMENTS

The poor visual prognosis in this disease is due in part to the frequently asymptomatic glaucoma early in life. Earlier surgical intervention would be beneficial, but the absence of a family history in this usually recessive inherited rare disorder has made early detection difficult. Certainly, all relatives of affected individuals should be evaluated thoroughly and treated appropriately. The high frequency of visual loss occurring before surgery, the fact that delay of surgery permits irreversible angle damage, and the potential favorable postoperative intraocular tension control emphasize the need for early diagnosis and surgical intervention in microspherophakic eyes with glaucoma.

References

Gorlin RJ, L'Heureux PR, Shapiro I: Weill-Marchesani syndrome of two generations: Genetic heterogeneity or pseudodominance? J Pediatr Ophthalmol 11:139–144, 1974.

Jensen AD, Cross HE, Paton D: Ocular complications in the Weill-Marchesani syndrome. Am J Ophthalmol 77:261–269, 1974.

Ritch R, Solomon LD: Argon laser peripheral iridoplasty for angle-closure glaucoma in siblings with Weill-Marchesani syndrome. J Glaucoma 1: 243–247, 1992.

Willi M, Kut L, Cotlier E: Pupillary-block glaucoma in the Marchesani syndrome. Arch Ophthalmol 90:504–508, 1973.

Wright KW, Chrousos GA: Weill-Marchesani syndrome with bilateral angle-closure glaucoma. J Pediatr Ophthalmol Strabismus 22:129–132, 1985.

SECTION 12

SKELETAL DISORDERS

ANKYLOSING SPONDYLITIS 720.0

DOUGLAS A. JABS, M.D.

Baltimore, Maryland

Ankylosing spondylitis is a chronic inflammatory disorder characterized by involvement of the cartilaginous joints of the axial skeleton. It is typically a disease of young people, with onset usually between 16 and 40 years of age. Although older studies suggested that men were affected far more often than women, it is now clear that women are affected nearly as often as men; however, women often have mild and/or atypical disease. Ankylosing spondylitis has a strong association with the histocompatibility antigen HLA-B27.

The susceptible joints in ankylosing spondylitis are the sacroiliac joints, the intervertebral spaces, and the apophyseal and costovertebral articulations. The most frequent manifestation is chronic low back pain. If the disease is persistent and untreated, it may progress over several years and cause loss of motion and fusion of involved joints. The end result is a fixed forward flexion of the spine and hips. Peripheral joints, particularly the shoulders, hips, and knees, can also be involved. A potentially severe manifestation of ankylosing spondylitis is cardiac involvement, which can result in heart block or hemodynamically significant aortic insufficiency.

The characteristic ocular manifestation of ankylosing spondylitis is recurrent acute iridocyclitis. Bouts of anterior segment inflammation usually involve only one eye at a time, and they often recur after a lapse of months to years. Both eyes may eventually be involved. In some patients, the repeated attacks of iridocyclitis are mild; in others, the attacks may be severe. Some patients develop a severe fibrinous exudate ("plastic iritis") or hypopyon. Posterior synechiae, band keratopathy, and rarely even phthisis bulbi can occur.

THERAPY

Systemic. Systemic antiinflammatory drugs are important in the treatment of ankylosing spondylitis. The most frequently used agent is indomethacin, at a dosage of 25 to 50 mg three times a day or as a 75-mg slow-release formulation once or twice daily. Phenylbutazone, at a dosage of 100 to 200 mg two times daily, is also very effective, but its use is limited due to its potential toxicity. A good therapeutic response to aspirin is unusual. If indomethacin is not tolerated, other nonsteroidal anti-inflammatory agents may be of value.

Ocular. The treatment of iridocyclitis associated with ankylosing spondylitis consists of local cycloplegics and topical corticosteroids. Cycloplegics are used to relieve ocular pain and to minimize the formation of posterior synechiae. Either a 1 per cent atropine or 0.25 per cent scopolamine ophthalmic solution, given two to four times daily, may be used. Topical corticosteroids are used to control inflammation. A suspension or solution of 1 per cent prednisolone seems to be most effective. One or two drops should be instilled in the affected eye to suppress the inflammation; generally the initial frequency is hourly or every 2 hours. Once the inflammation is quiet, topical corticosteroids should be tapered and discontinued.

Supportive. A daily exercise program designed to maintain chest expansibility, maximal spinal mobility, and a full range of motion of the proximal joints is the cornerstone of managing ankylosing spondylitis. Education of the patients and lifelong cooperative effort on their part are essential to successful therapy.

Ocular or Periocular Manifestations

Anterior Chamber: Aqueous flare and cells; hypopyon.
Cornea: Band keratopathy; keratic precipitates.
Iris: Anterior uveitis ("plastic iritis"); synechiae.
Other: Ocular pain; photophobia; scleritis; visual loss.

PRECAUTIONS

Topical steroids used to treat ocular inflammation should be tapered and withdrawn once the anterior chamber reaction clears and should be given again only if the inflammation recurs. Because the uveitis is usually acute and recurrent in nature, rather than chronic, long-term topical corticosteroid therapy can usually be avoided.

COMMENTS

A strong genetic component is present in the pathogenesis of ankylosing spondylitis, as demonstrated by the association of this condition with the antigen HLA-B27. Approximately 90 per cent of Caucasian patients and 50 per cent of African-American patients with ankylosing spondylitis are HLA-B27 positive, as compared to the 4 to 8 per cent prevalence of this gene in control populations. A similar relation with HLA-B27 antigen has been demonstrated for other spondylarthropathies, such as Reiter's syndrome and psoriatic spondylitis.

There is no clear evidence that systemic anti-inflammatory drugs alter the natural history of the disease; their major role is in the relief of pain and stiffness, thus allowing the patient to pursue an exercise program and maintain a normal lifestyle. For this reason, such drugs are valuable.

Iridocyclitis occurs in about 25 per cent of patients with ankylosing spondylitis. Furthermore, studies of patients with "idiopathic" acute nongranulomatous iridocyclitis demonstrate a high frequency (over 50 per cent) of subtle clinical, radiographic, or scintigraphic evidence of spondylarthropathy or the presence of HLA-B27 (about 50 per cent). Therefore, the possibility of ankylosing spondylitis should be considered in any young person presenting with acute iridocyclitis, and appropriate clinical and radiologic investigations should be obtained.

References

Calin A: Ankylosing spondylitis. In Kelley WN, Harris ED Jr, Ruddy S, Sledge CD (eds): Textbook of Rheumatology, 3rd ed. Philadelphia, WB Saunders, 1989, pp 1021–1037.
Jabs DA: The rheumatic diseases. In Tasman W, Jaeger EA (eds): Duane's Clinical Ophthalmology. Philadelphia, JB Lippincott, 1992, Vol 5, pp 1–39.
Kimura SJ, et al: Uveitis and joint diseases: A review of 191 cases. Trans Am Ophthalmol Soc 64: 291–310, 1966.
Russell AS, et al: Scintigraphy of sacroiliac joints in acute anterior uveitis. A study of thirty patients. Ann Intern Med 85:606–608, 1976.
Watson PG, Hazleman BL: The Sclera and Systemic Disorders. Philadelphia, WB Saunders, 1976, pp 246–252.

COCKAYNE'S SYNDROME 759.8

WILLIAM H. COLES, M.D., M.S.

Buffalo, New York

Although the condition can be present at birth or detected at exam in the first year of life, children with Cockayne's syndrome have a normal birth and normal development until the second year or later when their growth is retarded and the full syndrome becomes apparent. Dwarfism, with disproportionately large hands and feet, is the predominant feature; beak-like noses, sunken eyes, and the prominent jaws of prognathism with associated dental malocclusion and carious teeth are common manifestations. The head is microcephalic, and progressive retardation develops. Additional signs that are not present in all patients include photosensitivity, hypertension, and emphysema. By the second decade, these children appear severely aged. They rarely live beyond 20 years. Pneumonia is a common cause of death.

Although the condition is rare, reported cases have established an autosomal recessive inheritance from the following characteristics: frequent occurrence in siblings, an equal sex distribution, and a not infrequent history of parent consanguinity of affected children. Examination of the amniotic cells from the uterus of a high-risk mother may help in establishing a prenatal diagnosis of Cockayne's syndrome.

Cockayne's syndrome should not be confused with progeria (premature aging) or Seckel (bird-headed) dwarfism.

THERAPY

Ocular. If corneal changes occur that may be due to corneal drying, artificial tears or mild ophthalmic ointments are indicated.

Surgical. Both acquired and congenital cataracts of severe enough density to require surgery have been reported. No corneal transplant has been required for corneal changes. Cosmetic surgery is not indicated.

Supportive. Guidance and support help parents deal with the progressive retardation. The children usually have a pleasant and very social nature, and they can frequently be cared for at home until the very late stages of their disease, despite their retardation. Genetic counseling is also indicated if parents are planning to have other children.

Ocular or Periocular Manifestations

Cornea: Keratoconjunctivitis sicca; opacity.
Lens: Nuclear, zonular, and fleck cataracts.
Optic Nerve: Atrophy; pallor.
Retina: Attenuation of vessels; spotty "peppered" pigmentary degeneration of the posterior pole.
Other: Enophthalmos; exotropia; nystagmus (usually pendular).

PRECAUTIONS

Cataract extraction in the late stages of the disease should be considered carefully. Frequently, retinal and optic nerve changes contribute more to visual loss than do cataracts, and in many of these patients, cataract removal has a very poor visual prognosis. The emphysema and hypertension that occur in these patients also make them poor anesthesia risks, especially in the second decade of life.

COMMENTS

Cultured skin fibroblasts from patients with Cockayne's syndrome are hypersensitive to lethal effects of ultraviolet (UV) irradiation and UV-mimetic chemicals, a feature shared with xeroderma pigmentosa. Cells also show depressed RNA and DNA synthesis after UV irradiation. However, other features of cultured cells (fibroblasts and lymphocytes) differ between the two diseases; clinically, in Cockayne's syndrome patients, there is no increase in carcinogenesis, as is seen in xeroderma pigmentosa patients.

The pathology in the central nervous system is patchy tigroid demyelination similar to Pelizaeus-Merzbacher disease; however, there are few clinical similarities between these two conditions. Enlarged ventricles are also a feature of Cockayne's syndrome, but the clinical changes are not caused by hydrocephalus.

In Cockayne's syndrome, calcifications may be found in the basal ganglion, cerebellum, and cerebrum. Magnetic resonance imaging has recently been shown to be particularly effective in demonstrating central nervous system lesions. Also, tapering of the thoracic vertebral bodies and a steeping of the iliac crest in the small pelvis are seen as the disease progresses.

References

Boltshauser E, et al: MRI in Cockayne syndrome type I. Neuroradiology 31:276–277, 1989.

Cheng WS, et al: Ultraviolet light-induced sister chromatid exchanges in xeroderma pigmentosum and in Cockayne's syndrome lymphocyte cells lines. Cancer Res 38:1601–1609, 1978.

Coles WH: Ocular manifestations of Cockayne's syndrome. Am J Ophthalmol 67:762–764, 1969.

Jaeken J, et al: Clinical and biochemical studies in three patients with severe early infantile Cockayne syndrome. Hum Genet 83:339–346, 1989.

Lambert WC: Genetic diseases associated with DNA and chromosomal instability. Dermatol Clin 5:85–105, 1987.

Patton MA, et al: Early onset Cockayne's syndrome: Case reports with neuropathological and fibroblast studies. J Med Genet 26:154–159, 1989.

Pearce WG: Ocular and genetic features of Cockayne's syndrome. Can J Ophthalmol 7:435–444, 1972.

Riggs W Jr, Seibert J: Cockayne's Syndrome. Roentgen findings. Am J Roentgenol 116:623–633, 1972.

Schmickel RD, et al: Cockayne syndrome: A cellular sensitivity to ultraviolet light. Pediatrics 60:135–139, 1977.

Soffer D, et al: Cockayne syndrome: Unusual neuropathological findings and review of the literature. Ann Neurol 6:340–348, 1979.

Timme TL, Moses RE: Review: Diseases with DNA damage-processing defects. Am J Med Sci 295:40–48, 1988.

DOWN'S SYNDROME 758.0
(Mongolism, Trisomy 21)

EDWARD A. JAEGER, M.D.

Philadelphia, Pennsylvania

Down, in 1866, first ascribed the term "mongolism" to those with short stature, mental deficiency, and mongolian features. It was the first multisystem disease syndrome to be related to abnormal chromosome numbers. Several chromosome patterns are found in Down's syndrome. The most common is tripling of chromosome 21, which is found in 95 per cent of those with mongolism; hence, the more appropriate title, trisomy 21. A total chromosome number of 47 is present in all cells, rather than the normal 46. A second pattern, termed "translocation," occurs when the extra chromosome 21 becomes attached to another chromosome. In this case, the total number of chromosomes is 46. A third pattern results if the failure in chromosome separation occurs in a cell division after fertilization. Some cells then contain the normal 46 chromosomes, whereas others contain 47. These individuals are termed "mosaics." There are no significant clinical differences, including the eye findings, among these chromosomal patterns.

The physical appearance of those with Down's syndrome is easily recognizable and characteristic. Nonophthalmologic physical features include an anteriorly and posteriorly flattened head, fissured and protruding tongue, short broad neck, dry skin, shortened extremities and phalanges, simian palmar crease, cardiac disorders, and a wide variation in the degree of mental retardation (an I.Q. below 60 to 70). Premature aging is frequent, and Alzheimer's disease is not an uncommon finding.

The ocular findings in Down's syndrome include epicanthus, upward and outward slanting of palpebral fissures, external infections, keratoconus, Brushfield's spots, strabismus, high refractive errors, nystagmus, lacrimal obstruction cataracts, and an increase in the number of small retinal vessels radiating from the disc. Ocular abnormalities due to self-inflicted trauma may also be seen.

THERAPY

Ocular. The commonly encountered external ocular problems of blepharitis, styes, chalazions, and conjunctivitis are treated in the standard manner. In the therapy of these conditions, it is important to remember that the use of corticosteroids can contribute to the development of a herpes simplex keratitis in patients with Down's syndrome.

Surgical. Although surgical corrections of ocular manifestations of Down's syndrome may result in a more productive life for these individuals, there is no specific therapy.

Those with keratoconus must be watched for the development of hydrops and corneal perforation. Corneal transplant is indicated in impending perforation or severe scarring. Traumatic ocular injuries should be treated in the usual manner.

High refractive errors, such as myopia, hyperopia, and astigmatism, are common, but high myopia seems to be predominant. There is some evidence that early correction of high refractive errors leads to a better visual and neurosensory environmental adjustment.

Full hypermetropic correction should be tried in those cases of accommodative estropia. The surgical correction of nonaccommodative estropia is indicated in selected cases. However, bifoveal fixation is seldom achieved after surgery. Patching for amblyopia is difficult, but may be attempted in those patients with a strongly supportive environment. Fortunately, profound amblyopia secondary to strabismus is less frequent than might be anticipated in those with Down's syndrome.

Lacrimal surgery must be approached with caution as excessive bleeding in the immediate postoperative phase may be encountered.

The development of senile cataracts presents special problems in patients with trisomy 21. These patients seem to age more rapidly, and lens opacification is another manifestation of this process. Better general medical care, along with improved family and institutional awareness, has increased the life expectancy of many persons with Down's syndrome; hence, there is a greater incidence of cataracts in this group.

Cataract extraction is indicated when vision has deteriorated to the point that self-care and general function are significantly impaired. Since family members or attendants are often in the best position to evaluate visual function, the ophthalmologist should rely heavily on their input. Phacoemulsification with posterior chamber lens implantation offers the advantage of smaller incision size, although a standard extracapsular procedure with a secure wound is suitable. Some consideration should be given to posterior capsulotomy at the time of surgery as subsequent YAG laser capsulotomy may be difficult. The use of anterior chamber lenses presents some additional concerns. If an intraoperative complication has occurred and there is inadequate posterior capsule support, it may be best not to implant an intraocular lens. Many patients with Down's syndrome do well as aphakes, even without correction. Since general anesthesia is required, the presence of a close family member or familiar attendant is absolutely necessary for a reasonably calm pre- and postoperative period. Returning the patient to familiar surroundings, preferably the same day, is also helpful; likewise, a well-sutured wound provides for surgeon tranquility. It is surprising how well some of these patients tolerate the procedure. Careful planning is imperative, however.

Supportive. Those with Down's syndrome are susceptible to respiratory infections and cardiac problems and have a higher incidence of leukemia. The trend in management of multiple handicapped individuals is to return as many systems as possible to normal early in life. This philosophy holds true for those with Down's syndrome, although it must be judiciously applied to the individual.

The ophthalmologist often is asked to examine patients with Down's syndrome early in life because of manifest or pseudo strabismus. An awareness of the ocular and systemic problems is helpful in further counseling of parents.

There is some evidence that those persons with Down's syndrome who are raised in an understanding and supportive environment achieve a greater degree of adjustment and advancement than institutionalized persons. Day schools and work centers have also been quite successful in contributing to the development and social adjustment of these individuals.

Ocular or Periocular Manifestations

Cornea: Keratoconus.
Extraocular Muscles: Accommodative or nonaccommodative esotropia; nystagmus.
Eyelids: Blepharitis; chalazion; epicanthus; hordeolum; lateral upward slope of palpebral fissures; entropion; trichiasis; ectropion.
Iris: Brushfield's spots; hypoplasia.
Lacrimal System: Obstruction of nasolacrimal duct or canaliculi.
Lens: Cataracts.
Retina: Detachment; vascular proliferation (radiating in spoke-like fashion from the disc).
Other: Astigmatism; conjunctivitis; hyperopia; myopia; infantile glaucoma.

PRECAUTIONS

Persons with Down's syndrome have been thought to be unusually sensitive to atropine, which produces a rapid heart rate. However, this has not been found in controlled studies involving systemic and topically administered atropine. The possibility of unreported ocular trauma must be kept in mind. When ocular surgery is performed on patients with Down's syndrome, every contingency must be anticipated in the immediate pre- and postoperative periods. Familiar surroundings and attendants are the best precautions.

COMMENTS

Down's syndrome occurs once in every 600 to 700 live births; however, because of patients increased life span, the percentage of the population with Down's syndrome has increased. It has been associated with increased maternal age; in one study, the maternal age for Down's births was found to be 34.43 years compared to 28.17 years for normal births.

Recently discovered biochemical changes in the serum of mothers with a Down's syndrome fetus have improved the reliability of prenatal screening. Pregnant women with positive serum screening results, as well as those at significant risk of bearing a trisomy 21 child, should be offered amniocentesis. Improved techniques of amniocentesis with chromosomal mapping analysis and chorionic villus biopsy utilizing DNA analysis have resulted in safe and increasingly accurate diagnosis of Down's syndrome, as well as a wide variety of other genetic disorders.

References

Behrman RE, Kliegman RM: Nelson Textbook of Pediatrics, 14th ed. Philadelphia, WB Saunders, 1992, pp 282–284.

Caputo AR, et al: Down syndrome. Clinical review of ocular features. Clin Pediatr 28:355–358, 1989.

Down JL: Observations on the ethnic classification of idiots. London Hosp Rep, 3:259–262, 1866.

Frantz JM, et al: Penetrating keratoplasty in Down's syndrome. Am J Ophthalmol 109:143–147, 1990.

Haddiwm JE, et al: Prenatal screening for Down's syndrome with use of maternal serum markers. N Engl J Med 327:588–593, 1992.

Jaeger EA: Ocular findings in down's syndrome. Trans Am Ophthalmol Soc 78:808–845, 1980.

Nelson LB, Calhoun JH, Harley RD: Pediatric Ophthalmology, 3rd ed. Philadelphia, WB Saunders, 1991, pp 31–34.

Nelson LB, Jackson LG: Techniques in prenatal genetic diagnosis. *In* Tasman W, Jaeger EA (eds): Foundations of Clinical Ophthalmology. Philadelphia, JB Lippincott, 1992, Vol 3, pp 1274–1301.

Shapiro MB, France TD: The ocular features of Down's syndrome. Am J Ophthalmol 99:659–663, 1985.

ENGELMANN'S DISEASE 756.59

(Camurati-Engelmann's Disease, Diaphyseal Dysplasia, Hereditary Diaphyseal Dysplasia, Hereditary Multiple Diaphyseal Sclerosis, Hyperostosis Corticalis Generalisata Familiaris, Juvenile Paget's Disease, Osteopathia Hyperostotica Sclerotisans Multiplex Infantilis, Progressive Hyperostosis)

PETER H. MORSE, M.D., F.A.C.S.

Sioux Falls, South Dakota

Engelmann's disease is a rare, usually progressive bone dystrophy of unknown etiology that is included in a spectrum of disorders known as the craniotubular (osteosclerotic) dysplasias. Uncertainty in the diagnosis exists in some of the reported cases, and several diseases having similar manifestations may have been described under this eponym. Radiographs demonstrate a symmetric, spindle-shaped, sclerotic, cortical thickening of the intermediate segment of the shaft of the long tubular bones. With progression, the osteo sclerosis extends proximally and distally. The base of the skull, calvarium, mandible, cervical vertebrae, clavicles, and bones of the pelvis are often involved. The scapulae, ribs, and bones of the hands and feet are rarely affected.

The various clinical symptoms and signs are pain in the limbs, easy fatigability, delayed ambulation, generalized neuromuscular weakness, inability to run, broad-based waddling gait, thin legs, poor musculature and disproportionately long limbs, bowing of the tibiae, abnormal deep tendon reflexes, hepatosplenomegaly, failure to thrive, delayed puberty, hypogonadism, delay of secondary sex characteristics after apparent early sexual precocity, dry skin, absence of subcutaneous fat, delayed dentition, hypoplasia of the enamel of the upper front teeth, carious teeth, exophthalmos, papilledema, optic atrophy, and deafness.

The age of patients ranges from 3 months to 57 years with a mean age of 19.2 years. There is a slightly greater prevalence of males than females, and the disease is predominantly seen in Caucasians. Hereditary transmission is not definitely established and may be variable. Several families with an autosomal dominant pattern have been reported. The penetrance and expressivity, the spectrum of manifestations, the severity of the disease, and the rate of progression may vary. The severe form in older age may resemble myelosclerosis, chronic sclerosing osteitis, tertiary syphilis, or osteoblastic carcinomatosis.

THERAPY

Systemic. The progression and degree of activity of the disease should be determined by clinical, radiologic, and laboratory examination before any therapy is begun. Treatment should be directed toward the demonstrated activity or a dynamic process. Corticosteroids have been used in an attempt to suppress bone formation and increase resorption with a calciuric effect. The dosage is 0.5 to 2.0 mg/kg of oral prednisone daily. If there is evidence of abnormal phosphate metabolism, aluminum hydroxide or probenecid might be useful. In the absence of hypocalcemia, a diet low in calcium with cellulose phosphate may be tried. The rapid regrowth of bones may be controlled with diphosphonates. The use of calcitonin and etidronate disodium (EHDP) seems illogical unless the specific medication is used with respect to bone formation activity.

Ocular. Secondary glaucoma may be

treated with antiglaucomatous medications. One must be aware of the possibility of induced secondary glaucoma in patients undergoing corticosteroid therapy. If the glaucoma is caused by an increased pressure on the globe secondary to bony overgrowth that creates decreased orbital volume, a surgical decompression may be necessary.

Surgical. Luxation of the globe may require surgery. Lysis of the lateral canthal tendon and resection of Müller's muscle may prevent exposure of the cornea. With progression of the disease, these procedures may not be permanently effective. Orbital decompression may be necessary to counteract secondary glaucoma, and unroofing of the optic canal has been used to alleviate disc edema. However, the rapid regrowth of bone renders this surgical therapy only temporarily successful.

Ocular or Periocular Manifestations

Extraocular Muscles: Convergence insufficiency; diplopia; palsy of lateral rectus muscle.
Eyelids: Lagophthalmos; ptosis; skin atrophy.
Globe: Luxation.
Optic Nerve: Disc edema; pallor or atrophy; vascular tortuosity.
Orbit: Exophthalmos; proptosis; secondary hypertelorism.
Other: Cataracts; decreased visual acuity; epiphora; irritation; secondary glaucoma.

PRECAUTIONS

No specific etiology or effective therapy exists for Engelmann's disease. Patients being treated with systemic corticosteroids must always be observed for the potential complications of glaucoma or cataract.

COMMENTS

Despite the fact that the underlying metabolic defect in Engelmann's disease is unknown, most of the clinical signs and symptoms are a result of the osteosclerotic process and bony overgrowth. This is particularly true of the ocular manifestations, which are the consequence of the physical limitation of the size of the orbit and compression of the nerves.

References

Brodrick JD: Luxation of the globe in Engelmann's disease. Am J Ophthalmol 83:870–873, 1977.
Hundley JD, Wilson FC: Progressive diaphyseal dysplasia. Review of the literature and report of seven cases in one family. J Bone Joint Surg 55-A:461–474, 1973.
Krohel GB, Wirth CR: Engelmann's disease. Am J Ophthalmol 84:520–525, 1977.
Kumar B, Murphy WA, Whyte MP: Progressive diaphyseal dysplasia (Engelmann disease): Scintigraphic-radiographic-clinical correlations. Radiology 140:87–92, 1981.
Morse PH, Walsh FB, McCormick JR: Ocular findings in hereditary diaphyseal dysplasia (Engelmann's disease). Am J Ophthalmol 68:100–104, 1969.
Ramon Y, Buchner A: Camurati-Engelmann's disease affecting the jaws. Oral Surg 22:592–599, 1966.
Smith R, et al: Clinical and biochemical studies in Engelmann's disease (Progressive diaphyseal dysplasia). Q J Med 46:273–294, 1977.
Yoshioka H, et al: Muscular changes in Engelmann's disease. Arch Dis Child 55:716–719, 1980.

HALLERMANN-STREIFF-FRANCOIS SYNDROME 756.0
(Francois-Hallermann-Streiff Syndrome, Francois Syndrome, Hallermann-Streiff Syndrome, Mandibulo-Oculofacial Dyscephaly, Mandibulo-Oculofacial Dysmorphia)

DAVID J. HOPKINS, M.B., Ch.B., F.R.C.S., F.R.C.Ophth.

Bradford, England

The Hallermann-Streiff-Francois syndrome is characterized by dyscephaly with bird-like facies; atrophy of the skin; hypotrichosis; dental anomalies; proportionate dwarfism; cataract, and other ocular abnormalities. A well-documented problem is spontaneous cataract absorption leading to hypersensitivity to lens matter and loss of vision from chronic uveitis with severe secondary glaucoma.

THERAPY

Ocular. Miotics, 1 per cent epinephrine, and in older patients, beta blockers, may be used to reduce intraocular pressure. Corticosteroids are used if uveitis is present.

Systemic. A carbonic anhydrase inhibitor, such as acetazolamide, 25 mg/kg/day in divided doses, may be helpful if local medications do not control the glaucoma.

Surgical. Early bilateral lensectomy is recommended to reduce the risk of spontaneous cataract absorption and the loss of vision from uveitis with secondary glaucoma, and suppression amblyopia. Surgical treatment of established secondary glaucoma is unlikely to be successful. Strabismus may be treated surgically. Mandibular advancement may improve the airway and the patient's appearance.

Supportive. Patients who have had cataracts removed require frequent, regular follow-up examinations to ensure that if intraocular inflammation and secondary glaucoma occur, diagnosis and treatment are prompt. Spectacle and, where possible, contact lens correction of aphakia should be carried out as soon as possible after surgery. Orthoptic support is necessary to optimize visual acuity.

Ocular or Periocular Manifestations

Adnexae: Cutaneous atrophy; sparse eyebrows and eyelashes; antimongoloid slant.
Choroid: Coloboma; peripapillary choroidal atrophy.
Cornea: Microcornea; sclerocornea; keratoglobus.
Globes: Microphthalmos; occasional buphthalmos; blue scleral coloration; raised pressure.
Iris: Atrophy; coloboma; aniridia; granulomatous anterior uveitis; synechiae.
Media: Cataract; lens and capsular remnants; persistent pupillary membrane; vitreous degeneration.
Ocular Posture: Nystagmus; strabismus.
Orbit: Reduced intraorbital distance.
Retina: Folds; abnormal pigmentation.
Vision: Impaired.
Other: Abnormal anterior chamber angle; optic disc coloboma.

PRECAUTIONS

The ophthalmic surgeon should not delay intervention in the hope of a spontaneous cataract absorption occurring, because the attendant chronic uveitis and refractory secondary glaucoma will lead to the irreversible loss of sight. Airway management will present difficulties for the anesthesiologist.

COMMENTS

When the ocular manifestations of the Hallermann-Streiff-Francois syndrome are extensive, the therapeutic possibilities are limited and the visual prognosis is poor. Early cataract surgery is imperative to restore function and obviate blinding complications.

References

Cohen MM Jr: Hallermann-Streiff syndrome: A review. Am J Med Genet 41:488–499, 1991.
Francois J: A new syndrome: Dyscephalia with bird face and dental anomalies, nanism, hypotrichosis, cutaneous atrophy, microphthalmia and congenital cataract. Arch Ophthalmol 60:842, 1958.
Francois J: François dyscephalic syndrome. Birth defects. March of Dimes Birth Defects Foundation. Original article series 18:595–619, 1982.
Hopkins DJ, Horan EC: Glaucoma in the Hallermann-Streiff syndrome. Br J Ophthalmol 54:416–422, 1970.
Sataloff RT, Roberts BR: Airway management in Hallermann-Streiff syndrome. Am J Otolaryngol 5:64–67, 1984.
Schanzlin DJ, Goldberg DB, Brown SI: Hallermann-Streiff syndrome associated with sclerocornea, aniridia and a chromosomal abnormality. Am J Ophthalmol 90:411–415, 1980.
Sugar A, Bigger JF, Podos SM: Hallermann-Streiff-Francois syndrome. J Pediatr Ophthalmol 8:234–238, 1971.

MANDIBULOFACIAL DYSOSTOSIS 756.0
(Berry Syndrome, Franceschetti Syndrome, Treacher Collins Syndrome)

TREVOR H. KIRKHAM, M.D., D.O., F.R.C.S.

Montreal, Quebec

Mandibulofacial dysostosis is a congenital anomaly caused by the effects of an incompletely penetrant dominant autosomal gene with pleiotropic manifestations. The major effects of the gene are to retard fusion of the embryonic facial clefts and to inhibit development of the facial bones derived from the first branchial arch. The syndrome is characterized by hypoplasia of the maxilla and mandible, malformation of the pinnae, and a beaked nose. There is a marked antimongoloid obliquity of the palpebral fissures, characteristically with a pronounced coloboma of the outer third of the lower lids. The mouth appears wide and fishlike. The hairline projects prominently in front of the ears onto the cheeks. A high arched palate and dental abnormalities may be present. There are sometimes blind fistulas on the cheeks between the ears and the angles of the mouth. Conductive deafness resulting from malformation of the ossicular chain may be present. Less commonly, other skeletal anomalies occur. The ophthalmic problem is usually cosmetic. Recognition of the syndrome is clinical, and there are no reported biochemical or chromosomal abnormalities.

THERAPY

Surgical. A team approach of orbitocraniofacial surgery may produce dramatic cosmetic improvement in the facial appearance. Detailed preoperative ophthalmic examination, particularly of ocular alignment and the lacrimal system, is a medicolegal safeguard. Otolaryngologic reconstruction of the ossicular chain may be possible. The eyelid defects may be repaired at an early stage, sometimes after initial build-up of the hypoplastic maxilla by cartilage or other tissue. Various methods have been suggested for the repair of colobomas, including full-thickness skin grafts and transposition of flaps. Early repair of extensive colobomas is recommended to obviate corneal damage. Sometimes, the antimongoloid slant of the palpebral fissures may be lifted.

Supportive. The unusual facial appearance and possible deafness may lead to a mistaken diagnosis of mental retardation. Early evaluation of hearing is necessary; if there seems to be a speech problem, speech therapy is essential. Psychiatric help and genetic counseling are recommended for the patients and their families.

Ocular or Periocular Manifestations

Extraocular Muscles: Strabismus; underdeveloped orbicularis oculi muscle.
Eyelids: Antimongoloid slant; coloboma of temporal third of lower lid.
Lens: Cataract; ectopia.

PRECAUTIONS

Early recognition of the syndrome is important, since children born into affected families should be examined for deafness at an early age. A series of reconstructive procedures must usually be undertaken, some during infancy and childhood and others deferred until adolescence or adult life.

COMMENTS

Many incomplete forms of the syndrome have been described, and patients displaying all the manifestations of the syndrome are rare.

References

Kirkham TH: Mandibulofacial dysostosis with ectopia lentis. Am J Ophthalmol 70:947–949, 1970.
Rogers BO: The surgical treatment of mandibulofacial dysostosis (Berry syndrome: Treacher Collins syndrome; Franceschetti-Zwahlen-Klein syndrome). Clin Plast Surg 3:653–666, 1976.

OCULOAURICULO-VERTEBRAL DYSPLASIA
756.0
(Goldenhar's Syndrome)

CHARLES R. LEONE JR., M.D.

San Antonio, Texas

Oculoauriculovertebral dysplasia (Goldenhar's syndrome) is a disorder characterized by a triad of anomalies: epibulbar dermoids or dermolipomas, deformity of the ears, and vertebral skeletal defects. The syndrome does not seem to be inherited as most cases have been sporadic, with males being affected in 60 per cent of cases. The disease is usually unilateral, although the epibulbar dermoids may occur bilaterally in 25 per cent of patients. The epibulbar dermoids are typically located in the lower temporal limbal area and are present in 75 per cent of cases. The dermolipomas are less frequent, occupy the upper lateral fornix, and are usually unilateral. Rarely, they occupy the lateral fornix and distort the lateral canthal angle. Upper eyelid colobomas are present in 25 per cent of cases, are unilateral, and occur in the medial aspect of the upper lid. There is also a significant incidence of lacrimal obstruction of the affected side, usually in the nasolacrimal duct.

The ear deformity consists of preauricular appendages, misshapen ears due to hypoplasia of the pinna, and absent external auditory meati. There may also be a suggestion of hemifacial microsomia. Cervical vertebral anomalies consisting of fusion of the vertebrae, hemivertebrae, and occipitalization of the atlas may be present.

THERAPY

Ocular. Rarely, decreased corneal sensitivity may require ocular lubricants to moisten and lubricate the eyes. Either 0.5 per cent methylcellulose solution or petrolatum ointment may be applied several times daily.

Surgical. If the limbal epibulbar dermoids are producing visual disturbance or an obvious cosmetic blemish, they can be excised. It is important to keep in mind that limbal dermoids may involve the entire thickness of the cornea. Therefore, it is advisable to remove only the part that is elevated from the cornea, followed by the use of the diamond burr to smooth the surface flush with the normal cornea. If a large area of cornea is involved, it may be necessary to do a lamellar transplant.

Dermolipomas that bulge between the lids temporally should be removed with caution. If there is a pilosebaceous area with cilia present, it can be removed along with the lipomatous mass underlying the conjunctiva. Large excisions of the epidermalized conjunctiva should be avoided, as should excision of fat beyond the anterior orbit. Those lesions that distort the lateral canthal angle will require excision as well as canthoplasty to reform the canthus.

Repair of the upper eyelid coloboma is dependent on the size and degree of corneal exposure. Small colobomas are better left alone. If the defect involves the entire tarsus but the cornea is protected, the repair can be done when the child is a good anesthetic risk. If the cornea shows signs of mechanical injury or exposure keratopathy despite lubricants, repair should be undertaken. It is necessary to freshen the edges of the coloboma vertically to prevent notching, and possibly stay sutures should be used across the incision to prevent separation. With the large defects, it may be necessary to do a canthotomy and cantholysis in order to close the defect.

Lacrimal obstruction is usually not amenable to probing, and dacryocystorhinostomy is usually necessary.

Supportive. Parents should be aware that only 10 per cent of those affected with oculoauriculovertebral dysplasia may be retarded.

Ocular or Periocular Manifestations

Choroid: Coloboma.
Conjunctiva: Dermolipoma; epibulbar dermoid.
Cornea: Dermoid; hypesthesia; keratoconus; microcornea.
Extraocular Muscles: Duane's retraction syndrome; strabismus.
Eyelids: Coloboma (upper eyelid); ptosis.
Globe: Anophthalmos; exophthalmos; microphthalmia.
Iris: Atrophy; coloboma.
Lacrimal System: Dacryocystitis; obstruction of nasolacrimal duct; punctal or canalicular atresia or absence.
Orbit: Dermolipoma; hypoplasia.
Other: Amblyopia; astigmatism; cataract; persistent pupillary membrane.

PRECAUTIONS

Because of cervical vertebral abnormalities, the neck may not extend sufficiently, making intubation for general anesthesia very difficult. Tracheostomy may be necessary in these cases.

Care must be exercised in approaching limbal dermoids; since many of them involve full-thickness cornea, corneal perforation may result from attempting complete removal. It is far better to remove only the part that protrudes from the corneal surface. In some cases after surgery, there can be conjunctival overgrowth resembling a pterygium.

Radical excision of a dermolipoma could result in foreshortening of the lateral fornix, inadvertent removal of the palpebral portion of the lacrimal gland, or injury to the levator or lateral rectus muscles. Therefore, removal of only the part that is visible between the eyelids is recommended.

Although most colobomas will not produce exposure keratopathy, large colobomas must be watched closely for signs of exposure, especially those that are close to the midline. After repairing a coloboma, there can be tethering of the upper eyelid, which could result in a ptosis that may require correction in the future.

COMMENTS

Corneal dermoids cause a disturbance of vision by encroachment on the visual axis or distortion by the induced astigmatism. Despite removal, strabismus and amblyopia may follow and require further therapy.

The diagnosis of Goldenhar's syndrome should lead to complete examination for associated systemic abnormalities, especially cardiovascular, renal, genitourinary, and gastrointestinal defects.

References

Bowen DI, Collum LMT, Rees DO: Clinical aspects of oculo-auriculo-vertebral dysplasia. Br J Ophthalmol 55:145–154, 1971.
Geeraets WJ: Ocular Syndromes, 3rd ed. Philadelphia, Lea & Febiger, 1976, p 194.
Mortada A: Orbital dermo-lipoma with Goldenhar's syndrome and exophthalmos. Br J Ophthalmol 53:786–788, 1969.
Peyman GA, Sanders DR, Goldberg MF (eds): Principles and Practice of Ophthalmology. Philadelphia, WB Saunders, 1980, pp 2235, 2409.
Sargent RA, Ousterhout DK: Ocular manifestations of skeletal diseases. In Harley RD (ed): Pediatric Ophthalmology, 2nd ed. Philadelphia, WB Saunders, 1983, pp 1041–1044.
Zion VM, Billet E: Musculoskeletal disorders. In Duane TD (ed): Clinical Ophthalmology. Hagerstown, MD, Harper & Row, 1982, Vol V, pp 29: 1–20.

ORBITAL HYPERTELORISM 376.41
(Greig's Syndrome)

LOIS A. LLOYD, M.D., F.R.C.S.(C), *and* RAYMOND BUNCIC, M.D., F.R.C.S.(C)

Toronto, Ontario

Orbital hypertelorism is an abnormally increased distance between the orbits. It is an indicator of craniofacial anomaly and produces a significant cosmetic facial defect. Orbital hypertelorism can be classified on the basis of unilateral or bilateral orbital displacement, its severity of deformity, or axial rotation. Tessier has ranked the severity of deformity according to the interorbital distance: first degree, 30 to 34 mm; second degree, 34 to 40 mm; and third degree, greater than 40 mm. However, these distances are only applicable to adults and must be scaled downward for children and infants. The orbital displacement may be uniaxial in the lateral plane, but it is more frequently polyaxial with the lateral orbital wall rotated posteriorly. There may also be vertical rotation or displacement causing three-dimensional malposition of the orbit.

Orbital hypertelorism has been ascribed to arrested development of the first brachial arch. This produces a deficiency in the midline that allows the brain to herniate anteroinferior and to intrude between the orbits, preventing their forward growth during embryonic and fetal life. A facial cleft may also be present.

Hypertelorism seldom exists alone. Associated cranial anomalies include encephaloceles that deform the malar, sphenoidal, and frontal bones; brachycephaly that stretches the supraorbital arch and flattens the supraorbital rims; or gigantic frontal bone pneumatization and widened ethmoidal cells that displace the orbits laterally. Orbital hypertelorism may be associated with craniostenosis in which the volume of the cranial vault is decreased and intracranial pressure is occasionally increased. Crouzon's disease, Apert's syndrome, Englemann's disease, and Aarskrog's syndrome may manifest hypertelorism secondary to craniostenosis. Rarely, hypertelorism is secondary to fibrous dysplasia or trauma.

THERAPY

Surgical. Clinical measurements alone are inadequate criteria for recommending surgery. Roentgenographic methods of measuring hypertelorism are difficult if the dacryon is masked by ethmoidal air cells or basal tomograms are not available. Similarly, magnified photographs fail to demonstrate the facial midline accurately, making photographic intercanthal measurements unreliable. The real indications for cosmetic surgery are the relationship between the interorbital distance and width of the skull—that is, the general proportions of the child's head and face—the patient's social acceptance by others, as well as his or her success in maintaining binocular vision.

The clinical assessment and management of patients with hypertelorism should be done by a craniofacial reconstruction team consisting of the following: plastic surgeon, neurosurgeon, neuro-ophthalmologist, neuro-otologist, dentist, radiologist, psychiatrist, psychologist, geneticist, anthropologist, medical photographer, speech therapist, social worker, and cosmetologist. A medical illustrator projects possible changes by imposing an overlay on a photograph of the patient. A Styrofoam model of the patient's face outlines contours from the stereophotographs of the face, which are transferred to a terraced model done to actual scale. The model can be cut in all dimensions and the parts moved to correct the facial deformity. Once plans are complete and the social and psychologic factors are considered, correction is undertaken surgically by a team of neurosurgeon and plastic surgeon.

The operation is usually performed at the age of 2 years. In children younger than 2 years, the cranium is too small to produce successful results. The entire operation is done without external scars on the nose or cheeks. It is performed under hypotensive anesthesia in approximately 5 hours. The scalp incision is made from ear to ear, and skin is turned forward over the face. A frontal bone flap is raised by the neurosurgeon so that the frontal lobes can be retracted from the orbital roofs. The bony forehead can then be advanced or recessed as necessary. The plastic surgeon separates the orbital soft tissues from the bony orbits by subperiosteal dissection, using an incision through the lower fornices and proceeding as far back as the superior orbital fissures. The apex of the orbits and the orbital nerves remain untouched. The incisions through the bony orbital walls anterior to the superior orbital fissures allow displacement of the orbits as a bony box-like unit in any direction—medially, upward, downward, or obliquely.

The U-shaped osteotomy is used for minor corrections up to 15 mm. It mobilizes the lateral orbital wall, the inferior orbital rim and floor, and the medial orbital wall as a single block. Medial orbital wall migration can be augmented by medial movement of the lateral orbital wall or by insertion of a bone graft to the lateral orbital wall. The extracranial technique can be used only if there is no prolapse of the cribriform plate between the medial orbital walls. The intracranial technique of Tessier and Converse mobilizes the majority of the orbit as a box.

The predetermined width of the nasal bone and ethmoidal cells is removed. A glabellar part of the frontal bone and the anterior cranial fossa anterior to the cribriform plate are left intact. The reconstructed bony walls are wired together through the supraorbital ridges and to the frontal bone. Bone chips from the patient's own iliac crest fill any bony gaps in the orbital walls. The medial canthal ligaments are wired to each other by drilling through the anterior lacrimal crests, and the soft tissues are similarly wired. It is important to identify the medial canthal ligaments and perform transnasal canthoplasty after orbital depositioning by fixing the ligaments at the dacryon with a transnasal wire. Excess skin and tissue over the roof of the nose and glabellar areas are resected, and the upper canthal fold is corrected if necessary.

In patients with a recessed midface, the entire midfacial skeletal block may be freed, advanced, and rotated downward to repair maxillary malocclusion. The dentist wires the mandibular arch to the frontal bone to maintain the condyle in the glenoid fossa.

Ocular surgery to correct muscle imbalance follows in about 6 months if necessary.

Ocular. Primary therapeutic measures by the ophthalmologist include care of strabismus, treatment of lagophthalmos with tarsorrhaphy and medication, and both pre- and postoperative assessment and treatment of tearing, ptosis, and visual loss.

Ocular or Periocular Manifestations

Cornea: Microcornea.
Extraocular Muscles: Strabismus; vertical muscle imbalance; V-pattern exotropia.
Eyelids: Coloboma; ptosis.
Globe: Microphthalmos.
Optic Nerve: Atrophy; papilledema.
Orbit: Exophthalmos; lateral displacement of the eyes; misalignment.
Other: Dyschromatopsia; retinal anomalies (congenital); visual field defects; visual loss.

PRECAUTIONS

Telecanthus is a lateral displacement of the inner canthi seen in Waardenburg's syndrome. It is not true orbital hypertelorism.

The surgical excision of the bone in the midline produces an eso-movement of the globes, thereby improving any preoperative exotropia or producing a frank esotropia. The esotropia is caused by abduction difficulties secondary to medial movement of the anterior two-thirds of the orbits. The surgery is also associated with marked overaction of the inferior oblique muscles, underaction of the superior rectus muscles, and underaction of the superior oblique muscles.

Binocularity preoperatively may result in diplopia postoperatively. It is helped by alternate patching of the eyes. Narrowing of the palpebral fissure, lateral ptosis from eyelid tension, and incorrect alignment of the canthal regions are complications that are often difficult to avoid.

Advancement of the orbital bony rim ideally corrects any lagophthalmos, but overcorrection may produce lack of apposition of the ocular globe to the inner lid surface and occasionally tightness of the lid margins due to lateral tension, with resultant tearing.

After orbital dissection, an intraorbital hematoma occurring during the procedure may produce acute visual loss by optic nerve compression and ischemia. Once the visual loss is recognized, this uncommon complication responds to prompt evacuation of the hematoma before the child leaves the operating room.

COMMENTS

Pure cases of idiopathic orbital hypertelorism are rare. The condition may be inherited as an autosomal dominant or recessive condition, has an unknown sex ratio, and is usually detected early in life. Familial cases are not frequent.

Hypertelorism is one of the most difficult craniofacial problems to correct completely. These patients should be treated by experienced surgical teams located in only a few centers in the world. The risks include death, brain damage, blindness, and infection with osteomyelitis.

References

Buncic R, Lloyd LA: Treatment of craniofacial anomalies in pediatric ophthalmology. *In* Crawford JS, Morin JD (eds): The Eye in Childhood. New York, Grune & Stratton, 1983.
Hoffman WY, et al: Computerized tomographic analysis of orbital hypertelorism repair: Spatial relationship of the globe and the bony orbit. Ann Plast Surg 25/2:124–131, 1990.
Lloyd LA: Craniofacial reconstruction: Ocular management of orbital hypertelorism. Trans Am Ophthalmol Soc 73:123–140, 1975.
Posnick JC: Craniofacial dysostosis: Staging of reconstruction and management of the midface deformity. Neurosurg Clin North Am 2:683–701, 1991.
Tessier P: Orbital hypertelorism. I. Successive surgical attempts. Materials and methods. Causes and mechanisms. Scand J Plast Reconstr Surg 6:135–155, 1972.
Tessier P, Guiot G, Derome P: Orbital hypertelorism. II. Definite treatment of orbital hypertelorism (OR.H.) by craniofacial or by extracranial osteotomies. Scand J Plast Reconstr Surg 7:39–58, 1973.
Waitzman AA, Posnick JC: Craniofacial surgery: Correction of orbital hypertelorism. Univ Toronto Med J 69/1:12–12, 1991.
Walker JW: Hypertelorism. Br Orthopt J 48:13–15, 1991.

OSTEOPETROSIS 756.52
(Albers-Schönberg Disease, Marble Bone Disease, Osteosclerosis Congenita Diffusa, Osteosclerosis Fragilis Generalista)

JONATHAN D. WIRTSCHAFTER, M.D., F.A.C.S.

Minneapolis, Minnesota

Osteopetrosis describes a group of at least eight inherited disorders of reduced osteoclast function that result in failure of bone resorption and a generalized increase in bone density. The frequency of these disorders is 1 per 20,000 in Caucasians. Osteoclasts are derived from macrophage stem cells in the bone marrow. In some of these disorders there are abnormalities of cytokines produced by stromal cells, such as osteoblasts. Insufficient production of macrophage colony-stimulating factor (M-CSF) by osteoblasts may explain the absence of osteoclast production in the bone marrow. Moreover, abnormalities of macrophage differentiation partially explain the high susceptibility to infection. In some patients, osteoclasts are present, but do not function normally. For example, the absence of the c-src proto-oncogene may interfere with osteoclast tyrosine kinase production. In other cases, the osteoclasts have abnormalities of the H+ATPase proton pumps that produce the acid hydrolases necessary for the resorption of calcium from bone. Abnormal osteoclast numbers or function may result from micro-environmental products that influence cellular differentiation or regulation. Anemia, hepatosplenomegaly, and extramedullary hematopoiesis result from the reduced marrow space and replacement of its normal contents by chondro-osseous tissue in the sclerotic bones. Abnormal hematopoiesis occurs in the marrow of the skull base of infants and the calvaria of children even when these bones appear sclerotic or hyperosteotic. Pathologic fractures limit mobility.

Although the majority of patients are affected by the autosomal dominantly inherited disorders, most children presenting with osteopetrosis in infancy have the autosomal recessively inherited "infantile" or "malignant" form of the disease. These children have limited longevity due to hematologic and neurologic involvement. Juvenile-onset osteopetrosis has been subdivided into malignant (formerly "lethal"), nonlethal, carbonic anhydrase II (CAII) deficiency(ies), and inactive parathyroid hormone types. The most common forms of the disease (osteopetrosis tarda) are two autosomal dominantly inherited forms (I and II) that usually present in childhood, but may not be symptomatic until after the seventh decade. Some obligate carriers of the dominant type have no phenotypic features. Type II is associated with an elevated serum level of creatine kinase isoenzyme BB that may be a marker for immature osteoclasts. Some sporadic cases may be due to retroviral infection characterized by reverse transcriptase activity present in the supernatant from cultured white blood cells.

The radiographic examination of patients with the dominant forms may show pronounced sclerosis of the cranial vault (type I) or of the cranial base, vertebrae, and the pelvis (type II). Serial roentgencephalometry documents craniofacial abnormalities, including narrowed optic canals, orbital hypertelorism, defective growth of the middle and lower face, decreased intracranial volume, and calcified secondary cartilage. Cerebral calcifications are seen in the CAII disorder. Imaging findings consistent with narrowing of the petrous carotid canals or the cervical vertebral canal may explain transient, permanent, or positional neurologic dysfunction due to carotid or cerebral artery compression.

Visual loss may occur as a result of several mechanisms: compressive optic atrophy, hydrocephalus, papilledema, or a chorioretinal degeneration (infantile amaurosis simulating Leber's congenital amaurosis) characterized by a markedly abnormal electroretinogram (ERG) at the first examination and associated with degeneration of all layers of the neural retina. The chorioretinal degeneration may be associated as well with a diffuse central nervous system neuronal degeneration. Assessment of visual function is frequently difficult in affected children because of deafness and impaired communication skills. These problems and the effects of anticonvulsive medications compound structural causes of impaired mental function. Serial visual evoked potential (VEP) examinations may be the only objective measure of visual deterioration or improvement.

THERAPY

Ocular. Bony decompression of the superior half of the optic canal (with or without widening of the canal) may be indicated in those children where there is computed tomographic evidence (2 mm or thinner sections and bone window display) of narrowing of the optic canals, a normal ERG, and subjective and objective evidence (such as progressive abnormality on serial VEP examinations) of decreased optic nerve function. The VEP may show further deterioration in the first weeks after surgery and then improve. Intraoperative VEP monitoring is probably not indicated. Surgery was performed at age 8 months in the youngest reported case with a successful visual result. That patient had a mild systemic disease and did not require bone marrow transplantation. Bilateral decompression at a single sitting amounts essentially to sequential operations using the pterional approach and is not recommended for infants. Optic canal decompression is probably of no value for those patients whose osteopetrosis is associated with an extinguished ERG. Osteosclerosis of the nasolacrimal canal may require dacryocystorhinostomy, with modifications of technique appropriate to the increased density of the bone.

Systemic. Bone marrow transplantation is the only definitive therapy for the previously lethal infantile or malignant forms of the disease that are characterized by the presence of osteoclasts on bone marrow biopsy. Presumably, these osteoclasts are not working properly and might be replaced if a perfectly matched sibling donor is available. The success rate for at least partial engraftment is approximately 80 per cent. After successful transplantation, magnetic resonance (MR) of the spine shows that material of high signal intensity fills in the marrow cavity of the vertebrae where once there was a complete signal void. However, successful transplantation may not reverse optic canal compression in a timely manner or at all. Therefore, bone marrow transplantation may not greatly affect the indications for optic canal decompression nor for shunting patients with hydrocephalus.

In other infants, the bone marrow biopsy may show no osteoclasts, in which case it may be presumed that the abnormality lies in the osteoblasts or other stromal cells that have failed to secrete M-CSF and other factors required for differentiation of macrophages. Such patients may respond to recombinant human M-CSF. In patients in whom the above therapies have failed, one may attempt systemic treatment with recombinant human interferon gamma, a cytokine that enhances production of leukocytic superoxide and leukocytes, as well as bone resorption. Systemic therapies with vitamin D analogues are losing favor, but may play a role.

Supportive. Although the adult patient may require little or no support other than the treatment of an occasional fracture, the management of deafness, and the treatment of dental caries, the child may require extreme measures to maintain normal blood cell populations (splenectomy, corticosteroids, transfusions), to control infections (antibiotics and surgical drainage), to maintain weight gain, and to encourage normal psychologic development. There have been reports of hematologic improvement following the use of high-dose intravenous methylprednisolone or prednisone and a low-calcium/high-phosphate diet in juvenile osteopetrosis.

Surgical. Opening the Fallopian canal in the temporal bone, which decompresses the facial and vestibular nerves and the stylomastoid artery, is sometimes indicated.

Ocular or Periocular Manifestations

Extraocular Muscles: Paralysis of the third, fourth, or sixth cranial nerves.

Eyelids: Weakness due to recurrent facial nerve paralysis, ptosis.

Globe: Proptosis.

Lacrimal System: Nasolacrimal canal stenosis.

Lens: Congenital cataracts.

Optic Nerve: Ischemic swelling of the nerve head; papilledema; primary optic atrophy, which is associated with retinal degeneration; secondary optic atrophy, which is associated with compression, increased intracranial pressure, meningitis, or other infections.

Orbit: Hypertelorism.

Pupil: Anisocoria.

Retina: Primary degeneration; vascular dilation.

Other: Nystagmus; strabismus; trigeminal neuralgia; visual field constriction.

Precautions

The ophthalmic surgeon should be aware that the sclerotic bone encroaches on many structures and may cause unforeseen complications, such as hypopituitarism, sleep apnea, and foraminal occlusion of an internal jugular vein with dural sinus thrombosis. Some other problems not listed above include intracranial hemorrhage and seizures.

Comments

In addition to bone marrow transplantation and M-CSF treatments, other more specific therapies will be advocated in the future when more is known about the mechanisms of this heterogeneous group of disorders, particularly for those forms of the disease in which abnormal osteoclast numbers or function may result from local environmental products that influence cellular differentiation or regulation. The next candidates for therapeutic intervention may be drugs that correct abnormalities of the osteoclast proton pumps. The indications for optic canal decompression are still uncertain, but surgical intervention seems to be useful for selected patients within the first decade of life. Optic canal decompressions may be indicated shortly before or soon after bone marrow transplantation in infants with what was once a uniformly lethal disease.

References

Al-Mefty O, Fox JL, Al-Rodhan N, Dew JH: Optic nerve decompression in osteopetrosis. J Neurosurg 68:80–84, 1988.

Chatterjee D, Chakraborty M, Leit M, Neff L, Jamsa-Kellokumpu S, Baron R. Sensitivity to vanadate and isoforms of subunits A and B distinguish the osteoclast proton pump from other vacuolar H+ATPases. Proc Natl Acad Sci USA 89:6257–6261, 1992.

Coccia PF, Krivitt W, Cervenka J, et al: Successful bone marrow transplantation for infantile malignant osteopetrosis. N Engl J Med 302:701–708, 1980.

Ellis PP, Jawckson E: Osteopetrosis: A clinical study of optic nerve involvement. Am J Ophthalmol 53:943–953, 1962.

Haines SJ, Erickson DL, Wirtschafter JD: Optic nerve decompression for osteopetrosis in early childhood. Neurosurgery 23:470, 1988.

Hoyt CS, Billson FD: Visual loss in osteopetrosis. Am J Dis Child 133:955–958, 1979.

Key LL Jr, Carnes D, Cole S, et al: Treatment of congenital osteopetrosis with high-dose calcitriol. N Engl J Med 310:409–415, 1984.

Key LL Jr, Ries WL, Rodriguiz RM, Hatcher HC: Recombinant human interferon gamma therapy for osteopetrosis. J Pediatr 121:119–124, 1992.

Kodama H, Yamasaki A, Nose M, Niida S, Ohgame Y, Abe M, Kumegawa M, Suda T: Congenital osteoclast deficiency in osteopetrotic (op/op) mice is cured by injections of macrophage colony-stimulating factor. J Exp Med 173:269–272, 1991.

Labat ML, Bringuier AF, Chandra A, Einhorn TA, Chandra P: Retroviral expression in mononuclear blood cells isolated from a patient with osteopetrosis (Albers-Schonberg disease). J Bone Mineral Res 5:425–435, 1990.

Marks SC: Osteopetrosis: Multiple pathways for the interception of osteoclast function. Appl Pathol 5:172–183, 1987.

Merin S, Harwood-Nash DC, Crawford JS: Axial tomography of optic canals in diagnosis of children's eye and optic nerve defects. Am J Ophthalmol 72:1122–1129, 1971.

Orengo SD, Patrinely JR: Dacryocystorhinostomy in osteopetrosis. Ophthalmic Surg 22:396–8, 1991.

Ruben JB, Morris RJ, Judisch GF: Chorioretinal degeneration in infantile malignant osteopetrosis. Am J Ophthalmol 110:1–5, 1990.

Soriano P, Montgomery C, Geske R, Bradley A: Targeted disruption of the c-src proto-oncogene leads to osteopetrosis in mice. Cell 64:693–702, 1991.

Yarington CT Jr, Sprinkle PM: Facial palsy in osteopetrosis: Relief by endotemporal decompression. JAMA 202:549, 1967.

ROBIN SEQUENCE 756.0
(Pierre Robin Syndrome, Robin Anomalad)

STEPHEN P. CHRISTIANSEN, M.D.

Little Rock, Arkansas

The Robin sequence is a nonspecific disorder consisting of multiple abnormalities. The most characteristic of these abnormalities are micrognathia, a U-shaped cleft palate, and upper airway obstruction. It is thought that the initiating event is the arrest of mandibular development between 7 and 11 weeks gestational age. This event maintains the tongue in a high posterior position, interfering with fusion of the merging palatine shelves, which is normally complete by 11 weeks. This mechanism explains the absence of cleft lip in patients with Robin sequence.

Abnormal mandibular development may have several causes, which include (1) intrinsic hypoplasia of the mandible, which is seen in Stickler syndrome and results in a shortened ramus with antegonial notching of the body; (2) neurologic or neuromuscular abnormalities that prevent the tongue from descending between the palatal shelves and render the affected fetus incapable of normal intrauterine mandibular movements; and (3) positional deformation. Any disorder that abnormally flexes the head downward positions the chin against the prominent fetal chest, physically preventing normal mandibular growth. Oligohydramnios, uterine abnormalities, arthrogryposis, and the multiple pterygium syndrome may all contribute to the Robin sequence, at least in part, by this mechanism.

The small, retrodisplaced mandible in combination with a posteriorly positioned tongue decreases the volume of the pharynx and increases upper airway resistance. On inspiration, the tongue may actually occlude the oropharynx (glossoptosis). However, glossoptosis is not the only means of airway obstruction. Delayed maturation or neuromuscular compromise of the parapharyngeal muscles, mucosal edema and lymphoid hypertrophy secondary to upper respiratory tract infection, skull base anomalies, and nasal constriction may all contribute to respiratory embarrassment and pharyngeal collapse in these patients.

With a compromised airway, the infant with Robin sequence struggles to maintain a patent pharynx during feedings. This leads to difficult and extended feeding sessions, aspiration, poor weight gain, and a "failure to thrive." Relief of the upper airway obstruction usually resolves the feeding difficulties. Other serious complications of Robin sequence include aspiration pneumonitis, cor pulmonale, pulmonary edema, congestive heart failure, and right-sided cardiac enlargement.

Once the diagnosis of Robin sequence has been made, it is important to search for underlying syndromes. In a recently reported series of 100 patients with Robin sequence, only 17 per cent were nonsyndromic. Over one-third of the patients had Stickler syndrome. This autosomal dominant syndrome has been termed "hereditary progressive arthro-ophthalmopathy." In addition to the ocular findings described below, these patients have premature degenerative changes of the articular cartilage and may have midfacial flattening, mitral valve prolapse, and sensorineural hearing loss. The velocardiofacial syndrome, fetal alcohol syndrome, and Treacher Collins syndrome are also frequently seen in patients with Robin sequence. The syndromic association with Robin sequence is far higher than with cleft palate alone or with cleft lip.

THERAPY

Systemic. Depending on the severity of upper airway obstruction, respiratory distress or failure may occur any time between birth and 6 to 12 months of life. Therefore, immediate recognition of the disorder is mandatory. If respiratory and/or feeding difficulties occur, endoscopy of the nasopharynx will help establish the mechanism of airway obstruction and direct management. In mild cases, simply placing the infant in a prone position will decrease airway resistance by increasing pharyngeal dimensions. However, it is rarely effective in the long term and, worse, may hide signs of obstructive apnea, such as sternal and subcostal retractions. Nasopharyngeal intubation, glossopexy (moving the tongue anteriorly and attaching it to the lip or mandible), endotracheal intubation, and, as a last resort, tracheostomy can also be used to manage the airway in appropriate patients. Nasogastric feeding or gastrostomy should not be necessary once an adequate airway has been established. With time, the mandible grows, parapharyngeal neuromuscular maturation occurs, and upper airway dimensions increase. These developments make airway obstruction increasingly less likely as the affected infant matures.

Ocular. The ocular anomalies found in patients with Robin sequence are not therapeutically unique and are treated as if they were isolated findings. The glaucoma that occurs in affected children is typical of congenital glaucoma. Goniotomy or trabeculotomy are equally effective initial surgical procedures. Cataracts, if present, may be subtotal and should be removed only if visually significant.

Supportive. Perhaps the most important task of the health care team, once the Robin infant has been stabilized, is teaching the parents how to manage their child in the home environment. Discharge of the infant from the hospital should not occur until the parents have demonstrated proficiency with feedings and management of any airway devices. A visiting nurse is invaluable during the initial weeks at home. If a syndrome is identified, appropriate genetic testing and counseling also need to be instituted.

Ocular or Periocular Manifestations

Lens: Presenile nuclear sclerotic cataracts; wedge or comma-shaped cortical cataracts.

Retina: Chorioretinal degeneration; complicated retinal detachments; perivascular pigmentary changes; retinal holes or breaks.

Vitreous: Premature vitreous syneresis.

Other: Coloboma; congenital glaucoma; high myopia; microphthalmos; Mobius syndrome; ocular hypertension; ocular motor paresis; primary open-angle glaucoma; strabismus.

PRECAUTIONS

Because a large proportion of infants with the Robin sequence have Stickler syndrome, these children should all have a complete eye exam as early as permissible, using sedation or general anesthesia if necessary. Particular attention should be paid to the refractive status, clarity of the visual axis, intraocular pressure, and the condition of the vitreous and retina. Early recognition of Stickler syndrome may minimize or prevent visual loss. Periodic ocular follow-up of these patients is also important.

COMMENTS

Although Robin sequence is rare, occurring in about 1 in 8,500 live births, it remains a potentially fatal condition. A relatively recent study reported a 19 per cent mortality rate. This underscores the need for immediate recognition of the disorder, appropriate management of the airway, and intensive care monitoring. These measures should be followed by family teaching and support coupled with an interdisciplinary evaluation for associated syndromes. These interventions will help ensure accurate diagnosis and appropriate treatment and counseling.

References

Brown DM, Nichols BE, Weingeist TA, Sheffield VC, Kimura AE, Stone EM: Procollagen II gene mutation in Stickler syndrome. Arch Ophthalmol 110:1589–1593, 1992.

Bush PG, Williams AJ: Incidence of Robin anomalad (Pierre Robin syndrome). Br J Plast Surg 36:434–437, 1983.

Cohen MM Jr: The Robin anomalad—its nonspecificity and associated syndromes. J Oral Surg 34:587–593, 1976.

Couly G: Actes du seminaire sur les formes graves neonatales du syndrome de Pierre Robin. Rev Stomatol Chir Maxillofac 85:355–359, 1984.

Dykes EH, Raine PAM, Arthur DS, Drainer IK, Young DG: Pierre Robin syndrome and pulmonary hypertension. J Pediatr Surg 20:49–52, 1985.

Figueroa AA, Glupker TJ, Fitz MG, BeGole EA: Mandible, tongue, and airway in Pierre Robin sequence: A longitudinal cephalometric study. Cleft Palate Craniofac J 28:425–434, 1991.

Girard B, Topouzis F, Saraux H: Microphtalmie au cours du syndrome de Pierre Robin. Etude clinique et tomodensitometrique. Bull Soc Ophth (France) 12:1385–1390, 1989.

Sadewitz VL: Robin sequence: Changes in thinking leading to changes in patient care. Cleft Palate Craniofac J 29:246–253, 1992.

Sher AE: Mechanisms of airway obstruction in Robin sequence: Implications for treatment. Cleft Palate Craniofac J 29:224–231, 1992.

Shprintzen RJ: The implications of the diagnosis of Robin sequence. Cleft Palate Craniofac J 29:205–209, 1992.

Smith JL, Stowe FR: The Pierre Robin syndrome (glossoptosis, micrognathia, cleft palate): A review of 39 cases with emphasis on associated ocular lesions. Pediatrics 27:128–133, 1961.

WAARDENBURG'S SYNDROME 756.89
(Klein-Waardenburg Syndrome)

ANGELO M. DIGEORGE, M.D.

Philadelphia, Pennsylvania

Waardenburg's syndrome is a rare genetic disorder involving the pigmentary, auditory, and ocular systems. Three subtypes have been delineated; all are inherited in an autosomal dominant fashion. Hirschsprung's disease (aganglionic megacolon) has been reported in association with Waardenburg's syndrome in several dozen patients (both type I and type II). A few instances of atretic lesions of the gastrointestinal tract and one of atresia of the vagina have also been associated.

Type I is characterized by lateral displacement of the medial canthi (dystopia canthorum) and of the inferior lacrimal punctae. This leads to shortening of the palpebral fissures (blepharophimosis) and reduced visibility of the medial parts of the sclera, giving the mistaken impression of strabismus. The distance between the medial canthi is increased, but the distances between the pupils and between the lateral canthi are normal.

Other characteristics include partial or total heterochromia of the irides, a white forelock or premature graying of the hair, congenital sensorineural deafness, prominence of the nasal root, hyperplasia of the medial portions of the eyebrows, hypoplasia of the alae nasi, and full lips. Penetrance of the components of the syndrome varies. The laterally displaced medial canthus is present in virtually all patients who carry the gene for the type I disorder, whereas the manifestations of heterochromia iridum, white forelock, and deafness each occur in only about one-third of affected patients. Ptosis has been noted in six patients; in two instances, it was related to the Horner syndrome, and in two others, it was of the Marcus Gunn type.

Type II is characterized by the pigmentary disorder and the deafness, but lateral displacement of the medial canthi is absent. The prominence of the nasal root and synophrys occur less often, but the white forelock and heterochromia iridum develop in about the same percentage of patients as in type I. Deafness occurs in slightly over 50 per cent of affected patients and is usually bilateral.

Type III has been reported in only a few patients and consists of the type I syndrome in association with hypoplastic upper limb anomalies.

In 50 per cent of families with type I Waardenburg's syndrome, the gene has been localized to chromosome 2q37. The mutation of the gene has been characterized in two families thus far, and in each a different defect was found. The gene is designated Pax-3 because of its homology to the Pax 3 mutation, which causes the Splotch phenotype in mice, a disorder of pigmentation and dysgenesis of neural crest cells that is analogous to type I Waardenburg's syndrome. The long-held presumption that the congenital anomalies of this syndrome are caused by defective migration of neural crest cells is now firmly established. Genetic heterogeneity for the syndrome is increasingly apparent.

THERAPY

Supportive. All individuals with Waardenburg's syndrome should be subjected to careful audiometric studies. Unilateral or partial hearing loss may be easily overlooked in the absence of testing.

Other family members should be examined for evidence of the syndrome, and genetic counseling should be provided, particularly in regard to the risk of recurrence of deafness.

Surgical. The lateral displacement of the inferior lacrimal punctae occasionally leads to chronic dacryocystitis. Nasal transposition of the lacrimal punctae and medial canthi may be indicated to remedy this defect.

Ocular or Periocular Manifestations

Choroid or Retina: Hypopigmentation; hypoplasia.
Cornea: Cornea plana; microcornea.
Eyebrows: Hyperplasia of medial portion; poliosis; synophrys.
Eyelids: Blepharophimosis; caruncle hypoplasia; epicanthus; lateral displacement of medial canthi.
Lacrimal System: Lateral displacement of inferior punctae; lengthening of lacrimal canaliculi.
Lens: Lenticonus; microphakia.
Other: Heterochromia (partial or total).

PRECAUTIONS

One should be aware of the rare associations, such as Hirschsprung megacolon or genital anomalies.

COMMENTS

The type I disorder has been reported twice as frequently as type II. The laterally displaced canthi (in type I) are critical clues in the detection of affected infants who may not manifest heterochromia or the other pigmentary changes. Detection of this condition can lead to early recognition of deafness.

References

Baldwin CT, et al: An exonic mutation in the HuP2 paired domain causes Waardenburg syndrome. Nature 355:637–638, 1992.
Curri ABM, et al: Associated developmental abnormalities of the anterior end of the neural crest: Hirschsprung's disease-Waardenburg syndrome. J Pediatr Surg 21:248–250, 1986.
da-Silva EO: Waardenburg I syndrome: A clinical and genetic study of two large kindreds, and literature review. Am J Med Genet 40:65–74, 1991.
DiGeorge AM, Olmsted RW, Harley RD: Waardenburg's syndrome. A syndrome of heterochromia of the irides, lateral displacement of the medial canthi and lacrimal puncta, congenital deafness, and other characteristic associated defects. J Pediatr 57:649–669, 1960.
Foy C: Assignment of the locus for Waardenburg syndrome Type I to human chromosome 2q37 and possible homology to the Splotch mouse. Ann J Hum Genet 46:1017–1023, 1990.
Klein D: Historical background and evidence for dominant inheritance of the Klein-Waardenburg syndrome (Type III). Am J Med Genet 14:231–239, 1983.
Tassabehji M, et al: Waardenburg syndrome patients have mutations in the human homologue of the Pax-3 paired box gene. Nature 355:635–636, 1992.
Waardenburg PJ: A new syndrome combining developmental anomalies of the eyelids, eyebrows and nose root with pigmentary defects of the iris and head hair and with congenital deafness. Am J Hum Genet 3:195–253, 1951.

WERNER'S SYNDROME 259.8

JOHN D. BULLOCK, M.D., M.S., F.A.C.S.,
Dayton, Ohio
and STUART H. GOLDBERG, M.D.
Hershey, Pennsylvania

Werner's syndrome is a rare multisystem disorder described as either a partial phenocopy of aging or one of a group of chromosome instability syndromes. It is an autosomal recessive condition that becomes manifest in the second or third decade of life. Cardinal characteristics include short stature, premature graying and baldness, atrophic changes of the skin with the loss of underlying connective tissue and muscle, bilateral cataracts, trophic ulcers of the legs, and hypogonadism. The general picture is that of a prematurely aged, short patient with thin extremities, stocky trunk, and markedly atrophic skin. The characteristic facies—a "beaked" nose, thin lips, and sunken orbits—results from taut, adherent facial skin. Other features include Mönckeberg-type vascular calcification, which leads to diffuse arteriosclerosis; adult-onset diabetes mellitus; osteoporosis; increased consanguinity rates among affected families; and an increased incidence of neoplasia. Although the disease has been likened to premature aging, it is more likely a condition that merely displays features of normal aging.

The constant ocular manifestation is the development of bilateral cataracts early in the clinical course. These cataracts mature rapidly and are generally characterized by posterior subcapsular opacities that may appear striated or homogeneous. Another common finding is apparent proptosis that is secondary to the atrophy of circumorbital tissue. The incidence of retinopathy seems to be no greater and possibly less frequent in Werner's syndrome patients with diabetes mellitus compared with the general diabetic population.

THERAPY

Systemic. Diabetes mellitus in Werner's syndrome can generally be controlled by diet; however, insulin or oral hypoglycemics may be required. Insulin resistance is common, but ketoacidosis is rare. Diffuse arteriosclerosis may lead to development of a variety of problems (hypertension, coronary artery disease, nephropathy) necessitating appropriate medical therapy.

Surgical. Good visual results can be achieved with cataract extraction. Ulcerations of the legs and feet may benefit from treatment with skin grafting.

Supportive. No curative therapy for Werner's syndrome exists. Individual problems are treated palliatively. Genetic counseling should be offered to patients and their relatives. Management by dermatologic and orthopedic specialists is required for the treatment of the crippling ulcerations of the lower extremities that may occur.

Ocular or Periocular Manifestations

Cornea: Arcus senilis; keratoconjunctivitis; metastatic calcification.
Eyelids or Eyebrows: Madarosis; poliosis.
Globe: Apparent proptosis.
Iris: Telangiectasia.
Lens: Cataracts (usually posterior subcapsular).
Retina: Chorioretinitis; macular degeneration; pigmented retinal dystrophy.
Other: Scleral discoloration; decreased accommodation; decreased tear secretion.

PRECAUTIONS

A high incidence of postoperative complications following cataract extraction in patients with Werner's syndrome has been reported by several authors. Corneal endothelial decompensation, corneal ulceration, wound dehiscence, iris prolapse, and secondary glaucoma have occurred. The surgical approach should be individualized; technique and management should be directed at anticipating poor wound healing and minimizing endothelial cell damage.

COMMENTS

Ophthalmologic and dermatologic manifestations are the major sources of morbidity early in the course of the disease. Diffuse arteriosclerosis is the major cause of organ failure and mortality. Patients usually die of malignancy or myocardial or cerebrovascular accidents in the fourth or fifth decade.

The relationship of the pathologic process in Werner's syndrome to natural aging has prompted considerable research and debate. Recent cytogenetic and clinical observations in Werner's syndrome have led some to include this disorder in the category of autosomal recessive genetic diseases with chromosome instability and increased incidence of neoplasia. These genetic diseases include ataxia telangiectasia, Fanconi's anemia, Bloom's syndrome, and xeroderma pigmentosum. Patients with Werner's syndrome have been found to have hyaluronic aciduria; their abnormal connective tissue may be due to aberrations of collagen and/or proteoglycans. Fibroblast abnormalities are the subject of a large volume of current research. A recently proposed hypothesis is that the primary genetic abnormality of Werner's syndrome is a regulatory gene mutation.

References

Bullock JD, Howard RO: Werner syndrome. Arch Ophthalmol 90:53–56, 1973.

Epstein CJ: Werner's syndrome and aging: A reappraisal. Adv Exp Med Biol 190:219–228, 1985.

Epstein CJ, et al: Werner's syndrome: A review of its symptomatology, natural history, pathologic features, genetics and relationship to the natural aging process. Medicine 45:177–221, 1966.

Goldstein, Murano S, Shmookler Reis RJ: Werner syndrome: A molecular genetic hypothesis. J Gerontol 45:B3–8, 1990.

Jonas JB, et al: Ophthalmic surgical complications in Werner's syndrome: Report on 18 eyes of nine patients. Ophthalmic Surg 18:760–764, 1987.

Kremer I, Ingber A, Ben-Sira I: Corneal metastatic calcification in Werner's syndrome. Am J Ophthalmol 106:221–226, 1988.

Petrohelos MA: Werner's syndrome. A survey of three cases, with review of the literature. Am J Ophthalmol 56:941–953, 1963.

Salk D: Werner's syndrome: A review of recent research with an analysis of connective tissue metabolism, growth control of cultured cells, and chromosomal aberrations. Hum Genet 62:1–15, 1982.

PHAKOMATOSES

ANGIOMATOSIS RETINAE
759.6

(Angiomatosis of the Retina and Central Nervous System, Retinal and Optic Disc Capillary Hemangiomas, Retinal Capillary Hamartoma, Retinal Hemangioblastoma, von Hippel-Lindau Disease, von Hippel's Disease)

JOHN J. WEITER, M.D., Ph.D., *and* SHIYOUNG ROH, M.D.

Boston, Massachusetts

Angiomatosis retinae is characterized by congenital capillary angiomatous hamartomas of the retina and optic nerve. If there are associated central nervous system and visceral angiomas, the condition is called von Hippel-Lindau disease. The retinal angiomas are usually diagnosed when the patient is between 10 and 30 years old. Central nervous system and visceral tumors are frequently noted after the ocular symptoms become manifest. The mode of transmission of these angiomas is autosomal dominant with incomplete penetrance and variable expressivity. There is no well-established predilection for sex or race. The retinal tumors are often multiple and are bilateral in more than 50 per cent of the cases. Approximately 20 per cent of patients with retinal angiomas develop central nervous system tumors.

These ocular angiomas may develop in the retina, optic nerve head or peripapillary retina, or the retrobulbar portion of the optic nerve. The retinal angiomas usually arise from the inner (endophytic) layers of the retina and are discrete angiomas, whereas the peripapillary angiomas frequently arise from the outer (exophytic) retinal layers and are diffuse.

These angiomas consist of masses of capillaries that tend to exhibit an embryonic appearance (hemangioblastoma) and often have abnormal fenestrations. Glial proliferation (astrocytes) separates the vascular channels and frequently contains large lipid-filled vacuoles, most likely representing astrocytic phagocytosis of leaking plasma. The retinal tumors are usually located at the equator or in the peripheral retina and have a propensity for the temporal side. The tumor characteristically remains stable or grows very slowly. With the gradual growth of these tumors, arteriovenous shunting usually occurs within the tumor, resulting in an increasingly dilated, tortuous, feeding artery and draining vein. With time, subretinal fluid and yellow exudate begin to accumulate around the lesion. There is also a tendency for the exudate to accumulate in the macular region as the tumor enlarges. (The visual change resulting from this macular accumulation of exudation from a peripheral tumor is frequently the presenting sign). The endophytic tumors are frequently associated with vitreous traction that can lead to vitreous hemorrhage and a tractional retinal detachment that may be either rhegmatogenous or nonrhegmatogenous. The peripapillary angiomas tend to be endophytic and relatively flat, without feeding and draining vessels. Their clinical appearance is similar to outer retinal telangiectasia. Hemangiomas of the optic disc often clinically simulate papilledema or disc edema. Untreated retinal angiomatosis frequently leads to vitreous hemorrhage, total retinal detachment, secondary glaucoma, and phthisis bulbi.

THERAPY

Surgical. Since angiomatosis retinae is usually a progressive disease, therapy should be initiated as soon as the diagnosis is made. The treatment selected should depend upon the size and location of the tumor, the clarity of the ocular media, and the associated ocular complications. Argon laser photocoagulation has proven to be effective in the treatment of smaller tumors with a clear media. Treatment should consist of large spot size, low-intensity, and long-duration burns directed at the angioma itself. Multiple treatment sessions should be planned for all but the smallest tumors. The end point should be based on obliteration of the tumor by both clinical observation and fluorescein angiography. Once the tumor becomes yellowish in appearance secondary to gliosis and lipid ingestion, photocoagulation of the tumor becomes difficult because of poor penetrance of the laser light.

Anterior angiomas and larger posterior angiomas may be successfully treated by cryotherapy using a repetitive freeze-thaw technique. Only two to three freeze-thaw cycles should be used at each therapy session in order to minimize the risk of hemorrhage. Multiple treatment sessions are usually required. Eradication of the tumor by either photocoagulation or cryotherapy usually results in resolution of the macular edema and improved visual acuity.

For large angiomas, angiomas not responding to photocoagulation or cryotherapy, and angiomas associated with retinal detachment, penetrating diathermy under a lamellar scleral bed has proven effective. If there is extensive subretinal exudation, the fluid should be drained and a scleral buckling procedure considered.

Frequently, large tumors develop surface membranes and vitreous traction that can lead to vitreous hemorrhage and/or rhegmatogenous retinal detachments. These complications may be amenable to treatment using vitreous surgery techniques, endodiathermy, or scleral buckling procedures.

The peripapillary and optic disc angiomas are difficult to treat without destroying useful central vision. Diffuse exophytic peripapillary hemangiomas with associated visual loss may be considered for laser photocoagulation, using a wavelength that spares the inner retina and is absorbed well by blood. Treatment should be conservative and aimed at the foci of greatest leakage.

Ocular or Periocular Manifestations

Globe: Phthisis bulbi.
Optic Nerve: Angioma; disc edema; hard exudates.
Retina: Angioma; circinate exudative retinopathy; dilated tortuous vessels; epiretinal membranes; exudate; hemorrhages; macular star exudation; retinal detachment.
Vitreous: Hemorrhage; proliferative vitreoretinopathy.
Other: Secondary glaucoma; visual loss.

PRECAUTIONS

Since these tumors are highly vascular, any form of treatment may cause further leakage or hemorrhage before the vascular channels are obliterated. It may result in further loss of vision from macular exudation, vitreous hemorrhage, and retinal detachment. Proliferative vitreoretinopathy frequently occurs after treatment of large tumors. Most of these complications are only an exacerbation of the normal course of the disease process. Many complications can be avoided by treatment of the angioma in multiple sessions, rather than an aggressive single-session treatment.

Treatment is best accomplished when the tumor is small. The visual prognosis is related to the size, location, and associated complications at the time that therapy is initiated. Early detection of a peripheral tumor results in a good prognosis, whereas large tumors with an associated retinal detachment or angiomas of the optic nerve have a less favorable prognosis. Since these tumors tend to be multiple and/or bilateral, it is important to

have close follow-up once a tumor is diagnosed. Furthermore, since there is a familial tendency, other family members should be evaluated.

COMMENTS

Multiple tumors tend to occur frequently in the same quadrant of the retina. The earliest endophytic tumors tend to be in the peripheral retina. Subsequent tumors often occur proximally in the same quadrant, having the same feeding and draining vessels. Fluorescein angiography shows evidence of arteriovenous shunting of blood through the tumor with an associated relative hypoperfusion of the retina peripheral to the tumor, suggestive of a vascular steal syndrome. Although not proven, the subsequent, more proximal angiomas may very well represent a "neovascular angiomatous" reaction in a susceptible vascular bed.

Since approximately 20 per cent of patients presenting with retinal angiomas develop multiple systemic involvement including central nervous system tumors (von Hippel-Lindau syndrome), patients with angiomatosis retinae should have a thorough systemic evaluation. The cerebellar hemangioma is the typical central nervous system tumor in the von Hippel-Lindau syndrome and tends to occur somewhat later than the retinal angioma. The cerebellar tumor is similar to the retinal angioma in having large feeding and draining blood vessels and in histologic appearance. In the von Hippel-Lindau syndrome, angiomas may also be found in the medulla oblongata, spinal cord, liver, or kidney. Cysts of the liver, pancreas, kidney, and epididymus are occasionally found, as well as a higher incidence of pheochromocytoma and renal cell carcinoma. In patients with von Hippel-Lindau syndrome, renal cell carcinoma was the most frequent cause of death, followed closely by cerebellar hemangioblastoma.

The gene for von Hippel-Lindau disease has recently been mapped to the short arm of chromosome 3, and DNA markers that flank the von Hippel-Lindau disease locus have recently been identified. Early detection is important for genetic counseling and improves the visual prognosis by allowing early treatment of retinal angiomas. Diagnosis using DNA markers will allow relatives shown to be at low risk to be screened less frequently, thereby enabling a focus on affected individuals and high-risk relatives.

References

Annesley WJ Jr, et al: Fifteen-year review of treated cases of retinal angiomatosis. Trans Am Acad Ophthalmol Otolaryngol 83:446–453, 1977.

Font RL, Ferry AP: The phakomatosis. Int Ophthalmol Clin 12:1–50, 1972.

Gass JDM, Braunstein R: Sessile and exophytic capillary angiomas of the juxtapapillary retina and optic nerve head. Arch Ophthalmol 98:1790–1797, 1980.

Hardwig P, Robertson DM: von Hippel-Lindau disease: A familial, often lethal, multi-system phakomatosis. Ophthalmology 91:263–270, 1984.

Lindau A: Zur Frage der Angiomatosis Retinae and ihrer Hirnkomplikationen. Acta Ophthalmol 4:193–209, 1926.

Machemer R, Williams Sr. JM: Pathogenesis and therapy of traction detachment in various retinal vascular diseases. Am J Ophthalmol 105:170–181, 1988.

Machmichael IM: von Hippel-Lindau's disease of the optic disc. Trans Ophthalmol Soc UK 90:877–885, 1970.

Maher ER, Bentley E, Yates JRW, et al: Localization of the gene for von Hippel Lindau disease to a small region of chromosome 3 confirmed by genetic linkage analysis. Genomics 10:957–960, 1991.

Maher ER, Yates JRW, Harries R, et al: Clinical features and natural history of von Hippel-Lindau disease. Q J Med 77:1151–1163, 1990.

Moore AT, Maher ER, Rosen P, Gregor Z, Bird AC: Ophthalmological screening for von Hippel-Lindau disease. Eye 5:723–728, 1991.

Neumann HP, Wiestler OD: Clustering of features of von Hippel-Lindau syndrome: Evidence for a complex genetic locus. Lancet 337:1052–1054, 1991.

Nicholson DH, Green WR, Kenyon KK: Light and electron microscopic study of early lesions in angiomatosis retinae. Am J Ophthalmol 82:193–204, 1976.

Shields JA: Diagnosis and Management of Intraocular Tumors. St. Louis, CV Mosby, 1983, pp 534–556.

von Hippel E: Uber eine sehr seltene Erkrankung der Netzhaut; Klinische Beobachtungen. Albrect von Graefes Arch Ophthalmol 59:83–97, 1904.

Welch RB: von Hippel-Lindau disease: The recognition and treatment of early angiomatosis retinae and the use of cryosurgery as an adjunct to therapy. Trans Am Ophthalmol Soc 68:367–424, 1970.

Wing GL, Weiter JJ, Kelly PJ, et al: von Hippel-Lindau disease angiomatosis of the retina and central nervous system. Ophthalmology 88:1311–1314, 1981.

NEUROFIBROMATOSIS-1
237.7
(NF-1, von Recklinghausen's Disease)

RICHARD A. LEWIS, M.D., M.S.

Houston, Texas

Characterized as a distinct entity in 1882 by von Recklinghausen, classical neurofibromatosis, now designated NF1, is among the most common inherited disorders in humans, with an estimated frequency of approximately 1 per 3000. No racial or geographic biases are known. About half of the affected individuals clearly inherit the disease as an autosomal dominant trait from an affected parent, whereas the disease in the other half of affected individuals results from a new genetic mutation, which, once having occurred, will also be transmitted in that same fashion. For those afflicted individuals with a negative antecedent family history, as confirmed by normal outcomes of diligent clinical examinations of both parents, about half give a history of advanced paternal age at the time of the proband's birth. The NF1 gene has recently been localized to the pericentromeric region of chromosome 17 at 17q11.2. This gene encodes a GTP-ase activating protein that is termed "neurofibromin." Only 5 per cent of individuals with NF1 have gene mutations that are readily identifiable by molecular methods. Therefore, direct analysis is not feasible for prenatal diagnosis. However, analysis of linked markers on chromosome 17 is informative 95 per cent of the time if an unequivocally affected child and both parents are available.

The defining features of NF1 are (1) the presence (in room light) of six or more hyperpigmented skin macules over 5 mm in greatest diameter in prepubertal individuals and over 15 mm in postpubertal individuals, usually described as café-au-lait spots; (2) two or more cutaneous neurofibromata or one plexiform neurofibroma; (3) melanocytic hamartomata of the iris, eponymically termed Lisch nodules; (4) multiple "freckles" (in actuality, small café-au-lait spots) in the axillary, inframammary, inguinal, or gluteal creases; (5) distinctive osseous lesions, such as sphenoid dysplasia, thinning of the long bone cortex, or pseudoarthrosis; (6) glioma of the anterior visual pathway; and (7) a first-degree relative (sibling, parent, or offspring) with NF1 by these same criteria. NF1 is confirmed if three of these criteria are met. Other characteristic features may include areolar neurofibromata (in 85 per cent of postpubertal females), neural crest tumors (meningiomas, pheochromocytomas, neurofibrosarcomas, and malignant schwannomas), and cervicothoracic kyphoscoliosis. Both short stature and either relative or absolute (>97 percentile) macrocephaly may occur, as may seizure disorders, overt mental retardation, learning disabilities, and school behavior problems in children and adolescents.

Usually, only café-au-lait spots are present from birth into the first year of life, although they may become darker and more numerous with age. Congenital plexiform neurofibromata may appear anywhere on the body, but have significance if they occur across the midline, especially if they have an overlying "pancake" zone of hyperpigmentation or if the tumor involves the orbit. Cutaneous and deep neurofibromata may be undetectable or minimal until puberty ensues. They may be punctiform or nodular on the eyelids and face or may enlarge on the torso to be sessile or even pedunculated. Exacerbation of tumor growth also occurs in both puberty and pregnancy.

Ophthalmic features of NF1 may involve all tissues of the eyelid, orbit, and globe, except the crystalline lens. Extensive plexiform neurofibroma involving the lid and orbit may be associated with ipsilateral facial hemihypertrophy or asymmetric enlargement of orbital volume. Exophthalmos may occur either with diffuse orbital neurofibromatosis; with a tumor of specific tissue in the orbit, such as glioma of optic nerve or chiasm, meningioma, or astrocytoma; or with an occasionally pulsatile herniation of intracranial contents (meningocele or brain) into the orbit through a defect in the bony orbital wall, most often involving dysplasia of the sphenoid bone. Uncommonly, either pulsatile or nonpulsatile enophthalmos may occur.

Eyelids may show small café-au-lait spots or punctiform neurofibromata in about one-third of (adult) cases. Although thickening of the upper lid margin by plexiform neurofibroma with S-shaped configuration of the upper outer one-third is highly characteristic, it probably occurs in about 5 per cent of patients. The association of congenital glaucoma with neurofibromatosis is well established, but its occurrence in the absence of orbital or upper lid involvement is extremely rare. Lisch nodules occur in 95 per cent of NF1 individuals who have passed their sixth birthday. An experienced ophthalmologist will have no difficulty identifying Lisch nodules in adolescents and adults, but must discriminate them carefully from normal stromal variants, such as iris mammillations, to avoid misdiagnosis when he or she counsels geneticists and pediatricians.

THERAPY

Supportive. Once the diagnosis of NF1 is made, genetic counseling for recurrence of the trait follows the classical pattern for autosomal dominant transmission with 100 per cent penetrance of the phenotype. However, the patient must be advised of the markedly variable expressivity, with the risk that at least 25 per cent of affected individuals will have moderate or severe disease.

For a proband's first-degree relative (parent, sibling, offspring) who is postpubertal and has no café-au-lait spots, neurofibromas, or Lisch nodules, counseling is also uncomplicated. It is unlikely that the individual is afflicted, and therefore his or her risk of producing affected children is essentially that of the general population.

Problematic individuals should be studied carefully for both defining and other characteristic features and followed as necessary for evolving complications. That evaluation may include (1) a detailed history of cognitive or psychomotor deficiencies, constipation, pain, and vision problems; (2) a family history and examination of at least two antecedent generations (where appropriate and available); (3) a physical examination with attention to systemic hypertension, scoliosis, macrocephaly, proptosis, iris Lisch nodules, short stature, precocious puberty or hypogonadism, café-au-lait macules, and cutaneous neurofibromas; and (4) a contrast CT scan or paramagnetic contrast-enhanced MRI scans of the central nervous system.

Surgical. Close monitoring for early recognition of surgically amenable complications and surgical intervention at the earliest possible time are the only ways to minimize serious problems. Even then, surgery may not resolve the problem entirely, and at times surgery is not possible. Surgical removal of cutaneous neurofibromas should be reserved for those that are especially disfiguring or functionally compromising or both. In general, these tumors are progressive and radioresistant. Orbital tumors may mandate optic nerve section and a definitive sacrifice of vision. The management of intracranial tumors is more problematic. Many anterior optic gliomas identified on routine scanning may not grow.

Ocular or Periocular Manifestations

Choroid: Melanocytic hamartomas (typically in the posterior pole and best imaged by indirect ophthalmoscopy in fair-skinned races); melanoma; neurofibromata (exceedingly rare).

Conjunctiva or Episclera: Neurofibroma (uncommon).

Cornea: Prominent corneal nerves.

Eyelids: Café-au-lait spots or lentigines; plexiform neurofibroma; ptosis (usually secondary); punctate or nodular neurofibroma.

Globe: Buphthalmos (almost always associated with orbital plexiform neurofibromata); intermittent or pulsatile exophthalmos or enophthalmos.

Iris or Ciliary Body: Lisch nodules; ectropion uveae. (The relative risk of melanoma or neurofibroma compared to the general population is not established, although both have been reported rarely.)

Optic Nerve: Glioma; meningioma; dysgerminoma.

Orbit: Bony asymmetry (orbital neurofibroma); dysplasia of orbital bones (sphenoid); enlarged optic foramen (optic nerve glioma).

Retina: Astrocytic hamartoma (extremely rare); an historical association with congenital myelinated nerve fibers has not been substantiated.

PRECAUTIONS

No laboratory feature, including histopathologic details of the primary lesions, uniquely diagnoses NF1. Sequence-based DNA diagnosis is not yet available. In light of the defining features listed above, all persons afflicted with or at risk for NF1 should undergo a meticulous evaluation to define the diagnosis, to identify complications, and to monitor progression. That evaluation may include diligent examination of the entire cutaneous surface; cranial CT scan without or with contrast or paramagnetic contrast-enhanced MRI scan, including the orbits and the optic chiasm; ophthalmologic consultation with emphasis on biomicroscopy and indirect stereo-ophthalmoscopy; electroencephalography; audiometry; and psychometric testing. Ophthalmologists must respect not only the problems and complications within their purview but also must recognize a 6 per cent lifelong risk for development of malignancy associated with this disorder. However, significant and progressive disfigurement and a heavy psychosocial burden are the most significant long-term complications.

COMMENTS

Although NF1 (von Recklinghausen's disease) is the most recognized variant and comprises at least 95 per cent of all NF cases, several other entities can be confused. Bilateral acoustic neurofibromatosis, designated NF2, is characterized by bilateral eighth nerve masses imaged with appropriate techniques or at least two of the following hallmarks: a first-degree relative with NF2; either a unilateral eighth nerve mass or two of the following—neurofibroma, meningioma, glioma, schwannoma; or juvenile central posterior cortical lenticular opacities. Combined hamartomas of the retinal pigment epithelium and retina also occur. NF2 is also an autosomal dominant trait with a relative paucity of café-au-lait spots and cutaneous neurofibromas and has no other ocular signs except in the lens and, uncommonly, the retina. NF2 has been assigned to chromosome 22q2. Segmental neurofibromatosis, in which café-au-lait spots and neurofibromas are restricted to a single body segment and do not cross the midline, occurs presumably as a somatic (nonheritable) mutation. Multiple café-au-lait spots may occur as an autosomal dominant variant with no other systemic features. In addition, an "adult" neurofibromatosis, an apparently nonheritable variant, has neurofibromas, lipomas, other tumefactions, and no ocular features. This entity is still poorly understood and reported.

References

Destro M, D'Amico DJ, Gragoudas ES, et al: Retinal manifestations of neurofibromatosis: Diagnosis and management. Arch Ophthalmol 109:662–666, 1991.
Imes RK, Hoyt WF: Childhood chiasmal gliomas: Update on the fate of patients in the 1969 San Francisco study. Br J Ophthalmol 70:179–182, 1986.
Imes RK, Hoyt WF: Magnetic resonance imaging signs of optic nerve gliomas in neurofibromatosis 1. Am J Ophthalmol 111:729–734, 1991.
Lewis RA, Gerson LP, Axelson KA, Riccardi VM, Whitford RP: von Recklinghausen neurofibromatosis II: Incidence of optic gliomata. Ophthalmology 91:929–935, 1984.
Lewis RA, Riccardi VM: von Recklinghausen neurofibromatosis. Incidence of iris hamartomata. Ophthalmology 88:348–354, 1981.
Listernick R, Charrow J, Greenwald MJ, et al: Optic gliomas in children with neurofibromatosis type 1. J Pediatr 114:788–791, 1989.
Martuza RL, Eldridge R: Neurofibromatosis 2 (bilateral acoustic neurofibromatosis). N Engl J Med 318:684–688, 1988.
Miller RM, Sparkes RS: Segmental neurofibromatosis. Arch Dermatol 113:837–838, 1977.
Mulvihill JJ, Parry DM, Sherman JL, et al: Neurofibromatosis 1 (Recklinghausen disease) and neurofibromatosis 2 (bilateral acoustic neurofibromatosis). Ann Intern Med 113:39–52, 1990.
Riccardi VM: von Recklinghausen neurofibromatosis. N Engl J Med 305:1617–1627, 1981.

STURGE-WEBER SYNDROME 759.6
(Encephalotrigeminal Syndrome)

F. HAMPTON ROY, M.D., F.A.C.S.

Little Rock, Arkansas

The Sturge-Weber syndrome is a congenital malformation that is characterized by angiomatosis that involves the central nervous system, skin, and eye. The complete syndrome includes intracranial and facial hemangiomas with an ipsilateral choroidal hemangioma and often glaucoma. Along with epilepsy, hemiplegia, and hemangiomatosis must be also considered in this disorder. The port-wine nevus or nevus flammeus is generally distributed over the branches of the trigeminal nerve and is usually unilateral. The ocular significance of Sturge-Weber syndrome is its frequent association with glaucoma and choroidal hemangioma. Glaucoma is caused by high episcleral venous pressure, which results in arteriovenous shunting in episcleral and intrascleral hemangiomas.

THERAPY

Ocular. Because intraocular pressure is caused by high episcleral venous pressure, medical treatment to reduce aqueous formation or to improve aqueous outflow is not very effective. It can narrow the gap between the intraocular pressure and episcleral venous pressure, but cannot lower intraocular pressure below the episcleral venous pressure.

One per cent epinephrine twice daily or 4 per cent pilocarpine four times a day can improve aqueous outflow. Reduction of aqueous formation can be accomplished with a beta blocker, such as 0.5 per cent timolol twice daily. Oral administration of 5 mg/kg of acetazolamide four times daily in infants or young children or up to 1 gm daily in older children and adults may be indicated if topical ophthalmic therapy is inadequate.

Surgical. Trabeculectomy has been the treatment of choice when medical therapy of glaucoma proves inadequate and the optic disc is becoming damaged by the elevated intraocular pressure. A large choroidal effusion may form during surgery. It can be anticipated and treated by a posterior sclerotomy over the ciliary body for drainage before entering the anterior chamber. Recent studies suggest that a goniotomy controls the intraocular pressure as well as the trabeculectomy. Therefore, since goniotomy is such a safe procedure in skilled hands, it seems to be the rational choice for the management of glaucoma.

Goniotomy, trabeculectomy, and trabeculotomy are often ineffective. Cryotherapy may be used if those procedures fail.

Ocular or Periocular Manifestations

Anterior Chamber: Blood reflux in Schlemm's canal; wide angle.
Choroid: Hemangioma.
Conjunctiva: Episcleral and conjunctival hemangioma; increased vascularity.
Eyelids: Port-wine stain.
Globe: Buphthalmos.
Iris: Neovascularization.
Optic Nerve: Cupping.
Other: Anisometropia; facial port-wine stain; hemianopsia; increased corneal diameter; increased intraocular pressure; retinal detachment; visual loss.

PRECAUTIONS

The age of onset of glaucoma is unpredictable and seldom symptomatic. Therefore, frequent examinations are essential.

Port-wine nevus has no propensity to regress. Although cryosurgery is useful in treating some hemangiomas, it has proved inadequate for producing regression of the port-wine nevus.

COMMENTS

Early diagnosis and treatment of elevated intraocular pressures are essential and, if instituted early, can lower intraocular pressure to prevent visual loss. When the facial area supplied by both the ophthalmic and maxillary division of the trigeminal nerve is involved, there is a 15 per cent chance of glaucoma and a 30 per cent chance of the patient being a glaucoma suspect and having elevated intraocular pressure. Patients with only mandibular involvement seldom have glaucoma.

References

Cibis GW, Tripathi RC, Tripathi BJ: Glaucoma in Sturge-Weber syndrome. Ophthalmology *91:* 1061–1071, 1984.
Iwach AG, et al: Analysis of surgical and medical management of glaucoma in Sturge-Weber syndrome. Ophthalmology *97:*904–909, 1990.
Shihab AM, Kristan RW: Recurrent intraoperative choroidal effusion in Sturge-Weber syndrome. J Pediatr Ophthalmol Strabismus *20:*250–252, 1983.

SECTION 14

NEUROLOGIC DISORDERS

ACUTE IDIOPATHIC POLYNEURITIS 357.0
(Acute Febrile Polyneuritis, Acute Infectious Polyneuritis, Fisher's Syndrome, Guillain-Barré Syndrome, Inflammatory Polyradiculoneuropathy, Landry-Guillain-Barré-Strohl Syndrome, Landry's Paralysis, Postinfectious Polyneuritis)

KAY-UWE HAMANN, M.D.

Hamburg, Germany

The nosology of acute idiopathic polyneuritis remains obscure. It is a reversible paralytic disease of unknown etiology and pathogenesis, usually starting with complaints of symmetric bilateral weakness involving the extremities, most likely the legs, and emerging into an ascending type of paralysis involving the respiratory muscles and eventually causing bulbar paralysis. In about 35 per cent of all patients, a previous harmless viral infection can be traced, though this disease may follow a variety of other disorders. An inflammatory infiltration of the nerve roots suggesting a lymphocyte-mediated autoimmune reaction probably against the myelin of the peripheral nerve has been reported. On cerebrospinal fluid examination, a high protein level with poor cellular response confirms the diagnosis. However this finding is not a prerequisite to the diagnosis, though certain features of the syndrome are closely linked to the albuminocellular dissociation.

The ocular findings in the bulbar variant include a painless, rapidly progressive ophthalmoplegia with bilateral symmetric involvement, mimicking a supra- or internuclear disorder of ocular motility. The lid elevators are affected but to a lesser degree. The autonomic nervous system serving pupillary function, accommodation, and lacrimal secretion may or may not be spared, and corneal sensation may be reduced. The appearance of papilledema in inflammatory polyneuritis is rare. The different evolution of impairment of ocular motility in both eyes renders the diagnosis more difficult; however, the presence of facial diplegia virtually precludes other disorders. Fisher's syndrome comprises the ophthalmoplegic variant of acute idiopathic polyneuritis, including oculomotor palsies, areflexia, and ataxia.

THERAPY

Systemic. The vague knowledge of this syndrome makes an assessment of therapeutic trials difficult. The treatment that is most widely employed consists of corticosteroids in full doses with low-salt diets and precautions against peptic ulcerations. Although beneficial effects after steroid medication have been reported, oral administration of 45 to 60 mg of prednisone[‡] daily is still a matter of controversy, since controlled studies revealed the inefficacy of this drug, as well as detrimental side effects. Immunosuppressive drugs[‡] are used sparsely, but no affirmative report on this medication is available.

Ocular. In the patient with facial and trigeminal involvement, the cornea is threatened by the development of exposure and neuroparalytic keratitis. Lack of lacrimal secretion compounds the problem. To prevent ulceration of the cornea and epidermalization of the conjunctiva, precautions to moisten the cornea by using artificial tears, to shield the eye by producing a moist chamber, or to employ permanent or temporary tarsorrhaphies should be taken. Paresis or paralysis of one of the oculomotor nerves is treated by patching as soon as diplopia ensues. Strabismus surgery is not considered until the stability of the deviation is proven and prism balance is tolerated. Correction of the ptosis and the extraocular muscles should not be performed in one procedure. Decreased accommodation may require reading glasses employing convergence prisms. Papilledema resolves spontaneously.

Supportive. If the vital capacity declines below 800 to 1000 ml, mechanical respiratory assistance and tracheostomy are required to maintain oxygen supply with minimal positive-pressure breathing during mechanical ventilation. Secretions from the tracheobronchial tree are removed and pulmonary infections combatted. The support of blood pressure in the face of hypotension completes the therapeutic regimen. The best results are obtained in an intensive care unit under the surveillance of a skilled staff. Under these circumstances, the mortality rate can be reduced from 20 to 5 per cent. Physiotherapy and orthopedic procedures should be initiated for the long-term permanent muscle weakness and contractures.

Ocular or Periocular Manifestations

Cornea: Exposure keratitis; keratoconjunctivitis sicca; neuroparalytic keratitis.

Extraocular Muscles: Gaze paresis (in symmetric involvement); internuclear ophthalmoplegia of abduction; paresis or paralysis of the third, fourth, or sixth nerve.

Eyelids: Ectropion; lagophthalmos; ptosis.

Optic Nerve: Hemorrhages; papilledema.

Pupil: Anisocoria; dilation lag.

Other: Decreased accommodation; dyschromatopsia; photophobia; scotoma.

PRECAUTIONS

Patients with the tentative diagnosis of acute idiopathic neuropathy require prompt attention and surveillance. It is an anxiety-laden experience for the patient and the next of kin alike, and the approach to this patient should be thoughtful. The physician should not hesitate to admit the patient to an intensive care unit if the vital capacity drops. The clinical course is variable, and permanent paralysis ensues in 5 to 10 per cent of all patients. Children have a greater tendency for residual weakness; skeletal deformity before skeletal maturity is achieved presents a further hazard.

COMMENTS

Acute idiopathic polyneuritis causes long-term disability secondary to paresis and paralysis of various muscles. The various specialists—the neurologist, the plastic and orthopedic surgeons, and the ophthalmologist—should be consulted to elicit functional impairment, to initiate proper therapeutic procedures, and to mitigate permanent disability.

References

Asbury AK, Arnason BG, Adams RD: The inflammatory lesion in idiopathic polyneuritis. Its role in pathogenesis. Medicine 48:173–215, 1969.

Ashworth B: Ophthalmoplegia in the Guillain-Barré syndrome. Trans Ophthalmol Soc UK 93: 207–211, 1973.

Banerji NK, Millar JHD: Guillain-Barré syndrome in children, with special reference to serial nerve conduction studies. Dev Med Child Neurol 14: 56–63, 1972.

Behan PO, Geschwind N: The ophthalmoplegic form of the Guillain-Barré syndrome: An immunologic study. Acta Ophthalmol 51:529–542, 1973.

Grunnet ML, Lubow M: Ascending polyneuritis and ophthalmoplegia. Am J Ophthalmol 74: 1155–1160, 1972.

Hamann K-U: Die dissoziierte Ophthalmoplegie der Abduktion: hintere "internukleäre" Ophthalmoplegia im Rahmen eines Fisher-Syndroms. Ophthalmologica 178:365–372, 1979.

Hughes RAC, et al: Controlled trial of prednisolone in acute polyneuropathy. Lancet 2:750–753, 1978.

Morley JB, Reynolds EH: Papilledema and the Landry-Guillain-Barré syndrome. Brain 89:205–222, 1966.

Pollard JD, McLoad JG, Gatenby P, Kronenberg H: Prediction of response to plasma exchange in chronic relapsing polyneuropathy. J Neurol Sci 58:269–287, 1983.

Ravin H: The Landry-Guillain-Barré syndrome. A survey and a clinical report of 127 cases. Acta Neurol Scand 43:(Suppl) 9–64, 1967.

Sherman WH, Olarte MR, McKiermann G, Sweeney K, Latov N, Hays AP: Plasma exchange treatment of peripheral neuropathy associated with plasma cell dyscrasia. J Neurol Neurosurg Psychiat 47:813–819, 1984.

BELL'S PALSY 351.0
(Idiopathic Facial Paralysis)

THOMAS R. HEDGES, III, M.D.,

Boston, Massachusetts

and THOMAS R. HEDGES, JR., M.D.

Philadelphia, Pennsylvania

Bell's palsy is an acute, idiopathic, unilateral, peripheral facial nerve paralysis that gradually disappears over a period of time. Its cause is unknown, although ischemic, autoimmune, and viral etiologies are possible. Involvement of the nerve may occur in its proximal portion or within the fallopian canal, where the inability of the nerve to swell may limit the chances for recovery in affected patients. Definable causes of facial paralysis must be ruled out by a thorough examination of the ears, nose, throat, and cranial nerves. If there are any doubts about the clinical findings or if the paralysis lasts longer than 6 to 8 weeks, further investigations, including magnetic resonance imaging with gadolinium enhancement directed toward the temporal bones and the pons, should be considered.

Early symptoms of Bell's palsy include aching of the ear or mastoid (60 per cent), alteration of taste (57 per cent), hyperacusis (30 per cent), tingling or numbness of the cheek or mouth, epiphora, ocular burning, blurred vision, and weakness of the facial muscles. Ocular complications are caused by lagophthalmos, and ectropion of the lower lid, as well as decreased tear output, increased evaporation, and poor tear distribution further compounds the problem. Corneal erosion, infection, and ulceration may also occur.

Late ocular manifestations are caused by permanent damage and aberrant regeneration of the facial nerve. Motor synkinesis is characterized by reversed jaw winking, wherein contracture of the facial muscles with twitching of the corner of the mouth or dimpling of the chin occurs simultaneously with each blink. Autonomic synkinesis, or crocodile tears, is characterized by tearing with chewing. Several months after Bell's palsy, there may be mild, generalized mass contracture of the facial muscles, rendering the affected palpebral fissure more narrow than the opposite one.

Facial paralysis may also be caused by pontine lesions (stroke, multiple sclerosis, tumor), cerebellopontine angle disorders (tumor, sarcoidosis, meningitis); geniculate ganglion infection (herpes zoster oticus and herpes simplex), otitis media, parotid gland disease (tumor, inflammation), congenital malformation, syphilis, or Lyme disease, Melkersson-Rosenthal syndrome, Guillaine-Barré syndrome, and trauma.

THERAPY

Systemic. A short course of high-dose corticosteroids may relieve pain when it is present and may decrease the incidence of late complications, such as aberrant regeneration of the facial nerve in those patients with severe paralysis. A dose of 60 mg of prednisone given for 3 to 7 days tapered over the next 7 to 10 days is recommended. Because steroids have not been clearly shown to be beneficial in a randomized control study, one should consider withholding this form of therapy in diabetic patients who are predisposed to having Bell's palsy. One might use corticosteroids only if the pain accompanying the Bell's palsy is quite severe.

Ocular. In most cases of Bell's palsy, topical ocular lubrication is sufficient to prevent the complications of corneal exposure. An artificial tear preparation instilled frequently during the day and a lubricating ophthalmic ointment used at bedtime may be sufficient. Occasionally, an ointment must be instilled around the clock. Although ointment blurs the patient's vision, makes the lids sticky, and is messy, it is usually well tolerated for a few weeks. If an associated conjunctivitis should occur, an antibiotic ointment should be used. Hydrophilic soft contact lenses in conjunction with lubricating drops may assist in preventing corneal exposure.

Occluding the eyelids with tape or a pressure patch can be done for 1 or 2 days to help heal corneal erosions. Upper eyelid closure can also be accomplished with a lid suture placed in a mattress fashion to the skin of the upper lid, taping the ends firmly to the upper cheek to close the eyelid. Because of the danger of infection, the lid suture should be used only as a temporary measure. A final measure uses clear plastic wrap, cut 8 × 10 cm, and applied with generous amounts of ointment as a nighttime occlusive bandage.

Moisture chambers are bulky affairs and are seldom necessary. Wraparound sunglasses are useful for the patient who is comfortable indoors, but suffers outdoors because of wind exposure. Lower lid ectropion or droop can be temporarily helped by applying tape below the lid margin in the center of the lower lid, pulling the lid laterally and upward to anchor on the orbital rim.

Surgical. Surgery for Bell's palsy is done for three reasons: to decompress the facial nerve, to correct eyelid abnormalities, and to restore dynamic lid closure.

Surgery to decompress the facial nerve is controversial, based on experimental evidence that immediate facial nerve decompression prevents nerve degeneration. It is used in patients with complete Bell's palsy who have not responded to medical therapy and who show more than 90 per cent of axonal degeneration by facial nerve electroneurography within 3 weeks of the onset of the paralysis. In such patients localization of the problem must be performed by magnetic resonance imaging so that the surgeon can decide whether it is the maxillary segment that may be decompressed externally or whether the labyrinthine segment and geniculate ganglion must be decompressed by a way of a middle-fossa craniotomy. Obviously, this type of approach should be considered only in the most severe cases.

Surgery to correct lower lid droop and ectropion includes tarsorrhaphy, lid shortening, tarsoconjunctival ellipse, and canthoplasty. Lateral tarsorrhaphy is very useful in patients with mild orbicularis oculi palsy and lagophthalmos. It decreases horizontal lid opening, provides better support of the precorneal lake of tears, and provides better coverage of the eye during sleep. Horizontal lid wedge shortening accomplishes these same objectives, but it is not reversible, whereas lateral tarsorrhaphy can be easily separated in the office. In severe, permanent palsy, these procedures are not useful by themselves because lid laxity will progress.

Epiphora due to punctal eversion with mild laxity of the lower lid can be treated by excising a horizontal tarsoconjunctival ellipse of tissue inferior to the lower lid punctum (protecting the canaliculus with a probe) and suturing the edges of the ellipse together. Punctal eversion, associated with severe lid laxity, requires medial canthoplasty combined with horizontal shortening of the lower lid and a tarsoconjunctival ellipse. Severe lid laxity of a permanent nature often requires lateral canthoplasty, which supports the lower lid at the lateral orbital rim.

A host of ingenious devices have been invented to restore dynamic lid closure in cases of severe, symptomatic lagophthalmos. All overcome the elevator action of the levator palpebrae superioris muscle. A weight-adjustable magnet, Gold weights, palpebral springs, or silicone-encircling bands can be inserted into the eyelids. These devices require frequent patient examination for adjustment and are subject to infection, breakage, and extrusion.

Finally, temporal muscle implant or reinnervation of the facial nerve through cross-facial nerve grafting or hypoglossal-facial nerve anastomosis can be used in cases of significant, permanent paralysis to help restore relatively normal function to the orbicularis oculi muscle or eyelids.

Ocular or Periocular Manifestations

Cornea: Erosion; infection; ulcer.
Extraocular Muscles: Paresis or paralysis of orbicularis oculi muscles.
Eyelids: Ectropion; lagophthalmos; paralysis; ptosis.
Lacrimal System: Epiphora.
Other: Decreased visual acuity; diplopia; ocular irritation.

PRECAUTIONS

A careful clinical examination looking for possible causes of facial paralysis must be performed. Bell's palsy rarely occurs with other cranial nerve palsies or brainstem signs. Facial palsy in children may be caused by pontine glioma, whereas in young and middle-aged adults, facial palsy can be the early sign of a cerebellar pontine tumor. An MRI scan should be done in all atypical cases to rule out a tumor.

Aberrant regeneration of the facial nerve must be differentiated from spastic paretic facial contracture, spastic facial contracture, and myokymia associated with multiple sclerosis and hemifacial spasm. Aberrant regeneration of the facial nerve is recognized by the abnormal contracture of the facial muscles, usually a twitch at the corner of the mouth, that occurs simultaneously with every blink. Even if the history and physical findings are characteristic of aberrant regeneration of the facial nerve, a brainstem mass lesion must be ruled out by neuroradiologic investigation, especially if associated brainstem findings are present.

Lid taping and application of a loose pressure patch should be avoided in obtunded patients or those with pre-existing corneal hypesthesia. Even with the most diligent nursing, a loose patch or a loose tape will often move out of position and expose or abrade the cornea. A properly applied pressure dressing with lids firmly closed is an excellent temporary procedure, however.

COMMENTS

Bell's palsy is more common in adults, diabetics, and pregnant women. It recurs in 3 to 10 per cent of patients either on the same or opposite side. Prognosis for complete recovery of mild cases is almost universally good and occurs within days to weeks. In severe paralysis, recovery may be prolonged for several months, especially in the elderly. In 15 to 25 per cent of patients with severe involvement, permanent facial weakness and aberrant regeneration of the facial nerve may result. The treatment of Bell's palsy should be conservative, guided by the severity and probable prognosis in each particular case. Electrodiagnostic tests can help improve the accuracy of prognosis in problem cases. Such tests include the stapedius reflex test, evoked facial nerve electromyography, and audiography.

Topical ocular therapy is successful in all but severe, prolonged cases. In these individuals, the best procedure is lateral tarsorrhaphy. This procedure eliminates the necessity of constant drops and ointments, improves cosmesis by eliminating lid sag, and preserves vision on the affected side. Lateral tarsorrhaphy can be taken down wholly or in part whenever recovery occurs.

References

Adour KK, Byl FM, Hilsinger RL, et al: The true nature of Bell's palsy, analysis of 1000 consecutive cases. Laryngoscope 88:787–801, 1978.
Fisch U: Surgery for Bell's palsy. Arch Otolaryngol 107:1–11, 1981.
Jelks GW, Smith B, Bosniak S: The evaluation and management of the eye in facial palsy. Clin Plast Surg 6:397–419, 1979.
Mitchell JM, Smith JL: Spastic paretic facial contracture. In Smith JL (ed): Neuro-Ophthalmology Update. New York, Masson, 1982, pp 239–246.
Murphy TP: MRI of the facial nerve during paralysis. Otolaryngol Head Neck Surg 104:47–51, 1991.
Peitersen E: The natural history of Bell's palsy. Am J Otolaryngol 4:107–111, 1982.
Wepman B, Baum JL: Ocular findings in Bell's palsy. Ophthalmology 86:1943–1946, 1979.
Wolf SM, et al: A treatment of Bell's palsy with prednisone: A prospective randomized study. Neurology 28:158–161, 1978.

BLINDNESS 369.0

ROBERT L. BERRY, M.D.

Little Rock, Arkansas

Blindness is defined as correctable distant visual acuity of 20/200 or poorer in the better eye or a visual field of less than 20 degrees in its widest diameter. There are an estimated 15 million totally blind people in the world today.

The leading causes of blindness are trachoma, cataract, onchocerciasis, xerophthalmia, and leprosy. The World Health Organization (WHO) estimates that more than 6 million people are blind from trachoma, making it the major cause of worldwide blindness. WHO estimates that 2 million people are blinded by onchocerciasis, and 1.4 million are blinded by leprosy. The leading cause of childhood blindness is xerophthalmia secondary to vitamin A deficiency. It is estimated that some 20,000 children throughout the world become blind from this cause each year.

Within the United States, approximately 0.5 million people are considered legally blind. Of these, 53 per cent are 65 years of age or older. The prevalence of blindness among African-Americans is double the rate among whites. The rate of blindness is equal among men and women.

In order of decreasing frequency, the causes of legal blindness in the United States are glaucoma, macular degeneration, senile cataract, optic nerve atrophy, diabetic retinopathy, and retinitis pigmentosa. In total, these diagnoses account for 51 per cent of the blind persons. Trauma accounts for only 4 per cent of blindness in the United States, whereas hereditary or congenital conditions account for some 20 per cent. Retinitis pigmentosa is the most common hereditary condition, followed by prenatal cataract, congenital glaucoma, albinism, and congenital optic nerve atrophy. Genetic counseling is resulting in a gradual decrease in new hereditary cases of blindness.

THERAPY

Supportive. The main role of the ophthalmologist in the treatment of the newly blind patient is supportive, with appropriate referrals to low-vision rehabilitative services made as soon as practical. Psychiatric referral may be needed for severe depression. Genetic counseling is important when the cause of blindness is hereditary.

PRECAUTIONS

The psychologic reaction to blindness is often overwhelming, particularly if it has occurred suddenly. These patients are members of a psychiatrically high-risk population. Anxiety, low self-esteem, and depression may result in suicidal tendencies. An open and supportive relationship between physician and patient is essential for the promotion of good mental health. It is important that the physician not offer false hope to the patient or the family. It is also important that the physician ensure the patient and family that a blind person can live a full and productive life. Ophthalmologists may have unfounded feelings of guilt and consequently are uncomfortable when dealing with blind patients. It is essential that physicians accept that they cannot cure all blindness and that they learn to be more comfortable and communicate with their blind patients.

COMMENTS

The number of visually impaired or partially sighted persons in the United States is estimated to be 11 million. Of these, 3.4 million are monocularly blind, and a small proportion have a defective but not blind second eye. Because these individuals have the potential for improved vision, low-vision clinics

and optical aids should be recommended by ophthalmologists.

New devices are being developed every day to help blind persons live more normal and productive lives. Electronic devices, including talking calculators and watches, sonar sensor canes, and auditory aids, are now available; however, these aids may not be affordable by the majority of blind people.

References

Hiatt RL: World blindness. J Tenn Med Assoc 80: 403–406, 1987.
Lewallen S, et al: Ophthalmology in Ethiopia. Arch Ophthalmol 1099:1029–1031, 1991.
National Society to Prevent Blindness: Vision problems in the U.S. New York, National Society, 1980.
Perry EC, Roy FH: Light in the Shadows: Feelings about Blindness. Little Rock, AR, World Eye Foundation, 1982.
Smith GT, Taylor HR: Epidemiology of corneal blindness in developing countries. Refract Corneal Surg 7:436–439, 1991.
Tielsch JM, et al: Blindness and visual impairment in an American urban population. Arch Ophthalmol 108:286–290, 1990.

CEREBRAL PALSY 343.9
(Brain Damage Syndrome, Perinatal Encephalopathy)

P. D. BLACK B.Sc., F.R.C.S., F.R.C.Ophth.

Gorleston, Norfolk, England

Cerebral palsy is a group of conditions of widely diverse etiologies that arise as a result of brain damage occurring before, during, or within a relatively short time after birth. These disorders are not progressive, but are not unchanging and are dominated by the motor abnormality. Associated with the motor dysfunction are varying degrees of mental subnormalities, emotional instability, convulsive disorders, speech defects, and abnormalities of hearing and vision. Brain damage can occur in utero secondary to such infections as rubella or cytomegalovirus or to placental insufficiency. It may occur during birth or in the immediate perinatal period and be caused by such factors as prematurity, precipitate labor, neonatal asphyxia and hypoxia, hypoglycemia, hyperbilirubinemia, and accidents during labor and delivery. The brain damage may occur after birth, in particular in relation to meningitis, encephalitis, and injury both accidental and nonaccidental. Some 10 per cent of children with cerebral palsy have the condition for no known reason, in spite of extensive investigation. An extremely small number seem to have familial cerebral palsy. In any unselected population of children with this condition, such as those attending special schools, there will be a small number of children with well-defined, recognizable clinical syndromes.

Cerebral palsy is usually classified according to the motor abnormality and its topography. Spastic, ataxic, and athetoid forms are the most common, either in isolation or less commonly mixed. With the exception of athetoid cerebral palsy, it is rarely possible to localize the site of the causative lesion within the brain. The widely differing nature of the disabilities is a reflection of the diffuse and widespread nature of the central nervous system lesions. This is supported by postmortem studies. Abnormalities of the visual apparatus are common; the incidence of ocular changes has been reported at between 50 and 80 per cent. The range of disorders is wide, with refractive errors, squint, amblyopia, field defects, nystagmus, and optic atrophy being particularly common.

Spastic types of cerebral palsy are most likely to have an ocular abnormality associated with them and purely athetoid types the least. There is some evidence that the incidence of ocular abnormality rises with the degree of mental subnormality. However, an ocular abnormality rate of 70 per cent has been reported in children with cerebral palsy who have normal or near-normal intelligence. The problems caused by the ocular abnormalities are compounded by visuospatial and perceptual difficulties caused by the underlying brain damage.

THERAPY

Ocular. Refractive errors are common. Myopia tends to be associated with prematurity. In any series of children with cerebral palsy, if those whose refractive error is associated with prematurity are excluded, then there is a bias toward the hyperopic. Children with normal or near-normal intelligence should have a full correction of any refractive error after a subjective refraction. If that is not possible, which is the case in the majority of such children, then an objective refraction should be carried out after the instillation of a cycloplegic drug, i.e., atropine 1 per cent, or cyclopentolate 1 per cent, depending on the age of the child. The level at which refractive errors should be corrected in those who are severely subnormal has been the matter of some discussion within the literature. Small refractive errors should only be corrected in those who are likely to benefit from such corrections. Larger refractive errors should be corrected in all children with cerebral palsy in whom the acceptance of spectacle correction is usually very good. Those children at risk of amblyopia because of anisometropia or squint, should be identified at an early age so that appropriate therapy directed toward amblyopia can be carried out. At the same time, a

thorough examination of the fundus and the optic nerve can be carried out, particularly with the indirect ophthalmoscope.

Strabismus is detected in the usual manner. There is a far higher percentage of divergent and incomitant squints in a population of children with cerebral palsy than in a population of children who are neurologically normal. In addition, approximately 25 per cent of children with concomitant squint will have a retinal or optic nerve abnormality, which will preclude an improvement in visual acuity. Full correction of any refractive error based on a cycloplegic refraction must be given, followed by occlusion of the squinting eye and orthoptic treatment, if appropriate. Rarely, treatment may involve the use of prisms and occasionally anticholinesterase eyedrops, although one must guard against adverse reactions occurring with this group of compounds in such children. The aim of the treatment is to give the child binocularity or at least good vision in both eyes before surgery, if it is indicated. There is some evidence that successful treatment of squint may improve the coordination of such children. Defects of retina and optic nerve associated with squint must be identified so that conventional treatment of amblyopia is not applied to those eyes in which there is no hope of visual improvement.

Surgical. For nonaccommodative esotropia and exotropia, recession and resection of the appropriate muscles are usually adequate. The degree to which the horizontal muscles are weakened or strengthened must be determined by repeated observation because of the variable angles often found in squints in these children. Particularly when squints present a purely cosmetic problem, and one eye has a very poor vision that cannot be improved, the aim should be to undercorrect the deviation because overcorrections are said to be common. Vertical deviations are fairly common, most of which are manifest as overaction of the inferior oblique muscles for which there are several causes. In these cases, simple recession or myotomy of the inferior oblique muscle is satisfactory. In very young children, bilateral cataract, lens aspiration, or lensectomy/vitrectomy may be carried out. Subsequent optical correction with contact lens or spectacles may pose special problems and difficulties. In older children in whom cataracts develop, appropriate cataract surgery can be carried out with the insertion of a posterior chamber lens implant. Although while the use of intraocular lenses remains controversial in children, there may be a special place for their use in children who have severe behavioral, emotional, and motor disabilities. Rarely, other abnormalities amenable to surgical treatment, such as congenital glaucoma, may be seen and should be treated along conventional lines.

Supportive. The aim of examination is to identify at an early age, those ocular defects that are treatable and to undertake such treatment for them as if the child were otherwise normal. Many studies have shown that children with cerebral palsy have their ocular disabilities detected much later than children who are normal. Equally important is to identify those children with severe visual handicap that is not amenable to treatment. The ophthalmologist is then in a position to counsel the parents on the placement of the child in the correct educational environment. As well as the parents, those responsible for assessing the child's intellectual ability and those who will educate the child need to know of the child's visual status. Teachers in particular need to know the visual acuity, the size of the visual field, and the child's ability to match colors. Many of these children are deaf, and their education relies heavily on visual stimulation. The ophthalmologic findings cannot be taken in isolation. Assessment and treatment must be coordinated with other disciplines, and to this end the ophthalmologist should be part of a multidisciplinary team, which includes psychologists, teachers, and other physicians concerned with the welfare of the child. There is a continual need for reassessment as the child grows. Parents and teachers need constant reassurance. The aim of the ophthalmologist is to help provide the child with the best possible chance of attaining independence or at least minimizing the amount of institutional care required when the child leaves the shelter of school.

Ocular or Periocular Manifestations

Extraocular Muscles: Esophoria; esotropia; exophoria; exotropia; hypertropia; paralysis of the third, fourth, and sixth cranial nerves; gaze palsies.
Eyelids: Epicanthus; ptosis.
Iris: Coloboma; heterochromia.
Lens: Cataracts.
Optic Nerve: Atrophy; coloboma; hypoplasia.
Retina: Chorioretinal scars; coloboma; pigmentary degeneration; retinopathy of prematurity.
Other: Amblyopia; refractive errors; leukomas; microphthalmos; nystagmus; visual field defects.

PRECAUTIONS

Examination of these children is often difficult, particularly those with mental subnormality. Subjective tests, such as those for visual acuity, are unreliable, and the examination may need to be repeated on several occasions before the ophthalmologist can be sure of the findings. Newer methods of assessing visual acuity, such as the use of visual evoked potentials and the techniques of forced preferential looking, may be particularly useful in those who are mentally subnormal. It is easy to underestimate a child's visual performance, especially in those with gross disturbances of motility, such as athetosis, and in those with hemianopic field defects. Young, severely handicapped children should be examined in familiar surroundings, if possible with someone they know and trust alongside them. Doing so allays their fears and in some cases is necessary since such children with speech disorders and deafness may need to have their responses interpreted. Topical drugs with known systemic side effects should be used with caution. There are reports, largely anecdotal, that these children are unusually prone to develop adverse reactions to some eyedrops. It is important that surgical therapy, usually for squint, be planned in conjunction with the other disciplines concerned with the medical care of the child, since these children are often subjected to multiple surgical procedures, particularly for musculoskeletal problems. Few guidelines exist on the management of squint in these children, but what information there is available suggests that squints should be treated as if the child were otherwise normal.

COMMENTS

It is apparent from the literature that visual problems in children with cerebral palsy are either overlooked or ignored because they are overshadowed by the more dramatic musculoskeletal and intellectual problems. The diagnosis of cerebral palsy has usually been made by the time that such a child is 18 months of age. The initial ophthalmologic examination should also be made by then. At that time treatment for probable amblyopia can be started or planned; continued reassessment is necessary, particularly before the child starts his or her education and during schooling, so that appropriate decisions regarding training can be made at the earliest opportunity. The overall aim for medical care and training is to enable the child to become independent. This aim will not be possible in those who are severely handicapped, but this may not be apparent until the child reaches the second decade of life. All the help possible will be required by the child before then. To this end all treatable defects should be identified at a sufficiently early age to enable appropriate measures to be carried out.

References

Black PD: Visual disorders associated with cerebral palsy. Br J Ophthalmol 66:46–52, 1982.
Douglas AA: The eyes and vision in infantile cerebral palsy. Trans Ophthalmol Soc UK 80:311–325, 1960.
Fantl EW, Perlstein MA: Refractive errors in cerebral palsy. Am J Ophthalmol 63:857–863, 1967.
Harcourt B: Strabismus affecting children with multiple handicaps. Br J Ophthalmol 58:272–280, 1974.
Hiles DA, Wallar PH, McFarlane F: Current con-

cepts in the management of strabismus in children with cerebral palsy. Ann Ophthalmol 7:789–798, 1975.

Orel-Bixler D, Haagerstrom-Portnoy G, Hall A: Visual assessment of the multiply handicapped patient. Optometry Vis Sci 66:530–536, 1989.

Schiemann MM: Optometric findings in children with cerebral palsy. Am J Optometry Physiol Optics 61:321–323, 1984.

CHRONIC PROGRESSIVE EXTERNAL OPHTHALMOPLEGIA 359.1

(Abiotrophic Ophthalmoplegia, Chronic Progressive External Ophthalmoplegia with Ragged Red Fibers, Chronic Progressive Muscular Dystrophy, Kearns-Sayre-Daroff Syndrome, Kearns-Sayre Syndrome, Kearns-Sayre-Shy Syndrome, Ocular Myopathy, Oculocraniosomatic Neuromuscular Disease, Oculopharyngeal Muscular Dystrophy Syndrome, Oculoskeletal Myopathy, Olson's Disease, Ophthalmoplegia Plus, Progressive Dystrophy of the Extraocular Muscles)

JOSEPH ESHAGIAN, M.D.

Los Angeles, California

Chronic progressive external ophthalmoplegia (CPEO) encompasses a spectrum of diseases causing bilaterally impaired extraocular motility and blepharoptosis. It is called "external" ophthalmoplegia because the iris and ciliary body muscles are not affected. The onset of the disease may occur at any age, and about half of the cases are familial. These patients present with diplopia, blepharoptosis, poor vision, weakness, syncopal episodes, dysphagia and weight loss, or symptoms of exposure keratopathy. Chronic progressive external ophthalmoplegia usually has a slow, gradual onset with an insidious course. At the end stage, the eyes may be totally immobile, and there may be no levator action. Almost any of the body's skeletal muscles may be weak. When the face is involved, a myopathic or Hutchinson's facies occurs. A number of autopsy reports seem to indicate that people with CPEO generally tend to die at a younger age than the normal population.

The multitude of associated neurodegenerative disorders that may occur with CPEO include dysthyroid ophthalmopathy, myasthenia gravis, myotonic dystrophy, hereditary oculopharyngeal dystrophy, Bassen-Kornzweig syndrome, Refsum's syndrome, progressive supranuclear palsy, symptomatic focal (neurogenic) ophthalmoplegia, abiotrophic ophthal-

moplegia externa, muscular dystrophy, retinal pigmentary degeneration, retinitis pigmentosa with spastic quadriplegia or heart block, spongiform encephalopathy, and a generalized disorder of the nervous system, skeletal muscle, and heart resembling Refsum's disease and Hurler's syndrome (Shy). Some cases of double elevator palsy in which there is more involvement of the extraocular muscles than simply the muscles involved with upward gaze and some cases of congenital fibrosis of the extraocular muscles may mimic or present with CPEO.

Kearns and Sayre (1958) described the triad of retinitis pigmentosa, chronic progressive external ophthalmoplegia, and complete heart block. Daroff emphasized the spongiform encephalopathic aspects of this syndrome. A childhood onset, high cerebrospinal fluid proteins, abnormal muscle mitochondria, and ragged red fibers are associated with the Kearns-Sayre syndrome. Ragged red fibers are muscle fibers containing abnormal mitochondria and excessive amounts of subsarcolemmal and intermyofibrillar lipid droplets that stain red with the modified Gomori trichrome stain. Ragged red fibers represent abnormal mitochondria (mt) that have abnormal or partially deleted mt-DNA (and hence abnormal or partially deleted mtRNA) with abnormalities or deletions in the protein sequence of mt-DNA. These abnormalities lead to abnormal pyruvate-lactate levels; acid-base imbalances in both the peripheral blood and cerebrospinal fluid; and reduced NADH-dehydrogenase, rotenone-sensitive NADH-cytochrome c reductase, succinate-cytochrome c reductase, and cytochrome c oxidase—four enzymes of the mt respiratory chain containing subunits encoded by mt-DNA. However, no ragged red fibers were found in ophthalmoplegia patients with myasthenia gravis, myotonic dystrophy, thyrotoxicosis, or Mobius syndrome. Therefore, it seemed that the chronic progressive external ophthalmoplegia with ragged red fibers and no positive family history represented a distinct entity; namely, oculocraniosomatic neuromuscular (Olson's) disease, which may be differentiated histologically and clinically from the oculopharyngeal syndrome. Oculopharyngeal muscular dystrophy syndrome consists of progressive dysphagia and symmetric ptosis (usually of late onset, after the fourth decade); it is either sporadic or familial (autosomal dominant) and has an insidious onset with slow progression. The oculopharyngeal syndrome usually has rimmed vacuoles (on muscle biopsy) and does not have ragged red fibers. Unlike the Kearns-Sayre syndrome, oculopharyngeal "dystrophy" does not have central nervous system, retinal, or cardiac abnormalities.

THERAPY

Ocular. Certain ocular features of CPEO are remediable. The blepharoptosis may be treated with lid crutches, adhesive (Scotch) tape, or surgical repair. Yet, lid crutches may prevent the eyelid from closing and may cause exposure keratopathy. Scotch tape usually does not keep the eyelid· up because moisture causes the tape to slip. Therefore, most patients soon become unhappy with lid crutches and Scotch tape for treatment of the blepharoptosis. However, the advantage of lid crutches and/or adhesive (Scotch) tape is that they can easily be removed, whereas in cases of surgical overcorrection (leading to exposure keratopathy), another operation may be required either to lower the eyelids or perform a tarsorrhaphy.

Surgical repair of the blepharoptosis with a fascial (with either fresh homograft or preserved fascia lata) or alloplastic material sling brow suspension, or levator surgery, is usually the most satisfactory treatment in properly chosen patients. In patients with more than 5 mm of levator function, resection, tucking, or advancement of the levator aponeurosis usually yields excellent results. When levator function is less than 5 mm, lavatory surgery sufficient to lift the upper eyelid above the pupil may cause an inability of the eyelid to close fully; hence, exposure keratopathy may occur.

Exposure keratopathy may be aggravated at night, as many of these patients have poor Bell's phenomenon and some have dry eyes. Although these patients usually have weak orbicularis oculi muscles, they often have strong frontalis or brow muscles. Currently, it is generally felt that the best sling material for a suspension operation is autogenous fascia, which may be either obtained from the limb or from the temporalis. The usual measures of treating exposure keratopathy are advisable for chronic progressive external ophthalmoplegia and may include the use of artificial tears, bland ophthalmic ointment, humidification of the air, patching the eyes, swimmer's or protective goggles, closure of the lacrimal puncta (either by punctal plugs, laser, cautery, or surgery), and pyridostigmine.

Base-down reading prisms may be helpful if voluntary downward gaze is severely limited. These patients usually see better with two pairs of glasses (one for near and the other for distance), rather than with bifocals.

Supportive. The dysphagia and aspiration (usually associated with the oculopharyngeal form of CPEO) may be treated with cricopharyngeal myotomy. For heart block and Stokes-Adams attacks, which may be fatal, a pacemaker may be life saving. Genetic counseling should also be offered because some cases of CPEO are familial (either autosomal dominant or recessive or sex (X) linked. Some patients have undergone heart transplants for the cardiomyopathy that is not responsive to pacemakers. Treatment with coenzyme Q10 and succinate may improve clinical respiratory functions.

Ocular or Periocular Manifestations

Choroid: Atrophy.

Cornea: Exposure keratopathy; filamentary keratitis; keratoconjunctivitis sicca; scarring.

Extraocular Muscles: Esotropia; exotropia; gaze paresis or paralysis; low amplitude to no opticokinetic nystagmus; low amplitude or no response to caloric stimulate; ragged red fibers (mitochondrial abnormalities.)

Eyelids: Incomplete eyelid closure; levator paresis or paralysis; ptosis; weak orbicularis oculi muscles.

Lens: Posterior subcapsular opacity (rare).

Optic Nerve: Pallor or even atrophy.

Retina: Atypical pigmentary retinopathy (tapetoretinal degeneration).

Other: Constriction of visual fields; diplopia.

PRECAUTIONS

Properly establishing the diagnosis of CPEO is critical for management. A complete work-up of CPEO requires several clinical and laboratory tests that would delineate the amount of "ophthalmoplegia plus" and would rule out diseases that mimic the idiopathic form of CPEO. It should include a complete family history with examination of photographs of family members for blepharoptosis and strabismus, as well as a physical examination with review of systems, particularly neurologic and ophthalmic systems. A dilated funduscopic examination should be done to check for pigmentary retinopathy. Yearly electrocardiograms would rule out cardiac conduction defects, cardiomyopathy, and the need for a pacemaker. Electromyography, nerve conduction velocities, and repetitive stimulation tests may reveal a myopathy, neuropathy, neuromyopathy, myasthenia, or myotonia. Electroencephalography might reveal abnormalities that are not suspected clinically. The cerebrospinal fluid could be examined for an elevated protein, lactate, or pyruvate level, as commonly seen in the Kearns-Sayre syndrome. Muscle enzymes (aldolase, CPK), lactic acid, or pyruvic acid levels may be elevated as well. The dysphagia, which may be remediable, may be elucidated by a barium swallow or cinemography. Abetalipoproteinemia should be ruled out (lipoprotein electrophoresis, peripheral smear for acanthocytes). Refsum's disease should be ruled out (phytanic acid if motor nerve conduction velocities are slow). Dysthyroidism and myasthenia should be ruled out. Myasthenia gravis may be difficult to differentiate from CPEO (without myasthenia), since some patients with CPEO are supersensitive to edrophonium and curariform agents. Such hypersensitivity requires the administration of curare with great caution. Some patients with CPEO have been misdiagnosed for years as having myasthenia gravis or dysthyroidism. A limb muscle biopsy is helpful in categorizing better the type of CPEO. Ragged red fibers are usually found in the oculocraniosomatic neuromuscular (Olson) disease, whereas rimmed vacuoles are usually found in the oculopharyngeal syndrome.

COMMENTS

An ongoing controversy has raged over the basic nature of CPEO. The pendulum has swung back and forth between authorities supporting the nuclear-neuropathic, myopathic, and myoneuropathic schools. Later, slow viruses were proposed as the etiologic agent, and then biochemical defects in pyruvate-lactate metabolism were postulated to be responsible for the marked proliferation of abnormal mitochondria. Hyman et al. (1977) felt that abnormal mitochondria in CPEO were morphologic reflections of the metabolic defect. One cannot be certain that the syndromes described in the older literature are the same as those in the modern literature because of the different histochemical stains available. Drachman (1967) found so-called myopathic changes in patients with the chronic denervation of poliomyelitis and subsequently confirmed this finding experimentally. Alvarado found that denervation of a cat's rectus muscle led to so-called myopathic changes and ragged red fibers. Drachman (1969) concluded that electromyographic and histologic criteria to distinguish myopathic and neuropathic lesions in limb muscles do not apply to ocular muscles. Moreover, Rowland (1974) questioned whether the so-called muscular dystrophies are neurogenic. A myopathic hypothesis of CPEO does not explain abnormalities in liver functions and CSF enzymes. The vacuolation and ataxia of CPEO are similar to those of the spongiform encephalopathies of slow viral diseases.

Melmed et al. (1975) infused uncouplers of oxidate phosphorylation into rats and caused lactic acidosis. Muscle histochemistry showed ragged red fibers, and electron microscopy showed abnormal mitochondria. Reske-Neilson performed light and electron microscopy and found abnormal mitochondria and degeneration of muscle and nerve in patients with CPEO who had abnormal pyruvate or lactate levels. They therefore suggested that a biochemical defect in pyruvate-lactate metabolism could cause a proliferation of abnormal mitochondria.

In summary, the etiology of CPEO is disputed. It has been postulated to be a nuclear, neuropathic, myopathic, supranuclear, viral, metabolic, and/or autoimmune disease by different authorities. Most modern studies support a theory that the primary defect in CPEO with ragged red fibers is an abnormality of mt-DNA (and mt-RNA) with abnormal or deleted protein (amino acid) sequence of mt-DNA in muscle and other tissues of the body. The ragged red fibers contain abnormal

mt. The abnormal or deleted amino acid sequence of the mt-DNA leads to abnormal pyruvate-lactate levels and reduced coenzyme Q10, cytochrome oxidase, and respiratory enzyme levels. Some cases of CPEO are hereditary (either autosomal dominant or recessive) or sex (X) linked, whereas other cases appear to be sporadic. It is hoped that the future treatment of CPEO with ragged red fibers will involve the alteration or addition of the amino acid sequence of mt-DNA and/or DNA manipulation.

References

Anderson RL, Dixon RS: Neuromyopathic ptosis. A new surgical approach. Arch Ophthalmol 97: 1129–1131, 1979.

Bresolin N, et al: Progressive cytochrome c oxidase deficiency in a case of Kearns-Sayre syndrome: Morphological, immunological, and biochemical studies in muscle biopsies and autopsy tissues. Ann Neurol 21(6):564–572, 1987.

Carroll JE, et al: Depressed ventilatory response in oculocraniosomatic neuromuscular disease. Neurology 26:140–146, 1976.

Degoul F, et al: Deletions of mitochondrial DNA in Kearns-Sayre syndrome knight ocular myopathies: Genetic, biochemical, and morphologic studies. J Neurol Sci 101(2):168–177, 1991.

Drachman D, et al: "Myopathic" changes in clinically denervated muscle. Arch Neurol 16:14–24, 1967.

Drachman DA: Ophthalmoplegia plus: A classification of the disorders associated with progressive external ophthalmoplegia. In Vinken PJ, Bruyn GW (eds): Handbook of Clinical Neurology. New York, American Elsevier, 1975, Vol 22, pp 203–216.

Drachman DA, et al: Experimental denervation of ocular muscles: A critique of the concept of "ocular myopathy." Arch Neurol 21:170–183, 1969.

Eshagian J, et al: Orbicularis oculi muscle in chronic progressive external ophthalmoplegia. Arch Ophthalmol 98:1070–1073, 1980.

Hyman BN, Patten BM, Dodson RF: Mitochondrial abnormalities in progressive external ophthalmoplegia. Am J Ophthalmol 83:362–371, 1977.

Johnson CC, Kuwabara T: Oculopharyngeal muscular dystrophy. Am J Ophthalmol 77:872–879, 1974.

Kearns TP, Sayre GP: Retinitis pigmentosa, external ophthalmoplegia, and complete heart block: Unusual syndrome with histologic study in one of two cases. Arch Ophthalmol 60:280–289, 1958.

Larsson NG, et al: Progressive increase of the mutated mitochondrial DNA fraction in Kearns-Sayre syndrome. Pediatr Res 28(2):131–136, 1990.

Larsson NG, et al: Lack of transmission of deleted mtDNA from a woman with Kearns-Sayre syndrome to her child. Am J Hum Genet 50(2):360–363, 1992.

McShane MA, et al: Pearson syndrome and mitochondrial encephalomyopathy in a patient with a deletion of mtDNA. Am J Hum Genet (48)1: 39–42, 1991.

Melmed C, Karpati G, Carpenter S: Experimental mitochondrial myopathy produced by in vivo uncoupling of oxidative phosphorylation. J Neurol Sci 26:305–318, 1975.

Mita S, et al: Detection of "deleted" mitochondrial genomes in cytochrome-c oxidase-deficient muscle fibers of a patient with Kearns-Sayre syndrome. Proc Natl Acad Sci USA *86(23)*:9509–9513, 1989.

Moraes CT, et al: Mitochondrial DNA deletions in progressive external ophthalmoplegia and Kearns-Sayre syndrome. N Engl J Med *320(20)*:1293–1299, 1989.

Moraes CT, et al: Mitochondrial DNA deletion in a girl with manifestation of Kearns-Sayre and Lowe syndromes: An example of phenotypic mimicry? Am J Med *41(3)*:301–305, 1991.

Nakase H, et al: Transcription and translation of deleted mitochondrial genomes in Kearns-Sayre syndrome: Implications for pathogenesis. Am J Hum Genet *46(3)*:418–427, 1990.

Olson W, et al: Oculocraniosomatic neuromuscular disease with "ragged-red" fibers. Histochemical and ultrastructural changes in limb muscles of a group of patients with idiopathic progressive external ophthalmoplegia. Arch Neurol 26:193–211, 1972.

Ota Y, et al: Detection of platelet mitochondria DNA deletions in Kearns-Sayre syndrome. Invest Ophthalmol Vis Sci *32(10)*:2667–2675, 1991.

Phillips CI, Gosden CM: Leber's hereditary optic neuropathy and Kearns-Sayre syndrome: Mitochondrial DNA mutations. Surv Ophthalmol *35(6)*:463–472, 1991.

Ponzetto C, et al: Kearns-Sayre syndrome: Different amounts of deleted mitochondrial DNA are present in several autoptic tissues. J Neurol Sci *96(2-3)*:207–210, 1990.

Poulton J, et al: Germ-like deletions of mtDNA in mitochondrial myopathy. Am J Hum Genet *48(4)*:649–653, 1991.

Rivner MH, et al: Kearns-Sayre syndrome and complex II deficiency. Neurology *39(5)*:693–696, 1989.

Romero NB, et al: Immunocytological and histochemical correlation in Kearns-Sayre syndrome with mtDNA deletion and partial cytochrome c oxidase deficiency in skeletal muscle. J Neurol Sci *93(2-3)*:297–309, 1989.

Rowland LP: Trophic functions of the neuron. IV. Clinical disorders of trophic function. Muscular dystrophy? Are the muscular dystrophies neurogenic? Ann NY Acad Sci *228*:244–260, 1974.

Schon EA, et al: A direct repeat is a hotspot for large-scale deletions of human mitochondrial DNA. Science *244(4902)*:346–349, 1989.

Shanske S, et al: Widespread tissue distribution of mitochondrial DNA deletions in Kearns-Sayre syndrome. Neurology *40(1)*:24–28, 1990.

Shoffner JM, et al: Spontaneous Kearns-Sayre/chronic external ophthalmoplegia plus syndrome associated with a mitochondrial DNA deletion: A slip-replication model and metabolic therapy. Proc Natl Acad Sci USA *86(20)*:7952–7956, 1989.

Shy GM, et al: A generalized disorder of nervous system, skeletal muscle and heart resembling Refsum's disease and Hurler's syndrome. I. Clinical, pathologic and biochemical characteristics. Am J Med *42*:163–168, 1967.

Zeviani M, et al: Tissue distribution and transmission of mitochondrial DNA deletions in mitochondrial myopathies. Ann Neurol *28(1)*:94–97, 1990.

Zierz S, Jahns G, Jerusalem F: Coenzyme Q in serum and muscle of 5 patients with Kearns-Sayre syndrome and 12 patients with ophthalmoplegia plus. J Neurol *236(2)*:97–101, 1989.

Zupanc ML, et al: Deletion of mitochondrial DNA in patients with combined features of Kearns-Sayre and MELAS syndromes. Ann Neurol *29(6)*:680–683, 1991.

CLUSTER HEADACHE 346.2

(Benign Type of Raeder's Paratrigeminal Syndrome, Ciliary Neuralgia, Histamine Headache, Horton's Headache, Paroxysmal Nocturnal Cephalalgia, Periodic Migrainous Neuralgia)

BAIRD S. GRIMSON, M.D.

Chapel Hill, North Carolina

Cluster headaches are unilateral vascular headaches characterized by the sudden onset of severe, "burning," "boring," "pounding," or "throbbing" periorbital pain. The pain may radiate to the adjacent temple, jaw, upper neck, or nose and be accompanied by ipsilateral lacrimation, conjunctival hyperemia, and nasal stuffiness or rhinorrhea. The hemicephalgia usually is present for less than 2 hours, but often occurs several times a day during cluster periods that may last several weeks or months. The patient then has a headache-free interval before another series of cluster headaches begins. Occasionally, the cluster headaches become chronic, and these pain-free periods are absent.

Cluster headache usually occurs in young or middle-aged adults and is seen much more frequently in males than in females. A transient postganglionic Horner's syndrome can be seen during the attacks, and sometimes the Horner's syndrome becomes permanent. Often, the cluster headache awakens the patient in the middle of the night, although an attack can occur anytime during the day, sometimes with clock-like regularity. The ingestion of alcoholic beverages during the cluster period often precipitates a headache attack.

THERAPY

Systemic. Ergotamine is a mainstay in the abortive therapy of cluster headache. If used to stop the headache at its onset, inhalation becomes a practical method of quick drug delivery, with each inhalation containing 0.36 mg of ergotamine. However, no more than three inhalations several minutes apart should be used for each headache attack. Similarly, sublingual tablets containing 2 mg of ergotamine can be tried, but no more than three tablets taken 30 minutes apart are recommended over a 24-hour period. If the cluster headache occurs at regular times during the day, 1 or 2 mg of oral ergotamine taken 30 to 60 minutes before the attack can be effective in preventing the headache, as can bedtime ergotamine/caffeine suppositories for nighttime attacks. Suppositories have the advantage of reducing the nausea, vomiting, and elevated blood pressure that frequently accompany ergotamine preparations.

Prophylactic therapy, rather than abortive therapy, is the most widely used and practical approach to the management of cluster headache. Calcium channel blockers are particularly helpful in preventing cluster headache. Verapamil in its slow-release form can be started at 240 mg once a day or 120 mg twice a day orally and can be safely increased to a total daily dosage of 480 mg. Systemic corticosteroids are useful in relieving the pain of cluster headaches during the 1 to 3 weeks needed for verapamil to reach its maximum therapeutic effect. Prednisone, 60 to 80 mg once a day, can be given during the first week of verapamil therapy and then rapidly tapered. Methysergide, another effective prophylactic drug during cluster periods, may be given in dosages of 2 to 8 mg daily in divided doses, taken during meals. Methysergide should not be used continuously for longer than 4 months.

Ocular. When indicated, dilute solutions of phenylephrine (0.12 to 2.5 per cent) may be used for cosmetic relief of the postganglionic Horner's syndrome.

Supportive. The patient should be advised to avoid situations that precipitate attacks of cluster headache, such as the ingestion of alcoholic beverages or other agents known for their vasodilatory activity (e.g., nitroglycerin) during cluster periods. A careful history should be obtained to identify and avoid situations found to precipitate headache attacks; afternoon naps or other sudden alterations in the normal sleep-wake cycle are examples of such situations.

Ocular or Periocular Manifestations

Conjunctiva: Hyperemia.
Eyelids: Ipsilateral ptosis (postganglionic Horner's syndrome).
Lacrimal System: Increased lacrimation.
Pupil: Anisocoria; ipsilateral miosis (postganglionic Horner's syndrome).
Other: Periorbital pain; photophobia.

PRECAUTIONS

Ergotamine and methysergide are potent vasoconstrictors and are not recommended in patients with coronary artery disease, hypertension, peripheral vascular disturbances, thrombophlebitis, pregnancy, or impaired hepatic or renal function. A serious side effect of methysergide is the development of retroperitoneal, cardiac or pulmonary fibrosis. To help prevent this complication, methysergide should not be used for longer than 3 or 4 months without discontinuing therapy for at least several weeks. Another rare side effect of methysergide is the rapid development of an acute psychosis. Complications of short-term use of high doses of steroids include abrupt mood swings, insomnia, fluid retention, and increased appetite. The use of steroids for managing cluster headache is not recommended if the patient has diabetes mellitus, hypertension, peptic ulcer disease, or an active infection or has undergone recent immunization.

Side effects of verapamil include constipation, mild systemic hypotension and bradycardia, dizziness, lightheadedness, flushing, headache, nausea, weakness, and peripheral edema. Calcium channel blockers can precipitate or aggravate congestive heart failure. Verapamil should not be used in patients with left ventricular dysfunction or AV heart block.

COMMENTS

Cluster headache is a rewarding headache syndrome to recognize as management is often successful and the patient is extremely grateful for relief from the severe pain. However, ophthalmologists who take on the responsibility of managing these patients need to become thoroughly familiar with the side effects of ergotamine, methysergide, and calcium channel blockers. If a trial of these therapeutic agents proves unsuccessful or the cluster headaches become chronic, a neurologic consultation is recommended for confirmation of the diagnosis and consideration of a wide variety of alternative drugs now available for the treatment of cluster headaches. If the patient at any time develops a third, fourth, fifth, or sixth cranial nerve palsy, a work-up for a parasellar mass lesion including cranial CT, MRI, and possibly cerebral angiography should be initiated immediately.

References

Ekbom K: A Clinical comparison of cluster headache and migraine. Acta Neurol 41(Suppl):7–48, 1970.

Gabai IJ, Spierings ELH: Prophylactic treatment of cluster headache with verapamil. Headache 29: 167–168, 1989.

Graham JR, et al: Fibrotic disorders associated with methysergide therapy for headache. N Engl J Med 274:359–368, 1966.

Grimson BS, Thompson HS: Raeder's syndrome. A clinical review. Surv Ophthalmol 24:199–210, 1980.

Solomon SS, Lipton RB, Newman LC: Review: Prophylactic therapy of cluster headaches. Clin Neuropharmacol 14:116–130, 1991.

CREUTZFELDT-JAKOB DISEASE 046.1

ROBERT L. LESSER, M.D.

New Haven, Connecticut

Creutzfeldt-Jakob disease (CJD), a fatal, rapidly progressive disease of gray matter, is characterized by dementia, myoclonus, ataxia, and variable neurologic signs. Most patients range in age from 40 to 60 years, with equal frequency among the sexes. Five to 15 per cent of cases of Creutzfeldt-Jakob disease are familial. Most patients die within 15 months after the onset of symptoms.

Initial symptoms may include vertigo, blurred vision, anxiety, fatigue, difficulty in concentrating, hyperacusis, and dysarthria, followed by variable neurologic signs that may include the following: cortical blindness (Heidenhain's variant), pyramidal tract signs (weakness or stiffness of extremities with hyperreflexia), extrapyramidal tract signs (tremors, rigidity, dysarthria, slowness of movement, ataxia), and seizures. Myoclonus—rapid involuntary jerk-like movements of a muscle group—is seen in many cases and is diagnostic of Creutzfeldt-Jakob disease when present in an adult with dementia. Other signs include aphasia and cranial neuropathies. In some cases, brainstem and cerebellar signs are prominent.

In 1920, Creutzfeldt described a 23-year-old female with ataxia, ankle clonus, hyperreflexia, myoclonus, nystagmus, and dementia. In 1921, Jakob described five patients, all 40 years or older, who had dementia and pyramidal and extrapyramidal signs. Autopsy in all cases showed gray matter disease with neuronal degeneration. In 1928, Heidenhain described two similar patients, but with cortical blindness as an additional feature.

The electroencephalogram classically first shows slowing and triphasic waves, followed by periodic synchronous sharp wave complexes with low voltage background, and finally decreased voltage uniformly near death. CSF analysis using two-dimensional gel electrophoresis now identifies abnormal proteins that are found in patients with Creutzfeldt-Jakob disease. Routine testing of spinal fluid is usually within normal limits. MRI may show increased ventricular size with prominent sulci secondary to cortical atrophy; however, it is not unusual for the MRI to be negative. Definitive diagnosis is made with a brain biopsy.

THERAPY

Supportive. Treatment is primarily supportive. Antiviral agents have been unsuccessful. Phenytoin is used for seizures, and diazepam is used for myoclonus.

Ocular or Periocular Manifestations

Extraocular Muscles: Eye movement disorders; nystagmus, supranuclear gaze palsy.
Optic Nerve: Atrophy.
Other: Cortical blindness; dyschromatopsia; palinopsia; visual field defects, visual hallucinations.

PRECAUTIONS

Creutzfeldt-Jakob disease has been transmitted by corneal transplant. Two cases occurred in patients who had implants of cortical electrodes after the electrodes had been placed in patients with Creutzfeldt-Jakob disease. One neurosurgeon has developed the disease after exposure, although no reports of Creutzfeldt-Jakob disease have been reported in neuropathologists or general pathologists. Four per cent of the cases with Creutzfeldt-Jakob disease in one report had cranial or ocular surgery up to 3 years before the onset of symptoms. At least three patients have developed Creutzfeldt-Jakob disease after operation in the same neurosurgical unit. Creutzfeldt-Jakob disease has been reported in patients receiving pooled human growth hormone and dura mater grafts. Since 15 per cent of Creutzfeldt-Jakob disease is familial, it has been suggested that blood and organ donations should be avoided in family members of patients with Creutzfeldt-Jakob disease.

An association with intraocular pressure testing performed within 2 years of onset of Creutzfeldt-Jakob disease has been reported. Concern about the risk of applanation tonometry as a means of transmitting Creutzfeldt-Jakob agent and a suggestion that all patients with dementia should have their intraocular pressure taken with a sterile disposable tonometer or with a cover on the corneal surface of the tonometer have also been expressed.

Creutzfeldt-Jakob disease has been transmitted to laboratory animals by intracerebral, subcutaneous, intraperitoneal, intramuscular, or intravenous injection. Creutzfeldt-Jakob-like disease has been reported among primates after exposure to animals infected with Creutzfeldt-Jakob disease.

Any tissue being discarded from patients should be incinerated because its infectivity is not destroyed by storage either in formalin, glutaraldehyde, ethylene oxide, or alcohol. Care should be taken with electroencephalography, electromyography, or tonometry. No tissue of a patient with Creutzfeldt-Jakob disease should be used for transplantation.

Fully effective sterilization procedures for Creutzfeldt-Jakob disease tissues and contaminated materials are steam autoclaving for 1 hour at 132° C and immersion in 1N sodium hydroxide for 1 hour at room temperature. Partially effective procedures include steam autoclaving at either 121° or 132° C for 15 to 30 minutes, immersion in 1N sodium hydroxide for 15 minutes or in lower concentrations (less than 0.5N) for 1 hour, and immersion in hypochlorite (undiluted or up to 1:10 dilution) for 1 hour. Ineffective procedures include boiling, ultraviolet irradiation, ethylene oxide sterilization, and immersion in ethanol, formaldehyde solution, B-propiolactone, detergents, quaternary ammonium compounds, Lysol, alcoholic iodine, acetone, and potassium permanganate.

COMMENTS

Creutzfeldt-Jakob disease is found worldwide with an incidence of one to two cases per million. It is caused by a prion, which is a proteinaceous particle made up of minimal or no nucleic acid in which a protein is an important component. The term "prion" was coined by Prusiner to distinguish this infectious agent from viruses or viroids. Kuru, Creutzfeldt-Jakob disease, and Gerstmann-Straussler-Scheinker (GSS) syndrome are all human neurodegenerative diseases that are caused by prions and can be transmitted to laboratory animals. Familial Creutzfeldt-Jakob disease and GSS are genetically transmitted.

Recently, a mutation of the prion protein has been found in Libyan Jews, which accounts for the disease occurring a hundred times more frequently in this group than in the general population. Previously, it had been speculated that the habit of eating either sheep brain or sheep eyeballs was responsible for the increased incidence among Libyan Jews; however, the finding of a specific mutation of the prion protein at codon 200 adds strong support for a genetic cause. The incidence of Creutzfeldt-Jakob disease among Libyan Jews has increased from 31 to more than 75 cases per million. This rise is thought to be due to increased longevity, as well as the spread of this autosomal dominant disease by Libyan Jews marrying outside their ethnic community. Prenatal diagnosis testing has been proposed as a way to control this disease in high-risk groups.

References

Austin JH: Precautions in Creutzfeldt-Jakob disease. Ann Neurol 20:748, 1986.

Brown P, Cathala F, Castaigne P, Gajdusek DC: Creutzfeldt-Jakob disease: Clinical analysis of a consecutive series of 230 neuropathologically verified cases. Ann Neurol 20:597–602, 1986.

Centers for Disease Control: Human-to-human transmission of rabies via a corneal transplant—France. MMWR 29:25–26, 1980.

Committee on Health Care Issues, American Neurological Association: Precautions in handling tissues, fluids, and other contaminated materials from patients with documented or suspected Creutzfeldt-Jakob disease. Ann Neurol 19:75–77, 1986.

Harrington MG, Merril CR, Asher DM, et al: Abnormal proteins in the cerebrospinal fluid of patients with Creutzfeldt-Jakob disease. N Engl J Med 315:279–283, 1986.

Hsiao K, Prusiner SB: Inherited human prion diseases. Neurology 40:1820–1827, 1990.

Hsiao K, Meiner Z, Kahana E, et al: Mutation of the prion protein in Libyan Jews with Creutzfeldt-Jakob disease. N Engl J Med 324(16):1091–1097, 1991.

Korczyn AD: Creutzfeldt-Jakob disease among Libyan Jews. Eur J Epidemiol 7(5):490–493, 1991.

Manuelidis L, Manuelidis EE: Creutzfeldt-Jakob disease and dementias. Microb Pathogen 7(3):157–164, 1989.

Masters CL: Epidemiology of Creutzfeldt-Jakob disease: Studies on the natural mechanisms of transmission. In Prusiner SB, McKinley MP (eds): Prions—Novel Infectious Pathogens Causing Scrapie and Creutzfeldt-Jakob Disease. Orlando, FL, Academic Press, 1987, pp. 511–522.

Masters CL, Gajdusek DC, Gibbs CJ: The familial occurrence of Creutzfeldt-Jakob disease and Alzheimer's disease. Brain 104:535–558, 1981.

Prusiner SB: Novel proteinaceous infectious particles cause scrapie. Science 216:136–144, 1982.

Prusiner, SB: Molecular biology of prion disease. Science 252:1515–1522, 1991.

Rizzo M, Corbett JJ, Thompson HS: Is applanation tonometry a risk factor for transmission of Creutzfeldt-Jakob disease? Arch Ophthalmol 105:314, 1987.

Taylor DM: Inactivation of the unconventional agents of scrapie, bovine spongiform encephalopathy and Creutzfeldt-Jakob disease. J Hosp Infect 18(Suppl A):141–146, 1991.

Traub RD: Pathogenesis of Creutzfeldt-Jakob disease. Neurology 37:1821, 1987.

DYSLEXIA 784.61

MARSHALL P. KEYS, M.D.

Rockville, Maryland

Dyslexia, primary or specific reading disability, strephosymbolia, and congenital word blindness are just a few of the conditions affecting children or adults that cause a primary defect in their ability to read. In spite of intact senses, normal intelligence, and proper motivation, dyslexic individuals demonstrate various degrees of inability to interpret written symbols. A family history of reading problems is common. In general, the label "dyslexia" excludes all those learning disorders considered secondary to other recognizable entities, such as seizure states, emotional disorders, mental retardation, environmental deprivation, poor teaching, and physical handicaps (including eye and ear defects).

Boder's (1973) classification of dyslexia is based on three reading-spelling patterns and is helpful in understanding and planning remedial therapy. Children with *dysphonetic dyslexia* are unable to decipher a word phonetically. They lack word analysis skills and avoid interpreting words that are not part of their sight-memorized vocabulary. The second group labeled *dyseidetic dyslexia* demonstrates poor memory for whole words (gestalts) and has difficulty in discriminating similar letters. These children read by phonetic analysis and have a limited sight memory vocabulary. Spelling mistakes frequently make good phonetic sense, such as "laf" "for laugh." The third group is a mixture of the first two and is therefore the most difficult group to approach through usual remedial reading techniques.

In a broader sense, it is important to realize that children with dyslexia may fit into a syndrome with a variety of confusing labels. Minimal brain dysfunction syndrome (MBDS) is now usually referred to as attention deficit disorder (ADD) or attention deficit hyperactivity disorder (ADHD). Regardless of the labels, children with a learning disability present four areas of concern: (1) learning disability possibly affecting visual or auditory perception, sequencing ability, right/left orientation, memory, language, or motor skills; (2) distractibility or short attention span (3) hyperactivity; and (4) secondary emotional problems.

Inattention, distractibility, and impulsivity are characteristic of children or adults with ADD. Teachers report that children with ADD need a lot of supervision, call out in class, cannot get organized, and have difficulty waiting their turn in lines. They also have difficulty completing tasks, listening, and staying with play activity. Children with ADHD are described as being very physical and seem to be in perpetual motion with excessive running and fidgeting.

A child with normal or superior intelligence who is not reading at an adequate level will be aware of his or her poor school performance. Silver (1992) has drawn attention to the multiple psychologic problems that may develop due to ego damage and other factors related to school failure. In some cases, it may be difficult to determine whether school problems are causing emotional disorders or are resulting from emotional disorders. Psychiatric evaluation may be necessary for diagnosis and treatment of some poor readers. Other children may require evaluation for ADD and ADHD.

During routine ophthalmologic examination, a history of school difficulties, speech problems, defective memory, or poor coordination is common. Poor attention span and distractibility may be obvious. The afflicted child may have difficulty labeling letters on a vision chart yet be able to accurately trace them in the air.

Right/left disorientation may be exemplified by reading chart lines backward. During "E"-game testing, a weaker score on horizontal as compared to vertical characters may also reflect a right/left conflict. Attempts at reading graded paragraphs (Gilmore, Gray) can be quite revealing and should be part of routine near vision testing for elementary school students.

Although strabismus, amblyopia, and refractive errors may occur simultaneously with dyslexia, a cause-and-effect relationship should not be assumed. In a study of 1910 elementary school students, Helveston et al, (1985) found no difference in the incidence of ocular disorders and strabismus among above-average, average, and below-average readers. Hall and Wick (1991) reported on a study of 111 students evaluated by three optometrists looking for subtle defects in accommodation, motor control, and stereopsis. They concluded that there was no relationship between ocular functions and reading achievement.

A general examination should be performed to rule out underlying disease and neurologic disorders. Children should especially be screened for visual and auditory deficiencies. Neurologic or psychiatric consultation may be indicated. A specific educational evaluation is usually available through learning disability specialists within the school system. Independent diagnosticians are also frequently helpful.

THERAPY

Systemic. Medications, including psychostimulants, tranquilizers, and antidepressants, are used in the therapy of hyperactivity and should only be prescribed by physicians who are familiar with their effects. These drugs are used in specific cases to enhance attention so that acceptable *educational* techniques may be utilized. The treatment of dyslexia and other learning disabilities is the responsibility of educational specialists.

Controversial. Many other types of therapy have not been studied adequately. These controversial therapies include visual training, eye exercises, neurologic reorganization, megavitamins, motion sickness medication, colored lenses, and chiropractic skull manipulations.

PRECAUTIONS

Regardless of the method of treating learning disability, there are some children and adults who have almost no capacity for reading. These individuals can benefit from tape recorders and equipment used for the visually handicapped, such as "talking books for the blind."

Obviously, coexistent ocular disorders require customary treatment. However, parents must be warned that glasses or strabismus therapy will not correct deficiencies in right/left orientation, vision memory, and symbol interpretation. These concepts are emphasized in the recently revised joint organizational statement on dyslexia available from the American Academy of Ophthalmology.

COMMENTS

Above all, it is the physician's responsibility to provide adequate counseling so that families do not fall prey to the many cults offering quick cures. Specific referral to educational specialists using appropriate therapeutic programs is an acceptable and positive approach. In addition to testing and tutoring, experienced educational professionals can fulfill an advocacy role to ensure support for the child in the school system and provide counseling in preparation for college or vocational training.

References

Boder E: Developmental dyslexia: A diagnostic approach based on three atypical reading-spelling patterns. Dev Med Child Neurol 15:663–687, 1973.

Committee on Children With Disabilities, American Academy of Pediatrics, American Association for Pediatric Ophthalmology and Strabismus, and the American Academy of Ophthalmology: Learning disabilities, dyslexia and vision. Pediatrics 90:124–126, 1992.

Duane D, Rawson M (ed): Reading, Perception and Language. Papers from the World Congress on Dyslexia. Baltimore, York Press, 1975.

Gilmore JV: Oral Reading Test. Chicago, World Book, 1971.

Hall S, Wick B: The relationship between ocular functions and reading achievement. J Pediatr Ophthalmol Strabismus 28:17–19, 1991.

Hartstein J (ed): Current Concepts in Dyslexia. St. Louis, CV Mosby, 1971.

Helveston E, Weber D, Miller K, et al: Visual function and academic performance. Am J Ophthalmol 99:346–355, 1985.

Keys MP: Dyslexia and reading disorders. In Kelly VC (ed): Practice of Pediatrics. Hagerstown, MD, Harper & Row, 1977, Vol IV, pp 1–10.

Keys MP, Silver LB: Learning disabilities and vision problems: Are they related? Pediatrician 17: 194–201, 1990.

Levine MD: Reading disability: Do the eyes have it? Pediatrics 73:869–870, 1984.

Metzger RL, Werner DB: Use of visual training for reading disabilities: A review. Pediatrics 73:824–829, 1984.

Silver LB: The minimal brain dysfunction syndrome. In Noshpitz JD (ed): Basic Handbook of Child Psychiatry. New York, Basic Books, 1979, Vol II, pp 416–439.

Silver LB: Controversial approaches to treating learning disabilities and attention deficit disorder. Am J Dis Child 140:1045, 1986.

Silver LB: The Misunderstood Child. A Guide for Parents of Children with Learning Disabilities, 2nd ed. Blue Ridge Summit, PA, TAB Books, 1992.

Vellutino, F: Dyslexia. Sci Am 256:34, 1987.

FUNCTIONAL AMBLYOPIA 368.0

RONALD V. KEECH, M.D.

Iowa City, Iowa

Amblyopia is a decrease in vision in one or both eyes with no apparent organic abnormality that would account for the visual loss. The etiology is thought to be formed vision deprivation, competitive binocular interaction, or both of these factors. Some precipitating clinical conditions include strabismus, high hypermetropia, anisometropia, cataracts, and complete blepharoptosis. Amblyopia begins in early childhood and is corrected most successfully if treated soon after its onset. The prevalence is between 2 and 4 per cent of the general population.

THERAPY

Ocular. Although many therapeutic approaches for amblyopia have been suggested, the most effective treatment is occlusion of the dominant eye. The amount of occlusion required per day to correct amblyopia is unknown. Constant occlusion during all waking hours will result in the fastest recovery of vision. "High percentage" occlusion consisting of 75 to 90 per cent of the patient's waking hours may be nearly as effective and will reduce the chances of developing occlusion amblyopia. Occlusion therapy for less than 50 per cent of the day is unlikely to result in a significant improvement in vision.

Occlusion therapy is best accomplished with commercially available eye patches applied to the skin. An occluder placed over glasses should be avoided, since it requires more patient cooperation and is generally less effective. An opaque contact lens may be a useful alternative to a patch, especially if the patient is already wearing contact lenses for aphakia or anisometropia.

During occlusion therapy, the frequency of follow-up visits will vary depending on the patient's age and the severity of the amblyopia. A traditional guideline is one patching interval or 1 week of constant or nearly constant patching between examinations for every year of the patient's age. This is especially important with children under 2 years of age, in whom occlusion amblyopia is most likely to occur. The patching interval for older children is less critical and generally varies between 3 to 6 weeks, depending on the rate of visual improvement.

If for any reason the interval between examinations must be longer than suggested or the patient has previously demonstrated occlusion amblyopia, patching may be alternated between the dominant and the nondominant eye. The ratio of alternate patching will vary depending on the patient's age, follow-up interval, and level of amblyopia; usually a 2:1 to a 6:1 day ratio is used.

Treatment is continued until vision in both eyes is equal or until no significant improvement is noted after three intervals of full-time occlusion with good compliance. Once the best possible vision has been attained, patching may be discontinued or instituted on a part-time basis. One approach is to reduce the hours per day of patching by one half every few months until it is discontinued completely or the amblyopia recurs.

An alternative form of therapy for amblyopia is pharmacologic defocusing. This technique uses cycloplegics, long-acting miotics, and glasses in various combinations to alter accommodation. The purpose is to blur the dominant eye, thereby enhancing the use of the amblyopic eye. The best results are attained in moderate to high hypermetropes with mild amblyopia. In this case, atropine is administered to the undercorrected dominant eye while the amblyopic eye is given a full optical correction. It is helpful to test the effectiveness of the drug in reducing vision in the office before recommending this therapy for home use. Pharmacologic defocusing is most useful when occlusion therapy is not tolerated, as with skin allergies, and in patients requiring maintenance therapy after successful occlusion.

Anisometropic amblyopia may require occlusion therapy, as well as correction of the refractive error. If the vision in the amblyopic eye is better than or equal to 20/100 and there is no strabismus, glasses alone may, in time, restore vision to normal. With more severe amblyopia, patching and glasses are begun simultaneously. After the vision improves, a contact lens may be tried if the patient is symptomatic or has poor fusion due to aniseikonia.

Surgical. If deprivational amblyopia is a result of remedial ocular lesion, such as a cataract, persistent hyperplastic primary vitreous, or corneal opacity, surgical intervention should be considered. There is convincing evidence that very early surgery, optical correction, and aggressive amblyopia therapy can produce excellent visual results in selected cases.

Strabismus surgery is usually performed only after the amblyopia is resolved. Once resolution has been attained, the correction of any strabismus may aid in maintaining vision if fusion is present.

Supportive. Home exercises with graded sizes of letters and objects in combination with occlusion may offer psychologic support, as well as providing a real benefit. Treatment with pleoptics, prisms, and red filters is controversial and rarely recommended in this country.

Ocular or Periocular Manifestations

Cornea: Opacities.
Extraocular Muscles: Nystagmus; strabismus.
Eyelids: Hemangioma; ptosis.

Lens: Developmental or traumatic cataracts.
Vitreous: Persistent hyperplastic primary vitreous.
Other: Anisometropia; high hypermetropia or myopia.

PRECAUTIONS

An uncommon but serious complication of amblyopia therapy is the development of occlusion amblyopia, a reduction in vision of the patched eye. Children under 2 years of age and those with mild amblyopia are most susceptible. The best method to prevent occlusion amblyopia is to tailor the patching interval to the age of the patient, the severity of the amblyopia, the amount of recommended patching per day, and the speed of improvement.

If the amblyopia is slow to respond to treatment, a refractive or organic abnormality must be considered. Repeat refraction and ophthalmoscopy are indicated. Uncorrected or undercorrected refractive errors are an important cause of a poor response to amblyopia treatment. Most amblyopes will benefit from glasses if they have a refractive error equal to or greater than 2.00 diopters of hyperopia or 1.50 diopters of astigmatism. Uncorrectable organic abnormalities, such as retinal and optic nerve disorders, should not preclude attempts at visual rehabilitation; however, they may warrant a re-evaluation of the visual acuity goal.

Another potential problem is the development of a new strabismus or the deterioration of a pre-existent strabismus as a result of patching. Parents should be made aware of this possibility at the onset of treatment.

Skin irritation from a patch can be an obstacle to successful occlusion therapy. Tincture of benzoin applied to the involved areas and allowed to dry before applying the patch provides a protective coating for the skin. Another approach is to reduce the adhesiveness of the patch by applying cold cream to the patient's skin or applying the adhesive side of the patch several times to another surface, such as the hand, before placing it on the face.

COMMENTS

The greatest obstacle to effective occlusion therapy for amblyopia is poor compliance. This is especially prevalent in older children and children with dense amblyopia. In most instances compliance with occlusion therapy can be optimized by explaining clearly to the parents the nature of the condition and the rationale for treatment. If the child continues to remove the patch after a reasonable trial, other methods, such as the use of adhesive skin preparations or restraints, may reinforce compliance. Mittens for infants and elbow restraints for older children can be used to remind the child not to remove the patch. Restraints should be removed frequently during the day to assess the child's compliance. They are usually needed for only a few days with this approach.

Long-term follow-up is critical for the proper management of amblyopia. The response to therapy and the tendency for recurrence differ for each patient. After reaching equal vision in both eyes, approximately 50 per cent of amblyopia patients will require part-time occlusion during visual immaturity to maintain vision. After reaching visual maturity, approximately 25 per cent will still have a loss of one or more lines of vision in the amblyopic eye. Special care must be taken with strabismus patients after surgery; they may attain good alignment, yet still develop amblyopia.

The treatment of amblyopia requires a considerable amount of patient and parent cooperation. Parent participation by observing the child's fixation pattern when the patch is removed and involvement in visual games may enhance the results. Another useful measure is to write a "prescription" indicating the eye to be patched, the duration and frequency of patching, and the date for reassessment of vision.

References

Beller R, Hoyt CS, Marg E, Odom JV: Good visual function after neonatal surgery for congenital monocular cataracts. Am J Ophthalmol 91:559–565, 1981.

Bradford GM, Kutschke PJ, Scott WE: Results of amblyopia therapy in eyes with unilateral structural abnormalities. Ophthalmology 99:1616–1621, 1992.

Ching FC, Parks MM, Friendly DS: Practical management of amblyopia. J Pediatr Ophthalmol Strabismus 23:12–16, 1986.

Kutschke PJ, Scott WE, Keech RV: Anisometropic amblyopia. Ophthalmology 98:258–263, 1991.

Nucci P, Alfarano R, Piantanida A, Brancato R: Compliance in antiamblyopia occlusion therapy. Acta Ophthalmol 70:128–131, 1992.

Oliver M, Neumann R, Chaimovitch Y, Gotesman N, Shimshoni M: Compliance and results of treatment of amblyopia in children more than 8 years old. Am J Ophthalmol 102:340–345, 1986.

Oster JG, Simon JW, Jenkins P: When is it safe to stop patching? Br J Ophthalmol 74:709–711, 1990.

Scott WE, Dickey CF: Stability of visual acuity in amblyopic patients after visual maturity. Graefe's Arch Clin Exp Ophthalmol 226:154–157, 1988.

von Noorden GK: Application of basic research data to clinical amblyopia. Ophthalmology 85:496–504, 1978.

HEADACHE 784.0
(Migraine)

THOMAS R. HEDGES, JR., M.D.

Philadelphia, Pennsylvania

Migraine is commonly misdiagnosed by the ophthalmologist mainly because the examiner does not listen carefully to the patient's symptoms and does not ask pertinent questions. Ophthalmologists tend not to be familiar with the subject and consider it to be beyond their capabilities in management.

It is of primary importance to identify the type of *vascular headache* by taking a careful history, including the chief complaint and past history of headache, which are of equal importance. The most important characteristic identifying migraine or one of its equivalents is periodicity. Migraine occurs as a major or minor attack of cephalalgia depending on its severity, in contrast to tension headache, which does not follow such a pattern. The next major identifying feature is a preceding aura (usually visual), which is present in classic migraine but absent in common migraine. The aftermath of a migraine attack of any severity is lassitude or a feeling of being "washed out." A family history is of great help in diagnosing migraine headache. The age of the patient is very important. Pediatric, ophthalmoplegic, and basilar migraine occur in children and adolescents. Classic and common migraine are most common in adults between 20 and 40 years of age, and isolated ophthalmic migraine occurs mostly in older patients. Once one has identified the type of vascular headache, treatment or management can be pursued appropriately.

Classic migraine occurs in young and in middle-aged adults. It is easy to diagnose when it presents as a periodic episode characterized by a visual aura and a throbbing unilateral or generalized headache of variable duration and severity. The more severe the headache, the more it is accompanied by nausea and vomiting, postheadache lassitude, or complete exhaustion. Obtaining a family history is of great importance. One must above all emphasize any family history of significant headache often labeled "sinus headache" or "nerves."

A wide spectrum of symptoms may occur, which may vary in both severity and duration. A typical fortification scotoma of 20 minutes duration or any unformed visual hallucinations precede or overlap the onset of headache, which typically is a pounding hemicrania that builds to a peak, often becoming generalized.

The pathophysiology of this important entity is classically explained by vasoconstriction during the aura, which typically causes fortification scotoma or more rarely aphasia, numbness, or motor weakness. This lasts 10 to 30 minutes and either totally precedes or overlaps the vasodilative phase, which creates the headache.

Patients with classic migraine are most commonly seen by the ophthalmologist because of the visual episode that precedes or accompanies the headache. Therefore, it is the examiner's duty to inquire about all the symptoms stated earlier in order to make a proper diagnosis and direct the patient toward the best mode of treatment. The ophthalmologist may manage the patient him- or herself or refer the patient to an internist or headache specialist, depending on the severity of the headache problem.

Common migraine does not have an aura or vasoconstrictive prodrome. It begins with a buildup of headache and rises to a peak of pain. It is highly variable in severity, but is the most frequently encountered migraine syndrome, often beginning in the teens and lasting through the menopause in females. Its hallmarks are periodicity and postheadache fatigue. The severity of the headache dictates the amount of accompanying nausea, vomiting, and prostration. All migraine patients want to be alone or in a dark room.

Isolated ophthalmic migraine is commonly encountered in ophthalmic practice because of the alarming and often disabling attack of visual obscuration. The terms "isolated ophthalmic migraine," "migraine accompaniments," and "acephalgic migraine" have been used to describe these attacks. They occur in older patients with an average age of 55 years, but can occur in patients from 20 through 70 years of age. These patients usually have not had migraine headaches in the past.

In isolated ophthalmic migraine, the visual attack comes on suddenly as a typical fortification scotoma lasting 15 to 20 minutes. It appears much the same as the aura of classic migraine, but is not accompanied or followed by headache or other symptoms; thus, the appellation, isolated ophthalmic migraine. If the attacks are typically hemianopic with jagged lines of prisms of light, the origin is related to posterior cerebralcalcarine vascular insufficiency. Retinal migraine has been described as a unilateral attack of blurred vision lasting 10 to 30 minutes. It should not be confused with amaurosis fugax (lasting from seconds to 1 to 2 minutes). Even if monocularity is claimed by alternately covering the eyes, the author feels these are most commonly homonymous attacks in which the patient notices only the large temporal field affected, neglecting the smaller nasal field deficit on the other side. These attacks occur infrequently, but are very frightening. They are probably due to sludging or dysautoregulation in the terminal posterior cerebral or calcarine arteries, but the exact cause is unknown.

Pediatric migraine occurs in children usually between 6 and 14 years of age. Complaints of headache and blurred vision are ill defined, and one must take a very specific history to obtain the story of an episodic, often poorly defined headache. The headache is periodic. Head pain is accompanied by an atypical fuzzy vision and is therefore referred to by the term "fragmented" in comparison to adult migraine. Typically, the child comes home from school with a headache, may or may not have vague descriptions of unformed visual hallucinations, and then refuses supper because of mild nausea and goes to bed and sleeps. Thus, the classic combinations of episodic headache, blurred vision, nausea, and lassitude that are the hallmarks of the migraine syndrome are still present, but are more ill defined. Obtaining a family history of headache is most important in helping establish the diagnosis. Such questions as "Is anyone in the family headachy?" and "Did you or your spouse ever have headaches as a child?" are helpful. Many people forget that they had headache or were told they were nervous or had sinus problems as children. Females who have had headache at the time of their menstrual period do not realize that migraine commonly presents this way.

Ophthalmoplegic migraine is a very rare form of complicated migraine. Most of these patients are under 10 years of age. The patient first complains of lingering severe headache followed by ptosis and extraocular muscle paralysis; the pupil is usually involved as part of a third nerve paresis. This entity then emerges with the syndrome of painful ophthalmoplegia, which responds dramatically to oral steroids. The headaches preceding or accompanying the paresis in complicated migraine attacks are more severe and prolonged than usual. They may respond to ergotamine initially, but provoke concern regarding the differential diagnosis of aneurysms of the internal carotid-posterior communicating artery.

Cluster headache has been labeled as sphenopalatine, vidian and other neuralgias, and histamine cephalgia. Presently, it is most probably considered a migraine variant of vascular origin. It occurs more in males than females in contrast to true migraine, tends to be seasonal, and occurs in a series of episodes (clusters). Conversely, these attacks can often be quite isolated and infrequent. Cluster headache has no familial or constitutional background and is less responsive to routine migraine therapy.

These patients suffer from severe unilateral, periorbital headache with an onset in the early morning hours; it often awakens them from sleep. In contrast to migraineurs, these patients want to be active. In its extreme phase of severity, the pain generally lasts 20 to 30 minutes. The attack gradually subsides, but leaves the patient with pain in the eyeball or in and around the orbit. The eyeball usually remains white and quiet. Rhinorrhea and suffusions occur with severe attacks. A careful evaluation of the eye, including the cornea, the anterior chamber and its angle, the pupil, and intraocular tension, is vitally important in all cases. Horner's syndrome occurs infrequently in this entity. Chronic narrow-angle glaucoma must be ruled out.

Headache and *transient blurred vision* are so commonly seen in general ophthalmic practice that one cannot discuss one without the other. Even though at first one may wonder why migraine has anything to do with vascular disease of the carotid-ophthalmic or vertebral-basilar-posterior cerebral arteries, with experience one realizes that the visual prodroma of migraine and transient binocular attacks experienced without headache are so much alike they cannot be separated.

The term "transient blurred vision" covers a wide spectrum of conditions from short-lived unilateral transient ischemic attacks or transient monocular blur (TMB) to cerebral hemianopic episodes of transient binocular blur (TBB) of 20 to 30 minutes duration. Researchers have stated that any patient over 40 years of age with classic migraine should be considered a potential victim of vaso-occlusive disease. The author's personal clinical experience shows that patients over 40 years can have headaches of a classic migraine type and very rarely have a vaso-occlusive disease.

Any patient complaining of visual blurring should be asked the following questions: (1) Is the blur in one eye or to one side? (it should be remembered that patients tend to neglect the blurring in the small nasal field of the eye contralateral to the homonymous field loss), (2) How long does it last?, (3) Is there an association with any other vasomotor problems, such as hypertension or hematopoietic disorders (polycythemia, anemia, lipidemias, or platelet coagulability)?, (4) Are there cervical orthopedic problems, such as spondylitis?, and (5) Is there any association with stress?

Wavy vision is described as a homonymous hemianopic "spectral march" or fortification scotoma with or without lights and altitudinal "heat wave" type of blurring. It is a common complaint in middle-aged and older individuals. Although it may occur at any age, in the author's experience, the average age is about 52 years. These symptoms resemble in every way the aura or prodroma of migraine, but little or no headache accompanies this often frightening phenomenon. The more typical attacks vary in length from 10 minutes to as long as 2 hours, whereas the true fortification scotoma averages 20 minutes in duration. These patients may be reassured after a physical examination and other appropriate studies has ruled out sludging phenomenon due to hematopoietic disorders. It is particularly important to rule out hypertension and/or atherosclerotic disease, which must be treated accordingly.

Transient ischemic attacks occurring in one eye (amaurosis fugax) are very fleeting, lasting seconds to minutes. These patients readily identify the attacks as monocular, even when they do not cover one eye. They are most commonly caused by emboli from extracranial carotid atheromata.

Monocular attacks of long duration (i.e., several hours or days) are often associated with hypertension, diabetes, or hematopoietic disorders. Prolonged monocular blindness should be differentiated from transient visual obscurations that last only seconds and are seen in chronic papilledema usually caused by pseudotumor cerebri and anterior ischemic neuropathy or amaurosis fugax.

Transient blurred vision in young people may be due to the prolonged use of oral contraceptive pills, emboli from a prolapsed mitral valve (Barlow's syndrome), other cardiac abnormalities, or postoperative complications of surgery to correct these defects.

Tension headache is probably the most common headache encountered in clinical practice. It rarely occurs in the very young or very elderly. It is described typically as a band-like or pressure sensation in the frontal region, nuchal area, or top of the head. It follows no pattern, does not have periodicity as its hallmark, but when severe may simulate migraine because of the accompanying physical fatigue that is augmented by the emotional state of the patient. Tension headache occurs with migraine, even in young people, and is commonly concurrent in 60 to 70 per cent of migraineurs. These patients often cannot verbalize, recognize, or accept a cause for the tension state.

The ophthalmologist rarely sees patients with *cranial neuralgias* initially, but must be aware of trigeminal neuralgias. This unilateral, excruciating facial pain in the first, second, and third division of the fifth nerve is usually present in middle-aged patients and presents characteristically as acute lancinating pain of brief duration. It is triggered by stimulation of the skin and is repetitive over a period of minutes.

The most serious cause of secondary trigeminal neuralgia is herpes zoster ophthalmicus, which begins acutely with unilateral head pain. It can be a tricky diagnostic problem because erythema and vesicle formation may not appear for days. Ocular involvement may have a sudden onset, especially if the nasociliary branch is involved.

Multiple sclerosis and internal carotid artery occlusion can also produce unilateral neuralgic-type head pain.

Intracranial neoplasms and vascular lesions, such as aneurysms and arteriovenous malformations, often must be ruled out when unilateral facial pain is persistent, especially when accompanied by sixth nerve palsy, nasopharyngeal carcinoma, chordoma, or aspergillosis. For all of these conditions, appropriate studies must be pursued. MRI is most helpful in making the diagnosis, its value far exceeding that of any other study.

THERAPY

Systemic. Ergotamine and ergot-like drugs remain the cornerstone of migraine therapy. Treatment of common migraine depends on the severity of the attacks, the age of the patient, and any complicating medical or psychiatric problem. Each patient and each attack must be approached individually. Thus, patients often complain of failure when therapy has not been tailored to the type of attack and its severity. Sublingual ergotamine is good therapy for on-the-spot treatment of common migraine attacks. It is vital that the patient take the medication at the onset of the attack to cause vasoconstriction and to abort the vasodilative headache.

"Spot" treatment of classic migraine consists of ergotamine/belladonna/caffeine/pentobarbital combination administered at the onset of the visual aura, thus giving this oral medication sufficient time to cause vasoconstriction and to prevent the onset of the headache caused by vasodilation. Synthetic sympathomimetic drugs, such as isometheptene/dichloralphenazone combinations, can be used if the patient is sensitive to ergotamine. These medications are also valuable in treating migraine-tension headache. It must be remembered that 70 per cent of migraine sufferers also have tension headache.

Prophylactic treatment of classic migraine involves the use of a beta-blocker. It should be used when migraine attacks occur frequently (i.e., four to six times a month) and they become incapacitating. Prevention of classic migraine by digital massage of the superficial temporal arteries recently has been re-emphasized.

Carbon dioxide inhalation has also been used for many years to abort the visual attack of classic and isolated ophthalmic migraine, with a 50 to 60 per cent success rate in the latter. A small plastic sandwich bag should be available at *all* times. The patient should remain seated while rebreathing in the bag, and the opening of the plastic bag should be held over the mouth only. The patient should be instructed to exhale *fully* into the bag to fill it and then inhale and exhale deeply, rebreathing the air in the bag. This should be continued for 1.5 to 3 minutes at the most or until the visual disturbance begins to disappear. This procedure is to be performed as soon as possible after the onset of visual disturbance, not after 10 to 15 minutes have elapsed and definitely not after the onset of headache.

Recently, isoproterenol[‡] inhalation has been used successfully to abort the visual attack. Sublingual nitroglycerin[‡] also has been used with limited success.

Aspirin rarely helps an individual attack of common migraine, but it has been helpful in prophylaxis. Aspirin/caffeine/butalbital combinations are often helpful when stress is prominent. Isometheptene/dichloralphenazone contains a sympathomimetic plus a tranquilizer and is quite effective in prophylaxis of common migraine in many patients.

Patients with isolated ophthalmic migraines need careful ophthalmologic evaluation and medical referral when deemed necessary. Angiography is unnecessary, unless other neurologic signs are present. The administration of aspirin and carbon dioxide inhalation aborts isolated ophthalmic migraine in approximately 60 per cent of these patients.

Monocular attacks of transient visual loss of variable duration deserve much more concern. Carotid bruits, significant difference in ophthalmodynametric readings greater than 20 per cent, and ophthalmoscopic evidence of atheromatous embolic disease (Hollenhorst plaques) must be searched for diligently.

Treatment of pediatric migraine is usually unnecessary. Aspirin is usually sufficient, since the syndrome is so fragmented and mild. However, there are rare instances in which ergotamine is indicated in common or classic migraine in children. A careful eye examination is important to rule out refractive errors and muscle imbalance; although these conditions have little or nothing to do with the headache, they must be treated if present. The parents should be advised that any prescription for glasses may have no effect on the headache problem and if beneficial is only a dividend. Asthenopic or eye fatigue headaches should be clinically evident after a refraction is done.

Steroid therapy given at the onset of symptoms should be considered in all patients with ophthalmoplegic migraine, unless other neurologic signs indicate the presence of an aneurysm, in which case angiography should be done immediately. However, it would be most unusual to have an aneurysm in most patients with ophthalmoplegic migraine because of the young age group.

Cluster headache responds best to sublingual ergotamine used at the onset of the attack. It can be a serious, recurrent, incapacitating headache, which can be extremely difficult to control if severe. Prophylactic or interim headache treatment may require the use of steroids, as well as ergotamine therapy. Oxygen therapy at home or referral to a headache specialist may also be necessary.

Aspirin or dipyridamole therapy is indicated for all patients with transient blurred vision complaints. The use of carbon dioxide inhalation may also be a source of reassurance, but does not rule out other more serious causes of cerebral hypoxia. The inspiration of 1 per cent isoproterenol[‡] via a nebulizer in conjunction with aspirin treatment at the onset of visual symptoms may not only abort the visual attack but also prevent permanent visual loss that can occur in these patients. Patients with amaurosis fugax should be examined for carotid bruits, retinal emboli, and coronary, femoral, or aortic atheromatous disease. Ophthalmologists should perform ophthalmodynamometry and take blood pressure readings on all patients with these symptoms, in addition to ordering blood studies and a medical vascular work-up. These patients should also have arterial digital subtraction angiography. If carotid artery stenosis is discovered, endarterectomy should be considered. Despite current controversy, this operation has definite value, as judged after all data and arteriography results are studied individually. If negative, further investigation is necessary, especially regarding the heart.

Treatment of tension headache should start with aspirin and progress to a combination of aspirin/caffeine/butalbital or any adjunctive or psychiatric treatment when deemed necessary.

As in many other facial neuralgias, treatment with carbamazepine‡ can be successful in patients with cranial neuralgias, but often surgery of the fifth nerve, its ganglia, or tract is necessary for relief. Secondary trigeminal neuralgia due to herpes zoster ophthalmicus may be treated with 600 to 800 mg of acyclovir administered four times daily for 2 weeks in conjunction with 100 mg of prednisone daily, unless the patient is diabetic. Prophylactic cimetidine should also be used with the above regimen to prevent stomach ulcers. This is the most effective way of avoiding the dreaded ocular complications and postherpetic neuralgia. Steroids have also been successful in treating cranial oculomotor nerve palsies and uveitis, the common ocular complications of herpes zoster.

COMMENTS

The initial procedure for headache problems should be to listen carefully to the patient's symptoms, discern any headache or visual obscuration problems, and then put these in a diagnostic category to enable proper management by the ophthalmologist or referring physician. When this is not done, the patient may be misdiagnosed and poorly managed. When diagnosis is pursued in a knowledgeable, systematic fashion, the patient obtains the necessary relief and psychologic support. Patients appreciate the ophthalmologist's interest in their headache and hearing an explanation of the type of headache they have with some indication of the treatment or studies necessary. At this point, the physician can decide whether primary management or referral is the best course to follow. This decision is made depending on the personnel and facilities available. If no headache specialist is available, the primary care must of necessity be given by the ophthalmologist. Otherwise, a referring letter to the patient's general physician, internist, or neurologist will enable that physician to take over the procedures and treatment indicated. Indeed, the interested ophthalmologist can be the deciding factor in starting the headache patient on his or her course to treatment and long-term management.

References

Buci ER, Herlot CP, Rufflieux C: Oral acyclovir in the treatment of acute herpes zoster ophthalmicus. Am J Ophthalmol 102:531–532, 1986.
Cruciger HH: Ophthalmoplegic migraine. Am J Ophthalmol 86:414–417, 1978.
Fisher CM: Late life migraine accompaniments as a cause of unexplained transient ischemic attacks. Can J Neurol Sci 7:9–17, 1980.
Fisher CM: Late life migraine accompaniments—Further experience. Stroke 17:1033–1042, 1986.
Hachinski EH: Pediatric migraine. Neurology 23:570–579, 1973.
Hedges TR Jr: Terminology of transient visual loss due to vascular insufficiency. Stroke 15:907–908, 1984.
Hedges TR Jr, Lackman RD: Isolated ophthalmic migraine in the differential diagnosis of cerebro-ocular ischemia. Stroke 7:4, 1976.
Kupersmith MA, Hass WK, Chase NE: Isoproterenol treatment of visual symptoms in migraine. Stroke 10:299–305, 1979.
Kupersmith MA, Warren FA, Hass WK: The non-benign aspect of migraine. Neuro-Ophthalmol 7:1–10, 1987.
Lipton SA: Prevention of classic migraine headache by digital massage of the superficial temporal arteries during visual aura. Ann Neurol 19:515–516, 1986.
Prensky AL, Sommer D: Diagnosis and treatment of migraine in children. Neurology 29:506–510, 1979.

HYSTERIA, MALINGERING, AND ANXIETY STATES 300.10

AUGUST L. READER, III, M.D., F.A.C.S.

Los Angeles, California

Medical practitioners are often faced with patients whose ocular examination does not correlate with their complaints. These patients may be feigning ocular disease for psychologic or physical gain. Occasionally, organic disease can develop secondary to the stress accompanying a constant or periodically recurring emotional state.

Malingering may be defined as the willful exaggeration or simulation of symptoms of an illness, usually to obtain some physical gain (financial, evasion of military service). Occasionally, dissimulation occurs where the patient claims to be normal when disease or disability is present in order to obtain a goal, such as to qualify for a specific occupation (pilots, truck drivers). Hysteria is the feigning of disease or injury on an unconscious level in order to satisfy certain unconscious psychologic needs. There are three main groups of hysteric symptoms: conversion symptoms (aphonia, blindness, deafness, paralysis of a limb, hemiplegia), dissociative state (fugues, multiple personality), and somatic symptoms. Both hysteria and malingering may arise from and be complicated by a state of anxiety, which is characterized by a subjective feeling of fear and uneasy anticipation. These anxiety states may present separately from hysteria and malingering, with organic disease manifested periocularly from emotional stress (angioneurotic edema, rosacea). Certain psychosomatic symptoms are commonly associated with anxiety states and include irritability, fearfulness, disorientation, insomnia, tachycardia, shortness of breath, fatigue, vertigo, pains in the chest, and blurred vision. These symptoms may lead the patient to present to a physician with fears of a serious physical disorder and may account for the majority of the patient's symptoms.

THERAPY

Systemic. In acute anxiety states, temporary relief is usually obtained with benzodiazepines, such as diazepam, alprazolam, lorazepam, clorazepate, or oxazepam. Patients liable to sudden attacks of panic gain security from carrying capsules of a rapidly acting anxiolytic, such as 50 mg of amobarbital. For patients with depression and a sleep disorder associated with their disability, 25 to 75 mg of amitriptyline at bedtime can be of help. Newer and less toxic antidepressants, such as fluoxetine, bupropion, and trazodone, are also available. Patients with organic disease secondary to anxiety (blepharospasm) may be helped by biofeedback therapy or hypnotherapy. In all cases where the chronic use of any medication is indicated, evaluation and treatment should be under the direction of an internist, neurologist, or psychiatrist.

Supportive. A short discussion with the patient and family about the findings of the examination in a very frank and open manner is usually well accepted by patients who seem to have chronic complaints of a hysterical nature. In patients whose hysteria is mild, simple autosuggestion or pointing out inconsistencies in complaints may produce a normal examination. Hysterics are suggestible and may improve with placebo therapy. Malingerers, however, should be approached more cautiously since confrontation can be interpreted as an accusation of prevarication with ensuing hostility. Inconsistencies can be outlined to the patient, but conclusions should be generally communicated only to the referring physician or agency.

Removal of a patient from an anxiety-producing situation may alleviate anxiety-based complaints. Discussing the possible causes for the complaints may be the only therapy necessary. Reassurance is very important and therapeutic for these patients. If the anxiety state is severe and long standing, psychiatric help should be sought.

Ocular or Periocular Manifestations

Choroid or Retina: Anxiety-induced angiospastic or central serous retinopathy; anxiety-induced or aggravated posterior uveitis.

Conjunctiva: Conjunctivitis (self-induced); hyperemia; allergic.

Cornea: Epithelial erosions (traumatic); hypesthesia; phlyctenular keratitis; recurrent herpetic keratitis.

Eyelids: Angioneurotic edema; blepharospasm; chronic blepharitis; contact dermatitis; eczema; hordeolum and chalazion; loss of cilia; ptosis; recurrent herpetic vesicles; rosacea.

Pupil: Anisocoria; hippus; peculiar pupillary reflexes.

Other: Accommodative spasm; amaurosis fugax; anxiety-induced optic neuritis; disturbance of conjugate movement; dyschromatopsia; facial tic; hypersecretion glaucoma; induced or decreased tear secretion; night blindness; nystagmus; photophobia; strabismus; visual loss; visual field defects.

PRECAUTIONS

Moralizing about hysterical illness or exhortations to stop imagining symptoms should be avoided. Direct discussion of the nature and causation of the symptoms should be done carefully, stating unequivocally that physical illness has been excluded and giving firm reassurance that the condition "will improve." The medical examination of patients with presumed hysteria should be conducted and brought to an end quickly. In patients who are felt to be malingering, the examination should be extended or resumed another day to allow the patient to "maintain face." Ambitious medical or surgical intervention is contraindicated, since such measures tend to reinforce the patient's invalidism. Drugs have a limited role in the treatment of hysteria; if they are used, they should be kept under strict supervision, confined to a transitional period, and terminated within a few weeks.

In unmasking conscious or unconscious ocular fraud, the ophthalmologist should remember that hysterics will have positive tests, just as malingerers. Cases of the greatest difficulty to detect are patients with ocular diseases that cause anxiety and induce additional symptoms.

COMMENTS

In both hysteria and malingering, well-documented records and a complete examination to rule out disease are essential. Electrophysiologic testing can be of great help in differentiating organic visual loss. Completely normal pattern visual evoked potentials, electroretinography, and electro-oculography are strong evidence for normal visual function and functional visual loss. These tests should always be obtained in questionable cases or in cases where litigation (either malpractice or personal injury) is involved. Malpractice litigation in cases of feigned disease is difficult to defend unless the records explain the discrepancy between the complaints and the examination. Anxiety-induced ocular disease can respond to routine therapy, but will recur if the underlying stress is not treated.

References

Catalano RA, Simon JW, Krobel GB, et al: Functional visual loss in children. Ophthalmology 93: 385–390, 1986.

Keltner JL, May WN, Johnson CA, et al: The California syndrome: Functional visual complaints with potential economic impact. Ophthalmology 92:427–435, 1985.

Kramer KK, LaPiana FG, Appleton B: Ocular malingering and hysteria: Diagnosis and management. Ophthalmology 24:89–96, 1979.

Miller BW: A review of practical tests for ocular malingering and hysteria. Surv Ophthalmol 17: 241–246, 1973.

Smith CH, Beck RW, Mills RP: Functional disease in neuro-ophthalmology. Neurol Clin 1:955–971, 1983.

Thompson HS: Functional visual loss. Am J Ophthalmol 100:209–213, 1985.

IDIOPATHIC INTRACRANIAL HYPERTENSION AND PSEUDOTUMOR CEREBRI 348.2

(Benign Intracranial Hypertension)

MARK S. GANS, M.D.,

Montreal, Canada

RONALD M. BURDE, M.D.,

Bronx, New York

SATOSHI KASHII, M.D., Ph.D.,

Kyoto, Japan

and WILLIAM L. BASUK, M.D.

Atlanta, Georgia

The terms "pseudotumor cerebri" (PTC) and "benign intracranial hypertension" have been used interchangeably to describe a condition characterized by headaches and papilledema. The intracranial pressure (ICP) is elevated with normal cerebral spinal fluid (CSF) constituents, and there is an absence of hydrocephalus or a space-occupying lesion. The papilledema may be unilateral or bilateral, but the symptomatology or progression of the disease is independent of its laterality. ICP, when measured, is usually elevated, but if charted may vary from low to very high.

Over time, the term "idiopathic intracranial hypertension" (IIH) has become accepted, thus eliminating the implication of the term "benign" as these patients often experience loss of visual function. Four criteria are proposed for the diagnosis of IIH: (1) elevated CSF pressure (>200 mm Hg), (2) normal CSF composition (CSF protein concentration may be low, <20mg/dl), (3) symptoms and signs restricted to those of elevated ICP, and (4) normal neuroimaging studies, excluding nonspecific findings of increased ICP (scans may demonstrate small, slit-like ventricles, enlarged optic nerve sheath, reversal of the optic nerve head, and empty sella).

The use of certain medications has induced a disease state that mimics IIH. Similarly, IIH can be seen in patients with certain disease states. Since there is a hint of causality, the authors prefer to call this condition secondary IIH. Therapeutic use of drugs producing secondary IIH include systemic corticosteroids (use and withdrawal), nalidixic acid, nitrofurantoin, danazol, and lithium. In addition, tetracycline has been shown to result in secondary IIH in children and young adults. Hypervitaminosis A produced by the use of vitamin A or its congener, retinoic acid, used for treating various skin disorders, consistently produces secondary IIH. Systemic conditions, such as hypoparathyroidism, iron-deficiency anemia, systemic lupus erythematosus (SLE), periarteritis nodosa, sarcoidosis, thoracic outlet syndrome, and uremia, may produce secondary IIH. In addition, dural sinus thrombosis following such entities as middle-ear infection, the use of oral contraceptives, pregnancy, SLE with circulating cardiolipins, and protein S and C deficiency can produce secondary IIH.

The peak incidence of IIH occurs during the third decade. There is a significant predominance in women; the ratio of women to men ranges from approximately 2:1 to 10:1. Obesity is a common finding (44 to 90 per cent). The incidence of IIH in women in their third decade ranges from 3.5 to 19.3 per 100,000. Although the general incidence for women in the 15–44 year old age group was 3.5 per 100,000, it rose to 13 per 100,000 and 19.3 per 100,000 for females who were 10 per cent and 20 per cent above their ideal weight, respectively. Thus, the typical patient is a young obese female. Although the literature indicates that the condition is self-limited, lasting 3 to 9 months in most patients, IIH is now considered by many to be a chronic disease that requires careful follow-up to prevent devastating visual loss. Recurrence rate has been low, usually less than 10 per cent, but a recrudescence may occur many years later.

The mechanisms underlying increased ICP and IIH are unknown. Using the compartmental model of Foley; there are four possible mechanisms that could lead to elevated intracranial pressure: (1) increased blood volume, (2) increased CSF production, (3) decreased absorption, or (4) parenchymal brain edema. At the present time, decreased absorption of CSF is the most often evoked theory. It is postulated that in IIH there is a relative obstruction to CSF absorption across the arachnoid villi. Decreased absorption could be caused by increased resistance within the villi themselves or by an increase in the draining venous system. In the latter case, there is a reversed normal gradient between the sinus and subarachnoid space. Increased resistance to CSF outflow (absorption block) has been demonstrated by studies using intrathecal saline infusion and radioisotope cisternography. Thus, it would seem that IIH is somewhat analogous to primary open-angle glaucoma.

Similarly, it is believed that the secondary IIH associated with hypervitaminosis A and acute systemic corticosteroid withdrawal is caused by an increase in arachnoidal resistance. It can be argued that the finding of smaller-than-normal ventricles on CT scanning in primary or secondary IIH excludes an increase in resistance to CSF absorption as a possible mechanism. In fact, it has been shown that normalization of the CSF pressure is associated with an increase in ventricular volume into normal range. This finding suggests that parenchymal edema may be the underlying pathogenetic mechanism.

The supposition that parenchymal edema is the cause of IIH has been supported by altered cerebrovascular reactivity at the capillary-venule level, and it has been postulated that changes in vascular permeability result in parenchymal edema. However, a CSF absorption block could also result in cerebral interstitial edema. Elevated CSF pressure could produce an increase of transependymal transport of CSF fluid from ventricular spaces into brain tissues. Although a 33 per cent increase in cerebral blood volume was noted in one series, it was pointed out that this would produce a 1 per cent increase in intracranial contents, far less than needed to sustain an elevation in ICP. Some compensatory increase in cerebral blood volume would be expected as an autoregulatory response of the cerebral vasculature to elevated ICP. Evidence to support the theory that hypersecretion of CSF is the cause of IIH is contradictory. Individual patients may have different underlying causative mechanisms in primary or secondary IIH. Headache is the initial symptom in 99 per cent of the patients seen by neurologists, but in only 80 to 85 per cent of those who initially see an ophthalmologist. The headache is usually generalized in nature, is worse early in the morning, and is exacerbated by anything that produces a Valsalva maneuver and in some by head turning.

Other symptoms of IIH are related to the visual system. Transient visual obscurations (TVOs) are a presenting symptom in 46 to 72 per cent of patients. TVOs usually last between 1 and 5 seconds and rarely more than 30 seconds. It is postulated that the increased ICP produces a relative decrease in perfusion of the prelaminar disc, resulting in further compromise of capillary perfusion. This failure of perfusion is secondary to an increase in the intrinsic tissue pressure in the optic nerve. Superimposed upon this failure, a transient alteration of the perfusion pressure to the nerve head by suddenly standing up or bending over or a transient increase in the intraocular pressure by rubbing of the eyes will produce TVOs.

The only serious complications of this condition involve the visual system and include loss of visual field or loss of central vision. The characteristic visual field abnormalities in IIH are disc related and mimic those defects associated with glaucoma. Thus, if one single test is to be used to follow patients with this disease process, it would be a quantitative visual field, either kinetic or static. At this time, automated perimetry (static visual fields) is the preferred method of sequentially following the visual function of these patients, as the currently available statistical packages used for analysis of the visual field defects allow an objective comparison between subsequent and sequential visual fields.

Enlarged blind spots are found in virtually all patients with papilledema. These blind spots have been attributed to displacement and detachment of the peripapillary retina by the swollen axons. It has now been demonstrated that blind spot enlargement is a refractive perturbation. In addition, patients with papilledema often have peripapillary choroidal folds or striae that can increase the size of the blind spot, and it remains enlarged long after the papilledema has disappeared. Initially, peripheral nerve fiber involvement causes constriction of the visual field, progressing to nasal depression, nasal steps, and then to overt arcuate defects. When sufficient nerve fibers (axons) are lost, central visual acuity is affected. One study noted that 21 per cent of patients with IIH sustained loss of visual acuity (8 per cent less than 20/40), as well as severe visual field loss.

Occasionally, patients with papilledema may experience acute visual loss. Mechanical distortion of the peripapillary tissues can cause a break in Bruch's membrane, allowing the formation of the subretinal neovascular capillary net. Transudation or overt bleeding from this membrane can spread to the macular area. Central retinal vein occlusion has also been reported to cause acute visual loss in these patients. Superimposed anterior ischemic optic neuropathy with acute field defects has been reported to occur in patients with IIH. Whether this is a fortuitous occurrence or is pathogenetically associated is not known.

Diplopia, when present, is almost always horizontal and is due to unilateral or bilateral sixth nerve palsies. These cranial nerve palsies are a nonspecific sign of increased ICP. Rare reports of skew deviation and third and fourth nerve palsies are to be found. In addition, paralysis of the seventh nerve has also been reported. How these findings relate to the disease process is not clear, but they should place the diagnosis of primary IIH in question. Patients may experience dizziness, nausea, vomiting, and other nonspecific symptoms. None of these symptoms correlates well with recorded CSF pressure, appearance of the papilledema, or the ultimate prognosis.

If a patient presents with signs and symptoms of IIH and neuroimaging has excluded the presence of an intracranial mass lesion, a spinal tap is indicated to measure the ICP and to assess the constituents of the CSF. If the pressure is not elevated on one or two successive taps, 24-hour monitoring of the ICP is indicated. In IIH, there is free communication of spinal subarachnoid with the intracranial subarachnoid space. ICP can be monitored readily and simply by inserting a catheter into the lumbar subarachnoid space and connecting it to a transducer. Interestingly, patients with IIH and florid papilledema frequently have a normal ICP during the day, whereas during rapid eye movement (REM) sleep, their ICP reaches heights of systemic arteriolar pressure. Thus in patients suspected to have IIH whose ICP on spinal tap is normal, a baseline must be obtained over a 24-hour period, including REM sleep. Repeated CSF taps late in the course of the disease are only indicated in the face of progressive visual dysfunction despite appropriate intervention.

As mentioned previously, continuous monitoring of visual fields and measurement of visual acuity, as well as sequential fundus photographs, are fundamental in the follow-up care of patients with IIH. Because therapy for IIH is determined by the degree and progression of visual dysfunction, it has been suggested by some that specific visual field strategies should be employed. Because of the similarity of visual field loss in IIH and glaucoma, kinetic perimetry using the modified Armaly-Drance strategy has been recommended for routine examinations. Automated threshold static perimetry (i.e., Octopus program 32 or Humphey 30-1) has been advocated by others who feel that it may be a more sensitive methodology for detecting visual field change. Visual function testing should be carried out at regular intervals, the length of which should be determined by the patient's clinical condition. Slit-lamp examination with measurement of intraocular pressure is necessary at regular intervals if systemic corticosteroids are used.

THERAPY

Systemic. Severe and intractable headaches and evidence of optic neuropathy (i.e., visual dysfunction) are the primary reasons for initiating treatment. Visual loss when present at the time of the first examination is considered by some to be an indication for intensive therapy. No prospective randomized study comparing various treatments has been done. Although there are claims of a high spontaneous remission rate for IIH, there are no controlled data on the natural history of untreated IIH. Some patients only briefly experience symptoms of IIH that may disappear after the initial diagnostic tap, and it is difficult to know whether reported improvements are the result of treatment or simply represent the natural course of the disease.

The first line of therapy in the treatment of IIH is the systemic use of carbonic anhydrase inhibitors (CAIs). CAIs have been shown to decrease CSF secretion in humans after intravenous bolus injections of 1 gm of acetazolamide.[§] CSF production is inhibited for approximately 2 hours after such an injection. Daily doses of 60 mg/kg (2 to 4 gm) of acetazolamide[§] in its sustained-release form in divided doses effectively lower ICP, even in patients with mass lesions. The side effects from the use of acetazolamide are for the most part dose related and may be bothersome at a dose as little as 500 mg daily. These side effects include drowsiness; tingling of the fingers, toes, and circumoral region; metallic taste; nausea; and anorexia. The use of the drug is associated with a metabolic acidosis accompanied by an alkalization of the urine, reducing the solubility of oxylate and predisposing susceptible individuals to the development of calcium oxylate stones. Unfortunately, it has been shown that lower daily doses of acetazolamide (0.5 to 2.5 gm) are ineffective in lowering ICP or relieving symptoms. It is known that methazolamide penetrates the blood-brain barrier more readily, and it has been postulated to be effective in relatively lower doses, thus reducing some side effects but not the drowsiness. Although the use of CAIs reduces the serum concentration of potassium, total intracellular stores are not affected. The metabolic acidosis remains relatively constant.

CAIs are sulfonamides and therefore can produce an idiosyncratic agranulocytopenia or aplastic anemia; thus, a baseline complete blood count is indicated. In addition, the sulfonamides have been reported to be teratogenic and should be used with caution during pregnancy. In spite of apocryphal statements to the contrary, there is little available evidence demonstrating the efficacy of thiazide diuretics, furosemide, or ethacrynic acid in treating IIH. However, a recent paper has demonstrated that furosemide[‡] can be effective over a prolonged period of time. In an uncontrolled study, chlorthalidone,[‡] a long-acting thiazide, has been reported to be effective in treating IIH.

Oral hyperosmotic agents can acutely lower ICP. A single dose of 1 gm/kg of glycerol raises serum osmolality from 295 to 320 mosm/1 in 90 minutes and concomitantly reduces CSF pressure for 3 to 5 hours. Obviously, treatment would be required every 4 hours. Glycerin is extraordinarily fattening and can produce either ketoacidosis or nonketotic hyperosmolar coma. The taste of glycerin is terribly sweet and often so nauseates patients that they cannot swallow; it can be made more tolerable by diluting it with orange juice and serving it over ice. A reversed osmotic gradient and a rebound increase in ICP can occur. In addition, glycerin is metabolized and can have an adverse effect on serum glucose concentration. Isosorbide, which is not metabolized, can be substituted for glycerin at a dose level of 2 cc/kg. The use of hyperosmotics in IIH should be limited to a few days in an attempt to "break" the cycle.

Cardiac glycosides[†] have been reported to reduce CSF production, but the efficacy of such therapy has never been substantiated.

If CAIs do not relieve the symptoms or a patient cannot tolerate their side effects, a 2-week course of oral corticosteroids (60 mg of prednisone daily) may be instituted. If remission occurs, it is noted usually within 4 days of the start of prednisone therapy. If there is no response by the end of the first week, the corticosteroids should be discontinued. Prednisone treatment can be discontinued after 2 weeks of therapy without a recrudescence of the disorder. It is curious that both the use of and the withdrawal of systemic corticosteroids have been associated with the onset of IIH.

It is well known that long-term use of systemic corticosteroids can raise intraocular pressure and can cause posterior subcapsular cataracts, but such side effects are unlikely to occur with a short course. Yet, the increase in intraocular pressure caused by the use of orally administered corticosteroids for an injudicious amount of time may act as the final insult to produce ischemic damage of the optic nerve head. The systemic side effects are of greater importance. The immediate effects of systemic corticosteroids include aggravation of underlying hypertension and a disturbance in the control of serum glucose in susceptible individuals. They also have a profound effect on mentation, causing insomnia, a hyperactive state, or depression. The long-term effects of variably induced Cushing's syndrome are well known.

Surgical. Because no single drug or combination of medications has proven to be effective or tolerated in patients with IIH, surgical intervention should be contemplated before serious visual loss has developed. Most physicians choose to demonstrate progressive visual field loss before recommending surgery, but the finding of significant visual field loss at the time of the initial examination may itself prove to be an indication for intervention. Surgical intervention is indicated in patients with intractable headaches, progressive visual dysfunction as demonstrated by visual fields or Snellen visual acuities, significant visual dysfunction that does not improve with treatment, evidence of progressive nerve fiber bundle dropout or involutional atrophy, or "malignant" IIH.

Multiple or repeated spinal punctures are mentioned only for historical interest. A lumbar puncture has a short-lived effect on CSF pressure. The CSF pressure returns to "pre-tap" levels within 60 to 90 minutes, unless an inadvertent rip is made in the meninges at the time of the tap. Most patients find the experience of undergoing a lumbar puncture so unpleasant that the suggestion of multiple sequential taps causes them either not to seek help (thus, taking the chance of developing visual dysfunction) or seeking help elsewhere.

Subtemporal decompression has been generally abandoned because of significant morbidity and mortality. It has been replaced by CSF shunting procedures. Lumboperitoneal shunts are preferable to ventriculoatrial shunts because the ventricles are by definition normal or small in size in patients with IIH, making access technically difficult. A lumbar cisternogram is usually done before shunting to ensure patency of the subarachnoid space. The major problems associated with lumboperitoneal shunts are (1) a difficulty in testing their patency due to the presence of excess surrounding adipose tissue as these patients are usually obese and (2) the high rate of shunt failure caused by obstruction. In addition to the technical problem of obstruction, lumboperitoneal shunts have been reported to be ineffective in preventing progressive visual field loss in some series of patients. Cervicoperitoneal shunting has been proposed to solve this problem, but no large series measuring the efficiency of this technique has been forthcoming.

The visual function of patients with IIH stabilizes after an optic nerve sheath decompression. Optic nerve sheath decompression or fenestration is considered by many to be the procedure of choice in preventing or arresting the development of the visual dysfunction associated with papilledema. Until recently, this surgical intervention was reserved for patients who developed progressive visual dysfunction despite aggressive medical treatment for chronic papilledema. However, there are indications that patients with acute papilledema who undergo optic nerve sheath decompression have significantly better visual results than do patients with chronic atrophic papilledema. With the mounting evidence in the literature supporting the effectiveness of this procedure in visually compromised IIH patients, it is the belief of some that all patients with visual dysfunction, regardless of the presence of headache, should undergo an optic nerve sheath fenestration procedure.

Technically, there are two ways to approach the optic nerve: the medial and the lateral approach. The lateral approach may require a lateral orbitotomy with bone resection, although it has been recently suggested that this resection is not necessary in all cases to gain access to the optic nerve. The medial approach does not require any bone resection and is technically easier. Using the operating microscope, the medial approach has become the standard for most ophthalmic surgeons. This approach has a low operative morbidity, and by operating on the medial aspect of the optic nerve, the critical foveomacular projection is avoided. This approach can be used under a variety of circumstances to access the retrobulbar optic nerve safely in order to obtain tissue and CSF for chemical and cytologic analysis.

Under local anesthesia, a peritomy is made for approximately 180°, and the medial rectus muscle is detached from the globe. A baseball stitch is placed through the insertion of the medial rectus muscle, or posterior equatorial sutures are placed in the inferior and superior nasal quadrants. The globe is retracted anteriorly and laterally, which exposes the nerve as the fat either falls away or can be gently swept away with cotton-tipped applicators. A window is cut in the optic nerve dural sheath just posterior to the globe. Some surgeons prefer to make multiple longitudinal slits in the nerve sheath. The use of the operating microscope makes it easy for the surgeon to avoid the myriad of vessels in the immediate retrobulbar region where the nerve exits the globe. Some mechanical means is suggested to break subarachnoid trabeculations that tend to sequester CSF, thereby impeding the free flow of fluid. Improvement in disc edema may not occur for weeks, but visual function ordinarily begins to improve within days.

The presence of preoperative disc pallor (early optic atrophy) does not necessarily indicate a poor prognosis. This procedure rarely results in lowering of the ICP, but in some cases there is a bilateral deturgescence of the nerves, as well as a disappearance of the headache with a unilateral sheath decompression. Should papilledema recur in the operated eye, secondary and even tertiary decompression procedures are indicated. The mechanism by which the optic nerve sheath decompression is effective remains speculative. The possibilities include the development of a fistula from the subarachnoid space to the orbit in the vicinity of the fenestration site. Magnetic resonance imaging has been used to demonstrate a cyst-like structure contiguous to the fenestration site in a few patients, supporting such a mechanism. Other studies—both clinical and experimental—suggest that there is a collapse of the vaginal sheaths with scarring, sealing off the anterior optic nerve from communication with the subarachnoid space and thus protecting it from the ravages of raised pressure.

As previously mentioned there is substantial evidence both clinically and experimentally that unilateral optic nerve sheath decompression can effectively produce a bilateral deffervescence of papilledema. The variable results with respect to the contralateral side are thought to be caused by variations in the meshwork of the subarachnoid space at the optic canal that connects intracranial menin-gial space to intraorbital meningial space. The meshwork seems to play an important role in determining the extent to which the entire subarachnoid space is decompressed by unilateral or bilateral optic nerve decompression.

Optic nerve decompression is extraordinarily effective in preventing further deterioration of visual function, but has a variable effect on the headache. Complications include transient asymmetry of the pupils, probably due to trauma to the posterior ciliary nerves or the ciliary ganglion, horizontal motility disturbances from disinsertion of the medial rectus muscle, recurrence of papilledema due to obstruction of the fenestration site, chorioretinal scarring from excessive retraction of the globe, and occasional blindness due to a retinal artery occlusion despite a surgically acceptable procedure. Unfortunately, failure of this procedure can occur from months to years postoperatively in up to 32 per cent of patients who have undergone an initially successful operation. The subsequent prognosis with respect to the acute and chronic postoperative course in patients requiring reoperation is significantly poorer than in initial fenestration cases.

Ocular or Periocular Manifestations

Extraocular Muscles: Abducens nerve palsy.
Optic Nerve: Papilledema; optic nerve atrophy; opticociliary shunt vessels.
Retina: Choroidal folds; subretinal neovascular membrane.
Other: Visual field defect—enlargement of the blind spot and generalized constriction, nasal (especially inferonasal) loss; central, paracentral, and cecocentral scotomas in altitudinal patterns of loss.

PRECAUTIONS

The single most important risk factor associated with visual loss in a patient with IIH is systemic hypertension. Rapid lowering of an elevated blood pressure may contribute to ischemic damage of the optic disc in the presence of papilledema with compromised perfusion of the prelaminar nerve. Patients with secondary IIH undergoing hemodialysis for chronic renal failure, in whom hypotensive episodes are more common, are especially prone to such ischemic damage.

Obese hypertensive females seem to be at greatest risk for visual field defects. Weight reduction by diet has been advocated as a treatment of IIH. Others have suggested surgically induced weight loss by gastric exclusion to stabilize the visual function. The relationship of obesity to the pathogenesis of IIH is uncertain. It has been postulated that estrone produced exclusively by adipocyte (via the aromatization of circulating androstenedione) could increase the rate of CSF production. In obese females, who have reduced absorptive capacity of CSF, this combination of factors could result in IIH. It has been the experience of most physicians dealing with this patient population that dieting and weight loss are unachievable goals, thus leaving only the options of medical or surgical intervention.

COMMENTS

IIH may be benign from the standpoint that it is not life threatening, but it should not be considered benign in the functional sense because it can produce devastating visual loss. Permanent visual loss in adults with IIH occurs in from 6 to 25 per cent of patients. Moreover, permanent visual impairment can occur in children as well. Hypothalamic-hypophyseal dysfunction has been attributed to increased ICP. It is postulated that longstanding intracranial hypertension may weaken the diaphragm sellae and through uncertain mechanisms allow the pituitary gland to be flattened against the floor of the sella turcica, producing a so-called empty sella syndrome. Rare cases of chiasmal herniation into the sellae with concomitant visual field loss have been reported. Even when the pituitary gland is flattened against the floor of the sella, endocrine function seems to remain normal, although it is suggested that pituitary dysfunction may eventually develop.

Acknowledgment. Supported in part by an unrestricted Departmental grant from RPB, New York.

References

Amaral JF, et al: Reversal of benign intracranial hypertension by surgically induced weight loss. Arch Surg 122:926–949, 1987.

Beatty R: Cervical peritoneal shunt in the treatment of pseudotumor cerebri. J Neurosurg 57:853–855, 1982.

Brourman ND, Spoor TC, Ramocki JM: Optic nerve sheath decompression for pseudotumor cerebri. Arch Ophthalmol 106:1378–1383, 1988.

Burde RM: Surgical therapy of idiopathic intracranial hypertension. Presented at North American Neuro-Ophthalmology Society Annual Meeting, San Diego, California, February, 1992.

Corbett JJ: Problems in the diagnosis and treatment of pseudo-tumor cerebri. Can J Neurol Sci 10: 221–229, 1983.

Corbett JJ: Mechanisms of elevated ICP in IIH. NANOS 1992.

Corbett JJ, et al: Results of optic nerve sheath fenestration for pseudotumor cerebri. Arch Ophthalmol 106:1391–1397, 1988.

Digre KB: Epidemiology of idiopathic intracranial hypertension. NANOS 1992.

Foley J: Benign forms of intracranial hypertension—"toxic" and "otitic" hydrocephalus. Brain 18:1–41, 1955.

Hupp SK, Glaser JS, Frazier-Byrne S: Optic nerve sheath decompression. Arch Ophthalmol 105: 386–389, 1987.

Kaye AH, Galbraith JEK, King J: Intracranial pressure following optic nerve decompression for benign intracranial hypertension. J Neurosurg 55: 453–456, 1981.

Kilpatrick CJ, et al: Optic nerve decompression in benign intracranial hypertension. Clin Exp Neurol 18:161–168, 1981.

Plotnick JL, Kosmorsky GS: Operative complications of optic nerve sheath decompression. Ophthalmology 100:683–690, 1993.

Sergott RC, Savino PJ, Bosley TM: Modified optic nerve sheath decompression provides long-term visual improvement for pseudotumor cerebri. Arch Ophthalmol 106:1384–1390, 1988.

Spoor TC, McHenry JG: Long-term effectiveness of optic nerve sheath decompression for pseudotumor cerebri. Arch Ophthalmol 111:623–635, 1993.

Tse DT, et al: Optic nerve sheath fenestration in pseudotumor cerebri. Arch Ophthalmol 106: 1458–1462, 1988.

LOW VISION AIDS 369.0

K. NOLEN TANNER, M.D., Ph.D.

Portland, Oregon

About 80 per cent of the information received in our brains comes to us through our eyes. Obviously, loss of all or a significant part of this information is disabling. Of all the senses, loss of form perception is most disabling, except for loss of light sense itself. Clearly, impairment of color, space, direction, and motion sense will produce a disability, but it is loss or a threat of loss of form sense that brings patients to our attention. This loss is what we think of as "low vision." The diseases that impair form perception are many, and the patients so afflicted are indeed very numerous. According to a 1990 survey by the National Center for Health Statistics, there are in the United States almost 4.3 million people with *severe visual impairment* defined as the inability to read ordinary newsprint with glasses or contact lenses or, in the case of children, a parent's report that the child lacks useful vision. The rate is 17.3 per 1000 persons. About 2.9 million of these individuals are over the age of 65. Most of these older people have degenerative conditions, such as macular degeneration, cataract, keratopathy, and glaucoma, but inflammatory disease of the retina, choroid, optic nerve, or cornea afflicts a large number in all age groups. Trauma takes a heavy toll, as does metabolic disease in the form of diabetes. Many, if not most, of these afflicted patients should be given at least a trial of low vision aids.

Handicaps can be classified as to kind and degree. Loss of travel vision is the most severe, but accounts for a relatively small proportion of the visually handicapped. The degree ranges from no light perception to light perception with light projection, although a patient with severe field loss from advanced glaucoma or retinitis pigmentosa may have relatively good vision in a very small field and have a difficult time traveling. The aids available for this handicap are limited to canes and seeing-eye dogs.

The next kind of visual handicap is the inability to care for oneself—to dress, eat at table, and otherwise to attend to essential daily activities. Obviously, the presence of other physical disability enters into the equation and must be taken into account. Braille watches, "high Marks," a quick-drying plastic used to make tactile bumps; tactile controls for stoves and other equipment; and auditory signaling devices are available from organizations and companies, such as those listed below. The ability to drive a motor vehicle is of great importance to most people, especially the young. Unfortunately low vision aids are of no benefit since the requirements for a driver's license are fixed in the law. Any gain from telescopic devices will be offset by loss of field. Elderly people with other infirmities can usually accept this loss. By far, the greatest use for low vision aids is to enable reading by the use of magnification.

THERAPY

Ocular. The first and very important step is a thorough medical examination. If available and possible, such remedies as cataract extraction and keratoplasty should be exhausted. Treatable and chronic conditions, such as glaucoma, that result in progressive visual loss should be controlled. The patient's general physical and mental condition and their desires should be explored. Does the patient want to read? When this has been established, the best obtainable visual acuity and the refraction that will produce it are determined. The refraction is the diagnostic step that yields the degree of magnification necessary to accomplish the objective of enabling the patient to read newsprint. The refractive technique is essentially standard with a few modifications. Since visually handicapped persons are more comfortable in a near environment, the refraction should be done at 10 feet (3 meters), rather than the usual 20 feet (6 meters), although it can be done even at 5 feet. There are several acuity charts for 10-ft refraction available: Keeler, Sloan, Bailey-Lovey, Lighthouse, etc. The standard 20-ft Snellen chart is closely logarithmic, with a 25 per cent increase in letter size for each higher line, until about 20/80 when the logarithmic gaps become large. This of course is just where the visually handicapped will operate. The Sloan chart fills in these gaps with the same approximately 25 per cent logarithmic steps. The Keeler chart starts at 6/6, or 20/20, and steps the letter sizes up an exact 25 per cent per line to about 20/500 using "A" numbers to identify the lines. In general, a

"fogged" refraction in these higher lines can proceed in the same fashion as for the normally sighted. One click of the refractor, or 0.25 sphere diopter, will improve the acuity one line, and the refraction should stop when one, or at most two, clicks fail to improve the acuity. If possible the retinoscopy end-point of +1.50 fog should be used to begin. Retinoscopy also has the advantage of indicating the quality of the patient's optical system, i.e., does he or she have keratoconus or some other aberration? Any cylinder should be carefully determined, but the usual 0.25 or 0.37 cross cylinders will probably not be very helpful since these patients usually cannot detect the small swing in the conoid of Sturm. Cross cylinders of 0.5 or 1.0 diopter should be used. In the final prescription cylinder, corrections of less than 1.5 diopter will usually make little difference in the patient's "street" or reading acuity. The importance of the refraction cannot be overstated. Even an improvement of one line, say from 20/120 to 20/100, will be appreciated by these patients.

When the best distance acuity has been determined, the near acuity should be determined, and this is usually very consistent with the distance acuity. Near acuity charts by Keeler, Sloan, and others, when used with a suitable add if necessary, will quickly determine it. The Keeler chart is used at 25 cm with at most 2.50 to 3.00 add. The Sloan chart is used at 40 cm, with 2.00 to 2.50 add. These near charts will determine what magnification will be necessary to enable the patient to achieve the goal of reading newsprint. This magnification is usually printed on the chart itself. Newsprint is read at about the 20/50 level. Thus, the patient who can read the 20/100 line on the Keeler or Sloan chart will require 2X magnification to read newsprint. The magnification required is 20/50 divided by the patient's best acuity. The dioptric power of the lens required will be four times the magnification if the Keeler test distance of 25 cm is used or 2.5 times the magnification if the Sloan test distance of 40 cm is used. This magnification can be obtained either by bringing the print closer and keeping it in focus with the necessary add in a head-borne device or by creating an enlarged image at a more distant and perhaps more comfortable or convenient position. One way of creating this enlarged image is with a convex hand lens—a magnifier. Such a lens held at any distance from the eye but with the print just inside the focal distance will create an enlarged, erect, virtual image at a greater distance than the print, thus perhaps requiring little or no accommodation on the part of the patient's eye. It so happens that a plus lens will produce the same magnification whether used as a reading add in a frame with the print held close to the face or as a hand lens with the print held on the lap. In both cases, the print must be held at the same distance from the lens, just inside the focal point. Older patients are often uncomfortable with the print held close to their nose and prefer a hand lens. The field will be smaller, but the cost will be less. Young patients generally prefer a head-borne device with a larger field for more rapid reading and a free hand. Enlarged images can of course be produced by projection devices or closed-circuit television, and for some patients this is the best arrangement. With these devices, very large magnifications, 50X or more, can be obtained, but the cost is high. Simple hand lenses or spectacles with suitable reading adds are much less expensive and more portable, although the practical limit of magnification is about 12X. Most patients who can successfully use optical low vision aids need from 2X to 8X magnification. It is very important to remember that magnification is obtained at the expense of field. Patients who have severe peripheral field loss from glaucoma or retinitis pigmentosa will find it easy to magnify the print right out of the field so that sentences are fragmented, words become letters, and reading can become slow and tortured. Only the minimal degree of magnification necessary must be used.

Attention must be given to the degree of illumination of the print. Patients with macular degeneration or optic nerve disease usually benefit by high light levels, but a patient with cone dystrophy requires much reduced illumination to prevent his or her available rods from being dazzled out.

A few other devices that can facilitate reading should be mentioned. A simple straight edge under the line of print can make reading much easier since large magnification can make it very easy to get lost in the print. A cylinder lens that magnifies only the vertical dimension but that covers an entire line can be very effective, although only small degrees of magnification can be used. In teaching children to read with magnifying lenses, it would help if the material could be printed in small blocks covering the area of a single field. This would keep a phrase or sentence together, eliminating the extraneous and sometimes confusing material in the lines above and below and greatly reducing the movement of the lens. A good trick for patients with homonymous hemianopia is to turn the print sideways and read vertically.

Hand-held telescopes for distance vision of Galilean or terrestrial construction can be effective in enabling a patient to see bus signs or street signs. The practical limit of magnification, however, is generally less than 3X. Usually, a monocular device is preferred.

If binocular vision is possible, the patient may achieve a line or more better acuity than with either eye alone. This is especially true with macular degeneration. In this condition, macular vision is very spotty, with many small areas of reduced sensitivity. The relative blind spots, however, are not the same in both eyes, and when overlapped, the central field may be much better than expected. Binocular Galilean telescopes set for reading enable this binocular reading vision, but they are expensive. Simple high plus reading lenses cannot be used alone for binocular reading because of the high degree of convergence required. However base-in prism can be used to supply this convergence. Fonda's rule of thumb is to use 1 diopter of base-in prism in each lens for each diopter of plus spherical equivalent. For a patient with the average PD of 6 cm, this would supply one third of the necessary convergence. With a +10 lens with 10 diopter base-in prism for each eye, for example, this would leave 40 diopters for the patient or an equivalent convergence to 15 cm, about 6 inches. This is usually comfortable. With larger adds, however, the residual convergence is too much. Up to 1.5 diopters of base-in prism for each diopter of add in each lens can be used, but it should always be tried in a trial frame first. Plus 16 lenses with 24 prism diopters in each lens will leave 48 diopters of residual convergence or to 12 cm, which is less than 5 inches. Over 12 diopters of add is not often successful because the lenses are bulky (although Fresnel prisms can sometimes be used), and the focal distance becomes very critical. Fusion becomes very difficult. Even a small head tilt will induce enough vertical prism to break fusion. With high magnification monocular vision is preferred. Half eye glasses with base-in prism in a range of spherical powers are available from several commercial sources.

Finally, the physician should recommend large-print books and magazines, although there is reason to believe that children learn to read better and faster with a magnifying low vision aid. This material, which is especially published for the visually handicapped, is available from the Library of Congress, the Lighthouse in New York, the American Foundation for the Blind, Readers Digest, the *New York Times*, many local libraries, and other sources. Talking books—books and magazines on tapes and records—is also available from some of these sources. Many older people prefer the large-print or talking books. Braille and talking books, of course, will be the only reading material available to those who cannot see even the largest print.

Complex and expensive optical devices should be avoided in favor of simple and inexpensive ones. The elaborate and bizarre head-borne devices that are touted to relieve almost all visual handicap are inordinately expensive and rarely used very long in practice. The low vision patient cannot appreciate highly corrected and finely honed optical devices.

Loss of vision or of visual acuity, especially if rapid, is very debilitating and has serious psychologic effects. No patient should be told that "I can't do anything more for you." Such a statement will result in discouragement, depression, and ultimately resentment and even hostility. All ophthalmologists should be prepared to do some low vision aid work-up. The special charts are inexpensive, readily available, and easy to use. Only minor modifications to the standard comprehensive examination are required to arrive at a diagnosis, with little if any addition of time. Most of the time, the standard trial lens set with up to 20D of plus lenses will suffice. Trial sets with lenses to 10 or 12 power (about 48D) are available from Keeler and other suppliers, and most are relatively inexpensive. A small collection of hand-held and stand magnifiers from 6 to 28 diopters, such as those made by COIL in England and widely distributed in the United States, and one or two small high-power folding lenses, such as used by stamp and insect collectors, will suffice for almost all cases. A few hundred dollars worth of equipment will do the job very well. If ophthalmologists are unwilling to purchase this limited equipment and to do these simple tests, they should at least be prepared to refer the patient promptly to someone they know will do them and without discouraging the patient in the least. A discouraged and hopeless patient is much more difficult to treat than one who is hopeful and optimistic.

When the necessary magnification has been determined, it is very helpful if a knowledgeable technician is available to help the patient explore the various ways of obtaining this magnification—through hand lens, headborne, closed-circuit television, or projection—and to coach the patient on the best ways for their use. Each of these methods requires some skill and practice in their best use. At all times the patient should be encouraged and never discouraged. Most cities and states that have medical centers and universities with an ophthalmology and/or optometry department will have low vision clinic services with these technicians available to the community. Every ophthalmologist should know how to contact his or her state's Commission for the Blind. These agencies can usually be of great help. Support groups for the blind and visually handicapped are rapidly developing in many states, and their services should be sought as soon as possible for newly handicapped patients.

PRECAUTIONS

Patient counseling is very important. Loss of vision in whole or in part has been compared with dying, especially if the process has been sudden or rapid. The patient must then be reborn into a new world, that of the visually handicapped. The attending ophthalmologist is in the best position to help the patient through this traumatic experience, or he or she can make it much worse. Louis Cholden many years ago pointed out the harm that ophthalmologists can do by delaying, or even not allowing, the patient to progress through the normal psychologic stages of denial, an-

ger, grief, and finally acceptance of the condition, and the beginning of rehabilitation. By saying, "let's wait and see if another operation will restore your sight", the patient is placed in limbo and time passes, with more heroic medical and surgical efforts. In the meantime with each failure to achieve his or her hopes, which are always the complete restoration of vision, the patient becomes more depressed and dependent. He or she loses the attitude and the will that could carry him or her through a successful rehabilitation. The ophthalmologist must, gently and with real support, inform the patient of the most probable long-term condition at the earliest possible moment and start the rehabilitation, even if more medical or surgical efforts are to be made. Unless the loss of vision has been complete or almost so, optical low vision aids can be crucial in maintaining spirit and motivation. In using them, however, unrealistic expectations must be avoided. Without discouraging the patient it should be made clear that while low vision aids can do a great deal to help compensate for the handicap, no low vision aid can eliminate it.

If the disease and visual loss are not progressing rapidly, with practice and experience, the patient will use the aids to better and better effect. Macular degeneration is especially prone to cause conflict between direction sense and resolving power. If the patient looks "at" the word it disappears but by looking slightly to one side, he or she can see it. Eccentric fixation can be learned, and ultimately the clash between direction sense and resolving power will be resolved in favor of the latter. This author has no experience using prisms to obtain this eccentric fixation, but the technique of prismatic scanning described by Roymayananda et al. (1982) is certainly interesting and worth exploring.

COMMENTS

The exchange of letters between Stetten (1981) and Winer (1981) in the *New England Journal of Medicine* illustrates dramatically the lack of attention paid to low vision aids by the ophthalmic community and the great distress and frustration induced in the patient by being dismissed with the statement that "nothing more can be done." All visually handicapped deserve more. Such journals as the *Journal of Visual Rehabilitation* and the *Journal of Visual Impairment and Blindness* are available in libraries. The American Academy of Ophthalmology gives courses, as does the Lighthouse in New York, Pacific Presbyterian Medical Center in San Francisco, Pennsylvania College of Optometry, and others. Several very good books are in print and available in libraries on low vision aid work-up and treatment. There is no reason why residents in training and ophthalmologists in practice should have to neglect this very important subject.

The following is a short list of commercial and nonprofit organizations from which aids for the visually handicapped and the blind can be obtained. Many others exist.

Mons International, PO Box 91163; Atlanta, Ga 30364, (404)344-8805, (800)541-7903

LS&S Group PO Box 673, Northbrook, Il. 60065, (708)498-9777

Science Products, PO Box 888, Southeastern, Pa, 19399, (800)888-7400

Keeler Instruments Inc, 456 Parkway, Broom-all, Pa, (800)523-5620

Lighthouse, Inc., Low Vision Service, 800 2nd Ave, New York, NY 10017, (212)355-2200

American Foundation for the Blind, 15 West 16th St., New York, NY 10011, (212)620-2000, (800)829-0500 for catalog

Designs for Vision, Inc. 760 Koehler Ave., Ronkonkama New York, NY 11779, (516)585-3300

References

Cholden L: A Psychiatrist Works with Blindness. New York, American Foundation for the Blind, 1958.
Faye EE: Clinical Low Vision, 2nd ed. Boston, Little Brown, 1984.
Fonda G: Management of Patients with Subnormal Vision. St. Louis, CV Mosby, 1970.
Keeler CH: Visual aids for the pathological eye. Trans Ophthalmol Soc UK 76:605–614, 1956.
Nelson KA, Dimitrova E: Statistical brief #36. Severe visual impairment in the United States and in each state. J Vis Impair Blindness 3:80–84, 1993.
Rosenblum AA, Morgan MW (eds): Vision and Ageing, General and Clinical Perspectives. New York, Professional Press, 1986.
Roymayananda N, Wong SW, Elzeneiny IH, Chan GH: Prismatic scanning method for improving visual acuity in patients with low vision. Ophthalmology 89:937–945, 1982.
Stetten D Jr: Coping with blindness. N Engl J Med 305:458–460, 1981.
Winer M: Coping with blindness. N Engl J Med 305:1474–1475, 1981.

MULTIPLE SCLEROSIS 340

ANTHONY C. ARNOLD, M.D.

Los Angeles, California

Multiple sclerosis (MS) is a disease of undetermined etiology that results in multifocal demyelination within the white matter of the central nervous system. It attacks young adults most frequently, with a peak incidence at age 20 to 40 years; females are affected more often than males, with a ratio of about 1.5 to 1. Neurologic symptoms typically follow a pattern of exacerbation and remission, with acute episodes lasting weeks to months. There is a predilection for involvement of the corticospinal tracts and posterior columns of the spinal cord, the brainstem (particularly the medial longitudinal fasciculus [MLF]) and cerebellum, and the anterior visual pathway. The most common presenting features include weakness, numbness, and paresthesias of the extremities; ataxia; bulbar signs; and visual disturbance.

Involvement of the visual system usually takes the form of either ocular inflammation or eye movement disorder. Optic neuritis (ON) is the most frequently seen inflammatory manifestation, with rapid onset of a unilateral decrease in visual acuity, central visual field disturbance, pain on eye movement, afferent pupillary defect, and possible optic disc swelling; retinal periphlebitis, uveitis, and retinitis are other manifestations that are reported less often. Internuclear ophthalmoplegia (INO) is the most common abnormality of eye movement in MS, with slowed adducting saccades and possible limitation of range of adduction ipsilateral to the MLF lesion, in association with lateral-beating nystagmus of the contralateral abducting eye; other forms of nystagmus, defective ocular saccades and pursuit, and cranial nerve palsies are also noted routinely.

THERAPY

Systemic. The mainstay of therapy for the general neurologic manifestations of MS has been immunosuppressive agents, either adrenocorticotropic hormone (ACTH) or corticosteroids. For the exacerbating-remitting form of MS, flareups are currently most effectively treated with initial intravenous methylprednisolone at doses of 1 gm per day for up to 1 week, followed by several weeks of tapering oral prednisone beginning at 60 to 80 mg per day. Milder attacks are treated with oral medication alone. This regimen has been shown to be beneficial in speeding recovery from the acute episodes, but has not been proven to decrease the number of future attacks or to reduce progressive disability. For the chronic progressive form of MS, the same therapy may be tried initially, but long-term corticosteroid use is ineffective, and significant side effects are common. The addition of cyclophosphamide or azathioprine may have a beneficial effect in stabilizing the disease, but these medications are as yet unproven, and toxic effects are frequent. Other experimental immunosuppressive modalities, including Cop 1, interferons, cyclosporine A, total lymphoid irradiation, plasmapheresis, and various monoclonal antibodies, are currently under investigation.

Ocular. Therapy for optic neuritis has been controversial. Based on prior limited studies using intravenous ACTH and retrobulbar triamcinolone, it has been common practice to treat ON with oral prednisone, with the goal of speeding visual recovery and relief of pain, the long-term visual effect being unproven. The recently completed Optic Neuritis Treatment Trial (ONTT) has provided extensive data on the value of such therapy. The ONTT suggests that the use of oral prednisone alone is ineffective in the treatment of ON and that it increases the risk of developing new episodes of ON; therefore, it should not be used for this disease. For mild cases of ON, those with initial visual acuity of 20/40 or better and mild visual field loss, therapy is not required. In cases of more severe visual loss, an initial 3-day course of intravenous methylprednisolone at 1 gm per day followed by an 11-day course of oral prednisone tapering from 1 mg/kg body weight/day was shown to speed recovery in the first several weeks and to produce a mild improvement in visual function after 6 months. In this last group of patients, consideration of therapy is indicated, but cases must be evaluated individually. At present, there are no more well-defined guidelines available; in general, patients with most severe visual loss, the greatest need for a rapid return of vision, and the least systemic contraindications to the use of high-dose corticosteroids are most likely to undergo therapy.

The other ocular inflammatory conditions associated with MS most often require no therapy. Retinal periphlebitis and retinitis are typically focal and self-limiting, without progression to retinal vascular occlusive disease, neovascularization, or chorioretinal scarring. The most common form of uveitis in MS involves the ciliary body, with pars plana exudates and vitreous cells seen frequently, but such complications as scarring and macular edema are quite uncommon and treatment is usually unnecessary. Occasional cases involve more severe anterior uveitis, which may require standard topical corticosteroid and cycloplegic therapy.

The eye movement disorders seen in MS are often transient and require no long-term therapy other than that which may be administered for associated general neurologic symptoms. Bilateral INO may result in exotropia, with diplopia in the primary gaze position; it may be treated with temporary press-on prisms or, more commonly, by alternating occlusion. Unilateral INO typically does not result in diplopia in primary gaze, but may cause transient diplopia and oscillopsia as gaze is directed laterally into the field of action of the paretic medial rectus muscle; no effective treatment is available. Primary position nystagmus may result from brainstem or cerebellar dysfunction and may

occasionally produce prominent oscillopsia. Agents that augment the effects of gamma-aminobutyric acid (GABA) often decrease the amplitude and intensity of the nystagmus and reduce symptoms. Baclofen in oral doses up to 20 mg three times per day and clonazepam up to 0.5 mg two to three times per day have been used alone or in combination for various forms of nystagmus. Drowsiness and fatigue are the most common side effects and often limit the effectiveness of treatment.

Ocular or Periocular Manifestations

Extraocular Muscles: Internuclear ophthalmoplegia; nystagmus; oculomotor cranial nerve palsies.

Optic Nerve: Papillitis; retrobulbar neuritis; optic atrophy.

Pupil: Afferent pupillary defect.

Retina: Retinal periphlebitis; retinitis.

Uvea: Anterior and posterior uveitis.

Visual Fields: Central or cecocentral scotoma; altitudinal defect; generalized depression.

Other: Dyschromatopsia; retrobulbar pain with eye movement; diplopia; oscillopsia.

PRECAUTIONS

The therapy of optic neuritis must be undertaken with an important caveat in mind—that ON may be mimicked both by compressive lesions of the anterior visual pathway and by noncompressive optic neuropathies that may require specific therapy. First, then, it is essential to maintain a high index of suspicion for compressive optic neuropathy in cases of presumed ON that have an atypical presentation or clinical course, particularly those that may improve with steroid therapy, only to recur upon attempted tapering. It is generally not necessary to proceed to neuroradiologic imaging in each case; this is reserved for those with contralateral temporal visual field loss, visual loss that progresses or fails to improve after 3 to 4 weeks, or pain that does not resolve in 3 to 4 weeks. Second, it is important to screen for causes of acute optic neuropathy that may respond to specific therapy. Although the value of therapy is debatable in many cases of demyelinating ON, antibiotic therapy for syphilitic optic neuropathy and systemic corticosteroids for the optic neuropathies associated with sarcoidosis, systemic lupus erythematosus, or other connective tissue diseases are documented to be effective. The issue of whether other forms of optic nerve inflammation—for example, Leber's idiopathic stellate neuroretinitis and nonspecific postviral ON—require corticosteroid therapy is undecided.

COMMENTS

There continues to be debate as to whether all idiopathic ON is related to MS and thus whether each case of isolated ON should receive extensive neurologic evaluation, including MR scanning for periventricular plaques, cerebrospinal fluid examination for IgG synthesis and oligoclonal bands, HLA typing, and other sophisticated analysis to detect an increased risk of developing MS. In light of recent studies that suggest that nearly 60 per cent of patients with isolated ON will develop MS within 15 years, we discuss the possible implications with each patient, realizing that there is no definitive test for proving the diagnosis of MS. We attempt to involve each patient individually in an informed decision-making process in this regard.

References

Arnold AC: Ophthalmic manifestations of multiple sclerosis. Sem Ophthalmol 3:229–243, 1988.

Arnold AC, et al: Retinal periphlebitis and retinitis in multiple sclerosis. I. Pathologic characteristics. Ophthalmology 91:255–262, 1984.

Bamford CR, et al: Uveitis, perivenous sheathing, and multiple sclerosis. Neurology 28:119–124, 1978.

Beck RW, et al: A randomized, controlled trial of corticosteroids in the treatment of acute optic neuritis. N Engl J Med 326:581–588, 1992.

Carter JL, Rodriguez M: Immunosuppressive treatment of multiple sclerosis. Mayo Clin Proc 64:664–669, 1989.

Carter JL, et al: Immunosuppression with high dose IV cyclophosphamide and ACTH in progressive multiple sclerosis: Cumulative 6-year experience in 164 patients. Neurology 38 (Suppl 2):9–14, 1988.

Currie J, Matsuo V: The use of clonazepam in the treatment of nystagmus-induced oscillopsia. Ophthalmology 93:924–932, 1986.

Durelli L, et al: High dose intravenous methyl-prednisolone in the treatment of multiple sclerosis: Clinical-immunologic correlations. Neurology 36:238–243, 1986.

Lim JI, et al: Anterior granulomatous uveitis in patients with multiple sclerosis. Ophthalmology 98:142–145, 1991.

Rizzo JF, Lessell S: Risk of developing multiple sclerosis after uncomplicated optic neuritis: A long term prospective study. Neurology 38:185–190, 1988.

Yee RD, et al: Effect of baclofen on congenital nystagmus. In Lennerstrand G, Zee DS, Keller EL (eds): Functional Basis of Ocular Motility Disorders. Oxford, Pergamon Press, 1982, pp 151–157.

MYASTHENIA GRAVIS 358.0

NEIL R. MILLER, M.D.,
and DAVID R. CORNBLATH, M.D.

Baltimore, Maryland

Myasthenia gravis is an autoimmune disorder of the post synaptic neuromuscular junction characterized by weakness and fatigability. Ptosis and diplopia are frequent presenting symptoms because the extraocular muscles and elevators of the eyelids can be affected early in this disease. When the bulbar musculature is affected, there may be impairment of speech, chewing, swallowing, and facial expression. More generalized disease may affect the trunk and limb muscles. If the muscles of respiration or swallowing are affected, necessitating respiratory or nutritional assistance, the patient is said to be in "crisis." Symptoms are often least prominent in the morning and after rest, but they tend to worsen later in the day or after exercise.

Myasthenia gravis may begin at any age, but reaches a peak incidence in the third decade in females and in the fifth to sixth decades in males. A family history of myasthenia gravis is present in about 5 per cent of cases. Associated autoimmune disorders, particularly thyroid dysfunction, may also be present.

The basic abnormality in myasthenia gravis is a deficiency of acetylcholine receptors at neuromuscular junctions caused by an antibody-mediated autoimmune process. This deficiency causes muscle weakness and fatigue on repeated activity because of impaired neuromuscular transmission. The factors that trigger the production of autoantibodies in myasthenia gravis are not known, but the complex relationship of the thymus gland to myasthenia suggests that this organ may play a role in the pathogenesis of the disease.

THERAPY

Systemic. Although the basic autoimmune disorder is systemic, clinical weakness may remain confined to the extraocular muscles in up to 40 per cent of patients. If the symptoms are mild or intermittent, many patients prefer not to take medication. Such patients may be forced to patch one eye occasionally or to elevate one of the eyelids with tape.

Anticholinesterase agents continue to be the first line of treatment for most patients with myasthenia gravis. Pyridostigmine is the most widely used oral anticholinesterase drug. Its effects begin within 10 to 30 minutes, reach a peak at 1 to 2 hours, and decline within 3 to 4 hours. The correct dose must be determined empirically. The timing of doses should be adjusted to avoid fluctuations in symptoms and to anticipate periods of greatest need or weakness. The usual starting dose is 60 mg every 4 to 6 hours during the day. Side effects, such as gastric upset or diarrhea, are lessened by taking the medication with food. The dosage is then adjusted on the basis of an individual's requirements. It is unusual for a patient to benefit from more than 120 mg of pyridostigmine every 3 hours. Sustained-release preparations are available, but should be used only at bedtime. It is important to note that ocular symptoms of myasthenia are usually more refractory to anticholinesterase treatment than are systemic symptoms.

Thymectomy is used frequently in the treatment of systemic myasthenia gravis. It is usually performed in patients younger than 50 years of age whose systemic symptoms are not controlled by pyridostigmine. Thymectomy is best performed in centers with experience in the procedure and in caring for myasthenia gravis patients. The role of thymectomy in the treatment of myasthenia gravis in children is controversial. Similarly, there is divided opinion regarding whether patients whose symptoms are purely ocular should undergo thymectomy if they do not respond satisfactorily to anticholinesterase agents.

Any patient with myasthenia gravis whose weakness is not satisfactorily controlled by anticholinesterase medication, thymectomy, or both may be a candidate for immunosuppressive therapy. Adrenal corticosteroids are the immunosuppressive drugs most widely used in the treatment of myasthenia gravis. Both ocular and systemic symptoms of myasthenia gravis often respond dramatically to prednisone, especially when this drug is combined with optimum doses of anticholinesterase medication. Older patients are particularly good candidates for steroid treatment, since they usually respond well to this therapy. Before beginning steroid therapy, however, patients should be told of the serious side effects that may occur, including cataracts, osteoporosis, reduced resistance to infection, gastrointestinal ulceration, systemic hypertension, exacerbation of diabetes mellitus, and salt and fluid retention. Relative contraindications to prednisone treatment include pre-existing diabetes mellitus, systemic hypertension, and ulcer disease, although these problems can often be controlled. Patients who are unable or unwilling to be followed at regular intervals by their physician should never be treated with steroids.

When treatment is begun with high doses of steroids, such as prednisone, a proportion of patients will experience exacerbation of myasthenic weakness within the first weeks of treatment. A gradually increasing dosage schedule (sometimes with observation in the hospital) usually avoids this problem. When the daily goal of 50 mg of oral prednisone is reached or when a satisfactory result has been achieved at a lower dose, administration of prednisone is then gradually shifted toward an alternate-day treatment schedule. The drug is then tapered slowly to establish the minimum dose required by the individual patient.

Azathioprine[‡] has been used frequently in myasthenia gravis, mainly as a "steroid-sparing" agent. It is less satisfactory as primary therapy since it requires months to take effect. Hematologic and liver toxicity mandate frequent monitoring of the blood count and liver function of patients treated with this drug.

Cyclosporine is an effective agent in the treatment of myasthenia gravis. Its time to onset of action is similar to that of prednisone; however, it is expensive and requires frequent monitoring of blood levels to avoid nephrotoxicity.

Other immunosuppressive drugs, such as cyclophosphamide,[‡] have been used in the treatment of myasthenia gravis. However, the beneficial effects of these drugs may take from several months to a year to appear, and the toxicity limits their use to severely affected patients cared for in institutions with special expertise.

Plasmapheresis may be temporarily beneficial in some cases of myasthenia, but is usually not needed or useful for long-term treatment. In general, it is useful in improving the clinical condition quickly and getting the patient through such difficult periods as a myasthenic crisis, preparation for thymectomy, or the initiation of immunosuppressive therapy.

Ocular. Although attempts have been made to treat purely ocular myasthenic patients with prisms, ptosis crutches, or both, these devices are generally ineffective. The incomitance of the strabismus often precludes successful therapy, and ptosis crutches often cause severe exposure keratopathy. Strabismus surgery may occasionally be useful in patients on maximum therapy whose ocular deviation and alignment have been stable for many months or years.

Ocular or Periocular Manifestations

Extraocular Muscles: Generalized limitation of ocular motility; pseudogaze palsy; pseudointernuclear ophthalmoplegia; pseudo-Parinaud's syndrome, may mimic sixth nerve paresis, fourth nerve paresis, or pupil-sparing complete or incomplete third nerve paresis.

Eyelids: Cogan's lid twitch; orbicularis oculi weakness; paradoxic lid retraction; ptosis.

Other: Accommodative insufficiency (rare); monocular or binocular conjugate or dysconjugate nystagmus.

PRECAUTIONS

If surgery is needed, oral medication may have to be discontinued. Anticholinesterase medication may be given by intravenous infusion pump. A dose of 60 mg of oral pyridostigmine is equivalent to 1 to 2 mg of intravenous neostigmine. If prednisone has been used before surgery, parenteral hydrocortisone and methylprednisolone should be maintained as a daily dose equivalent to the "on" day dose of oral prednisone.

Curare and its analogues should never be used during surgery on patients with myasthenia gravis because they produce profound and lasting weakness of the voluntary muscles. Certain other drugs are also contraindicated in myasthenic patients because they increase weakness. These drugs include quinine, quinidine, and procainamide. Aminoglycoside antibiotics may increase weakness, but may be used when necessary provided the patient is monitored closely.

Patients with myasthenia gravis should be allowed to regulate their own activity levels. The effects of overexertion are reversible, and each patient soon learns his or her own limitations. These patients should be instructed to contact their physicians immediately if infections of any sort develop. Overdosage of anticholinesterase compounds can cause symptoms similar to worsening of myasthenia gravis, but rarely result in worsening of eye movement or alignment.

COMMENTS

Before initiating or modifying treatment in a patient with presumed myasthenia gravis, it is necessary to establish the diagnosis unequivocally, to document the severity of myasthenia gravis, and to evaluate the possibility of related or unrelated intercurrent conditions. The diagnosis of myasthenia gravis may be suspected from a typical history of fluctuating symptoms that become worse with fatigue. On physical examination, the strength of the orbicularis oculi should be tested, since this is the most consistently involved muscle. The combination of both ptosis and orbicularis oculi weakness is highly suggestive of the disease. Quantitative movements of ocular motility and eyelid function with evaluation of fatigue are also useful. Observation of Cogan's lid twitch may help confirm the diagnosis. The time at which ptosis develops while the patient is attempting to maintain upward gaze is a useful objective measurement that may be used to evaluate the success of later treatment. Other quantitative tests of systemic muscle function and fatigue, such as the arm abduction time and the vital capacity, are also useful.

Once myasthenia is suspected, several diagnostic maneuvers may be carried out to confirm the diagnosis. Pharmacologic testing using edrophonium or neostigmine is often performed. These tests are most reliable when an alternative placebo treatment is also given, evaluation of the patient is carried out by a blinded observer, and quantitative measurements of the patient's function are carried out before and after each medication. Patients whose medical health precludes pharmacologic testing (e.g., patients with cardiac disease) may be given a "sleep test." In this test, the patient's ocular motility, ocular alignment, and degree of ptosis are assessed by measurement and photography. The patient is then taken to a quiet room with a bed, stretcher, or lounge chair and is permitted to sleep for 30

to 60 minutes. The patient is subsequently awakened, and the same parameters are immediately reassessed. An improvement in ocular motility, alignment, ptosis, or a combination of these are highly suggestive and probably pathognomonic of myasthenia gravis. Other diagnostic tests on patients suspected of having myasthenia gravis may include repetitive nerve stimulation, single fiber electromyography, and measurement of anti-acetylcholine receptor antibodies. Conditions that may exacerbate myasthenia gravis and should be searched for in every patient include intercurrent infection, thyroid disease, and thymoma. Most patients should also be screened for the presence of other autoimmune diseases, and a careful drug history should be taken.

References

Acheson JF, Elston JS, Lee JP, Fells P: Extraocular muscle surgery in myasthenia gravis. Br J Ophthalmol 75:232–235, 1991.

Chaudhry V, Cornblath DR: Treatment of myasthenia gravis. *In* Lisak RP (ed): Handbook of Myasthenia Gravis. Toronto, M. Decker, 1993.

Drachman DB: The biology of myasthenia gravis. Annu Rev Neurosci 4:195–225, 1981.

Drachman DB: Present and future treatment of myasthenia gravis. N Engl J Med 316:743–745, 1987.

Grob D: Myasthenia gravis: Pathophysiology and management. Ann NY Acad Sci 377:1–898, 1981.

Miller NR: Walsh and Hoyt's Clinical Neuro-Ophthalmology, 4th ed. Baltimore, Williams & Wilkins, 1985, Vol 2, pp 841–866.

Odel JG, Winterkorn JMS, Behrens MM: The sleep test for myasthenia gravis. A safe alternative to Tensilon. J Clin Neuro-ophthalmol 11:288–292, 1991.

Toyka KV: Myasthenia gravis. *In* Johnson RT (ed): Current Therapy in Neurologic Disease—3, 3rd ed. Philadelphia, BC Decker, 1990, pp. 385–391.

PARKINSON'S DISEASE 332.0

STEPHEN GANCHER, M.D.

Portland, Oregon

Parkinson's disease (PD) is a slowly progressive, degenerative neurologic illness. It most typically affects middle-aged or elderly individuals although it may occur in young adults. It usually starts insidiously and progresses at a variable rate. Typical symptoms are resting tremor, rigidity, a flexed posture, postural instability, and bradykinesia. Bradykinesia, which produces difficulty in initiating and maintaining movement, can be the most disabling yet least obvious aspect of the disease. The most severe neurochemical abnormality is a deficiency of dopamine in the basal ganglia caused by loss of pigmented, dopaminergic neurons in the substantia nigra, although other neurotransmitter systems, such as serotonin and norepinephrine, are also affected.

There is considerable overlap with other, related degenerative disorders that cause bradykinesia, and early in its course, it may be difficult to separate these other disorders from idiopathic parkinsonism. The most common related illness, progressive supranuclear palsy (PSP), may present with very similar symptoms initially before the supranuclear vertical ophthalmoplegia becomes apparent. Multiple system atrophy (Shy-Drager syndrome), which causes dysautonomia and parkinsonism, can also be confused with idiopathic parkinsonism early in its course.

A variety of ocular abnormalities, chiefly involving the eyelids and eye movements, may be observed in PD and related conditions. Common to PD, PSP, and other disorders causing bradykinesia are a loss of facial expression and infrequency of blinking, giving rise to the typical "parkinsonian stare." Blepharoclonus, tremor of the eyelids with gentle eye closure, is also common, especially if there is associated head or chin tremor, and apraxia of eye opening may occasionally occur. Myerson's sign, an inability to suppress blinking following tapping on the nasion, is also very common. Uncommonly, symptomatic blepharospasm may occur in parkinsonism, most typically as a dyskinetic phenomenon due to chronic L-dopa treatment. Seborrhea is also common in PD and may lead to recurrent hordeola and blepharitis.

A variety of eye movement disturbances also occur in PD. An increase in saccadic latency, hypometric saccades, a mild degree of saccadic slowing, and a breakdown in smooth pursuit are the most common abnormalities. A mild degree of limitation in upgaze also occurs, but is also common with "normal" aging. Other eye movement disturbances, such as nystagmus, horizontal or marked vertical ophthalmoplegia, or apraxia of eye opening, may occur, but are uncommon and should suggest an alternative diagnosis. Oculogyric crises do not occur in idiopathic parkinsonism, but are common in postencephalitic parkinsonism and also occur as an acute dystonic reaction to neuroleptics.

Other abnormalities in the visual pathway, including visual neglect, prolonged latency of visual evoked response, and elevated threshold in foveal contrast sensitivity, may also occur, but are rarely symptomatic. In fact, prominent visual complaints are rare in idiopathic parkinsonism and should suggest an alternative diagnosis.

THERAPY

Systemic. Drug treatment of Parkinson's disease is chiefly symptomatic. Selegiline is commonly prescribed as initial therapy in mild patients in the hope that disease progression is slowed, but this is uncertain. Levodopa replacement (usually combined with a peripheral decarboxylase inhibitor, such as carbidopa) is initially very effective and a mainstay of therapy in most patients. However, diurnal fluctuations in motor state and drug-induced choreoathetosis or dystonia commonly emerge with chronic treatment, especially in younger patients. Thus, levodopa is usually reserved for those patients who are refractory to other medications or have moderately severe disease at presentation. For patients with predominant tremor, anticholinergics may be effective, but are limited by accommodative paralysis, miosis, dry mouth, and memory loss. Other useful medications include amantadine, pergolide, bromocriptine, propranolol,[‡] and antidepressants.[‡] Unfortunately, some degree of residual parkinsonism is nearly always present, despite the above treatments.

Ocular. Infrequent blinking may necessitate the use of artificial tears. Ocular secretions tend to be greasy and may lead to blepharitis and hordeola, which may be avoided by good lid hygiene.

Supportive. Psychologic support, with reassurance, encouragement, and supportive counseling, is very useful in managing the major symptoms of parkinsonism. Patient support groups may provide considerable practical advice, as well as emotional support for the patient and caregiver. Adult day care may also be very helpful to avoid caregiver "burnout."

Ocular or Periocular Manifestations

Extraocular Muscles: Decreased convergence; hypometric saccades; limited upgaze (especially in PSP); oculogyric crises (postencephalitic); saccadic pursuit.

Eyelids: Blepharoplegia; blepharospasm, hordeolum; infrequent blinking; seborrheic blepharitis.

Pupils: Normal in idiopathic parkinsonism; tonic or Argyll Robertson pupils may be seen in patients with Shy-Drager syndrome.

Other. Abnormal visual evoked responses; increased foveal threshold; visual neglect.

PRECAUTIONS

Confusion with PSP and multiple system atrophy (Shy-Drager syndrome) is a common problem, even in clinics specializing in Parkinson's disease. Early recognition of these diseases, which have a worse prognosis, will avoid presenting an incorrect prognosis to the patient and family. Avoidance of anticholinergics in the patient with memory impairment is also crucial. Other side effects seen with anticholinergics, including decreased accommodative ability and miosis, are important to recognize. Drug-induced dyskinesias may also interfere with treatment.

COMMENTS

Ophthalmic evaluation and treatment, such as slit-lamp examination or surgery, may be difficult either because of parkinsonian tremor or head and neck dyskinesias, and evaluation of the patient both before and after a dose of levodopa may be needed. Narcotics or benzodiazepines typically do not markedly affect the tremor, although deep sedation with any drug usually suppresses tremor or dyskinesia. Intravenous diphenhydramine, administered in 25-mg increments, has been found to be useful. Before general anesthesia, it is best to avoid levodopa for at least 4 to 6 hours, as the risk of cardiac arrhythmias may be increased with increased plasma dopamine levels due to the incomplete inhibition of levodopa decarboxylase.

References

Bodis-Wollner I, Onofrj M: The visual system in Parkinson's disease. Adv Neurol 45:323–327, 1986.

Kupersmith MJ, et al: Visual system abnormalities in patients with Parkinson's disease. Arch Neurol 39:284–286, 1982.

Lesser RP, et al: Analysis of the clinical problems in parkinsonism and the complications of long-term levodopa therapy. Neurology 29:1253–1260, 1979.

Stone DJ, DiFazio CA: Sedation for patients with Parkinson's disease undergoing ophthalmologic surgery. Anesthesiology 68:821, 1988.

Villardita C, Smirni P, Zappala G: Visual neglect in Parkinson's disease. Arch Neurol 40:737–739, 1983.

White OB, et al: Ocular motor defects in Parkinson's disease. II. Control of the saccadic and smooth pursuit systems. Brain 106:571–588, 1983.

TOLOSA-HUNT SYNDROME 378.9
(Painful Ophthalmoplegia)

WILLIAM T. SHULTS, M.D.

Portland, Oregon

The Tolosa-Hunt syndrome is a painful ophthalmoplegia caused by a nonspecific steroid-sensitive granuloma in the cavernous sinus. A steady pain, frequently described as "gnawing" or "boring," may precede the ophthalmoplegia by days or even weeks or may not appear until cranial nerve deficit is seen. The third, fourth, or sixth nerves and the ophthalmic or, rarely maxillary divisions of the fifth nerve may be involved. There may be balanced or unbalanced loss of the parasympathetic and sympathetic pupillomotor fibers. Symptoms may last for weeks or months. Spontaneous remission may occur, sometimes with residual neurologic deficits. Recurrences are found at intervals of months to years. Rarely, the syndrome may alternate sides, or a single attack may have bilateral but asymmetric findings.

Diagnosis of the Tolosa-Hunt syndrome is made by exclusion after other causes of subacute painful ophthalmoplegia have been thoroughly ruled out. This requires neuroimaging of the orbits and the cavernous and paranasal sinuses. Cerebral angiography or MRI is necessary to rule out aneurysms, arteriovenous malformations, and carotid cavernous fistulas. Infrequently, orbital venography may be deemed necessary to show stenosis of the third segment of the superior orbital vein. Bloodwork for systemic infections, inflammations, or hematologic malignancies should be done, including complete blood counts, erythrocyte sedimentation rates, protein studies, and vasculitis markers (ANA, rheumatoid factor, angiotensin-converting enzyme). The causes of the Tolosa-Hunt syndrome are still unknown, but probably include dysfunction of the delayed cell-mediated immunity system.

THERAPY

Systemic. After excluding other disorders, corticosteroids are the treatment of choice for the Tolosa-Hunt syndrome, and an immediate response is expected when large doses are prescribed. The usual oral adult dose is 80 to 100 mg of prednisone daily. Although there may be a rapid initial response to therapy (within hours), recurrences do not respond as well and require larger doses. Therefore, corticosteroids should be tapered to a maintenance level and gradually discontinued when the pain has abated. The ophthalmoplegia may not resolve for some weeks after clearing of the painful inflammation if severe nerve damage has occurred.

If treatment is prolonged, steroid dependency may be a problem, accompanied by all the Cushingoid side effects. This complication is usually avoided by the practice of tapering medication within a week of the subsidence of pain. If response is poor, reinvestigation to rule out neoplasm should be undertaken. Immunosuppression with 1 to 3 mg/kg of oral cyclophosphamide[‡] daily may be used to diminish the steroid requirements.

Ocular or Periocular Manifestations

Extraocular Muscles: Paralysis of third, fourth, or sixth nerve.
Eyelids: Ptosis.

Globe: Proptosis (rare).

Pupil: Anisocoria; relative afferent pupillary defect; sympathetic and/or parasympathetic paralysis.

Other: Decreased visual acuity; diplopia; ocular and periocular pain; orbital inflammatory signs (rare); scotoma.

PRECAUTIONS

Prompt relapse may follow corticosteroid withdrawal in some patients. Patients treated with corticosteroids for any length of time should be appropriately evaluated before therapy and carefully followed for the complications of this treatment. Cyclophosphamide in child-bearing women should be avoided. Careful monitoring for hepatotoxicity and hematopoietic toxicity is necessary.

COMMENTS

Prednisone may produce its effect by reducing edema and inflammation of the granulomatous tissue in the cavernous sinus, thereby relieving pressure on the adjacent cranial nerves. This generally requires a 3-week or longer course. Although rapid improvement after corticosteroid therapy may be highly suggestive of the Tolosa-Hunt syndrome, it must be remembered that temporary remission may also be seen when the pain and ophthalmoplegia are of neoplastic origin or are caused by aneurysms in a growth or leak phase, cavernous sinus fistulas, or other such steroid-sensitive processes as granulomatous infections, Wegener's granulomatosis, lymphoma, and infiltrative leukemias.

The Tolosa-Hunt syndrome and orbital pseudotumor (idiopathic, noncaseating, granulomatous inflammation of the orbit) may be the same disease process on two sides of the superior ophthalmic fissure.

References

Glaser JS: Infranuclear disorders of eye movements. *In* Duane TD (ed): Clinical Ophthalmology. Hagerstown, MD, Harper & Row, rev ed, 1991, Vol II, pp 12:24–25.

Hoes MJAJM, Bruyn GW, Vielvoye GJ: The Tolosa-Hunt syndrome—literature review: Seven new cases and a hypothesis. Cephalalgia 1:181–194, 1981.

Hunt WE: Tolosa-Hunt syndrome: One cause of painful ophthalmoplegia. J Neurosurg 44:544–549, 1976.

Hunt WE et al: Painful ophthalmoplegia. Its relation to indolent inflammation of the cavernous sinus. Neurology 11:56–62, 1961.

Roca PD: Painful ophthalmoplegia: The Tolosa-Hunt syndrome. Ann Ophthalmol 7:828–834, 1975.

Schatz NJ, Farmer P: Tolosa-Hunt syndrome: The pathology of painful ophthalmoplegia. *In* Smith JL (ed): Neuro-Ophthalmology. St. Louis, CV Mosby, 1972, Vol VI, pp 102–112.

Smith JL, Taxdal DSR: Painful ophthalmoplegia. The Tolosa-Hunt syndrome. Am J Ophthalmol 61:1466–1472, 1966.

Tolosa E: Periarteritic lesions of the carotid siphon with the clinical features of a carotid infraclinoidal aneurysm. J Neurol Neurosurg Psychiatry 17:300–302, 1954.

TRIGEMINAL NEURALGIA 350.1

(Tic Douloureux)

BAIRD S. GRIMSON, M.D.

Chapel Hill, North Carolina

Trigeminal neuralgia is a brief, sharp, unilateral facial pain that usually occurs in the middle or lower face within the distribution of the second or third division of the trigeminal nerve. Occasionally, the first division of the trigeminal nerve is involved with the cephalalgia occurring in or around the eye. The "stabbing," "searing," "lightning-like," or "electrical" pain most often occurs in patients over 40 years of age and is experienced more frequently by females than males. The right side of the face is involved more often than the left. Characteristically, this memorable pain is precipitated by mechanical stimulation of trigger zones within the ipsilateral face or mouth during such activities as chewing, swallowing, laughing, brushing teeth, combing one's hair, or shaving. Each attack of trigeminal neuralgia usually lasts for only several seconds or minutes, often presenting intermittently at first, but the frequency can increase to many episodes per day. Spontaneous exacerbations and remissions of tic douloureux are not uncommon and can complicate judgments on the efficacy of therapeutic measures for controlling the pain. If the pain presents bilaterally, the rare occurrence of multiple sclerosis as an underlying etiology of trigeminal neuralgia should be suspected.

THERAPY

Systemic. Carbamazepine or phenytoin[‡] is particularly useful when started shortly after the onset of tic douloureux. Although carbamazepine usually proves more effective, prolonged use of either of these drugs is limited because of their side effects and the tendency for trigeminal neuralgia to become refractory to medical management. Baclofen[‡] is also useful in the management of trigeminal neuralgia.

Carbamazepine is initiated in dosages of 100 mg orally twice a day after meals, with subsequent increments of 100 mg every 12 hours until the pain is relieved or toxic side effects are observed. The total daily dose of carbamazepine usually ranges between 400 and 800 mg, but should never exceed 1.2 gm. Between 300 and 700 mg of phenytoin[+] per day are required daily for adequate relief from trigeminal neuralgia. Baclofen should be started at 5 mg orally three times a day for 3 days, then increased to 10 mg three times a day for 3 days, and then 20 mg three times a day. The total dosage should not exceed 80 mg of baclofen.

Surgical. Surgical intervention for tic douloureux is reserved for those patients who have become refractory to medical management. Numerous surgical procedures have been tried in the past, but radiofrequency trigeminal gangliolysis and microsurgical decompression of the trigeminal nerve rootlet are the current procedures of choice, as they provide the best chance for permanent relief of pain while producing minimal postoperative complications. Thermal trigeminal gangliolysis is performed by the percutaneous insertion of the radiofrequency needle through the foramen ovale directly into the trigeminal nerve rootlet. After radiofrequency stimulation locates the rootlets responsible for the trigeminal pain, the needle tip is heated for thermocoagulation. This procedure does not require a craniotomy, but occasionally produces disagreeable subjective sensations within the trigeminal nerve distribution and sometimes objective trigeminal involvement (hypalgesia, neuroparalytic keratitis, weakness of the jaw muscles). A significant rate of recurrence of the trigeminal neuralgia does occur over time, but radiofrequency thermocoagulation can then be repeated without difficulty. Microsurgical decompression of the trigeminal nerve root near the brainstem does require a suboccipital craniotomy, but this has proved to be a relatively safe procedure associated with a low incidence of postoperative trigeminal nerve dysfunction and rare return of pain in the postoperative period.

Ocular or Periocular Manifestations

Conjunctiva: Ipsilateral hyperemia accompanying the pain.
Lacrimal System: Ipsilateral lacrimation during the pain.
Other: Periorbital pain.

PRECAUTIONS

Among the common side effects of carbamazepine therapy are lightheadedness, drowsiness, and lethargy. Ataxia, nausea and vomiting, and skin rashes can also occur. Cardiac arrhythmias and congestive heart failure may develop, and carbamazepine should be used with caution in patients with heart disease. A rare, but serious drug reaction is the development of leukopenia, thrombocytopenia, or aplastic anemia. A complete blood and platelet count is recommended before starting carbamazepine, every week or two after its initiation for several months, and then every 3 or 4 months during maintenance therapy.

Side effects of phenytoin include nystagmus, ataxia, slurred speech, dizziness, nausea, vomiting, and epigastric pain. Gingival hyperplasia, peripheral neuropathy, hirsutism, skin rashes, and a generalized lymphadenopathy may also develop. Liver dysfunction occasionally occurs, and rarely leukopenia, agranulocytopenia, thrombocytopenia, or pancytopenia have been observed.

Baclofen is usually well tolerated, but can cause drowsiness, weakness, fatigue, headache, dizziness, nausea, and hypotension.

Although carbamazepine, phenytoin, and baclofen are very successful at first in controlling the pain, the trigeminal neuralgia often becomes refractory to systemic treatment. When this happens, surgical management is quite successful and should not be delayed.

COMMENTS

If objective trigeminal nerve involvement is detected on the initial evaluation or if other parasellar cranial nerve palsies (third, fourth, or sixth) are found, the diagnosis of trigeminal neuralgia is in question, and an investigation for a parasellar mass lesion, including CT, MRI, and possible cerebral angiography, should be initiated. However, if these ipsilateral parasellar cranial nerve palsies are documented soon after surgery for trigeminal neuralgia, no further investigation is indicated as these findings most likely represent postoperative sequelae.

References

Bederson JB, Wilson CB: Evaluation of microvascular decompression and partial sensory rhizotomy in 252 cases of trigeminal neuralgia. J Neurosurg 71:359–367, 1989.

Fromm GH, Terrence CF, Chattha AS: Baclofen in the treatment of trigeminal neuralgia: Double-blind study and long-term follow-up. Ann Neurol 15:240–244, 1984.

Grimson BS, Boone SC: Sixth nerve palsy complicating percutaneous thermal ablation of the trigeminal nerve rootlet. Am J Ophthalmol 92:225–229, 1981.

Hart RG, Easton JD: Carbamazepine and hematological monitoring. Ann Neurol 11:309–312, 1982.

Klun B: Microvascular decompression and partial sensory rhizotomy in the treatment of trigeminal neuralgia: Personal experience with 220 patients. Neurosurgery 30:49–52, 1992.

Rovit RL: Trigeminal neuralgia. Compr Ther 18:17–21, 1992.

SECTION 15

NEOPLASMS

Benign

ACTINIC AND SEBORRHEIC KERATOSIS
702

RONALD R. LUBRITZ, M.D.

New Orleans, Louisiana

Actinic keratosis (solar keratoma) is a precancerous lesion that appears as an erythematous, scaly patch and occurs most commonly on sunlight-exposed areas of the skin, such as the face, neck, and dorsa of the hands. It is more common in middle-aged or older individuals and is pre-eminently noted in fair-complexioned individuals.

Seborrheic keratosis is a benign epithelial tumor that appears predominantly on the trunk and head. It is rare in children, but very common in adults over 40 years of age.

Seborrheic keratoses can occur both on the eyebrows and eyelids. The upper lids are more often involved than the lower. When on the lids, seborrheic keratoses can occasionally be somewhat pedunculated. Actinic keratoses most often involve the eyebrows. Although they can occur on the eyelids, this is uncommon because the eyelids, especially the upper eyelids, are usually protected from sunlight.

THERAPY

Surgical. Cryosurgery is a natural choice as a primary method of therapy for keratoses. These lesions are superficial and as such do not have to be treated deeply for eradication. Although use of a cotton-tipped applicator saturated with liquid nitrogen may possibly be indicated for certain areas of the skin, it is not indicated for treatment around the eyes because of potential drip problems. For single multiple lesions of actinic keratosis, freezing with a portable liquid nitrogen spray unit is effective for clinical cure of these growths. No local anesthetic is necessary. When treating multiple lesions, it is sometimes advisable to mark them for therapy; because of the short freeze and thaw times, edema and erythema occasionally cannot be relied on to flag the treated sites. For most lesions, the spray tip is placed at the center of the target site and then

carried in an ever-widening circle or spiral pattern until the entire lesion is covered. If the lesion is linear, a back-and-forth paint-brush pattern may be utilized. The keratoses should be frozen just outside the border. Timing the thaw period is an effective means of judging the adequacy of the freeze. The thaw time is defined as the elapsed time from the last application of the spray or probe until the entire lesion is thawed. This end point is detected by the disappearance of the white frosted appearance of the surface or of any hard area on palpation. A thaw time of 20 to 30 seconds is usually sufficient. Within a few days, the lesion will undergo a vesicular crusted stage; and by the tenth to fourteenth day, the eschar will usually slough off, leaving a residual smooth cutaneous surface usually pinkish or reddish in color that fades with time.

Flat seborrheic keratoses may be treated in a manner similar to that for actinic keratoses. However, raised lesions do not respond adequately to simple freezing. For these, a light spray is employed first. While the lesion is still superficially frozen, a sharp curette is then used to remove the raised tumor level with the skin. If the seborrheic keratosis is raised and on loose periorbital skin, the above two methods may not be able to be used. Instead, local anesthetic injection is used followed by light electrodesiccation and curettage. If the lesion is somewhat pedunculated, a small curved iris scissors may be used to remove the tumor mass from the skin, rather than a curette. Hemostasis is effected with Gelfoam or a similar dressing. A bandage can then be applied if the area permits.

Periocular Manifestations

Seborrheic keratoses are usually asymptomatic but can become large enough to interfere with vision. They usually occur as brownish or black, somewhat verrucous excrescences. In the periocular area they are usually somewhat small, being only several millimeters to a centimeter is size. They can be somewhat larger around the eyebrow and outer canthi.

Actinic keratoses, on the other hand, are usually flatter, more reddish brown in color and usually present with some degree of hyperkeratosis or scaling. Although most are asymptomatic, some can become inflamed or irritated and then cause burning or stinging. They will become more noticeable if the patient is exposed to heavy sunlight. When occurring on the upper lid they can be confused with contact dermatitis; biopsy may thus sometimes be necessary.

PRECAUTIONS

Care should be taken with cryosurgical procedures around the eye lest the global structures be harmed unnecessarily. When using the technique described for raised seborrheic keratoses, one should be cautious not to freeze too hard. If this happens, the operator must wait until the lesion is partially thawed before continuing. Also, clinical experience is necessary to judge the degree of freezing required for these techniques; too much freezing can result in scarring or pigmentary changes out of proportion to the tumor being treated. Patients should be informed of the possibility that pigmented lesions may not lose all their color after cryosurgical treatment.

COMMENTS

Some lesions may recur and must be retreated. This is not a frequent occurrence, however, and is usually limited to large or hypertrophic sites. The cosmetic results in these cases are usually excellent.

References

Lubritz RR: Cryosurgery of benign lesions. Cutis 16:426–432, 1975.
Lubritz RR: Cryosurgery for benign and malignant skin lesions: Treatment with a new instrument. South Med J 69:1401–1405, 1976.
Lubritz RR: Cryosurgery of benign and premalignant cutaneous lesions. In Zacarian SA (ed): Cryosurgical Advances in Dermatology and Tumors of the Head and Neck. Springfield, IL, Charles C. Thomas, 1977, pp 55–73.
Lubritz RR: Cryosurgery of nonmalignancies. In Zacarian SA (ed): Cryosurgery for Skin Cancer and Cutaneous Disorders. St. Louis, CV Mosby, 1985, pp 49–58.
Torre D, Lubritz RR, Kuflik E (eds): Practical Cutaneous Cryosurgery. East Norwalk, CT, Appleton & Lange, 1988, pp 61–86.

CAPILLARY HEMANGIOMA 228.01

(Angioblastic Hemangioma, Benign Hemangio-Endothelioma, Hemangioblastoma, Strawberry Hemangioma)

BARRETT G. HAIK, M.D.

New Orleans, Louisiana

Capillary hemangiomas are among the most common orbital tumors in the pediatric population. They are not true neoplasms, but seem to be hamartomatous proliferations of primitive vasoformative tissues. These tumors consist of anastomosing blood-filled endothelial-lined channels and typically have an infiltrative growth pattern with no true encapsulation. With rare exception, these tumors present in the first 6 months of life, and one-third are clinically obvious at birth. They follow a characteristic clinical course with a period of rapid hypertrophy for 3 to 12 months followed by a period of stabilization and then involution. The major degree of involution takes place by 5 years of age, although smaller degrees of tumor regression may be noted until the end of the first decade. Involution is complete with no significant cosmetic sequelae in the majority of cases. However, in some larger lesions, especially those with a combined subcutaneous superficial component, it is not uncommon to observe cosmetically disturbing defects. Additionally, ocular complications, primarily in the form of amblyopia, have been noted in 50 to 75 per cent of cases with orbital and adnexal hemangiomas. Rarer dermatologic and systemic complications may occur secondary to this vascular mass.

THERAPY

Supportive. The great majority of capillary hemangiomas undergo significant spontaneous regression. Although it is well established that therapy can speed regression of these tumors, it will not significantly affect the final amount of tumor involution and the cosmetic result. Therefore, unless there are specific ocular, dermatologic, or systemic indications for rapid resolution, treatment should be withheld, since all of the available therapeutic modalities have significant real or theoretic risks. It is generally of great value to discuss the natural history of the tumor with the family and explain the advantages and disadvantages of administering or withholding therapy in any particular case. Likewise, parents of these patients often find it advantageous to study photographs of children who have undergone spontaneous regression and to speak with parents of children who have reached the stage of maximal tumor regression.

Systemic. Corticosteroids have been shown to be effective in significantly speeding natural tumor involution. Details of their inhibitory effects are not definitely known, but they seem to be related to a vasoconstrictor effect. The typical oral administration of corticosteroids is either 2 mg/kg of prednisone daily or 4 mg/kg on an alternate daily basis. Most patients show a significant decrease of tumor size within 1 week after administration. Unfortunately, this involution does not persist in many cases when the steroid level is discontinued or reduced significantly. Because of this rebound growth, it can therefore be difficult to taper corticosteroids in these patients, and corticosteroid complications are a threat after extended use in this infantile population. The use of intralesional corticosteroid injections is an excellent method of maximizing the steroid effect in the area of the tumor mass while minimizing systemic absorption levels. Both rapidly acting steroid and deposteroid are injected under low pressure into the tumor mass with a small-gauge needle, often at several different sites in order to distribute the medication throughout the tumor. Recent reports suggest that interferon alpha-2a has antiangiogenic activity and may be valuable in the treatment of recalcitrant tumors.

Irradiation. Radiation has been shown to be effective in creating microembolic episodes in these vascular tumors, thus leading to hemangioma regression. Superficial or orthovoltage radiotherapy may be administered in a single treatment of 200 rads, with appropriate shielding of the globe and adjacent uninvolved tissues. The involutionary response usually is noted in 1 to 2 weeks, and these treatments may be repeated up to two times, if necessary.

Surgical. Various surgical modalities attempt to reduce tumor size through compromise of the major arterial feeding vessels, constriction and sclerosing of the smaller vascular channels, or primary surgical excision of the mass. Ligation of afferent vessels surgically or through intra-arterial embolization can be an effective means of decreasing blood flow to the tumor mass, therefore stimulating further involution or decrease of vascularity before excisional surgery. Such treatments require accurate radiographic visualization of the major vascular channels supplying the tumor in order to enable selective interference with the tumor's vascular supply. This visualization is often difficult because of the complex configurations and anastomoses assumed by major feeding vessels to such tumors. Attempts to stimulate the natural involutionary process by destroying smaller vascular channels and stimulating thrombosis include cryotherapy, diathermy, and injections of sclerosing solutions or boiling water. These procedures certainly can speed tumor involution, but often result in more significant cosmetic and functional deformities than would have occurred with natural involution or alternative forms of therapy.

Primary surgical excision of tumors has limited value because of the diffusely infiltrative nature of these masses, lack of encapsulation, and the resultant difficulty in differentiating them from adjacent or infiltrative critical orbital structures. When surgery is necessary for diagnosis or therapy, it is strongly recommended that one obtain an arteriogram or digital intravenous angiogram before surgery, so that the major vascular channels of the tumor are delineated. When surgery is performed, hypotensive anesthesia is recommended to aid in minimizing the volume of blood loss from these infants and to permit

more accurate visualization of orbital structures during surgery.

Laser. Argon, neodymium yag, and carbon dioxide lasers have been used with moderate success in attempts to ablate abnormal tumor blood vessels. The most promising results are from flash lamp-pumped pulsed dye laser treatments.

Ocular or Periocular Manifestations

Conjunctiva: Hemangioma.
Eyelids: Hemangioma; ptosis.
Globe: Displacement; proptosis.
Lacrimal System: Hemangioma of lacrimal gland or sac.
Optic Nerve: Secondary optic atrophy.
Other: Amblyopia (refractive, occlusive, strabismus); anisometropia (astigmatism, or relative myopia in affected eye); diplopia; exposure keratitis; strabismus.

PRECAUTIONS

Potential complications of the prolonged administration of systemic corticosteroids in infants include delayed growth, iatrogenic Cushing's syndrome, and adrenal suppression. Ocular and systemic complications from corticosteroid usage generally follow relatively high-dose, long-term use, but should not accompany "pulse" treatment of several weeks. Complications reported from intralesional corticosteroid injections at this time include mild pigmentary disturbances in the overlying skin, especially in darkly pigmented children, and the persistence of solid corticosteroid and carrier complexes beneath the skin for several months after injection. Central retinal artery occlusion, eyelid necrosis, and linear subcutaneous atrophy have also been detected. Systemic absorption has resulted in transient adrenal suppression, growth retardation, and Cushingoid symptoms. All children receiving systemic or intralesional corticosteroids should avoid routine pediatric immunizations with live attenuated viruses during and for 2 weeks before and after administration of corticosteroids.

Radiation precautions include shielding of radiation-sensitive ocular structures, such as the lens, uninvolved adjacent tissues, and the thyroid gland, even if the tumor extends to the neck area. There is a real risk of radiation oncogenesis when the thyroid is inadvertently exposed to low levels of radiation and a theoretic but unproven risk of radiation oncogenesis in the orbital area after low-dosage irradiation.

Because surgical embolization and ligation techniques can be associated with damage to adjacent crucial structures secondary to inadvertent ischemia following occlusion, they should be reserved for masses causing significant functional complications that are resistant to other forms of therapy.

Destructive techniques, such as diathermy, cryotherapy, and the injection of sclerosing solutions, often cause significant scarring and deformity of the treated area and are rarely indicated in the orbital region. Surgical excision of hemangiomatous tissue is rarely indicated because it involves sacrificing critical orbital structures infiltrated with hemangiomatous tissue that are impossible to surgically distinguish or separate. Surgery is occasionally effective in small, relatively localized adnexal hemangiomas and for excision of fibrovascular remnants after regression. Complications of surgery include the inevitable creation of surgical scars and excision of critical vascular, muscular, and neurogenic components of the orbit.

COMMENTS

Clinically, these tumors may be detected in the orbit and periocular area in three ways. Most commonly, a bluish-purple subcutaneous mass with normal overlying skin is noted in the anterior orbit. Second, approximately one-third of the patients have an obvious superficial component consisting of an overlying strawberry hemangioma. Lastly, 5 per cent of patients present with a deep orbital mass and have no signs that suggest the diagnosis. This last group of patients is by far the most clinically perplexing and diagnostically important, since the differential diagnosis of deep orbital tumors in a young infant includes such malignancies as rhabdomyosarcoma and metastatic neuroblastoma. Fortunately, the diagnosis of capillary hemangioma can usually be made on clinical grounds alone, and biopsy will not be necessary.

Although clinical examination of the cutaneous and subcutaneous lesions usually leads to the diagnosis, several associated clinical findings can be supportive in establishing a secure diagnosis. Approximately one-third of all patients have obvious hemangiomatous involvement of the palpebral or fornical conjunctiva or lacrimal gland. One-fourth of patients have superficial strawberry hemangiomas on other portions of the body. It is also quite common to observe an increase in the size of a subcutaneous hemangiomatous tumor when the child undergoes a Valsalva maneuver, such as crying.

There are many ancillary tests available to aid in the diagnosis, treatment plan, and subsequent management of this condition. Plain radiographs and computed tomography reveal diffuse enlargement of the orbit without evidence of bony erosion. CT and MR studies with contrast, angiography, and digital intravenous angiography reveal the existence and the extent of the diffusely infiltrating vascular tumor, as well as outline the major feeding vessels supplying this tumor. Ultrasonographic studies are valuable in determining the presence and extent of orbital involvement and permit a safe noninvasive method of monitoring tumor growth and regression.

The most important factors governing the management of capillary hemangiomas are treatment indications. Children afflicted with this condition may not ultimately be helped cosmetically by treatment and may indeed be cosmetically disfigured by surgical scars or may develop systemic or local complications from corticosteroids or radiotherapy. Therefore, treatment should be reserved for those patients in whom the rapidity of tumor regression will significantly influence the clinical outcome. Ocular indications for treatment include threatened amblyopia from mechanical occlusion of the palpebral aperture and, more rarely, exposure keratitis or optic nerve compression from the expanding orbital mass. A high degree of both myopia and astigmatism is noted in the globe of the affected orbit, and evidence now exists that these changes are partially reversible if treated early. Systemic indications for treatment include oral or nasopharyngeal obstruction from extensive hemangiomatous tissue, high output congestive heart failure caused by the multiple vascular shunts in extensive masses, thrombocytopenia, hemolytic anemia, and disseminating intravascular coagulation. All forms of treatment must include periodic evaluation of refractive errors and amblyopia therapy, when indicated.

References

Bilyk JR, Adamis AP, Mulliken JB: Treatment options for periorbital hemangioma of infancy. Int Ophthalmol Clin: Orbital Dis 32:95–109, 1992.

deVenecia G, Lobeck CC: Successful treatment of eyelid hemangioma with prednisone. Arch Ophthalmol 84:98–102, 1970.

Glassberg E, Lask G, Rabinowitz LG, Tunnessen WW: Capillary hemangiomas: Case study of a novel laser treatment and a review of therapeutic options. J Dermatol Surg Oncol 15:1214–1223, 1989.

Guyer DR, Adamis AP, Gragoudas ES, et al: Systemic antiangiogenic therapy for choroidal neovascularization. Arch Ophthalmol 110:1383–1384, 1992.

Haik BG: Vascular tumors of the orbit. In Hornblass A (ed): Ophthalmic and Orbital Plastic and Reconstructive Surgery. Baltimore, Williams & Wilkins, 1989, pp 509–517.

Haik BG, et al: Capillary hemangioma of the lids and orbit: An analysis of the clinical features and therapeutic results in 101 cases. Ophthalmology 86:760–789, 1979.

Hobby LW: Further evaluation of the potential of the argon laser in the treatment of strawberry hemangiomas. Plast Reconstr Surg 74:481–489, 1991.

Loughnan MS, Elder J, Kemp A: Treatment of a massive orbital-capillary hemangioma with interferon alfa-2b: Short term results. Arch Ophthalmol 110:1366–1367, 1992.

CAVERNOUS HEMANGIOMA 228.01

BARRETT G. HAIK, M.D.

New Orleans, Louisiana

Cavernous hemangiomas are among the most common orbital tumors of adults. They are benign vascular hamartomas that occur more commonly in females and usually present in the third to fifth decade of life. Although multiple tumors have been reported simultaneously or sequentially separated by long intervals, the majority of cavernous hemangiomas are single lesions and are unassociated with vascular lesions in the eye or elsewhere in the body. These masses can occur in any portion of the orbit, but usually develop in the muscle cone; they are usually spheral or ovoid in shape with a nodular surface and a purplish-red color. The tumor is typically well circumscribed and contained within a firm fibrous capsule, with only small vessels penetrating the tumor surface. Microscopically, cavernous hemangiomas are composed of large blood-filled vascular channels that are lined by flattened endothelial cells and are often separated by multiple fibrous septae.

A characteristic clinical course of slow progressive enlargement typically occurs and may be associated with ophthalmologic findings related to compression or displacement of ocular or orbital structures.

THERAPY

Surgical. The primary treatment modality available is surgical excision. Nonsurgical means of treatment, such as radiation or pharmacologic therapy, have been ineffective. Surgical therapy optimally consists of total excision of the tumor mass through whichever standard orbital approach is dictated by tumor location. In certain cases where the tumor abuts the optic nerve or other critical structures in the orbital apex, incomplete excision may be acceptable in order to avoid damage to these structures. Cavernous hemangiomas rarely recur even after incomplete excision, and it is generally assumed that the residual mass of incompletely excised tumor is obliterated by postsurgical fibrosis.

Ocular or Periocular Manifestations

Choroid: Striae.
Conjunctiva: Subconjunctival hemorrhages.
Globe: Displacement; proptosis.
Optic Nerve: Secondary edema or atrophy.
Other: Anisometropia (astigmatism or relative hyperopia in affected eye); diplopia; exposure keratitis; strabismus.

PRECAUTIONS

In the rare cases in which a secure clinical diagnosis can be established without surgery and the tumor is adjacent to critical orbital structures, observation alone may be indicated. In these cases, even subtotal excision may present a significant risk of visual com-

plications, thus outweighing the benefit of surgery. This period of observation should include not only clinical examination but also serial imaging studies and visual fields to dictate if and when surgical intervention should take place.

COMMENTS

The clinical symptoms and signs at the time of diagnosis are generally proptosis of the affected eye. It is usually axial proptosis, but occasionally can present with associated horizontal or vertical displacement. Additionally, the tumor can exert sufficient pressure on the posterior sclera to cause hyperopia and choroidal folds. Restriction of extraocular motility may be present, as well as diplopia in extreme positions of gaze. There are rare reports in which headaches have existed on the side of the orbital tumor, as well as recurrent subconjunctival hemorrhages in the affected eye.

Several ancillary diagnostic tests may aid in differentiating cavernous hemangiomas from other benign and malignant orbital conditions. Plain orbital x-rays may show an increase in soft tissue density and, more rarely, phlebolith formation. Additionally, orbital asymmetry secondary to diffuse orbital enlargement, local fossa formation, or hyperostosis may be detected following chronic pressure on the orbital bone. A- and B-scan ultrasonography can reveal the presence and location of a circumscribed mass in the orbit. Sound transmission through the tumor is usually good, with a high degree of internal reflectivity produced by the blood septae interfaces of these vascularized lesions. On CT scan, a discrete circumscribed orbital mass may be detected and localized. The rounded or oval contour of this mass is well portrayed. When the mass is adjacent to the optic nerve, distinct separation may not be possible. Internal heterogeneity and loculation of the mass are often noted. Enhancement of the tumor mass after intravenous contrast injection is usually present, but can be totally absent in some cases. Magnetic resonance studies reveal a well-circumscribed mass that is hypointense on T1-weighted sequences and hyperintense on T2-weighted sequences. The mass becomes hyperintense on T1-weighted images following Gadolinium-DTPA contrast enhancement and may blend into the orbital fat if fat suppression is not employed.

References

Coleman DJ, Jack RL, Franzen LA: II. Hemangiomas of the orbit. Arch Ophthalmol 88:368–374, 1972.
Haik BG: Vascular tumors of the orbit. *In* Hornblass A (ed): Ophthalmic and Orbital Plastic and Reconstructive Surgery. Baltimore, Williams & Wilkins, 1989, pp 509–517.
Harris GJ, Jakobiec FA: Cavernous hemangiomas of the orbit: A clinicopathologic analysis of sixty-six cases. *In* Jakobiec FA (ed): Ocular and Ad-

nexal Tumors. Birmingham, Aesculapius, 1978, pp 741–781.

Henderson JW: Orbital Tumors, 2nd ed. New York, Brian C Decker, 1980, pp 128–133.

Henderson JW, Farrow GM, Garrity JA: Clinical course of an incompletely removed cavernous hemangioma of the orbit. Ophthalmology *97*: 625–628, 1990.

McNab AA, Wright JE: Cavernous hemangioma of the orbit. Aust NZ J Ophthalmol 17:337–345, 1989.

Orcutt JC, Wulc AE, Mills RP, Smith CH: Asymptomatic orbital cavernous hemangiomas. Ophthalmology 98:1257–1260, 1991.

Reese AB: Tumors of the Eye, 3rd ed. Hagerstown, MD, Harper & Row, 1976, p 272.

CRANIOPHARYNGIOMA 237.0

HAROLD J. HOFFMAN, M.D., B.Sc. (Med), F.R.C.S.(C)

Toronto, Ontario

Craniopharyngiomas are benign congenital tumors arising from epithelial remnants of Rathke's pouch. They are the most common nonglial, intracranial tumor in childhood. These slowly growing tumors of squamous epithelium arise in the pituitary stalk and infundibulum and encroach and compress adjacent structures. In general, they compress the optic chiasm in front, the diaphragm and pituitary gland below, and the cavity of the third ventricle above, which frequently results in hydrocephalus. In most cases, cysts form in the center of the tumor. The tumor may project extensively enough to cause varied pituitary and hypothalamic constitutional symptoms, including infantilism diabetes insipidus, and abnormal sexual development.

Craniopharyngiomas can be divided into three anatomic subtypes. The sellar tumors are relatively small tumors that enlarge the sella tursica and encroach on the pituitary gland. Patients with sellar tumors therefore present with endocrine deficiency symptoms and headache. The prechiasmatic tumors protrude forward between the two optic nerves. These tumors push back on chiasm, producing severe visual loss that usually affects one optic nerve more than the other. The patients with prechiasmatic tumors rarely have raised intracranial pressure, but do have headaches and frequently have endocrine symptomatology. The retrochiasmatic tumors protrude upward into the third ventricle and push the chiasm forward. As they fill the third ventricle, they produce hydrocephalus and thus raised intracranial pressure. These patients present with papilledema, may have endocrine problems, but rarely do they have visual sympto-

matology other than papilledema. About 5 per cent of craniopharyngiomas are sellar in location, 35 per cent are prechiasmatic, and 60 per cent are retrochiasmatic.

THERAPY

Surgical. Surgical removal of a craniopharyngioma was regarded as a discouraging proposition in the past owing to the nature of the surrounding structures and its anatomically remote location. In recent years, sophisticated endocrinologic management, the new imaging facilities of CT and MRI scanning that enable earlier diagnosis, the development of the operating microscope and its accompanying armamentarium of elaborate surgical instrumentation, and the development of surgically destructive tools, such as the cavitron and the laser beam, that can deal with solid tumors in delicate locations, have evolved. The availability of these tremendous clinical and technologic advances has greatly reduced operative morbidity and permitted a much higher incidence of complete excision of tumor.

When a tumor has reached a size where it has obliterated the foramen of Monro and has produced significant hydrocephalus with grossly raised intracranial pressure (typically a retrochiasmatic tumor), a bypass diversionary shunt may be necessary as an initial step before removal of the tumor. However, in most cases, this shunt is not necessary since the tumor removal will usually resolve the disturbed cerebrospinal fluid dynamics.

Irradiation. Radiotherapy seems to have some destructive influence on craniopharyngioma epithelium. However, unlike conventional radiosensitive tumors, craniopharyngiomas never completely resorb after radiation. Furthermore, radiotherapy is not completely benign. There are numerous reports of parenchymal damage to the brain, as well as damage to brain vasculature, caused by radiotherapy. There is also a risk of a radiation-induced tumor, the most common of which is a sarcoma. For these reasons, radiation is used only when surgery has failed to control the tumor.

Supportive. Since more than half of the patients with craniopharyngiomas present with endocrine deficiency, a preoperative endocrine work-up should be done, and specific endocrine deficiencies, particularly those of corticosteroids and electrolyte abnormalities, should be corrected.

Dexamethasone in a dosage of 1 to 4 mg every 6 hours should be started immediately preoperatively and continued postoperatively for 48 to 72 hours, at which point maintenance doses of cortisone (25 mg/square meter) are substituted. Eventually, the cortisone should be reduced to the lowest effective level, with a warning to the patient that an increase in dosage may be necessary to avoid possible addisonian crisis during periods of stress or infection.

Total removal of a craniopharyngioma usually results in diabetes insipidus, a condition that typically is manifested during the first 24 to 48 hours postoperatively. Treatment with desmopressin administered by nasal instillation in doses of 5 to 20 μg every 12 to 24 hours is used for management of this disorder.

Because of surgical retraction of the frontal lobe during surgery, prophylactic doses of 5 to 7 mg/kg of phenytoin should be administered daily for a period of 7 to 10 days postoperatively.

Ocular or Periocular Manifestations

Extraocular Muscles: Paresis of third or sixth nerve.
Optic Nerve: Atrophy; optic neuritis; pallor; papilledema.
Pupil: Abnormal response to light; dilation.
Other: Diplopia; hemianopsia; nystagmus; ocular pain; scotoma; visual field defects; visual loss.

PRECAUTIONS

Any episode of sudden blindness in otherwise healthy individuals, especially children, should be suspected of being caused by craniopharyngioma. Plain skull x-rays show calcification of craniopharyngioma in 26 per cent of the cases, but the CT scan is a far more definitive investigative tool. Angiography has largely been replaced by the MRI scan, which provides an accurate picture of the relationship between tumor and cerebral vessels.

Physicians should be aware of the difficulties associated with total removal of the tumor, particularly when it is adherent to the internal carotid arteries. If part of the tumor is left behind, careful follow-up becomes necessary. However, MRI scanning has made this follow-up a matter of relative ease.

COMMENTS

The unusual feature of craniopharyngiomas in children, and particularly in adults, is the frequency of finding normal optic discs when there may be extensive loss of visual fields and sometimes visual acuity. A retained pupillary response in the presence of total blindness may also occur, suggesting that only pupillomotor fibers have remained functional. After surgical removal of the tumor, an almost blind eye may recover a remarkable amount of vision.

Although craniopharyngiomas are benign, they will recur in a significant proportion of patients if any portion of tumor is left behind. Late diagnosis may not preclude total removal of the tumor, but can certainly lead to more advanced compression of the optic apparatus and a poor visual prognosis. In the

era before corticosteroid replacement therapy, the mortality rate of patients with craniopharyngiomas was extremely high. The present availability of replacement endocrine medication, the use of CT and MRI scanning for early diagnosis, and the development of better neurosurgical instruments have resulted in far better management of these tumors and a tremendously improved outlook for patients with this disorder.

References

Adams RD, Hochberg F, Webster H deF: Neoplastic disease of the brain. In Isselbacher KJ et al (eds): Harrison's Principles of Internal Medicine, 9th ed. New York, McGraw-Hill, 1980, p 1957.
Amacher AL: Craniopharyngioma: The controversy regarding radiotherapy. Child's Brain 6: 57–64, 1980.
Hoffman HJ: Craniopharyngioma in children. In Ransohoff J (ed): Modern Technics in Surgery: Neurosurgery. Mt Kisco, NY. Futura, 1979, pp 5: 1–6.
Hoffman HJ, Buncic JR: Craniopharyngioma in children. In Smith JL: Neuro-Ophthalmology Update. New York, Masson, 1977, pp 241–252.
Hoffman HJ, et al: Management of craniopharyngioma in children. J Neurosurg 47:218–227, 1977.
Matson DD, Crigler JF Jr: Management of craniopharyngioma in childhood. J Neurosurg 30:377–390, 1969.
Ross HS, Rosenberg S, Friedman AH: Delayed radiation necrosis of the optic nerve. Am J Ophthalmol 76:683–686, 1973.
Sweet WH: Radical surgical treatment of craniopharyngioma. Clin Neurosurg 23:52–79, 1975.
Waga S, Handa H: Radiation-induced meningioma: With review of literature. Surg Neurol 5:212–219, 1976.
Walsh FB, Hoyt WF: Clinical Neuro-Ophthalmology, 3rd ed. Baltimore, Williams & Wilkins, 1969, pp 2157–2162.
Waltz TA, Brownell B: Sarcoma: A possible late result of effective radiation therapy for pituitary adenoma. Report of two cases. J Neurosurg 24: 901–907, 1966.

DERMOID 224.9
(Dermoid Choristoma, Dermoid Cyst, Dermolipoma, Lipodermoid)

ARTHUR S. GROVE, JR., M.D.

Boston, Massachusetts

Dermoids are benign tumors that are usually considered to be choristomas, rather than neoplasms. A choristoma is a growth that arises during embryologic development from tissue elements that are not normally present in the location of the lesion. Most dermoids are cystic and are believed to be caused by developmental sequestrations of surface epidermis, frequently adjacent to bony suture lines around the orbit. Some dermoids are chiefly solid with large quantities of fatty tissue, in which case they are described as dermolipomas or lipodermoids.

Histologically, dermoids are composed of epidermal tissue together with one or more dermal adnexal structures and skin appendages, such as hair follicles, sebaceous glands, and sweat glands. The cystic component is lined by keratinizing epidermis and may be filled with keratin, hairs, and fatty material. If these contents are released into the orbit either spontaneously or during surgery, an inflammatory reaction may result. Dermolipomas are usually found beneath the conjunctiva over the surface of the globe. Hairs may arise from these solid tumors and irritate the eye.

Anatomically, dermoids can be classified into three groups: superficial subcutaneous dermoids, deep orbital dermoids, and subconjunctival dermoids. Superficial dermoids are usually found during childhood, when they appear as painless subcutaneous nodules that often occur beneath the lateral brow. Deep orbital dermoids may not be discovered until maturity, since a long period of slow growth may precede displacement of the eye and exophthalmos. Subconjunctival dermoids are frequently dermolipomas, which are usually located on the temporal surface of the globe and may extend far into the posterior orbit.

Orbital x-rays are usually normal in patients with superficial subcutaneous dermoids and subconjunctival dermoids or dermolipomas. However, deep orbital dermoids often displace the orbital walls or cause sharply marginated defects in the orbital bones adjacent to the lesion. Ultrasonography and CT scanning usually demonstrate a cyst, and sometimes an adjacent solid component may be seen as well.

THERAPY

Surgical. Superficial subcutaneous dermoids can usually be removed through a skin incision directly over the lesion. The deep surface of the tumor is nearly always adherent to periosteum, from which it must be sharply divided. The diagnosis of these lesions can commonly be made from their clinical appearance, and excision may be delayed when the abnormality is discovered in young children.

Deep orbital dermoids are often located in areas that cannot be visualized adequately without removing the lateral orbital rim. If the lesion is located in the upper orbit, a superolateral approach similar to that described for removal of lacrimal gland tumors may be used. Deep dermoid cysts located in the lower orbit may be removed using an inferolateral approach. Excision is sometimes made easier by careful removal of the contents before dissection of the cyst wall. Some deep orbital dermoids extend through the orbital bones

and involve the intracranial space in which case they should usually be removed through a neurosurgical approach.

Subconjunctival dermoids or dermolipomas can also be recognized by their location and appearance in most instances. These lesions are usually located adjacent to the temporal surface of the globe and are commonly yellow or white. Hairs may project from the surface of the tumor and irritate the eye. Solid epibulbar dermoids may occur in Goldenhar's syndrome together with eyelid colobomas and auricular appendages. Subconjunctival dermoids may have deep orbital extensions that lie near the levator and extraocular muscles. Excision of these tumors may be complicated by damage to the eye, decreased lacrimal secretion, restricted eye movement, and ptosis. Because of the potential for complications, excision of subconjunctival dermoids or dermolipomas should usually be avoided if possible. If excision is necessary because of enlargement, cosmetic deformity, or irritation, surgery should be performed with great care.

Ocular or Periocular Manifestations

Conjunctiva: Dermoid.
Cornea: Dermoid; exposure keratitis (secondary to dermolipoma surgery).
Extraocular Muscles: Paresis or paralysis.
Eyebrows or Eyelids: Dermoid; ptosis.
Orbit: Exophthalmos.
Other: Astigmatism (caused by pressure against the cornea); visual loss (rare).

PRECAUTIONS

Cystic dermoids should be removed with care to avoid spilling their potentially irritating contents into the orbit or beneath the skin. If some spillage occurs, it is usually adequate to irrigate the area thoroughly to remove debris. Solid dermoids and dermolipomas are often located near the levator and extraocular muscles. Excision of these tumors should either be avoided or performed with great care to avoid such damage to the eye as ptosis or restricted extraocular muscle movement.

COMMENTS

The diagnosis and localization of dermoids can usually be made on the basis of clinical findings and CT scanning. X-rays and ultrasonography may contribute to the evaluation of these lesions. Since dermoids are benign, the benefits of surgery should be balanced against the risks of operation. Cystic dermoids commonly enlarge progressively and therefore should usually be completely removed, if possible. Solid dermoids (most often subconjunctival dermolipomas) may remain relatively stable in size. Therefore, dermolipomas are frequently observed without surgery, since excision may be complicated by damage to surrounding tissues.

References

Grove AS Jr: Giant dermoid cysts of the orbit. Ophthalmology 86:1513–1520, 1979.
Grove AS Jr: Surgery of the orbit. *In* Spaeth GL (ed): Ophthalmic Surgery: Principles and Practice. Philadelphia, WB Saunders, 1982, pp 431–546.
Henderson JW: Orbital Tumors, 2nd ed. New York, Brian C Decker, 1980, pp 75–114.
Paris GL, Beard C: Blepharoptosis following dermolipoma surgery. Ann Ophthalmol 5:697–699, 1973.

JUVENILE XANTHOGRANULOMA 224.0
(JXG, Nevoxanthoendothelioma)

PAUL E. ROMANO, M.D., M.S.O.,

Gainesville, Florida

Juvenile xanthogranuloma is a disease of infancy and childhood of unknown etiology that is characterized by multiple benign tumors. The skin is most frequently involved, with yellow, elevated, papular, sharply demarcated lesions singly or in groups that have a predilection for the head or neck. These lesions spontaneously regress over several years.

Ocular and adnexal juvenile xanthogranuloma has been recognized since 1949 and may occur independently of concurrent skin lesions. The iris or ciliary body is commonly affected, and the typical presentation in an infant is a salmon or darkly pigmented solitary iris lesion with spontaneous unilateral hyphema. Orbital, corneal, epibulbar, and lid lesions as well as bilateral iris involvement have been described. Although most eye lesions manifest in infancy (85 per cent at age less than 1 year, 64 per cent at age less than 7 months), adult cases have also been reported.

THERAPY

Supportive. The natural course of juvenile xanthogranuloma of the iris and ciliary body in infancy is spontaneous regression punctuated by one or more episodes of spontaneous bleeding. Whether juvenile xanthogranuloma iris lesions occur without bleeding is currently unknown, as eye involvement is usually recognized only after spontaneous hyphema. Such hyphemas may progress to secondary glaucoma. Therefore, prophylactic therapy may be advisable. Experience with other ocular lesions is very limited, but suggests self-limited disease, if not spontaneous regression. The following treatment modalities have been used or advocated by numerous authors; none has had the benefit of controlled studies.

Systemic. Topical, subconjunctival, systemic or combination route corticosteroids should be given to promote involution of the ocular lesions. Oral prednisone[‡] in a daily dosage of 2 mg/kg may be given in divided doses for no more than 4 to 6 weeks. In patients with corneal or intraocular lesions, one drop of topical ophthalmic 1 per cent prednisolone[‡] solution may be applied several times daily. However, such therapy should not be administered for more than a few weeks. Orbital disease responds well, but steroids alone may not stabilize intraocular lesions.

Irradiation. Many authors consider radiation therapy to be the most effective treatment modality. Though even smaller doses are advocated, most authors report regression of lesions with a total dose of between 250 and 500 rads, given in divided doses of 150 to 200 rads to minimize cataractogenic effects. Cataract has not to date been reported following such a dosage.

Surgical. Iridectomy and iridocyclectomy have been used for both diagnosis and therapy. However, the location of the lesions, their friability, and the propensity to bleed make such procedures technically difficult, and some authors caution against surgical intervention. Large incisions in infantile eyes are hazardous, and refractive and other changes following surgery may cause a functional amblyopia, with a poor visual prognosis akin to a unilateral infantile cataract.

Ocular or Periocular Manifestations

Conjunctiva: Epibulbar mass (very rare).
Cornea: Blood-stained (from hyphema); edema (from glaucoma).
Eyelids: Yellow to brown papules or nodules.
Iris or Ciliary Body: Heterochromia; salmon-colored lesion; uveitis.
Pupil: Oval and/or eccentric.
Other: Proptosis (rare); spontaneous hyphema (common).

PRECAUTIONS

Prolonged use of either topical or systemic corticosteroids may cause glaucoma, cataract, or iatrogenic Cushing's syndrome. Fluorinated corticosteroids should not be used in children.

COMMENTS

When ocular juvenile xanthogranuloma occurs with typical skin lesions, diagnosis can be confirmed by skin biopsy. In about 50 per cent of cases, however, ocular juvenile xanthogranuloma presents without such lesions. Iris lesions may present as unilateral glaucoma, spontaneous hyphema, uveitis, or heterochromia. In such cases, ultrasonic echography or examination under anesthesia or both are indicated to rule out retinoblastoma. Anterior chamber tap for cytology may be useful, though not without some hazard. When glaucoma secondary to hyphema does occur, standard medical and surgical therapy may not control progression to a blind, painful eye. Thus, steroid and radiation therapy is especially important early in the disease process to accelerate natural involution and regression.

References

Hadden OB: Bilateral juvenile xanthogranuloma of the iris. Br J Ophthalmol 59:699–702, 1975.

Harley RD, Romayananda N, Chan GH: Juvenile xanthogranuloma. J Pediatr Ophthalmol Strabismus 19:33–39, 1982.

Sanders TE: Infantile xanthogranuloma of the orbit. A report of three cases. Am J Ophthalmol 61:1299–1306, 1966.

Schwartz LW, Rodrigues MM, Hallett JW: Juvenile xanthogranuloma diagnosed by paracentesis. Am J Ophthalmol 77:243–246, 1974.

Smith JLS, Ingram RM: Juvenile oculodermal xanthogranuloma. Br J Ophthalmol 52:696–703, 1968.

Treacy KW, Letson RD, Summers CG: Subconjunctival steroid in the management of uveal juvenile xanthogranuloma: A case report. J Pediatr Strabismus 27:126–127, 1990.

Zimmerman LE: Ocular lesions of juvenile xanthogranuloma. Nevoxanthoendothelioma. Am J Ophthalmol 60:1011–1035, 1965.

KERATOACANTHOMA 224.4

J. BROOKS CRAWFORD, M.D.

San Francisco, California

Keratoacanthoma is a benign epithelial tumor that arises in hair follicles in exposed skin of Caucasian patients of middle or old age. Most are solitary. The majority of these tumors occur on the face (including the eyelids and rarely the conjunctiva), where they may be unusually aggressive, and on the hands.

Multiple keratoacanthomas are rare and occur in several different subtypes. The Ferguson Smith type consists of multiple self-healing keratoacanthomas of the skin that may appear in childhood or early adolescence. The Grzybowski type are smaller (2 to 3 mm in diameter) and do not appear until adult life. The Witten Zak variant is a combination of both the larger self-healing type of Ferguson Smith and the multiple miliary keratoacanthomas of Grzybowski. A giant massive or confluent keratoacanthoma is believed to result from the fusion of small, closely spaced keratoacanthomas. In the multinodular variant (keratoacanthoma centrifugum marginatum), multiple keratoacanthomas occur at the periphery of the progressively expanding lesion with central scar formation; unlike the usual solitary keratoacanthomas, this variant has no tendency to involute spontaneously.

The Muir-Torre syndrome is an autosomal dominant genodermatosis consisting of multiple keratoacanthomas and sebaceous skin tumors associated with an up to 40 per cent incidence of internal malignancies, especially adenocarcinoma of the colon. Multiple keratoacanthomas may be the only skin manifestation of this syndrome, but they are not a marker for the syndrome. On the other hand, the presence of even a solitary benign or transitional sebaceous neoplasm, such as a sebaceous adenoma or sebaceous differentiation in a basal cell carcinoma, may be a marker for the syndrome and should prompt the physician to search for internal malignancies (especially adenocarcinoma of the colon) in the patient and blood relatives.

Keratoacanthomas may occur in patients with xeroderma pigmentosum; in immunologically compromised patients (such as recipients of renal transplants, patients with metastatic cancer, and patients with leukemia and lymphoma); in industrial workers exposed to mineral oils, pitch, or tar; and in patients treated with psoralen plus ultraviolet A (PUVA) light therapy.

The usual solitary keratoacanthoma is a raised, dome-shaped tumor with rolled lateral borders and a central keratin core. It is characterized by an abrupt onset and rapid growth. Most reach a maximum size of 1 to 2 cm in 6 to 8 weeks and then spontaneously involute over a period of months. Some lesions, particularly those on the face, may grow larger and regress more slowly. In most patients, the presence of a rapidly growing lump is the main symptom, but occasionally pain, discomfort, or irritation may occur.

THERAPY

Surgical. Despite the tendency for these tumors to involute spontaneously, surgery is usually the treatment of choice. Small lesions can be excised completely; a biopsy can be taken of larger lesions, biopsied, after which they often undergo an accelerated rate of involution.

There are several reasons why surgery is

generally preferred over observation. Keratoacanthomas are benign, but may closely resemble squamous cell carcinomas, which are malignant and can metastasize. Lesions on the face are usually disfiguring, and many patients prefer not to wait for spontaneous involution. Small lesions can be removed before they enlarge and produce destruction of cosmetically and functionally important areas. Basal cell carcinomas and squamous cell carcinomas may occur at the base or edges of a true keratoacanthoma. Some keratoacanthomas never regress. In addition to excision, other surgical measures include curettage with electrocoagulation, cryotherapy, and treatment with the argon laser. Nonsurgical treatments include radiation therapy; the use of fluorouracil, which can be injected into the lesion or applied as a cream or ointment; the intralesional injection of methotrexate; and the intralesional injection of interferon. Synthetic retinoids, taken orally, have been used successfully for both solitary and multiple keratoacanthomas that failed to resolve or recurred after conventional surgery or the use of antimetabolites. In patients who refuse surgery or for whom surgery is contraindicated, these alternative modalities may be effective. However, if the lesions do not regress as expected with these methods, a biopsy should be performed to be certain that the lesion is not a basal or squamous cell carcinoma.

Ocular or Periocular Manifestations

Conjunctiva: Nodules.
Eyelids: Nodules.
Other: Irritation; ocular pain.

PRECAUTIONS

An adequate biopsy is essential to rule out the possibility of squamous cell carcinoma, which keratoacanthoma resembles closely. Occasional progression and malignant change of keratoacanthomas, especially in immunosuppressed patients, have been documented. However, most reports of these benign tumors that later undergo malignant change and metastasize are probably cases of carcinomas that are not recognized initially, either because of an inadequate biopsy or because it is occasionally impossible to differentiate a keratoacanthoma from a squamous cell carcinoma on histologic evaluation alone. The biopsy should include a spindle-shaped portion across the entire lesion including the center, subcutaneous tissue beneath the lesion, and normal tissue at both edges of the lesion. Many large tumors undergo an accelerated rate of spontaneous involution after such a biopsy. Recurrences of keratoacanthomas are rare, but occur occasionally; some keratoacanthomas, particularly those on the eyelids and face, have an especially aggressive behavior.

COMMENTS

The etiology of keratoacanthomas is unknown. Since most occur on sun-exposed areas of light-skinned individuals and may occur in patients with xeroderma pigmentosum, ultraviolet radiation has been implicated. Exposure to some chemical carcinogens has also been suspected in the etiology of some cases. Immunologic depression may play a role in some patients. Multiple keratoacanthomas occasionally have a hereditary component.

References

Boniuk M, Zimmerman LE: Eyelid tumors with reference to lesions confused with squamous cell carcinoma. III. Keratoacanthoma. Arch Ophthalmol 77:29–40, 1967.
Boynton JR, Searl SS, Caldwell EH: Large periocular keratoacanthoma: The case for definitive treatment. Ophthalmic Surg 17:565–569, 1986.
Caccialanza M, Sopelana N: Radiation therapy of keratoacanthomas: Result of 55 patients. Int J Radiat Oncol Biol Phys 16:475–477, 1989.
Chuang TY, Heinrich LA, Schulz MD, et al: PUVA and skin cancer. A historical cohort study on 492 patients. J Am Acad Dermatol 26:173–177, 1992.
Donahue B, Cooper JS, Rush S: Treatment of aggressive keratoacanthomas by radiotherapy. J Am Acad Dermatol 23:489–493, 1990.
Eliezri YD, Libow L: Multinodular keratoacanthoma. J Am Acad Dermatol 19:826–830, 1988.
Finan MC, Connolly SM: Sebaceous gland tumors and systemic disease: A clinicopathologic analysis. Medicine 63:232–242, 1984.
Font RL: Eyelids and lacrimal drainage system. In Spencer WH (ed): Ophthalmic Pathology. Philadelphia, WB Saunders, 1986, Vol 3, pp 2151–2155.
Goldberg LH, Rosen T, Becker J, Knauss A: Treatment of solitary keratoacanthomas with oral isotretinoin. J Am Acad Dermatol 23:934–936, 1990.
Grossniklaus HE, Martin DF, Solomon AR: Invasive conjunctival tumor with keratoacanthoma features. Am J Ophthalmol 109:736–738, 1990.
Hamed LM, Wilson FM, Grayson M: Keratoacanthoma of the limbus. Ophthalmic Surg 19:267–270, 1988.
Haydey RP, Reed ML, Dzubow LM, Shipack JL: Treatment of keratoacanthomas with oral 13-cis retinoic acid. N Engl J Med 303:502–505, 1980.
Jakobiec FA, Zimmerman LE, Piana FL, et al: Unusual eyelid tumors with sebaceous differentiation in the Muir-Torre syndrome. Ophthalmology 95:1543–1548, 1988.
Lever WF, Schaumberg-Lever G: Histopathology of the Skin, 7th ed. Philadelphia, JB Lippincott, 1990.
Melton JL, Nelson BR, Stough DB, et al: Treatment of keratoacanthomas with intralesional methotrexate. J Am Acad Dermatol 25:1017–1023, 1991.
Neumann RA, Knobler RM: Argon laser treatment of small keratoacanthomas in difficult locations. Int J Dermatol 29:733–736, 1990.
Parker CM, Hanke CW: Large keratoacanthomas in difficult locations treated with intralesional 5-fluorouracil. J Am Acad Dermatol 14:770–777, 1986.
Poleksic S, Yeung KY: Rapid development of keratoacanthoma and accelerated transformation into squamous cell carcinoma of the skin. Cancer 41:12–16, 1978.

Popkin GL, et al: A technique of biopsy recommended for keratoacanthomas. Arch Dermatol 94:191–193, 1966.

Rook A, Whimster I: Keratoacanthomas—a thirty year retrospect. Br J Dermatol 100:41–47, 1979.

Rothenberg J, Lambert WC, Vail JT, et al: The Muir-Torre (Torre's) syndrome: The significance of a solitary sebaceous tumor. J Am Acad Dermatol 23:638–640, 1990.

Schwartz RA: The keratoacanthoma: A review. J Surg Oncol 12:305–317, 1979.

Shaw JC, White CR Jr: Treatment of multiple keratoacanthomas with oral isotretinoin. J Am Acad Dermatol 15:1079, 1082, 1986.

Shimm DF, Duttenhavar JR, Doucette J, et al: Radiation therapy of keratoacanthomas. Int J Radiat Oncol Biol Phys 9:759–761, 1983.

Street ML, White JW, Gibson LE: Multiple keratoacanthomas treated with oral retinoids. J Am Acad Dermatol 23:862–866, 1990.

Wickramasinghe L, Hindson TC, Wacks H: Treatment of neoplastic skin lesions with intralesional interferon. J Am Acad Dermatol 20:71–74, 1989.

LEIOMYOMA 224.1

DAVID SEVEL, M.D., Ph.D., F.A.C.S.

La Jolla, California

Leiomyoma is a rare, benign tumor that arises from smooth muscle; it comprises only 2 to 14 per cent of all primary iris tumors. It may be located in the iris, the ciliary body, or the orbit and originates in these structures from the sphincter or dilator pupillae muscle, the ciliary muscle, and Müller's or capsulopalpebral muscle, respectively.

Leiomyoma of the iris is reported most frequently in white female subjects and occurs in a wide age group, ranging from 10 to 80 years of age. This white or pink tumor commonly involves the inferior temporal iris and is well circumscribed and elevated. A presenting feature may be a distorted pupil, ectropion uveae, or hyphema. Vision is not affected unless there is a complication of glaucoma or cataract. Clinically, a leiomyoma of the iris cannot be differentiated from an amelanotic malignant melanoma. Fine-needle aspiration biopsy of the tumor may help with the differential diagnosis.

Leiomyoma of the ciliary body usually presents as a pigmented mass of the ciliary body that slowly increases in size and may distort the iris, compress the lens, or locally occlude the filtration angle. Clinically, it cannot be differentiated from a malignant melanoma of the ciliary body.

A leiomyoma of the orbit is an extremely rare, well-encapsulated, vascular tumor that is usually located in an extraconal position. Regardless of the primary site of the tumor, the diagnosis of leiomyoma is only made on histologic examination. Although local recurrences may occur if the tumor is not completely removed, distant metastases have not been described.

THERAPY

Supportive. Leiomyomas of the iris and ciliary body are only excised if the tumors increase in size, bleed, or cause complications, such as glaucoma or cataract. Repeated frequent examinations (every 6 months) should include photography of the tumor to aid in the assessment of the size, gonioscopy, and fluorescein iridography.

Surgical. The tumor should be removed in toto, as local recurrences may occur if the tumor is excised incompletely. Fluorescein iridography helps determine the actual tumor size, which may extend beyond that noted on clinical observation. In addition, the blood supply of the tumor may be ascertained preoperatively. Radioactive phosphorus uptake may be done preoperatively to help assess the vascularity of the tumor. Perhaps of greater importance, the extension of the tumor in the filtration angle can be determined, helping one decide whether or not an iridectomy or iridocyclectomy is required. A tumor of the ciliary body is treated by an iridocyclectomy, which can involve up to a quarter of the ciliary body circumference. A leiomyoma of the orbit is well encapsulated and is removed easily.

Ocular or Periocular Manifestations

(C) refers to ciliary body leiomyoma; (I) indicates iris leiomyoma; (O) refers to orbital leiomyoma.

Anterior Chamber: Hyphema (I); shallow angle (C).

Ciliary Body: Pigmented tumor (C).

Globe: Proptosis (O).

Iris: Distorted pupil (I); ectropion uveae (I); pale tumor (I).

Other: Glaucoma (C, I); localized cataract (C, I).

PRECAUTIONS

An iris or ciliary body leiomyoma cannot be differentiated clinically from a malignant melanoma and is diagnosed on histologic examination. The tumor must be removed totally; otherwise, recurrences are inevitable.

Orbital leiomyoma is localized and well encapsulated and usually shells out without difficulty. The tumor is removed in toto. Patients may experience intermittent episodes of pain, a feature not common with other benign orbital growths. This symptomatology may be related to the vascularity of the tumor.

COMMENTS

Leiomyoma has a propensity for slow growth. Although degeneration may occur within its substance, resulting in hemorrhage and local necrosis, spread by continuity, contiguity, or metastasis has not been recorded.

Histologically, a leiomyoma is composed of interlacing, tightly arranged spindle-shaped cells with oval nuclei and blunted ends. There is only a moderate amount of eosinophilic cytoplasm. Longitudinal fibrils are noted within the cells and are best seen with phosphotungstic acid hematoxylin stain. With light microscopy, a leiomyoma can be difficult to differentiate from a neurofibroma, an amelanotic spindle-shaped malignant melanoma, or a neurilemoma, especially as phosphotungstic acid hematoxylin stain does not differentiate myofibrils from neurofibrils. Electron microscopy may be the only means of differentiating these tumors from a leiomyoma.

It has also been suggested that oxytalan fiber demonstration can differentiate between a leiomyoma and a spindle-cell malignant melanoma of the iris. However, in the diagnosis of leiomyoma of the ciliary body, oxytalan fiber demonstration is not of use because these fibers are normally present in the ciliary body.

References

de Buen S, Olivares ML, Charlin VC: Leiomyoma of the iris. Report of a case. Br J Ophthalmol 55: 353–356, 1971.

Grossniklaus HE: Fine-needle aspiration biopsy of the iris. Arch Ophthalmol 110:969–976, 1992.

Henderson JW, Harrison EG Jr: Vascular leiomyoma of the orbit: Report of a case. Trans Am Acad Ophthalmol Otolaryngol 74:970–974, 1970.

Meyer SL, et al: Leiomyoma of the ciliary body. Electron microscopic verification. Am J Ophthalmol 66:1061–1068, 1968.

Sevel D, Tobias B: The value of fluorescein iridography with leiomyoma of the iris. Am J Ophthalmol 74:475–478, 1972.

Sunba MSN, et al: Tumours of the anterior uvea. III. Oxytalan fibers in the differential diagnosis of leiomyoma and malignant melanoma of the iris. Br J Ophthalmol 64:867–874, 1980.

LYMPHANGIOMA 228.1

IRA SNOW JONES, M.D.,
and MICHAEL KAZIM, M.D.

New York, New York

Lymphangiomas are benign, congenital tumors most commonly affecting the head and neck. When present within the orbit, they produce slowly progressive proptosis that may be punctuated by explosive episodes of proptosis. Acute proptosis may be associated with upper respiratory infections or spontaneous intralesional hemorrhages. The histopathology is controversial and has been discussed at length in recent reviews of the subject. It is currently held that these lesions represent the inappropriate differentiation of vascular mesenchyme originally destined for normal vascular channels into lymphatic spaces without adequate connection to normal circulation. The presence of lymph-like fluid within fine endothelially lined channels and the presence of lymphoid follicles in many lesions support this theory. It is the lymphoid elements that are felt to proliferate in response to upper respiratory tract infections and thereby to produce rapid growth of the tumor. In addition, the modest response of some tumors to systemic corticosteroids or radiotherapy is felt to represent a modulation of the intrinsic lymphoid elements. In some cases the lesions become secondarily blood vascularized. This too can result in rapid growth and potentiate internal hemorrhage, producing what appears clinically as a "chocolate cyst." In cases of secondary arterialization the lesions may be imaged by angiography, and selective embolization of feeder vessels may shrink the tumor and simplify surgical excision if it becomes necessary. Some would alternatively classify the vascularized lesions as primary orbital varices, the result of differentiation of the pluripotential mesenchymal cell into a venous system and therefore subject to a different pattern of clinical presentation, growth, and management. Although most of these lesions are first detected by the second decade, smaller, deeper lesions may go unnoticed in unusual cases until the seventh decade. In the deeper lesions, optic neuropathy or paralytic strabismus may dominate the clinical picture, and proptosis may be modest or nonexistent.

Recent advances in noninvasive imaging of the orbit have produced substantial improvement in the diagnosis and management of lymphangiomas. Ultrasound imaging of the orbit with a 10-mHz probe produces excellent images of the anterior two-thirds of the orbital soft tissues. Ultrasound is particularly sensitive to the presence of soft tissue lesions within the orbit and provides excellent imaging of cystic structures within lymphangiomas. However, it is limited in its ability to image the posterior one-third of the orbit with standard probes and lacks specificity. Computed tomography provides excellent soft tissue and superior bony imaging of the orbit and periorbital tissues. It provides superlative detail of the extent of orbital lesions, but is lacking in soft tissue detail of the internal structures of lymphangiomas. MRI provides the best soft tissue detail of all noninvasive techniques and has been shown to delineate clearly the presence and contents of cysts with lymphangiomas. It more clearly details the invasiveness of lesions into and around surrounding tissues and has the advantage of multiplanar imaging without the need for ionizing radiation. Angiography is most useful in defining the feeder vessel if arterialization is suspected. It can also provide an alternative to open surgical treatment.

THERAPY

Supportive. In view of the many difficulties of managing these lesions, an attempt is made to allow the lesion to resolve spontaneously in all cases except those involving compressive optic neuropathy. Lymphoid proliferation resulting from upper respiratory tract infections and spontaneous hemorrhages tend in most cases to resolve. During the period of resolution, supportive care to treat the complications of corneal exposure is necessary. Corticosteroids are sometimes useful in producing resolution of these lesions.

Surgical. Surgical intervention is limited to those cases in which there is compressive optic neuropathy, disabling strabismus, or significant cosmetic deformity. In cases of orbital hemorrhage, percutaneous needle aspiration of the cystic fluid with CT or ultrasound guidance remains fraught with potential risks, including globe perforation and secondary hemorrhage. In such cases, after appropriate imaging, we would favor an open orbital exploration and decompression of the chocolate cyst. Of particular advantage has been the combined use of a neurosurgical operating microscope and a carbon dioxide laser with a micromanipulator. This procedure is particularly helpful in cases in which the tumor is not well encapsulated and interdigitates itself with critical orbital structures. The combination of these two tools allows for superior visualization and differentiation of normal from tumor tissue and facilitates the ablation of tumor tissue while preserving normal tissue. The CO_2 laser is particularly suited to this task as its depth of penetration is quite superficial, which prevents the collateral spread of laser energy to normal surrounding structures. The CW neodymium yag laser is avoided in such cases since it produces significant amounts of collateral damage.

The surgical approach is chosen based on the location of the lesion. In selected cases, a transcranial approach has been necessary to gain access to lesions in the superior orbit and in one case in which the tumor was invading intercranially through the superior orbital fissure.

Ocular or Periocular Manifestations

Conjunctiva: Chemosis; hemorrhage; lymphangioma; prominent blood vessel channels.
Extraocular muscles: Strabismus; restricted motility.
Eyelids: Lymphangioma; edema; ptosis; hemorrhage.

Globe: Exophthalmos (stable, variable, rapidly, or slowly progressive).
Optic nerve: Compressive optic neuropathy.
Orbit: Bony asymmetry; cystic, solid, or mixed solid and cystic; invasive or well-circumscribed lymphangioma.
Other: Amblyopia secondary to mass effect and induced astigmatism; facial and nasopharyngeal lymphangioma; choroidal striae.

COMMENTS

Orbital and periorbital lymphangiomas remain among the most difficult lesions to characterize pathologically and to treat clinically. The growth rate of these lesions is unpredictable, and although most often they progress slowly, the lesions can produce explosive episodes of proptosis resulting in compressive optic neuropathy. Urgent management can be anticipated in a small fraction of such cases; however, the vast majority respond well to supportive care. The great advances in noninvasive imaging have provided greater accuracy and a higher level of surgical proficiency. These lesions can be present at any level within the orbit, and the deeper, more critically placed lesion can produce an occult form of compressive optic neuropathy. Intraoperatively, they present a varied morphologic picture. Lesions may be predominantly solid or cystic; however, they are most often mixed in pattern. Most are invasive, although some are well circumscribed. Ultimately, surgical management may require multiple procedures over the course of years, producing an uncertain functional and cosmetic result.

References

Graeb DA, Rootman J, Robertson WD, Lapointe JS, Nugent RA, Hay EJ: Orbital lymphangiomas: Clinical, radiologic, and pathologic characteristics. Radiology 175:417–421, 1990.

Harris GJ, Sakol PJ, Bonavolenta G, DeConciliis C: An analysis of thirty cases of orbital lymphangioma. Ophthalmology 97:1583–1592, 1990.

Hornblass A: The use of YAG-tipped contact laser in removing orbital lymphangiomas. Plast Reconstr Surg 83:397, 1989.

Jones IS: Lymphangiomas of the ocular adnexa: An analysis of sixty-two cases. Am J Ophthalmol 51:481–509, 1961.

Kazim M, Kennerdell J, Rothfus W, Marquardt M: Orbital lymphangioma: Correlation of magnetic resonance images and intraoperative findings. Ophthalmology 99:1588–1594, 1992.

Kennerdell J, Maroon JC, Garrity JA, Abla AA: Surgical management of orbital lymphangioma with the carbon dioxide laser. Am J Ophthalmol 102:308–314, 1986.

Rootman J, Hay E, Graeb D, Miller R: Orbital-adnexal lymphangiomas. A spectrum of hemodynamically isolated vascular hamartomas. Ophthalmology 93:1558–1570, 1986.

Skalka HW, Callahan MA: Ultrasonically-aided percutaneous orbital aspiration. Ophthalmic Surg 10:41–43, 1979.

MEDULLOEPITHELIOMA 225.0
(Diktyoma)

LEONARD APT, M.D.

Los Angeles, California

Medulloepithelioma is a rare congenital tumor that arises from the primitive, nonpigmented medullary epithelium of the ciliary body before differentiation into its various derivatives (sixth week of gestation). Occasionally, the tumor originates in the iris, the retina, and the optic nerve. Medulloepithelioma formerly was called "diktyoma" (from the Greek diktyon, meaning net) because, at times, it has a lace- or net-like appearance.

These tumors are classified into nonteratoid and teratoid types, and each is further divided into benign and malignant varieties. Nonteratoid medulloepitheliomas contain tissue resembling medullary epithelium, but may also contain tissue derived from secondary optic vesicle, such as retinal pigment epithelium, ciliary epithelium, vitreous, and neuroglia. The teratoid group exhibits heteroplasia; that is, it contains tissues not normally present in the eye, such as cartilage, brain tissue, and striated muscle. The teratoid types are more likely than the nonteratoid to be malignant. Criteria for malignancy in these tumors include (1) local invasion of other ocular tissues with or without extraocular extension, (2) many poorly differentiated neuroblastic cells that may resemble retinoblastoma, (3) increased pleomorphism or mitotic activity, and (4) appearance of sarcomatous areas. Medulloepitheliomas are locally destructive, but also may metastasize. They should be considered potentially malignant tumors.

Medulloepitheliomas tend to affect children in the first decade of life, commonly between 2 and 4 years of age. The tumor, however, has been observed in young infants and occasionally in adults, the oldest being in a 79-year-old individual. In one large series of cases, the first clinical manifestation was noted at an average age of 3.8 years, and the average time of final diagnosis by enucleation was 5 years of age. Medulloepitheliomas almost always are unilateral, with no laterality preference, and they exhibit no hereditary, racial, or sexual predilection. These tumors occur spontaneously and are not related to any predisposing condition, such as trauma or inflammation.

The clinical course of medulloepitheliomas is not uniform; most often they grow as a localized, relatively benign tumor in the ciliary body and iris, proceed to cover the lens surface and posterior surface of the iris, and then may fill the anterior chamber or even extend posteriorly to detach the retina. More often, the lesion is recognized inferiorly. Medulloepitheliomas may occur as a solid or cystic tumor or as a net-like mass that extends into adjacent cavities. Although these tumors are slow growing, they may crowd the anterior chamber angle and cause secondary glaucoma.

The color of the tumor varies, appearing as white, gray, yellow, pigmented or brown in the center, or fleshy pink. In some cases, cysts dislodge from the tumor and float freely in the anterior chamber or enter the posterior chamber and vitreous cavity. If the lens appears colobomatous in the area of the tumor in a child with neovascular glaucoma and rubeosis iridis but the retina and choroid are normal, the diagnosis of medulloepithelioma should be considered. The colobomatous defect is the result of partial resorption of the lens in the area of the tumor.

Differential diagnosis includes retinoblastoma, persistent hyperplastic primary vitreous (sometimes coexists with medulloepithelioma), peripheral uveitis (pars planitis, cyclitis), nematode granuloma (usually *Toxocara canis*), iris cyst, nevus, amelanotic and melanotic melanoma, leiomyoma, glioneuroma, neurofibroma of the iris or ciliary body, juvenile xanthogranuloma, and primary tumors of the pigmented or nonpigmented ciliary epithelium, e.g., adenoma and adenocarcinoma.

The clinical diagnosis of medulloepithelioma usually is based on (1) the tumor's appearance on indirect ophthalmoscopy and slit-lamp biomicroscopy and (2) familiarity with the tumor's growth pattern. Correct clinical diagnosis before microscopic tissue study, however, has been infrequent. Fluorescein angiography, ultrasonography, computed tomography, and magnetic resonance imaging have not been diagnostic. Because of the cystic component of some medulloepitheliomas, ultrasonography possibly could be of some diagnostic assistance if the globe is so positioned as to permit proper placement of the instrument's probe. Definitive diagnosis of medulloepithelioma is made by light and electron microscopy examination of material obtained on aspiration, biopsy, or excision.

Ocular or Periocular Manifestations

Anterior Chamber: Shallow; hyphema; medulloepithelioma (rare).

Conjunctiva: Hyperemia.

Cornea: Breaks in Descemet's membrane; tumor infiltration.

Globe: Exophthalmos; buphthalmos (infants, young children); perforation.

Iris or Ciliary Body: Heterochromia; medulloepithelioma (solid or cystic); iritis; rubeosis iridis; synechiae.

Lens: Cataract; colobomatous in tumor area; subluxation.

Optic Nerve: Medulloepithelioma (rare).

Orbit: Medulloepithelioma extension.

Pupil: Fixed or deformed; abnormal reflexes; leukocoria.

Retina: Detachment; medulloepithelioma (rare).

Vitreous: Retrolental membrane with dilated blood vessels; net-like strands; hemorrhage.

Other: Visual loss; pain; strabismus; secondary glaucoma.

THERAPY

Surgical. Treatment of medulloepitheliomas is based on early recognition and surgical management. If the tumor is confined to the iris and growth is documented, excisional biopsy (iridectomy) is indicated. If the tumor is small, well circumscribed, and confined to the ciliary body, cyclectomy or iridocyclectomy is recommended; unfortunately, tumors in the ciliary body usually are large before clinical manifestations lead to their detection. Enucleation generally is required for most medulloepitheliomas because of one or more of the following reasons: tumor size, location, encroachment on or destruction of adjacent ocular tissues, pain, secondary glaucoma, incomplete excision or local recurrence of tumor, malignant changes observed in an excised histopathologic specimen, or failure to exclude an intraocular malignancy, such as retinoblastoma. Orbital exenteration should be considered in patients with advanced extrascleral extension of the tumor.

PRECAUTIONS

Since medulloepithelioma is slow growing, early enucleation generally results in a high survival rate. Spread may lead to fatality, however, since the tumor then grows into the orbital bones and brain and may metastasize to the regional lymph nodes and lungs. After enucleation the patient should be observed closely for local recurrences or metastases. If extraocular extension has occurred, exenteration of the orbit is necessary. The rare optic nerve medulloepithelioma, because of its location and invasive tendency, requires enucleation with long sections of the optic nerve or exenteration; removal of the intracanalicular and intracranial portions of the optic nerve may also be necessary.

COMMENTS

Treatment of medulloepithelioma with radiotherapy or chemotherapy has been used too infrequently to judge its true value. Medulloepitheliomas are likely to be radiosensitive as are most embryonic tumors, such as retinoblastoma and neuroblastoma. The actual radiation response of ocular medulloepithelioma, however, is unknown because of the lack of experience with this method of treatment. The probable radiation dose for tumor ablation by conventional external beam techniques might produce serious ocular complications. Whether newer approaches, such as radioisotope applicators or particle beams, could eliminate the tumor without undue morbidity remains unanswered. In cases with local recurrence of tumor or metastasis to distant organs, the use of irradiation and chemotherapy should be considered.

References

Anderson SR: Intraocular epithelial tumors and cysts. *In* Garner A, Klintworth GK (eds): Pathology of Ocular Disease. A Dynamic Approach. New York, Marcel Dekker, 1982, pp 635–650.

Apt L, et al: Diktyoma (embryonal medulloepithelioma). Recent review and case report. J Pediatr Ophthalmol 10:30–38, 1973.

Broughton WL, Zimmerman LE: A clinicopathologic study of 56 cases of intraocular medulloepitheliomas. Am J Ophthalmol 85:407–418, 1978.

Canning CR, McCartney ACE, Hungerford J: Medulloepithelioma (diktyoma). Br J Ophthalmol 72:764–767, 1988.

Floyd BB, Minckler DS, Valentin L: Intraocular medulloepithelioma in a 79-year-old man. Ophthalmology 89:1088–1094, 1982.

Green WR, Iliff WJ, Trotter RR: Malignant teratoid medulloepithelioma of the optic nerve. Arch Ophthalmol 91:451–454, 1974.

Jakobiec FA, et al: Electron microscopic diagnosis of medulloepithelioma. Am J Ophthalmol 79:321–329, 1975.

Shields JA, Shields CL: Intraocular Tumors. Philadelphia, WB Saunders, 1992, pp 465–481.

MENINGIOMA 225.2

DUNCAN P. ANDERSON, M.D., F.R.C.S(C)

Vancouver, B.C., Canada

Meningiomas are generally benign, slow-growing tumors that arise from the arachnoid matter, the middle layer of meninges that lies inside the dura mater, and outside the pia mater. They comprise about 15 per cent of adult intracranial tumors and 2 per cent of pediatric intracranial tumors. They are three times more common in females than males and reach a peak incidence in the seventh decade of life, although those arising from the sphenoid bone resulting in visual complaints usually present in the fifth to sixth decades of life.

Meningiomas are seldom invasive. They produce signs and symptoms by compressing adjacent structures; these signs and symptoms depend on the site of origin of the tumor. Because of the characteristic slow tumor growth, the clinical findings have usually been present for a long time before correct diagnosis is made. It is important to recognize these signs and symptoms because surgery performed early in the course of the tumor generally has good results, whereas surgery performed late is fraught with complications.

Approximately half of all meningiomas occur parasagittally or over the convexity of the cerebral hemispheres. Those tumors that arise anteriorly present with a long history of headache, mental change, and chronic papilledema as a result of longstanding increased intracranial pressure. Those that arise posteriorly present more acutely with seizures, hemiplegia, or homonymous hemianopsia from compression of motor and sensory cortical areas.

Approximately one-third of meningiomas arise from the arachnoid over the sphenoid bone, and their clinical presentations are almost exclusively neuro-ophthalmic. Those arising from the lateral third of the sphenoid wing are usually of the en plaque type and produce slowly progressive, painless exophthalmos and fullness in the temporal fossa, with relative preservation of vision and ocular motility. Middle third sphenoid wing meningiomas present with signs of increased intracranial pressure (headaches, vomiting, papilledema) and few cranial nerve signs. Those arising from the inner one-third of the sphenoid wing produce early symptoms due to involvement of cranial nerves II, III, IV, V, and VI, resulting in slowly progressive visual loss, decreased corneal reflex, and disorders of ocular motility.

Meningiomas that arise from the tuberculum sellae of the sphenoid bone (anterior wall of sella turcica) produce early and isolated symptoms of visual loss and/or field defect because the optic nerves and chiasm are immediately above and behind this structure. Those tumors more centrally located will cause slowly progressive asymmetric bitemporal field defects. Those that arise slightly more laterally will present with slowly progressive monocular visual loss, afferent pupil defect, color vision defect, central scotoma and, in the early stages, a normal-appearing disc. If the diagnosis is delayed the second eye is eventually involved with a junctional scotoma (superotemporal defect in contralateral eye), and optic atrophy will eventually supervene. Associated neurologic signs and symptoms are invariably absent. Meningiomas arising slightly more anteriorly from the planum sphenoidale and olfactory groove (floor of anterior fossa) present late with anosmia, mental changes, and papilledema.

Sphenoid meningiomas may also arise from or invade the optic canal and spread down the optic nerve sheath into the orbit, causing optic atrophy, opticociliary shunt vessels, and proptosis.

Less than 1 per cent of meningiomas arise primarily from the arachnoid of the optic nerve sheath, but these patients present exclusively with visual complaints. Those that arise anteriorly in the orbit present with decreased vision, proptosis, mechanical restriction of ocular motility, and choroidal folds. Those arising in the apex of the orbit or in the optic canal produce visual loss early because minimal growth of even a very small tumor compresses the optic nerve against unyielding bony structures. These patients have no other neurologic or ophthalmologic findings apart from failing vision, optic atrophy, and occasional opticociliary shunt vessels.

THERAPY

Surgical. Since most meningiomas are encapsulated and noninvasive early in their course, surgical excision at this time is usually curative. Those involving the convexity of the cerebral hemispheres are usually excised easily with little morbidity. Those that arise from the sphenoid bone are more difficult to excise, but are usually amenable to surgery in their early stages. As the tumor grows, it surrounds vital neural and vascular structures and grows down the foramina, so that in the late stages a surgical cure is almost impossible. When diagnosed late, partial removal of the tumor and adjacent bony structures in an effort to decompress the anterior visual system will usually give many years of useful visual function. Attempted complete excision of a large tumor surrounding the optic nerve or chiasm usually has devastating visual results because removal of the tumor is invariably accompanied by removal of most of the blood supply of these vital structures.

The optimal management of patients with primary optic nerve sheath meningioma has yet to be determined. These tumors have unpredictable biologic activity, and surgical excision usually results in blindness. There are occasional anecdotal reports of preservation of vision with complete excision, but these are rare.

In general, meningioma surgery is the domain of the neurosurgeon. Even in primary optic nerve sheath meningioma, a combined intracranial-orbital approach is preferred as many of these tumors extend into the orbital apex and optic canal. Some anterior optic nerve sheath meningiomas may be excised via a lateral orbital approach by the orbital surgeon. The ophthalmologist's main role is in early diagnosis and rapid referral to the neurosurgeon so that he or she may operate early while the tumor is still resectable.

Irradiation. Although meningiomas are generally regarded as insensitive to radiotherapy, there are increasing reports in the literature of its stabilizing effect on those cases in which the risks of surgery are unacceptable. There is also some evidence that radiation reduced the recurrence rate in those meningiomas that can only be partially resected surgically.

Systemic. Meningiomas are generally resistant to standard chemotherapy; however, hormonal therapy has shown some promising effects more recently. Estrogen and progesterone receptors have been found in as many as 70 per cent of human meningiomas, which is why the tumor may rapidly progress in pregnancy, the luteal phase of the menstrual cycle, and with breast feeding. Hormonal therapy using estrogen or progesterone antagonists has been successful in controlling the growth of meningiomas in a number of cases.

Supportive. Elderly meningioma patients with unilateral, slowly progressive visual symptoms may be better left alone. Isolated optic nerve sheath meningiomas that are not causing progressive visual decline or have caused complete blindness may also best be observed because of their extreme biologic variability. Hormonal therapy and/or irradiation may be tried in these cases, but if there is progressive growth resulting in blindness, the meningioma and optic nerve should probably be removed en bloc.

Ocular or Periocular Manifestations

Cornea: Exposure keratopathy; hypesthesia (fifth nerve).
Extraocular Muscles: Imbalance or paralysis (third, fourth, or sixth nerve).
Globe: Proptosis.
Optic Nerve: Atrophy; opticociliary shunts; papilledema.
Other: Afferent pupil defect (second nerve); choroidal folds; hyperopia; ocular and facial pain (fifth nerve); visual field defect; visual loss (second nerve).

PRECAUTIONS

The signs and symptoms of meningiomas occasionally improve with systemic steroids; one must not misdiagnose these cases as optic neuritis or multiple sclerosis. Pregnancy occasionally results in worsening of these signs and symptoms.

COMMENTS

Early diagnosis and rapid referral are of utmost importance so that the neurosurgeon may excise the meningioma before it has compromised vital neural and vascular structures. Early diagnosis is brought about by having a strong clinical suspicion that there is a compressive lesion and then insisting on appropriate neuroimaging to define it. Plane skull films are often negative unless there is associated bony hyperostosis. High-resolution CT scanning and MRI will almost always show even the smallest meningioma as long as the suspected site is well defined for the neuroradiologist. Selective internal and external carotid angiography should be performed preoperatively.

Once patients have undergone partial or total excision of the tumor, they should be watched carefully for signs and symptoms of recurrence and followed for life with repeated evaluations of visual acuity, color vision, visual fields, exophthalmometry, corneal sensation, and ocular motility. Periodic repeat neuroimaging should also be performed.

References

Anderson D, Khalil M: Meningioma and the ophthalmologist. A review of 80 cases. Ophthalmology 88:1004–1009, 1981.
Andrews BT, Wilson CB: Suprasellar meningiomas: The effect of tumor location on postoperative visual outcome. J Neurosurg 69:523–528, 1988.
Barbaro NM, Gutin PH, Wilson CB, et al: Radiation therapy in the treatment of partially resected meningiomas. Neurosurgery 20:525–528, 1987.
Capo H, Kupersmith MJ: Efficacy and complications of radiotherapy of anterior visual pathway tumors. Neurol Clin 9:179–203, 1991.
Clark WC, Theofilos CS, Fleming JC: Primary optic nerve sheath meningiomas. J Neurosurg 70:37–40, 1989.
Finn JE, Mount LA: Meningiomas of the tuberculum sellae and planum sphenoidale. A review of 83 cases. Arch Ophthalmol 92:23–27, 1974.
Jane JA, McKissock W: Importance of failing vision in early diagnosis of suprasellar meningiomas. Br Med J 2:5–7, 1962.
Kennerdell JS, Maroon JC, Malton M, et al: The management of optic nerve sheath meningiomas. Am J Ophthalmol 106:450–457, 1988.
Knight CL, Hoyt WF, Wilson CB: Syndrome of incipient prechiasmal optic nerve compression. Progress toward early diagnosis and surgical management. Arch Ophthalmol 87:1–11, 1972.
Kupersmith MJ, Warren FA, Newall J, Ransohoff J: Irradiation of meningiomas of the intracranial anterior visual pathway. Ann Neurol 21:131–137, 1987.
Miller N (ed): Walsh and Hoyt's Clinical Neuro-Ophthalmology, 4th ed. Baltimore, Williams & Wilkins, 1988, Vol 3, pp 1325–1379.
Newell FW, Beaman TC: Ocular signs of meningioma. Am J Ophthalmol 45:30–40, 1958.
Wan WL, Jessica L, Geller BA, et al: Visual loss caused by rapidly progressive intracranial meningiomas during pregnancy. Ophthalmology 97:18–21, 1990.
Wilson WB: Meningiomas of the anterior visual system. Surv Ophthalmol 26:109–127, 1981.
Wright JE: Primary optic nerve meningiomas: Clinical presentation and management. Trans Am Acad Ophthalmol Otolaryngol 83:617–625, 1977.
Wright JE, Call NB, Liaricos S: Primary optic nerve meningioma. Br J Ophthalmol 64:553–558, 1980.

MUCOCELE 376.81
(Pyocele)

IRA A. ABRAHAMSON, M.D.

Cincinnati, Ohio

Mucocele is an accumulation and retention of mucoid material within the sinus as a result of continuous or periodic obstruction of the sinus osteum. X-ray studies may show the frontal sinus completely obliterated by bone density with no bone erosion or destruction. The occurrence of mucocele involving the paranasal sinuses is not as rare a condition as previously reported. The literature reveals many reports of mucoceles involving the various paranasal sinuses.

A gradual onset of headaches, orbital or forehead pain unilateral proptosis, and limited ocular motility should make the physician suspicious of a paranasal sinus mucocele. The patient may also complain of decreased or blurred vision or diplopia, which may be the presenting symptom.

The frontal and ethmoid sinuses are the two most common locations of the mucocele. The least common location is in the maxillary sinus where the mucocele produces bulging of the turbinates with subsequent occlusion of the nasal passages, loosening of the teeth, erosion of the orbital floor, and compression of the orbital fissure. Proptosis, diplopia, and even blindness may result on the involved side.

In the frontal sinus, erosion of the anterior wall results in a tender fluctuant mass beneath the periosteum of the frontal bone, commonly known as a Pott's puffy tumor or a subcutaneous abscess, which requires local drainage or exenteration of the sinus. Erosion of the posterior sinus wall may produce an epidural abscess, subdural empyema, meningitis, or brain abscess.

Ethmoid sinus mucoceles encroach upon the medial wall of the orbit and the orbital fissure, producing proptosis and ocular motility disturbances.

Mucocele of the sphenoid sinus occurs less frequently than in frontal and ethmoid sinuses and can produce variable clinical pictures. It must be differentiated from retrobulbar neuritis, pituitary tumors, and ophthalmoplegic migraine.

THERAPY

Surgical. A team approach to complete surgical drainage and removal of the tumor and diseased mucous membrane should be used. An osteoplastic anterior wall approach to the frontal sinus is performed with obliteration of the sinus cavity by abdominal wall fat. Under general anesthesia, both the face and abdominal wall are prepared. Bilateral eyebrow butterfly-type incisions are made, and the superior flap is elevated. The periosteum is left attached to the cranium. A previously sterilized precut template of the Caldwell view of the frontal sinus is outlined on the periosteum over the sinus. A Stryker saw is used to cut the bone after incising the periosteum, and flap bone is hinged inferiorly upon entering the frontal sinus. After aspirating the contents of the sinus cavity and the cyst and removing the sinus mucosa, the inside of the sinus wall is drilled with a cutting burr of the Jordan Day drill until all the inner periosteum is removed. A tantalum mesh is fashioned to replace the deficient orbital roof. The frontal sinus cavity is then obliterated with the fat obtained from the abdominal wall. The bone flap is then repositioned, and the periosteum is closed. The skin flap is laid back and closed in layers, and a pressure-type dressing may be applied.

Ocular or Periocular Manifestations

Extraocular Muscles: Paralysis.
Globe: Exophthalmos; proptosis.
Lacrimal System: Lacrimation.
Orbit: Erosion of bony walls; mucocele.
Other: Decreased visual acuity; diplopia.

PRECAUTIONS

The diagnosis of a frontal sinus mucocele is established by laminographic radiography. However, this clinical picture may also be caused by several other conditions. Included in a differential diagnosis are thyroid disease, retrobulbar tumor, retrobulbar neuritis, pseudotumor, temporal arteritis, acute or chronic sinusitis, and sinus, nasal, or pharyngeal tumors. Tomography is essential in investigating this lesion and establishing a diagnosis.

COMMENTS

The diagnosis and management of mucoceles have improved greatly over the past few years. The use of laminograms has greatly aided the diagnosis. However, a team approach (ophthalmologist, radiologist, otorhinolaryngologist, and neurosurgeon) is essential for an accurate diagnosis and therapeutic approach to this problem. A precut template from the Caldwell projection is a very useful device to outline the contours of the frontal sinus during surgery. The not-so-frequent use of abdominal fat to fill the frontal sinus cavity has resulted in no apparent postoperative fat necrosis.

References

Abrahamson IA Jr, et al: Frontal sinus mucocele. Ann Ophthalmol 11:173–178, 1979.
Evans C: Aetiology and treatment of fronto-ethmoidal mucocele. J Laryngol Otol 95:361–375, 1981.
Feldman M, Lowry LD, Rao VM, et al: Mucoceles of the paranasal sinuses. Trans PA Acad Ophthalmol 39:614–617, 1987.
Gillespie RP, Marshall A, Ludlow P: Use of the CUSA in removal of a recurrent intraorbital mucocele. Otolaryngol Head Neck Surg 99:71–72, 1988.
Jones JL, Kaufman PW: Mucopyocele of the maxillary sinus. J Oral Surg 39:948–950, 1981.
Kaufman SJ: Orbital mucopyoceles. Two cases and a review. Surv Ophthalmol 25:253–262, 1981.
Lund VJ: Anatomical considerations in the aetiology of fronto-ethmoidal mucoceles. Rhinology 25:83–88, 1987.
Schaefer SD, Anderson RG, Carder HM: Epidural mucopyocele: Diagnosis and management. Otolaryngol Head Neck Surg 89:523–527, 1981.

Stankiewicz JA: The endoscopic approach to the sphenoid sinus. Laryngoscope *99*:218–221, 1989.

Weinstein GS, Biglan AW, Patterson JH: Congenital lacrimal sac mucoceles. Am J Ophthalmol *94*: 106–110, 1982.

NEURILEMOMA 215.9
(Neurinoma, Schwannoma)

NORMAN S. LEVY, M.D., Ph.D., F.A.C.S.

Gainesville, Florida

Neurilemoma is a slow-growing encapsulated neoplasm arising from the Schwann cells of nerves. Some are malignant. These tumors have been found diffusely throughout the body in both the sensory and motor nerves, but their frequency in sensory nerves is several hundredfold greater than in motor nerves. Neurilemomas have been documented as arising from each of the nerves within and around the eye. They have been reported within the uveal tissues and sclera. They account for 2 per cent of orbital tumors.

Involvement of any branch of the trigeminal nerve is the most common periocular presentation. Retro-orbital headaches, facial numbness, progressive proptosis, lid swelling, intermittent pain, numbness or paresthesias in the distribution of the appropriate sensory nerve branch, or atypical trigeminal neuralgia have been described as initial signs. The presenting findings in neurilemomas of the third, fourth, and sixth cranial nerves include diplopia or blurring of vision. The proximity of the optic nerve to the expanding tumor within the orbit has occasionally resulted in loss of vision.

CT scanning of the suspected tumor can be extremely helpful in characterizing its size and extent. Magnetic resonance imaging (MRI) has high sensitivity in defining the nature and invasiveness of the tumor. In vivo differential diagnosis of the tumor type may be achieved with localized H-1 magnetic resonance spectroscopy. Positron-emitting tracers (PET) have been used to image malignant schwannomas, but their clinical utility is still under evaluation. Orbital and ocular echography can also be helpful, characteristically showing a sharply outlined capsule, well-defined central cystic space, slight compressibility, and blood flow.

THERAPY

Surgical. The tumor must be anatomically defined by appropriate radiographic studies. Preoperatively, fine-needle aspiration may be diagnostically helpful through immunocytochemical and electron microscopic evaluation of the specimen. Dissection of the tumor from the adjacent tissues is facilitated by careful preoperative planning based upon the above studies and intraoperative microscopic surgical control. Complete surgical excision is the therapy of choice. Tumors are not highly vascular so that bleeding is rarely a problem. Occasionally, the extent and location of the tumor prevent complete excision or cause damage to the nerve and adjacent tissues. In such cases, incomplete excision may be required. If growth continues, repeated excision, radiation, or chemotherapy are indicated.

Irradiation. When histologic examination of the tissue confirms malignancy or radiographic recurrence has been documented, focal application of up to 6000 rads of 10 MeV photons may be employed for local treatment.

Systemic. Intravenous combination chemotherapy consisting of 2 mg of vincristine,[‡] 100 mg of doxorubicin,[‡] 1 gm of cyclophosphamide,[‡] and 500 mg of dacarbazine[‡] has been employed. This therapy should be undertaken over a 5-day intensive course, followed by the weekly administration of vincristine. Dactinomycin has also been employed. Recurrent courses may be required based upon clinical response to therapy. Such chemotherapy should only be undertaken by a physician trained in these procedures.

Ocular or Periocular Manifestations

Conjunctiva: Localized swelling or mass.
Cornea: Discrete mass.
Extraocular Muscles: Diplopia or blurring.
Eyelids: Horner's syndrome; localized mass; ptosis.
Globe: Proptosis.
Sclera: Discrete mass.
Uvea: Discrete mass.
Other: Visual loss.

PRECAUTIONS

Accurate diagnosis of the tumor is only achieved histologically, although radiographic studies can be suggestive. The histologic evaluation must be done by a pathologist who is extremely familiar with this type of tumor. Studies indicate that the morphology and histology of the collagen of such tumors can be useful in their differentiation. Electron microscopy is often useful when standard histologic techniques are not definitive. Human glia-specific proteins, S100 and GFA, have been useful in characterizing the malignancy of these tumors.

The importance of a surgically aggressive approach to patients with malignant neurilemomas cannot be overemphasized. The 5-year survival in one study was 48 per cent. Even tumors initially classified as low grade histologically often eventually metastasize and cause death. Prognosis of any lesion is dependent upon its location, size, the adequacy of excision, and the malignant potential of that particular neurilemoma.

COMMENTS

The increased incidence of malignant neurilemomas in sites of prior irradiation and in patients with von Recklinghausen's disease must be recognized. Melanotic neurilemoma of the orbit has been reported and can grossly mimic a malignant melanoma.

References

Bickler-Bluth ME, Custer PL, Smith ME: Neurilemoma as a presenting feature of neurofibromatosis. Arch Ophthalmol 106:665–667, 1988.

Bojen-Miller M, Myhre-Jensen D: A consecutive series of 30 malignant schwannomas. Survival in relation to clinico-pathological parameters and treatment. Acta Pathol Microbiol Immunol Scand 92:147–155, 1984.

Bruhn H, Frahm J, Gyngell ML, et al: Noninvasive differentiation of tumors with use of localized H-1 MR spectroscopy in vivo: Initial experience in patients with cerebral tumors. Radiology 172:541–548, 1989.

Byrne BM, van Heuven WAJ, Lawton AW: Echographic characteristics of benign orbital schwannomas (neurilemomas). Am J Ophthalmol 106:194–198, 1988.

Capps DH, Brodsky MC, Rice CD, et al: Orbital intramuscular schwannoma. Am J Ophthalmol 110:535–539, 1990.

Jacque CM, et al: GFA and S100 protein levels as an index for malignancy in human gliomas and neurinomas. J Natl Cancer Inst 62:479–483, 1979.

Leone CR Jr, Wissinger JP: Surgical approaches to diseases of the orbital apex. Ophthalmology 95:391–397, 1988.

Leskinen-Kallio S, Huovinen R, Nagren K, et al: 11C Methionine quantitation in cancer PET studies. J Comput Assist Tomogr 16:468–474, 1992.

Mafee MF, Putterman A, Valvassori GE, et al: Orbital space-occupying lesions: Role of computed tomography and magnetic resonance imaging. An analysis of 145 cases. Radiol Clin North Am 25:529–559, 1987.

Ron E, Modan B, Boice JD, et al: Tumors of the brain and nervous system after radiotherapy in childhood. N Engl J Med 319:1033–1039, 1988.

Rose GE, Wright JE: Isolated peripheral nerve sheath tumours of the orbit. Eye 5:668–673, 1991.

Smith PA, Damato BE, Ko MK, et al: Anterior uveal neurilemoma; a rare neoplasm simulating malignant melanoma. Br J Ophthalmol 71:34–40, 1987.

Zbieranowski I, Bedard YC: Fine needle aspiration of schwannomas—Value of electron microscopy and immunocytochemistry in the preoperative diagnosis. Acta Cyto 33:381–384, 1989.

OPTIC GLIOMAS 225.1

BRIAN R. YOUNGE, M.D.

Rochester, Minnesota

Optic gliomas are intrinsic tumors of the optic nerve, chiasm, or tract that may involve any or all of these structures and extend beyond into the hypothalamus and ventricles. They are generally low-grade astrocytomas, usually are apparent within the first two decades of life, and grow slowly, permitting survival for many years. There are, however, many exceptions, and these have stirred controversy for nearly 100 years, both in terms of their nature and the best treatment. Clearly, the patient with a unilateral tumor of a single optic nerve has the best chance of survival with surgical resection. Conversely, an untreated glioma of either the nerve or chiasm has a much poorer prognosis, but again survival can be long.

There remain several questions today about the nature and management of these tumors. Are these tumors hamartomas and do they grow along the optic pathways? What is the natural history of these tumors? What is the best means of monitoring patients—computed tomography (CT) or magnetic resonance imaging (MRI). What treatment is best in unilateral cases—radiation or surgery? Does radiation help in chiasmal cases? Finally, does chemotherapy help? These and other questions will probably continue to haunt the clinician for years because each new case is unique and likely to be unpredictable.

There is no way to conduct a randomized treatment protocol for this disease because there are so few cases and very long follow-up is needed, in the order of 20 years or more. Nonetheless, some basic facts can be ascertained from the literature, from which the author has drawn, as well as from his fairly extensive experience at the Mayo Clinic. It is convenient to divide the location of these tumors into two main groups: (1) unilateral optic nerve and (2) all the others, which will be called chiasmal gliomas, with the realization that there may be multiple sites and extensive involvement of neighboring structures.

Optic Nerve Gliomas

These tumors present most often within the first few years of life with unilateral proptosis. The proptosis often has been present for some time, ranging from a month to a year. There is little evidence of visual loss until later in the evolution of the tumor, not only because of the child's age but also because vision persists at fairly good levels for a long time. Strabismus may ensue, but more often the globe is axially displaced forward in the orbit without other deviation until later. Retropulsion of the globe is met with resistance, but the tumor itself is usually not palpable externally. Motility is often good, becoming limited with the further protrusion. Often there is a relative afferent pupil defect, and if testable, color vision is mildly reduced (as with the Ishihara plates). The optic nerve head may be moderately pale, with some evidence of swelling, and occasionally there are shunt vessels similar to those typical of optic nerve meningioma. Choroidal folds are not typical, despite the obvious displacement of the eye forward. Foreshortening of the globe may induce hyperopia.

Chiasmal Gliomas

In contrast to unilateral optic nerve gliomas, chiasmal gliomas present at a later age, and visual loss is the key symptom. Because of the obscure and slowly progressive nature of the visual loss, it is often several months to a year or more before the diagnosis is established. Behavioral changes, seizures, headaches, or even a fortuitous detection of pale optic nerve heads during routine examination of the fundi may be the first clue to the abnormality. Optic atrophy is often pronounced by the time the symptoms become manifest, and it is not accompanied by disk swelling. Field defects, when plottable, are of the chiasmal type, but are rarely of a classic nature. Symptoms of obstructive hydrocephalus may ensue if the tumor involves the hypothalamus and third ventricle. Other developmental delays may result from involvement of contiguous hypothalamic structures.

The multicentric origin of these tumors is suggested by the rare occurrence of bilateral optic nerve tumors and of tumors of the orbit and chiasm together. That one is the extension of another is a more likely explanation, even to the nerve of the other side. The optic tract may be involved primarily, as may the optic radiations by extension. Recent studies of patients with type I neurofibromatosis have offered some evidence that other tumors may be more common elsewhere in the brain, along with optic gliomas; yet, it should be emphasized that acoustic neuroma and optic glioma do not coexist because they are manifestations of two different types of neurofibromatosis (Riccardi, 1987).

It is of value to inspect the skin for patches of brownish pigmentation (café-au-lait spots) and to examine the pupil for pigmented nodules (Lisch nodules) because many affected children have neurofibromatosis. Other skin manifestations of this disorder include cutaneous tumors, subcutaneous neurofibromas, plexiform neuromas, and axillary freckling, which is quite characteristic.

Radiologic Features. Even before the advent of modern CT and MR scanning, there were sophisticated means of examining the area of the optic canal and chiasmal region. Plain skull films and optic canal views were the simplest means of study, and they showed an abnormality in more than half of the patients studied. Hypocycloidal axial polytomography of the optic canals became a most sensitive means for detecting minor bony changes along the canals and into the chiasmal region. When CT became available, these tumors suddenly became visible to the neuroradiologist, and a wholly new era of diag-

nostic imaging changed our approach to these tumors, along with our ability to find other lesions, characterize changes over time, and tailor therapy to individual cases. MRI has added the latest dimension to studying these tumors and has suggested other abnormal findings not seen on CT. The role of gadolinium-enhanced MRI has not yet been determined. Positron emission tomography also promises to be helpful for delineating newer aspects of these lesions, but it may have limited application because of cost factors.

THERAPY

Surgical. Unilateral optic nerve gliomas are best treated by complete excision. However, if there is useful vision, not much proptosis, no evidence of extension into the intracranial area, and an opportunity for adequate follow-up of the patient, a period of careful observation may be indicated. In contrast, the child with unilateral proptosis whose vision is compromised and who has a tumor of the optic nerve should have complete excision of the tumor. Although many approaches to the tumor have been advocated, it is important to obtain free margins of optic nerve behind the tumor. In many cases doing so requires unroofing of the optic canal and excision of the nerve just anterior to the chiasm. In a few cases in which orbitotomy has been the primary approach, incomplete excision has resulted, and recurrence intracranially has ensued. In only one case has "pathologically proven" complete excision resulted in death, whereas incompletely excised tumors have sometimes recurred and been the cause of death.

Bilateral tumors of each optic nerve invariably involve the optic chiasm and may extend into the tract as well. These and frank chiasmal gliomas are not amenable to complete excision, and surgery is palliative for relief of obstructive hydrocephalus and tumor compression of nearby vital structures.

Irradiation. Radiation therapy has proved in many cases to be of value, even to the point of improving vision and fields, at least for a time. Because of the slow growth of these tumors, long survival is possible even in the absence of any treatment; most experts agree that radiation does prolong useful vision and life in chiasmal glioma. No useful data link any form of chemotherapy to improvement of either visual function or prognosis for life.

References

Alvord EC Jr, Lofton S: Gliomas of the optic nerve or chiasm: Outcome by patients' age, tumor site, and treatment. J Neurosurg 68:85–98, 1988
Glaser JS, Hoyt WF, Corbett J: Visual morbidity with chiasmal glioma: Long-term studies of visual fields in untreated and irradiated cases. Arch Ophthalmol 85:3–12, 1971.
Hoyt WF, Baghdassarian SA: Optic glioma of child-

hood: Natural history and rationale for conservative management. Br J Ophthalmol 53:793–798, 1969.

Lloyd LA: Gliomas of the optic nerve and chiasm in childhood. Trans Am Ophthalmol Soc 71:488–535, 1973.

Miller NR, Iliff WJ, Green WR: Evaluation and management of gliomas of the anterior visual pathways. Brain 97:743–754, 1974.

Packer RJ, Savino PJ, Bilaniuk LT, Zimmerman RA, Schatz NJ, Rosenstock JG, Nelson DS, Jarrett PD, Bruce DA, Schut L: Chiasmatic gliomas of childhood: A reappraisal of natural history and effectiveness of cranial irradiation. Childs Brain 10: 393–403, 1983.

Riccardi VM: Neurofibromatosis. In Gomez MR (ed): Neurocutaneous Diseases: A Practical Approach. Boston, Butterworths, 1987, pp 11–29.

Rush JA, Younge BR, Campbell RJ, MacCarty CS: Optic glioma: Long-term follow-up of 85 histopathologically verified cases. Ophthalmology 89: 1213–1219, 1982.

Wilson WB, Feinsod M, Hoyt WF, Nielsen SL: Malignant evolution of childhood chiasmal pilocytic astrocytoma. Neurology 26:322–325, 1976.

Wilson WB, Lloyd LA, Buncic JR, Younge BR, Grimson BS, Shults WT, Lubow M, Slamovits TL, Wirtschafter JD, Kupersmith M, Lessell S: Tumor spread in unilateral optic glioma—I. Neuro-Ophthalmology 7:179–184, 1987.

Wilson WB, Lloyd LA, Buncic JR, Younge BR, Grimson BS, Shults WT, Lubow M, Slamovits TL, Wirtschafter JD, Kupersmith M, Lessell S: Tumor spread in unilateral optic glioma—II. Neuro-Ophthalmology 89(2):195–203, 1992.

PAPILLOMA 078.1
(Verruca, Wart)

FRED M. WILSON II, M.D.

Indianapolis, Indiana

A papilloma is a cutaneous or mucosal tumor that consists of a cluster of finger-like projections of proliferating epithelial and fibrovascular tissues. Each projection is composed of hypertrophic (and sometimes hyperkeratotic) epithelium, subepithelial connective tissue stroma, and a central vascular core. A papilloma is recognized clinically by its mulberry-like or cauliflower-like appearance on the cutaneous or mucosal surface. Mucosal papillomas may be sufficiently translucent that their frond-like vascular cores are visible.

Papillomas may be of viral etiology, caused by the human papilloma (wart) virus, or of a noninfectious etiology, representing primary squamous neoplasia (conjunctival or corneal intraepithelial neoplasia; CIN). Papillomas of viral origin include verrucae (common cutaneous warts), condylomata acuminata (anogenital warts), and laryngeal papillomas. Noninfectious papillomas include all cutaneous and mucosal squamous neoplasms, whether benign or malignant, that happen to have papillomatous configurations.

Papillomas can be encountered on the eyelids, conjunctiva, cornea, or mucosa of the lacrimal system. Common infectious warts occur most commonly on the palpebral conjunctiva and the eyelids. Viral papillomas are usually asymptomatic, but low-grade chronic papillary conjunctivitis or punctate epithelial keratitis may result. Noninfectious papillomas may involve the eyelids, bulbar conjunctiva, limbus, or cornea. They are usually encountered in older adults and are not multiple or associated with cutaneous warts. They may be benign, premalignant, or malignant. Papillomas of the lacrimal mucosa, whether viral or noninfectious, can cause bleeding from the puncta.

THERAPY

Supportive. Conservative treatment is advised for viral papillomas because they are likely to disappear spontaneously, usually within a period of 2 years or less. Every effort should be made to await these spontaneous cures because the attempted excision or ablation of a single lesion may result in the subsequent appearance of several lesions.

The successes of "wart charmers" have been touted for generations. Whether these successes relate only to coincidental spontaneous regressions or to some obscure psychogenic effect on the body's immune system is unclear. In any case, warts (viral papillomas) may disappear after such apparently worthless efforts as the reciting of chants or the performance of rituals.

Surgical. Excisional biopsy is currently the mainstay of treatment for noninfectious papillomas. Excisional biopsy of either kind of papilloma provides a histopathologic diagnosis and a good chance for elimination of the lesion, although recurrences are possible. Excision should be sufficiently wide as to include some normal tissue. A viral papilloma should not be removed by cutting across its stalk; the head of the lesion, the stalk, and some normal tissue surrounding the base of the stalk should be excised.

Cryotherapy is useful as an adjunct to excision of viral papillomas. However, when cryotherapy is used as the sole method of treatment, there is always the danger that incomplete destruction of virus or proliferating cells will result in recurrence. Cryotherapy with a cryoprobe or cryospray following excisional biopsy is probably of value for reducing the likelihood of recurrence. A viral papilloma of the eyelid or conjunctiva may be treated with application of a cryoprobe at −70° to −100°C for 30 to 60 seconds. The lesion can be expected to disappear in 10 to 30 days if cryoablation has been successful. Despite extensive dermatologic experience with liquid nitrogen spray in the treatment of cutaneous papillomas, it probably should be regarded only as an experimental method for treating viral papillomas of the conjunctiva. Cryotherapy for *noninfectious* papillomas of the eyelid or eye must presently be considered to be only in the experimental stages of development, but it may very well reduce the probability of recurrence when it is used immediately after surgical excision.

After excision of either a viral or noninfectious papilloma, the remaining cut edges of conjunctiva and the tissues underlying the site of the tumor (sclera, limbus, cornea, or tarsus) may be treated with contiguous or slightly overlapping, superficial, 1- to 2-second applications of a cryoprobe. A double freeze-thaw technique (two consecutive applications of the cryotherapy) might be more efficacious than a single treatment.

Electrodesiccation is essentially equal in efficacy to cryotherapy. It is used mainly for the treatment of verrucae of the eyelids, although it could be used cautiously for treating viral papillomas of the conjunctiva. After local anesthesia, the electric needle is inserted into the lesion and kept in place until the tissue begins to bubble. The wart is then curetted away. Care must be taken to minimize scarring by not inserting the needle too deeply. As is the case with cryotherapy, electrodesiccation can be followed by recurrence. Electrodesiccation should not be used for noninfectious papillomas.

Although not widely available to ophthalmologists, the carbon dioxide (CO_2) laser seems to be very effective for treating viral papillomas of the eye and other sites, with or without surgical excision and cryotherapy, even when all other current methods of treatment have been unsuccessful. The emission wavelength of the laser corresponds to the absorption band of water, so water-containing tissue can be vaporized rapidly, as well as carbonized and coagulated. The causative virus seems also to be readily destroyed, thus helping greatly to protect against recurrence. Low energy levels and short exposure times are advised for treating ocular lesions, e.g., 5 watts of energy for 0.2 seconds in a spot size of 2 mm.

Irradiation. Radiotherapy is rarely, if ever, indicated as primary treatment for viral papillomas. It might possibly be considered when there is extensive involvement of the eyelid or conjunctiva or when there have been multiple recurrences after surgery. Even in these trying circumstances, however, consideration should probably be given first to CO_2 laser therapy, cryotherapy, or immunotherapy.

However, beta irradiation can be used rather safely in difficult cases as an adjunct to surgical excision. After excision of a wart of the eyelid, 1000 to 2500 rads of beta radiation may be applied in the hope of reducing the likelihood of recurrence. A dosage of 1000 to 2000 rads may be used after excision of a viral papilloma of the conjunctiva. Especially recalcitrant viral papillomas of the eyelids or conjunctiva may be treated with a combination of excision, cryotherapy, and beta irradiation. Beta rays may also be used after excision of a neoplastic papilloma of the eyelid or conjunctiva, but they should not be relied upon as a primary means of therapy.

Topical. Immunotherapy is a promising, but still experimental method of therapy. Dinitrochlorobenzene[†] has been used successfully to eradicate multiple and recurrent papillomatous squamous tumors of the conjunctiva and lacrimal mucosa that had previously resisted all conventional forms of therapy. It was unclear whether these lesions were infectious or noninfectious papillomas. By applying dinitrochlorobenzene repeatedly to the skin, the patient is made sensitive ("allergic") to this agent, which is a potent contact sensitizer. The chemical is then given topically to the ocular tumor, whereupon a type IV (thymus-derived, lymphocyte-mediated) hypersensitivity reaction occurs and destroys the tumors. This type of treatment causes considerable inflammation of the ocular surface.

Ocular or Periocular Manifestations

Conjunctiva: Follicular or papillary conjunctivitis; hemorrhages; hyperemia keratinization; papilloma (noninfectious, viral); pseudopterygium.

Cornea: Infiltration; keratinization; opacity; papilloma (noninfectious); pseudopterygium; punctate epithelial keratitis; vascularization.

Eyelids: Hemorrhages; papilloma (noninfectious; viral); ulcer.

Lacrimal System: Hemorrhages; obstruction; papilloma (noninfectious, viral).

PRECAUTIONS

Papillomas are fundamentally epithelial lesions; subepithelial fibrovascular proliferation probably occurs only because the proliferating epithelium requires a vascular supply. To minimize the chance of recurrence, it is necessary only to remove the epithelial component of the lesion. It is quite permissible for the surgical plane in the conjunctiva to extend down to the level of Tenon's capsule or even to sclera because these tissues heal rapidly with relatively little scarring and it is difficult to remove only the epithelial layer of the conjunctiva. However, surgical planes in the eyelid or cornea should be superficial so as to avoid unnecessary scarring and loss of tissue. Corneal papillomas, in fact, should merely be scraped gently from the corneal surface, leaving Bowman's layer intact except in the rare instance in which a frankly carcinomatous papilloma has invaded the deeper layers.

Care must be taken when using cryotherapy not to freeze too deeply. It is mainly the epithelial layer of the conjunctiva that should be frozen, although no harm is done by allowing the freeze to enter Tenon's layer. Overzealous freezing of sclera, however, can occasionally cause scleral thinning. Inadvertent freezing of the ciliary body and processes can cause uveitis and hypotony. Freezing of the corneal endothelium can cause endothelial dysfunction and corneal edema. Excessive freezing of the eyelid may cause necrosis, scarring, notching, and trichiasis.

Intact human papilloma virus DNA can be liberated into the air during CO_2 laser treatment. Practitioners should realize that the liberated smoke and vapor might be infectious and should take precautions to avoid being infected themselves by these emissions by using gloves, masks, goggles, and proper suctioning apparatus.

COMMENTS

Viral papillomas tend to occur mainly in children and young adults and are transmissible by direct or indirect contact and auto-inoculation. These lesions may be multiple and are self-limited. They undergo malignant transformation very rarely, if ever. Whether, after apparent resolution, these lesions might years later lead to squamous dysplasia or carcinoma is unknown, but the DNA of human papilloma virus types 6, 11, 16, 18, 31, 33, 35, and 51 has been found both in papillomas and squamous neoplasms of the genital tract. Types 6, 11, and 13 have been associated with mild or moderate dysplasia in the cervix, vulva, penis, and anus, whereas types 16, 18, 31, 33, 35, and 51 have been associated with severe dysplasia and with in situ and invasive carcinoma. The time between infection and malignant transformation seems to be about 30 years. Altogether, more than 50 distinct types of human papilloma virus have been differentiated by DNA molecular hybridization techniques. Types 6 and 11, both of which

seem to be able to cause dysplasia in the genital tract, have so far been found in conjunctival and lacrimal sac papillomas.

Noninfectious papillomas have a predilection for older individuals and are neither transmissible nor multiple. They are not self-limited and frequently undergo malignant transformation. Such lesions (CIN) have sometimes revealed DNA of papilloma virus types 16 and 18.

Common cutaneous warts are usually caused by type 2 virus.

References

Dunlap EA (ed): Gordon's Medical Management of Ocular Disease, 2nd ed. Hagerstown, MD, Harper & Row, 1976, pp 126, 165–166.
Ferry AP, Meltzer MA, Taub RN: Immunotherapy with dinitrochlorbenzene (DNCB) for recurrent squamous cell tumor of conjunctiva. Trans Am Ophthalmol Soc 74:154–171, 1977.
Gal AA, Meyer PR, Taylor CR: Papillomavirus antigens in anorectal condyloma and carcinoma in homosexual men. JAMA 257:337–340, 1987.
Garden JM, et al: Papillomavirus in the vapor of carbon dioxide laser-treated verrucae. JAMA 259:1199–1202, 1988.
Holmes KK: Infectious diseases. JAMA 254:2254–2257, 1985.
Jackson WB, Beraja R, Codere F: Laser therapy of conjunctival papillomas. Can J Ophthalmol 22:45–47, 1987.
Nelson JH Jr, Averette HE, Richart RM: Dysplasia, carcinoma in situ, and early invasive cervical carcinoma. Ca-A Cancer J Clinicians 34:306–327, 1984.
Pearce WB, et al: Conjunctival papillomas in northern Canadian natives. Can Med J 112:1423–1426, 1975.
Reese AB: Tumors of the Eye, 3rd ed. Hagerstown, MD, Harper & Row, 1976, pp 54–56.
Schachat A, Iliff WJ, Kashima HK: Carbon dioxide laser therapy of recurrent squamous papilloma of the conjunctiva. Ophthalmic Surg 13:916–918, 1982.

Malignant

BASAL CELL CARCINOMA 173.1

JOHN L. WOBIG, M.D.

Portland, Oregon

Basal cell carcinoma is the most common malignant neoplasm of the eyelids. The lesion is locally infiltrative and only rarely metastasizes. Basal cell carcinoma may be classified as nodular, ulcerative, syringoid, adenoid, basosquamous, multicentric, recurrent, morpheaform, or sclerosing. Nodular basal cell

carcinomas are generally easy to treat, whereas sclerosing and morpheaform basal cell carcinomas are difficult to cure.

Clinically, approximately 90 per cent of the malignant neoplasms of the eyelid are basal cell carcinomas. The lesion is primarily found in the lower lid and medial canthus, with less frequent occurrence in the lateral canthus and upper lid. Variation is typical in the clinical course of a basal cell carcinoma. Initially, the lesion is usually a discrete nodule with or without ulceration and distinct margins. Eventually, the central area becomes ulcerated with rolled waxy borders.

Histologically, the tumor is composed of solid masses of uniform cells with basophilic nuclei and scanty cytoplasm. Palisading of the peripheral cells of tumor lobules is characteristic. Squamoid differentiation can be present in basal cell carcinomas.

THERAPY

Irradiation. Irradiation should be used with caution in the medial canthus, since permanent scarring of the canalicular system can result. If irradiation is used, silicone intubation should be placed in the lacrimal excretory system before any such therapy. Radiotherapy is effective only in the early stages of basal cell carcinoma; however, it makes surgical repair more difficult in the reconstructive phase.

Surgical. Mohs' fresh tissue, microscopically controlled surgery gives the highest success rate for cure. The tumor removal can be done as an outpatient under local anesthesia with surgical reconstruction following. The excised tumor mass is based on clinical margins. The base and sides remaining are cut into 2-mm strips and divided into portions that are placed on a glass slide. All edges are marked with different colored dyes. Frozen sections are made, and residual tumor is marked on a map. Residual tumor is then resected until the lesion is tumor-free, proven microscopically.

Electrodesiccation and curettage are occasionally used for removal of basal cell carcinomas. All the tumor is curetted away, and the base and sides are electrodesiccated. Since only the medial canthus tends to heal by granulation without significant scarring, this method is not used for most eyelid lesions.

Cryosurgery for the management of basal cell carcinomas of the eyelids has had increasing use, probably more so in dermatology than in ophthalmology. Both in cure rates and cosmetic results, carefully performed cryosurgery by an experienced physician is probably equally effective compared to other modalities, especially for lesions less than 1 cm in diameter. However, other forms of therapy should be considered for lesions larger than this size and for those without raised margins, which make it difficult to ascertain the extent of the edge of the tumor. After outlining 3 to 4 mm of normal tissue around the suspected tumor edge, equal parts of bupivacaine and lidocaine are injected around the involved area. The edge of the tumor can be seen best under a slit lamp by pulling on the skin adjacent to the tumor. If any of the skin's stress lines are distorted, then the tumor probably involves that area. A thermocouple needle is placed within 1 to 2 mm inside of the black felt pen outline, and the tumor is frozen to −25° C. It is allowed to completely thaw to 30° C, and then this is repeated. Whenever the tumor is located near the eye, a bone plate should be inserted in the cul-de-sac to protect the globe.

PRECAUTIONS

It seems that larger lesions are best treated by Mohs' technique. Nodular lesions, which are small, can be controlled by almost any technique. Sclerosing lesions need careful monitoring because it is impossible to determine clinically the free margins.

Complications of cryosurgery and irradiation include the difficulty of late repair to tissue treated by those methods. Extreme care must be taken in the medial canthus to preserve the canalicular system. This may include silicone intubation prior to the above treatment. Pigmentary changes and loss of eyelashes with occasional tissue loss are also complications that must be considered.

The low cost of cryotherapy is certainly an advantage. However, it is important not to use cryotherapy without a thermocouple to monitor the tissue temperatures. The tissue does not need to be frozen beyond −25° C. Also, the freezing of lid tissue must be observed, since defense against infection of the lid is reduced in the initial healing period.

The reconstructive surgery must be well conceived because occasionally more tissue than anticipated is removed. The lid surgery repair may include rebuilding a total lid and canthus, and a physician experienced in this procedure should be available.

COMMENTS

Basal cell carcinoma is a malignant tumor that needs to be treated accordingly. Local infiltration in the periorbital region can extend to the globe, bone, and surrounding sinuses. The reconstruction of the lids and lacrimal apparatus is important in the functional as well as the cosmetic result. For recurrences, the best approach is Mohs' microscopically controlled excision. These patients should especially be examined for tumors of the skin and other regions, as well as for recurrence in the eyelids. Any lid lesion that does not heal should arouse suspicion of a tumor.

References

Domonkos AN: Treatment of eyelid carcinoma. Arch Dermatol 91:364–371, 1965.

Fraunfelder FT, et al: The role of cryosurgery in external ocular and periocular disease. Trans Am Acad Ophthalmol Otolaryngol 83:713–724, 1977.

Jones LT, Wobig JL: Surgery of the Eyelids and Lacrimal System. Birmingham, Aesculapius, 1976.

Older JJ, Quickert MH, Beard D: Surgical removal of basal cell carcinoma of the eyelids utilizing frozen section control. Trans Am Acad Ophthalmol Otolaryngol 79:658–663, 1975.

Payne JW, et al: Basal cell carcinoma of the eyelids. A long-term follow-up study. Arch Ophthalmol 81:553–558, 1969.

CONJUNCTIVAL OR CORNEAL INTRAEPITHELIAL NEOPLASIA (CIN) AND SQUAMOUS CELL CARCINOMA 234.
(Invasive Neoplasm)

F. T. FRAUNFELDER, M.D.

Portland, Oregon

Conjunctival or corneal intraepithelial neoplasms are not uncommon tumors that include all dysplastic lesions of the conjunctival and corneal epithelium, regardless of their severity. Clinical and laboratory investigations have led to a simple classification of the intraepithelial process, ranging from mild dysplasia (partial-thickness intraepithelial neoplasia) to severe dysplasia (full-thickness intraepithelial neoplasia). If the dysplastic process breaks through the basement membrane, the end stage of this process is invasive neoplasia or squamous cell carcinoma. This terminology replaces such previously used terms as Bowen's disease of the eye, carcinoma in situ (CIS), intraepithelial epithelioma, intraepithelioma, and intraepithelial dysplasia.

Conjunctival or corneal intraepithelial neoplasia (CIN) has a distinctive clinical course, which is characterized by slow growth and a relatively low malignancy potential. The most common cell types comprising dysplastic processes of the conjunctiva and cornea are elongated spindle cells with a monotonous appearance and epidermoid cells; these atypical cells grow upward from an initial basal location. The clinical appearance of the lesions is that of an elevated, gelatinous, leukoplakic, or papilliform limbal mass. The lesions are almost always unilateral and generally unifocal; they are primarily located at the nasal or temporal limbus, although some may involve the cornea only or conjunctiva only. CIN more often affects males than females and is predominantly a disease of the sixth and seventh decades. Intraocular extension and metastatic disease may occur secondary to developing squamous cell carcinoma.

THERAPY

Surgical. Local surgical excision of CIN lesions combined with cryotherapy use a double-cycle freeze-thaw-refreeze technique has been found to yield the lowest recurrence rate. Since the margins of the tumor are indistinct because of the root-like subepithelial extension, lesions may not always stain with rose bengal; individual or multiple conjunctival scrapings with Papanicolaou stain can often aid in outlining the area to be excised. Topical ocular anesthetics, such as proparacaine or cocaine, are instilled, and the conjunctiva under and around the lesion is elevated with subconjunctival injection of 1 per cent lidocaine with epinephrine. The conjunctiva will elevate easily in cases not previously treated. If the conjunctiva does not elevate in eyes without prior treatment, the diagnosis of squamous cell carcinoma may be suspected. Multiple conjunctival cautery applications 1.5 to 2 mm from the suspected tumor margin are used to outline the area to be excised. An incision is then made through these marks down to bare sclera. The conjunctival and episcleral tissues are then surgically dissected to the limbus. In areas where the conjunctiva is adherent to the episcleral area, a superficial sclerectomy may be necessary. The area of corneal involvement must be outlined by retroillumination before surgery. Multiple applications of a local anesthetic are then used to soften the corneal epithelium. Using a No. 64 Beaver blade, 1 mm of normal epithelium and the involved corneal epithelium are removed by simply "bulldozing" the epithelium to the limbus. A superficial limbal keratectomy is not usually performed because a pannus may form postoperatively, although areas with prior surgical keratectomies or suspected tumor invasion may require a superficial keratectomy. Simple excision of the conjunctiva flush with the limbus is all that is required.

A Brymill CryAc unit with either a 2- or 4-mm liquid nitrogen cryoprobe tip is used to freeze the limbal area. The most important area in which to obtain adequate freezing is at the limbus, since this is the site of most recurrences. The end point of the freeze is a 1-second application that, on removal of the probe, causes a white circular imprint of the probe tip on the eye. Multiple overlapping imprints are done to cover the entire surgical limbus twice. If a scleral or limbal area of inadequate dissection is suspected, a triple freeze-thaw technique should be performed; however, an attempt should be made not to freeze more than 1 mm of peripheral clear cornea. No suturing is necessary. A topical antibiotic-corticosteroid preparation may be given three times daily for 3 days.

Other cryoprobes using other cryogens are satisfactory; however, the contact time is doubled. Remember, this is a very superficial dysplasia and requires only a very superficial freeze.

Squamous cell carcinoma is treated in the same manner, but more aggressive cryotherapy (triple freeze-thaw) with wider margins around the tumor and deeper sclerectomy and keratectomy are recommended. Deep invasion of the sclera and cornea requires full eye wall resection. Lamellar transplants are seldom used, since they cover the signs of an early recurrence. Small intraocular extension can be treated with iridocyclectomy, whereas larger intraocular extensions may require enucleation.

PRECAUTIONS

Although deep cryotherapy may result in severe iritis, posterior synechiae, and corneal scarring, the complications of superficial cryosurgery are minimal, even when the cornea is treated. To avoid adherence of the cryoprobe, it is of utmost importance to have the probe completely frozen before ocular application. If the probe is applied warm and then frozen, it will cause a tight ocular adherence that is not easily removed without a sterile liquid and may result in excessive freezing.

Squamous cell carcinoma of the conjunctiva with regional or distant metastasis may be life threatening if it is not treated. Biopsy of the excised tissue is essential, with special attention paid to the surgical margins and base of the tumor. Careful clinical follow-up examination after resection of such lesions is further recommended for the detection of early signs of recurrence.

COMMENTS

An obvious advantage of cryosurgery over other modalities for CIN is that "root tips" missed by surgery alone, especially at the limbus, can be treated. This procedure results in a higher cure rate and avoids grafting and symblepharon formation. To date, surgical excision combined with cryotherapy has almost tripled previous cure rates with surgery alone.

Despite the low virulence of CIN, it can be difficult to cure. CIN recurrence has been found to be dependent on the status of the surgical bed and margins and not on the clinical appearance, presence of invasion, degree of dysplasia, or cell types. However, not all incompletely excised lesions recur, and some may revert to normal. Recurrence most often develops in the first 2 years postoperatively; thus, close follow-up is suggested. The histopathologic features of recurrence may or may not show the same cell pattern.

The highest recurrence rates are in lesions involving over two-thirds of the limbus and in reoperations.

References

Campbell RJ, Bourne WM: Unilateral central corneal epithelial dysplasia. Ophthalmology 88: 1231–1238, 1981.
Divine RD, Anderson RL: Nitrous oxide cryotherapy for intraepithelial epithelioma of the conjunctiva. Arch Ophthalmol 101:782–786, 1983.
Dutton JJ, Anderson RL, Tse DT: Combined surgery and cryotherapy for scleral invasion of epithelial malignancies. Ophthalmic Surg 15:289–294, 1984.
Erie JC, Campbell RJ, Liesegang TJ: Conjunctival and corneal intraepithelial and invasive neoplasia. Ophthalmology 93:176–183, 1986.
Fraunfelder FT, Wingfield D: Management of intraepithelial conjunctival tumors and squamous cell carcinomas. Am J Ophthalmol 95:359–363, 1983.
Geggel HS, Friend J, Boruchoff SA: Corneal epithelial dysplasia. Ann Ophthalmol 17:27–31, 1985.
Tabbara KF, et al: Metastatic squamous cell carcinoma of the conjunctiva. Ophthalmology 95:318–321, 1988.
Waring GO III, Roth AM, Ekins MB: Clinical and pathologic description of 17 cases of corneal intraepithelial neoplasia. Am J Ophthalmol 97:547–559, 1984.

EWING'S SARCOMA 170

DAVID J. WILSON, M.D.

Portland, Oregon

Ewing's sarcoma, a small round-cell neoplasm, is a family of tumors of parasympathetic nerve origin with a spectrum of neural differentiation. It usually originates in bone, but may arise in soft tissues. The most commonly involved bony sites are the femur, pelvis, tibia, humerus, fibula, scapula, and ribs. The bones of the head and neck account for only 2 to 3 per cent of cases of Ewing's sarcoma.

Ewing's sarcoma generally presents in the first or second decade of life. Males are affected more commonly than females, and this tumor is rare in African Americans. The usual presenting symptoms are pain and swelling, or both. In the orbit, the presenting symptoms are proptosis, swelling of orbital tissues, or decreased vision. The orbit is much more likely to be involved in metastatic disease than as a primary site.

The diagnosis of Ewing's sarcoma is made by biopsy of affected tissues. Electron microscopy and immunohistochemistry are essential to differentiate this tumor from other similar-appearing tumors, including lymphoma, rhabdomyosarcoma, neuroblastoma, and primitive round-cell sarcoma of bone.

THERAPY

Proper treatment for Ewing's sarcoma requires multimodality therapy. Local treatment with radiation or surgery alone results in abysmal 5-year survival rates of approximately 10 per cent. Consequently, current approaches to treating Ewing's sarcoma combine chemotherapy regimens for systemic control with radiation therapy or surgery for local control.

Systemic. Combination chemotherapy regimens usually incorporate four drugs: vincristine, actinomycin-D, cyclophosphamide, and doxorubicus. Other chemotherapeutic agents, including ifosfamide and etoposide, are being investigated for use in Ewing's sarcoma.

Irradiation. Radiation therapy combined with multiple drug chemotherapy may afford the best chance for cure. Local radiotherapy of 4000 to 4500 rads to the entire diseased bone with a booster of 1500 rads to a small field of primary tumor is effective in controlling local disease. The suggested therapy for orbital Ewing's sarcoma is high-dose radiation therapy to orbital bone, delivered over a 5- to 6-week period.

Surgical. There are a number of settings in which surgery should be considered the primary local control modality: (1) small rib lesions that can be completely resected with a margin of normal tissue; (2) primary tumors in expendable bones (clavicle, body of the scapula, small confined lesions of the ileum, and proximal fibula); and (3) tumors of the weight-bearing bones in young children where radiation therapy would include one of the major growth sites.

Ocular or Periocular Manifestations

Globe: Exophthalmos; proptosis.
Optic Nerve: Edema.
Orbit: Soft tissue mass; exostosis.

PRECAUTIONS

Because of the poor prognosis and the tendency for the lesions to be multicentric, wide surgical excision is generally discouraged. Widespread metastases follow both aggressive surgery and irradiation, when used without adjunctive chemotherapy.

High-dose irradiation of an epiphyseal plate arrests bone growth and may produce ankylosis when administered to the full width of a joint. Therefore, careful irradiation technique is required to minimize bone and joint deformity and to avoid irradiation to the entire width of an extremity with the subsequent production of lymphatic obstruction. Prophylactic pulmonary irradiation is of doubtful value, since the disease metastasizes as frequently to other bones as to the lungs. Radiation therapy in combination with chemotherapy can cause lethal pulmonary fibrosis. Irradiation of large volumes of bone marrow should be avoided because it may compromise the value of chemotherapy.

COMMENTS

Surgery and radiotherapy seem to be equally effective for small lesions; however, a trend toward a better prognosis has been seen in surgically treated patients with large lesions. The failure rate is higher in patients undergoing irradiation alone. The majority of relapses occur within the first year of diagnosis, and recurrence after 3 years of disease-free interval is unlikely.

Disease-free survival rates have improved dramatically with aggressive combinations of radiation therapy and multiple chemotherapy with or without surgery. Although the cure rates for localized Ewing's sarcoma of a distal extremity are quite respectable, the prognosis for axial tumors remains poor. Among concepts being explored to improve these results are aggressive induction chemotherapy, irradiation to the bulky site of disease, and surgical resection of persistent pulmonary nodules.

References

Halperin EC: Pediatric radiation oncology. Invest Radiol 21:429–436, 1986.

Horowitz HE, Tsokos MG, DeLaney TF: Ewing's sarcoma. CA Cancer J Clin 42:300–320, 1992.

Jakobiec FA, Rootman J, Jones IS: Secondary and metastatic tumors of the orbit. *In* Duane TD (ED): Clinical Ophthalmology. Hagerstown, MD, Harper & Row, 1982, Vol II, pp 46:51–52.

Jurgens H, et al: Multidisciplinary treatment of primary Ewing's sarcoma of bone. A 6-year experience of a European Cooperative Trial. Cancer 61:23–32, 1988.

Rosen G: The current management of malignant bone tumors: Where do we go from here? Med J Aust 148:373–377, 1988.

Sauer R, et al: Prognostic factors in the treatment of Ewing's sarcoma. The Ewing's sarcoma study group of the German Society of Paediatric Oncology CESS 81. Radiother Oncol 10:101–110, 1987.

Woodruff G, Thorner P, Skarf B: Primary Ewing's sarcoma of the orbit presenting with visual loss. Br J Ophthalmol 72:786–792, 1988.

FIBROSARCOMA 171.9

F. HAMPTON ROY, M.D., F.A.C.S.

Little Rock, Arkansas

Fibrosarcoma is a malignant tumor that is most common in adults aged 30 to 70 years. Most tumors arise in the soft tissue of extremities, but some arise in the bone. Those that arise in the bone are more likely to involve the knee region and may be the delayed result of radiation exposure. The usual symptoms of fibrosarcoma include the presence of a mass with gradually progressive pain and variable swelling.

Primary fibrosarcoma of the orbit is unusual, but most often occurs secondary to invasion from nearby paranasal sinuses or adjacent bones. Another source of fibrosarcoma includes irradiation of sarcomas after extensive radiotherapy for prior malignancies of the eye or adnexa, which are most commonly retinoblastoma. The most common age of onset for primary orbital fibrosarcoma is 55 to 60 years, but 30 to 50 years would be the expected age of onset of a secondary orbital fibrosarcoma. When a mass is found in the soft tissue of the orbit or the area of the lacrimal sac, primary fibrosarcoma should be strongly considered. It can, however, occur on the eyelid, sclera, or conjunctiva.

THERAPY

Surgical. Complete excision is the only hope for survival. Total removal may be possible without the undue sacrifice of tissue in those rare cases where the tumor is located on or near the surface of the eyelid, eyeball, or in the area of the lacrimal sac. The complete removal of those growths primary in the orbital cavity is more difficult. In these situations, surgical manipulations affecting the integrity of ocular functions and the psychologic impact of visual loss on the patient are subtle barriers to adequate excision. In addition, some fibrosarcomas in this area are partially circumscribed, rather than grossly infiltrative. This feature provides an easier anatomic plane for surgical dissection and may lull the surgeon into the mistaken belief that the neoplasm has been completely removed. Nevertheless, the patient should still be advised to undergo an orbital exenteration. Most complex is the surgical eradication of the secondary fibrosarcomas from the maxilla, nasal cavity, or paranasal sinuses. These neoplasms are infiltrative. Widespread excision of affected soft tissues and bold sacrifice of underlying bone are recommended. Although the recurrence rate of these secondary tumors is high, repeated radical surgery may result in the rare survival of an affected patient. Surgical management of those fibrosarcomas induced by prior irradiation or of those located in the deeper recesses of the face and orbit adjacent to the intracranial foramina is almost hopeless. Chemotherapy and radiotherapy are ineffective, except as palliative or psychologically directed measures.

Ocular or Periocular Manifestations

Extraocular Muscles: Paralysis.
Eyelids: Fibrosarcoma.
Globe: Proptosis.
Lacrimal Sac: Fibrosarcoma.
Orbit: Edema; erosion of bony walls; fibrosarcoma; increased intraorbital pressure.
Sclera: Fibrosarcoma.

PRECAUTIONS

Once the diagnosis is established by incisional or excisional biopsy, the patient should be informed of the malignant nature of the neoplasm, and plans should be made for a more radical removal, such as maxillectomy or exenteration. The longer the duration of symptoms or the greater the interval before definitive surgery, the greater is the chance of a fatal outcome. When radical surgery is undertaken, it should be done in a facility with expertise in frozen-tissue examination to provide on-the-spot information of the extent of neoplastic cells in the periphery of the surgical specimen.

COMMENTS

Although orbital fibrosarcomas develop at a slower rate and the interval between recurrences is longer than in many other sarcomas, they should not be regarded as benign on the basis of this less aggressive behavior. Recurrences, metastases, or intracranial extensions of the neoplasm usually develop within 6 to 8 years from the time of definitive surgery, but it is unwise to consider a cure until 10 to 12 years have passed from the last operation.

The histologic diagnosis of fibrosarcoma is not as easy as once believed. The examiner should be aware of the capabilities of the malignant fibrocyte to merge with or develop into one of the other related tumors of supportive tissue, such as may arise from Schwann cells, histiocytes, lipoblasts, and rhabdomyoblasts. Also, care should be taken to differentiate these tumors from an aggressive type of tumor that is classified as a fibromatosis, rather than a sarcoma. When in doubt, electron microscopy of the tissue specimen may be helpful. With this medium, the true fibroblast has a highly developed, rough-surfaced endoplasmic reticulum, a prominent Golgi apparatus, poorly developed desmosomes, and no basement membrane formation.

References

Jakobiec FA: Ocular and Adnexal Tumors. Birmingham, Aesculapius, 1978.
Jones LT, Wobig JL: Surgery of the Eyelids and Lacrimal System. Birmingham, Aesculapius, 1976.
Scott SM, et al: Soft tissue fibrosarcoma. A clinicopathologic study of 132 cases. Cancer *64*:925–931, 1989.

HODGKIN'S DISEASE 201.9

GLENN J. LESSER, M.D.,
STUART A. GROSSMAN, M.D.,
and NEIL R. MILLER, M.D.

Baltimore, Maryland

Hodgkin's disease is a malignant lymphoma of unknown cause that generally arises in the lymph nodes. Involved tissues are characterized by the presence of the pathognomonic, malignant, Reed-Sternberg cell. The clinical course of this disease is quite variable. It may present with relatively localized infiltration of cervical, supraclavicular, or mediastinal lymph nodes, or multiple contiguous lymph node areas may be affected by disease. Extension beyond the lymph nodes to the lung, liver, spleen, bones, bone marrow, orbit, and brain may also occur. Patients with early-stage Hodgkin's disease are often asymptomatic, whereas systemic or "B" symptoms, including fever, night sweats, and weight loss, are frequently present in advanced-stage disease.

The ocular manifestations of Hodgkin's disease may result from damage to the eye, orbit, or intracranial visual sensory and ocular motor systems by the neoplasm or its treatment. Infiltration of orbital and intracranial structures is exceedingly rare and usually occurs in patients who have already developed systemic relapse of their disease. However, in rare instances a discrete orbital or subconjunctival mass may be the initial manifestation of the disease. Also, infiltration or compression of the optic nerves or chiasm can occur. Central and peripheral nervous system damage in Hodgkin's disease may result in papilledema from increased intracranial pressure, optic neuropathy, optic atrophy, visual field defects, cortical blindness, and ocular motor nerve paresis. Horner's syndrome can occur when the cervical lymph nodes are affected. Motor, sensory, and autonomic peripheral neuropathies may occur in patients with Hodgkin's disease. They are usually caused by infiltration of peripheral nerves by the tumor. In extremely rare cases, central nervous system dysfunction will include a generalized encephalopathy and cerebellar degeneration as a result of a paraneoplastic syndrome. In general, damage to the central nervous system in Hodgkin's disease occurs late in the course of the disorder, but cases of primary intracranial Hodgkin's disease occasionally occur.

THERAPY

Irradiation. Radiation therapy with megavoltage equipment is a major form of treatment for early-stage (local) Hodgkin's disease. Radiation therapy is usually delivered to affected nodes, to adjacent draining nodal groups, and to areas of potential contiguous nodal involvement. Appropriate shielding of surrounding organs and tissues is essential. Doses of 4000 to 4500 cGy are usually required to eradicate permanently any site of infiltration. As carefully planned radiation therapy has the potential to cure this neoplasm, it should be administered at centers that have substantial experience in treating Hodgkin's disease.

Systemic. Combination chemotherapy is the treatment of choice for advanced-stage Hodgkin's disease. The introduction of combination chemotherapy with MOPP (mechlorethamine, vincristine (Oncovin), procarbazine, prednisone) in 1964 was a breakthrough in the therapy of Hodgkin's disease. Complete remission rates of 70 to 90 per cent have been described with MOPP and similar combination chemotherapy regimens. A cure can be expected in over 65 to 75 per cent of patients with advanced disease. Further improvements in survival are expected with chemotherapy in patients with less advanced disease, with combined radiation and chemotherapy in patients with bulky disease, with alternating non-cross-resistant chemotherapy regimens, with and aggressive salvage protocols including bone marrow transplantation.

Ocular or Periocular Manifestations

Anterior Chamber: Uveitis.
Choroid: Infiltration.
Conjunctiva: Infiltration.
Cornea: Keratitis.
Extraocular Muscle: Lymphomatous infiltration; Graves' disease.
Iris: Posterior synechiae.
Lacrimal Gland: Infiltration.
Lens: Cataract.
Lid: Infiltration; ptosis.
Optic Nerve: Infiltration; paraneoplastic optic neuropathy; papilledema.
Orbit: Infiltration; tumor mass; exophthalmos.
Retina: Exudates; hemorrhages; ischemia; perivascular sheathing; vasculitis; serous macular detachment.
Sclera: Episcleritis.
Other: Cortical blindness; Horner's syndrome; ocular motor nerve paresis; visual field defects; opportunistic infections; Vogt-Koyanagi-Harada syndrome; Sjögren's syndrome.

PRECAUTIONS

Considerable experience is required to deliver antineoplastic agents properly and safely because of their effects on normal hematopoiesis, the immune system, the gastrointestinal tract, and the cardiorespiratory system. Patients vary greatly in their tolerance to antineoplastic agents and should be evaluated frequently for clinical manifestations of drug toxicity. Chronic drug and radiation toxicity, such as secondary cancers, sterility, and the side effects of systemic corticosteroids, are of as much importance as acute drug toxicity. Patients receiving antineoplastic drugs are also more likely to develop systemic infections from opportunistic organisms during therapy. Finally, patients who receive radiation therapy to the mediastinum may become hypothyroid from the effects of the radiation.

COMMENTS

Advances in the use of combination chemotherapy and radiation therapy in Hodgkin's disease have increased the importance of accurate pathologic subclassification and staging of the extent of the disease. Staging procedures include a meticulous history (looking for such predisposing factors as AIDS or the presence of "B" symptoms) and physical examination, a complete blood count, tests of renal and hepatic function, as well as serum uric acid and calcium levels. A chest x-ray; computed tomographic scanning of the chest, abdomen, and pelvis; lymphangiography; and bone marrow aspiration and biopsy are also important. In some patients, bone scans, Gallium scans, or a staging laparotomy and splenectomy are helpful in accurately assessing the extent of disease.

The optimum therapy for Hodgkin's disease is continuously changing and is an area of extensive research. Advances in diagnostic and therapeutic techniques have resulted in an improved prognosis. Cure is attainable for most patients with early-stage Hodgkin's disease, and even patients with advanced and recurrent disease have a significant chance of cure or long-term, disease-free survival. Treatment of these patients is best performed at a center where surgeons, medical oncologists, radiation therapists, and pathologists work closely together as a team.

References

Case records of the Massachusetts General Hospital. Weekly clinicopathological exercises. Case 7-1989. Unilateral exophthalmos three years after treatment of cervical and mediastinal Hodgkin's disease. N Engl J Med 320:447–457, 1989.

Chuah SY, Lyne AJ, Dronfield MW: Vogt-Koyanagi-Harada syndrome, a rare association of Hodgkin's disease. Postgrad Med J 67:476–478, 1991.

Hellman S, Jaffe ES, DeVita VT Jr: Hodgkin's disease. In DeVita VT Jr, Hellman S, Rosenberg SA (eds.): Cancer: Principles and Practice of oncology, 3rd ed. Philadelphia, JB Lippincott, 1989, pp 1696–1740.

Fratkin JD, Shammas HF, Miller SD: Disseminated Hodgkin's disease with bilateral orbital involvement. Arch Ophthalmol 96:102–104, 1978.

Hancock SL, Cox RS, McDougall IR: Thyroid diseases after treatment of Hodgkin's disease. N Engl J Med 325:599–605, 1991.

Hoppe RT: Radiation therapy in the management of Hodgkin's disease. Sem Oncol 17:704–715, 1990.

Kielar RA: Orbital granuloma in Hodgkin's disease. Ann Ophthalmol 13:1197–1199, 1981.

Kremer I, Loven D, Mor C, Lurie H: A solitary conjunctival relapse of Hodgkin's disease treated by radiotherapy. Ophthalmic Surg 20:494–496, 1989.

Kumar H, Garg SP, Kumar A, Gupta P: Serous macular detachment in lymphoproliferative disorders. Can J Ophthalmol 26:280–282, 1991.

Litvak J, Leder MM, Kauvar AJ: Hodgkin's disease involving optic nerve and brain. J Neurosurg 21: 798–801, 1964.

Longo DL: The use of chemotherapy in the treatment of Hodgkin's disease. Sem Oncol 17:716–735, 1990.

McFadzean RM, McIlwaine GG, McLellan D: Hodgkin's disease at the optic chiasm. J Clin Neuro-ophthalmol 10:248–254, 1990.

Miller NR: Clinical Neuro-Ophthalmology, 4th ed. Baltimore, Williams & Wilkins, 1988, Vol 3, pp 1588–1596.

Miller NR, Iliff WJ: Visual loss as the initial symptom of Hodgkin's disease. Arch Ophthalmol 93: 1158–1161, 1975.

Rowland KM Jr, Murthy A: Hodgkin's disease: Long-term effects of therapy. Med Pediatr Oncol 14:88–96, 1986.

Urba WJ, Longo DL: Hodgkin's Disease. N Engl J Med 326:678–687, 1992.

Vivancos J, Bosch X, Grau JM, Coca A, Font J: Development of Hodgkin's disease in the course of primary Sjögren's syndrome. Br J Rheumatol 31: 561–563, 1992.

Vose JM, Bierman PJ, Armitage JO: Hodgkin's disease: The role of bone marrow transplantation. Sem Oncol 17:749–757, 1990.

Wessel K, Diener HC, Schroth G, Dichgans J: Paraneoplastic cerebellar degeneration associated with Hodgkin's disease. J Neurol 235:122–124, 1987.

KAPOSI'S SARCOMA
171.9
(Idiopathic Multiple Pigmented Sarcoma)

BIJAN SAFAI, M.D., D.S.C.,
and BEATRICE M. DIAS, M.D.

New York, New York

Kaposi's sarcoma (KS) is a multicentric disease that generally presents as red-purple macules, plaques, or nodules on the lower extremities, but may appear anywhere in skin, mucous membrane, lymph nodes, or internal organs. The disease is primarily seen in males (15:1) and is rare except in certain endemic pockets, including Eastern Europe, Italy, Equatorial Africa, and North America. The course of the disease ranges from slow and indolent to rapid and fulminant, with the average survival time in American series ranging from 8 to 13 years. In Africa, a lymphadenopathic form of the disease, which is highly fatal, is seen in children. Furthermore, a more aggressive form of Kaposi's sarcoma has been observed in kidney transplant recipients and in patients with a variety of immunologic disorders who have been on immunosuppressive therapy. Kaposi's sarcoma has been seen more frequently among individuals who are infected with the human immunodeficiency virus (HIV), specifically among homosexual and bisexual men. Since the beginning of the AIDS epidemic, 31,140 cases of AIDS-associated KS have been reported. Of these, 423 have been described in women. The victims of this epidemic have been shown to suffer from a profound cellular immune deficiency and usually succumb to death from opportunistic infection(s). Kaposi's sarcoma in these patients may have an aggressive course; when involving the skin it usually occurs on the upper extremities, trunk, head, and neck. It can also be limited to lymph nodes as well as involve the mucocutaneous membranes and/or visceral organs. An increased incidence of second primary malignancies, especially that of lymphoma, has been observed in patients with Kaposi's sarcoma. AIDS-associated Kaposi's sarcoma seems to be a growth-factor-driven proliferative process involving the spindle cell, progenitor cells, and lymphatic vessels in a localized manner of distribution. Three different histopathologic types of ophthalmic Kaposi's sarcoma have been described and are believed to be part of a continuum involving vascular channels and endothelial and spindle cells.

Kaposi's sarcoma may involve the ocular adnexa, including the eyelids, conjunctiva, lacrimal glands, and orbit. Ocular lesions usually develop after the appearance of tumors on the extremities, but conjunctival tumors have been reported in the absence of other manifestations. Such involvement has been seen more frequently in patients with the epidemic form of Kaposi's sarcoma. Conjunctival involvement by this tumor is characteristically more evident in the inferior fornix. It is also seen in other areas of the palpebral and bulbar conjunctiva. Ophthalmic Kaposi's sarcoma lesions are usually slowly progressive, although in rare cases they have a rapidly progressive course. Conjunctival lesions usually appear red with tissue thickening and may be associated with subconjunctival hemorrhage. Kaposi's sarcoma may develop into circumscribed subepithelial nodules or diffuse infiltrative lesions of the conjunctiva. Palpebral involvement usually appears purple in color and may be flat or elevated. Ophthalmic Kaposi's sarcoma does not usually interfere with visual function. Exceptions are those cases in which edema secondary to lymphatic obstruction or extensive sarcoma of tissues causes closure of the palpebral fissure.

THERAPY

Irradiation. The treatment of choice for the isolated nonaggressive lesions of Kaposi's sarcoma of the ocular adnexa has been radiation therapy. Low-dose x-ray treatment ranging from a few hundred to a few thousand rads has been given in divided doses over 3 to 8 weeks and has been shown to be effective. Recurrences are, however, common.

Surgical. Isolated conjunctival or orbital lesions of Kaposi's sarcoma may also be surgically excised or treated with electrosurgery or cryotherapy.

Systemic. Single or combination chemotherapy is generally used for aggressive Kaposi's sarcoma with visceral involvement. Recombinant alpha-interferon has been used in the treatment of Kaposi's sarcoma with limited success. Approximately one-third of treated patients have had complete response. Newer treatment modalities, including the use of growth factors and related antibodies, as well as an anti-TAT compound, may be developed in the next few years.

Topical. Immunotherapy with topical agents, such as dinitrochlorobenzene[†] or intralesional purified protein derivative,[†] has been used for localized disease. More recently, superficial Kaposi's sarcoma lesions of the conjunctiva have been treated with strontium-90 with an ophthalmic applicator. Initial reports indicate that this simple form of treatment has been effective and well-tolerated.

PRECAUTIONS

Since most ocular lesions in Kaposi's sarcoma are indolent, conservative management is recommended unless there is clear evidence of aggressive disease.

COMMENTS

In the new epidemic of Kaposi's sarcoma, more than half of the patients have exhibited intraretinal exudates, nerve fiber layer hemorrhages, and cotton-wool spots on ocular examination. Cytomegalovirus retinitis has also been described. These lesions were usually adjacent to and sometimes obscured the vessels in the peripapillary retina. The cotton-wool spots are seen in a variety of illnesses, such as diabetes mellitus, systemic lupus erythematosus, dermatomyositis, hypertension, anemia, and leukemia. They seem to be the result of focal retinal ischemia and are histologically and morphologically identical to cotton-wool spots seen in the fundi of patients with Kaposi's sarcoma. Although the cause of the cotton-wool spots in these patients is unclear, infections with cytomegalovirus or high levels of circulating immune complexes should be considered. The cotton-wool spots do not correlate with the course of the systemic disease.

References

Brunt AM, Phillips RH: Strontium-90 for conjunctival AIDS-related Kaposi's sarcoma: The first case report. Clin Oncol 2:118–119, 1990.

DiGiovanna JJ, Safai B: Kaposi's sarcoma. Retrospective study of 90 cases with particular emphasis on the familial occurrence, ethnic background and prevalence of other diseases. Am J Med 71:779–783, 1981.

Dugel PU, et al: Ocular adnexal Kaposi's sarcoma in acquired immunodeficiency syndrome. Am J Ophthalmol 110:500–503, 1990.

Dugel PU, et al: Particles resembling retrovirus and conjunctival Kaposi's sarcoma. Am J Ophthalmol 110:86–87, 1990.

Epidemiologic aspects of the current outbreak of

Kaposi's sarcoma and opportunistic infections. N Engl J Med 306:248–252, 1982.

Giraldo G, Beth E, Huang ES: Kaposi's sarcoma and its relationship to cytomegalovirus (CMV). III. CMV, DNA and CMV early antigens in Kaposi's sarcoma. Int J Cancer 26:23–29, 1980.

Giraldo G, et al: Antibody patterns to herpes viruses in Kaposi's sarcoma. II. Serological association of American Kaposi's sarcoma with cytomegalovirus. Int J Cancer 22:126–131, 1978.

Harwood AR, et al: Kaposi's sarcoma in recipients of renal transplants. Am J Med 67:759–765, 1979.

Heinemann MH: Ophthalmic problems. Med Clin North Am 76:83–97, 1992.

Howard GM, Jakobiec FA, DeVoe AG: Kaposi's sarcoma of the conjunctiva. Am J Ophthalmol 79:420–423, 1975.

Jakobiec FA, Jones IS: Vascular tumors, malformations, and degenerations. In Duane TD (ed): Clinical Ophthalmology. Hagerstown, MD, Harper & Row, 1982, Vol II, pp 37:27–31.

Lieberman PH, Llovera IN: Kaposi's sarcoma of the bulbar conjunctiva. Arch Ophthalmol 88:44–45, 1972.

Myskowshi PL, Niedzwiecki D, Shurgot BA, et al: AIDS-associated Kaposi's sarcoma: Variables associated with survival. J Am Acad Dermatol 18:1299–1306, 1988.

Nadji M, et al: Kaposi's sarcoma. Immunohistologic evidence for an endothelial origin. Arch Pathol Lab Med 105:274–275, 1981.

Nicholson DH, Lane L: Epibulbar Kaposi sarcoma. Arch Ophthalmol 96:95–96, 1978.

Safai B: Pathophysiology and epidemiology of epidemic Kaposi's sarcoma. Sem Oncol 6:7–12, 1987.

Safai B, Good RA: Kaposi's sarcoma: A review and recent developments. Cancer J Clin 31:2–12, 1981.

Safai B, Lynfield R, Lowenthal DA, Koziner B: Cancers associated with HIV infection. Anticancer Res 7:1055–1068, 1987.

Safai B, et al: Association of Kaposi's sarcoma with second primary malignancies. Possible etiopathogenic implications. Cancer 45:1472–1479, 1980.

Shuler JD, et al: Kaposi sarcoma of the conjunctiva and eyelids associated with the acquired immunodeficiency syndrome. Arch Ophthalmol 107:858–862, 1989.

Siegal FP, et al: Severe acquired immunodeficiency in male homosexuals, manifested by chronic perianal ulcerative herpes simplex lesions. N Engl J Med 305:1439–1444, 1981.

Taylor J, et al: Kaposi's sarcoma in Uganda: A clinicopathological study. Int J Cancer 8:122–135, 1971.

Urmacher C, et al: Outbreak of Kaposi's sarcoma with cytomegalovirus infection in young homosexual men. Am J Med 72:569–575, 1982.

LIPOSARCOMA 190.1

RICHARD M. CHAVIS, M.D., and RONALD E. DEI CAS, M.D.

Washington, District of Columbia

Liposarcoma is the most common soft tissue malignancy of the body, accounting for approximately 16 per cent of sarcomas. This aggressive tumor arises from primitive mesenchymal cells, rather than mature adipose tissue. Liposarcomas show a marked predilection for the intermuscular fascial planes of deeper soft tissues, such as the thigh, retroperitoneum, leg, and groin, although such tumors may arise anywhere in the body that fat is found. Relapse despite adequate treatment is common, either from local recurrence or metastasis, most frequently to the lungs, liver, lymph nodes, and periosteum. The tumor can occur at any age; however, for nonorbital liposarcomas, the average age of presentation is in the fifth decade. A slight male predominance has been noted.

Liposarcomas may be divided into groups by histologic type. The most currently accepted typing system is that of Enzinger and Winslow with four groups: well-differentiated, myxoid, round cell, and pleomorphic tumor types. Some current authors, however, argue that the round cell group should be eliminated, and two additional types, lipoblastic and fibroblastic, should be added. Common to all the histologic groups is the presence of lipoblasts. The well-differentiated and myxoid groups are considered less malignant than the other types. Pleomorphic-type liposarcoma is marked by extreme cellular atypia, and it is often difficult to differentiate this tumor from other mesenchymal tumors.

With nonorbital liposarcomas, the prognosis depends on the following features: histologic subtype, with the well-differentiated and myxoid types less apt to metastasize than the other types; location, with extremity tumors having a better prognosis than retroperitoneal tumors; overall tumor volume; presence or absence of mitotic figures; and the adequacy of local excision. The prognostic factors related to orbital liposarcomas are less well defined, largely because of the small number of cases.

To date, less than 20 cases of primary orbital liposarcoma have been reported in the literature. The vast majority of these were of the myxoid type. The cases reported represent patients of all age groups with no clear predilection for older patients or men; however, this distribution may be secondary to the low number of cases. Diplopia and proptosis are the most common clinical manifestations, with visual acuity generally well maintained. Because of the rarity of this tumor, it is often not considered in the differential of orbital masses. Prompt diagnosis is especially possible in the orbit, with resulting early therapy and increased chance for survival. In addition to primary orbital liposarcoma, metastatic lesions to the orbit, as well as one patient with primary conjunctival liposarcoma, have been reported.

Recent studies have demonstrated a nonrandom aberration of chromosome 12 in liposarcoma. A translocation between chromosomes 12q13 and 16p11 seems to be specific for the myxoid type. Although chromosomal aberrations have also been seen in the other types of liposarcoma, none seems to be as type-specific as the t(12;16)(q13;p11).

Both computed tomography and magnetic resonance imaging seem to be useful in imaging liposarcomas. In some cases of orbital liposarcomas, the CT appearance was deceptively cystic; however, in such cases both ultrasound and MR imaging were able to depict the solid nature of the tumor. No radiologic imaging technique is able to make a histologic diagnosis clearly. Thus, the role of radiologic imaging is to discern the size and extent of the tumor and to aid in the preoperative plan.

The small number of primary orbital liposarcomas, limited follow-up, and the varying methods by which they were treated (i.e., local excision versus exenteration; with and without irradiation) makes definitive information on the prognosis of orbital liposarcomas difficult. Regarding nonorbital liposarcomas, it is known that all types of liposarcomas are prone to local recurrence, especially those located in the retroperitoneum, while the more malignant types (round cell, lipoblastic, fibroblastic, and pleomorphic, depending on classification scheme) are those most likely to metastasize. Studies generally demonstrate 5-year survival rates close to 100 per cent for the well-differentiated liposarcomas and 70 to 90 per cent for the myxoid tumors. Five-year survival rates for the other types are considerably less ranging from 40 to 60 per cent.

THERAPY

Surgical. Complete surgical excision with wide margins is desirable. A wide excision must be emphasized; reliance on frozen section diagnosis of clear margins is condemned since many liposarcomas are irregularly encapsulated, and their margins lack in diagnostic lipoblasts, despite their malignant nature. For small low-grade orbital tumors, particularly those in elderly patients, local tumor excision may be justifiable. However, in many patients the need for a wide excision will necessitate exenteration.

Irradiation. Prophylactic irradiation after local excision seems to increase the survival rate. This combination of treatment modalities should be considered in patients with orbital liposarcoma, especially of the myxoid type, which is known to be radiosensitive. Irradiation alone should be used only in cases of inoperable tumors.

Chemotherapy. Although some authors have reported attempts at treating liposarcomas with adjunct chemotherapy, the results have been disappointing and do not support chemotherapy as an adequate treatment modality for this malignancy.

Ocular or Periocular Manifestations

Extraocular Muscles: Paresis.
Eyelids: Edema.

Globe: Proptosis.
Orbit: Liposarcoma.

References

Abdalla MI, Ghaly AF, Hosni F: Liposarcoma with orbital metastases. Case report. Br J Ophthalmol 50:426–428, 1966.
Bartley GB, et al: Spindle cell lipoma of the orbit. Am J Ophthalmol 100:605–609, 1985.
Chang HR, et al: Prognostic value of histologic subtypes in primary extremity liposarcoma. Cancer 64:1514–1520, 1989.
Dooms GC, et al: Lipomatous tumors and tumors with fatty component: MR imaging potential and comparison of MR and CT results. Radiology 157:479–483, 1985.
Enzinger FM, Weiss SW: Soft Tissue Tumors. St. Louis: CV Mosby, 1983, pp 242–280.
Enzinger FM, Winslow PJ: Liposarcoma: A study of 103 cases. Virchows Arch 335:376–388, 1962.
Henderson JW: Orbital Tumors, 2nd ed. New York, Brian C Decker, 1980, pp 253–258.
Jakobiec FA, et al: Primary liposarcoma of the orbit. Ophthalmology 96:180–191, 1989.
Karakousis CP, et al: Chromosomal change in soft-tissue sarcomas. Arch Surg 122:1257–1260, 1987.
Lane CM, Wright JE, Garner H: Primary myxoid liposarcoma of the orbit. Br J Ophthalmol 72:912–917, 1988.
London J, et al: MR imaging of liposarcomas: Correlation of MR features and histology. J Comput Assist Tomogr 13:832–835, 1989.
Mandahl N, et al: Liposarcomas have characteristic structural chromosomal rearrangements of 12q13-q14. Int J Cancer 39:685–688, 1987.
McNab AA, Moseley I: Primary orbital liposarcoma: Clinical and computed tomographic features. Br J Ophthalmol 74:437–439, 1990.
Miser JS, Pizzo PA: Soft tissue sarcomas in childhood. Pediatr Clin North Am 32:779–800, 1985.
Miyashita K, Abe Y, Ozamura Y: Case of conjunctival liposarcoma. Jpn J Ophthalmol 35:207–210, 1991.
Mortada A: Rare primary orbital sarcomas. Am J Ophthalmol 68:919–925, 1969.
Nasr AM, et al: Standardized echocardiographic-histopathologic correlations in liposarcoma. Am J Ophthalmol 99:193–200, 1985.
Orson GG, et al: Liposarcoma of the musculoskeletal system. Cancer 60:1362–1370, 1987.

LYMPHOID TUMORS 202.8
(Inflammatory Pseudotumor, Malignant Lymphoma, Neoplastic Angioendotheliomatosis, Pseudolymphoma, Pseudotumor, Reactive Lymphoid Hyperplasia)

MICHAEL D. EICHLER, M.D.,
and F. T. FRAUNFELDER, M.D.

Portland, Oregon

Ocular lymphoid tumors are an intriguing, diverse, and controversial area of ophthalmology. A variety of pathology can be seen with unique natural histories and response to treatment. Areas of overlap create diagnostic challenge, though immunotyping has greatly improved this effort. Lymphoid tumors typically occur in the sixth and seventh decades of life and affect males and females equally. These neoplasms can be divided into three main categories based on their natural history: orbital inflammatory pseudotumor; periocular (ocular adnexal) lymphoid tumors—hyperplasia and lymphoma; and intraocular lymphoid tumors—hyperplasia and lymphoma.

Idiopathic orbital inflammation is a localized orbital disease frequently referred to as pseudotumor because it causes proptosis due to diffuse multifocal infiltration of lymphocytes and only rarely forms a discrete localized mass. The clinical disease is typified by the acute onset of pain, hyperemia, chemosis, periocular edema and erythema, extraocular motility disturbances, and the rapid development of proptosis. Inflammatory involvement adjacent to the optic nerve may produce visual disturbances. There is a light dispersal of lymphocytes, plasma cells, and occasionally eosinophils (particularly in children) around blood vessels and interstitially within the orbital fat, extraocular muscles, Tenon's space, and lacrimal gland. The involved tissue is variably fibrotic, and the lymphoid component is not hyperplastic or sheet-like. Systemic disease is rarely associated (less than 5 per cent of cases); associated diseases are either endocrinopathy, neoplasm, or vasculitis.

Ocular adnexal lymphoid tumors encompass both reactive lymphoid hyperplasia (RLH) and lymphoma as both share similar natural histories, histologic features, and response to therapy. Periocular lymphomas are rare. Approximately 1.5 to 4.0 per cent of systemic lymphomas involve the eye, and less than 1 per cent of patients have ocular involvement as the initial presentation. Non-Hodgkin's lymphomas (NHLs) compromise 99 per cent of these lesions; essentially, all are of B-cell origin. Only one case exists in the literature of a T-cell periocular lymphoma, though mycosis fungoides affecting the skin of the eyelid does occur but typically is not considered as periocular lymphoma.

Reactive lymphoid hyperplasia and non-Hodgkin's lymphoma have variable presentations depending on the site of involvement. Conjunctival lesions are usually asymptomatic, with patients seeking medical attention because of cosmetic considerations or fear of an unknown disease. Flesh or salmon-pink patches or masses are often incidentally noticed. The forniceal, bulbar, and palpebral conjunctiva all can be affected, with a predilection for the fornices. Involvement of the orbit generally results in painless, slowly progressive proptosis with or without diplopia and visual impairment. There is a distinct propensity for anterior orbital involvement with a palpable rubbery mass. CT scan reveals a mass lesion that displays a tendency to conform to pre-existing anatomic structures or tissue planes without bone destruction.

The pathologist is challenged when diagnosing lymphoid tumors. Malignant lymphomas are composed of cytologically malignant and immature lymphocytic cells, whereas clearly benign RLH lesions appear as polymorphic proliferations of small lymphocytes and intermixed plasma cells, immunoblasts, histiocytes, and endothelial cell proliferations. Difficulty results from the similar appearance of small lymphocytic lymphoma (SLL) and diffuse hyperplasia, both of which are sheet-like, hyperplastic, hypercellular accumulations of lymphocytes devoid of stroma. The presence of germinal centers and of mature lymphocytes and plasma cells thought to represent benignity is now recognized in both lesions. Advances in immunotyping with flow cytometry or immunofluorescence staining have greatly improved diagnostic accuracy with immunologically heterogeneous (polyclonal) lesions classified as benign and immunologically homogeneous (monoclonal) as malignant.

The natural history of periocular lymphoid tumors is controversial. Some authors feel that polyclonal RLH and monoclonal NHL have clearly distinct natural histories, whereas others feel they follow the same course. Knowles et al. (1990) and Jakobiec et al. (1986) have shown that both RLH and SLL have approximately a 30 per cent association with prior, concurrent, and/or future systemic lymphoma (dissemination). However, Medeiros et al. (1989) report that polyclonal RLH lesions had no dissemination and yielded 100 per cent disease-free survival through 7 years of follow-up. Variable accuracy in monoclonal detection may explain this difference. It is proposed that RLH lesions may initially contain a very small clonal subpopulation that is undetectable by immunotyping; it will eventually expand to encompass the lesion, thereby creating the potential for dissemination. There may be a spectrum of disease from RLH to NHL. This has been supported by DNA analysis showing monoclonal cells within RLH lesions and progression to systemic lymphoma. Because of this potential dissemination of RLH lesions, they are evaluated and treated in a similar manner to NHL lesions. Atypical lymphoid hyperplasia, a diagnosis made less commonly due to immunotyping, falls within this spectrum of disease between RLH and NHL and is treated similarly.

The clinical course and prognosis of periocular lymphoid tumors depend on three major factors: histology, stage at diagnosis (dissemination), and anatomic site of involvement. Controversy remains a part of each factor. Knowles et al. (1990) report a 27 per cent versus 46 per cent dissemination of low- versus high-grade lymphomas. Most authors agree that higher-grade lymphomas have increased rates of advanced stage disease and poorer prognoses compared to low-grade lymphomas or RLH. Interestingly, this is actually opposite of nodal disease. Nodal low-grade lymphomas are more often at an advanced stage at diagnosis. This may be explained by the premise of ocular lesions being truly primary disease with an equal frequency of early detection of both low- and high-grade lesions. Nodal disease—in particular, low-grade indolent tumors—may go undetected for longer periods of time, allowing for advanced stages at diagnosis.

The stage of disease at diagnosis has significant survival implications. Knowles et al. (1990) report that 86 per cent of stage IE (localized, extranodal) patients were disease free after radiation therapy, with an average 51 months of follow-up. However, 32 per cent of patients at advanced stages (dissemination) had progressive disease resulting in death. Interestingly, regardless of histology, all stage IE lesions carried good prognoses, with 10 to 20 per cent dissemination after treatment. With localized disease, histology does not have prognostic significance, as all grades develop extraocular disease with the same frequency.

Anatomic site is the third major prognostic factor. Medeiros et al. (1989) found no difference in survival and rate of dissemination between the conjunctiva, orbit, or eyelid. Knowles et al. (1990) however, report a significant difference. They found prior, concurrent, and/or future extraocular disease in 20 per cent of conjunctival lesions, 35 per cent of orbital lesions, and 67 per cent of eyelid lesions. Many other reports report better prognoses of conjunctival lesions than in those in other sites. As the conjunctiva contains indigenous lymphoid elements and the other sites do not, it is postulated that the presence of lymphoid elements creates the potential for development of primary tumors with a lower chance of extraocular disease. Bilateral versus unilateral disease is also a controversial prognostic factor. Several publications report that bilateral disease is associated with a poorer prognosis, as opposed to data from McNally et al. (1987), which show no difference in prognosis between the two groups. Overall, for localized (stage IE) lymphoid tumors, the site of involvement is the most significant prognostic factor.

A specific type of orbital lymphoma is Burkitt's lymphoma. This is the only lymphosarcoma that is likely to involve the orbits of children. In the African type, there tends to be involvement of the maxilla, with secondary encroachment on the orbit; hepatosplenomegaly and central nervous system involvement are also typical, with relative sparing of the superficial lymph nodes. This form of lymphoma is curable with chemotherapy, provided that therapy is introduced before evidence of central nervous system disease develops.

Intraocular lymphoid tumors fall into four groups: primary malignant lymphomas, malignant lymphomas of the uvea, reactive lymphoid hyperplasia of the uvea, and neoplastic angioendotheliomatosis. Primary malignant lymphomas (reticulum cell sarcoma or microgliomatosis) of the central nervous system mainly involve the retina and optic nerve; a dispersion of cells into the vitreous is often associated with these tumors. The patient often has cerebral lesions, but only exceptionally are the lymph nodes or other noncentral nervous system tissues affected. Malignant lymphomas of the uvea occur most frequently in patients who have involvement of the lymph nodes, liver, spleen, or other viscera, but rarely is the central nervous system affected. Lymphoid hyperplasias of the uvea are typically isolated lesions that are not associated with malignant lymphomas in the central nervous system or other viscera. Neoplastic angioendotheliomatosis is a variant of large-cell malignant lymphoma with widespread intravascular proliferation of malignant cells of endothelial origin. Although the most common signs and symptoms relate to skin and central nervous system involvement, ophthalmic manifestations of neoplastic angioendotheliomatosis may include decreased vision, iridocyclitis, vitritis, retinal vascular alterations, papilledema, and visual field defects.

The presence of lymphoid tumors necessitates proper evaluation before therapy. Because there is no clinical way of being absolutely certain that one is dealing with a benign or a malignant discrete lymphoid tumor, and because CT scan results are similar to those of metastatic carcinomas and infiltrating primary neoplasms of the orbit, a biopsy is required. An incisional biopsy should not be overly aggressive; because of the radiosensitivity of these tumors, one need not attempt to remove the mass in total. A surgical pathologist should be consulted before performing the biopsy since most require fresh tissue, special fixatives, and/or formalin.

THERAPY

There are presently three major modalities of therapy for idiopathic orbital inflammation: systemic steroids, surgery, and radiotherapy. Because of the tendency of pseudotumor toward spontaneous remission, it is probably inaccurate to ascribe all of the improvement noted to the efficacy of treatment.

Systemic. Systemic steroids seem to be most helpful in patients with acute or subacute lesions and are least effective in those lesions exhibiting histologic features of a chronic phase. High doses of prednisone, 80 mg daily, should be continued for a total of 3 weeks and tapered over a 2- to 3-week period to prevent a rebound. Radiotherapy is felt to be quite effective for steroid-resistant lesions, with typically 2000 cGy providing nearly 100 per cent local control. Repeated and extensive surgical intervention seems to be harmful.

When the diagnosis of periocular lymphoid tumor is made, a thorough evaluation is required for systemic disease. Approximately 20 to 30 per cent of patients will have prior or concurrent systemic lymphoma. After therapy of limited stage disease, dissemination rates are 10 to 20 per cent. Staging evaluation should include consultation with an internist/oncologist with laboratory tests (CBC, SPEP, chemistries), CT scan of chest rather than a chest x-ray, CT scan of abdomen, and bone marrow biopsy. After therapy, patients should be followed every 6 months by an ophthalmologist and internist/oncologist to monitor for local or systemic disease.

Therapy of advanced stage lymphoma is variable depending on the histologic grade and whether a patient is symptomatic. Chemotherapy should be entrusted to a general oncologist, and although periocular lesions can be expected to shrink during chemotherapy, adjuvant radiotherapy or cryotherapy may be required, especially if visual impairment is present.

Irradiation. Radiotherapy is considered the standard treatment of localized disease. General doses are 2000 to 3000 cGy for RLH and low-grade lymphomas, and 3000 to 4000 cGy for higher grades. Side effects vary from self-limited conjunctivitis and erythema to potentially severe dry eye syndrome, symblepharon, and cataracts. Side effects are dose dependent, and with the low doses required for lymphoid tumors, they are infrequent. With aggressive radiotherapy, nearly 100 per cent local control can be expected; however, 10 to 20 per cent of patients will develop systemic lymphoma, regardless of histology.

Cryotherapy has been employed for conjunctival lymphoid lesions, as surgery alone is less likely to remove all of the tumor. One limited study of its use exists.

For suspected intraocular reticulum cell sarcoma (microgliomatosis), a diagnostic vitrectomy with cytologic evaluation can establish the diagnosis. Radiotherapy to the globe and neuraxis is the chief form of therapy for intraocular reticulum cell sarcoma and neoplastic angioendotheliomatosis. For cases of suspected reactive lymphoid hyperplasia of the uvea, a diagnostic iris biopsy (if heterochromia is present) or a transcleral needle biopsy with cytologic studies may enable diagnosis, which can be extremely elusive. Prolonged doses of 80 to 100 mg of prednisone daily can shrink the choroidal masses; if this form of therapy should fail, 2500 cGy of radiotherapy might be tried.

PRECAUTIONS

When orbital pseudotumors are bilateral, the chances that a systemic disorder will subsequently be discovered are greatly increased, especially in adults. The ocular signs of hyperthyroidism not only mimic or produce the clinical picture of an orbital pseudotumor but also the histopathologic appearance is remarkably similar to that of inflammatory pseudotumor. Likewise, pseudotumor of the orbit can occur as the initial manifestation of Wegener's granulomatosis. Orbital cellulitis of bacterial origin can usually be ruled out by obtaining sinus x-rays to demonstrate the absence of a primary sinus infection.

Topical ophthalmic corticosteroid eyedrops are relatively ineffective in melting large conjunctival lymphoid masses. Intralesional injections of 110 mg of triamcinolone acetonide in aqueous suspension in four divided doses over a 10-week period may cause some tumors to regress. However, because of the potential malignant transformation and dissemination of these lesions, steroid therapy is not recommended. Instead, biopsy and definitive treatment with radiotherapy or cryotherapy are recommended.

Conjunctival lymphoid tumors involving a fornix need to be treated with caution. These lesions are associated with higher rates of recurrence and dissemination after cryotherapy compared to bulbar and palpebral lesions. Orbital ultrasound or CT scan should be obtained to rule out orbital extension. Radiotherapy should be initiated if orbital disease is present and should be considered for large forniceal conjunctival lesions.

References

Char DH, et al: Primary intraocular lymphoma (ocular reticulum cell sarcoma): Diagnosis and management. Ophthalmology 95:625–630, 1988.
Dunbar SF, et al: Conjunctival lymphoma: Results and treatment with a single anterior electron field. A lens-sparing approach. Int J Radiat Oncol Biol Phys 19(2):249–257, 1990.
Erickson BA, et al: Periocular lymphoproliferative diseases: Natural history, prognostic factors, and treatment. Radiology 185(1):63–70, 1992.
Jakobiec FA, et al: Ocular adnexal monoclonal lymphoid tumors with a favorable prognosis. Ophthalmology 93(12):1547–1557, 1986.
Jereb B, et al: Radiation treatment of orbital lymphoid tumors. Int J Radiat Oncol Biol Phys 10:1013–1022, 1984.
Knowles DM, et al: Lymphoid hyperplasia and malignant lymphoma occurring in the ocular adnexa (orbit, conjunctiva, and eyelids). Hum Pathol 21(9):959–973, 1990.
McNally L, et al: Clinical, morphologic, immunophenotypic, and molecular genetic analysis of bilateral ocular adnexal lymphoid neoplasms in 17 patients. Am J Ophthalmol 103:555–568, 1987.
Medeiros LJ, et al: Immunohistologic features predict clinical behavior of orbital and conjunctival lymphoid infiltrates. Blood 74(6):2121–2129, 1989.
Medeiros LJ, et al: Lymphoid infiltrates of the orbit and conjunctiva. Am J Surg Pathol 13(6):459–471, 1989.
Medeiros LJ, et al: Immunohistologic analysis of small lymphocytic infiltrates of the orbit and conjunctiva. Hum Pathol 21(11):1126–1131, 1990.

Minehan KJ, et al: Local control and complications after radiation therapy for primary orbital lymphoma: A case for low-dose treatment. Int J Radiat Oncol Biol Phys 20(4):791–796, 1991.

Orcutt JC, et al: Treatment of idiopathic inflammatory orbital pseudotumors by radiotherapy. Br J Ophthalmol 67:570–574, 1983.

Paryani SB, et al: Analysis of non-Hodgkin's lymphomas with nodular and favorable histologies, stages I and II. Cancer 52:2300–2307, 1983.

Takano Y, et al: Molecular-genetic analysis of ocular adnexal benign lymphoid hyperplasias by a two-step polymerase chain-reaction. J Cancer Res Clin Oncol 118:581–586, 1992.

Trudeau M, et al: Intraocular lymphoma: Report of three cases and review of the literature. Am J Clin Oncol 11:126–130, 1988.

Vogiatzis KV: Lymphoid tumors of the orbit and ocular adnexa: A long-term follow-up. Ann Ophthalmol 16:1046–1055, 1984.

MYCOSIS FUNGOIDES
173.9
(Cutaneous T-Cell Lymphoma, Lymphomatoid Papulosis, Sézary Syndrome, T-Cell Lymphoma-Leukemia)

F. T. FRAUNFELDER, M.D.

Portland, Oregon

Mycosis fungoides is a cutaneous T-cell lymphoma that can progress to involve multiple extracutaneous tissue. Sézary syndrome is the rare leukemic form of this disease in which the lymphomatous process originally starts in the skin. Mycosis fungoides may involve the viscera, especially the lung, spleen, and liver. Although lymphoids may be involved, the central nervous system is rarely involved. Ocular findings are most commonly found in the eyelids; however, intraocular involvement has been reported. Ocular findings include keratitis, uveitis, papilledema, optic atrophy, and conjunctival and orbital involvement.

This disease is rare, with only two new cases per million seen each year. The course is chronic; commonly, its duration is 10 to 20 years. The process begins in the skin, remaining there for long periods of time. Eventually, extracutaneous organ involvement develops. Once this occurs, the prognosis is poor, with 50 per cent of patients dying in 1 to 2.5 years.

THERAPY

Topical. Topical nitrogen mustard is effective in the plaque stage. Application of 10 to 40 mg of mechlorethamine* dissolved in 40 ml water may be made to the entire skin. Photochemotherapy with psoralens‡ and ultraviolet light (PUVA) is apparently of equal efficacy in early stages of the disease. There is no uniformly accepted method of PUVA therapy because of the lack of long-term outcomes. Combination PUVA with nitrogen mustard has been advocated for eyelid involvement. Electron beam is used in plaque and tumor stages with doses of 2.5 to 4.0 MeV for a total dose of 3000 rads. Conventional x-rays can be used on isolated tumors.

Systemic. Extracutaneous stages are treated with chemotherapy, usually in combination with topical therapy. The chemotherapeutic agents are usually given in combination, and the most effective regimen includes cyclophosphamide, methotrexate with leucovorin, bleomycin,‡ doxorubicin, and prednisone. Maintenance therapy should be given for at least 1 year.

Ocular. Intraocular involvement may be treated with x-rays in dosages dependent on the size of the tumors. These tumors often respond to low doses of radiation. The least amount of radiation should be applied in order to prevent radiation damage. Tumors on the lids may be irradiated or removed by plastic surgery with transplantation. Liquid nitrogen cryotherapy will also melt these lesions. One should treat these lesions the same degree as a basal cell carcinoma, but only a single freeze-thaw cycle should be used.

Ocular or Periocular Manifestations

Conjunctiva or Cornea: Chemosis; marginal interstitial keratitis; opacity; tumor.

Eyelids: Ectropion; edema; necrosis; nodules; plaques; tumor.

Optic Nerve: Papilledema.

Orbit: Exophthalmos; necrosis.

Retina: Edema; exudates; hemorrhages; vascular engorgement.

Other: Endophthalmitis; scleritis; uveitis.

PRECAUTIONS

Contact allergy frequently develops after the topical use of nitrogen mustard. When the solution is applied to the skin, contact of the eye with the solution should be avoided by the use of protective glasses.

There is a risk of cataract development in patients receiving PUVA. Therefore, ultraviolet-blocking glasses should be worn outdoors during the day of treatment, as well as indoors. An increased risk of squamous cell carcinoma has also been reported with PUVA therapy.

Side effects of electron beams may include erythema and edema of the skin with chronic radiation damage. The eyes should be shielded during treatment periods.

COMMENTS

In many Western countries, cooperative mycosis fungoides study groups have been established, and these groups should be consulted concerning evaluation of the patient and the appropriate treatment modality. However, it should be emphasized that treatment of extracutaneous stages of mycosis fungoides is still very difficult, although early stages can be controlled by effective topical measures.

References

Catovsky D, et al: Adult T-cell lymphoma-leukaemia in blacks from the West Indies. Lancet 1:639–643, 1982.

Cox NH, Jones SK, Downey DJ, et al: Cutaneous and ocular side-effects of oral photochemotherapy: Results of an 8-year follow-up study. Br J Dermatol 116:145–152, 1987.

Edelson RL: Cutaneous T-cell lymphoma: Mycosis fungoides, Sézary syndrome, and other variants. J Am Acad Dermatol 2:89–106, 1980.

Erny BC, Egbert PR, Peat IM, et al: Intraocular involvement with subretinal pigment epithelium infiltrates by mycosis fungoides. Br J Ophthalmol 75:698–701, 1991.

Gupta AK, Anderson TF: Psoralen photochemotherapy. J Am Acad Dermatol 17(5):703–734, 1987.

Jimbow K, Takami T: Cutaneous T-cell lymphoma and related disorders. J Int Dermatol 25:485–497, 1986.

Lange Wantzin G: Cutaneous T-cell lymphomas and retrovirus infection. Dermatology 176:221–223, 1988.

Zachariae H, Threstrup-Pedersen K: Combination chemotherapy with bleomycin, cyclophosphamide, prednisone and etretinate in advanced mycosis fungoides: A six-year experience. Acta Dermatol Venereol 67:433–437, 1987.

Zackheim HS: Cutaneous T-cell lymphomas. A review of the recent literature. Arch Dermatol 117:295–304, 1981.

Zucker JL, Doyle MF: Mycosis fungoides metastatic to the orbit. Arch Ophthalmol 109:688–691, 1991.

NEUROBLASTOMA 194.0

DEVRON H. CHAR, M.D.

San Francisco, California

Neuroblastoma is a neoplasm derived from immature sympathetic ganglion cells; it can develop anywhere that this primitive neural tissue is located. Metastatic orbital disease is the most common ophthalmic manifestation of neuroblastoma; however, there are isolated case reports of primary neuroblastoma involving the ciliary ganglion.

Neuroblastoma has the highest incidence of spontaneous regression of any human malignancy. It is estimated that as many as 1 in 200 neonates may have an in situ tumor that regresses spontaneously. Previous studies may have overestimated this occurrence because immature neuroblasts are present in the fetal adrenal gland.

Neuroblastoma is one of the three most common malignancies in young children. There are approximately 500 new cases annually in the United States. There is no sexual predilection. More than 50 per cent of cases develop in children younger than 2 years of age, with a range from birth to 62 years of age.

The vast majority of metastatic orbital neuroblastomas present after the discovery of the primary neoplasm. In approximately 3 per cent of cases, orbital metastases may be the first manifestation of the disease; often, the characteristic puffy lids with ecchymosis can mimic a battered child syndrome. Orbital metastases in neuroblastoma can be either unilateral or bilateral, but there is a slight predominance of bilateral involvement. The differential diagnosis of orbital proptosis in this age group includes sinusitis and contiguous orbital involvement, leukemia, lymphoma, rhabdomyosarcoma, and the orbital spread of retinoblastoma.

Metastatic neuroblastomas have increased our understanding of the potential prognostic import of tumor oncogenes; amplification is observed in poor-risk tumors.

THERAPY

Surgical. The diagnosis of orbital neuroblastoma can often be made presumptively if the patient has known metastatic neuroblastoma. All patients require a medical evaluation if there is no history of neuroblastoma. Body CT/MRI, bone scan, and bone marrow aspiration are the initial studies necessary in a patient suspected of having neuroblastoma. In patients who present first with an orbital metastasis, a fine-needle aspiration biopsy or an incisional biopsy is indicated. Since the vast majority of patients with ophthalmic involvement have widespread disease, the mainstay of palliation is chemotherapy and irradiation. Total resection of an orbital metastasis does not improve survival. In the extremely rare situation in which there is a primary neuroblastoma of the ciliary ganglion, local surgical resection with adjunct chemotherapy may be useful.

Irradiation. Irradiation is a useful palliative adjunct therapy in the management of neuroblastoma. Most patients with orbital metastases respond to 1500 to 3000 rads given over a 2-week period. The effect of radiation on survival is minimal.

Systemic. Combination chemotherapy seems to have greater efficacy than single drug treatment in the management of metastatic neuroblastoma. Current chemotherapeutic agents used in the management of neuroblastoma include cyclophosphamide, vincristine, decarbazine,[‡] doxorubicin, cisplatin,[‡] mechlorethamine,[‡] papaverine,[‡] teniposide,[‡] and trifluridine. Usually these agents are given in cycles. The two most commonly used drugs are vincristine and cyclophosphamide. Vincristine is used intravenously at a dose of 1.5 mg/square meter for 2 days of every month along with 750 mg/square meter of cyclophosphamide for 1 day of every month. There is also some experimental therapy being performed using monoclonal antibodies and antibodies to ferritin.[†] Other newer therapies include high-dose chemo/radiotherapy followed by bone marrow transplantation and ^{131}I-methiodobenzylguanidine (MIBG); both approaches have produced improvement in short-term survival, although longer follow-up is necessary. In most studies long-term survival has been about 11 per cent, but short-term remissions are produced in as many as 55 per cent of cases.

Ocular. The use of artificial tears after orbital irradiation may be useful in patients who develop dry eye.

Ocular or Periocular Manifestations

Conjunctiva: Chemosis; subconjunctival hemorrhages.

Eyelids: Ecchymosis; edema; ptosis.

Globe: Exophthalmos; proptosis.

Optic Nerve: Atrophy; edema; optic neuritis; papilledema.

Orbit: Metastatic or rarely primary tumor.

Retina: Dilated veins; edema; exudates; hemorrhages; striae.

Other: Absent pupillary reaction to light; convergent strabismus; mydriasis; paralysis of the sixth or seventh nerve.

PRECAUTIONS

The response of patients with metastatic orbital neuroblastoma to either chemotherapy or radiation is transient; there is less than 15 per cent long-term survival in children older than 2 years of age. Children less than 1 year old with stage IV-S do quite well. The chemotherapeutic agents used have marked hematologic and, in the case of doxorubicin, cardiac toxicities. In addition, rapid destruction of tumor cells by these agents may produce high blood or renal levels of uric acid, which can result in subsequent renal shutdown and death. Ocular changes secondary to irradiation of the orbit include erythema, loss of eyelashes or eyebrows, conjunctivitis, conjunctival contraction, keratitis, lens opacities, uveitis, vitreous hemorrhage, retinal pigment epithelial hyperplastic changes, and secondary glaucoma.

COMMENTS

Although it is unusual for neuroblastoma patients to present first to the ophthalmologist because of an orbital mass, unilateral or bilateral orbital swelling and lid ecchymosis in a young child should be evaluated for neuroblastoma. Children with orbital neuroblastoma should have an extensive metastatic evaluation because over 70 per cent of these patients have widespread disease at the time of diagnosis. This evaluation should include a general physical examination, complete blood count and SMA-12 bone marrow aspirate and biopsy, brain and body CT scans, urinary catecholamine levels, bone scan, skeletal bone survey, and an intravenous pyelogram. In some centers, metaiodobentylguanidine (MIBG), a norepinephrine analogue, scans are also used.

The prognosis in neuroblastoma is dependent on the age and stage of disease. Patients younger than 1 year of age or those older than 6 years of age at the time of diagnosis have a substantially better prognosis than children between the ages of 1 and 5. Although chemotherapy and radiation have had a palliative effect on metastatic disease, they do not seem to have improved the prognosis of widespread neuroblastoma. The mean survival after the diagnosis of orbital neuroblastoma metastases is approximately 3.5 months. Although results with early, localized neuroblastoma (stage I and II) are promising, the prognosis for survival with advanced disease remains dismal.

References

Albert DA, Rubenstein RA, Scheie HG: Tumor metastasis to the eye. Part II. Clinical study in infants and children. Am J Ophthalmol 63:727–732, 1967.

Alfano JE: Ophthalmological aspects of neuroblastomatosis: A study of 53 verified cases. Trans Am Acad Ophthalmol Otolaryngol 72:830–848, 1968.

Bowman LC, Hancock ML, Santana VM, Hayes FA, Kun L, Parham DM, Furman WL, Rao BN, Green AA, Crist WM: Impact of intensified therapy on clinical outcome in infants and children with neuroblastoma. J Clin Oncol 9:1599–1608, 1991.

Breslow N, McCann B: Statistical evaluation of prognosis for children with neuroblastoma. Cancer Res 31:2098–2103, 1971.

Coldman AJ, et al: Neuroblastoma: Influence of age at diagnosis, stage, tumor site, and sex on prognosis. Cancer 46:1896–1901, 1980.

OCULAR METASTATIC TUMORS 198.89

FREDERICK H. DAVIDORF, M.D.

Columbus, Ohio

Metastatic disease to the eye is a grave prognostic sign, with death commonly occurring within 2 years after the ocular involvement. Breast cancer, being the most common primary malignancy, represents 60 to 70 per cent of all metastatic tumors to the choroid and occurs in approximately 30 per cent of these individuals. In females, metastatic carcinoma of the breast accounts for nearly 90 per cent of choroidal metastases. In males, the most common neoplasm is lung cancer, representing nearly 50 per cent of the metastatic tumors to the eye. Genitourinary and gastrointestinal metastases each represent approximately 13 per cent of the metastatic tumors to the choroid in males. The route of metastasis is via blood. Therefore, the uveal tract is the site of the majority of ocular metastasis because of its rich blood supply. Usually, uveal metastasis is unilateral, but bilateral tumors occur approximately 25 per cent of the time. Although most of the metastases to the eye occur in the choroid, rarely do we see retinal metastasis, with only 12 cases reported in the literature, of which 7 arose from cutaneous melanoma. Metastases to the optic nerve are also very rare.

The time between the diagnosis of the primary malignancy and the discovery of ocular metastasis varies. Uveal metastasis usually occurs within 2 years, but there are reports in the literature of metastatic uveal disease occurring as long as 22 years after treatment for the primary tumor. Rarely are metastatic lesions diagnosed without symptoms. Although pain, inflammation, and glaucoma may occur with ocular metastatic disease, the usual presenting symptoms are photopsia and decreased vision.

A typical metastatic tumor to the uvea presents as a pale choroidal elevation with an irregular undulating surface. The overlying pigment epithelium is destroyed, and a retinal detachment is present with shifting subretinal fluid.

Since the most common primary tumor of the choroid is a malignant melanoma, the distinction between these two lesions is important. The clinical appearance of these two tumors differs in many respects. Although most choroidal melanomas are at least partially pigmented, ocular metastases are generally amelanotic. Since metastatic tumors usually grow more rapidly than primary choroidal melanomas, which may lie dormant in the eye for many years, the pigment changes in the metastatic lesions are more pronounced than in the melanomas. The pigment epithelium and choriocapillaris overlying the metastatic lesion undergo more complete destruction, and the pigment disruption is profound. A malignant melanoma produces gradual destruction, manifested by islands of pigmented atrophy adjacent to areas of completely intact pigment epithelium.

The vasculature of these two lesions also appears different clinically. Virtually all melanomas have an intrinsic blood supply, and frequently these vascular channels can be seen on ophthalmoscopy and with fluorescein angiography. Because metastatic lesions grow more rapidly, their vasculature is usually not as prominent. Finally, the two lesions differ in their growth patterns. Melanomas have two growth phases. During the slow growth phase, the lesion appears dome shaped; the rapid phase is characterized by a collar button lesion produced as the tumor breaks through Bruch's membrane and the pigment epithelium. Metastatic lesions, although dome shaped when small, are characterized by an irregular surface as the tumor enlarges.

Ophthalmoscopy is the best clinical means to distinguish melanomas from metastatic lesions, but other diagnostic modalities also are beneficial in differentiating these lesions. Quantitative A-scan ultrasonography is one of the most useful tests available. Since melanomas are composed of tightly packed, homogeneous cells, there is minimal internal reflectivity to sound as it passes through the tumor. Metastatic lesions are composed of much more heterogeneous cells that are less tightly packed. As sound passes through these tumors, there is much more interference, resulting in significant internal reflectivity.

THERAPY

Systemic. The treatment of choroidal metastasis depends on the type of the tumor and whether there is other evidence of metastatic disease. If the patient has recently begun chemotherapy for metastatic disease at other sites, the choroidal mass should be monitored every 3 to 4 weeks. In this situation, the choroidal metastasis frequently responds to systemic treatment.

Irradiation. Irradiation of the globe should be considered if metastasis occurs in spite of chemotherapy. In individuals whose ocular lesion is the only site of active metastasis, local radiotherapy is recommended. Administration of 4000 cGy over a 3-week period (20 treatments with 200 cGy) is a sufficient dose to destroy a metastatic breast tumor in the choroid, with usually minimal complications. Generally, metastatic breast carcinoma is quite radiosensitive, whereas metastatic lung lesions are relatively radioresistant.

COMMENTS

Cancer of the breast is the most common source of metastatic disease to the eye, representing over 80 per cent of the cases, whereas in 10 per cent of the cases the primary site is the lung. In females, metastatic carcinoma of the breast accounts for nearly 90 per cent of choroidal metastasis. When confronted with a choroidal mass, metastatic disease should always be considered, and a metastatic evaluation should be performed. The differentiation between a metastatic mass and a malignant melanoma of the choroid on the basis of ophthalmoscopy and quantitative ultrasound studies is 98 per cent reliable. If the choroidal mass is an isolated metastasis, the treatment of choice is local radiation therapy. If the patient has other evidence of metastasis and is on chemotherapy, the mass should be observed at monthly intervals. Frequently, the uveal metastasis will respond in a similar manner as the other sites. If it fails to regress, radiation therapy is recommended.

References

Char DH, et al: Ocular metastases from systemic melanoma. Am J Ophthalmol 90:702–707, 1980.

Dobrowsky W: Treatment of choroid metastases. Br J Radiol 61:140–142, 1988.

Ferry AP, Font RL: Carcinoma metastatic to the eye and orbit. I. A clinicopathologic study of 227 cases. Arch Ophthalmol 92:276–286, 1974.

Ferry AP, Font RL: Carcinoma metastatic to the eye and orbit. II. A clinicopathological study of 26 patients with carcinoma metastatic to the anterior segment of the eye. Arch Ophthalmol 93:472–482, 1975.

Freedman MI, Folk JC: Metastatic tumors to the eye and orbit: Patient survival and clinical characteristics. Arch Ophthalmol 105:1215–1219, 1987.

Halpern J, et al: Choroidal metastases arising from carcinoma of the breast. Review and analysis of five cases. J Med 17:1–11, 1986.

Jeager EA, et al: Effects of radiation therapy on metastatic choroidal tumors. Trans Am Acad Ophthalmol Otolaryngol 75:94–101, 1971.

Letson AD, Davidorf FH, Bruce RA Jr: Chemotherapy for treatment of choroidal metastases from breast carcinoma. Am J Ophthalmol 93:102–106, 1982.

Maor M, Chan RC, Young SE. Radiotherapy of choroidal metastases. Breast cancer as a primary site. Cancer 40:2081–2086, 1977.

Merrill CF, Kaufman DI, Dimitrov NV: Breast cancer metastatic to the eye is a common entity. Cancer 68:623–627, 1991.

Mewis L, Young SE: Breast carcinoma metastatic to the choroid: Analysis of 67 patients. Ophthalmology 89:147–151, 1982.

Shields JA, Young SE: Malignant tumors of the uveal tract. Curr Probl Cancer 5:1–35, 1980.

Young SE: Retinal metastases. In Schachat AP (ed): Retina. St. Louis, CV Mosby, 1989, pp 321–338.

ORBITAL METASTASES
198.89

DEVRON H. CHAR, M.D.

San Francisco, California

Metastases to the orbit are uncommon and account for only 10 to 15 per cent of ophthalmic metastases. In either adults or children, orbital metastases are often the initial presentation of a systemic malignancy. In children, orbital metastases usually occur before the age of two years. In the United States, the most frequent cause of pediatric orbital metastases is neuroblastoma, which is discussed on page 347. Acute myelomonocytic leukemia (AMML), although a disseminated disease process and not truly a metastatic tumor, can also present in the orbit of infants or young children as the initial sign of malignancy. Other neoplasms including Wilm's tumor and Ewing's sarcoma can secondarily involve the pediatric orbit, but they are much less common. Involvement of orbital bones is common with metastatic pediatric tumors, especially neuroblastoma; the differential diagnosis of orbit bony destruction in this age group also includes primary orbital rhabdomyosarcoma and the histiocytosis syndromes.

Approximately 3 to 7 per cent of adult orbital biopsies demonstrate metastatic tumors. The orbit is approximately ten times less frequently involved than the choroid as a site for adult metastatic disease. Metastases to the orbit can involve the extraocular muscles, the intraconal space, the globe and contiguous orbit, the orbital bones, or the orbit and contiguous central nervous system or sinus structures. Overall, approximately 50 per cent of orbital metastases are the initial sign of the systemic neoplasm; however, in women usually the primary tumor is a previously treated breast carcinoma. In adult males, the most common primary neoplasms include lung carcinoma, renal carcinoma, and gastrointestinal tract tumors. In the former two tumors, as many as 85 per cent of patients present to the ophthalmologist with ocular or orbital symptoms before the diagnosis of the primary neoplasm. Rarer causes of orbital metastases include pancreatic carcinoma; hepatoma; pheochromocytoma; testicular carcinoma; carcinoid, prostate, and bladder carcinomas; cardiac myxoma; bile duct carcinoma; and squamous cell carcinoma. Although metastases to the orbit can be the initial sign of systemic disease, there are reports with a latency as long as 30 years between primary tumor treatment and development of orbital disease.

CT and MRI are the diagnostic modalities of choice to demonstrate orbital metastases. Metastases in the orbit often produce bone involvement, although they can produce focal enlargement of an extraocular muscle or a more diffuse pattern that can simulate a pseudotumor. In adults, other causes of orbital bony destruction include infection, mucocele, midline lethal granuloma, Wegener's granuloma, histiocytosis syndromes, sarcomas, hematic cysts, epithelial lacrimal gland tumors, lymphoid lesions, and sinus carcinomas. Less commonly, enophthalmos, usually occurring in association with either a scirrhous breast or gastric carcinoma, occurs.

In approximately 50 per cent of orbital metastases, an elevation of the plasma CEA (>10 mg/ml), is found, which is consistent with the diagnosis of a metastasis, especially if there is a typical CT/MRI pattern or a history of a known primary tumor. In older patients, it is usually not possible to differentiate idiopathic orbital inflammation (pseudotumor) from metastatic tumors on MR or CT if there is no bone involvement. We have observed metastatic tumors that perfectly mimic the imaging findings of a pseudotumor, including the production of fluid in Tenon's space. Sometimes the T_1 or T_2 pattern on MRI is useful to differentiate these two processes. Inflammatory (pseudotumor) orbital masses usually are isodense with respect to muscle on a T_1-weighted scan and isodense with respect to fat on the T_2-weighted image. In contrast, metastases are isodense to muscle on T_1-weighted images, but hyperintense to central nervous system on T_2-weighted scans.

Fine-needle aspiration biopsy is the most useful ancillary diagnostic modality in uncertain cases. Usually, fine-needle aspiration biopsy under CT control is diagnostic for a metastatic tumor. Rarely, a false-negative biopsy can occur in a patient with either scirrhous carcinoma or in those with a marked lymphocytic infiltration of a metastatic tumor. This technique using both CT guidance and documentation is especially important in posterior orbital tumors and in lesions with a presumed false-negative result. If the needle is in the tumor on CT, yet insufficient material is obtained, an open biopsy is indicated.

If a metastatic orbital tumor is diagnosed, consultation with an oncologist is mandatory. If the orbital lesion represents either the first evidence of widespread disease or disease recurrence after a quiescent period, a thorough metastatic evaluation is indicated, including central nervous system imaging and cerebral spinal fluid cytology. We have observed a few disastrous cases in which subtle simultaneous frontal lobe metastases were not recognized at the time of diagnosis of an orbital metastasis. In both cases external beam irradiation was given at other institutions, and the failure to image and recognize the CNS disease resulted in two courses of radiation with significantly increased, unnecessary morbidity.

THERAPY

Surgical. If a focal symptomatic lesion is found, it can be removed surgically. However, most commonly, patients have either diffuse or nonresectable orbital tumors.

Systemic. Some patients with diffuse orbital tumors respond to chemotherapy, since there is no blood-brain or blood-ocular barrier present. If an orbital lesion is discovered and there is new or progressive systemic disease, chemotherapy is often a reasonable first option.

Irradiation. External beam irradiation is useful for many orbital metastases. If there is no other site of metastasis and a nonresectable orbital lesion is symptomatic or if the patient is not responsive to chemotherapy, radiation is indicated. The radiation dose and fraction

schedule depend on the tumor type and disease status. Generally, patients receive approximately 40 Gy of photon irradiation over a 5-week period. In some malignancies, especially melanoma and Kaposi's sarcoma, higher daily fractions (>400 cGy) are more effective. Similarly, if a patient has a life expectancy of less than 6 months, large daily fractions can decrease the number of times a patient must return for radiation with acceptable morbidity in a shortened life span. Although the risk of ocular radiation vasculopathy is increased with daily fractions above 200 cGy, the mean latency for radiation retinopathy and similar complications is 18 months. Diabetic patients and those on chemotherapy are at greater risk for ocular radiation complications. Orbital metastases are associated with poor survival, and in our experience these patients have a mean survival of 8 months after diagnosis of a metastatic orbital tumor.

References

Albert DM, Rubenstein RA, Scheie HG: Tumor metastasis to the eye. II. Clinical study in infants and children. Am J Ophthalmol 63:727–732, 1967.

Bullock JD, Yanes B: Ophthalmic manifestations of metastatic breast cancer. Ophthalmology 87:961–973, 1980.

Char DH: Clinical Ocular Oncology. New York, Churchill Livingstone, 1988.

Char DH, Unsold R: Ocular and orbital pathology. Clinical aspects. In Newton TH, Hasso AN, Dillon WP (eds): Modern Neuroradiology, Vol 3, Computed Tomography of the Head and Neck. New York, Clavadel Press, 1988, pp 212–238.

Font RL, Ferry AP: Carcinoma metastatic to the eye and orbit. III. A clinicopathologic study of 28 cases metastatic to the orbit. Cancer 38:1326–1335, 1976.

Huh SH, Nisce LZ, Simpson LD, Chu FCH: Value of radiation therapy in the treatment of orbital metastasis. Am J Roentgenol Radium Ther Nucl Med 120:589–594, 1974.

PERIOCULAR MERKEL CELL CARCINOMA 173.9
(Cutaneous Neuroendocrine Carcinoma, Endocrine Carcinoma of the Skin, Small-Cell Skin Carcinoma, Trabecular Carcinoma)

TERO KIVELÄ, M.D.

Helsinki, Finland

Merkel cell carcinoma is a newly recognized, relatively rare but important, highly malignant primary cutaneous neoplasm. It frequently involves the eyelids or periocular region, which account for about one-tenth of all Merkel cell carcinomas. During the last 10 years, about 70 primary periocular Merkel cell carcinomas have been reported. Most of them occurred in the eyelids, preferentially the upper one, whereas the rest arose in the canthal or eyebrow region. Metastatic Merkel cell carcinomas to the eyelids, choroid, ciliary body, and orbit have also been described.

Merkel cell carcinoma preferentially affects elderly patients, and those with eyelid tumors are on an average 75 years old. It practically never occurs in the African-American population. The tumor is a solitary, painless, and nontender dermal skin nodule that is bulging and protuberant in shape. It arises close to the lid margin, tends to spare the eyelashes, and may be pedunculated. A reddish or purplish erythematous hue and telangiectatic small vessels, which probably result from the associated inflammatory infiltration and invasion of local lymphatic vessels, are highly characteristic features. The tumor typically invades the orbicularis muscle, but spares the tarsal plate. The overlying skin is generally not ulcerated. The tumor may imitate a chalazion.

Local recurrence has been reported in one-third of patients and may be multiple. About two-thirds develop regional lymph node metastases at some time during the disease. Systemic metastases ultimately develop in up to one-half of cases. They are most common in the liver, bone, lungs, skin, and brain, but may occur in any location and are generally heralded by regional lymph node metastases. Disseminated Merkel cell carcinoma nearly always proves fatal. The estimated 5-year survival for all patients is less than 50 per cent. The above figures are based on Merkel cell carcinomas in general. Preliminary evidence suggests that eyelid tumors may have a somewhat better prognosis than Merkel cell carcinomas located elsewhere, including other periocular sites.

THERAPY

Surgical. Merkel cell carcinoma demands prompt initial therapy for a favorable outcome. Wide surgical excision and full thickness resection of the eyelid should be done whenever possible, with a suggested margin of 5 mm. Frozen section control is helpful in ensuring the deep margin of excision, but does not guarantee complete removal due to frequent early lateral spread through lymphatic vessels. Exenteration may be considered for recurrent tumors extending to the orbit in the absence of evidence of metastatic disease.

When regional lymph node metastases are detected, radical neck dissection either with or without irradiation is recommended and may result in permanent cure, even though many patients eventually develop systemic metastases.

Irradiation. Merkel cell carcinomas are ra-

diosensitive. In carefully selected cases, irradiation has been used successfully as primary therapy to avoid extensive plastic surgery in elderly and debilitated patients.

The frequent lymphatic invasion, the high risk of regional metastases, and the poor prognosis of disseminated disease have led many authors to recommend prophylactic treatment of regional lymph nodes. Even though prophylactic dissection of lymph nodes does not seem to be justified at the present stage of knowledge, and the efficacy of adjuvant radiotherapy has not been formally studied, serious consideration should be given to irradiation of tissues between the tumor and the regional lymph nodes, particularly when it is not limited to the eyelids. The dose most frequently used has been 50 to 60 Gy in 20 to 25 fractions over 4 to 6 weeks.

Radiotherapy is also an effective treatment for regional and systemic metastases, but it is associated with a high incidence of relapse. Nevertheless, it is a valuable palliative modality with less complications than chemotherapy. Irradiation with an iodine plaque may be used to eradicate a uveal metastasis.

Systemic. Chemotherapeutic agents have been used to treat extensive local or recurrent, as well as metastatic, Merkel cell carcinoma. So far, no treatment protocol has been found to be superior to others, and treatment regimens are constantly evolving. Consequently, the choice of treatment should be delegated to experts in cancer chemotherapy. Most Merkel cell carcinomas respond initially to chemotherapy, but the disease tends to recur rapidly after the cessation of treatment. However, long-term cures have also been reported.

Ocular or Periocular Manifestations

Choroid: Metastatic Merkel cell carcinoma.
Eyelids: Reddish or purplish skin nodule; telangiectatic vessels; partial loss of eyelashes; infrequently ulcerated skin; primary or metastatic Merkel cell carcinoma.
Iris or Ciliary Body: Metastatic Merkel cell carcinoma.
Orbit: Exophthalmos; metastatic Merkel cell carcinoma.
Other: Reddish or purplish skin nodule; telangiectatic vessels; primary Merkel cell carcinoma close to the eyebrows or orbital rim.

PRECAUTIONS

Merkel cell carcinoma has been clinically misdiagnosed as chalazion. Chalazia are very rare in the elderly population and should always undergo biopsy to exclude the possibility of either sebaceous or Merkel cell carcinoma.

Merkel cell carcinoma metastasizes frequently, and it is important to exclude the possibility that a periocular tumor is a manifestation of systemic disease. The lesions may be confused with other neuroendocrine small-cell carcinomas and lymphomas by the pathologist. Moreover, it is not uncommon that the patient has an unrelated second primary tumor. A careful systemic work-up is thus always mandatory before therapy to exclude the possibility of a primary malignancy elsewhere.

Most patients with Merkel cell carcinoma are elderly and are likely to have intercurrent diseases. When planning treatment, it is important to weigh the benefits against the potential hazards of aggressive surgery and chemotherapy. With current chemotherapeutic regimens, a significant proportion of patients have died of treatment complications. Irradiation may be a better mode of palliative therapy in selected cases.

Patients with Merkel cell carcinoma must be followed carefully for evidence of recurrent disease and regional and systemic metastases. Regional metastases affect the ipsilateral preauricular, submandibular, and cervical lymph nodes.

COMMENTS

Merkel cells are specialized epidermal cells of probable epithelial origin. They have neuroendocrine features, are associated with nerve endings, and are thought to form part of a touch receptor. In the eyelids, single Merkel cells occur in the epidermis, the outer root sheath of hairs and eyelashes, and in the dermis. Aggregates of Merkel cells, called touch spots, occur regularly at the palpebral margin between successive eyelashes. The origin of Merkel cell carcinoma has not been definitely resolved. Most authors currently ascribe it to an epidermal stem cell common to keratinocytes and Merkel cells.

In histopathologic examination, Merkel cell carcinomas consist of round cells of intermediate size, with vesicular nuclei mimicking large-cell lymphoma or oat-cell carcinoma. Some tumors additionally show adnexal or squamous differentiation. The neoplastic cells are either arranged in cords and nests or infiltrate diffusely. Early invasion of lymphatic vessels and an inflammatory reaction consisting of plasma cells and lymphocytes occur very frequently. A definite diagnosis may require demonstration of dense core neurosecretory granules or perinuclear whorls of intermediate filaments by electron microscopy, or simple epithelial cytokeratins, epithelial membrane antigen, neurofilaments, chromogranin, synaptophysin, and neuron-specific enolase by immunohistochemistry.

References

Alexander E III, et al: Merkel cell carcinoma. Long term survival in a patient with proven brain metastasis and presumed choroid metastasis. Clin Neurol Neurosurg 91:317–320, 1989.

Bourne RG, O'Rourke MGE: Management of Merkel cell tumour. Aust NZ J Surg 58:971–974, 1988.

Cotlar AM, Gates JO, Gibbs FA Jr: Merkel cell carcinoma: Combined surgery and radiation therapy. Am Surg 52:159–164, 1986.

Crown J, et al: Chemotherapy of metastatic Merkel cell cancer. Cancer Invest 9:129–132, 1991.

Goepfert H, et al: Merkel cell carcinoma (endocrine carcinoma of the skin) of the head and neck. Arch Otolaryngol 110:707–712, 1984.

Hitchcock CL, et al: Neuroendocrine (Merkel cell) carcinoma of the skin. Its natural history, diagnosis, and treatment. Ann Surg 207:201–207, 1988.

Kivelä T, Tarkkanen A: The Merkel cell and associated neoplasms in the eyelids and periocular region. Surv Ophthalmol 35:171–187, 1990.

O'Brien PC, Denham JW, Leong AS-Y: Merkel cell carcinoma: A review of behaviour patterns and management strategies. Aust NZ J Surg 57:847–850, 1987.

Redmond J III, et al: Chemotherapy of disseminated Merkel-cell carcinoma. Am J Clin Oncol (CCT) 14:305–307, 1991.

Rubsamen PE, et al: Merkel cell carcinoma of the eyelid and periocular tissues. Am J Ophthalmol 113:674–680, 1992.

Shaw JHF, Rumball E: Merkel cell tumour: Clinical behaviour and treatment. Br J Surg 78:138–142, 1991.

Yiengpruksawan A, et al: Merkel cell carcinoma. Prognosis and management. Arch Surg 126:1514–1519, 1991.

PERIOCULAR SQUAMOUS CELL CARCINOMA 173.1

ROBERT M. DRYDEN, M.D., F.A.C.S.,

Tucson, Arizona

and PETER J. WONG, M.D.

Redwood City, California

Although squamous cell carcinoma of the eyelids is a relatively rare tumor, it must be diagnosed as early as possible and managed correctly. This tumor accounts for approximately 7 to 9.2 per cent of all eyelid malignancies and 1 to 2 per cent of all eyelid lesions. It tends to occur in fair-skinned, older patients with a history of sun exposure and is found in association with actinic keratoses and in areas exposed to (ultraviolet and x-ray) irradiation. Total sun exposure in a predisposed individual is of prime importance in the production of squamous cell carcinoma of the eyelid. This neoplasm is much less common in younger adults and is rare in children. In children, squamous cell carcinoma of the eyelid is usually associated with a premalignant condition, such as irradiation, radiation dermatitis, or xeroderma pigmentosum.

The most common periocular location for squamous cell carcinoma is the lower lid.

There is also a high incidence in the canthal areas, particularly the medial canthus. Some authors have noted that squamous cell carcinoma has a predilection for the eyelid margin.

Squamous cell carcinoma of the periorbital region may arise from a precancerous solar (actinic) dermatosis or de novo. Clinically, the lesion appears as a discrete, flat, infiltrative, faintly erythematous lesion with overlying telangiectatic vessels and epidermal scaling. Crusting erosions and fissures tend to develop over a period of months. Later, the tumor develops a shallow ulcer surrounded by a wide, indurated, and elevated border. Cilia are frequently lost in the involved area, and bleeding may occur with minor trauma. Growth of the neoplasm is fairly rapid, and local destruction of tissue may occur with possible extension into the surrounding connective tissue and ocular structures. Although squamous cell carcinoma may metastasize to regional lymph nodes and internal organs (0.5 per cent), metastasis rarely occurs in carcinomas arising in the skin of sun-damaged areas. However, tumors arising in areas of previous irradiation or osteomyelitis have a higher incidence of metastasis.

The clinical presentation of squamous cell carcinoma, especially early in its course, may be very similar to actinic keratosis, basal cell carcinoma, or other benign or malignant skin lesions. Diagnosis therefore depends on a high index of suspicion followed by a careful biopsy and histologic examination. Histologically, this carcinoma of the epidermis contains abnormal cells of varying degrees of differentiation with hyperchromatic nuclei and abnormal keratinization invading the dermis. The diagnosis must be confirmed before management can be determined.

THERAPY

Surgical. The treatment of choice for periocular squamous cell carcinoma is surgical excision. The fresh tissue technique of modified Mohs, in which control of the tumor margin is monitored by frozen section, gives the best chance of complete tumor resection. After excising the entire tumor mass, including a generous margin of normal tissue, a thin layer of tissue approximately 2 mm thick is excised from the entire base and edges of the resected tissue or from the remaining wound. If the lesion is tissue other than a full thickness eyelid resection, the deep base of the tumor should also be examined for deep extension. Histologic examination is performed on each specimen using frozen sections. The specimens are sectioned in the plane parallel to the outer painted edge so that the entire periphery is microscopically examined. Margins containing tumor are marked on a map depicting the area of resection, and further specimens are obtained in the involved area until all margins are free of tumor. The success rate of this method directly relates to the care devoted by the surgeon and the pathologist. Reconstruction of the wound is not considered until all margins are determined to be free of tumor.

If the tumor is extensive, orbital invasion may have occurred. Preoperative radiologic examination with CT scanning helps determine the extent of tumor involvement. Exenteration is indicated for orbital extension. If metastasis to regional lymph nodes has occurred, a radical neck dissection should be considered along with adjunctive chemotherapy or irradiation.

Cryosurgery of eyelid squamous cell carcinoma is indicated only when the patient is unable to withstand surgical excision. Based on clinical experience with the fresh tissue technique of modified Mohs, clinical accuracy in determining the amount of tissue involved with tumor is poor. Frequently, a much larger surgical resection must be performed than anticipated on preoperative clinical examination. Cryosurgical technique requires freezing the tumor and a 5- to 6-mm margin of surrounding normal tissue to a temperature of $-40°$ to $-50°C$ and then allowing it to thaw before refreezing. The surgeon must rely entirely on clinical impression in determining the extent of the tissue to be frozen. Not only is this an inaccurate method of determining the extent of the tumor involvement but cryosurgery also frequently produces a poorer functional and cosmetic result than surgical excision with frozen section control followed by plastic reconstruction.

Irradiation. Squamous cell carcinoma is relatively radioresistant. A control rate of 93.3 per cent at 5 years has been reported with radiation therapy doses of 20 to 60 Gy in the treatment of periocular squamous cell cancer. This form of therapy should be reserved for extensive tumors that are surgically inaccessible, usually after tumor debulking.

Systemic. Systemic chemotherapy using cisplatin (Platinol) and doxorubicin (Adriamycin) has been reported to be effective as adjunctive therapy when integrated with surgery or radiation therapy in two patients who had extensive squamous cell carcinomas of the periorbital region. Each patient received four courses of cisplatin 25 mg/m^2 and doxorubicin 50 mg/m^2 as chemotherapy in addition to radiation therapy. One of the patients required surgical excision. Both patients were noted to be recurrence free. Although a study with a larger series of patients with longer follow-up is needed, this form of adjunctive therapy may be useful in treating extensive tumors.

Ocular or Periocular Manifestations

Conjunctiva: Squamous cell carcinoma.
Cornea: Exposure keratitis; hypopyon ulcer; squamous cell carcinoma.

Eyelids: Chronic inflammation; ectropion; hemorrhages; madarosis; pain; squamous cell carcinoma.
Other: Fixed globe; pain (rare); vision loss; diplopia.

PRECAUTIONS

As does basal cell carcinoma, squamous cell carcinoma often presents as a benign-appearing lesion. Such lesions are often overlooked by the physician unless his or her clinical suspicion for malignancy is high. Any unknown lesion on the periocular skin should undergo biopsy to determine its nature. Only an adequate biopsy of a representative portion of an epidermal tumor can provide the information required to make an accurate diagnosis. A relatively quick and easy means of obtaining a tissue specimen is to perform a shave biopsy. Shave biopsies are allowed to re-epithelialize; thus, they do not need surgical closure nor do they leave a scar. Shave biopsies usually provide enough tissue for the pathologist to make a diagnosis. If, however, a specimen proves to be inadequate for diagnosis, a larger deeper biopsy that requires surgical closure can be performed.

Topical fluorouracil‡ should not be used to treat squamous cell carcinoma. Although it is an effective medication to treat solar keratosis, it is rarely curative in squamous cell carcinoma and may mask deep extension.

Patients who have had one skin malignancy are at greater risk of having a new primary malignancy and are at constant risk of recurrence. Patients must be encouraged to limit their ultraviolet exposure (sunshine particularly) and must be re-evaluated periodically for the remainder of their lives.

COMMENTS

The goals of periocular skin cancer surgery in descending order of preference are complete tumor elimination, maintenance of periocular and ocular function, and obtaining satisfactory cosmesis. Although other modalities of therapy have been reported to achieve acceptable cure rates, complete tumor resection with appropriate reconstructive repair provides the highest cure rate and best functional maintenance and cosmetic appearance.

References

Anderson RL, Ceilley RI: A multispecialty approach to the excision and reconstruction of eyelid tumors. Ophthalmology 85:1150–1163, 1978.
Aurora A, Blodi F: Lesions of the eyelids: A clinicopathologic study. Surv Ophthalmol 15:94, 1970.
Beard C: Management of malignancy of the eyelids. Am J Ophthalmol 92:1–6, 1981.
Fitzpatrick PJ, et al: Basal and squamous cell carcinoma of the eyelids and their treatment by radiotherapy. Int J Radiat Oncol Biol Phys 10:449–454, 1984.
Lederman M: Radiation treatment of cancer of the eyelids. Br J Ophthalmol 60:794–805, 1976.
Lever WF, Schaumburg-Lever G: Histopathology of the Skin, 5th ed. Philadelphia, JB Lippincott, 1975.
Lund HZ: How often does squamous cell carcinoma of the skin metastasize? Arch Dermatol 92:635–637, 1965.
Luxenberg MN, Guthrie TH: Chemotherapy of basal cell and squamous cell carcinoma of the eyelids and periorbital tissues. Ophthalmology 93:504–510, 1986.
Reifler DM, Hornblass A: Squamous cell carcinoma of the eyelid. Surv Ophthalmol 30:349–365, 1986.
Wilkes TDI, Fraunfelder FT: Principles of cryosurgery. Ophthalmic Surg 10:21–30, 1979.
Zacarian SA (ed): Cryosurgical Advances in Dermatology and Tumors of the Head and Neck. Springfield, IL, Charles C Thomas, 1977.

RETINOBLASTOMA 190.5

ROBERT M. ELLSWORTH, M.D.,
and COREY M. NOTIS, M.D.

New York, New York

Retinoblastoma is the most common intraocular malignancy of childhood; it arises from one or both retinas, usually by the age of 2 years. The incidence of the tumor is 1 in 18,000 for 30,000 births, with an estimated 300 new cases each year in the United States; it occurs bilaterally in approximately 30 per cent of cases. Trilateral retinoblastoma refers to bilateral disease associated with a tumor of the pineal gland. Recent genetic advances have identified the retinoblastoma gene at band 14 on the long arm of chromosome 13 (13q14). The retinoblastoma gene product, or retinoblastoma protein, seems to control differentiation of the retinal cell, whereby absence of the protein leads to the formation of the retinoblastoma tumor. In two-thirds of cases this tumor is due to a somatic mutation in a retinal cell that presents as a unifocal tumor in one eye, usually by 2 years of age. Although the majority of these tumors are nonhereditary, approximately 10 per cent of unifocal tumors represent new germinal mutations and can be passed on to offspring.

The remaining one-third of cases are due to germinal mutations, all of which are heritable. Twenty-five per cent of these germinal cases will have a positive family history for the tumor, whereas the remainder of cases are new germ-line mutations, often derived from the paternal genome. Hereditary retinoblastoma includes multifocal tumors, unifocal tumors with a positive family history, and unifocal tumors with a secondary malignancy associated with retinoblastoma. These cases usually present by 1 year of age. On a cellular level the retinoblastoma gene functions in an autosomal recessive manner as a recessive oncogene, in that only one functioning gene is required to control retinal cellular growth, thereby preventing tumor formation. However, since the mutation rate for the retinoblastoma gene is estimated at one in ten million, and one hundred million cell divisions are required to form the mature retina, the tumor manifests itself in an autosomal dominant manner with 90 per cent penetrance. Current techniques for genetic diagnosis of retinoblastoma-predisposing mutations include the use of Southern blotting with DNA probes detecting intragenic restriction fragment length polymorphisms with primer-directed enzymatic amplification. In most families with retinoblastoma, these methods can indirectly detect tumor-predisposing mutations with 99 per cent accuracy.

The most common presenting sign of retinoblastoma is leukokoria, which is seen in more than 60 per cent of cases. Patients present with strabismus in about 20 per cent of cases, caused by macular involvement of the tumor. Less common presenting signs include an inflamed, painful eye, with or without glaucoma. When the tumor is encountered initially in an older individual, a spontaneous regression is suspected. Overall, spontaneous regressions occur in 1.8 per cent of patients.

Tumor growth may be exophytic toward the subretinal space, endophytic toward the vitreous cavity, or a combination of both. Exophytic retinoblastoma leads to progressive retinal detachment, is more likely to invade the choroid, and is more often associated with glaucoma. Endophytic retinoblastoma is more common in patients with a positive family history. The tumor within the eye has a poorly developed collagenous structure and vascular stroma, which tends to break apart with seeding into the vitreous as the tumor becomes larger. These seeds then multiply on the retinal surface and establish implantation growths, often near the ora serrata. When untreated, retinoblastoma usually remains confined to the eye for a relatively long period of time, several months to years, but it may then metastasize rapidly by various routes. These routes include (1) direct extension through the optic nerve to gain access to the subarachnoid space, with subsequent spread in the CSF, (2) spread to the base of the brain, producing a variable picture of basal meningitis, or (3) hematogenous spread, commonly to the bone marrow. In addition, the tumor may extend through the sclera to the orbit and then through lymphatics to the regional lymph nodes. If untreated, the tumor is almost uniformly fatal. The most significant factor for the prognosis of retinoblastoma is the stage of the disease at the time treatment is undertaken. The Reese-Ellsworth classification is most commonly used to compare treatment results. Group I includes solitary (A) and multiple (B) tumors less than 4 disc diameters (dd) in size, located at or behind the equator.

Group II includes solitary (A) and multiple (B) tumors between 4 to 10 dd, located at or behind the equator. Group III includes any tumor anterior to the equator (A), and solitary tumors greater than 10 dd behind the equator (B). Group IV includes multiple tumors greater than 10 dd (A) and any tumors extending to the ora serrata (B). Group V includes massive tumor involvement of over half of the retina (A) and vitreous seeding (B).

THERAPY

The primary goal of therapy is directed toward decreasing mortality of the retinoblastoma tumor and late secondary neoplasms. All attempts are made to preserve as much vision as possible.

Systemic. Systemic work-up includes a thorough physical examination, head CT scan, lumbar puncture, and bone marrow studies, the latter of which may be done concurrently at the time of diagnosis while the patient is under anesthesia.

Orbital and CNS disease, including trilateral retinoblastoma, is treated with a combination of radiation therapy and both systemic and intrathecal chemotherapy. The current regimen includes the use of systemic vincristine,[‡] doxorubicin,[‡] and cyclophosphamide, in conjunction with intrathecal methotrexate[‡] and cytosine arabinoside. Systemic carboplatin and etoposide are added in the presence of hematogenous metastasis. Enucleation is reserved for most cases of advanced unilateral disease, when there is no evidence of systemic disease. In bilateral retinoblastoma, one eye will generally have far advanced disease, often requiring enucleation, with subsequent treatment then directed at the remaining eye.

Irradiation. External beam irradiation is currently the mainstay of treatment for most cases of retinoblastoma. It is the treatment modality that is least likely to damage normal retina and is therefore used in all cases of macular and peripapillary tumors. The radiation treatments are given 5 days a week with a daily dose of 250 cGy. The total tumor dose ranges from 3500 to 4500 cGy given over a 4-week period.

Patients are then followed at 6- to 8-week intervals to observe tumor regression. Five regression patterns have been described for irradiated retinoblastomas after treatment. In type 0, the tumor completely regresses without any subsequent visible pathology. In the type I pattern, the tumor shrinks in size dramatically, taking on a mulberry cauliflower-like appearance that has been described as cottage cheese calcification. These patterns are not associated with tumor regrowth. Tumors of the type II pattern contain no calcium after radiation, lose their vascularity, and resemble the appearance of cooked fish flesh. Type III is a combination of type I and II and is the most common pattern seen. Recently, a type

IV pattern has been described in which bare sclera underlies an obliterated retina and choroid. Tumor regrowth has been shown to be inversely proportional to the age at diagnosis. Regrowth is managed by cryotherapy, photocoagulation, or brachytherapy, and then followed at 3- to 4-week intervals. Cryotherapy may also be used as a primary treatment modality for group I tumors, as well as small tumors anterior to the equator. The technique consists of triple freeze-thaw cycles. Photocoagulation with the indirect ophthalmoscope may also be used in similar circumstances. Direct photocoagulation using the Xenon arc may be used for group I tumors. The technique is to destroy the blood supply to the tumor without treating the tumor directly. Episcleral plaque therapy using Iodine 125 can be used for solitary tumors, especially when choroidal extension is suspected. The tumor apex receives a dose of 4000 cGy. The end point of treatment is reached when the tumors become completely flat scars, as any residual height may be a sign of incomplete treatment.

Ocular or Periocular Manifestations

Anterior Chamber: Hyphema; pseudohypopyon.
　　Choroid: Extension of retinoblastoma.
　　Cornea: Tumor cells on the endothelium.
　　Eyelids: Edema (if inflammatory signs are present).
　　Globe: Endophthalmitis; exophthalmos; intraocular calcification.
　　Iris: Heterochromia; neovascularization; retinoblastoma cells.
　　Optic Nerve: Papilledema; retinoblastoma.
　　Orbital: Panophthalmitis; orbital cellulitis; retinoblastoma extension.
　　Pupil: Leukokoria; mydriasis.
　　Vitreous: Tumor seeding; hemorrhage.
　　Other: Esotropia; exotropia; ocular pain; secondary glaucoma; visual loss.

PRECAUTIONS

Because of the strong hereditary factors involved in retinoblastoma, all siblings, parents, and children of survivors must have a thorough retinal evaluation with full mydriasis by an ophthalmologist. These examination are conducted at birth, at 6 weeks of age, and then at 3- to 4-month intervals during the first 2 years of life. If no tumor is present by age 3, it is unlikely that one will arise.

One course of external beam irradiation with a tumor dose below 4500 cGy is attended by few significant complications. If a second course of radiation is necessary, with a cumulative dose of 8000 cGy, there is at least a 90 per cent chance that the eye function will be lost as a result of the radiation vascular complications. When the retina is detached at the time of radiation, marked salt-and-pepper pigmentary changes supervene, although the retina usually functions well when it spontaneously reattaches. Arrest of bone centers is unusual at dosage levels of 3500 to 4500 cGy, but does occasionally occur, especially in the younger treated patients. The most serious complication of radiation is the induction of late tumors in children with the germinal mutation. It is estimated that 50 per cent of children carrying the germinal mutation will eventually develop either a radiation-induced tumor, most commonly osteogenic sarcoma or fibrous histiocytoma, or a second primary tumor related to the retinoblastoma gene. The immediate complications of cryotherapy or photocoagulation are retinal edema, hemorrhage, and detachment. The complications of systemic chemotherapy have been markedly reduced in recent years as clinicians have become more familiar with the use of these highly toxic agents. Trepidation persists as these medications may predispose to secondary malignancies in hereditary cases.

COMMENTS

The management of retinoblastoma patients and families requires a team approach. The ophthalmologist and ocular oncologist, pediatrician and pediatric oncologist, radiation oncologist, as well as genetic counselor, social worker, and ocularist all play an important role. The distinction between nonhereditary and hereditary retinoblastoma is critical, as the latter commonly carries the chromosomal 13q14 deletion. This deletion contributes to an increased incidence of secondary tumors and may be passed on to further offspring. The treatment of retinoblastoma must be tailored to the individual patient, depending on the size, location, and extent of the tumor. The goal of this treatment is to decrease any tumor-associated mortality while maintaining as much visual function as possible.

References

Abramson DH, Ellsworth RM: The surgical management of retinoblastoma. Ophthalmic Surg *11*: 596–598, 1980.

Abramson DH, Ellsworth RM, Rozakis GW: Cryotherapy for retinoblastoma. Arch Ophthalmol *100*:1253–1256, 1982.

Abramson DH, et al: Retreatment of retinoblastoma with external beam irradiation. Arch Ophthalmol *100*:1257–1260, 1982.

Abramson DH, et al: The management of unilateral retinoblastoma without primary enucleation. Arch Ophthalmol *100*:1249–1252, 1982.

Abramson DH, Ellsworth RM, Palazzi M: Endophytic vs exophytic unilateral retinoblastoma: Is there any real difference? J Pediatr Ophthal Strabismus *27(5)*:255–258, 1990.

Abramson DH, Ellsworth RM, et al: Retinoblastoma. The long term appearance of radiated ocular tumors. Cancer *67*:2753–2755, 1991.

Abramson DH, Ellsworth RM, et al: Cobalt 60

plaques in recurrent retinoblastoma. Int J Radiat Oncol Biol, Phys 21:625–627, 1991.

Abramson DH, Greenfield DS, Ellsworth RM: Bilateral retinoblastoma: Correlation between age at diagnosis and time course for new intraocular tumors. Ophthalmol Pediatr Genet 1:7, 1992.

Dryja TP, et al: Parental origin of mutations of the retinoblastoma gene. Nature 339:556–558, 1989.

Ellsworth RM: Current concepts in the treatment of retinoblastoma. In Peyman GA, et al (eds): Intraocular Tumors. New York, Appleton-Century-Crofts, 1977, pp 335–355.

Ellsworth RM: The practical management of retinoblastoma. Trans Am Ophthalmol Soc 67:462–533, 1969.

Grabowski EF, Abramson DH: Retinoblastoma. In Fernback and Vlietti (eds): Clinical Pediatric Oncology. New York, Saunders, 1991, pp 427–435.

Kopelman JE, et al: Multivariate analysis of risk factors for metastasis in retinoblastoma treated by enucleation. Ophthalmology 94:371–377, 1987.

Reese AB: Tumors of the Eye, 3rd ed. Hagerstown, MD, Harper & Row, 1976, pp 89–132.

Wiggs JL, Dryja TP: Predicting the risk of hereditary retinoblastoma. Am J Ophthalmol 106:346–351, 1988.

RHABDOMYOSARCOMA 143.9

HILARY J. RONNER, M.D.,
and IRA SNOW JONES, M.D.

New York, New York

Although rhabdomyosarcoma represents only 4 per cent of all orbital tumors, it is the most common malignant orbital neoplasm of childhood and accounts for 4 to 8 per cent of all childhood malignancies. At present, a 90 per cent 2-year survival rate can be expected if the neoplasm is limited to the orbit. The tumor characteristically produces rapidly evolving proptosis. It may also present as a palpable nodular subconjunctival or lid mass with injection of the eye and edema of the lids. Most rhabdomyosarcomas occur in children under the age of 10 years. Several cases of congenital and infantile orbital rhabdomyosarcomas have also been reported. The lesion is more commonly seen in males with a sex ratio of 5:3.

Four major histologic types of rhabdomyosarcoma are recognized: pleomorphic, embryonal, alveolar, and botryoid. Most cases of orbital rhabdomyosarcomas are embryonal tumors, frequently located superonasal to the globe or in the retrobulbar space and resulting in a forward, downward, and outward proptosis of the affected eye. The alveolar variety has a predilection for the inferior orbit; any quadrant, however, may be involved in orbital rhabdomyosarcoma. The majority of orbital rhabdomyosarcomas seem to arise from connective tissue planes within the orbit, rather than from an already differentiated extraocular muscle. Retinal changes produced by the tumor include hyperemia of the optic nerve head with fullness of the retinal veins. Optic atrophy is usually never seen initially because of the rapidity with which the neoplasm progresses.

A tissue diagnosis of orbital rhabdomyosarcoma is essential before initiation of therapy and should be obtained as quickly as possible after the patient is examined and the diagnosis is suspected. It should be stressed that the clinical picture of this disease is so typical that the diagnosis should be suspected at first presentation. In certain cases, growth is truly rapid and grossly obvious over a period of days. After an examination has taken place, the patient should undergo a CT or MRI scan, which would reveal a lesion and perhaps also subtle signs of bone erosion and destruction, which are highly suggestive of a malignant process. Benign lesions, such as lymphangioma and hemangioma, may rapidly enlarge in the orbit, but rarely produce destruction of bone. A chest x-ray should be performed to disclose any possible metastases, and careful inspection and palpation of the cervical and preauricular lymph nodes should be carried out. A bone marrow biopsy is also indicated.

The biopsy of the lesion should be performed as quickly after presentation as possible. To achieve access to an anterior lesion, a brow incision should be performed. If the mass is retrobulbar, the approach should be via a lateral orbitotomy. No attempt should be made to remove all of the suspected tumor, and all maneuvers should be performed as delicately as possible.

THERAPY

Radiotherapy and chemotherapy are the preferred modes of therapy for the majority of cases of primary orbital rhabdomyosarcoma. Because the function of the eye is at stake and because the tumor is highly radiosensitive, most ocular oncologists believe that prompt biopsy should be followed by 2 weeks of chemotherapy and then radiotherapy should be instituted.

Irradiation. Most radiotherapists treating this disease now try to give patients under the age of 6 years less than 4200 rads delivered from combined lateral and anterior portals. Patients who are 6 and older are given up to 4500 rads delivered in the same manner. In those patients whose primary tumor exceeds 5 cm in diameter, 5000 rads should be utilized. The eye can generally handle this amount of radiation without devastating complications. The radiotherapy is delivered in divided doses of 200 rads for 5 days a week over a 6-week period. Two patterns of response to the radiotherapy have been clinically recognized: a rapid resolution of the tumor over a period of days or weeks, and a slower response in which gradual shrinkage of the lesion is detected over several months.

Systemic. In addition to radiotherapy, adjuvant chemotherapy is now given to all patients for 1 year. The current protocol for children with orbital rhabdomyosarcoma consists of only two-drug chemotherapy using dactinomycin and vincristine. It must be emphasized that these agents should be administered at a major oncology center by a pediatric oncology team in conjunction with an ophthalmologist and a radiotherapist. It is mandatory that patients be carefully monitored with respect to their hemoglobin, leukocyte, and platelet counts. The role of chemotherapy in destroying cryptic micrometastases is encouraging, but its ability to control established metastatic disease is inadequate at the present time.

Surgical. In the past, exenteration of the orbit was the favored treatment of choice for orbital rhabdomyosarcoma. When this mode of treatment was used, survival rates of patients ranged between 30 and 40 per cent. With the introduction of radiotherapy and chemotherapy, local cure has increased to over 90 per cent of cases, and 5-year survival is up to 80 per cent. Exenteration, obviously, is no longer the preferred mode of therapy and should be reserved for current tumor formation.

Ocular or Periocular Manifestations

Choroid: Folds.
Conjunctiva: Chemosis; hyperemia.
Cornea: Edema; exposure keratitis.
Extraocular Muscles: Paralysis; rhabdomyosarcoma.
Eyelids: Ecchymosis; edema; ptosis; rhabdomyosarcoma.
Globe: Decreased motility; proptosis.
Optic Nerve: Hyperemia.
Orbit: Edema; enlarged optic foramen; erosion of bony walls; rhabdomyosarcoma.
Pupil: Irregularity.
Other: Decreased visual acuity; headache; increased intraocular pressure.

PRECAUTIONS

Irreversible radiation complications are common and include keratopathy, cataract, retinopathy, and optic neuropathy. When massive proptosis prevents lid closure, exposure keratitis may lead to corneal ulceration with resultant perforation and loss of the globe. The orbital bones also may be retarded in their growth after radiotherapy, leading to a sunken socket and atrophy of the brow region. Cataract formation caused by radiotherapy is a virtually unavoidable consequence, but one that may be treated several years after the exposure with excellent results.

Local recurrence of orbital rhabdomyosarcoma after treatment has been completed indicates a poor prognosis. Survival after metastasis also carries a very poor prognosis.

COMMENTS

Other etiologies in addition to rhabdomyosarcoma should certainly be considered as the cause of a rapidly progressive proptosis in children. Pediatric orbital pseudotumor and orbital cellulitis are two entities that are more commonly seen than rhabdomyosarcoma and may be confused with the more serious lesion. Pediatric pseudotumor and orbital cellulitis commonly exhibit erythema and painful inflammation of the lids and extraocular muscles, which are not usually seen in patients with rhabdomyosarcoma. X-rays of the orbit in a patient with cellulitis often shows infection in adjacent sinuses. Metastatic tumors to the orbit, including neuroblastoma and Ewing's sarcoma, are rare, but should nonetheless be considered. Abdominal examination and a MRI scan looking for a mass in the area of the adrenal glands generally disclose the primary tumor. A bone scan should reveal the primary tumor in the case of Ewing's sarcoma. Leukemia and lymphoma may also involve the orbit and produce proptosis in children. A complete blood count discloses the cause of proptosis in the case of leukemia. Lymphoma of the orbit in children is rare and may be verified by employng a Leder stain on biopsied material. Rapidly progressive proptosis may also be produced by orbital hemorrhage caused by trauma or within a pre-existing lymphangioma. Additionally, rupture of a dermoid cyst may elicit a fulminating proptosis. Ultrasound or MRI scan will reveal a subperiosteal hematoma, and one may often see a bony defect that is well corticated in the case of a dermoid cyst.

References

Abramson DH, et al: The treatment of orbital rhabdomyosarcoma with irradiation and chemotherapy. Ophthalmology 86:1330–1335, 1979.

Crist WM, et al: Prognosis in children with rhabdomyosarcoma: A report of the Intergroup Rhabdomyosarcoma Studies I and II. J Clin Oncol 8:443–452, 1990.

Ellsworth RM: Discussion of localized orbital rhabdomyosarcoma: An interim report of the Intergroup Rhabdomyosarcoma Study Committee. Ophthalmology 94:254, 1987.

Fiorillo A, et al: Multidisciplinary treatment of primary orbital rhabdomyosarcoma. Cancer 67:560–563, 1991.

Jakobiec FA, Font RL: Orbit. *In* Spencer WH (ed): Ophthalmic Pathology. Philadelphia, WB Saunders, 1986, Vol 3, pp 2556–2568.

Jones IS, Reese AB, Kraut J: Orbital rhabdomyosarcoma: An analysis of 62 cases. Am J Ophthalmol 61:721–736, 1966.

Knowles DM II, et al: Ophthalmic striated muscle neoplasms. Surv Ophthalmol 21:219–261, 1976.

Knowles DM II, et al: The diagnosis and treatment of rhabdomyosarcoma of the orbit. *In* Jakobiec FA (ed): Ocular and Adnexal Tumors. Birmingham, Aesculapius, 1978, pp 708–734.

Wharem M, et al: Localized orbital rhabdomyosarcoma: An interim report of the Intergroup Rhabdomyosarcoma Study Committee. Ophthalmology 94:251–253, 1987.

SEBACEOUS GLAND CARCINOMA 173.9

ROGER A. DAILEY, M.D.,

Portland, Oregon

and GRANT GILLILAND, M.D.

Dallas, Texas

Sebaceous gland carcinoma is a rare epithelial tumor with a proclivity for occurring on the eyelids. It accounts for less than 1 per cent of all eyelid tumors and 1.5 to 5 per cent of malignant epithelial eyelid neoplasms in the United States. This low rate is in contrast to a 28 per cent incidence of lid cancers that are sebaceous carcinomas in Shanghai and reports of sebaceous carcinomas being the second most common eyelid malignancy in Singapore. Sebaceous carcinoma of the eyelid occurs most often in women beyond the sixth decade, with an average age of onset being 61 years of age. It occurs twice as often on the upper as the lower eyelid, which reflects the predominance of meibomian glands in the upper eyelid. In addition to the meibomian glands, the ocular adnexae contain several different types of sebaceous glands, all of which may be involved with sebaceous carcinoma. The most common presentation of sebaceous carcinoma is a localized nontender tumefaction of the eyelid. Rarely, pagetoid changes similar to those seen in Paget's disease of the breast are noted in the epithelium of the eyelid overlying the sebaceous carcinoma. Sebaceous carcinoma has the ability to masquerade as many different diseases and may mimic chalazion, carcinoma-in-situ, blepharoconjunctivitis, cutaneous horn, squamous cell carcinoma, or basal cell carcinoma.

THERAPY

Surgical. Surgery is the preferred mode of therapy for these tumors. Wide local excision with frozen section analysis of the surgical margins is the initial therapy of choice for sebaceous gland carcinomas confined to the eyelid. Because sebaceous carcinomas are commonly multicentric, conjuctival map biopsies may be used to determine pagetoid spread. Adjunctive cryotherapy may be useful in the treatment of residual intraepithelial pagetoid spread within the conjunctival sac. Recently, Moh's micrographic surgery has been used in the initial therapy of sebaceous carcinomas. With suspected orbital invasion, excision of the tumor with exenteration of the orbit is effective treatment. After initial excision, patients should be observed carefully for local recurrences, regional lymph node metastasis, and distant metastasis. Sebaceous carcinoma of the eyelid with regional lymphadenopathy is best treated by local excision, radical neck lymph node dissection, parotidectomy, and postoperative radiation therapy.

Irradiation. Radiation therapy is rarely reliable in the primary management of sebaceous carcinoma. It should be considered palliative therapy in those patients who are not surgical candidates. Occasional cures have been reported with the use of as much as 9,800 rads. However, sebaceous carcinomas are generally considered radioresistant.

Ocular or Periocular Manifestations

Eyelids: Blepharitis; madarosis; meibomianitis; sebaceous carcinoma; thickening.

Orbit: Edema; proptosis; sebaceous carcinoma.

Other: Chronic conjunctivitis; superficial keratitis.

PRECAUTIONS

Because of the heterogeneous clinical features of sebaceous carcinoma, many errors and delays in diagnosis occur. Sebaceous gland carcinoma may simulate a chalazion, chronic blepharoconjunctivitis, cutaneous horn, squamous cell carcinoma, basal cell carcinoma, and an orbital tumor. Tumors occurring in the caruncle may be overlooked and result in orbital extension. Because histologic sections may be misinterpreted as squamous cell or basal cell carcinoma, it is therefore important that fat stains be used in the pathologic diagnosis. In addition, sebaceous carcinoma and metastatic breast cancer may share similar histologic characteristics, with the exception of lack of estrogen receptor protein expression in sebaceous carcinoma. Sebaceous carcinoma may be associated with Torre-Muir syndrome (sebaceous gland tumors and visceral malignancy).

COMMENTS

The incidence of sebaceous gland carcinoma seems to be increasing in recent years. This increase may be due to a better awareness of the manifestations of this disease and to improved diagnostic techniques. Sebaceous gland carcinoma must be suspected in atypical cases of blepharoconjunctivitis (unilateral), atypical or recurrent chalazion, yellowish tumors of the lid margin, and diffuse or nodular tumors involving the upper and lower lids. In addition, any orbital tumor occurring after excision of an eyelid or caruncle lesion should make one suspicious of sebaceous carcinoma. In these cases, full-thickness eyelid surgery should be performed. Radiation therapy to the eyelids is also a risk factor for the development of sebaceous carcinoma. It is important in any of these situations to obtain a pathologic specimen for definitive diagnosis. If possible, excisional biopsy with wide local margins and frozen sections should be obtained and special stains for fat made. In patients not considered surgical candidates, fine-needle aspiration may be a useful diagnostic tool.

Despite the fact that sebaceous carcinoma can arise from a variety of eyelid sebaceous glands, the site of origin of the sebaceous carcinoma does not seem to be of prognostic significance. Poor prognostic factors include vascular or lymphatic invasion, orbital extension, poor differentiation, involvement of both the upper and lower eyelids, multicentric origin, duration of symptoms longer than 6 months, highly infiltrative pattern, tumor diameter greater than 10 mm, and involvement limited to the conjunctiva alone. It is unclear whether pagetoid invasion of the overlying epithelia is a poor prognostic factor. It may represent invasion of the epithelium from the underlying malignancy or signify in situ transformation of epithelial cells. Rao reported a 50 per cent mortality in cases with pagetoid involvement and an 11 per cent mortality in those without pagetoid disease. Recent DNA studies confirm that sebaceous tumors with pagetoid involvement demonstrate aneuploidy, which is characteristic of highly aggressive tumors.

Previously, mortality rates for sebaceous gland carcinoma ranged from 24 to 40 per cent. With improved diagnostic techniques, increased awareness of the manifestations, and more aggressive therapy, the mortality rate has been significantly decreased in recent years. In a study of patients with primary eyelid sebaceous carcinoma with metastatic disease, the mortality rate approached 50 per cent 8 years after diagnosis. Interestingly, lower eyelid lesions have not been reported to cause mortality.

References

Arora R, Rewari R, Betheria SM: Fine needle aspiration cytology of eyelid tumors. Acta Cytol 34(2):227–232, 1990.

Doxanas MT, Green R: Sebaceous gland carcinoma. Arch Ophthalmol 102:245–249, 1984.

Epstein GA, Putterman AM: Sebaceous adenocarcinoma of the eyelid. Ophthalmic Surg 14:935–940, 1983.

Khan JA, Grove AS, Joseph MP, Goodman M: Sebaceous carcinoma. Ophthalmic Plast Reconst Surg 5(4):227–234, 1989.

Lisman RD, Jakobiec FA, Small P: Sebaceous carcinoma of the eyelids. Ophthalmology 96:1021–1026, 1989.

Nunery WR, Welsh MG, McCord CD: Recurrence of sebaceous carcinoma of the eyelid after radiation therapy. Am J Ophthalmol 96:10–15, 1983.

Putterman AM: Conjunctival map biopsy to determine pagetoid spread. Am J Ophthalmol 102:87–90, 1986.

Sakol PJ, Simons KB, McFadden PW, Harris GJ, Massaro BM, Koethe S: DNA flow cytometry of sebaceous cell carcinomas of the ocular adnexa: Introduction to the technique in the evaluation of periocular tumors. Ophthalmic Plast Reconstr Surg 8:77–87.

Shields JA, Shields CL: Sebaceous carcinoma of the glands of Zeis. Ophthalmic Plast Reconst Surg 4(1):11–14, 1988.

Swanson PE, Mazoujian G, Mills SE, Campbell RJ, Wick MR: Immunoreactivity for estrogen receptor protein in sweat gland tumors. Am J Surg Pathol 15(9):835–841, 1991.

Tillawi I, Katz R, Pellettiere EV: Solitary tumors of meibomian gland origin and Torre's syndrome. Am J Ophthalmol 104(2):179–182, 1987.

Wolfe JT, Yeatts RP, Wick MR, Campbell RJ, Waller RR: Sebaceous carcinoma of the eyelid. Am J Surg Pathol 8:597–606, 1984.

Yeatts RP, Waller RR: Sebaceous carcinoma of the eyelid: Pitfalls in diagnosis. Ophthalmic Plast Reconstr Surg 1:35–42, 1985.

SECTION 16

MECHANICAL AND NONMECHANICAL INJURIES

Burns

ACID BURNS 940.9

HARVEY H. SLANSKY, M.D.

Boston, Massachusetts

Acid burns of the eye produce a relatively uniform clinical picture of a sharply demarcated area of damage. Since the corneal epithelium is immediately coagulated and opacified by contact with an acid, further penetration of the acid is slowed, unlike with alkaline burns. Unless the injury destroys the cornea throughout its whole thickness, the damaged epithelium will gradually slough and be replaced by new transparent cells. The acute phase of an acid burn lasts for about 3 days after the injury, and the eye presents with chemosis and injection, possible limbal blanching, denuded corneal epithelium, and decreased corneal transparency. The patient complains of severe ocular pain, photophobia, and impaired visual acuity. In the intermediate phase from 3 to 7 days after the injury, there may be a prolonged period of active inflammation with an anterior uveitis. If the burn is severe, corneal ulceration and subsequent perforation may occur. In the chronic phase, which occurs in severe burns, vascularization of the cornea and cicatrix formation between the globe and lids may occur.

THERAPY

Ocular. The single most important treatment in the management of the eye injured by acid is copious irrigation immediately after the injury with the closest available water. Irrigation should then be continued with saline or Ringer's solution until litmus paper indicates neutrality when touched to the fornix. Continuous irrigation of the conjunctival sac can be accomplished by an intravenous delivery system. Both the upper and lower fornices should be irrigated, and eversion of the upper lid should be done, whenever possible.

Since bacterial infection (especially by *Staphylococcus* and *Pseudomonas*) is often a

problem after chemical burns to the eye, topical antibiotics, such as 0.3 per cent gentamicin solution every 3 hours and 0.5 per cent erythromycin or bacitracin ointment four times daily, should be applied at least until epithelialization is complete. Systemic antibiotics are not usually necessary in mild burns, but may be required in burns with severe ocular infections.

Cycloplegics, such as 1 per cent cyclopentolate or atropine, should be given several times daily to minimize posterior synechiae that may accompany iritis.

Several daily applications of 0.1 per cent dexamethasone will help control anterior uveitis during the first 3 or 4 days after a chemical burn. Initial dosage should depend on the severity of the burn.

Re-epithelialization of the corneal epithelium may be enhanced by using a therapeutic soft contact lens that is large enough to cover the entire cornea. The epithelium grows beneath the lens, free from trauma caused by the burned lids.

If corneal perforation threatens, a cyanoacrylate adhesive has proved useful in emergency sealing of the performation. The bed of the corneal ulcer adjacent to the thin area should be débrided of necrotic material before the adhesive is applied.

The use of collagenase inhibitors is still under investigation, but a 20 per cent solution of acetylcysteine* can be added to the regimen in desperate situations to retard ulceration.

Surgical. If corneal thinning occurs, a lamellar keratoplasty may be performed. The procedure should not be viewed as an attempt to restore lasting vision, but rather as a preparatory step for later surgery. Penetrating keratoplasty can be performed to restore vision. The results have been only fair owing to wound healing problems, but with the use of postoperative soft lenses, collagenase inhibitors, and new suture materials, the results are improving.

If frank corneal perforation has occurred, a blowout patch of preserved or fresh cornea may be applied. The patch is sutured in place and covered by a silicone membrane. This is a temporary procedure to maintain the integrity of the anterior chamber until more definitive surgery can be done. Mucosal grafts can likewise be performed to maintain the integrity of the fornices.

PRECAUTIONS

Topical corticosteroids should be used with caution in the acid-burned eye, since they retard wound healing and may enhance ulceration. If the corneal epithelium has not managed to spread over existing defects by the end of the fifth to seventh day after the injury, corticosteroids should be withheld or used with caution.

COMMENTS

Acid burns of the eyes are generally less severe than alkali burns. Since acids have less ability to penetrate, the overall prognosis in mild to moderate acid burns is good. The most important therapeutic measure is prompt and copious irrigation to dilute the offending agent.

References

Duke-Elder S (ed): System of Ophthalmology. St. Louis, CV Mosby, 1972, Vol XIV, pp 1055–1064.
Paton D, Goldberg MF: Management of Ocular Injuries. Philadelphia, WB Saunders, 1976, pp 163–171.
Ralph RA, Slansky HH: Therapy of chemical burns. Int Ophthalmol Clin 14:171–191, 1974.
Zagora E: Eye Injuries. Springfield, IL, Charles C Thomas, 1970, pp 290–307.

ALKALINE INJURY 940.9

ROSWELL R. PFISTER, M.D.

Birmingham, Alabama

Splash of an alkaline solution into the eye causes an immediate rise in the pH, resulting in damage and death of the external ocular tissues (corneal and conjunctival epithelium), the protective envelope (cornea and sclera), and the intraocular tissues (trabecular meshwork, iris, and ciliary body and lens). Alkalis rapidly penetrate cornea and sclera, causing saponification and lysis of cell membranes and denaturation of collagen. The severity of the burn is dependent on the anion concentration, the duration of exposure, and the pH of the solution. It is important to document exactly the degree of injury with respect to the extent of epithelial loss on cornea and conjunctiva, as well as the corneal stromal opac-

ity and perilimbal whitening. Accurate classification of the burn is the key to prognosis.

THERAPY

Ocular. The eyes should immediately be irrigated with copious volumes of an innocuous aqueous solution available at the scene of the injury and on the way to the hospital. Ocular irrigation with lactated Ringer's or other available intravenous solutions should be continued in the emergency facility for at least 2 hours or until the pH of the cul-de-sac is returned to neutrality. The intravenous tubing may be hand-held, or alternately, a scleral shell with an inflow tube (Mediflow lens) may provide a more efficient method to deliver fluid to the eye.

The sticky paste of lime (calcium hydroxide) may be removed from the conjunctiva with cotton-tipped applicators soaked in 0.01 M edentate calcium disodium.* Mydriasis and cycloplegia should be induced with 1 per cent atropine instillation twice a day. Antibiosis is effected by topical application of a broad spectrum of antibiotics four times a day as long as an epithelial defect persists. Analgesics and sedatives may be required for patients who sustain a severe burn.

The pressure rise occurring after the burn frequently responds to the oral administration of carbonic anhydrase inhibitors, such as 125 mg of acetazolamide four times a day, or topical 0.5 per cent timolol twice daily. Extensive burns of the palpebral conjunctiva or eyelid skin may cause lagophthalmos, a condition poorly tolerated by the burned cornea. In these cases, coverage of the affected eye with Saran wrap or a bubble provides a moist chamber to protect the cornea. Patching is only occasionally helpful in less severe burns, when the redevelopment of epithelial defects simulates recurrent corneal erosions. The persistence of corneal epithelial defects enhances the incidence of ulcerations and increases the likelihood of infection. Soft contact lenses may facilitate re-epithelialization by acting as a bandage to protect fresh epithelium from exposure to the air and by reducing the shearing stress of blinking. Disposable or extended wear soft contact lenses are preferred. The use of 0.5 N saline drops hourly and lubricants four times daily helps maintain adequate hydration and lens mobility. If the epithelium can be encouraged to re-cover the cornea, stromal healing is accelerated and the incidence of corneal ulceration is reduced.

In experimental animal studies, inhibitors of collagenase applied topically to the cornea reduced the incidence of corneal ulceration from 80 to 20 per cent. In extreme injuries acetylcysteine has not had any effect Although cysteine† and acetylcysteine* are both effective inhibitors of this enzyme, the latter is more desirable because of its stability, efficacy, and availability. Although it is suspected that 20 per cent acetylcysteine has a favorable effect in the human alkaline-burned cornea, this has not been proved by a clinical trial.

Early insertion of a methylmethacrylate ring designed to fit into the cul-de-sacs may prevent fibrinous adhesions and reduce subsequent fibrotic contracture of the conjunctiva. An alternate approach is to suture Saran wrap over the palpebral and fornix conjunctiva. Such treatments are not clearly advantageous, since it is not unusual for severely burned eyes to undergo total ankyloblepharon. Later lysis of these adhesions with or without mucous membrane grafts, insertion of a symblepharon ring, and placement of intermarginal lid adhesions can restore the cul-de-sacs, improve lid mobility, and reduce or eliminate corneal exposure.

Surgical. Animal studies by Grant have suggested that early paracentesis of the eye did not alter the outcome after an alkaline burn. However, the finding of a severely elevated pH in the aqueous humor of rabbits up to 2 hours after a 2 N sodium hydroxide burn seems to offer a compelling reason for removal of aqueous humor and reformation of the anterior chamber with a buffered solution. This procedure may be performed safely under topical anesthesia by an ophthalmologist. A No. 11 Bard-Parker blade is initially used to facilitate entry of a 27- or 30-gauge needle into the eye.

If an epithelial defect persists in a monocular injury, transplantation of limbal stem cells is indicated to stabilize and renew the corneal surface. Removal of the residual epithelium, peritomy and conjunctival recession, and, if necessary, superficial keratectomy prepare the recipient eye. Three conjunctival autographs from the uninjured eye are delineated with a wet field cautery 3 mm on a side and equally based around the limbus. The autographs are oriented the same way they were in the donor eye and are evenly spaced and sutured around the recipient limbus. This procedure is required before corneal transplantation if 5 mm or more of limbal epithelium has been lost 360°.

There is no medical way known to re-establish cornea clarity after a moderately severe, severe, or very severe alkaline injury. Extensive scarring and vascularization of the cornea, without other complications, are the best possible outcome. Corneal transplantation with fresh tissue may be considered no sooner than 12 to 18 months after injury. Such a transplant cannot survive without the normal blink mechanism and an adequate tear film. For this reason, operative procedures to lyse symblephera, expand cul-de-sacs, and eliminate lagophthalmos are often required to re-establish a more normal external anatomy and physiology before transplantation.

The success of transplants in alkaline-burned eyes is lower than usual (3 to 50 per cent) because of the high incidence of secondary glaucoma, immunologic rejections, and recurrent epithelial erosions. The necessity for cataract extractions and glaucoma filtering procedures in these eyes after multiple procedures often complicates management.

Ocular or Periocular Manifestations

Conjunctiva: Edema; ischemia; necrosis; scarring; symblepharon.

Cornea: Edema; infiltration; neovascularization; opacity; perforation; ulcer.

Eyelids: Lagophthalmos; scarring.

Iris or Ciliary Body: Chemical mydriasis; hypopyon; iridocyclitis; ischemic necrosis; phthisis bulbi.

Other: Cataract; secondary glaucoma.

PRECAUTIONS

Topical ophthalmic application of steroids after alkaline burns is extremely controversial. In mild or moderate ocular burns, the anti-inflammatory effects may be beneficial throughout the acute phase without enhancing the chance for corneal ulceration. The use of topical steroids in these cases, as well as the more severe burns, for the first 7 days after injury might decrease the inflammatory reaction of the entire anterior segment, possibly reducing some of the late side effects, such as glaucoma. The advantages of such treatment, however, must be weighed against the retardation of wound healing, a consequence of fibroblast inhibition. Topical steroids interfere with the repair process and result in corneal ulcerations and perforations when used for longer than 7 days after a severe injury. It seems most reasonable to avoid topical steroids if possible, but especially later than 7 to 10 days after the burn. The use of systemic steroids soon after the burn has certain theoretic advantages, but its efficacy is unproved.

COMMENTS

It may take 48 to 72 hours after the burn to correctly assess the degree of ocular damage and to offer an accurate prognosis. The basis of such an evaluation is the degree of corneal opacification and perilimbal whitening. If mild corneal epithelial erosion, faint anterior stromal haziness, and no ischemic necrosis of perilimbal conjunctiva or sclera are present, healing with little or no corneal scarring will result, and the visual loss will usually be no greater than 1 to 2 lines. When moderate corneal opacity and little or no significant ischemic necrosis of perilimbal conjunctiva result, the epithelium will slowly heal with moderate scarring and peripheral corneal vascularization, and a visual loss of 2 to 7 lines may occur. Moderate to severe damage following an alkaline burn is noted by corneal opacity, blurring iris details, and ischemic necrosis of conjunctiva limited to less than one-third of perilimbal conjunctiva. Corneal healing will be prolonged with significant corneal vascularization and scarring; the prognosis for visual acuity will usually be limited to 20/200 or less. Blurring of pupillary outline, ischemia of approximately one-third to two-thirds of perilimbal conjunctiva, and often marbleized cornea indicate severe damage. Very prolonged corneal healing with inflammation and a high incidence of corneal ulceration and perforation are common. In the best cases, severe corneal vascularization and scarring will result in counting-finger vision. When the pupil is not visible, greater than two-thirds of perilimbal conjunctiva is ischemic, and the cornea is completely marbleized, a very poor prognosis results. Corneal healing may be prolonged with frequent conversion of stroma into necrotic sequestrum and very severe corneal vascularization and scarring. Corneal ulceration and perforation are frequent. Phthisis bulbi may occur.

Promising new research focuses on orthomolecular approaches, including supplemental sodium ascorbate[‡] to stimulate collagen production from corneal fibroblasts and sodium citrate[‡] to inhibit the respiratory burst, enzyme release, and superoxide radical production from the invading polymorphonuclear leukocytes. A randomized clinical trial of sodium ascorbate and sodium citrate in the treatment of the alkaline burned eyes is currently in progress.

An alternative technique is to excise the fat from an internal lower lid approach. An incision is made through conjunctiva, Muller's muscle, and capsulopalpebral fascia just above the inferior fornix. Orbital fat is removed from the three lower lid pockets, and the conjunctiva is reapproximated with one to three sutures.

References

Donshik PC, et al: Effect of topical corticosteroids on ulceration in alkali-burned corneas. Arch Ophthalmol 96:2117–2120, 1978.

Kramer S: Late numerical grading of alkali burns to determine keratoplasty prognosis. Trans Am Ophthalmol Soc 81:97–106, 1983.

Paterson CA, Pfister RR, Levinson RA: Aqueous humor pH changes after experimental alkali burns. Am J Ophthalmol 79:414–419, 1975.

Pfister RR, Paterson CA: Ascorbic acid in the treatment of alkali burns of the eye. Ophthalmology 87:1050–1057, 1980.

Thoft RA: Conjunctival transplantation as an alternative to keratoplasty. Ophthalmology 86:1084–1092, 1979.

ELECTRICAL INJURY 940.1

F. T. FRAUNFELDER, M.D.

Portland, Oregon

Electrical injury occurs when an electric current passes through the body. The current may arc between an electrode and the body at voltages ranging from that of lightning, which may be 100 million volts, to as low as 380 volts. Contact with a conductor has also caused electrical burns at potentials less than 6 volts. However, significant ocular injuries have not occurred at potentials of less than 200 volts.

The size of the burn has minimal relationship to the long-term outcome. Small skin burns may cause severe multisystem injury, involving the cardiovascular, central nervous, and musculoskeletal systems as well. Extensive tissue necrosis and vascular injury can also result from small entry wounds.

The most common ocular injury from electricity seems to be opacity of the crystalline lens, which often appears after current flow through the head with the input either at or near the eye. The cataract formation is usually unilateral on the side proximal to the point of contact, but the contralateral eye may also be involved.

THERAPY

Supportive. Treatment for electrical burns includes relief of pain, strict asepsis and care of the wound, prevention or relief of shock, and control of infection. Analgesia is best provided by meperidine. The usual dose is 25 to 100 mg, which may be repeated every 3 to 4 hours as necessary. Some patients may need psychiatric support with tranquilizers.

Prophylactic treatment of a major burn wound should include an injection of 0.5 ml of absorbed tetanus toxoid to all patients who have not had a booster within the past year. In nonvaccinated subjects, immunization will be completed by two further injections at 4 to 6 weeks and then at 6 months.

Systemic. While dead tissue remains, bacterial activity is heightened, and while the wound remains open, bacterial invasion may occur. *Pseudomonas aeruginosa* and *Staphylococcus aureus* are the predominant organisms present in the majority of significant burn wound infections; streptococci and *Proteus* are less frequent. The administration of gentamicin is recommended for the treatment or prevention of burn infections. The usual daily dosage is 3 mg/kg given intravenously or intramuscularly in three divided doses.

Ocular. If the burn wound is around the eye, exposure is the most practical, efficient, and effective means of yielding a cool, dry, and clean wound environment. A topical antibacterial ointment, such as gentamicin, should generally be applied after an initial gentle cleansing with a dilute solution of soap and normal saline, rinsing-irrigation of the burned surface with saline, and gentle drying with sterile cotton-free gauze pads or lint-free sterile towels. Such gentle washing is done two to three times a day. Crust formation may be anticipated in the superficial injury, and crust separation and spontaneous healing may be completed within 2 to 4 weeks after injury. Eschar development, accompanied later by curling, cracking, and separation with thick drainage, occurs in deep wounds. At this point, exposure may need to be abandoned, and daily surgical débridements, washing, and dressing procedures should be instituted. Every 4 hours, the sterile cotton-free gauze dressing with topical antibiotics is changed to maintain free drainage of infected material and promote eschar separation. This process is continued until satisfactory granulation tissue is achieved.

Depending on the severity of the electrical injury, an attack of anterior uveitis may develop. Anterior uveitis may be treated by an application of 1 or 2 per cent atropine one to four times daily. Early and constant pupillary dilation lessens the likelihood of synechiae. One drop of 0.1 per cent dexamethasone may be applied two to four times daily in severe uveitis.

Surgical. If a cataract develops, lens extraction may be necessary. The same operative procedures as for nontraumatic cataracts of particular age groups apply to electrical cataracts.

A split-thickness skin graft may be necessary for achieving burn wound closure of the eyelids. The transplanted skin provides the essential epithelial cover for the granulating surface from which no spontaneous re-epithelialization is possible.

Ocular or Periocular Manifestations

Choroid: Atrophy; rupture.
Cornea: Cicatrization; necrosis; perforation.
Eyelids: Blepharospasm; burns; necrosis.
Lens: Anterior or posterior subcapsular cataract; anterior or posterior subcapsular vacuoles.
Optic Nerve: Atrophy; optic neuritis.
Retina: Attenuated arteries; cysts; dilation of retinal veins; edema; exudates; hemorrhages; holes; pigmentary degeneration.
Other: Anterior uveitis; hyphema; hypotony; increased intraocular pressure; night blindness; nystagmus; paralysis of extraocular muscles; photophobia; visual field defects; visual loss.

PRECAUTIONS

The best treatment for electrical injury to the eye is prevention; actual treatment is supportive and aimed at preventing infection and tissue loss. Surgical procedures are performed as indicated to restore the eye as nearly as possible to its original state.

COMMENTS

Initial changes in the formation of electrical cataracts are multiple vacuoles beneath the anterior chamber. These vacuoles are replaced by anterior subcapsular streaks in an irregular pattern. Scale-like gray opacities may appear in the subcapsular layers of the extreme anterior cortex. Vesicles and amorphous opacities, as well as crystalline formations, may also appear in the posterior subcapsular area. Although the lens changes may appear to resolve, they are generally progressive. The onset of cataracts may be almost immediate, or several years may elapse; the average time of onset is 2 to 6 months after injury. If only a few vacuoles are present in the anterior lens cortex within the first few postinjury weeks, there is a high probability that no significant cataract requiring surgery will occur.

Part of the injury may be heat-related as much as true electrical damage. Retinal damage is more likely to be a thermal injury unless the exit point of the electrical injury indicated that the electrical current passed through the posterior segment of the eye.

References

Alexandridis A, et al: Electrophysiological and CT findings in a case of optic neuropathy caused by lightning. Klin Monatsbl Augenheilkd 190:56–58, 1987.
Al Rabiah SM, et al: Electrical injury of the eye. Int Ophthalmol 11:31–40, 1987.
Andrews CJ, et al: Pathophysiology of lightning injury. In Andrews CJ, Cooper MA, Darveniza M, Mackerras D (eds): Lightning Injuries: Electrical, Medical, and Legal Aspects. Ann Arbor, CRC, 1992, pp 92–96.
Cooper MA, et al: Treatment of lightning injury. In Andrews CJ, Cooper MA, Darveniza M, Mackerras D (eds): Lightning Injuries: Electrical, Medical, and Legal Aspects. Ann Arbor, CRC, 1992, pp 130–132.
Gans M, Glaser JS: Homonymous hemianopia following electrical injury. J Clin Neuro-Ophthalmol 6:218–221, 1986.
Saffle JR, Crandall A, Warden GD: Cataracts: A long-term complication of electrical injury. J Trauma 25:17–21, 1985.
Van Johnson E, Kline LB, Skalka HW: Electrical cataracts: A case report and review of the literature. Ophthalmic Surg 18:283–285, 1987.

HYPOTHERMAL INJURY 991.6
(Cryoinjury, Frostbite)

F. W. FRAUNFELDER, M.D.,
and F. T. FRAUNFELDER, M.D.

Portland, Oregon

Localized frostbite results from exposure to extremely low temperatures, and the severity of injury depends on four factors: (1) duration of exposure, (2) actual temperature of exposure, (3) the degree of protection that one's circulation provides, and (4) individual tissue susceptibility. Clinically and pathologically, localized cold injury resembles heat injury although the treatment differs for the two entities. On initial presentation, the clinician can only evaluate the depth of an injury due to frostbite, and over the next few days, four degrees of severity can be used to categorize the insult to tissues. In first-degree frostbite, hyperemia and edema are present. Second-degree frostbite includes hyperemia and edema; in addition, large clear blisters may become extensive. In third-degree frostbite, along with hyperemia and edema the vesicles are filled with hemorrhagic fluid. These vesicles are usually smaller than those in second-degree frostbite. Fourth-degree frostbite includes necrosis and gangrene with loss of affected tissues.

THERAPY

Systemic. Ibuprofen, a prostaglandin inhibitor, and a topical antithromboxane agent, aloe vera, are used to prevent progressive tissue injury by cutting off production of these mediators that cause dermal ischemia. Tetanus prophylaxis is useful because frostbite is considered a *Clostridium tetani*-prone wound. Institution of prophylactic antibiotics is a questionable measure and should be reserved for specific infectious complications.

Cold injuries induce intense vasoconstrictive effects due to increased sympathetic tone. Intra-arterial drugs, such as tolazoline (Priscoline), or surgical sympathectomy may offset these vasospastic effects. Both of these measures can be started prophylactically in subjects whose occupation or cold sensitivity dictates a need.

Ocular. The eyelids have a rich vascular supply that helps protect the eye from cold injuries. The cornea, however, is avascular, and its forward position is the most exposed part of the eye. Corneal ulceration and epithelial desquamation have been reported in patients with hypothermal injury to the eye.

Prophylactic treatment in which measures are taken to protect the eye from the cold is most effective. Eye goggles and sunglasses, which filter out UV rays reflecting off snow, ice, or water, are important when exposure to the elements is anticipated. If mild injury occurs to the eyelids or around the eyes, simple techniques of rewarming include placing warm towels over the periocular area. In more severe cases, keratitis and corneal opacification may require management as outlined elsewhere for corneal erosion, ulcerations, and infections.

Supportive. For mild types of frostbite, simple rewarming of affected parts should suffice. For severe injuries, warming of body temperature is important before treatment of localized frostbite is undertaken. Rapid rewarming is the mainstay of treatment, preferably in a water bath at 39 to 42°C (102 to 108°F). This rewarming procedure should continue until the injured tissue has a flushed appearance signifying circulatory re-establishment. This whole process is uncomfortable for the patient and may require narcotics over the 35- to 45-minute period. After rewarming, the periocular tissues should be dried carefully and dressed with sterile dressing. Physiotherapy should be a daily measure to ensure the adequate debridement of wounds and blisters and to help maintain a sterile environment.

Ocular or Periocular Manifestations

Choroid or Retina: Atrophy; exudative posterior uveitis; hemorrhages; hyperpigmentation.

Conjunctiva or Cornea: Edema; endothelial damage; epithelial dysplasia; erosion; folds in Descemet's membrane; immune ring; neovascularization; subconjunctival hemorrhage.

Eyelids: Bullae; cicatrization; contracture deformity; depigmentation; discharge; ectropion; edema; hemorrhages; hyperemia; hypesthesia; madarosis; pseudoepitheliomatous hyperplasia.

Other: Anterior uveitis; iris atrophy; paresis of extraocular muscles.

PRECAUTIONS

Because hypothermal injury is, in most cases, preventable, advice to patients about prophylactic measures is of paramount importance. These measures include wearing warm, loose-fitting clothing and protective eyewear when exposure to cold is expected. In addition, counseling individuals on the vasospastic effects of nicotine in cigarettes is beneficial.

Cryotherapy actually attempts to induce a freeze and subsequent destruction of tissue. Patients undergoing this type of procedure should expect hyperemia, edema, bullae, eschar formation, and a serous or serosanguineous discharge over the course of the next few days. Patients should be advised that this process may occur and last approximately 2 weeks.

In cases of potential frostbite, field treatment should not include rubbing the extremities or increasing physical exertion to warm the individual. Cold extremities are more prone to mechanical injury than under normal circumstances. Also, rewarming techniques should be limited to controlled settings (i.e., the hospital emergency room) because refreezing is a definite risk.

COMMENTS

In most cases of hypothermal injury, no treatment is necessary, but the therapy can prevent loss of viable tissue, especially in the more severe degrees of frostbite. Ocular frostbite can result in corneal erosion and opacity, especially in cases where blinking is diminished.

References

Britt LD, Dascombe WH, Rodriguez A: New horizons in management of hypothermia and frostbite injury. Surg Clin North Am 71:345–370, 1991.

Edlich RF, Chang DE, Birk KA, Morgan RF, Tafel JA: Cold injuries. Compr Ther 15:13–21, 1989.

Fraunfelder FT, et al: The role of cryosurgery in external ocular and periocular disease. Trans Am Acad Ophthalmol Otolaryngol 83:713–724, 1977.

McCauley RL, Heggers JP, Robson MC: Frostbite. Methods to minimize tissue loss. Postgrad Med 88:73–77, 1990.

RADIATION 990
(Gamma Rays, X-rays, Infrared Waves, Microwaves, Radiowaves)

BUDD APPLETON, M.D.

St. Paul, Minnesota

The shortest wavelengths of electromagnetic radiation (gamma rays, x-rays, and short ultraviolet rays) possess very high photon energies (6 electron volts and greater). This level of photon energy is sufficient to cause ionization in biologic tissues; consequently, this range is referred to as ionizing radiation. The longest wavelengths (infrared, microwaves, and radiowaves) possess very low photon energies (1 electron volt and less) and are capable only of causing molecular agitation (heating). Therefore, they are considered to have only thermal effects in biologic tissues; these wavelengths are referred to as nonionizing radiation. Wavelengths lying in between (long ultraviolet and visible light) have photon energies that, although too weak to cause ionization, are capable of rupturing certain chemical bonds, so these wavelengths are referred to as photobiologically active.

Strongly ionizing radiations (gamma rays and x-rays) are well known for their ability to cause human cataract. Whether such cataract has a characteristic form is unclear. Early reports by ophthalmologists examining the eyes of atomic bomb survivors indicated that there was a "bivalve" configuration of the opacities. Recently, however, one ophthalmologist hypothesized that cataracts caused by ionizing radiation are morphologically no different from posterior subcapsular cataracts from other causes.

There is some evidence that the weakly ionizing short ultraviolet rays may play some role in the causation of human cataract, but little is known about thresholds or susceptibility, and the correlation is not dramatic. A similar generalization can be made about the role of ultraviolet radiation in the causation of lid cancers, although the evidence is much more convincing for this type of lesion.

Ionizing radiation usually has a latent period for biologic effects and can cause a variety of lesions in the eye, depending on the dose. Radiation retinopathy after therapeutic radiation of orbital malignancies has been reported. Atrophy of the meibomian glands and decreased lacrimal secretion have also been reported after irradiation, and localized poliosis has been observed.

Infrared radiation can cause thermal burns, for which there is no latency. However, there is some support for the concept of cumulation. Infrared has been implicated in a specific type of occupational cataract called "glassblower's cataract." This cataract starts in the posterior subcapsular region and is often associated with a splitting off of the anterior lamella of the anterior capsule, called true exfoliation (as distinguished from the syndrome of pseudoexfoliation). It is an unusual form of cataract and is said to be caused by many years of exposure to intense levels of infrared radiation for prolonged periods. Because workers subject to such occupational exposure are now required to wear protective eyewear with appropriate filtering lenses, this has now become a very rare disease.

The question of "microwave cataracts" has received much attention in recent years, especially in connection with allegations that human cataracts have resulted from microwave ovens and from radar. Although it is possible to cause cataracts in anesthetized rabbits and dogs using microwave energy at extremely high levels (hundreds of milliwatts per square centimeter) these cataracts seem to be exclusively thermal effects. By contrast, attempts to cause comparable effects in awake rhesus monkeys, using the same exposure levels, have been unsuccessful. As to microwave cataracts in humans, there is no valid evidence that this condition actually exists, and all the evidence to date indicates that it does not.

Longer wavelengths, including those in the short wave and long wavelength radio bands, seem to have no identifiable ocular effects. The ocular effects of visible light and a more detailed discussion of the ocular effects of ultraviolet light are covered separately under sections on solar retinopathy and ultraviolet radiation, respectively, by other authors.

THERAPY

Supportive. The best form of therapy for ocular injuries from energies in the electromagnetic spectrum is prevention. Despite the theoretical value of substances that might protect the lens and skin enzyme systems from radiation damage, there is not yet available "an ionizing radiation protection pill" for this purpose. In the case of occupational exposure to infrared, the use of infrared-absorbing lenses has become an occupational requirement. Treatment of thermal burns from infrared radiation exposure is described in the following section on thermal burns.

Surgical. The only known treatment of radiation cataract is surgical removal of the opaque lens.

Ocular or Periocular Manifestations

Conjunctiva: Cicatrization; hyperemia; symblepharon.

Cornea: Epithelial loss; keratoconjunctivitis sicca; necrosis; opacity; punctate keratitis; ulcer; vascularization.

Eyebrows or Eyelids: Blepharitis; carcinoma (?); depigmentation; ectropion; entropion; madarosis; poliosis.

Iris or Ciliary Body: Anterior uveitis; ciliary spasm.

Lacrimal System: Atrophy of lacrimal gland.

Lens: Cataracts; true exfoliation of lens capsule.

Orbit: Necrosis.

Retina: Burns; exudates; hemorrhages; macular degeneration; macular holes; neovascularization; vascular occlusion.

Other: Secondary glaucoma.

PRECAUTIONS

Without any doubt, the lens of the eye is one of the most radiosensitive tissues and therefore can be damaged by relatively low doses of conventional radiation. Other parts of the eye may also become injured as a result of inadequate protection during radiotherapy or by direct exposure after irradiation for intraocular malignancy and for lesions located adjacent to the eye. To avoid such complications, eliminating or at least minimizing radiation exposure of the eyes is of decisive importance.

COMMENTS

Because many of the radiation cataracts are situated near the posterior pole of the lens, the opacity has a very damaging effect on vision. Fortunately, since the ocular tissues are otherwise healthy, the postoperative results of cataract extraction are usually good.

References

Appleton B, et al: Microwave lens effects in humans. II. Results of five-year survey. Arch Ophthalmol 93:257–258, 1975.

Bagan SM, Hollenhorst RW: Radiation retinopathy after irradiation of intracranial lesions. Am J Ophthalmol 88:694–697, 1979.

Geeraets WJ: Radiation effects on the eye. Ind Med 39:441–450, 1970.

Karp LA, Streeten BW, Cogan DG: Radiation-induced atrophy of the Meibomian glands. Arch Ophthalmol 97:303–305, 1979.

Macfaul PA, Bedford MA: Ocular complications after therapeutic irradiation. Br J Ophthalmol 54: 237–247, 1970.

THERMAL BURNS 940.9

ARDEN H. WANDER, M.D.

Cincinnati, Ohio

The thermally burned patient may present a difficult and challenging management problem for the ophthalmologist. Although many seriously burned individuals with large, total body burns may initially escape direct damage to the globe, complications from the overall injury can have a devastating effect on the ocular system. Many severely burned patients may well escape direct injury to the cornea and conjunctiva because of the Bell's phenomenon and protection from the eyelids. On the other hand, many do suffer direct corneal and conjunctival injuries that may be thermal in nature from the flame itself or from hot gases. Some corneal injuries may also be toxic in nature from the combustion of toxic chemicals that are released when synthetic materials burn. Finally, severe corneal and ocular injuries may occur if hot liquids or molten metal explode into the eye. These more severe, direct ocular injuries behave much like toxic alkaline burns, with resultant avascular necrosis in some cases and symblepharon formation as well. These more severe, direct ocular injuries are managed similarly to those of toxic chemical injuries.

THERAPY

Supportive. It is imperative to analyze the extent of the ocular injury itself and assess the patient's overall condition and degree of the total body burn. The ophthalmologist must assume that the patient will survive the injury, no matter how severe it appears. Initial supportive therapy is directed at resuscitation. This includes maintenance of the airway, management of shock, and replacement of fluids.

Systemic. Severely burned victims are susceptible to endogenous endophthalmitis from bacterial or fungal septicemia. Hence, the fundi should be checked periodically, especially if blood cultures for fungus or bacteria are positive. *Candida albicans* is a common invader of the bloodstream in such patients because they are often on hyperalimentation, have many open areas, and often are on broad-spectrum antibiotics. Early detection of intraocular infection with *Candida* helps facilitate treatment of the ocular infection, as well as the potential meningitis and encephalitis that may develop. If the funduscopic examination is not possible because of tarsorrhaphies, B-scan ultrasound can be performed periodically if blood cultures become positive. Mucormycosis may also occur in these patients, especially when acidosis is present. One should be alert to this possibility if orbital cellulitis or proptosis occurs. Cultures and biopsy should be performed to make this diagnosis so that systemic therapy with amphotericin B can be initiated.

Ocular. With respect to the ocular injury, the major goal of therapy is to promote the re-epithelialization of the corneal and conjunctival epithelium and then maintain its health and integrity. To accomplish this goal, initial examination is important to determine the state of each eye. The eyelids may be swollen shut initially, but may be examined with the use of local anesthetics and Desmarres lid retractors, even when severe chemosis is present. The cornea should be evaluated with the application of fluorescein instilled into the conjunctival sac. Foreign bodies need to be removed. Gentle débridement of devitalized lid epithelium may be helpful. Assessment of the lid is very important because both ectropion and spastic entropion may occur. For spastic entropion, a soft bandage contact lens may be used to protect the cornea from the eyelashes until resolution of the edema and reassessment of the lid function are achieved. Thermal corneal and conjunctival burns may be pressure patched daily over antibiotic ointment until re-epithelialization is complete. If facial, brow, or eyelid burns are also present, pressure patching may not be possible. Bandage contact lenses may be used to promote epithelial healing in this situation. When the lids are swollen closed, the eye becomes in essence patched, which is helpful for a corneal burn that should be treated like a corneal abrasion.

First- and second-degree burns to the eyelids and face should be treated with a conservative approach with sterile wet compresses and antibiotic ointment. Third-degree burns to the eyelids will lead to cicatricial contractures of the lids and cicatricial ectropion. These conditions result in exposure keratitis, which by itself can lead to scarring of the cornea, as well as serious corneal infection. Such contractures are best treated with skin grafting after relaxing incisions are made to replace the lost tissue. In large severe burns, split-thickness grafting is recommended for this purpose.

If the total body burn is more than 50 to 60 per cent and mostly third degree, there may not be enough normal skin to allow initial eyelid skin grafting, since the burned area must be replaced with skin from the unburned areas. In such cases, a large, almost total tarsorrhaphy should be performed early, allowing healing time before the onset of contractures. It is wise to leave an opening of several millimeters at the medial aspect of each eye for examination and to allow cross-fixation for children who may be in the amblyopic age group. If contractures have already developed before tarsorrhaphy, sufficient relaxing incisions in the contracted tissue will allow the eyelid margins to come together without traction so that tarsorrhaphy may be performed successfully. Split-thickness skin grafts can be put into the tarsal bed thus created. If not enough skin is available from the patient to perform this lid grafting, time may be bought to allow the tarsorrhaphy to heal by placing either donor skin or pigskin into the tarsorrhaphy defect. Later, during the reconstructive phase of therapy, the tarsorrhaphies may be released as the eyelids are rebuilt. It must be emphasized that although the corneas may not be injured initially, serious third-degree burns of the face and eyelids in the presence of a large, total body burn can lead to severe cicatricial contractures and ectropion. Exposure keratitis can ensue if tarsorrhaphy is not performed. *Pseudomonas* or other bacteria, as well as fungus, on many of the burned areas may find their way to the exposed cornea and cause serious corneal infection. This infection may be prevented by the use of aggressive early tarsorrhaphies. Prophylactic antibiotics do not always prevent corneal infections in such a case. This is especially true when the patient is upside down on a rotating bed when minimal therapy can be given to the eyes. A good tarsorrhaphy will protect the corneas during this phase of the therapy in a severely burned patient.

During the initial assessment of the injury, associated ocular injuries, such as corneal lacerations and intraocular foreign bodies, must also be assessed and treated. This is especially true in explosive-type injuries.

For severe conjunctival burns caused by exploding liquids or molten metal, severe necrosis of the conjunctiva may occur. Local mucosal grafts may be applied in such cases, and the use of symblepharon rings may also help prevent symblepharon. These cases are similar to severe chemical burns, and the articles on acid burns and alkaline burns will provide further information on the management of such injuries.

Ocular or Periocular Manifestations

Conjunctiva: Avascular necrosis; chemosis; symblepharon.
Cornea: Avascular necrosis; cicatrization; exposure keratitis (secondary to ectropion); infection; lacerations and foreign bodies; ulcer (secondary to infection).
Eyelids: Avascular necrosis; cicatricial ectropion; contracture deformity; edema; spastic entropion.

Globe: Endophthalmitis; intraocular foreign bodies; proptosis.

Lacrimal System: Chronic epiphora; dacryocystitis; occlusion of the puncta.

Orbit: Cellulitis.

PRECAUTIONS

Scar tissue that may result from the burned cornea will not be prevented by corticosteroids. Furthermore, corticosteroids may delay the re-epithelization and increase the chance of secondary infection.

COMMENTS

In large, total body burns, the acute phase of the injuries requires frequent operations for débridement, as well as skin grafting. Until these patients are totally covered with skin, they are susceptible to infections both systemically and topically. The patients need very frequent follow-up care after the application of large tarsorrhaphies. Once tarsorrhaphies are healed, examinations may be less frequent, provided the blood cultures remain negative and signs of orbital cellulitis do not occur. When the entire burned area is covered, the reconstructive phase of therapy can begin. When reconstruction of the eyelids with skin grafting is successful, tarsorrhaphies may be released. Significant corneal

complications, such as *Pseudomonas* corneal ulcers, may be prevented by tarsorrhaphies; this technique is preferable to treating such an infection, especially in combination with lid retraction and exposure keratitis. For this reason, the need for adequate and early tarsorrhaphies to protect the corneas in the severely burned patient cannot be overemphasized.

References

Asch MJ, et al: Ocular complications associated with burns: Review of a five-year experience including 104 patients. J Trauma *11*:857–861, 1971.
Bloom SM, Gittinger JW Jr, Kazarian EL: Management of corneal contact thermal burns. Am J Ophthalmol *102*:536, 1986.
Deutsch TA, Feller DB: Paton and Goldberg's Management of Ocular Injuries, 2nd ed. Philadelphia, WB Saunders, 1985, pp 99–103.
Duke-Elder S (ed): System of Ophthalmology. St. Louis, CV Mosby, 1972, Vol XIV, pp 747–774.
Guy RJ, et al: Three-years' experience in a regional burn center with burns of the eyes and eyelids. Ophthalmic Surg *13*:383–386, 1982.
Huang TT, Blackwell SJ, Lewis SR: Burn injuries of the eyelids. Clin Plast Surg *5*:571–581, 1978.
Kaufman HE, Thomas EL: Prevention and treatment of symblepharon. Am J Ophthalmol *88*: 419–423, 1979.
Silver B (ed), et al: Ophthalmic Plastic Surgery, Rochester, NY, American Academy of Ophthalmology and Otolaryngology, 1977, pp 116–123.
Zagora E: Eye Injuries. Springfield, IL, Charles C Thomas, 1970.

Foreign Body

INTRAOCULAR FOREIGN BODY—COPPER* 871.6
(Chalcosis)

FLEMING D. WERTZ, M.D.,
and THOM S. THOMASSEN, M.D.

Washington, District of Columbia

The incidence of copper-containing intraocular foreign bodies has risen as a result of the increased use of nonmagnetic metal in industries, warfare, and recreation. The presence of an intraocular copper-containing foreign body can cause suppurative endophthalmitis, recurrent nongranulomatous inflammation, fibrous encapsulation, and dissemination of copper throughout the intraocular structures. The inflammatory response may be acute and suppurative or more chronic and less intense. Either the intensity or the chronicity of the inflammation can cause disorganization and atrophy of the ocular structures, resulting in

phthisis. However, not all eyes develop inflammation as a sequela of a copper intraocular foreign body. In those that do not develop inflammation, copper ions may be disseminated throughout the eye, particularly in the limiting membranes of the eye. The deposition of copper produces the clinical picture of chalcosis.

The influence of copper ion in the eye may be extensive. Copper ion participates in two basic processes. The first is a result of copper's tendency to be a reagent for and catalyst of oxidation-reduction reactions. Copper, which has a relatively low Redox potential, has the tendency to remove electrons from appropriate organic donors. An example of this is the oxidation of ascorbic acid by cuprous ion to produce hydrogen peroxide. In addition, copper participates in superoxide and hydrogen peroxide chemistry, resulting in the formation of superoxide and hydroxyl radicals. These attack polyunsaturated fatty acids, resulting in lipid peroxidation and the formation of alkoxy and peroxy radicals. This reaction may simultaneously lead to (1) the initiation of arachidonic acid metabolism that produces prostaglandins and leukotrienes resulting in inflammation, and (2) the incapac-

*The opinions contained herein are the private views of the authors and are not to be construed as official or as reflecting the views of the Department of the Army or the Department of Defense.

itation and death of cells resulting from the radicals' attack on lipid-containing membranes. The second process involves the complexing of critical enzymes with copper ion, which either displaces key molecules or distorts their stereo configuration, rendering them unable to participate in intracellular metabolism. An example of this process is copper's ability to inactivate carbonic anhydrase, producing a persistent reduction in ocular pressure as long as the copper ion is present.

Patients who retain small copper intraocular foreign bodies and do not have recurrent intraocular inflammation may have a relatively benign course. Several benign functional effects may be noted. These sequelae need not be permanent, as removal of the foreign body will be followed by clearing of copper from the ocular structures.

THERAPY

Ocular. The need to administer ocular therapy depends on the purity of the copper foreign body, its location in the eye, its size and shape, and the associated ocular damage. Alloyed copper foreign bodies in which the copper content is less than 85 per cent do not incite as severe an intraocular inflammatory response as those containing more than 85 per cent copper. The location of the foreign body is critical. If placed in the anterior midvitreous where the oxygen tension is low, it may not incite an inflammatory response. As the location moves progressively toward the ocular coat, the probability of a severe inflammatory response increases. Those foreign bodies adjacent to or in contact with the anterior or posterior segment structures induce an inflammatory or encapsulating fibrotic response in nearly all cases. Finally, the associated ocular damage may well direct the initial therapy. Eyes in which the anterior and posterior segments are disrupted require repair. Lensectomy and vitrectomy, as well as closure of a primary wound, may be required in addition to removal of the foreign body. However, if there is little in the way of ocular damage, the therapy may be directed solely at the presence of inflammation. As in the management of any trauma case, precautions are required to prevent endophthalmitis. These may range from cultures of the ocular fluids to the application of intraocular, periocular, and systemic antibiotics.

After primary repair, therapy should be directed at the copper-induced intraocular inflammation. Small visible shiny foreign bodies in the midvitreous may not induce an inflammatory response; therefore, these cases need not be treated. Systemic steroids, such as prednisone in the range of 60 to 100 mg per day, will suppress the general inflammatory response and inhibit migration of polymorphonuclear leukocytes. Periocular steroids have been shown to be effective in suppressing intraocular inflammation in general. Specifically, periocular injection of dexamethasone* has been shown to retard both inflammation and encapsulation.

Surgical. The therapeutic plan should be flexible. First, the steps necessary to ensure the short-term retention of the eye should be undertaken. Open wounds should be closed, and mixtures of lens, hemorrhage, and vitreous should be removed as the situation dictates. Depending on the location, size, and shape of the foreign body, it may be removed immediately. Further surgical procedures should be directed at repair of ocular damage (cataract, retinal detachment) or removal of the foreign body if serious sequelae follow. Accurate localization of the intraocular foreign body is now possible using the Berman locator, ultrasound devices, computed tomography, and x-ray localization techniques. After the appropriate preoperative maneuvers, bimanual vitrectomy techniques with modern instrumentation can be utilized to remove most intraocular foreign bodies safely.

Subsequent surgical intervention is undertaken if the surgeon judges that the foreign body is inciting a severe inflammatory response that if left unchecked could produce ocular destruction or the foreign body is producing functional impairment (decreased visual acuity, visual field changes, electrophysiologic changes) from the dissemination of copper within the ocular structure. If the foreign body is small and located in the midvitreous with little concomitant ocular damage, serial observation every 3 to 6 months with measurement of the visual acuity, color vision, intraocular pressure, visual field, and ERG may be all that is required. If there is intraocular dissemination of copper or the foreign body is inciting destructive or recurrent inflammation or is adjacent to the ocular coat, the foreign body should be removed by modern surgical techniques.

In those patients who are followed, the foreign body should be watched closely for corrosion or tarnishing of the surface and migration of the foreign body. One may be able to predict whether copper is being deposited in the eye from the appearance of the foreign body. Corrosion or tarnishing of its surface has been associated with an increased aqueous copper level and heavy generalized deposition of intraocular copper. In those eyes that harbor an encapsulated foreign body, softening of the capsule and migration or release of the foreign body from the capsule must be watched for and subsequent action taken.

Supportive. Either therapeutic plan—observation or surgery—may be associated with complications, and the patient should be counseled accordingly. The patient who is observed should be made aware that the potential exists for subsequent cataract, hypotony, uveitis, decreased visual function, and migration of the foreign body with subsequent acute inflammation or copper deposition. If the patient undergoes surgery, the procedure and its complications of cataract, aphakia, retinal breaks, retinal detachment, intraocular hemorrhage, and infection should be carefully explained. The patient should be made to feel like an integral part of the managing team, and that ultimately, the decision for enactment of any plan will rest with him or her.

Systemic. Experimental long-term penicillamine[‡] has been reported to be of some benefit in reducing the amount of copper deposited intraocularly. If treatment is undertaken, serum and urinary copper levels, renal function tests, and ceruloplasmin levels should be monitored carefully.

Ocular or Periocular Manifestations

Anterior Chamber: Cells and flare/hypopyon; hyphema; multitude of floating metallic particles.

Cornea: Deep stromal deposits; Kayser-Fleischer ring (usually superior and/or inferior but may be circumferential).

Globe: Endophthalmitis; phthisis bulbi.

Iris: Greenish tinge; poor response to mydriatics.

Lens: Brownish-red, small, round deposits on zonules; displacement; sunflower cataract; yellowish opacity (with intraocular lenticular copper foreign body).

Optic Nerve: Papillitis.

Retina: Copper-colored macular sheen; detachment; edema; gliosis; "gold-leaf" granular deposits in macula or adjacent vessels in the posterior pole; hemorrhages.

Sclera: Abscess; softening.

Vitreous: Abscess; fibrillar degeneration; greenish-brown or reddish-brown deposits; opacity; organization.

Other: Decreased visual acuity; encapsulation of foreign body with possible simulation of growing intraocular tumor with or without evidence of chalcosis; nonspecific color vision defect; ocular hypotension (secondary to possible carbonic anhydrase inhibition from metallosis); secondary glaucoma; subconjunctival foreign body from intraocular extrusion (rare); sympathetic ophthalmia (rare); variable disturbance in ERG amplitude; variable elevation in dark adaptometry rod and cone thresholds; variable isopter constriction in visual field testing.

Precautions

Those foreign bodies containing a high percentage of copper (usually greater than 85 per cent) often cause a severe suppurative response leading to phthisis bulbi, unless surgical intervention is performed swiftly. Less pure copper-containing foreign bodies can cause severe retinal toxicity if located near the wall of the eye, or they may become encapsulated and cease to be toxic. Encapsulated foreign bodies may migrate and produce a suppurative reaction long after the original injury. A pure or alloy copper foreign body may remain free of inflammation for an indefinite period if located anteriorly in the midvitreous. In such cases, a conservative policy of observation for macular changes and vitreous opacification is probably justified before attempting the difficult surgical removal of a nonmagnetic foreign body, with the possibility of eventual loss of vision as a direct result of the surgical maneuver. Even after the foreign body has been extracted, an intensification of the chalcosis may occur due to dissemination from microfragmentation of the particle. Use of penicillamine[‡] has yielded equivocal results, and if used, the patient must be observed for possible serious hematologic and renal adverse reactions. In diagnostic dilemmas, the presence of abnormal amounts of intraocular copper can be determined by diagnostic x-ray spectrometry, which may also prove advantageous over conventional electrophysiologic tests in the early detection of chalcosis.

Comments

The clinical course of chalcosis can be highly variable, being dependent on the copper content, as well as the location of the foreign body. Increased use of alloys as opposed to the pure form may make the chronic form of chalcosis more common in the future. In chronic chalcosis, inevitable blindness, as is the rule in siderosis, tends not to occur, owing to the fact that deposition of copper in the eye is primarily extracellular. However, the tendency is for gradual diminution of vision and for the clinical picture of chalcosis to occur over a period of months or years. Recent advances in surgical technique have made the removal of such foreign bodies less hazardous than in the past. Nonetheless, surgical removal of these nonmagnetic foreign bodies is difficult and potentially fraught with serious complications and is best left to surgeons experienced in the latest technique of their removal.

References

Gorodetsky R, et al: Noninvasive copper measurement in chalcosis. Comparison with electroretinography and ophthalmoscopy. Arch Ophthalmol 95:1059–1064, 1977.

McGahan MC, Bito LZ, Myers BM: The pathophysiology of the ocular microenvironment. II. Copper-induced ocular inflammation and hypotony. Exp Eye Res 42:595–605, 1986.

Mittag T: Role of oxygen radicals in ocular inflammation and cellular damage. Exp Eye Res 39:759–769, 1984.

Neubauer H: The Montgomery Lecture, 1979. Ocular metallosis. Trans Ophthal Soc UK 99:502–510, 1979.

Paton D, Goldberg MF: Management of Ocular Injuries. Philadelphia, WB Saunders, 1976, pp 134–137.

Peyman GA, Schulman JA: Intravitreal Surgery Principles and Practice. New York, Appleton-Century-Crofts, 1986, pp 239–278.

Rosenthal AR, Eckhert C: Copper and zinc in ophthalmology. *In* Karcioglu ZA, Sarper RM (eds): Zinc and Copper in Medicine. Springfield, IL, Charles C Thomas, 1980, pp 595–609.

Rosenthal AR, et al: Chalcosis: A study of natural history. Ophthalmology *86*:1956–1969, 1979.

Soyeux, A: Traitement de corps étrangers intraoculaires cuivriques par la D.-pénicillamine (dans deux cas avec 1 et 2 ans $^1/_2$ de recul). Bull Soc Ophthalmol Fr *80*:727–729, 1980.

Zeimer R, et al: Experimental chalcosis. A comparison between in vivo and in vitro findings. Arch Ophthalmol *96*:115–119, 1978.

INTRAOCULAR FOREIGN BODY—NONMAGNETIC CHEMICALLY INERT 871.6

JOSEPH E. ROBERTSON, JR., M.D.

Portland, Oregon

The evaluation of a patient with a suspected intraocular foreign body has three components. The first obligation is to evaluate the extent of ocular damage that is a direct result of the physical forces of the injury. The second responsibility is to determine whether an intraocular foreign body is present and, if so, to define its location. Finally, an assessment of the potential toxicity from the foreign body must be completed.

The initial evaluation of the globe is no different from those methods used for any ocular injury. Either the physical findings or more often the history may lead one to suspect that an intraocular foreign body is present. In some instances the foreign body may be visualized directly, and no ancillary studies are necessary. If visualization of any portion of the globe is obscured and a foreign body is suspected, then imaging studies must be undertaken.

X-rays of the globe and orbit are useful for screening purposes and will determine the presence of most metallic and many nonmetallic foreign bodies. Ultrasonography is extremely sensitive in locating foreign bodies, but requires a skilled examiner and special precaution if an open globe is suspected. An open globe does not necessarily preclude ultrasonography as stand-off techniques that transmit minimal or no pressure to the eye may be employed. When performing ultrasonography the examiner may slowly advance a strong magnet toward the globe to determine whether the foreign body is magnetic or nonmagnetic.

Computed tomography is atraumatic but relatively expensive and may actually fail to detect small foreign bodies, especially if they are nonmagnetic. Magnetic resonance imaging has been used in only a limited manner in this type of evaluation partly because of the concern about the potential for injury from a foreign body that unexpectedly proved to be magnetic. Sensitivity is probably greatest when ultrasound and CT studies are used together.

Once a foreign body has been discovered and localized, a preliminary assessment of its potential to cause toxic damage must be made. In most instances this determination can be made from the historical account of the events transpiring at the time of injury. If only a small piece of an object has entered the eye, then an analysis of the remaining object reveals its chemical composition.

Such materials as glass, lead, silicone, polymethyl methacrylate, and plastic are generally considered nonreactive. As a customary guideline if an item would be relatively undamaged from lying exposed to the weather for 5 years it is considered chemically nonreactive in the eye. Such substances as porcelain, silver, platinum, aluminum, stainless steel, tantalum, and pottery fragments are usually placed in this category.

THERAPY

Ocular. All open globes need to be closed. If a foreign body is nonreactive, does not interfere with the visual axis, and is not in a position to cause ongoing mechanical injury, then the most prudent course of management may be to leave such an object in the globe. If doubt persists and removal seems to be straight-forward, then surgical extraction of the foreign body at the time of primary closure is appropriate.

In addition to closure of open wounds, all patients with intraocular foreign bodies require evaluation of their tetanus immunization status, treatment of the accompanying traumatic uveitis, vigilant observation for the possible development of endophthalmitis, and an ongoing evaluation for possible late sequelae of their injury, including but not limited to cataract, retinal detachment, and unexpected toxicity from a foreign body previously considered to be inert. All patients with intraocular foreign bodies, even small ones, will have an accompanying uveitis. In all instances the uveitis should be treated with topical steroids and cycloplegics. Even though steroids may increase the risk of infection, the potential sequelae from the marked inflammation that accompanies these injuries mandate the use of such agents. Topical cycloplegics are also beneficial as they reduce vascular permeability, as well as place the ciliary body at rest.

Endophthalmitis is a constant threat during the initial period of follow-up. Topical prophylactic antibiotics are indicated for all patients. An agent providing gram-positive and gram-negative effectiveness is appropriate. The new broad-spectrum topical cephalosporins are preferred over chloramphenicol because of its risk of bone marrow suppression. Prophylactic intravitreal antibiotics are not routinely used but some authors feel that they are indicated if the wound is particularly dirty or the foreign body originated from the soil or in a farm environment. In this setting the antibiotic(s) selected for intravitreal use should specifically be effective against *Bacteroides fragilis.*

One must always be aware of the risks associated with intravitreal injection and that these intravitreal agents themselves are potentially toxic. Intravitreal injection must not be administered unless there is excellent visualization of the needle tip at all times during the procedure. A slow injection with the stream of fluid directed away from the macula is recommended. Increasing inflammation may be an indicator of incipient endophthalmitis. Fibrin, vitreous organization, and hypopyon are suggestive. The first posterior signs include a slight whitening of the retina and a subtle retinal vasculitis. Even though the actual incidence of endophthalmitis is low, the effects are often devastating. Therefore, a high index of suspicion must be maintained in all cases. This necessitates that cultures be taken at the time of primary closure. All foreign bodies that are removed from the globe should also be sent for culture and identification.

Surgical. Sound, basic principles of closure apply. If a decision is made to remove the foreign body, then the removal should be undertaken only under conditions that provide excellent visualization. The foreign body is grasped directly with the forceps and removed either through the original injury site or through a separate incision in the pars plana. Obviously great care must be exercised to avoid injury to other intraocular structures, such as the lens and the retina. If the foreign body is thought to be inert and there is any concern about causing further tissue damage during its attempted removal, then it should be left in place and the patient's status monitored carefully regarding toxic or mechanical damage. Removal is frequently easier during a secondary procedure when visualization is good and conditions for hemostasis have improved. Even so-called inert foreign bodies may become encapsulated when left in the globe. If secondary removal is eventually attempted, great care must be taken to ensure that the foreign body is dissected free from such encapsulating material before any attempt is made to withdraw it. Otherwise strong tractional forces may be transmitted to adjacent structures, and significant iatrogenic injury may occur.

PRECAUTIONS

These cases demand a combination of conservatism and vigilance. Because removal may entail high-risk surgery, early management should be biased toward leaving small inert foreign bodies alone. One must be aware that the label of inert is a tentative one until the foreign body has been observed for an extended period of time. Any contamination with wood or vegetative material is tolerated poorly. Chemical additives may make plastics reactive. In contrast, cilia that may be swept into the globe at the time of injury are often well tolerated. A foreign body that has not caused any reaction after several years may generally be considered as safe and inert. However, even these objects may cause some fibrous tissue proliferation with late contraction, resulting in such late complications as epimacular proliferation or retinal detachment. An eye not initially suspected of having a foreign body may harbor a small object over the ciliary body or pars plana where visualization is difficult. If this material should prove to be toxic, severe ocular injury or even blindness may result from what was initially felt to be a relatively minor injury. If the history provides any clue that a foreign body may be present, a complete foreign body evaluation with use of appropriate ancillary studies must be completed.

COMMENTS

The management of nonmagnetic chemically inert intraocular foreign bodies requires a complete and comprehensive evaluation, proper surgical closure of any open wounds, and long-term follow-up to monitor any late sequelae. Endophthalmitis can cause devastating destruction from a seemingly minor wound. A diagnosis of inert foreign body is always tentative until it has been observed for several years. One should temper any tendency to remove the intruding object with the realization that surgical intervention may cause greater damage than the natural course of leaving such a foreign body in the globe.

References

Duke-Elder S (ed): System of Ophthalmology. St. Louis, CV Mosby, 1972, Vol XIV, pp 459–460, 500–508.

Fisher YL: Advances in contact ophthalmic ultrasonography: Ocular trauma and intraocular foreign body patients. Dev Ophthalmol *18*:69–74, 1989.

Havener WH: Ocular Pharmacology, 5th ed. St. Louis, CV Mosby, 1983.

Havener WH, Gloeckner SL: Atlas of Diagnostic Techniques and Treatment of Intraocular Foreign Bodies. St. Louis, CV Mosby, 1969, pp 168–175.

Joondeph BC, Flynn HW Jr: Management of subretinal foreign bodies with a cannulated extrusion needle. Am J Ophthalmol *110*(3):250—253, Sep 15, 1990.

Williams DF, Mieler WF, Abrams GW: Intraocular foreign bodies in young people. Retina *10*(Suppl 1):S45–S49, 1990.

INTRAOCULAR FOREIGN BODY—STEEL OR IRON 871.5

(Siderosis)

DAVID W. JOHNSON, M.D.,
and PHILIP P. ELLIS, M.D.

Denver, Colorado

Penetrating ocular trauma often involves the presence of an intraocular foreign body. Steel or iron-containing fragments are the most common type of intraocular foreign bodies found in this setting. These particles may lodge in the anterior or posterior segment of the eye, are usually magnetic, and generally result from hammering metal-on-metal or machine injuries. Most foreign bodies are small and travel at a high rate of speed into the eye. Although hemorrhage, tissue disruption, and inflammation may occur, mechanical damage from the foreign body is usually limited. Retained iron foreign bodies may cause siderosis and ultimate blindness.

Siderosis may occur in nearly all ocular structures. It is the process of chronic intracellular damage resulting from electrolytic dissociation or oxidation of elemental iron to ferrous (Fe^{2+}) and ferric (Fe^{3+}) ions. These ions are toxic to intracytoplasmic enzyme systems, causing damage to vital cell function and structure. Ferritin deposits also are seen in the cell cytoplasm in phagosomes, which may rupture and release toxic products, thereby resulting in cell disruption. The degree of siderotic change in the eye depends upon the percentage of iron contained in the foreign body and its location. Intravitreal foreign bodies can produce siderotic changes, whereas some intraretinal foreign bodies may become encapsulated and functionally inert. Small intralenticular foreign bodies may not lead to cataract and can be retained on a long-term basis without sequelae.

Patients with an intraocular foreign body may present shortly after injury with an awareness of a fragment flying into the eye, foreign body sensation, or decreased vision. A scleral or corneal perforation may be apparent. Some patients may not be aware of the initial injury and may present weeks to months later with decreased vision and signs of siderosis. Anterior segment signs raising one's suspicion of an intraocular foreign body include scleral or corneal perforation with a positive Seidel's test, conjunctival laceration, hemorrhage or edema, hyphema, iris defect or transillumination, or lens disruption with or without cataract formation. Examination of the posterior segment may reveal vitreous strands or hemorrhage, air bubbles, retinal hemorrhage, inflammation or edema related to an impact site, or an encapsulated or visible foreign body. Retinal tears or detachment are rare initially. Chronic siderotic changes are listed below under ocular and periocular manifestations.

THERAPY

Surgical. Most iron-containing intraocular foreign bodies should be removed as soon as possible to eliminate the possibility of siderosis. In some instances, however, removal may be more dangerous to the eye than leaving the intraocular foreign body in place, and these cases can be managed conservatively.

The evaluation of a patient with a suspected intraocular foreign body should include a history of the circumstances of the injury, including the type of material involved. This history can help determine the extent of injury and influence the urgency and choice of management. Visual acuity measurement and examination of the fellow eye should not be overlooked. For patients with an anterior segment intraocular foreign body, slit-lamp examination is the most useful diagnostic technique since most anterior segment foreign bodies are visible directly. Intracorneal and intralenticular foreign bodies can be diagnosed in this manner. Occasionally, gonioscopy is useful in diagnosing a foreign body lodged in the anterior chamber angle. Radiologic studies may be helpful in selected cases.

The removal of an anterior segment intraocular foreign body usually is best accomplished with the patient under general anesthesia. If the foreign body is anterior to the lens, preoperative or intraoperative miotic therapy may help protect the lens. If a corneoscleral laceration is present, it should be repaired first to restore the integrity of the globe. The anterior segment intraocular foreign body should be approached through a limbal incision, either over the area of the foreign body or in a meridian 180° away. The anterior segment foreign body can be dislodged with a bent needle or a fine intraocular pick and can be removed with a 20-gauge rare earth magnet or 20-gauge fine intraocular forceps.

An intralenticular foreign body with cataract formation can be managed by extracapsular lens extraction, phacoemulsification, or intracapsular lens extraction. If the posterior capsule of the lens is ruptured, a mechanical anterior vitrectomy is recommended to eliminate the possibility of vitreous incarceration in the wound. The decision to implant an intraocular lens at the time of primary repair should be made on an individual basis with regard to other anatomic disruptions caused by the injury. Options for correction of the aphakic refractive error include posterior chamber intraocular lens implant in an intact capsular bag, scleral or iris suture-fixated posterior chamber intraocular lens, anterior chamber intraocular lens, contact lens correction, or later implantation of an intraocular lens.

Patients with a posterior segment intraocular foreign body can be evaluated best by indirect ophthalmoscopy. Timely examination is important since cataract formation or the spread of vitreous hemorrhage may obscure the view of the intraocular foreign body. If the media are opaque, ancillary studies can be helpful to determine the location of the foreign body. Ultrasonography can accurately detect and localize intraocular foreign bodies, but can be hazardous with an open globe. Computed tomography is the radiologic study of choice to image a metal intraocular foreign body. One disadvantage of the CT scan is a scattering artifact due to the presence of the metal intraocular foreign body, making precise localization difficult in some instances. Magnetic resonance imaging is contraindicated as it may cause a shift in position of a magnetic intraocular foreign body.

Posterior segment foreign bodies may be visible or obscured by media opacities, such as a vitreous hemorrhage. If a foreign body is visible and magnetic, it may be extracted by an external magnet. When the foreign body is intravitreal, the extraction should be made via the pars plana. If the foreign body is intraretinal and in an accessible location, a magnet extraction can be performed through a scleral "trapdoor" or direct cutdown. Extraction of an intraretinal foreign body by this method is often hazardous due to the possibility of retinal tear, incarceration, or hemorrhage. If a posterior segment foreign body is obscured by hemorrhage, is posterior in location, or is encapsulated, pars plana vitrectomy should precede the foreign body extraction, which may be accomplished using a variety of instruments including fine intraocular forceps, bent needles or blades, and a 20-gauge rare earth magnet.

In cases requiring pars plana vitrectomy, removal of the posterior hyaloid to prevent epiretinal membrane formation has been emphasized. Retinopexy around the impact site and the need for fluid-gas exchange in the absence of retinal detachment are controversial. Retinal tears associated with retinal detachment after foreign body extraction should be treated with scleral buckling and fluid-gas exchange with retinopexy. All cases of foreign body extraction requiring pars plana vitrectomy should receive a prophylactic scleral buckle to offset late vitreous base contraction and retinal tear formation.

Large intravitreal foreign bodies usually are associated with greater tissue disruption and a poorer prognosis. Extraction may be accomplished via a limbal incision after lensectomy has been performed. If corneal damage necessitates a penetrating keratoplasty, an open-sky vitrectomy with foreign body removal also can be effective.

Not all steel or iron-containing intraocular foreign bodies require removal. Intralenticular or encapsulated intraretinal foreign bodies may be observed and the patient followed for the onset of siderosis. The most sensitive clinical measure of siderotic change is the electroretinogram. Typical changes include a normal or supernormal a-wave initially, followed by a slow decrease in b-wave amplitude over time. The rod ERG seems to be the most affected and shows the most predictable decline over time. The b-to-a wave ratio is also useful when comparing responses to the fellow eye over time and multiple tests. Early receptor potentials remain normal, indicating that siderotic damage is largely confined to the inner retina until very late in the disease. Up to a 50 per cent reduction in b-wave amplitude is believed to be reversible with recovery after foreign body removal.

Systemic. Intravenous antibiotics are routinely given in the acute phase of management of patients with intraocular foreign bodies as prophylaxis against endophthalmitis. Broad-spectrum coverage with cephalosporin and aminoglycoside antibiotics is recommended. If endophthalmitis is suspected, clindamycin should be added to cover *Bacillus cereus*, which is estimated to cause 25 per cent of cases of trauma-related endophthalmitis. Intravitreal antibiotics generally are not used prophylactically, but are indicated when concurrent endophthalmitis is strongly suspected.

Deferoxamine* is an effective iron-chelating agent that has been used successfully in systemic iron-storage diseases. It combines with iron to form a stable chelate that prevents the iron from entering into further chemical reactions. The chelate is readily soluble in water and excreted in urine. The use of deferoxamine in ophthalmology has been controversial. Experimental evidence in animals has shown that subconjunctival deferoxamine causes a slowing of siderotic damage and a diminution of ERG changes with intravitreal iron foreign bodies. Systemic use in humans has been reported to improve rust discoloration and glaucoma associated with siderosis. The ability of systemic deferoxamine to reverse ERG changes in siderosis is doubtful. The usual systemic dose is 1 gm intramuscularly followed by 500 mg intramuscularly every 4 hours for two doses. Topical administration of a 10 per cent solution of deferoxamine* or a 5 per cent ointment formulation may improve superficial corneal iron deposits. Subconjunctival injections* of 0.5 ml of a 10 per cent solution two times a week for 8 to 10 weeks may improve deeper corneal, iris, or lens deposits.

Ocular or Periocular Manifestations

Anterior Chamber: Cells and flare; hypopyon.
Conjunctiva: Rusty discoloration; subconjunctival hemorrhages.
Cornea: Edema; Fleischer's ring; Hudson-Stähli line; interstitial keratitis; neovascularization; opacity.

Iris: Iridoplegia; rusty discoloration; synechiae; uveitis.

Lens: Brown discoloration; cataract and subanterior capsular deposits; luxation or subluxation.

Retina: Detachment; macular edema; pigmentary degeneration; rusty discoloration; arteriolar narrowing.

Other: Secondary glaucoma; syneresis; dyschromatopsia; night blindness; visual loss; phthisis bulbi.

PRECAUTIONS

With current surgical techniques, it is possible to safely remove the majority of steel intraocular foreign bodies, thereby preventing siderosis. Most intraocular foreign bodies should be removed emergently as soon as it is feasible to do so safely. The onset of siderotic damage can occur within a few weeks and may not be reversible after the intraocular foreign body removal.

A high index of suspicion for endophthalmitis must always be maintained when evaluating a patient with an intraocular foreign body. Foreign bodies may carry bacteria and fungi into the eye, as well as other foreign bodies, such as bone or eyelashes. Inflammatory reactions to intraocular foreign bodies can be intense and may mimic endophthalmitis.

Deferoxamine is contraindicated in patients with severe renal disease and should not be administered to women in early pregnancy because of possible teratogenic effects. The long-term use of deferoxamine for the treatment of iron-storage disease has been linked with the development of retrobulbar neuritis. This visual loss is usually reversible after the medication is discontinued.

COMMENTS

In industry, most of the foreign bodies that enter the eye are particles from highly tempered steel tools. These particles strike the eye with great force, accounting for the fact that 85 per cent of iron-containing intraocular foreign bodies are found in the posterior segment of the globe. Siderosis is not inevitable if the steel intraocular foreign body is retained. Different types of steel are not equally destructive, owing to their lower ferrous content. Occasionally, steel fragments remain in the posterior segment of the eye for months without the patient being aware of their presence until impaired vision forces them to seek medical advice. In other cases, encapsulated intraocular metallic foreign bodies that have long remained dormant may shift location and cause an inflammatory reaction resulting in hypopyon, plastic endophthalmitis, and atrophy of the globe.

References

Ambler JS, Meyers SM: Management of intraretinal metallic foreign bodies without retinopexy in the absence of retinal detachment. Ophthalmology 98:391–394, 1991.

DeBustros S: Posterior segment intraocular foreign bodies. *In* Shingleton BJ, Hersh PS, Kenyon KR (eds): Eye Trauma. St. Louis, CV Mosby, 1990.

DeClercq SS: Desferrioxamine in ocular siderosis: A long term electrophysiological evaluation. Br J Ophthalmol 64:626–629, 1980.

Gardner HB: Deferoxamine: Effects on intravitreal iron. Exp Eye Res 23:333–339, 1976.

Schechner R, Miller B, Merksamer E, Perlman I: A long term follow up of ocular siderosis: Quantitative assessment of the electroretinogram. Doc Ophthalmol 76:231–240, 1991.

Smiddy WE, Stark WJ: Anterior segment intraocular foreign bodies. *In* Shingleton BJ, Hersh PS, Kenyon KR (eds): Eye Trauma. St. Louis, CV Mosby, 1990, pp 331–347.

Sneed SR: Ocular siderosis. Arch Ophthalmol 106(7):997, 1988.

Sternberg P Jr: Trauma: Principles and techniques of treatment. *In* Ryan SJ (ed): Retina. St. Louis, CV Mosby, 1989.

Tawara A: Transformation and cytotoxicity of iron in siderosis bulbi. Invest Ophthalmol Vis Sci 27: 226–236, 1986.

ORBITAL IMPLANT EXTRUSION 996.59

MARK R. LEVINE, M.D.

Cleveland, Ohio

Loss of an eye from enucleation is emotionally traumatic. Subsequent extrusion of the orbital implant complicates the problem even more. Extrusions may occur early or many years after the initial implant. The causes of early extrusions are edema, infection, hemorrhage, too large an implant, and faulty surgical technique. Late extrusion occurs because of erosion of tissue covering the anterior surface of the implant from friction by a rough prosthesis. This erosion causes either (1) a secondary infection and extrusion or (2) epithelialization of the cavity around the implant and contraction of the orbital tissues that then result in extrusion. The most recent advance in orbital implant surgery is the hydroxyapatite implant. This rough surface spherical implant is a complex-calcium phosphate salt that promotes vascular ingrowth and therefore enhances motility. Once exposed, the blood supply within the implant supports tissue growth over the implant so that it is resurfaced with normal tissue and epithelium. A secondary implant is always desirable to maintain orbital volume, minimize supratarsal sulcus deformity, promote motility, and maximize cosmetic acceptability.

THERAPY

Surgical. For implant replacement after complete extrusion, the method of choice is immediate replacement with patching, unless the socket is infected. If the socket is infected, it is packed with antibiotic-impregnated gauze that is replaced often until the socket infection has been resolved, which may take 7 to 10 days. A secondary implant is then placed. The conjunctiva is dissected from the rest of the orbital contents, taking care not to injure the superior or inferior rectus muscles. A cavity may be present within the muscle cone if the extrusion occurred within 2 to 3 weeks of the implant; however, the extraocular muscles and Tenon's capsule will usually have retracted into a small fibrotic mass. A cavity is created in this mass by sharp dissection only in the oblique meridian to avoid severing the rectus muscle, which may or may not be visualized. Excision of scar tissue posteriorly or posterior dissection is carried out until Tenon's capsule and the muscles can stretch easily over the implant. For the patch itself, autogenous fascia lata femoris taken from the lateral thigh is wrapped around a 16- to 18-mm spherical implant and sutured together with 4-0 Vicryl. This adds 2 mm more to the 16- or 18-mm implant. Sutures of 4-0 double-armed Vicryl are placed in each of four quadrants of the fascia-enveloped sphere. The implant is placed in the socket, and the sutures are brought out from each socket quadrant between the rectus muscle and fixed externally. Doing so helps position the implant. Tenon's capsule posterior to the recti is sutured over the fascial ball with interrupted 5-0 Vicryl, taking bites of the fascia lata, creating a barrier, and centrally fixing the implant. The recti are gently approximated with 5-0 Vicryl suture, and the anterior Tenon's capsule is closed with 6-0 Vicryl suture. The conjunctiva is closed with a continuous locking 6-0 chromic catgut suture. A conformer is inserted that is of sufficient size so that the incision is under no tension. Two 4-0 silk suture tarsorrhaphies are performed. A pressure patch is then applied that is not removed for 3 days. If a hydroxyapatite implant is inserted, it too is wrapped in fascia lata or sclera. Multiple window defects made in the wrapped sphere combined with multiple small drill holes in the hydroxyapatite enhance vascular ingrowth and healing.

An alternate method is the use of a dermis fat graft that is obtained from the lateral thigh near the buttock. A dermatome is used to remove the epidermis, and the dermis fat graft is then fashioned to the appropriate size (25 mm by 25 mm) and placed into the orbital socket with the dermis facing anteriorly. The dermis is then sewn to the rectus muscles and Tenon's capsule. If there is sufficient conjunctiva, it may be closed over the dermis, but if conjunctiva is in short supply, the dermis may be left bare. The conjunctiva will migrate over the dermis in 4 to 6 weeks. The donor site is closed by using 5-0 Vicryl sutures to close the dermis and 5-0 nylon to close the skin.

The treatment of hydroxyapatite implant extrusions is inconclusive. It seems that small tissue defects of 2 to 3 mm will granulate in. Larger defects require a patch of sclera or fascia lata over the implant, which is sewn to Tenon's capsule and covered with a bipedicle conjunctival flap from the fornix.

PRECAUTIONS

Any implant not covered by conjunctiva will ultimately extrude if not repaired. Also, any oversized or irregularly placed implant is bound to extrude eventually. The exposure of an orbital implant should be repaired immediately unless it is a 2 to 3 mm defect over a hydroxyapatite implant. Generally, freshening the edges of conjunctiva and Tenon's capsule and resuturing them are only temporary measures in early extrusion. Autogenous fascia lata remains the safest and most convenient wrapping material, particularly with the increasing rise in AIDS.

COMMENTS

Implant extrusion is prevented by using basic surgical principles and good surgical technique. Meticulous hemostasis is essential to prevent hematoma formation and tension on the suture line. A well-positioned, centrally placed implant with layered closure (fascia lata, posterior Tenon, rectus muscle, anterior Tenon, and conjunctiva) will act as a barrier to early and late extrusion and will enhance motility and cosmesis. In the case of hydroxyapatite implants, a vaulted prosthesis will minimize friction between the prosthesis and the rough surface of the implant.

References

Buettner H, Bartley G: Tissue breakdown and exposure associated with orbital hydroxyapatite implants. Am J Ophthalmol 113:669–673, 1992.

Goldberg RA, Holds JB, Ebrahimpour J: Exposed hydroxyapatite orbital implant. Ophthalmology 99:824–830, 1992.

Levine MR: Extruding orbital implant: Prevention and treatment. Ann Ophthalmol 12:1384–1386, 1980.

Levine MR, Older JJ: Enucleation surgery and treatment of the extruding orbital implant. In Stewart WB, et al: Ophthalmic Plastic Surgery. A Manual Prepared for the Use of Graduates in Medicine, 4th ed., San Francisco, American Academy of Ophthalmology, 1983, pp 43–47.

Fractures

EXTERNAL ORBITAL FRACTURES 802.8

RICHARD D. LISMAN, M.D., F.A.C.S.,
and MARK H. WEINER, M.D.

New York, New York

External fractures of the orbit involve direct disjunction of any portion of the orbital rim and may also involve the walls of the orbit. Naso-orbital fractures are one of the most common external orbital fractures; these fractures of the medial aspect of the orbit commonly involve the lacrimal system. Trauma in this region usually includes the severance of the medial canthal tendon, which displaces and widens the medial canthus and severs the lacrimal excretory apparatus by direct laceration or bony fragments. As a consequence of damage to the medial canthal tendon, the lid margins may relax and evert the lacrimal punctum away from the globe. This results in epiphora caused by the abnormal evacuation of tears. A direct injury to the lacrimal sac or nasolacrimal duct caused by displaced bony fragments results in a more serious disturbance of the lacrimal outflow system. Repeated bouts of acute dacryocystitis often follow such injuries.

Orbital rim fractures commonly occur through bony suture lines. The zygomaticofrontal suture superolaterally and the zygomaticomaxillary suture infranasally are the weakest portions of the orbital rim. Fractures through these sites and the zygomatic arch produce a displaced zygoma, often referred to as a tripod fracture. Zygomatic fractures present clinically as a flattening of the malar prominence. Often, gaps or step deformities of the rim can be palpated easily. Separation at the zygomaticofrontal suture results in inferior displacement of the lateral canthal tendon. Separation at the zygomaticomaxillary suture can result in lower eyelid retraction as the orbital septum is pulled downward with the inferiorly displaced orbital rim. A depressed zygomatic arch may press on the coronoid process of the mandible, creating pain and problems with mastication. Zygomatic fractures are also frequently associated with infraorbital hypesthesias and orbital floor fractures.

Fractures to the supraorbital rim are usually seen with severe head trauma and accompanying cerebral injury. The orbital roof is quite thin and can be penetrated by any long sharp foreign bodies that pass through the upper eyelid avoiding the globe.

THERAPY

Supportive. External orbital fractures can occur in the setting of multiple injuries, and their evaluation remains secondary to management of more life-threatening injuries. Orbital roof and nasoorbital fractures are often associated with intracranial injuries and cerebrospinal fluid rhinorrhea, which require urgent neurosurgical evaluation. It is not unusual for external orbital fractures to be associated with severe injury to the globe. A complete ophthalmic examination should be performed promptly. Plain films and CT scanning with axial and coronal views are useful for localizing fracture sites, assessing the degree of displacement, and in surgical planning.

The only midfacial fractures that involve the orbit are LeFort II and LeFort III fractures. "Pure" LeFort fractures are rare in ophthalmologic practice. More commonly, they involve naso-orbital fractures, classically obtained during automobile accidents when the victim's face hits the dashboard of the car. Medial canthal deformities, lacrimal obstruction, and a widened interpalpebral distance are often repaired late. Zygomatic fractures are more easily repaired after resolution of the edema that occurs during the acute phase of the injury. Supportive therapy in all external orbital fractures should include broad-spectrum antibiotics.

Surgical. Only those fractures that produce cosmetic deformities or functional defects are explored and repaired. The more serious of the external orbital fractures are those involving the medial and lateral canthal regions. Fractures through these extremities of the orbit require a significant restoration of orbital contour, as well as functional components of the orbit. Repair of both medial canthal and lacrimal defects are performed through vertical or curvilinear skin incisions made over the frontal process of maxilla. The dissection is carried down through subcutaneous tissue and a periosteum. The periosteum should be raised from the bone with a small elevator along the medial orbital wall over the lacrimal groove and across the lamina papyracea. Bony fragments that protrude are resected; the lacrimal sac or its remnants are elevated and retracted laterally. If the medial orbital wall is excessively thickened by overlapping or malunion of bony fragments, it is thinned with a Hall drill to allow repositioning of the medial canthal structures. Next, the medial canthal tendon should be isolated and the lacrimal system reconstituted. Severed canaliculi may be repaired with silicone intubation and a nasolacrimal duct obstruction restored with a dacryocystorhinostomy. The medial canthal tendon should be reinserted at the level of the posterior lacrimal crest. Repair of the medial canthal tendon may require transnasal wiring or miniplate fixation.

Depressed zygomatic fractures with smooth

edges may be approached through a Gillies incision. The incision is made temporally, parallel and posterior to the hair line, and is carried down to the temporal fascia. The temporal muscle is exposed, and a surgical plane is dissected bluntly between the temporal fascia and the temporal muscle deep to it, usually with a Bristoe elevator. This elevator is pushed through this surgical space down to the overhanging bone of the zygoma, and minimal pressure is exerted on the temporal bone, lifting the fractured zygoma into place. This is usually performed as a bimanual procedure. The surgeon's hand is used over the zygoma to push the fractured bone up into position while the Bristoe elevator is used from beneath and above.

If there is significant displacement of the fracture or the fragments are comminuted, direct visualization and internal fixation are preferable. The zygomaticofrontal and zygomaticomaxillary fracture sites can be exposed with combined subciliary and superotemporal subbrow incisions. A more favorable cosmetic approach to these fracture sites is through a lateral canthotomy and transconjunctival approach. With reduction of the zygomatic fracture, a floor fracture may become evident and require attention. Reduction and internal fixation may be required only at the zygomaticofrontal fracture site. Internal fixation is best achieved with miniplates. After accurate reduction of the fracture, a miniplate is bent to conform to the curvature of the bone as it straddles the fracture site. Two drill holes are created on either side of the fracture. Stainless steel screws then result in rigid fixation, which resists rotation better than wiring.

Ocular or Periocular Manifestations

Extraocular Muscles or Eyelids: Displacement; downward displacement of the lateral canthus; ecchymosis; edema; laceration; ptosis; telecanthus.

Lacrimal System: Avulsion; dacryocystitis; epiphora; laceration; mucocele; obstruction.

Orbit: Cicatrization; damage of soft tissue; edema; enophthalmos; emphysema; exophthalmos; fracture; hemorrhages; step deformity of the inferior orbital rim.

PRECAUTIONS

Contusion and orbital hemorrhage may mimic orbital fracture. In these patients, careful observation frequently reveals marked improvement within a week. Failure to diagnose fractures that require early treatment may result in complications caused by fibrosis, con-

tracture, and malunion. The mere presence of an orbital fracture without a functional or cosmetic defect is not necessarily an indication for surgery. In many cases, a surgeon can be of greatest assistance to the patient by conservatively following the clinical findings to determine whether surgery may become necessary later.

COMMENTS

Orbital fractures are of particular interest to the ophthalmologist because of the frequency with which the eye and ocular adnexa are damaged. Fractures in the orbital region are unique; the bones are closely associated with many fragile anatomic structures. These areas of bone are subject to severe comminution. Orbital fractures are usually in close approximation to the paranasal sinuses, which compounds the clinical problems for the surgeon.

Solitary rim fractures may be plated if the cosmetic defect is significant. Exploration of an orbital roof with a communication superiorly should be performed in conjunction with a neurosurgeon.

References

Bedrossian EH, Della Rocca RC: Management of zygomaticomaxillary (tripod) fractures. *In* Smith BC (ed): Ophthalmic Plastic and Reconstructive Surgery. St. Louis, CV Mosby, 1987, pp 506–522.
Converse JM, Smith B: Naso-orbital fractures and traumatic deformities of the medial canthus. Plast Reconstr Surg 38:147–162, 1966.
Converse JM, Smith B, Lisman RD: Differential diagnosis and its influence on the treatment of orbital blow-out fractures. *In* Aston SJ, et al (eds): Third International Symposium of Plastic and Reconstructive Surgery of the Eye and Adnexa. Baltimore, Williams & Wilkins, 1982, pp 96–104.
Dortzbach RK, Soll DB, McCord CD: Orbital fractures. *In* Silver B (ed): Ophthalmic Plastic Surgery. Rochester, NY, American Academy of Ophthalmology and Otolaryngology, 1977, pp 177–194.
Freeman LN, Seiff SR, Aguilar GL, Rathbun JE, Sullivan JH: Self compression plates for orbital rim fractures. Ophthalmic Plast Reconstr Surg 7(3):198–207, 1991.
Jackson IT, Somers PC, Kjar JG: The use of champy miniplates for osteosynthesis in craniofacial deformities and trauma. Plast Reconstr Surg 77(5):729–736, 1986.
Nunery WR: Lateral canthal approach to repair of trimalar fractures of the zygoma. Ophthalmic Plast Reconstr Surg 1:175–183, 1985.
Smith B, Lisman RD: Blow-out fractures of the orbit. *In* Harley RD (ed): Pediatric Ophthalmology, 2nd ed. Philadelphia, WB Saunders, 1983, pp 388–395.
Smith B, Nightingale JD: Fractures of the orbit: Blow-out and naso-orbital fractures. Int Ophthalmol Clin 18:137–147, 1978.

INTERNAL ORBITAL FRACTURES 802.6
(Blowout Fractures)

RICHARD D. LISMAN, M.D., F.A.C.S.,
and STEPHEN SOLL, M.D.

New York, New York

An internal orbital fracture, commonly called a blowout fracture, involves the roof, floor, or walls of the orbit, but does not include an orbital rim fracture in isolation. Blowout fractures frequently occur as an isolated event, but they can be seen in conjunction with naso-orbital, zygomatic, or rim fractures. These fractures can be divided into "pure" blowout fractures, which involve only the internal orbital bony structure, and "impure" blowout fractures, which have associated rim fractures. As with any bony injury, fractures may be displaced, compounded, or telescoped. A keen understanding of the mechanism and theory underlying this unique type of fracture is important in predicting the outcome of the injury; further, a good understanding of the anatomy of this region is essential.

A "pure" blowout fracture can be produced when the orbit is struck by an object of greater diameter than the interior orbital bony dimension. Circular objects, such as a fist or a ball, of a dimension larger than the horizontal diameter of the anterior opening of the orbit are typical of the type of objects that can increase intraorbital pressure and produce fractures at the weakest point of the bony orbit.

The orbital rims are quite strong, but the walls of the orbit are mostly comprised of thin bones. The most common site of a blowout fracture is the ethmoidal plate or that part of the floor weakened by the infraorbital groove, which is directly in front of the inferior orbital fissure. If the fracture is located lateral to this groove, the muscles may not be affected. The medial wall is by far the thinnest of the orbital walls; fractures through the medial walls produce variable amounts of inflammation and hemorrhage. After such fractures, the possible sequelae are enophthalmos, cranial nerve dysfunction, ptosis, disruption of ocular motility, and superior sulcus deformities.

THERAPY

Supportive. Although the radiographic analysis is most important, it is secondary to clinical impressions. The Caldwell frontal view is most helpful in evaluation of margin walls, superior orbital fissure, sphenoid ridges, and temporal, ethmoidal, frontal and nasal fossae. The Waters' view shows the orbital floor and roof, the zygomatic bone, and temporal arch. The lateral view is used to interpret the anteroposterior relationships. Optic canal views (Rhese) may define optic canal contours and fractures. Localization of a fracture is enhanced by the use of serial tomography; however, this has been largely replaced by CT. In evaluating fractures by CT, both coronal and axial views are taken to evaluate fully the extent of injury. This is necessary, especially in the evaluation of medial orbital wall fractures that may extend to the optic canal. Occasionally radiographic studies do not confirm clinical findings of a blowout fracture, despite appropriate history and clinical examination. In such circumstances a so-called trap door fracture may have resulted. In this situation, the fractured bones have realigned themselves and in so doing have incarcerated tissue; namely, the inferior rectus and/or surrounding tissue.

Patients are managed by x-ray studies, repeated exophthalmometry, repeated diplopia fields, and repeated muscle measurements. Obviously, forced ductions play a significant role in the establishment of the diagnosis, and measurement of the interpalpebral distances can be a useful adjunct to exophthalmometry. All patients present with a variable amount of edema and ecchymosis, depending on soft tissue damage.

The management of blowout fractures is somewhat controversial. No two fractures are alike; the first 7 to 14 days after the fracture are usually spent in conservative management. All patients are symptomatic to some degree on initial presentation. Patients with persistent diplopia in primary position, which has not improved by direct diplopia field examinations, are also explored at that time. Patients with an increasing amount of enophthalmos over a period of 10 to 14 days fall into the same category. The most difficult patients to manage are those who have no diplopia, but have noticeable enophthalmos that has not improved during the initial 7 to 14 day period. The surgical possibilities should be presented to these patients so they understand that the enophthalmos will remain and possibly worsen without surgical intervention. It is further noted that surgery may produce the complication of diplopia, which is not present at initial presentation. Finally, "old" blowout fractures without diplopia, but with significant enophthalmos, are a most vexing problem. Bone is grafted to the orbital floor of these patients only after a guarded prognosis is given. Obviously, patients without diplopia or enophthalmos or those with improving diplopia or stable enophthalmos are not surgically explored. Patients with diplopia in upward gaze only are not subjected to surgery.

Surgical. Fracture reduction and plating of the inferior floor defects are done only within the above general guidelines. A subciliary or lateral canthal approach is cosmetically superior to incisions directly over the inferior orbital rim. A skin or skin-orbicularis flap is created in the fashion of a blepharoplasty. The inferior orbital rim is identified, and the periosteum is incised and elevated to explore the orbital floor. A hand-over-hand method is used to free the orbital contents from the defect and elevate the contents from the maxillary antrum. If necessary, the rim is mobilized and wired. The orbital floor can be restored with cartilage, bone graft, or inorganic implants. Gel film has been used for small defects; Teflon, Silastic, or supramid are preferred as implants. Additionally, rigid fixation of internal orbital fractures with such materials as titanium or vitallium alloy may be performed.

The inferior rectus muscle is identified, and forced ductions document that the inferior rectus muscle is free from entrapment. After the implant is placed, periosteum is closed; care is taken not to include the orbital septum in the skin closure. A modified Frost lid suture is used to prevent eyelid retraction; it is taped to the skin above the brow and removed after a few days.

Ocular or Periocular Manifestations

Extraocular Muscles: Pain; positive forced duction test; restriction of elevation and depression.
Eyelids: Hypesthesia; ptosis.
Globe: Enophthalmos; exophthalmos.
Orbit: Ecchymosis; edema; emphysema; pain; retro-orbital hemorrhage.
Pupil: Mydriasis.
Other: Decreased vision; diplopia; infraorbital anesthesia.

PRECAUTIONS

Visual acuity should be checked frequently during the postoperative period. Significant decreases in vision should be explored for evidence of postoperative hemorrhage into the orbit. Late permanent muscle imbalances are observed until measurements are consistent and stabilized for a period of at least 3 months. Surgery is advocated for muscles that control motility in the field of action of greatest deviation. Most often, the operation is performed on the sound eye.

Contraction of the inferior rectus is almost invariably responsible for limitation in the fields of monocular fixation. Retraction of the globe may occur when the patient looks upward. Resection of the antagonistic superior rectus in the presence of a fibrotic inferior rectus may create or augment the extent of the enophthalmos. Horizontal and vertical deviations are less troublesome than torsional deviations. Fortunately, most patients with persistent diplopia learn to cope by the acquisition of monocular suppression. Contracture of the extraocular muscles other than the inferior rectus or inferior oblique occurs less frequently. The anatomic relationship of the muscles near the floor of the orbit renders them more vulnerable to ischemic involvement.

If pseudoptosis is present, it is not treated until maximal muscle recovery has been obtained. Levator resection or tarsal shortening usually rectifies the residual lid problems. Severe enophthalmos requires orbital floor implantation; excellent results with bone grafting are obtained, even in seeing eyes. Mild enophthalmos can be cosmetically corrected with implants into the upper lids, such as scleral strips or collagen injections, to augment and create the appearance of a lid fold in an enophthalmic socket.

Although orbital hemorrhage is dreaded, a defect in the inferior floor remains with most floor implant procedures. This defect allows drainage through the maxillary antrum, leaving the orbit decompressed. Infection and allergy to the implant are rare. More common, though, is displacement or migration of the implant. Ectropion, entropion, or vertical shortening of the lower lid is possible. Muscle deviation may be improved or exacerbated by the surgery; visual disturbances are caused by the pressure to the plate upon the optic nerve or tissue in the apex of the orbit. Late complications include enophthalmos, pupillary abnormalities, blepharoptosis, ptosis of the globe, abnormalities of the interpalpebral fissure, sinus disease, lacrimal obstruction, and chronic lid edema.

COMMENTS

It has long been recognized that the inferior rectus muscle is quite fibrotic in some patients with "old" blowout fractures. An ischemic type of contraction has been postulated as responsible for this finding. This is similar to Volkmann's ischemic contracture, which orthopedic surgeons have long recognized. With some defects of the inferior orbital floor, not only is the inferior rectus muscle entrapped in the bony fragments and maxillary antrum but also hemorrhage and edema within the compartment of the inferior rectus muscle are responsible for the eventual infarction and fibrosis. Blowout fractures with large floor defects may produce a ptotic globe, but if the globe is well supported by the periorbita, diplopia may not be present.

Without entrapment of the inferior rectus, hemorrhage and edema apparently expand into the maxillary antrum. However, in small defects of the orbital floor, the osseofascial planes around the inferior rectus form a compartment. Edema and hemorrhage reside in this compartment, and pressure increases; this is similar to Volkmann's contractures in the small muscles of the hands or limbs. The vascular supply to the extraocular muscles is both from distal and proximal; these fine vessels can be occluded when the pressure in the inferior rectus "compartment" rises from 20 to 40 mm Hg. Normal and fibrotic inferior recti muscles have low compartment pressures, 0 to 2 mm Hg. In acute blowout fractures, pressure rises from 2 to 60 mm Hg. This is a useful adjunct to management of blowout fractures. There is a definite group of patients with minimal diplopia or enophthalmos and high inferior rectus pressures who should be explored within 7 days. This group with small floor defects is the one that may go on to inferior rectus fibrosis. Systematic steroids normally are indicated in this small group. Patients with small floor defects and high inferior rectus pressure are given 100 mg of systemic steroids daily for short duration.

Not every practitioner has the equipment to measure the pressure within the inferior rectus muscle sheath. However, systemic steroids are helpful in patients with small floor fractures and an excessive amount of edema and ecchymosis; the ophthalmologist should be wary of the possibility of compartment syndrome and resultant inferior rectus fibrosis.

References

Converse JM, Smith B: Enophthalmos and diplopia in fractures of the orbital floor. Br J Plast Surg 9: 265–274, 1957.

Converse JM, Smith B: Blowout fracture of the floor of the orbit. Trans Am Acad Ophthalmol Otolaryngol 64:676, 1960.

Converse JM, Smith B, Lisman RD: Differential diagnosis and its influence on the treatment of orbital blow-out fractures. In Aston SJ, et al (eds): Third International Symposium of Plastic and Reconstructive Surgery of the Eye and Adnexa. Baltimore, Williams & Wilkins, 1982, pp 96–104.

Lisman RD, Smith B, Rodgers R: Volkmann's ischemic contractures and blowout fractures. Adv Ophthalmol Plastic Reconstr Surg 7:117–131, 1988.

Nathog RH: Traumatic enophthalmos. In Smith BC (ed): Ophthalmic Plastic and Reconstructive Surgery. St. Louis, CV Mosby, 1987, pp 491–505.

Putterman AM, Smith BC, Lisman RD: Blowout fractures. In Smith BC (ed): Ophthalmic Plastic and Reconstructive Surgery. St. Louis, CV Mosby, 1987, pp 477–490.

Putterman AM, Stevens T, Urist MJ: Nonsurgical management of blow-out fractures of the orbital floor. Am J Ophthalmol 77:233–239, 1974.

Smith B, Lisman RD: Blow-out fractures of the orbit. In Harley RD: Pediatric Ophthalmology, 2nd ed. Philadelphia, WB Saunders, 1983, pp 388–395.

OPTIC FORAMEN FRACTURES 802.8

ROGER A. DAILEY, M.D.,
and PETER B. MARSH, M.D.

Portland, Oregon

Fractures of the optic foramen are usually seen in the context of a nonpenetrating blow to the head (usually frontal but occasionally temporal), with subsequent transfer of force to the optic canal and its contents. The optic nerve may be damaged directly by a displaced fracture within the foramen, but it can also be damaged in the absence of fracture by other mechanisms including hematoma and crush injury. Pial vessels supplying the optic nerve may be severed as the result of shearing forces. All of these mechanisms may result in edema formation, ischemia, and indirect traumatic optic neuropathy. Therefore, the absence of an optic foramen fracture seen on imaging studies does not rule out the diagnosis of traumatic optic neuropathy, nor does it lessen the severity of the diagnosis.

Traumatic optic neuropathy is most commonly seen in a young person who has suffered a closed head injury in a moving vehicle accident. Bicycle and motorcycle accidents are the most frequent causes of injury. The patient typically presents with loss of consciousness, making the diagnosis difficult. A conscious patient will complain of loss of vision in the eye ipsilateral to the head trauma. Ipsilateral epistaxis may also be present.

The clinical picture is important and will often suggest the diagnosis. In both unconscious and conscious patients, a relative afferent pupillary defect (Marcus Gunn pupil) may point to the diagnosis of traumatic optic neuropathy. Once the diagnosis is suspected, a complete ophthalmologic exam should be performed to rule out other causes of visual loss and a Marcus Gunn pupil (i.e., significant retinal injury). Plane films may reveal optic foramen or other orbital fractures. A direct coronal CT scan of the head and orbits using 1.5 or 2 mm cuts is currently the best imaging technique and may show fracture, perineural nor subperiosteal hematoma, or transsection of the optic nerve. Axial cuts with coronal reconstruction are satisfactory if direct coronals cannot be obtained. A normal appearing eye, both externally and funduscopically, is consistent with acute indirect injury to the optic nerve.

THERAPY

Treatment of optic foramen fractures in the setting of indirect traumatic optic neuropathy is controversial. The question is which treatment is appropriate for each clinical setting. Unfortunately, since optic nerve injury is relatively uncommon, there have been no large clinical trials. Current treatment options include giving intravenous steroids alone or in conjunction with optic canal decompression. It is estimated that between 30 and 50 per cent of patients will improve without any therapy. However, it is not currently possible to identify this group of patients.

The choice of therapy is dependent not so much on the presence of a fracture seen on imaging studies as it is on the clinical picture. Patients who have no light perception from the time of injury have a poor prognosis, and it is unlikely that any treatment will make a difference in their clinical course. Patients who have a delayed onset of visual loss or who lose vision on the withdrawal of steroids are thought to benefit from aggressive medical and surgical treatment.

Ocular. Optic nerve decompression may be performed by either transcranial or transethmoidal routes. Transcranial decompression has been the traditional technique, but requires a craniotomy and retraction of the frontal lobe. Transethmoidal decompression, although technically more difficult, seems to be gaining popularity. It is possible to perform transethmoidal decompression under local anesthesia, during which the medial wall of the optic canal is removed. Visualization of orbital structures is more difficult when this route is chosen.

We recommend the treatment plan first suggested by Spoor. Accordingly, every patient is first given a loading dose of methylprednisolone (30 mg/kg) followed by a 15 mg/kg dose 2 hours later and then 15 mg/kg every 6 hours. Conscious patients are checked for improvement in visual acuity and/or pupillary defect in 48 to 72 hours. If there is no improvement, the steroids are discontinued. If there is any improvement, steroids are continued for 5 days and then tapered rapidly. Any decline in visual acuity, visual field, or pupillary response on withdrawal of steroids warrants repeating a CT scan, restarting steroids, and considering decompression. The treatment of the unconscious patient is identical, except only the pupillary response can be followed clinically.

The presence of an optic foramen fracture may influence treatment in one clinical setting—when a patient has delayed loss of vision and an obvious foramen fracture impinging the optic nerve. In this setting, we recommend starting the above steroid protocol immediately, followed by surgical decompression as soon as possible.

Ocular or Periocular Manifestations

Extraocular Muscles: Paralysis secondary to third, fourth, or sixth nerve injury.

Optic Nerve: Usually normal early; swelling; hemorrhages; pallor; atrophy.
Pupil: Marcus Gunn pupil (relative afferent pupillary defect).
Other: Visual loss ipsilateral to trauma; scotoma; hemianopsia.

COMMENTS

The ideal treatment for traumatic optic neuropathy has yet to be determined. The presence or absence of an optic foramen fracture is less important in determining prognosis than is the clinical picture. Complete, immediate visual loss is a poor prognostic sign, and it is likely that any improvement seen after therapy in this setting would also have occurred in the absence of treatment as well. Nevertheless, intravenous steroids, by possibly reducing swelling in the injured tissue, preventing cell degeneration, and increasing blood supply to the affected area, might somehow improve outcome in these patients. Given the risks associated with optic nerve decompression, we feel it is only justified in patients with delayed loss of vision or visual deterioration on withdrawal of steroids.

References

Braughler JM, Hall ED: Current applications of "high dose" steroid therapy for CNS injury. J Neurosurg 62:806–810, 1985.
Joseph MP, Lessel S, Rizzo J, Momose KJ: Extracranial optic nerve decompression for traumatic optic neuropathy. Arch Ophthalmol 108:1091–1093, 1990.
Kline LB, Morawetz RB, Swaid SN: Indirect injury of the optic nerve. Neurosurgery 14:756–764, 1984.
Spoor TC, Hartel WC, Lensink DB, Wilkinson MJ: Treatment of traumatic optic neuropathy with corticosteroids. Am J Ophthalmol 110:665–669, 1990.
Spoor TC, Kwitko GM, Ramocki JM: Traumatic optic neuropathies. In Linberg JV (ed): Oculoplastic and Orbital Emergencies. Norwalk, CT, Appleton & Lange, 1990, pp 199–213.

Laceration, Tear, or Contusion

CHORIORETINAL CONCUSSIONS AND LACERATIONS 921.3

DAVID J. WILSON, M.D.

Portland, Oregon

A concussion is a condition that results from a violent shake or jar of a tissue; in the case of the eye, it usually results from the contact of some type of missile with the globe. A concussion may result in a contusion, an injury without rupture of the tissue, or it may result in a laceration, which is defined as a tear.

When a missile strikes the globe, the amount of damage that is done is dependent on the kinetic energy transferred to the globe. The kinetic energy is a function of the mass of the missile and the square of the velocity of the missile. The perturbations of the globe after missile impact have been described in four stages: compression, decompression, overshooting, and oscillation. During compression, the cornea indents and pushes the lens posteriorly. The anterior sclera expands to compensate for the decrease in volume caused by the corneal indentation. Decompression follows as the cornea or sclera pushes the missile outward. The equatorial diameters continue to expand, and the vitreous moves posteriorly. During compression and decompression, the combined effects of the expanding anterior and equatorial sclera and posterior movement of the lens and vitreous result in traction on the retina at the vitreous base. During overshooting, the anteroposterior diameter exceeds its original dimension, and the equatorial diameter decreases. A series of oscillations follow, during which the anteroposterior and equatorial diameters expand and contract periodically.

THERAPY

Surgical. Retinal tears are a well-known complication of concussive injuries. The most common type of tear is a retinal dialysis, which may occur anterior or posterior to the vitreous base. Also, large ragged retinal holes with pieces of necrotic retina in the adjacent vitreous may result from retinal necrosis at the site of severe retinal contusion. In addition, horseshoe tears may occur at sites of vitreous attachment, and macular holes may develop secondary to contrecoup forces. The treatment of retinal tears without detachment is cryopexy or laser photocoagulation. When an associated retinal detachment is also present, a retinal reattachment operation is indicated.

Choroidal damage following concussive injuries usually takes the form of subretinal hemorrhage or choroidal rupture. Choroidal ruptures appear as white curvilinear streaks concentric to the optic nerve head. They occur more commonly on the temporal side of the optic nerve head. If the choroidal rupture occurs directly beneath the fovea, the visual prognosis is poor. However, if the fovea is spared, central vision may be unaffected. There is no treatment for choroidal ruptures, but choroidal neovascular membranes can develop as a late complication of choroidal rupture. If recognized early, these membranes may be amenable to treatment with laser photocoagulation.

Ocular or Periocular Manifestations

Anterior Chamber: Hyphema.
Choroid: Hemorrhage; rupture.
Ciliary Body: Cyclodialysis.
Lens: Cataract.

Retina: Commotio retinae; dialysis; hemorrhage; tears.
Sclera: Laceration.
Vitreous: Detached vitreous base; hemorrhage.
Other: Decreased vision; pain.

PRECAUTIONS

At the time of the initial examination, care should be taken to document the full extent of the injury. If no initial treatment is required, the patient should be warned about the symptoms of possible late complications, such as retinal detachment and choroidal neovascular membranes.

COMMENTS

A thorough examination of both the injured and fellow eye should be accomplished to ascertain the extent of the injury. The initial visual acuity should be recorded, and appropriate x-rays, CT, or MRI scanning should be obtained to evaluate for associated orbital or head injuries and for intraocular foreign bodies. In the presence of vitreous hemorrhage, ultrasonography may be helpful in delineating the extent of the ocular damage. It is essential to determine if a scleral rupture is present; if this is suspected, an exploration of the globe and repair of the laceration should be performed.

The most common retinal injury after nonpenetrating blunt trauma is commotio retinae (Berlin's edema). The milky-white appearance of the retina in this condition has been shown experimentally to be caused by disruption of the photoreceptor outer segments. There is no treatment. RPE hyperplasia occurs in response to the disruption of the photoreceptor outer segments, which may result in a corpuscular intraretinal pigmentary pattern similar to that seen in retinitis pigmentosa. The visual prognosis after commotio retinae depends on the location and the extent of the photoreceptor outer segment regeneration.

References

Bloome MA, et al: Acute retinal necrosis. Ann Ophthalmol 11:723–728, 1979.
Cox MS, Stephens CI, Freeman HM: Retinal detachment due to ocular contusion. Arch Ophthalmol 76:678–685, 1966.
Delori F, Pomerantzeff O, Cox MS: Deformation of the globe under high speed impact: Its relation to contusion injuries. Invest Ophthalmol 8:290–301, 1969.
Kelley JS, Hoover RF, George T: Whiplash maculopathy. Arch Ophthalmol 96:834–835, 1978.
Russell SR, Olsen KR, Folk JC: Predictors of scleral rupture and the role of vitrectomy in severe blunt ocular trauma. Am J Ophthalmol 105:253–257, 1988.
Sipperley JO, Quigley HA, Gass JDM: Traumatic retinopathy in primates, the explanation of commotio retinae. Arch Ophthalmol 96:2267–2273, 1978.

CILIARY BODY CONCUSSIONS AND LACERATIONS 921.3

IGOR WESTRA, M.D.

Wilmington, North Carolina

Ciliary body concussions and lacerations are injuries that usually accompany damage to other structures of the eye. Mild blunt trauma may produce a transient iritis with cells and flare in the anterior chamber and anterior vitreous, as well as a relative hypotony. More severe blunt trauma may result in pupillary sphincter rupture, iridodialysis, angle recession, and cyclodialysis. Cyclodialysis is defined as separation of the ciliary body from the scleral spur and may be associated with hyphema, choroidal detachment, hypotony, and inflammation. Once the choroid is separated from the sclera, aqueous may drain into the suprachoroidal space and commonly results in profound hypotony. Prolonged hypotony may result in irreversible complications, including iris atrophy, angle-closure glaucoma, cataract, loss of retinal pigment epithelium from crests of choroidal folds, cystoid macular edema, optic atrophy, or phthisis bulbi. Decreased function of the ciliary body may also lead to difficulty with accommodation. Other late manifestations of blunt trauma include secondary glaucoma associated with major circumferential areas of angle recession. Extensive ciliary body injuries may involve necrosis of major portions of the pars plicata and lead to extensive fibrosis or atrophy. Massive fibrosis and organization of the vitreous may follow with subsequent retinal detachment.

Lacerations of the ciliary body usually result from perforations or penetrations of the cornea or anterior sclera. However, some penetrating objects that have their initial injury site through the skin of the lid at or even outside the orbital rim may bypass the conjunctival sac and produce scleral and uveal penetration more posteriorly. Penetrating injuries caused by small projectiles may create anterior as well as posterior lacerations. Indirect ophthalmoscopy, orbital x-rays, computed tomography scan, and ultrasound evaluation may be used to locate the foreign body.

THERAPY

Supportive. The ciliary body injured by blunt trauma should be protected from further injury by using a Fox shield. Topical cycloplegics, such as atropine 1 per cent twice per day or cyclopentolate 1 per cent four times per day, may be administered. Topical corticosteroids may be given two to six times per day to limit the inflammatory reaction. In the presence of hyphema, bedrest and administration of aminocaproic acid every 4 hours for 5 days decrease the occurrence of recurrent hemorrhage. Initial studies recommended a dose of 100 mg/kg of aminocaproic acid every 4 hours up to a maximum of 30 gm per day, but a substantial number of patients treated at this dosage develop nausea, vomiting, dizziness, and postural hypotension; reducing the dose to 50 mg/kg often reduces these side effects without reducing the therapeutic effect. Sedation and pain medication may be necessary for patient comfort.

Ocular. Eyes injured by blunt trauma require gonioscopic evaluation. When there is a hyphema present, the exam is carried out after it clears. If a hypotonous cyclodialysis cleft is suspected, use of the Goldmann three-mirror lens is recommended. If a cyclodialysis cleft is found, medical treatment with atropine 1 per cent twice a day for 2 to 6 weeks is used in an attempt to approximate the ciliary body and sclera. Unless a marked uveitis necessitates their use, corticosteroids are avoided because they inhibit the scarring necessary for cleft closure. Spontaneous closure seldom occurs after 6 weeks. Review of the literature suggests that reversal of hypotony by any means within 2 months results in best visual acuity. Delay in treatment results in loss of one to three Snellen lines of ultimate visual acuity.

If the ciliary body concussion has resulted in a shallow anterior chamber, a hypotonous cyclodialysis cleft is suspected. The chamber can be deepened by making a stab incision and infusing sodium hyaluronate intracamerally. In this situation, pilocarpine 2 per cent is first administered to maximize pupil constriction and open clefts. Then, under retrobulbar anesthesia, a stab incision is made at the limbus, sodium hyaluronate is injected through the incision, and the pressure is adjusted to between 10 and 20 mm Hg by releasing aqueous humor. The stab incision is then closed with a single 10-0 nylon. The angle can then be examined by gonioscopy, and argon laser photocoagulation can be performed. To avoid postoperative ocular hypertension, the anterior chamber is irrigated with balanced salt solution through the reopened limbal incision, and sodium hyaluronate is aspirated out through a second stab incision. These incisions are subsequently closed with 10-0 nylon taking care to bury the knots. A subconjunctival injection of an antibiotic such as cefuroxime 125 mg, should be given. Atropine 1 per cent, one drop twice a day, and an antibiotic drop, such as ciprofloxacin, one drop four times per day are given. Corticosteroids are avoided. In a few cases, hidden clefts may be found by injecting fluorescein into the anterior chamber and making sclerostomies over the ciliary body in all four quadrants. Detection of fluorescein in the suprachoroidal fluid confirms the presence of an occult cyclodialysis cleft. Immersion b-scan ultrasound may also be helpful.

Surgical. If medical treatment of the hypotonous cyclodialysis cleft has failed, laser treatment is administered. After expansion of the anterior chamber with sodium hyaluronate as described above, contiguous rows of argon laser burns causing bubble formation are delivered to the scleral surface. A Goldmann lens, 100 to 200 μm spot size, 0.1 second time setting, and high power settings of 2000 to 3000 mW are recommended. The uveal surface is also treated, but with a lower power setting of 1000 mW, which causes an intense blanching. In cases in which prelaser anterior chamber deepening is not required, retrobulbar anesthesia is recommended for patient comfort. Atropine 1 per cent drops twice a day are used for several weeks. Laser treatment is usually effective, but if several laser sessions have proved to be unsuccessful, surgery may be necessary. Techniques include ciliochoroidal diathermy, cycloplexy, cryoablation, and an anterior scleral buckling procedure.

When surgical repair of a ciliary body laceration is performed, cultures should be taken of the wound. Because the traumatized eye does not tolerate a cyclectomy well, ciliary body tissue is excised only if it is necrotic, severely traumatized, or grossly contaminated. If a cyclectomy is necessary, encircling transscleral diathermy may be indicated to decrease bleeding and subsequent ciliary body detachment. Meticulous reconstruction of corneal and scleral lacerations by microsurgical techniques should be undertaken as soon as possible after careful evaluation. The surgical goals are maintaining the contour of the eye and obtaining a liquid-tight seal. Loss of corneal or scleral tissue may require replacement with patch grafting. For corneal closure, 10-0 nylon sutures are used; 7-0 or 8-0 nonabsorbable sutures are preferred for scleral repair. Suturing of the ciliary body laceration is rarely indicated.

After primary repair of the lacerations, secondary repair may be necessary for the management of associated injuries, such as disrupted lens, vitreous hemorrhage, vitreous traction, retinal breaks, or retinal detachment. Although some authors feel that immediate vitrectomy is preferable, a 7- to 10-day interval allows for choroidal hemorrhages to recede, decreases the risk of intraoperative hemorrhage, and allows for spontaneous separation of the posterior hyaloid, which makes the procedure safer. Safety is also enhanced by preoperative ultrasound evaluation of eyes where the view of the posterior pole is limited. Delay of secondary repair past 2 weeks runs the risk of severe intraocular proliferative membranes. Vitrectomy is carried out under controlled conditions with an infusion line keeping the intraocular pressure constant and instrumentation that passes through 0.88 mm sclerostomies. Scleral buckling may be required for retinal pathology or is prophylactically placed by some surgeons. Postoperative medications consist of topical antibiotics, such as gentamicin or ciprofloxacin four times per day for 1 week, prednisolone acetate 1 per cent four times per day for several weeks depending on inflammation, and scopolamine 0.25 per cent twice a day for several weeks.

Ocular or Periocular Manifestations

Anterior Chamber: Angle recession; hyphema; shallow; Tyndall effect and cellular debris.
Choroid: Detachment; rupture; choroidal folds.
Ciliary body: Cyclodialysis cleft; hemorrhage or exudative detachment.
Iris: Atrophy; iridodialysis; sphincter rupture; uveitis.
Lens: Decreased accommodation; cataract.
Optic nerve: Papilledema; optic nerve atrophy.
Retina: Berlin's edema; dialysis; retinal hemorrhages; vitreous hemorrhage; macular edema.
Other: Hypotony; secondary glaucoma; phthisis bulbi.

PRECAUTIONS

When faced with a ciliary body laceration associated with a severely traumatized eye, the question of primary enucleation may arise. Primary enucleation of traumatized eyes should be avoided, especially if there is any visual function. Patients appreciate that everything possible has been done to save their eye. Often, traumatized eyes appear less gruesome and less hopeless after primary and secondary repair, and occasionally remarkable recoveries occur. Sympathetic ophthalmia is a remote possibility and probably should be discussed with the patient. If secondary repair has failed, enucleation can still be performed within the 2-week time period that is thought to be protective from sympathetic ophthalmia.

COMMENTS

Since concussions and lacerations of the ciliary body usually accompany injuries to other ocular structures, an exam that is as complete as possible should be carried out as promptly as feasible without exacerbating the injury. Delay in exam may allow hemorrhage and inflammation to obscure intraocular details. Ophthalmic ultrasound can be a valuable adjunct. Lacerations need immediate treatment, and hypotonous cyclodialysis clefts should be treated within a 2-month period. Patients with ciliary body injuries generally need long-term follow-up to watch for complications, such as cataract and angle recession resulting in glaucoma.

References

Kutner R, et al: Aminocaproic acid reduces the risk of secondary hemorrhage in patients with traumatic hyphema. Arch Ophthalmol 105:206–208, 1987.

Ormerod LD, Baerveldt G, Green RL: Cyclodialysis clefts: Natural history, assessment and management. *In* Weinstein GW (ed): Open-Angle Glaucoma. New York, Churchill Livingstone, 1986, pp 201–225.

Ormerod LD, Baerveldt G, Sunalp MA, Riekhof FT: Management of the hypotonous cyclodialysis cleft. Ophthalmology 98:1384–1393, 1991.

Palmer DJ, et al: A comparison of two-dose regimens of epsilon aminocaproic acid in the prevention and management of secondary traumatic hyphemas. Ophthalmology 93:102–108, 1986.

Read JE, Crouch ER: Trauma: Ruptures and bleeding. *In* Tasman W, Jaeger EA (eds): Clinical Ophthalmology. Philadelphia, JB Lippincott, 1992, Vol. 4, pp 1–18.

Sternberg P: Trauma: Principles and techniques of treatment. *In* Ryan SJ (ed): Retina. St. Louis, CV Mosby, 1989, pp 469–495.

CONJUNCTIVAL LACERATIONS AND CONTUSIONS 921.1

L.F. RICH, M.D., M.S.

Portland, Oregon

Traumatic injuries to the conjunctiva are usually not serious in themselves. However, they may mask an underlying ocular injury or retained foreign body. Puncture of the eyelid associated with a conjunctival laceration suggests the possibility of ocular penetration. Edema or hemorrhage may obscure the scleral or corneal entry site, so every conjunctival laceration must be explored for deeper trauma. Surgical evaluation may be done under topical or local anesthesia if the patient is cooperative. Careful dissection of conjunctiva and Tenon's capsule from the sclera will permit visualization of the sclera. Without direct visualization, vitreous, uveal, retinal, or even lens material may be overlooked beneath conjunctival edema and associated blood. Complications may occur if a conjunctival laceration contains an embedded foreign body that goes unnoticed. Such an occurrence may result in corneal erosion, tissue reactions, conjunctival cysts or granuloma, and membrane formation. Likewise, contusion injuries of the conjunctiva are seldom of major clinical importance. However, late sequelae from extensive necrosis may occur, including loss of fornices or changes in the tear film.

THERAPY

Supportive. Because conjunctival hemorrhage and chemosis following contusions are usually not serious, treatment requires only supportive therapy, such as ice packs to minimize swelling in the acute phase. Subconjunctival hemorrhage following contusive injuries may at times result in a chemosis so severe that the conjunctiva balloons out between the lids. In this situation, treatment does not relieve the edema, but may be directed at relief of discomfort. This distended conjunctiva should be covered with ointment or a plastic sheet until swelling subsides. At some point, the use of a muscle hook may allow an infolding of the conjunctiva into the fornices to a degree that will allow a pressure patch. Rarely is it necessary to attempt to find the source of hemorrhage.

In the case of conjunctival laceration, the wound should be examined carefully, usually under topical anesthesia, to determine the extent of injury and to search for retained foreign bodies. Any foreign bodies that are found and removed should be cultured for bacterial and fungal growth. Dental film is most useful for detecting nonmetallic foreign bodies. A Berman metal locator is also of value in selected instances. Prophylactic use of topical antibiotic solutions is advisable for all conjunctival lacerations.

Surgical. Surgical repair is rarely necessary if the laceration is less than 1 cm in length. If surgical reapproximation of a gaping wound is deemed necessary, interrupted or continuous 6-0 or 7-0 gut sutures are sufficient for this purpose. Careful attention should be given to reapproximation of lacerated conjunctival edges in order to exclude Tenon's capsule from the wound. If Tenon's fascia is included in a sutured conjunctival laceration, a chalky-white herniation will result. On rare occasions, extensive loss of conjunctiva may require a conjunctival graft from the fellow eye or a mucous membrane graft from the mouth. However, even injuries that have resulted in loss of a considerable amount of tissue can usually be closed satisfactorily because of the elasticity of the conjunctiva.

If tissue necrosis has resulted from a severe contusive injury, excision of the necrotic tissue will facilitate more rapid wound healing and will also decrease the possibility of infection.

Ocular or Periocular Manifestations

Conjunctiva: Chemosis; cicatrization; cysts; granulation; hemorrhages; hyperemia; keratinization; necrosis; nodules; pseudomembranous conjunctivitis.

PRECAUTIONS

In the exploration of conjunctival lacerations, care must be taken to eliminate any pressure on the globe, as it may cause the prolapse of intraocular contents through an unsuspected scleral penetration. If laceration of the globe is detected at the time of this exploration, it is desirable to proceed immediately with all necessary surgical repairs. A fracture of one of the paranasal sinuses allows air to be trapped within the conjunctival tissues, which can be diagnosed by crepitus, as well as a roentgenographic study. Fractures involving the ethmoidal sinuses are probably the most common cause of traumatic conjunctival emphysema. Care must be taken to ensure that any prolonged course of conjunctival edema is not associated with an infectious process, a retained subconjunctival or orbital foreign body, or even a scleral rupture.

Knowledge of the normal anatomy of the plica semilunaris and the caruncle is required to prevent an unsightly surgical repair. Traction on the plica by tight closure to inadequately mobilized bulbar conjunctiva may produce a disfiguring appearance of the eye caused by persistent redness of the conjunctiva. The implantation of conjunctival epithelium in the subconjunctival space may produce inclusion cyst formation.

COMMENTS

Most conjunctival wounds involve the bulbar conjunctiva in the interpalpebral zone. Less frequently, the superior and inferior palpebral areas are lacerated, and in these instances, painstaking inspection must be performed. These tears are commonly seen in association with lid lacerations or perforations, and meticulous examination of the underlying sclera and a thorough fundus examination are essential. The possibility of scleral perforation always exists in these cases, and proper management depends on an immediate and accurate diagnosis.

References

Norton AL, Green WR: Foreign bodies as a cause of conjunctival pseudomembrane formation. Br J Ophthalmol 55:312–316, 1971.
Paton D, Goldberg MF: Management of Ocular Injuries. Philadelphia, WB Saunders, 1976, pp 181–190.
Runyan TE: Concussive and Penetrating Injuries of the Globe and Optic Nerve. St. Louis, CV Mosby, 1975, pp 1–7.

CORNEAL ABRASIONS, CONTUSIONS, LACERATIONS, AND PERFORATIONS 871.4

ROGER L. HIATT, M.D.

Memphis, Tennessee

The most important corneal injury is an epithelial abrasion following a contusive force or a direct contact injury to the epithelium. It is associated with pain, lacrimation, blepharospasm, and photophobia. Concussive injuries involving the cornea may result in either localized or generalized edema. Folds may be present at the level of Bowman's or Descemet's membrane or both. A contusive injury of the cornea may result in multiple focal areas of corneal erosion associated with epithelial and endothelial edema but without observable stromal changes. Late recurrent corneal erosion may result and should be anticipated. If the blow is severe enough, hyphema may result from associated uveal tract injury.

Compression injuries are the most common corneal injuries associated with birth. Usually, the localized edema or corneal clouding disappears within a few hours. More severe trauma causes a residual astigmatism or even tears in Descemet's membrane running in a parallel fashion, usually vertical, across the posterior corneal surface. These tears may result in marked visual loss and persistent cloudiness because of the irregular refraction produced.

Superficially embedded bodies generally produce no lasting symptoms other than transient irritation. Corneal scarring results only when a foreign body has penetrated Bowman's membrane. A partial-thickness corneal laceration involving the stroma is frequently the result of a tangentially directed cutting force, such as a fingernail. If infection does not supervene and the laceration does not involve the visual axis, the only sequela is usually a minimal linear corneal scar. However, many severe complications may be associated with penetrating corneal lacerations, including loss of the anterior chamber, penetration of the lens capsule, cataract, vitreous hemorrhage, iris incarceration, uveal prolapse, epithelial or stromal ingrowth, corneal astigmatism, corneal opacities, and endophthalmitis.

THERAPY

Ocular. With any corneal abrasion or laceration, meticulous inspection of the eye for the presence of a foreign body is necessary. A topical anesthetic, such as 0.5 per cent proparacaine, may be needed for the examination but not for therapy. The cornea should be examined with a biomicroscope using oblique illumination. This exam should be attempted even in a child, but direct focal illumination with magnification obtained from a head loop may have to be substituted in some patients. A hand-held microscope and slit lamp are helpful in examining children. All damage to intraocular structures should be documented and treated promptly. Pressure should never be applied to the globe. Desmarres retractors, sterile bent paper clips, or a small wire speculum may be used to retract the lids. In a cooperative patient with severe blepharospasm, a modified lid block, such as that performed by the Atkinson's technique, may be necessary to facilitate examination and treatment. Foreign bodies should be removed with a moistened cotton-tipped applicator or a fine sterile hypodermic needle attached to a syringe. Foreign bodies embedded in the cornea should be removed with care so as not to disrupt the deeper layers of the cornea, thereby producing unnecessary scarring. If no foreign body can be found, fluorescein staining may locate an abrasion.

Treatment of a corneal abrasion consists of a topical broad-spectrum antibiotic ointment followed by firm patching for 24 to 48 hours, depending upon the size of the epithelial defect. If ocular discomfort or inflammation is significant, a drop of a cycloplegic, such as 2 per cent homatropine, will relieve ciliary spasm until the patient can be seen again the following day. Significant abrasions should always be re-examined within 24 to 48 hours to ensure that epithelium healing is complete and that no infection, iritis, or other complication develops. If a rust ring is present on re-examination, it may be removed with a fine needle or peeled from the cornea with fine forceps. Again, topical antibiotics and patching are applied. A central deep rust ring may be allowed to work its way to the surface until it extrudes spontaneously. Another alternative is to try to remove it with an electrically powered burr applied to the site of the rust ring with the aid of the slit lamp. This should be treated with antibiotic drops or ointments several times a day and followed at frequent intervals until the epithelium is healed completely. Antibiotic drops or ointments should be continued for several days after surface healing, as much for their lubricating properties as for their antibacterial properties.

Surgical. Partial-thickness corneal lacerations with well-apposed margins and no tendency toward gaping may be managed by placement of an ultra-thin bandage soft contact lens over the cornea. Antibiotic coverage and careful follow-up are essential. Full-thickness lacerations larger than 2 or 3 mm or irregular lacerations usually require direct suturing under a microscope. A leak can be detected by placing sterile fluorescein in the eye and observing the "water fall" under the slit lamp. General anesthesia is employed to obviate the necessity for retrobulbar injections, particularly if the laceration is large or possible expulsion of the internal contents is anticipated. After careful scrupulous cleaning of the skin and lids and copious irrigation of the fornices, any prolapsed uveal or lenticular tissue should be excised to free the wound margins. The wound should then be sutured with interrupted 10-0 silk or nylon sutures, avoiding placement of sutures across the visual axis and by burial of knots in the central cornea, if possible. Jagged irregular lacerations may occasionally be closed with 10-0 nylon sutures. An initial suture well placed in the center of the laceration stabilizes the wound so that less prolapse of eye contents will occur as the wound is sutured. After the wound has been sutured, the anterior chamber should be reformed by introducing saline between the sutures with a 30-gauge irrigating needle or through a paracentesis tract in the periphery and the cornea. If iris or lens material is adherent to the back of the wound, the injection of a large air bubble and a sweep of the anterior chamber with a very fine cyclodialysis spatula may be required. The spatula should be introduced through a paracentesis site usually placed across from the wound at right angles to the line of the laceration. The sutures should be left in place until wound healing is certain. In general, fine corneal sutures should be left for at least 2 to 3 months before being removed, particularly if the eye is quiet and uninflamed. The sutures should be removed only if they become loose, if the vessels bridge the wound, if they irritate the lid, or if the wound develops the characteristic scar of healing.

Extensive perforating injuries with avulsion or melting of tissue may require lamellar or penetrating keratoplasty. A blowout patch or modified keratoplasty may be required when other methods are contraindicated or the peripheral cornea or limbus is involved. The decision to remove traumatized iris at the same time must be made on an individual basis. Vitreous cutting instruments, such as the ocutome, should be available in such cases for use in the anterior segment. Systemic broad-spectrum antibiotics should be considered in all such wounds. Viscous material, such as sodium hyaluronate, should also be available to maintain the anterior chamber during repair. Secondary surgery may be required, such as in cataract formation and progression.

PRECAUTIONS

Topical corticosteroids should not be used in the eye with a corneal abrasion, since these medications allow for delayed wound healing and overgrowth of fungal and bacterial infections. Topical anesthetics should not be given to the patient suffering from corneal abrasion or a foreign body, since they can retard healing, aggravate the keratitis, and cause the patient to become dependent upon the drug.

No matter how severe or penetrating a corneal laceration, primary repair should be attempted. Enucleation should not be done until it is obvious that the eye will not have any function. A traumatic blind eye may have better appearance than the best prosthesis that can be fitted. However, primary enucleation is justified when the globe is totally disorganized, the retina has prolapsed, or other more severe signs exist.

COMMENTS

The sooner surgery is performed in patients with corneal lacerations, the better the chance of good recovery. Corneal wounds rapidly become edematous, making strict anatomic repair more difficult. Iris prolapse and lens damage result in an increasingly fibrinous reaction and inflammation, and scleral and uveal wounds may ooze blood into the vitreous. Chronic inflammation may further irritate and scar internal tissues.

References

Boruchoff SA: Corneal surgery. In Duane TD (ed): Clinical Ophthalmology. Hagerstown, MD, Harper & Row, 1982, Vol V, pp 6:1–10.

Duke-Elder S (ed): System of Ophthalmology. St. Louis, CV Mosby, 1972, Vol XIV, pp 313–321.

Paton D, Goldberg MF: Management of Ocular Injuries. Philadelphia, WB Saunders, 1976, pp 193–225.

Read JE: Trauma: Ruptures and bleeding. In Duane TD (ed): Clinical Ophthalmology. Hagerstown, MD, Harper & Row, 1982, Vol IV, pp 61:1–16.

Runyan TE: Concussive and Penetrating Injuries of the Globe and Optic Nerve. St. Louis, CV Mosby, 1975, pp 8–23.

Schlaegel TF Jr, Giles CL: Trauma: Inflammations. In Duane TD (ed): Clinical Ophthalmology. Hagerstown, MD, Harper & Row, 1982, Vol IV, pp 62: 1–4.

Stamper RL, et al: Glaucoma, Lens and Anterior Segment Trauma. Basic and Clinical Science Course, Section 8. San Francisco, American Academy of Ophthalmology, 1987–1988.

Wilson FM II, et al: External Disease and Cornea. Basic and Clinical Science Course, Section 7. San Francisco, American Academy of Ophthalmology, 1987–1988.

DETACHMENT OF DESCEMET'S MEMBRANE 371.33

(Stripping of Descemet's Membrane)

R. BRUCE WALLACE, III, M.D., F.A.C.S.

Alexandria, Louisiana

Fortunately, central corneal clarity is rarely affected by focal detachments of Descemet's membrane after anterior segment surgery. The most common clinical finding associated with this condition is transient localized corneal edema along the site of corneal entry after cataract surgery. Early work by Monroe (1971) showed an 11 per cent incidence of detached Descemet's membrane after cataract extraction as measured by gonioscopy. With normal healing, neighboring endothelial cells cover these defects and, over time, secrete a thin new layer of Descemet's membrane.

Modern cataract surgery has not eliminated Descemet's membrane detachment, yet smaller wound sizes may have reduced its incidence. Faulty wound construction and improper instrument manipulation are still recognized offenders. With phacoemulsification, tips are commonly inserted "bevel down" to reduce iris trauma. This maneuver can increase the risk of the phaco tip coming into contact with the edge of Descemet's membrane. Poorly tapered silicone sleeves around the tip may also contribute to this risk. Sutureless wounds dictate more anteriorly placed corneal entry sites, making Descemet's membrane even more vulnerable. Constant downsizing of wounds means less room for instrumentation and intraocular lens placement. Folding IOL injectors can traumatize wound sites if adequate space for their insertion is not provided. In most cases, this dissection of Descemet's membrane is so temporary and peripheral, especially if a temporal wound is made, that little if any harm results.

Possibly a greater threat is that of central endothelial trauma, which can be caused by a sudden thrust of a keratome when first entering the anterior chamber or by inadvertent anterior "hops" of intraocular instruments, such as the cystotome. Surgical separation of Descemet's membrane can also occur during or after keratoplasty procedures. Dull trephines and poor alignment of corneal scissors may introduce small detachments that can enlarge with postoperative stromal edema.

Site-threatening disruption of Descemet's membrane can also be associated with various types of corneal trauma, especially birth trauma with the use of delivery forceps. Due to the remarkable health of neonatal endothelium, these injuries can go undetected for many years.

THERAPY

Surgical. When severe detachments do occur, surgical repair can be a challenge. Descemet's membrane may not readily return to its original position after detachment principally due to the rather weak bonds that exist between this membrane and overlying stroma. Simple injections of air and/or viscoelastic agents can be beneficial if performed soon after detection. Viscoelastics should be used with caution, and careful monitoring of postoperative intraocular pressure is important in the early postoperative period. Suturing with interrupted 10-0 nylon may be necessary to maintain opposition for large detachments. Zusman et al. (1987) have reported the benefit of injecting sulfur hexafluoride gas into the anterior chamber for intractable cases. This method is advised only for those detachments that are not remedied with standard surgical methods, such as air injections or full-thickness corneal sutures. Sulfur hexafluoride gas does not expand, lasts longer than air and, in animal studies, shows the same endothelial toxicity as air.

COMMENTS

Improved surgical techniques and better instrumentation have helped reduce the incidence of Descemet's membrane detachments. The transient nature of most separations reduces the clinical significance of the majority of these cases. However, when these detachments seem to affect the central visual axis and visual acuity, careful inspection to determine the limits of the detachment is important. The surgeon must make certain that the etiology of the central keratopathy is a Descemet's detachment and not endothelial dysfunction related to other causes. Once this is ascertained, spontaneous reattachment and proper functioning of corneal endothelium may not occur. Timely surgical intervention may be necessary to restore corneal integrity.

References

Dowlut SM, Brunet M: Detachment of Descemet's membrane in cataract surgery. Can J Ophthalmol 15:122–124, 1980.

Makley TA Jr, Keates RH: Detachment of Descemet's membrane (an early complication of cataract surgery). Ophthalmic Surg 11:189–191, 1980.

Makley TA Jr, Keates RH: Detachment of Descemet's membrane with insertion of an intraocular lens. Ophthalmic Surg 11:492–494, 1980.

Monroe WM: Gonioscopy after cataract extraction. South Med J 64:1122–1124, 1971.

Waring GO, Laibson PR, Rodrigues M: Clinical and pathologic alterations of Descemet's membrane: With emphasis on endothelial metaplasia. Surv Ophthalmol 18:325–368, 1974.

Zusman NB, Waring GO, Najarian LV, et al: Sulfur hexafluoride gas in the repair of intractable Descemet's membrane detachment. Am J Ophthalmol 104:660, 1987.

EXTRAOCULAR MUSCLE LACERATIONS 871.4

EUGENE M. HELVESTON, M.D.

Indianapolis, Indiana

Laceration of an extraocular muscle without globe or eyelid involvement is rare; most injuries of this nature also involve adjacent structures. The inferior rectus muscle is the most frequently injured extraocular muscle. The rectus muscles are injured more frequently than the oblique muscles, probably because there is less protective anatomy separating the rectus muscles from the environment. In addition, when the eye is threatened, forced eyelid closure is accompanied by upward and usually outward movement of the eyes. This places the inferior and medial rectus muscles more anteriorly, causing them to be more prone to injury. The superior oblique may be lacerated along with the upper lid if it is avulsed by an object, such as a store display hook.

THERAPY

Surgical. Surgical treatment consists of reattachment of the lacerated ends of the muscles or tendon as soon as possible after exploration of the injury site. When a muscle is lacerated either at or near the insertion, the muscle capsule and attachment to the posterior Tenon's capsule prevent the muscle from retracting deeply into the orbit. If no muscle tissue can be found for reattachment to the insertion or cut end of the muscle, a muscle transfer may be indicated.

Full tendon transfer of the two adjacent rectus muscles may be done with retention of the anterior ciliary artery in the remaining rectus muscles. If any reason exists for concern about postoperative anterior segment ischemia, a muscle tendon splitting technique with the muscle bellies joined by a slip of proline-reinforced bank sclera might be indicated. If the passive duction test is restricted, disinsertion of the antagonist of the transected muscle, followed by a scleral augmented muscle transfer, should be done, even in a young patient. This allows retention of at least one anterior ciliary artery. Injection of 2.5 to 10 units of botulinum A toxin may be made at the myoneural junction of the antagonist muscle instead of carrying out a recession. Laceration of the superior oblique tendon may be treated as a superior oblique paralysis.

Ocular or Periocular Manifestations

Anterior Chamber: Abnormal angle; hyphema.
Conjunctiva: Chemosis; laceration; subconjunctival hemorrhages.
Cornea: Edema; opacity.
Extraocular Muscles: Paralysis of third or sixth nerve.
Eyelids: Blepharospasm; ecchymosis; edema.
Other: Blowout orbital fracture; cataract; diplopia; ocular pain; optic nerve or retinal hemorrhages; photophobia; strabismus.

PRECAUTIONS

Dilation of the pupil and meticulous examination of the globe are necessary to rule out associated injury to the globe. Determination of visual acuity and retinal examination should always be done. If foreign bodies or fractures are suspected, x-ray studies should be considered.

COMMENTS

One of the major problems facing an ophthalmologist in the diagnosis of extraocular muscle laceration is whether a muscle is lacerated or trauma to the nerve has occurred. A lacerated muscle requires immediate attention. On the other hand, trauma to the nerves may spontaneously recover with time. Patients who have normal binocular cooperation before extraocular muscle injury can withstand significant insult to motility and retain good fusion if alignment is re-established in a portion of the field.

References

Helveston EM: Atlas of Strabismus Surgery, 2nd ed. St. Louis, CV Mosby, 1977, p 96.
Helveston EM, Grossman RD: Extraocular muscle lacerations. Am J Ophthalmol 81:754–760, 1976.
Helveston EM, Merriam W, Ellis FD: Extraocular muscle-tendon transfer with scleral augmentation. Am J Ophthalmol 89:819–823, 1980.
Mailer CM: Avulsion of the inferior rectus. Can J Ophthalmol 9:262–266, 1974.

EYELID CONTUSIONS, LACERATIONS, AND AVULSIONS 870.8

ROBERT C. DELLA ROCCA, M.D., F.A.C.S.,
and JOHN NASSIF, M.D.

New York, New York

Eyelid contusions, lacerations, and avulsions associated with blunt or sharp trauma to the adnexa and orbital region may result in permanent and severe functional or structural abnormalities. Prompt evaluation, recognition, and treatment will allow for appropriate repair, satisfactory healing, renewed lid function, and ocular protection.

Lacerations or avulsion of the lids and canthi can lead to sequelae, such as lid malposition, severe scarring, lacrimal dysfunction, ptosis, and chronic ocular problems. Effective treatment may minimize these secondary problems. Definitive repair of traumatic ptosis, lacrimal obstruction, and motility problems can be delayed up to 6 to 12 months after injury because partial or complete resolution may occur during this period. If motility abnormalities or globe malposition is seen, an orbital floor fracture should be suspected and managed appropriately.

THERAPY

Supportive. A careful history determining the time, circumstances, and type of injury is first obtained. Associated injury to the globe must be suspected in all cases of eyelid trauma. Ocular evaluation is essential. Evaluation of visual acuity, pupillary reaction, motility status, intraocular pressure, slit-lamp microscopy, and ophthalmoscopy should be completed. Suspicion of an ocular or orbital foreign body should prompt evaluation with ultrasonography, radiography, and CT scanning. To rule out orbital fractures, orbital x-rays, including Waters' and intermediate views are done when periorbital and adnexal trauma is severe.

Although each wound is somewhat different, the application of a few basic principles of wound management is useful. Initially, attempts to alleviate pain, reduce swelling, and prevent drying of the wound should be made. Plain gauze moistened with saline is useful in preventing dryness of the wound; detergent solutions should be avoided.

With a relatively clean wound, débridement can be accomplished with irrigation, using copious amounts of saline. The heavily contaminated wound (with debris) may be cleaned with saline and perhaps a small brush. Foreign material should be removed from the wound. Irregularities at the wound margin should be smoothed. Doing so may require excision of a small amount of tissue and should be done judiciously when the laceration is near important structures, such as the lacrimal gland or canaliculi.

It is necessary to ask the patient or family when tetanus immunization was last received. Tetanus may occur even in patients with minor lesions, but is more common after contamination of deep wounds that contain devitalized tissue. The need for active immunization with tetanus toxoid or passive immunization with tetanus immune globulin is determined both by the patient's immunization history and nature of the wound. Except in individuals with three or more doses of recent tetanus immunization, tetanus toxoid is administered when the wound is cleaned and relatively minor. It is combined with tetanus immune globulin when the wound is severe. If it has been 5 years since the last immunization, tetanus toxoid should be given again after injury, even though the patient has received three or more doses of tetanus immunization in the past.

Human and animal bites that cause lacerations of the adnexa present special problems. Primary repair of the laceration or avulsion should be performed without delay, but only after thorough irrigation of the wound. Broad-spectrum antibiotics and tetanus prophylaxis should be administered. The local public health department should be consulted regarding the need for rabies prophylaxis.

Surgical. Surgical technique should include adequate subcutaneous closure, careful eversion of the skin edges, and good approximation of the wound margins. Tension at the wound surface should be avoided.

Whenever possible, primary repair is recommended. If significant bacterial contamination is evident, delayed primary repair is advised. In this instance, the wound is cleaned with forced saline irrigation, left open, and dressed. Three to four days later, surgical débridement and delayed primary repair are completed. If marked lid edema or facial swelling obscures the extent and details of the injury, delayed repair is considered. Secondary repair allowing for the formation of granulation tissue may be necessary when there is extensive tissue loss. Secondary reconstruction can be delayed if the globe is protected appropriately.

Partial-thickness lid lacerations are repaired with 6-0 silk or 6-0 nylon interrupted sutures. Rarely is it necessary to suture lacerated orbicularis muscle or orbital septum. Vertical traction near the lid margin should especially be avoided to limit the possibility of late ectropion.

Full-thickness lid lacerations through the margin require meticulous repair to prevent notching. First, the lid margin is repaired with three 6-0 silk sutures. The first suture is placed near the mucocutaneous junction to approximate the posterior aspect of the lid margin. The meibomian gland orifices can be used as an anatomic landmark for the placement of this suture. The second suture is placed anteriorly in the lash line. The third suture is placed centrally through the gray line. The tarsus is approximated with partial-thickness 5-0 absorbable sutures. The sutures are knotted anteriorly to prevent corneal irritation. The skin is closed with 6-0 silk sutures. The ends of the margin sutures should be tied in the knot of the first skin suture. The skin sutures are removed at 5 days, and the margin sutures after 10 to 14 days.

Although full-thickness tissue loss is uncommon, it may be simulated by edema and contraction of the wound margins. Direct closure can often be accomplished after a lateral canthotomy and cantholysis. Tissue loss involving more than one-third of the lid may require a temporal semicircular myocutaneous flap after cantholysis. Pedicle lid grafts (modified Hughes or Beard procedures) may be necessary if there has been more extensive loss of eyelid tissue. The modified Hughes and Beard procedures are used for reconstruction of the lower and upper lids, respectively.

Late contracture and secondary lid malposition of the lids after the repair of complicated lacerations can be avoided. With extensive lid lacerations, a temporary tarsorrhaphy or modified Frost suture passed through the involved lid margin for traction may be helpful in maintaining fornix depth while limiting lid retraction. The tarsorrhaphy or sutures may be left in place for 14 to 21 days as indicated.

If there is minimal postoperative wound elevation or irregularity, massaging the wound with a steroid ointment can be helpful. If scar hypertrophy or perhaps early keloid formation is detected, the use of intradermal steroids can be effective. When intralesional injection with steroids is indicated, triamcinolone is used (40 mg/ml for lesions involving the lids). For 5 mm of scar, 0.1 ml of steroid is injected with a tuberculin syringe. It may be necessary to repeat the injection up to five times, once every 3 to 4 weeks. Treatment of the scar should be uniform. Depigmentation is a complication of this treatment, and darkly pigmented individuals should be alerted to this possibility. The results of steroid injection, sometimes combined with surgical scar removal, can be rewarding.

Lacerations in the medial canthal region are repaired primarily with 5-0 nylon or silk sutures. Inferior traction on the medial aspect of the lid or commissure should be avoided. If this should develop, the use of full skin grafts from the upper lids or postauricular region is necessary. Subcutaneous cicatricial tissue must be excised before the graft can be sutured into position. A succession of Z-plasties is useful in treating scars that are away from the lid margin.

If the lid is avulsed medially, the avulsed portion should be attached to the deep limb of the medial canthal tendon or the periosteum with a 4-0 Polydek suture. If associated with a nasal fracture, stabilizing the lid position medially may require transnasal wiring or miniplate fixation.

Lacrimal sac or canalicular injury is suspected with severe eyelid contusions, lacerations, or avulsions that occur medially. After assessing the degree of injury and anatomic disruption, the lacrimal system is evaluated. Canalicular lacerations are repaired with the aid of a surgical microscope by monocanalicular or bicanalicular intubation. With monocanalicular intubation, the tubing is passed through the identified margins of the lacerated canaliculus and into the lacrimal sac. It is then fixed in position. Repair of the lid laceration is completed after the intubation has been completed.

Definitive repair of lacrimal sac obstruction secondary to trauma is delayed until at least 4 to 6 months after injury. Of course, the onset of recurrent acute dacryocystitis may require earlier repair. A dacryocystorhinostomy or perhaps conjunctival dacryocystorhinostomy may be necessary at that time.

If a laceration through the upper lid has involved the levator aponeurosis, immediate repair of the aponeurosis should be attempted. Careful separation of the anatomic layers and identification of the medial and lateral horns of the superior transverse (Whitnall's) ligament are helpful in completing this repair. If the patient with ptosis is evaluated several weeks after injury, delayed repair of ptosis is advised. It should be done at least 6 months after injury.

If there is extensive or deep tissue loss in the medial canthal region, advancement glabella flaps or combined advancement and rotation myocutaneous flaps are useful. If tissue loss extends down to bone, median frontal flaps are reasonably effective.

Laceration or avulsion of the lateral aspect of the lower lid may lead to severe ectropion and displacement of the lids. Restoration of lid position is contingent upon re-establishing lateral support. When the injury is extensive, it is very difficult to identify the torn lateral canthal tendon. A substitute tendon can be made by reflecting a tongue of periosteum from the zygoma at a level above the lateral commissure and attaching the lateral lid margin to the periosteum with 4-0 Polydek suture. The repaired lateral canthal angle may initially be higher than normal, allowing for some sagging within a few months.

The establishment of satisfactory medial and lateral canthal position is very important. This is a necessary step in the reconstruction process and will avoid such problems as ectropion, lid retraction, and possibly epiphora.

Ocular or Periocular Manifestations

Eyelids: Edema; lid malposition and globe exposure; scarring; traumatic ptosis.
Other: Keratoconjunctivitis sicca; lacrimal obstruction; orbital hemorrhage; restricted motility.

PRECAUTIONS

Careful suturing techniques with good wound approximation are of paramount importance in limiting unsatisfactory scarring and perhaps secondary lid deformities. Initially, sacrificing tissue should be avoided, although its vitality may be questionable.

Orbital compression secondary to hemorrhage must be treated promptly. A lateral canthotomy, allowing for some relaxation of the lids, may not be completely successful. If there is marked or resistant compression, a 1.5-cm incision extending laterally from the lateral commissure is made down to the periosteum.

The periosteum over the anterior aspect of the zygoma is incised vertically. An incision is made through the periorbita, and the retrobulbar hemorrhage and clot are evacuated.

COMMENTS

When significant injury to the lids has occurred, the extent of tissue loss should be determined first. Although avulsed lid tissue may be discolored and appear devitalized, it can usually be grafted back into the lid. Fortunately, adnexal circulation is excellent, thereby enhancing lid reconstruction even when the tissues have been traumatized severely. If avulsions or lacerations are extensive, the use of 4-0 silk sutures to fix tissue in proper position is helpful in an emergency room setting. The wound should be covered with a slightly moistened dressing (sterile saline) before definitive surgery is scheduled.

Protection of the globe, maintenance of tissue vitality, and re-establishment of lid function are important priorities. Further reconstructive and cosmetic procedures, such as skin grafting, scar revision, and ptosis repair, can be scheduled at a later date as indicated.

References

Chang WHJ: Wound management. *In* Chang WHJ (ed): Fundamentals of Plastic and Reconstructive Surgery. Baltimore, Williams & Wilkins, 1980, pp 9–63.

Linberg JV (ed): Oculoplastic and Orbital Emergencies. Norwalk, CT, Appleton & Lange, 1990, pp 1–14, 215–228.

Smith BC, et al (eds): Ophthalmic Plastic and Reconstructive Surgery. St. Louis, CV Mosby, 1987, pp 417–472.

Tessier P, et al: Symposium on Plastic Surgery in the Orbital Region. St. Louis, CV Mosby, 1976, pp 8–17, 39–78, 129–140.

Tessier P, et al: Plastic Surgery of the Orbit and Eyelids. New York, Masson, 1981, pp 328–362.

INDIRECT GLOBAL RUPTURES AND SHARP SCLERAL INJURIES 871.0

WILLIAM H. COLES, M.D., M.S.

Buffalo, New York

Indirect scleral rupture results from concussive injuries to the globe with subsequent tears in the ocular coats, usually the sclera. The presence of hyphema (especially if the blood has clotted), increased depth of the anterior chamber, and low intraocular pressure are important signs in the diagnosis of indirect scleral ruptures. Low intraocular pressure may be variable, and the presence of normal or high intraocular pressure does not rule out the possibility of a scleral rupture if other signs are present. Other important signs include limitation of gaze in the field of rupture near the rectus muscle insertion, which is a common site for rupture, and chemosis of the conjunctiva, which may be localized or generalized. This chemosis is fairly distinctive and is usually not associated with direct trauma to the conjunctival area. Ultrasound and CT scanning can help locate the site of rupture and degree of associated damage. With CT scans, signs of a flattening of the normal curved posterior globe, a thickened sclera, intraocular air, vitreous hemorrhage and opacification, or disruption of the scleral coat should be sought.

Direct scleral injuries are the result of penetrating injuries from a sharp or pointed object. Penetrating scleral wounds are usually accompanied by a history of trauma that the patient readily provides. Penetration of the globe by objects most commonly occurs anteriorly because the orbital bones protect posteriorly. Posterior penetrating injuries can occur from bones fractured in the surrounding orbit. Penetrating objects through the brow or lids or from gunshot wounds to the temple region may be responsible for posterior wounds.

THERAPY

Supportive. Immediate management of scleral injuries includes protection of the eye by a firm shield until repair is possible; tetanus protection if indicated; and systemic antibiotics, although the need for them is not proved.

Surgical. After the initial suturing, surgical therapy for blunt injuries with rupture usually requires a secondary procedure. The extent of retinal and choroidal damage is determined, and repair is undertaken if the prognosis indicates the need. If vitreous hemorrhage is present, aggravation of the fibrotic process may make surgery more urgent. These operations require vitrectomy instrumentation inserted through a pars plana approach.

Sharp penetrating injuries anterior to the equator are always repaired. In double perforating injuries with small posterior exit wounds, after suturing the anterior wounds, repair is frequently not necessary if the posterior wound is smaller than 2 to 3 mm. Scleral wounds are usually sutured with nonabsorbable sutures.

Systemic. Systemic steroids to delay reaction are used in injuries with high risk of complications from fibrotic contraction.

PRECAUTIONS

The most important precaution in both penetrating and blunt injury is recognition of the presence of hemorrhage as a poor prognostic factor. Hemorrhage is both a source of fibrosis and an aggravating influence on fibrosis in the posterior part of the eye. If this dense contracting fibrosis is not treated, it can cause total disruption of the structural integrity of the eye and eventual visual loss.

COMMENTS

Penetrating and blunt trauma with rupture of the globe can be a devastating process. In both types of injury, the initial insult is followed by a healing process. Excessive healing with destructive fibrosis may eventually cause loss of vision or the eye. Tracks from injury through the vitreous, for example, provide sources of fibroblast growth and a framework for subsequent organization. This process can be significantly established within a few weeks. If the vitreous is not removed sooner than 14 days postinjury, the technical aspects of removal become more difficult because of this progressive fibrosis.

Whether immediate or delayed vitrectomy is correct for penetrating injuries is controversial. In penetrating injuries where there is little associated contusive injury, immediate surgery can be done with few risks of complications. However, when a significant contusive injury has occurred, as in a blunt rupture or penetrating injury with a blunt foreign object, early surgery can be complicated by bleeding during the surgery. The vitreous detachment that will occur in these injuries after a few days can make removal of the vitreous technically easier, especially in younger patients. In these cases, waiting up to 10 days is advised before initiating surgery.

Injury in children can be more devastating than in adults. The fibrosis can be far more massive and develop more rapidly than in adults, and the risk of amblyopia is high. The need is urgent to establish the best visual stimulus for prevention of amblyopia. In children, aggressive therapy without delay is often indicated.

When a suspicion of rupture or penetration is present, operation to explore the globe may be indicated. Even with advanced imaging techniques, exploratory surgery is often needed. If a penetration or rupture is found, the possibility of a second noncontiguous site should not be ignored.

Surgical procedures on the globe may predispose the eye to rupture with less severe injury. Radial keratotomy, cataract, and corneal and glaucoma surgery all weaken the integrity of the globe.

References

Abrams GW, Topping TM, Machemer R: Vitrectomy for injury. The effect on intraocular proliferation following perforation of the posterior segment of the rabbit eye. Arch Ophthalmol 97: 743–748, 1979.

Cherry PMH: Indirect traumatic rupture of the globe. Arch Ophthalmol 96:252–256, 1978.

Cleary PE, Ryan SJ: Experimental posterior penetrating eye injury in the rabbit. II. Histology of wound, vitreous and retina. Br J Ophthalmol 63: 312–321, 1979.

Cleary PE, Ryan SJ: Vitrectomy in penetrating eye injury. Results of a controlled trial of vitrectomy in an experimental posterior penetrating eye injury in the rhesus monkey. Arch Ophthalmol 99: 287–292, 1981.

Coles WH, Haik GM: Vitrectomy in intraocular trauma. Its rationale and its indications and limitations. Arch Ophthalmol 87:621–628, 1972.

Conway BP, Michels RG: Vitrectomy techniques in the management of selected penetrating ocular injuries. Ophthalmology 85:560–583, 1978.

Kylstra JA: Management of suspected ocular laceration or rupture. Can J Ophthalmol 26:224–228, 1991.

Meredith TA, Gordon PA: Pars plana vitrectomy for severe penetrating injury with posterior segment involvement. Am J Ophthalmol 103:549–554, 1987.

Pilkerton AR, et al: Experimental vitreous fibroplasia following perforating ocular injuries. Arch Ophthalmol 97:1707–1709, 1979.

Russell SR, Olsen KR, Folk JC: Predictors of scleral rupture and the role of vitrectomy in severe blunt ocular trauma. Am J Ophthalmol 105:253–257, 1988.

IRIS LACERATIONS, 871.4 HOLES, AND IRIDODIALYSIS 364.76

HELLMUT F. NEUBAUER, M.D.

Cologne, West Germany

Iris lacerations, holes, and iridodialysis usually occur secondary to concussive or penetrating injuries. Although tears or holes in the stromal or interstitial tissues of the iris are frequent, they are often difficult to locate unless they are at least 1 mm in size and the defect includes the pigment epithelium. These tears or holes are usually of little clinical significance unless they are of considerable size. If bleeding should occur in conjunction with the tear, it is often minimal and self-limited. Wounds in the iris form fibrous tissue slowly after trauma; therefore, healing is minimal and occurs primarily when the wound margins are in apposition. Tears or lacerations in the pupillary zone most commonly involve the sphincter, stromal, and pigmented epithelial layers. If only the stromal layer is torn, no permanent pupillary dysfunction will result, and only a few residual iris frills or tags will be detected. However, if the sphincter is involved, a characteristic triangular defect will be seen, with the apex toward the periphery. The pupil is typically irregular, is dilated or semidilated, and has abnormal sphincter reactions to stimulation. The portion of the sphincter not involved in the laceration functions normally. Hyphema may be associated with a tear of the sphincter, but if this is the sole origin of bleeding, it usually causes no major problems. A flattened or misshapen pupil results from iridodialysis. Severe hemorrhages may be associated with iridodialysis, resulting from tears in the iris feeder vessels, which cross this zone in a radial fashion, or from extension of the laceration into the ciliary body. Iridodialysis may be small and slit-like or large, and single or multiple. Areas of iris atrophy may accompany these tears.

THERAPY

Supportive. Rest and observation are preliminary measures in patients with iridodialysis. The iridodialysis itself seldom requires treatment, unless the dialysis is of sufficient size to cause visual confusion owing to the irregular diffusion of light or unless the dialysis, acting as a second pupil, allows the formation of a second image, with the development of uniocular diplopia. In these patients, operative measures may be indicated, but such corrective measures should be deferred until the vision is stable. Since McCannel's technique for refixation of the iris has only minor risks, this operation may also be done for cosmetic reasons in special cases. However, an opaque contact lens with clear optic may be tried before surgical measures are undertaken.

Surgical. Treatment depends on the individual situation and the extent of tissue damage. However, in all cases one needs to restore optimal optic conditions. Reposition of the iris is certain in the smaller fresh incarceration without basic tissue damage. If the iris continues to incarcerate in the limbal area after an otherwise favorable reposition, a small basal iridectomy should be done in that area.

A primary iris suture without tissue excision should be considered when a smooth radial laceration is present. If the iris injury is irregular and a large portion of the iris tissue is damaged with loss of the pigment layer, the iris suture should be performed after excision of the damaged tissue. The purposes of these measures are to restore a reasonably useful pupil and avoid constant blurring.

The sector iridectomy should be considered only when a large iris incarceration persists for longer than 24 hours. Considerable loss of pigment and the impossibility of restoration of a useful pupil should also be evident. The decision is easier when a sector iridectomy occurs under the upper lid. Iris bleeding can be controlled either by wet-field cautery, by grasping the small vessel with Barraquer iris forceps and touching the forceps with diathermy, or by a 10-0 nylon suture.

For iridodialysis occurring in a blunt injury without cataract, McCannel's operation should be performed secondarily, when the eye has recovered from the injury. A repair can be made by passing a 10-0 monofilament suture on its needle into the iris angle under a small conjunctival flap opposite the dialysis tear. The needle is continued from the angle root, into the posterior chamber, and under the edge of the torn iris and proceeds vertically across the anterior chamber and through the cornea. A small, narrow limbal keratome incision is made beside the suture, just at the corneoscleral junction. A small blunt iris hook is slipped through this incision and moved across the anterior chamber to engage the previously placed vertical suture, which is drawn out in a loop. The corneal suture is then cut flush at its exit, and its loop is pulled out in a single strand. The two ends are then tied, and as the knot is drawn down firmly, it pulls the torn edge of the iris securely into the iris root cleft. A second suture can be placed in a similar manner, and even a third and fourth if the iridodialysis is large. If the distance between the iris root and the natural place of its fixation is large, the filling of the anterior chamber by transient sodium hyalonurate will stretch the iris and facilitate the maneuver. This technique may also help in primary wound surgery (e.g., in closing a subconjunctival scleral rupture) to bring the incarcerated iris into its normal position by a spatula.

If a contusion cataract is present, iridopexy is performed together with the cataract extraction. Only in corneoscleral lacerations with or without cataract should one consider performing the iridopexy at the same time as the wound is treated.

Ocular or Periocular Manifestations

Anterior Chamber: Cells and flare; hyphema.
Iris or Ciliary Body: Anterior uveitis; atrophy; hemorrhages; iridoplegia; pigmentary deposits; sphincter stromal tear.
Lens: Pigmentary deposits; Vossius' ring.
Pupil: Constriction; cycloplegia; deformed margins; dilation; notching.
Other: Corneal pigmentary deposits; decreased accommodation; diplopia; photophobia.

PRECAUTIONS

Often, injuries resulting in a torn or lacerated iris also involve other areas of the eye. These areas must be identified. In the case of serious damage to the anterior segment, injuries involving the cornea, sclera, iris, lens, vitreous, and even the retina must be handled in the correct order. The surgeon must be able to devise a plan for each individual case.

The presence and exact location of an iridodialysis should be noted in the record, since recurrence of bleeding or hyphema may arise from the ciliary body at the site of the iridodialysis. One should be certain to perform McCannel's operation for iridodialysis only after the eye has recovered from the injury, because functional success is endangered by the traumatic iritis. In treating iridodialysis, there is a risk of producing a recurrent hyphema, since the incision may have to pass through a proliferative scar from the original injury. A period of observation is usually necessary after iridodialysis to determine if associated ocular injuries are present. The iridodialysis itself rarely causes problems; however, recessed-angle glaucoma may occur months or years after the initial injury.

COMMENTS

The mechanism of the production of iris lacerations after contusions involves several factors. The most important of these are dilation of the corneoscleral ring occurring in compensation for the anteroposterior compression of the globe; the prompt and marked contraction of the sphincter of the iris, which occurs immediately on the application of blunt trauma to the cornea whether or not a posttraumatic mydriasis develops; the impact of the compression wave of aqueous that forces the iris into the lens and the lateral displacement of the aqueous; and possibly a rebound of the lens from the vitreous against which it is thrust, an action that may distend the iris. It is possible that some or all of these forces acting simultaneously and momentarily may produce different end results, depending on the relative strength of each in a particular case.

One should not forget that even cyclodialysis may be observed after concussive injury. In cases of marked hypotony, refixation of the ciliary body could become necessary.

References

Foster CS, Mark DB: Uveal prolapse. *In* Heilmann K, Paton D (ed): Atlas of Ophthalmic Surgery, Vol II, New York, Thieme Medical Publishers, 1987, pp 5.23–5.25.

Hanna C, Roy FH: Iris wound healing. Arch Ophthalmol 88:296–304, 1972.

Mackensen G: Repair of a postcontusional iridodialysis. *In* Blodi F, Mackensen G, Neubauer H (eds): Surgical Ophthalmology. Berlin, Springer, 1991, Vol I, pp 567–570.

McCannel MA: A retrievable suture idea for anterior uveal problems. Ophthalmic Surg 7:98–103, 1976.

Neubauer H: Treatment of major trauma of the anterior segment: With a discussion of more radical primary surgery. Trans Ophthalmol Soc UK 95: 322–325, 1975.

Neubauer H, Paulmann H: Replantation of one third of the ciliary body after severe impalement injury. Ophthalmologica (Basel) 181:1–10, 1983.

Paton D, Craig J: Management of iridodialysis. Ophthalmic Surg 4:38–39, 1973.

Runyan TE: Concussive and Penetrating Injuries of the Globe and Optic Nerve. St. Louis, CV Mosby, 1975, pp 61–63.

Waubke TN, Mellin KB: Treatment of iris injuries. *In* Blodi F, Mackensen G, Neubauer H (eds): Surgical Ophthalmology. Berlin, Springer, 1992, Vol II, pp 516–518.

LACRIMAL SYSTEM CONTUSIONS AND LACERATIONS 871.0

BENJAMIN MILDER, M.D.

St. Louis, Missouri

Because of the superficial location of the lacrimal canaliculi, any traumatic insult to the medial canthal area may interrupt the lacrimal drainage system. Any laceration of the nasal one-third of the eyelids may likewise impair tear drainage as a result of direct injury to the puncta, the canaliculi, or the lacrimal sac. Eyelid injuries may also disrupt lacrimal excretion indirectly by interfering with the pumping action of the orbicularis muscle or by altering the position of the punctum in relation to the globe. Cicatrization following injuries to the lids may produce ectropion or stenosis of the punctum. Fractures of the orbit may result in deformity or obliteration of the lacrimal sac or nasolacrimal duct, with subsequent obstructive dacryocystitis. About 20 per cent of naso ethmoidal and maxillofacial fractures cause disruption of the nasolacrimal duct and, sooner or later, purulent dacryocystitis. Such a discontinuity of the membranous nasolacrimal duct may also result in the formation of fistulas to the skin surface or into the antrum or the nasal cavity. Although occasional cysts or fistulas occur in the lacrimal gland, such injury is rare, since the gland is protected by the bony orbital rim.

THERAPY

Systemic. Although the principal concern of the surgeon is the repair of damaged tissues and restoration of function, appropriate triage should be the first consideration in severe trauma. Urgent medical needs should precede surgical intervention. In grossly contaminated injuries, prophylactic broad-spectrum antibiotics should be administered at the outset. A suitable broad-spectrum program would include daily intravenous administration of 5 mg/kg of gentamicin. This should be combined with 250 mg of oral cephalexin four times daily. The surgeon must judge whether 0.5 ml of tetanus toxoid is indicated.

Surgical.

CANALICULUS: If a torn canaliculus is not repaired, an occasional patient may escape troublesome epiphora. However, since the patient with such good fortune cannot be identified in advance, it is necessary to repair all severed canaliculi using fine sutures under microscopic control and a stent. Silicone tubing is currently favored for this purpose. It is not essential that a lacerated canaliculus be repaired immediately. In fact, waiting for 6 to 24 hours may allow for reduction of edema and some retraction of tissue so that the medial cut end of the canaliculus is better exposed to view. Anastomosis is usually successful even if performed as much as 3 to 5 days after the injury. If this proximal end of the canaliculus cannot be identified readily with the operating microscope, the intact canaliculus may be irrigated with a fluorescein solution instilled under increased pressure. Reflux of the fluorescein solution can be facilitated by simultaneous digital pressure on the lacrimal sac. Air instillation and sodium hyaluronate have also been employed for this purpose.

When silicone tubing is employed as a stent, the tube is passed through the punctum and distal end of the cut canaliculus, across the defect, through the proximal end of the cut canaliculus, and down the nasolacrimal duct emerging in the inferior meatus of the nose. The free upper end of the silicone tube is then threaded through the intact canaliculus into the nasal cavity, creating a loop between the two puncta at the nasal canthus. The two ends of the tube are then tied and cut just within the external naris. If the free end of the stent cannot be drawn through the intact canaliculus, it may be fastened to the end emerging from the naris, at the nasolabial fold. The stent should be left in place for 2 months to ensure lasting patency of the surgical anastomosis. However, the silicone is relatively inert and can be left for as much as 6 months.

After this silicone stent is in position, the severed ends of the canaliculus are approximated under microscopic control, using three interrupted 8-0 or 9-0 sutures. The lid margin is then sutured, and the posterior and skin surfaces of the lid laceration are then closed. Finally, a mattress suture may be threaded across the laceration from the nasal end of the tarsus to the insertion of the medial canthal tendon to reduce the tension on the anastomosis. It should remain in place for 3 weeks.

Stenosis of the canaliculus may result from an injury or from an unsuccessful attempt to repair it. If the axial extent of the stenosis is minimal, it may be possible to penetrate the occluded area with a punctum dilator, insert a stent, and leave it in place for 1 to 2 months in order to ensure continued patency. If the stenosis is more extensive, the scarred portion should be resected and a fresh anastomosis attempted. With more than 3 mm of the canaliculus absent, reconstructive surgery is rarely successful. If the patient is relatively symptom-free, with adequate outflow through the intact canaliculus, and if outflow function can be confirmed using the fluorescein dye disappearance or other functional tests, no intervention is necessary. In the symptomatic patient, an alternate route for tear elimination must be established. The preferred procedure is conjunctivo-dacryocystorhinostomy after the method of Jones, with insertion of a Pyrex glass tube as a permanent stent.

If the canaliculus is lacerated at or near the punctum, a functional restoration is rarely successful. The preferred approach is to provide access to the tear lake by marsupialization of the canaliculus on the conjunctival surface along the horizontal limb.

PUNCTUM. If the punctum is lacerated and the canaliculus is otherwise intact, careful repair around a stent should be undertaken. Compression of the canaliculus in the act of blinking is a more significant physiologic element in tear excretion than is the capillary action at the punctum. Thus, a patent punctum, even if patulous, will be adequate to restore function. If the punctum cannot be repaired, the horizontal limb of the canaliculus may be marsupialized.

In patients with stenosis of the punctum and a relatively intact canaliculus, every effort should be made to re-establish patency of the punctum. Once again, the silicone stent is indicated. If it is unsuccessful in keeping the punctum open, a punctumplasty should be performed using the three-snip method or the punch technique. In the three-snip operation, the punctum is dilated and a snip 2 mm long is made with scissors in the vertical limb of the canaliculus. A second cut is made along the ampulla, parallel with the lid margin, and the third snip joins the first two. This three-snip procedure results in a gaping opening on the posterior surface of the eyelid, including the punctum and the vertical limb of the canaliculus; the opening is in contact with the tear lake. The same result can be achieved using a Holth scleral punch, inserting the male blade of the punch into the vertical limb of the canaliculus and the female blade on the conjunctival side of the lid.

If the lower punctum is everted, with or without stenosis, the three-snip or Holth punch punctumplasty may be sufficient to restore adequate tear drainage. More pronounced degrees of punctal eversion will require excision of an elliptical or diamond-shaped segment of conjunctiva and tarsal plate below the ampulla of the canaliculus. The excised segment should be 8 mm long and 5 mm wide and the defect closed with 6-0 sutures. However, if the eversion is the result of an eyelid cicatrix, primary attention should be given to the scarred area.

COMMON CANALICULUS. Stenosis of the common canaliculus is confirmed by instilling an irrigating solution into one canaliculus and confirming reflux from the opposite canaliculus, without distention of the lacrimal sac or passage of the fluid into the nasal cavity. After opening the stenotic area with a slender punctum dilator or a stainless steel lacrimal probe, silicone tubing is employed to maintain patency. It should be left in place for an extended period, usually 3 to 8 weeks. If the common canaliculus closes after removal of the stent, it can be reinserted for an additional period.

If the medial canthal tendon is avulsed and displaced in a fracture, it should be reattached either by direct or transnasal wiring. After restoration of the medial canthus, lacrimal drainage function should be tested. If a functional block is present (i.e., patency with persistent epiphora) and confirmed with dacryocystography, a dacryocystorhinostomy should be performed.

NASOLACRIMAL DUCT. Obliteration of the nasolacrimal duct as a result of trauma will always eventuate in dacryocystitis, managed by dacryocystorhinostomy. Initially, at the time of reduction of the facial and/or nasal fracture, a probe should be passed through the upper canaliculus, tear sac, and nasolacrimal duct and identified in the inferior meatus. This method aids in determining whether the bones are positioned adequately.

The surgical treatment of traumatic lacrimal fistula is dacryocystorhinostomy with excision of the fistulous track. Traumatic fistulas or diverticulae require careful contrast dacryocystography to establish the site of obstruction and the course of the fistula.

Ocular or Periocular Manifestations

Lacrimal System: Avulsion of medial canthal tendon; cicatrization; cyst of lacrimal gland; dacryocystitis; disruption of nasolacrimal duct; ectropion of puncta; epiphora; fistula of lacrimal gland or sac; stenosis of canaliculi or puncta.

PRECAUTIONS

Interruption of the nasolacrimal duct may occur in any injury involving the middle third of the face, especially the ocular adnexa. Early recognition and prompt treatment are the keys to successful results. In particular, any injury in the medial canthal area should be carefully inspected for canalicular damage. The disturbance caused by complete stenosis of the lacrimal canaliculus may be minimal in elderly persons, and if this is confirmed by low Schirmer readings, surgery may not be required.

COMMENTS

Because injury to the lacrimal apparatus usually produces gross abnormality of the tissue or obvious functional disturbances, the sensitive tests of drainage function are not often required for immediate diagnosis. Repair of a canaliculus should always be undertaken. The more remote the laceration is from the nasal angle, the higher the likelihood of a successful result. It is true that, in some patients, one functioning canaliculus may ensure adequate drainage. However, appropriate surgical management of the lacerated canaliculus is indicated if it is feasible.

References

Aguirre Vila-Coro A, Zaragoza Garcia P: Hyaluronate in the identification of the cut end in lacerations of the lacrimal canaliculi. Am J Ophthalmol 105:214–251, 1988.
Bennett JE: The lacrimal drainage system. *In* Duane TD (ed): Clinical Ophthalmology. Hagerstown, MD, Harper & Row, 1982, Vol V, 11:1–8.
Bohigian GM: Handbook of External Diseases of the Eye. Fort Worth, Alcon, 1980, p 163.
Haik BG: Teflon sleeve canalicular. AJO 106:367, 1988.
Harris GJ, et al: Lacrimal intubation in the primary

repair of midfacial fractures. Ophthalmology 94: 242–247, 1987.

Hurwitz JJ, Archer KF, Gruss JS: Double stent intubations in difficult post-traumatic dacryocystorhinostomy. Ophthalmic Surg 19(1):33–36, 1988.

Kennedy RH, May J, Dailey J, Flanagan JC: Canalicular laceration. An eleven-year epidemiologic and clinical study. Ophthalmic Plast Reconstr Surg 6(1):46–53, 1990.

Nagashima K, et al: Relative roles of upper and lower lacrimal canaliculi in normal tear drainage. Jpn J Ophthalmol 28:259–262, 1984.

Paton D, Goldberg MF: Management of Ocular Injuries. Philadelphia, WB Saunders, 1976, pp 52–58.

Reifler DM: Management of canalicular laceration. Surv Ophthalmol 36(2):113–132, 1991.

Romano PE: Single silicone intubation for repair of single canaliculus laceration. Ann Ophthalmol 18:112, 1986.

Wulc AE, Arterberry JF: The pathogenesis of canalicular laceration. Ophthalmology 98(8):1243–1249, 1991.

Zagora E: Eye Injuries. Springfield, IL, Charles C Thomas, 1970, pp 164–168.

TRAUMATIC CATARACT 366.20

GEORGE M. GOMBOS, M.D., F.A.C.S.

Brooklyn, New York

Cataract is by far the most common complication causing loss of vision after any type of ocular injury. Traumatic cataract may result from nonperforating and perforating injury to the globe. Nonperforating trauma to the eye includes contusive or concussive injuries. Cataract development after such injuries is not unusual and may occur without any detectable damage to the lens capsule. The exact mechanism of this type of cataract is not known. Contusive or concussive forces produce waves of pressure changes that may injure the epithelial cells, lens capsule, lens fibers, or zonules. Lenticular opacifications present in a variety of forms, such as discrete, punctate, scattered subepithelial changes or rosette-shaped opacities. Most commonly, the location of these changes is anterior, frequently segmental or localized. Occasionally, late rosette opacities deep in the cortex may occur many years after the acute trauma. Contusive injury may cause a full or partial circle of iris pigment on the anterior surface of the lens capsule, which is called the Vossius ring. Opacities caused by concussive or contusive injury may be transient, static, or progressive. Such cataracts may mature suddenly any time.

Traumatic cataract may also result from electric shock or radiation. In addition to the lens opacities, blunt trauma to the globe can cause subluxation or complete luxation of the lens. The striking force tears the zonules holding the lens in place behind the iris. Any contusive or concussive injury may cause instant rupture of the lens capsule, which will result in a rapid development of cataractous changes.

Perforating injury of the lens always involves other tissue injury, such as corneal or scleral perforation. Injury to any other intraocular tissue is a possibility, although perforating injury of the globe may rupture the anterior lens capsule only. Needles, wires, darts, and other sharp objects can cause puncture wounds of the eyeball, with minimal evidence of entry and anterior lens capsule damage. Occasionally, such injury causes partial opacity of the lens material, but it is not progressive in nature, and the eye may retain very good visual acuity. If both the anterior and the posterior capsules are damaged, full-blown cataract formation is a strong likelihood. The progress is usually rapid. Sudden deterioration of vision to hand movement or light perception can be expected.

Traumatic cataract may present as the only significant pathology (simple traumatic cataract) or as part of an overall perforating ocular injury (complicated traumatic cataract). In the latter case, lens material is mixed with vitreous or blood or both. A secondary inflammatory process develops in almost every case. Swelling of the lens material may induce pupillary-block glaucoma. Also, lens material causes a characteristic macrophage reaction in the anterior segment of the globe. Proteinaceous material and cellular debris clog the outflow channels of the aqueous humor and raise the intraocular pressure. This condition, the combination of severe uveitis and extremely high intraocular pressure, is called phacolytic glaucoma. Rapid development of infection, endophthalmitis, may be part of the clinical picture, which may alter the overall prognosis.

THERAPY

Supportive. If the visual acuity is 20/40 or better, the cataract is nonprogressive, and the eye is quiet, no specific treatment is required. Periodic re-evaluations are suggested.

Surgical. Traumatic cataract should be operated on if visual acuity deteriorates or ocular complications exist. In cases where the traumatic cataract is part of an extensive perforating injury, immediate surgical intervention is essential. Extracapsular cataract extraction or manual or automated irrigation-aspiration techniques are the procedures of choice. However, these simple surgical techniques are not always feasible. If the lens capsule is badly ruptured and the lens material is mixed with vitreous and blood, complete lensectomy and anterior vitrectomy are indicated. The "open sky" approach or pars plana techniques are equally acceptable; however, the open sky approach in experienced hands results in less postoperative morbidity and better visual acuity. Limbal lens extraction may be employed when the cataractous lens is subluxated or dislocated. If vitreous is present in the anterior chamber, anterior vitrectomy in conjunction with cataract extraction is the preferred surgical approach.

The use of an intraocular lens after traumatic cataract surgery is controversial. As most traumatic cataracts occur in young patients, lens implantation might be hazardous because biodegradation of the plastic material may cause the UGH (uveitis, glaucoma, hemorrhage) syndrome in later life. Such advances as epikeratophakia and keratomileusis in surgical techniques and new generations of contact lenses have resulted in excellent visual results in unilateral aphakia, and the newer contact lenses could be excellent substitutes for an intraocular lens. However, in some selected cases, an intraocular lens is the only alternative enabling both rapid visual rehabilitation and treatment of amblyopia, especially in children younger than 7 years of age.

In conclusion, one should remember that each traumatic injury is different, and therefore, no dogmatic techniques or rules could apply to cataract surgery in cases of trauma.

Ocular or Periocular Manifestations

Anterior Chamber: Flare and cells; lens particles; shallow anterior chamber.
Conjunctiva: Chemosis; hemorrhage; hyperemia.
Cornea: Corneal edema; possible perforation site.
Pupil: Leukokoria; irregular pupil.
Sclera: Possible perforation site.

PRECAUTIONS

A complete history and circumstances of the trauma must be obtained. Documentation of the place, date, and time of the injury, as well as the visual acuity, is important for medical and medicolegal purposes. The possibility of an intraocular foreign body should always be considered. Therefore, appropriate x-ray films and CT scans have to be per-

formed when the clarity of the media does not allow complete evaluation or the history suggests an intraocular foreign body. The potential of an intraocular infection and the proper attention to this problem should always be kept in mind by the physician.

COMMENTS

In severe or extensive injury to the eye, almost all structures of the eye (cornea, sclera, lens, uvea, vitreous, and retina) can be involved. A recent concept, the so-called primary overall repair, is considered an important development in the management of ocular trauma. It seems to be an obsolete idea that trauma of the eyeball or traumatic cataract must be handled first by a so-called cataract specialist and that later the case is referred to a retinal or a "foreign body" specialist. The ophthalmologist who handles the anterior segment should take care of the entire eye as soon as possible. All necessary repairs should be treated in one surgical session, if feasible.

References

Bellows JG, Bellows RT: Cataract due to trauma, cataracta complicata, and displacement of the lens. A. Traumatic cataract. *In* Bellows JG (ed): Cataract and Abnormalities of the Lens. New York, Grune & Stratton, 1975, pp 265–272.

Bhatia IM, Panda A, Sood NN: Management of traumatic cataract. Ind J Ophthalmol *31*:290–293, 1983.

Bienfait MF, et al: Intraocular lens implantation in children with unilateral traumatic cataract. Int Ophthalmol *14*:271–276, 1990.

Billore OP, Shroff AP, Dubey AK: Evaluation of lensectomy in traumatic cataract with perforated and nonperforated eye injuries. Ind J Ophthalmol *31*:585–587, 1983.

Charles S: Vitreous Microsurgery. Baltimore, Williams & Wilkins, 1981, pp 33–42.

Gombos GM: Handbook of Ophthalmologic Emergencies. New Hyde Park, NY, Medical Examination Publishing, 1977, pp 112–113, 168–169.

Jain IS, et al: Prognosis in traumatic cataract surgery. J Pediatr Ophthalmol Strabismus *16*:301–305, 1979.

Jones WL: Traumatic injury to the lens. Optometry Clin *1*:125–142, 1991.

Morgan KS, et al: Epikeratophakia in children with traumatic cataracts. J Pediatr Ophthalmol Strabismus *23*:108–114, 1986.

Paton D, Goldberg MF: Management of Ocular Injuries. Philadelphia, WB Saunders, 1976, pp 239–254.

Venom

BEE STING OF THE CORNEA 989.5

IRA G. WONG, M.D.,
and GILBERT SMOLIN, M.D.

San Francisco, California

Bee sting of the cornea occurs when the toothed lancet of the stinging apparatus penetrates the cornea. Attached to the stinger are poison sacs containing as much as 0.3 mg venom, which can produce both a toxic and immunologic reaction in the cornea. The venom contains toxin, such as melittin, apamin, and formic acid, and a potent allergen, phospholipase A.

The corneal response depends upon the amount of venom and the patient's immunologic reaction to the venom. When free of venom, the stinger is inert and can be tolerated for a long period of time. If a small amount of venom penetrates the cornea, the reaction may be minimal corneal edema and conjunctival chemosis, and hyperemia. If a large amount of venom is introduced or the patient has a hypersensitivity to the venom, a dense cellular infiltration may occur at the sting site, as well as an iritis and iridoplegia.

THERAPY

Systemic. A systemic reaction to a bee sting of the cornea has not been reported. However, a patient may have additional stings elsewhere and develop a systemic reaction. If anaphylaxis or laryngeal edema develops in a hypersensitive patient, 0.5 ml of 1:1000 epinephrine should be given intramuscularly and repeated in 5 minutes for as often as necessary. In severe reactions, the same dosage of epinephrine may be given intravenously in 10 ml of saline. Intravenous administration of 5 to 20 mg of diphenhydramine may be given after the epinephrine. Patients with severe laryngeal edema should be given 500 mg of hydrocortisone intravenously every 6 hours, and tracheostomy should be strongly considered. The patient is placed in shock position and kept warm.

Ocular. Topical instillation of one drop of 0.1 per cent epinephrine and one drop of 1 per cent prednisolone solution in the conjunctival sac should be made immediately. The prednisolone drops are continued every 2 to 3 hours, and cold compresses are applied to the eye. The stinger should be removed from the wound, with care not to express more venom into the wound by squeezing the poison sac. A prophylactic topical antibiotic may also be prescribed.

Ocular or Periocular Manifestations

Anterior chamber: Cells and flare; hyphema.
Cornea: Abscess; epithelial and stromal keratitis.
Eyelids: Edema; induration.
Iris: Depigmentation; iridoplegia; iritis.
Lens: Cataract; subluxation.
Others: Internal ophthalmoplegia; optic neuritis.

PRECAUTIONS

If the stinger cannot be removed from the cornea or is in the anterior chamber, surgical intervention may not necessarily be needed, as the stinger is inert when free of venom. Intensive anti-inflammatory therapy should be given to treat the effects of the venom.

COMMENTS

The order Hymenoptera contains over 60,000 species that are found throughout the world. All insects of this order have a stinging apparatus located at the rear of the abdomen, through which venom is ejected. In some species, such as the honey bee, the venom apparatus may be torn away from the insect's body and remain in the prey. Stings from other Hymenoptera, such as wasps, hornets, and ants, may be treated in the same manner.

References

Chen C, Richardson C: Bee sting-induced ocular changes. Ann Ophthalmol 18:285–286, 1986.
Duke-Elder S (ed): System of Ophthalmology. St. Louis, CV Mosby, Vol XIV, 1972, pp 1204–1207, 1346–1348.
Smolin G, Wong I: Bee sting of the cornea: Case reports. Ann Ophthalmol 14:342–343, 1982.
Song H, Wray S: Bee sting optic neuritis. J Clin Neuro-Ophthalmol 11:45–49, 1991.

SPIDER BITES 989.5

F. HAMPTON ROY, M.D., F.A.C.S.

Little Rock, Arkansas

The bite of several different spiders can cause severe, even fatal systemic poisoning in humans. The most numerous of the venomous spiders are members of the genus *Latrodectus*. The venom of this genus (which includes the American black-widow spider) and of the genus *Phoneutria* is a nonhemolytic, noncytotoxic neurotoxin that produces diffuse central and peripheral nervous excitement, autonomic activity, muscle spasm, hypertension, and vasoconstriction in humans. Other symptoms may include marked abdominal rigidity, intense pain, paresthesia, headache, sweating, nausea, and facial congestion.

The venom of spiders of the *Loxosceles* genus (which includes the brown recluse spider) is a mixture of hemolysin and cytotoxin that causes ischemic necrosis at the site of the bite. The bite is often relatively painless, and the lesion is initially surrounded by a bluish-white halo of vasoconstriction that may later develop extensive gangrene. Systemic symptoms may include chills, malaise, or a scarlatiniform rash. In cases of severe envenomation, massive intravascular hemolysis, convulsions, hemoglobinuria, and acute renal failure may occur. Bites from spiders of the genus *Chiracanthium* cause similar, though milder symptoms. Tarantulas or wolf spiders of various genera, including *Lycosa* and *Phidippus*, may also cause local necrosis and ulceration in humans.

Severe systemic envenomation by the black-widow spider occasionally results in edema of the eyelids, ptosis, conjunctivitis, and constriction of the pupils. The venom of spiders of the *Phoneutria* genus may cause visual disturbances, including blindness. The bite of Australian funnel-web spiders (*Atrax robustus* and *A. formidabilis*) also results in pupillary constriction. A unique type of ocular injury is the ejection of venom into the eye by the green lynx spider (*Peucetia viridans*).

THERAPY

Supportive. For *Latrodectus* poisoning, measures should include a hot tub bath, which provides prompt, though temporary relief. Intravenous injection of 10 ml of 10 per cent calcium gluconate may relieve muscle cramps. However, the action of this drug is often brief, and subsequent doses have less effect than the first dose. Alternative intravenous treatment with 10 to 20 ml of methocarbamol, followed by oral administration, has been indicated. In some cases, if pain is severe, opiates may be necessary.

Persons bitten by *Loxosceles* spiders should be observed carefully and should be hospitalized if severe sequelae develop. Administration of 100 mg of hydroxyzine four times a day may alter the necrotic local lesions. Renal functions, white count, and abnormalities in coagulation should be followed. If severe hemolysis develops, renal dialysis should be begun within the initial 48 to 72 hours. Maintenance of an alkaline urine and transfusion may also be beneficial in patients with hemolysis. Broad-spectrum antibiotics given early may help localize inflammation and control secondary infection.

Nonspecific treatment consists of broad-spectrum antibiotics (systemic and local) after the wound is cleaned. Tetanus prophylaxis is indicated.

Surgical. Surgery should be considered only for large (greater than 1 cm) and deep necrotic bites of the *Loxosceles* genus, especially those extending into fat. The affected area should be excised and saucerized. Excision at the fascial level is usually sufficient. Resurfacing with split thickness grafts, skin flaps, or pedicles is seldom indicated in orbital or lid lesions. Plastic surgery may be performed if the bite results in a cosmetically disfigured area.

Systemic. Systemic treatment of *Latrodectus* or *Loxosceles* envenomation consists of the administration of 2.5 ml of reconstituted antiserum. This is usually quite effective within a few hours.

For *Loxosceles* bites for which antivenin is unavailable, 100 mg of prednisone or 16 mg of dexamethasone should be given orally for large bites and always at the first indication of systemic envenomation. This dosage may be used daily for the first 3 days, with gradual tapering. In severe cases, an intralesional injection of 2.5 mg/ml of triamcinolone may be administered; no more than 5 mg should be infiltrated into the lesion. Antihistamines may be useful for milder lesions. The administration of heparin seems to give some protection against disseminated intravascular coagulation.

Ocular or Periocular Manifestations

Conjunctiva: Chemosis; conjunctivitis; cyanosis; edema; subconjunctival hemorrhages.
Eyelids: Edema; gangrene; necrosis; paralysis; ptosis; purpura.
Pupil: Constriction.
Retina: Cyanosis.
Other: Visual disturbances, visual loss.

PRECAUTIONS

Early excision of spider bites should only be undertaken when the spider has been identified as a brown recluse. However, only few cases require surgical care. For early surgery to be acceptable, it must be proven that the bite is destined to become one of the very rare, large, deep bites.

Potential problem cases should be recognized early. Patients at risk, such as older hypertensive patients and young children, should be hospitalized and expectantly treated with antivenin. Close supervision during the first 12 hours after the bite is important in this high-risk group; deaths due to cardiac or respiratory failure have occurred.

Because of the excellent blood supply to the eyelids, the lid margin may be spared in gangrenous eyelid processes. There is sparing of the marginal lid strip and a propensity for self-repair for lid bites.

COMMENTS

Most spiders bite humans defensively. Only a few types, including the black widow, the wandering spider, and the funnel-web spider, seem to be aggressive to any degree.

The brown recluse spider is the most dangerous of North American arachnoids and seems to be most abundant in the mid-Southern states of the United States. Bites cause only local itching without systemic signs, or there may be a local vesicle with an area of necrosis. If the area of necrosis is greater than 1 cm, there usually are mild to moderate systemic signs; if the area of necrosis is greater than 4 cm, there is definite systemic envenomation and sometimes secondary infection.

References

Edwards JJ, Anderson RL, Wood JR: Loxoscelism of the eyelids. Arch Ophthalmol 98:1997–2000, 1980.

Grant WM: Toxicology of the Eye, 3rd ed. Springfield, IL, Charles C Thomas, 1986.

Wilson DC, King LE: Spiders and spider bites. Dermatol Clin 8:277–286, 1990.

Zeligowski AA, Peled IJ, Wexler MR: Eyelid necrosis after spider bite. Am J Ophthalmol 15:101:254–255, 1986.

SECTION 17

UNCLASSIFIED DISEASES OR CONDITIONS

AMYLOIDOSIS 277.3

STEVEN P. DUNN, M.D.,

Southfield, Michigan

and JAY H. KRACHMER, M.D.

Minneapolis, Minnesota

Amyloidosis is a disease complex resulting in the accumulation of an extracellular amorphous eosinophilic substance that is readily identified by its staining with Congo Red, associated apple-green birefringence under polarized light, and distinctive fibrillar ultrastructure. In recent years, the study of amyloid fibrils has led to the classification of amyloid on the basis of the biochemical composition of its subunit proteins. Currently, 13 molecular species have been described.

Amyloidosis has been classified into two main groups, primary and secondary, each of which is subdivided into systemic and localized forms.

Six types of primary familial amyloidosis have now been described and seem to be related to an abnormality in transthyretin (prealbumin) or apolipoprotein A-I. Amyloid deposits from these conditions have been designated "AF" and are usually associated with an autosomal dominant form of inheritance. Multisystem involvement is characteristic, with progressive peripheral polyneuropathy, cardiomyopathy, and gastrointestinal and skin involvement being seen most frequently. The eye may be involved in several ways; linear and veil-like vitreous opacities associated with slowly progressive visual loss, however, are virtually diagnostic of this disease. Discrete, bilateral yellow-white xanthoma-like nodules, occasionally with petechiae and hemorrhage, may be the initial findings. Involvement of the lacrimal and parotid glands may produce dryness of the eyes and mouth. Proptosis and external ophthalmoplegia have been attributed to amyloid deposits in the extraocular muscles. Pupillary abnormalities are thought to be due to amyloid neuropathy or possibly secondary to deposits in the iris sphincter and dilator muscles. Neurotrophic keratopathy and glaucoma are probably secondary to intraocular tissue deposition.

Localized, primary amyloidosis may also be found in the eye in the form of small pink-red nodules in the lids or conjunctiva. This form of the disease is usually bilateral in nature and affects young adults in their twenties and thirties. Several forms of primary corneal amyloidosis exist. The most recognized is lattice corneal dystrophy, which has now been broken down into three subtypes based on inheritance pattern and clinical findings. Type I lattice corneal dystrophy is the classic form with autosomal dominant inheritance and central anterior and midstromal lattice lines, dots, and stromal haze. It is not associated with any systemic disorders and typically presents in the 10- to 40-year age range. Type II lattice corneal dystrophy, also known as Meretoja's syndrome, is also autosomal dominant. It is actually a manifestation of a form of primary systemic amyloidosis known as Finnish hereditary amyloidosis. It is generally associated with blepharochalasis, bilateral facial nerve palsies, and peripheral neuropathy. Clinically, both peripheral and central lattice lines are found in the anterior stroma. Occasionally, conjunctival and adnexal deposits of amyloid may be seen. Recently, molecular genetics research has isolated a point mutation on the gelsolin gene in patients with clinical findings quite similar to those seen in Finnish hereditary amyloidosis. Type III lattice corneal dystrophy typically presents in an older age group (70–90 years of age) and is felt to be a recessive disorder characterized by markedly thickened lattice-like lines involving the anterior stroma centrally and paracentrally. This condition is not associated with any systemic problem. Primary gelatinous drop-like keratopathy is a rare, amyloid disorder seen most frequently in individuals of Japanese ancestry. The inheritance pattern is felt to be autosomal recessive with a low degree of penetrance. Clinical findings consist primarily of numerous small to moderate-sized subepithelial gelatinous excrescences that give the corneal surface a "mulberry-like" or "toad skin" appearance. Patients with this disorder tend to present before the age of 20 with symptoms of photophobia, lacrimation, redness, and foreign body sensation. No systemic disorders are associated with this condition. As of yet, the precise type of amyloid has not been elucidated.

Secondary systemic amyloidosis may accompany a variety of chronic systemic disorders, including pyogenic or granulomatous infections, arthritis, malignancy (i.e., multiple myeloma), or chronic inflammatory disease of the intestine. Except for myeloma-associated amyloid, most of the secondary systemic forms of amyloid are composed of fibrils made up of a non-immunoglobulin-related protein, amyloid A protein (AA). Deposits are chiefly found in the spleen, kidney, and liver. The eyelids may be involved occasionally.

Localized secondary amyloidosis may present as clinically detectable deposits in the lids, conjunctiva, and cornea. Clinically unrecognizable microdeposits of amyloid have been found in association with such conditions as basal cell carcinomas of the lid margin, conjunctival intraepithelial neoplasia, and conjunctival sarcoidosis. Microdeposits within the cornea have been seen with retrolental fibroplasia, phlyctenular keratoconjunctivitis, trachoma, keratoconus, and penetrating ocular trauma. Polymorphic amyloid degeneration, a condition typically seen in older patients without a history of ocular disease, is probably a form of primary localized amyloidosis.

THERAPY

Supportive. The treatment of systemic amyloidosis is presently unsatisfactory. The disease is almost invariably fatal. Because some amyloid fibrils have an immunologic origin, therapeutic trials using melphalan-prednisone[‡] have been tried. Preliminary reports have been unimpressive. Similarly, studies with dimethyl sulfoxide (DMSO),[‡] an amyloid-fibril denaturing agent, and colchicine[‡] have been discouraging.

Supportive medical care thus becomes very important. All patients in this group deserve a thorough evaluation and search for an underlying cause of their amyloidosis. Partial or complete resorption of amyloid deposits with improvement of symptoms has been reported with treatment of the underlying inflammatory or neoplastic process.

Surgical. The surgical management of amyloidosis is usually directed at a localized disease. There is a strong tendency, however, for recurrence to occur, and this should be explained to the patient. Local discomfort, marked proptosis, diplopia, and poor vision are the usual reasons for surgical therapy. Excision of orbital amyloid is useful in cases where it is well circumscribed. In most cases, however, the infiltration is diffuse and impossible to remove completely. Surgical therapy often proves more diagnostic than therapeutic. Mucous membrane grafting is frequently necessary after the excision of conjunctival amyloid deposits. Reduced vision often leads to penetrating keratoplasty by the fourth or fifth decade in patients with lattice dystrophy. Though the success rate of penetrating keratoplasty exceeds 90 per cent in this group, re-

currences may occur. Keratoplasty may be helpful in patients with gelatinuous drop-like dystrophy and diffuse familial amyloidosis as well. Polymorphic amyloid degeneration does not usually require therapy. Total vitrectomy seems to be the treatment of choice for amyloid patients with dense vitreous opacities interfering with vision.

Ocular or Periocular Manifestations

Ciliary Body: Fuchs' epithelioma.
Conjunctiva: Amyloid deposits; hemorrhages.
Cornea: Polymorphic amyloid degeneration; lattice corneal dystrophy (Classic type—type I, Meretoja's syndrome [type II], type III); gelatinous, drop-like dystrophy; familial amyloidosis; secondary amyloid deposits.
Extraocular Muscles: Convergence insufficiency; restriction; paralysis.
Eyelids: Amyloid deposits; thickening; swelling; petechial hemorrhages; ptosis.
Orbit: Amyloid deposits, proptosis.
Pupil: Anisocoria; irregularity.
Retina: Perivascular sheathing; arterial occlusion; hemorrhage.
Sclera: Amyloid deposits.
Uvea: Amyloid deposits; perivascular sheathing; choriocapillaris occlusion.
Vitreous: Pseudopodia lentis; glass-wool/sheet-like opacities.

PRECAUTIONS

A high incidence of recurrent amyloid deposits after surgery should be borne in mind by the ophthalmologist and patient. This is particularly important when cosmetic surgery is planned. Regrafting and repeat vitrectomy are options available to the patient with recurrent corneal and vitreal amyloidosis and visual deterioration.

COMMENTS

Localized amyloid deposits are by far the most common form of ocular amyloidosis. In some cases, amyloid deposits involving the eye may actually be an early localized manifestation of a generalized amyloidosis. This is particularly true with eyelid and vitreal amyloid deposits. The possibility that these deposits may be associated with an underlying disease process or immunologic abnormality must always be considered.

References

Doughman DJ: Ocular amyloidosis. Surv Ophthalmol 13:133–142, 1969.
Gertz MA, Kyle RA: Primary systemic amyloidosis—a diagnostic primer. Mayo Clin Proc G4:505–519, 1989.
Gorevic PD, Muroz PE, Gorgone G, et al: Amyloidosis due to a mutation of the gelsolin gene in

an American family with lattice corneal dystrophy, Type II. N Engl J Med *325*:1780–1785, 1991.

Henderson JW: Orbital Tumors. Philadelphia, WB Saunders, 1973, pp 602–608.

Hitchings RA, Tripathi RC: Vitreous opacities in primary amyloid disease. A clinical, histochemical, and ultrastructural report. Br J Opththalmol *60*:41–54, 1976.

Knowles DM II: Amyloidosis of the orbit and adnexae. Surv Ophthalmol *19*:367–384, 1975.

Mannis MJ, et al: Polymorphic amyloid degeneration of the cornea. A clinical and histopathologic study. Arch Ophthalmol *99*:1217–1223, 1981.

Meretoja J: Familial systemic paramyloidosis with lattice dystrophy of the cornea, progressive cranial neuropathy, skin changes and various internal symptoms. A progressive unrecognized heritable syndrome. Ann Clin Res *1*:310, 1969.

BEHÇET'S DISEASE 136.1
(Silk Road Disease)

KANJIRO MASUDA, M.D.

Tokyo, Japan

Behçet's disease is a systemic disease of unknown etiology, and its diagnosis is based on a combination of major and minor symptoms. The major symptoms are recurrent aphthae in the mouth; skin lesions, such as erythema nodosum, acne, and subcutaneous thromboangiitis; ocular lesions, such as hypopyon iritis and retinal vasculitis with hemorrhages and exudates; and genital ulcer. During the chronic course of the disease, these major symptoms recur as attacks, but not necessarily together. The minor symptoms include arthritis, epididymitis, intestinal lesions, and vascular, neuropsychologic, lung, or kidney involvement.

The disease has been seen all over the world, but it is especially frequent in Japan, the eastern Mediterranean, and the Middle East, where it is known as the Silk Road disease. Immunogenetically, HLA-B51 is closely related to this disease.

The onset of the disease usually occurs in the third and fourth decades. Its course shows exacerbations and remissions, and symptoms may subside within several years or linger for more than 20 years.

The visual prognosis is usually poor. From the ophthalmologic point of view, Behçet's disease may be classified into two groups: the anterior type, which chiefly involves the anterior segment of the eye (iridocyclitic type), and the posterior type involving the posterior segment of the eye (fundus type).

THERAPY

Ocular. A good visual acuity can be maintained in the anterior type of Behçet's disease for a much longer time than in the posterior type. At the time of attack, 1 per cent atropine once or twice a day and topical corticosteroids two to four times daily should be used. After severe attacks showing distinct hypopyon iritis, subtenon injection* of corticosteroids is indicated.

Systemic. Long-term systemic administration of corticosteroids results in an unfavorable visual prognosis. Consequently, immunosuppressive agents are the main drugs currently used in the posterior type of Behçet's disease. Systemic steroids should be used only in cases with macular involvement and only for a short period of time (7 days). As soon as the attacks subside, corticosteroids must be tapered. The immunosuppressive agents are used both to treat the attacks and to reduce the number of attacks. A daily dosage of 0.5 to 1.5 mg of colchicine[‡] or 50 to 150 mg of cyclophosphamide[‡] or both is recommended. Oral administration of chlorambucil[‡] has also been reported to be beneficial. Newly developed immunosuppressive agents such as cyclosporine and FK506 are used with an initial dose of 5 mg/kg daily or 0.15 mg/kg daily, respectively. The dose may be increased or decreased according to the clinical manifestations and side effects, such as kidney or liver dysfunction.

Ocular or Periocular Manifestations

Anterior Chamber: Angle hypopyon; cells and flare; hypopyon.
Choroid: Cell infiltration; choroiditis.
Cornea: Keratic infiltration; keratic precipitates.
Globe: Phthisis.
Iris or Ciliary Body: Iridocyclitis; posterior synechia.
Lens: Cataracts.
Optic Nerve: Atrophy.
Retina: Cystoid macular edema; exudates; hemorrhages; macular hole; thromboangiitis.
Sclera: Episcleritis; scleritis.
Vitreous: Cells; hemorrhages; opacity.
Other: Glaucoma.

PRECAUTIONS

Side effects of the immunosuppressive agents must be checked carefully. Cyclophosphamide induces azoospermia, which may continue for a long time even after cessation of its use. Colchicine and chlorambucil also have toxic effects on reproductive cells and bone marrow. Regular blood cell counts must be carried out, and the dosage of these drugs should be controlled, depending on the results. Cyclosporine causes liver and kidney dysfunction. Therefore, kidney and liver function and blood pressure must be checked regularly. FK506 also causes liver, kidney, and pancreas dysfunction. Regular checks must be made on these organs. Cyclosporine and

FK506 sometimes induce mental and neurologic disorders.

COMMENTS

Before the introduction of immunosuppressive agents, the visual prognosis of Behçet's disease had been very poor. In more than 80 per cent of the cases with ocular involvement, particularly those involving the posterior segment, severe decrease in vision occurred within 5 years after onset. However, use of the immunosuppressive agents has greatly improved the visual prognosis; only 5 per cent of cases now show severe visual acuity loss 5 years after the onset. In males, 84 per cent of cases are of the posterior type, whereas 36 per cent of cases in females are of the anterior type. Consequently, visual prognosis is usually better in females than in males. The cause of death is often neuropsychologic, intestinal, or cardiovascular involvement.

References

Graham E, et al: Cyclosporin A in the treatment of severe Behçet's uveitis. *In* Lehner T, Barnes CG (eds): Recent Advances in Behçet's Disease, New York, Royal Society of Medicine Services, 1986, p 351.
Hayashi K, et al: Long-term treatment of severe Behçet's disease with cyclosporin A. *In* Lehner T, Barnes CG (eds): Recent Advances in Behçet's Disease, New York, Royal Society of Medicine Services, 1986, p 347.
Masuda K, et al: A nation-wide survey of Behçet's disease in Japan. 2. Clinical survey. Jpn J Ophthalmol *19*:278–285, 1975.
Masuda K, et al: Cyclosporin A treatment of Behçet's disease—A multicentre double-masked trial. *In* Lehner T, Barnes CG (eds): Recent Advances in Behçet's Disease. New York, Royal Society of Medicine Services, 1986, pp 327–331.
Mishima S, et al: Behçet's disease in Japan: Ophthalmologic aspects. Trans Am Ophthalmol Soc *77*:225–279, 1979.
Pisanti S, et al: Oral health parameters in Behçet's disease. A comparison between conventional therapy and cyclosporin A treatment. *In* Lehner T, Barnes CG (eds): Recent Advances in Behçet's Disease. New York, Royal Society of Medicine Services, 1986, pp 337–341.

COGAN'S SYNDROME
370.52

REX M. McCALLUM, M.D.

Durham, North Carolina

Cogan's syndrome is a rare clinical entity of unknown etiology first described by David Cogan in 1945. It occurs primarily in young adults, with an average age of onset of 28.6 years in 47 patients evaluated at the National Institutes of Health and Duke University Medical Center. The syndrome is characterized by inflammatory eye disease, typically nonsyphilitic interstitial keratitis, and vestibuloauditory dysfunction, typically Meniere's-like. Presenting ocular complaints are ocular discomfort (90 per cent), redness (79 per cent), and photophobia (68 per cent). Ocular examination reveals interstitial keratitis in 72 per cent, conjunctivitis in 34 per cent, iritis in 32 per cent, and episcleritis/scleritis in 28 per cent of cases. Presenting vestibuloauditory symptoms are vertigo (85 per cent), sudden hearing loss (79 per cent), sudden nausea and vomiting (70 per cent), tinnitus (53 per cent), ataxia (45 per cent), and gradual decrease in hearing (17 per cent). Vestibuloauditory features include Meniere's-like symptoms with hearing loss in 92 per cent, nystagmus in 32 per cent, oscillopsia in 15 per cent, Meniere's-like symptoms without hearing loss in 4 per cent, and hearing loss in 4 per cent. Ocular symptoms and signs develop initially in 50 per cent, with vestibuloauditory complaints initially and both within 1 month of one another in 25 per cent each. Half of patients have an antecedent upper respiratory illness.

The primary ocular manifestation, interstitial keratitis, is either acute and recurrent or chronic. It may vary in intensity from day to day and from eye to eye. In the acute stages, conjunctival hyperemia and patchy white infiltrates of the subepithelial are noted more often than deep or midcorneal stroma. Corneal infiltrates are more prominent at the periphery. In the later stages, corneal vascularization and opacity may be noted, typically at the corneal periphery. Posterior uveitis and other forms of ocular inflammation are found rarely.

Laboratory studies reveal WBC > 11,000 in 50 per cent, ESR of > 20 in 40 per cent, rheumatoid factor ≥1:80 in 10 per cent, and elevated CSF protein and/or WBC in 25 per cent of patients studied. The primary systemic complication is the development of aortitis and/or large vessel (Takayasu-like) vasculitis in 10 to 20 per cent of patients. Vascular complications may be more frequent in patients with ocular inflammation other than interstitial keratitis.

Ocular outcome is excellent with only 6 per cent of patients having a visual acuity of greater than 20/30 in either or both eyes. The auditory outcome is frequently permanent loss of hearing and is dependent upon oral corticosteroid therapy. Seventeen per cent of patients not treated with oral corticosteroids had an auditory threshold of <60 db, whereas 81 per cent of patients treated with oral corticosteroids had an auditory threshold of >60 db.

THERAPY

Ocular. Topical 1 per cent mydriatic solution or ointment is appropriate for the management of acute anterior uveitis. Topical corticosteroids are indicated for the control of corneal and ocular inflammation. One per cent prednisolone is a frequently used topical corticosteroid. It may be applied every 1 to 2 hours during the acute stages of inflammation and then tapered after an appropriate response. Between flares of interstitial keratitis, no topical ophthalmic therapy is usually necessary. Systemic corticosteroids are rarely necessary to control the symptoms and signs of acute interstitial keratitis, but they may be appropriate for the rare patient with posterior ocular inflammation associated with Cogan's syndrome.

Systemic. Systemic corticosteroids are immediately indicated in the treatment of hearing loss associated with Cogan's syndrome. Hearing loss may respond to corticosteroids with significant improvement. An initial trial of daily oral corticosteroid at a dose of 1 to 2 mg/kg/day prednisone-equivalent therapy is instituted. It can be started in divided doses for 3 to 5 days in severely symptomatic patients, with subsequent consolidation to a single daily morning dose. If hearing improves, then a once-daily regimen over 4 to 6 weeks followed by the tapering off to corticosteroids over the subsequent 6 to 8 weeks, while monitoring the patient's clinical status, is indicated. Such clinical parameters as auditory symptoms, ESR, ocular inflammatory disease, and audiogram establish the efficacy of therapy. If no response is noted in 2 to 3 weeks, then the patient should be rapidly tapered off corticosteroids, and a trial of immunosuppressive therapy should be considered. The effectiveness of such immunosuppressive treatment has never been established. Immunosuppressive therapy does seem effective for "steroid sparing" in some patients whose hearing loss responds to corticosteroid therapy but who cannot be tapered to an acceptably low dose or who suffer unacceptable steroid side effects.

Later in the course of Cogan's syndrome, if the patient does not respond to steroids and there is no clear evidence of inflammatory activity, hearing fluctuations may represent cochlear hydrops secondary to cochlear damage from previous episodes of inflammation. Fluctuation with changes in fluid status may be seen, such as vacillations that increase during the time around menses in women. Salt restriction and/or diuretic therapy may be effective in the treatment of hearing fluctuation secondary to cochlear hydrops. Commonly used diuretics are hydrochlorothiazide and chlorthalidone.

If aortitis with aortic insufficiency or large vessel (Takayasu's-like) vasculitis develops, treatment should be instituted with prednisone[‡] at 1 to 2 mg/kg/day and immunosuppressive therapy. Cyclophosphamide[‡] at 2 mg/kg/day with appropriate monitoring of the WBC has been used for aortitis. Cyclosporine[‡] at 5 mg/kg/day with appropriate monitoring of blood pressure and renal function is chosen for large vessel vasculitis. If one form of immunosuppressive therapy proves ineffective, the other should be tried. Aortic valve replacement should be considered in patients with hemodynamically significant aortic insufficiency. Aortitis can make this procedure technically challenging, and the cardiovascular surgeon should be made to understand the inflammatory nature of the problem. Ideally, the operation should occur after a period of treatment that is deemed effective. Vascular bypass procedures may be indicated to prevent ischemic tissue damage. Operating at a time of active inflammation can complicate such procedures; therefore, surgery should be postponed until effective treatment has been established, if possible. Prednisone is tapered to once-daily therapy after 4 to 6 weeks with subsequent tapering off in 2 to 3 months. Prolonged remission of both aortitis and large vessel vasculitis has been accomplished by the judicious use of the above treatment protocols in patients with the inflammatory vascular complications of Cogan's syndrome.

Ocular or Periocular Manifestations

Conjunctiva: Catarrhal conjunctivitis; chemosis; hyperemia.
Cornea: Stromal infiltration; interstitial keratitis; epithelial defects; vascularization.
Iris: Anterior uveitis.
Other: Nystagmus; pain, photophobia; rare posterior inflammation.

PRECAUTIONS

Corticosteroids are potentially dangerous medications, patients must be closely supervised and have the dosage individualized in accordance with the severity of the Cogan's syndrome, therapeutic response, side effects evident (if any), and the anticipated duration of therapy. Corticosteroids should be given as a single morning dose except for the initial few days when starting therapy or when there is an active inflammatory exacerbation of the disease. The least effective dose that controls the specific manifestation being treated should be sought and used for the shortest amount of time possible. The use of alternate-day regimens can frequently give therapeutic benefit while minimizing significant side effects. Tapering of corticosteroids should be performed gradually and cautiously while monitoring clinical parameters of disease activity. The side effects of systemic corticosteroids are numerous, potentially serious, and occur frequently in patients receiving prolonged therapy. They include osteoporosis, susceptibility to infections, weight gain, rounded facies, cataracts, increased intraocular pressure, proximal muscle weakness, easy bruisability, striae, and psychosis. Given the potential for side effects, trials of corticosteroid therapy should be administered with therapeutic goals, therapeutic end points, and criteria for monitoring established at the onset of the trial. The best indicators for corticosteroid therapy are hearing loss and the development of inflammatory vascular complications.

The most common side effects of hydrochlorothiazide and chlorthalidone are volume and potassium depletion. Potassium replacement therapy may be necessary. Unusual side effects of these drugs include leukopenia, allergic problems, and rashes.

Cyclosporine is a potent immunosuppressive agent that profoundly inhibits normal T-cell activation and function, in part through effects on interleukin-2. The primary clinically significant toxic manifestations of cyclosporine are renal dysfunction and hypertension. Renal dysfunction has four primary mechanisms. The first three are reversible and the last is not: (1) tubular dysfunction, (2) proximal tubulopathy, (3) vascular dysfunction, and (4) striped renal fibrosis (vasculopathy). Therefore, careful monitoring of both the blood pressure and renal function is necessary. Baseline serum creatinine should be established before instituting therapy, with subsequent monthly monitoring. Serum creatinine should not be allowed to rise greater than 30 per cent above the baseline. If this occurs, the cyclosporine dose should be decreased by 50 mg/day, and repeat monitoring should be undertaken in 2 weeks. The usual starting dose of cyclosporine is 2.5 to 5.0 mg/kg/day in two equally divided doses 12 hours apart. Doses of $\leq$ 5.0mg/kg/day and through levels of $\leq$ 400mg/ml may be associated with less renal dysfunction. If therapy is required for longer than 18 months, consideration of renal biopsy to assess any irreversible cyclosporine-induced changes is appropriate. Other potential cyclosporine side effects include hirsutism, infection, tremulousness, hypomagnesemia, hepatic dysfunction, nausea, and lymphorecticular neoplasm.

Cyclophosphamide, an alkylating agent, is also a potent immunosuppressive drug. Its potential side effects include bone marrow suppression, hemorrhagic cystitis, bladder cancer, nausea, infection (particularly herpetic), gonadal dysfunction, pulmonary and hepatic reactions, and lymphoreticular neoplasm. The drug is usually given each morning with breakfast and with forced fluids of 1 to 2 liters from breakfast to lunch to minimize the risk of bladder irritation. Initial doses are 2 mg/kg/day, unless severe inflammatory vascular disease is present; then, doses can begin at 4 mg/kg/day with careful monitoring. Blood counts are monitored every 1 to 2 weeks initially, and drug doses are adjusted to keep the WBC in the 3500 to 4000 cells/mm^3 range with an absolute neutrophil count $\geq$1000 cells/mm^3. Use of cyclophosphamide longer than 1 to 1$^1/_2$ years of continuous therapy should be considered only with the utmost care.

COMMENTS

The etiology of Cogan's syndrome is unknown, and the clinical course is extremely variable. Most often, the syndrome seems to be characterized by an acute phase lasting months to years followed by a low-grade, chronic phase that may persist forever, eventually become quiescent, or become intermittently active. Rare patients have died within months of disease onset, typically from associated systemic vasculitis. Topical ophthalmic corticosteroid therapy usually controls the symptoms of interstitial keratitis and seems to prevent the corneal vascularization noted in early untreated patients. It can be used intermittently for flares of ocular inflammation. Systemic corticosteroids are effective in preventing deafness, but some degree of loss of auditory acuity is the rule. Only two patients in our series were without any hearing loss. Most patients require steroids for only the first 2 to 6 months of their disease. Regular attempts must be made to taper the corticosteroid dose to the least effective level. Every other day and the intermittent use of steroids are effective in some patients. If a patient is unable to taper to an acceptable dose of steroids and/or significant steroid side effects develop, cyclophosphamide is capable of steroid-sparing activity in some patients, and a well-conceived therapeutic trial is recommended.

Inflammatory vascular complications occur in 10 to 12 per cent of patients. Periodic monitoring for signs and symptoms of a systemic vasculitis is essential. It should include carefully palpating all pulses and listening for the murmur of aortic insufficiency. Periodic two-dimensional echocardiographic monitoring of the aortic valve could be considered.

References

Allen NB, et al: Use of immunosuppressive agents in the treatment of severe ocular and vascular manifestations of Cogan's syndrome. Am J Med 88:296–301, 1990.

Cobo LM, Haynes BF: Early corneal findings in Cogan's syndrome. Ophthalmology 91:903–907, 1984.

Cogan DG: Syndrome of nonsyphilitic interstitial keratitis and vestibuloauditory symptoms. Arch Ophthalmol 33:144–149, 1945.

Haynes BF, et al: Cogan syndrome: Studies in thirteen patients, long term follow-up, and a review of the literature. Medicine 59:426–441, 1980.

Haynes BF, et al: Successful treatment of sudden hearing loss in Cogan's syndrome with corticosteroids. Arthritis Rheum 24:501–503, 1981.

Mason J: Renal side-effects of cyclosporine. Transplant Proc 22:1280–1283, 1990.

McCallum RM, et al: Cogan's syndrome: Clinical features and outcomes. Arthritis Rheum 35:S51, 1992.

FAMILIAL DYSAUTONOMIA 742.8

(Riley Day Syndrome)

FELICIA B. AXELROD, M.D.,
and ROBERT A. D'AMICO, M.D.

New York, New York

Familial dysautonomia is a congenital condition of autonomic dysfunction and decreased sensory appreciation. It is inherited as an autosomal recessive trait and occurs almost exclusively among Jews of Eastern European ancestry (Ashkenazi).

Consistent neuropathologic findings include low populations of sympathetic neurons and terminals, severe depletion of parasympathetic neurons in sphenopalatine ganglia but minimal depletion in ciliary ganglia, and a paucity of unmyelinated sensory neurons in sural nerves and dorsal root ganglia. Biochemical data indicate diminished norepinephrine and epinephrine excretion, but normal amounts of dopamine products.

Clinical manifestations of familial dysautonomia are caused by deficits in autonomic homeostatic function and sensory appreciation of peripheral pain and temperature. Prominent early manifestations include feeding difficulties, hypotonia, delayed developmental milestones, labile body temperature and blood pressure, absence of overflowing tears and corneal hypesthesia, marked diaphoresis with excitement, and breath-holding episodes. Gastroesophageal reflux is also common. Recurrent pneumonias are frequent and are caused by repeated aspiration. Intractable vomiting crises occur in 40 per cent of patients on a cyclical basis and are associated with hypertension, tachycardia, diffuse sweating, personality changes, and, occasionally, hyperpyrexia. Spinal curvature occurs in 95 per cent of patients by adolescence. Ocular complications occur primarily as a result of decreased lacrimation and corneal hypesthesia and often worsen during acute illnesses because of hypertension, fever, and dehydration. Convergence insufficiencies and exodeviations are frequently associated with familial dysautonomia, and there is a higher-than-normal incidence of myopia. Optic pallor and abnormal visual evoked potentials have also been noted and indicate further involvement of cranial sensory nerves. The optic neuropathy worsens with age and is compatible with a progressive neurologic disorder.

Diagnosis is confirmed by lack of an axon flare following the intradermal injection of histamine phosphate (1:10,000), miosis with dilute parasympathomimetic agents, decreased or absent deep tendon reflexes, and absence of fungiform papillae on the tongue.

THERAPY

Systemic. Treatment is directed to specific symptoms and complications. For infants with feeding problems, dietary therapy and thickened foods are used. In many cases, gastrostomy with fundoplication is indicated to maintain nutrition, avoid dehydration, correct gastroesophageal reflux, and prevent aspiration. Pulmonary hygiene, consisting of postural drainage, is helpful for children who have had recurrent pneumonias. Suctioning of tracheal secretions may be needed because of ineffective cough. Inhalation with bronchodilators and prophylactic antibiotics are used in selected cases.

Vomiting crises are managed in the hospital with intravenous fluids and parenteral diazepam. Diazepam[‡] at 0.2 mg/kg is given intravenously every 3 hours until the crisis is resolved. Induction of a deep sleep is necessary for resolution of the crisis. Chloral hydrate (30 mg/kg) can be given as a rectal suppository with diazepam to induce sleep and can be repeated every 6 hours as needed. For children with a gastrostomy, a crisis can often be managed at home. However, hospitalization is indicated if the crisis is not resolved by 12 hours, if serious infection is suspected because of high fever or uncharacteristic behavior, if blood or coffee-ground material is vomited, or if dehydration is suspected.

Ocular. Fundamental to the therapy of all dry eye syndromes is the regular use of tear substitutes. Frequency of instillation depends on the child's own baseline eye moisture, environmental conditions, and whether the child is febrile or dehydrated. Tear substitutes may be required as frequently as every half-hour. When more than 10 drops are necessary in a day, the toxicity of preservatives in a compromised epithelium should be considered. Use of a nonpreserved solution in unit-dose packaging is preferred. The wetting effect of saline solutions may be prolonged by the addition of viscosity-increasing, large molecular weight polymers, such as methylcellulose or polyvinyl alcohol. Increasing corneal surface wettability by the addition of mucomimetic polymers also may be beneficial. Lubricant rod inserts designed to thicken the precorneal tear film may not dissolve uniformly in an eye with a shallow lacrimal lake and a reduced blink rate, causing transient blurring of vision. Ointments are preferred for nighttime application.

Corneal hypesthesia compounds the problem, as it results in decreased blink frequency and indifference to corneal trauma. Epithelial erosions of the exposed cornea and conjunctiva are the hallmarks of dry eye states. These lesions may become confluent, leading to patchy areas of de-epithelialization. Early treatment of corneal epithelial erosions includes increased use of tear substitutes, prophylactic topical antibiotics, patching the eye, attention to the general state of hydration, and a search for a precipitating systemic factor that may have disturbed the patient's fragile catecholamine homeostasis. Persistent erosions or ulcerations may require more vigorous and innovative approaches, such as moisture chamber spectacle attachments, swim goggles or taped-on "bubbles" for sleep, bandage lenses, occlusion of the lacrimal puncta, or small lateral tarsorrhaphies that limit the area exposed to surface evaporation. Temporary narrowing of the palpebral fissures may limit progression of a surface defect and allow re-epithelialization while the patient's homeostasis is restored.

Temporary tarsorrhaphies can be obtained by adhesion of the outer lid margins without denuding of the opposing surfaces. Bipedicled tarsorrhaphies and conjunctival flaps are disfiguring and visually limiting. These procedures should be reserved for unresponsive cases in which the integrity of the globe is threatened. If tarsorrhaphy is required, eyelash destruction can be avoided by splitting the lid at the gray line and suturing only the posterior halves of the lids. Corneal epithelial repair may be encouraged by the use of a collagen shield hydrated in antibiotic solution. A therapeutic soft contact lens may also be used if there is no sign of infection and if tear supplementation and close monitoring are continued.

All epithelial defects are at risk for secondary infection, and corneal and conjunctival cultures should be obtained when clinical signs suggest contamination. In addition, lack of the irrigating function of tear flow and its bacteriostatic elements predisposes the eye to chronic blepharitis.

Calcium deposition in the region of the palpebral fissure may be seen in persistent corneal ulcerations. Dense, white, anterior stromal infiltrates accompanied by interstitial vascularization are noted occasionally. These infiltrates are sterile, seem to be caused by tissue anoxia, and usually respond to a short course of topical steroids. A dry eye is often a congested eye, and topical steroids may give a false picture of improvement by their anti-inflammatory action. The risks of long-term steroid therapy, such as lens opacification, secondary glaucoma, and susceptibility to infection, far outweigh any symptomatic benefits derived.

The dry anesthetic cornea is an unfavorable environment for a corneal graft. Delayed re-epithelialization, recurrent erosions, and late opacification frequently complicate and limit the fine visual result. The importance of restoring the patient's homeostasis when treating ocular complications in familial dysautonomia cannot be overemphasized. Failure to correct dehydration or even a low-grade systemic infection can thwart the most heroic efforts at ocular therapy.

Ocular or Periocular Manifestations

Cornea: Hypesthesia; ulcer.
Eyelids: Blepharitis.
Lacrimal System: Decreased tear secretion.

Other: Hyperreactivity to sympathetic and parasympathetic agents; myopia; optic pallor; sensitivity to preservatives; strabismus.

PRECAUTIONS

Systemic dehydration compounds the problem of the dry eye. Vomiting crises, febrile episodes, and severe diarrhea should be considered situations that pose potentially increased risk to the cornea.

If surgical procedures are performed, special precautions are required in the administration of anesthesia. Dysautonomic patients have labile blood pressures and diminished responsiveness to variations in blood bases. Local anesthesia is preferred. However, if general anesthesia is indicated, the patient should be hydrated preoperatively, as well as intraoperatively, and there should be constant intraoperative monitoring of blood pressure and heart rate.

COMMENTS

Cornea pathology is complicated. The relatively dry eye and corneal hypesthesia predispose to de-epithelialization, but systemic autonomic dysfunction and disturbed catecholamine homeostasis may precipitate acute problems, complicate management, and inhibit normal healing processes.

Vigorous attention to systemic problems, avoiding chronic and acute dehydration, and early attention to corneal problems through education of parents and patients have helped preserve corneal integrity and resulted in a decreased need for tarsorrhaphies.

References

Axelrod FB: Familial dysautonomia. *In* Gellis SS, Kagan BM (eds): Current Pediatric Therapy 13. Philadelphia, WB Saunders, 1990, pp 94–96.

Axelrod FB, Nachtigal R, Dancis J: Familial dysautonomia: Diagnosis, pathogenesis and management. Adv Pediatr 21:75–96, 1974.

Brunt PW, McKusick VA: Familial dysautonomia. A report of genetic and clinical studies, with a review of the literature. Medicine 49:343–374, 1970.

Diamond GA, D'Amico RA, Axelrod FB: Optic nerve dysfunction in familial dysautonomia. Am J Ophthalmol 104:645–648, 1987.

Ginsberg SP, et al: Autonomic dysfunction syndrome. Am J Ophthalmol 74:1121–1125, 1972.

Goldberg MF, Payne JW, Brunt PW: Ophthalmologic studies of familial dysautonomia. The Riley-Day syndrome. Arch Ophthalmol 80:732–743, 1968.

Howard RO: Familial dysautonomia (Riley-Day syndrome). Am J Ophthalmol 64:392–398, 1967.

Pearson J, Axelrod F, Dancis J: Current concepts of dysautonomia: Neuropathological defects. Ann NY Acad Sci 228:288–300, 1974.

Rizzo JF III, Lessell S, Liebman SD: Optic atrophy in familial dysautonomia. Am J Ophthalmol 102: 463, 1986.

Smith AA, Dancis J, Brienin G: Ocular responses to

autonomic drugs in familial dysautonomia. Invest Ophthalmol 4:358–361, 1965.

HISTIOCYTOSIS X 277.8
(Eosinophilic Granuloma, Hand-Schüller-Christian Disease, Letterer-Siwe Disease)

DAVID J. APPLE, M.D.,
TIMOTHY P. POWERS, M.D.,
HUGH L. HENNIS, M.D., Ph.D.,

Charlotte, North Carolina

and KEVIN N. MILLER, M.D.

Las Vegas, Nevada

The term "histiocytosis X" refers to a spectrum of diseases of unclear etiology that are characterized by an abnormal proliferation of histiocytes. These histiocytic syndromes have been recently reorganized into three groups based primarily on their pathologic features. The first of these three groups includes the Langerhans' cell histiocytes. Included under this category are Letterer-Siwe, Hand-Schüller-Christian syndrome, and eosinophilic granuloma. Until recently, these three diseases were referred to as histiocytosis X, a term first proposed by Lichtenstein in 1952. These entities are currently considered part of a continuous clinical spectrum and are classified as acute disseminated Langerhans' histiocytosis, multifocal, and unifocal Langerhans' cell histiocytosis, respectively. The second category includes histiocytes that are not Langerhans' cells. Included in this group is juvenile xanthogranuloma. The final group encompasses malignant disorders of histiocytes, including histiocytic lymphoma and acute monocytic leukemia.

Langerhans' cells are derived from bone marrow and are characterized by a dendritic pattern, clear cytoplasm, and ultrastructurally by Birbeck granules. Birbeck granules are pentalamer, rodlike, tubular structures with a characteristic periodicity and sometimes a dilated terminal end that resembles a tennis racket. By studying cell surface markers, these cells have been identified as belonging to the monocyte/macrophage group. They may be detected in tissue sections by monoclonal antibodies directed against cell-surface antigens including T_4 and T_6 markers, class II histocompatibility antigens, and an intracytoplasmic marker, the S100 protein. These immunologic markers and ultrastructural features are present in the histiocytosis X cells that infiltrate organs involved in these disorders.

The widespread location of the histiocytic system in the human body explains the numerous clinical manifestations of this disease. Letterer-Siwe disease, also termed "acute disseminated Langerhans' cell histiocytosis," is typically much more "malignant" than the former two entities in a clinical sense. Some authors consider eosinophilic granuloma and Hand-Schüller-Christian disease as variants of the same disease process, i.e., unifocal and multifocal Langerhans' cell histiocytosis. However, highly disseminated forms of Hand-Schüller-Christian disease may occur that may more closely resemble the findings of Letterer-Siwe disease. Therefore, since histiocytosis X may exhibit such a wide variety of clinical manifestations, it does not always fit precisely into one of the above three categories. Some authors have assumed eosinophilic granuloma to be characterized by well-differentiated histiocytes contrasted to poorly differentiated histiocytes in Letterer-Siwe disease. Others have concluded that the lesions are basically similar in appearance regardless of clinical course. In a detailed study of the atypia in mitotic activity in histiocytosis X, the authors were unable to predict clinical outcome from the histopathologic findings. Additionally, flow cytometric studies have shown conflicting results. Euploidy has been demonstrated in the majority of cases. However, aneuploidy has also been reported. It is not known whether aneuploidy portends a poor prognosis. The most significant prognostic factors are thus clinical: the age of onset of disease, extent of involvement, rapidity of progression, and presence or absence of visceral involvement.

Eosinophilic granuloma of bone (unifocal Langerhans' cell histiocytosis), the most "benign" disease in this group, may occur over a wide age range, from the preschool years to adulthood. Most cases are diagnosed before the age of 10, but onset well into adult life is not unusual; therefore, these patients are on the average slightly older than those in the other two categories. The hallmark of the disease is bone infiltrates, which may be unifocal or multifocal. They most commonly affect the skull, ribs, vertebrae, pelvis, scapula, and proximal long bones. These lesions may be visible or palpable and may be associated with pain or tenderness. So-called extraosseous forms of eosinophilic granuloma, most commonly affecting the gastrointestinal tract and lung, have also been described.

Unifocal eosinophilic granuloma behaves almost invariably as a benign lesion and responds readily to excision or radiation therapy. With multifocal disease, there is a clear overlap in symptoms with Hand-Schüller-Christian disease, and the two entities may be difficult to separate by either clinical or histologic criteria.

Hand-Schüller-Christian disease (multifocal Langerhans' cell histiocytosis) is an intermediate form between eosinophilic granuloma and Letterer-Siwe disease. It includes a combination of the bony lesions that are more typically associated with eosinophilic granuloma and some of the visceral and soft tissue lesions that are the hallmark of Letterer-Siwe disease. Typically, patients have fever; a diffuse, scaly, seborrhea-like eruption, particularly on the scalp and in the ear canals; and frequent bouts of otitis media, mastoiditis, and upper respiratory infections, as well as gingival inflammations. Lymphadenopathy, hepatomegaly, splenomegaly, and pneumonitis may be present. Granulomatous involvement of the posterior pituitary stalk or hypothalamus leads to diabetes insipidus. Orbital lesions may induce exophthalmos. The classic clinical triad of Hand-Schüller-Christian disease comprises bony lesions in the skull, exophthalmos, and diabetes insipidus. Actually, the full triad occurs in only a small percentage of patients. This disease occurs during childhood, usually presenting before the age of 4 years. This is a slightly older age group than that seen in Letterer-Siwe disease, which typically occurs in infancy. As one might expect, it often has a clinical course intermediate in character between that of Letterer-Siwe disease and eosinophilic granuloma.

The most severe form of histiocytosis X, Letterer-Siwe disease (acute differentiated histiocytosis), is usually seen in children under 2 years of age. In addition, congenital forms have been described. The disease is rapidly progressive, often fatal, and characterized by widespread tissue involvement with cellular infiltration. Most commonly involved are the skin, lungs, lymph nodes, liver, spleen, bone marrow, and gingival mucosa. The disease is not uniformly fatal, however. In one series, a mortality rate of 70 per cent in children under the age of 6 months was reported. In general, the younger the child at the onset of the disease, the worse the prognosis. The bony involvement, typically seen in eosinophilic granuloma, is less prominent. These patients may develop liver, lung, or bone marrow dysfunction, all of which are poor prognostic signs. Most deaths are secondary to hepatic or lung failure or complications, such as bleeding or infection.

The widespread effects of histiocytosis X sometimes result in infiltration of ocular and periocular structures. Several studies have shown that the incidence of orbital involvement is about 20 per cent. In addition, only about half of these developed proptosis. The most commonly seen signs of eye involvement include unilateral and bilateral proptosis and, less frequently, papilledema with optic atrophy.

Exophthalmos is usually caused by involvement by lytic lesions of the orbital bones, but rarely may be due to involvement of the orbital soft tissues. On rare occasions, the globe may be directly involved by infiltrates as with the choroidal infiltrates seen in Letterer-Siwe disease. In addition, secondary open-angle glaucoma, bilateral perforating corneal ulcers, nystagmus, secondary intracranial palsies, posterior scleritis, eyelid infiltration, and secondary infection all have been reported.

When confronted with a questionable case of histiocytosis X, appropriate studies include a complete blood count with differential, liver function tests (SGOT, SGPT, alkaline phosphatase, bilirubin, total protein, and albumin), coagulation studies, chest x-ray, skeletal radiograph survey, urine osmolality measurement after overnight water deprivation, and bone marrow biopsy. Other studies, such as liver biopsy, dental radiography, and endocrine evaluation, should be performed for specific indications, and consultation with a pediatric oncologist should be sought. Orbital x-rays may reveal evidence of a lytic lesion that frequently shows a narrow zone of sclerosis. The gold standard of diagnosis is still a detailed histopathologic examination of appropriate biopsy specimens.

THERAPY

Irradiation. Single bony lesions and even cases with multifocal lesions affecting the bone have an excellent prognosis. Spontaneous clearing may actually occur in some cases. When therapy is required, lesions are often best treated with curettage or local low-dose irradiation or both. If a lesion is easily accessible and asymptomatic, a diagnostic biopsy followed by a simple curettage or excision is often all that is needed. If the lesion recurs or does not improve clinically or radiographically, local irradiation is indicated.

If curettage is difficult or is required in a location that may result in dysfunction or disfigurement, a diagnostic biopsy followed by irradiation is the preferred initial treatment. Biopsy with irradiation is also preferred over curettage for large lesions in weight-bearing bones because it lessens the likelihood of pathologic fractures.

Vertebral lesions present a special situation and may require radiation therapy if there is partial collapse or lytic involvement. Only low-dose irradiation is needed for bony lesions. A dose of 400 to 600 rads given in 150- to 200-rad fractions daily is usually effective.

The most common ophthalmic complications of histiocytosis X are localized orbital and periorbital lesions with or without exophthalmos. These complications can be treated much like other localized lesions. Low-dose radiation therapy with 300 to 600 rads or curettage or both are often effective. Additionally, intralesional injection of 125 mg methoprednisolone sodium with or without computed tomographic guidance has been reported to be effective.

Systemic. The optimum treatment regimen for disseminated histiocytosis X (usually connoting severe forms of the Hand-Schüller-Christian disease variant, as well as Letterer-Siwe disease) has not been established. The variable clinical presentation or course and the fact that this disease sometimes undergoes spontaneous remission have made evaluation of therapy difficult. Evaluation has been further complicated by the disease's response to a wide variety of therapeutic modalities. These include steroids, vinca alkaloids (vincristine or vinblastine), alkylating agents, antimetabolites, antibiotics, radiation, and thymic extract.[†]

It remains to be determined what drug or drug combination will be most effective for a given patient with disseminated histiocytosis X. Some authors have shown that vinblastine used as a single agent can be effective in treating severe forms of this disease. It may be given intravenously once a week at an initial dose of 0.15 mg/kg. This dose is increased by 0.05 mg/kg weekly until the white blood cell count drops below 3000/mm³. Thereafter, the maximum dose that does not cause leukopenia is given weekly. If the disease clears in 12 weeks, the medication is discontinued and the patient observed. If there is improvement in the majority of the initial organs involved but not complete remission, the patient continues with the maximum tolerated dose given every 2 weeks for 3 to 6 months. If the patient is started on vinblastine and there is no improvement or improvement in less than 50 per cent of the initial organs involved after 12 weeks of therapy, the patient should be started on another regimen.

Prednisone may be administered in conjunction with the above regimen for vinblastine. Prednisone has often been helpful in reducing exophthalmos. It is administered orally in a daily dosage of 2 mg/kg in three divided doses for 6 weeks. This is followed by 1 mg/kg daily for 4 weeks, and it is then gradually reduced over a 2-week period and discontinued.

More aggressive therapy is justified in patients with the most severe forms of disseminated histiocytosis X, particularly infants with Letterer-Siwe disease and severe organ dysfunction. A few of these patients have been treated with a combination of vinblastine, prednisolone, methotrexate[‡], and cyclophosphamide.[‡] Vinblastine is given in an intravenous dose of 6.5 mg/m² once a week for 8 weeks. The daily dose of prednisolone is 40 mg/m², given orally once a day for 6 weeks. The weekly dose for methotrexate is 20 mg/m², administered once a week 1 day after vinblastine for 8 weeks. Administration of 200 mg/m² of cyclophosphamide once a week for 8 weeks may be given 2 days after methotrexate. After this 8-week induction phase is completed, weekly cyclophosphamide and methotrexate are continued in the above doses. The patient is also given consolidation courses of vinblastine; this is defined as daily doses of 6.5 mg/m² for 1 week and is repeated every 4 weeks. The therapy is discontinued if all measurable lesions disappear. If there is resolution of 50 per cent or more of the initial lesions, the treatment is continued for 6 more months.

Irradiation can be combined with chemotherapy in treating disseminated histiocytosis X. The severity of gingival and cutaneous lesions may be reduced by giving 450 to 600 rads in 2 or 3 fractions during the time period while the response to chemotherapy is being evaluated.

Ocular. Intraocular infiltrates, usually manifested as an anterior or posterior uveitis or less commonly as a scleritis, must be treated according to the standard regimens that are well known to ophthalmologists. In addition, the cornea must be protected from exposure by frequent instillation of lubricants and ointments, cellophane patching, or lateral tarsorrhaphy.

Supportive. Supportive care is also very important in treating disseminated histiocytosis X. Appropriate antibiotics, blood products, nutrition, skin care, physical therapy, and orthopedic care are often required.

Ocular or Periocular Manifestations

Anterior Chamber: Cells and flare due to anterior uveitis; hypopyon; spontaneous hemorrhage.

Choroid: Extramedullary hematopoiesis (rare); infiltration by histiocytic cells leading to a rather diffuse, flat thickening.

Conjunctiva: Chemosis; dilated vessels.

Cornea: Bullous keratopathy; endothelial atrophy; infiltration; pannus; perforation; scarring; ulcer; vascularization.

Eyelids: Edema; infiltration; rash; xanthoma, especially in patients with icterus.

Globe: Exophthalmos; luxation.

Iris or Ciliary Body: Cellular infiltration with possible secondary increased intraocular pressure; infiltration; iridocyclitis or cyclitis with possible formation of a cyclitic membrane; nodular lesions mimicking tumors or juvenile Xanthogranuloma; pigmentary changes, including heterochromia; secondary atrophy; uveitis or iridocyclitis with potential for synechiae formation.

Lens: Cataract.

Optic Nerve: Atrophy and gliosis; infiltration of surrounding meninges; papilledema.

Orbit: Infiltrates; periorbital bone lesions.

Retina: Degeneration; detachment and retinal folds; edema; histiocytic infiltration.

Sclera: Episcleritis; scleritis.

Vitreous: Histiocytic infiltration, often leading to liquefaction.

Other: Glaucoma; nystagmus; phthisis bulbi; poor pupillary dilation with mydriatics; visual loss.

PRECAUTIONS

Although many of the chosen therapeutic agents have significant associated morbidity, the severe forms of histiocytosis X may show such severe extremes of morbidity and mortality that radical treatment may be required. Therapy should be undertaken only by physicians experienced in the use of such chemotherapeutic agents (usually pediatric oncologists) and should be monitored closely with frequent blood counts and periodic evaluations of liver and renal function.

Systemic steroids are also useful in reducing exophthalmos. Nevertheless, depending on the severity of the disease, the side effects associated with their use must be considered carefully.

Low-dose irradiation of the eye carries the risk of producing radiation cataracts.

COMMENTS

Diabetes insipidus is a classic complication of histiocytosis X, and local radiation therapy may be beneficial in preventing its progression. This treatment is most effective in patients with at least partial urinary-concentrating ability. Low doses of 800 to 1200 rads delivered to the hypothalamic-pituitary region are probably sufficient for this treatment. Vasopressin is important in the management of patients who retain some degree of pituitary dysfunction. Intrathecal methotrexate has also been used to treat diabetes insipidus, but the results have been disappointing.

Some patients have been shown to have decreased levels of human growth hormone associated with impaired linear growth. Therapy with human growth hormone is therefore indicated in selected patients.

Infections are common in patients with histiocytosis X, both because of the nature of the disease and its treatment. Otitis media is a frequent complication and may result in the loss of hearing. The physician should watch for and be prepared to treat these infections. However, prophylactic antibiotics are not useful because they predispose the patient to opportunistic infections.

References

Cotran RS, Kumar V, Robbins SL: Robbins Pathologic Basis of Disease, 4th ed. Philadelphia, WB Saunders Co, 1989, pp 745–747.

Favara BE: Langerhans' cell histiocytosis: Pathobiology and pathogenesis. Sem Oncol 18:3–7, 1991.

Greenberger JS, et al: Results of treatment of 127 patients with systemic histiocytosis (Letterer-Siwe syndrome, Hand-Schüller-Christian syndrome and multifocal eosinophilic granuloma). Medicine 60:311–338, 1981.

Harrist TJ, Bhan AK, Murphy GF: Histiocytosis X: In situ characterization of cutaneous infiltrates with monoclonal antibodies. Am J Clin Pathol 79:294–300, 1983.

Jakobiec FA, Jones IS: Lymphomatous, plasmacytic, histiocytic, and hematopoietic tumors. In Duane TD (ed): Clinical Ophthalmology. Hagerstown, MD, Harper & Row, 1982, Vol II, 39:28–37.

Kindy-Degnan NA, Laflamme P, Duprat G, Allaire GS: Case reports. Intralesional steroid in the treatment of an orbital eosinophilic granuloma. Arch Ophthalmol 109:617–618, 1991.

Lahey ME: Prognostic factors in histiocytosis X. Am J Pediatr Hematol Oncol 3:57–60, 1981.

Moore AT, Pritchard J, Taylor DSI: Histiocytosis X: An ophthalmological review. Br J Ophthalmol 69:7–14, 1985.

Ornvold K, Carstensen H, Larsen JK, Christensen IJ, Ralfkiaer E: Flow cytometric DNA analysis of lesions from 18 children with Langerhans cell histiocytosis (Histiocytosis X). Am J Pathol 136:1301–1307, 1990.

Osband ME: Histiocytosis X: Langerhans cell histiocytosis. Hematol Oncol Clin North Am 1(4):737–751, 1987.

Richter MP, D'Angio GJ: The role of radiation therapy in the management of children with histiocytosis X. Am J Pediatr Hematol Oncol 3:161–163, 1981.

Risdall RJ, Dehner LP, Duray P, Kobrinsky N, Robison L, Nesbit ME: Histiocytosis X (Langerhans' cell histiocytosis). Prognostic role of histopathology. Arch Pathol Lab Med 107:59–63, 1983.

Starling KA: Chemotherapy of histiocytosis. Am J Pediatr Hematol Oncol 3:157–160, 1981.

The Clinical Writing Group of the Histiocyte Society: Broadbent V, Gadner H, Komp DM, Ladisch S: Histiocytosis syndromes in children: II. Approach to the clinical and laboratory evaluation of children with Langerhans cell histiocytosis. Med Pediatr Oncol 17:492–495, 1989.

Wood CM, Pearson ADJ, Cratt AW, Howe JW: Globe luxation in histiocytosis X. Br J Ophthalmol 72:631–633, 1988.

INTERSTITIAL NEPHRITIS 583.89

JAMES T. ROSENBAUM, M.D.

Portland, Oregon

Acute tubulointerstitial nephritis is a form of renal inflammation characterized by the presence of a mononuclear infiltrate in the interstitium and tubules of the kidney. Patients display variable degrees of azotemia along with sterile pyuria. Eosinophils may be present in the urine. Hypertension, oliguria, hematuria, and marked proteinuria, which are characteristic of glomerular disease, are less common in interstitial nephritis. In addition to the renal disease, patients are often systemically ill with fever, anemia, mildly abnormal liver function tests, and abdominal pain. Although an antecedent event for interstitial nephritis is often not found, it may be precipitated by drugs, infections, and immunologic diseases, such as Sjogren's syndrome. Medications that may trigger an acute tubulointerstitial nephritis include antibiotics, such as cephalosporins, or nonsteroidal anti-inflammatory drugs, such as ibuprofen. The disease is more common in children than adults and in women than men. A definitive diagnosis is established by renal biopsy. Chronic interstitial nephritis is characterized primarily by fibrosis rather than interstitial edema. The differential diagnosis for chronic interstitial nephritis includes Alport's syndrome, multiple myeloma, gout, and heavy metal poisoning.

Acute interstitial nephritis may be accompanied by a bilateral, acute onset, anterior uveitis. The eye disease usually occurs subsequent to the renal disease by several months, but instances in which the eye disease precedes or accompanies the kidney involvement have also been described. Although an anterior uveitis is characteristic, cells in the vitreous humor and intraretinal hemorrhage have been described. Synechiae, keratic precipitates, and increased intraocular pressure may complicate the iritis. Although interstitial nephritis with uveitis is considered a rare disease, it is probably underrecognized and should be suspected in patients with a bilateral iritis in association with a systemic illness.

THERAPY

Systemic. For all patients, the use of potential triggering medications, such as ibuprofen, should be stopped. Patients with mild disease may respond without specific therapeutic intervention. Patients with an increasing creatinine level or with systemic symptoms usually respond promptly to systemic corticosteroids. For example, an initial starting dose of 20 to 60 mg per day of prednisone or its equivalent will usually result in a rapid therapeutic response. After renal function has improved and reached a plateau, corticosteroids can usually be withdrawn gradually without loss of the achieved therapeutic benefit.

Ocular. Topical or periocular corticosteroids and dilating drops should be used as is appropriate for any noninfectious form of anterior uveitis. A brief course of oral corticosteroids in doses similar to what might be used for the renal disease will generally result in a rapid response. For most patients, the eye disease will resolve completely, and all medications can be withdrawn completely without recurrence, although the eye disease may persist or recur after the resolution of the renal disease.

Ocular or Periocular Manifestations

Iris: Iridocyclitis.

References

Cameron JS: Allergic interstitial nephritis: Clinical features and pathogenesis. Q J Med 66:97, 1988.
Rosenbaum JT: Bilateral anterior uveitis and interstitial nephritis. Am J Ophthalmol 105:534, 1988.
Salu P, Stempels N, Vanden Houte K, Verbeelen D: Acute tubulointerstitial nephritis and uveitis in the elderly. Br J Ophthalmol 74:53, 1990.
Toto RD: Review: Acute tubulointerstitial nephritis. Am J Med Sci 299:392, 1990.

REITER'S DISEASE 099.3
K. MATTI SAARI, M.D.

Turku, Finland

Reiter's disease is a symptom complex with varying degrees of expression. Patients have a high incidence of HLA-B27 antigen. The disease has been reported more frequently in males than in females during the years of maximum sexual activity. It may occur as a complication of nonspecific urethritis, postgonococcal urethritis, or dysentery and after *Yersinia*, *Salmonella*, or *Campylobacter* infection. Commonly, a first attack in the male consists of nonspecific urethritis (with or without complications of hemorrhagic cystitis or epididymitis), conjunctivitis, anterior uveitis, latex negative erosion polyarthritis with marked periarthritis, and fascitis. Characteristic keratodermic involvement of skin and mucous membrane occurs in about 25 per cent of patients. Circinate balanitis may develop first after the nonspecific urethritis and is a sign that arthritis is about to develop. There may also be cardiac or neurologic involvement. Sequelae may include painful deformed feet, ankylosing spondylitis, and, rarely, aortic incompetence or amyloid disease. In recurrent attacks of the venereal form, genital infection may sometimes be absent after systemic treatment. *Chlamydia* has been isolated from urethral material in about 50 per cent of the cases.

Ocular manifestations in Reiter's disease are common and nonspecific; over 50 per cent of patients develop eye lesions. The conjunctivitis, which is usually bilateral and mucopurulent, occurs in 30 to 50 per cent of patients and is occasionally the presenting complaint, but usually causes little discomfort. Anterior uveitis occurs in severe attacks, which may last 6 weeks or longer; although the disease usually follows a self-limiting course, recurrences are common. Corneal complications are rare and consist of epithelial edema and erosions, superficial punctate keratitis, and anterior stromal infiltrates affecting mainly the peripheral cornea. The infiltrates disappear generally during several weeks without any permanent scar or residua.

THERAPY

Systemic. The urethritis associated with Reiter's disease warrants administration of a

3- to 4- week course of oral tetracyclines. The usual adult dosage of tetracycline or oxytetracycline is 250 to 500 mg, given four times daily after meals. Alternatively, 100 mg of doxycycline can be given one to two times daily after meals; this drug is well absorbed and causes little gastrointestinal upset. While urethritis persists, other manifestations remain or may recur. Tests of overnight urethral secretion will show when the urethritis has cleared. It is epidemiologically vital that all sexual partners be examined for genital infection. If treatment is necessary, it should be given concurrently to prevent "ping-pong" reinfection. When *Chlamydia* infection is affecting the whole family, oral erythromycin is the drug of choice for children (daily dosage 40 mg/kg) and for pregnant women (500 mg administered every 8 hours).

Septic cases of *Salmonella, Shigella,* and *Yersinia* infections triggering Reiter's disease can be treated with a mixture of trimethoprim and sulfamethoxazole; the suggested adult oral dosage is 160 mg of trimethoprim and 800 mg of sulfamethoxazole twice daily. The recommended daily dose for children is 6 mg/kg of trimethoprim and 30 mg/kg of sulfamethoxazole. *Yersinia* infection in adults is usually treated with 250 mg of oral tetracycline every 6 hours for 10 days. *Campylobacter* infection is treated, when needed, with erythromycin; the oral dosage for adults is 250 to 500 mg every 6 hours and 40 mg/kg daily for children.

Ocular. The anterior uveitis usually responds gradually to standard therapy with cycloplegics and corticosteroids. This regimen usually includes topically administered corticosteroids, such as 0.1 per cent dexamethasone or 0.5 to 1.0 per cent prednisolone, every hour daily and corticosteroid ointment for the night, and 1 per cent atropine or 0.25 per cent scopolamine three times daily. In severe cases with fulminant onset of intraocular inflammation, 60 mg of oral prednisolone daily with subsequent lowering of dosage or anterior subconjunctival depot corticosteroid injection* (into the lower fornix or beneath Tenon's capsule) may be used. Another alternative in severe cases is the anterior subconjunctival injection of a soluble corticosteroid, such as 1 ml of dexamethasone* solution containing 4 mg/ml, which is repeated every 1 to 2 days. Conjunctivitis does not usually require treatment, but the lubricating action of 1 per cent chlortetracycline ophthalmic ointment is comforting. Keratitis is often self-limited during the systemic therapy. Corneal erosions can be treated with 0.5 per cent chloramphenicol eye drops four times daily and the subepithelial infiltrates with 0.1 per cent dexamethasone or 0.5 to 1.0 per cent prednisolone eye drops four times daily.

Supportive. The patient with arthritis and a high erythrocyte sedimentation rate should be admitted to the hospital for rest. Symptomatic therapy for arthritis associated with Reiter's disease includes nonsteroidal anti-inflammatory drugs and modalities of physical therapy. Indomethacin is the agent of choice, administered in a dosage of 25 to 50 mg three times daily. If indomethacin is not tolerated, other nonsteroidal anti-inflammatory drugs can be used. These agents relieve pain, reduce swelling and tenderness of the joints, and increase grip strength.

Ocular or Periocular Manifestations

Anterior Chamber: Cells and flare; fibrinous exudate.
Conjunctiva: Chemosis; follicles; hyperemia; mucopurulent conjunctivitis; subpalpebral papillary conjunctivitis.
Cornea: Anterior stromal infiltrates, edema; epithelial erosion; fine keratic precipitates; punctate keratitis.
Iris: Acute anterior uveitis; posterior synechiae; vasodilation of iris vessels.
Optic Nerve: Disc edema; optic neuritis.
Other: Cells in vitreous; macular edema.

PRECAUTIONS

Photosensitivity may follow the intake of tetracyclines, particularly doxycycline; therefore, patients taking such drugs should limit their exposure to the sun. Any product containing aluminum, magnesium, or calcium ions (antacids, milk, and milk products) should not be taken 1 hour before or 2 hours after an oral dose of a tetracycline, since it can decrease the absorption by as much as 25 to 50 per cent. An exception to this is doxycycline, which is well absorbed in the presence of milk and milk products and is best taken with milk after meals. Tetracyclines should be avoided during pregnancy and in children younger than 8 years of age because of irreversible deposition of the substance in growing teeth and bones.

Local side effects of topical corticosteroids may include a rise in intraocular pressure. This rise can usually be handled by the addition of topically administered 1 per cent epinephrine or 0.5 per cent timolol eyedrops twice daily or by oral carbonic anhydrase inhibitors. Fluorometholone is of value in such patients, since it rarely causes an increase in intraocular pressure.

In Reiter's disease, the urethritis, balanitis, conjunctivitis, and mouth ulcers are often clinically silent, and these components of the disease are frequently missed. "Formes frustes" of the syndrome are becoming more clearly recognized, and the condition will be diagnosed more often also in females. In children, the diagnosis may be made during an epidemic of dysentery or enteritis, with Reiter's syndrome affecting many members of the family.

COMMENTS

Recurrences without urethritis should probably still be treated with tetracycline. The conjunctivitis is usually painless, clears by itself within days, and is not affected by treatment. The keratitis, although self-limited, may be temporarily incapacitating.

Many individuals develop an exacerbation or relapse without obvious reason, and the disease is frequently disturbing for the patient producing feelings of guilt and anxiety about sexual misconduct. Therefore, one of the major considerations in treatment is explanation of the recurrent nature of the condition: the patients have a genetically determined susceptibility to develop Reiter's disease after contact with an unrecognized (or recognized) precipitating event.

References

Calin A: Reiter's syndrome. Med Clin North Am 61:365–376, 1977.

Lee DA, et al: The clinical diagnosis of Reiter's syndrome. Ophthalmology 93:350–356, 1986.

Ostler HB, et al: Reiter's syndrome. Am J Ophthalmol 71:986–991, 1971.

Rowson NJ, Dart JKG: Keratitis in Reiter's syndrome. Br J Ophthalmol 76:126, 1992.

Saari KM: Reiter's syndrome: Ocular features. *In* Bialasiewicz AA (ed): Update on Infectious Diseases of the Eye. New York, Springer, 1993, pp 833–841.

Saari KM, Kauranen O: Ocular inflammation in Reiter's syndrome associated with *Compylobacter jejuni* enteritis. Am J Ophthalmol 90:572–573, 1980.

Saari KM, et al: Ocular inflammation in Reiter's disease after *Salmonella* enteritis. Am J Ophthalmol 90:63–68, 1980.

Wiggins RE, Steinkuller PG, Hamill MB: Reiter's keratoconjunctivitis. Arch Ophthalmol 108:280–281, 1990.

SARCOIDOSIS 135

DANIEL H. GOLD, M.D.,
and ERNESTO I. SEGAL, M.D.

Galveston, Texas

Sarcoidosis is a systemic inflammatory disease characterized by the development of noncaseating epitheliod cell granulomas in tissues and organs throughout the body. It may take an acute or chronic course and is often a benign self-limited disorder. Its clinical manifestations are protean and depend upon the specific site(s) of inflammation in any given patient. Intrathoracic involvement occurs in close to 90 per cent of cases, with granulomas in the lungs or intrathoracic lymphoid tissue. Ocular involvement occurs in about 25 per cent of cases and produces some of the most serious complications of this disorder.

Although its etiology is unknown, sarcoidosis is associated with several immunologic abnormalities. Immunohistopathologic studies have demonstrated a high ratio of T-helper to T-suppressor lymphocytes in the lungs, lymph nodes, and eyes of patients with active sarcoidosis. Lymphokines produced by these activated T-helper cells may attract other inflammatory cells, resulting in the subsequent development of a typical granuloma. They may also affect the humoral immune system by stimulating B-lymphocytes to produce a polyclonal increase in circulating immunoglobulins, as well as a variety of autoantibodies.

THERAPY

Ocular. Most of the ophthalmologic complications of sarcoidosis are secondary to inflammatory involvement of ocular or periocular structures and respond quite well to steroid therapy. Topical steroids may suffice in the treatment of anterior uveitis. During waking hours, 1 per cent prednisolone eyedrops are used every 1 to 2 hours, with gradual tapering of the dose as the inflammation subsides. This treatment must be combined with mydriatic/cycloplegic drops to avoid development of posterior synechiae with a small bound-down pupil. Long-acting drugs, such as 1 per cent atropine twice daily or 2 to 5 per cent homatropine four times daily, are preferred in acute or severe uveitis, whereas shorter-acting mydriatics (1 per cent tropicamide) can be used once daily to keep the pupil moving in patients with low-grade, chronic inflammatory disease. A combination of mydriatic agents, including 2.5 or 10 per cent phenylephrine, may be used in an attempt to break pre-existent posterior synechiae.

When anterior segment inflammation is very severe or does not respond quickly to topical medication, this treatment should be supplemented by anterior subtenon steroid injection; 40 mg of triamcinolone,* 40 mg of methylprednisolone,* 24 mg of dexamethasone*, or 20 mg of betamethasone may be used. Triamcinolone has the greatest anti-inflammatory activity, is well absorbed, produces little discomfort when injected, and lasts 2 to 3 weeks. The periocular injection may be repeated in 3 to 4 weeks, if needed. In the presence of posterior segment disease topical corticosteroids are rarely effective, and posterior subtenon injection or systemic corticosteroids are indicated. Intralesional steroid injections can be used for the treatment of sarcoidosis lesions of the eyelid skin.

Glaucoma may develop as a result of the underlying disease or may occur as a response to the topical steroid therapy. If the patient is a steroid responder, fluorometholone drops may produce a sufficient anti-inflammatory response without as much pressure-elevating effect as topical prednisolone. Regardless of its etiology, the glaucoma may be treated with topical 0.25 or 0.5 per cent timolol every 12 hours or carbonic anhydrase inhibitors, such as 250 mg of acetazolamide four times daily or long-acting 500 mg sequels two times a day.

Systemic. Systemic steroid therapy is indicated for control of posterior segment inflammation, orbital disease, eyelid lesions, the neuro-ophthalmologic complications of sarcoidosis, or anterior segment inflammatory disease that is not responsive to topical or periocular steroids. Treatment should begin with 60 to 80 mg of prednisone daily (or equivalent doses of prednisolone or dexamethasone). The drugs may be given as a single daily dose before breakfast or in divided doses four times daily. The dosage should be slowly tapered as the inflammation subsides. Alternate-day therapy with twice the usual daily dose may avoid some of the complications of prolonged systemic steroid therapy. It may be useful in patients requiring long-term treatment for chronic inflammatory disease, but should not be employed in the initial stages of treatment when rapid control of significant inflammation is desired.

No other drugs can approach the effectiveness of systemic steroids in the treatment of sarcoidosis. In patients requiring treatment and in whom strong contraindications to the use of systemic steroids are present, who are resistant to steroid therapy, or who develop intolerable side effects to them, immunosuppressive therapy with chlorambucil*, azathioprine*, methotrexate* or cyclosporine may be of value, either alone or in combination with systemic steroids. The drugs are given orally in daily doses. They should be considered only under unusual circumstances and given in consultation with physicians thoroughly familiar with their use. Nonsteroidal anti-inflammatory agents, such as oxyphenbutazone‡ or indomethacin,‡ may be of value in selected patients with ocular or systemic inflammation but are not widely used. Oral chloroquine phosphate* has been used in the treatment of cutaneous sarcoidosis, including eyelid lesions. Chloroquine has also been used as adjunctive therapy for extracutaneous systemic sarcoidosis and to control the hypercalcemia and hypercalcinuria associated with this disease.

Irradiation. High-voltage radiation therapy has been used in the treatment of anterior visual pathway sarcoidosis in patients who are intolerant to systemic steroid treatment. Temporary beneficial response was seen, and subsequent immunosuppressive therapy was necessary.

Surgical. Since the initial ocular complications of sarcoidosis are inflammatory in nature, surgery plays little role in their management. However, surgery may be required in the management of late complications, such as cataract formation that occurs secondary to the chronic uveitis or steroid therapy. Surgical

or laser iridectomy may be needed to relieve pupillary block with iris bombé if the synechiae cannot be broken with mydriatic therapy. Filtering surgery is a last resort in uncontrolled glaucoma secondary to chronic angle closure with peripheral anterior synechiae, though the inflammatory nature of the underlying disease decreases the chance of a successful outcome.

Argon laser photocoagulation is of value in treating the retinal neovascularization seen in sarcoid patients. Scatter (modified panretinal) photocoagulation to areas of retinal nonperfusion can produce regression of the neovascularization. Focal treatment directly to the neovascular fronds has also been effective, although more widespread photocoagulation is preferred in the presence of significant zones of nonperfused retina. Disc neovascularization, without extensive areas of peripheral retinal vascular nonperfusion, may regress promptly with systemic steroid therapy. A 4- to 6-week trial of systemic steroids is appropriate before attempting laser photocoagulation.

Vitrectomy may be required for nonclearing vitreous opacities, hemorrhage, or traction retinal detachment.

Ocular or Periocular Manifestations

Choroid: Chorioretinal scarring; granuloma; subretinal neovascular membranes (juxtapapillary and macular).
Ciliary Body: Intermediate uveitis (snowbank).
Conjunctiva: Granuloma; nonspecific conjunctivitis; phlyctenules.
Cornea: Band keratopathy; hypesthesia (secondary to fifth nerve paralysis); interstitial keratitis; keratoconjunctivitis sicca.
Extraocular Muscles: Granulomatous infiltration of muscles; paralysis of third, fourth, or sixth cranial nerve with diplopia.
Eyelids: Cutaneous granuloma (lupus pernio); paralysis (secondary to seventh nerve palsy); ptosis (secondary to paralysis of third nerve).
Iris: Anterior and/or posterior synechiae; anterior uveitis (usually chronic granulomatous, but may be acute nongranulomatous); nodules (intrastromal lesions or surface keratic precipitate-like deposits).
Lacrimal System: Dacryoadenitis; dacryocystitis (may produce obstructive disease of lacrimal drainage system); lacrimal gland enlargement.
Lens: Cataracts.
Optic Nerve: Atrophy; neovascularization over disc; papilledema (secondary to elevated intracranial pressure); retrobulbar or optic neuritis (usually associated with granuloma formation within the optic nerve).
Orbit: Granuloma; proptosis.
Pupil: Amaurotic pupillary signs; internal ophthalmoplegia.
Retina: Detachment; edema; granuloma;

hemorrhages; neovascularization; perivasculitis; pigmentary loss, clumping, or mottling (gross or subtle change); retinal vein occlusions (usually peripheral); superficial exudative "candle-wax" lesions.

Sclera: Episcleritis; scleritis; scleral thinning; anterior staphyloma.

Vitreous: Granulomas (snowball or string of pearls configuration, usually inferior); hemorrhages; vitreitis (associated with inflammation of adjacent structures).

Other: Phthisis; secondary glaucoma (may be due to peripheral anterior synechiae, iris bombé, or nodular infiltration of trabecular meshwork); visual field defects (secondary to granulomatous involvement of optic nerves, chiasm, or tracts).

PRECAUTIONS

The major complications of the treatment of sarcoidosis are related to the adverse effects of steroid therapy. Systemic steroids produce a host of potentially serious side effects and should be used in consultation with the patient's internist. Salt and water retention may cause problems in patients with cardiac disease or hypertension. Potential aggravation or unmasking of diabetes mellitus, peptic ulcer, gastritis, esophagitis, or chronic infections (especially tuberculosis) requires particular attention. Other serious side effects include steroid-induced myopathy, osteoporosis with vertebral collapse, psychiatric problems, and adrenal insufficiency secondary to rapid withdrawal of the drugs after prolonged treatment. Ocular complications of both systemic and topical therapy include the development of posterior subcapsular cataracts and elevated intraocular pressure. The use of intralesional corticosteroids for eyelid lesions may create some degree of skin atrophy.

Chloroquine can produce macular pigmentary changes progressing to bull's eye maculopathy with loss of central vision. A baseline ophthalmologic exam with subsequent follow-up, including visual acuity testing, funduscopic examinations, and central visual field studies with an Amsler grid should be performed on patients receiving chloroquine. Fluorescein angiography, color vision testing, and electro-oculography may also be useful in following these patients. Corneal deposits, usually reversible and asymptomatic, are often seen in patients treated with chloroquine.

Sarcoid inflammatory disease tends to be recurrent, especially as therapy is decreased or withdrawn. Both the patient and the treating physician must be aware of this pattern, and careful follow-up evaluations are essential. Synechiae and their complications may develop fairly rapidly; if significant inflammation is present, weak mydriatics, such as tropicamide, are not strong enough to prevent their development or to break them once they occur. Patients should be encouraged to seek attention at the first sign of a change in their ocular status. At the same time, the physician must not "overtreat" the disease. Many uveitis patients develop a chronic "breakdown" in their blood-ocular barrier, with mild flare and an occasional cell in the anterior chamber. Distinguishing this situation from a chronic, active, ongoing inflammatory process may be difficult. The absence of new synechiae, keratic precipitates, and increasing anterior chamber reaction allows the ophthalmologist to observe the patient without reinstituting or increasing the therapy.

Every patient with anterior segment sarcoidosis should be carefully evaluated for posterior segment disease. Care must be taken to avoid a situation in which topical therapy is producing a satisfactory regression of anterior uveitis while leaving a serious, progressive, posterior inflammatory process untouched. Although most patients have bilateral ocular disease, the extent of involvement and degree of inflammation may be quite asymmetric. Both eyes must be carefully evaluated.

COMMENTS

The ocular complications of sarcoidosis are part of a *systemic* disorder, and a coordination of effort between the ophthalmologist and other physicians caring for the patient is essential. Almost all patients with ocular sarcoidosis have evidence of active disease elsewhere in the body. Although there has been widespread debate in the medical literature as to when sarcoidosis should be treated, the presence of ocular inflammatory disease is almost universally accepted as an absolute indication for initiating therapy.

The diagnosis of sarcoidosis is made on the basis of three main criteria: compatible clinical and radiologic evidence, histopathologic demonstration of noncaseating epithelioid-cell granulomas in affected tissues, and negative results of bacterial and fungal studies of tissues or body fluids. The tests and diagnostic procedures used to confirm this diagnosis include typical chest x-ray findings; elevated serum levels of angiotensin-converting-enzyme (ACE); positive Gallium 67 head, neck, and chest scan; elevated serum lysozyme levels; bronchoalveolar lavage with an increased number of T-lymphocytes and elevated T-helper/T-suppressor ratio (highly suggestive of sarcoid alveolitis and tissue biopsy obtained from superficial or palpable lesions in the skin, lymph nodes, conjunctiva, lacrimal gland, any mucosa, or lung tissue. Cerebrospinal fluid analysis, computed tomography, and MRI can be helpful in the diagnosis of central nervous system sarcoidosis. A positive Kveim-Siltzbach skin test and nonreactive PPD and other delayed hypersensitivity skin tests are also characteristic.

Conjunctival biopsy may reveal typical sarcoid granulomas. Although the incidence of positive biopsies varies greatly among series reported in the literature, biopsies of visible conjunctival nodules may be more likely to demonstrate granulomas than blind biopsy. It has been suggested that either technique may yield more positive results in patients with advanced chest x-ray findings or ocular abnormalities.

ACE concentration and ACE/protein ratio in tears are elevated in patients with sarcoidosis, but this elevation seems to be independent of any ocular involvement. Bronchoalveolar lavage not only has proven its importance in the diagnosis of pulmonary sarcoidosis but also seems to be of value in the diagnosis of patients with ocular disease, even when chest x-rays and ACE levels are normal.

Although anterior uveitis is the most common clinically observed manifestation of ocular sarcoidosis, conjunctival biopsy studies and lacrimal gland gallium uptake studies suggest that asymptomatic lacrimal gland and conjunctival granulomas are actually the most common forms of ocular involvement. Ocular changes are more likely to occur in patients with sarcoidosis of the skin, peripheral lymphadenopathy, hypercalcemia, neurologic involvement, parotid enlargement, and joint disease. Band keratopathy is strongly associated with an underlying hypercalcemia. Other reported associations include posterior segment inflammation (especially optic nerve involvement) with central nervous system sarcoidosis, and upper respiratory involvement with sarcoidosis of the lacrimal sac.

There are, within the broader clinical spectrum of sarcoid disease, several widely recognized syndromes with ocular components. These include Heerfordt's syndrome (uveitis, parotid enlargement, a chronic febrile course, and cranial nerve palsies, especially seventh) and Löfgren's syndrome (erythema nodosum, bilateral hilar adenopathy, acute iritis, and parotitis). Löfgren's syndrome is generally considered to have a relatively benign, self-limiting course. Another sarcoid "syndrome" includes chronic uveitis, cutaneous sarcoidosis, bone cysts, and pulmonary fibrosis and is considered a more persistent and troublesome clinical complex. There has been some controversy about a syndrome characterized by granulomatous arthritis-uveitis-rash described in children, since some of the clinical features are similar to those seen in early-onset sarcoidosis ("preschool sarcoidosis"), and some authors suggest that both are part of the same clinical spectrum. It is also important at this age to consider juvenile rheumathoid arthritis in the differential diagnosis, and in either case early ophthalmologic examination and long term follow-up are indicated.

Treatment of ocular sarcoidosis requires both diligence and patience. Therapy in this condition is seldom a quick "one-shot" proposition. The patient's clinical response is the ultimate determinant in making decisions as to the type, route, and duration of therapy. Recurrences may develop after long periods of quiescence, and these patients must be followed indefinitely.

References

Bienfait MF, et al: Diagnostic value of bronchoalveolar lavage in ocular sarcoidosis. Acta Ophthalmol 65(6):745–748, 1987.

Brownstein S, et al: Sarcoidosis of the eyelid skin. Can J Ophthalmol 25(5):256–259, 1990.

Gelwan MJ, et al: Sarcoidosis of the anterior visual pathway: successes and failures. J Neurol Neurosurg Psychiatry 51(12):1473–1480, 1988.

Immonen I, et al: Concentration of angiotensin-converting enzyme in tears of patients with sarcoidosis. Acta Ophthalmol 65(1):27–29, 1987.

Jordan DR, et al: The diagnosis of sarcoidosis. Can J Ophthalmol 23(5):203–207, 1988.

Mader TH, et al: The treatment of an enlarged sarcoid iris nodule with injectable corticosteroids. Am J Ophthalmol 106(3):365–366, 1988.

Mayers M: Ocular sarcoidosis. Int Ophthalmol Clin 30(4):257–263, 1990.

Rose CD, et al: Early onset sarcoidosis with aortitis—juvenile systemic granulomatosis? J Rheumatol 17(1):102–106, 1991.

Sahn EE, et al: Preschool sarcoidosis masquerading as juvenile rheumathoid arthritis: Two case reports and a review or the literature. Pediatr Dermatol 7(3):208–213, 1990.

Spaide RF, Ward DL: Conjunctival biopsy in the diagnosis of sarcoidosis. Br J Ophthalmol 74(8):469–471, 1990.

Zeiter JH, et al: Ocular sarcoidosis manifesting as an anterior staphyloma (Letter). Am J Ophthalmol 112(3):345–347, 1991.

Zic JA, et al: Treatment of cutaneous sarcoidosis with cloroquine. Arch Dermatol 127(7):1034–1040, 1991.

VOGT-KOYANAGI-HARADA SYNDROME
364.24
(Harada's Syndrome, Uveitis-Vitiligo-Alopecia-Poliosis Syndrome, Vogt-Koyanagi Syndrome)

ALAN H. FRIEDMAN, M.D.

New York, New York

The Vogt-Koyanagi-Harada (VKH) syndrome is a multisystem disorder characterized by headache, fever, bilateral uveitis (granulomatous or nongranulomatous), vitiligo, poliosis, alopecia, tinnitus, neck stiffness, loss of hearing, and pleocytosis of the cerebrospinal fluid. The etiology of the VKH syndrome is unknown, despite reports implicating viruses, bacteria, and fungi. A genetic predisposition has been suggested by the finding of the syndrome in three siblings. The syndrome has a definite predilection for darkly pigmented races or those with Oriental ancestry and affects adults, usually between 20 and 50 years of age. The first symptoms of the disease may be headache, nausea, vomiting, stiffness, and pain in the back of the neck that is sometimes associated with a meningeal syndrome or encephalitic signs. In the later stage, there is a hearing decrease or tinnitus, which is often caused by involvement of the eighth cranial nerve. Skin involvement manifested by poliosis, alopecia, or vitiligo may occur after the central nervous system and ocular signs of the disorder have subsided. This is usually within 2 to 3 months after onset, but the earliest signs of depigmentation can be found in the perilimbal area about 1 month after onset.

Initially, ocular involvement is characterized by posterior uveitis, which is manifested by bilateral serous retinal detachment with congestive papillary edema that rapidly becomes severe. As the inflammation progresses, the retinal detachment tends to predominate in the inferior segment of the eye. Fluorescein angiography reveals characteristic leakage of the dye from the choroid into the subretinal space. Subsequently, inflammatory reaction spreads toward the anterior uvea and produces various signs of anterior uveitis, such as flare and cells in the anterior chamber, mutton-fat keratic precipitates, and iris nodules. The severity of the anterior segment reaction varies from almost no reaction (Harada type) to severe reaction (Vogt-Koyanagi type). Marked decrease in visual acuity is noted early in the course of the disease. Impairment of visual fields is variable and corresponds to the extent of the retinal detachment. Rarely, cataracts or secondary glaucoma may develop. The usual course of events with prompt and adequate therapy is for the vision to return eventually to normal. However, many patients have some permanent impairment of vision. After resolution of the retinal detachments, a diffuse depigmentation of the entire fundus is seen that has been characterized in the choroid as "the sunset glow" sign with associated changes at the level of the retinal pigment epithelium, namely depigmentation and hyperpigmentation.

THERAPY

Systemic. In the VKH syndrome, systemic corticosteroid therapy is the most effective agent. One regimen is to prescribe 100 mg of prednisone orally at breakfast each day for the first week and then to decrease the dosage to 100 mg at breakfast every other day during the second week. The dosage should be tapered according to the therapeutic response. Particular attention should be directed toward detection of acute ocular inflammatory recurrence, which is liable to occur as early as 3 to

6 weeks or up to 9 months after systemic corticosteroid therapy has been discontinued. The clinical signs during the flare-up are almost identical to those during the initial attack. In the case of such a flare-up, the same therapeutic regimen should be reinstituted.

Ocular. The cornerstone of ocular therapy is systemic and local corticosteroids. One per cent prednisolone drops are instilled hourly during the first several days (while awake), with tapering to four to six times daily. Concomitant periocular injection of dexamethasone* or methylprednisolone* should be given.

Ocular or Periocular Manifestations

Choroid: Edema: exudative choroiditis; depigmentation (sunset glow fundus); multiple area of leakage on fluorescein angiography.
Conjunctiva: Perilimbal vitiligo (Sugiura's sign).
Eyelids: Poliosis; vitiligo.
Iris: Anterior uveitis; nodules.
Optic Nerve: Edema; hemorrhages; optic disc hyperemia.
Retina: Exudative retinal detachment; macular edema; macular scarring; retinal pigment epithelial depigmentation and hyperpigmentation; retinal vascular sheathing; subretinal neovascularization.
Vitreous: Exudates; haze.
Other: Cataracts; mutton-fat keratic precipitates; phthisis bulbi; secondary glaucoma.

PRECAUTIONS

The ocular inflammatory reactions in this disease are severe and can be chronic. Unless adequately treated, they often result in severe visual impairment or blindness.

Corticosteroids should be used cautiously to avoid the side effects of these drugs. The lowest possible dosage should be utilized to control the inflammation; when reduction in dosage is possible, the reduction should be gradual.

COMMENTS

In the VKH syndrome, the retinal detachments usually start in the macular area, extend inferiorly, and finally extend to involve the entire retina. Without treatment, the neuroretinitis and posterior uveitis regress slowly, taking from 6 to 12 months. Visual prognosis is poor without treatment. Less than 30 per cent of patients who have not been treated regain useful vision because of secondary glaucoma, cataract, or phthisis bulbi. Although varying in intensity, the clinical signs and symptoms closely simulate those occurring in the sympathized eye in sympathetic ophthalmia.

References

Friedman, AH, Deutsch-Sokol RH: Sugiura's sign: Perilimbal vitiligo in the Vogt-Koyanagi-Harada syndrome. Ophthalmology 88:1159–1165, 1981.

Ohno S, et al: Vogt-Koyanagi-Harada syndrome. Am J Ophthalmol 83:735–740, 1977.

Shimizu K: Harada's Behcet's, Vogt-Koyanagi syndromes—Are they clinical entities? Trans Am Acad Ophthalmol Otolaryngol 77:281–290, 1973.

Snyder DA, Tessler HH: Vogt-Koyanagi-Harada syndrome. Am J Ophthalmol 90:69–75, 1980.

Sugiura S: Vogt-Koyanagi-Harada disease. Jpn J Ophthalmol 22:9–35, 1978.

PART II

EYE AND ADNEXA

SECTION 18

ANTERIOR CHAMBER

EPITHELIAL INGROWTH
379.8
(Epithelial Downgrowth)

PATRICIA W. SMITH, M.D.,

Raleigh, North Carolina

and WALTER J. STARK, M.D.

Baltimore, Maryland

Sheet-like epithelial invasion of the anterior chamber is a rare, dreaded complication of ocular trauma or anterior segment surgery. Its diagnosis, often delayed, is based on a constellation of signs and symptoms together with an awareness of the disease. Its presence should be suspected after surgery or trauma complicated by wound leak, hypotony, persistent inflammation, and, later, intractable glaucoma.

Fortunately, the incidence of epithelial ingrowth after cataract surgery seems to have decreased from an incidence of 1.1 per cent reported 40 years ago to less than 0.2 per cent in recent reports. The onset of symptoms of epithelial ingrowth—usually within 3 years after surgery—may be insidious, with the patient complaining of tearing, dull aching pain, photophobia, and blurred vision. On examination, wound gap, a bleb, or a fistula may be seen with judicious pressure on the globe. These conditions are sometimes seen more clearly after instillation of 2 per cent fluorescein. On retroillumination, the ingrowth itself appears as a translucent posterior corneal membrane demarcated by a gray line. This leading gray line is often scalloped, with focal pearl-like areas of thickening. No keratic precipitates are present. Diminished corneal sensation, corneal edema overlying the ingrowth, stromal vascularization, and striae are variably present. Glaucoma is present in half of the cases. Gonioscopy may show wound-incarcerated tissue, a fistula or suture tract, and obliteration of the angle by the epithelial sheet or by peripheral anterior synechia. Anterior chamber cells-and-flare are frequently present. Involvement of the iris is more extensive than that of the cornea and is seen clinically as an immobile, distorted area with obscured details. Precise delineation of iris involvement using the argon laser (500-μm spot, 100 mW, 0.1 second) can be done preoperatively; the normal iris sustains a well-demarcated slight burn, whereas epithelium overlying iris shows a characteristic fluffy white appearance. Iris biopsy or corneal endothelial curettage provides histologic confirmation of the diagnosis. Membranes over the pupil, over the vitreous face, and enveloping the intraocular lens may be seen in advanced cases.

THERAPY

Supportive. There is no effective medical treatment for epithelial ingrowth. Topical corticosteroids may suppress inflammation and its symptoms indefinitely, but do not prevent progression of the ingrowth. To date, antimetabolites have not proven useful.

Surgical. Surgical intervention for epithelial ingrowth has been reported to result in the retention of good vision in 25 per cent of eyes (greater than 20/40). Before operation, the site of invasion, any fistula or bleb, and the extent of iris involvement are determined. At surgery, a peritomy is performed, and any leaking fistula is closed using a partial-thickness, limbus-based scleral flap dissected just posterior to the site, reflected anteriorly, and secured with 10-0 nylon suture. Vitrectomy instruments are introduced using a pars plana approach, and involved iris and vitreous tissues are excised. If present, the capsular bag should be removed completely. The anterior vitreous is then removed as well to provide space for the subsequent fluid-gas exchange. With a sterile air bubble in the anterior segment, any retinal breaks are localized and treated. Cryotherapy is then applied in a transcorneal and transcleral fashion to devitalize any epithelium remaining on the posterior cornea, in the angle, and on the ciliary body. On the cornea, a single freeze-thaw is applied sufficient to form ice crystals on the posterior surface of the cornea. The air bubble is replaced, if it is not needed to tamponade any retinal breaks.

Ocular or Periocular Manifestations

Conjunctiva: Bleb; ciliary flush; fistula.
Cornea: Edema; hypesthesia; neovascularization; posterior corneal membrane.
Iris: Corectopia; decreased mobility iritis; loss of details; peripheral anterior synechiae.
Vitreous: Epithelial sheet covering; inflammation; intraocular lens cocoon.
Other: Blur; glaucoma; pain; photophobia.

PRECAUTIONS

Closure of a leaking fistula in an eye thought otherwise inoperable may lead to intractable glaucoma.

On operative evaluation, photocoagulation of the iris to delineate its involvement is done within 24 hours of surgery, since it produces moderate anterior chamber inflammation.

Cryotherapy will destroy corneal endothelium so the freeze should be limited to the involved area of cornea. The presence of air in the anterior chamber enables such precise treatment. Penetrating keratoplasty may be needed later for visual rehabilitation if extensive corneal cryotherapy is required.

COMMENTS

The differential diagnosis of epithelial ingrowth includes (1) an anteriorly shelved cataract incision, seen as a diagonal, posterior-to-anterior intrastromal line on careful slit lamp examination; (2) fibrous ingrowth, distinguished by its slow growth and vascularity; (3) vitreocorneal adhesions, which may cause corneal edema and have a grayish appearance; (4) detachment of Descemet's membrane; (5) peripheral corneal edema caused by surgical or traumatic endothelial damage; and (6) reduplication of Descemet's membrane over the cornea, angle, and iris ("glass membrane"), in which the photocoagulation test is negative.

Once epithelial ingrowth is proven by biopsy or photocoagulation, early treatment is recommended because the necessary surgery is often less extensive and its results may be better at that stage. Observation of the corneal area of involvement is not advocated, since it may remain stationary while angle, iris, and ciliary body involvement progresses.

A recent review noted that patients treated surgically underwent fewer enucleations than those treated medically, or not treated (Weiner, et al., 1989).

References

Bernardino VB, Kim JC, Smith TR: Epithelialization of the anterior chamber after cataract extraction. Arch Ophthalmol 82:742–750, 1969.

Calhoun FP Jr: An aid to the clinical diagnosis of epithelial ingrowth into the anterior chamber following cataract extraction. Am J Ophthalmol 61:1055–1059, 1966.

Maumenee AE, et al: Review of 40 histologically proven cases of epithelial downgrowth following cataract extraction and suggested surgical management. Am J Ophthalmol 69:598–603, 1970.

Schaeffer AR, Nalbandian RW, Brigham DW, O'Donnell FE, Jr: Epithelial downgrowth following wound dehiscence after extracapsular cataract extraction and posterior chamber lens implantation: Surgical management. J Cat Refr Surg 15:437–441, 1989.

Smith PW, et al: Epithelial, fibrous, and endothelial proliferation. In Ritch R, Krupin T, Shields MB (eds): The Glaucomas. St. Louis, CV Mosby, 1989, pp 1299–1335.

Stark WJ, et al: Surgical management of epithelial ingrowth. Am J Ophthalmol 85:772–780, 1978.

Weiner JJ, Trentacoste J, Pon DM, Albert DM: Epithelial downgrowth: a 30-year clinicopathological review. Br J Ophthalmol 73:6–11, 1989.

Portions of this chapter were excerpted from Smith PW, Stark WJ, Maumenee AE, Green WR: Epithelial, fibrous, and endothelial proliferation. In Ritch R, Krupin T, Shields MB (eds): The Glaucomas. St. Louis, CV Mosby, 1989. Used with permission.

FIBROUS INGROWTH
379.8
(Fibroblastic Ingrowth, Fibrocytic Ingrowth, Fibrous Metaplasia, Stromal Ingrowth, Stromal Overgrowth)

KENNETH C. SWAN, M.D.

Portland, Oregon

Fibrous ingrowth is a condition in which connective tissue grows into the anterior chamber during abnormal wound healing following penetrating wounds in the cornea or limbus. The connective tissue invasion may clothe the back of the cornea, the chamber angle, the surface of the iris, and the anterior face of the vitreous. It may infiltrate the vitreous and even adhere to the retina. Factors predisposing the eye to this complication include poor wound apposition, recurrent hemorrhage, uveitis, tissue incarceration, and bulky, poorly placed, or tight sutures. Retrocorneal membranes are not uncommon after penetrating keratoplasty. Clinically, fibrous membranes appear to be frayed, gray or white, mesh-like structures, with irregular tongue-like strands on the advancing edge. Associated findings may include detachment of Descemet's membrane, bullous keratopathy, corneal edema, glaucoma, or phthisis bulbi, and retinal detachment may result in severe impairment of vision. Frequently, the patient experiences little discomfort, although chronic irritative changes may eventually ensue. Contraction of this newly formed tissue may pull upon the corneal scar and deform the globe until the eye becomes atrophic or until recalcitrant secondary glaucoma appears.

THERAPY

Ocular. There is no specific treatment for fibrous ingrowth into the anterior chamber. Although topical ocular corticosteroids are frequently prescribed, they seldom are of significant value. Currently available antimetabolites[†] exert toxic effects of the endothelium, but new agents hold promise. Some manifestations of fibrous ingrowth may be treated. For example, the thin fibrous membrane covering the pupillary aperture may be surgically excised or penetrated by YAG laser; however, this manipulation should be undertaken only if there is little evidence of continuing fibrous ingrowth. Otherwise, it may aggravate the process and cause increased proliferation. If the fibrous ingrowth extends posteriorly into the vitreous and causes retinal detachment by direct traction, the prognosis generally is unfavorable, but an effort should be made to save these globes by removing the traction employing vitreous surgery techniques.

Ocular or Periocular Manifestations

Cornea: Bullous keratopathy; detachment of Descemet's membrane; edema; retrocorneal membrane.
Globe: Atrophy; deformity; phthisis bulbi.
Other: Pupillary distortion; retinal detachment; secondary glaucoma.

PRECAUTIONS

Proper operative and postoperative techniques are important in minimizing fibrous ingrowth. Endothelial bridging of the inner wound after cataract surgery seems to block migration of fibroblasts in the eye; therefore, care must be taken not to injure this layer, especially in those patients with an endothelial dystrophy. During the critical period when the limbal wound is fragile, a precisely closed flap that contains both conjunctiva and Tenon's capsule provides considerable support. These layers seal down rapidly. Secondly, the limbal incision should be directed to enter the anterior chamber in the region of the Schwalbe line. Incisions that enter posteriorly are more likely to result in serious bleeding and to heal with more proliferative reactions than are anterior incision. Limbal wound closure should be precise; multiple bulky knots incite undue fibroplasia. Improperly placed sutures actually may hold the wound edges apart. Too tightly tied sutures exaggerate errors made in placement, as well as incite reaction caused by pressure necrosis.

COMMENTS

The pathogenesis of fibrous ingrowth is not fully understood. The most likely sources are subepithelial connective tissue, corneal or limbal stroma, and metaplastic endothelium. Fibrous ingrowth is often confused with epithelial downgrowth, although the appearance of the membrane is different. Fibrous ingrowth tends to be self-limiting in many cases. Estimating the incidence of fibrous ingrowth is difficult, since many of these cases remain unrecognized until the globe is enucleated.

References

Friedman AH, Henkind P: Corneal stromal overgrowth after cataract extraction. Br J Ophthalmol 54:528–534, 1970.
Jaffe NS: Cataract Surgery and Its Complications, 2nd ed. St. Louis, CV Mosby, 1976, pp 428–441.
Jaffe NS: Fibrous ingrowth. *In* Jaffe NS (ed): Cataract Surgery and Complications, 3rd ed. St. Louis, CV Mosby, 1981, pp 537–550.
Smith PW, Stark WJ, Maumenee AE, Green WR: Fibrous ingrowth. *In* Ritch R, Shields MB, Krupin T (eds): The Glaucomas. St. Louis, CV Mosby, 1989, pp 1321–1329.
Swan KC: Fibroblastic ingrowth following cataract extraction. Arch Ophthalmol 89:445–449, 1973.
Yanoff M, Fine BS: Stromal ingrowth. *In* Ocular Pathology, 2nd ed. Philadelphia, Harper & Row, 1983, pp 157–159.

INTRAOCULAR EPITHELIAL CYSTS 379.8

PATRICIA W. SMITH, M.D.,
Raleigh, North Carolina
and WALTER J. STARK, M.D.
Baltimore, Maryland

Cystic invasion of the anterior chamber may occur after trauma, cataract surgery, penetrating keratoplasty, or perforating corneal ulcer. Delayed or inadequate wound closure, perhaps complicated by incarceration of the iris, lens capsule, or vitreous, predisposes to cyst formation.

Clinically, it is important to differentiate epithelial cysts from sheet-like epithelial ingrowth, since their courses and prognoses differ greatly. The translucent or gray epithelial cyst appears to connect at one end with the wound. Transillumination and tremulousness, as well as lack of vascularity, which is demonstrable on fluorescein angiography, attest to its cystic nature. The cyst appears on the iris surface, in contrast to the stromal or iris pigment epithelial origin of primary iris cysts; however, a cyst that has grown through a peripheral iridectomy and presents in the posterior chamber may appear to arise from the iris stroma. Pupillary distortion, iridocyclitis, glaucoma, and encroachment on the visual axis may accompany growth of the cyst and indicate treatment. The course of these lesions varies tremendously; some lie dormant for years before enlarging, and others grow to considerable size before stabilizing.

THERAPY

Supportive. If periodic observation of the epithelial cyst shows sight-threatening complications, antiglaucoma and anti-inflammatory medication are used as temporizing measures before definitive treatment.

Surgical. Intervention is warranted only when growth, glaucoma, or iritis affect vision, because the cyst can recur as sheet-like epithelial ingrowth.

The current surgical technique is wide excision of the intact cyst, if possible. If the cyst is adherent to the cornea, iris, or vitreous face, it is first collapsed by aspiration, using a 25-gauge needle through the limbus at the cyst attachment. A vitreous sweep through a separate limbal wound may be used to peel the cyst away from the cornea. If small, the collapsed cyst is frozen through the cornea and limbus after an insulating air bubble is introduced into the anterior chamber. Larger cysts may require the use of vitrectomy instruments, introduced through the limbus or the pars plana, to excise iris and vitreous that are firmly adherent to the cyst. Freezing over air is then performed that is sufficient to cause the brief formation of an ice ball involving the adherent epithelial cells. Corneal edema may ensue after cyst excision and freezing; penetrating keratoplasty has been done to restore good vision in some of these cases.

Photocoagulation has been used to puncture and shrink epithelial cysts, although multiple applications are necessary. In one report, three cases of epithelial cysts were treated with sessions of photocoagulation to the pigmented base; four to six sesions were required before rapid movement of fine particles within the cyst or iris constriction was noted. The three cysts resolved without sequelae, except for updrawn pupils, at less than 1-year follow-up. Other authors have reported cyst resolution in small series with up to 5-year follow-up. Photocoagulation has the advantage of being relatively less invasive than some surgical procedures. However, when the cyst is not pigmented, is firmly adherent to cornea or vitreous, or presents in the posterior chamber, photocoagulation may not be useful.

Ocular or Periocular Manifestations

Anterior Chamber: Cells-and-flare; cyst; obliteration of angle.
Conjunctiva: Bleb; ciliary flush; fistula.
Cornea: Edema.
Iris: Corectopia; immobility; mass (if presenting from posterior chamber).
Other: Blur; glaucoma; photophobia.

PRECAUTIONS

Cryotherapy should be limited to the cornea involved with adherent cyst, since it will destroy endothelium, as well as epithelium. Air tamponade enables precise treatment of the intended area and insulates other anterior segment structures. A single freeze-thaw, suf-

ficient to form ice crystals on the posterior surface of the cornea, is recommended.

In treating a cyst with laser, care should be taken not to perforate the cyst, since externalizing it may convert it into sheet-like epithelial ingrowth.

COMMENTS

Cystic and sheet-like epithelial invasion of the anterior chamber differs only in mechanical factors, with epithelial cysts entering the anterior chamber as a loop and expanding in a balloon fashion in the anterior chamber. Clinically, evidence for this theory is found in the conversion of cyst to sheet-like ingrowth after surgical intervention. Occasionally, the cyst may be free floating within the anterior chamber, which is thought to result from implantation of viable epithelial cells by anterior segment instrumentation.

References

Harbin TS, Jr, Maumenee AE: Epithelial downgrowth after surgery for epithelial cyst. Am J Ophthalmol 78:1–4, 1974.

Okun E, Mandell A: Photocoagulation treatment of epithelial implantation cysts following cataract surgery. Trans Am Ophthalmol Soc 72:170–183, 1974.

Scholz RT, Kelley JS: Argon laser photocoagulation treatment of iris cysts following penetrating keratoplasty. Arch Ophthalmol 100:926–927, 1982.

Smith PW, et al: Epithelial, fibrous, and endothelial proliferation In Ritch R, Krupin T, Shields MB (eds): The Glaucomas. St. Louis, CV Mosby, 1989, pp 1299–1335.

Portions of this chapter were excerpted from Smith PW, Stark WJ, Maumenee AE, Green WR: Epithelial, fibrous, and endothelial proliferation. In Ritch R, Krupin T, Shields MB (eds): The Glaucomas. St. Louis, CV Mosby, 1989, pp 1299–1335. Used with permission.

POSTOPERATIVE FLAT ANTERIOR CHAMBER 360.34

E. MICHAEL VAN BUSKIRK, M. D.

Portland, Oregon

Collapse of the anterior chamber is a serious complication of anterior segment surgery that may lead to corneal decompensation, cataract, or intractable glaucoma due to peripheral anterior synechiae. It may immediately follow glaucoma or cataract surgery or may be delayed for days, weeks, or even months into the postoperative period. Shallowing of the anterior chamber is relatively more common after glaucoma-filtering surgery, particularly when the full-thickness procedures are chosen over the partial-thickness "trabeculectomy" procedures. The latter technique reduces the incidence, but does not eliminate the flat chamber as a complication. Contemporary use of releasable sutures may prevent or only delay the onset of this complication. The flat anterior chamber almost invariably results from one or a combination of the following events: wound leak, serous or hemorrhagic choroidal detachment, pupillary block and posterior misdirection, or entrapment of aqueous humor (malignant glaucoma or ciliary-block glaucoma). Identification of the pathogenesis is essential to plan the safest and most effective therapy. Occasionally, the appropriate etiologic diagnosis only becomes clear during operative intervention so that the surgeon must be prepared to follow a logical series of surgical steps to do the least necessary to correct the problem and prevent its recurrence.

The wound should be examined carefully to identify any possible leak. In an eye that does not appear to be extremely soft, the intraocular pressure can be carefully measured using a sterilized applanation tonometer. A hypotonous eye suggests a wound leak or choroidal detachment, whereas a normotensive or firm eye is more suggestive of pupillary block or posterior aqueous misdirection. However, pupillary block can also occur with a soft eye if wound leak or choroidal detachment coexists. Prolonged shallow or flat anterior chamber, initially arising from a wound leak or excess filtration, may eventually develop posterior aqueous misdirection as the associated inflammation blocks the access of aqueous humor to the anterior chamber.

Excess aqueous runoff through the filtration site commonly occurs during the first few days after filtering procedures, resulting in shallowing of the anterior chamber and choroidal detachment, which, in turn, lead to further flattening of the anterior chamber. Pupillary block rarely follows filtration surgery if an adequate iridectomy has been performed. This condition occurs more commonly after cataract surgery, especially with anterior chamber intraocular lenses, when vitreous or lens material can block one or more iridectomies. With the contemporary practice of "no-stitch" cataract surgery, we are now beginning to see more postoperative wound leaks, inadvertent filtering blebs, and their attendant flat anterior chambers. In some cases, particularly when pupillary block has been allowed to persist, the aqueous humor may be misdirected into the vitreous cavity, driving the vitreous forward and blocking access to both the anterior and posterior chambers, leading to so-called malignant glaucoma.

Hemorrhagic choroidal detachment also occasionally follows any intraocular procedure, but it is more common in eyes that have had multiple intraocular procedures. It may occur intraoperatively and be heralded by rapid shallowing of the anterior chamber and prolapse of ocular contents into the wound site. Even patients under local and retrobulbar anesthesia will complain of pain. After filtration surgery, hemorrhagic choroidal detachment more commonly occurs during the early postoperative period, rather than during surgery, and again is heralded by severe pain and loss of vision with flattening of the anterior chamber. These postoperative suprachoroidal hemorrhages are now seen more frequently than in previous decades, because more high-risk eyes are being subjected to filtration surgery with the availability of adjunctive chemotherapy or tube implants. Aphakic eyes that have undergone vitrectomy are especially prone to suprachoroidal hemorrhage after filtration surgery. Although most suprachoroidal hemorrhages will absorb spontaneously, prompt diagnosis will permit the institution of appropriate therapy that can save vision.

THERAPY

Ocular. Therapy for the flat anterior chamber is entirely dependent upon the correct determination of its pathogenesis. Wound leaks usually require surgical repair, but very tiny wound leaks sometimes heal spontaneously with a pressure dressing and administration of systemic carbonic anhydrase inhibitors used to reduce aqueous flow. Absorbable collagen shields or large-diameter soft contact lenses may sometimes successfully tamponade a slowly leaking bleb until it heals with endogenous fibrosis.

When a flat anterior chamber results from excess filtration, tamponade with a Simmons scleral shell or hydrogel large-diameter contact lens applied with a pressure dressing often proves useful if applied before extensive choroidal detachment is well established. The anterior chamber usually deepens within 2 to 3 hours, but the Simmons shell should then be left in place for at least 48 hours, "weaning away" first the pressure dressing and then the shell tamponade. Mydriasis and cycloplegia are also helpful to retrodisplace the lens-iris diaphragm and prevent complicating pupillary block.

Pupillary block rarely follows filtration surgery if an adequate iridectomy has been performed, but more commonly occurs after cataract surgery or after filtration in aphakic or pseudophakic eyes. These eyes invariably require a laser or surgical iridectomy, but the attack should initially be broken medically to reduce the intraocular pressure and to allow clearing of the cornea. Mydriasis should be achieved using 1 per cent cyclopentolate in combination with 2.5 per cent phenylephrine In some cases, a combination of 4 per cent cocaine and 1 per cent epinephrine may augment mydriasis. Vitreous dehydration with osmotic agents, such as oral glycerin, oral isosorbide, or intravenous mannitol, is useful in combination with ocular mydriatic/cycloplegics to reverse some cases of pupillary block and posterior entrapment of aqueous humor.

A flat anterior chamber, associated with visible patent iridectomy, a high intraocular pressure, and a visible red fundus reflex, should raise the specter of posteriorly entrapped aqueous humor (aqueous misdirection) or malignant glaucoma. In previous years, these cases required surgical intervention, and the diagnosis was often made on the operating table. With the current availability of the neodymium YAG laser, malignant glaucoma in the aphakic or pseudophakic eye can often be treated without returning to the operating room. In the aphakic or pseudophakic eye with malignant glaucoma, the vitreous face appears to be tightly adherent to the entire posterior surface of the posterior capsule, the intraocular lens, and the iris. The iris appears to be bulging forward into the anterior chamber as though under posterior tension. Vitreous is seen bulging forward through a patent iridectomy. Careful slit-lamp examination of the vitreous cavity reveals vitreous fibrils densely compacted against the posterior capsule or anterior hyaloid face, with clear fluid-containing space entrapped posteriorly. These findings can be confirmed by ultrasonic examination in some cases. Disruption of the anterior and posterior vitreous surface with the YAG laser allows a pathway for posteriorly entrapped aqueous humor to enter the anterior chamber and exit the eye. This Nd-YAG laser "vitrotomy" results in a dramatic deepening of the anterior chamber and lowering of intraocular pressure. Malignant glaucoma in the phakic eye is more difficult to treat with YAG vitrotomy because of poor visibility; it usually requires surgical intervention.

Vitreous dehydration with osmotic agents, such as oral glycerin, oral isosorbide, or intravenous mannitol, is useful in combination with ocular mydriatic/cycloplegic agents to reverse some cases of pupillary block and posterior aqueous entrapment.

Surgical. Wound leaks should usually be repaired surgically. If the wound is present within an otherwise intact conjunctival flap, it may sometimes be sealed with cryosurgery or various chemical agents, such as trichloracetic acid (100 per cent solution applied with an orange stick barely moistened with the acid).

Small focal or diffusely oozing leaks from filtering blebs may be tamponaded temporarily with the large soft contact lenses or collagen shields while natural wound healing mechanisms fill in the offending defects. Substantially leaking filtration blebs with a flat anterior chamber usually need to be repaired surgically. Tapered noncutting needles with 10-0 suture permit surgical closure with minimal further disruption of delicate conjunctiva. Leaking cystic blebs at the limbus may be excised locally, sliding adjacent conjunctiva over to cover the resultant defect. To provide a smooth limbal area and to anchor the new conjunctiva firmly, a very small corneoscleral groove can be prepared to recess the conjunctival flap edge for suturing.

In the absence of a wound leak, surgical anterior chamber reformation after filtering surgery almost always includes drainage of suprachoroidal fluid from a choroidal detachment. Most moderately shallow anterior chambers after filtering surgery will reform spontaneously without any intervention. Deepening the chamber at the slit lamp is rarely necessary and subjects the patient to the risk of infection and lens injury.

If surgical intervention must be undertaken, it is best performed with good anesthetic control and visibility in an operating room. After surgically reforming the anterior chamber through a corneal paracentesis wound, suprachoroidal fluid should be drained completely from two inferior posterior sclerotomies. If no suprachoroidal fluid is present and the anterior chamber remains flat, especially with increased intraocular pressure, pupillary block or posterior misdirection of aqueous humor is likely to be present. In this case, an additional peripheral iridectomy should be performed. If the anterior chamber remains shallow even after peripheral iridectomy, malignant glaucoma from posterior diversion of aqueous humor is the most likely diagnosis. In this case, liquid vitreous may be aspirated through the pars plana as described by Simmons (1972) and Chandler (1949). Alternatively, a vitrectomy may be performed via the pars plana in phakic eyes if visibility permits or through the limbus in the aphakic eye.

If pupillary block is strongly suspected, probably the safest procedure is laser iridotomy. An incomplete iridectomy is readily opened with argon laser applied to the underlying intact iris pigment epithelium. An occluded iridectomy requires additional laser iridotomies to be placed. Two iridotomies, one on each side of the intraocular lens, should be performed in patients with pupillary block associated with anterior chamber intraocular lenses.

Ocular or Periocular Manifestations

Conjunctiva: Filtering bleb with or without leakage of aqueous humor.

Corneoscleral Limbus: Possible wound separation.

Iris or Ciliary Body: Anterior displacement of iris; ciliary body detachment.

Vitreous: Anterior displacement; hemorrhages.

Other: Choroidal detachment; nonrhegmatogenous retinal detachment; orbital hemorrhages; scleral invagination.

PRECAUTIONS

The flat anterior chamber should not be allowed to persist longer than 14 days, depending on its etiology and the degree of intraocular inflammation. Surgical wound leaks, increased intraocular pressure, collapse of the filtration bleb, lens-corneal touch, "kissing" choroidal detachments, or excess inflammation all mandate earlier surgical intervention. Their absence permits watchful waiting. Eyes with wound leaks usually require surgical repair if other measures do not correct the problem promptly. Pupillary block requires prompt iridectomy to prevent the development of permanent angle-closure glaucoma from peripheral anterior synechiae. Laser iridotomy should be performed away from the visual axis to reduce the possibility of macular laser burns.

After filtration surgery, the surgeon should eschew the temptation to operate simply because the anterior chamber is shallow. Nearly all shallow anterior chambers related to excess aqueous runoff, even with choroidal detachment, resolve spontaneously over 7 to 10 days. Management during this critical period is designed to prevent compromise of the other intraocular structures. Usually, watchful waiting is the safest course. Adjunctive antimetabolite therapy may prolong postoperative hypotony and delay spontaneous resorption of suprachoroidal fluid. Deepening of the anterior chamber at the slit lamp is almost never necessary. If the chamber is shallow enough to threaten the lens or cornea, such deepening under poorly controlled conditions runs a significant risk of lens injury and, with lesser degrees of shallowing, is unnecessary.

COMMENTS

Closing trabeculectomy split-thickness scleral flaps with mechanically releasable sutures or cutting them with laser provides an extra measure of security against flat chamber in the immediate postoperative period. However, doing so may merely delay the onset of the complication until after the sutures are removed.

During draining of either serous or hemorrhagic choroidal detachment, one must ensure as much of the suprachoroidal fluid as possible is removed to prevent rapid recurrence of large choroidal detachment and flattening of the anterior chamber. After initial drainage of suprachoroidal fluid from both sclerotomy sites, the anterior chamber should be reformed to greater than normal depth through a corneal paracentesis wound. The sclerotomy sites should then be reinspected with further drainage of any additional fluid. At the conclusion of the procedure, the anterior chamber should again be deepened to slightly greater than normal depth and the eye left tacitly normotensive.

If the hemorrhage is more than a few hours old, it may be expected to have layered out within the suprachoroidal space, with the red cells most dependent. Hence, any xanthochromic fluid may at first appear, with thick wine-colored material following later. In many of these cases, a large portion of the blood dissects interstitially within the choroid, making its complete removal technically impossible. Hence, a large, choroidal, hemorrhagic mass with obscuration of the red fundal reflex may be present, even after all suprachoroidal blood has been removed. The blood-engorged choroid will be visible at the sclerotomy site. At that stage, no further attempts should be made for fluid drainage, and the overlying Tenon's and conjunctival incisions should be closed. The interstitial blood will gradually absorb with time.

References

Bellows AR, Chylack LT Jr, Hutchinson TT: Choroidal detachment. Clinical manifestation, therapy and mechanism of formation. Ophthalmology 88:1107–1115, 1981.

Brubaker RF: Intraocular surgery and choroidal hemorrhage. Arch Ophthalmol 102:1753–1754, 1984.

Brubaker RF, Pederson JE: Ciliochoroidal detachment. Surv Ophthalmol 7:281–289, 1983.

Chandler PA: V. Complications of surgery. Causes of failures and methods of prevention and correction. Trans Am Acad Ophthalmol Otolaryngol 53:224–231, 1949.

Chandler PA, Maumenee AE: A major cause of hypotony. Am J Ophthalmol 52:609–618, 1961.

Cohen JS, Osher RH: Releasable scleral flap suture. Ophthalmol Clin North Am 197, 1988.

Gressel MG, Parris RK II, Heurer DK: Delayed nonexpulsive suprachoroidal hemorrhage. Arch Ophthalmol 102:1757–1760, 1984.

Shields MB: Trabeculectomy vs. full-thickness filtering operation for control of glaucoma. Ophthalmic Surg 11:498–505, 1980.

Simmons RJ: Malignant glaucoma. Br J Ophthalmol 56:263–272, 1972.

Simmons RJ, Kimbrough RL: Shell tamponade in filtering surgery for glaucoma. Ophthalmic Surg 10:17–34, 179.

Watkins PHR, Brubaker RF: Comparison of partial-thickness and full-thickness filtration procedures in open-angle glaucoma. Am J Ophthalmol 86: 756–761, 1978.

RECURRENT LATE HYPHEMA FROM FOCAL WOUND VASCULARIZATION 364.41

KENNETH C. SWAN, M.D.

Portland, Oregon

Focal vascularization of the stromal wound may result in recurrent hyphema months to as long as 15 years (mean, 4 to 5 years) after cataract or glaucoma surgery. It results from the ingrowth of episcleral vessels that terminate in capillaries at the inner edge of the incision site. In one series, this ingrowth was observed in 12 per cent of 58 eyes examined 5 to 10 years after cataract extraction. Bleeding from these capillaries may occur spontaneously or result from physical strain or minimal trauma, such as gonioscopy or insertion of contact lenses. Bleeding usually is minimal and therefore is easily overlooked or mistaken for iridocyclitis. Blurred vision is the major symptom, but occurs only during the bleeding episode, unless the blood extends into the anterior vitreous. Pain is minimal or absent. During bleeding episodes, blood cells can be observed streaming down through the anterior chamber or on the iris. Enough blood may accumulate to produce a visible hyphema, but the diagnosis usually requires gonioscopy. Collections of old or new blood cells or their pigmented remnants in the lower chamber angle confirm that bleeding has occurred. A tuft of capillaries visible in the lips of the wound identifies the bleeding site. The entity may be innocuous, but recurring hyphemas may lead to angle-closure glaucoma or serious visual disturbance, if there is recurrent bleeding into the anterior vitreous. Patients who have had bleeding only after physical strain or trauma have the best prognosis.

THERAPY

Supportive. Initially, treatment should be by conservative measures, including protecting the eye from trauma, avoiding the prone position in sleep, wearing a protective shield at night, and discontinuation of contact lenses if insertion or removal precipitates bleeding.

Surgical. Recurrent bleeding, especially into the vitreous, requires intervention, but no form of treatment has been universally successful. Argon laser applications applied through a gonioscope and surface applications with the cryoprobe have been most useful, but recurrences have been reported with both techniques. Identification and surgical excision or direct coagulation of the indipping vessel should be reserved for recalcitrant bleeding.

Ocular or Periocular Manifestations

Anterior Chamber: Angle-closure glaucoma; floating cells (red blood cells); hyphema; pigment and synechiae in lower angle.
Cornea: Focal tufts of capillaries in inner edges of old wound.
Vitreous: Old and new collections of blood cells on surface or in anterior vitreous.
Other: Transient blurring of vision.

PRECAUTIONS

To avoid alarm, patients suspected of having this condition should be warned that gonioscopy may precipitate bleeding and transitory blurring of vision. If cryotherapy is used, the probe should be applied and withdrawn gently; otherwise, significant bleeding may be precipitated.

COMMENTS

The pathogenesis of wound vascularization has not been fully established, but poor wound apposition, especially gapping of the interior edges of the wound at the bleeding site, has been observed in many patients. Posterior placement of the incision in the sclera may also predispose to wound vascularization, but this has not been well documented. Although most cases have been observed after intracapsular extraction, wound vascularization with late hyphema is now appearing in patients who have had extracapsular extractions through relatively small incisions, as well as after iridectomy, filtrations, and trabeculectomies. The entity should be suspected in patients who have recurrent transitory blurring of vision after operative procedures requiring incisions in the limbal area.

References

Jarstad JS, Hardwig PW: Intraocular hemorrhage from wound vascularization years after anterior segment surgery. (Swan Syndrome) Can J Ophthalmol 22:271–275, 1987.

Swan KC: Hyphema due to wound vascularization after cataract extraction. Arch Ophthalmol 89:87–90 1973.

Swan KC: Late hyphema due to wound vascularization. Trans Am Acad Ophthalmol Otolaryngol 81:138–144, 1976.

Watzke RC: Intraocular hemorrhage from wound vascularization following cataract surgery. Trans Am Ophthalmol Soc 72:242–252, 1974.

Watzke RC: Intraocular hemorrhage from vascularization of the cataract incision. Ophthalmology 87:19–23, 1980.

TRAUMATIC HYPHEMA
921.3

PAUL E. ROMANO, M.D., M.S.O., *and* JERRY N. SHUSTER, M.D.

Gainesville, Florida

Hyphema, an accumulation of blood within the anterior chamber, is most commonly the result of trauma. The typical injury is a direct blow to the cornea from a fist or low-velocity missile. The force is transmitted to the aqueous humor, pushing the iris-lens diaphragm posteriorly, which results in a tear in the root of the iris or the face of the ciliary body. Bleeding that follows from torn blood vessels is usually self-limited because of the tamponade of such bleeding into the closed space of the anterior chamber. The intraocular pressure may be elevated acutely due to the mechanical block of the trabecular meshwork by the blood.

Approximately 2 days after the onset of the hyphema, the clot begins to retract, and the risk of rebleeding begins. With recurrent hemorrhage, the risks of such complications as elevation of intraocular pressure, corneal endothelial decompensation, and progressive blood staining of the corneal stroma increase. Additionally, the indications for surgical intervention are more likely to be encountered with a secondary hemorrhage.

THERAPY

Before undertaking therapy, sickle cell anemia (including trait) must be ruled out because the patient who also has that blood dyscrasia must be treated much more carefully and at times more aggressively. (See below under Surgical Therapy and under Precautions.)

Supportive. The patient with *initial bleed* should be hospitalized at bedrest for 6 days, which covers the period of greatest risk of rebleeding—days 2 through 5; the patient should be allowed progressive ambulation on the sixth day in preparation for discharge. Hospitalization *is* cost effective because it protects the young patient from further or repeat trauma, facilitates the frequent observations that are appropriate, ensures the administration of systemic treatment, and seems to produce better overall results. The head of the bed may be elevated to facilitate settling of the hyphema, clearing of the superior filtering angle, and earlier visualization of the fundus. Allowing bathroom privileges seems not to affect the situation deleteriously.

The size of the hyphema does not alter these recommendations; most studies suggest that the rebleeding rate is the same regardless of the size of the initial hyphema. Although small hyphemas (less than one third) show no greater rebleed rate with modest ambulation than bedrest, larger ones do. In addition, bedrest seems to accelerate clearing of the hyphema.

Ocular occlusion seems unnecessary. Certainly, it has been demonstrated that binocular occlusion has no advantage over monocular, and the former is hazardous psychologically. Likewise as seen in more recent studies, patching does not seem to have any effect at all on the outcome.

A perforated aluminum shield should be prescribed to prevent accidental reinjury of the eye. Otherwise limiting the use of the eyes seems a futile exercise and has not been demonstrated as having any effect upon the outcome.

Although some studies have suggested that the rebleed rate is higher for children and African-Americans, and the inference has been made that different age and ethnic groups might therefore be treated differently, that evidence is weak and far from providing any definitive medical indication for treating these different groups differently. For the present, then, all traumatic hyphemas should be treated identically, as above and as follows.

Sedatives or tranquilizers may be useful in some patients. However, aspirin is contraindicated, as its antiplatelet action may facilitate a rebleeding episode.

Systemic. Recent studies strongly support the use of systemic antifibrinolytic agents, such as corticosteroids and aminocaproic acid, (and tranexamic acid where available), and one of these should be given for 5 days in all cases. Systemic treatment should be initiated as soon as the diagnosis is made in the emergency room or clinic. The recommended daily dose of prednisone is the equivalent of 40 mg for an adult or 0.6 mg/kg for children, given in divided doses. Aminocaproic acid should be given in dosages of 50 mg/kg every 4 hours, not to exceed 30 g/day, for 5 days. Both drugs may be discontinued at that time without tapering dosages, if there has been satisfactory resolution of the initial bleed. Both drugs have been demonstrated to reduce the rebleeding rate to virtually zero in this condition. Prednisone and aminocaproic acid are equally effective. However, corticosteroids are favored over aminocaproic acid because most physicians are intimately familiar with prescribing steroids, undesirable side effects from aminocaproic acid have been reported occasionally, and aminocaproic acid has also been demonstrated to retard clot reabsorption slightly. Steroids also have an anti-inflammatory effect not found in aminocaproic acid.

If there is *rebleed*, the foregoing treatment is simply continued for an additional 5 days, with closer observation for complications (glaucoma and corneal blood staining) that occur much more frequently after rebleeds than after primary bleeds.

Significant pressure evaluation of greater than 50 mm Hg for more than 5 days or 35 mm Hg for more than 7 days may increase the possibility of optic nerve damage. A healthy, normal, young eye can withstand the following pressures without damage to the optic nerve: 50 mm Hg for 5 days, 45 mm Hg for 7 days, or 35 mm Hg for 14 days. Since the pressure will go down when the angle clears, it is not necessary therefore to treat elevated pressure per se. However, if treatment is needed, 250 mg of oral acetazolamide may be given four times daily (30 mg/kg daily in divided doses in children, total dose not to exceed 1000 mg/day). In addition, topical ophthalmic 0.25 or 0.5 per cent timolol or 1 to

2 per cent epinephrine may be applied twice daily. Osmotic agents may be added, if necessary. A 50 per cent solution of glycerin may be administered orally in a dosage of 2 to 3 ml/kg, or a 20 per cent solution of mannitol may be given intravenously in a dosage of 1 to 2 gm/kg.

Surgical. There is rarely an indication for surgical intervention before the fourth day after the initial bleed, except for patients with sickle cell anemia. Increased intraocular pressure in these patients may be a result of increased sickling of red blood cells in the anterior chamber, which blocks the trabecular meshwork and renders medical therapy ineffective. Therefore, the optic nerve can be damaged at lower pressures because of sickling, and earlier surgical intervention is needed. The rule for patients with sickle cell anemia is "24 × 24": any pressure elevation greater than 24 mm Hg for 24 hours is cause for aggressive treatment because of danger to the optic nerve.

Otherwise, the indications for surgical intervention in patients with hyphema include (1) sustained pressure elevation that is unacceptable given the baseline health of the optic nerve or is unresponsive to medical management, (2) early corneal blood staining demonstrated by an orange granular appearance to the posterior corneal stroma, or (3) a greater than 50 per cent hyphema that shows no evidence of clearing after 4 days because the risk of peripheral anterior synechiae and secondary glaucoma increases.

Many techniques have been advocated, and all are hazardous because blood clots and uveal tissue are easily confused and the hyphema limits visibility. We advocate trabeculectomy. Trabeculectomy provides quite adequate exposure and control of intraocular pressure postoperatively. An irrigating and aspirating technique may be used to wash out free blood. This may be combined with the use of fibrinolysins. An ocutome may be used to aspirate and cut the clot from the anterior chamber. Sears (1970) described a technique to express the clot in toto on the fourth day, at which time the clot begins to retract. A cryoprobe or forceps has also been recommended to extract the clot; these procedures have the disadvantage of necessitating a large incision and involving the risk of loss of lens, uvea, and vitreous. Removing the blood from the anterior chamber usually halts corneal blood staining and alleviates the glaucoma. If persistent bleeding occurs during the procedure, the involved area of the ciliary body can be treated transclerally with diathermy.

Ocular or Periocular Manifestations

Anterior Chamber: On presentation may be clear or contain various quantities and forms and colors of either or both clotted and unclotted blood; from and including a small dark horizontally layered, almost invisible clot at the bottom of the chamber, to larger layered amounts of dark blood; to a chamber completely filled with almost black clot, the so-called eight ball hyphema. The blood may also be unclotted bright red and diffusely fill the chamber. Combinations of the above may be seen. Later, residuae of clots may be seen, including whitish fibrin membranes.

Conjunctiva: Injected secondary to initial trauma; iritis and uveitis from hyphema.

Cornea: On presentation, clear; or with manifestations of blunt or abrading trauma, such as an epithelial abrasion. After one or more days, corneal blood staining, manifest initially by a translucent diffuse reddish granular appearance to the posterior stroma; changing with time to an opaque green (bile-colored) stain that may last for a year or two.

Iris: Obscured anterior chamber blood; traumatic lesions, such as dialysis or recession of the angle; pupil occluded or secluded by fibrin; iritis; peripheral anterior and posterior synechiae.

Vitreous and Retina: Usually uninvolved but may have suffered any of a variety of traumatic lesions from the initial trauma. Even when directly untraumatized, in severe hyphemas, blood often enters and fills the vitreous body, as well as the anterior chamber, viz. "eight ball hyphema."

Other: Ocular pain, secondary glaucoma (until hyphema clears or permanently secondary to angle recession and scarring); visual loss.

PRECAUTION

There is no specific indication for any topical ocular medication in the management of the initial bleed. Contraindications include rapidly acting cycloplegics and mydriatics that may occasionally precipitate rebleeding episodes and the use of miotics that may cause vascular dilation and congestion in the iris and ciliary body, thereby increasing the risk of rebleeding.

It is usually neither necessary nor possible to examine the posterior pole ophthalmoscopically in most hyphemas. Although postponement of pupillary dilation for this is recommended, there may be reasons, such as scleral rupture, intraocular foreign body, or retinal detachment, when atropine only should be used. Atropine seems to have no deleterious effect on the course of traumatic hyphema. The less manipulation of the eye, the better. Daily tonometry and slit lamp examination are not required unless one has reason to suspect a significant elevation of pressure or blood staining. This is especially true for the young patient in whom sedation may be required or a struggle may be anticipated. Some pressure elevation on the first day should be expected, but it is usually transient and not very high and does not specifically require treatment. Acetazolamide should not be given routinely because it slows clot reabsorption and may facilitate rebleeding by lowering intraocular pressure too far. Acetazolamide may be contraindicated in children with sickle cell disease because it lowers the blood pH, which facilitates sickling. Methazolamide may be better if such a drug must be used as it raises pH.

If the clot reabsorbs without complication, no further therapy is necessary. Eye examination is completed 2 weeks after discharge. Gonioscopy, which can be traumatic, must be performed at some point to identify angle recession. The timing of gonioscopy depends on the instrument to be used, the skill of the examiner, the cooperation of the patient, and the fact that early gonioscopy most reliably identifies angle recession. Regular long-term follow-up of all hyphema patients is indicated for the detection of late-onset secondary glaucoma.

All persons who might have sickle cell anemia should have the appropriate studies performed on admission because the management of these patients with traumatic hyphema has much narrower limits with regard to elevated pressure. Use of acetazolamide in patients with sickle cell diseases is contraindicated because of its concomitant acidosis, which may trigger sickling.

COMMENTS

Significant pressure elevation or blood staining of the cornea occasionally occurs with a severe initial bleed, but usually follows a rebleed. Additional treatment may be required; however, both pressure elevation and corneal blood staining tend to be self-limiting or transient.

Corneal blood staining is more significant in the child under 6 years of age, as a functional amblyopia is likely to result. In addition, the probability of developing secondary strabismus is greater in the child under 8 or 10 years of age who will have more difficulty regaining fusion when the blood has cleared months or years later. The blood staining itself is a significant cosmetic defect as well.

Since the pressure will go down when the angle clears, it is not necessary therefore to treat elevated pressure per se. This is an especially important principle when almost every agent used to lower pressure may have a deleterious effect on the primary problem, delaying clot reabsorption, removing the tamponade effect of elevated pressure, or promoting rebleeding episodes through iris vascular congestion and engorgement.

References

Crouch ER Jr, Frenkel M: Aminocaproic acid in the treatment of traumatic hyphema. Am J Ophthalmol 81:355–360, 1976.

Edwards WC, Layden WE: Monocular versus binocular patching in traumatic hyphema. Am J Ophthalmol 76:359–362, 1973.

Farber MD, Fiscella, R, Goldberg MF: Aminocaproic acid versus prednisone for the treatment of traumatic hyphema. Ophthalmology 98:279–286, 1991.

Goldberg MF: The diagnosis and treatment of sickled erythrocytes in human hyphema. Trans Am Ophthalmol Soc 76:481–501, 1978.

Rakusin W: Traumatic hyphema. Am J Ophthalmol 74:284–292, 1972.

Read J, Goldberg MF: Comparison of medical treatment for traumatic hyphema. Trans Am Acad Ophthalmol Otolaryngol 78:799–815, 1974.

Romano PE: Pro steroids for systemic antifibrinolytic treatment for traumatic hyphema. In Rosenbaum AL (ed): Controversies in Pediatric Ophthalmology, Vol 23, No 2, pp 92–95, 1982.

Rynne MV, Romano PE: Systemic corticosteroids in the treatment of traumatic hyphema. J Pediatr Ophthalmol Strabismus 17:141–143, 1980.

Sears ML: Surgical management of black ball hyphema. Trans Am Acad Ophthalmol Otolaryngol 74:820–826, 1970.

Wilson FM II: Traumatic hyphema: Pathogenesis and management. Ophthalmology 87:910–919, 1980.

Yasuna E: Management of traumatic hyphema. Arch Ophthalmol 91:190–191, 1974.

SECTION 19

CHOROID

ANGIOID STREAKS 363.43

ROY D. ALTMAN, M.D.

Miami, Florida

The description of angioid streaks of the fundus by Doyne in 1889 was followed by an association with a variety of illnesses but is generally most commonly associated with pseudoxanthoma elasticum (Grönblad-Strandberg syndrome, present in 85 per cent of patients), sickle cell anemia (overall 1.5 per cent of patients, but particularly common hemoglobinopathy in SC disease) and osteitis deformans (Paget's disease of bone, present in 5 to 15 per cent of patients). However, there continues to be patients with no known associated illness to their angioid streaks.

The angioid streaks are usually visualized in patients over age 25 equally in both sexes, and appear as bilateral irregular linear streaks radiating from a peripapillary ring. They are most commonly narrow, are not branched and taper at the periphery of the posterior polar region of the eye. The color is somewhat dependent on the color of the fundus, being brown in heavily pigmented and red in more lightly pigmented people.

On histopathologic examination the streaks coincide with disruptions in Bruch's membrane, bridged by a thin hypopigmented epithelium. Subsequent ingrowth of fibrous and perhaps fibrovascular tissue from the choroid may lead to lessening of the color with broadening and blurring of the margin of the streak. The bridges between the capillaries of Bruch's membrane may become thickened and calcified. Fibrovascular ingrowth can lead to serous and/or hemorrhagic detachment of the retinal pigmented epithelium and retina; depending on the severity, field cuts or even blindness can occur.

Identification of angioid streaks is facilitated by fluorescein angiography. When serous or hemorrhagic detachment occurs, the angiography may have the appearance of macular degeneration or a related syndrome.

Although the reason for the association to medical illnesses is unclear, the pathogenesis of mechanical breaks in the brittle Bruch's membrane due to the associated illness remains the most likely cause of the angioid streaks.

The association of angioid streaks to Paget's disease of bone has been recently questioned on the basis of finding angioid streaks in only 1 of 70 unselected patients with Paget's disease. In a critique of this argument, Clarkson pointed out that in his previously studied patients, 5 of 50 had angioid streaks associated with skull involvement of the Paget's disease. These patients had active Paget's disease by serum alkaline phosphatase and a number of involved sites. Clarkson also reported 2 patients with angioid streaks without skull involvement for an overall prevalence of angioid streaks in Paget's disease of 14 per cent. The unselected patients of Dabbs assuredly had less active Paget's disease. It should be also noted that in a condition as rare as angioid streaks, even one patient in 70 with Paget's disease may suggest an association.

Another common finding in Clarkson's patients was the presence of disc drusens. Mansour has also noted this association.

Occasional cases, such as abetalipoproteinemia, continue to be reported as associations to angioid streaks.

THERAPY

Presently, no therapy is recommended other than addressing the underlying illness. Photocoagulation of the neovascular membranes is of uncertain value.

Ocular or Periocular Manifestations

Choroid: Atrophy; neovascularization; vascular sclerosis.

Retina: Focal chorioretinal lesions (salmon spot); hemorrhages; macular degeneration (exudative or nonexudative); pigmentary mottling (peau d'orange).

Other: Visual loss.

References

Clarkson JG: Paget's disease and angioid streaks: One complication less. Br J Opthalmol 75, 1991.
Clarkson JG, Altman RD: Angioid Streaks. Surv Ophthalmol 26:235–246, 1982.
Dabbs TR, Skjodt K: Prevalence of angioid streaks and other ocular complications of Paget's disease of bone. J Ophthalmol 74:579–582, 1990.
Dieckert JP, White M, Christmann L, Lambert HM: Angioid streaks associated with abetalipoproteinemia. Ann Ophthalmol 21:173–179, 1989.
Doyne RW: Choroidal and retinal changes—the result of blows to the eye. Trans Ophthalmol Soc UK 9:128–140, 1889.
Mansour AM: Is there an association between optic

disc drusen and angioid streaks. Graefe's Arch Clin Exp Ophthalmol 230:595–596, 1992.

Smith JL, Gass JDM, Justice J Jr: Fluorescein fundus photography of angioid streaks. Br J Ophthalmol 517–521, 1964.

CHOROIDAL DETACHMENT 363.70
(Ciliochoroidal Detachment)

PAUL H. KALINA, M.D.,
and A. ROBERT BELLOWS, M.D.

Boston, Massachusetts

Choroidal detachment is the clinical term used to describe fluid accumulation in the potential space between the choroid and sclera. Anatomically, the suprachoroidal space is limited anteriorly by the scleral spur and posteriorly in the region of the four vortex veins. As fluid accumulates in this space, anterior displacement of the ciliary body and lens-iris diaphragm often also occurs and frequently can be associated with anterior chamber shallowing. Some clinicians prefer the term "ciliochoroidal detachment," implicating both the ciliary body and the choroid. The terms are used interchangeably.

The initial description of a choroidal detachment by Zinn was substantiated with histopathology by Waltrop in 1818. In 1858, Von Graefe first described the clinical characteristics as viewed through the direct ophthalmoscope. Ten years later, Knapp reported enucleating an eye after cataract surgery because he suspected malignant melanoma, but the intraocular brown mass proved to be a benign choroidal detachment.

The mechanism of this disorder is not understood completely. In 1900, Fuchs believed that the aqueous contributed to a choroidal detachment through an unsuspected cyclodialysis cleft. A few years later, Meler and Verhoeff each suggested that, after surgery or trauma, intraocular pressure decreased and remained sufficiently low to encourage a fluid transudation from the choroidal venous circulation into the suprachoroidal space, resulting in the development of a choroidal detachment. This altered physiology during hypotony is thought to be a major contributor to choroidal detachment. The mechanism by which aqueous secretion is decreased or absent when the ciliary body is detached, thereby prolonging the hypotony and permitting more transudation from the vascular network, was not explained. Capper and Leopold (1956) have demonstrated that surgical trauma and hypotony are necessary to produce suprachoroidal fluid accumulation in experimental rabbits. Pederson and associates (1979) created experimental choroidal effusion in monkeys, suggesting that the aqueous may contribute to the mechanism of uveal scleral flow.

In humans, when the intraocular pressure is dropped to zero, osmotic pressure alone cannot prevent the transudation of fluid from the choroidal capillaries into the suprachoroidal space. A dynamic example of this process occurs during glaucoma surgery in patients with elevated episcleral venous pressure. In these patients, when the intraocular pressure has been lowered to zero intraoperatively, elevated venous pressure creates a large transcapillary pressure differential in the ciliary body and choroid and results in profound egress of fluid out of the vascular network into the suprachoroidal space. This effusion can occur rapidly and acutely during the operative course and tends to mimic the dreaded surgical complication of expulsive suprachoroidal hemorrhage. Fluid analysis by Chylack and Bellows (1978) demonstrated very few small molecular-weight protein particles, principally albumin, with little evidence of other serum proteins, suggesting that the mechanism of molecular sieving contributed to the rapid fluid formation in the suprachoroidal space. It is possible to postulate that the differential created by the elevated episcleral venous pressure when the intraocular pressure is lowered creates a pressure differential across an intact isosporous membrane that produces this rapid fluid accumulation.

Choroidal detachment can occur shortly after intraocular surgery when the intraocular pressure is low and inflammation is prominent, or many years postoperatively. Cataract, glaucoma, and retinal detachment surgery have been associated with the development of choroidal detachment. It also occurs as a result of ocular and periocular trauma, in the presence of ocular tumors, nanophthalmos, uveal effusion syndrome, local inflammatory processes (choroiditis and scleritis), systemic inflammatory disorders (Vogt and Koyanagi-Harada syndromes), systemic vascular disorders (carotid-cavernous fistula, Sturge-Weber, and eclampsia), and with the reinstitution of aqueous suppressants after failed filtration surgery.

Several surgical advances have decreased the incidence of hypotony, thereby reducing the frequency of choroidal detachment; these advances include the use of the operating microscope, which provides excellent visualization for tissue manipulation and apposition. In addition, the use of microsurgical techniques and multiple fine sutures decreases the incidence of wound leakage and shallow anterior chambers. Glaucoma surgery also has been improved with the development of guarded filtration procedures (trabeculectomy).

When fluid accumulates in the suprachoroidal space, it produces a characteristic internal ballooning of the choroid that appears as a large, brown, quadratic mound delimited posteriorly by the vortex veins ampullae. Common locations are the nasal and temporal quadrants. Minimally elevated anterior choroidal detachments are often difficult to identify by ophthalmoscopy, but can be associated with anterior displacement of the ciliary body and lens-iris diaphragm, leading to significant shallowing and anterior chamber. The development of lens-corneal touch is a serious complication and can result in corneal decompensation, cataract formation, peripheral anterior synechia, and the failure of filtration surgery.

Aphakic and postvitrectomized eyes are most susceptible to choroidal detachment. The other potential risk factors include postoperative hypotony and inflammation, elevated intraocular pressure, axial myopia, advanced age, hypertension, and hypotony associated with the use of antimetabolites during glaucoma filtration surgery.

The three distinct forms of choroidal detachment are serous choroidal detachment, hemorrhagic choroidal detachment, and intraoperative choroidal effusion.

Serous choroidal detachment, the most common form of choroidal effusion, occurs approximately 2 to 7 days after glaucoma surgery, 10 days or longer after combined glaucoma and cataract surgery, and 2 to 4 weeks after routine cataract surgery. Patients are usually asymptomatic except for visual symptoms related to hypotony or a shallow anterior chamber. At the time of choroidal tap, suprachoroidal fluid has been shown to contain approximately two-thirds of the proteins seen in serum. Normal distributions of electrolyte and ascorbic acid concentrations are recognized, and there is an absence of high-molecular-weight proteins. This mechanism is thought to develop when the intraocular pressure is low postoperatively and the pressure differential across the capillary bed permits fluid to escape, with small- and medium-sized protein molecules forming the major portion of the transudation. This fluid passes through an isosporous membrane and collects in the interstitium of the choroidal as well as the suprachoroidal space.

Hemorrhagic choroidal detachment, one of the most serious ocular surgical or postoperative complications, occurs after cataract extraction, combined cataract and glaucoma surgery, or filtering surgery alone in patients who are often hypertensive and have microvascular abnormalities, with a higher incidence occurring in myopic eyes. The spontaneous development of suprachoroidal hemorrhage is rare; intra- and postoperative occurrences are usually the rule and are often associated with profound hypotony. The more dramatic and usually intraoperative expulsive hemorrhage is associated with an arterial defect including the long or short posterior ciliary artery. Venous disruption is more often the cause of the controlled intraoperative or localized postop-

erative form of hemorrhagic choroidal detachment.

The dramatic, massive, expulsive suprachoroidal hemorrhage, the most severe form of hemorrhagic choroidal detachment, is fortunately not common. It is characterized by arterial bleeding and extrusion of intraocular contents during surgery. All efforts are made to close the wound and salvage the eye, but all too frequently the condition has devastating consequences. Intervention by pars plana vitrectomy with infusion of air, balanced salt solution, or gas and concomitant choroidal drainage has improved the prognosis in these cases.

Delayed postoperative suprachoroidal hemorrhage is more common than the expulsive form. Characteristically, the patient reports a sudden onset of excruciating pain during the early postoperative stage that is often accompanied by anterior chamber flattening, ocular congestion, and frequently elevated intraocular pressure. Hemorrhage most often occurs after an increase in orbital venous pressure associated with the Valsalva maneuver, vomiting, coughing, or straining at stool. The hemorrhage, which may be large or extremely localized, appears as a dark, balloon-like elevation of the choroid and can be characterized more completely with B-scan ultrasonography. When blood exists in the suprachoroidal space, it is often accompanied by increased ocular inflammation and rotation of the ciliary body forward to create peripheral anterior synechia. The inflammation results in failure of a glaucoma filtration bleb. When surgical drainage is indicated, the suprachoroidal space often is filled with dark unclotted blood with small collections of xanthochromic fluid.

The development of an *intraoperative choroidal effusion* is a dramatic event that can occur during cataract extraction, penetrating keratoplasty, or glaucoma surgery. It most often is observed in patients with prominent episcleral vessels and elevated episcleral venous pressure. This intraoperative event can mimic an expulsive suprachoroidal hemorrhage because of rapid fluid accumulation after the commencement of surgery, but differs, because if the suprachoroidal space is evacuated, clear, copious amounts of fluid are found and the eye can be transiently decompressed.

THERAPY

Ocular. Serous, or small hemorrhagic suprachoroidal detachment is usually self-limited. With normal ocular architecture, surgical therapy is not indicated. Spontaneous reabsorption of fluid and blood products within the first few postoperative days often results in improved clinical status.

A clinically significant serous choroidal detachment with anterior chamber shallowing creates the potential for lens-corneal touch, prominent ocular inflammation, and retinal apposition. Medical management with topical cycloplegic/mydriatic drops and frequently applied steroids should be initiated. Some believe that a short course of high-dose systemic steroids is helpful in decreasing the inflammatory component of suprachoroidal hemorrhage and diminishing the amount of fluid in the suprachoroidal space. Changing the capillary permeability of the blood-retinal barrier may diminish the fluid accumulation in the suprachoroidal space and hasten reabsorption. The role of nonsteroidal anti-inflammatory medications has not been clinically evaluated, but may be helpful. When excessive filtration results in profound hypotony or an active wound leak is discovered, suturing the wound leak or diminishing filtration with a firm pressure patch, bandage contact lens, or even a compressive shell may enhance ciliary body reattachment and decrease the complications of a choroidal effusion.

Suprachoroidal hemorrhage is difficult to predict and prevent. Preoperatively, systemic hypertension should be controlled meticulously and the administration of anticoagulants or aspirin-containing medications avoided if possible. Preoperatively, the intraocular pressure can be lowered with digital massage or osmotic agents, or intraoperatively by paracentesis and very slow lowering of the intraocular pressure. The anesthetic choice is not often related to the development of this complication, because it occurs with both general and local anesthesia. Postoperatively, prolonged hypotony should be avoided if possible, with efforts taken to minimize coughing, straining, and vomiting; increasing orbital venous pressure should also be avoided. Stool softeners, laxatives, and antiemetics are recommended.

Surgical. Intraoperative choroidal detachment is a surgical problem. When serous or delayed choroidal detachment occurs, surgical intervention involves drainage of the suprachoroidal space and anterior chamber reformation. The procedure, called "choroidal tap," can be performed under local or general anesthesia. Paracentesis is necessary to reform the anterior chamber, and use of a pre-existing paracentesis incision is preferable. The conjunctiva and Tenon's capsule are incised circumferentially approximately 3.5 mm from the visible limbus in the inferotemporal and inferonasal quadrants. It is advisable to tap both infusion quadrants to remove fluid, since one may be inadequate. Cauterization is often necessary, and a radial incision to the suprachoroidal space is made with a scratch-down maneuver. When the suprachoroidal space has been entered, a serous detachment is characterized by copious amounts of clear xanthochromic fluid; with a hemorrhagic choroidal detachment, dark, unclotted blood with xanthochromic fluid is released. Elevation alternating with depression of each side of the wound facilitates release of the suprachoroidal fluid. This procedure is alternated with repeated reformation of the anterior chamber through the paracentesis incision. It is important not to allow the eye to become too soft during the evacuation phase, because then reformation becomes more difficult. After drainage completion, there is usually little or no further fluid evacuation. It is important to continue the procedure until as much fluid as possible is released, and the anterior chamber is reformed. The sclerostomy is left unsutured, but the conjunctiva is closed over the sclera. The indications for surgical intervention in the presence of a choroidal detachment include (1) lens-corneal touch; (2) progressive corneal edema or rapid cataract formation; (3) a flat anterior chamber with inflammation and a failing filtration bleb; (4) hemorrhagic choroidal detachment with a flat anterior chamber; (5) intraocular inflammation, a flat anterior chamber, and aphakia or pseudophakia with no improvement in 3 to 5 days; (6) a large, pronounced choroidal detachment with appositional ("kissing") choroidals for longer than 48 hours; and (7) wound leak with a flat anterior chamber and prominent choroidal detachment.

Mild, nonexpulsive suprachoroidal hemorrhages usually resolve spontaneously and are treated by observation. Larger hemorrhages require surgical intervention. Management includes par plana vitrectomy with continuous infusion of air, balanced salt solution, or perfluorocarbin liquids plus choroidal drainage. A coexisting retinal detachment may require a scleral buckle. Collaboration with a retinal specialist is strongly recommended because surgical evacuation of blood and retinal vitreous techniques can save the eye and even visually rehabilitate the patient.

A posterior sclerostomy performed preoperatively in patients with increased episcleral venous pressure minimizes intraoperative complications. Recognition of an intraoperative choroidal effusion with prompt management by posterior sclerostomies may allow repositioning of the intraocular contents and even completion of the procedure. Complications of a choroidal tap include intensification of intraocular inflammation and the potential for endophthalmitis. Decompression may result in papillary or large vessel bleeding with recurrence of suprachoroidal hemorrhage and anterior chamber flattening. The creation of a cyclodialysis cleft with forceful deepening of the anterior chamber is unusual, but can occur. Cataract development occurs more frequently in patients who undergo choroidal tap. Bleb survival in patients undergoing choroidal tap seems to be unaltered compared to the control group.

COMMENTS

Development of intra- or postoperative choroidal detachment is usually associated with ocular hypotony. The spontaneous occurrence of a choroidal effusion is puzzling and unsolved. The contribution of aqueous hyposecretion is significant and remains a mystery. The role of uveal scleral flow, as well as the capacity for bulk flow across the sclera, is being actively investigated. Elucidating these mechanisms could result in more effective noninvasive methods to prevent and treat choroidal effusion. Efforts to decrease the chance of profound intraoperative or postoperative hypotony seem to reduce the incidence of serous choroidal effusion and clinically significant choroidal detachment or hemorrhage.

References

Abrams GW, Thomas MA, Williams GA, Burton TC: Management of postoperative suprachoroidal hemorrhage with continuous-infusion air pump. Arch Opthalmol 104:1455–1458, 1986.

Bellows AR, Chylack LT, Hutchinson BT: Choroidal detachment. Clinical manifestation, therapy and mechanism of formation. Ophthalmology 88:11107–1115, 1981.

Bellows AR, et al: Choroidal effusion during glaucoma surgery in patients with prominent episcleral vessels. Arch Ophthalmol 97:493–497, 1979.

Berke SJ, et al: Chronic and recurrent choroidal detachment after glaucoma filtering surgery. Ophthalmology 94:154–162, 1987.

Brubaker RF, Pederson JE: Choroidal detachment. Surv Ophthalmol 27:281–289, 1983.

Burton TC, Stevens TS, Harrison TJ: The influence of subconjunctival depot corticosteroid or choroidal detachment following retinal detachment surgery. Trans Am Acad Ophthalmol Otolaryngol 79:845–850, 1975.

Cantor LB, Katz LJ, Spaeth GL: Complications of surgery in glaucoma. Suprachoroidal expulsive hemorrhage in glaucoma patients undergoing intraocular surgery. Ophthalmology 92:1266–1270, 1985.

Capper SA, Leopold IH: Mechanism of serous choroidal detachment. A review and experimental study. Arch Ophthalmol 55:101–113, 1956.

Chandler PA, Maumenee AE: A major cause of hypotony. Am J Ophthalmol 52:609–618, 1961.

Chylack LT, Bellows AR: Molecular sieving in suprachoroidal fluid formation in man. Invest Ophthalmol Vis Sci 17:420–427, 1978.

Desai UR, et al: Use of perfluorohydrophenanthrene in the management of suprachoroidal hemorrhages. Ophthalmology 99:1542–1547, 1992.

Fluorouracil Filtering Study Group: Risk factors for suprachoroidal hemorrhage after filtering surgery. Am J Ophthalmol 113:501–507, 1192.

Frenkel REP, Shin DH: Prevention and management of delayed suprachoroidal hemorrhage after filtration surgery. Arch Ophthalmol 104:1459–1463, 1986.

Givens K, Shields MB: Suprachoroidal hemorrhage after glaucoma filtering surgery. Am J Ophthalmol 103:689–694, 1987.

Gressel MG, Parrish II RK, Heuer DK: Delayed nonexpulsive suprachoroidal hemorrhage. Arch Ophthalmol 102:1757–1760, 1984.

Lakhanpal V, et al: A new viteroretinal surgical approach in the management of massive suprachoroidal hemorrhage. Ophthalmology 96:793–800, 1989.

Peyman GA, et al: Computed tomography in choroidal detachment. Ophthalmology 91:156–162, 1984.

Pederson JE, Gaasterland DE, MacLellan HM: Experimental ciliochoroidal detachment. Effect on intraocular pressure and aqueous humor flow. Arch Ophthalmol 97:536–541, 1979.

Reynolds MG, et al: Suprachoroidal hemorrhage. Clinical features and results of secondary surgical management. Ophthalmology 100:460–465, 1993.

Ruderman JM, Harbin Jr TS, Campbell DG: Postoperative suprachoroidal hemorrhage following filtration procedures. Arch Ophthalmol 104:201–205, 1986.

Ruiz RS, Salmonsen PC: Expulsive choroidal effusion. A complication of intraocular surgery. Arch Ophthalmol 94:69–70, 1976.

Sugar HS: Postoperative cataract in successfully filtering glaucomatous eyes. Am J Ophthalmol 69:740–746, 1979.

CHOROIDAL FOLDS 363.8

AMY R. JEFFERY, M.D.,

Philadelphia, Pennsylvania

and JOHN D. BULLOCK, M.D., M.S., F.A.C.S.

Dayton, Ohio

Choroidal folds, first described by Nettleship in 1884, are alternating light and dark striae in the posterior pole. They usually radiate horizontally from the optic nerve, but may be vertical or oblique. Choroidal folds are of variable number, length, and width. They never extend beyond the equator and are more often on the temporal side of the disc. It is important to distinguish between choroidal folds and the more common retinal folds. Retinal folds are ophthalmoscopically finer, are usually associated with vitreoretinal disease, are associated with a normal fluorescein angiogram, and usually radiate from visible pathology in the retina. Choroidal folds, in contrast, have a distinctive fluorescein angiographic pattern first described by Norton in 1969. Early in the angiogram, alternating lines of hypofluorescence and hyperfluorescence are seen. The density of the retinal pigment epithelium at the peaks and valleys allows greater or lesser transmission of choroidal fluorescence, respectively. No leakage is seen. One is often able to see more folds with a fluorescein angiogram than can be appreciated ophthalmoscopically.

The mechanism responsible for choroidal folds may be folding of Bruch's membrane and/or traction on the optic nerve in the absence of scleral touch. Choroidal folds are usually caused by an expanding orbital mass, but the folds can occur in many other ocular and/or systemic conditions.

THERAPY

Ocular. One can diagnose choroidal folds on a biomicroscopic exam with fluorescein angiographic confirmation. The management of such a patient must be individualized since there is an extensive differential diagnosis. The most commonly associated entities are orbital tumors (hemangioma, meningioma), hypotony (fistulizing surgery), swelling of the optic nerve, orbital and scleral inflammation (posterior scleritis, orbital pseudotumor), severe hyperopia, previous scleral surgery, thyroid eye disease, or idiopathic disease. Intraocular neoplasms, choroidal neovascularization (folds radiating from the macula), trauma, uveitis, choroidal edema, sinusitis, orbital cellulitis, central serous choroidopathy, diode endolaser photocoagulation, and dural sinus fistula are infrequently associated with choroidal folds. If a cause is not apparent or needs to be defined, a CT or MRI scan should be performed. An ultrasound is important if a diagnosis of posterior scleritis is being entertained. The location of the folds does not always represent the location of the pathology. Treatment of the underlying condition usually results in resolution of the choroidal folds, albeit slowly. Persistent or recurrent choroidal folds can form characteristic pigmentation pattens: bead-like pigmentation lines on the slope of the fold are described most commonly.

Ocular or Periocular Manifestations

Choroid: Neovascularization; choroidal inflammation.
Extraocular Muscles: Enlargement of muscle bellies.
Globe: New or increased hyperopia; proptosis.
Optic Nerve: Swelling.
Orbit: Inflammation; mass.
Retina: Macular degeneration; central serous chorioretinopathy; vasculitis.
Sclera Scleritis (anterior and posterior).
Uvea: Uveitis; hypotony.

PRECAUTIONS

Choroidal folds can occur in normal eyes and can be overlooked easily. One reason may be that choroidal folds do not necessarily interfere with good visual function. On occasion a person may complain of blurry vision or metamorphopsia. It is important to distinguish between retinal and choroidal folds since the entities associated with each are usually very different and rarely present together. The position of choroidal folds are of no value in localizing pathology. Most orbital tumors do not present with choroidal folds.

COMMENTS

Once a patient is diagnosed with choroidal folds, a thorough work-up is necessary; the etiology is usually discovered then. Symptoms are usually secondary to the etiology of the choroidal folds.

References

Bullock JD, Egbert PR: Experimental choroidal folds. Am J Ophthalmol 78:618–523, 1974.
Bullock JD, Egbert PR: The origin of choroidal folds: A clinical, histopathological, and experimental study. Documenta Ophthalmol 37(2):261–293, 1974.
Bullock JD, Waller RB: Choroidal folding in orbital disease. In Proceedings of the Third International Symposium on Orbital Disorders. Amsterdam, 1977, pp 483–488.
Cangemi FE, Trempe CL, Walsh JB: Choroidal folds. Am J Ophthalmol 86:380–387, 1978.
Newell FW: Choroidal folds. Am J Ophthalmol 75:930–939, 1973.
Newell FW: Fundus changes in persistent and recurrent choroidal folds. Br J Ophthalmol 68:32–35, 1984.
Norton EWD: A characteristic fluorescein angiographic pattern in choroidal folds. Proc Roy Soc Med 62:119, 1969.

CHOROIDAL NEOVASCULAR MEMBRANES 362.16
(Disciform Macular Degeneration, Hemorrhagic Disciform Detachment, Subretinal Neovascularization)

ROBERT E. KALINA, M.D.

Seattle, Washington

Choroidal neovascularization is a sheet of new capillaries, with or without a fine connective tissue network, that extends from the choroid either through a break in Bruch's membrane or around the peripapillary end of Bruch's membrane into the subretinal pigment epithelial or subretinal space. Although neovascular membranes may occur anywhere in the fundus, they are most common in the posterior pole and often cause permanent loss of central vision secondary to serous and hemorrhagic detachment of the macula. Clinical examination reveals a dirty gray or yellow subretinal membrane or a pigmented mound beneath the retina. Subretinal blood or exudate may be present.

If a pigmented ring can be seen, the neovascular membrane often is confined to the ring. Fluorescein angiography permits accurate localization of the extent of the neovascular membrane, except when it is obscured by blood or other opacity. The membrane often assumes the configuration of a wheel, including radial vessels and larger peripheral arcades.

Choroidal neovascularization is associated with a wide variety of clinical syndromes affecting Bruch's membrane and adjacent tissues. Most important among these associations are macular drusen and presumed ocular histoplasmosis. Less common, but still important, predisposing causes are angioid streaks, choroidal ruptures, myopia, drusen of the optic disc, choroidal tumors, and many other inflammatory or degenerative disorders of the posterior pole of the eye. Idiopathic cases are not rare.

THERAPY

Systemic. A wide variety of vitamin[‡] and mineral preparations[‡] have been advocated for macular diseases, but there is no generally accepted scientific or clinical evidence to suggest that these are beneficial. Anticoagulants[‡] have been advocated by some authorities based on the mistaken belief that the observed process is related to circulatory deficiency, but these agents actually may be harmful by predisposing to intraocular hemorrhage. Oral corticosteroids[‡] often have been prescribed, but there is no evidence that the final visual result is altered by such therapy.

Surgical. Choroidal neovascular membranes can be destroyed by laser photocoagulation. Uniformly white burns must be applied to cover the entire neovascular network. The side of the neovascular membrane closest to the fovea should be treated first. Small (50- or 100-μm) spots may be used to outline the margin of the area to be treated, but the entire membrane should be treated with larger (200- to 500-μm) spots at up to 0.5-second exposures. Treatment should extend beyond the edge of the membrane by at least 100 μm in all directions. The surgeon must make reference to a recent fluorescein angiogram, and retrobulbar anesthesia and akinesia often are required. The patient should be re-examined at intervals to detect persistence or recurrence. Fluorescein angiography should be repeated at about 3 weeks or with any change in symptoms.

Although photocoagulation of choroidal neovascular membranes is often beneficial, treatment is not without risk, and some cases may undergo spontaneous involution. In general, the prognosis for vision in eyes with choroidal neovascular membranes improves with increasing distance of the membranes from the center of the macula with or without treatment. Also, the prognosis with or without treatment is worse for choroidal neovascular membranes due to age-related macular degeneration than for those due to other causes.

Subretinal surgery to remove blood and choroidal neovascular membranes has been attempted, but visual results are often disappointing, particularly in age-related macular degeneration. Complications include recurrence, retinal detachment, proliferative vitreoretinopathy, and cataract.

Supportive. Choroidal neovascular membranes are a leading cause of visual loss. Fortunately, peripheral vision is retained in most patients, and total blindness does not ensue, a prognostic fact that can be comforting to the patient and that should be stressed by the ophthalmologist. The responsibility of the physician does not end with such reassurance for bilaterally affected patients, but should include assessment of the potential usefulness of low-vision aids and services for the partially sighted.

Ocular or Periocular Manifestations

Retina: Chorioretinal scars; detachment of retinal pigment epithelium or retina; drusen; subretinal hemorrhage or lipid.

Other: Central scotoma; metamorphopsia; micropsia.

PRECAUTIONS

Since photocoagulation of choroidal neovascular membranes can contribute to visual loss, patients should be selected carefully for treatment. Choroidal neovascular membranes farther than 2500 μ from the center of the fovea probably do not require treatment. Although treatment of choroidal neovascularization in all other locations generally is associated with a better long-term visual result than the natural history, treatment closer than 200 μm to the center of the fovea often results in immediate visual loss. Use of the argon blue-green laser may result in sensory retinal damage due to absorption of blue light by macular xanthophyll pigment. Photocoagulation in the papillomacular bundle may produce nerve fiber layer damage, particularly if the retina is not elevated by serous fluid. Partial treatment of a choroidal neovascular membrane generally is unsuccessful and is not recommended.

Neither treatment nor study by fluorescein angiography is indicated for advanced stages of macular scarring caused by choroidal neovascularization. Treatment should be considered only for symptomatic eyes in which there is reasonable hope of preserving vision. Since recurrence in the treated eye or involvement of the fellow eye is common, patients should report promptly if new symptoms are observed. Home use of an Amsler grid may be helpful for early detection. Ophthalmoscopic or fluorescein angiographic detection of a pigment epithelial defect in the foveal area of the fellow eye in the presumed ocular histoplamosis syndrome is a risk indicator for that eye.

COMMENTS

Choroidal neovascular membranes always should be suspected when detachment of the macula occurs. Their presence is particularly likely when the subretinal fluid contains blood or lipid.

Photocoagulation of choroidal neovascular membranes became possible after the introduction of fluorescein angiography permitted their precise localization. The xenon arc photocoagulator was used initially, but soon was supplanted by the argon laser. Argon blue-green laser no longer is used for photocoagulation in the macula because absorption of blue light by xanthophyll pigment may result in damage to the sensory retina. Lasers emitting longer wavelengths (red or yellow) have theoretical advantages, including reduced damage to retinal blood vessels, reduced absorption by lens and macular pigments, and deeper penetration. Although widely used, other wavelengths have not been shown conclusively to effect better visual results than argon green.

References

Bressler NM, et al: Age-related macular degeneration. Surv Ophthalmol 32:375–413, 1988.
Gass JDM: Stereoscopic Atlas of Macular Diseases: Diagnosis and Treatment, 3rd ed. St. Louis, CV Mosby, 1987.
Macular Photocoagulation Study Group: Argon laser photocoagulation for neovascular maculopathy. Three-year results from randomized clinical trials. Arch Ophthalmol 104:694–701, 1986.
Macular Photocoagulation Study Group: Krypton laser photocoagulation for neovascular lesions of ocular histoplasmosis. Results of a randomized clinical trial. Arch Ophthalmol 105:1499–1507, 1987.
Macular Photocoagulation Study Group: Laser photocoagulation of subfoveal neovascular lesions in age-related macular degeneration. Arch Ophthalmol 109:1220–1231, 1991.
Macular Photocoagulation Study Group: Subfoveal neovascular lesions in age-related macular degeneration. Arch Ophthalmol 109:1242–1257, 1991.

CHOROIDAL RUPTURES 363.63

ROBERT C. WATZKE, M.D.

Portland, Oregon

Rupture of the choroid causing immediate subretinal and retinal hemorrhage and edema and late chorioretinal scarring is common after severe ocular trauma. This injury is most frequent in young men and is usually sport, assault, or work related.

Punch-related choroidal ruptures are usually peripapillary, temporal, and concentric with the disc. Projectile-related ruptures are usually caused by direct deformation of the exposed sclera. Typically, they are anterior, inferior, irregular, and multiple. The peripapillary choroidal ruptures are thin, vertically oriented streaks of exposed sclera with reactive pigment epithelial pigmentation. Anterior ruptures are usually ragged, irregular patches of exposed sclera and retinal pigment epithelial scars. Both are first covered with retinal and vitreous hemorrhage that gradually clears during the first month after the injury.

THERAPY

Ocular. There is no immediate treatment for choroidal ruptures except to examine the anterior type closely and frequently to detect surrounding retinal detachment. Ocular inflammation usually requires mydriatics. If there is anterior segment inflammation, topical steroids should be prescribed. Unilateral patching is only necessary for temporary comfort. Bedrest is not necessary.

Retinal detachment occasionally occurs after anterior choroidal ruptures. Detachment of the surrounding retina is difficult to differentiate from severe retinal edema in the first week after injury. Even if a detachment is present, it should not be treated surgically while the eye is inflamed and hemorrhagic. In fact, progressive scar formation may limit the detachment, and surgery may not be necessary. Retinal detachment surgery should be done when the detachment is shown to be progressive and the ocular inflammation has subsided.

Subretinal neovascularization at the margin of posterior choroidal rupture scars is a late complication of indirect choroidal ruptures. The incidence is unknown, but is frequent enough that patients should be warned of symptoms of central visual blurring or metamorphopsia. These vessels can occur many years after the injury, but the highest incidence is within the first 6 months and patients should be followed monthly for this period. If the scars are inspected carefully by slit-lamp biomicroscopy with a contact lens, a fluorescein angiogram is unnecessary unless the characteristic serous retinal detachment and pigment epithelial thickening and discoloration are detected. A fluorescein angiogram should then be done.

The value of laser photocoagulation for subretinal neovascular membranes associated with choroidal ruptures has not been proven. Nevertheless, if these vessels are within one disc diameter of the center of the fovea, enlarge in size, and cause a serous retinal detachment involving the fovea, argon laser photocoagulation should be considered.

Indirect choroidal ruptures usually cause permanent visual loss only if the rupture involves the fovea or subsequent subretinal neovascularization does so. Occasionally, visual loss occurs from pigmentary scarring in the macula subsequent to traumatic macular edema. For medical/legal reasons the visual prognosis of these injuries should not be stated until at least 6 months after the injury. When the ocular inflammation has subsided, a complete ocular examination should be done that includes gonioscopy, indirect ophthalmoscopy of the peripheral retina, and careful examination of the macula and choroidal ruptures in the posterior pole.

References

DeLaey JJ: Choroidal neovascularisation after traumatic choroidal rupture. Bull Soc Belge Ophthalmol *220*:53–59, 1986.

Duke-Elder S (ed): System of Ophthalmology. St. Louis, CV Mosby, 1972, Vol XIV, pp 151–158.

Luxenberg MN: Subretinal neovascularization associated with rupture of the choroid. Arch Ophthalmol *104*:1233, 1986.

Smith RE, Kelley JS, Harbin TS: Late macular complications of choroidal ruptures. Am J Ophthalmol 77:650–658, 1974.

Wood CM, Richardson J: Chorioretinal neovascular membranes complicating contusional eye injuries with indirect choroidal ruptures. Sunderland Eye Infirmary, Tyne. Br J Ophthalmol 74:93–96, 1990.

Wood CM, Richardson J: Indirect choroidal ruptures: Aetiological factors, patterns of ocular damage, and final visual outcome. Sunderland Eye Infirmary. Br J Ophthalmol 74:208–211, 1990.

Wyszynski RE, Grossniklaus HF, Frank KE: Indirect choroidal rupture secondary to blunt ocular trauma. A review of eight eyes. Retina 8:237–243, 1988.

Zagora E: Eye Injuries. Springfield, IL, Charles G Thomas, 1970, pp 21–23.

EXPULSIVE HEMORRHAGE 363.62

(Subchoroidal Expulsive Hemorrhage)

DANIEL M. TAYLOR, M.D., F.A.C.S.

New Britain, Connecticut

Expulsive hemorrhage may take the form of a localized subchoroidal hemorrhage, a massive subchoroidal hemorrhage with a break into the vitreous, or a hemorrhage that proceeds to extrusion of the contents of the globe. It is the most serious and devastating complication of intraocular surgery, but fortunately is uncommon with an incidence of approximately 0.20 per cent. The author has experienced 22 expulsive hemorrhages in over 9,000 intraocular procedures performed from 1951 through 1991. It is most often encountered during cataract extraction in elderly patients with arteriosclerosis and/or hypertension and glaucoma, but may also occur

in young patients, particularly when glaucoma is present. The author has experienced a high incidence of expulsive hemorrhage during extensive keratoplasty procedures with a total of 9 occurrences in some 1,800 keratoplasties. The eye is most vulnerable and treatment is least effective when the hemorrhage occurs during penetrating keratoplasty. The author has also experienced extensive subchoroidal bleeding during the first 24 hours after filtering surgery for uncontrollable glaucoma.

The *immediate cause* of expulsive hemorrhage during intraocular surgery is a sudden change in the intraocular pressure gradient when the eye is opened. These changes will be greater if the arterial pressure is chronically elevated due to hypertensive cardiovascular disease or is acutely elevated at the time of surgery due to anoxia, CO_2 build-up, pressor drugs, or venous obstruction (Valsalva—vomiting, bucking, coughing). The underlying or contributing cause is the presence of arterial necrosis of the short and long posterior ciliary arteries. The most common site is just after the vessel emerges from the scleral wall to enter the subchoroidal space. The arterial necrosis may be due to degenerative vascular disease, such as hypertensive arteriosclerotic cardiovascular disease and diabetes. It may also occur on a nutritional basis in an otherwise normal eye, since the vessel walls of the small arterials are nourished by filtration only. The average filtration pressure of 30 mm Hg is the difference between the average intraocular arterial pressure of approximately 50 mm Hg minus the intraocular pressure of 20 mm Hg. Chronic glaucoma, by reducing the differential between the intraocular arterial pressure and the intraocular pressure, may result in inadequate nutrition of the vascular wall and subsequent arterial necrosis. It is estimated that expulsive hemorrhage occurs ten times more frequently in glaucomatous eyes than in nonglaucomatous eyes.

The first signs of this complication are a sudden shallowing of the anterior chamber, firmness of the globe, and the unexplained presentation of vitreous from the wound. A choroidal bulge or shadow can be seen forming deep within the eye that rapidly moves forward. The choroid and retina may bulge through the incision. Ultimately the hemorrhage breaks through the retina and choroid, with massive outpouring of blood through the wound. If the subchoroidal bleeding spontaneously stops or is exteriorized by sclerotomy, the choroid and the retina may not rupture. If it continues, the entire contents of the eye may extrude. With severe arterial bleeding the condition rapidly becomes irreversible. In my experience, 75 per cent of expulsive hemorrhages occurred at the time of surgery and 25 per cent during the first 24 hours after surgery. Some of the postoperative cases may represent hemorrhages of small magnitude that require additional time to manifest changes or in the case of glaucoma filtering procedures, to prolonged hypotony.

THERAPY.

Surgical. Immediate and rapid closure of the corneal scleral wound with temporary 7-0 or 8-0 interrupted black silk sutures is mandatory to permit a rapid build-up of the intraocular pressure, which, in turn, tends to tamponade bleeding from the ruptured arterial vessel. Modern small incision scleral tunnel wounds may be self-sealing or require only a single suture to permit tight closure, thus checking the progression of the hemorrhage as the intraocular pressure rises. In those cases where rapid closure is impossible (keratoplasty, large incision cataract surgery) or the hemorrhaging is particularly severe, a posterior sclerotomy should be done approximately 8 to 10 mm behind the limbus over the site of the suspected subchoroidal hemorrhage. This opening should be kept open until bleeding stops. A T- or Y-shaped sclerotomy is preferred, as it results in more adequate drainage. The lips of the wound may be cauterized to cause shrinkage, thereby keeping the wound open, possibly for days, to allow continuous drainage. If the first sclerotomy does not find the bleeding site, a second or third sclerotomy should be done in the opposite quadrants. This will usually provide adequate drainage of the subchoroidal space to prevent massive prolapse and rupture of the choroid and retina. When the bleeding is extremely brisk, it may be necessary to aspirate the subchoroidal blood with a syringe and a cannula for as long as 1 hour. On occasion, the blood loss may exceed 100 ml.

When the bleeding stops, the initial operative incision can be reopened and a vitrectomy performed to carefully remove all formed vitreous from in front of the iris and from the wound. These steps should be performed meticulously to prevent shallowing of the anterior chamber with peripheral anterior synechiae formation and severe secondary angle-closure glaucoma. The cataract incision can then be carefully reclosed with nonabsorbable sutures consisting of nylon and interrupted silk. The globe should be reformed with an anterior chamber or intravitreal injection of viscolelastics or balanced salt solution to increase the intraocular pressure. This maneuver may also result in the expression of residual blood through the sclerotomy site. Before closure, it may even be possible to insert an intraocular lens if the bleeding seems to be completely under control. If the hemorrhage occurs during keratoplasty, shortly after removal of the button, it will be impossible to close the eye quickly enough. Under these circumstances, the assistant can place a thumb over the keratoplasty opening to tamponade the eye while the surgeon performs the posterior sclerotomy. When all bleeding

has ceased, it will then be possible to suture in the donor button. With these techniques, the author has salvaged 62 per cent of all eyes experiencing expulsive hemorrhage during surgery. Evisceration or enucleation may be necessary in rare instances if the contents of the eye have been extruded and the bleeding cannot be stopped.

Systemic. After the surgical treatment of an expulsive hemorrhage, systemic and topical ophthalmic corticosteroids may be given to control inflammation and suppress secondary uveitis and vitreitis. Daily oral administration of 40 mg of prednisone and 1 per cent topical ophthalmic prednisolone solution four times daily is helpful. Cycloplegics, consisting of atropine 1 per cent or homatropine 5 per cent, may be given twice daily.

PRECAUTIONS

Any procedure that reduces intraocular pressure abruptly may precipitate expulsive hemorrhage. Patients with hypertension should be well controlled with their blood pressure lowered before surgery. Patients with chronic glaucoma should also have their intraocular pressures under control with the usual glaucoma medications. Patients on anticoagulants or acetylsalicyclic acid should refrain from using these medications at least 5 days before surgery. Epinephrine and other pressor agents should be avoided. Immediately before surgery, the intraocular pressure should be reduced to a minimum, and the globe and orbit should be decompressed by a mercury bag or through massage. The use of intravenous hypotensive agents, such as 150 to 250 ml of 20 per cent mannitol, given 1 hour before surgery is helpful. The head of the operating table can be elevated slightly to avoid elevation of venous pressure. General anesthesia should be avoided whenever possible to eliminate the possibility of a Valsalva effect produced by bucking on the tube, coughing, or vomiting. Postoperatively, if the chamber remains shallow and peripheral anterior synechiae develop, intractable glaucoma may occur with ultimate loss of the eye. Trabeculectomy, laser sclerostomy, or cyclocryotherapy may prove effective in controlling postoperative angle-closure glaucoma.

COMMENTS

Unfortunately, there is no way to completely avoid an expulsive hemorrhage. They will occur in spite of our best efforts. However, a heightened index of suspicion does permit one to operate more efficiently and effectively should an expulsive hemorrhage occur. One must be particularly wary of any patient who has had a previous expulsive hemorrhage, as it has been amply documented that expulsive hemorrhages can occur in both eyes on successive occasions. Under these circumstances, small incision surgery with phacoemulsification would be the procedure of choice for the fellow eye. In the author's experience, the presence of an intact lens capsule is not an effective barrier against the development of an expulsive hemorrhage. The incidence of this complication should be the same whether intracapsular or extracapsular technique is employed. One must be willing to accept the risk of a higher incidence of expulsive hemorrhage with extensive reconstructive procedures, including total penetrating keratoplasties on seriously diseased eyes, triple procedures, and the like, in which the eye is permitted to remain open for prolonged periods of time.

In surgical management, speed is more important than accuracy. A few moments of delay may be the difference between success and failure. Unfortunately, the neophyte surgeon is usually ill prepared to cope with a sudden massive expulsive hemorrhage. Late recognition and inability to perform the proper surgical maneuvers efficiently and effectively will usually result in total loss of the eye. With experience, it is possible to salvage the eye in approximately two-thirds of the cases and to even obtain useful or excellent vision. Early recognition and immediate steps to close the eye and to externalize the bleeding are mandatory. On the positive side, it seems predictable that the increased use of small, self-sealing scleral incisions and phacoemulsification will not only reduce the incidence of expulsive hemorrhage through better control of intraocular pressure during surgery but will also render management far more effective. Utilizing this technique, the author was easily able to control a recent expulsive hemorrhage with return of vision to 20/30.

References

Freiwald MJ: Recovery from severe traumatic ocular hemorrhage. J Albert Einstein Med Center 20:87–90, 1972.

Gerard LJ, et al: Expulsive hemorrhage during intraocular surgery. Trans Am Acad Ophthalmol Soc 77:119–125, 1973.

Payne JW, Kameen AJ, Jensen AD, Christy NE: Expulsive hemorrhage: Its incidence in cataract surgery and the report of four bilateral cases. Trans Am Ophthalmol Soc 83:181–196, 1985.

Shaffer RN: Posterior sclerotomy with scleral cautery in the treatment of expulsive hemorrhage. Am J Ophthalmol 61:1307–1311, 1966.

Speaker MG, Guerriero PM, Met JA, Coad CT, Berger A, Marmer M: A case-control study of risk factors for intraoperative suprachoroidal expulsive hemorrhage. Ophthalmology 98:202–210, 1991.

Taylor DM: Expulsive hemorrhage. Am J Ophthalmol 78:961–966, 1974.

Taylor DM: Expulsive hemorrhage: Some observations and comments. Trans Am Ophthalmol Soc 72:157–169, 1974.

Taylor DM: Discussion of Payne et al: Expulsive hemorrhage: Its incidence in cataract surgery and the report of four bilateral cases. Trans Am Ophthalmol Soc 83:198–201, 1985.

MALIGNANT MELANOMA OF THE POSTERIOR UVEA 190.6

(Choroidal Melanoma, Ciliary Body Melanoma)

JERRY A. SHIELDS, M.D.,
and CAROL L. SHIELDS, M.D.

Philadelphia, Pennsylvania

Malignant melanoma of the uvea is the most common primary intraocular malignancy. This tumor arises from the uveal melanocytes, which are derived embryologically from the neural crest. Melanomas that occur in the ciliary body and peripheral choroid frequently attain a large size before they are diagnosed clinically. Choroidal melanomas that arise in the macular region, however, are usually smaller at the time of diagnosis because they produce earlier visual symptoms.

In the past a patient with a fundus lesion suspected to be a posterior uveal melanoma was promptly managed by enucleation of the affected eye, often by the local ophthalmologist. More recently, ophthalmic oncology has emerged as an established subspecialty of ophthalmology. Hence, more patients with uveal melanomas are referred to centers where physicians specialize almost exclusively in the diagnosis and management of patients with ocular tumors. Consequently, the diagnosis and management of ocular tumors, particularly uveal melanoma, have become more refined and the quality of patient care has improved. Today, there are often several reasonable options to enucleation in the management of uveal melanoma.

The goal of the ophthalmologist in the management of a patient with a posterior uveal melanoma is to control the tumor and to salvage the patient's vision when this can be achieved without endangering the patient's overall health. The method of treatment should be selected carefully so as to meet these goals. Important considerations that should be taken into account when recommending specific management for a patient with a malignant melanoma of the posterior uvea include the size, extent, location, and activity of the tumor; the condition of the opposite eye; and the patient's age, general health, and psychologic status. Once all of the factors that influence the therapeutic choice have been assessed thoroughly, the patient with a posterior uveal melanoma can be managed by any of several methods, depending upon the overall clinical situation.

THERAPY

Supportive. Some authorities recommend only *periodic observation* to initially manage selected melanomas of the posterior uvea. This approach may be justifiable in the case of a small melanocytic tumor that has dormant characteristics on ophthalmoscopic examination. Such a lesion should be carefully examined two or three times a year, and some form of active treatment should be instituted if growth of the tumor is documented subsequently.

The diagnostic tests used and the frequency of follow-up examinations depend upon the size, category, and apparent activity of the tumor. If a patient has a tumor that is classified as a suspicious nevus, he or she should have fundus photographs and be re-examined in 3 months. If no growth is detected, examination should be repeated every 6 months thereafter. If a lesion is classified as a small melanoma that has dormant characteristics, the patient should have baseline fundus photographs, fluorescein angiography, and A-scan and B-scan ultrasonography. The photographs should be repeated in 3 to 4 months. If the lesion shows no apparent change at that time, fundus photography should then be repeated every 6 months. If growth is suspected on the basis of clinical examination, then fundus photography, fluorescein angiography, and ultrasonography should be repeated to confirm any change, and the patient should be considered for one of the therapeutic methods described below.

Surgical. *Photocoagulation* is another method of treating selected small choroidal melanomas. However, it cannot be used in the treatment of ciliary body melanomas. The relative indications for treatment of a choroidal melanoma by photocoagulation are as follows: (1) a small melanoma that shows unequivocal evidence of growth by both serial photography or ultrasonography; (2) some small melanomas that have not necessarily been documented to grow but that show features of activity on the initial examination, particularly if the tumor margin is more than 3 mm from the foveola or optic disc margin; and (3) selected medium-sized melanomas that are more than 2 mm from the optic disc or fovea. To use photocoagulation, the ocular media should be clear, and retrobulbar anesthesia is usually preferable. Argon laser, using either the slit-lamp delivery system or the indirect ophthalmoscopy delivery system, is generally used.

During the first treatment session, laser is applied in two confluent rows around the margins of the tumor. The settings necessary to obtain adequate burns around the tumor vary with the degree of fundus pigmentation. Using the argon laser, a spot size of 200 to 500 μm, an intensity of 500 to 1000 mW, and duration of 0.5 second will usually suffice.

About 3 weeks later, the tumor is surrounded again using similar settings. After two or three surrounding treatments, most of the choroidal vessels around the tumor become obliterated or incorporated into scar tissue. Afterward, in subsequent sessions about 3 to 5 weeks apart, the surrounding area is retreated, and the surface of the tumor is treated heavily. It may require up to 1500 mW with a duration of 1 to 10 seconds to obtain sufficient destruction of the tumor. After a total of four to ten treatments, the area of the tumor is usually replaced by a depressed scar consisting of a thin layer of fibroglial tissue overlying the bare sclera. In many cases treated by this method, a central area of flat pigmentation is left in the center of the scar. It is not necessary to continue treatment once the central pigment is flat, less than 1.5 mm in diameter, and hypofluorescent with fluorescein angiography.

With the advent of low-energy radioactive plaques, photocoagulation is rarely used today in the management of choroidal melanomas. Treatment of small uveal melanoma by primary photocoagulation is used less frequently because techniques of radiotherapy have been greatly improved. However, it is being employed in selected patients as supplemental treatment to plaque radiotherapy.

Although *radiotherapy* was once believed to be ineffective in the treatment of uveal melanomas, it has recently become the most widely employed method in the management of melanomas of the choroid and ciliary body. In view of the recent controversy regarding enucleation for posterior uveal melanomas, the indications for radiotherapy are increasing. The relative indications will probably continue to change as more follow-up data on treated patients become available. The most widely used method of radiotherapy has been the application of an episcleral radioactive plaque. Iodine-125 is the isotope that is most often employed today. Charged particle radiotherapy, using proton beam or helium ions, also has advocates. However, the authors believe that the overall complications are fewer when radioactive plaques are employed.

The current indications for treating a posterior uveal melanoma with an episcleral plaque are as follows: (1) selected small melanomas that are documented to be growing; (2) most medium-sized and large choroidal and ciliary body melanomas that are less than 10 mm in thickness and that show evidence of growth in an eye with useful or salvageable vision; and (3) most medium-sized and large melanomas that occur in the patient's only useful eye, regardless of the visual acuity. Initially, the use of episcleral plaque radiotherapy was confined to medium-sized melanomas that were located in the nasal portion of the fundus and that were at least 3 mm from the optic disc. More recently, selected larger melanomas and those located closer to the disc and fovea have been treated successfully by episcleral plaque radiotherapy. Today, specially designed episcleral plaques can be used for juxtapapillary melanomas and subfoveal melanomas. For patients who have a large melanoma located in their only eye, episcleral plaque radiotherapy is generally used, in spite of the large size of the tumor. More recently, radioactive plaques have been used to treat selected patients with extraocular extension of uveal melanoma and patients with growing iris melanomas that are considered too large to resect locally.

The surgical application of an episcleral plaque should be performed as gently as possible to minimize the theoretical possibility of systemic dissemination of tumor cells during the surgical manipulations. The current policy is to gently expose and inspect the sclera to detect any extrascleral extension of the tumor and then to localize the lesion with transcleral transillumination. The shadow of the tumor is outlined on the sclera with a sterile marking pencil, and a dummy plaque is used to align the scleral sutures. The dummy plaque is then removed and the radioactive plaque is inserted and tied securely in position. The plaque is left in position long enough to deliver about 8,000 to 10,000 cGy to the tumor apex, after which it is removed under local anesthesia and the patient discharged.

Theoretically, an ideal approach to the management of a melanoma of the ciliary body or choroid is to perform *local resection* to remove the tumor and salvage the eye, particularly if this can be achieved without worsening the patient's prognosis. In recent years a technique of partial lamellar sclerouvectomy has been popularized. This technique involves removing the tumor and inner sclera while leaving the retina and outer sclera intact. This procedure is described in the recent literature.

The relative indications for local resection of a posterior uveal melanoma are as follows: (1) a growing ciliary body melanoma or a ciliochoroidal melanoma that does not cover more than one-third of the pars plicata, and (2) a choroidal melanoma that is not greater than 12 mm in diameter, is centered near the equator, and is documented to be growing. It should be emphasized that melanomas that meet these criteria can also be managed by episcleral plaque radiotherapy in most instances. The preferred method of therapy in these instances is unresolved, and each case must be evaluated individually.

As mentioned earlier, the role of *enucleation* in the management of patients with posterior uveal melanomas remains controversial. There are definite indications for enucleation, although they are fewer than in the past. Current indications for enucleation to treat posterior uveal melanomas are as follows: (1) most ciliary body or choroidal melanomas that have produced visual loss, but that are too large to manage with either radiotherapy or local resection; (2) most posterior uveal melanomas that have produced total retinal detachment or severe secondary glaucoma; and (3) most small and medium-sized choroidal melanomas that are documented to be growing and that are invading the tissues of the optic nerve.

The so-called no-touch technique is used less frequently today in enucleation. The value of this technique in reducing the mortality rate from uveal melanomas remains unproven, although some believe that adherence to this technique does reduce the mortality rate. We believe that a gentle enucleation with minimal manipulation of the globe is adequate.

In the last few years, pre-enucleation radiotherapy (PERT) has been employed by some clinicians in hopes of decreasing the chances of metastasis. Recent studies have suggested that PERT is of little or no value, and the technique has been largely abandoned. However, PERT is being evaluated in prospective study as part of the Collaborative Ocular Melanoma Study (COMS).

Exenteration of the orbital contents is considered by some authorities to be an acceptable method of treating uveal melanomas with extraocular extension into the orbit. Others believe that orbital exenteration does not improve the patient's life-span in such cases. The current indications for orbital exenteration for a uveal melanoma are extensive extraocular involvement by the melanoma at the time of initial presentation (provided there is no evidence of systemic metastasis) or orbital recurrence of a uveal melanoma some time after enucleation (provided there is no evidence of systemic metastasis). An eyelid-sparing technique has been popularized for treating patients with massive orbital extension of posterior uveal melanoma. With improved diagnostic techniques and earlier recognition of uveal melanomas, it has become uncommon for patients to present initially with extensive extraocular involvement.

Ocular or Periocular Manifestations

Choroid: Tumor.
Ciliary Body: Tumor.
Conjunctiva: Injection.
Episclera: Extrascleral extension; sentinel vessels (ciliary body tumor).
Iris: Neovascular glaucoma; tumor-induced dialysis (from ciliary body tumor).
Optic Nerve: Atrophy.
Retina: Nonrhegmatogenous retinal detachment, hemorrhage.

PRECAUTIONS

There seems to be little or no danger in close observation of small melanomas that have dormant features. Most of these tumors have little, if any, tendency to grow and a low potential to metastasize. Lesions located within 2 mm of the optic disc or foveola should be followed more frequently. If growth toward either of these structures is documented, either plaque radiotherapy or photocoagulation should be considered.

The complications of photocoagulation for choroidal melanomas include branch retinal vein obstruction, cystoid macular edema, preretinal membrane formation with retinal traction, choroidovitreal neovascularization, vitreous hemorrhage, and retinal detachment. Treatment of choroidal melanomas by photocoagulation is most often successful if the tumor is in the small size category, being less than 3 mm in thickness as measured by ultrasonography.

There are very early complications of episcleral plaque radiotherapy, including ocular irritation and diplopia. Diplopia can occur if a rectus muscle is disinserted to properly position the plaque. Later potential complications of episcleral plaque radiotherapy include radiation retinopathy, radiation papillopathy, neovascular glaucoma, vitreous hemorrhage, radiation cataract, punctal occlusion with epiphora, keratoconjunctivitis sicca, radiation anterior uveitis, sclera necrosis, and persistent diplopia.

Tumors treated by episcleral plaque radiotherapy can sometimes show a rather dramatic response to treatment. Most posterior uveal melanomas show either stabilization or a decrease in tumor size during a follow-up period of 2 to 6 years. The visual results have been satisfactory, and the complications have been relatively few. The mortality rate during this relatively short follow-up period seems to be the same for patients treated with episcleral plaques and those with comparable-sized tumors treated with enucleation.

Episcleral plaque radiotherapy usually is not associated with immediate visual morbidity. The early complications of local tumor resection, however, are greater than those of plaque radiotherapy. The most important potential early surgical complications of local resection are hypotony, wound leak, vitreous bleeding, and retinal detachment. Potential late complications of local resections include vitreous fibrosis, cataract, and ischemic inflammation in the anterior segment. The vitreous fibrosis can lead to chronic traction on the retina and a delayed retinal detachment. In many cases, removal of a ciliochoroidal tumor necessitates removal of a large portion of the zonular support to the lens. This can lead to postoperative shifting of the lens, with inflammation, corneal edema, or glaucoma. To avoid this complication, the lens should generally be removed at the time of surgery when the tumor covers more than 4 clock hours of the pars plicata.

COMMENTS

The management of malignant melanoma of the posterior uvea has recently become a topic of great controversy. The traditional treatment of enucleation of the tumor-containing eye has recently been challenged by a number of authorities, and clinicians are more frequently using alternative methods of management when possible. Current management can range from periodic observation and fundus photography of selected small lesions that appear dormant to photocoagulation, radiotherapy, or local resection in the case of growing tumors in eyes with useful or salvageable vision. In cases where the tumor is far advanced and there is no hope of useful vision, enucleation is generally advisable.

The choice of therapy is a complex issue, and each case must be individualized. In selecting a therapeutic approach, certain factors must be weighed carefully: the size of the melanoma, its extent and location, its apparent activity, the status of the opposite eye, and the age, general health, and psychologic status of the patient.

Periodic observation can be cautiously employed for selected small choroidal melanomas that have dormant characteristics. If such lesions are documented to grow or if they show ophthalmoscopic evidence of progressive growth on the initial examination, then active treatment, usually in the form of episcleral plaque radiotherapy, may be employed. Laser photocoagulation may be an option if the tumor is not greater than 10 mm in diameter or 3 mm in thickness. In the case of medium-sized or large tumors that are growing, the patient can be managed with either scleral plaque radiotherapy or local resection of the tumor. Because radiotherapy has less immediate visual morbidity than local resection, more patients are being managed today by radiotherapy, most commonly in the form of a radioactive plaque.

Patients with large tumors that have produced severe visual loss are currently managed by enucleation. It seems that the so-called no-touch technique of enucleation and preenucleation radiotherapy do not favorably alter the prognosis. If there is extrascleral extension on initial examination or orbital recurrence after enucleation, exenteration of the orbit or one of its modifications seems advisable.

Patients who have known systemic metastases, either before or after enucleation or other treatment, have a poor prognosis. In such cases, palliative irradiation, chemotherapy, or immunotherapy may be employed.

The management of posterior uveal melanoma will probably remain controversial for several years. It is hoped that with the accumulation of further knowledge of the various therapeutic alternatives, the physician will be able to recommend a specific form of therapy in an individual case with more certainty and confidence. Although randomized clinical trials are difficult to accomplish for treatment of uveal melanomas, the COMS should provide additional valuable information for management of patients with posterior uveal melanoma. Until then, each case should be evaluated independently, and the physician should recommend the form of therapy that seems most appropriate in view of the overall clinical situation.

References

Char DH, et al: Helium ion therapy for choroidal melanoma. Ophthalmology 90:1219–1225, 1983.

Fraunfelder FT, et al: No-touch technique for intraocular malignant melanomas. Arch Ophthalmol 95:1616–1620, 1977.

Gragoudas ES, et al: Current results of proton beam radiation of melanomas. Ophthalmology 92:284–291, 1985.

Manschot WA, van Peperzeel HA: Choroidal melanoma: Enucleation or observation? A new approach. Arch Ophthalmol 98:71–77, 1980.

Shields JA: Counseling the patient with posterior uveal melanoma. (Editorial). Am J Ophthalmol 106:88–91, 1988.

Shields JA, Shields CL: Surgical approach to lamellar sclerouvectomy for posterior uveal melanomas. The 1986 Schoenberg Lecture. Ophthalmic Surg 19:774–780, 1988.

Shields, JA, Shields CL: Management of posterior uveal melanoma In Shields JA, Shields CL (eds): Intraocular Tumors. A Text and Atlas. Philadelphia, WB Saunders, 1992, pp 171–205.

Shields JA, Glazer LC, Mieler WF, Shields CL: Comparison of xenon arc and argon laser photocoagulation in the treatment of choroidal melanomas. Am J Ophthalmol 109:647–655, 1990.

Shields JA, Shields CL, Donoso LA: Management of posterior uveal melanoma. Surv Ophthalmol 36:161–195, 1991.

Shields JA, Shields CL, Shah P, Sivalingam V: Partial lamellar sclerouvectomy for posterior uveal tumors. Ophthalmology 98:971–983, 1991.

Shields JA, Shields CL, Suvarnamani C, Tantasira M, Shah P: Orbital exenteration with eyelid sparing: Indications, technique and results. Ophthalmic Surg 22:292–297, 1991.

Shields CL, Shields JA, De Potter P: Hydroxyapatite orbital implant after enucleation. Experience with initial 100 consecutive cases. Arch Ophthalmol 110:333–338, 1992.

Wilson WS, Fraunfelder FT: "No touch" cryosurgical enucleation. A minimal trauma technique for eyes harboring intraocular malignancy. Ophthalmology 85:1170–1175, 1978.

Zimmerman LE, McLean IW: An evaluation of enucleation in the management of uveal melanomas. Am J Ophthalmol 87:741–760, 1979.

Zimmerman LE, McLean IW, Foster WD: Does enucleation of the eye containing a malignant melanoma prevent or accelerate the dissemination of tumor cells? Br J Ophthalmol 62:420–425, 1978.

SYMPATHETIC OPHTHALMIA 360.11
(Sympathetic Uveitis)

GEORGE E. MARAK, JR., M.D.

Alexandria, Virginia

Sympathetic ophthalmia is a bilateral non-necrotizing uveitis that is believed to represent an autoimmune response to an unidentified ocular antigen suspected to be of retinal or retinal pigment epithelial origin. A penetrating wound is important in the pathogenesis of the disease, since it allows antigens to escape from the "immunologic privilege" of the intraocular compartment. The contamination introduced with a perforating wound may have an adjuvant effect that helps account for the 30 to 50 times more frequent incidence of sympathetic ophthalmia after accidental compared to surgical penetrating wounds.

Sympathetic ophthalmia, as with any inflammatory disease, may present with varying degrees of severity. This creates problems in the differential diagnosis. The textbook description of sympathetic ophthalmia is well recognized and need not be repeated; however, it may also present as a mild anterior uveitis, pars planitis, peripapillitis, or focal choroiditis, which is not easily confused with multifocal placoid pigment epitheliopathy (in the author's experience).

Fluorescein angiography presents a characteristic picture in sympathetic ophthalmia. Ultrasonography can demonstrate choroidal thickening. A peau d'orange appearance seen on slit-lamp examination indicates variations in the choroidal infiltrate that may be helpful in distinguishing sympathetic ophthalmia from bilateral phacoanaphylactic endophthalmitis.

THERAPY

Systemic. The objective of therapy in sympathetic ophthalmia is to control the inflammation as quickly as possible. A combination of systemic, subtenon,* and topical corticosteroids in doses proportionate to the severity of the inflammation is the treatment of choice. Severe disease may require initial daily doses of 200 mg of oral prednisone. This is given as a single morning dose for 3 to 10 days. Depending upon the patient's response, alternate-day therapy may be initiated. The steroids may be gradually tapered with clinical monitoring of the inflammation. In the absence of systemic complications, treatment should be maintained 3 to 6 months after all signs of inflammation have cleared. Exacerbations are unpredictable and may occur several years after a preceding episode of inflammation. Regular lifetime observation of the patient is necessary.

Patients unresponsive or intolerant of steroids require highly individualized management. A variety of anti-inflammatory agents have been employed with irregular success. Combinations of steroids and immunosuppressive drugs are the most promising alternative approach in difficult cases. Various immunosuppressive drugs have been employed alone in systemic treatment of sympathetic ophthalmia with anecdotal success in problem patients. Most recently, cyclosporine† has been fashionable, but it may cause permanent renal damage, and it is a potential neoplastic agent. Appropriate precautions and patient consent are essential in problem cases when individualized management includes treatment with immunosuppressive drugs.

Ocular. Subtenon injections of soluble steroids, such as 4 mg of dexamethasone,* may be employed several times a week in the initial treatment of severe disease. Topical corticosteroids can be used hourly in severe disease and reduced as the inflammation resolves.

Careful attention should be given to mydriasis. In severe uveitis, long-acting agents, such as atropine and scopolamine, often do not provide adequate dilation to prevent posterior synechia formation. Moving the pupil with pilocarpine and obtaining maximum dilation with phenylephrine and cyclopentolate should be done at office visits to ensure against synechia formation.

Surgical. Cataract surgery has been performed successfully in a number of patients with sympathetic ophthalmia. There seem to be no unusual risks if it is done during a remission. Additional steroid coverage has conventionally been employed when cataract surgery is performed on patients with sympathetic ophthalmia.

The success of glaucoma surgery in uveitis is not widely discussed. Many enucleated eyes have had previous glaucoma surgery, but there are no reliable data on the complications of glaucoma surgery in either sympathetic ophthalmia or other forms of severe uveitis.

Ocular or Periocular Manifestations

Choroid: Chorioretinal scarring and adhesions; focal obliteration of choriocapillaris.

Iris: Focal to diffuse nonnecrotizing granulomatous uveitis.

Optic Nerve: Edema; infiltration around pia septa; meningeal inflammation; perivasculitis.

Retina: Dalen-Fuchs' spots; exudative detachment; inflammation; perivasculitis.

Other: Cataracts; focal scleritis; phthisis bulbi; poliosis; secondary glaucoma; vitiligo.

PRECAUTIONS

Continued lifelong observation of patients with sympathetic ophthalmia is necessary. Relapses occur in most patients, and the interval between relapses has been as long as 13 years.

It is important not to produce an exacerbation of the inflammation by tapering medication too rapidly. Patients should be reexamined within a few days after any medication reduction. Continuing systemic or topical medication for 3 to 6 months after all inflammation has cleared is important in avoiding exacerbations.

The usual complications and ocular side effects of systemic steroids are to be anticipated, and therapy should be modulated accordingly. Immunosuppressive agents are reserved for those patients who cannot tolerate or do not respond to steroid treatment.

COMMENTS

Although two recent reports resurrect the idea that early enucleation of the injured eye is helpful to the sympathizing eye, this conclusion is not supported by the author's own data. As in all other reports, no statistically significant difference in the visual outcome of the sympathizing eye is related to the time of enucleation of the inducing eye once sympathetic ophthalmia has been developed.

One would not treat glomerulonephritis or multiple sclerosis by removing one kidney or half of the brain. The idea of removing a noxious influence by enucleating the sympathizing eye is of historic interest, but is inconsistent with current concepts of autoimmunity. It is not justifiable to remove a potentially functional eye in established cases of sympathetic ophthalmia for the purpose of improving the prognosis of the sympathizing eye. The injured eye may eventually achieve better vision.

Every attempt should be made to save potentially useful eyes. However, with the development of sympathetic ophthalmia in eyes after vitrectomy, those eyes that have no hope for useful vision in the opinion of the surgeon should be enucleated after discussion with the patient.

The only known prevention for sympathetic ophthalmia is enucleation within 2 weeks of injury (before the development of the autoimmune response). Prophylactic steroids do not prevent sympathetic ophthalmia. The potential increased incidence of infection outweighs any potential benefit of prophylactic steroids.

References

Andrasch RH, Pirofsky B, Burns RP: Immunosuppressive therapy for severe chronic uveitis. Arch Ophthalmol 96:247–251, 1978.

Ben Ezra D, Nussenblatt RB, Timonen P: Optimal Use of Sandimmune in Endogenous Uveitis. Berlin, Springer-Verlag, 1988.

Croxatto JO, et al: Atypical histopathologic features in sympathetic ophthalmia. A study of a hundred cases. Int Ophthalmol 4:129–135, 1982.

Makley TA, Azar A: Sympathetic ophthalmia. A long-term follow-up. Arch Ophthalmol 96:257–262, 1978.

Marak GE Jr: Recent advances in sympathetic ophthalmia. Surv Ophthalmol 24:141–156, 1979.

Rao NA, et al: The role of the penetrating wound in the development of sympathetic ophthalmia. Arch Ophthalmol 101:102–104, 1983.

SECTION 20

CONJUNCTIVA

ALLERGIC CONJUNCTIVITIS 372.05
(Atopic Conjunctivitis, Hay Fever Conjunctivitis, Acute Allergic Catarrhal Conjunctivitis)

ROBERT ABEL, JR., M.D.,
and KHALAD A. NAGY, M.D

Wilmington, Delaware

Several types of hypersensitivity disorders cause conjunctival and external ocular symptomatology, including atopic conjunctivitis, hay fever conjunctivitis, acute allergic catarrhal conjunctivitis, atopic eczema, and vernal keratoconjunctivitis. The natural history of each of these disorders is different, just as individual response is different. They bear in common a variable inflammatory response that may be acute, subacute, or chronic and may be triggered by specific ocular atopic phenomena. Atopic conjunctivitis is acute/chronic conjunctival inflammation manifested by vascular engorgement, chemosis, and a papillary reaction. It is provoked by specific allergens, including pollens, inhalants, vegetable substances, animal dander, and dust. There may be an associated punctate keratopathy.

Hay fever conjunctivitis has been extensively investigated by Allansmith and colleagues (1988) and found to be IgE-mediated and to involve the release of histamine through the degranulation of the millions of conjunctival mast cells; prostaglandins and leukotrienes are other intermediaries of inflammation. Hay fever conjunctivitis is a type I hypersensitivity response that is seasonal in origin and found in a large number of patients. It is possible to know when the pollen count is high by looking at the eyes. Many patients do not recognize the initial findings of itching, swelling, photophobia, and epiphora until the conjunctivitis is full blown. With vernal catarrh, the inflammatory process may extend to the globe as well (bulbar type and a mixed type), producing greater photophobia, mucoid discharge, and Trantas' dots near the limbus. Cobblestone-papillae are caused by cellular infiltration of lymphocytes, plasma cells, and eosinophils, with proliferation of the epithelium. Tobgy has classified vernal catarrh and documented progressive corneal tenons. Keratoconus has been found in some young boys suffering from spring catarrh.

THERAPY

Systemic. Pharmacologic therapy is the mainstay of treatment and has arisen from both physician and patient expectations. Patients prefer a quick response, but a long-term management program is more important. Rapid diagnosis allows for the use of 4 per cent cromolyn sodium four times daily that will stabilize mast cells before degranulation. Topical antihistamines and vasoconstrictors also must be applied immediately for therapy to be efficacious. Topical steroids (of various strengths) may reduce the inflammatory processes, but require frequent administration early on. Fluorometholone or other weak topical steroids are advisable for chronic use because of the reduction of possible complications, such as cataract and glaucoma. Oral antihistamines or corticosteroids are last choices of therapy because of their debilitating side effects. Newer products, such as cyclosporine, lodoxamide 0.1 per cent, and levacobastine, are showing promise as replacements for cromolyn sodium, which has been off the market.

Surgical. Silver nitrate and direct curettage of large papules may be helpful in patients with significant sensitivity. A recent report of a saphenous vein graft to replace the superior tarsal conjunctiva deserves future investigation.

Supportive. The most successful long-term treatment for allergic conjunctivitis patients is minimizing contact with the allergens in question. Changing the air filter system in the house, removing rugs and drapes, minimizing cutting the grass and sweeping the basement, and the like can be very helpful. In conjunction, hyposensitization therapy may reduce the ocular signs and symptoms in a large number of people. This of course requires 3 months of advanced therapy before that particular allergen season begins.

Ocular or Periocular Manifestations

Conjunctiva: Chemosis; superficial, conjunctival erythema; glistening appearance to the conjunctiva; thickened tear film meniscus.

Cornea: Superficial punctate keratitis; Trantas' dots.

Eyelids: Hyperkeratosis; erythema and edema of lid skin; occasional maceration of lateral and medial canthi.

456

Other: Anterior uveitis; cataracts (unusual).

PRECAUTIONS

Long-term use of any topical medication may have significant side effects; (in addition, vasoconstrictors may cause tachyphylaxis, and elevated intraocular pressure and posterior subcapsular cataracts are side effects of stronger corticosteroids). Long-term objectives must be established with these patients, and they cannot be lost to follow-up. Contact lens wearers, who will often do anything to maintain their lens wear, must develop an appropriate long-term program of topical medication to minimize symptoms. Other types of keratoconjunctivitis must be excluded from the differential diagnosis: phlyctenular keratoconjunctivitis, staphylococcal hypersensitivity, erythema multiforme (Stevens-Johnson syndrome), and acne rosacea keratoconjunctivitis.

References

Allansmith MR: Immunologic effects of extended wear contact lenses. Ann Ophthalmol 21:465, 1989.

Allansmith MR, Ross RN: Ocular allergy. Clin Allergy 18:1, 1988.

Ayoub M: Different causes of allergic conjunctivitis. *In* Osman A (ed): The Pathology of the Eye, 2nd ed. Cairo, Arab Contractor Press, 1989, pp 39–41.

Buckley RJ: Vernal keratoconjunctivitis. Int Ophthalmol Clin 28:303, 1988.

Caldwell DR, Verin P, Young RH, Meyers SM, Darke ML: Efficacy and safety of lodoxamide 1% vs cromolyn sodium 4% in patients with vernal keratoconjunctivitis. Am J Ophthalmol 113:632–637, 1992.

Dart JKC, Buckley RJ, Monnickenda M, Prasad J: Perennial allergic conjunctivitis. Definition, indications characteristics and prevalence. A comparison of seasonal allergy conjunctivitis. Trans Ophthalmol Soc UK 105:513, 1986.

Langston DP: Manual of Ocular Diagnosis and Therapy, 2nd ed. Boston, Little Brown and Co., 1985, pp 98–100.

Verin PC, Fritsch DS: Lodoxamide, a maintenance preventive agent for management of vernal keratoconjunctivitis. Ophthalmology 96 (Suppl):120, 1989.

BACTERIAL CONJUNCTIVITIS 372.03

(Mucopurulent Conjunctivitis, Purulent Conjunctivitis)

DOUGLAS J. COSTER, F.R.C.S., and PAUL R. BADENOCH, Ph D

Adelaide, Australia

Bacterial infection of the conjunctiva usually produces a purulent or mucopurulent conjunctivitis. Most but not all cases of purulent conjunctivitis are caused by bacteria. The infective process is usually of an acute nature, but occasionally, bacteria produce a low-grade chronic reaction. For the most part, the condition is a mild affliction.

A wide range of bacterial species can infect the conjunctiva. There is considerable variation in causative organisms with the age of the patient, the locality, and the season. *Staphylococcus aureus, Streptococcus pyogenes, Pseudomonas aeruginosa,* and enteric gram-negative bacilli are common causes of purulent conjunctivitis. In most developed countries, *Neisseria gonorrhoeae* is an unusual cause of ophthalmia neonatorum; *Chlamydia trachomatis* is the usual agent. Between the ages of 3 months and 8 years, pneumococcal infection is frequent. *Hemophilus influenzae* conjunctivitis also occurs most commonly in this age group, presumably associated with the decline of maternally transferred antibody and a delay in the development of specific mucosal immunity. *Moraxella* conjunctivitis is often seen in the elderly or infirm.

The only certain way to implicate an etiologic agent is to isolate it in the laboratory. Management of bacterial conjunctivitis involves recognition of the disease at a clinical level, identification of the etiologic agent, appreciation of the importance of the case from a public health point of view, and the administration of antimicrobial chemotherapy.

THERAPY

Ocular. Broad-spectrum antibiotics are often used before laboratory results are known or, in most cases, without collecting material for microbiologic assessment. Commonly used topical ophthalmic agents include sulfacetamide 10 per cent, chloramphenicol 0.5 per cent, tobramycin 0.3 per cent eyedrops, and bacitracin 0.5 per cent, chloramphenicol 1 per cent, and erythromycin 0.5 per cent ointments. The combination neomycin-polymyxin B-gramicidin is still widely used as either a drop or as an ointment. The ointments are useful with children or for overnight use in adults. A satisfactory agent would be active against expected pathogens, have low local and systemic toxicity, and be nonallergenic. Adverse effects to topically applied agents are not common, however, the prolonged use of bacitracin or polymyxin B may be toxic at the site of delivery, neomycin is allergenic to the corneal epithelium, and chloramphenicol drops have been implicated in fatal aplastic anemia.

Most cases of bacterial conjunctivitis respond to a low dose of any broad-spectrum antibiotic applied topically. Severe fulminating cases, cases not responding to initial therapy, and all conjunctivitis in children deserve bacteriologic investigation. Purulent conjunctivitis failing to respond to initial antimicrobial measures should have medication withdrawn for 24 hours after which material should be collected for cytologic and microbiologic examination. On the basis of these cultures, specific chemotherapy should be instigated.

Patients infected with *N. gonorrhoeae, N. meningitidis,* or streptococci should be treated with penicillin G eyedrops in a concentration of 100,000 units/ml. If there is an allergy to penicillin or if the gonococci produce penicillinase, chloramphenicol 0.5 per cent eyedrops may be substituted. Those with *Hemophilus* or *Moraxella* infection should also receive chloramphenicol eyedrops. Infections with other gram-negative bacilli are best treated with gentamicin 0.3 per cent eyedrops until susceptibility tests (tube dilution method) suggest otherwise. Topical therapy for conjunctivitis should be given every 2 hours for 2 to 3 days until the process is controlled and then four times a day for another week.

Recently, ciprofloxacin 0.3 per cent eyedrops and ointment have become available. This quinolone has excellent activity against most strains of *S. aureus, P. aeruginosa,* and enteric gram-negative bacilli. Subject to further evaluation, ciprofloxacin is likely to become a popular broad-spectrum agent for bacterial conjunctivitis.

Systemic. Systemic treatment should be considered in cases of neonatal gonococcal conjunctivitis and *H. influenzae* Type B conjunctivitis in children in whom the instillation of drops may be difficult. For gonococcal conjunctivitis, a suggested regimen is 50,000 units/kg/day intravenous aqueous penicillin G in two doses, or 300,000 units/kg/day intramuscular in four doses, for 7 days. For penicillinase-producing gonococci, intravenous or intramuscular ceftriaxone (25–50 mg/kg/day) for 7 days is advocated. Infants of low birthweight should receive a single dose only. Children from whom *H. influenzae* Type B is isolated should be treated with systemic ampicillin: (25–50 mg/kg/day) in two or three divided doses for 5 days to a maximum daily dose of 1.5 gm. If the strain is ampicillin resistant, chloramphenicol (80–100 mg/kg/day in four divided doses for 5 days) is recommended.

PRECAUTIONS

A patient with purulent conjunctivitis may fail to respond to topical medication for several reasons. The disease may be due to an intracellular bacterial infection, such as *C. trachomatis,* or to a noninfective process, that occurs with erythema multiforme or Reiter's syndrome. If the condition is due to bacterial infection, the agent may not be susceptible to the drug used. Alternatively, the conjunctival sac may be loaded with organisms from the lacrimal sac or from other nonocular sites under various circumstances. A persistent, uniocular, purulent discharge should alert the

ophthalmologist to the possibility of a foreign body. Another reason for treatment failure is poor patient compliance. Occasionally, in mucopurulent disease, mucus may protect organisms from chemotherapeutic agents. This can be overcome by the combined use of topical antibodies and mucolytic agents. Ten per cent acetylcysteine eyedrops* used twice a day are very effective in this uncommon situation.

COMMENTS

The need for bacteriologic investigation is debatable. Two approaches to bacterial conjunctivitis can be followed. A broad-spectrum antibiotic may be administered on suspicion of bacterial infection, with laboratory investigations reserved for refractive cases. Alternatively, more specific chemotherapy can be prescribed based on the bacteria isolated if cultures are initiated as a first step. In favor of broad-spectrum therapy is the excellent response achieved in most cases with simple treatment. Against this approach is the fact that not all purulent conjunctivitis is due to bacteria and not all bacteria will respond to simple broad-spectrum therapy. When a case has not responded to a trial of chemotherapy, the chances of achieving a microbiologic diagnosis may have been lost. In most situations, broad-spectrum antibiotics are used based on a clinical diagnosis of bacterial conjunctivitis. Severe purulent conjunctivitis, however, requires initial laboratory investigation.

References

Baum J, Barza M: Infections of the Eye. *In* Gorbach SL, Bartlett JG, Blacklow NR (eds): Infectious Diseases. Philadelphia, WB Saunders, 1992, pp 1134–1151.

Fraunfelder FT, Bagby GC, Kelly DJ: Fatal aplastic anemia following topical administration of ophthalmic chloramphenicol. Am J Ophthalmol *93:* 356–360, 1982.

Leibowitz HM: Antibacterial effectiveness of ciprofloxacin 0.3% ophthalmic solution in the treatment of bacterial conjunctivitis. Am J Ophthalmol *112:*29S–33S, 1991.

CICATRICIAL PEMPHIGOID 372.04
(Benign Mucous Membrane Pemphigoid, Ocular Cicatricial Pemphigoid)

LYNNE H. MORRISON, M.D., *and* KENNETH C. SWAN, M.D.

Portland, Oregon

Cicatricial pemphigoid is a relatively rare, chronic inflammatory disease affecting primarily the mucous membranes. Patients are usually 60 years of age or older, and females are more frequently affected than males. The conjunctiva and oral mucosa are the most frequently affected areas, but the oropharynx, nasopharynx, esophagus, genitalia, and rectal mucosa may also be involved. Cutaneous lesions are present in up to 25 per cent of cases. Although the primary lesions are subepithelial bullae that heal with scarring, erythema and erosions, rather than blisters, are most frequently observed in the mucous membranes. Ocular involvement of cicatricial pemphigoid often begins with a conjunctivitis accompanied by subepithelial fibrosis. Progressive fibrosis results in foreshortening of the fornices and eventually leads to the development of symblepharon. The fibrotic process can cause trichiasis and entropion. Reduced numbers of conjunctival goblet cells produce altered tear composition, which, combined with tear insufficiency caused by lacrimal duct compromise, contributes further to corneal exposure, resulting in corneal ulcerations, keratinization, and neovascularization. Blindness has occurred in approximately 25 to 33 per cent of patients with ocular involvement. The disease is chronic, with only rare cases of spontaneous remission noted.

Cicatricial pemphigoid is thought to be mediated by autoantibodies directed against an antigen in the basement zone. These antibodies are detectable in the majority of cases in conjunctival or other mucous membrane biopsies processed for immunofluorescent studies. Direct immunofluorescent studies are the most reliable means of establishing a diagnosis.

THERAPY

Systemic. The disease is best controlled with systemic therapy. Topical treatment alone provides little benefit. Most experience has been gained with systemic corticosteroids, usually in the form of prednisone. Starting doses are usually in the range of 40 to 60 mg of prednisone daily. After initial control, the dose is tapered to the lowest level possible, with the goal of achieving alternate-day therapy. Steroids act as a suppressive agent and do not produce long-term remission of the disease. When they are discontinued or tapered, the process is likely to be reactivated. Unfortunately, high doses of prednisone are often required on a long-term basis to maintain control, although some patients can be tapered to low doses. Maintenance doses range from 2.5 to 60 mg of prednisone daily. Another problem with the use of prednisone as sole therapy is its possible failure to halt the progression of disease. In one series, 25 per cent of patients on systemic corticosteroids progressed to blindness. Despite these problems, prednisone can be considered for patients with mild, nonprogressive, early ocular disease. If they show evidence of contin-

ued scarring, require high doses of prednisone for control, or manifest unacceptable steroid side effects, alternate therapy should be considered.

The sulfone derivative dapsone[+] has been shown to be effective in controlling cicatricial pemphigoid. It is a reasonable therapeutic choice for mild to moderately active cicatricial pemphigoid that is not rapidly progressive. It is effective in oral lesions, but also has been found to stop progression of ocular disease. In one series, 88 per cent of patients with mild to moderately active ocular cicatricial pemphigoid responded to dapsone with evidence of improvement in 4 weeks. An usual and expected side effect of dapsone is hemolytic anemia, which is dose dependent and is accompanied by a compensatory reticulocytosis. To allow time for this compensation to occur and to allow for assessment of drug tolerance, dapsone is started at a low dose and then increased to the therapeutic range. The usual starting dose is 50 mg daily for 1 to 2 weeks; the dose is then increased to 50 mg twice a day and is adjusted thereafter based on the therapeutic response and level of anemia. Successful maintenance doses range from 50 to 150 mg of dapsone daily. Patients should have glucose-6-phosphate dehydrogenase levels checked before starting therapy. If these levels are deficient, marked degrees of hemolysis can occur with the use of dapsone.

In patients with rapidly progressive or extremely active ocular disease or potentially life-threatening manifestations of the disease, more aggressive therapy should be considered. A very successful form of treatment seems to be the use of immunosuppressive drugs either alone or in combination with prednisone. Cyclophosphamide[+] in combination with prednisone has been shown to be highly effective for suppressing disease activity. Rather than simply suppressing disease activity, this regimen has the potential to induce a sustained remission. Azathioprine[*] can be used as an alternative immunosuppressive agent, but may be less effective than cyclophosphamide and is less likely to induce a long-term remission. Cyclophosphamide is started at a dose of 1 to 2 mg/kg daily together with prednisone 1 mg/kg daily. Prednisone may be deleted if there are contraindications to its use, but control of the disease activity will be slower. The patients are treated with this combination of drugs for 1 month and then re-evaluated clinically. If significant disease activity is still present, the dose of cyclophosphamide can be increased in 25-mg amounts monthly as tolerated. The prednisone dose is tapered rapidly to 40 mg daily and then over the course of a month is tapered to 40 mg every other day. The alternate-day dose is then tapered and finally discontinued over the course of about 2 months. Once the disease is well controlled, the cyclophosphamide is continued for another 12 months. Usually a total of 18 months is required to complete the course of therapy.

Ocular. Ocular surface lubrication is an important part of therapy in patients with sicca syndrome secondary to advanced ocular cicatricial pemphigoid. Ointment lubricants without preservatives are preferred and should be used frequently enough to provide surface protection (every 2 to 4 hours and at bedtime). Artificial tears without preservatives can be used between ointment applications as needed.

Routine lid hygiene is useful adjunctive therapy, especially in patients with chronic blepharitis.

Surgical. Corneal clarity and integrity are best preserved by control of entropion and trichiasis, adequate lubrication, and prevention of infection. Destruction of aberrant lashes is an important part of patient management because it not only reduces the damage to the ocular surface epithelium but it also removes a source of ocular inflammation, which may be confused with inflammation caused by the underlying immunologic disease. The aberrant lashes are best removed by cryotherapy. This should be performed precisely, and freezing should be limited to the lid margin, since freezing of the conjunctival surface may incite a marked inflammatory reaction. Punctal occlusion is essential in cases where tear flow is deficient.

Oculoplastic procedures may be useful to correct conjunctival shrinkage and thereby minimize corneal exposure and blinding sequelae. These procedures can exacerbate the existing inflammation and therefore should generally be deferred until the disease activity has been adequately controlled. Incisions made directly through the contractured conjunctiva into the fornices have been disappointing, even with stents and grafts. Cicatricial entropion generally can be corrected by sliding the conjunctiva off the tarsal plates into the fornices. Although this procedure can be performed under topical anesthesia, subconjunctival injections of anesthetic solution serve the dual purpose of deep anesthesia and establishment of a line of dissection. The addition of epinephrine minimizes the bleeding. Under the operating microscope, an incision is made through the conjunctiva at the lid margin. Thickened conjunctiva is dissected off the tarsus and allowed to retract into the fornices. This allows the lids to return to their normal positions and leaves the bulbar conjunctiva undisturbed. The tarsus re-epithelializes rapidly. During healing, patients are instructed to stretch the skin of the lids over the orbital margins while rotating their eyes. This maneuver helps preserve the fornices.

Both lamellar and penetrating keratoplasties have been used to restore clarity and substance to the cornea, but the outcome may be disappointing. Cataracts are also common in these patients and may progress to maturity. Cataract extractions have been performed through limbal incisions under limbal base flaps on patients with ocular pemphigoid. Such surgical procedures can exacerbate disease activity and in general are best performed once the disease activity has been brought under control.

Ocular or Periocular Manifestations

Conjunctiva: Chronic inflammation with cicatrization and symblepharon; keratinization.

Cornea: Mechanical irritation and infection; pannus; recurrent keratitis secondary to exposure; stromal thinning; ulcers.

Eyelids: Ankyloblepharon; entropion; trichiasis.

Lacrimal System: Cicatricial closure of the ducts.

PRECAUTIONS

Several diseases may mimic cicatricial pemphigoid. Severe conjunctival inflammation caused by erythema multiforme, toxic epidermal necrolysis, or alkali burns may result in a scarring conjunctivitis similar to what is seen with cicatricial pemphigoid. Additionally, topical application of ocular medication, such as echothiophate, pilocarpine, epinephrine-containing compounds, and idoxuridine, can produce toxic effects to the conjunctival epithelium that are difficult to distinguish from cicatricial pemphigoid. These cases of pseudopemphigoid are best distinguished from idiopathic cicatricial pemphigoid by direct immunofluorescent studies. A biopsy taken from uninvolved tissue immediately adjacent to a lesion shows linear deposition IgG and C3 along the basement membrane zone in cases of cicatricial pemphigoid, but not in pseudopemphigoid. A conjunctival biopsy is preferred when ocular involvement is present, but a biopsy from other perilesional sites may also be equally useful.

Patients in whom long-term use of systemic steroids is contemplated should be questioned regarding the presence of diabetes mellitus, hypertension, history of peptic or duodenal ulcers, and history of tuberculosis, since high doses of corticosteroids can exacerbate these conditions. A chest x-ray, skin test for tuberculosis, and fasting blood sugar should be obtained before placing patients on long-term high-dose corticosteroids. Additionally, blood pressure, fasting glucose and weight should be monitored periodically while patients are on corticosteroids. Management in association with an internist or endocrinologist who can provide preventive measures for and evaluation of osteoporosis would be appropriate.

The side effects of cyclophosphamide include: hemorrhagic cystitis, alopecia, leukopenia, anemia, thrombocytopenia, and possibly an increased risk of developing a malignancy. The most common side effect is leukopenia. It may be helpful to manage the patient in conjunction with an internist, oncologist, or rheumatologist familiar with the use and side effects of this drug. Patients should have a weekly complete blood cell count with differential, platelet count, and urinalysis. If the dose of cyclophosphamide is unchanged after several months, these parameters may then be monitored every 2 weeks and then subsequently every month if parameters remain stable. The white blood cell count should not fall below 3000 cells/ml,[3] with at least 1500 granuloctyes/ml[3] while on immunosuppressive agents. Azathioprine has the same adverse effects as cyclophosphamide, except that it has not been associated with hemorrhagic cystitis; however, it has been associated with hepatic damage. Initially, patients on azathioprine should have a complete blood cell count with differential, platelet count, and liver functions monitored weekly.

The most common adverse effects of dapsone are hemolytic anemia and methemoglobinemia. The anemia is dose related, generally occurring in patients taking 50 mg or more daily, and is compensated by a reticulocytosis. Although the anemia is usually well tolerated by most patients, it may cause problems for those with cardiopulmonary disease. Patients should have G-6-PD levels checked before starting dapsone; if they are deficient in this enzyme, a marked hemolytic anemia may occur. Less common side effects include peripheral neuropathy and toxic hepatitis. Complete blood cell counts should be done routinely in patients on dapsone.

COMMENTS

The natural history of untreated cicatricial pemphigoid is that of a progressive disease, which generally does not have a spontaneous remission. It most frequently affects ocular and oral mucous membranes, but may involve the skin, esophagus, or rectal, vaginal, or pharyngeal mucous membranes. Because of the chronic nature of the disease and the potential for various organ system involvement, these patients require long-term care that may involve a variety of specialists, including dermatologists, gastroenterologists, and otorhinolaryngologists. The disease activity may be suppressed by corticosteroids or dapsone, but cytotoxic agents offer the possibility of disease remission. Because of the potentially serious adverse effects associated with these medications, patient management is best done in conjunction with an internist, dermatologist, or rheumatologist familiar with their use.

References

Camisa C, Meisler DM: Immunobullous diseases with ocular involvement. Dermatol Clin 10:555–570, 1992.
Fiore PM, Jacobs IH, Goldberg DB: Drug-induced pemphigoid. A spectrum of diseases. Arch Ophthalmol 105:1660–1663, 1987.
Foster CS: Cicatricial pemphigoid. Trans Am Ophthalmol Soc 84:527–663, 1986.
Mondino BJ: Cicatricial pemphigoid and erythema multiforme. Ophthalmology 97:939–952, 1990.
Rogers RS, Seehafer JR, Perry HO: Treatment of cicatricial pemphigoid with dapsone. J Am Acad Dermatol 6:215–223, 1982.

CONJUNCTIVAL MELANOTIC LESIONS 224.3
(Benign Congenital Melanosis, Benign Nevi, Melanoma, PAM, Precancerous and Cancerous Melanosis, Primary Acquired Melanosis)

DAVID J. WILSON, M.D.

Portland, Oregon

Melanotic conjunctival lesions can be divided into benign epithelial melanosis, benign melanocytic nevi, primary acquired melanosis with or without atypia, and melanoma. Primary acquired melanosis was formerly known as Reese's precancerous melanosis, benign acquired melanosis, idiopathic acquired melanosis, and intraepithelial atypical melanocytic hyperplasia. Recent major contributions in this confusing and controversial area have been made by Folberg, Jakobiec, Zimmerman, and their co-workers.

Benign congenital melanosis simply denotes the increased production of melanin granules, which are distributed by normal numbers of melanocytes to the surrounding epithelial cells of the conjunctiva. Clinically, they are brown flat macules or patches without thickening or vascularity. These lesions occur most frequently in African-American patients near the limbus in the interpalpebral space because their melanocytes can readily produce extramelanin granules when irritated by external stimulation. In Caucasians, similar lesions can develop idiopathically. In skin pathology, such lesions are called ephelides (freckles) or lentigines, the latter implying a mild increase in the number of benign melanocytes in addition to increased pigment production.

Benign nevus is the most common melanocytic tumor of the conjunctiva. Nevi are characteristically located in the interpalpebral space from the limbus to the caruncle, but they may rarely arise anywhere in the palpebral conjunctiva or the lid margins. Nevi commence generally within the first two decades of life; they almost always make their appearance by the end of the third decade. These lesions begin as intraepithelial nests of benign melanocytes (junctional nevi). During the second and third decades, the intraepithelial cells drop off into the connective tissue of the substantia propria (compound nevi). During the third and fourth decades of life, the intraepidermal nests cease to proliferate and leave nests of subepithelial melanocytes (subepithelial nevi). Epithelial inclusion cysts, which become more prominent with expansion of the subepithelial component, are a helpful diagnostic finding. Nevi are not necessarily pigmented, and up to 30 per cent of them are poorly pigmented or nonpigmented so that identification of the typical inclusion cysts is valuable clinically. It is worth emphasizing that any melanocytic lesion that first appears after the third or fourth decade and that was assuredly not present during the first two should be regarded with suspicion.

Primary acquired melanosis (PAM) is a condition that is most common in the middle-aged Caucasian population. It usually appears as a unilateral, multifocal, flat pigmentation in various patterns and colors. In contrast to junctional nevi, which are almost always found only in childhood, PAM is acquired after childhood. Primary acquired melanosis can be histologically differentiated into presence (high risk) or absence (low risk) of atypia; however, these two subgroups cannot be differentiated clinically. The recognition and management of acquired pigmentation in middle age are critical. Primary acquired melanosis may result in malignant melanoma if not treated accurately and promptly, as seen in some series that report a 25 per cent mortality rate with this disease.

Malignant melanoma of the conjunctiva is a rare disease. Conjunctival melanomas may arise in one of three ways: as a de novo lesion, probably springing up from the malignant transformation of an individual intraepithelial melanocyte; as a malignant degeneration within a pre-existent benign nevus; or as a nodule arising from PAM.

When a melanoma arises de novo, there is presumably a period of intraepithelial horizontal proliferation of atypical melanocytes, followed by an invasive vertical growth phase into the underlying connective tissue of the substantia propria. This type of melanoma often develops on the epibulbar surface, frequently next to the limbus.

The second type of melanoma, that arising in a nevus, also tends to be a localized lesion, but one will often obtain the history of a pre-existent pigmented lesion developing in childhood that was stationary for many years. In this case, it is presumed that persistent junctional intraepithelial nests, which are a site of ongoing mitotic activity, were the site of malignant transformation. In excised specimens of such cases, one can see a mixture of the benign pre-existent nevus cells in the substantia propria and the new clone of cells proliferating both within the epithelium and as an invasive melanoma component.

The third type of conjunctival melanoma develops in primary acquired melanosis. In this disease, there is widespread radial intraepithelial proliferation of melanocytes that progresses slowly over large geographic regions of the conjunctiva for many years and sometimes for decades. The lesion is granular brown in coloration, and at its outset is flat. With progression of primary acquired melanosis to malignant melanoma, there is invasion of atypical melanocytes into the substantia propria. This invasion is evident clinically as the appearance of a nodule in a previously flat area of pigmentation.

Although malignant melanomas arising without PAM seem to grow more rapidly than those with primary acquired melanoma, the mortality rates are the same. Approximately 75 per cent of malignant melanomas occur with PAM, and 20 to 30 per cent occur in prior nevi with or without primary acquired melanosis. The average age of patients with this condition is 52 to 53 years. Conjunctival melanomas are extremely rare in African-Americans and in those younger than 20 years of age. Regardless of the site of origin, the approximate 5-year mortality rate is 75 per cent.

THERAPY

Supportive. Benign congenital melanoses do not require therapy unless the patient desires their removal for cosmetic reasons.

Surgical. Because of the persistence of junctional activity and the drop-off of melanocytes into the connective tissue in the formation of compound and subepithelial nevi, it is part of the natural history of nevi to enlarge and acquire thickness. However, nevi should be excised only if they become so large as to produce foreign body sensations or corneal wetting problems, are cosmetically undesirable, or their enlargement leads one to suspect a possible malignant degeneration into a melanoma. A malignant degeneration will be signalled by increased vascularity around the lesion, homogeneous nodule formation within it, fixation to underlying sclera, or hemorrhage and bleeding. A biopsy should be performed on any suspicious conjunctival nevus for histopathologic evaluation because it has been shown that nevi are potential precursor lesions; 20 to 30 per cent of conjunctival melanomas arise from nevi. The development of a conjunctival melanoma in the first or second decade is fortunately rare; suspicious lesions in this age group generally turn out be be nevi, which can grow rapidly at this point in development.

The management of primary acquired melanosis requires close cooperation with a pathologist familiar with ophthalmology. Excisional biopsy is preferred for small lesions. If a quadrant of conjunctiva is involved, a biopsy should be done of the central area, especially the thickest area. Biopsies may be required in multiple areas to evaluate large lesions fully. PAM with atypia requires complete eradication of the entire lesion. Small areas are surgically excised and treated with cryotherapy to the surgical bed to produce a superficial freeze. Large lesions may not be amenable to surgical resection due to the likely production of symblepharon, as well as the migration of atypical melanocytes from adjacent unresected areas. Large lesions may be treated more successfully with cryotherapy or laser ablation. A quadrant of PAM can be treated with cryotherapy by ballooning up the conjunctiva with a local anesthetic and lightly freezing the involved area with cryogen spray; freezing should not be deep enough to touch the sclera. Treatment of more than one quadrant at a time is seldom helpful because sicca and significant symblepharon may occur. The carbon dioxide laser can also be used to eradicate superficial juxtalimbal disease without causing untoward damage. If there is evidence postoperatively of intraocular inflammation, administration of 80 mg of oral prednisone daily for 1 to 2 weeks helps suppress the potentially damaging inflammation and cataractogenic effects. Since new lesions of PAM without atypia may appear, close observation with drawings to map the areas of pigmentation and examination with a Wood's light two to three times yearly are essential.

The management of malignant melanoma of the conjunctiva requires total eradication followed by close observation (three to four times yearly). The treatment of choice is wide surgical excision with cryotherapy of the surgical bed. Enucleation is rarely indicated because the bulk of the conjunctiva still remains. Exenteration is usually reserved for bulky tumors of the anterior segment and often is only palliative. Regional spread is usually to the preauricular or submandibular lymph nodes and may be successfully treated surgically. Systemic metastasis may occur to any site, and no effective form of treatment is available.

PRECAUTIONS

Pigment surrounding the lacrimal duct or punctum suggests the spread of tumor cells along these ducts and indicates that cancer is more extensive than clinically apparent. In the management of conjunctival melanotic lesions with corneal involvement, care is required not to damage Bowman's layer, unless the lesion is a malignant melanoma, since this layer may act as a barrier to PAM invasion. In this situation, superficial abrading with secondary cryotherapy or chemical cautery may suffice. Although palpebral lesions may be flat in appearance, they may in reality have undergone significant vertical growth because the conjunctiva is adherent to the tarsal plate, thereby fooling the unwary clinician. Since nevi are rare in the fornix and palpebral conjunctiva,

pigmented lesions in these areas are more prone to be malignant.

COMMENTS

Primary acquired melanosis with atypia and malignant melanoma of the conjunctiva may be managed best by the collaborative efforts of an ophthalmic oncologist and an experienced ophthalmic pathologist. Familiarity with the use of cryotherapy is essential in achieving the best cure rates. Clearly, there is no place for observation of conjunctival melanomas as is possible in the management of small choroidal melanomas.

References

Buckman G, Jakobiec FA, Folberg R, McNally LM: Melanocytic nevi of the palpebral conjunctiva. Ophthalmology 95:1053–1057, 1988.
Cochran AJ, et al: Assessment of immunological techniques in the diagnosis and prognosis of ocular malignant melanoma. Br J Ophthalmol 69:171–176, 1985.
Codere F, et al: Carbon dioxide laser treatment of the conjunctiva and the cornea. Ophthalmology 95:37–45, 1988.
Dutton JJ, Anderson RL, Tse DT: Combined surgery and cryotherapy for scleral invasion of epithelial malignancies. Ophthalmic Surg 15:289–294, 1984.
Folberg R, Jakobiec FA, Bernadino VB, Iwamoto T: Benign conjunctival melanocytic lesions. Clinicopathologic features. Ophthalmology 96:436–461, 1989.
Folberg R, McLean IW, Zimmerman LE: Conjunctival melanosis and melanoma. Ophthalmology 91:673–678, 1984.
Folberg R, McLean IW, Zimmerman LE: Malignant melanoma of the conjunctiva. Hum Pathol 16:136–143, 1985.
Jakobiec FA: The ultrastructure of conjunctival melanocytic tumors. Trans Am Ophthalmol Soc 82:599–752, 1984.
Jakobiec FA, et al: Unusual melanocytic nevi of the conjunctiva. Am J Ophthalmol 100:100–113, 1985.
Jakobiec FA, et al: Secondary and metastatic tumors of the orbit. In Duane TD (ed): Clinical Ophthalmology. Philadelphia, WB Saunders, 1987, Vol 2, pp 46:23–65.
Jakobiec FA, et al: Cryotherapy for conjunctival primary acquired melanosis and malignant melanoma. Experience with 62 cases. Ophthalmology 95:1058–1070, 1988.
Jakobiec FA, Folberg R, Iwamoto T: Clinicopathologic characteristics of premalignant and malignant melanocytic lesions of the conjunctiva. Ophthalmology 96:147–166, 1989.
Jeffrey IJ, et al: Malignant melanoma of the conjunctiva. Histopathology 10:363–378, 1986.
Lederman M, Wybar K, Busby E: Malignant epibulbar melanoma: Natural history and treatment by radiotherapy. Br J Ophthalmol 68:605–617, 1984.
Spencer WG, Zimmerman LE: Conjunctiva: Neoplasm and related conditions. In Spencer W (ed): Ophthalmic Pathology: An Atlas and Textbook, 3rd ed. Philadelphia, WB Saunders, 1985, Vol 2, pp 192–228.

CORNEAL AND CONJUNCTIVAL CALCIFICATIONS 371.43

KERRY K. ASSIL, M.D.,
and DAVID J. SCHANZLIN, M.D.

St. Louis, Missouri

Corneal and conjunctival calcification may occur as isolated conditions or in association with a variety of disease entities. The source and mechanism of the calcium deposits are not always clear. The corneal involvement is described as calcific band keratopathy because of the band-like distribution of the deposits across the interpalpebral zone.

Although the exact cause of calcific band keratopathy is not known, a combination of factors is thought to be responsible. One theory suggests that the combination of a metabolically altered tissue from mechanical or chemical trauma in the presence of local alkalosis and chronic exposure facilitates precipitation of calcium with the deposition of salts in the interpalpebral fissure. Elevated serum calcium and phosphorus concentrations may also result in tissue deposition of calcium phosphate salts. Histologically, calcium salts are deposited in the extracellular space when the condition is secondary to local ocular disease and in the intracellular space when the condition is secondary to systemic alterations of calcium metabolism. The epithelial basement membrane, Bowman's layer, and superficial stroma are involved.

Band keratopathy is associated with local ocular and systemic disease. Chronic uveitis of any etiology and ocular trauma, along with its accompanying chronic inflammation, are the most common ocular causes of band keratopathy. Systemic disease with altered calcium metabolism, such as hyperparathyroidism, vitamin D toxicity, and uremia, is also commonly associated with calcific band keratopathy. Calcific band keratopathy has also been described in individuals treated with or exposed to organomercurials, such as phenylmercuric nitrate or thimerosal. Band keratopathy has recently been reported after the use of Viscoat (chondroitin sulfate, sodium hyaluronate, and phosphate buffer) during routine cataract extraction. Inborn errors of metabolism, such as hyper- and hypophosphatemia, may also predispose patients to develop corneal and conjunctival calcification. Calcified deposits may also occur within the palpebral conjunctiva. These generally represent chronic degenerative changes and are often observed in patients with chronic blepharitis or other external eye disease.

Clinically, calcific band keratopathy appears as a superficial corneal opacity resembling frosted or ground glass, with "white flecks" and "clear spots" interspersed within the band, giving it a "Swiss cheese" appearance. The opacity is covered by a clear epithelium and is usually localized to the area of exposed cornea in the interpalpebral fissure. The band is concentric with the limbus, but is separated from it by a clear interval.

As calcification progresses, fragmentation and even destruction of Bowman's membrane may ensue. Early in its course, before the calcific band approaches the pupillary area, there is no immediate effect on visual acuity. With progression, however, plaques composed of coalesced calcium replace the subepithelial layers of the cornea, resulting in epithelial erosions, accompanied by marked irritation and pain. Eventual involvement of the central cornea and pupillary axis results in decreased visual acuity. A fibrous pannus may also develop.

Conjunctival calcification appears as small, hard, white, or yellow elevated concretions in the palpebral conjunctiva. These concretions are usually products of cellular degeneration, but may also be associated with any chronic conjunctival inflammation. They may be accompanied by hyperemia and symptoms of irritation.

Unlike calcific band keratopathy, calcareous degeneration usually spares the basement and Bowman's membranes and is characterized by clumps of calcium salts in the superficial and deep stroma. Calcareous degeneration can occur rapidly, especially with anterior segment ischemia. Band keratopathy associated with hyperuricemia can occur and is differentiated based upon historical data, its golden-brown color on examination, and elevated uric acid levels.

The causes of calcific band keratopathy can be divided into five categories: (1) chronic keratitis or uveitis (the most common causes); (2) degenerative calcium deposition associated with chronic damage from mercurial preservatives in many ophthalmic preparations; (3) hypercalcemia secondary to milk alkali syndrome, vitamin D toxicity, sarcoidosis, hyperparathyroidism, lytic lesions affecting the bones, and other systemic diseases; (4) chronic renal failure or other conditions that may cause a rise in serum phosphorus levels; and (5) heredity.

Patients should be questioned concerning excessive vitamin D ingestion. Although corneal and conjunctival calcification may be reversible with discontinuation of the vitamin, nephrocalcinosis may still develop. A general medical workup is advisable. Laboratory tests may include renal function test; serum calcium, phosphorus, uric acid, parathyroid hormone, and angiotensin-converting enzyme levels; and a search for lytic lesions affecting the bones. Clearly, testing should be focused toward uncovering diagnoses suggested from the history and examination.

THERAPY

Surgical. Treatment of band keratopathy is indicated in patients with symptomatic irritation or decreased vision. The success of therapy in restoring vision may be limited if the underlying disease process has produced decreased acuity. Also, unless the underlying disease process is controlled, calcium deposition may recur after therapy. In this situation, treatment may need to be repeated. The surgical goal is to remove the opaque calcium deposits without producing stromal scarring. The initial approach is to attempt chelation of the calcium salt deposits with edentate sodium (EDTA).

Topical anesthetic instilled into the conjunctival cul-de-sac is sufficient for achieving intraoperative anesthesia, however, due to the frequent incidence of severe postoperative discomfort, many surgeons elect to use supplemental retrobulbar anesthesia with 0.5 per cent marcaine. Next, the epithelium is mechanically removed. The distal end of a Weck-Cel sponge is saturated with 0.5 per cent EDTA (prepared by mixing a 20 per cent stock of NaEDTA with 0.9 per cent sodium chloride) and held against the area of calcium deposition. A "to-and-fro" abrasive action is used to help remove the calcium deposits; this is best accomplished at the slit lamp. If significant clearing has not occurred after 10 minutes of treatment, one should move to higher concentrations of EDTA (1.0 or 1.5 per cent). Sometimes, the treatment must be continued for 20 to 30 minutes. In refractory cases, gentle curettage with a scalpel may be necessary. An antibiotic solution and weak cycloplegic are then instilled. A patch or bandage lens may be used for comfort and to facilitate epithelial healing.

If the opacification cannot be removed by chelation or curettage, lamellar keratoplasty should be considered. A technique using EDTA and a diamond burr on a Fisch drill has been shown to be effective in removing deposits without significant scarring. The excimer laser has also been applied for removal of band keratopathy. Excimer keratectomy alters the corneal curvature with a shift toward hyperopia. In addition, the more peripheral deposits cannot be removed without inducing even greater changes in refraction.

Conjunctival concretions causing irritation and a foreign body sensation can often be shelled out with a sharp pointed knife or broad needle. On occasion, this procedure may be difficult, and if so, it should be reserved for symptomatic lesions.

Ocular or Periocular Manifestations

Conjunctiva: Palpebral conjunctival calcific deposits or concretions.
Cornea: Calcific band-shaped keratopathy; opacity.
Other: Decreased visual acuity; irritation.

References

Bokosky JE, Meyer RK, Sugar A: Surgical treatment of calcific band keratopathy. Ophthalmic Surg 16: 645–647, 1985.

Duffey RK, LoCascio JA: Calcium deposition in a corneal graft. Cornea 6:212–215, 1987.

Galin MA, Obstbaum SA: Band keratopathy in mercury exposure. Ann Ophthalmol 6:1257–1261, 1974.

Kennedy RE, Roca PD, Landers PH: Atypical band keratopathy in glaucomatous patients. Am J Ophthalmol 72:917–922, 1971.

Kennedy RE, Roca PD, Platt DS: Further observations on atypical band keratopathy in glaucoma patients. Trans Am Ophthalmol Soc 72:107–122, 1974.

Lembach RG, Keates RH: Band keratopathy: Its significance and treatment. Perspect Ophthalmol 1:13–16, 1977.

Lemp MA, Ralph RA: Rapid development of band keratopathy in dry eyes. Am J Ophthalmol 83: 657–659, 1977.

Lessell S, Norton EWD: Band keratopathy and conjunctival calcification in hypophosphatasia. Arch Ophthalmol 71:497–499, 1964.

O'Connor GR: Calcific band keratopathy. Trans Am Ophthalmol Soc 70:58–81, 1972.

Schecter EL, Keates RH: Treatment of band keratopathy. Ophthalmic Surg 2:75, 1971.

FILTERING BLEBS 997.9
(Leaking and Inadvertent Nonleaking)

GISSUR J. PETURSSON, M.D.

Little Rock, Arkansas

A filtering bleb is a blister-like postoperative scar through which aqueous drains from the anterior chamber to the subconjunctival space. Often, such a scar is created after glaucoma surgery to allow a permanently open channel for drainage. However, a filtering bleb can be a complication of cataract surgery, although it is more rare with modern techniques. Such blebs usually resolve spontaneously in weeks or few months. If not, grave consequences may occasionally follow and include delayed endophthalmitis, problems and added risk of contact lens wear, and possibly maculopathy from bleb-induced hypotony. Normally, filtering blebs of any etiology are asymptomatic and without noteworthy manifestations.

A leaking filtering bleb can occur immediately, such as in incomplete repair of conjunctival flap buttonholing or closure, or it can be delayed, wherein a thin-walled bleb or flap incision ruptures at a later time. Leaking blebs symptoms are usually those associated with extreme hypotony. Additionally, excessive precorneal "tear" pooling is frequently seen. Hypotony, with the absence or near absence of the anterior chamber with no visible filtering bleb after glaucoma surgery, is highly suggestive of a leak.

THERAPY

Surgical. Buttonholing during the filtering glaucoma procedure, when close to the limbus, requires peritomy and suturing of the conjunctiva onto the cornea. The use of 10-0 nylon mattress suture is recommended after the corneal epithelium is abraded in the area. Direct suturing of a leaking bleb away from the limbus can be tricky. If the conjunctiva is very thin in the hole area, this procedure may fail unless suture material and needle are selected carefully. The tapered point needles, BV100-4 or BV75-4, make a very tight tract that will hold a leak in the most delicate tissue. This needle is intended for microsurgery and is labeled as such, but is not listed with ophthalmic sutures. The needle comes with black monofilament 9-0 or 10-0 nylon or prolene sutures. Owing to the delicate nature of the needle, a delicate needle holder is necessary. The suture can be left in place indefinitely or removed as needed. Another way to deal with such holes is to close with a suture and then use the wing suture of Chandler and Grant.

For the nonleaking bleb with extreme hypotony or a risk of infection, trichloroacetic acid and argon laser shrinkage can be successful in reducing it. However, cryosurgery for these blebs is more practical. Three freeze-thaw applications with the retina or preferably the glaucoma probe at temperature of -65 to $-80°C$ for 5 seconds each time seem to be effective. Tenon's and episcleral tissue of the entire bleb area must be involved in the freezing. Up to 8 weeks must be allowed for full results.

For stubborn persistent blebs, the following suturing method seems to work. One 7-0 chromic catgut suture is passed to the cornea, deep across the corneoscleral wound, and either beyond or through the bleb, depending on its size. The suture is tied snugly, compressing the bleb beneath the knot. In the same manner, 8-0 or 7-0 black silk can be used and left in place for 2 to 4 weeks until the bleb has disappeared. This suture method is felt to work largely by virtue of its inflammatory response. The patient is placed on topical cycloplegics and antibiotics. This procedure is performed under microscopic control after either local subconjunctival injection* of 2 per cent lidocaine with epinephrine in the adjacent area or, alternatively, retrobulbar block.* For the immediate large bleb with obvious wound dehiscence, direct surgical revision is required.

Supportive. For a delayed leak discovered postoperatively, which is often intermittent or only seen with 2 per cent fluorescein, conservative treatment consisting of topical antibiotics, pressure dressings, and oral acetazolamide may be indicated initially. This treatment sometimes enables spontaneous closure of the fistula in 1 to 2 days. Tissue adhesives have also been used successfully, sometimes aided by use of a collagen shield or large-diameter therapeutic soft contact lens. The glaucoma tamponade shell is also a helpful tool in the management of early and late small leaks, and symblepharon rings have also been used successfully.

Ocular or Periocular Manifestations

Conjunctiva or Sclera: Marked uniformly diffuse hyperemia.

Cornea: Edema; folds in Descemet's membrane.

Lacrimal System: Increased lacrimation; precorneal accumulation of "tears."

Other: Irritation; markedly decreased intraocular pressure or frank hypotony; photophobia; shallow or flat anterior chamber.

PRECAUTIONS

Acid and heat cautery of postcataract blebs may cause tissue necrosis. In some instances, heat or acid cautery of a bleb has resulted in endophthalmitis, originating at the site of the bleb in a bed of tissue necrosis.

Surgical revision of leaking blebs sometimes involves major mobilization and pull-down of conjunctiva, especially if the leaky area is very thin walled and ischemic. Leaks, sometimes intermittent, are not commonly caused by inadequately closed conjunctival incisions of limbal-based or poorly fixed fornix-based flaps.

COMMENTS

True postcataract filtering blebs should be distinguished from the occasional cystic, sterile, inflammatory reaction surrounding sutures, especially 8-0 virgin silk and chromic catgut. The true postcataract filtering bleb always resembles the bleb created intentionally in glaucoma surgery.

When compared to other methods of bleb elimination, such as heat cautery or chemical cauterization, cryotherapy seems to be preferable. With cryosurgery, tissue destruction is minimal. Thus, one avoids the problems of aqueous leakage and necrosis, which may predispose the eye to more dreaded complications, such as loss of the anterior chamber, epithelial downgrowth, and intraocular infection. However, there may be mild anterior chamber cellular reaction after cryotherapy.

References

Bruner WE, Maumenee AR: A simple method of repairing inadvertent filtering blebs after cataract surgery. Am J Ophthalmol 91:794–796, 1981.

Coyle JT: Outpatient repair of unintentional filtering blebs. Ocul Ther Surg 1:35, 1982.

Hoskins H Jr, Kass M: Becker-Shaffer's Diagnosis and Therapy of Glaucomas, 6th ed. St. Louis, CV Mosby, 1989, pp 583–586.

Kirk HW: Cauterization of filtering blebs following cataract extraction. Trans Am Acad Ophthalmol Otolaryngol 77:573–580, 1973.

O'Connor DJ, Tressler CS, Caprioli J: A surgical method to repair leaking filtering blebs. Ophthalmic Surg 23:336–338, 1992.

Petursson GJ, Fraunfelder FT: Repair of an inadvertent buttonhole or leaking filtering bleb. Arch Ophthalmol 97:926–927, 1979.

Thomas JV, Belcher CD III, Simmons RJ: Glaucoma Surgery. St. Louis, CV Mosby, 1992, pp 44–50.

Zalta AH, Weider RH: Closure of leaking filtering blebs with cyanoacrylate tissue. Br J Ophthalmol 75:170–175, 1991.

GIANT PAPILLARY CONJUNCTIVITIS 372.12

THOMAS L. STEINEMANN, M.D.

Little Rock, Arkansas

Giant papillary conjunctivitis (GPC) is a condition characterized by inflammation of the tarsal conjunctiva and is usually associated with contact lens wear. After the first report by Spring in 1974, Allansmith and coworkers in 1977 described a syndrome of contact lens intolerance, ocular itching, mucus discharge, hyperemia, blurred vision, and eruption of giant papillae in the upper tarsal conjunctiva. These symptoms, which may resemble vernal conjunctivitis, are often seen in patients wearing soft gas-permeable or hard contact lenses. GPC is estimated to affect 10 per cent of the nearly 20 million contact lens wearers in the United States; contact lens wear is clearly the most common factor in the development of this syndrome. Identical findings may, however, be seen in other patients in conjunction with a variety of external ocular foreign bodies, including exposed monofilament suture ends, keratoprostheses, artificial eyes, corneal-scleral shells, cyanoacrylate glue, and extruded scleral buckles.

The syndrome presents a spectrum of clinical signs and symptoms. Abnormally large papillae (diameter greater than 0.3 mm) are diagnostic and best visualized by using fluorescein and the cobalt blue light. Giant papillae are classically described as 1 mm or larger in diameter and are concentrated in the superior tarsal conjunctiva. However, they are usually not seen except in advanced cases. Increased production of mucus results in strings or sheets that coat the contact lens and may cloud vision.

Giant papillary conjunctivitis can resemble vernal conjunctivitis. In fact, similar immunologic processes may be involved in both diseases. Both conditions present with ocular itching and mucoid discharge. However, the itching of GPC is usually milder than vernal conjunctivitis. Also, unlike vernal conjunctivitis, GPC is not associated with atopy. GPC occurs in all age groups and both sexes, whereas vernal conjunctivitis is more common in young males. Vernal conjunctivitis usually displays seasonal variation, worsening in warm weather. Patients with GPC experience a rapid relief of symptoms upon discontinuation of contact lens wear, whereas vernal conjunctivitis patients do not have a dramatic response with any one treatment.

In early stages, GPC patients may note itching when the contact lenses are removed, mucus accumulation in the inner corners of the eyes upon awakening, and slight blurring of vision. These symptoms are so common that patients are not likely to report them. As GPC progresses, patients may report blurring of vision after wearing the contact lenses for several hours, excessive movement of the contact lenses, mucus discharge, and contact lens awareness. The examination may reveal mucus strands and mild hyperemia of the upper tarsal conjunctiva. In early to moderate cases, the conjunctiva is usually translucent, but may be somewhat thickened.

As inflammation increases, the conjunctiva may become opaque. In late stages of GPC, patients develop contact lens intolerance and describe dryness, foreign body sensation, or pain when wearing the lens. Sheets or ropes of mucus are usually present, contributing to sticking of the eyelids upon awakening. Hyperemia is marked, and pseudoptosis may appear in some patients.

Concurrent with the opacification of the upper tarsal conjunctiva, enlarged collagen structures (papillae) begin to emerge from the tarsal plate. As they grow, they push aside the normal smaller papillae, and their apexes flatten gradually. The overlying conjunctiva may break down, resulting in fluorescein staining, which is a critical sign of moderate-to-severe disease. In soft contact lens wearers, papillae appear on the upper tarsal conjunctiva and advance to the lid margin. In rigid gas-permeable contact lens wearers, papillae are fewer in number and smaller and appear first on the lid margin.

The etiology and pathogenesis of GPC are not fully understood. Evidence suggests that GPC may be the result of mechanical trauma combined with a hypersensitivity reaction to antigenic proteins trapped on the roughened surface of a worn contact lens, prosthesis, or suture ends. Because GPC occurs in wearers of soft, hard, and rigid contact lenses, it is unlikely that the lesions associated with contact lens wear are caused by a reaction to the lens material itself. The observation that not all patients with contact lens deposits develop GPC indicates that an individual's immunologic response to protein deposits is a key factor in the development of GPC.

It is recognized that increased coatings on worn contact lenses exacerbate signs and symptoms of existing cases of GPC and may contribute to the onset of the disease. Conditions that favor the development or exacerbation of GPC include: (1) wearing contact lenses for long periods during the day, (2) continued use of worn contact lenses for months or years without replacing them with new lenses, (3) larger diameter contact lenses (presenting a greater area to which adherent antigenic material can react with the conjunctival epithelium), and (4) inadequate cleaning and enzyming of the lenses.

THERAPY

The primary treatment of GPC involves removal of the foreign body and treatment of inflamed conjunctiva with pharmacotherapy. Removal of a prosthesis or contact lens or trimming of an offending suture barb usually results in prompt resolution of the problem. Most contact lens patients, however, wish to continue wearing their lenses.

Supportive. In severe cases, patients must stop wearing their contact lenses until such symptoms as hyperemia and mucus discharge resolve and the eye is quiet. Fluorescein staining of the apexes of papillae, copious mucus discharge, tarsal hyperemia, and decentering of the contact lens are all indications for lens removal. Lenses should be discontinued for at least 4 weeks and may be reintroduced several days after signs and symptoms have resolved. Patients should be free of injection, mucus discharge, and punctate keratopathy before being fitted with a new contact lens. Enlarged papillae may take months or years to regress.

Some patients will be able to continue contact lens wear without stopping, provided certain strategies are followed. First, lens replacement (with a new and preferably different type of contact lens) is recommended. A smaller diameter, thinner-edge lens should be fit. Also, meticulous attention to lens hygiene is essential. Contact lens cleaners should be free of preservatives, such as thimerosol. Nonpreserved saline in an aerosol can is recommended. These steps will help minimize antigenic exposure. Sterilization by hydrogen peroxide has been found to be the best tolerated disinfection method. Weekly enzymatic cleaning to remove deposits is necessary.

The patient should understand that regular replacement of contact lenses should occur every 6 to 12 months or at the first sign of any significant lens coating or mucus discharge. In some soft contact lens patients, a switch to a rigid gas-permeable contact lens may be the only alternative to increase contact lens tolerance.

Frequent replacement (disposable) contact lenses are an important addition to the supportive treatment regimen for GPC patients. Disposable contact lenses obviate the need for enzymatic cleaning; deposits are minimized since the contact lenses are discarded and replaced every 1 to 2 weeks. In the treatment of GPC, disposable contact lenses should be worn on a daily basis with daily cleaning.

Ocular. After the discontinuation of contact lens wear, topical lubrication may be the only therapy required. In cases of advanced GPC in which inflammation is marked, a short course of topical corticosteroids may be appropriate to quiet the eye before initiating further treatment. However, corticosteroids have not proven particularly effective in the long-term management of GPC.

Cromolyn sodium, a mast cell stabilizer, has had a beneficial effect in the management of GPC. In conjunction with lens replacement and rigorous lens hygiene, 4 per cent cromolyn sodium ophthalmic solution applied four times daily (even while the lens is in place) may help resolve early GPC before it progresses. More advanced cases of GPC are not amenable to treatment with cromolyn sodium alone. However, once the signs and symptoms of GPC are brought under control with supportive therapy, cromolyn sodium may be introduced as part of regular maintenance therapy.

Ocular or Periocular Manifestations

Conjunctiva: Macropapillae (0.3 to 1.0 mm diameter); giant papillae (greater than 1.0 mm diameter); fluorescein staining of papillae; tarsal and bulbar conjunctival injection; tarsal conjunctival thickening and opacity; mucus strands, Horner-Trantas' dots; gelatinous limbal nodules.

Cornea: Superficial punctate keratopathy.

Eyelid: Pseudoptosis.

Other: Mucus coating of contact lenses; protein deposits on contact lenses.

PRECAUTIONS

Successful treatment of GPC depends upon the earliest possible recognition of the disease process and initiation of appropriate therapy. The symptoms of GPC usually precede the earliest subtle signs. Therefore, proper diagnosis requires careful examination and a high index of suspicion. Patient education regarding the nature of GPC is crucial to the successful continuation or resumption of contact lens wear. Patients should thoroughly understand the importance of meticulous lens care and frequent lens replacement, as well as such alternatives as disposable contact lenses.

COMMENTS

To follow the progression or regression of the clinical signs of GPC with contact lens wear and therapy, it is necessary to describe accurately the appearance of the upper tarsal conjunctiva at each visit. A record should be made indicating the zones of involvement, size and elevation of the papillae, fluorescein staining pattern of the tops of papillae, and the presence of mucus. The progression of these signs and symptoms in the initial disease state has some prognostic value. The earlier that GPC is treated, the more likely treatment will arrest progress of the disease while maintaining long-term tolerance of the contact lens.

References

Allansmith MR, Ross RN: Ocular allergy and mast cell stabilizer. Surv Ophthalmol 30:229–244, 1986.

Allansmith MR, Ross RN: Giant papillary conjunctivitis. In Duane TD, Jaeger EA (eds): Clinical Ophthalmology. Philadelphia, Harper & Row, 1987, Vol 4, pp 1-10.

Allansmith MR, et al: Giant papillary conjunctivitis in contact lens wearers. Am J Ophthalmol 83:697–708, 1977.

Driebe WT Jr: Disposable contact lenses. Surv Ophthalmol 34:44–46, 1989.

Ehlers WH, Donshik PC: Allergic ocular disorders: A spectrum of diseases. Contact Lens Assoc Ophthalmol J 18:117–124, 1992.

Griener JV, et al: Giant papillary conjunctivitis. In Dabezies OH Jr (ed): Contact Lenses. The CLAO Guide to Basic Science and Clinical Practice. Orlando, Harcourt Brace Jovanovich, 1984, pp 43.1–43.16.

Spring TF: Reaction to hydrophilic lenses. Med J Aug 1:449, 1974.

Srinivasan BD, et al: Giant papillary conjunctivitis with ocular prostheses. Arch Ophthalmol 97:892–895, 1979.

IRRITATIVE CONJUNCTIVITIS 372.14
(Toxic Conjunctivitis)

MICHAEL C. ROBERSON, M.D.

Little Rock, Arkansas

A variety of chemicals and pollutants in the environment, as well as topical ophthalmic drugs, can cause acute and chronic conjunctivitis. More commonly, the conjunctivitis is of a milder chronic type, but acute, severe reactions with conjunctival necrosis can occur. Both acute and long-term exposure to these irritants can cause conjunctival and corneal scarring.

Symptoms generally include those associated with chronic irritation. Burning, dryness, and photophobia are common complaints. If a superficial punctate keratitis is present, varying amounts of blur may be noted. The lid margins may be hyperemic, and the skin of the lids may have edema. Usually a minimal mucus discharge is present. For the most part, the conjunctival reaction is usually a fine papillary one. In the case of toxicity to reactions, frank conjunctival ulceration and necrosis may occur. Corneal scarring may accompany severe or prolonged cases.

THERAPY

The most effective therapy is to identify and remove the offending agents. This may be difficult to do when the agent is an environmental one. Investigation into patterns of worsening and improvement of the condition may give clues to its cause. Identification of chemical exposure in the workplace is important. The use of cosmetics and personal hygiene articles should also be examined. One should consider topical ophthalmic drugs as an etiology if the patient has been using them.

Supportive. Supportive therapy must be used if the offending agents cannot be identified or removed. In moderate to severe reactions, topical corticosteroids, such as flouromethalone 1 per cent four times a day, can be used. Irrigation of the conjunctival sac with nonpreserved saline may be helpful. Topical astringents and vasoconstrictors, as well as artificial tears, may be needed for long-term therapy. One should consider using nonpreserved preparations. The prolonged use of corticosteroids is contraindicated because of the potential for causing glaucoma, cataracts, and lowered resistance to infection.

Ocular or Periocular Manifestations

Conjunctiva: Edema; follicles and papillae; hyperemia; necrosis (rare); watery discharge.

Cornea: Epithelial erosion and punctate staining; late scarring and vascularization with severe irritants (rare); mild epithelial and rarely stromal edema; stromal infiltration and ulceration in severe cases (rare).

Other: Foreign body sensation; irritation; photophobia.

References

Berdy G, Abelson M, Smith L, George M: Preservative-free artificial tear preparations—assessment of corneal epithelial toxic effects. Arch Ophthalmol 110:528–532, 1992.

Friedlander M: Contact allergy and toxicity in the eye. Int Ophthalmol Clin 29:317–3320, 1988.

Leibowitz HM, et al: Human conjunctivitis. II. Treatment. Arch Ophthalmol 94:1752–1756, 1976.

Lubniewski A, Nelson J: Diagnosis and management of dry eye and ocular surface disorders. Ophthalmol Clin North Am 3:575–594, 1990.

Schwab I, et al: Foreshortening of the inferior conjunctival fornix associated with chronic glaucoma medications. Ophthalmology 99:197–202, 1992.

LIGNEOUS CONJUNCTIVITIS 372.10

JOHN R. BIERLY, M.D.

Lexington, Kentucky

Ligneous conjunctivitis is a rare cause of membranous conjunctivitis that most commonly afflicts children. It is more prevalent in females and usually is bilateral, although often it is asymmetric. Although patients often present acutely, they can present as a chronic conjunctivitis with a prolonged history of red eyes and a mucoid discharge. In some chronic cases, the patients are relatively asymptomatic. The most important finding is a membrane formation on the tarsal conjunctiva that can cause the lid to lose its flexibility. This firm, woody induration of the tarsal conjunctiva and lid is what the adjective ligneous describes. In some patients the lesion can approach tumor-like proportions. Although either the inferior or superior lid can be involved, more often the superior lid has the greater involvement. Eversion of the upper lid reveals a thick (1 to 2 mm) white or yellowish-white membrane that is firmly adherent to the underlying tarsal conjunctiva with a free peripheral margin. The membrane bleeds if removed from its base. Corneal complications are uncommon, but may include opacification, vascularization, and keratomalacia with possible perforation.

The disease often begins in infancy, although it may present in patients anytime from birth until age 85. The duration of the disease can range from several months to 44 years. It has been reported as persisting in a mild form without impairing vision for 35 years in one patient. Recurrence of the membranes is common after their removal. In addition, patients may experience periods where they are free of conjunctivitis only to have a relapse at a later date. Relapse has been recorded up to 25 years after spontaneous resolution. Patients may have acute systemic signs and symptoms that either precede or occur at the same time as their initial ocular findings. These symptoms include upper respiratory tract infections, urinary tract infections, middle ear infections, tonsillitis, sinusitis, cervicitis, and vulvovaginitis. In addition, patients have been reported to have chronic involvement of other mucous membranes besides the conjunctiva. In patients who develop lesions in the larynx or tracheobronchial tree, there is a potential for life-threatening tracheobronchial obstruction.

Histopathologically, the membranes are thick plaques of amorphous, eosinophilic, hyaline material that are localized to the subepithelial conjunctival stroma in association with vascularization and granulation tissue. There also are areas of mixed cellular infiltration that include plasma cells, eosinophils, lymphocytes, neutrophils, and mast cells. Immunohistochemistry has demonstrated that T lymphocytes are a prominent component of the cellular infiltrate. The hyaline material has been shown to be comprised of a hyaluronidase-sensitive acid mucopolysaccharide in some cases. However, the hyaline material may be composed primarily of fibrin, and the acid mucopolysaccharide is found only in the granulation tissue adjacent to the hyaline plaque. Immunofluorescence studies have been performed in other cases and have demonstrated that IgG is the prominent component of the amorphous hyaline material.

The pathogenesis of ligneous conjunctivitis remains unknown. Several predisposing factors have been implicated, including bacterial and viral infections, trauma, hypersensitivity reactions, a genetic metabolic disorder, and abnormally increased vascular permeability. One possibility is that a conjunctival epithelial injury is followed by an exaggerated localized inflammatory immune response. Subsequently, there is excessive permeability of the blood vessels in the area of the injury that leads to a serofibrinous exudate composed of albumin, immunoglobulins, and fibrin. With time, this material coagulates and hardens, resulting in the accumulation of the hyaline material. In support of this theory, electron microscopy of the membranes shows that they contain abnormal capillaries with unusually wide gaps between the endothelial cells and multilaminar basement membranes. The disease is sometimes seen within families, which has led to speculation that it is an autosomal recessive genetic disorder. Numerous mast cells and eosinophils have been seen in some patients, which would support the theory that the disease represents a hypersensitivity response.

THERAPY

Systemic. Marked improvement has been reported with the administration of systemic steroids in a dosage of 1 mg/kg/day in patients who fail to respond to other therapies. Systemic antibiotics may be necessary in patients who have an associated upper respiratory tract infection.

Ocular. Foremost, the use of vasoconstrictor drops, mucolytics (acetyl cysteine), and topical antibiotics seems to have little effect on the natural history of the conjunctivitis in most cases. However, some patients may have a concomitant bacterial infection and should be treated with an appropriate broad-spectrum topical antibiotic several times a day to the conjunctival sac. In addition, topical steroids have not usually been of benefit.

Enzymatic treatment with either hyaluronidase* or chymotrypsin* has been reported to be successful in many cases. Hyaluronidase should be used at a concentration of 1.5 mg (750 IU) in 1 ml of saline either topically every hour, or alternatively 1 cc may be injected directly into the eyelid. Similarly, chymotrypsin may be applied either topically or injected at a concentration of 0.2 mg/cc. If there is improvement the dosage may be tapered to topical administration four times a day. A low level of administration (two to three times a day) may be required indefinitely.

Some patients may respond to topical therapy with sodium cromoglycate 4 per cent solution applied four times daily. This regimen can be instituted after surgical excision of the membrane and may be required indefinitely.

Fibrinolysin* has been utilized as 1000 U/ml eye drops with some success. Therapy should begin with two drops applied to the patient's eyes every hour. This therapy decreases the viscosity of the discharge and improves the ability to keep the eyes clean.

Favorable responses have been obtained with surgical excision followed by topical administration of 2 per cent (20 mg/ml in oil) cyclosporine drops. With resolution of the membranes, small atrophic scars may be seen in the areas of the previous ligneous lesions. Dosage may begin at one drop four times daily, which may be increased up to hourly administration if necessary. This schedule may be tapered to less frequent administration, although recurrence is possible after the cyclosporine is discontinued. Serum cyclosporine levels do not seem to be significant during treatment.

Surgical. Before instituting medical treatment, it is advisable to excise and debulk the membranes and associated granulomatous tissue. Pathology can be performed on the excised material, which will help support the diagnosis of ligneous conjunctivitis. Diathermy coagulation may be applied to help control bleeding. Cryosurgery may be attempted, although it has not had consistent success. Mucous membrane grafts, autologous conjunctival grafts, and donor sclera grafting have all been attempted after excision of the membranes with variable success.

Ocular or Periocular Manifestations

Conjunctiva: Fibrosis; membrane and pseudomembrane.
Cornea: Clouding; keratomalacia; opacity; perforation; vascularization.
Eyelids: Induration; ligneous membrane.

PRECAUTIONS

Even with the use of overlying grafts, surgical stripping of the membrane in ligneous conjunctivitis uniformly results in severe bleeding and prompt recurrence, even as early as 48 hours. Removal alone without medical treatment may be of little benefit.

The topical administration of cyclosporine may result in very low serum levels of cyclosporine. Although this does not seem to be a concern in most patients, those with any history of renal disease deserve special attention and should have serum creatinine and creatinine clearance monitored during therapy.

COMMENTS

The treatment of patients with ligneous conjunctivitis is often frustrating because of the poor response to therapy and the tendency for the lesions to recur after their excision. Most patients fail to improve with commercially available medications, such as topical steroids, antibiotics, and vasoconstrictors. However, they may respond to other topical medications such as cromolyn, cyclosporine, hyaluronidase, and fibrinolysin, that require preparation by a pharmacist. Since none of these therapies is uniformly successful, it may require more than one medication to achieve an improvement in the patient's condition.

The choice of medication may be guided in part by the findings on pathology, if they are available. Enzymatic therapy was the first therapy demonstrated to be effective and is recommended especially in cases that demonstrate mucopolysaccharide. In cases that demonstrate mast cells, cromolyn has been shown to be of benefit. Since cromolyn inhibits mast cell degranulation, the success of this therapy supports the suggestion that in certain cases mast cells are involved in the pathogenesis of the conjunctivitis. Other cases may respond to topical cyclosporine, which suggests that T-cell-mediated immunity is an important factor.

Finally, despite a chronic conjunctivitis that is unresponsive to therapy, patients may maintain good visual acuity. Only in severe cases with impending blindness from corneal complications or those in danger of tracheobronchial obstruction should one consider the use of systemic immunosuppressive agents.

References

Bateman JB, Pettit TH, Isenberg SJ, Simons KB: Ligneous conjunctivitis. An autosomal recessive disorder. J Pediatr Ophthalmol Strabismus 23:137, 1986.
Chambers JD, et al: Ligneous conjunctivitis. Trans Am Acad Ophthalmol Otolaryngol 73:996–1004, 1969.
Cohen SR: Ligneous conjunctivitis: An ophthalmic disease with potentially fatal tracheobronchial obstruction. Laryngeal and tracheobronchial features. Ann Otol Rhinol Laryngol 99:509–512, 1990.
Cooper TJ, Kazdan JJ, Cutz E: Ligneous conjunctivitis with tracheal obstruction. A case report, with light and electron microscopy findings. Can J Ophthalmol 14:57–62, 1979.
Eagle RC Jr, Brooks JSJ, Katowitz JA, et al: Fibrin as a major constituent of ligneous conjunctivitis. Am J Ophthalmol 101:493, 1986.
Firat T: Ligneous conjunctivitis. Am J Ophthalmol 78:679–688, 1974.
Francois J, Victoria-Troncoso V: Treatment of lig-

with light and electron microscopy findings. Can J Ophthalmol 14:57–62, 1979.

Eagle RC Jr, Brooks JSJ, Katowitz JA, et al: Fibrin as a major constituent of ligneous conjunctivitis. Am J Ophthalmol 101:493, 1986.

Firat T: Ligneous conjunctivitis. Am J Ophthalmol 78:679–688, 1974.

Francois J, Victoria-Troncoso V: Treatment of ligneous conjunctivitis. Am J Ophthalmol 65:674–678, 1968.

Girard IJ, Veselinovic A, Font RL: Ligneous conjunctivitis after pingueculae removal in an adult. Cornea 8:714, 1989.

Hidayat AA, Riddle PJ: Ligneous conjunctivitis: A clinicopathologic study of 17 cases. Ophthalmology 94:949, 1987.

Holland EJ, et al: Immunohistologic findings and results of treatment with cyclosporine in ligneous conjunctivitis. Am J Ophthalmol 107:160–166, 1989.

Kanai A, Polack FM: Histologic and electron microscopic studies of ligneous conjunctivitis. Am J Ophthalmol 72:909–916, 1971.

Marcus DM, et al: Ligneous conjunctivitis with ear involvement. Arch Ophthalmol 108:514–519, 1990.

McGrand JC, Rees DM, Harry J: Ligneous conjunctivitis. Br J Ophthalmol 53:373–381, 1969.

Melikian HE: Treatment of ligneous conjunctivitis. Ann Ophthalmol 17:763, 1985.

Rubin BI, et al: Response of reactivated ligneous conjunctivitis to topical cyclosporine. Am J Ophthalmol 112:95–96, 1991.

Spencer LM, Straatsma BR, Foos RY: Ligneous conjunctivitis. Am J Ophthalmol 80:365–367, 1968.

OPHTHALMIA NEONATORUM 771.6
(Conjunctivitis of Newborns, Neonatal Ophthalmia)

LAURIE E. CHRISTENSEN, M.D.

Portland, Oregon

Although the term "ophthalmia neonatorum" connotes gonorrheal infection, it designates a syndrome including any conjunctivitis, affecting one or both eyes, that occurs during the first month of life. Thus, it is not a single disease. Frequently, purulent exudate occurs out of proportion to erythema and edema; hence, comes the pediatric colloquialism, "sticky eye." This syndrome varies in severity from the mild chemical conjunctivitis caused by instillation of prophylactic 1 per cent silver nitrate to the fulminating corneal perforation and panophthalmitis that can complicate infection with *Neisseria gonorrhea* or *Pseudomonas aeruginosa*. Even mild or moderate eye infection in the newborn may be rarely associated with grave systemic complications.

Inclusion conjunctivitis (inclusion blennorrhea) caused by *Chlamydia trachomatis* is the most common infectious ophthalmia neonatorum seen in the United States. The majority of bacterial cases, in contrast, result from infection with *Staphylococcus aureus, Pneumococcus*, or species of *Neisseria* or *Hemophilus*. One of an assortment of general saprophytic organisms may be occasionally isolated from milder cases. Anaerobic organisms may be more commonly at fault than is generally appreciated. Even herpes simplex virus can infect the newborn eye.

Infectious keratitis may produce visual damage through corneal scarring. Bacterial keratitis (especially *Pseudomonas* or gonococcal) may perforate to cause endophthalmitis. Herpes simplex keratoconjunctivitis may accompany an encephalitis that can produce brain damage. Chlamydial (inclusion) conjunctivitis is associated with a neonatal pneumonia syndrome, prominent tachypnea, absent febrile response, and diffuse infiltrates on x-ray. Thus, chlamydial conjunctivitis in a newborn is an indication for systemic treatment, even though the conjunctivitis may respond well to topical therapy. Neonatal infection may be derived in utero, during passage through the birth canal, or postpartum from external fomites and personal contact. Several pyogenic organisms are dangerous to the newborn because they may be associated with septicemia. These include gram-positive diplococci (*Pneumococcus*), and gram-negative diplococci (*N. gonorrhea* and *N. meningitidis*). Newborn infants may not show a febrile response to sepsis and have an immature microbial defense system.

THERAPY

Ocular. Specific treatment depends upon knowledge of the infecting agent. Therefore a culture for sensitivity should be obtained in case the chosen treatment proves ineffective. A gram-stained smear should be examined microscopically to guide initial therapy. If no organisms are found, a Giemsa preparation may show the intracytoplasmic inclusions of chlamydial infection.

Bacterial cultures should include reduced blood agar, thioglycolate broth, Thayer-Martin media, and chocolate agar. Viral cultures should be prepared only if indicated clinically. Chlamydia can be detected by culture using McCoy cell culture. A more rapid diagnosis can be made using an ELISA (enzyme-linked immunosorbent assay) or a direct immunofluorescent monoclonal antibody stain. These tests have excellent sensitivity and specificity.

The following pertinent subjects are discussed elsewhere in this volume: bacterial conjunctivitis; candidiasis; *Escherichia coli*; gonorrhea; *Hemophilus influenzae*, herpes simplex; inclusion conjunctivitis; irritative conjunctivitis; Koch-Weeks bacillus; *Pneumococcus*; *Proteus*; *Pseudomonas aeruginosa*; *Staphylococcus*; and *Streptococcus*.

Chemical conjunctivitis caused by 1 per cent silver nitrate prophylaxis is typically rigations, and any synechiae should be broken with a glass rod as they form.

Candida conjunctivitis of the newborn may be suggested by associated thrush of the oral cavity and a thrush-like pseudomembrane on the conjunctiva. It may be substantiated by microscopic examination of a scraping. The condition is usually self-limited.

In acute purulent conjunctivitis caused by coliform organisms, topical gentamicin is usually suitable. The drops or ointment should be instilled every hour on the first day and then every 4 hours for the next 10 to 14 days. Since corneal invasion and perforation can result from *Pseudomonas* conjunctivitis, treatment must be initiated rapidly and aggressively, especially in the premature infant. Topical gentamicin or tobramycin instilled every 30 to 60 minutes is recommended. The frequency of drops is gradually reduced to every 4 hours as inflammation subsides. The eyelids may be cleansed or gently irrigated with saline as often as necessary. Coliform organisms can invade the bloodstream of newborns, particularly premature infants, and result in death, with or without meningitis.

Hemophilus species may be treated with either topical 10 or 15 per cent sulfacetamide or 0.3 per cent gentamicin drops instilled each hour until clinical resolution begins and then tapered to every 4 hours for about another 5 days.

Conjunctivitis caused by gram-positive cocci and diplococci is treated with 0.5 per cent erythromycin ointment every 2 hours the first day and four times a day for the next 7 days.

Herpes keratoconjunctivitis in newborn infants is sometimes associated with a severe systemic illness with a high mortality rate. Effective treatment for the disseminated infection is still being sought. Intravenous acyclovir is usually given if there is evidence of systemic disease. When conjunctivitis occurs in an infant born to a mother with genital herpes, topical prophylactic trifluridine instilled five times daily should be strongly considered. Treatment of herpetic keratitis is discussed elsewhere.

Inclusion conjunctivitis is treated systemically as noted in the following section.

Systemic. Where systemic complications occur, care should be directed by a pediatrician. The systemic drug dosages in newborn infants may vary depending upon renal or hepatic function, level of maturity, concomitant medications, state of hydration, and other systemic variables that are best evaluated by the pediatrician.

Chlamydial inclusion conjunctivitis is treated with oral erythromycin 50 mg/kg daily in four divided doses for 14 days. Topical erythromycin does not improve the response rate. Recurrent or persistent disease should be treated with an additional 1 to 2 weeks of oral erythromycin. In addition, the mother of the affected infant and all her sexual partners need evaluation and treatment for chlamydia, as well as other possible venereal infections. Prophylaxis of the newborn with topical erythromycin is effective in preventing chlamydial conjunctivitis, but does not prevent nasopharyngeal infection or chlamydial pneumonia.

Gonorrheal ophthalmia neonatorum signifies probable venereal disease in the mother. Possible complications include disastrous invasion of the globe, septicemia, arthritis, and meningitis. It typically appears as an acute purulent conjunctivitis between 24 hours and 72 hours after birth. It may, however, be acquired prenatally by ascending invasion. A culture with sensitivities is initiated. After treatment has begun, hospital care under isolation for 24 hours is indicated. Aqueous crystalline penicillin G is given intravenously for 7 days at a dose of 100 mg/kg daily in four divided doses. A single intramuscular dose of ceftriaxone 125 mg or cefotaxine 100 mg has been shown to be highly effective in treating neonatal conjunctivitis when dealing with strains of *Neisseria* that are resistant to penicillin. Topical antibiotics may be superfluous in the absence of corneal ulceration. Exudates should be removed gently with saline periodically.

Supportive. All newborn infants should receive the benefit of prophylactic treatment. Good prepartum care of the mother is the first step. For the infant, treatment is logically directed against gonorrhea, but ideally, as many other microbes as possible should also be covered. The following alternatives have been found to be highly effective. A 1 per cent silver nitrate solution (from a single-use ampule and not rinsed out), 1 per cent tetracycline, or 0.5 per cent erythromycin ophthalmic ointment should be instilled as soon as practical after delivery, ideally in the first 15 minutes and whenever possible within the first hour postnatally. Even infants born by cesarean section should receive prophylaxis. An infant born to a mother known to be infected with gonorrhea should be given a single dose of parenteral aqueous crystalline penicillin G: 50,000 units for full-term infants and 20,000 units if birthweight is under 2000 grams.

Ocular or Periocular Manifestations

Conjunctiva: Bloody discharge; catarrhal, membranous, or pseudomembranous conjunctivitis; chemosis; cicatrization; follicles; hyperemia; mucopurulent or purulent exudates; necrosis.

Cornea: Infiltration; keratitis; micropannus; necrosis; perforations; staphyloma; ulcer.

Eyelids: Blepharitis; edema; hyperemia; vesicles.

Globe: Endophthalmitis; panophthalmitis.

Others: Iris atrophy; peripheral posterior uveitis; photophobia; visual loss; vitreitis.

PRECAUTIONS

The appearance of localized or generalized corneal haze in this condition should be taken as a serious sign of potential corneal ulceration.

Silver nitrate prophylaxis is safe unless untrained personnel erroneously administer a solution not intended for the eye. No silver nitrate solution more concentrated than 2 per cent should be placed in the eye; 1 per cent concentration is sufficient.

Systemic infection with herpes simplex can be thoroughly devastating and is often fatal to the newborn. Fortunately, this is rare as there is no proven effective treatment. Herpetic keratoconjunctivitis can rarely be present at birth, although more typically it is acquired during passage through an infected birth canal. Thus, even infants born by cesarean operation can exhibit this entity.

The "venereal" causes of ophthalmia neonatorum also require treatment of the parents. These causes include gonorrhea, herpes simplex type 2, and *Chlamydia trachomatis*.

COMMENTS

The exact time of onset may be helpful in clinically distinguishing among the causes of ophthalmia neonatorum. Silver nitrate irritation is evident within hours after the drops are instilled, but abates dramatically within 24 hours and disappears within 72 hours.

Gonorrheal conjunctivitis is most likely to appear in newborns at 2 to 6 days of age. A severe purulent conjunctivitis appearing at this time should suggest gonorrhea. Inclusion conjunctivitis develops from 5 to 14 days postnatally; herpetic keratoconjunctivitis follows about the same pattern, but can appear even earlier. *Pseudomonas* conjunctivitis or corneal ulcer may appear acutely at any time in debilitated infants, particularly premature infants on mechanical ventilation.

References

Beem MO, Saxon EM: Respiratory-tract colonization and a distinctive pneumonia syndrome in infants infected with *Chlamydia trachomatis*. N Engl J Med *196*:306–310, 1977.

Burns RP, Rhodes DH: *Pseudomonas* eye infection as a cause of death in premature infants. Rach Ophthalmol *65*:517–525, 1961.

Chandler JW, Rapoza PA: Ophthalmia neonatorum. Int Ophthalmol Clin *30*:36–38, 1990.

Hammerschlag MR, et al: Erythromycin ointment for ocular prophylaxis of neonatal chlamydial infection. JAMA *244*:2291–2293, 1980.

Hammerschlag MR: Chlamydial infections. J Pediatr *114*:727–734, 1989.

Hammerschlag MR, et al: Efficacy of neonatal ocular prophylaxis for the prevention of chlamydial and gonococcal conjunctivitis. N Engl J Med *320*:769–772, 1989.

Laga M, et al: Single-dose therapy of gonococcal ophthalmia neonatorum with ceftriaxone. N Engl J Med *315*:1382–1385, 1986.

Laga M, Meheus A, Piot P: Epidemiology and control of gonococcal ophthalmia neonatorum. Bull WHO *67*:471–477, 1989.

Miller ME, Stiehm ER: Introduction. Host defenses in the fetus and neonate. Pediatrics *64* (Suppl): 708, 1979.

Nahmias AJ, et al: Eye infections with herpes simplex viruses in neonates. Surv Ophthalmol *21*: 100–105, 1976.

Nishida H, Risemberg HM: Silver nitrate ophthalmic solution and chemical conjunctivitis. Pediatrics *56*:368–373, 1975.

Oriel JD: Ophthalmia neonatorum: Relative efficacy of current prophylactic practices and treatment. J Antimicrob Chemother *14*:209–219, 1984.

Sexually transmitted disease treatment guidelines. MMWR *34* (Suppl):75S–108S, 1985.

Whitley RJ, Ch'ien LT, Alford CA Jr: Neonatal herpes simplex virus infection. Int Ophthalmol Clin *15*:141–149, 1975.

Zanoni D, Isenberg SJ, Apt L: A comparison of silver nitrate with erythromycin for prophylaxis against ophthalmia neonatorum. Clin Pediatr *31*: 295–298, 1992.

PTERYGIUM AND PSEUDOPTERYGIUM 372.40

L.F. RICH, M.D., M.S.

Portland, Oregon

A pterygium is a triangular elevated mass of thickened bulbar conjunctiva that extends onto the cornea in the interpalpebral zone. Its name is derived from the Greek word meaning wing, which describes its characteristic shape. Within the interpalpebral fissure, a pterygium is most commonly found on the nasal aspect of the globe and less often on the temporal aspect. If present outside the interpalpebral fissure area, it is considered an atypical pterygium, and other diagnoses, such as phlyctenular keratoconjunctivitis or malignancies, must be considered.

Environment and heredity are thought to play important roles in the pathogenesis of pterygium. Its incidence is higher in tropical or subtropical areas of the world and in individuals frequently exposed to sunlight, airborne allergens, wind, dust, fumes or other noxious stimuli. Frequently, a pingueculum precedes the pterygium. The elevated conjunctival tissue may lead to tear film defects and may form a dellen or an area of dryness in the adjacent tissue. Inflammation and vascularization are thereby initiated, and the patient may have symptoms of irritation or itching. Recurrent episodes of exposure may irritate the mass of tissue, enlarge it, and produce another dellen, which continues the advancement. Eventually, the lesion grows beyond the limbus, invades the cornea, may progress into or beyond the visual axis, and may result in blindness.

Pseudopterygium is similar in appearance to a true pterygium, but bridges the limbus so that a probe may be passed beneath the lesion at the limbus. It is often the result of damage to the cornea with a chemical, thermal or physical insult. Pseudopterygium is more likely to occur in atypical locations (i.e., outside the interpalpebral fissure area) than a true pterygium. As with a true pterygium, recurrences are more aggressive than the primary lesion.

THERAPY

Supportive. Unless the patient specifically requests surgery, it is best to avoid intervention and limit treatment to medical modalities. Advice can be given to help minimize the progression of the pterygium. Specifically, protection against sunlight and dryness is important. Episodes of irritation should be treated with topical lubricants, such as artificial tears or ointments; if inflammation and edema occur, a mild vasoconstrictor drop may prevent elevation and dellen formation. Punctal occlusion may ameliorate the symptoms of dryness and/or retard the progression of the pterygium. Mild corticosteroids, such as medrysone, can be prescribed for short-term usage. More potent steroids, particularly those with good ocular penetration, should be avoided if possible to minimize complications associated with corticosteroid use.

When outdoors, the patient should be encouraged to wear sunglasses or protective goggles. Occlusive goggles are of value in dusty windy environments. If a patient has a known sensitivity to an air-borne allergen and anticipates exposure to it, systemic antihistamines before exposure may prevent an allergic response. Once the response has occurred, however, antihistamines are of little value.

Surgical. Surgical intervention is indicated when the patient requests removal of the pterygium for cosmetic reasons, the progression of the lesion threatens vision, or symblepharon limits ocular motility. If none of these indications exists, it is best to treat the pterygium medically, because if the pterygium recurs after surgery, it is often worse than the primary lesion.

There are multiple surgical techniques for removal of pterygium. Avulsion of the head of the pterygium from the cornea may be possible if the lesion is attached loosely. This technique has the advantage of being relatively noninvasive to corneal tissue. Leaving a smooth area with little or no removal of corneal and limbal tissue may lessen the chances of recurrence. Many surgeons smooth the base of the cornea where the pterygium had been removed, using a diamond burr or scalpel blade. If the pterygium is firmly attached and cannot be avulsed from the cornea, a delimiting keratotomy with partial lamellar keratectomy will aid removal. This procedure is best done under the microscope to minimize removal of corneal tissue and to avoid perforation into the anterior chamber. Once the head of the pterygium has been removed from the cornea and is beyond limbus, its body and tail should be excised to avoid the insertion of the rectus muscle. Some surgeons prefer to remove as little of the body of the pterygium as possible and attach the cut ends of conjunctiva to the sclera or to one another. Others prefer to leave the sclera bare. Control of bleeding is essential, and all feeder vessels should be cauterized.

Local anesthesia is preferred over general anesthesia unless the patient is unable to cooperate or is extremely anxious about ocular surgery. Subconjunctival injection* of lidocaine without hyaluronidase is preferred. Epinephrine may be added to the anesthetic to inhibit bleeding. A topical anesthetic, such as cocaine, may also be used to prevent pain when the eye is grasped in an area other than where the lidocaine had been injected. Occasionally, retrobulbar anesthesia is necessary if the patient is unable to control ocular movements. In such patients, akinesia of the eyelids may be necessary as well.

After the lesion has been excised, it is wise to submit it to the pathologist for evaluation. Occasionally, malignancies may mimic a pterygium; in these cases, surgery may stimulate growth.

Several postoperative adjunctive measures lower the recurrence rate after pterygium excision, but each has significant drawbacks. Strontium[90] beta irradiation, applied to the limbus and the adjacent sclera in divided doses totalling 1000 to 1500 reps, decreases the rate of recurrence. However, significant complications may occur, including scleral necrosis, infection, and cataract. Triethylene thiophosphoramide‡ (Thiotepa) applied as eye drops four to six times daily for 6 to 8 weeks postoperatively, also decreases the probability of recurrence, but depigmentation of the skin and eyelashes around the treated eye limits its use, particularly in dark-skinned individuals. More recently, mitomycin‡ (mitomycin-C), used as a 0.02 per cent to 0.04 per cent eyedrops twice daily for 5 to 14 days postoperatively, has been advocated. Recurrence rates between 0 to 11 percent have been reported, but serious, blinding complications are now recognized. Sequelae of scleral and corneal ulcers with perforation, glaucoma, sudden onset of cataract, corneal edema, and uveitis caution against this treatment.

Primary excision of pterygium is followed by recurrence in 40 to 50 per cent of cases. Recurrent pterygium is more difficult to treat and is more likely to recur after a second excision than a primary pterygium. If symblepharon is present or the remaining conjunctiva is insufficient to permit adequate ocular motility, a mucous membrane or conjunctival graft may be needed to cover the bare area. A conjunctival graft may be used from the same or the fellow eye and is preferably taken from a vicinity outside the interpalpebral fissure area. Although perhaps slightly less successful at preventing recurrence than adjunctive antimetabolite therapy, autologous conjunctival transplantation often provides a significantly better cosmetic result and a much lower incidence of complications. It is becoming the treatment of choice for recurrent pterygium.

Corneoscleral grafts with or without mucous membrane or conjunctival grafts have been advocated in cases of recurrent pterygium. Their use is advised in cases where the limbal architecture has been disturbed by one or more surgical interventions. They are best accomplished with partial-thickness grafts incorporating corneal and scleral donor tissue in the same configuration as the tissue resected from the recipient eye. The grafted area can be trephined or cut freehand and the donor tissue similarly dissected to fit the outline. If cornea and scleral tissue is used, it can be incorporated as a single graft to maintain the architecture of the limbal sulcus. A clear corneal graft that bridges the limbus has also been advocated, but it has the disadvantage of producing a single contour without providing a limbal sulcus. A corneal graft alone is likely to allow vascularization at the graft-host interface, so it is probably best to avoid leaving the edge of the graft at the limbus. Grafting is necessary if multiple excisions have left the corneal tissue thin, and perforation or ocular weakness is imminent.

Ocular or Periocular Manifestations

Conjunctiva: Temporal displacement of semilunar fold; symblepharon; wing-shaped fleshy, vascularized growth.
Cornea: Conjunctival (encroachment); gray infiltrates; elevated mass; keratitis; iron pigment line.
Other: Astigmatism; decreased visual acuity; diplopia; restriction of ocular motility.

PRECAUTIONS

Surgical excision of a pterygium is the most common form of therapy employed today. The surgical process and the pterygium itself destroy limbal tissue and predispose the eye to recurrence of the lesion. In addition, the elevation of conjunctiva and the irregular corneal and limbal tissue resulting from surgery may reinitiate the pathologic process of localized dryness, vascularization, and regrowth. Furthermore, an acute inflammatory process after surgery may produce granulation tissue that can contract and stimulate conjunctivalization of the limbus and cornea. Excessive postoperative inflammation and irritation from exposure during the early postoperative period encourage regrowth. Recurrences may be seen as early as 2 weeks or several years after excision. The size of the original lesion may play a role in the probability of recurrence. A large, fleshy, vascularized, primary pterygium with inflammation indicates activity and should not be approached surgically until the inflammation has been minimized. In addition, large pterygia require more extensive surgery, which produces greater injury to underlying and surrounding tissue than occurs when smaller lesions are removed.

COMMENTS

Each surgical intervention may produce a greater cosmetic blemish and a more difficult management situation than the previous lesion. A pterygium is more likely to return after a recurrence than after removal of a primary lesion. Symblepharon is often a sequela of pterygium surgery; restriction of ocular motility and pain with extraocular movements, particularly abduction of the globe, may result.

References

Bahrassa F, Datta R: Postoperative Beta radiation treatment of pterygium. Int J Rad Oncology Biol Phys 9:679–684, 1983.

Ehrlich D: The management of pterygium. Ophthalmic Surg 8:23–30, 1977.

Howitt D, Karp E: Side effects of topical Thiotepa. Am J Ophthalmol 68:473, 1969.

Kleis W, Picó G: Thio-tepa therapy to prevent postoperative pterygium occurrence and neovascularization. Am J Ophthalmol 76:371–373, 1973.

Rubinfeld RS, et al: Serious complications of topical mitomycin-C after pterygium surgery. Ophthalmology 99:1647–1654, 1992.

Singh G, et al: Long-term follow-up study of mitomycin eyedrops as adjunctive treatment for pterygia and its comparison with conjunctival autograft transplantation. Cornea 9:331–334, 1990.

Talbot AN: Complications of beta ray treatment of pterygia. Trans Ophthalmol Soc NZ 31:62–63, 1979.

Tarr KH, Constable IJ: Late complications of pterygium treatment. Br J Ophthalmol 64:496–505, 1980.

Vastine DW, et al: Reconstruction of the periocular mucous membrane by autologous conjunctival transplantation. Ophthalmology 89:1072–1081, 1982.

Vorkas AP: Pterygium. Choice of operation. Trans Ophthalmol Soc UK 101:192–194, 1981.

VERNAL KERATOCONJUNCTIVITIS 370.40

MEDHAT M. EL HENNAWI, M.Ch.(Ophth.)

Alexandria, Egypt

Vernal keratoconjunctivitis is a severe perennial form of allergic conjunctivitis involving the cornea and conjunctiva. The condition is found predominantly in children or young adults and commonly in atopic individuals, who may also suffer from eczema, asthma, or hay fever. It is characterized by intermittent exacerbations, which are often seasonal.

The disease generally affects the upper tarsal conjunctiva, which shows a papillary hypertrophy and has a cobblestone appearance in severe cases. The limbal conjunctiva may also be affected, either as localized edema and hyperemia or as fleshy isolated vegetations. The main symptoms are intense photophobia, severe itching, and the production of tenacious stringy mucous discharge. It is considered to be an atopic disease and has been classified as a type I allergic disease of the outer eye.

THERAPY

Supportive. Desensitization to inhalant allergens has been used in the treatment of this disease, but has not generally been found to be helpful. Iced compresses and dark glasses may produce marked amelioration of ocular symptoms in most cases.

Systemic. Corticosteroid therapy is of great help in severe perennial cases. In addition, long-acting antihistamines may be required. Sustained-release preparations of pheniramine may be used for administration once daily at bedtime.

Ocular. Cromolyn sodium is a valuable drug both in the prophylaxis and treatment of vernal keratoconjunctivitis. As a prophylactic agent, a 2 per cent solution of cromolyn sodium may be used three times daily for 1 month before the expected season of exacerbation. As a therapeutic agent, marked improvement is attained with administration four times daily in mild and moderate cases. In severe cases or acute exacerbation, additional therapy is recommended. Topical ophthalmic corticosteroids are very effective in the treatment of vernal keratoconjunctivitis. Prednisolone or dexamethasone may be required three or four times daily. Dosages are applied according to severity; in acute exacerbation, steroid eyedrops may be required very frequently, every 2 or 3 hours during the day. Vasoconstrictors may also be helpful in decreasing hyperemia.

Surgical. Shaving of papillae, combined excision of tarsus and conjunctiva, and cryotherapy have been used, but none seems to give longlasting relief. Plano-T contact lenses may be helpful in persistent epithelial keratitis. In epithelial plaques, superficial keratectomy and iodine cautery usually result in healing of the epithelium.

Ocular or Periocular Manifestations

Conjunctiva: Cobble-stone appearance; palpebral hyperemia; perilimbal hyperemia; stringy mucous discharge; "Tranta's spots"; vegetations that encroach to the cornea.
Cornea: Erosion; keratitis epithelialis vernalis; plaques; vernal ulcer.
Other: Decreased visual acuity; persistent lacrimation; photophobia.

PRECAUTIONS

Although stinging may occur as an adverse reaction to cromolyn sodium, the eyedrops do not cause significant adverse effects, such as the increase in ocular tension found with steroid eyedrops. In addition to reducing the risk of steroid-induced glaucoma, cromolyn sodium also reduces the possibility of herpetic keratitis or cataract.

If increased intraocular pressure persists in chronic topical corticosteroid users, the optic nerve may become damaged, and severe or total loss of sight may result from steroid-induced glaucoma. Periodic measurement of the intraocular pressure is obligatory in those patients using corticosteroids.

COMMENTS

Chronic vernal keratoconjunctivitis in children is usually one of the very difficult problems of management. Continuous and persistent observation is very essential, especially in children receiving chronic steroid therapy.

This risk of steroid-induced glaucoma should always be considered. Although the various forms of therapy available may ameliorate symptoms markedly in most cases, they are not curative. Further research is needed to clarify the etiology of vernal keratoconjunctivitis and to establish a more effective, safer, and curative therapy. As an experimental procedure, some researchers are using excimer laser photoablation for the papillae of vernal keratoconjunctivitis.

References

Dart JKG, Buckley RJ, Monnickenda M, Prasad J: Perennial allergic conjunctivitis: definition, clinical characteristics and prevalence. A comparison with seasonal allergic conjunctivitis. Trans Ophthalmol Soc UK 105:513–520, 1986.

El Hennawi M: Thesis. Study of the effect of disodium cromoglycate in spring cattarh as compared with other certain anti-allergic drugs. The effect of disodium cromoglycate on locally administered radioactive histamine concentration. Alexandria, University of Alexandria, 1974.

El Hennawi M: Clinical trial with 2% sodium cromoglycate (Opticrom) in vernal keratoconjunctivitis. Br J Ophthalmol 64:483–486, 1980.

Jones BR: Allergic disease of the outer eye. Trans Ophthalmol Soc UK 91:441–447, 1971.

Rice NSC, et al: Vernal kerato-conjunctivitis and its management. Trans Ophthalmol Soc UK 91:483–489, 1971.

SECTION 21

CORNEA

BACTERIAL CORNEAL ULCERS 370.00
(Bacterial Keratitis)

DOUGLAS J. COSTER, F.R.C.S.,
and PAUL R. BADENOCH, Ph.D.

Adelaide, Australia

Bacterial infection of the cornea is a sight-threatening process. Corneal ulceration, stromal abscess formation, and anterior segment inflammation are features of the disease. Similar findings may result from infection with fungi or amoebae. Keratitis induced by herpes simplex virus or toxic chemicals may resemble bacterial disease. A particular feature of bacterial keratitis is its rapid progression; corneal destruction may be complete in 24 to 48 hours. However, less pathogenic bacteria may induce a slower disease process than that induced by virulent strains of fungi, such as those of *Fusarium solani*. A large number of pathogens have been implicated; commonly *Staphylococcus aureus, Staphylococcus epidermidis, Streptococcus pneumoniae, Pseudomonas aeruginosa,* and *Moraxella spp.* are found. Suspicion of an infective process demands careful microbiologic assessment.

THERAPY

Ocular. The objectives of treatment of bacterial keratitis are to eliminate the replicating etiologic agent with specific chemotherapy, to suppress destructive inflammation, and then to withdraw therapy so as not to hinder repair of the cornea.

Initial antimicrobial selection is based on the gram stain result. When gram-positive cocci are seen, a cephalosporin is the standard treatment. Topical or subconjunctival delivery of medication may be necessary. Cefazolin* at a concentration of 50 mg/ml can be given topically each hour, or even more frequently, for the first 24 hours. Subconjunctival injections of 100 mg of cefazolin* may produce higher peak levels, but therapeutic levels only persist for 6 to 7 hours; therefore, adjunctive topical delivery for round-the-clock coverage is necessary. Systemic administration is indicated only when the underlying uvea is directly involved in the process. If gram-positive bacilli are seen, the administration of topical cefazolin* or penicillin G* (50 mg/ml)

in artificial tears is appropriate. For gram-negative cocci, ceftriaxone or chloramphenicol is normally effective. For gram-negative bacilli, the administration of gentamicin or tobramycin either topically (10 mg/ml) or subconjunctivally* (20 mg) is indicated. If no organisms are seen but the clinical picture suggests an active infection, the concomitant use of a cephalosporin and aminoglycoside is advocated. The antibiotics chosen as initial therapy may be changed in response to the culture result or the in vitro susceptibility profile.

Recently, topical quinolone preparations have become available for ophthalmic use. These agents have a wide antimicrobial spectrum. Ciprofloxacin 0.3 per cent, for example, has excellent activity against most strains of staphylococci, *P. aeruginosa,* and enteric gram-negative bacilli. Subject to further evaluation, these agents may gain acceptance as single-agent therapy for bacterial keratitis. However, as they are not universally effective, the need for accurate microbiologic diagnosis remains.

In addition to these specific measures, effective mydriasis is necessary. Administration of 1 per cent atropine eyedrops two to four times daily is required.

Supportive. Close observation is mandatory. Progression of the condition may be rapid and blinding. Punctilious attention to treatment schedules is demanded. For these reasons, hospital admission is usually necessary.

Surgical. If perforation of the cornea should occur during the course of the disease, penetrating keratoplasty is indicated if the area of necrosis is resectable. In other situations where there is extensive peripheral corneal necrosis, a conjunctival flap after a period of intensive specific chemotherapy is often the safest course of treatment.

PRECAUTIONS

The suppression of inflammation with topical corticosteroids in this condition is a controversial issue. Polymorphonuclear leukocytes contribute to corneal destruction by delivering enzymes capable of degrading collagen and other tissue components. The recruitment of these cells can be inhibited with topical corticosteroids. Studies in animal models suggest that this inhibition can be achieved without adversely affecting the clearance of organisms from the cornea, provided an appropriate antibiotic is used con-

478

currently. No controlled clinical data on this subject exist. It is probably safe to suppress anterior segment inflammation with topical steroids after the effectiveness of the antimicrobial therapy has been suggested by a non-progressive clinical course.

COMMENTS

Epithelial closure may be inhibited by continuing inflammation or the prolonged use of topical antibiotics. Intensive medication should only be maintained when indicated for the suppression of growth micro-organisms. Usually, only 2 or 3 days of intensive therapy is necessary, with careful reduction of medication over the next week. It is often possible to take patients with a healing epithelial and stromal defect off the medication but under close supervision within 10 days.

References

Badenoch PR, Hay GJ, McDonald PJ, Coster DJ: A rat model of bacterial keratitis. Effect of antibiotics and corticosteroid. Arch Ophthalmol *103*: 718–722, 1985.

Jones DB: Initial therapy of suspected microbial corneal ulcers. II. Specific antibiotic therapy based on corneal smears. Surv Ophthalmol *24*: 105–116, 1979.

Leibowitz HM: Clinical evaluation of ciprofloxacin 0.3% ophthalmic solution for treatment of bacterial keratitis. Am J Ophthalmol *112*:34S–47S, 1991.

Stern GA, Schemmer GB, Farber RD, Gorovoy MS: Effect of topical antibiotic solutions on corneal epithelial wound healing. Arch Ophthalmol *101*: 644–647, 1983.

CONGENITAL HEREDITARY ENDOTHELIAL DYSTROPHY 371.50
(CHED)

IRENE E.H. MAUMENEE, M.D.

Baltimore, Maryland

Two types of congenital hereditary endothelial dystrophy (CHED) are recognized. The hereditary disorder can either occur as an autosomal recessive disorder at birth or as an autosomal dominant disorder during early to late childhood or even early adolescence. The clinical symptoms are similar and consist of diffuse corneal haze with significant thickening of the cornea secondary to dysfunction of the endothelium. In this disorder, the corneal endothelium is severely attenuated and may be totally absent. The disorder may be slowly progressive and lead to bullous epithelial changes in adulthood. The visual acuity varies between 20/40 and finger-counting vision. Otherwise, the eyes are normal, and the corneal diameter and the intraocular pressure are normal. There is no excess tearing. These features should help in the differential diagnosis from congenital glaucoma, which is commonly confused with CHED.

THERAPY

Surgical. In patients with severely reduced vision caused by corneal opacification or in those with a painful eye with bullous epithelial changes, corneal grafting is indicated. In milder cases, this procedure should be delayed.

Ocular or Periocular Manifestations

Cornea: Clouding; diffuse thickening or extreme thinness of Descemet's membrane; endothelial dysgenesis; stromal edema; stromal thickening.
Other: Amblyopia; nystagmus, visual loss.

PRECAUTIONS

The differential diagnosis of congenital corneal clouding includes congenital glaucoma, corneal dysgeneses (Peters' anomaly, sclerocornea, anterior staphyloma), posterior polymorphous dystrophy, birth trauma with rupture of Descemet's membrane, metabolic diseases (mucopolysaccharidoses, mucolipidoses), and interstitial keratitis (luetic, herpetic).

COMMENTS

Congenital hereditary endothelial dystrophy is a disorder that is commonly misdiagnosed as congenital glaucoma, resulting in unnecessary surgical intervention in these patients. Given that there are two genetic types, the existence of two different pathogenetic mechanisms has to be assumed. However, the basic mechanisms are not known to date.

References

Antine B: Histology of congenital hereditary corneal dystrophy. Am J Ophthalmol *69*:964–969, 1970.

Judisch GF, Maumenee IH: Clinical differentiation of recessive congenital hereditary endothelial dystrophy and dominant hereditary endothelial dystrophy. Am J Ophthalmol *85*:606–612, 1978.

Kenyon KR, Antine B: The pathogenesis of congenital hereditary endothelial dystrophy of the cornea. Am J Ophthalmol *72*:787–795, 1971.

Maumenee AE: Congenital hereditary corneal dystrophy. Am J Ophthalmol *50*:1114–1124, 1960.

Pearce WG, Tripathi RC, Morgan G: Congenital endothelial corneal dystrophy. Clinical, pathological, and genetic study. Br J Ophthalmol *53*:577–591, 1969.

CONJUNCTIVAL, CORNEAL, OR SCLERAL CYSTS 372.75

(Acquired Epithelial Inclusion Cysts, Epithelial Cysts)

F. T. FRAUNFELDER, M.D.

Portland, Oregon

Although conjunctival cysts are not uncommon, corneal and scleral cysts are rare. The most common cause of all these cysts is trauma. Conjunctival cysts are most often seen after strabismus surgery and conjunctival flaps. Henle's folds and cysts are secondary to chronic conjunctivitis and are usually left alone. If calcium concretions erode through the cyst wall, these concretions are usually removed manually. Traumatic cysts of the conjunctiva, cornea, or sclera usually result from proliferation of the epithelial cells that have been entrapped within the tissue. The cysts may develop along any part of the injury track. In the sclera, traumatic cysts are usually found anteriorly in the exposed area near the limbus or beneath the bulbar conjunctiva. Congenital corneal or scleral cysts occur most commonly near the limbus and are usually less than 1 mm in size. Scleral cysts may send extensions within the globe, causing ocular pain. Although most cysts are asymptomatic, some conjunctival cysts are so large that they interfere with blinking.

THERAPY

Surgical. The treatment of choice for extraocular cysts is chemical cautery. A local anesthetic, such as three to four applications of one drop of cocaine 5 minutes apart, is preferred. A 30-gauge needle attached to a 1- or 2-ml syringe containing 0.5 ml of 20 per cent trichloroacetic acid is readied. It is important to allow this solution to attain room temperature; if this liquid was refrigerated, just handling the syringe could warm the fluid and cause the acid to drop from the tip of the needle. Any spillage should be absorbed immediately with a cotton swab and irrigated by an assistant. The contents of the cyst are then aspirated until the cyst walls have collapsed. The partially diluted fluid containing cyst fluid plus 20 per cent trichloroacetic acid is then reinjected to fill the cyst. Care should be taken during this procedure not to overinflate and rupture the cyst but to fill it to approximately three-quarters of its original size. The cyst wall immediately turns white, and the cyst should be reaspirated flat and the needle removed. While removing the needle, the exit wound should be irrigated by an assistant so that the damage from the trichloroacetic acid to the surrounding tissue is minimized. It is important to maintain suction while removing the needle to avoid spread of the acid into the surrounding tissue. If some coagulation of the conjunctiva occurs at the puncture site, it is a transient effect, and the tissue will clear within a day. These patients may be given postoperative topical steroids.

Chemical cautery is a highly satisfactory method of treatment, and many cysts can be treated in one sitting. The only restriction is that the cyst must be large enough to be entered clearly by a needle.

Cryosurgery is another successful method of destroying conjunctival cysts; however, this technique is not recommended for scleral or corneal cysts. The roof of the cyst is usually removed, although successful results have been obtained without removing the "roof." A local anesthetic, such as 1 per cent lidocaine, is injected under the cyst, and forceps and scissors are used to surgically unroof the top of the cyst. Using a liquid nitrogen probe, the probe is applied to the base of the cyst area, and the epithelium within the cyst is destroyed by freezing. As soon as probe contact is obtained, the conjunctiva is pulled away from the eye and frozen for 2 to 3 seconds. Irrigation with a sterile solution and counterpressure with a swab are used to break the probe's contact to the base of the cyst.

Simple excision of conjunctival, corneal, or scleral cysts is also successful; however, not infrequently, the cyst is inadvertently ruptured. If this occurs, one can cauterize the base of the cyst with either cryosurgery as outlined above or chemical cautery, such as 20 per cent trichloroacetic acid or 1 per cent tincture of iodine. Within a few moments after cauterization, this area should be irrigated with saline. Some have advocated fine sutures to hold the cyst walls together until scarring has permanently sealed them, but this is seldom necessary.

Another alternative to treatment of conjunctival cysts is the use of the YAG laser with topical anesthesia. Numerous applications of laser are placed on the surface of the cyst at an energy level of 5mJ. The wall of the cyst should be opened, allowing the cyst to collapse.

In large corneal cysts involving the visual axis, lamellar or penetrating keratoplasty may be the procedure most likely to remove the cyst and restore vision. Lamellar keratoplasty may be difficult in deep cysts, but penetrating keratoplasty has given successful results in intrastromal epithelial corneal cysts.

Ocular or Periocular Manifestations

Conjunctiva: Calcium deposits; opacity.
Cornea: Opacity.
Other: Astigmatism; loss of vision; ocular pain.

PRECAUTIONS

If any cyst enters the intraocular structures, the use of chemical cautery, especially trichloroacetic acid, can cause the formation of cataracts. Although aphakic eyes are not affected, chemical cautery is a satisfactory method of management for anterior chamber cysts in some phakic eyes. In eyes with good vision and a cyst that is deep within the stroma requiring extensive surgical manipulation, it is best to document a progressive change in the cyst before doing a procedure that may cause astigmatism and endanger visual acuity or the corneal endothelium. Simple drainage procedures or aspirations are seldom of any benefit in the destruction of corneal, conjunctival, or scleral cysts, since they usually recur. Cysts at the limbus need to be evaluated for anterior chamber communication; gonioscopy or insertion of a needle into the cyst and aspiration will demonstrate any effect on the depth of the anterior chamber. In a few cases, a "cyst" may in fact be a filtering bleb. Therefore, if the "cyst" was unroofed, it would just allow a track of aqueous to come out through the eye. Simple cauterization of a scleral or limbal cyst is ideal, if superficial; however, because of the thinness of the globe in these situations, partial- or full-thickness corneoscleral grafting may be necessary.

COMMENTS

Corneal intrastromal cysts have been reported after lamellar keratoplasties. They can be treated by making an incision toward the cyst area, entering the cyst with a 30-gauge needle, and cauterizing it with trichloroacetic acid. This method can be used for peripheral cysts; however, those near the visual axis need other management due to possible chemical-induced corneal opacities.

There is disagreement whether intracorneal or corneoscleral cysts are indeed traumatic or congenital in origin. This disagreement is of academic interest, because the management in either case is the same. However, with congenital cysts seen shortly after birth, one needs to be aware that other congenital abnormalities may also be present within the eye.

References

DeBustros S, Michels RG: Treatment of acquired epithelial inclusion cyst of the conjunctiva using the YAG laser. Am J Ophthalmol 98:807–808, 1984.

Jahnle RL, et al: Conjunctival inclusion cyst stimulating malignant melanoma. Am J Ophthalmol 100:483–484, 1985.

McCarthy RW, et al: Conjunctival cysts of the orbit following enucleation. Ophthalmology 88:30–35, 1981.

Newton JC, et al: Giant cysts of the conjunctiva following scleral buckling. Ophthalmic Surg 18:295–298, 1987.

Panda A, Arora R, Mohan M: Cystic lesions of conjunctiva. Ann Ophthalmol 19:60–62, 1987.

Purcell JJ Jr, Brady HR: Intrastromal epithelial corneal cyst. Ophthalmic Surg 14:491–493, 1983.

Rosenquist RC, Fraunfelder FT, Swan KC: Treatment of conjunctival epithelial inclusion cysts with trichloroacetic acid. J Ocular Ther Surg 4:51–53, 1985.

CORNEAL EDEMA 371.20
(Bullous Keratopathy, Epithelial Edema, Stromal Edema)

JOEL SUGAR, M.D.

Chicago, Illinois

Corneal edema is caused by altered fluid transport across the cornea. Epithelial edema has the greatest effect on visual acuity because it induces anterior irregular astigmatism. Fluid accumulation begins within basal cells, then settles between cells, and ultimately gathers subcellularly, lifting up the corneal surface and forming bullae. Stromal edema has a less detrimental effect on acuity and is manifested as thickening and hazy opacification, with folding of Descemet's membrane. Early epithelial edema presents as blurred vision, often most severe on awakening and decreasing as the day goes on. As the edema increases in severity, the acuity deficit becomes persistent, and blinking across the bullae or their rupturing leads to irritation, pain, redness, and photophobia. Rupture of bullae may lead to anterior chamber inflammation, including sterile hypopyon, or may predispose to secondary corneal infection. Frequent causes of corneal edema are endothelial dysfunction and elevated intraocular pressure. Fuchs' dystrophy and aphakic (pseudophakic) bullous keratopathy are the most common endothelial disorders associated with edema that require treatment. One-third or more of patients requiring keratoplasty suffer from those disorders. Angle-closure glaucoma causes significant endothelial cell loss, and silicone oil in contact with a significant area of the cornea excludes nutrients and leads to endothelial damage. Inflammation, such as herpetic disciform keratitis, may also produce corneal edema. Prolonged edema of any cause may lead to pannus formation and stromal vascularization. Corneal edema seems to be associated with the loss of stromal glycosaminoglycans.

THERAPY

Ocular. The treatment of corneal edema depends in part on its etiology. When edema is associated with stromal inflammation or uveitis, treatment of the underlying cause is essential. When elevated intraocular pressure causes corneal edema, the treatment of the pressure elevation is primary. However, when corneal edema is caused by endothelial dysfunction, as in Fuchs' dystrophy and aphakic bullous keratopathy, initial treatment is with topical hyperosmotic agents. The most readily available of these agents is 5 per cent sodium chloride. This solution is used as often as necessary to relieve visual blurring associated with mild or moderate edema. Because symptoms are usually greatest in the morning due to the retention of fluid during sleep, drops may be necessary as frequently as every 15 minutes on awakening and less often as the day goes on. Five per cent sodium chloride ointment at bedtime may also be beneficial. A hair dryer directed at the eyes held at arm's length may also help dehydrate the cornea.

In patients with irritation induced by ruptured bullae, cycloplegic agents may aid comfort. Soft contact lenses that provide a smooth surface for the cornea may provide some improvement in vision in patients with early decompensation, but, in general, soft contact lenses are more useful to reduce painful rupture of bullae when worn continuously for palliation.

Surgical. Surgical therapy with penetrating keratoplasty is the treatment of choice for visual restoration. In the presence of cataract, combined keratoplasty and lens extraction with or without intraocular lens implantation are the treatments of choice. In aphakic bullous keratopathy with vitreous in the anterior chamber, anterior vitrectomy is combined with keratoplasty. In pseudophakic bullous keratopathy, the implant may be left in place at the time of keratoplasty if it is stable and positioned away from the cornea. However, it may be better to remove a poorly positioned or unstable implant, and all closed loop anterior chamber lenses and iris supported lenses should be removed. Fortunately, the success rate of keratoplasty for corneal edema is very high, although in aphakic and pseudophakic patients, acuity may be limited by macular edema. In patients with good vision in the contralateral eye, comfort may be all that is desired. If an extended-wear soft contact lens does not provide comfort, a conjunctival flap or cautery to Bowman's layer usually eliminates painful rupture of bullae and restores patient comfort.

Ocular or Periocular Manifestations

Cornea: Pannus; recurrent epithelial erosion; stromal vascularization.
Other: Cystoid macular edema; glaucoma; ocular pain; uveitis.

PRECAUTIONS

Patients with corneal endothelial disease are at higher risk of developing bullous keratopathy after intraocular surgery. Patients who have developed edema, however slight, invariably have progression of their edema after cataract surgery, so that combined lens removal and corneal grafting are warranted. Patients with endothelial guttata but no edema, however, may do well with lens removal alone and should not have a combined surgical procedure.

References

Bahn CF, Sugar A: Endothelial physiology and intraocular lens implantation. Am Intraocular Implant Soc J 7:351–364, 1981.
Kangas TA, Edelhauser HF, Twining SS, O'Brien WJ: Loss of stromal glycosaminoglycans during corneal edema. Invest Ophthalmol Vis Sci 31: 1994–2002, 1990.
Levenson JE: Corneal edema: Cause and treatment. Surv Ophthalmol 20:190–204, 1975.
Lindquist TD, McGlothan JS, Rotkis WM, Chandler JW: Indications for penetrating keratoplasty: 1980–1988. Cornea 10:210–216, 1991.
Price FE, Whitson WE, Makrs RG: Graft survival in four groups of patients undergoing penetrating keratoplasty. Ophthalmology 98:322–328, 1991.
Smith PW, et al: Complications of semiflexible, closed-loop anterior chamber intraocular lenses. Arch Ophthalmol 105:52–57, 1987.
Sternberg P, Hatchell DL, Foulks GN, Landers MB: The effect of silicone oil on the cornea. Arch Ophthalmol 103:90–94, 1985.
Waring GO, et al: The corneal endothelium: Normal and pathologic structure and function. Ophthalmology 89:531–590, 1982.
Waring GO, Stulting RD, Street D: Penetrating keratoplasty for pseudophakic corneal edema with exchange of intraocular lenses. Arch Ophthalmol 105:58–62, 1987.

CORNEAL MUCOUS PLAQUES 371.44
(Keratitis Mucosa)

RAMESH C. TRIPATHI, M.D., Ph.D., F.A.C.S.

Columbia, South Carolina

Corneal mucous plaques are abnormal collections of a mixture of mucus, epithelial cells, and proteinaceous and lipoidal material that adhere firmly to the corneal surface. The plaques may also enmesh calcareous granules and bacteria, as well as dust particles and other foreign bodies. The mucous plaques are translucent to opaque and may vary in size and shape from multiple small islands to bizarre patterns that may involve more than half the corneal surface. An abnormality of the exposed surface of the superficial corneal epithelial cells, excessive mucus formation, and the presence of epithelial receptor sites for the plaque elements predispose to this condition. The normal desquamation of epithelial cells beneath the plaque is thus retarded. The plaque is formed when high-viscosity mucus and proteinaceous material become adherent to the deeper squamous cells of the cornea or even to Bowman's layer through the intercellular spaces, as well as through abnormally formed transcellular apertures; because of its physicochemical property, this material enmeshes the desquamated epithelial cells. The viscosity of the mucus may increase due to dehydration, an increase in its sialomucin component, or secondarily because of infection by staphylococci, the enzymes of which can destroy the mucoprotein and mucopolysaccharide components of normal mucus produced by the conjunctival goblet cells. Corneal mucous plaques occur primarily in patients with keratoconjunctivitis sicca, but may also be seen with herpes zoster keratitis and after local radiation exposure. Ciliary or conjunctival injection, mild iritis, profuse keratic precipitates, and epithelial and stromal edema are associated findings.

Symptoms associated with the plaques vary from blurring of vision to foreign body sensation and marked pain; except when severe, they are often indistinguishable from the symptoms of keratoconjunctivitis sicca with or without Sjögren's syndrome. These symptoms may also occur with herpes zoster keratitis and in patients using extended-wear soft contact lenses. There seems to be an association of the entity with systemic disease, primarily rheumatoid arthritis or other collagen diseases.

THERAPY

Ocular. Topically applied 10 to 20 per cent acetylcysteine drops*, one to four times daily, usually prevent corneal mucous plaques. Existing plaques can also often be loosened rapidly and dissolved with this treatment. Mucous plaques causing severe symptoms may be removed surgically by scraping, followed by a bandage soft contact lens. In some patients, a soft contact lens is also of therapeutic or preventive value.

Staphylococcal blepharitis may occur in association with corneal mucous plaques and may predispose patients to this condition. Therefore, treatment should also include the control of associated local microbial infections.

Artificial tear preparations may be indicated for the treatment of dry eye. In the presence of filamentary keratitis and the formation of excessive mucus, hypotonic artificial tear substitutes (rather than the mucoid type of tear substitutes) may be combined with acetylcysteine. Because preservatives, such as benzylkonium chloride, chlorobutanol, and thymersol, affect adversely the corneal epithelium, the use of preservative-free tear substitutes or lubricants is preferable.

Ocular or Periocular Manifestations

Conjunctiva: Conjunctivitis; fornix filaments; hyperemia; mucoid discharge.
Cornea: Filamentary keratitis; keratoconjunctivis sicca; mucous plaques.
Eyelids: Chronic blepharitis; blepharospasm.

PRECAUTIONS

Because of variations in the frequency and severity of corneal mucous plaques, the use and concentration of topical mucolytic agents, such as acetylcysteine, should be individualized.

The bandage soft contact lense may often be subject to deposit formation and spoilage secondary to alterations in tear function (including rapid tear break-up time), associated necrosis of keratoconjunctival tissue, and the plaque exposure. Periodic cleaning or change of the soft contact lens may be required.

COMMENTS

In some cases, corneal mucous plaques recur when the mucolytic agent is discontinued. Plaques may occur even in those patients receiving acetylcysteine, but usually the mucous adherences are smaller or remain on the cornea for shorter periods of time than in patients who did not receive therapy. In some patients, plaques may recur if the soft contact lens is discontinued.

Multiple plaques, which are frequently bilateral, are common. When a plaque has adhered to the cornea, it remains for a few days or weeks; recurrences may appear but seldom in the same location. Thickened plaques with a dry surface may appear elevated well above the tear film and may even cause dellen formation.

References

Fraunfelder FT, Wright P, Tripathi RC: Corneal mucus plaques. Am J Ophthalmol 83:191–197, 1977.
Marsh RJ, Fraunfelder FT, McGill JI: Herpetic corneal epithelial disease. Arch Ophthalmol 94: 1899–1902, 1976.
Shaw EL, Gasset AR: Management of an unusual case of keratitis mucosa with hydrophilic contact lenses and N-acetyl-cysteine. Ann Ophthalmol 6: 1054–1056, 1974.
Tripathi BJ, Tripathi RC, Kolli SP: Cytotoxicity of ophthalmic preservatives on human corneal epithelium. Lens Eye Tox Res 9:361–374, 1993.

CORNEAL NEOVASCULARIZATION 370.60

KARL G. STONECIPHER, M.D., F.A.A.O.

Greensboro, North Carolina

The normal cornea is devoid of any blood vessels, and this characteristic, combined with some other structural facts in the anatomy of the cornea, is responsible for the transparency of this tissue. Corneal neovascularization can be defined as a pathologic state in which new blood vessels extend from the limbus into the superficial or deep areas of the cornea and is the result of various causes. In humans, corneal neovascularization can be associated with inflammatory states, such as keratitis and graft rejection, but can also be a response of the cornea to traumatic or toxic corneal injuries, such as those seen in penetrating lacerations of the cornea and alkali burns. Various dry eye states, as well as nutritional disorders, have been associated with corneal neovascularization. Neovascularization can be as simple as a micropannus, which is defined as a superficial, fibrovascular proliferation that extends one to two ml beyond the normal vascular arcade. It is most commonly seen in contact lens wearers, but can also occur in infections associated with *Chlamydia*, blepharitis, superior limbic keratoconjunctivitis, vernal keratoconjunctivitis, and rheumatoid keratoconjunctivitis. In contrast, a superficial vascular pannus that extends more than 2 mm beyond the normal vascular arcade is defined as a gross pannus. Etiologies associated with this extent of corneal neovascularization include trachoma, phlyctenulosis, rosacea keratitis, contact lens wear, atopic keratoconjunctivitis, chemical keratitis, toxic keratitis, herpetic keratitis, severe blepharoconjunctivitis, and corneal graft rejections.

Klintworth and associates (1983) have proposed three potential mechanisms for the pathogenesis of corneal neovascularization. First, a corneal injury inactivates a restraint that the normal cornea exerts on cell division and migration of the vascular cells of the pericorneal plexus. Second, corneal edema loosens corneal stromal tissue and therefore permits the ingrowth of vessels normally restrained by its compact composition. Third, corneal neovascularization is related to production of locally generated angiogenic factors. The most noted of these angiogenic factors are epidermal growth factor, fibroblast growth factor, urokinase-like plasminogen activator, and interleukin II. More and more basic science research has been aimed at the identification of these angiogenic factors and those cells producing these substances in attempts to treat corneal neovascularization.

As well, polymorphonuclear leukocyte invasion, traumatic disruption of the corneal architecture, and oxygen deprivation have a key definitive role to play in corneal neovascularization. Prostaglandin E has been implicated as a potent mediator of inflammatory reactions associated with angiogenic activity. In a model of corneal neovascularization associated with chemical cautery, the time of events shows that, within the first few hours, dilation of pericorneal blood vessels and the influx of polymorphonuclear leukocytes are associated with increased vascular permeability and dilation of pericorneal lymphatics. Within 24 to 48 hours, invasion of the cornea proper by buds from pericorneal venules and capillaries occurs and is associated with vascular loop formation from the superficial limbal plexus. Superficial corneal vascularization can run irregular courses; however, interstitial neovascularization is usually associated with vessels that are not anastomosing, but are rather straight and follow corneal planes. Slit-lamp evaluation of the depth of corneal neovascularization can be beneficial in the ultimate definition of etiologic mechanisms.

Corneal neovascularization associated with contact lenses has been studied extensively. The various lens components can produce relative hypoxia, which results in corneal neovascularization. Theoretically, the increased lactic acid present in the cornea resulting from corneal hypoxia may cause corneal neovascularization. Those patients using extended-wear contact lenses are more prone to develop severe corneal neovascularization; however, even daily-wear lens users are not excluded from this process. With the advent of new contact lenses and increased oxygen permeabilities, many of the complications associated with contact lenses have been reduced. It is also important to pay particular attention to lens fitting to prevent improper venting of the lens and decentration of the lens.

THERAPY

Supportive. Particularly in those patients with a micropannus, observation rather than treatment of the underlying condition is indicated. It is when the micropannus proceeds to gross corneal neovascularization that treatment alternatives may be instituted other than simply treating the underlying disease process.

Ocular. Various regimens have been proposed for the treatment of active, corneal vascularization. The mainstay of the current ocular armamentarium is corticosteroid therapy. Topically applied prednisolone acetate may be given liberally, except when used in cases with infectious causes. Its judicious usage is indicated in infectious cases to prevent collagenase activation and the associated melting of the cornea. In severe cases, subconjunctival injections of corticosteroids may be considered, but their benefit over and beyond topical administration is limited and the potential complications associated with subconjunctival injections may be potentiated by this therapeutic modality. Vascularization that has been present for a long time, particularly when located in the deeper layers of the cornea, is usually resistant to any form of treatment.

Surgical. Various surgical modalities have been recommended in the treatment of corneal neovascularization. Initially, diathermy of large feeding vessels into the cornea has been advised by some clinicians. More recently, corneal laser photocoagulation for the treatment of neovascularization has included the argon and the yellow dye laser. Both of these modalities depend primarily on energy absorption by hemoglobin and oxyhemoglobin. Results from these studies show that many subsets of patients with corneal neovascularization may be treated effectively with laser photocoagulation; however, recurrence of the neovascularization has been a problem associated with this modality. Penetrating keratoplasty in vascularized corneas can be very difficult. Pretreatment of the recipient bed with diathermy of large feeder vessels into the cornea has been advised by some authors. As well, diathermy of the inside graft edge must be done with extreme caution so as to prevent induced postoperative astigmatism. Early suture removal has been advocated, as sutures have been implicated as a source of irritation and increased neovascularization with associated corneal graft rejection. In the past, the use of beta irradiation was advocated; however, this practice has been abandoned as the use of corticosteroids and current immunosuppressive agents achieves better results. Lipman and associates (1992) have demonstrated the suppression of corneal neovascularization with topical cyclosporine. They suggest that this action is probably secondary to a reduction in interleukin II activity. Recently, the Collaborative Corneal Transplantation Study showed that neither HLA-A-B nor HLA-DR antigen matching substantially reduced the likelihood of corneal graft failure, but that ABO blood group matching did so. Therefore, appropriately tissue-matched transplantation may be indicated in recipient corneas that are highly vascularized and at increased risk for graft failure.

Ocular or Periocular Manifestations

Cornea: Cicatrization; edema; exudates; infiltration; injection; opacity.

Other: Anterior uveitis; irritation; loss of vision.

PRECAUTIONS

It is important to keep in mind that prolonged, topical ophthalmic treatment with corticosteroids can increase intraocular pressure and cataract formation. Therefore, it is essential to follow these patients closely. As mentioned, treatment of certain infectious states with corticosteroids alone can potentiate collagenase activity and in fact exacerbate corneal melting. Radiation therapy, diathermy, and cryotherapy have all been used in an attempt to treat corneal neovascularization, but none of these methods has been found to be any more effective than corticosteroids. In the cases of deep, long-standing, corneal neovascularization, most of these modalities are, in fact, unsuccessful.

COMMENTS

As our knowledge of the biochemical pathogenesis of corneal neovascularization improves, so will our treatment of this devastating ocular process. Current research in arachidonic acid metabolism has shown that corticosteroids and cyclo-oxygenase inhibitors, when topically applied, can decrease significantly the neovascular response to various insults. Attempts to use lipo-oxygenase inhibitors and combined cyclo-oxygenase and lipo-oxygenase inhibitors have not proved as successful in decreasing the neovascular response in an animal model of corneal revascularization. Our understanding of interleukin and T cell associations has led to the use of cyclosporine to suppress corneal neovascularization. Also, current evaluation of collagenase inhibitors in alkali burns has shown that reducing the initial injury and the body's associated response can limit the associated disruption of normal corneal architecture. Usage of tissue-matched corneas in corneal transplantation has shown success in ABO-matched tissue, but not with the HLA-associated markers. Finally, extended contact lens wear usage, either in the disposable or nondisposable form, will continue to cause corneal neovascularization by the mechanisms of hypoxia and lactic acid accumulation. Identifying these problematic patients early can be rewarding when closer follow-up of these patients is then implemented. In addition, contact lens technology continues to change rapidly, thereby reducing the problems associated improving on past with its usage.

The response of the cornea to injury or inflammation and the associated corneal neovascularization that may follow have plagued the ophthalmic surgeon and diagnostician for years. Continued research and development of new topically applied agents as well as preventive mechanisms should reduce the prevalence of this potentially devastating ocular pathologic process.

References

Baer JC, Foster S: Corneal laser photocoagulation for treatment of neovascularization: Efficacy of 577 NM yellow dye laser. Ophthalmology 99: 173–179, 1992.

Boyd BF (ed): Highlights of Ophthalmology. New York, Arcata Book Group, 1988.

Collaborative Corneal Transplantation Studies: Effectiveness of histocompatibility matching in high risk corneal transplantation. Arch Ophthalmol 110:1392–1403, 1992.

Dabezies DH Jr (ed): Contact Lenses—The CLAO Guide to Basic Science and Clinical Practice. Boston, Little, Brown, 1988.

Haynes WL, Proia AD, Klintworth GK: Effect of inhibitors of arachidonic acid metabolism on corneal neovascularization in the rat. Invest Ophthalmol Vis Sci 30:1588–1593, 1989.

Klintworth GK. Corneal Angiogenesis: A Comprehensive Critical Review. New York, Springer-Verlag, 1991.

Klintworth GK, Burger PC: Noninfectious inflammation of the anterior segment. Neovascularization of the cornea: Current concepts of its pathogenesis. Int Ophthalmol Clin 23:27–39, 1983.

Lipman RM, Epstein RJ, Hendricks RL: Suppression of corneal neovascularization with cyclosporine. Arch Ophthalmol 110:405–407, 1992.

Schanzlin DJ, Cyr RJ, Friedlaender MH: Histopathology of corneal neovascularization. Arch Ophthalmol 101:471–472, 1983.

CRYSTALLINE CORNEAL DYSTROPHY 371.56
(Schnyder's Crystalline Corneal Dystrophy)
MALCOLM N. LUXENBERG, M.D.

Augusta, Georgia

Schnyder's crystalline corneal dystrophy is a rare bilateral disease that is often progressive. It is inherited as an autosomal dominant trait, and onset occurs in early life. The lesions are oval or round with irregular borders, and the margins tend to be denser than the center of the lesion. The opacities are usually located in the central cornea and grossly appear yellowish-white. On slit-lamp examination, many fine, needle-shaped, colored crystals are seen in the anterior stroma with some involvement of Bowman's membrane, and crystals often extend into the deeper stroma. The surrounding cornea is usually clear, especially in younger patients, but in some reported cases there has been considerable stromal haze, which usually worsened with increasing age. The presence and nature of the corneal crystals can be determined by specular microscopy. The epithelium, endothelium, and Descemet's membrane are usually normal. A dense corneal arcus is frequently present, and corneal sensation is occasionally decreased; this decrease may accelerate in older patients. There are usually no edema, abnormal vascularization, or signs of previous inflammation. Xanthelasma has been noted in some patients, and rarely there may be associated skeletal abnormalities. Visual acuity is usually good, particularly in younger patients, but in some cases, vision has decreased significantly in older patients and can warrant keratoplasty. Except for decreased vision, the lesions are usually asymptomatic. Hyperlipidemia and hyperlipoproteinemia are often present, but this is not a universal finding. There is a suggestion, but no firm evidence, of a direct relationship between abnormal elevation of serum lipids and development of the lesions. Histologic studies have shown that the crystalline material is cholesterol, and in addition, there may be a deposition of neutral fats in the corneal stroma. The pathogenesis of the corneal changes is unknown.

THERAPY

Systemic. Dietary measures and drug therapy to lower serum lipids have not been shown to have any beneficial effects on the lesions.

Surgical. In the majority of patients, especially younger ones, surgical treatment is not necessary as visual acuity is good. However, if vision is significantly decreased by the corneal lesions, keratoplasty can be performed. However, crystals may recur postoperatively.

Ocular or Periocular Manifestations

Cornea: Arcus; hypesthesia; stromal haze and opacities.
Eyelids: Xanthelasma.

PRECAUTIONS

Crystalline corneal dystrophy must be differentiated from other crystalline deposits in the cornea that may be seen in association with cystinosis, the dysproteinemias, multiple myeloma, porphyria, hyperuricemia, primary or secondary lipid keratopathy, and various inborn errors of metabolism.

COMMENTS

The etiology of crystalline corneal lesions is unknown. They are most likely the result of a local defect in corneal lipid metabolism. The changes noted may be modified by abnormalities of the plasma lipoproteins.

References

Bron AJ: Corneal changes in the dislipoproteinaemias. Cornea. 8:135–140, 1989.

Bron AJ, Williams HP, Carruthers ME: Hereditary crystalline stromal dystrophy of Schnyder. I. Clinical features of a family with hyperlipoproteinaemia. Br J Ophthalmol 56:383–399, 1972.

Brooks AMV, Grant G, Gillies WE: Determination of the nature of corneal crystals by specular microscopy. Ophthalmology 95:448–452, 1988.

Delleman JW, Winkelman JE: Degeneratio corneae cristallinea hereditaria. A clinical, genetical and histological study. Ophthalmologica 155:409–426, 1968.

Ehlers N, Matthiessen ME: Hereditary crystalline corneal dystrophy of Schnyder. Acta Ophthalmol 51:316–324, 1973.

Garner A, Tripathi RC: Hereditary crystalline stromal dystrophy of Schnyder. Histopathology and ultrastructure. Br J Ophthalmol 56:400–408, 1972.

Luxenberg M: Hereditary crystalline dystrophy of the cornea. Am J Ophthalmol 63:507–511, 1967.

Rodrigues MM, et al: Unesterified cholesterol in Schnyder's corneal crystalline dystrophy. Am J Ophthalmol 104:157–163, 1987.

Weiss JS: Schnyder's dystrophy of the cornea. A Swede-Finn connection. Cornea 11:93–101, 1992.

Weller RO, Rodger FC: Crystalline stromal dystrophy: Histochemistry and ultrastructure of the cornea. Br J Ophthalmol 64:46–52, 1980.

Williams HP, et al: Hereditary crystalline corneal dystrophy with an associated blood lipid disorder. Trans Ophthalmol Soc UK 91:531–541, 1971.

EPITHELIAL BASEMENT MEMBRANE DYSTROPHY
371.52
(Cogan's Microcystic Corneal Dystrophy, Map, Dot, Fingerprint Dystrophy)

and RECURRENT EROSION
371.42
(Recurrent Epithelial Erosion)

PETER R. LAIBSON, M.D.

Philadelphia, Pennsylvania

Corneal erosion and recurrent corneal erosion are common ocular disorders that are sometimes preceded by trauma, but at other times occur spontaneously. In the spontaneous cases of corneal erosion, the underlying disease process may be an epithelial basement membrane corneal dystrophy.

Epithelial basement membrane dystrophy is usually a bilateral epithelial disorder characterized by various patterns of intraepithelial dots, linear changes that mimic the appearance of maps, and other corneal irregularities, such as parallel lines, which may bring to mind fingerprints. The intraepithelial dots consist of opaque putty-gray intraepithelial cysts that are located usually in the central two-thirds of the cornea. These cysts, called Cogan's cysts, are made up of cytoplasmic and nuclear debris and range in size from a pinpoint lesion to a cyst measuring up to 2 mm across. They may be oval, oblong, or comma shaped and are associated with the map and the fingerprint patterns in most cases. Microcysts are rarely found alone, but map and fingerprint changes are commonly seen without the presence of microcysts (dots).

This disorder occurs in adults of both sexes, although somewhat more commonly in females and usually after the fourth decade. It is probably hereditary, with variable penetrance, although in 6 per cent of a large study population, these changes were present in some form.

Map and fingerprint alterations are not rare and can be found in asymptomatic individuals without prior history of trauma or ocular disease. They are frequently seen in conditions where there is corneal edema, such as near the healing incision of a cataract wound or in the central cornea in Fuchs' corneal dystrophy.

Fingerprint lines histologically are similar to map-like changes, since both have an aberrant or multilaminar basement membrane produced by the basal epithelial cells of the corneal epithelium. At least 80 to 90 per cent of patients who have epithelial basement membrane dystrophy are asymptomatic. Symptoms, when they are present, consist of slightly blurred vision when the epithelial and basement membrane changes are in the visual axis or of foreign body sensation with recurrent erosion when the epithelium is loose.

Recurrent corneal erosions may follow corneal trauma that involves the epithelium and basement membrane. Recurrent epithelial erosions probably occur as a result of inadequate basement membrane healing, either because the basal epithelial cells fail to produce proper basement membrane complexes that attach to Bowman's membrane and stroma or because of faulty basement membrane adherence.

Recurrent epithelial erosions tend to recur in the early morning during sleep and often awaken the patient with a sharp pain. In rare cases, patients so fear the pain on awakening that they are unable to sleep well at night. The very common sharp pain on opening the eyelids either during sleep or on awakening in the morning may be fleeting, lasting only seconds, or it may last for minutes to an hour or two. In most cases, this sharp pain is only fleeting and is a warning that the epithelium is not completely healed. Continued use of precautionary measures, such as not rubbing the eyes through the lids on awakening and medications to prevent recurrent erosion, are necessary as long as the fleeting, sharp pain occurs in the morning.

THERAPY

Ocular. The greatest problem facing patients with epithelial basement membrane dystrophy is pain from recurrent corneal erosion. If the erosion is small, it will usually heal spontaneously or with the aid of a pressure patch placed on the eye for a day or two. Usually, a lubricating or an antibiotic ointment, such as bacitracin or erythromycin, is used beneath the pressure patch. Resistant cases may well require mechanical debridement, depending on the size of the defect or the amount of ocular irritation. Local cycloplegics may be necessary. The minor corneal erosion may be treated with lubricating ointments alone for several weeks to several months to control symptoms.

Soft contact lenses have been helpful in cases with multiple recurrent corneal erosions. However, concern about extended soft contact lens use persists because of the fear of corneal infectious disease.

In some cases, very mild corneal erosion may be prevented by using 2 or 5 per cent sodium chloride drops during the day and 5 per cent sodium chloride ointment at bedtime. Many patients believe that sodium chloride ointment is no more effective than a lubricant ointment or an ointment without preservatives. Each person must establish a regimen of drug use that seems to control symptoms most effectively. It might involve the use of medication only when symptoms recur or, in some instances, daily application for many months after the termination of a recurrent episode to prevent further recurrences.

With the more severe cases of recurrent corneal erosion that do not seem to heal with any of the above regimens, the use of anterior stromal puncture has been advocated. This procedure may be used for patients with severe multiple erosions that fail to heal with all previous therapeutic regimens. Forty to fifty puncture marks through the epithelium and Bowman's membrane are created into the anterior stroma, using a sharp 23- or 25-gauge needle. The needle is inserted through loosened epithelium and indents the cornea in order to enter the stroma. Patients who have had multiple recurrences and were not helped by debridement alone or debridement with cautery showed significant improvement with anterior corneal puncture.

When used correctly, anterior corneal puncture is effective in recalcitrant recurrent erosion in 90 per cent of cases with the first application. A few patients may require a second application of anterior corneal puncture.

Surgical. Excimer laser photoablation of the very superficial epithelium, basement membrane, and just into Bowman's membrane has been done for spontaneous recurrent erosion and erosions secondary to dystrophies. These dystrophies include epithelial basement dystrophy, superficial variant of granular dystrophy, Reis-Bücklers' dystrophy, and lattice dystrophy. The Food and Drug Administration has not yet approved the excimer laser for this use, but early promising results with little, if any, visual loss and long-term cure of recurrent erosion hold promise for this treatment in the future.

The use of fibronectin[†] epidermal growth factor[†] or other locally active macromolecules is still experimental.

Ocular or Periocular Manifestations

Cornea: Epithelial blebs; opacity (punctate, striate, map, dot, geographic, fingerprint).
Other: Astigmatism; irritation; visual loss.

PRECAUTIONS

Treatment should be as simple as possible with as few drugs as necessary. Some drugs, such as local anesthetics, have been shown to delay epithelial wound healing. For this reason, it is imperative never to prescribe a topical anesthetic for the patient's own use, even when symptoms are severe.

Indications for chemical cautery or lamellar keratectomy for resistant erosions have become almost nonexistent with the advent of therapeutic soft contact lenses and now anterior stromal puncture. Owing to the cost of the lens and frequent follow-up visits, the use of long-term therapeutic soft contact lenses should be delayed, and anterior corneal puncture should be relied on for treatment of the most severe cases. Excimer laser holds promise for the future.

COMMENTS

Systemic disease does not seem to play a role in epithelial basement membrane dystrophy or recurrent corneal erosion.

References

Laibson PR: Microcystic corneal dystrophy. Trans Am Ophthalmol Soc 74:488–531, 1976.
McDonnell PJ, Seiler T: Phototherapeutic keratectomy with excimer laser for Reis-Bücklers' corneal dystrophy. Refract Corneal Surg 8:306–310, 1992.
McLean EN, MacRae SM, Rich LF: Recurrent erosion. Treatment by anterior stromal puncture. Ophthalmology 93:784–788, 1986.
Trobe JD, Laibson PR: Dystrophic changes in the anterior cornea. Arch Ophthalmol 87:378–382, 1972.

FILAMENTARY KERATITIS 370.23

WILLIAM R. MORRIS, M.D.,
and THOMAS O. WOOD, M.D.

Memphis, Tennessee

Filamentary keratitis is a condition of unknown origin in which fine filaments develop on the anterior surface of the cornea. These filaments may occur singly or in great numbers; the process may be acute or chronic.

In vivo specular microscopy of filaments reveals that they are composed of cellular and mucoid debris. Their base is triangular, with elongation and stretching of the epithelial cells toward the filament. In most cases, the epithelial cells in the filament do not appear to be attached to the corneal epithelium. In eyes with an abnormal tear film, epithelium exposed to the surface may serve as a receptor site for mucous adherence and filament formation. Elevated epithelial receptor sites may develop in some cases secondary to inflammatory damage to the basal epithelial cells or epithelial basement membrane. When excess mucus occurs, such as in keratoconjunctivitis sicca, desquamated epithelial cells, lipids, and other foreign matter become entrapped in the mucus.

Filaments have the appearance of gelatinous, refractile objects adhering to the anterior surface of the cornea, moving with each blink, but staying attached at their bases. They may vary in length from 0.5 to 10.0 mm. Epithelial defects are sometimes present adjacent to the filaments, and at the base of a filament, there may be a gray subepithelial opacity.

Symptoms can vary from mild to severe foreign body sensation with photophobia, blepharospasm, and epiphora. Filamentary keratitis tends to be chronic and recurrent when not associated with an acute pathologic process.

Numerous diseases have been associated with filamentary keratitis. A frequent cause is keratoconjunctivitis sicca, with or without Sjögren's syndrome. Sarcoidosis, trachoma, ocular pemphigoid, and radiation therapy are causes of secondary keratoconjunctivitis sicca, which may lead to filamentary keratitis. Recurrent corneal erosion, numerous types of epithelial keratitis, soft contact lenses, corneal edema, superior limbic keratoconjunctivitis (SLKC), ligneous conjunctivitis, carcinoma of the conjunctiva, virtually all types of intraocular and extraocular surgery, epidemic keratoconjunctivitis, nodular degeneration, prolonged lid closure, ptosis, large-angle strabismus (presumably caused by corneal occlusion), and beta irradiation have all been associated with filamentary keratitis. Patients with systemic diseases, such as diabetes mellitus, ectodermal dysplasia, psoriasis, brainstem injury, neurotrophic keratitis, atopic dermatitis, and hereditary hemorrhagic telangiectasia, have also been found to have filamentary keratitis. Antihistamines, which decrease tear production, as well as other topical medications, especially antivirals, can also cause filamentary keratitis.

THERAPY

Ocular. The use of 5 per cent sodium chloride eye drops four times daily has been shown to reduce symptoms and significantly eliminate filaments in 89 per cent of patients within 1 month of initiating treatment and in 95 per cent of patients within 8 months. Filamentary keratitis of an acute or traumatic origin usually responds to hypertonic saline within a few days. Hypertonic saline ointment at bedtime is also helpful. When the filaments are associated with keratoconjunctivitis sicca from any cause, the average response time is 1 month. In eyes with filaments secondary to keratoconjunctivitis sicca, punctal occlusion may be required. The hypertonic saline can eventually be discontinued in patients with filamentary keratitis associated with acute or traumatic origin, but usually must be continued in patients with chronic disease processes.

Hypotonic tears should be used frequently if hypertonic saline does not improve the keratitis. Sometimes, combining hypotonic tears with acetylcysteine may help dissolve filaments; equal amounts of hypotonic tears and 20 per cent acetylcysteine* are recommended. Eledoisin†, which stimulates tear production, has also been successful in long-term treatment of filamentary keratitis associated with keratoconjunctivitis sicca.

Other treatments for filamentary keratitis are directed at treating the underlying etiology. Soft contact lenses have been used in filamentary keratitis following cataract extraction, corneal transplant surgery, or brainstem injury. In patients with epithelial keratitis associated with herpes simplex or recurrent corneal erosion, curing the underlying pathologic condition usually resolves the filamentary keratitis. Patients with SLKC (of other than soft contact lens origin) respond to conjunctival resection.

Ocular or Periocular Manifestations

Conjunctiva: Chronic mild hyperemia; increased mucus in the tear film and inferior cul-de-sac; in SLKC, may be filaments on the superior bulbar conjunctiva or cornea even after conjunctival resection.

Cornea: Filaments; punctate keratitis; neovascularization in filamentary keratitis associated with brainstem injury; nodular degeneration secondary to chronic filamentary keratitis; subepithelial granular opacity beneath the filaments.

Eyelids: Blepharospasm; chronic blepharitis; increased blink rate.

Other: Epiphora; irritation; ocular pain; photophobia.

PRECAUTIONS

Acetylcysteine can cause conjunctival irritation and burning in the 20 per cent concentration. A 10 per cent solution may be prepared by diluting 20 per cent acetylcysteine with an equal amount of hypotonic tears or antibiotic drops. The application of a contact lens, particularly in patients with keratoconjunctivitis sicca or Stevens-Johnson syndrome, may precipitate a bacterial ulcer. Silver nitrate, which has been used to reduce goblet cells and thereby reduce mucus production, has only a temporary effect that lasts about 3 weeks.

COMMENTS

Five per cent hypertonic saline solution is beneficial in approximately 95 per cent of the patients with filamentary keratitis. In addition to treating the filaments, any underlying etiology should also be treated.

Punctal occlusion in cases of severe keratoconjunctivitis sicca may be useful adjunctive therapy. In patients with keratoconjunctivitis sicca, the histologic appearance of the conjunctival epithelium returns to normal after punctal occlusion.

One should inquire into the use of systemic drugs that may decrease tear production, e.g., antihistamines or diuretics.

References

Coster DJ: Superficial keratopathy. In Duane TD (ed): Clinical Ophthalmology. Philadelphia, Harper & Row, 1980, Vol IV, 71:5–6.

Davis WG, Drewry RD, Wood TO: Filamentary keratitis and stromal neovascularization associated with brain-stem injury. Am J Ophthalmol 90:489–491, 1980.

Good WV, Whitcher JP: Filamentary keratitis caused by corneal occlusion in large-angle strabismus (Letter). Ophthalmic Surg 23:66, 1992.

Hamilton W, Wood TO: Filamentary keratitis. Am J Ophthalmol 93:466–469, 1982.

Jaeger W, Gotz ML, Kaercher T: Eledoisin—A successful therapeutic concept for filamentary keratitis. Trans Ophthalmol Soc UK 104:496, 1985.

Lemp MA, et al: An in vivo study of corneal surface morphologic features in patients with keratoconjunctivitis sicca. Am J Ophthalmol 98:426–428, 1984.

Lohman LE, Rao GN, Aquavella JV: In vivo microscopic observations of human corneal epithelial abnormalities. Am J Ophthalmol 93:210–217, 1982.

Maudgal PC, Missotten L (eds): Superficial Keratitis. The Hague, W Junk, 1981, pp 41–48.

Rotkis WM, Chandler JW, Forstot SL: Filamentary keratitis following penetrating keratoplasty. Ophthalmology 89:946–949, 1982.

Seedor JA, et al: Filamentary keratitis associated with diphenhydramine (Benadryl). Am J Ophthalmol 101:376–377, 1986.

Theodore FH: Filamentary keratitis. Contact Intraocular Lens Med J 8:138–146, 1982.

Tuberville AW, Frederick WR, Wood TO: Punctal occlusion in tear deficiency syndromes. Ophthalmology 89:1170–1172, 1982.

Wood TO: Salzmann's nodular degeneration. Cornea 9:17–22, 1990.

Zaidman GW, et al: The histopathology of filamentary keratitis. Arch Ophthalmol 103:1178–1181, 1985.

FUCHS' CORNEAL DYSTROPHY 371.57
(Combined Dystrophy of Fuchs, Endothelial Dystrophy of the Cornea, Epithelial Dystrophy of Fuchs, Fuchs' Epithelial-Endothelial Dystrophy)

WILLIAM M. BOURNE, M.D.

Rochester, Minnesota

Fuchs' combined corneal dystrophy is a bilateral, slowly progressive corneal disease. It is characterized by endothelial degeneration that allows accumulation of water in the cornea and is followed by the development of dystrophic changes in the epithelium and eventually in the substantia propria. The condition is usually transmitted dominantly and occurs in elderly females two times as often as in males. All elements of the disease are ultimately caused by endothelial dysfunction that starts very early in life, but this dysfunction may not be manifest itself until the third to sixth decade of life. The first stage is an uncomplicated central endothelial dystrophy (cornea guttata), which progresses in disciform fashion toward the periphery and may extend from limbus to limbus. Fine pigment granules may be found centrally on the posterior surface of the cornea and within the endothelial cells. Symptoms are often absent. The second stage is characterized by edema of the stroma and the epithelium wherein bullae may be formed. Vision becomes affected, and haloes that are usually more serious in the morning may occur. The third stage of subepithelial connective tissue formation with vascularization and scarring may result in a completely opaque cornea and loss of large superficial areas of epithelium. The final stage is one of complications, particularly glaucoma or infection.

THERAPY

Ocular. In early instances of epithelial edema, 5 per cent sodium chloride drops administered six to eight times a day and at bedtime may be used to decrease corneal edema and allow the patient to see better for a short period of time. This hyperosmotic agent acts primarily on the epithelial edema and has little or no influence on the stromal edema. It is especially useful in the morning when epithelial edema has accumulated during the night as the closed eyes have prevented evaporation. A hair dryer held at arm's length from the corneal surface may help decrease stromal edema. If discomfort is present as a result of bulla formation or rupture, a bandage soft contact lens may be beneficial.

The degree of edema that may appear in a cornea with Fuchs' dystrophy is in direct relation to the level of intraocular pressure. Incipient Fuchs' dystrophy in which the failure of endothelial function is just beginning to produce stromal and endothelial edema may sometimes be controlled temporarily by a reduction in the intraocular pressure, even though it is within normal limits. This reduction may be achieved by the use of miotics, such as 1 per cent pilocarpine three to four times daily or 0.25 per cent timolol twice daily.

These topical ophthalmic measures do not affect the progression of the endothelial dysfunction, however. They are useful as temporary therapy during the early stages of epithelial edema. Eventually, these measures offer no improvement, and keratoplasty offers the only hope for good vision.

Surgical. Over 90 per cent of penetrating corneal transplants for Fuchs' dystrophy are successful, resulting in clear grafts. Even corneas in the most advanced stages of the disease can be successfully operated on. Keratoplasty employing a 7.5- to 8.5-mm graft is the treatment of choice when the visual function is irreversibly compromised and no longer fulfills the patient's needs. Each case must be considered separately. A healthy active individual may merit keratoplasty when the visual acuity has decreased to 20/70 in the worse eye or to 20/40 (the visual acuity needed to drive an automobile) in the better eye when both eyes are affected. On the other hand, an old, infirm, or inactive individual may not benefit from keratoplasty until the visual acuity is less than 20/200 in both eyes. In some patients, a Gundersen-type, thin, conjunctival flap or even cauterization of superficial cornea may be helpful.

Ocular or Periocular Manifestations

Cornea: Bullous keratopathy; cicatrization; endothelial degeneration; epithelial and stromal edema; folds in Descemet's membrane; pigment on posterior surface; striae; vascularization; vesicles.

Other: Irritation; ocular pain; secondary glaucoma.

Precautions

Anything that damages corneal endothelial cells, such as iridocyclitis or cataract extraction, can lead to more rapid progression of Fuchs' dystrophy and corneal decompensation.

Any corneal transplant is susceptible to immune rejection episodes that, if not controlled, lead to graft failure and a permanently cloudy cornea. Transplant failures, however, may be regrafted with success. Rejection episodes should be treated with hourly administration of prednisolone eyedrops for several days, tapering the dosage over the next few weeks. If treated early, most transplants will clear.

Comments

Penetrating keratoplasty is an effective treatment for Fuchs' dystrophy because it replaces the diseased corneal endothelial cells with normal cells. Lamellar corneal transplants are not indicated in this disease because they do not replace the dystrophic endothelial cells that are its cause.

Fuchs' dystrophy progresses slowly over many years, rather than in days or months. Therefore, the conservative topical ocular therapies mentioned earlier may suffice in the early stages of the disease for a year or more, and it may be several more years before keratoplasty is indicated.

References

Bourne WM, Johnson DH, Campbell RJ: The ultrastructure of Descemet's membrane. III. Fuchs' dystrophy. Arch Ophthalmol *100*:1952–1955, 1982.

Davison JA, Bourne WM: Results of penetrating keratoplasty using a double running suture technique. Arch Ophthalmol 99:1591–1595, 1981.

Fine M, West CE: Late results of keratoplasty for Fuchs' dystrophy. Am J Ophthalmol 72:109–114, 1971.

Kenyon KR, Fogle JA, Grayson M: Dysgeneses, dystrophies, and degenerations of the cornea. *In* Duane TD (ed): Clinical Ophthalmology. Hagerstown, MD, Harper & Row, 1982, Vol IV, pp 16:33–35.

Krachmer JH, et al: Corneal endothelial dystrophy. A study of 64 families. Arch Ophthalmol *96*: 2036–2039, 1978.

Olson RJ, et al: Visual results after penetrating keratoplasty for aphakic bullous keratopathy and Fuchs' dystrophy. Am J Ophthalmol *88*:1000–1004, 1979.

Waring GO III, Rodrigues MM, Laibson PR: Corneal dystrophies. II. Endothelial dystrophies. Surv Ophthalmol 23:147–168, 1978.

Wilson SE, Bourne WM: Fuchs' dystrophy. Cornea 7:2–18, 1988.

FUCHS' DELLEN 371.41
(Facets, Fuchs' Dimples)

FRANCOISE LAGOUTTE, M.D.

Cedex, France

Dellen are paralimbal corneal ulcerations occurring at the base of abnormal conjunctiva or corneal elevations. These ellipsoid depressions or dells in the cornea are a quite common but not well-known phenomenon. Dellen are usually elliptical and saucer-shaped with clearly defined edges. Although transient dellen are superficial and purely epithelial, they may last several weeks and sometimes become deep. Cicatrization normally follows, often with reduction of corneal thickness (facets). Abnormal paralimbic conjunctival elevation most commonly is associated with filtering bleb, hematoma, chemosis, conjunctival tumor, rectus muscle surgery, conjunctival autograft, or pterygium. Abnormal corneal elevations can be seen secondary to localized graft displacement or edema, too tight corneal sutures, or corneal tumor. Poor palpebral congruence prevents the lids from normally spreading the tears, which causes a break in the oily film. This break and the resulting dessication can be aggravated by a trapped air bubble that sometimes bursts when the lids open.

THERAPY

Ocular. Treatment consists of elimination of the cause. In most cases, a pressure dressing is sufficient to control any abnormal conjunctival or corneal elevation. Rarely, an elevated growth may require conjunctival surgery. If there is an inflammatory elevation (such as a granuloma), topical corticosteroids may be of value, but should be used with caution because of the corneal ulcer.

Further treatment should be directed toward the secondary complications that may result. The area of dellen formation should be treated three times daily with ocular lubricants, preferably in ointment form; drops are less effective because they do not maintain prolonged protective coating over the dellen. Antibiotics may be necessary to avoid secondary infections.

Recently, the depression of the cornea has been "filled" with a fibrin sealant, i.e., TISSUCOL®. The sealant is covered with a bandage lens, and the cicatrization forms in a few days.

Ocular or Periocular Manifestations

Conjunctiva: Ectasia.
Cornea: Cicatrization; keratoconjunctivitis sicca; marginal keratitis; paralimbal elevation; thinning; ulcer.

PRECAUTIONS

Elimination of the cause of the elevation should be the primary focus of therapy. Use of corticosteroids should be limited and closely supervised because of the possibility of corneal ulcer.

COMMENTS

Dellen are more frequent than is commonly thought. They are usually benign, but occasionally present difficulties. In almost all cases, they heal well with the use of the simple techniques described earlier.

References

Baum JL, Mishima S, Boruchoff SA: On the nature of dellen. Arch Ophthalmol 79:657–662, 1968.
Fuchs A: Pathological dimples ("dellen") of the cornea. Am J Ophthalmol 12:877–883, 1929.
Insler MS, Tauber S, Packer A: Descemetocele formation in a patient with a postoperative corneal dellen. Cornea 8:129–130, 1989.
Lagoutte F, Gauthier L, Comte P: A fibrin sealant for perforated and preperforated corneal ulcers. Br J Ophthalmol 73:757–761, 1989.
Lagoutte F, Lebur J: Un phénomène méconnu: Les ulcérations cornéennes à l'aplomb des reliefs conjonctivaux exagérés ("dellen de Fuchs"). A propos de 7 cas. Bull Soc Ophthalmol Fr 80:1033–1035, 1980.
Mackie IA: Localized corneal drying in association with dellen, pterygia and related lesions. Trans Ophthalmol Soc UK 91:129–145, 1971.
Nauheim JS: Marginal keratitis and corneal ulceration after surgery on the extraocular muscles. Arch Ophthalmol 67:708–711, 1962.
Tragakis MP, Brown SI: The tear film alteration associated with dellen. Ann Ophthalmol 6:757–761, 1974.

FUNGAL KERATITIS 111.1
(Fungal Corneal Ulcer, Keratomycosis)

MICHAEL C. ROBERSON, M.D.

Little Rock, Arkansas

The incidence of fungal keratitis seems to have increased over the past few years. This increase is probably due to an increased awareness of the disease, better diagnostic techniques, and the widespread use of topical antibiotics and corticosteroids. Over 100 species of fungi have been reported as corneal pathogens. The frequency of fungal keratitis and the fungi causing infections have a geographic distribution. In the southern United States, as high as 33 per cent of microbial corneal ulcers may be fungal. Filamentous fungi, such as *Fusarium*, *Aspergillus*, *Penicillium*, and *Curvularia* spp., predominate. These infections are frequently associated with trauma, especially with vegetable matter. The overall incidence of fungal keratitis is less in the northern United States. *Candida* spp. are the main cause of these infections, and they are more commonly associated with pre-existing corneal disease. If the integrity of the corneal epithelium is breached by any number of insults including trauma, pre-existing disease, and lid abnormalities, fungal keratitis may occur. Contact lens wear and the use of contaminated eyedrops may also play a role in causing fungal keratitis. Local immunosuppression through the use of topical corticosteroids and general host immunosuppression can enhance the fungal infection. Spontaneous fungal keratitis has been reported in AIDS patients.

Fungal infections are frequently more indolent processes than bacterial ones. The cornea has an epithelial defect overlying a slightly raised stromal infiltrate with feathery edges. Occasionally, the epithelium is edematous, but intact over the infiltrate. Accompanying features may include satellite corneal lesions, immune stromal rings, endothelial plaques, and hypopyon. *Candida* tends to produce more discreet abscess lesions. Fungal hyphae can extend through Descemet's membrane and into the anterior chamber without evidence of perforation. The diagnosis is made by recovering the organism on smears and cultures. Scrapings should be taken from both the center and the edges of the ulcer. Stains to be used include Giemsa, gram, PAS, and methenamine silver. Cultures should be done at room temperature (30°C) on blood agar and Sabouraud's without cycloheximide. Usually, the fungi grow on culture in 72 hours, but it may be necessary to allow a longer time. In deep infections, corneal biopsy may be needed to recover the organism. Biopsy should be done in suspicious cases with negative initial scrapings and cultures.

THERAPY

Ocular. The mainstay of therapy in fungal keratitis is topical antifungal agents. In severe cases, subconjunctival, oral, and even intravenous therapy may be considered. There are three groups of antifungal agents available: polyenes, imidazoles, and fluorinated pyrimidines.

Since fungal sensitivities are difficult to obtain and imprecise, the choice of antifungal agents is empiric and based on prior experience and published studies. Three agents are available in the polyene group. Natamycin 3 per cent suspension is the only commercially available topical antifungal ophthalmic agent in the United States. It has a broad spectrum of activity, and in vitro, it is active against 70 to 90 per cent of corneal fungal isolates. It and all topical antifungal agents should be used one drop every 15 minutes for the first few hours and then hourly for the next week. Further adjustment of the dosage must be based on the clinical response. Amphotericin B* 0.05 to 1.0 per cent solution can be used topically. It is the drop of choice in *Candida* infections. Subconjunctival amphotericin B* injections are very irritating and cause conjunctival necrosis. Intravenous amphotericin B has poor ocular penetration and is not useful in treating fungal keratitis. Nystatin is a polyene antifungal agent that has been supplanted by natamycin. Miconazole, clotrimazole, and ketoconazole are imidazole antifungal agents available in the United States. All have a broad spectrum of antifungal activity. Miconazole is available in a 10 mg/ml intravenous solution that can be used topically*. It may be given subconjunctivally in 5- to 10-mg doses. Clotrimazole* 1 per cent solution can be made in arachis oil for topical use. The 1 per cent clotrimazole dermatologic cream is also well tolerated on the eye. Dermatologic lotions containing alcohol are to be avoided. Ketoconazole* may be used topically in 1 per cent solution.

Oral ketoconazole in a 200 to 400 mg daily dose has been reported to be effective in fungal keratitis. Flucytosine is the only fluorinated pyrimidine in common use. This drug has a limited spectrum of activity and is used primarily in combination with amphotericin B for *Candida* infections. It can be given orally at 150 mg/kg and used as a 1 per cent solution topically. In general, topical therapy should be maintained for 6 weeks. Evaluation of the clinical response will dictate the need for further therapy. Negative corneal scrapings and cultures may not indicate a cure, as viable fungus may persist in the deep stroma.

Surgical. Surgical intervention is necessary if the response to medical therapy is inadequate. Response to medical therapy is usually slow, but if there seems to be a worsening of the infection or if perforation is threatening or present, surgical intervention may be warranted. There are reports of curing fungal ulcers with conjunctival flaps. Yet, the infection may progress beneath the flap, and the flap itself may be a barrier to topical therapy. Excisional penetrating keratoplasty is the procedure of choice. In an inflamed eye, it will be difficult to perform. Adequate tissue margins must be obtained since fungal elements may extend beyond the visible limits of the infiltrate. Deep extension of fungi makes lamellar keratoplasty inadvisable.

COMMENTS

The corneal epithelium is a barrier to the penetration of antifungal agents. If the epithelium is intact, it should be debrided to enhance the penetration of the drugs. Physically scraping the ulcer to debulk the fungus present can be of value. Combinations of antifungal agents may enhance their activity, but most of the positive studies are in vitro. There is, however, a risk of antagonistic effect in combining antifungal agents. Corticosteroids are to be avoided until the fungus has been eradicated. Corticosteroids can potentiate fungal growth. In the future, newer and perhaps more effective agents will be available. Several triazole antifungal agents, such as intraconazole and fluconazole, show promise.

References

Hyndiuk R, Tee R: Antifungal agents. *In* Tabbara K, Hyndiuk R (eds): Infections of the Eye. Boston, Little Brown and Co., 1986, pp 239–256.
Ingram H, Starr M: Bacterial and fungal keratitis. Ophthalmol Clin North Am 3:545–362, 1990.

Johns K, O'Day D: Pharmacologic management of keratomycoses. Surv Ophthalmol 33:178–188, 1988.

Jones D: Decision making in the management of microbial keratitis. Ophthalmology 88:814–820, 1981.

O'Day D: Selection of appropriate antifungal therapy. Cornea 6:238–245, 1987.

Oliver D: Microbial contamination of in-use ocular medications. Arch Ophthalmol 110:82–85, 1992.

Ostler B: Diseases of the External Eye and Adnexa. Baltimore, Williams & Wilkins, 1993, pp 186–193.

Santos C, Parker J, Dawson C, et al: Bilateral fungal corneal ulcers in a patient with AIDS-related complex. Am J Ophthalmol 102:118–119, 1986.

GRANULAR CORNEAL DYSTROPHY 371.53

(Bücklers' Type I, Groenouw's Type I)

KAMAL F. NASSIF, M.D.,
and ROBERT A. HYNDIUK, M.D.

Milwaukee, Wisconsin

Granular dystrophy is an autosomal dominant inherited dystrophy that tends to affect both eyes symmetrically. It becomes apparent in the first decade of life as superficial stromal and central irregular white opacities. These opacities, most of which are located under Bowman's membrane, assume different shapes and sizes that do not usually exceed 0.5 mm in diameter. They are nontransparent in direct and retroillumination. At this stage, the intervening stroma is clear, and the epithelium is regular and uninvolved; these patients are therefore asymptomatic. Early in the first and second decade, the visual acuity is normal.

As the affected individual ages, the opacities enlarge and increase in number and may even coalesce, with loss of the characteristically clear intervening stroma. A diffuse, superficial stromal, ground glass haze develops during the fourth and fifth decades, and visual acuity starts to decline. The opacities progressively involve the deeper stroma and the midperiphery, whereas the far periphery is characteristically clear even late in the disease. A less common confluent superficial form may be confused with the geographic type of Reis-Bücklers' dystrophy, with opacification extending beyond the central area leaving only a peripheral clear vein of uninvolved clear cornea.

The epithelium and basement membrane are usually not clinically affected. When such involvement occurs, it is usually late in the disease and produces an irregularity of the surface with a resultant irregular astigmatism and decreased visual acuity. Depending on the extent of involvement of the epithelium,

recurrent erosions may result, causing pain, foreign body sensation, and photophobia.

The lesions of granular dystrophy are eosinophilic accumulations of noncollagenous proteins that histologically stain intensely red with Masson's trichome stain and fail to do so with periodic acid-Schiff. They are sharply demarcated and interdigitate with the collagen fibrils, which retain their normal structure and organization. The lesions appear to concentrate around keratocytes, which often show nonspecific changes consisting of either degenerative or active intracellular changes. This has prompted some investigators to assume that the pathology lies within the keratocytes.

Ultrastructurally, electron-dense, rod-shaped crystals have been found that are 100 to 500 μm in diameter and of variable morphologic organization. Recent reports have shown these rod-shaped granules to be surrounded by microfibrils. The granules stain with protein stains and with Luxol fast blue, suggesting a phospholipid composition possibly from abnormal degradation of corneal epithelial cell membranes containing specific phospholipid-protein complexes. The stromal deposits could result from a genetic defect in processing or assembly of membrane-derived corneal epithelial proteins and phospholipids. Also immunohistologic stains show that the deposits react at the edges with antibodies to form microfibrillar protein. These granules have been noted not only in the superficial stroma but also in the epithelial and subepithelial layers. An epithelial etiology has been suggested by the detection of these granules intraepithelially as well in both primary and recurrent dystrophy.

Granular corneal dystrophy is localized in the cornea without associated ocular or systemic disease. It has, however, been noted to occur coincidentally in a family with retinal degeneration and albinism and in another family with ectodermal dysplasia.

THERAPY

Supportive. Granular dystrophy has variable expressivity and therefore may remain asymptomatic in some patients. Even when it progresses, it does so late in life, starting during the fifth or sixth decade. Recurrent erosions are rare, but when they do occur, they do so late in the disease and are treated symptomatically with lubrication, patching, or even soft contact lenses. The lenses may control the recurrence of the erosions and may help improve visual acuity, as they mask the epithelial irregularity.

Surgical. When the opacities progress and coalesce and the visual acuity decreases sufficiently to interfere with the patient's lifestyle, surgical treatment is recommended. Since the opacities usually lie in the superficial stroma, Descemet's membrane and endothelium remain unaffected even when the opacities extend deep into the stroma. Therefore, a lamellar keratoplasty should be adequate to achieve a clear cornea devoid of opacities. However, since the visual results obtained with penetrating keratoplasty are superior to those after lamellar keratoplasty, penetrating keratoplasty has become the procedure of choice. The success rate of clear grafts maintained for over 10 years after penetrating keratoplasty for granular dystrophy is over 90 per cent.

PRECAUTIONS

Although uncommon, granular dystrophy may recur in either a lamellar or penetrating graft between 1 and 19 years after the surgical procedure. This recurrence may be related to repopulation of the donor cornea with "diseased" host epithelium or keratocytes. It most commonly occurs as a deposition of the hyaline opacities between the epithelium and Bowman's membrane. These subepithelial deposits often can be shaved off with a Bard-Parker blade in the office, with prompt healing following pressure patching in 2 to 3 days.

COMMENTS

The hyaline deposits may represent a metabolic product of corneal epithelial cells, rather than a product of collagen breakdown, since the hyaline material is a noncollagenous protein with an amino acid composition that is similar to keratohyaline. However, these deposits fail to react with antibodies to keratin. They have recently been shown to contain phospholipids and microfibrillar proteins. The location of the deposits, the chemical composition, and the recent demonstration of intracellular changes in the overlying epithelium in primary and recurrent granular dystrophy support the concept that the epithelium, rather than the keratocytes, may be the source of this abnormal material.

The best criterion at present for a definite diagnosis of granular dystrophy is transmission electron microscopy, which reveals the characteristic electron-dense, crystalline, rod-shaped bodies.

References

Akiya S, Brown SI: Granular dystrophy of the cornea, characteristic electron microscopic lesion. Arch Ophthalmol 84:179–192, 1970.

Brownstein S, et al: Granular dystrophy of the cornea. Light and electron microscopic confirmation of recurrence in a graft. Am J Ophthalmol 77:701–710, 1974.

Rodrigues MM, Krachmer JH: Recent advances in corneal stromal dystrophies. Cornea 7:19–29, 1988.

Rodrigues MM, Gaster RN, Pratt MV: Unusual superficial confluent form of granular corneal dystrophy. Ophthalmology 90:1507–1511, 1983.

Rodrigues MM, et al: Microfibrillar protein and phospholipid in granular corneal dystrophy. Arch Ophthalmol 101:802–810, 1983.

Spencer WH: Ophthalmic Pathology. Philadelphia, WB Saunders, 1985, Vol. I, pp 320–325.

Waring GO III, Rodrigues MM, Laibson PR: Corneal dystrophies. I. Dystrophies of the epithelium, Bowman's layer and stroma. Surv Ophthalmol 23:71–122, 1978.

Supported in part by an unrestricted grant from Research to Prevent Blindness, Inc. and supported in part by Ophthalmic Research Core Grant EY-01931.

INFECTIOUS CRYSTALLINE KERATOPATHY 371.40

ROGER H. S. LANGSTON, M.D., C.M., F.A.C.S.

Cleveland, Ohio

Infectious crystalline keratopathy is an unusual disease characterized by snowflake-like or crystalline-appearing infiltrates in the corneal stroma. There is no corneal inflammation and a variable amount of associated conjunctival or uveal inflammation. It is progressive, usually at a slow rate, and leads to significant permanent corneal scarring.

The usual cause of infectious crystalline keratopathy is *Streptococcus viridans*, although the condition has been caused by other varieties of streptococcus, *Hemophilus aphrophilus*, and *Staphylococcus aureus*. It seems that most of the cases have occurred postkeratoplasty. Predisposing influences seem to be a history of corneal edema and the use of topical steroids. Most cases also have had an epithelial defect, although some have not. In those cases without an epithelial defect, the access of the organism seems to have been through a suture track.

THERAPY

Ocular. All cases of infectious crystalline keratopathy known to the author have been sensitive to a wide variety of antibiotics in vitro, but have proved to be quite treatment resistant, with limited response to topical antibiotics alone. However, intensive topical ophthalmic therapy is appropriate. The author's best results have been obtained with cefazolin* (50 mg/ml) and gentamicin§ (14 mg/ml), one drop of each at hourly intervals for a week, and then tapering doses.

Topical steroids should be continued in a sufficient dose to suppress uveitis.

Surgical. Definitive treatment is by keratectomy. A successful outcome is achieved when the procedure is performed either as a simple keratectomy or as a penetrating keratoplasty. Since *Streptococcus viridans* is capable of causing endophthalmitis, penetrating keratoplasty should be preceded by intensive topical antibiotics.

Successful excimer laser phototherapeutic keratectomy has recently been described in a case that did not respond to topical antibiotic therapy.

Ocular or Periocular Manifestations

Conjunctiva: Variable bulbar injection; watery discharge.

Cornea: Crystalline-appearing infiltrates, sometimes multifocal, in the anterior stroma, may be under or near an epithelial defect or at the margin of a corneal transplant, may slowly increase in size or may rapidly increase in size and be associated with an endothelial plaque and hypopyon.

Other: Variable amounts of uveitis and sequelae of uveitis.

PRECAUTIONS

Although most cases of infectious crystalline keratopathy have been caused by *Streptococcus viridans*, it has been seen with other organisms. A similar picture can be seen in fungal infections and, rarely, with postkeratoplasty calcium deposition. Hence, isolation of the organism for culture and sensitivities is appropriate. Since the infection is intracorneal and not suppurative, biopsy rather than scraping may be necessary to establish the etiology.

Although topical steroid usage seems to predispose to this infection, the temptation to discontinue steroids should be resisted. In the author's experience, two eyes were lost to secondary glaucoma from uveitis when steroids were discontinued. Both patients, who had a history of herpes simplex keratitis, had a dense endothelial plaque and hypopyon. Other patients with identical findings have responded well to continuation of topical steroids plus addition of topical antibiotics, though some eventually required a keratectomy.

COMMENTS

Almost all cases of infectious crystalline keratopathy have occurred in corneas that were once edematous or in patients on topical steroids. Several cases have occurred in patients with ocular herpes simplex disease, and a few cases have been seen concomitant with corneal *Acanthamoeba* infections. These conditions and epithelial defects seem to predispose to crystalline keratopathy. One can postulate that the previous corneal edema has caused potential spaces in the corneal stroma that the organisms then invade. Compromise of the immune system in the cornea may also play a role in the pathogenesis. It is less clear why the disease is so resistant to topical antibiotic treatment and, in fact, has occurred in patients while they were taking antibiotics to which the organism was found to be sensitive. In some patients, the strain of *Streptococcus viridans* was a dextran former, which may make the organism more treatment resistant in vivo.

The goals of treatment of infectious crystalline keratopathy are multiple: control of the infectious process, control of associated uveitis, and restoration of vision. It is not easy to tell when the infection is adequately controlled. In one patient, a pathology specimen taken after 2 weeks of hourly topical antibiotic treatment showed viable replicating organisms. In another patient, the crystalline pattern persisted for months, although in most patients it fades to a stromal scar over a period of weeks. Loss of crystalline pattern and decreasing uveitis suggest successful control of the infection and should be used as a guide in tapering antibiotic treatment.

A successful routine for treating this disease is intensive topical antibiotics plus topical steroids (as indicated earlier) for approximately 1 week. If there has not been a dramatic response, then partial keratectomy is performed. Unless penetrating keratoplasty is contraindicated for some reason, it is performed when anterior uveitis is controlled.

References

Davis RM, et al: Acanthamoeba keratitis and infectious crystalline keratopathy. Arch Ophthalmol 105:1524–1527, 1987.

Eiferman RA, Ogden LL, Snyder J: Anaerobic peptostreptococcal keratitis. Am J Ophthalmol 100: 335–336, 1985.

Eiferman RA, et al: Excimer laser ablation of infectious crystalline keratopathy. Arch Ophthalmol 110:18, 1992.

Gorovoy MS, et al: Intrastromal noninflammatory bacterial colonization of a corneal graft. Arch Ophthalmol 101:1749–1752, 1983.

Groden LR, Pascucci SE, Brinser JH: *Haemophilus aphrophilus* as a cause of crystalline keratopathy. Am J Ophthalmol 104:89–90, 1987.

Kincaid MC, Snip RC: Antibiotic resistance of crystalline bacterial ingrowth in a corneal graft. Ophthalmic Surg 18:268–271, 1987.

Meisler DM, et al: Infectious crystalline keratopathy. Am J Ophthalmol 97:337–343, 1984.

Nanda M, et al: Intracorneal bacterial colonization in a crystalline pattern. Graefes Arch Clin Exp Ophthalmol 224:251–255, 1986.

Weisenthal RW, et al: Postkeratoplasty crystalline deposits mimicking bacterial infectious crystalline keratopathy. Am J Ophthalmol 105:70–74, 1988.

JUVENILE CORNEAL EPITHELIAL DYSTROPHY 371.51
(Meesman's Corneal Dystrophy)

PETER R. KASTL, M.D., Ph.D.

New Orleans, Louisiana

Meesman's corneal dystrophy has autosomal dominant inheritance, as do most corneal dystrophies. This rare disease causes infrequent discomfort and minimal (if any) visual loss. However, mild discomfort and slightly decreased vision may occur in later life. Slit-lamp findings include epithelial bleblike lesions that appear to direct illumination as whitish-gray, small punctate opacities, but which on retroillumination appear as clear, spherical vesicles. The overlying epithelium is clear. Histopathologically, small cysts are found throughout the epithelium, which are the vesicles seen on retroillumination. These contain debris and are most numerous in the anterior third of the epithelium. Electron microscopy demonstrates a "peculiar substance" in the cytoplasm, seen more often in the basal cells. This substance appears to be fibrillo-granular material, probably derived from degeneration of cytoplasmic filaments.

THERAPY

Ocular. Treatment is not usually called for. Bandage soft contact lenses can reduce any symptoms that may occur. If vision is decreased markedly, debridement or even lamellar keratoplasty can be done.

Ocular or Periocular Manifestations

Cornea: Epithelial cysts; irregular astigmatism; superficial haze.
Other: Decreased vision; irritation.

PRECAUTIONS

Corneal debridement has its own attendant complications, including scarring and infection. Prolonged wear of soft contact lenses also may result in infection; patients placed on long-term soft lens wear should be examined periodically for side effects of lens wear.

COMMENTS

The exact mechanism of this disease process has not been elucidated. The material in the cysts stains with Alcian blue and colloidal iron, indicative of glycosaminoglycans. This substance appears to be degenerated cellular material. Increased glycogen is present.

References

Alkemade PP, Balen AT: Hereditary epithelial dystrophy of the cornea: Meesman type. Br J Ophthalmol 50:603–605, 1966.

Bourne WM: Soft contact lens wear decreases epithelial microcysts in Meesman's corneal dystrophy. Trans Am Ophthalmol Soc 84:170–182, 1986.

Burns RP: Meesman's corneal dystrophy. Trans Am Ophthalmol Soc 66:530–635, 1968.

Fine BS, Yanoff M, Pitts E, Slaughter FD: Meesman's epithelial dystrophy of the cornea. Am J Ophthalmol 83:633–642, 1977.

Nakanishi I, Brown SI: Clinicopathologic case report: Ultrastructure of the epithelial dystrophy of Meesman. Arch Ophthalmol 93:259–263, 1975.

Pülhorn G, Thiel HJ: Light and electron microscope studies of cyst formation in Meesman-Wilke hereditary corneal epithelial dystrophy. Ophthalmologica 168:348–359, 1974.

Roca PD: Meesman's hereditary epithelial dystrophy (differential diagnosis). Eye Ear Nose Throat Monthly 48:424–425, 1969.

Thiel HJ, Behnke H: On the extent of variation of hereditary epithelial corneal dystrophy (Meesman-Wilke type). Ophthalmologica 155:81–86, 1968.

Tremblay M, Dube I: Meesman's corneal dystrophy: Ultrastructural features. Can J Ophthalmol 17:24–28, 1982.

Wittebol-Post D, van Bijsterveld OP, Delleman JW: Meesman's epithelial dystrophy of the cornea. Biometrics and a hypothesis. Ophthalmologica 194:44–49, 1987.

KERATOCONJUNCTIVITIS SICCA 370.33
(Dry Eye Syndrome, KCS, Keratitis Sicca, Sjögren's Syndrome [710.2])

MOGENS S. NORN., M.D., Ph.D.

Copenhagen, Denmark

In a dry eye, the exposed part is deficiently covered by a liquid film. The precorneal film does not fully cover the underlying epithelium. The intervals between two blinks leave dry spots in the film. The epithelium dries up before the next blink rewets the area concerned.

A diagnosis of dry eye can be made objectively by controlling the break-up time (BUT). A BUT below 10 seconds is regarded as pathologic, this period being shorter than the interval between two blinks. The procedure presupposes, however, the use of correct BUT technique (correct fluorescein concentration [0.125 per cent], no touching of the lid, no previous tests, etc.) or of special nontouch techniques without fluorescein.

The BUT depends on the composition of the precorneal film. A thin layer of fat is found superficially, which reduces evaporation of the underlying layer of fluid. Under this layer is a layer of mucus, which the lid movements cause to be rubbed in between the villi of the epithelial cells and which covers the epithelium. Hence, it follows that dry eyes may be due to abnormalities of the layers of fat, fluid, or mucus.

A reduced superficial fatty layer of the precorneal film may enhance evaporation and thus cause dry eyes. A reduced layer of fat has been observed in cases of recurrent corneal erosions. The composition of fat breakdown products immediately below this layer is perhaps of greater importance to the surface tension of the precorneal film. In sick building syndrome (pollution keratoconjunctivitis), the fat layer, influenced by volatile organic compounds or surface active substances in the environment, is reduced.

A deficient tear secretion is the essential cause of dry eyes. It may be caused by the congenital absence of lacrimal glands or arrested innervation or form part of the sicca syndrome. Keratoconjunctivitis sicca is a condition marked by dry eyes and is diagnosed by a pathologic BUT (less than 10 seconds), pathologic rose bengal staining of exposed area (with Bijsterveld score greater than 3.5 out of 9 possible), and pathologic Schirmer test I (below 5 mm in 5 minutes for elderly persons and below 10 mm for younger patients).

In Sjögren's syndrome, keratoconjunctivitis sicca is associated with general disorders. In primary Sjögren's syndrome, dryness of the oral cavity is a typical sign. In so-called secondary Sjögren's syndrome, rheumatoid arthritis or another connective tissue disease, presumably with an autoimmune basis, is also present.

Altered mucus production may be the cause of dry eyes. In keratoconjunctivitis sicca, a greatly enlarged thread is found in the fornix conjunctiva, partly owing to a slow mucous thread flow and partly caused by increased numbers of desquamated epithelial cells. In addition, filiform formations (corneal mucous plaques) may occur on the cornea. These phenomena all indicate an abnormally viscous mucus, which perhaps may be regarded as an inconvenient compensation for the reduced tear secretion.

A reduced amount of mucus is seen in xerophthalmia (vitamin A deficiency). This form of dry eye is one of the most frequent causes of blindness all over the world. Xerophthalmia is treated with vitamin A (see the section, Hypovitaminosis A).

The amount of mucus is also reduced in conjunctival pemphigoid, in which the mucosa keratinizes and the number of goblet cells declines drastically. In such cases, the lacrimal puncta may gradually become occluded, and the tear secretion declines correspondingly.

In addition to the stated causes of dry eyes due to altered contents of the precorneal film (fat, tears, and mucus), abnormal eyelid positions (ectropion, lagophthalmos with a fairly pronounced closing defect exophthalmos), defective blinking reflex action in its widest sense, palpebral coloboma, and denervated cornea are also possible causes. These abnormalities render the concept of dry eyes more comprehensive. Permanently dry spots (BUT = zero) occur in cases of epithelial bullae on the cornea (Fuchs' endothelial dystrophy, granulated cornea in acute glaucoma, graft complications). This phenomenon may be explained as dry eye-induced uneven epithelial surface. In addition, actual systemic treatment can be the cause of reduced tear production (beta blockers, psychopharmacologic drugs, antidepressives, atropine, and some antiestrogens). Thus, dry eyes have many causes and, of course, must be treated differently dependent on the cause.

Symptoms are not always expressed by the patient as a sensation of dryness. The complaints may include smarting pain, itching, a feeling of grains of sand in the eyes, irritation, photophobia, and dimness of vision. The symptoms are often intermittent, with periods of improvement during some of which there may paradoxically be complaints of epiphora!

THERAPY

Ocular. In some cases, the precorneal film can be stabilized in such a manner that the BUT is prolonged, preferably so much as to prevent the epithelium from drying up before it is covered again by tears on the next blinking. Desiccation of the epithelial cells is thereby avoided, and the rose bengal stainability decreases. Unfortunately, most drops have no effect after 30 to 60 minutes. Frequent instillations are therefore required. Their effect may be difficult to assess, because the syndrome may alter spontaneously in severity.

Local treatment of the sicca syndrome may either aim at increasing the aqueous phase, reducing the outflow of the aqueous phase, or acting on the mucous or lipid phase. The simplest agents having the least side effects should be employed in attempts to eliminate the symptoms or render them bearable.

INCREASING THE AQUEOUS PHASE. The simplest procedure is to instill sodium chloride, either physiologic (0.9 per cent) or the even more physiologic balanced salt solution, which is a little more expensive. Since the lacrimal fluid of sicca patients is hyperosmotic, it seems reasonable to employ a hypo-osmotic fluid (0.45 per cent sodium chloride). This treatment "cleanses" the eye. Having no side effects, it is agreeable to the patient, but its effect is too short-lived.

Efficient therapy is made possible by special rinsing apparatuses attached to spectacles or a contact lens; however, this equipment is not commercially available. A dry eye irrigation system, consisting of a 40-ml circular plastic container to be worn under the clothes, can supply about 10 ml of fluid under pressure every 24 hours and is adjustable (4 to 20 ml) by means of a screw. The fluid is led to the inner canthus through PVS tubing fastened with adhesive tape on the forehead. In addition, tight-fitting swimmer's goggles with a humid atmosphere produced by a wet tuft of cotton inside the goggles can be worn. These arrangements are troublesome, and the goggles get steamy. Their use is therefore limited to desperate cases.

REDUCING THE OUTFLOW OF TEARS. It is possible to economize on the scant amount of tears by reducing or completely obstructing the outflow. Doing so, however, results in a reflectorily reduced tear secretion; in other words, the reverse of the desired effect. The lacrimal puncta can be closed temporarily by a gelatin rod, plugs, or tissue glue; however, experience with gelatin rods has been disappointing. Occlusion of both puncta is required to obtain a good effect. Permanent occlusion by cautery is only indicated, if at all, in quite desperate, maximally pronounced cases, after temporary occlusion of both lacrimal puncta of the same eye with objective evaluation of the result. This surgical intervention must be undertaken with great care right into the canaliculus and on the lacrimal puncta to ensure a permanent result.

Mucomimetics, or artificial tears with methylcellulose or polyvinyl alcohol, are muciform agents of high molecular weight that retain the lacrimal fluid in their meshes, thus retarding the outflow. The BUT is prolonged as a result. Although the favorable response is of longer duration than that of sodium chloride, typically lasting 30 to 60 minutes, frequent instillations six to twelve times daily or more often are often necessary. The drops have no side effects other than disagreeable plastic-like films along the palpebral ciliary margins. The favorable effect can be increased by raising the concentration of the active agent to a certain maximum; however, the inconvenient film will likewise increase. Therefore, in a mild case of keratoconjunctivitis sicca, a low concentration should be instilled. The grave cases should be treated frequently with gradually increasing concentrations, and different mucomimetics should be tried. Experience has shown that these agents are of no use in chronic simple conjunctivitis. A patient with a normal BUT gains nothing by having it prolonged, but will be troubled by drying up of the viscous fluid along the ciliary margins.

Methylcellulose and similar agents (hydroxypropyl methylcellulose) are to be used initially in a concentration of 0.5 per cent. These solutions are excellent media for bacterial growth; therefore, preservatives should usually be added, although allergies commonly develop. The concentration may be raised to 1.5 per cent, at which level the BUT improves maximally (BUT prolonged four times). At higher concentrations, the methyl-

cellulose becomes too stiff to be supplied in a tube and can be spread less readily over the precorneal film. The BUT will then be inconveniently shortened.

Polyvinyl alcohol (PVA) is less viscous than methylcellulose. Many, therefore, prefer PVA, whereas others give definitive preference to methylcellulose. No explanation can be given for this difference of opinion. PVA is usually used in a concentration of 1.4 per cent; in severe cases, 3 per cent or even higher concentrations are used. Maximum BUT response is obtained using 10 per cent PVA (BUT prolonged seven times). At higher concentrations, the BUT will fall again.

Viscoelastic Substances. In cataract extraction, sodium hyaluronate* in a 1 per cent concentration has a better protective effect on the cornea than the above mucomimetics. Sodium hyaluronate, a long, nonramified molecular chain, is viscoelastic in aqueous solution. Sodium hyaluronate 0.2 per cent is more effective than sodium hyaluronate 0.1 per cent in the treatment of keratoconjunctivitis sicca. Chondroitin sulfate is another viscoelastic substance with a great affinity for the cornea; it is more effective than polyvinyl alcohol in keratoconjunctivitis sicca, but is not yet available (Marquardt, 1991).

Many lubricating and rewetting solutions for use with conventional hard contact lenses, soft (hydrophilic) contact lenses, and contact lenses made with other new polymers are mucomimetics. These solutions also can be tried in cases of keratoconjunctivitis sicca. Other muciform agents—dextran, carbomer (polyacryl acid gel), and gelatin—may have a favorable effect.

A drug-release system that liberates a mucomimetic for 8 to 16 hours has been invented. A hydroxypropyl cellulose ophthalmic insert, supplied in aluminum foil, is placed on the inferior tarsal conjunctiva by the aid of a special applicator.

A soft contact lens can maintain the aqueous phase in the same manner as mucomimetics. Unfortunately, the sicca patient is often exposed to secondary bacterial infection, owing to reduced amounts of lysozyme, lactoferrin, and other bactericides in the scant lacrimal fluid. Therefore, these patients are badly suited for wearing contact lenses, and this treatment is hazardous because of keratitis. As a general rule, a BUT below 10 seconds should be a relative contraindication to wearing contact lenses.

Epithelial-Protecting Topical Treatment. SUCRALFATE (sodium-aluminium-sucrose-sulfate) is a well known gastric mucosal protectant with a possible growth-factor-promoting effect. In an open study, the rose bengal score improved after topical treatment. As expected, the Schirmer test and BUT were not changed (Prause, 1991).

Tear-Stimulating Polypeptides. Tachykinins (peptides consisting of 11 amino acids) can stimulate tear secretion by vasodilation, perhaps also with other favorable effects on the tear film. Physalaemine was first obtained from the skin of a South American toad (physalaemus fuscumaculatus). Eledoisin was extracted from the salivary gland of the mediterranean octopus (Eledona moschata) and has now been synthesized. It has been useful in some pronounced cases that were treated topically three times daily for more than 10 years (Marquardt, 1991). Systemic levels of pilocarpine may increase the tear secretion, though hardly efficiently and without causing too pronounced general side effects.

Prolactin and estrogens are modulating hormones of lacrimal gland function. Oophorectomy in the rat causes atrophic changes in the lacrimal gland (Lemp, 1992). Perhaps systemic or topical treatment with one of these hormones could be used in the future.

The patient may be advised to stay in a moist room. Unfortunately, very few evaporators and air-conditioning plants are sufficiently efficient to yield a high enough degree of moisture to be of any aid to the patient with keratoconjunctivitis sicca. Transplantation of small pieces of salivary gland in humans has succeeded subjectively and objectively as judged by vital staining, Schirmer test, and ptyalin in tears and biopsy (Murube, 1992).

ALTERING THE MUCOUS PHASE. Doubleblind tests with bromhexine,[‡] a cough mixture that reduces the viscosity of mucous sputum and bronchial exudates in vivo though not in vitro, have shown that this agent has a favorable effect in some cases of keratoconjunctivitis sicca. The bromhexine seems to alter the mucous phase in keratoconjunctivitis sicca. BUT and Schirmer I tests have shown improvement. Bromhexine is recommended in a daily dose of 24 to 48 mg, distributed over three doses. If no improvement is registered within 2 or 3 weeks, the daily dose should be increased to 96 mg divided into three doses and given for 1 or 2 weeks. This is an expensive treatment, which, if effective, should be continued for years under regular control. Bromhexine is contraindicated in patients with peptic ulcer. The possibility of topical ocular bromhexine[*] treatment is currently being studied.

Acetylcysteine acts enzymatically on sputum in vitro, opening disulfide compounds in the sulfhydryl groups of mucoproteins with a consequent reduction of the viscosity. In keratitis sicca, filiform formations (corneal mucus plaques) on the cornea can possibly be improved by treatment with 10 per cent acetylcysteine.[*] However, the eyedrops have a nasty smell (like a rotten egg), and the shelf-life is limited. Removal of these mucous-covered cell strands can also be attempted by a few instillations of 0.67 per cent silver nitrate at intervals of some weeks.

Many sicca patients prefer alkaline eyedrops combined with methylcellulose. These solutions contain 0.6 per cent sodium chloride, 0.45 per cent sodium bicarbonate, 0.5 per cent sodium carboxymethylcellulose, 0.005 per cent chlorhexidine, and water and have a pH of approximately 8.45. The rationale for the use of the alkaline drops is unknown, but a modification of the properties of the conjunctival mucus is a possibility.

ALTERING THE LIPID PHASE. When the lipid phase is reduced, evaporation of the precorneal film will increase. However, the lipid phase is not reduced in keratoconjunctivitis sicca. Accordingly, treatment with ointment or drops is not indicated. Such treatment is, in fact, contraindicated, as it shortens the BUT. In sick building syndrome (pollution keratoconjunctivitis), the treatment is prophylactic (ventilation, temperature, cleaning, etc.) to avoid diminished lipid phase in the tear film. Trials with lipids (topic emulsions, "intralipid" moisture) are in progress.

Ocular or Periocular Manifestations

Conjunctiva: Hyperemia (secondary to bacterial infection); retarded mucous flow; thick and viscous mucous threads.

Cornea: Complicating keratitis; epithelial defects from which filaments may proceed; leukoma; pannus; ulcer.

Eyelids: Chronic, squamous blepharitis.

PRECAUTIONS

Many patients have conjunctival complaints; however, only few of these patients suffer from the dry eye syndrome. It is of decisive importance to establish the diagnosis, because mucomimetics are beneficial for patients with the syndrome, whereas patients with other disease are greatly troubled by such viscous drugs.

Treatment of the ciliary margin with ointment is difficult because ointment shortens the BUT. By blinking, ointment passes into the precorneal film, even though it is applied on the palpebral ciliary margins alone. Intense ointment massage (80 per cent petroleum jelly and 20 per cent liquid paraffin) is recommended, but only at night. Ointment and oil drops (fats) are contraindicated in keratitis sicca during the day, because blinking spreads fat over the precorneal film with consequent shortening of the BUT and thus further drying of the eye.

In the treatment of keratoconjunctivitis sicca, it is advisable to start with the simplest therapy possible having the least side effects. The response is evaluated more on the basis of the subjective improvement than by objective criteria, because the objective methods (BUT, Schirmer I, rose bengal vital staining, tear ferning) are unfortunately not fully reliable.

Occlusion of the lacrimal puncta may cause a reflectory reduction of the existing scant tear secretion.

The treatment of keratitis sicca is lifelong.

Consequently, allergies, especially to the preservatives employed, have a considerable chance of development. Use of mucomimetics without a preservative may be required. However, they require frequent changes of eye drop bottles to avoid contamination. The reduced tear secretion in KCS, with consequently decreased amounts of lysozyme, lactoferrin, and other bactericidal principles in the tears, will often give rise to secondary bacterial infections. One is therefore often forced to use antimicrobial therapy with the risks involved—the development of resistant microorganisms, allergy, and toxic side effects.

Topical ophthalmic steroid treatment is contraindicated owing to a risk of bacterial infection. General steroid treatment and antimetabolic treatment of Sjögren's syndrome have been tried; however, controlled tests have not substantiated any effectiveness of these agents thus far.

Blink-instructions may be of benefit in contact lens wearers with inadequate blinking and dry eye feeling provocated by the use of contact lens.

COMMENTS

Dry eyes may have many causes—vitamin A deficiency, pemphigoid, lagophthalmos, etc.—and must accordingly be treated differently dependent on the cause. If, for example, the dry eye syndrome is caused by treatment with beta blockers, such as timolol, discontinuation of this agent should be considered. In most cases, however, the dryness is a transitory phenomenon, and the beta blocker can be continued.

Keratoconjunctivitis sicca is the most frequent form, particularly among elderly patients; it is sometimes included in Sjögren's syndrome. The shortened BUT is treated primarily with the simplest drug that is sufficiently effective (1.4 per cent PVA or a 0.5 per cent methylcellulose derivative). At the same time, one should bear in mind that the disease is cyclic, with alternate improvement and aggravation. During periods of aggravation, the therapy may be intensified (higher concentration, use of other mucomimetics, or other principles), with the pathology of the precorneal film (lacrimal and mucous phases) being taken into consideration.

References

Dohlman CH: Punctal occlusion in keratoconjunctivitis sicca. Ophthalmology 85:1277–1281, 1978.

Jones BR, Coop HV: The management of keratoconjunctivitis sicca. Trans Ophthalmol Soc UK 85:379–390, 1965.

Lemp M: Dry eye treatment strategies. Dacriology News 7. International Symposium on the Lacrimal System. Bruxelles, May 23–24, 1992, pp 14–15.

Lemp MA, Hamill JR Jr: Factors affecting tear film breakup in normal eyes. Arch Ophthalmol 89:103–105, 1973.

Lindahl G, Calissendroff R, Carle B: Clinical trial of sustained-release artificial tears in keratoconjunctivitis sicca and Sjögren's syndrome. Acta Ophthalmol 66:201–205, 1988.

Mackie IA, Seal DV: The questionably dry eye. Br J Ophthalmol 65:2–9, 1981.

Marquardt R, Lemp MA (eds): Das trochkene Auge in Clinik und Praxis. Berlin, Springer-Verlag, 1991.

Murube del Castillo J: Lacrimal gland surgical management. Dacriology News 7. International Symposium on the Lacrimal System. Bruxelles, May 23–24, 1992, p 18.

Norn MS: Treatment of keratoconjunctivitis sicca with liquid paraffin or polyvinyl alcohol in double-blind trials. Acta Ophthalmol 55:945–950, 1977.

Norn MS: Quantitative tear ferning. Acta Ophthalmol 66:201–205, 1988.

Norn MS: Pollution keratoconjunctivitis: A review. Acta Ophthalmol 70:269–273, 1992.

Norn MS, Opauski A: Effects of ophthalmic vehicles on the stability of the precorneal film. Acta Ophthalmol 55:23–34, 1977.

Poirier RH, Ryburn FM, Isreal CW: Swimmer's goggles for keratoconjunctivitis sicca. Arch Ophthalmol 95:1405–1406, 1977.

Prause JU: Beneficial effect of sodium sucrose sulfate on the ocular surface of patients with severe KCS in primary Sjögren's syndrome. Acta Ophthalmol 69:417–421, 1991.

Prause JU, Norn MW: Relation between blink frequency and break-up time? Acta Ophthalmol 65:19–22, 1987.

Ruben M, Trodd C: Constant perfusion for dry eyes and sockets. Br J Ophthalmol 62:268–270, 1978.

van Bijsterveld OP: Diagnostic tests in the sicca syndrome. Arch Ophthalmol 82:10–14, 1969.

KERATOCONUS 371.60

KHALAD A. NAGY, M.D.,
and ROBERT ABEL, JR., M.D.

Wilmington, Delaware

Keratoconus is a noninflammatory thinning and ectasia of the cornea of unknown course. It tends to be bilateral, involving the inferocentral portion of the cornea. It affects central vision relatively early, becomes manifest in the first three decades, and results in progressive visual impairment due to highly irregular myopic astigmatism. In advanced cases, the involved area takes the shape of a truncated cone and can be seen as Munson's sign on downgaze. Keratoconus is usually an isolated finding, but may be seen in certain systemic diseases, such as Down's syndrome, Marfan's syndrome, Leber's familial amaurosis, Ehlers-Danlos syndrome, and mitral valve prolapse. It has also been noted in people with atopic allergies and those individuals who rub their eye vigorously.

The ectasia usually starts around puberty and progresses slowly for 5 to 10 years, often becoming stationary. Diagnostic findings include subepithelial scarring, vertical striae in the deep stroma, Fleischer's ring, a progressive irregularity of the corneal mires, and abnormal corneal and retinoscopic reflexes. Corneal thinning is usually confined to the central two-thirds of the cornea, but may progress to the limbus in cases of keratoglobus. There is often photophobia and decreasing corneal sensation; rarely there is increased visibility of the corneal nerves. Occasionally, there is a rupture in Descemet's membrane, giving rise to acute hydrops.

THERAPY

Ocular. Usually by the time keratoconus is diagnosed, the K readings have changed and the myopic astigmatism has increased to a point that special correction is difficult. Some people stabilize in the early stages (form fruste). However, the majority of people require special rigid gas-permeable lenses to correct the highly irregular astigmatism; these must be fit very carefully so as to maintain some movement and yet vault the core without being ejected by routine blinking. Usually the steep-fitting lens may contribute to subepithelial scarring and recurrent corneal erosion. When vision is compromised or contact lenses can no longer be tolerated, then keratoplasty must be considered.

Surgical. Penetrating keratoplasty remains the definitive therapy for keratoconus. Such alternatives as thermokeratoplasty, lamellar keratoplasty, and epikeratoplasty have been tried in the past two decades as alternatives to intraocular surgery. However, these less invasive procedures have fallen short of producing the potential 20/20 visual acuity that is possible with full-thickness corneal transplantation. The success rate of penetrating keratoplasty is 90 to 95 per cent, but this procedure carries with it associated complications, the most frequent being high postkeratoplasty astigmatism (requiring contact lens wear). The authors are currently evaluating a bevel-edged surgical technique that has limited the amount of astigmatism and has provided the opportunity for postkeratoplasty spectacle correction in our first ten patients.

Ocular or Periocular Manifestations

Cornea: Inferocentral corneal steepening and thinning; subepithelial or anterior stromal scarring; Fleischer's ring; decreased corneal sensation and rarely acute hydrops.

Other: Photophobia; mild conjunctival erythemia; Munson's sign; progressive myopic astigmatism and occasionally association with other systemic diseases.

PRECAUTIONS

The rapid diagnosis of keratoconus minimizes patient uncertainty and allows for appropriate selection of the options. Keratometry becomes highly irregular and provides limited information. The placido disk, keratoscope, and now computerized corneal topography provide increasing information about the surface of the cornea. Corneal mapping through computerized photokeratoscopy detects even subclinical cases, provides a diopter plot in all cases, and suggests more accurate information for contact lens fitting of the keratoconus patient. It is also wise to perform corneal topography in order to avoid inadvertent refractive surgical procedures (radial keratotomy, photorefractive ablation) on the early cases.

COMMENTS

It is difficult to know the progression of keratoconus when the patient presents initially. It is also possible that contact lens wear may aggravate keratoconus. In fact, polymethylmethacrylate (PMMA) wear in the past has been associated with the development of keratoconus in a limited number of cases; these individuals usually do not have the typical iron line in the basal epithelial cells. The rare congenital cavity in the posterior keratoconus has no relationship with the current discussion. On the other hand, progressive thinning to and beyond the limbus (keratoglobus) may be seen in extreme cases of the disease. In these cases, large tetanic lamellar grafts are required to stabilize the cornea before any refractive penetrating graft can be performed. Patients with keratoconus should be instructed about trauma and continuous eye protection.

References

Arentsen JR, Laibson PR: Thermokeratoplasty for keratoconus. Am J Ophthalmol 82:447–449, 1976.

Ayoub M: The pathology of the eye. *In* Ectatic Corneal Dystrophy, 2nd ed. Osman, Cairo-Arab Contractor Press, 1990, pp 76–77.

Boger WP III, Petersen RA, Robb RM: Keratoconus and acute hydrops in mentally retarded patients with congenital rubella syndrome. Am J Ophthalmol 91:231–233, 1981.

Burato L, Ferrari M, Rama P: Excimer laser intrastromal keratomileusis. Am J Ophthalmol 113: 291–295, 1992.

Frangieh GI, Kwitko S, McDonnell PJ: Prospective corneal topographic analysis in surgery for postkeratoplasty astigmatism. Arch Ophthalmol 109: 506–510, 1991.

Gittinger JW, Asdwrian GK: Manual of Clinical Problems in Ophthalmology. Boston, Little, Brown, 1988, pp 43–45.

Goosey JD, Prager TC, Goosey CB, Bird EF, Sanderson JL: Comparison of penetrating keratoplasty to epikeratoplasty in the surgical management of keratoconus. Am J Ophthalmol 111:145–151, 1991.

Kennedy RH, Bourne WM, Dyer JA: A 48-year clinical and epidemiologic study of keratoconus. Am J Ophthalmol 101:267–273, 1986.

Kirkness CM, Ficker LA, Steele AD, Rice NS: Refractive surgery for graft induced astigmatism after penetrating keratoplasty for keratoconus. Ophthalmology 98:1786–1792, 1991.

Langston DP: Manual of Ocular Diagnosis and Therapy, 2nd ed. Boston, Little, Brown, 1985, p 104.

Smiddy WE, et al: Keratoconus: Contact lens or keratoplasty? Ophthalmology 95:487–492, 1988.

Tabbara KF, Butrus SI: Vernal keratoconjunctivitis and keratoconus. Am J Ophthalmol 95:704–705, 1983.

LATTICE CORNEAL DYSTROPHY 371.54
(Lattice Dystrophy Type I, Lattice Dystrophy Type II, Lattice Dystrophy Type III, LCD-I, LCD-II, LCD-III, Meretoja's Syndrome)

ROBERT A. HYNDIUK, M.D., and ERIN S. FOGEL, M.D.

Milwaukee, Wisconsin

Lattice corneal dystrophy type I (LCD-I) is an autosomal dominant dystrophy that usually affects both eyes symmetrically. It is characterized by a localized corneal deposition of amyloid that is unrelated to systemic disease. It appears in the first or second decade of life as characteristic refractile anterior stromal branching filamentous lines, focal white dots or dashes, or faint central stromal opacities. The deposits are prominent centrally and spare the peripheral 2 to 3 mm of cornea. The dystrophy is slowly progressive, with the lesions involving deeper cornea and the opacity becoming denser and visually disabling usually by the third or fourth decade. Occasionally, the first symptoms of the disease may be noted in childhood or in the sixth or seventh decade; there is a considerable variation among different families in the age at which symptoms appear. Symptoms of photophobia, foreign body sensation, and pain from recurrent corneal epithelial erosions may be prominent in some patients. As corneal sensation decreases, the recurrent epithelial erosions become less painful. Irregular surface corneal astigmatism further decreases functional vision. Clinically, some forms of LCD-I have been misdiagnosed as herpes simplex keratitis during erosion episodes.

The characteristic microscopic finding in the stroma is a fusiform deposit of amyloid that pushes aside the collagen lamellae, probably corresponding to the lattice lines and dots seen clinically. Portions of Bowman's membrane are replaced by the deposits and irregular connective tissue. These changes are associated with recurrent erosions clinically.

The stromal deposits appear pink histologically with Congo red and exhibit dichroism and increased birefringence. Electron microscopy of the lesions shows a felt-like mass of fine (8- to 10-mm diameter), nonbranching short fibrils without periodicity that are approximately half the size of adjacent collagen and are sometimes associated with amorphous, electron-dense elastoid material. The keratocytes often have prominent endoplasmic reticulum, and they show degeneration. Immunohistochemical studies have detected lectin receptors, suggesting a variety of amyloid glycoconjugates. The source of amyloid accumulation is unknown, but could be related to keratocytes or activated mononuclear cells.

Lattice corneal dystrophy type II (LCD-II, Meretoja's syndrome) is an autosomal dominant form of LCD with an onset of clinical signs in the third decade. It is associated with systemic amyloidosis, including signs of progressive cranial and peripheral nerve palsies, dry skin, blepharochalasis, protruding lips, a "mask-like" facies, and bundle branch block. It is more common in Scandinavian countries, and only a few cases have been reported in the United States. The vision is usually not reduced significantly as it is in LCD-I. Also, the corneal lattice lines are fewer in number and are densest in the midperiphery with relative axial sparing; most reach the limbus. The cornea is usually clearer between the lattice lines than in type I. Histologically, the corneal deposits are similar to those of LCD-I, with amyloid often surrounding nerve axons in peripheral stroma. Amyloid deposits are also found in conjunctiva below epithelium, in skin often around adnexal appendages, and in subepidermal areas. Recently, LCD-II has been shown to be due to a mutation in the gelsolin gene.

Lattice corneal dystrophy type III (LCD-III) has an adult onset, autosomal recessive inheritance. The lattice lines are thick and ropey, extending from limbus to limbus, and are easy to see with direct illumination. LCD type III-A may be a variant of type III. It occurs in Caucasians, is associated with corneal erosions, and has an autosomal dominant inheritance pattern.

THERAPY

Ocular. Epithelial irregularities may result in recurrent erosions and cause additional visual loss from the irregular surface. Artificial tears, lubricating ointments, intermittent pressure patching, and soft contact lenses help control the recurrent erosions. Therapeutic soft contact lenses may also be helpful in improving vision, sometimes dramatically, by correcting the irregular surface.

Surgical. Penetrating keratoplasty has become the procedure of choice with a high success rate (approximately 90 per cent). However, the dystrophy may recur in up to 48 per cent of grafts after periods ranging from 3 to 26 years postoperatively; the recurrences usually take the form of subepithelial opacities or anterior stromal haze, and rarely lattice figures. In one large series, regrafting was necessary to restore vision in 15 per cent of penetrating keratoplasties for LCD-I.

Ocular or Periocular Manifestations

Cornea: Central stromal opacity; decreased corneal sensitivity; pseudodendritic staining; recurrent epithelial erosion; refractile anterior stromal lines; white stromal dots.

Other: Epiphora; irritation; ocular pain; photophobia; visual loss from opacity and irregular surface.

PRECAUTIONS

Diagnosis may occasionally be a problem, especially in some children. Examination of the child's parents may be helpful. Pseudodendritic corneal lesion during erosion episodes may be misdiagnosed as herpes simplex keratitis.

The patient should be advised about the risk of postoperative recurrence of dystrophy in the graft. Lattice corneal dystrophy recurs more commonly than macular or granular corneal dystrophy.

COMMENTS

Some investigators consider the lattice lines to represent degenerated corneal nerves, but in typical LCD-I, there is no clear relationship between the corneal nerves and the amyloid deposits. The electron microscopic findings of a felt-like mass of short, fine, nonbranching fibrils are diagnostic for amyloid. Lattice dystrophy is unrelated to primary or secondary amyloidosis of the cornea. Keratocytes and possibly also corneal epithelial cells may have the ability to elaborate the amyloid material.

References

Dubord PJ, Krachmer JH: Diagnosis of early lattice corneal dystrophy. Arch Ophthalmol 100:788–790, 1982.

Gorevic PD, et al: Amyloidosis due to a mutation of the gelsolin gene in an American family with lattice corneal dystrophy type II. N Engl J Med 325:1780–1785, 1991.

Hida T, et al: Clinical features of a newly recognized lattice corneal dystrophy. Am J Ophthalmol 104:241–248, 1987.

Hida T, et al: Histopathologic and immunochemical features of lattice corneal dystrophy type III. Am J Ophthalmol 104:249–254, 1987.

Klintworth GK: The cornea—structure and macromolecules. Am J Pathol 89:719–808, 1977.

Meisler DM, Fine M: Recurrence of the clinical signs of lattice corneal dystrophy (type I) in corneal transplants. Am J Ophthalmol 97:210–214, 1984.

Meretoja J: Lattice corneal dystrophy—two different types. Ophthalmologica 165:15–37, 1972.

Panjwani N, et al: Lectin receptors of amyloid in corneas with lattice dystrophy. Arch Ophthalmol 105:688–691, 1987.

Purcell JJ, et al: Lattice corneal dystrophy associated with familial systemic amyloidosis (Meretoja's syndrome). Ophthalmology 90:1512–1517, 1983.

Rodrigues MM, Krachmer JH: Recent advances in corneal stromal dystrophies. Cornea 7:19–29, 1988.

Spencer WH: Ophthalmic Pathology. Philadelphia, WB Saunders, 1985, Vol I, pp 320–325.

Starck T, et al: Clinical and histopathologic studies of two families with lattice corneal dystrophy and familial systemic amyloidosis (Meretoja syndrome). Ophthalmology 98:1197–1206, 1991.

Stock EL, et al: Lattice corneal dystrophy type IIIA. Clinical and histopathologic correlations. Arch Ophthalmol 109:354–358, 1991.

Sturrock GD: Lattice corneal dystrophy: A source of confusion. Br J Ophthalmol 67:629–634, 1983.

Waring GO III, Rodrigues MM, Laibson PR: Corneal dystrophies. I. Dystrophies of the epithelium, Bowman's layer and stroma. Surv Ophthalmol 23:71–122, 1978.

Supported in part by an unrestricted department grant from Research to Prevent Blindness, Inc., New York, New York, and NEI core grant EY01931.

Macular Corneal Dystrophy 371.55
(Fehr's Macular Dystrophy, Groenouw's Type II)

PETER R. KASTL, M.D., Ph.D.

New Orleans, Louisiana

Macular corneal dystrophy is one of the three "classical" stromal dystrophies; it differs from granular and lattice dystrophies by being autosomal recessive. Stromal opacities of mucopolysaccharide appear in the first decade of life, affecting the central anterior layers of the stroma. These opacities come into view as diffuse, grayish-white spots with blurry edges. By the third decade these opacities become more confluent and extend posteriorly to the endothelium and laterally to the limbus. Late in the disease subepithelial opacities cause irregularities of the epithelial surface. Recurrent erosions can occur with decreased corneal sensation. Visual loss progresses to legal blindness by age 40 to 50.

THERAPY

Surgical. Definitive therapy requires a corneal transplant, but the disease may recur in the graft. Before a graft is considered, a contact lens may improve vision by "smoothing" the irregular corneal surface.

Ocular or Periocular Manifestations

Cornea: Grayish stromal opacities with indistinct margins; irregular surface (late); corneal leukoma (late).
Other: Loss of vision; photophobia.

PRECAUTIONS

Corneal transplantation may result in graft rejection. Lamellar keratoplasty is not successful, as diseased stroma forms the bed of the graft; thus, corneal opacities can rapidly extend into a lamellar graft.

COMMENTS

The clinical diagnosis of macular corneal dystrophy is not that difficult, as the stromal opacities have fuzzy borders. As the disease progresses, the entire stroma is affected, causing irregularities of Descemet's membrane and epithelial irregularities. Treatment eventually requires a corneal transplant. The disease may recur in the graft.

The lesions of macular corneal dystrophy stain with Alcian blue and colloidal iron and have been identified as an abnormal glycosaminoglycan similar to keratan sulfate. This compound accumulates intracellularly in keratocytes and endothelium, but extracellularly in the stroma.

References

Akova YA, Kirkness CM, McCartney AC, Ficker LA, Rice NS, Steele AD: Recurrent macular corneal dystrophy following penetrating keratoplasty. Eye 4:698–705, 1990.

Edward DP, Thonar EJ, Srinivasan M, Yue BJ, Tso MO: Macular dystrophy of the cornea. A systemic disorder of keratan sulfate metabolism. Ophthalmology 97:1194–1200, 1990.

Jonasson F, Johannsson JH, Garner A, Rice NS: Macular corneal dystrophy in Iceland. Eye 3:446–454, 1989.

Li YP, Yi YZ, Zheng HL: Macular, lattice and granular dystrophy of the cornea: ultra-histochemistry and ultrastructure study. Yen Ko Ksueh Pao 5:122–126, 1989.

Meek KM, Quantock AJ., Elliott GF, et al: Macular corneal dystrophy: The macromolecular structure of the stroma observed using electron microscopy and synchroton X-ray diffraction. Exp Eye Res 49:941–958, 1989.

Midura RJ, Hascall VC, MacCallum DK, et al: Proteoglycan biosynthesis by human corneas from patients with types 1 and 2 macular corneal dystrophy. J Biol Chem 265:15947–15955, 1990.

Quantock AJ, Meek KM, Ridgway AE, Bron AJ, Thonar EJ: Macular corneal dystrophy: Reduction in both corneal thickness and collagen interfibrillar spacing. Curr Eye Res 9:393–398, 1990.

Quantock AJ, Meek KM, Thonar EJ: Analysis of high-angle synchrotron x-ray diffraction patterns obtained from macular dystrophy corneas. Cornea 11:185–190, 1992.

MOOREN'S ULCER 370.07

WILLIAM R. MORRIS, M.D.,
and THOMAS O. WOOD, M.D.

Memphis, Tennessee

Mooren's ulcer is a chronic painful ulceration of the cornea that begins in the periphery with an elevated, de-epithelialized leading edge and progresses centrally and circumferentially. If untreated, it is usually relentlessly progressive and may invade the entire cornea. As the ulcer progresses, a vascularized pannus forms in its wake. Perforation may occur spontaneously or as a result of minor trauma. Iritis can be severe enough to result in posterior synechiae, cataracts, and secondary glaucoma.

Two types of Mooren's ulcer are recognized: (1) unilateral ulcers that tend to be mild and responsive to therapy and (2) bilateral ulcers occurring simultaneously or nonsimultaneously that generally are more severe and less responsive to treatment. Bilateral simultaneous ulcers are the most refractory to therapy.

Associated trauma or corneal inflammation, such as caused by corneal foreign body, abrasion, or cataract surgery, is antecedent in about one-third of cases. Patients with herpes simplex keratitis, herpes zoster ophthalmicus, chemical burns, hidradenitis suppurativa, and connective tissue/vasculitis diseases, such as rheumatoid arthritis and polyarteritis nodosa, may also have Mooren's or Mooren's-like ulcers.

The basic etiology of Mooren's ulcer is unknown. Recent evidence indicates, however, that autoimmune processes, both humoral and cell mediated, may play a role. Accidental or surgical trauma, which is often the precipitating event, may alter a portion of the cornea (probably the epithelium) and cause it to become recognized as foreign tissue. The finding of many plasma cells and lymphocytes in the adjacent conjunctiva is supportive of an autoimmune etiology.

THERAPY

Ocular. The use of frequent topical steroids (initially every 30 to 60 minutes) and tapering over 2 months as the ulcer heals are of benefit. If there is no response to topical steroids, conjunctival resection should be considered.

Mooren's ulcer that develops after cataract surgery may respond to soft contact lens therapy. Some cases require topical steroids and soft contact lenses. Many cases are precipitated by a loose suture at the limbus; suture removal and topical steroid therapy are usually curative.

Topical antibiotics may be used to protect the eye from secondary infection while the ulcer is healing.

Surgical. Conjunctival excision is the therapeutic procedure of choice if topical steroids and soft lens therapy have failed. A 3-mm conjunctival resection adjacent to the ulcer with debridement of the ulcer bed and the leading epithelial edge is usually adequate. Tarsorrhaphy may be combined with conjunctival resection to assist epithelial healing. Surgery performed at an early stage of the disease may preserve vision.

Cyanoacrylate glue or lamellar grafting may be necessary if the ulcer perforates. Autogenous periosteal grafts have been used successfully in some cases in which the ulcer recurred after lamellar keratoplasty. In end-stage ulcers, removal of the remaining central island of stroma can facilitate healing.

Systemic cyclosporine or immunosuppression should be considered when local therapy fails.

PRECAUTIONS

Although a few cases of successful penetrating keratoplasty have been reported, Mooren's ulcer is often reactivated after keratoplasty or cataract surgery.

COMMENTS

The visual acuity in patients with Mooren's ulcer that has progressed across the central cornea may improve when the disease becomes inactive. The eyes develop a vascularized flap of conjunctival origin covering a markedly thinned stroma. Because of the risk of reactivating the ulcer in the graft after surgery, these patients are usually best served with the vision provided by their thin vascularized cornea.

References

Berkowitz PJ, et al: Presence of circulating immune complexes in patients with peripheral corneal disease. Arch Ophthalmol 101:242–245, 1983.

Brown SI, Mondino BJ: Penetrating keratoplasty in Mooren's ulcer. Am J Ophthalmol 89:255–258, 1980.

Brown SI, Mondino BJ: Therapy of Mooren's ulcer. Am J Ophthalmol 98:1–6, 1984.

Dingeldein SA, Insler MS, Barron BA, Kaufman HE: Mooren's ulcer treated with a periosteal graft. Ann Ophthalmol 22:56–57, 1990.

Foster CS: Systemic immunosuppressive therapy for progressive bilateral Mooren's ulcer. Ophthalmology 92:1436–1439, 1985.

Gottsch JD, Liu SH, Stark WJ: Mooren's ulcer and evidence of stromal graft rejection after penetrating keratoplasty. Am J Ophthalmol 113:412–417, 1992.

Hill JC, Potter P: Treatment of Mooren's ulcer with cyclosporin A: Report of three cases. Br J Ophthalmol 71:11–15, 1987.

Martin NF, Stark WJ, Maumenee AE: Treatment of Mooren's and Mooren's-like ulcer by lamellar keratectomy: Report of six eyes and literature review. Ophthalmic Surg 18:564–569, 1987.

Mahmood MA, Pillai S, Limaye SR: Peripheral ulcerative keratitis associated with hidradenitis suppurativa. Cornea 10:75–78, 1991.

Murray PI, Rahi AHS: Pathogenesis of Mooren's ulcer: Some new concepts. Br J Ophthalmol 68:182–187, 1984.

Smolin G, O'Connor GR: Ocular Immunology. Philadelphia, Lea & Febiger, 1981, pp 171–178.

Wakefield D, Robinson LP: Cyclosporin therapy in Mooren's ulcer. Br J Ophthalmol 71:415–417, 1987.

Wood TO, Tuberville AW, Murrah W: Corneal problems following cataract surgery. In Emery JM, Jacobsen AC (eds): Current Concepts in Cataract Surgery. New York, Appleton-Century-Crofts, 1981, pp 193–199.

NEUROPARALYTIC KERATITIS 370.35
(Neurotrophic Keratitis, Trigeminal Neuropathic Keratopathy)

IAN A. MACKIE, F.R.C.S., F.R.C.Ophth.

London, England

Neuroparalytic keratitis is a potential sequel to trigeminal anesthesia. The three most common causes of trigeminal anesthesia are surgery of the trigeminal neuralgias, surgery of acoustic neuromata, and herpes zoster ophthalmicus. In the latter disease, about 8 per cent of patients develop neuroparalytic keratitis. Other infrequent causes are trauma, tumors, multiple sclerosis, toxic chemical reactions, leprosy, and brainstem hemorrhages. Congenital forms, occurring notably in familial dysautonomia, may also be found. An idiopathic form has also been described.

There is a notion that the disease is caused by dust and foreign matter lodging in an anesthetic eye, and protective spectacles are often fitted. These contribute very little to the management of the disease. A number of studies have shown that about 15 per cent of patients with anesthetic eyes develop serious complications, and these complications may develop soon or many years after the initiation of trigeminal insensitivity. It is important to realize that the potentiality of having neuroparalytic keratitis can wax and wane, and this is an important concept in the long-term management of these patients.

Probably to develop a true neuroparalytic keratitis, one must have an insensitive eye in an insensitive environment. Sensation in either the cornea or conjunctiva, which may occur after gasserian ganglion destruction and which is often present after herpes zoster, spares the patient from the disease. Conjunctival sensation should be tested by applying a hypodermic needle to the palpebral conjunctiva above and below. This test, together with the assessment of corneal sensitivity with a wisp of cotton wool, has important practical considerations in diagnosis and prognosis. It is, for example, sometimes difficult to differentiate the viral epitheliopathy of zoster from that of neuroparalytic keratitis. In this case, the demonstration of sensation in either cornea or conjunctiva implies a viral etiology. Furthermore, the prognosis after an attack of herpes zoster or after a neurosurgical procedure can be established.

All patients with trigeminal anesthesia have excess mucus, or excess "sleep" in the morning to a greater or lesser extent. The discharge often clings to the lashes. It is important to recognize this mucus as a feature of the condition. It does not imply infection and it does not seem to be related to keratopathy. The entire palpebral conjunctiva may stain with rose bengal after gasserian ganglion destruction. This staining is an index of increased conjunctival epithelial cell death, but does not mean that an eye is dry and it does not seem to be related to the development of keratopathy. About 50 per cent of patients with trigeminal anesthesia have abnormalities of the tear film and cornea, and with fluorescein, geographic drying areas are often seen.

Transient blurring of vision is common at this level of the disease. Punctate epitheliopathy is also common. It may have a geographic distribution and be extensive enough to lead to a drop in visual acuity.

The signs so far described can be considered stage I of the disease. Stage II develops as an acute episode and is characterized by epithelial detachment. The patient is usually first aware of a marked drop in visual acuity and the eye may be somewhat hyperemic. Such epithelial detachments often occur in an area of cornea covered by the top lid. A gap is seen in the epithelium that is surrounded by an area of undermined epithelium extending some distance beyond the gap. Folds develop rapidly in Descemet's membrane, and aqueous flare and cells may be present. Stage III develops when stromal lysis is involved.

THERAPY

Ocular.

STAGE I. When severe, the punctate epitheliopathy is best treated with intermittent patching of the eye with tape, such as Blenderm, for one-third of the waking day. The patient picks the time period to fit his or her social schedule, for this patching may have to be continued for many months. In more severe epitheliopathy, the portion of the day during which the eye is covered may have to be increased. The tape used should be 2.5 cm wide and 3.75 cm long. The eye is shut by closing it with the top lid only, and the patient is carefully instructed not to squeeze the eye shut. The tape is applied to the top lid (not to the superior orbital margin) and is brought down to the lower lid. Cutting the lashes helps in the proper application of the tape.

The patient is told to carry a mirror for periodic inspection of the closure. Mucomimetics do not have any influence on the punctate keratopathy, but they do seem to have some action in preventing the onset of the acute stage II of the disease. For some reason, oral administration of 250 mg of oxytetracycline[‡] twice daily diminishes the amount of excess mucus produced by these eyes and may be continued for long periods.

Contact lenses have been advocated to control keratopathy at this stage. However, they have several disadvantages: patients often lose their lenses during sleep, the keratopathy is difficult to assess under a lens, and fluorescein may produce marked staining of the lens. The overwhelming disadvantage is the common incidence of severe "apparent" infection with the development of corneal abscesses, including ring abscesses. The word "apparent" was used because it is often difficult to grow organisms from these corneas. Hypopyons may develop with great rapidity. Many people with neuroparalytic keratitis are elderly, and there is often a delay before help is sought. Slight or increased redness of the eye may not be noticed.

Untreated, stage I of the disease can become chronic and lead to epithelial hyperplasia and underlying stromal nebulae, which are often vascularized. Band keratopathy can develop. At this stage of epithelial hyperplasia, considerable resolution can be brought about by total daily closure over a number of weeks, and this should always be tried before a corneal transplant is contemplated.

STAGE II. This stage can be reached on the same day as a destructive procedure on the trigeminal nerve. It is an indication for urgent treatment. Atropine should be instilled, and the eye should be closed with Blenderm or a temporary central tarsorrhaphy, using 5-0 black braided silk and rubber tubing. This second stage should *not* be treated with a therapeutic soft lens. If it is, within 12 hours a very red eye, a massive hypopyon, and very thick aqueous flare may be present.

STAGE III. The principal treatment is closure, and tape closure is appropriate only if there is adequate supervision. A temporary tarsorrhaphy may again have to be used. Atropine should be instilled and appropriate wide-spectrum antibiotic treatment instituted topically, and perhaps systemically, if the severity of the condition warrants it. Corticosteroids are contraindicated because they potentiate collagenase activity.

Permanent tarsorrhaphy is rarely necessary in neuroparalytic keratitis, although chronic and relapsing disease sometimes make it necessary for economic reasons. A thin central pillar that can be later thinned even further to about 2 mm wide is ideal, this is known as the "elastic band" tarsorrhaphy. In this way, the eye can still see when looking to either side and may have some acuity looking straight ahead.

A further method of closing an eye and obviating tarsorrhaphy has been found to be effective, and it can be used in all three stages of the disease. A dose of 6.25 to 12.5 $\times$ 10^{-5} μg of botulinum A toxin[†] is injected into the levator palpebrae superioris. This is reached by passing a 25-gauge long needle through the skin of the upper lid midway and just under the superior orbital rim. The needle is directed straight back as far as it will go. This procedure produces a profound ptosis in 3 to 4 days that lasts up to 6 weeks.

COMMENTS

Neuroparalytic keratitis is probably a disease of abnormal cell turnover. Epithelial thinning, but not stromal thinning, has been shown in monkeys after the destruction of the nerve or its ganglion. This did not occur with tarsorrhaphy alone. The thinned epithelium had fewer cells. Scanning electron microscopy of the conjunctiva has shown irregularity of the epithelial cells and abnormalities of the epithelial microvilli. The corneal microvilli may similarly be abnormal. It has been suggested that the cyclic nucleotides, the "second messengers" of hormone action, are involved in the regulation of corneal epithelial cell turnover and that there is an imbalance in the anesthetic eye leading to a decreased cellular turnover. Cyclic AMP has been shown to produce quiescence in cells. Cyclic GMP has been shown to initiate mitosis. Cholinergic stimulation has been shown to be associated with rapid accumulation of cellular cyclic GMP. The normal corneal epithelium is rich in acetylcholine, but the anesthetic corneal epithelium has been shown to have depleted acetylcholine. If this hypothesis is correct, it raises exciting possibilities for topical treatment with drugs that influence the cyclic nucleotide imbalance. Blockage at the level of adenylate cyclase, which catalyzes the formation of cyclic AMP, is a possibility. Beta-adrenergic blocking drugs are obvious choices for investigation. The beta receptor blocking agent, pindolol, has been reported to accelerate the healing of corneal epithelial defects in rabbits. This drug has been used in several corneal conditions (including neuroparalytic keratitis) with claimed success. Timolol was apparently ineffective in this respect. Antiprostaglandins may also work at this level. Another avenue of approach may be the cyclic nucleotide phosphodiesterases, which degrade cyclic nucleotides. This may be a more fertile approach owing to the apparent sensitivity of the phosphodiesterases to a wider selection of chemical structures.

References

Adams GGW, Kirkness CM, Lee JP: Botulinium toxin A induced protective ptosis. Eye 1:603–608, 1987.
Kahan A, Hammer H: Pindolol in the treatment of corneal disorders. *In* The Cornea in Health and Disease. (VIth Congress of the European Society of Ophthalmology). Royal Society of Medicine International Congress and Symposium Series No. 40. London, Academic Press, 1981, pp 1073–1075.
Mackie IA: Neuroparalytic (neurotrophic) keratitis. *In* Black CJ, et al. (ed): Symposium on Contact Lenses. St. Louis, CV Mosby, 1973, pp 125–142.
Mackie IA: The role of the corneal nerves in destructive diseases of the cornea. Trans Ophthalmol Soc UK 98:343–347, 1978.

PELLUCID MARGINAL CORNEAL DEGENERATION 371.48
(Corneal Piriformis)

MARK S. DRESNER, M.D., F.A.C.S., and DAVID J. SCHANZLIN, M.D.

St. Louis, Missouri

Pellucid marginal corneal degeneration or corneal piriformis affects the inferior peripheral cornea bilaterally and results in marked thinning of the cornea. There is usually no evidence of scarring, infiltration, vascularization, iron ring, or lipid deposition. This condition is most commonly diagnosed between the ages of 20 and 40 years and occurs equally in males and females. Patients usually present with high degrees of irregular astigmatism. The 1- to 2-mm wide band of corneal thinning is characteristically located near the inferior limbus, causing an area of cylindrical protrusion of the cornea. Concentric Descemet's folds can develop near the inferior limbus, and acute hydrops is an infrequent complication.

The etiology of pellucid marginal corneal degeneration is unknown; however, heredity does seem to be a factor. Recently, similar changes in the epithelium and basement membrane have been reported in pellucid marginal corneal degeneration and keratoconus; similarly, collagen, such as the fibrous long-spacing (FLS) type with a periodicity of 100 to 110 nm versus 60 to 64 nm in normals, is seen in this entity, as well as advanced keratoconus. Some authors suggest that the pellucid marginal corneal degeneration most likely represents a peripheral form of keratoconus. Bowman's layer may be normal, focally disrupted, or completely absent in the area of the thin band. Descemet's membrane and endothelium are usually normal.

THERAPY

Ocular. Spectacle correction is usually unsatisfactory because of the irregular and high astigmatism. Contact lenses are difficult to fit because of the degree of astigmatism; however, when they can be worn, their use results in good vision. When the disease has progressed to such an extent that hard contact lenses cannot be worn, fitting with a piggy-back contact lens system (therapeutic bandage lens with overlying hard lens) is frequently successful.

Surgical. Penetrating keratoplasty has provided good results for the treatment of the cylindrical corneal protrusion and, for this reason, is considered a viable treatment in advanced cases of pellucid marginal degeneration of the cornea. Alternative modes of therapy include corneal wedge resection and thermokeratoplasty. Additionally, inferior lamellar patch grafts have been successful in reducing the inferior ectasia of the cornea, which results from the marked corneal thinning, and have not only allowed patients to resume contact lens wear but have also reduced the degree of high astigmatism.

PRECAUTIONS

Penetrating keratoplasty frequently tends to be accompanied by more complications when performed for pellucid marginal corneal degeneration than when used for keratoconus, primarily because of the larger, at times, eccentric graft that must be positioned to reach the limbus inferiorly. Surgery with such large penetrating grafts has a greater tendency to vascularize and results in erosion of the sutures. Thermokeratoplasty remains an unproven procedure for this disorder; this technique should be approached with caution, since it has been shown to cause endothelial damage, as well as persistent epithelial healing problems. In cases where there has been contact lens failure, an inferior lamellar patch graft to stabilize the structurally weakened inferior cornea and to steepen the flat vertical meridian should be considered.

COMMENTS

Pellucid marginal corneal degeneration is an infrequently diagnosed disorder. The condition is rare, and most of the literature on this condition is from Europe. Pellucid degeneration of the cornea affects the inferior portion of the cornea and does not extend into the limbus; it is without vascularization or lipid infiltration, and the cornea retains normal sensitivity, thus differentiating it from other peripheral corneal thinning diseases, such as Terrien's marginal degeneration, Mooren's ulceration, or senile marginal degeneration. The central cornea retains normal thickness, and the high astigmatism results from the inferior weakening and bowing forward of the inferior cornea, also serving to differentiate this condition from other corneal disorders that result in high irregular astigmatism and corneal thinning, such as central

keratoconus, posterior keratoconus, keratoglobus, and keratotorus.

References

Cameron JA: Results of lamellar crescentic resection for pellucid marginal corneal degeneration. Am J Ophthalmol 113:296–302, 1992.
Carter JB, Jones DB, Wilhelmus KR: Acute hydrops in pellucid marginal corneal degeneration. Am J Ophthalmol 107:167–170, 1989.
Kolker AE, Hetherington J Jr: Becker-Shaffer's Diagnosis and Therapy of the Glaucomas. 4th ed, St. Louis, CV Mosby, 1976, p 397.
Krachmer JH: Pellucid marginal corneal degeneration. Arch Ophthalmol 96:1217–1221, 1978.
Krachmer JH, Feder RS, Belin MW: Keratoconus and related non-inflammatory corneal thinning disorders. Surv Ophthalmol 28:293–322, 1984.
Petursson GJ, Fraunfelder FT: Repair of an inadvertent buttonhole or leaking filtering bleb. Arch Ophthalmol 97:926–927, 1979.
Rodrigues MM, et al: Pellucid marginal corneal degeneration: A clinicopathologic study of two cases. Exp Eye Res 33:277–288, 1981.
Varley GA, Macsai MS, Krachmer JH: The results of penetrating keratoplasty for pellucid marginal corneal degeneration. Am J Ophthalmol 110:149–152, 1990.
Yannuzzi LA, Theodore FH: Cryotherapy of postcataract blebs. Am J Ophthalmol 76:217–222, 1973.

PHLYCTENULOSIS 370.31
(Phlyctenular Keratoconjunctivitis)

MICHAEL D. WAGONER, M.D.,
ANN M. BAJART, M.D., F.A.C.S.,
and MATHEA R. ALLANSMITH, M.D.

Boston, Massachusetts

Phlyctenular keratoconjunctivitis is a nodular inflammation of the paralimbal tissues that occurs mainly in children and young adults as an allergic hypersensitivity response in the conjunctiva or cornea to some antigen to which it has become sensitized. The disease has a worldwide distribution and is particularly common in areas where there are crowded and impoverished living conditions. In such areas, there is a higher incidence among females (60 to 70 per cent) than males. It occurs more often in spring and summer. In regions where phlyctenular keratoconjunctivitis is endemic, it is believed to be caused by sensitization to tuberculin antigen. In these regions, a very high percentage of patients with corneal opacities caused by recurrent phlyctenular disease show a positive reaction to 10 tuberculin units of purified protein derivative i.e., intermediate-strength tuberculin. In nonendemic areas, phlyctenular keratoconjunctivitis occurs somewhat less commonly and is almost always associated with sensitization to *Staphylococcus aureus*. It can be seen either in association with acne rosacea keratitis or seborrheic staphylococcal blepharoconjunctivitis. Determination that *S. aureus* is the sensitizing antigen in these cases is partially supported by reproduction of phlyctenulosis in rabbit models, with rabbits immunized and boosted with phenol-inactivated *S. aureus*. Phlyctenulosis has been described with infestation by intestinal parasites (Metazoa), *Candida albicans*, *Chlamydia*, coccidioidomycosis, herpes simplex virus, and gonococci. Rarely, phlyctenular keratoconjunctivitis can occur idiopathically.

The symptoms of conjunctival phlyctenulosis are usually mild to moderate itching, tearing, and irritation. A mucopurulent discharge may be seen if secondary bacterial infection has occurred. A rope-like tenacious mucus may be seen when the underlying cause is staphylococcal blepharoconjunctivitis. Although conjunctival phlyctenules may be found anywhere on the bulbar conjunctiva, they typically occur near the interpalpebral limbus as a small pinkish-white nodule in the center of a hyperemic area. In a few days, the superficial part of the nodule becomes gray and soft, the necrotic center sloughs, and the lesion clears rapidly. No scar remains.

The symptoms of corneal phlyctenulosis are usually much more severe. There is extreme photophobia, blepharospasm, foreign body sensation, and tearing. Corneal phlyctenulosis usually begins at the limbus; it rarely develops in the cornea itself. The corneal lesions can be classified into two main groups: corneal (nonvascularized) and limbal (vascularized). The corneal lesions tend to be bilateral. They occur as either a solitary opacity or a generalized nebular opacity. The limbal lesions are usually triangular in shape, with the base at the limbus. In the majority of cases, they occur inferiorly. The old, inactive lesions or scars may be wedge shaped, fascicular, or trapeziform. The typical active limbal phlyctenule lies astride the limbus as a pinkish-white mound bordered on the conjunctival side by a fan of dilated vessels. It may remain at this position and evolve through stages of necrosis, shelling out, and healing. It may also wander toward the center of the cornea as a progressively developing gray, necrotic, superficial ulcer surrounded by a white infiltrated area. The end stage of multiple attacks of phlyctenulosis is a confluent pattern of more or less vascularized superficial corneal scars. Scars on the visual axis may severely limit vision and occasionally produce blindness. Corneal perforation is rare.

Histologic examination of the phlyctenule shows lymphocytes, histiocytes, and plasma cells. Polymorphonucleocytes are found in necrotic lesions. Bacteria are not found in the lesion itself.

The diagnosis of phlyctenulosis is based upon identification of the typical morphologic features. Phlyctenular keratoconjunctivitis can be a potentially serious condition that can, in some cases, result in severe visual impairment or blindness. Therefore, it is the responsibility of the physician to provide adequate, quick diagnosis and, if possible, etiologic identification at the time of presentation. Mucopurulent material should be cultured so the appropriate antibiotic may be selected for treatment of the suprainfection. In endemic areas, a thorough tuberculosis workup is mandatory. Because of the relative infrequency of tuberculosis, evaluation for systemic tuberculosis is not necessary for patients in nonendemic areas if the underlying etiology is obvious.

The diagnosis of *Chlamydia* is suggested by the history of persistent, usually unilateral chronic conjunctivitis in a young, sexually active adult. The diagnosis of herpes simplex virus is usually established by the previous history. The hyperacute onset of gonococcal conjunctivitis usually makes this diagnosis obvious and requires immediate smears, cultures, and treatment. Coccidioidomycosis is usually found only in endemic areas and has distinctive systemic symptomatology.

The diagnosis of acne-rosacea-associated keratitis or staphylococcal blepharoconjunctivitis is usually obvious. If all of the preceding diagnoses can be excluded, the stools of the patient should be examined for intestinal parasites or their ova by direct or flotation method. In some cases, serologic tests for parasites may be helpful.

THERAPY

Ocular. For *phlyctenulosis associated with tuberculosis*, systemic antituberculous therapy should be given if tuberculosis is diagnosed as the primary cause (family history, physical examination, skin tests, and chest x-ray). The treatment for the ocular lesion is the application of topical corticosteroids. Until the lesions subside, 1 per cent prednisolone or 0.1 per cent dexamethasone may be administered every 2 hours for the first 2 to 4 days, followed by rapid tapering once improvement begins to occur. A prophylactic broad-spectrum antibiotic, such as bacitracin-polymyxin B ointment, is used topically two or three times daily while steroids are being used.

For *phlyctenulosis associated with acne rosacea* keratitis, the mainstay of therapy in adults and children over the age of 10 is orally administered tetracyclines. The use of 250 mg of oral tetracycline three or four times daily or 100 mg of oral doxycycline two times daily for approximately 2 to 4 weeks is recommended until the patient is less symptomatic. Then a maintenance dose of 250 mg of tetracycline or 100 mg of doxycycline every day is given as long as the patient tolerates the medication. The lesions tend to be quite sensitive to topical corticosteroids; patients usually respond to 1 per cent prednisolone or 0.1 per cent dexamethasone drops four to six times a day for several days, with rapid tapering as the response to therapy permits. An antistaphylococcal antibiotic, such as bacitracin ointment, is applied topically two to four times daily. Although it is quite unusual to see children with phlyctenular keratoconjunctivitis on the basis of acne rosacea alone, it is recommended that children under 8 years of age be treated with erythromycin systemically, rather than tetracycline, to avoid staining of the enamel of the developing permanent teeth that may occur with tetracycline drugs.

In *staphylococcal-induced phlyctenulosis*, the corneal lesions usually respond to topical steroid treatment as outlined for acne rosacea. It is helpful to use a topical antistaphylococcal antibiotic ointment, such as bacitracin, administered initially two to four times daily followed by tapering to bedtime use only. If the lid changes are sufficiently severe, systemic tetracycline or doxycycline should be used. The mainstay of therapy and future prevention is a vigorous program of warm compresses to the lids combined with generous lid hygiene. The lid margins may be cleaned up to four times daily initially with a cotton-tipped applicator moistened either with water or preferably baby shampoo diluted with water 1:5. With the eyes closed, the lids should be scrubbed with a cotton ball and rinsed with water. Hot compresses should be applied for at least 5 minutes after the cleaning. This should be done initially four times a day, but rapidly tapered to one or two times daily to encourage continued patient compliance.

If the patient is infested with *intestinal parasites*, the specific anthelminthic treatment should be given. Once again, the topical steroid regimen is dictated by the severity of the pathology and the rapidity of response. The appropriate treatment for *chlamydial keratoconjunctivitis with phlyctenulosis* is a 3-week course of oral tetracyclines (250 mg of tetracycline four times daily or 100 mg of doxycycline two times daily) combined with topical steroids that are tapered as soon as the phlyctenular component improves. Treatment for *gonococcal-related phlyctenulosis* consists of proper and rapid diagnosis from conjunctival smears and scrapings combined with the appropriate systemic antigonococcal therapy, as well as intensive topical tetracycline ointment or aqueous penicillin G[§] drops (100,000 units/ml). Steroids should be withheld until the ocular surface has been adequately sterilized. *Herpes simplex virus* is treated by the judicious concomitant use of topical steroids and topical antivirals. Topical steroids alone are usually sufficient to eradicate and control *idiopathic phlyctenulosis*.

One of the most serious complications of phlyctenular keratoconjunctivitis is frequent recurrent disease with significant corneal scarring and visual disability. Usually, the eradication of the offending organism, such as tuberculosis, Metazoa, *Chlamydia*, or gono-cocci, is sufficient to prevent subsequent recurrences. More troublesome is the recurrent disease that is often seen in patients with acne rosacea keratitis or staphylococcal blepharoconjunctivitis in which eradication of the sensitizing antigen is impossible. Patients with acne rosacea keratitis require maintenance on systemic tetracycline to prevent progressive corneal vascularization and scarring, as well as recurrent phlyctenulosis. If blepharitis is a significant component, meticulous attention to lid hygiene is necessary. Patients with staphylococcal blepharoconjunctivitis should be maintained on lid hygiene and warm compresses at least once a day indefinitely, supplemented with a topical antistaphylococcal antibiotic during exacerbations. Short-term or long-term tetracycline use may be necessary in some recalcitrant cases. The use of topical steroids should not be advocated for the long-term suppression of blepharitis-related disease, inasmuch as the possibility of cataract formation and increased intraocular pressure may result in more morbidity than the disease itself.

If significant corneal scarring and visual impairment occur, penetrating keratoplasty may be required for visual rehabilitation. Persistence of the underlying disease complicates the postoperative course and limits the prognosis. The goal of therapy for phlyctenular keratoconjunctivitis is to prevent the disease from progressing to this point.

Ocular or Periocular Manifestations

Conjunctiva: Hyperemia; infiltration; necrosis; nodules; ulcer.

Cornea: Cicatrization; infiltration; perforation; ulcer; vascularization.

Eyelids: Blepharospasm; chronic staphylococcal blepharitis; meibomianitis.

Other: Irritation; lacrimation; ocular pain; photophobia; pruritus; visual loss.

PRECAUTIONS

All patients receiving tetracycline should be warned of potential gastrointestinal disturbances, phototoxicity, and the risk of oral or genital candidiasis. The risks of topical steroid use should be discussed in advance. Penetrating keratoplasty for visual rehabilitation should be performed only when the ocular surface condition has stabilized and the eye has been noninflamed for several months.

COMMENTS

Acne rosacea keratitis and staphylococcal blepharoconjunctivitis are chronic conditions that are difficult or impossible to eradicate. Both diligent attention by the physician and compliance by the patient are required to maximize comfort, prevent recurrence of phlyctenular keratoconjunctivitis, and minimize long-term disability.

References

Allansmith MR, Ross RN: Phlyctenular keratoconjunctivitis. *In* Duane TD (ed): Clinical Ophthalmology. Philadelphia, Harper & Row, 1986, Vol IV, 8:1–6.

Beauchamp GR, Gillette TE, Friendly DS: Phlyctenular Keratoconjunctivitis. J Pediatr Ophthalmol Strabismus 18:220–228, 1981.

Duke-Elder S: System of Ophthalmology. St. Louis, CV Mosby, 1965, Vol VIII, pp 461–475.

Jakobiec FA, Lefkowitch J, Knowles DM: B- and T-lymphocytes in ocular disease. Ophthalmology 91:635–654, 1984.

Mandino BJ, et al: Rabbit model of phlyctenulosis and catarrhal infiltrates. Arch Ophthalmol 99: 891–895, 1981.

Zaidman GW, Brown SI: Orally administered tetracycline for phlyctenular keratoconjunctivitis. Am J Ophthalmol 92:173–182, 1981.

POSTERIOR POLYMORPHOUS CORNEAL DYSTROPHY 371.58
(Hereditary Deep Dystrophy, Hereditary Mesodermal Dystrophy, Keratitis Bullosa Interna, Koeppe's Posterior Polymorphous Degeneration, Schlichting's Dystrophy)

S. ARTHUR BORUCHOFF, M.D., *and* ROGER F. STEINERT, M.D.

Boston, Massachusetts

Posterior polymorphous dystrophy is an uncommon congenital corneal condition that is bilateral but not symmetric. It is characterized by vesicles at the level of Descemet's membrane, which often occur in groups or in a linear-oriented distribution and are surrounded by gray haze. Intervening areas of cornea appear normal. Descemet's membrane is thickened, and localized excrescences project into the anterior chamber or form bands or lines. White patches may be localized, or the entire posterior cornea may appear opacified. Most cases have clear stroma and epithelium, with little or no effect on vision.

Autosomal dominant inheritance with high penetrance and variable expression is suggested by most pedigrees; however, sporadic cases do occur, and pedigrees consistent with autosomal recessive inheritance have also been reported. The condition is generally stable or slowly progressive. Rarely, epithelial and stromal edema may occur and may lead to loss of vision.

Many cases are associated with anomalies of the iris and angle. Glaucoma may occur in association with angles that may appear either normal or abnormal. Posterior polymorphous dystrophy may thus be classified as a mesodermal dysgenesis (anterior cleavage disorder).

THERAPY

Ocular. Patients should be followed for glaucoma and treated appropriately. If corneal edema occurs, topical hypertonic sodium chloride is of little benefit for the edema, but no other medical measures are indicated.

Surgical. Epithelial and stromal edema and opacification of Descemet's membrane sufficient to cause marked impairment of vision are indications for penetrating keratoplasty.

Supportive. The patient and family should be reassured that most cases are mild and nonprogressive, with little or no effect on vision.

Ocular or Periocular Manifestations

Cornea: Band keratopathy; epithelial and stromal edema; focal or diffuse gray-white opacity in Descemet's membrane; linear bands in Descemet's membrane; sclerocorneal posterior embryotoxon; vesicles and excrescences with areolar haze protruding into the anterior chamber.

Eyebrows or Eyelashes: Heterochromia (rare).

Eyelids: Vitiligo.

Iris: Atrophy; corectopia; "glassy" iris membrane; heterochromia; iridocorneal adhesions to Schwalbe's ring or peripheral cornea; prominent iris processes; prominent Schwalbe's ring.

PRECAUTIONS

Because of the frequent association with glaucoma, periodic examinations of the patient are indicated. Elevated intraocular pressure may precipitate edema, which may be reversible with control of pressure. Family members should likewise undergo ophthalmologic evaluation.

COMMENTS

Significant visual impairment in the absence of edema is rare. Periodic examination with pachymetry reveals, whether the condition is progressive. Severe edema can obscure the posterior changes, and examination of family members may suggest the diagnosis in such cases. The condition may recur after keratoplasty.

References

Boruchoff SA, Kuwabara T: Electron microscopy of posterior polymorphous degeneration. Am J Ophthalmol 72:879–887, 1971.

Boruchoff SA, Weiner MJ, Albert DM: Recurrence of posterior polymorphous corneal dystrophy after penetrating keratoplasty. Am J Ophthalmol 109:323–328, 1990.

Cibis GW, et al: The clinical spectrum of posterior polymorphous dystrophy. Arch Ophthalmol 95: 1529–1537, 1977.

Grayson M: The nature of hereditary deep polymorphous dystrophy of the cornea: Its association with iris and anterior chamber dysgenesis. Trans Am Ophthalmol Soc 72:516–559, 1974.

Johnson BL, Brown SI: Posterior polymorphous dystrophy: A light and electron microscopic study. Br J Ophthalmol 62:89–96, 1978.

REIS-BÜCKLERS' SUPERFICIAL CORNEAL DYSTROPHY 371.52
(BÜCKLERS' ANNULAR CORNEAL DYSTROPHY)

FRANK M. POLACK, M.D., F.A.C.S.

Gainesville, Florida

Reis-Bücklers' dystrophy is a corneal disease characterized by recurrent epithelial erosions that start early in life, irregular corneal opacities, thickening of Bowman's membrane and the progressive reduction of visual acuity. It has a dominant mode of transmission, becomes evident in the first years of life, and has typical symptoms of foreign body sensation or pain related to corneal erosions. Vision is not affected until individuals are in their late twenties. Slit-lamp examination shows an irregular corneal surface with epithelial changes over areas of thickened Bowman's membrane. With diffuse illumination, opacities are detected at the level of Bowman's membrane and may extend toward the limbus. The opacities have initially a diffuse granular appearance that evolves to whitish interwoven ring-like opacities and occasionally may acquire a honeycomb appearance (different from honeycomb dystrophy). Corneal opacities vary with the age of the patient. Optical sections show normal stroma and endothelium. There is fluorescein staining of the corneal surface and decreased corneal sensitivity. Histology shows destruction of Bowman's membrane with replacement by fibrous tissue. This fibrous tissue is localized initially between the basal epithelial layer and Bowman's membrane. Except for fibroblastic proliferation and collagen deposition in the anterior third of the cornea, most histological studies found no anomalies in the stroma or endothelium. Electron microscopic studies show an abnormal epithelial layer with an irregular basement membrane. The fibrous subepithelial tissue is a mixture of normal collagen and an abnormal fibrous material that is called "curly collagen." This is considered typical of Reis-Bücklers' dystrophy. In some areas, Bowman's membrane is replaced by fibrous material and proliferation of keratocytes. This fibrous tissue may invade the stroma. Recent studies show that the "curly collagen" material has immunofluorescent staining for laminin and bullous pemphigoid antigen. The identification of this protein in the abnormal tissue suggests that it originates from the epithelial tissue, a concept that has been suggested in the older literature. The recurrent erosions are due to areas of epithelial breakdown because of an abnormal basement membrane and the destruction of hemidesmosomes.

THERAPY

Ocular. The treatment of Reis-Bücklers' dystrophy in early stages consists of the use of ocular lubricants and patching during the episodes of recurrent erosion. The use of soft (bandage) contact lenses with a high water content is not only helpful in some patients with frequent episodes of erosion but also improves their vision.

Surgical. When vision is compromised, a superficial keratectomy is preferable to a lamellar corneal graft. If the opacities are very superficial, this keratectomy sometimes can be performed at least twice before keratoplasty. Lamellar keratoplasty has a good prognosis. Recurrence of the disease may occur after keratectomy and keratoplasty, but may take several years.

PRECAUTIONS

Penetrating keratoplasty is not indicated as a primary procedure in this type of dystrophy.

COMMENTS

On the basis of electron microscopic findings and the immune histochemistry, it is believed that this disease is caused by the secretion of an abnormal protein from epithelial cells. An abnormal fibrillary material or "curly collagen" seems to be characteristic of this disease. The presence of laminin and bullous pemphigoid antigen within this material suggests that it may be an epithelial product. The proliferation of fibroblasts and fibrous tissue may be a secondary process. Some authors have proposed that the disease is caused by primary degeneration of Bowman's membrane, whereas others suggest that Reis-Bücklers' dystrophy, honeycomb dystrophy, and granular dystrophy are variants of the same disease.

References

Hogan MJ, Wood I: Reis-Bücklers' corneal dystrophy. Trans Ophthalmol Soc UK 91:41–57, 1971.

Lohse E, Stock EL, Jones JCR, et al: Reis-Bücklers' corneal dystrophy: Immunofluorescent and electron microscopic studies. Cornea 8:200–209, 1989.

Malbran ES: Corneal dystrophies: A clinical, pathological and surgical approach. Am J Ophthalmol 74:771–809, 1972.

Moller HU: Granular dystrophy Groenouw type 1 (Grl) and Reis-Bücklers' corneal dystrophy (R-B). One entity? Acta Ophthalmologica 67:678–684, 1989.

Olson RJ, Kaufman HE: Recurrence of Reis-Bücklers' corneal dystrophy in graft. Am J Ophthalmol 85:349–351, 1978.

Perry HD, Fine BS, Caldwell DR: Reis-Bücklers' dystrophy. A study of eight cases. Arch Ophthalmol 97:644–670, 1979.

Wood TO, et al: Treatment of Reis-Bücklers' corneal dystrophy by removal of subepithelial fibrous tissue. Am J Ophthalmol 85:360–362, 1978.

Yamaguchi T, Polack FM, Valenti J: Electron microscopic study of recurrent Reis-Bücklers' corneal dystrophy. Am J Ophthalmol 90:95–101, 1980.

SUPERIOR LIMBIC KERATOCONJUNCTIVITIS 370.32

(SLK, Theodore's Superior Limbic Keratoconjunctivitis)

ARDEN II. WANDER, M.D.

Cincinnati, Ohio

Superior limbic keratoconjunctivitis (SLK) is a puzzling entity first described by Theodore in 1963. The disease is characterized by inflammation of the upper palpebral conjunctiva that is manifested clinically by a papillary reaction. The upper bulbar conjunctiva becomes thickened and inflamed. Fine punctate fluorescein or rose bengal staining occurs on the upper cornea, limbus, and adjacent conjunctiva. Filaments occur at the superior limbus and cornea in about one-third of the cases. The condition is usually bilateral, but may be unilateral and occurs in all age groups. It lasts anywhere from weeks to many years with a characteristic course of remissions and exacerbations; at times it is worse in one eye and at times worse in the other eye. This characteristic history makes evaluation of therapy quite difficult.

The symptoms include burning, foreign body sensation, pain, epiphora, photophobia, blepharospasm, mild decrease in vision, and a pseudoptosis. Some patients also complain of a dry feeling in the eyes. Mucous discharge may also occur. The symptoms are significantly worse when filaments are present. Although superior limbic keratoconjunctivitis is not reported to be associated with dry eyes, 5 of Theodore's original 11 patients with SLK

did in fact have diminished tearing. Later, he reported in another study that perhaps 25 per cent or more of his cases had decreased tear secretion. He further reported one case of a patient with keratitis sicca who had filaments of the superior cornea from the SLK and of the inferior cornea from the keratitis sicca. Punctal occlusion cured the lower corneal staining, and the filaments disappeared from the lower portion but not the upper portion of the cornea. In the author's series, this association has been found in about 30 per cent of the cases.

The cause, and thus the definitive treatment, is unknown. There is an associated increased incidence of dysthyroid disease. Diagnosis may be confusing and at times difficult, but is important so that ineffective and often dangerous therapy may be avoided. The diagnosis is made by the characteristic history and clinical findings. In addition, scrapings of the involved bulbar conjunctiva help make the diagnosis. Theodore and Ferry (1970) verified Thygeson's observation that Giemsa-stained scrapings demonstrate keratinized epithelial cells. Scrapings of the upper palpebral conjunctiva show polymorphonuclear leukocytes. The author has observed a unique nuclear serpiginous change in Papanicolaou-stained cells scraped from the superior bulbar conjunctiva of patients with typical superior limbic keratoconjunctivitis. Within the preserved nuclear membrane, there is an unusual arrangement of chromatin condensation in the form of a coil or in the shape of the letters S or M. Biopsy of the involved bulbar conjunctiva reveals keratinization, dyskeratosis, acanthosis, balloon degeneration of the nuclei, and some cells with swollen pale-staining cytoplasm. Serpiginous changes in the nuclei are also seen in histologic sections.

THERAPY

Ocular. Treatment remains a significant problem. Silver nitrate in concentrations from 0.25 to 0.50 per cent applied by cotton-tipped applicators to the upper tarsal conjunctiva and at times the upper bulbar conjunctiva has remained the treatment of choice. This has been the time-honored therapy and may dramatically improve the patient symptomatically. Unfortunately, the signs and symptoms may recur anywhere from a few days to several months later. This therapy can be repeated. Scraping the superior bulbar conjunctiva and tarsal conjunctiva with a platinum spatula seems to accomplish the same purpose. Scraping may relieve symptoms for up to several weeks to a few months.

Pressure patching the worse eye daily for a full week at a time may relieve the symptoms in some patients. The following week, the nonpatched eye may be patched for a week at a time, changing the patch each day. This alternate patching technique has also been used successfully in conjunction with the use of a bandage contact lens in the nonpatched eye.

One drop of 10 or 20 per cent acetylcysteine* three to five times a day can be used for the excess mucus that is related to the filament formation. It may help decrease the symptoms when mucus and filaments are prominent. Bandage contact lenses may also be used when the filaments predominate.

Topical application of one drop of 4 per cent cromolyn‡ to the involved eye or eyes every 3 hours has been reported to be beneficial for some patients with SLK. When successful, treatment must be continued on a long-term basis because recurrences may occur upon discontinuing the medication.

Because associated problems, such as chronic blepharitis, may increase the symptoms, these problems should also be treated. Those patients who also have decreased tear secretion and inferior corneal staining should certainly be treated with artificial tears and advised to avoid contributing environmental factors, such as wind, smoke, and polluted environments. Patients with associated significant decreased tearing with inferior corneal staining and filaments may be helped from a symptomatic point of view by hydroxylpropyl cellulose ophthalmic insert used once or twice a day. However, these inserts do not help the superior punctate staining or the superior filaments. Punctal occlusion may also help these patients.

Surgical. A recession or resection of the involved superior bulbar conjunctiva has been recommended for more severe cases. An arcuate segment of conjunctiva and Tenon's is removed from the 10 to 2 o'clock meridian superiorly for 2 to 5 mm after a peritomy incision. The remaining superior edge of the conjunctiva may be sutured to the episclera with interrupted sutures or left alone. Unfortunately, the symptoms may recur as the conjunctival epithelium grows over the resected area. Cryotherapy to the involved superior bulbar conjunctiva has also been advocated for relief of symptoms. As with the use of the silver nitrate and surgical resection, however, the symptoms may recur in days to months after this treatment.

Ocular or Periocular Manifestations

Conjunctiva: Filaments; mucous discharge; punctate staining; thickened; upper bulbar hyperemia.

Cornea: Filaments; pannus; punctate staining.

Eyelids. Blepharospasm; pseudoptosis; upper palpebral conjunctival papillary reaction.

Other: Burning; decreased visual acuity; foreign body sensation; irritation; lacrimation; photophobia.

PRECAUTIONS

Because this condition is chronic, corticosteroids, which have little effect, should be avoided. The condition does not respond to antibiotics or antivirals, and these should also be avoided because of their potential toxic nature. Ptosis surgery performed on SLK patients with pseudoptosis may cause a significant increase in the patient's symptoms. Hence, care should be taken before surgery in the evaluation of all ptosis cases to ensure that the ptosis is not a pseudoptosis secondary to SLK.

Extra precautions must be maintained when treating patients who have associated decreased tear production. Close follow-up is necessary when bandage contact lenses are used because the complications from bandage contact lenses are significantly higher in patients with dry eyes. It has also been found that conjunctival recession or resection may not be as successful in patients who also have significantly reduced tearing. A scleral melt may occur in the exposed portion of the sclera after a conjunctival resection in patients with severe dry eyes. Hence, one should be more conservative in managing patients with SLK who also have dry eyes.

COMMENTS

Because the definitive cause of the condition is unknown, definitive therapy is lacking. Therapy is difficult. Also, because of the characteristic natural history of the disease, which includes periods of exacerbation and remission, care and caution must be taken in the evaluation of the therapy for this condition. This is especially true because the condition can in fact disappear without treatment. Because these patients often live in pain and discomfort for many years, the ophthalmologist must treat them with strong supportive efforts both medically and psychologically. These patients often become incapacitated from their condition and need back-up and support from their physician.

References

Cher I: Clinical features of superior limbic keratoconjunctivitis in Australia. A probable association with thyrotoxicosis. Arch Ophthalmol 82: 580–586, 1969.

Confino J, Brown SI: Treatment of superior limbic keratoconjunctivitis with topical cromolyn sodium. Ann Ophthalmol 19:129–131, 1987.

Donshik PC, et al: Conjunctival resection treatment and ultrastructural histopathology of superior limbic keratoconjunctivitis. Am J Ophthalmol 85: 101–110, 1978.

Grayson M: Diseases of the Cornea. St. Louis, CV Mosby, 1979, pp 86–92.

Mondino BJ, Zaidman GW, Salamon SW: Use of pressure patching and soft contact lenses in superior limbic keratoconjunctivitis. Arch Ophthalmol 100:1932–1934, 1982.

Passons GA, Wood TO: Conjunctival resection for

superior limbic keratoconjunctivitis. Ophthalmology 91:966–968, 1984.

Tenzel RR: Comments on superior limbic filamentous keratitis: Part 2. Arch Ophthalmol 79:508, 1968.

Tenzel RR: Resistant superior limbic keratoconjunctivitis. Arch Ophthalmol 89:439, 1973.

Theodore FH: Superior limbic keratoconjunctivitis. Eye Ear Nose Throat Monthly 42:25–28, 1963.

Theodore FH: Further observations on superior limbic keratoconjunctivitis. Trans Am Acad Ophthalmol Otolaryngol 71:341–351, 1967.

Theodore FH: Superior limbic keratoconjunctivitis. A summary. Mod Probl Ophthalmol 9:23–26, 1971.

Theodore FH, Ferry AP: Superior limbic keratoconjunctivitis. Clinical and pathological correlations. Arch Ophthalmol 84:481–484, 1970.

Wander AH, Masukawa T: Unusual appearance of condensed chromatin in conjunctival cells in superior limbic keratoconjunctivitis. Lancet 2:42–43, 1981.

Wright P: Superior limbic keratoconjunctivitis. Trans Ophthalmol Soc UK 92:555–560, 1972.

TERRIEN'S MARGINAL DEGENERATION 371.48
(Furrow Dystrophy, Marginal Ectasia, Peripheral Furrow Keratitis)

THOMAS L. STEINEMANN, M.D.

Little Rock, Arkansas

Terrien's marginal degeneration is an uncommon, slowly progressive thinning of the peripheral cornea. First described by Terrien in 1881 as a noninflammatory degeneration, its etiology is still unknown. Subsequent reports have described an "inflammatory" type of Terrien's degeneration that may occur in up to one-third of affected individuals. The disease is commonly bilateral, but may be asymmetric. It occurs more often in males. Patients may become symptomatic at any age, but the older literature has described more cases occurring in middle-aged and older patients. More recent series suggest that the disease is more common in the 20- to 40-year-old age group. It has even been described in children under 10 years of age. It is usually asymptomatic unless astigmatism develops.

Progression of the marginal ectasia usually occurs gradually over many years. Initially, the disease process is noted superonasally, heralded by fine peripheral superficial vessels and punctate stromal opacities that coalesce gradually. At this stage no thinning is usually noted, and it may resemble arcus senilis. An atypical pterygium occurring in an unusual oblique axis (pseudopterygium) has also been described as an early clinical sign in Terrien's degeneration.

Gradually the stroma starts to thin in a clear zone of cornea between the marginal opacities and the limbus, forming a gutter-like furrow. The furrow remains covered with epithelium and has a sloping peripheral edge and a steep central edge. Yellow-white deposits, which appear to be lipid, are seen at the edge of the deepening furrow. The paralimbal thinning often progresses across the superior cornea. It may extend into the inferior cornea or even circumferentially, but usually spares the interpalpebral cornea. The epithelium remains intact throughout the progression of thinning, and patients do not typically complain of pain. Patients become symptomatic as the ectasia results in astigmatism, which is usually against-the-rule, and causes blurred vision. In 10 to 15 per cent of cases, severely thinned areas may perforate, either spontaneously or with minor trauma. Occasionally, patients experience pain associated with episodic inflammation that resembles conjunctivitis, episcleritis, or scleritis.

THERAPY

Supportive. No medical therapy is effective in preventing the progression of corneal thinning. In the early stages, supportive therapy consists of spectacle correction of astigmatic refractive errors. With the progression of astigmatism, rigid contact lenses or "piggyback" soft/rigid lens systems may be necessary.

Surgical. In advanced cases of Terrien's marginal degeneration, contact lens fitting may no longer be possible. In addition, ectatic areas may become dangerously thin. At this stage, surgical repair may be indicated both to decrease visually handicapping astigmatism and to prevent the rupture of ectatic areas through tectonic reinforcement. Various surgical techniques have been suggested. One approach involves the excision of ectatic tissue followed by suturing of the freshened edges of normal-thickness stroma. In another technique a large eccentric penetrating keratoplasty is placed, although the increased possibility of graft rejection in such large transplants increases the chance of graft failure. An annular peripheral penetrating keratoplasty technique has also been described. More recently, inlay lamellar crescentic keratoplasty has been used to treat severe thinning or perforation. In this technique, donor lamellar tissue—stroma, Bowman's layer, and, in some cases, epithelium—may be obtained by hand dissection from a whole eye. Alternatively, donor lamellar tissue may be obtained as a commercially available precarved lyophilized tissue (Keratopatch,[R] Allergan Medical Optics, Irvine, CA). A lamellar keratectomy is first performed in the area of thinning. The lamellar graft is then anchored to one edge of the keratectomy bed and alternately cut free hand and sutured in a step-wise fashion in order to fill the defect.

Ocular or Periocular Manifestations

Cornea: Flattening of the corneal curvature in the vertical meridian; perforation (usually following minor trauma); peripheral thinning and ectasia; peripheral vascularization and lipid deposition; corneal hydrops; pseudopterygium.

Other: Episodic inflammation resembling conjunctivitis, episcleritis, or scleritis; high astigmatism with blurred vision.

PRECAUTIONS

In the majority of cases, conservative management is indicated. Because of the thinning and ectasia in more advanced cases, mild trauma can result in rupture of the cornea. Such patients should therefore be instructed to avoid situations in which the eye might be traumatized. The dispensing of protective eyewear may be warranted. Patients should be cautioned to seek attention for any abrupt change in their visual status or for the development of pain in the eye. Because of the high risk of corneal perforation, surgeons should avoid excising a pseudopterygium in Terrien's degeneration. Also, surgery for corneal ectasia should be restricted to those cases in which astigmatism is severe and disabling or if perforation occurs or is imminent.

COMMENTS

Although a rare disorder, Terrien's degeneration typically presents either when the patient becomes visually symptomatic because of progressive astigmatism or after recurrent episodes of ocular irritation. This slowly progressive, generally noninflammatory disease can usually be managed conservatively, but must be followed periodically for progression to thinning, which might threaten the integrity of the globe.

References

Caldwell DR, et al: Primary surgical repair of severe marginal ectasia in Terrien's marginal degeneration. Am J Ophthalmol 97:332–336, 1984.

Goldman KN, Kaufman HE: Atypical pterygium: A clinical feature of Terrien's marginal degeneration. Arch Ophthalmol 96:1027–1029, 1978.

Insler MS, et al: Terrien's marginal degeneration. *In* Brightbill FS (ed): Corneal Surgery—Theory, Technique, and Tissue, 2nd ed. St. Louis, CV Mosby, 1993, pp 325–328.

Kaufman HE, McDonald MB, Barron BA, Wilson SE: Color Atlas of Ophthalmic Surgery—Corneal and Refractive Surgery. Philadelphia, JB Lippincott, 1992, pp 147–166.

Robin JB, et al: Peripheral corneal disorders. Surv Ophthalmol 31:1–36, 1986.

THYGESON'S SUPERFICIAL PUNCTATE KERATOPATHY 370.21

HUGH P. WILLIAMS, F.R.C.S., F.R.C.Ophth.

London, England

Thygeson's superficial punctate keratopathy (TSPK) is a bilateral, coarse, punctate epithelial keratopathy occurring without ocular inflammation. The disease is very uncommon and runs a chronic course with exacerbations and remissions. Typically, the patient is young, usually under 40 years of age, and small children may be affected. The symptoms are of foreign body sensation, photophobia, and tearing. The coarse punctate epithelial lesions are faint gray in color, oval and irregular in shape, and may be seen with magnification. They appear anywhere on the cornea, but commonly in the central area. The lesions are slightly elevated and are composed of a multitude of tiny gray dots. There is never any stromal, anterior chamber, or conjunctival involvement. Each lesion is transient, undergoing a cyclic enlargement and diminution. Corneal sensation and tear lysozyme concentration are normal. Attacks usually undergo spontaneous remission in days to weeks, only to recur again within weeks or months. Recurrences may develop over any period of time, and this prolonged morbidity has been observed in patients for over 30 years. There are no residual abnormalities between attacks. The etiology of the disorder is not known; no pathogens have been proved to be causative, and in particular there is no substantiated evidence for a viral infection.

THERAPY

Ocular. There is no specific treatment for this disorder, but symptomatic relief provided by the use of topical ocular corticosteroids is dramatic. The lesions and symptoms begin to clear after 2 to 3 days of treatment. An effective regimen is administration of 0.1 per cent betamethasone* or 0.5 per cent prednisolone five times daily for 5 days, thereafter reducing the treatment in potency and frequency of daily applications until ocular comfort is achieved. Nonsteroidal anti-inflammatory eyedrops, such as fluorometholone or clobetasone†, are helpful. Soft therapeutic contact lenses worn on daily demand can relieve symptoms and avoid complications associated with continuous-wear lenses.

Ocular or Periocular Manifestations

Cornea: Punctate epithelial opacities.
Other: Decreased visual acuity; irritation; lacrimation; photophobia.

PRECAUTIONS

Corneal scraping with or without chemical cauterization is ineffective in this disorder, as the lesions recur quickly. The keratopathy does not respond to antimicrobials or antiviral therapy. The potential hazards of topical ophthalmic corticosteroid therapy as used in this disorder must always be borne in mind.

COMMENTS

Thygeson's superficial punctate keratopathy is not a common or communicable condition. It is misdiagnosed most frequently as herpes simplex, trachoma-inclusion conjunctivitis, adenoviral keratitis, keratoconjunctivitis sicca, and staphylococcal keratoconjunctivitis. Such misdiagnoses, together with the fact that TSPK is a periodically remitting disorder, have resulted in the use of numerous ocular drugs with unmerited successes and not unexpected failures.

Characteristically, there is no residual scarring, but it has been observed in coincidental association with vernal keratoconjunctivitis and may occur with other external eye diseases capable of causing corneal scarring. The misuse of idoxuridine eyedrops may result in subepithelial opacities. The rapid response to corticosteroid therapy suggests a hyperimmune or dyskeratotic mechanism, although this has not been proved.

The decrease in visual acuity is usually minimal; however, exacerbations may reduce it to 20/60. Between attacks, it returns to normal.

References

Abbott RL, Forster RK: Superficial punctate keratitis of Thygeson associated with scarring and Salzmann's nodular degeneration. Am J Ophthalmol 87:296–298, 1979.

Goldberg DB, Schanzlin DJ, Brown SI: Management of Thygeson's superficial punctate keratitis. Am J Ophthalmol 89:22–24, 1980.

Jones BR: Thygeson's superficial punctate keratitis. Trans Ophthalmol Soc UK 83:243–245, 1963.

Thygeson P: Clinical and laboratory observations on superficial punctate keratitis. Am J Ophthalmol 61:1344–1349, 1966.

van Bijsterveld OP, Mansour KH, Dubois FJ: Thygeson's superficial punctate keratitis. Ann Ophthalmol 17:150–153, 1985.

Williams HP, Mackie IA: Current management of Thygeson's superficial punctate keratopathy. In The Cornea in Health and Disease (VIth Congress of the European Society of Ophthalmology). London, Academic Press, 1981, pp 693–698.

EXTRAOCULAR MUSCLES

ABDUCENS (SIXTH NERVE) PARALYSIS
378.54

EUGENE M. HELVESTON, M.D.

Indianapolis, Indiana

Abducens nerve abnormalities produce weakness or paralysis of the lateral rectus muscle, depending upon the extent of involvement of the nerve. The condition may be unilateral or bilateral, causing absence or reduction of lateral rectus function, esotropia, and homonymous or uncrossed diplopia. With total paralysis of the sixth nerve, esotropia is usually present in the primary position. Single binocular vision may be present in such a unilateral involvement if the eyes are directed maximally away from the field of action of the paretic muscle. In some cases, "single" vision occurs because the nose blocks the adducted eye. Bilateral sixth nerve palsy produces diplopia in all fields of gaze. Congenital sixth nerve palsy is rare, but acquired transient sixth nerve palsy in childhood may be more common than has been suspected. Because the long intracranial course of the abducens nerve makes it vulnerable, acquired sixth nerve palsy is not uncommon. It may result from generalized intracranial hypertension, direct pressure caused by space-occupying lesions, localized edema, inflammation, toxic substances, demyelinating diseases, and viruses. Acute sixth nerve palsy can be transient, with recovery occurring in weeks to months. Usually, a period of 6 months is required to ensure maximum recovery. Any deviation from an acquired sixth nerve palsy that is present 6 months after the incident can be considered permanent. Acquired sixth nerve palsy can be aggravated by contraction of the antagonist medial rectus. Hypoplasia of the abducens nucleus has been described at autopsy in cases with a clinical diagnosis of type I Duane's retraction syndrome.

THERAPY

Ocular. Unilateral sixth nerve palsy may be compensated for by assuming a head posture with the face turned toward the involved side and the eyes directed toward the side opposite the lesion. With bilateral sixth nerve palsy, diplopia can be relieved only by suppressing or closing one eye. The use of base-out prisms can be effective in helping the patient maintain fusion in unilateral sixth nerve palsy. The use of a base-out prism over the sound eye has been suggested as a temporizing technique, which can be effective in reducing the degree of contracture of the antagonist medial rectus on the involved side. Occlusion can also be applied to eliminate the diplopia.

The use of attenuated botulinum A toxin[†] has been suggested for treatment of acute sixth nerve palsy. In this pharmacologic approach, between 2.5 and 5 units are injected into the antagonist medial rectus muscle after localization of the myoneural junction with an EMG electrode. This treatment weakens the injected muscle for several weeks to months and prevents contraction. When lateral rectus function returns, the recovered muscle works against a normal antagonist.

Surgical. The surgical treatment of sixth nerve palsy should be undertaken only after an adequate workup has been completed. In cases of acquired sixth nerve palsy, a sufficient time, usually 6 months, should elapse before the condition can be considered stable. The deviation is usually incomitant, but does tend to become comitant with time.

The deviation should be measured carefully in the primary position, right gaze, and left gaze. In addition, up- and downgaze should be measured to determine the presence or absence of vertical incomitance. Saccadic velocity testing of the action of the paretic muscle and the antagonist, done either by observation or with an EOG recording device, can be compared to assess the degree of lateral rectus palsy. In cases where significantly limited abduction is present and sixth nerve palsy is suspected, differential intraocular pressure testing can be carried out. When intraocular pressure increases in the field of *limited* action, intact agonist function can be inferred. If no increase in intraocular pressure is found in the presence of limited ductions, absence of agonist contraction can be diagnosed. Passive ductions, carried out either in the office after the use of topical anesthetic or in the operating room, can determine the presence or absence of mechanical restriction of the antagonist.

With knowledge of the angle of deviation, the degree of weakness of the paretic lateral rectus, and the presence or absence of restriction of the antagonist, surgery may be carried out. In cases where the medial rectus is contracted, it may be recessed. In most instances, this means that the medial rectus should be recessed maximally (to a point approximately 11.0 mm from the limbus), and the overlying conjunctiva and anterior Tenon's capsule should be recessed to the muscle's original insertion. If some lateral rectus function is present, an 8- to 10-mm resection of the lateral rectus muscle in addition to the medial rectus recession may suffice. If no lateral rectus function is present, a muscle transfer procedure may be used to shift action of the superior rectus and the inferior rectus to the lateral rectus. This full tendon transfer should be accompanied by oculinum injection to the medial rectus. This procedure can produce straight eyes in the primary position and improved but never normal abduction in the involved eye. With surgically treated unilateral sixth nerve palsy, some range of fusion with single binocular vision can be obtained. In cases of bilateral sixth nerve palsy, even with successful surgical treatment and straight eyes in the primary position, troublesome diplopia invariably persists. This diplopia is caused by unresolvable and constant recurrent secondary deviations or a poorly understood condition called central disruption of fusion. This latter condition can accompany severe head trauma, which in turn is often a precursor of bilateral sixth nerve palsy.

PRECAUTIONS

The differential diagnosis of sixth nerve palsy includes several relatively uncommon conditions. Extraocular muscle fibrous syndrome is characterized by esotropia that increases on upgaze, bilateral ptosis, a chin-up position, and autosomal dominant inheritance. In this condition, passive elevation and abduction are restricted. Möbius syndrome is characterized by an esotropia, flat lower face, and atrophy of the distal third of the tongue. It occurs as a result of bilateral sixth and seventh nerve palsy. Class I Duane's syndrome is characterized by unilateral or bilateral esotropia, decreased abduction, and enophthalmos on abduction. It has been shown in certain cases to be associated with hypoplasia of the abducens nerve nucleus. Thyroid ophthalmopathy may involve the medial rectus muscles and produce a unilateral or bilateral mechanical esotropia. Myasthenia gravis may be associated with unilateral or bilateral esotropia. Blowout fracture of the medial wall of the orbit with entrapment of the medial rectus produces limited abduction with or without esotropia in the primary position. Certain cases that have been diagnosed in the past as congenital esotropia may be acquired sixth nerve palsy that has stabilized as an esotropia. Viral illness in childhood or prolonged anesthesia in infancy and childhood has been noted to cause transient sixth nerve palsy.

COMMENTS

Sixth nerve palsy in general does not constitute a diagnostic mystery. Careful evaluation of the patient in the office can usually provide enough information for an accurate diagnosis. Occasionally, an endrophonium test may be employed to rule out myasthenia gravis. However, in most cases of myasthenia, other extraocular muscles are involved. Also, the extraocular muscle response to myasthenia is usually less dramatic than the response of the levator palpebrae or facial muscles. In relatively rare cases for which no satisfactory explanation can be found, further neurologic workup, including CAT scan, may be employed.

References

Ellis FD, Helveston EM: Special considerations and techniques in strabismus surgery. Int Ophthalmol Clin 16:247–254, 1976.
Helveston EM: Atlas of Strabismus Surgery, 2nd ed. St. Louis, CV Mosby, 1977.
Hotchkiss MG, et al: Bilateral Duane's retraction syndrome. A clinical-pathologic case report. Arch Ophthalmol 98:870–874, 1980.
Metz HS, Mazow M: Botulinum toxin treatment of acute sixth and third nerve palsy. Graefes Arch Clin Exp Ophthalmol 226:141–144, 1988.
Scott AB: Botulinum toxin injection of eye muscles to correct strabismus. Trans Am Ophthalmol Soc 79:734–770, 1981.

ACCOMMODATIVE ESOTROPIA 378.35
EDWARD L. RAAB, M.D.
New York, New York

Accommodative esotropia is among the most common forms of acquired strabismus. Intermittency and a variable angle of deviation at onset in a child with no generalized neurologic abnormality are characteristic of this condition. The most common age of appearance is between 24 and 30 months, although onset before 1 year of age has been documented. Because presumably there has been an interval of normal binocular visual experience early in life before onset, some degree of fusion capacity usually can be demonstrated by the appropriate clinical office tests. Amblyopia may develop once the deviation becomes constant, but usually it is not severe unless there is anisometropic hyperopia that has gone untreated. Several series have shown that excessive hyperopia and a high AC/A ratio are equally prevalent as etiologic factors. Cases showing both features tend to pose more troublesome management problems.

Accommodative esotropia traditionally has been considered an essentially self-limited condition that subsides in the great majority of cases by about age 10 years. Recent reports have indicated that there is a high rate of persistence well beyond that age and that neither this outcome nor the deterioration to a partially or completely nonaccommodative component can be predicted from the presence or absence of any of several associated clinical features, such as family history of strabismus, inferior oblique overaction, or progressive increases in hyperopia.

THERAPY

Ocular. The basic objectives of treatment are to maintain straight eyes by discouraging excessive accommodative convergence, to prevent or eliminate amblyopia, and to remove or compensate for coexisting misalignments (e.g., oblique muscle dysfunctions) that can act as obstacles to fusion despite adequate control of the esotropia.

A decrease in accommodative convergence can be provided by reducing the accommodation requirement through optical or pharmacologic means. Generally, spectacles that compensate for the full hyperopic refractive error are well accepted for full-time wear immediately or after a brief period of adjustment. Although for ongoing management, the goal is to provide the *least* assistance that will keep the eyes straight in binocular viewing to encourage and expand fusional divergence, usually it is best to gain the fullest control possible at the initial treatment, with subsequent tapering as seems opportune.

Bifocals are given for residual esotropia at near greater by 10 or more prism diopters than the distance deviation with hyperopia compensated, provided that the eyes are realigned at distance to less than 10 prism diopters of residual deviation. Here too, although the minimally necessary addition is to be desired, rapid control of the case involving a high distance/near comparison calls initially for the full add of +2.50 or +3.00 diopters. Since in a one-visit initial examination/treatment scheme the cycloplegic determination usually is performed after alignment measurements have been completed, obviously it is desirable to estimate in advance the possible need for a bifocal even before it can be known that the esodeviation is entirely accommodative in nature. Generally, it is safe to assume that this requirement exists if the esotropia angle at near is greater than at distance by at least 20 prism diopters with no compensation for hyperopia and before any cycloplegic is administered. The need for a bifocal in patients with differences between 10 and 20 prism diopters is more difficult to predict, but in the author's experience it is required in at least half of such cases (although when later adjusted, usually in less than full

strength). When in doubt, it is probably best for this group to receive the bifocal initially and to remove or reduce it rapidly based on the examiner's subsequent experience with the case. The less desirable alternative of omitting the bifocal until the case is re-evaluated would result in a large number of automatic prescription changes.

Well-controlled patients are seen at intervals of 4 to 6 months, unless their schedule must be more frequent because of amblyopia treatment.

Once accommodative convergence is controlled, the distance and near (if any) powers can be reduced at intervals of several months by an amount determined by office trial to maintain at least peripheral fusion. The cover/uncover test may show no refixation shift for either eye, or there may be a small refixation (less than 10 prism diopters with the simultaneous prism/cover test) of the nonpreferred eye. The alternate cover test may, of course, show a larger deviation, e.g., an eso*phoria* response. Unless there has been surgery for a nonaccommodative portion of the deviation, such reductions in spectacle power before age 5 years usually are not possible. Generally, it is best not to prescribe a reduction in power greater than 0.75 diopters at one time, regardless of what may seem to be indicated. It is not necessary to verify such a change by a cycloplegic refraction that is otherwise unneeded at that visit, since the least assistance possible is intended, regardless of the total hyperopia or whether it shows a commensurate change.

Anticholinesterase drugs applied topically act by facilitating accommodative effort for a given level of innervational output. The usually employed agents are 0.06 or 0.125 per cent echothiophate (Phospholine) iodide, one drop in each eye once daily, and DFP (Floropryl) ointment 0.025 per cent applied once daily. In actual practice, these drugs are considered less reliable than optical correction for both diagnosis and treatment. The "indeterminate" case usually is not better detected by these agents.

Amblyopia is managed by conventional occlusion programs. If on initial evaluation it appears as though the eyes will be straightened successfully by glasses or miotics, it is permissible to defer occlusion temporarily in children who are old enough that their visual acuity can be monitored accurately. The restoration of proper alignment has been observed to result in some degree of spontaneous visual improvement in several cases. A short delay of 2 or 3 months could lessen considerably the duration of a subsequently employed occlusion regimen and avoid the interruption of the opportunity for fusion that patching would cause.

Surgical. There is a general agreement that during childhood an operation is an inappropriate substitute for optical or pharmacologic control of accommodative convergence. However, some patients with fully compensated accommodative esotropia gradually develop a constant nonaccommodative component as well. There are no reliable predictors of this sequel; various series indicate its occurrence rate to be 13 to 48 per cent. Surgery is necessary once this complication is present and should be planned for only the residual deviation that is no longer influenced by accommodation.

Comitant vertical deviations less than 10 prism diopters can be managed by incorporating vertical prism power in the spectacle prescription. Larger deviations, prominent inferior oblique overaction, and dissociated vertical deviation require surgery, occasionally even when the horizontal alignment has been controlled successfully.

Supportive. Formal orthoptic exercises to reduce dependency on glasses or miotics do not play a prominent role in the treatment of accommodative esotropia. Progressively reduced hyperopia correction or a schedule of decreasing miotic administration is in effect a training of fusional divergence under more natural circumstances. However, the assistance of the orthoptist in the other aspects of management of these patients, such as amblyopia monitoring and treatment reduction, is both appropriate and highly valuable.

PRECAUTIONS

There is controversy as to which of several available cycloplegic agents is best in determining the refractive error. Many ophthalmologists insist that atropine, as the most powerful of the group, is the only suitable drug for this purpose. However, the extra visit to accomplish the refraction, the multiple-dose regimen, the duration of side effects in predisposed individuals, and the prolonged wear-off time with its residual (although temporary) visual handicap suggest the need for an effective compromise.

The unreliability attributed to cyclopentolate for refraction in esotropia cases may be due to the common practice of refracting after only 25 to 30 minutes, as is generally done in routine situations. A 45- to 60-minute interval is more suitable and is in keeping with the described properties of this drug. The power of cyclopentolate to "uncover" additional hyperopia on serial determinations, when used in this manner, is similar to that of atropine. The ability to arrive at a definitive treatment plan, which with either agent often requires a subsequent adjustment of the prescription, in one visit is the overriding advantage of this suggested regimen. Studies have shown that it is not necessary to discontinue miotics to obtain reliable refraction data with this dosage and schedule.

An important limitation to miotic treatment is that these drugs do not substitute for glasses when the refractive errors are anisometropic, and they therefore do not remove a prominent predisposing factor in amblyopia development. In particular, the author has not found them to be useful in place of glasses in noncompliant children; the parent unable or unwilling to enforce firmly the wearing of spectacles is not likely to prevail in the comparably difficult conflict resulting from frequent drop instillation. Anticholinesterase agents also cannot replace glasses if prisms are to be part of the treatment program. If these agents are employed, it is likely that patients unresponsive to three or four doses weekly will not improve with more frequent use.

The patient (if old enough) and the responsible adult must be cautioned that succinylcholine employed as a muscle relaxant during general anesthesia can result in apnea if anticholinesterase agents have been taken within the previous several weeks.

COMMENTS

Despite its conceded shortcomings when compared to the gradient method of determination, the distance/near fusion-free alignment comparison remains the most practical method of estimating the AC/A ratio. Apparent changes in this determination often are noted over several examinations and usually are due to unappreciated variations in accommodative effort. This artifact can be minimized in measuring alignment by employing fixation targets that require accurate and clear observation of fine detail by the patient.

The natural history of accommodative esotropia is marked by two issues that are of particular concern to ophthalmologists and to the parents of these patients. One is whether surgery will be required. Operation should be reserved for those who, either through delayed or inadequate treatment or in many cases even despite timely and conscientious measures, deteriorate to a partially or completely nonaccommodative deviation. There is some evidence indicating that this outcome is more likely to occur in the patients with earliest onset. Surgery can restore straight eyes, but usually not without the need for continuing accommodation control.

The other familiar dilemma concerns the likelihood of spontaneous improvement of the condition so that treatment is no longer required. Conventional belief has held that most cases of accommodative esotropia subside uneventfully by about age 10 years. Recent scrutiny of this question has indicated that the age of disappearance is quite variable, that some cases persist indefinitely, and that, as with deterioration, there are no reliable predictive clues.

Accommodative esotropia has been noted as an accompanying feature to many other forms of strabismus. The most important of these combinations occurs in the infant with congenital esotropia. Although accommodative esotropia as a pure deviation occurs infrequently in the early months of life, many authors have described what seems to be a predisposition of the congenitally esotropic infant toward developing a simultaneous or subsequent accommodative strabismus, even after successful surgery for the former condition. It is particularly important that parents of these infants be forewarned of this prominent possibility.

Many parents are under the misconception that accommodation-controlling measures cure this condition. It is vital that they be educated to understand that these treatments compensate rather than cure, that they are effective only when used, and that they are meant to tide the child over until the condition (it is hoped) subsides naturally.

References

Baker JD, De Young-Smith M: Accommodative esotropia following surgical correction of congenital esotropia, frequency and characteristics. Graefe Arch Clin Exp Ophthalmol 226:175–177, 1988.

Dickey CF, Scott WE: The deterioration of accommodative esotropia: Frequency, characteristics, and predictive factors. J Pediatr Ophthalmol Strabismus 25:172–175, 1988.

Parks MM: Abnormal accommodation in squint. Arch Ophthalmol 19:364–380, 1958.

Raab EL: Etiologic factors in accommodative esodeviation. Trans Am Ophthalmol Soc 80:657–694, 1982.

Raab EL: Cycloplegic refraction after echothiophate iodide. J Pediatr Ophthalmol Strabismus 20:141–144, 1983.

Raab EL: Persisting accommodative esotropia. Arch Ophthalmol 104:1777–1779, 1986.

ACCOMMODATIVE INSUFFICIENCY 367.51
(Accommodative Effort Syndrome, Ill-Sustained Accommodation)

K. NOLEN TANNER, M.D., Ph.D.

Portland, Oregon

Asthenopia is a very frequent complaint heard by all general ophthalmologists, and all ophthalmologists know that it has a myriad of causes. One common cause, which is so easily treated with great patient satisfaction and has such characteristic features that it deserves a name as a special entity, is accommodative insufficiency. Unfortunately, this cause of asthenopia has not received the attention it deserves in the literature and in ophthalmic training programs. As a result, it is far more often missed than detected, and most patients with this condition either receive no treatment or inadequate treatment.

Stated simply, accommodative insufficiency is the inability to accommodate without the help of convergence. In other words, these patients have almost no accommodative reserve. On the classical accommodative-convergence graph plotted in diopters of accommodation versus meter angles of convergence, the comfortable function zone is narrow and lies almost entirely below the 1: 1 accommodative-convergence line.

The patient may be a male or female from about 10 to 35 years of age. In general, the symptomatology and the physical findings change little, if any, over this age range. Over 35 years of age, the condition of accommodative insufficiency begins to blend into presbyopia. The patients are not dyslexic; they can and do read well. Generally, however, prolonged and intensive reading is disliked, and these individuals tend to gravitate to outdoor activities and occupations that require little prolonged close work. Patients often seek help when their job situation changes, and they are suddenly required to spend much of their working day at intensive close work, such as examining computer printouts, or when beginning a course of study in college or graduate school. They typically complain of asthenopic symptoms—headaches, eyestrain, and intermittent blurring after 20 to 40 minutes of reading. If the asthenopic symptoms begin in less than 15 minutes or after an hour or so, they generally do not fit into this classical picture.

On examination patients generally have 20/20 visual acuity without correction, and their refractive error is negligible, ranging from about −0.50 diopters to about +0.75 diopters with no more than 0.50 diopters of cylinder. Over the years, this refractive error changes very little, if at all. Children who are found to be myopic at 8 to 10 years of age and who become increasingly myopic as they go through adolescence rarely, if ever, are found to have accommodative insufficiency. The typical accommodative-insufficient patient is able to read Jaeger 2 print easily, but may be noticed to squint or frown when reading. In making this diagnosis, the first specific test is applied while the patient is reading Jaeger 2. When +1.00 or +1.25 diopter spheres are placed in front of each eye in the form of loose lenses, an immediate positive response will be elicited from the accommodative-insufficient patient. Sometimes, the patient is seen to relax the facial muscles. If the patient says that +1.00 diopter spheres make the print "a little better," this test is considered negative.

After determining that the patient has little, if any, refractive error, the patient is placed behind the refractor with a reading card placed at 35 cm for the second test. With Risley prisms present over both eyes while reading Jaeger 2 print, base-in prisms are slowly wound in over both eyes. The typical accommodative-insufficient patient finds that the print blurs with approximately 2 to 4 diopters of base-in prism over each eye. The blur is relieved by adding bilateral +0.25 to +0.50 diopter spheres in the refractor. As the reading continues, additional prism is turned in. As the print blurs out, it is brought back with plus spheres, +0.25 diopters at a time, until 8 diopters of base-in prism are before each eye for a total of 16 diopters. A patient who has a pupillary distance of exactly 60 mm naturally viewing an object at 33 cm is converging 18 prism diopters. Thus, a patient with approximately 60 mm pupillary distance viewing an object at 35 cm and with 16 diopters of base-in prism has the eyes almost completely straight and with very little remaining convergence. Almost invariably under these conditions, the accommodative-insufficient patient requires +1.00 to +1.50 diopter (usually +1.25 diopter) spheres over each eye to be able to read Jaeger 2 print.

The third test is to place the patient in the refractor without prisms but with −3.00 diopters before each eye gazing at a Snellen chart 20 feet away. The typical accommodative-insufficient patient is unable to resolve any better than 20/100, in spite of all his or her efforts.

THERAPY

Ocular. A patient who is found to have markedly improved vision with +1.00 or +1.25 diopter spheres over both eyes when reading Jaeger 2 print, requires +1.25 diopter sphere to read Jaeger 2 at 35 cm with 16 diopters of base-in prism, and is unable to read better than 20/100 at 20 feet with −3.00 diopter spheres before each eye can certainly be said to have accommodative insufficiency. This patient will benefit greatly with reading glasses. They are usually given as simple half-eye reading glasses, with +1.00 to +1.25 diopter spheres and occasionally +1.50 diopters. The patient should be instructed that the benefit of these glasses will be apparent only after approximately 20 minutes or so of reading. Shorter periods of reading can usually be done comfortably without the reading glasses.

COMMENTS

When all of the features are present as described, there is little doubt as to the diagnosis and treatment. A number of patients, however, as might be expected, show the accommodative insufficiency syndrome to a somewhat lesser degree. If two of the three tests are positive, one can say the patient will benefit substantially with reading glasses for intensive reading. If only one of the three tests is positive, reading glasses probably will not prove sufficiently beneficial to justify their purchase.

Occasionally, patients complain of asthenopic symptoms, and when the base-in prism is turned in while they are reading at 35 cm,

they state that the print actually becomes sharper, blacker, and easier to read. These patients probably should be classified as having convergence insufficiency. Relaxing their convergence not only does not seem to impair their accommodation but actually seems to improve it. In the author's experience, this has proved to be quite infrequent. The obvious answer for these patients is base-in prisms in their reading glasses.

Another group of patients who complain of asthenopia with reading give negative responses to the base-in prism test and the −3.00 sphere test, but under cycloplegia they are found to have 2 diopters or more of hypermetropia. These individuals will be unlikely to wear glasses consistently for all purposes, unless the hypermetropia is of 3 or 4 diopters or more or they are over 30 years of age. However, their asthenopia on near work will be helped by correcting the hypermetropia with plus lenses set at the normal pupillary distance.

References

Duke-Elder S (ed): System of Ophthalmology. St. Louis, CV Mosby, 1970, Vol V, pp 463–464.
Hill RV: The accommodative-effort syndrome: Pathologic physiology. Am J Ophthalmol 34:423–429, 1951.

ACQUIRED NONACCOMMODATIVE ESOTROPIA 378.00

STUART R. DANKNER, M.D., F.A.C.S.

Baltimore, Maryland

Acquired nonaccommodative esotropia is a convergent deviation with onset after the age of 6 months. This deviation is most often concomitant; that is, its angle is approximately the same in all directions of gaze. It is not significantly affected by accommodation. Incomitant esodeviations of paretic or mechanical origin are discussed elsewhere. Since normal binocular vision often exists before the onset of this disease, the prognosis for binocular function in patients with acquired nonaccommodative esotropia is better than for those with congenital esotropia. One eye may prefer fixation in this condition. Amblyopia will develop if the deviation is unilateral and the onset occurs in childhood.

The etiology of nonaccommodative acquired esodeviation is believed to be both neurogenic and anatomic. The neurogenic or innervational cause may be excessive tonic convergence or deficient tonic divergence.

Anatomic factors may be anomalous medial recti insertions. Other causes of acquired non-accommodative esotropia include stress, organic lesions, and anisometropia. Stress-induced acquired esodeviation may be precipitated by illness and emotional factors that cause a breakdown of previously adequate fusional divergence. Patients under stress may also undergo spasm of the near synkinetic reflex, resulting in sustained convergence with accommodative spasm and miosis. Certainly, any monocular organic lesion, such as cataract, optic atrophy, or corneal scarring, may result in an esodeviation, especially if the onset occurs before 4 years of age. Amblyopia secondary to an asymmetric refractive error (anisometropia) may result in a secondary esodeviation. An acutely acquired esodeviation that is worse at distance should be suspected for divergence paralysis and may indicate an early lateral rectus palsy secondary to underlying neurologic disease, such as pontine tumor or head trauma. Acquired esotropia may rarely even be cyclic in pattern, i.e., every other day.

THERAPY

Ocular. If amblyopia is present, occlusion therapy is indicated. This therapy is accomplished best at an early age (less than 7 years old). As a general rule, the schedule for rechecking patients after patching should be one week per year of life to ensure that amblyopia does not develop in the patched eye. Any refractive errors that may further disrupt fusion should be corrected with glasses. Asymmetric refractive errors (anisometropia) may require contact lenses to reduce image disparity. Such underlying organic lesions as congenital cataracts that occlude vision should be treated as early as possible and be followed by aggressive amblyopia therapy. Orthoptics may be indicated to eliminate sensory adaptations, such as suppression or abnormal retinal correspondence, that may have developed secondary to the esodeviation.

Surgical. Any significant esodeviation that is still present after the completion of amblyopia therapy, refractive lens correction, and orthoptics is best treated with eye muscle surgery. Either unilateral or bilateral surgery may be performed, depending on the surgeon's preference. Unilateral surgery consists of a weakening (recession) of the medial rectus muscle and strengthening (resection) of the lateral rectus muscle. Some surgeons prefer performing unilateral surgery in those patients who have a strong preference for fixation in one eye. In these cases, surgery is usually performed on the nonfixating eye. Other surgeons always prefer bilateral weakening of the medial recti.

Deviations of less than 15 prism diopters may require a recession of only one medial rectus muscle. For deviations between 15 and 45 prism diopters, it is usually necessary to operate on two muscles (recess/resect on one eye or bilateral recessions). In deviations over 45 prism diopters, it may be necessary to operate on three or four muscles. However, some surgeons prefer to operate only on two muscles for the initial operation, regardless of how large the deviation may be.

Generally, the goal in strabismus surgery is to align the eyes in the initial postoperative period with the hope of allowing the patient long-term fusion. Some surgeons, however, feel that a small intentional surgical overcorrection (an exodeviation) in the initial postoperative period is desirable and produces a better long-term fusional result. This theory applies only to patients with acquired nonaccommodative esotropia who have no other significant factors disrupting fusion, such as amblyopia and organic or neurologic disease.

The use of adjustable sutures in strabismus surgery on older children and adults has significantly improved the postoperative results. This can be done with topical anesthesia at the time of surgery or within 1 day after the surgical procedure.

The injection of botulinum A toxin[†] (oculinum) into an ocular muscle to create an intentional temporary paralysis has resulted in improved alignment in carefully selected cases.

Prism adaptation therapy (PAT), in which prisms are used preoperatively, has been found to improve the results of surgery for acquired esotropia. Fresnel prisms are placed on eyeglasses until the angle of deviation is neutralized and/or fusion is obtained. This "adapted" angle becomes the goal for a surgical correction and may reduce the reoperation rate.

PRECAUTIONS

Early detection of strabismus and amblyopia is vitally important. Children treated at an early age for amblyopia respond better to occlusion therapy than older children. If amblyopia cannot be reversed, the prognosis for alignment of the eyes and fusion is worsened significantly.

In those patients requiring surgery, fusional results are significantly better in those children operated on at earlier ages. In addition, obvious psychologic sequelae have been noted in children with late surgical treatment of a long-standing and cosmetically displeasing esodeviation. However, no surgery should be attempted unless preoperative measurements are accurate and consistent. At least three sets of measurements should be taken before any strabismus operation is undertaken.

COMMENTS

Treatment of acquired nonaccommodative esotropia requires a specific management plan to achieve the best possible fusional results.

This plan should include a thorough ophthalmologic and strabismic evaluation, early amblyopia detection and therapy, orthoptics, and if needed, strabismus surgery.

References

Abel LA, Troost BT: Acquired cyclic esotropia in an adult eye. Am J Ophthalmol 91:805–806, 1981.

Biglan AW, Burnstine RA, Rogers GL, Saunders RA: Management of strabismus with botulinum A toxin. Ophthalmology 96:935–943, 1989.

Dankner SR, Mash AJ, Jampolsky A: Intentional surgical overcorrection of acquired esotropia. Arch Ophthalmol 96:1848–1852, 1978.

Delisle P, Strasfeld M, Pelletier D: The prism adaptation test in the preoperative evaluation of esodeviations. Can J Ophthalmol 23:208–212, 1988.

Helveston EM: Atlas of Strabismus Surgery, 4th ed. St. Louis, CV Mosby, 1992.

Jampolsky A: Current techniques of adjustable strabismus surgery. Am J Ophthalmol 88:406–418, 1979.

Kraft SP, Enzenauer RW, Weston B: Stability of the postoperative alignment in adjustable-suture strabismus surgery. J Pediatr Ophthalmol Strabismus 28:206–211, 1991.

Metz HS: Acquired cyclic esotropia in an adult eye. Am J Ophthalmol 91:804–805, 1981.

Parks MM, Mitchel PR, Wheeler MB: Ocular motility and strabismus. In Duane TD (ed): Clinical Ophthalmology. Philadelphia, JB Lippincott, 1990, Vol 1.

Prism Adaptation Study Research Group: Efficacy of prism adaptation in the surgical management of acquired esotropia. Arch Ophthalmol 108:148–1256, 1990.

Repka MX, Wentworth D: Predictors of prism response during prism adaptation. J Pediatr Ophthalmol Strabismus 28:202–205, 1991.

Scott AB: Botulinum toxin injection into extraocular muscle as an alternative to strabismus surgery. J Pediatr Ophthalmol Strabismus 17:21–25, 1980.

von Noorden GK: Binocular Vision and Ocular Motility. Theory and Management of Strabismus, 4th ed. St. Louis, CV Mosby, 1990.

A-PATTERNS 378.06, 378.12
(A-Pattern Esotropia—378.06, A-Pattern Exotropia—378.12)

HENRY S. METZ, M.D.

Rochester, New York

A-patterns are an incomitant deviation in which a greater amount of esotropia is demonstrated in upgaze than in downgaze or a greater amount of exotropia is found in downgaze than in upgaze. By convention, a 10 prism diopter difference between upgaze and downgaze is required to make this diagnosis. Superior oblique overaction and inferior oblique underaction are noted frequently. Some patients may have normal rotations in the field of action of the oblique muscles. An upward slant of the lid fissures has sometimes been described. A-patterns are somewhat less common than V-patterns and are seen more commonly in children with hydrocephalus. Longstanding, large-angle exotropia can sometimes be associated with A-patterns, but X-patterns with all overactive obliques may be the more common finding.

THERAPY

Ocular. Correction of the refractive error, prisms, or orthoptics do not have a beneficial effect on the A-pattern.

Surgical. When the A-pattern is large (40 prism diopters or more) and both superior obliques are overacting, a large bilateral superior oblique weakening procedure (tenotomy, tenectomy) can be considered. With smaller patterns (e.g., 20 prism diopters), marginal tenotomies may be an option. If fusion is present preoperatively, many surgeons feel that the superior oblique tendon should not be weakened because of the fear of inducing symptomatic torsional diplopia. In addition, if the inferior obliques are even mildly overactive preoperatively, superior oblique surgery should be avoided. Horizontal rectus surgery to correct the deviation in primary position should be performed at the same time.

In patients without superior oblique overaction and with a smaller A-pattern (e.g., 10 to 20 diopters), vertical transposition of the horizontal recti combined with recession or resection surgery can be useful. If both medial recti are to be operated on, the insertions should be elevated. When both lateral recti are to be operated on, the insertions should be depressed. If monocular surgery is planned, the medial rectus insertion is elevated while the lateral rectus insertion is depressed. Vertical transpositions vary between a half and a full tendon width displacement, depending upon the size of the pattern.

Horizontal transposition of the vertical recti (superior recti moved temporally or inferior recti moved nasally) is rarely recommended because of the lack of good predictability of the results.

Ocular or Periocular Manifestations

Extraocular Muscles: Inferior oblique palsy, rare; superior oblique overaction and inferior oblique underaction, frequent.

Other: Chin-up position to minimize or eliminate the deviation in downgaze in A-pattern esotropia; chin-down position to minimize or eliminate the exotropia in A-pattern exotropia; craniofacial dysostosis, perhaps because these patients have shallow orbits resulting anatomically in greater exotropia in downgaze.

PRECAUTIONS

If inferior oblique overaction is noted, superior oblique tenotomies may lead to an overcorrection with a resulting V-pattern. Although small amounts of torsion have been measured after monocular surgery with displacement of the horizontal recti, these have not been symptomatic. Patients who have fusion preoperatively in upgaze or downgaze may notice excyclotorsion after superior oblique tenotomies or tenectomies.

COMMENTS

Patients with A-pattern esotropia may have a satisfactory appearance in downgaze where the deviation is least. However, the upper lids usually cover the eyes in this position of gaze. In upgaze, where the esotropia is greatest, the ocular position is easily visible.

A patient with a chin-up position to fuse has a good prognosis for improved head position if the A-pattern is collapsed by vertical displacement of the horizontal recti along with horizontal rectus recession or resection or both.

A-pattern exotropes have the largest deviation in downgaze where the lids usually cover the eyes and make the exotropia less noticeable in this gaze position.

When fusion is present in upgaze with a chin-down head position, collapsing the A-pattern can improve this abnormal head position. The prognosis in such cases is good if superior oblique tenectomies are avoided.

References

France TD: Strabismus in hydrocephalus. Am Orthop J 25:101–105, 1975.

Goldstein JH: Monocular vertical displacement of the horizontal rectus muscles in the A and V patterns. Am J Ophthalmol 64:265–267, 1967.

Helveston EM: A-exotropia, alternating sursumduction and superior oblique overaction. Am J Ophthalmol 67:377–380, 1969.

Jampolsky A: Oblique muscle surgery of the A and V patterns. J Pediatr Ophthalmol 2:31–36, 1965.

Knapp P: A and V patterns. In Symposium on Strabismus. Transactions of the New Orleans Academy of Ophthalmology. St. Louis, CV Mosby, 1971, pp 242–254.

Metz, HS, Schwartz L: The treatment of A and V patterns by monocular surgery. Arch Ophthalmol 95:251–253, 1977.

BASIC EXOTROPIA 378.10

ANDREA CIBIS TONGUE, M.D.

Lake Oswego, Oregon

Basic exotropia refers to a divergent deviation of the visual axes of equal or nearly equal magnitude for distance and near fixation. It differs from divergence excess exotropia (deviation greater at distance than at near) and convergence insufficiency exotropia (deviation greater at near than at distance). Pseudodivergence exotropia mimics divergence excess because the deviation at near is less than that at distance due to accommodative convergence. Patients with pseudodivergence excess exotropia have a high AC/A ratio. Their deviation at distance and near is equal or nearly equal when accommodative convergence is suspended (measured without accommodative target or with +3.00 lenses at near).

Prism alternate cover measurements should be performed with the patient's refractive error corrected and with an accommodative fixation target. Patients with basic exotropia have nearly equal deviations with an accommodative target at distance and near. If the deviation is significantly greater in down- or upgaze, it falls into the categories of A- or V-pattern exotropia.

The etiology of basic exotropia is generally unknown. It may be congenital or acquired. In some cases orbital anomalies are identified (craniofacial disorders). Monocular vision loss is a predisposing factor leading to basic exotropia. Basic exotropia may also gradually evolve from basic esotropia, particularly when associated with amblyopia or vision loss, or from an exophoria or intermittent exotropia. Consecutive exotropia may be the result of surgical correction of esotropia. Patients with nonalternating exotropia require careful evaluation for conditions that may cause monocular visual loss.

THERAPY

Surgical. The treatment of basic exotropia is generally surgical when the deviation is cosmetically unacceptable or when fusion is a possibility. Deviations less than 18 diopters may be amenable to orthoptics if fusion capacity is present. In cases of acquired monocular visual impairment with a good chance of restoration of vision, treatment should be directed toward correction of vision first and strabismus second. Bilateral myopic refractive errors should be corrected before surgery. Hyperopic refractive errors may not require correction if the visual acuity is normal, but the deviation should be measured with the hyperopic correction in place whenever possible. It is important to measure the deviation in lateral gaze, since a significant number of patients show a decrease in the deviation in these positions. Knapp (1971) has pointed out that a 20 per cent greater decrease of the deviation in lateral gaze is associated with a high incidence of overcorrections, particularly if bilateral lateral rectus recessions are performed. For some reason, these patients obtain a much greater correction for each millimeter of lateral rectus recession than expected. Knapp suggests that not only should bilateral recessions be avoided but that a marginal tenotomy is preferable over a recession, even in unilateral surgery. Adjustable suture technique for the recessed muscle provides an excellent alternative and should be considered whenever lateral incomitance is present. The specific surgical procedure when there is good visual acuity in each eye is the surgeon's choice. Some prefer to perform a lateral rectus recession and medial rectus resection, whereas others prefer bilateral lateral rectus recessions. If the visual acuity is impaired in one eye, it is in general advisable to perform a recession/resection operation on that eye.

It is best to aim for small undercorrections in adult patients with longstanding exotropia, since postoperative diplopia may be intolerable in this group. Furthermore, many of these patients are used to the exotropic appearance, and even orthotropia may be interpreted as esotropia or crossed eyes to them. In young children, a small postoperative overcorrection is desirable. Deviations of 15 diopters or less may be managed conservatively for even months if fusion is not jeopardized, such as in infants or very young children, or if diplopia is manageable. Conservative management of consecutive esotropia includes correction of hyperopic refractive errors, bifocals, patching, miotics, and prism. In many patients the esotropic deviation gradually decreases, and the patient ultimately has a good and stable outcome. Reoperation should be undertaken if there is concern about a slipped muscle, increasing esotropia, unmanageable and intolerable diplopia, or concern about the loss of fusion ability in the visually immature child.

Small undercorrections in patients who are expected to have fusion may be managed with prism therapy, orthoptics, or minus lenses if accommodative convergence is sufficient to overcome the exotropia. If the patients are not expected to have fusion, then no further treatment is indicated if the deviation is cosmetically acceptable. Further surgery may be required if the deviation is sufficiently large and bothersome to the patient.

PRECAUTIONS

Nonalternating basic exotropia requires evaluation for visual loss of the nonfixating eye. Amblyopia treatment or correction of the visual loss should be instituted as soon as possible in infants and young children. Assessment of the deviation requires measurements in the cardinal directions of gaze, with particular attention paid to measurements in lateral gaze. If lateral incomitance is present, recession of the lateral rectus muscle is associated with a greater degree of correction than the norm. A- and V-patterns need to be identified, because they may be associated with marked abnormalities of the oblique muscle function. Routine horizontal muscle surgery may be associated with over- or undercorrections when the incomitancy of the deviation in up- and downgaze is greater than 20 or 25 diopters. Proper surgical management may require oblique muscle surgery or vertical displacement of the horizontal recti.

Overcorrection of exotropia is poorly tolerated by adults, who usually find prolonged periods of diplopia annoying. These patients may even be unable to tolerate diplopia on lateral gaze, especially if it interferes with driving or their professional or sports activities. If orthotropia is not attained, undercorrection rather than overcorrection is preferable in adults. Adjustable sutures are indicated in the surgical management of the adult exotropic patient at risk for postoperative diplopia.

COMMENTS

Basic exotropia may be congenital or acquired, alternating or unilateral. The deviation should be measured with an accommodative target both for distance and near fixation and with the patient's basic refractive error corrected. Measurements thus obtained are equal or nearly equal for distance and near fixation. Since the AC/A ratio is normal in these patients, optical treatment with minus lenses is not indicated unless the deviation is sufficiently small and fusion is likely. Prism treatment and orthoptics may be attempted in patients who have fusion potential and a small deviation. Surgery is necessary for larger deviations and those that are cosmetically unacceptable. Before surgical correction of exotropia is considered, treatment of conditions causing monocular vision loss, such as removal of acquired cataract, correction of refractive errors, or treatment of amblyopia, should be undertaken when the restoration of vision is likely. The extent and type of procedure are dictated by the age of the patient, absence or presence of fusion potential, cosmetic goals, magnitude of the deviation, and the presence or absence of any lateral or vertical incomitance.

References

Cibis GW: Post-surgical strabismus management. *In* Cibis GW, Tongue AC, Stass-Isern M (eds): Decision Making in Pediatric Ophthalmology. St. Louis, CV Mosby, 1992.

Hurtt J, Rasicovici A, Windsor CE: Orthoptics and Ocular Motility. St. Louis, CV Mosby, 1972, pp 71–73.

Knapp P: Management of exotropia. *In* Burian HM,

et al (eds): Symposium on Strabismus. St. Louis, CV Mosby, 1971, pp 242–245.

Parks MM: Atlas of Strabismus Surgery. Philadelphia, Harper & Row, 1983.

von Noorden GK: Binocular Vision and Ocular Motility: Theory and Management of Strabismus, 3rd ed. St. Louis, CV Mosby, 1985.

BROWN'S SYNDROME 378.61

(Superior Oblique Tendon Sheath Syndrome)

AMY AIELLO, M.D.,
and EARL A. PALMER, M.D.

Portland, Oregon

Brown's syndrome is an ocular motility deficit manifested by an inability of the adducted eye to elevate actively or passively above the midhorizontal plane. Typically, there is less elevation restriction in the midline and an even smaller limitation to elevation in abduction. There may be a widening of the palpebral fissure and a slight downshoot of the involved eye in adduction. A relative exodeviation is present on upgaze. Most patients maintain alignment in the primary position, but in some the involved eye is hypotropic and fusion only occurs in downgaze. This causes a compensatory chin-up posture with face turn toward the opposite eye, which is consistent with an inferior oblique palsy. Amblyopia may or may not be present.

Brown (1973) attributed this condition to congenital shortening of the sheath surrounding the reflected tendon of the superior oblique. The anomaly is now generally believed to be a congenitally tight superior oblique tendon. Brown's syndrome includes a spectrum of clinical severity, and the definition is often expanded to include numerous causes. Thus, it may be congenital, as classically described by Brown, or acquired. It may be permanent, transient, or intermittent. Acquired or simulated Brown's syndrome has been described after tucking or other surgical procedures on the superior oblique, blepharoplasty, or scleral buckling procedures. It may also be due to focal metastases to the superior oblique muscle, orbital trauma with formation of a blood cyst in the superior oblique sheath, frontal sinus osteoma, or an anomalous insertion of the superior oblique muscle in the superior nasal quadrant. Inflammation in the trochlear region causing Brown's syndrome has been described in patients with both juvenile and adult rheumatoid arthritis. More remote causes of a simulated Brown's syndrome include orbital floor fracture with entrapment of the inferior oblique, dense fibrous adhesions of the insertion of the inferior oblique muscle to the lateral orbital wall, or other fibromuscular adhesions in the nasal part of the orbit.

THERAPY

Surgical. Patients who are fusing in the primary position without an anomalous head posture are best managed without surgery. Such patients may experience diplopia in up-oblique gaze with the involved eye adducted, but learn to avoid that position of gaze.

If the eye is hypotropic in the primary position or if there is significant ocular torticollis, surgery is indicated to restore binocular function in the primary position. The treatment of choice is to weaken the superior oblique. Although doing so effectively eliminates the restriction to elevation, it results in the need for a second procedure in a significant number of cases. However, if fusion is present before surgical intervention, vertical fusional amplitudes may have increased with time so that the deviation can remain latent and a second surgical procedure for the superior oblique palsy may not be necessary. When fusional reserves fail to control the cyclovertical deviation, a second surgical procedure is usually necessary. Patients with relatively marked preoperative restriction seem to have an increased risk for a decompensated superior oblique palsy. Two solutions have been advocated by Parks and Eustis (1987): (1) perform tenotomy at the insertion, preserving intermuscular septum, for a milder effect and (2) combine the tenotomy with inferior oblique weakening initially in those with marked preoperative restriction.

To avoid superior oblique palsy, the superior oblique tendon can be lengthened (Wright et al., 1992) with a spacing element. This produces a graded weakening effect through calibrating the separation of the ends of the tendon. A nasal superior oblique intrasheath tenotomy is performed, followed by insertion of a segment of No. 240 silicone retinal band secured by horizontal mattress sutures to the cut ends of the tendon. This procedure has the advantage of being reversible.

Ocular or Periocular Manifestations

Extraocular Muscles: Decreased elevation in adduction; downshoot of the affected eye on adduction; positive forced duction in the direction of limitation.

Eyelids: Widening of the palpebral fissure on adduction.

PRECAUTIONS

If a horizontal deviation coexists or binocular vision is absent, successful realignment may be more difficult.

Overaction of the ipsilateral inferior oblique may occur after cutting the superior oblique tendon. Other complications of superior oblique weakening procedures include residual superior oblique overaction or persistent Brown's syndrome caused by missed tendon fibers, inadvertent injury to the superior rectus, iatrogenic superior oblique palsy, orbital hematoma due to damage to a vortex vein, and transient or permanent ptosis. Restricted movement of the globe may result when posterior dissection is carried into Tenon's capsule, allowing fat to prolapse into the wound. This complication can be avoided by a careful dissection close to the superior rectus muscle.

When the silicone expander procedure is used, gentle forced ductions should be performed after the silicone band is in place to estimate the tightness of the tendon. If a significant restriction remains, the implant should be lengthened. Long-term tissue acceptance of the silicone band for this purpose has not yet been demonstrated.

COMMENTS

Superior oblique tenotomy is an effective treatment for Brown's syndrome, but the surgeon must be prepared to deal with a possible iatrogenic superior oblique palsy. A graded weakening effect of the superior oblique tendon by use of the silicone expander technique facilitates effective elimination of the deviation while reducing the risk of consecutive superior oblique palsy.

References

Brown HW: True and simulated superior oblique tendon sheath syndromes. Doc Ophthalmol 34: 123, 1973.

Crawford JS, Orton RB, Labow-Daily L: Late results of superior oblique muscle tenotomy in true Brown's syndrome. Am J Ophthalmol 89: 824–829, 1980.

Goldhammer Y, Smith JL: Acquired intermittent Brown's syndrome. Neurology 24:666, 1974.

Goldstein JH: Intermittent superior oblique tendon sheath syndrome. Am J Ophthalmol 67:960–962, 1969.

Moore AT, Morin JD: Bilateral acquired inflammatory Brown's syndrome. J Pediatr Ophthalmol Strabismus 22:26, 1985.

Parks MM, Eustis HS: Simultaneous superior oblique tenotomy and inferior oblique recession in Brown's syndrome. Ophthalmology 94:1043, 1987.

von Noorden GK, Oliver P: Superior oblique tenectomy in Brown's syndrome. Ophthalmology 89:303, 1982.

Wright KW, Min BM, Park C: Comparison of superior oblique tendon expander to superior oblique tenotomy for the management of superior oblique overaction and Brown's syndrome. J Pediatr Ophthalmol Strabismus 29:92–97, 1992.

CONGENITAL ESOTROPIA
743.69
(Infantile Esotropia)

EUGENE M. HELVESTON, M.D.

Indianapolis, Indiana

The clinical picture of congenital or infantile esotropia is not present at birth, but a study of normal newborns suggests that an inborn defect causes inaccurate motor fusion leading to esotropia and subsequent sensory defects. Whether some inborn underlying defect in the sensory fusion mechanism is also present is not known at this time. However, otherwise normal parents of infants with congenital esotropia have a significantly higher incidence of subtle defects in stereopsis.

Congenital esotropia accounts for about 50 per cent of all strabismus treatment. These patients usually have a moderate angle, averaging between 40 and 60 prism diopters with a range from 10 to 90 diopters. In general, the only abnormality noted is the esotropia, and children are otherwise physically normal and neurologically sound.

Workup of the patient with congenital-infantile esotropia should include a detailed history. The age of a child at the onset of esotropia should be established. In addition, fixation preference, stability of angle, birth weight, any important milestones, a general family history, and a family history of hyperthermia are helpful in evaluating any child considered for surgery. The physical examination should include appraisal of the lids, lashes, and lacrimal apparatus; examination for versions and ductions; and an estimation of angle by interpretation of pupillary light reflex (Hirshberg) or centering of light reflex with prism (Krimsky). Prism and cover testing at distance and near fixation using an accommodative target should be done on children who will cooperate with these procedures. Other associated ocular findings, such as amblyopia, cross-fixation, abduction nystagmus and convergence to block nystagmus, A- or V-pattern, oblique palsy, dissociated vertical deviation, palpebral fissure narrowing on attempted adduction (Duane's syndrome), and facial paralysis with sixth nerve palsy (Möbius syndrome), should also be sought. Evaluation of cycloplegic retinoscopy (using 0.5 per cent cyclopentolate for children under 1 year, 1.0 per cent cyclopentolate for children over 1 year, and 0.5 to 1.0 per cent atropine twice a day for 3 days in darker-pigmented children), and of the ocular media, the fundus, and passive ductions is also helpful. The differential diagnosis of congenital-infantile esotropia should include refractive esotropia, accommodative esotropia, type I Duane's syndrome, sixth nerve palsy (congenital or acquired, unilateral or bilateral), fibrosis syndrome, sensory esotropia, and Möbius syndrome.

THERAPY

Surgical. Congenital (infantile) esotropia is treated surgically after amblyopia is treated by patching of the sound eye and after any refractive component (+3.00 diopters or greater) is treated. It is useful to have loaner glasses available in +3.00, +3.50, and +4.00 diopters because these glasses are often ineffective and use of loaner glasses reduces the financial strain on families. If competent anesthesia is available, surgery should be done as soon as possible after these conditions have been treated. The earliest surgery for essential-infantile esotropia is usually at 4 months, although any surgery done before 12 months of age is considered early. Surgical treatment may be recession of both medial recti, recession of one medial rectus and resection of the antagonist lateral rectus, recession of both medial recti with resection of one lateral rectus, or bilateral recession-resection. The number of muscles to be operated upon and the amount of surgery to be done are not universally agreed on.

One scheme for surgical treatment of essential-infantile esotropia is a graded bimedial rectus recession done with measurements carried out from the limbus. The rationale for this procedure is that the medial rectus has a variable insertion site between 3.0 and 6.0 mm from the limbus with an average of 4.4 mm. The insertion site has no relationship to the angle of deviation. At the same time, the anteroposterior diameter of the infant's eye and the corneal diameter are age related, and both of these are fairly constant. Therefore, the limbus seems to be a more reliable anatomic point for measurement than the muscle's original insertion site. Doing bimedial recession with measurement from the limbus, the following scheme for bimedial rectus recession can be employed for *children under 1 year of age*. For a deviation of 25 prism diopters, the medial rectus muscles are recessed to a point 8.5 mm from the limbus. For a deviation of 35 prism diopters, the medial rectus muscles are reattached 9.5 mm from the limbus. For deviations of 45 prism diopters and greater, the medial rectus muscles are reattached at 10.5 mm from the limbus. In *children over 1 year of age*, 0.5 mm is added to each medial rectus recession measurement because the globe is larger in older children. Using this scheme, it is not necessary to employ three or four muscle surgeries.

COMMENTS

Using the recession of the medial recti according to the above scheme, between 70 and 80 per cent of patients are corrected to within ±10 diopters of being straight after one procedure. About 10 per cent of the patients will need an additional procedure for an unacceptable over- or undercorrection in the first 3 to 6 months. An additional 10 per cent of

patients will require secondary surgery for late over- or undercorrection, and another 10 per cent will require surgery for dissociated vertical deviation in 2 to 5 years or later.

Even though congenital-infantile, esotropia is common, several aspects of this condition are not well understood and require further study. It is generally agreed that unless a contraindication exists, early surgery for congenital-infantile esotropia should be done. Evidence that early surgery for congenital-infantile esotropia produces better fusional results is accumulating at the present time. In addition, the benefits obtained from having straighter eyes earlier seems justification enough for this surgery.

References

Helveston EM: Origins of congenital esotropia. Am Orthop 36:40–48, 1986.
Helveston EM, Ellis FD: Pediatric Ophthalmology Practice. St. Louis, CV Mosby, 1980, pp 34–38.
von Noorden GK: Binocular Vision and Ocular Motility. Theory and Management of Strabismus, 2nd ed. St. Louis, CV Mosby, 1980, pp 294–301.
von Noorden GK: Reassessment of infantile esotropia. Edward Jackson Memorial Lecture. Am J Ophthalmol 105:1–9, 1988.

CONGENITAL FIBROSIS OF THE EXTRAOCULAR MUSCLES 378.62
(Congenital Enophthalmos with Ocular Muscle Fibrosis of the Inferior Rectus with Ptosis, General Fibrosis Syndrome, Strabismus Fixus, Vertical Retraction Syndrome)

R. D. HARLEY, M.D., Ph.D., F.A.C.S.

Philadelphia, Pennsylvania

Congenital fibrosis of the extraocular muscles is characterized by a replacement of normal contractile muscle tissue by fibrous tissue, dense collagen, lipid material, and vascular degeneration in various degrees. The clinical picture depends on the number of muscles involved, the degree of fibrosis, and whether involvement is unilateral or bilateral.

Several forms of congenital fibrosis can be recognized, including the general fibrosis syndrome and congenital fibrosis of the inferior rectus muscle. In the general fibrosis syndrome, patients exhibit a marked bilateral ptosis and underaction of all the extraocular muscles, although the inferior recti are usually more involved, causing the eyes to be fixed in a downward position. A chin-up head position is usually assumed in order to fixate objects straight ahead. In some individuals an anomalous convergent movement occurs on attempted upgaze. Forced ductions demonstrate a marked reduction to passive movement. Binocular vision is rare, and exotropia is common. The condition is present at birth, and several large pedigrees suggest an autosomal inheritance. Autosomal recessive and sporadic cases are much less common.

In congenital fibrosis of the inferior rectus muscles, there is a characteristic marked chin elevation because the eyes are held in a downward position by tight, inelastic inferior recti muscles. Exotropia is common, but variable. Either one or both inferior rectus muscles may be involved. A bilateral lid ptosis is present, which may be a pseudoptosis or a partial true ptosis.

THERAPY

Surgical. The goal of surgical management of congenital fibrosis of the extraocular muscles is functional readjustment of the ocular and lid position, as well as the abnormal head position. In those patients with pronounced backward head tilt and chin-up position, a maximal recession of the inferior rectus muscle relieves the exaggerated, uncomfortable position. However, elevation of a hypotropic eye accentuates the ptosis problem to the extent that a frontalis suspension may be required at the same time or soon after the motility correction. The horizontal deviation can be adjusted subsequently.

Levator resection or tucking for ptosis correction is effective only in mild cases; therefore, a frontalis suspension using fascia lata is generally the procedure of choice. Ptosis correction by brow suspension for patients without Bell's phenomenon produces a significant lagophthalmos, which can cause corneal complications. In such cases, the lid should be elevated only to the upper pupillary border so that complications may be avoided with this procedure.

Fibrosis of the superior rectus muscle is seen rarely in which the eye is markedly elevated under the upper lid. Tenotomy of the superior rectus permits the eye to resume the primary position. Early surgery and patching are advisable to help eliminate amblyopia.

Ocular or Periocular Manifestations

Eyelids: Ptosis.
Globe: Endophthalmos.
Optic Nerve: Disc hypoplasia.
Other: Astigmatism; esotropia; exotropia; hypotropia; nystagmus; visual loss.

PRECAUTIONS

Ptosis correction by brow suspension for patients without Bell's phenomenon may result in a significant lagophthalmos, which can cause such corneal complications as exposure keratopathy or corneal leukoma.

COMMENTS

The general fibrosis syndrome is the most severe form of congenital fibrosis of the extraocular muscles. All muscles, including the levator, are involved in this bilateral condition. Congenital fibrosis of the inferior rectus alone or with the levator is probably a variant of the general fibrosis syndrome. Strabismus fixus is a rare congenital disorder in which the eyes are observed in a markedly fixed position of esotropia or, less commonly, exotropia. The vertical retraction syndrome is the ability to depress either eye in abduction, with resistance encountered on attempted elevation. It may be an additional expression of the congenital fibrosis syndrome.

Three cases of congenital unilateral orbital fibrosis were reported with complete restriction of ocular motility caused by orbital defects, including adhesive bands, bone defects, or a mass lesion. The possibility of prenatal orbital penetration was considered.

In addition, a patient with bilateral congenital ocular fibrosis syndrome associated with Prader-Willi syndrome has been described. Although no abnormality was discovered with the long arm of chromosome 15 in this case, as has been reported with the Prader-Willi syndrome, the association suggested a possible linkage of the two disorders on the same chromosome.

Operative procedures of various types offer much hope for the patients. However, the responsibility of the ophthalmologist is not only strabismus and ptosis correction. Many of these individuals require genetic counseling as well, and this service should be made available.

Other ocular and systemic anomalies have been noted in patients with the general fibrosis syndrome. Ocular anomalies observed were the Marcus Gunn jaw wink, choroidal coloboma, pendular nystagmus, and optic nerve hypoplasia. Systemic abnormalities included ventricular septal defect, talipes equinovalgus, unilateral facial palsy, and facial asymmetry.

References

Apt L, Axilrod RN: Generalized fibrosis of the extraocular muscles. Am J Ophthalmol 85:822, 1978.

Brodsky MD, Pollock SC, Buckley EG: Neural misdirection in congenital ocular fibrosis syndrome: Implications and pathogenesis. J Pediatr Ophthalmol Strabismus 26:159, 1989.

Duke-Elder S (ed): System of Ophthalmology, St. Louis, CV Mosby, 1964, Vol III, pp 984–997; 1973, Vol VI, pp 736–752.

Effron L, Price RL, Berlin AJ: Congenital unilateral fibrosis with suspected prenatal orbital penetration. J Pediatr Ophthalmol Strabismus 2:133–136, 1985.

Harley RD, Rodrigues MM, Crawford JS: Congenital fibrosis of the extraocular muscles. J Pediatr Ophthalmol Strabismus 15:346–358, 1978.

Hiatt RL, Halle AA: General fibrosis syndrome. Ann Ophthalmol 15:1103, 1983.

Kalpakian B, et al: Congenital ocular fibrosis syndrome with the Prader-Willi syndrome. J Pediatr Ophthalmol Strabismus 23:170–173, 1986.

Khodadoust AA, von Noorden GK: Bilateral vertical retraction syndrome. Arch Ophthalmol 78: 606, 1967.

Leone CR, Weinstein GW: Orbital fibrosis with enophthalmos. Ophthalmic Surg 3:71, 1972.

Takeda K, Sakurai I: A general fibrosis syndrome. Folia Ophthalmol Jpn 28:1475–1480, 1977.

CONVERGENCE INSUFFICIENCY 378.83

(Asthenovergence of Stutterheim)

MALCOLM L. MAZOW, M.D.

Houston, Texas

Reading easily and comfortably is of paramount importance in the intellectual development of the child and young adult. It is a relative facility of accommodation and convergence that allows the young person to read at close range. When these mechanisms fail, reading becomes tiring, frequently producing headaches and even diplopia.

Asthenopia in a school-aged individual can be a significant handicap to learning. An inability to concentrate on written material creates frustration, impeding the learning process. Once the refractive error has been corrected and the symptoms persist, evaluation of the patient for mechanisms of binocular dysfunction is carried out.

Convergence insufficiency is a term for a group of common symptoms that, when occurring together, represent a syndrome. Without limitation of the lateral adduction, the eyes fail to converge fully, and only one eye appears to fixate when looking at a near point. The symptoms are similar to those of asthenopia and may include burning, tearing, blurred vision, diplopia, headaches, and difficulty in following moving objects. An absolute insufficiency exists when the near point (in the absence of presbyopia) is greater than 11 cm from the intraocular baseline (9.5 cm from the baseline of the cornea) or when there is difficulty in attaining 30 degrees of convergence. These criteria measure involuntary convergence, but voluntary convergence is also frequently disturbed. Relative insufficiency is for a particular working distance and is of more clinical importance. In this case, more than one-third of the total convergence cannot be used for any length of time without fatigue. Anatomic conditions, such as a wide interpupillary distance, may cause these convergence difficulties, but delayed development of a recent acquired function is apparently the most common etiologic factor. The diagnosis is based on the presence of orthophoria or a small phoric imbalance at distance, the periodic increase of divergence with subsequent phoria as the near point is approached, low prism convergence, and normal prism divergence.

Accommodative insufficiency combined with convergence insufficiency has been an often overlooked cause of asthenopic symptoms in children and young adults. There are now three major studies in the ophthalmologic literature with a total of 38 patients having significant accommodative and convergence insufficiency. In addition, attention must be paid to the presbyopic loss of accommodation in these prepresbyopic patients. This loss usually develops over a long period of time and must be recognized before proper therapy can be instituted. In both of the aforementioned groups, poor recovery of fusion, once broken, may be the most dramatic finding. Measurements of amplitudes of convergence with recovery are mandatory to ensure the diagnosis.

THERAPY

Ocular. Orthoptics is the treatment of choice. Both the facilitation of the reflexes mediating reflex convergence and the encouragement of this process by enlisting the aid of voluntary convergence are necessary to elicit satisfactory results. Before the institution of therapy, patching of one eye should be done. If symptoms persist, then the therapy for fusional deficiencies will not give the desired results. An adequate trial of patching with the assurance of clarity, accommodation, or its equivalent will then determine the need for the fusional amplitude therapy. Near-point exercises with a flashlight and red filter are suggested. The subjective near point should be brought into the break point, where the patient then backs up, fuses, and holds. The patient then gradually moves in, holding the two images as one, until 10 cm is reached or the symptoms have diminished. This is done on a sustained, rather than a short-time, basis.

Antisuppression techniques, including physiologic diplopia, are helpful in order to force the patient to appreciate diplopia. In conjunction with the exercises glasses may be required to stimulate accommodation and convergence. Hypermetropes should be given undercorrection, and myopes should be corrected fully, especially if reading.

If the symptoms are not sufficiently relieved by the above therapy, stereograms of the base-out type are employed. In conjunction with stereograms or instead of these instruments, the patient must attempt to build up amplitudes using base-out prisms. The base-out prism stimulates convergence, requiring fusional amplitudes. Gradual build-up resulting in the base-out prism convergence capabilities at near of three times distance will provide great relief of symptoms. An average end point is 35 to 40 prism diopters base-out at near. Once this is accomplished, the stereograms become much easier to do, with more desired results. Base-in prism spectacles will relieve symptoms, eliminating the patient's need and demand for convergence, which he or she is incapable of handling. They are especially beneficial in the presbyope who has insufficient convergence powers for near.

It was felt for many years that base-in prism was contraindicated because of the increase in deviation by decreased convergence demand. Time has not borne this out, and those individuals with both accommodative and convergence insufficiency may well use the base-in prism as the treatment of choice. If, however, the reverse is true, the deviation will worsen, necessitating surgery for correction.

Surgical. In patients who exhibit a large deviation for near (over 18 prism diopters), a remote near point of convergence, and intermittency, resection of the medial recti may be advisable, since the deficiency of the near point is corrected at the cost of esophoria or intermittent esotropia. Therefore, surgery is contraindicated, except when the defect is merely part of an exophoria of the convergence weakness type of sufficient severity to warrant it.

Ocular or Periocular Manifestations

Lacrimal System: Increased tear secretion.
Other: Astigmatism, decreased visual acuity; diplopia; exotropia; hypermetropia; irritation; orthotropia.

PRECAUTIONS

The physician should realize that much of the problem is psychogenic in origin. Any time the patient is debilitated for any reason, the conditions may be exacerbated. Symptoms of the syndrome frequently cause a neurosis that may persist after the condition has been corrected. Some patients need phenobarbital or other medications to calm them sufficiently to handle the exercises. However, certain medications, such as chlordiazepoxide and diazepam, worsen the condition by suppressing midbrain activity and should therefore not be used during therapy.

The correct diagnosis is often missed owing to the administration of cycloplegics before an ophthalmic examination. When they are given, the proper measurements cannot be made.

COMMENTS

There are two peaks in the incidence of convergence insufficiency. Although the disorder is seen throughout adult life, an initial peak may occur in the high school, college, or graduate student who is required to use the eyes for concentrated prolonged near work. The second peak is reached when an individual approaches early bifocal age and must learn to use bifocals to see clearly at near.

References

Chrousos GA, O'Neill JF, et al: Accommodative deficiency in healthy young adults. J Pediatr Ophthalmol Strabismus 25:176–179, 1988.

Duke-Elder S (ed): System of Ophthalmology. St. Louis, CV Mosby, 1973, Vol VI, pp 566–572.

Mazow ML: The convergence insufficiency syndrome. J Pediatr Ophthalmol 8:243–244, 1971.

Mazow ML, France TD, et al: Acute accommodative and convergence insufficiency. Trans Am Ophthalmol Soc 77:158–173. 1989.

von Noorden GK, Brown DJ, Parks M: Associated convergence and accommodative insufficiency. Doc Ophthalmol 34:393–403, 1989.

DISSOCIATED VERTICAL DEVIATION 378.31
(Alternating Sursumduction, Dissociated Vertical Divergence, Double-Dissociated Hypertropia, Occlusion Hypertropia)

RONALD V. KEECH, M.D.

Iowa City, Iowa

Dissociated vertical deviation is an ocular misalignment characterized by elevation, abduction, and excyclotorsion that may affect one eye or alternate between both eyes. It is generally comitant, bilateral, and asymmetric. Dissociated vertical deviation may present as an intermittent or constant tropia or as a phoria that occurs only when fixation is disrupted. Innervational, muscular, and sensory abnormalities have all been considered as possible causes, but the etiology is currently unknown. Dissociated vertical deviation may be distinguished from other vertical strabismus by the lack of a corresponding hypodeviation of the contralateral eye on alternate cover testing.

Dissociated vertical deviation is almost always associated with other forms of infantile strabismus. The incidence of dissociated vertical deviation in congenital esotropia is between 40 and 90 per cent, although it is rarely observed before 1 year of age. Other frequently accompanying abnormalities include inferior oblique overactions, head tilts, and latent nystagmus. It is less commonly associated with exotropia, heterophorias, and other vertical deviations.

THERAPY

Ocular. Correction of any ocular abnormality that limits binocular vision may improve a coexisting dissociated vertical deviation; occlusion for amblyopia, glasses or surgery for horizontal strabismus, and orthoptics for heterophorias can be beneficial in selected cases.

If the vision in each eye is nearly equal and the dissociated vertical deviation is asymmetric, switching fixation to the dissociated eye is sometimes effective. This may be accomplished with patching or by overcorrecting or undercorrecting a refractive error with glasses or contact lenses.

Surgical. If a dissociated vertical deviation is unresponsive to conservative treatment and the appearance is unsatisfactory, surgery to restore more normal ocular alignment should be considered. Good results have been achieved with a superior rectus recession of 5 to 16 mm. For small recessions, the muscle is sutured directly to the sclera. With larger recessions, the suture is attached to the original muscle insertion, allowing the muscle to recess the desired amount. Although problems with elevation of the eye, lid changes, and interference with the superior oblique muscle action might be expected to occur, they have not proven to be significant.

Another technique is a 2- to 6-mm recession of the superior rectus muscle combined with a posterior fixation suture placed 12 to 15 mm behind the original muscle insertion. Although technically more difficult, this procedure has the theoretical advantage of limiting the elevation of the eye without changing its position in primary gaze.

It is not clear whether surgery should be performed on one or both eyes. Limiting surgery to the worst eye is effective, except for the patient who alternates fixation between eyes. If the operated eye takes up fixation after unilateral surgery, a large vertical deviation will result in the opposite eye. Under these circumstances bilateral surgery may be a better choice. When the size of the dissociated vertical deviation is very asymmetric, however, bilateral surgery may leave the worse eye significantly undercorrected.

Dissociated vertical deviations are frequently associated with overaction of the inferior oblique muscles. In this situation, a recession and anterior displacement of the inferior oblique muscle have been effective in improving both conditions. The disinserted inferior oblique muscle is resutured to the globe laterally and sometimes anteriorly to the lateral pole of the insertion of the inferior rectus muscle.

Ocular or Periocular Manifestations

Extraocular Muscles: Congenital esotropia; inferior oblique overaction.

Other: Amblyopia; nystagmus; abnormal head position.

PRECAUTIONS

Accurate assessment of dissociated vertical deviation can be difficult. If the dissociated eye has dense amblyopia, a prism light reflex test (Krimsky test) should be used. If the vision is good, the deviation can be measured by a modified prism cover test. The deviated eye is occluded and a base-down prism added until no downward movement of the deviated eye is seen when the occluder is transferred to the opposite eye.

It is important to distinguish a dissociated vertical deviation from an overacting inferior oblique muscle. Doing so can be especially difficult because the two conditions frequently occur together. Overaction of the inferior oblique muscle is characterized by an incomitant deviation that is greater in adduction than abduction, a V-pattern strabismus, and the presence of a corresponding hypodeviation on alternate cover testing.

Although uncommon, possible complications from surgery for dissociated vertical deviation include limitation of elevation, overcorrection, abnormal torsion, change in eyelid position, and secondary overaction of the contralateral inferior oblique muscle.

COMMENTS

An unusual variation of a dissociated vertical deviation is a dissociated horizontal deviation. It is thought to be a type of dissociated vertical deviation in which the horizontal component predominates. A lateral rectus recession of the involved eye or eyes has proved beneficial in these cases.

Most dissociated vertical deviations are latent or of a small magnitude and do not require surgical intervention. However, when surgery is indicated, complete elimination of the deviation is difficult.

References

Esswein MB, von Noorden GK, Coburn A: Comparison of surgical methods in the treatment of dissociated vertical deviation. Am J Ophthalmol 113:287–290, 1992.

Helveston EM: Dissociated vertical deviation—A clinical and laboratory study. Trans Am Ophthalmol Soc 78:734–779, 1980.

Kratz RE, Rogers GL, Bremer DL, Leguire LE: Anterior tendon displacement of the inferior oblique for DVD. J Pediatr Ophthalmol Strabismus 26:212–217, 1989.

Magoon E, Cruciger M, Jampolsky A: Dissociated vertical deviation: An asymmetric condition treated with large bilateral superior rectus recession. J Pediatr Ophthalmol Strabismus 19:152–156, 1982.

Mallett RA, Repka MX, Guyton DL: Superior rectus suspension-recession for dissociated vertical deviation. Binocular Vision 2:209–215, 1987.

Schwartz T, Scott WE: Unilateral superior rectus re-

cession for the treatment of dissociated vertical deviation. J Pediatr Ophthalmol Strabismus 28: 219–222, 1991.
Wilson ME, McClatchey SK: Dissociated horizontal deviation. J Pediatr Ophthalmol Strabismus 28: 90–95, 1991.

DUANE'S RETRACTION SYNDROME 378.71

HENRY S. METZ, M.D.

Rochester, New York

Duane's retraction syndrome is a congenital disorder of ocular motility that is caused by an abnormal innervational pattern. Characteristically, abduction is limited or absent, with mild to moderate limitation of adduction (type 1). On adduction, there is retraction of the globe and a narrowing of the palpebral fissure; on attempted abduction, the palpebral fissure is noted to widen. Upshoot or downshoot of the eye or both frequently occur on adduction.

The majority of patients have a relatively small degree of esotropia in the primary position (less than 30 prism diopters), whereas some are orthotropic and a few exotropic. A habitual face turn toward the side of the underacting lateral rectus muscle may be done to provide fusion. Diplopia is an unusual complaint, although it can be demonstrated by appropriate testing. The condition is bilateral in 15 to 20 per cent of cases. The left eye is more often involved in unilateral cases, and Duane's syndrome occurs more commonly in females. Hereditary patterns are infrequent. Amblyopia secondary to strabismus is unusual, although anisometropia is common and may cause some decrease in vision. Binocular function is often good because of the ability to fuse in gaze opposite the Duane's involved eye.

Less common forms of Duane's syndrome include a type with marked limitation of adduction (and retraction) with only modest abduction deficiency and exotropia in primary gaze (type 2) and another form with significant abduction and adduction limitations (type 3).

THERAPY

Supportive. If there is no deviation in primary gaze or no habitual head turn, treatment is unnecessary. Glasses for correction of any significant refractive error or anisometropia can be beneficial. Orthoptics are generally not of value. Occlusion therapy for strabismic amblyopia is rarely needed.

Surgical. The goal of surgery should be straight eyes in the primary position without a head turn. Full abduction is not possible and does not seem to be a realistic aim of treatment.

Recession of the medial rectus muscle in the eye involved with Duane's syndrome can reduce both the esotropia and the head turn, but limited abduction cannot be improved. For larger amounts of estropia, bilateral medial rectus recession can be helpful. Resection of the involved lateral rectus is contraindicated, as it worsens the retraction of the globe on attempted adduction.

If adduction limitation and retraction of the globe with adduction are marked, lateral rectus recession in the Duane's eye along with medial rectus recession bilaterally is a useful option.

Lateral transposition of the insertions of the vertical recti has been described. Although some modest improvement of abduction was noted, some patients became exotropic, and this procedure is not recommended.

A "Faden"-type procedure on the lateral rectus muscle has been reported to minimize or eliminate the upshoot and downshoot that are sometimes seen on adduction. Splitting and recessing the lateral rectus, with attachment of the upper half of the insertion superiorly on the globe and the lower half of the insertion inferiorly on the globe, have also been reported to eliminate the upshoot or downshoot on adduction.

In type 2 Duane's syndrome, lateral rectus recession can both improve the exotropia and reduce the retraction of the globe on attempted adduction.

Ocular or Periocular Manifestations

Extraocular Muscles: Marked limitation of abduction; mild limitation of adduction with retraction of the globe; overshoot in the field of action of the inferior and superior oblique muscles.

Eyelids: Widening of the lid fissure on abduction and narrowing on adduction.

Other: Amblyopia; anisometropia; hearing deficits; coloboma of iris and choroid; corneal dermoid; head and neck malformations; association with the fetal alcohol syndrome.

PRECAUTIONS

Occasionally, patients with Duane's syndrome are misdiagnosed as having sixth nerve palsies because of the marked limitation of abduction. The surgical treatment for lateral rectus palsy often involves medial rectus recession and lateral rectus resection for the esotropia. If this plan is followed in Duane's syndrome, especially in a patient with marked retraction of the globe on adduction, a significant problem may result. On gaze to the side opposite the Duane's syndrome, the contralateral eye will abduct; the Duane's eye, instead of adducting in a conjugate fashion, may also abduct (the "splits"). Transposition of the vertical rectus insertions to the lateral side of the globe will usually limit adduction further and can result in an overcorrection in primary gaze (exotropia), as well as an induced vertical deviation.

COMMENTS

The constellation of findings noted in Duane's syndrome are caused by electrical silence of the lateral rectus muscle on attempted abduction with co-contraction of the medial and lateral rectus muscles on attempted adduction. These electromyographic findings explain the retraction of the globe and the lid fissure changes on horizontal gaze. Saccadic velocity testing can also assist in diagnosis. Abduction saccades are extremely slow (as in sixth nerve palsy), whereas adduction saccades are only modestly reduced in speed (due to lateral rectus contraction on adduction).

There has been a recent report of abnormal brainstem auditory evoked potentials in a group of patients with Duane's syndrome, indicating a pontine abnormality. A clinicopathologic report of a case of bilateral Duane's syndrome demonstrated the absence of both abducens nuclei and nerves. The lateral rectus muscles were partially innervated by branches of the oculomotor nerves.

Duane's syndrome may be caused by a teratogenic stimulus during the first trimester of pregnancy. Many of the anomalies that have been associated with the retraction syndrome share a common critical time of embryologic development.

References

Duane A: Congenital deficiency of abduction, associated with impairment of adduction, retraction movements, contraction of the palpebral fissure and oblique movements of the eye. Arch Ophthalmol 34:135–159, 1905.
Gobin MH: Surgical management of Duane's syndrome. Br J Ophthalmol 58:301–306, 1974.
Holzman AE, Chrousos GA, Kozma C, Trabulsi EI: Duane's retraction syndrome in the fetal alcohol syndrome. Am J Ophthalmol 110:565–566, 1990.
Hotchkiss MG, et al: Bilateral Duane's retraction syndrome: A clinical-pathologic case report. Arch Ophthalmol 98:870–874, 1980.
Huber A: Electrophysiology of the retraction syndromes. Br J Ophthalmol 58:293–300, 1974.
Isenberg S, Urist MJ: Clinical observations in 101 consecutive patients with Duane's retraction syndrome. Am J Ophthalmol 84:419–425, 1977.
Jay WM, Hoyt CS: Abnormal brain stem auditory-evoked potentials in Stilling-Turk-Duane retraction syndrome. Am J Ophthalmol 89:814–818, 1980.
Kirkham TH: Anisometropia and amblyopia in Duane's syndrome. Am J Ophthalmol 69:774–777, 1970.
Kraft SP: A surgical approach for Duane syndrome.

J Pediatr Ophthalmol Strabismus 15:119–130, 1988.
MacDonald AL, Crawford JS, Smith DR: Duane's retraction syndrome: An evaluation of the sensory status. Can J Ophthalmol 9:458–462, 1974.
Metz HS, Scott AB, Scott WE: Horizontal saccadic velocities in Duane's syndrome. Am J Ophthalmol 80:901–906, 1975.
Molarte AB, Rosenbaum AL: Vertical rectus muscle transposition surgery for Duane's syndrome. J Pediatr Ophthalmol Strabismus 27:171–177, 1990.
O'Malley ER, Helveston EM, Ellis FD: Duane's retraction syndrome—plus. J Pediatr Ophthalmol Strabismus 19:161–165, 1982.
Raab EL: Clinical features of Duane's syndrome. J Pediatr Ophthalmol Strabismus 23:64–68, 1986.

ESOTROPIA—HIGH AC/A RATIO 378.35

ARTHUR L. ROSENBAUM, M.D.

Los Angeles, California

The AC/A ratio is a measure of responsiveness of convergence for each diopter of accommodation. A high AC/A ratio is characterized by an excess of accommodative convergence for the amount of accommodation required to focus clearly at a given distance. This excessive accommodative convergence can result in an esophoria or an intermittent or constant esotropia, depending on the amount of fusional divergence available to each particular patient.

Clinically, the patient demonstrates an esodeviation that is greater at near than at distance fixation. Asthenopic symptoms of eyestrain, headaches, and even diplopia at near may occur. This type of esotropia may develop at any age, but is commonly seen in young children between ages 1 and 7 years. Parks (1958) reported a high AC/A ratio in almost 50 per cent of a population of childhood esotropes. The condition may be asymptomatic until the child is faced with stressful reading demands; it is especially common in students. Ludwig et al. (1988) determined that the rate of deterioration of esotropia after successful alignment with spectacles was greater in patients with a high AC/A ratio and less in patients with high hyperopia.

Von Noorden (1986) has pointed out that factors other than excessive accommodative convergence may cause a significant increase in esotropia at near fixation. He suggests the term "nonaccommodative convergence excess" to describe a condition in which the patient has orthotropia or a small angle esotropia at distance fixation and at near has an esotropia of 15 prism diopters or greater than the distance deviation. The patient with nonaccommodative convergence excess shows no reduction of the deviation at near with additional spherical plus lenses. This lack of reduction with plus spheres differentiates this type of patient from one with a high AC/A ratio. The AC/A ratio in patients with non-accommodative convergence excess is normal, and tonic convergence is suspected of causing this increased esotropia at near.

THERAPY

Ocular. When diplopia is present, the full cycloplegic spectacle correction should be prescribed if the patient is young enough to tolerate it. If the child is older than 7 years of age, a postcycloplegic refraction may be required. If moderate hyperopia is present, this spectacle correction will reduce the esotropia at both distance and near and may reduce the esotropia at near to an esophoria or infrequent intermittent tropia with few or no symptoms.

If little or no hyperopia is present or a single vision correction is unsuccessful, bifocals or miotics may be necessary. Bifocals are useful only when there is evidence of fusion at distance but the patient remains esotropic at near. Nothing is gained by adding bifocals if the distance esotropia remains larger than 10 to 15 prism diopters. The goal of bifocals is to create a fusional situation at near. The bifocal segment in children should be an executive type, which bisects the pupil to ensure that the bifocal is used for near fixation. In adults, the bifocal height may be lowered. The bifocal power usually varies between +1.50 and +3.00 diopters. The amount required can be determined by office trials of incremental increases in power until the esotropia at near is abolished or converted to a small phoria. Fresnel membrane spheres may be used as bifocal trials to determine effectiveness and power requirements, since a few days may be required to see whether the deviation may actually be reduced.

Pratt-Johnson and Tillson (1985) reported the long-term follow-up of esotropic patients with a high AC/A ratio, some of which were treated with bifocals. No significant difference in sensory fusion results was recorded in those patients wearing bifocals compared to those who did not wear bifocals. Miotic therapy was not particularly helpful in the long term.

If spectacle correction is only partially successful, orthoptics may be tried in an effort to increase fusional divergence amplitudes. In patients over the age of 12 years, an attempt should be made to reduce gradually the bifocal power, with the goal of eliminating the segment.

If bifocals are unsuccessful, miotics may be used. Some ophthalmologists actually prefer miotics as the first line of therapy, since some children object to bifocals and the possibility of prolonged hypoaccommodation exists with bifocals. Miotics may be especially useful in

young esotropia patients with a high AC/A ratio who do not otherwise require spectacles. Again, they should only be used when the goal is to eliminate the deviation at near and to create a fusional situation. The miotics used in esotropia with a high AC/A ratio are usually those of the anticholinesterase type that reduces the need for innervationally produced cholinesterase in the ciliary body. This reduction in required innervation reduces the accommodative effort required, thereby lowering the accommodative convergence. Miotics also cause pupillary constriction and accommodative spasm. These effects usually are intolerable in older children and adults. Administration of 0.30 to 0.125 per cent echothiophate solution daily or 0.025 per cent isoflurophate ointment every other day is effective. Both drugs are administered at bedtime to reduce symptoms of accommodative spasm.

Surgical. Surgery may be required if symptoms persist despite the above ocular measures and fusion exists at distance. In these cases, recession of each medial rectus muscle has a good chance of reducing the near deviation without causing an overcorrection at distance. Some success has been reported using posterior fixation sutures, the Faden procedure, on each medial rectus muscle. If the patient is older than 11 years of age, an adjustable recession procedure should be considered. Amblyopic treatment is essential before making a surgical decision.

Kushner et al. (1987) performed a prospective randomized trial of symmetric medial rectus recession with posterior fixation sutures versus symmetric augmented medial rectus recessions without posterior fixation sutures. A higher percentage of the augmented recession group achieved satisfactory alignment and were able to discontinue wearing bifocals postoperatively than those receiving posterior fixation sutures and recession. The number of patients surgically overcorrected was greater in the posterior fixation suture treated group.

Procianoy and Justo (1991) reported a series of patients treated with 6 to 8 mm unilateral medial rectus recession. Based on the near deviation, 96 per cent of the patients were aligned within 10 prism diopters.

The postoperative sensory status of treated patients with a high AC/A ratio has been analyzed by Leitch et al. (1990). Even though most patients have excellent bifoveal fixation at distance, only 16 per cent achieved bifoveal fusion at near. Seventy-one per cent had varying degrees of peripheral fusion, and a few had no detectable binocularity in the near range.

Ocular or Periocular Manifestations

Extraocular Muscles: Diplopia; esophoria; esotropia.
Other: Amblyopia; hyperopia; myopia.

PRECAUTIONS

It is imperative that the patient or the parents of the child on miotics be aware that the anesthesiologist must be warned of their use before any routine or emergency surgery. If the anesthesiologist uses muscle relaxants, such as succinylcholine, in a patient on anticholinesterase inhibitors or one who has been on these medications for several weeks before the anesthesia, prolonged respiratory paralysis may result. The anticholinesterase inhibitors lower blood cholinesterase levels, and muscle relaxants, such as succinylcholine, require cholinesterase for inactivation. Therefore, the anesthesiologist who is told about the use of miotics can then choose to use muscle relaxants that do not depend on cholinesterase for inactivation.

Iris cysts develop frequently with the use of miotics, but are only rarely large enough to warrant discontinuing the drug. Their incidence and size may be reduced with the concomitant use of 2.5 per cent phenylephrine drops. Miotic drugs may produce cataracts in adults, but only one case of transient lens changes has been reported in children. Retinal detachment and the precipitation of acute angle-closure glaucoma have been reported, but occur very rarely in children. Systemic side effects of miotics may include abdominal cramps, micturition, diarrhea, nausea, and vomiting.

COMMENTS

Esotropia with a high AC/A ratio may develop in hyperopic, myopic, and emmetropic subjects. The diagnosis is made by cover-uncover testing at distance and near with the full hyperopic or myopic refractive error corrected and with the patient focused on an accommodative target to avoid the possibility of hypo- or hyperaccommodation that may lead to variable and spurious measurements. Measurements at near should be made in the primary rather than in the reading position to avoid the error of actually detecting a V-pattern esotropia.

References

Breinin GM: Accommodative strabismus in the AC/A ratio. Am J Ophthalmol 71:303–311, 1971.

Kushner, BJ, Preslan M, Morton G: Treatment of partially accommodative esotropia with a high accommodative convergence-accommodation ratio. Arch Ophthalmol 105:815–818, 1987.

Leitch RJ, Burke JP, Strachan I: Convergence excess esotropia treated surgically with Faden operation and medial rectus muscle recessions. Br J Ophthalmol 74:278–279, 1990.

Ludwig I, Parks M, Getson P, Kammerman L: Rate of deterioration in accommodative esotropia correlated to the AC/A relationship. J Pediatr Ophthalmol Strabismus 25:8–12, 1988.

Parks MM: Abnormal accommodative convergence in squint. Arch Ophthalmol 59:364–380, 1958.

Pratt-Johnson JA, Tillson G: The management of esotropia with high AC/A ratio. J Pediatr Ophthalmol Strabismus 22:238–242, 1985.

Procianoy E, Justo D: Results of unilateral medial rectus recession in high AC/A ratio esotropia. J Pediatr Ophthalmol Strabismus 28:212–214, 1991.

Rosenbaum AL, Jampolsky A, Scott AB: Bimedial recession in high AC/A esotropia. A long-term follow-up. Arch Ophthalmol 91:251–253, 1974.

Sears M, Guber D: The change in the stimulus AC/A ratio after surgery. Am J Ophthalmol 64:872–876, 1967.

von Noorden G, Avilla C: Nonaccommodative convergence excess. Am J Ophthalmol 101:70–73, 1986.

INTERMITTENT EXOTROPIA 378.23

HIRAM H. HARDESTY, M.D.

Cleveland, Ohio

Because of its high recurrence rate, intermittent exotropia is often a frustrating strabismus to manage. This frustration is minimized by having realistic expectations for correcting this type of strabismus with one surgical procedure and by having a plan for the effective management of recurrences. Persistent overcorrections, although less common, can be very distressing to both the ophthalmologist and the parents. However, it is comforting to know that with proper care even large overcorrections have an excellent prognosis.

Nearly all patients with intermittent exotropia have some degree of fusion or at least a fusion potential. With proper management, even patients who can straighten their eyes only momentarily have a good prognosis. Since these patients have severely compromised fusion, a larger percentage require more than one operative procedure.

There are few published series with adequate follow-up of patients undergoing surgery for intermittent exotropia. However, the studies that do exist reveal that, with one operation, at best 40 to 50 per cent of the patients are immediately undercorrected or recur with time. Five to ten per cent remain permanently overcorrected unless further treatment is instituted. With some series, the success rate is as low as 25 per cent.

Not only is it important to be aware of these facts, but it is also important that the parents be made aware of these possible undesirable responses to surgery. In the author's office, the parents are told that such problems may follow surgery and that patching, special glasses, and even more than one operation may be necessary to effect a complete cure. Once we all understand that careful, well-selected initial surgery will correct approximately half of the patients and that proper management of under- and overcorrections is the key to a high success rate, intermittent exotropia loses much of its frustration.

The literature provides little information on the management of either under- or overcorrection of intermittent exotropia. Few investigators have stressed the role of fusion. It is not rare for a patient to overcorrect immediately, become straight for a time, and then recur after several months or years. In those cases, the problem is not too little surgery, but rather too little fusion.

Pratt-Johnson is one of the few investigators who has stressed the role and importance of fusion. The author wholeheartedly agrees that fusion plays an extremely important part in effecting a cure as defined in this article. Operating in the presence of severely compromised fusion usually results in recurrence. Unless attention is directed toward improving the fusion status of such patients, even multiple surgical procedures usually fail to effect a cure.

One no longer needs to be reluctant to operate on young children, even those under 2 years of age. It is often stated that operating on a young child frequently results in a small-angle esotropia that may lead to amblyopia. With proper management of overcorrections, this complication is no longer a significant danger. In over 300 cases with an average follow-up of over 5 years, the author has found no true small-angle esotropia. Even monofixation syndromes have been rare, and none of these children has developed amblyopia that was not then treated successfully.

Before proceeding to the discussion of surgery for intermittent exotropia, the term "cure" is defined. Cure means a *functional* cure, for which the patient must meet the following criteria: (1) there is no tropia, constant or intermittent, at either distance or near; (2) all supplementary therapy, such as prisms, orthoptics, and anticholinesterase medications have been discontinued; (3) the patient and the parents are unaware of any manifest deviation, even with extreme fatigue; and (4) the patient must demonstrate some degree of stereopsis on the Titmus stereotest.

THERAPY

Surgical. Not all surgeons agree on the proper surgical procedure for intermittent exotropia. Nearly all prefer a bilateral recession of the lateral recti for all patients with divergence excess type of intermittent exotropia. Many prefer a recess-resect procedure for basic and convergence insufficiency types. Few advocate bilateral resection of the medial recti as an initial procedure, even with the convergence insufficiency type.

The author's choice is to perform a bilateral recession of the lateral recti for all types. In a previous study, it was found that bilateral recession of the lateral recti did not affect the distance measurement more than the near measurement. Furthermore, no long term study has established the efficacy of a recess-resect procedure over a bilateral recession of the lateral recti for any type of intermittent exotropia.

Table 1 suggests guidelines for initial surgery.

Occasionally patients have a lesser degree of exodeviation on lateral gaze than in primary position. The author finds this to be less common than reported by other investigators. However, when such incomitance does occur to a significant degree, these patients have a good prognosis if the amount of recession of the lateral recti is reduced slightly.

It is necessary to weaken the inferior obliques when they are overactive, but with intermittent exotropia, such overactions are uncommon. Although this subject is controversial, the author agrees with Parks and others that tenotomy of the superior obliques should be reserved for *constant* A-pattern exotropia. This procedure for *intermittent* A-pattern exotropia may result in a vertical deviation with distressing torticollis.

Surgery should be advised whenever it becomes evident to both the parents and the ophthalmologist that the intermittent exotropia is definitely present and shows no sign of improvement. Delaying beyond this time results in deepening of suppression, as well as in lessening of fusional amplitudes. It results in a higher percentage of failures.

The patient who is operated on early before fusion is compromised severely, needs to be overcorrected very little or not at all. It is the longstanding exotrope with poor fusion that needs to be overcorrected up to 20 prism diopters. In this case, a large overcorrection is the only chance of effecting a cure with a single surgical procedure.

UNDERCORRECTIONS. As soon as an undercorrection is noted, the patient should be placed in base-in prisms to effect constant binocularity. If the child is seen soon after the recurrence of intermittent exotropia, one should prescribe an amount of prisms midway between the distance and near measurements. Since these children will be wearing prisms for several months, it is advisable to have the prisms ground into regular spectacle

TABLE 1. Bilateral Recession of Lateral Recti For X (T) (Based on Distance Measurement)*

20 prism diopters	4.0 mm OU
25 prism diopters	5.0 mm OU
30 prism diopters	5.5 mm OU
35 prism diopters	6.0 mm OU
40 prism diopters	6.5 mm OU

*If near measurement exceeds the distance measurement by more than 5 prism diopters, add 1 mm OU.

lenses. Fresnel press-on prisms are difficult to keep clean and become cloudy with the passage of time. In the author's experience, patients with prisms up to 10 diopters (each lens) are pleased when shifted from Fresnel press-on prisms to prism glasses. A small frame should be selected and the optician instructed to grind the prisms as thin as possible. Any significant refractive error should be incorporated in the glasses.

If the prism glasses are found to be of inadequate strength, a press-on prism can be added to the lens of the *preferred* eye. This usually requires a prism of low power, and the optics of the lower power press-on prism are superior to optics of higher powers.

The glasses should be worn at all times. Small children should be fitted with frames that hook firmly behind the ears. Once the glasses are made as suggested and the parents are firmly impressed with the importance of constant wear, there is little difficulty with compliance. If, after wearing the prism glasses for 6 months, the intermittent exotropia cannot be detected with the prism glasses removed, the child is usually given a trial without prisms. With cases that recur after removal of the prisms, the parents are given a choice between proceeding with surgery or having their child wear the prisms for another 6 months. Although surgery is offered at this time, it is not strongly urged unless the child is showing resistance to wearing prisms. Surgery is not urgent so long as the prisms are worn constantly. If compliance is excellent, surgery can be delayed as long as the parents wish. If, however, 6 months of wearing prisms has not resulted in constant binocularity, most parents are ready to discuss further surgery.

Originally, base-in prisms were prescribed for patients with recurrent intermittent exotropia solely for the purpose of improving the prognosis for a second surgical procedure. It was surprising to find that, with some patients, fusion was improved to such a degree that a functional cure resulted, making further surgery unnecessary.

The records of 268 private patients of the author who have undergone bilateral recession for intermittent exotropia between the years of 1964 and 1984 were reviewed. The follow-up range was from 1 to 15 years with an average of 5.4 years. Prisms were worn by 105 patients whose intermittent exotropia recurred. Of these 105 patients, 34 met the criteria for cure from just wearing the prisms alone. The same number of patients have undergone bilateral resection of the medial recti during this same period. It was found that children under six years of age, especially those with divergence excess type intermittent exotropia, have the best prognosis for a prism cure.

It is the exception for an older child with a longstanding intermittent exotropia to be cured solely by wearing prisms. Still, it is im-

portant for these children to wear prisms after recurrence of their intermittent exotropia because of their great need for improved fusion before their second surgery. In the author's study, some of these patients wore prisms for over a year, especially those who had an associated vertical deviation.

In addition, it was observed that, once patients wore prisms constantly, exotropia drift was rare. The exodeviation lessened more frequently than it worsened. Perhaps this result should not have been a surprise. If patients who have never had strabismus do not undergo an exoshift with the passage of time, why should the postsurgical patient manifest such a shift when fusing constantly with the assistance of prisms? It is the constant binocularity in either case that maintains stability of alignment.

Bilateral resection of the medial recti is the procedure of choice for recurrent intermittent exotropia up to 30 prism diopters. The author has completed a study of 56 patients who have undergone bilateral resection of the medial recti for recurrent intermittent exotropia. In each instance, the initial procedure was bilateral recession of the lateral recti. A cure rate of 70 per cent was obtained. Of those patients who did not meet the criteria for a cure, most either did not cooperate or are still wearing prisms and are potential cures. Table 2 establishes guidelines for selecting the proper amount of bilateral resection of the medial recti for varying amounts of recurrent intermittent exotropia.

Close observation immediately after surgery is extremely important. An immediate overcorrection up to 20 prism diopters is desirable. If the eyes are not at least intermittently straight after 3 weeks, the overcorrection should be managed in the same manner as overcorrections following initial surgery.

OVERCORRECTIONS. Although overcorrections are less common, they can be even more disconcerting than recurrences. All experienced surgeons have had a few marked consecutive esotropias. One child treated by the author developed 50 prism diopters of esotropia, and two developed over 40 prism diopters. With further surgery, these patients now meet the criteria for cure. Overcorrections have an excellent prognosis with proper management.

If the patient remains constantly esotropic for longer than 3 weeks, the following steps

TABLE 2. Bilateral Resection of Medial Recti For Recurrent X (T) (Based on Distance Measurements)*

15 prism diopters	4.5 mm OU
20 prism diopters	5.0 mm OU
25 prism diopters	6.0 mm OU
30 prism diopters	7.0 mm OU

*If the near measurement exceeds the distance measurement by more than 5 prism diopters, add 1 mm OU.

should be taken. If the patient has hypermetropia of $1^1/_2$ diopters or over, glasses should be prescribed. However, most of these patients are not hypermetropic. Constant patching should be started and continued for 3 to 4 weeks. The preferred eye should be patched unless the patient alternates, in which case the patch should be alternated. If, at the end of this time, the patient is constantly esotropic, prisms are prescribed. The prism strength should be equal to or should slightly exceed the greater measurement, whether this greater measurement is at distance or near. Prisms of inadequate strength may cause the esotropia to worsen.

When consecutive esotropia is managed in this manner, constant binocular vision with the prisms is restored promptly. Compliance is seldom a problem, especially if the child is diplopic when not wearing the glasses. The parents should be told that under these circumstances, diplopia is desirable.

If, after surgery, consecutive esotropia is permitted to remain for several weeks or months, nasal suppression occurs. Once nasal suppression becomes well established, usually the child will adapt to the prisms so that a greater strength of prism will be necessary to effect constant binocularity. If the required prism strength is small, the prisms can usually be discontinued in 6 to 12 months. With larger amounts of esotropia, surgery may be necessary, but should not be performed until the prisms have been worn for at least 6 months. Guidelines that have been found to be effective for consecutive esotropia are listed in Table 3.

PRECAUTIONS

No matter what the distance/near measurement relationship is, the author believes bilateral recession of the medial recti to be the procedure of choice. Surgery for consecutive esotropia should be conservative as these patients overcorrect easily. Overcorrection is indeed unfortunate because having now operated on all four horizontal muscles, the physician is back where he or she started. Further surgery is now even more unpredictable, not only because one must operate on scarred muscles but also because there are no longer guidelines for proper surgery.

COMMENTS

This described method of management of intermittent exotropia is based on known principles of pathophysiology of binocular vision. With either undercorrections or persistent overcorrections, fusion is restored as soon as possible by nonsurgical means. This requires minimal effort since nearly all of these patients can be restored to constant fusion by wearing prisms. Hence, with undercorrections, the worsening of old sensory defects is prevented, and with overcorrections, the development of new sensory defects is prevented. The fact that many undercorrections were corrected solely by wearing prisms certainly supports the observation that the described prism treatment significantly improves fusion status.

The author is aware that the management outlined in this chapter requires a little more attention to detail and is *slightly* more time consuming for those who work without the assistance of an orthoptist. Yet, often the alternative is multiple surgeries, and all too often a functional cure is still not the final result.

A study of 100 cases managed according to these guidelines and followed for 6.1 years was reported by the author in 1978. A functional cure rate of 78 per cent was found. These patients have since been followed for a total of 10.2 years. With the continued use of prisms and/or further surgery, the cure rate has improved to 81 per cent. If patients who did not cooperate with the recommended therapy were eliminated from the series, the cure rate would have been over 90 per cent.

References

Burian HM, Spivey BE: The surgical management of exodeviations. Am J Ophthalmol 59:603–620, 1965.

Burian HM, von Noorden GK: Binocular Vision and Ocular Motility, 3rd ed. St. Louis, CV Mosby, 1985, pp 304–315.

Clintic M, McNeer K: Postoperative drift rate of exotropia. Orthopt J 30:60, 1980.

Dunlap EA, Gaffney RB: Surgical management of intermittent exotropia. Am Orthopt J 13:20–33, 1963.

Folk ER: Surgical results in intermittent exotropia. Arch Ophthalmol 55:484–487, 1956.

Hardesty HH: Treatment of recurrent intermittent exotropia: A preliminary report. Am J Ophthalmol 60:1036–1046, 1965.

Hardesty HH: Treatment of overcorrected intermittent exotropia. Am J Ophthalmol 66:80–86, 1968.

Hardesty HH: Treatment of under and overcorrected intermittent exotropia with prism glasses. Am Orthopt J 19:110–119, 1969.

Hardesty HH: Prisms in the management of intermittent exotropia. Am Orthopt J 22:22–30, 1972.

Hardesty HH: Treatment of intermittent exotropia. Arch Ophthalmol 96:268–274, 1978.

Hardesty HH: Major review: Management of intermittent exotropia. Binocular Vision 5:145–152, 1990.

Jampolsky A: Management of exodeviations. *In* Haik GM (ed): Strabismus Symposium of the New Orleans Academy of Ophthalmology. St. Louis, CV Mosby, 1962, pp 140–156.

Knapp P: Management of exotropia. *In* Symposium on Strabismus. Transactions of the New Orleans

TABLE 3. Bilateral Recession of Medial Recti For Consecutive ET

20 prism diopters	2.5 mm OU
30 prism diopters	3.0 mm OU
40 prism diopters	4.0 mm OU

Academy of Ophthalmology. St. Louis, CV Mosby, 1971, p 236.

Moore S: The prognostic value of lateral gaze measurements in intermittent exotropia. Am Orthopt J *19*:69, 1969.

Parks MM: Ocular Motility and Strabismus. New York, Harper & Row, 1975, pp 113–121.

Pratt-Johnson JA, Barlow JM, Tillson G: Early surgery in intermittent exotropia. Am J Ophthalmol *84*:689–694, 1977.

Raab EH, Parks MM: Recession of the lateral recti. Arch Ophthalmol *82*:203, 1969.

Scott WE, Keech R, Mash A: The postoperative results and stability of exodeviations. Arch Ophthalmol *99*:1814–1818, 1980.

von Noorden GK: Simulated divergence excess diagnosis and surgical management. Doc Ophthalmol *26*:719–728, 1969.

MONOFIXATION SYNDROME 378.34

(Microstrabismus, Microtropia, Monofixational Orthophoria, Monofixational Phoria)

MARSHALL M. PARKS, M.D.

Washington, District of Columbia

A collection of patients from different sources manifest the monofixation syndrome, presenting with straight eyes or almost straight eyes, extramacular binocular vision but the absence of macular binocular vision, and with either equal visual acuity in each eye or a minimal difference. Since the patients are devoid of macular binocular vision, they must fixate with but one eye at a time; hence, the reason for the term "monofixation." Monofixating patients with extramacular normal retinal correspondence binocular vision may tolerate a manifest deviation of 8 prism diopters or less, which may be recognized as a tropia by the cover test. This explains why patients with this syndrome are referred to as having microstrabismus. However, approximately one-third of patients with this syndrome have no overt strabismus as recognized by the cover test. Therefore, a small angle deviation is not the essential finding in diagnosis of the monofixation syndrome. The syndrome is most frequently encountered as the end stage in the treatment of strabismus, in anisometropia, and a unilateral or bilateral macular anomaly. However, it may not be associated with any of these disorders, but rather may occur as a primary condition in otherwise normal eyes. It is most often found in family members of patients with congenital esotropia.

The inability to bifixate in a monofixating patient is proved by a demonstrable macular scotoma in the nonfixating eye during binocular visual field assessment. The macular scotoma vanishes during monocular visual field investigation.

A Worth 4 light test, Bagolini striated glasses test, or a more subtle vectographic Polaroid overlay test will easily disclose the 3 degree scotoma projecting from the nonfixating macula. A poor stereoacuity is another indicator of monofixation since bifixation is required to simultaneously perceive the small horizontal disparity of the identical retinal images on the maculas, which provides the perception of stereopsis. Stereo images having gross horizontal disparity are perceived by the lower resolving extramacular macular areas. All bifixators easily perceive stereopsis from 40 seconds of arc of disparity or better, but monofixators never perceive stereopsis from less than 60 seconds of arc of disparity. Therefore, the stereoacuity test is a rapid and accurate screening method to infer the presence or absence of the macular scotoma that is always found in the monofixator.

Unless the child alternates fixation, monofixation syndrome usually leads to amblyopia in the nonpreferred eye. Overcoming the amblyopia with treatment does not produce bifixation; hence, amblyopia is prone to recur after discontinuing treatment.

The monofixating patient rarely becomes bifixating, and therapy other than for amblyopia is usually unjustified. Possibly, the development of bifixation would occur in some anisometropic patients with the prevention of amblyopia, if the diagnosis and treatment of anisometropia were accomplished very early in life. Although all children should have an ophthalmologic examination by the age of 4 years whether or not symptoms are present, the discovered anisometropic amblyopia may be correctable, but the monofixation syndrome is permanent by this age.

THERAPY

Ocular. Patients with monofixation syndrome are refractory to learning to recognize diplopia by using the established orthoptic therapeutic approach for overcoming the suppression scotoma caused by tropias greater than 10 prism diopters. The scotoma in the monofixating patient's binocular field is not the suppression adaptation to single binocular vision in strabismus; rather, it is an absence of macular binocular vision. The patient with monofixation syndrome experiences physiologic diplopia or diplopia induced by displacing the image outside the scotoma with prisms. Inasmuch as these patients have adequate fusional vergence amplitudes, there is rarely a need to prescribe fusional vergence exercise. However, if the exercises are prescribed, the amplitudes increase with the same ease as in bifixating patients.

Unless the monofixating child alternates fixation from one macula to the other, the nonpreferred eye will become amblyopic. Occlusion therapy is indicated; however, the monofixation will persist despite the elimination of the amblyopia. If amblyopia tends to return when occlusion therapy is terminated, partial occlusion should be maintained until the patient is 9 years old.

Anisometropic patients may be converted to alternating the use of their monofixating maculas by the appropriate optical correction. Supplying equally clear images simultaneously to each macula usually does not improve the chance for bifixation any more than compensating for the small deviation with prism spectacles.

Surgical. Those few patients with an alternate cover test horizontal deviation of upward to 20 diopters or an alternate cover test vertical deviation of upward to 10 diopters may benefit from surgery designed to eliminate the deviations. However, these patients are rarely encountered.

COMMENTS

Some monofixating patients have a trivial deviation disclosed by the cover-uncover test, ranging from 1 to 8 prism diopters of horizontal deviation and 2 to 3 prism diopters of vertical deviation. About one-third of the patients manifest no detectable deviation of either eye by the cover-uncover test. Approximately one-third of the patients have a larger deviation disclosed by the alternate cover test. Monofixating patients usually are capable of easily overcoming their larger alternate cover deviations with their fusional vergences, reducing the deviation to 8 prism diopters or less as disclosed by the cover-uncover test.

The most impressive prognostic feature of patients with the monofixation syndrome is their static alignment state, regardless of the associated factors of strabismus, anisometropia, a unilateral macular lesion, or the absence of all three. Extramacular fusion alone seems to be just as effective as the combination of extramacular and macular fusion in maintaining straight eyes.

References

Helveston EM, von Noorden GK: Microtropia. A newly defined entity. Arch Ophthalmol 78:272–281, 1967.
Parks MM: The monofixation syndrome. Trans Am Ophthalmol Soc 67:609–657, 1979.

NYSTAGMUS 379.50
(Congenital Nystagmus, Downbeat Nystagmus, Periodic Alternating Nystagmus, Saccadic Oscillations, Vestibular Nystagmus)

ROBERT D. YEE, M.D., F.A.C.S.

Indianapolis, Indiana

Pathologic nystagmus and saccadic, oscillations are fixation instabilities that prevent the eyes from maintaining gaze steadily on targets. Abnormal eye movements move the image of the target away from the fovea. In nystagmus the abnormal movements are smooth or slow eye movements, and fast eye movements (saccades) usually bring the eyes back toward the target. Defects in various smooth eye movement systems, such as the vestibulo-ocular reflex, smooth pursuit, and optokinetic nystagmus, have been postulated as causes of nystagmus. In saccadic oscillations, fast eye movements carry the eyes away from the target, and corrective saccades attempt to bring the eyes back toward the target. Involuntary saccadic oscillations include macrosquare wave jerks, ocular flutter, and opsoclonus. Voluntary "nystagmus" consists of saccadic oscillations that some normal persons can generate volitionally. Neurons (burst cells) in the paramedian pontine reticular formation (PPRF), which discharge at high rates to generate saccades, are normally inhibited by other neurons (pause cells) until normal voluntary or involuntary saccades are made. Saccadic oscillations may be caused by the failure of pause cells to inhibit burst cells normally.

Although the types of pathologic nystagmus and saccadic oscillations are numerous, relatively few are frequently encountered by ophthalmologists among outpatients. Most fixation instabilities can be detected and classified adequately by the examiner's unaided eye. Their clinical significance, the need for additional diagnostic tests, and the drug, ocular, or surgical therapy can then be determined.

The important observations necessary to classify nystagmus include examinations for (1) waveform, (2) direction, (3) effect of visual fixation, (4) effect of gaze position, and (5) binocular symmetry. The examiner should ask the following questions: Are there slow movements in one direction and fast movements in the opposite direction (jerk waveform), or do movements in both directions have equal velocity (pendular)? Is the direction horizontal, vertical, oblique (combination of horizontal and vertical), or rotatory (torsional)? Does the amplitude or direction of the nystagmus change in different positions of gaze? If fixation is blocked by high plus lenses (Frenzel goggles), does the amplitude and frequency increase or decrease? Are the amplitude and direction of the nystagmus the same in both eyes?

The presence of associated signs and symptoms should be sought since fixation instabilities are often caused by damage to the vestibular apparatus and its pathways, brainstem, and cerebellum. Hearing loss, tinnitus, vertigo, ear pain, limb weakness or incoordination, sensory loss or paresthesias of the body, and imbalance may be accompanying symptoms. The reader can consult sources listed in the references for detailed information about the types and etiologies of fixation instabilities. A few types of nystagmus, for which medical and/or surgical therapy, have been useful are discussed below.

Vestibular nystagmus results from damage to the vestibular end organs, vestibular nerves, or their central connections in the lower brainstem and vestibulocerebellum (flocculonodular lobes). It has a jerk waveform and is horizontal, oblique, and torsional in direction. Fixation suppresses nystagmus caused by peripheral lesions (e.g. damage to one labyrinth from a viral labyrinthitis), but does not suppress nystagmus from lesions in the central pathways. Acute damage to one labyrinth or vestibular nerve produces an imbalance in the tonic innervation to the brainstem from both ears. This imbalance produces an intense nystagmus (fast components toward the undamaged side) and severe vertigo and oscillopsia. However, a compensatory process of the CNS rapidly decreases the nystagmus over several days such that it is detectable only when fixation that inhibits the nystagmus is blocked (closed eyelids, dark or Frenzel goggles). A simple technique can be used in the ophthalmologist's office to block fixation and detect the nystagmus. While one eye is occluded a direct ophthalmoscope or an indirect ophthalmoscope is used to visualize the fundus of the other eye. The ophthalmoscope's light effectively "occludes" the illuminated eye, and the instrument's angular magnification makes fixation instabilities of even less than 1 degree in amplitude visible. The examiner should note that the direction of the abnormal eye movements is in the *opposite* direction to that of the fundus if a direct ophthalmoscope is used and is in the *same* direction with an indirect ophthalmoscope. Instructing the patient to rapidly shake the head back-and-forth horizontally with the eyelids closed for several seconds, to stop the head movements, and to open the eyelids can enhance vestibular nystagmus.

Positional vestibular nystagmus is found only when the patient's body is moved from the upright sitting or standing positions to a supine position. The paroxysmal form requires a rapid positioning into a backward, head-hanging position (Barany-Nylen or Dix-Hallpike maneuver). Patients often report that similar movements of the head and body precipitate vertigo and oscillopsia. The nystagmus is initially intense, but quickly fatigues over several seconds. *Benign paroxysmal positional nystagmus* is probably caused by degenerative changes in the utricles in which otoconia from the utricular macule fall on the cupula of the posterior semicircular canal, making that cupula sensitive to linear acceleration. These changes can follow viral labyrinthitis, trauma, and vascular occlusion to the end organs or can be idiopathic. The jerk nystagmus is not inhibited by fixation and is disconjugate. It is usually induced by turning the head to the side of the damaged ear in the head-hanging position. The nystagmus in the eye on that side ("lower" eye) is oblique and torsional; the nystagmus in the other eye ("upper" eye) is upbeating. Rapid positioning can also induce other types of pathologic nystagmus, e.g., downbeat nystagmus. However, these types of nystagmus usually are not disconjugate.

Sustained positional nystagmus can be caused by damage to the end organs, vestibular nerves, or central vestibular pathways. The jerk nystagmus is less intense than in benign paroxysmal positional nystagmus, is inhibited by fixation, and persists as long as the supine position is maintained. It has been thought that a direction-changing positional nystagmus (direction of fast component changes from left lateral position to right lateral position) signifies that a central pathway lesion is present, whereas, a direction-fixed positional nystagmus (same direction in right and left lateral positions) indicates that a peripheral lesion is present. However, many patients with CNS lesions have direction-fixed nystagmus, and patients with peripheral lesions can have direction-changing nystagmus.

Congenital nystagmus (CN), in contrast to vestibular nystagmus, is decreased by blocking fixation and is intensified by the effort to fixate and see clearly. CN is not usually associated with other neurologic defects, and its etiology is essentially unknown, except for a hereditary basis in some families and associations with some ocular disorders, such as ocular albinism and aniridia. The nystagmus has pendular, jerk, and other complex waveforms; is almost always horizontal (even in vertical gaze); and has a high frequency. A null zone of gaze, in which the intensity of the nystagmus is least and visual acuity is greatest, and a neutral point, at which gaze farther to the right induces a jerk waveform with saccades to the right and gaze farther to the left produces a jerk left waveform, are often found. An associated habitual horizontal face turn places the eyes in the null position. Convergence usually dampens the nystagmus. Habitual head nodding might be present. The head oscillations help stabilize fixation, but not by generating vestibulo-ocular responses opposed to the nystagmus. An uncommon presentation of CN is as an apparently acquired nystagmus that was not identified in early childhood. Relatively good visual acuity in the null zone, dampening of nystagmus with convergence (obviating the need to use large-print schoolbooks), and a small amplitude explain how the nystagmus might not have been noticed previously. Identification of the congenital nature of the nystagmus should be possible by the characteristics noted above and the absence of oscillopsia. Few patients with congenital nystagmus spontaneously complain of oscillopsia, whereas most patients with acquired nystagmus do. High-resolution, electronic recordings of CN show characteristic waveforms—curved slow components with increasing velocity, braking saccades that seem to terminate run-away slow components, and foveating saccades followed by short periods of relatively stable eye position called "extended foveation"—that differentiate CN from acquired nystagmus.

Downbeat nystagmus is a vertical jerk nystagmus with fast components beating downward. It is one of the most localizing ocular motor signs. The amplitude is usually greatest in lateral gaze. Convergence often increases the nystagmus. The nystagmus might not be seen in some patients until rapid positioning of the head (Dix-Hallpike maneuver) is performed. A lesion at the level of the craniocervical junction, involving the cerebellum or lower brainstem, is usually present (Arnold-Chiari malformation, basilar impression, platybasia, multiple sclerosis, cerebellar degenerations, and infarction). Toxicity from carbamazepine, phenytoin, lithium, and amiodarone and deficiencies of thiamine or magnesium can cause downbeat nystagmus.

Periodic alternating nystagmus is a horizontal jerk nystagmus in the primary position with fast components alternately beating in opposite directions. The amplitude of right-beating nystagmus increases and decreases gradually (about 90 seconds). The phase of right-beating nystagmus is followed by a null phase (about 10 seconds) in which no nystagmus is present. A phase of left-beating nystagmus with increasing and decreasing amplitude (about 90 seconds) follows. The cycling of phases is repetitive and regular. This type of nystagmus usually results from lesions of the lower brainstem or cerebellum. Alternating nystagmus can be a form of congenital nystagmus or can be caused by acquired bilateral blindness. However, the phases are usually asymmetric and variable in these types of alternating nystagmus.

Superior oblique myokymia represents pendular and jerk, torsional, and oblique oscillations of one eye, producing transient diplopia and oscillopsia. The amplitude of the pendular component is very small, and its frequency is high. The jerk component has a lower frequency, and the fast component often intorts the eye. A tonic intorsion, responsible for the diplopia, is sometimes present. Observation of conjunctival vessels or iris with the slit lamp and examination of the fundus with an ophthalmoscope help detect the oscillations. The episodes of oscillopsia can last from a few to several seconds and can occur many times

each day. They usually affect otherwise healthy individuals and are caused by discharge of motor units of the superior oblique muscle at very high frequencies (35 cycles/sec). Superior oblique myokymia can resolve spontaneously. However, in other individuals it recurs many times over a period of several years. It has rarely been described in patients with CNS lesions.

The most common and significant ocular effects of nystagmus are reduction of visual acuity, as in congenital nystagmus, and oscillopsia, as in acquired forms of nystagmus. The motion of images across the fovea (retinal slip) at velocities of 4 degree/sec or higher due to instability of fixation decreases visual acuity. Therefore, therapy that reduces the slow component velocity of nystagmus improves visual acuity. The velocities of slow components in CN are very high. However, visual acuity can be normal or nearly normal. The amount of time in the nystagmus waveform during which the image is stationary at the fovea (foveation time) is correlated with visual acuity. Fixation instability and oscillopsia make orientation in space and executing saccades effectively during reading difficult.

Visual acuity is usually normal in the presence of macrosquare wave jerks since there is sufficient foveation time between saccades (intersaccadic interval) to maintain images on the fovea without retinal slip. Visual acuity is reduced by ocular flutter and opsoclonus. Large-amplitude to-and-fro saccades do not have intersaccadic intervals. Macrosquare wave jerks and ocular flutter are usually horizontal. Saccades in opsoclonus are horizontal, vertical, and oblique and often have curved trajectories. Saccadic fixation instabilities are often associated with disorders of the cerebellum.

THERAPY

Systemic. The most effective therapy for nystagmus and saccadic oscillations is treatment of the underlying disorder before irreversible damage to the CNS occurs. Detection and identification of the oscillations by the ophthalmologist, referral for neurologic evaluation when indicated, and obtaining appropriate laboratory tests are required. Improved techniques of neuroradiology, especially magnetic resonance imaging (MRI), enhances identification of CNS lesions. MRI is particularly useful in detecting abnormalities of the brainstem and cerebellum because the bones around the posterior fossa do not interfere with visualization of the soft tissues. Arnold-Chiari malformations can be detected easily by MRI. Scans with and without intravenous contrast (gadolinium) should be ordered when neuroimaging is indicated. Downbeat nystagmus, ataxia, cranial nerve palsies, and other defects caused by these and other malformations can resolve after surgical decompression of the foramen magnum.

Treatment for patients with vestibular nystagmus is usually aimed at alleviating vertigo. Antiverginous medications include several classes of drugs: anticholinergics (scopolamine and atropine), monoaminergics (amphetamine and ephedrine), antihistamines (meclizine, cyclizine, demenhydrinate, and promethazine), phenothiazines (prochlorperazine and chlorpromazine), benzodiazepines (diazepam), and butyrophenones (haloperidol and droperidol). The dosage and route of administration (oral, parenteral, and transdermal) vary according to the severity and chronicity of vertigo. Benign paroxysmal positional vertigo (nystagmus) has been treated successfully with positional exercises that induce the vertigo. Anticholinergic drugs have also been used to treat patients with other acquired forms of nystagmus. In a cross-over, double-blind study, trihexyphenidyl, a competitive agonist at muscarinic receptors, did not decrease pendular nystagmus caused by multiple sclerosis in most patients (five of six patients). Tridihexethyl chloride, a quaternary anticholinergic that does not cross the blood-brain barrier, decreased nystagmus in most patients (four of six patients). However, both drugs produced bothersome side effects.

Gamma-aminobutyric acid (GABA) is an inhibitory neurotransmitter in the CNS. Baclofen, an analogue of GABA, is absorbed after oral administration and has been used to treat spasticity caused by disorders of the spinal cord. Its therapeutic effects might result from inhibiting the release of glutamate, an excitatory CNS neurotransmitter, rather than from augmentation of GABA-ergic pathways. Baclofen[‡] has been used to treat several types of nystagmus and has been found to decrease nystagmus amplitude and oscillopsia. It is effective in treating patients with acquired periodic alternating nystagmus. It has also been reported to be effective for some patients with congenital periodic alternating nystagmus or acquired, nonperiodic alternating nystagmus. The dosage is usually 5 to 20 mg three times daily. Improvement in vision and decreased oscillopsia are noticed several minutes after taking the medication and regress after a few to several hours. Medications should not be administered at bedtime or at other times when use of the eyes is not anticipated. Common side effects include drowsiness, fatigue, nausea, headache, and confusion. It has not been recommended for children under age 12.

Adult patients with CN have also been treated with baclofen.[‡] In one study, nystagmus intensity (frequency × amplitude) decreased and vision improved subjectively in four of seven patients. However, only one patient chose to continue the medications for longer than 6 months. Baclofen has been reported to be effective in some patients with congenital or acquired see-saw nystagmus, although it was not found to be helpful in patients with downbeat nystagmus. Baclofen alone or in combination with clonazepam was not effective in patients with oculopalatal myoclonus.

Clonazepam is an anticonvulsant that augments GABA-ergic activity in the central nervous system. It has been reported to decrease the amplitude and oscillopsia of downbeat nystagmus. A test dose of 1 to 2 mg of clonazepam given orally can reduce downbeat nystagmus in 45 to 60 minutes. Sustained therapy with 0.25 to 0.50 mg several times a day has been used successfully by several patients. Drowsiness was the most common adverse effect. Cessation of drugs causing downbeat nystagmus and supplementation with thiamine or magnesium when deficiencies exist should be considered. The combination of baclofen and clonazepam has reduced see-saw nystagmus. Clonazepam has also been reported to be effective in treating opsoclonus. Corticosteroids[‡] and corticotropin[‡] can decrease opsoclonus in children with myoclonus of the limbs and ataxia due to a postinfectious encephalitis, and corticotropin can also reduce opsoclonus in children with neuroblastoma. Clonazepam has been successful in treating myoclonic ocular jerks, but was not useful in treating a few patients with oculopalatal myoclonus.

Carbamazepine[‡] is an anticonvulsant and an analgesic for trigeminal neuralgia. It can be effective in treating patients with superior oblique myokymia. The initial dosage might be 100 mg twice daily and can be increased by 200 mg daily until a maximum dose of about 1200 mg, in adults is reached. Drowsiness, dizziness, and confusion can occur. Lower maintenance dosages, as in the management of trigeminal neuralgia (400 to 800 mg daily), might be effective. The drug can cause bone marrow suppression and damage to the liver. Therefore, pretreatment complete blood count, platelet count, and liver function tests should be obtained and repeated periodically. Baclofen and clonazepam have also been used to treat superior oblique myokymia.

Ocular. Prisms in spectacle lenses can be useful in improving vision in CN. Several prism diopters of base-out prism in each lens induce convergence and can decrease nystagmus (increase foveation time). Prisms with bases oriented in the same direction can move the eyes toward a null position and reduce CN. However, the weight and blurring of prisms that are strong enough to affect the nystagmus can discourage their use. Hard and soft contact lenses can be worn successfully by patients with CN and can cause fewer optical aberrations than spectacles. Some studies have claimed that they also decrease intensity of the nystagmus. One mechanism by which contact lenses might decrease nystagmus is by sensory stimulation of the inner surface of the eyelids. Sensory stimulation of the ophthalmic division of the fifth nerve by pressure on the skin might decrease CN in some patients by a similar mechanism. Auditory biofeedback and acupuncture have been reported to decrease CN in the laboratory. However, it is not certain if the reduction in nystagmus persists outside the laboratory setting.

An optical method of stabilizing images on the retina has been described. A high plus spectacle lens focuses light rays at the center of rotation of the eye. A high minus contact lens moves the focal point to the retina. This method has improved vision in some patients with acquired forms of nystagmus. The method is used for one eye for a few hours at a time. Large-diameter, hard contact lenses made of PMMA were used originally, but often caused ocular discomfort and corneal edema. A smaller, gas-permeable, rigid lens has been used successfully. Stabilization of images improves visual acuity, but patients are cautioned not to walk because of interference with the vestibulo-ocular reflex and impairment of balance. Patients with CN do not usually complain of oscillopsia. However, this optical method has induced oscillopsia in some patients.

Surgical. Extraocular muscle surgery can improve visual function in patients with CN and eccentric null zones. A patient assumes a habitual face turn to place the eyes in a null zone located away from primary gaze. Large-amplitude face turns and eccentric gaze positions (30 deg or greater) can interfere with the patient's effective use of his or her best visual function. Improvement in visual acuity should be demonstrable in the null position. Patients with CN can have associated ocular disorders that are primarily responsible for impaired vision. In such patients, reduction of the nystagmus might not significantly improve visual function. The null positions at distance and at near are often different and can be in opposite directions. The author has not found that surgery based on the null position at distance has interfered with visual function at near. Recession and resection procedures on the four horizontal rectus muscles are performed to rotate the eyes in the direction opposite to that of the horizontal component of the null position. In most instances, maximal amounts of recession and resection are used to move the null zone toward the primary position. Various schemes for calculating the amounts of recession and resection have been used. Simultaneous correction of a horizontal strabismus can also be attempted. Correction of eccentric, vertical null zones can also be tried. Successful surgery can also enlarge the null zone. However, the null zone can gradually return toward its preoperative position after many months.

Recessions of all four horizontal rectus muscles to positions at or behind the equator of each eye (about 11.5 mm from medial and 13.0 mm behind lateral limbus) have been reported to be effective in reducing CN and abolishing eccentric null zones. A slight improvement in visual acuity has been reported. Limitation of ductions has not been significant. Manifest latent nystagmus (MLN) can be converted to latent nystagmus (LN) with strabismus surgery or treatment of accommodative esotropia with spectacles. Binocular visual acuity can be improved if the MLN is converted to LN or if MLN persists but is decreased.

Retrobulbar injection of botulinum toxin* into the muscle cone of one eye has been reported to decrease acquired nystagmus markedly and to improve vision. Its drawbacks are the need for repeated injections, diplopia, and the possibility of ptosis. Injections into the horizontal rectus muscles can reduce nystagmus in the horizontal direction, but persistent vertical and torsional nystagmus in the same patient can prevent improvement in vision. Increased nystagmus in the noninjected eye can occur. This phenomenon probably results from plastic-adaptive changes within the CNS in response to paresis of the injected eye.

PRECAUTIONS

To date, the author does not know of serious adverse effects of drug treatment for nystagmus. However, such drugs as baclofen and clonazepam have been used in relatively few patients. Too, numerous side effects have been reported when drugs have been used for other medical conditions, some of which can be life threatening, e.g., bone marrow suppression secondary to carbamazepine. Ophthalmologists should be familiar with these side effects. Developmental anomalies in fetuses of rats given more than the maximal human dose of baclofen and carbamazepine have been described. Reports have suggested that the use of clonazepam for epilepsy might be associated with an increased incidence of birth defects. Therefore, the author does not use baclofen, clonazepam, or carbamazepine to treat nystagmus in women with childbearing potential or in children.

COMMENTS

The ophthalmologist's contribution to the management of nystagmus usually is to identify the type of nystagmus and its diagnostic localizing value. Doing so can lead to the effective use of other diagnostic tests (neuroradiology), early diagnosis of CNS disorders before permanent damage occurs, and effective medical or neurosurgical management. In some types of acquired nystagmus, the ophthalmologist can improve visual function with systemic therapy. He or she can significantly improve visual function in some patients with CN using optical or surgical procedures.

References

Currie J, Matsuo V: The use of clonazepam in the treatment of nystagmus-induced oscillopsia. Opthalmology 93:924–932, 1986.

Dieterich M, Straube A, Brandt T, Paulus W, Buttner U: The effects of baclofen and cholinergic drugs on upbeat and downbeat nystagmus. J Neurol Neurosurg Psychiatry 54:627–632, 1991.

Epley JM: The canalith repositioning procedure: For treatment of benign paroxysmal positional vertigo. Otolaryngol Head Neck Surg 107:339–404, 1992.

Flynn JT, Scott WE, Kushner BJ, et al: Large rectus muscle recessions for the treatment of congenital nystagmus (Letter). Arch Opthalmol 109:1636–1638, 1991.

Golubovic S, Marjanovic S, Cvetkovic D, Manic S: The application of hard contact lenses in patients with congenital nystagmus. Fortschr Ophthalmol 86:535–539, 1989.

Helveston EM, Pogrebniak AE: Treatment of acquired nystagmus with botulinum A toxin. Am J Ophthalmol 106:584–586, 1988.

Helveston EM, Ellis FD, Plager DA: Large recession of the horizontal recti for treatment of nystagmus. Ophthalmology 98:1302–1305, 1991.

Herishanu YO, Zigoulinski R: The effect of chronic one-eye patching on ocular myoclonus. J Clin Neuro-ophthalmol 11:166–168, 1991.

Leigh RJ, Rushton DN, Thurston SE et al: Effects of retinal image stabilization in acquired nystagmus due to neurologic disease. Neurology 38:122–127, 1988.

Leigh RJ, Tomsak RL, Grant MP, et al: Effectiveness of botulinum toxin administered to abolish acquired nystagmus. Ann Neurol 32:633–642, 1992.

Mezawa M, Ishikawa S, Ukai K: Changes in waveform of congenital nystagmus associated with biofeedback treatment. Br J Ophthalmol 73:472–476, 1990.

Miller BA, Younger DA, Friendly DS: Treatment of acquired intermittent horizontal jerk nystagmus with baclofen (Letter). Am J Ophthalmol 114:336–337, 1992.

Parnes LS, Price-Jones RG: Particle repositioning maneuver for benign paroxysmal positional vertigo. Ann Otol Rhinol Largyngol 102:325–331, 1993.

Pratt-Johnson JA: Results of surgery to modify the null-zone position in congenital nystagmus. Can J Ophthalmol 26:219–223, 1991.

Rushton D, Cox N: A new optical treatment for oscillopsia. J Neurol Neurosurg Psychiatr 50:411–415, 1987.

von Noorden GK, Sprunger DT: Large rectus muscle recessions for the treatment of congenital nystagmus. Arch Ophthalmol 109:221–224, 1991.

Yaniglos SS, Leigh RJ: Refinement of an optical device that stabilizes vision in patients with nystagmus. Optom Vis Sci 69:447–450, 1992.

Yee RD, Baloh RW, Honrubia V: Effect of baclofen on congenital nystagmus. In Lennerstrand G, Zee DS, Keller EL (eds): Functional Basis of Ocular Motility Disorders. Oxford, Pergamon Press, 1982, pp 151–157.

Zubcov AA, Reinecke RD, Gottlob I, et al: Treatment of manifest latent nystagmus. Am J Ophthalmol 110:160–167, 1990.

Zubcov AA, Stark N, Weber A, Wizov SS, Reinecke RD: Improvement of visual acuity after surgery for nystagmus. Ophthalmology 100:1488–1497, 1993.

This work was supported by an Unrestricted Grant from Research To Prevent Blindness, Inc., New York, New York, to the Department of Ophthalmology, Indiana University School of Medicine.

OCULOMOTOR (THIRD NERVE) PARALYSIS 378.51

HOWARD M. EGGERS, M.D.

New York, New York

Paralysis of the oculomotor nerve may be congenital or acquired. It typically presents with symptoms of heteronymous diplopia with or without blurred vision. The findings are ipsilateral to the lesion and include paralysis of four of the six oculorotary muscles (the superior rectus, medial rectus, inferior rectus, and inferior oblique), which produces an exotropia, hypotropia, and incyclotropia of the involved eye; paralysis of the ciliary muscle and iris sphincter, resulting in absent accommodation and a dilated pupil; and paralysis of the levator, resulting in blepharotosis. A partial form, or paresis, produces any intermediate degree of weakness of these muscles. The upper division can be involved, producing a double elevator paresis with true or pseudoptosis. The lower division may be selectively involved, sparing the superior rectus and levator. A diabetic oculomotor paresis frequently partially involves pupillary function. A sufficiently discrete nuclear lesion may involve the contralateral instead of the ipsilateral superior rectus and may produce bilateral partial ptosis, although these findings are exceedingly rare.

Whenever an oculomotor palsy is present, a trochlear nerve palsy must be looked for as well. It is significant both diagnostically and in the choice of surgical procedure.

THERAPY

Supportive. Accurate diagnosis and appropriate medical treatment are necessary. Prism therapy is generally of limited benefit because of the marked incomitance. The involved eye is occluded, if necessary, for relief of diplopia. Because spontaneous recovery may occur up to 6 or 9 months after the onset of the paralysis, surgery should be deferred this long. If any recovery occurs, it must be followed to its end; surgery should only be considered for the remaining deviation.

Ocular. Bifocal correction for near vision may be needed. If amblyopia is present at a treatable age, patching is required. Because of the importance of adequate amblyopia therapy, surgical realignment is best deferred until after amblyopia therapy is completed.

The deformity resulting from anisocoria is particularly troubling to blue-eyed patients. It may be treated by wearing a contact lens with a pupil and iris painted on the surface.

Surgical. The goal of surgery is to realign the eye close to the primary position. The choice of procedure depends on which muscles are involved and the completeness of the paralysis. In partial paralysis there may be sufficient medial rectus function to respond well to a resection of the medial and recession of the antagonist lateral rectus.

In complete paralysis of the third nerve, the transposition of a sound superior oblique tendon should be considered. A viable muscle will then oppose the action of the recessed lateral rectus and keep the eyes aligned better than without any adducting force. The tendon can be released from the trochlea by cutting the trochlea with scissors or popping it with a hemostat. This should be done with as little trauma as possible. If the tendon is severed, then one goes ahead as though the superior oblique muscle also were paralyzed. If the tendon is freed, it is resected until it is snug and sutured to the insertion of the medial rectus, which then does not require any surgery. An alternative approach to transposition of the superior oblique is to leave the trochlea intact and to relocate the superior oblique tendon 2 to 3 mm anterior to the medial end of the superior rectus tendon, accompanied by the right amount of resection.

There is no value to resecting the medial rectus unless there is a small amount of residual function in it or the superior oblique tendon is lost. The lateral conjunctiva and Tenon's capsule are recessed from the vertical corneal meridian all the way to the orbital margin and the lateral rectus recessed as far as practically possible. The eye may then also be anchored in a slightly adducted position for 2 weeks.

Surgical elevation of the lid may be required if ptosis is severe enough; however, ptosis repair should be deferred until after the eye is aligned. A maximal levator resection using a transcutaneous approach can suspend the upper lid. However, a frontalis sling is preferred, as it is easier to set the correct lid height. The ptosis should only be corrected to cover half of the cornea with the brow relaxed because the eye cannot rotate upward with a protective Bell's reflex. Frequent blinking and moisturizing drops must be relied on to prevent corneal drying. Children adapt better than adults to this corneal exposure.

In double elevator paresis with a negative traction test for elevation, a transposition of the full tendons of the medial and lateral recti to the corners of the superior rectus is the operation of choice. The ptosis should not be corrected, for it may be a pseudoptosis caused by the hypotropia. If it is a real ptosis, elevation of the eye will aggravate the ptosis; therefore, the patient or family should be warned preoperatively.

A paralysis of the lower division of the third nerve (affecting the medial rectus, inferior rectus, and inferior oblique) is treated by transferring the functioning superior rectus to the medial rectus, the lateral rectus to the inferior rectus, and tenectomizing the superior oblique.

Ocular or Periocular Manifestations

Extraocular Muscles: Paralysis of superior rectus, medial rectus inferior rectus, and inferior oblique muscles.

Eyelids: Ptosis.

Other: Decreased visual acuity, diplopia; internal ophthalmoplegia (paralysis of pupillary sphincter and ciliary muscle); mydriasis; paralysis of accommodation.

PRECAUTIONS

Because of the severe loss of function of the oculorotary muscles in third nerve paralysis, the only attainable goal is realignment of the eye in primary position. Cases with incomplete paralysis may obtain a small horizontal and vertical range of fusion. Care must be taken not to elevate the lid too far and thereby compromise corneal function. Children learn to suppress the double image; however, adults frequently require an opaque contact lens because of the absence of fusion anywhere except in one direction of gaze.

COMMENTS

Total third nerve paralysis is devastating to oculomotor function, and even the limited goal of repositioning the eye near primary position is no small achievement. Useful function of the eye in a binocular context can only be obtained in some cases of partial paralysis. Accurate diagnosis and the ruling out of other neurologic involvement are essential before any consideration is given to surgical repair.

References

Glaser JS: Infranuclear disorders of eye movements. *In* Duane TD (ed): Clinical Ophthalmology. Hagerstown, MD, Harper & Row, 1982, Vol II, pp 12:1–38.

Gottlob I, Catalano RA, Reinecke RD: Surgical management of oculomotor nerve palsy. Am J Ophthalmol *111*:71–76, 1991.

Helveston EM: Atlas of Strabismus Surgery, 2nd ed. St. Louis, CV Mosby, 1977, pp 176–179.

SLIPPED EXTRAOCULAR MUSCLE 378.9

DAVID A. PLAGER, M.D.

Indianapolis, Indiana

An extraocular (rectus) muscle is said to be slipped when the skeletal muscle/tendon fibers have retracted posteriorly away from the intended insertion site on the globe while the "empty" muscle capsule remains attached to the sclera approximately at the intended point of insertion. A slipped muscle should be differentiated from "lost" muscle. A lost muscle refers to a rectus muscle that has been disinserted from the globe and has lost all direct connection to the sclera. A slipped muscle occurs almost exclusively as a complication of strabismus surgery, but can result any time a muscle is detached.

When a muscle has slipped, the patient will have a large overcorrection after a recession. A slipped muscle after resection usually results in a paradoxically larger deviation after surgery. In addition, the patient will have a decreased excursion in the field of action of the slipped muscle ranging from a subtle decrease to severe limitation. Widening of the palpebral fissure with attempted fixation in the field of action of the slipped muscle is often seen.

THERAPY

Surgical. Strabismus caused by a slipped muscle requires resection and/or advancement of the involved muscle for correction. Failure to correct a slipped muscle with or without weakening the antagonist at the time of surgery will result in failure to realign the eyes successfully.

When a slipped muscle is suspected preoperatively, care should be exercised during surgical manipulation of the muscle, particularly when identifying the empty muscle capsule. This tissue should be engaged with a muscle hook and held gently while it is freed from surrounding attachments. In cases of extensive slippage where the true tendon/muscle has retracted through the Tenon's penetration site into the extraconal space, the friable empty capsule can be used as a trail to follow from the insertion to the actual muscle tissue. In this case, the muscle fibers are usually found just at or beyond the Tenon's penetration site. Other, less severely slipped muscles may be found with anywhere from 2 to 10 mm or more of empty capsule between the insertion and the muscle fibers. There is typically a fusiform-shaped expansion in the width of the muscle just posterior to the transition area from empty capsule to muscle.

When identified, the muscle should be secured on a double arm suture if possible, or it should be grasped with a hemostat and carefully brought forward where it can be secured with a suture. Muscles that have been slipped for more than a few weeks are invariably tight, making it difficult to advance them very far anteriorly. In addition, the antagonist of the slipped muscle often is restricted, making recession of that muscle necessary.

Ocular or Periocular Manifestations

Extraocular Muscles: Subtle or marked decreased duction in the field of action of the involved muscle; vertical or horizontal strabismus depending on which muscle is slipped.
Eyelids: Variable widening of the palpebral fissures on attempted duction toward the involved muscle, particularly in severe cases.

PRECAUTIONS

If a slipped muscle is present it must be repaired by advancement and resection if the strabismus is to be corrected. Operating on antagonist or yoke muscles will be less effective.

The friable empty capsule should be handled with care until the muscle itself is secured; otherwise, the slipped muscle can be unfortunately converted into a lost muscle.

COMMENTS

A slipped muscle is a frequently overlooked cause of unsuccessful strabismus surgery. The misalignment caused by a slipped muscle can be evident in the early postoperative period, but it often becomes gradually more evident over a period of months or years. It is seen most commonly as a sequelae of medial rectus recession, but this may only be a reflection of the relative frequency that medial rectus recession is performed. This complication can probably be avoided by ensuring that solid, full-thickness locking bites around the skeletal muscle/tendon fibers are secured at the time the muscle is reattached to the sclera.

A slipped muscle should be ruled out in all patients undergoing strabismus reoperation, but especially in those patients with a large overcorrection after rectus muscle recession. A careful assessment of versions and ductions should be made, including both active and passive duction testing. If any limitation of excursion is noted in the field of action of the previously operated muscle, surgical exploration of that muscle is indicated.

Definitive diagnosis of a slipped muscle is made only at the time of surgery. The slipped muscle is identified by finding an empty muscle capsule extending from the intended insertion on the globe posteriorly to where the true skeletal muscle/tendon fibers are found. The empty capsule can be a few millimeters to 18 millimeters or more in length, depending on how far posteriorly the muscle has slipped.

Since the "empty capsule" is the principal attachment of the slipped muscle to the globe, it should be handled very carefully lest the attachment be severed and the muscle "lost" into the extraconal space. The empty capsule should be used more as a guide to find the muscle than as a handle to pull it up.

References

Bloom JN, Parks MM: The etiology, treatment and prevention of the "slipped muscle." J Pediatr Ophthalmol Strabismus 18:6–11, 1981.

Parks MM, Bloom JN: The "slipped" muscle. Ophthalmology 86:1389–1396, 1979.

Plager DA, Parks MM: Recognition and repair of the slipped rectus muscle. J Pediatr Ophthalmol Strabismus 25:270–274, 1988.

Plager DA, Parks MM: Recognition and repair of the "lost" rectus muscle. Ophthalmology 97:131–137, 1990.

SUPERIOR OBLIQUE MYOKYMIA 379.58

WILLIAM T. SHULTS, M.D.

Portland, Oregon

First described by Duane as unilateral rotary nystagmus, superior oblique myokymia is a benign disorder of ocular stabilization. It is characterized by recurrent episodes of monocular vertical and rotary microtremor and is accompanied by torsional shimmering oscillopsia. The affected eye phasically intorts for seconds during each episode. Although episodes may occur without a provoking change in ocular position, they may be precipitated by downward gaze or lateral head tilts in susceptible patients. There are no known associations with other neurologic disease. Disordered activation or inhibition at the level of the trochlear nucleus or both have been proposed as the mechanisms of production of this unique ocular dyskinesia.

THERAPY

Systemic. Carbamazepine[‡] in a dosage from 100 mg twice daily to 200 mg three times daily has provided dramatic relief of symptoms in most patients. The duration of therapy for superior oblique myokymia is rarely longer than 2 or 3 years.

Surgical. Those cases unresponsive to medical therapy have responded to intrasheath tenotomy of the superior oblique muscle and recession of the inferior oblique muscle of the involved eye.

Ocular or Periocular Manifestations

Extraocular Muscles: Vertical and rotary microtremor.

Other: Oscillopsia; sensation of eye movement; torsional diplopia.

PRECAUTIONS

Use of carbamazepine requires periodic laboratory evaluation of various hematologic parameters, as aplastic anemia, agranulocytosis, thrombocytopenia, and leukopenia are rare associated side effects. Before initiating therapy a pretreatment hematologic battery with the following tests should be obtained: complete blood count, platelet count, reticulocyte count, and serum iron. These tests should be repeated monthly for as long as therapy is continued.

COMMENTS

The symptom of episodic monocular torsional oscillopsia is so distinctive for this disorder that the diagnosis can literally be made over the phone. A slit-lamp examination is sometimes needed to see the fine tremorous ocular movements of this benign condition. Referral is unnecessary and, in fact, contraindicated lest the patient be subjected to a major battery of unnecessary neurodiagnostic tests by a consultant unfamiliar with this condition.

References

Duane A: Unilateral rotary nystagmus. Ophthalmol Rec 15:465–468, 1906.

Hoyt WF, Keane JR: Superior oblique myokymia. Report and discussion on five cases of benign intermittent uniocular microtremor. Arch Ophthalmol 84:461–467, 1970.

Palmer E, Shults WT: Superior oblique myokymia: Preliminary results of surgical treatment. J Pediatr Ophthalmol Strabismus 21:96–101, 1984.

Susac JO, Smith JL, Schatz NJ: Superior oblique myokymia. Arch Neurol 29:432–434, 1973.

SUPERIOR OBLIQUE PALSY 378.53

EUGENE M. HELVESTON, M.D.

Indianapolis, Indiana

Superior oblique palsy is the most commonly occurring cranial nerve palsy. It occurs so often because the trochlear nerve rootlets exit the tentorium as fragile threads that may be ruptured by the edge of the dura (tentorium) as the brain shifts and resettles after closed head trauma. Superior oblique palsy may be unilateral or bilateral, congenital or acquired. The superior oblique tendon is also the most frequently noted tendon to be congenitally anomalous or absent.

The symptoms of unilateral superior oblique palsy are abnormal head posture in childhood and both intermittent diplopia (both vertical and horizontal) and abnormal head posture in the adult. In bilateral superior oblique palsy, the chin is depressed to avoid diplopia. The head is tilted to the side opposite the involvement in unilateral superior oblique palsy. Spontaneous torsional diplopia is reported with horizontal displacement of the tilted images in many cases of bilateral superior oblique palsy. As with other cranial nerve palsies, acquired superior oblique palsy (bilateral or unilateral) may resolve in weeks to months after the onset. However, any deviation that persists after 6 months may be considered permanent.

Evaluation of the patient suspected of superior oblique palsy should begin with a careful history. Frequently, a history of trauma is elicited, but often it is not. Questions should be directed toward presence or absence of abnormal head posture, vertical diplopia, and torsional diplopia. An initial qualitative evaluation is carried out following a simple two-step test.

Step 1: The patient is asked to look far to the right and then far to the left. In the lateral version of greater vertical tropia, the adducted eye points to the oblique on the same side or the rectus muscle on the opposite side as the two vertically acting muscles that could be paretic.

Step 2: The head is tilted 45° to one side and then 45° to the other side (Bielschowsky head tilt test). If the vertical deviation increases when the head is tilted toward the higher eye, the oblique arrived at in Step 1 is considered paretic. If the vertical deviation increases when the head is tilted to the side of the lower eye, the rectus muscle arrived at in Step 1 is considered paretic.

This simple test combining lateral versions and the Bielschowsky head tilt test is a satisfactory method for diagnosing a paresis of any of the vertically acting muscles.

Prism and cover testing should then be carried out in the nine diagnostic positions to provide a quantified evaluation. An essential part of evaluation of the patient with suspected superior oblique palsy is the Maddox double rod test. A red Maddox rod, with the cylinders vertically oriented, is placed in front of the right eye, and a white Maddox rod, similarly oriented, is placed in front of the left eye. The patient is asked to view a point source of light in a darkened room. The Maddox rods are then adjusted if necessary so that red and white lines are parallel. The ocular torsion expressed in degrees is read directly from the trial frame holding the Maddox rods.

Superior oblique palsy without measurable torsion and without spontaneous complaint of torsional diplopia is considered congenital or early acquired; superior oblique palsy with measurable torsion less than 15° and without complaint of spontaneous torsional diplopia is acquired unilateral superior oblique palsy; and spontaneous complaint of torsional diplopia indicates bilateral superior oblique palsy. Also, any measured cyclotropia greater than 15° indicates bilateral superior oblique palsy. Facial asymmetry is seen frequently in congenital superior oblique palsy. The fuller face is on the involved side. No good reason has been found for this manifestation.

THERAPY

Surgical. The prism and cover measurements obtained in the nine diagnostic positions in a patient with superior oblique palsy can be recorded and interpreted according to a scheme devised by Knapp. *Class I* superior oblique palsy has the greatest vertical deviation in the field of action of the antagonist inferior oblique muscle. It is treated with inferior oblique weakening. *Class II* superior oblique palsy has the greatest vertical deviation in the field of action of the underacting paretic superior oblique. It is treated with superior oblique strengthening. *Class III* is an equal vertical deviation in the field of action of the inferior oblique antagonist and the paretic superior oblique. Deviations of less than 20 prism diopters are treated with inferior oblique weakening, and deviations over 20 prism diopters are treated with inferior oblique weakening combined with superior oblique strengthening. As an alternate to superior oblique strengthening, recession of the contralateral inferior rectus or the ipsilateral superior rectus may be carried out. The pattern in *Class IV* superior oblique palsy is characterized by an "L" shape with a vertical deviation in the field of action of the paretic superior oblique, the antagonist inferior oblique, and also the ipsilateral inferior rectus. It is treated with superior oblique strengthening, inferior oblique weakening, and, if needed, at a second procedure, strengthening of the ipsilateral inferior rectus. As an alternative to superior oblique strengthening, the contralateral superior rectus may be recessed. *Class V* superior oblique palsy is characterized by a greater vertical deviation in all fields of downgaze according to Knapp's classification. It may be treated by strengthening the paretic superior oblique and weakening the contralateral superior oblique. Appropriate vertical rectus surgery or superior oblique strengthening and appropriate vertical rectus surgery may represent a prudent alternative. *Class VI* superior oblique palsy is bilateral superior oblique palsy. It is characterized by a 'V'-pattern, chin depression, bilaterally positive Bielschowsky test, right hyper in left gaze, left hyper in right gaze, and complaints of torsional diplopia with the tilted images separated horizontally. Also, measured cyclotropia is often greater than 15°. It is treated with bilateral superior oblique strengthening. *Class VII* superior oblique palsy—canine tooth syndrome—is characterized by underaction of the superior oblique and of the inferior oblique on the same side. It can be caused by one or three conditions: trauma to the trochlear area, producing a "double Brown's syndrome"; iatrogenic causes, such as an acquired Brown's syndrome secondary to strengthening the superior oblique along with a residual superior oblique palsy; or a combination of local trauma to the trochlea causing restriction to upgaze along with closed head trauma producing a fourth nerve palsy. *Class VII* superior oblique palsy is extremely difficult to treat. If the patient is able to fuse in the primary position and has some range of fusion above and below, probably no treatment is indicated. If the Brown's syndrome is the most severe problem, an attempt may be made to relieve surgically the trochlear restriction with or without recession of the yoke and contralateral inferior rectus to treat the superior oblique palsy. Iatrogenic Brown's syndrome may require reduction of the tuck or recession of the resected superior oblique tendon along with recession of the contralateral inferior rectus.

Certain types of superior oblique palsy are characterized by fairly severe torsional defects with very little vertical tropia. They may occur unilaterally or bilaterally. In such a case, the patient may benefit from anterior transposition of the superior oblique tendon. It may be done by shifting the whole tendon or just the anterior fibers; an adjustable suture may be used in this procedure.

In cases where the superior oblique reflected tendon is absent, recession of the antagonist inferior oblique, recession of the ipsilateral superior rectus, and, if necessary, appropriate treatment of any coexisting horizontal deviation are done. Congenital absence of the superior oblique should be suspected if congenital superior oblique palsy is associated with a significant horizontal deviation, amblyopia, ptosis, or bony asymmetry of the orbits or face. A new classification of superior oblique palsy based on anatomic findings separates acquired superior oblique palsy from congenital anatomic superior oblique palsy.

Precautions

Strengthening procedures of the superior oblique frequently produce an iatrogenic mechanical limitation of elevation in adduction or Brown's syndrome. For this reason, shortening of the superior oblique tendon by tuck or resection and advancement should be done in fairly small amounts and should be graded according to the redundance or laxity of the tendon noted at surgery.

In cases of superior oblique palsy after closed head trauma, a high index of suspicion regarding bilateral superior oblique palsy should be maintained. If unsuspected bilateral superior oblique palsy is treated as unilateral superior oblique palsy, a second procedure for superior oblique palsy will invariably be required on the second eye. Because of the complicated nature of the vertical or torsional diplopia associated with superior oblique palsy, prism therapy is often ineffective. Generally, nearly every case of superior oblique palsy can be classified as either congenital, congenital absence, or traumatic acquired. Other causes for superior oblique palsy, such as tumor, vascular abnormalities, toxins, or inflammation, are rarely implicated. A reliable guideline is to suspect a redundant or anomalous tendon in cases of congenital superior oblique palsy. On the other hand, acquired superior oblique palsy is more likely to have a more normal-appearing tendon. The condition of the reflected tendon can be assessed accurately in most cases using the superior oblique traction test. In the former case, superior oblique tendon tuck, resection, or redirection are frequently indicated. In acquired superior oblique palsy, alternatives to superior oblique strengthening should be considered.

Occasionally, patients may present with intermittent symptomatic oscillopsia. Careful evaluation may reveal rhythmic intorsion of one eye accompanied by cyclodiplopia. This condition has been called superior oblique myokymia. It may be transient, or it may be persistent and extremely troublesome. Superior oblique tenectomy has been suggested as a suitable treatment, but such treatment may in turn result in troublesome superior oblique underaction. In this case, inferior oblique weakening may be done at the time of superior oblique myectomy or during a second procedure.

Comments

Superior oblique palsy is not uncommon and is usually a result of trauma or congenital unknown causes. These congenital causes are now thought to be physical anomalies of the tendon. Significant systemic disease is rarely associated with this condition, and therefore, extensive workup is not indicated unless other neurologic complaints warrant it. Surgical treatment can be very successful, and the scheme devised by Knapp has been very useful.

References

Ellis FD, Helveston EM: Superior oblique palsy: Diagnosis and classification. Int Ophthalmol Clin 16:127–135, 1976.

Helveston EM: Atlas of Strabismus Surgery, 3rd ed. St. Louis, CV Mosby, 1985.

Helveston EM, Birchler CCO: Class VII superior oblique palsy: Subclassification and treatment suggestions. Am Orthopt J, 1990.

Helveston EM, Giangiacomo JG, Ellis FD: Congenital absence of the superior oblique tendon. Trans Am Ophthalmol Soc 79:123–135, 1981.

Helveston EM, Krach D, Plager DA, Ellis FD: A new classification of superior oblique palsy based on congenital variations in the tendon. Ophthalmology 99:1609–1615, 1992.

Knapp P: Classification and treatment of superior oblique palsy. Am Orthopt J 24:18–22, 1974.

Metz HS, Lerner H: The adjustable Harada-Ito procedure. Arch Ophthalmol 99:624–626, 1981.

Plager DA: Traction testing in superior oblique palsy. J Pediatr Ophthalmol Strabismus 27:136–140, 1990.

von Noorden GK: Binocular Vision and Ocular Motility. Theory and Management of Strabismus, 2nd ed. St. Louis, CV Mosby, 1980, p 371.

von Noorden GK, Murray E, Wong SY: Superior oblique paralysis: A review of 270 cases. Arch Ophthalmol 109:1171–1176, 1986.

THYROID EXTRAOCULAR MUSCLE DISORDERS 246.9

(Graves Ophthalmopathy, Thyroid Related Ophthalmopathy, Dysthyroid Ophthalmopathy, Thyroid Autoimmune Disease, Thyroid-Associated Ophthalmopathy, Endocrine Orbitopathy, Exopthalmic Ophthalmoplegia, Infiltrative Ophthalmopathy, Dysthyroid Myositis)

DEREK T. SPRUNGER, M.D., and EUGENE M. HELVESTON, M.D.

Indianapolis, Indiana

Thyroid related ophthalmopathy, which can be part of a multisystem autoimmune inflammatory disease, may cause a variety of eye signs including proptosis, lid retraction, tearing, dry eye, exposure keratopathy and optic neuropathy in addition to strabismus and diplopia.

The diagnosis of thyroid related opthalmopathy is generally made by clinical impression and supported by other studies including CT scan, thyroid function tests and antibody tests. Some affected patients may have normal thyroid function tests. Others may have abnormal tests with active and changing "thyroid disease." The patient's internist is critical in evaluation, diagnosis, and treatment of the systemic aspect of the disease.

Patients with extraocular muscle involvement usually complain of diplopia which in most cases has a gradual onset. The diplopia results from restricted ocular motility caused initially by interstitial edema and round cell infiltration followed by fibrotic changes of the muscle fibers. The most commonly affected muscle is the inferior rectus followed by the medial rectus, superior rectus and the lateral rectus. The restriction is often asymmetric and in some instances, unilateral. There is debate as to whether eyelid retraction is the result of increased sympathetic stimulation or a primary muscle involvement. The specific diagnosis of eye muscle disorder in the disease complex is made by demonstrating thickening of muscles on radiography, restricted forced duction testing or differential intraocular pressure testing.

Differential intraocular pressure testing is done by checking the pressure in primary position of gaze and then rechecking the pressure in the field of restriction. An increase in pressure of more than 10mmHg is indicative of a restrictive process.

THERAPY

Systemic. Ocular motility has been shown to improve in patients after high doses of corticosteroids are administered systemically. However, this most likely affects only the acute orbital congestive aspect of the disease and not the longstanding restrictive problem.

Ocular. Orbital radiation has improved motility during the acute congestive phase of the disease. Its efficacy for longstanding diplopia is in question. Oculinum toxin injection[+] to the inferior rectus muscle for hypotropia has also been used in the acute stage of the disease.

Supportive. Once the diagnosis of thyroid extraocular muscle disorder in the presence of diplopia is made, prism therapy or occlusion therapy are the treatments of choice. Prism correction is used to alleviate diplopia, most notably for the primary and reading positions. This therapy is temporary since the angle of deviation may change or additional muscles may become involved over time. Prisms may be permanent for long term treatment but more often press-on prisms are used since the angle of deviation is large and patients usually require surgical correction later.

Surgery. The most effective treatment of thyroid eye muscle disease, once the deviation has been stable, is surgery. The eye muscle surgery is generally performed prior to eyelid surgery for retraction.

Recession of the restricted muscle(s) can be performed by standard scleral fixation of the muscle, hang back recession or by adjustable suture. Surgery is often bilateral and may involve multiple muscles. The amount of recession is generally larger than in nonrestrictive eye muscle problems. Care should be taken to dissect the muscle fully so that surrounding tissue does not interfere with passive movement of the eye. The goal of surgery is single binocular vision in the largest area of viewing with straight ahead and reading positions being the most critical. It is not uncommon for a patient to require more than one extraocular muscle procedure since the amount of surgery needed is not as quantifiable in restrictive eye muscle problems and also additional muscle involvement may become apparent later, after the initial procedure. Resections of muscles for this disorder are generally *not* advised and free tenotomy is no longer employed. Eye muscle surgery should not be performed until stability of the orbital findings and the strabismus are confirmed. Stability of the findings should also be confirmed after radiation treatment or orbital decompression which if performed, should precede eye muscle surgery.

Ocular or Periocular Manifestations

Conjunctiva: Chemosis; hyperemia.
Extraocular Muscles: Myositis (edema, lymphoid infiltration and necrosis of fibers) involving inferior rectus, medial rectus, superior rectus and lateral rectus in order of decreasing frequency; restriction of extraocular movements.
Eyelids: Edema; lag; retraction.
Optic nerve, Apical: Optic nerve compression (secondary to enlarged muscles); disc swelling; disc atrophy.
Orbit: Axial proptosis, decreased retropulsion of globe.
Other: Increased intraocular pressure in field of restricted gaze; positive forced ductions.

PRECAUTIONS

When making the diagnosis of thyroid eye muscle disorder one must remember that this disease process may occur simultaneously with other disorders affecting the eyes, most notably, myasthenia gravis.

The relevance of each factor contributing to the patient's problem must be ascertained.

Surgical treatment, the treatment of choice in longstanding diplopia from the disease, may be difficult. In cases of extremely tight muscles, rotating the globe to dissect and eventually disinsert the muscle from the globe can be nearly impossible. Care should be taken when applying tension to the muscle hook so as not to tear the muscle belly or tear the muscle from its insertion. One may consider disinsertion of the muscle from the globe by a scalpel blade cutting "metal on metal" against the muscle hook which engages the insertion rather than scissors in these extreme cases. In conjunction with longstanding muscle restriction, retracted conjunctiva is also often found. The conjunctiva is usually recessed in these cases.

With large recessions as are often needed, lid lag after inferior rectus recession can occur, even after extensive dissection of the inferior rectus muscle. Advancement of the capsulopalpebral head of the lower eyelid at the time of surgery can prevent this problem.

Late overcorrection after inferior rectus recession on adjustable suture has been reported and has dissuaded some strabismus surgeons from using this technique. To avoid this, recession of the other inferior rectus muscle should be performed in cases of bilateral unequal involvement.

Two muscles of a previously unoperated upon eye may be safely recessed. Three muscles operated upon simultaneously is generally not recommended. Four muscles operated on at one time is *never* advised as anterior segment circulation would be at great risk for compromise with a potential for blinding anterior segment ischemia.

COMMENTS

A stepwise approach to management of thyroid extraocular muscle disorders should be taken. Prior to eye muscle surgery the orbital and eye muscle finding must be *stable*.

Eye muscle surgery should not be undertaken during the acute congestive phase of the disease even if the patient is extremely anxious for definitive treatment. Before surgery is performed one may temporize with occlusion or more preferably press on prisms. If the angle of deviation is small, yet stable, and the patient is satisfied, ground in prism can be the definite treatment. More often surgery is undertaken and often is quite challenging, yet a rewarding outcome can be expected.

References

Burde RM: Grave's ophthalmopathy and the special problem of concomitant ocular myasthenia gravis. Am Orthoptic J *40*:37–50, 1990.

Helveston EM: Atlas of Strabismus Surgery, 3rd ed. St. Louis, CV Mosby, 1985.

Kushner BJ: A surgical procedure to minimize lower lid retraction with inferior rectus recession. Arch Ophthalmol *110*:1011–1014, 1992.

Sprunger DT, Helveston EM: Progressive overcorrection after inferior rectus recession. J Pediatr Ophthalmol Strabismus *30*:145–148, 1993.

von Noorden GK: Binocular Vision and Ocular Motility; Theory and Management of Strabismus, 4th ed. St. Louis, CV Mosby, pp 410–413, 1990.

V-PATTERNS 378.03, 378.12

(V-Pattern Esotropia 378.03, V-Pattern Exotropia 378.12)

HENRY S. METZ, M.D.

Rochester, New York

V-pattern esotropia is an incomitant esotropia in which the deviation is greater in downgaze than in upgaze. V-pattern exotropia is an incomitant exotropia in which the deviation is greater in upgaze than in downgaze. By convention, there should be a 15 prism diopter difference between up- and downgaze measurements to classify the patient as having a V-pattern. Many cases are associated with overaction of the inferior oblique muscles and underaction of the superior oblique muscles. Increased abduction in upgaze secondary to inferior oblique overaction may be the cause of the V-pattern. In some patients, oblique muscle function appears normal. A downward slant of the lid fissures has also been noted in some cases.

The V-pattern may be associated with any type of esotropia, including accommodative or paralytic varieties. Patients with superior oblique palsy often demonstrate a V-pattern, most likely secondary to superior oblique weakness and thus diminished abduction effect in downgaze. Brown syndrome patients also frequently have a V-pattern.

The V-pattern may be seen with intermittent or constant exotropia. It has also been noted with large-angle longstanding exotropia in which the lateral rectus muscle has become contracted with time, although an X-pattern with all obliques overacting may also be seen.

THERAPY

Ocular. Neither prisms nor orthoptics can be expected to eliminate the V-pattern.

Surgical. When the inferior oblique muscles overact, inferior oblique weakening surgery (recession, myectomy, disinsertion) can collapse the V-pattern. Appropriate surgery on the horizontal recti to correct the esotropia or the exotropia in primary gaze should be planned at the same time.

In cases in which the inferior oblique muscles do not overact, vertical transposition of the horizontal recti, along with recession or resection for the horizontal deviation, can be successful. When planning bilateral surgery, both medial recti should be depressed or both lateral recti elevated. If monocular surgery is performed, the medial rectus insertion should be depressed and the lateral rectus insertion elevated. Less than one-half tendon width transposition is usually ineffective, whereas more than one tendon width transposition is rarely indicated. Horizontal transposition of the vertical recti for V-pattern (superior recti moved nasally, inferior recti moved temporally) has been described, but is not commonly used because of the lack of good predictability of the results.

Ocular or Periocular Manifestations

Extraocular Muscles: Inferior oblique muscle overaction and superior oblique muscle underaction; V-pattern esotropia following superior oblique palsy with antagonist muscle (inferior oblique) overaction. Brown syndrome where there is restriction to elevation of the globe in adduction; Duane's syndrome, probably due to lateral recti co-contraction; inferior oblique overaction and superior oblique underaction.

Other: Chin-down position for upgaze for V-pattern esotropia. Chin-up position for V-pattern exotropia.

PRECAUTIONS

In the presence of superior oblique overaction (even mild overaction), it may be unwise to perform inferior oblique myectomies or large recessions as an A-pattern may result.

Some degree of torsion may result from monocular transposition of the horizontal rectus insertions (1 to 1.5°), but are not symptomatic. However, in patients with superior oblique palsy and excyclotorsion, this added cyclotorsion may add to the problem. Therefore, monocular horizontal rectus transpositions are best avoided. With bilateral superior oblique palsy V-pattern and symptomatic cyclotorsion, a bilateral superior oblique tuck may be the surgery of choice.

Occasionally, accommodative esotropes with fusion at distance fixation and esotropia at near fixation are mistaken for a V-pattern esotropia. This occurs because the near deviation is measured in downgaze instead of in primary gaze. Attention to proper measurement technique can help avoid this confusion.

COMMENTS

V-patterns are not only cosmetically unsatisfactory but are also a barrier to fusion (both central and peripheral) because of the incomitance of the deviation. Surgery for the deviation alone usually does not collapse the "V," so that oblique muscle surgery or vertical transposition of the horizontal rectus insertions is useful. Less than 10 prism diopters of V-pattern rarely require attention in surgical planning. Tilting the chin 30 degrees upward and downward for measurement has been seen to be equally as accurate as moving the target above and below primary gaze.

References

Costenbader F: Symposium: The A and V patterns in strabismus. Trans Am Acad Ophthalmol Otolaryngol 76:354, 1964.

Goldstein JH: Monocular vertical displacement of the horizontal rectus muscles in the A and V patterns. Am J Ophthalmol 64:265, 1967.

Jampolsky A: Oblique muscle surgry of the A and V patterns. J Pediatr Ophthalmol 2:31, 1965.

Knapp P: A and V patterns. *In* Symposium on Strabismus. Transactions of the New Orleans Academy of Ophthalmology. St. Louis, CV Mosby, 1971, p 242.

Metz HS, Schwartz L: The treatment of A and V

patterns by monocular surgery. Arch Ophthalmol 95:251, 1977.

Parks MM: The weakening surgical procedures for eliminating overaction of the inferior oblique muscle. Am J Ophthalmol 73:107, 1972.

Scott AB: V-pattern exotropia. Electromyographic study of an unusual case. Invest Ophthalmol 12: 232, 1973.

Scott AB, Stella SL: Measurement of A and V patterns. J Pediatr Ophthalmol 5:181, 1968.

Taylor J: The management of A and V patterns in strabismus. Aust J Ophthalmol 4:165, 1976.

SECTION 23

EYELIDS

ANKYLOBLEPHARON
374.46

David W. Vastine, M.D.,
and Robert L. Stamper, M.D.

San Francisco, California

Ankyloblepharon is an adhesion between the upper and lower lids along the palpebral margin that varies from a single filamentous band to a rather extensive adhesion. This condition is either congenital or secondary to severe inflammatory conditions of the lid margins. The pathogenesis is related to the apposition of two raw epithelial surfaces. The usual site of fusion is the outer canthus, in which case the condition is called external ankyloblepharon. An internal form, with fusion at the inner canthus, is less common. The condition is frequently associated with symblepharon and obliteration of the conjunctival fornices. Both forms give the appearance of a pseudostrabismus.

THERAPY

Surgical. Surgical therapy is aimed at separating the disturbed epithelial surfaces until re-epithelialization and healing can occur. Usually the eyelids may be separated with scissors. However, if the involvement is extensive, the separation is more effectively done with a scalpel while supporting the underside of the eyelid with a ribbon retractor or similar instrument to protect the cornea and to facilitate the dissection. The marginal surfaces may be separated by a thin, soft plastic or silicone sheet sutured in place until the margins have re-epithelialized. In severe cases, a marginal conjunctival graft and reconstruction of the palpebral conjunctiva by autologous conjunctival transplantation are indicated. The margins are lined with conjunctiva, the raw skin and conjunctival edges are sutured, and the lids are held apart to prevent new adhesions. If the canthus is involved, a medial or lateral canthoplasty may also be required.

Ocular or Periocular Manifestations

Eyelids: Adhesion; fusion; symblepharon.
Globe: Anophthalmos; microphthalmos; pht hisis bulbi.
Lacrimal System: Punctal occlusion.

PRECAUTIONS

Bands of scar tissue form most commonly at the outer canthus, but they may also form at the inner canthus. Bands may also bridge the palpebral aperture. In severe cases, scar tissue may significantly hinder eye opening and may even interfere with vision. In the most severe cases, ankyloblepharon is usually associated with symblepharon. However, the symblepharon must take operative priority. Nasal scarring may incorporate the puncta and canalicular apparatus. In this instance, reconstructive nasolacrimal procedures may be required to re-establish the integrity of the lacrimal drainage system.

COMMENTS

The inheritance pattern of congenital ankyloblepharon has been described as dominant in some patients and sporadic in others. Intrauterine injury or inflammation as well as a primary aberration of growth at either canthus have been postulated as potential causes of the congenital variety.

Acquired forms of ankyloblepharon may occur during healing of destructive processes involving the palpebral margins. Apposition of upper and lower marginal surfaces denuded of epithelium plays a key role in the pathogenesis of secondary ankyloblepharon. Some of the more common causes of acquired ankyloblepharon are trauma, caustic and thermal burns, ulcerative blepharitis, impetigo, cicatricial pemphigoid, and epidermolysis bullosa. Lupus vulgaris of the skin and eyelids, diphtheritic conjunctivitis, trachoma, vaccinia, smallpox, and other skin and mucous membrane disorders may also result in ankyloblepharon.

References

Beard C: Diseases of the lids. In Dunlap EA (ed): Gordon's Medical Management of Ocular Disease, 2nd ed. Hagerstown, MD, Harper & Row, 1976, pp 110–135.

Duke-Elder S. (ed.): System of Ophthalmology. St. Louis, CV Mosby, 1963, Vol III, pp 867–871; 1974, Vol. XIII, pp 590–591.

Vastine DW, Stewart WB, Schwat IR: Reconstruction of the periocular mucous membrane by autologous conjunctival transplantation. Ophthalmology 89:1072–1081, 1982.

BENIGN ESSENTIAL BLEPHAROSPASM 333.81

JOHN R. SAMPLES, M.D.

Portland, Oregon

Benign essential blepharospasm is a potentially disabling disorder that affects primarily older individuals and is often associated with other evidence of orofacial dyskinesia. It is an involuntary tonic, often forceful closure of the eyelids that may be either intermittent or continuous. Symptoms are typically made worse by stress, fatigue, bright lights, and driving, although this varies among affected individuals. They may be relieved by sleep and relaxation. In some instances, patients may be distracted from their blepharospasm by being given tasks to perform that require a fair amount of concentration. The disease is usually slowly progressive, but a variety of courses may be seen. It is almost always bilateral, although one side may be worse than the other. Involvement of the lower face and the oropharynx, termed Meig's syndrome, is surprisingly common and often overlooked.

It is helpful to differentiate the syndrome of benign essential blepharospasm from other causes of blepharospasm. A thorough neurologic and ophthalmologic examination is required before making the diagnosis. Some individuals have a psychogenic etiology for their blepharospasm. Such individuals are typically young and do not present with a true tonic closure of the eyelids, but rather a flutter or a voluntary squeezing. The chronic closing of the protractor muscles (orbicularis oculi, corrugator, and procerus) in patients with benign essential blepharospasm can lead to dermatochalasis, brow ptosis, and blepharoptosis. These patients are prone to developing entropion and ectropion. The differential diagnosis also includes dry eye conditions, other types of keratitis, apraxia of lid opening in which the patient is unable to initiate the opening of the eyes, hemifacial spasm, tardive dyskinesia, postencephalic parkinsonism, and other movement disorders. Since some patients with blepharospasm may have Parkinson's disease, referral to a neurologist to rule out that disease may be an important part of the initial evaluation. The pathophysiology of blepharospasm remains uncertain.

THERAPY

Systemic. A large variety of drugs have been recommended or tried for benign essential blepharospasm. Pharmacologic trials need to be limited because many patients will become frustrated after trying several drugs. However, if the patient is found to have diseases or disorders that mimic Parkinson's disease, treatment with a dopamine agonist, such as a carbidopa/levodopa combination, bromocriptine, or amantadine, may be effective.

It is usually best to start with an anticholinergic/antispasmodic, such as trihexyphenidyl, and to increase the doses slowly. Many patients will obtain control of their blepharospasm, but will not tolerate the associated systemic side effects, including dry mouth, that are seen with the use of trihexyphenidyl. After anticholinergic therapy, a trial with a benzodiazapine, such as clonazepam, may be worthwhile. Antidepressants have been useful in a very limited number of patients. No medication has been identified as specifically curative for this condition.

Ocular. Some patients who present with blepharospasm have keratitis or evidence of dry eyes. It is important therefore to rule out the presence of a dry eye or blepharitis. These patients may be particularly prone to both of these conditions. In particular, patients are prone to keratitis after surgery or botulinum A toxin injections for this condition.

Botulinum A toxin[+] injections provide effective relief for most patients with benign essential blepharospasm. The toxic works by interfering with acetylcholine release from nerve terminals. It may provide relief from spasm for 3 months or longer. It is generally well tolerated, although some patients develop ptosis or diplopia. A typical pattern of injection is to place 5 units subcutaneously at each of the two sites over the brow, the upper lid, and the lower lid on one side, for a total of six injections per side. Many patterns are used, and these should be tailored to the patient's spasm.

Surgical. Surgery should be reserved for individuals who have failed trials with medication and botulinum A toxin. Older procedures involved sectioning the seventh cranial nerve either at its main trunk or along the peripheral branches. Reinnervation was a frequent problem, and as a result resection of the orbicularis oculi muscles has become more popular using the technique described by Gillum and Anderson (1981). This technique involves the meticulous extirpation of all of the accessible orbicularis oculi, procerus, corrugator, superciliaris, and fascial nerves in postorbicular fascia.

Supportive. A foundation exists to deal with the problem of benign essential blepharospasm (Benign Essential Blepharospasm Research Foundation, Inc., 755 Howell Street, Beaumont, TX 77706). These patients are often helped by support groups, although a few patients have been adversely affected by participation when they have been exposed to patients with disease that is far more advanced than their own. Because there is substantial variability in the severity of blepharospasm, some patients may develop increased anxiety as the result of participating in support groups that include patients with severe truncal ataxia. Therefore, referral of patients needs to be individualized.

Ocular or Periocular Manifestations

Cornea: Keratitis.
Lids: Blepharospasm; dermatochalasis; ectropion; entropion.
Other: Dystonias of the head, neck, and whole body.

PRECAUTIONS

Knowledge and familiarity with the drugs used to treat this condition are essential. The effective use of botulinum A toxin requires experience tailoring the injections to each individual in order to obtain a desirable effect with minimal complications. Every patient receiving the toxin should have a complete eye examination before treatment, since baseline parameters are essential before ptosis or diplopia develops. Patients undergoing botulinum A toxin therapy should be closely monitored for ophthalmic complications, including ptosis and keratitis. Obtaining a careful and appropriate consent before using botulinum A toxin injections is mandatory.

COMMENTS

A therapeutic approach to the patient with benign essential blepharospasm should include a trial of medications before consideration of botulinum A toxin injections or surgery. Rarely, patients respond to medication and require no further therapy. Several patients have been observed to do extremely well with an anticholinergic alone. If systemic medications are ineffective in controlling the medicine, then a trial with botulinum A toxin injections is indicated. The efficacy of such injections has been demonstrated. Repeated injections and the patient's lack of acceptance of them are indications for proceeding with surgery. A variety of surgical approaches have been described. The most effective may be the removal of orbicularis oculi, procerus, and corrugator muscles to limit the effect and extent of the disease.

References

Freuh BR, et al: Treatment of blepharospasm with botulinum toxin. A preliminary report. Arch Ophthalmol *102*:1464–1468, 1984.

Gillum WN, Anderson RL: Blepharospasm surgery. An anatomical approach. Arch Ophthalmol *99*: 1056–1062, 1981.

Jankovic J: Clinical features, differential diagnosis and pathogenesis of blepharospasm and cranial cervical dystonia. *In* Bosniak SL, Smith BC (eds): Advances in Ophthalmic Plastic and Reconstructive Surgery—Blepharospasm. New York, Pergamon Press, Vol. *4*, 1985.

Jones FTW, Samples JR, Waller RR: The treatment of essential blepharospasm. Mayo Clin Proc *60*: 663–666, 1985.

Lingua RW: Sequelae of botulinum toxin injection. Am J Ophthalmol *100*:305–307, 1985.

BLEPHAROCHALASIS
374.34

JOHN H. SULLIVAN, M.D.

San Francisco, California

Blepharochalasis is characterized by bilateral episodic swelling of the eyelids and periorbital areas, lasting up to several days and resulting in progressive damage to the eyelid structures. It is sometimes familial, affecting both sexes, with the onset of symptoms usually between the ages of 7 and 20.

As a result of repeated attacks, the skin loses its elasticity, becomes thin, and resembles parchment. Stretching and thinning of the orbital septum cause the preaponeurotic fat and occasionally the orbital lobe of the lacrimal gland to prolapse into the eyelid. The upper nasal fat pad often atrophies, and the overlying skin retracts, causing a typical depression and pseudoepicanthal fold. Moderate to severe ptosis can result from progressive damage to the levator aponeurosis. The lateral canthal tendons may also deteriorate, resulting in horizontal phimosis of the lid slits and rounded lateral canthi.

THERAPY

Supportive. In the acute phase, treatment is symptomatic. If a specific factor that triggers an acute attack can be identified, the only treatment necessary is avoidance. Unfortunately, this is seldom possible. Cold compresses during the acute phase may reduce swelling and tissue damage. Local and systemic corticosteroids are of limited value. Fortunately, the frequency and severity of attacks lessen with age.

Surgical. Surgery is usually necessary to repair damaged eyelid tissue. Removal of redundant skin by blepharoplasty is beneficial. Prolapsed preaponeurotic fat may be excised, and the lacrimal gland may be sutured to the periorbita of the lacrimal fossa if it has been displaced. Horizontal phimosis is treated by reattaching the lateral canthal tissues to the periosteum anterior to the orbital tubercle with a nonabsorbable suture material.

Ptosis repair is frequently necessary and often difficult. The Fasanella-Servat procedure is sufficient to correct minimal ptosis. Disinsertion or dehiscence of the levator aponeurosis is best managed by reattachment or levator tuck. Surgery is often unsatisfactory because recurrent attacks of edema destroy the result. For this reason, ptosis surgery should be delayed until the frequency and severity of attacks have diminished. This is not always possible, particularly if the ptosis is disabling. Delayed repair, although preferable, may be complicated by the presence of severely damaged tissues. Reapproximation or repair of a markedly thinned levator complex can be very challenging and unfortunately is apt to be followed by recurrence.

PRECAUTIONS

The term "blepharochalasis" is frequently misused by ophthalmologists and plastic surgeons to indicate any of the conditions characterized by "baggy eyelids." Aging, redundant eyelid skin is more accurately termed "dermatochalasis." True blepharochalasis is a very rare cause of baggy eyelids.

COMMENTS

The etiology of this rare condition remains unknown. In the acute phase, it resembles angioneurotic edema, which is more common and believed to be allergic in origin. Blepharochalasis has not been shown to be an allergic reaction, although factors that seem to precipitate an acute attack, such as fever or exposure to sunlight, have been observed in some patients. Eosinophilia, urticaria, visceral involvement, laryngeal edema, and respiratory distress are rarely observed. Therefore, blepharochalasis seems to represent a specific localized disease entity that is not the same as angioneurotic edema.

References

Alvis BY: Blepharochalasis. Report of a case. Am J Ophthalmol 18:238–245, 1935.
Collin JRO, et al: Blepharochalasis. Br J Ophthalmol 63:542–546, 1979.
Custer PL, Tenzel RR, Kowalczyk AP: Blepharochalasis syndrome. Am J Ophthalmol 99:424–428, 1985.
Jordan DR: Blepharochalasis syndrome. Can J Ophthalmol 27:10–15, 1992.
Stieglitz LN, Crawford JS: Blepharochalasis. Am J Ophthalmol 77:100–102, 1974.
Sunder TR, Balsam MJ, Vengrow MI: Neurological manifestations of angioedema. Report of two cases and review of the literature. JAMA 247:2005–2007, 1982.

BLEPHAROPHIMOSIS 374.46

JAY JUSTIN OLDER, M.D., F.A.C.S.

Tampa, Florida

Blepharophimosis is the condition in which the palpebral aperture is decreased in height and width. The dominantly inherited tetrad of ptosis, epicanthus inversus, telecanthus, and blepharophimosis is referred to as the blepharophimosis syndrome. Patients with the blepharophimosis syndrome have small palpebral apertures associated with an increased width between the inner canthi (telecanthus) and a fold of skin from the lower lid extending toward the bridge of the nose (epicanthus inversus). The narrow palpebral aperture is a result of the ptosis, which is usually severe. Dominant inheritance with essentially 100 per cent penetrance has been well documented. There seem to be no other associated systemic findings, and intelligence is normal. Ectropion, punctal displacement, low-set ears, strabismus, and optic nerve colobomata have been reported in a few patients with this syndrome. The individual features of short palpebral apertures, telecanthus, and ptosis are sometimes seen as part of the following syndromes: fetal alcohol, Dubowitz, trisomy 18, Williams, cerebro-oculo-facial-skeletal, Carpenter, oral-facial-digital, and Waardenburg. These possibilities should be considered in the absence of a definite dominant pedigree or in the presence of other anomalies, particularly mental retardation.

Lack of support at the lateral canthus may also give rise to a senile or spastic blepharophimosis. Cicatricial blepharophimosis may follow destructive lesions, such as trachoma, or may occur after trauma.

THERAPY

Surgical. The goal of therapy is to create a more normal appearing eye with functional eyelids. It is usually preferable to reconstruct the medial canthal deformities 6 to 12 months before repair of the ptosis.

The upper canthal fold can be eliminated by Mustarde's double Z plasties, in which flaps are formed as rectangles and closed as triangles. This method provides needed tissue in the vertical direction. An alternative method for correction is the Y to V operation of Verwey, in which an incision in the medial canthus is created in the form of a horizontal Y and closed in the shape of a horizontal V. A modification of this technique is to place double opposing plasties on the apex of the V.

If telecanthus is present, the medial canthus can be shortened before closure of the flaps in either of these procedures. To advance the angle medially, a section of the canthal tendon can be excised and the remaining edges reapproximated with a permanent suture. For larger amounts of telecanthus, transnasal wiring can be performed by creating osteotomies in the area of both anterior lacrimal crests. The medial canthal tendons are attached to each other, using wires that pass through the osteotomies and the nasal septum. The wires are tightened until the desired amount of telecanthus repair is accomplished.

Since the levator muscle is usually weak, ptosis repair is best accomplished by a tarsofrontalis suspension. Autogenous fascia lata, removed from the patient's leg and placed as a double rhomboid or double triangle, gives the best chance for permanent repair. Good alternative materials are preserved fascia lata or silicone rods.

Some types of blepharophimosis have a skin shortage instead of epicanthal folds. In these cases, full-thickness skin grafts from the retroauricular area should be placed in all four lids 6 to 12 months before the other abnormalities are corrected. Some degrees of lower lid ectropion can be repaired with rotation flaps or free skin grafts in association with the medial canthal repair.

If the lateral canthus is medially placed, a lateral canthoplasty may be required to move the lateral canthus outward. A lateral canthotomy with advancement of the conjunctiva to the new skin edges is often sufficient to increase the horizontal direction of the palpebral fissure.

Surgical repair of acquired blepharophimosis is directed at the underlying disease. Medial and lateral canthoplasties or ectropion repair may be required.

Ocular or Periocular Manifestations

Conjunctiva: Scarred or contracted in secondary blepharophimosis because of ocular pemphigus or trachoma.

Eyelids: Ectropion; epicanthus inversus; lacrimal puncta displacement; ptosis; telecanthus.

PRECAUTIONS

Some families may desire only the ptosis repair, since reconstruction of the medial canthus would cause the child to look different from other family members. Careful evaluation of eyelid excursion is important because levator function is usually so minimal that a levator resection would be insufficient to elevate the eyelids. The possibility of severe congenital deformities should be investigated in the absence of a clear dominant pedigree or if there are associated malformations or mental retardation.

COMMENTS

Congenital blepharophimosis comprises 3 to 6 per cent of congenital ptosis. The eyelid and canthal deformities can be improved by the treatment described. Repair should be done at age of 5 years or any time thereafter.

References

Anderson RL, Nowinski TS: The five-flap technique for blepharophimosis. Arch Ophthalmol 107:448–452, 1989.

Beard C: Ptosis, 3rd ed. St. Louis, CV Mosby, 1981, pp 41–46, 211–225.

Callahan MA, Callahan A: Ophthalmic Plastic and Orbital Surgery. Birmingham, Aesculapius, 1979, pp 36–40.

Duke-Elder S (ed): System of Ophthalmology. St. Louis, CV Mosby, 1974, Vol XIII, pp 589–590.

Grizard WS, O'Donnell JJ, Carey JC: The cerebro-oculo-facio-skeletal syndrome. Am J Ophthalmol 89:293–298, 1980.

Kohn R, Romano PE: Blepharoptosis, blepharophimosis, epicanthus inversus, and telecanthus—A syndrome with no name. Am J Ophthalmol 72:625–632, 1971.

Mustardé JC: Repair and Reconstruction in the Orbital Region. Edinburgh, E & S Livingstone, 1966, pp 338–352.

Owens N, Hadley RC, Kloepfer HW: Hereditary blepharophimosis, ptosis, and epicanthus inversus. J Int Coll Surg 33:558–574, 1960.

Sacrez R, et al: Le blépharophimosis compliqué familial. Etude des membres de la famille. Ble Ann Pediatr 10:493–501, 1963.

Smith DW: Recognizable Patterns of Human Malformation: Genetic, Embryologic, and Clinical Aspects. Philadelphia, WB Saunders, 1970, pp 10–11, 54–55, 62–63, 122–125, 144–145, 240–241, 336–337, 447.

CHALAZION 373.2

HERBERT J. GERSHEN, M.D.

San Francisco, California

A chalazion is a chronic granuloma of a meibomian gland and may result from an inflammation of this gland. There is characteristic swelling caused by the retention of secretions and the formation of granulation tissue. As the gland fills with secretions and granulation tissue, it forms a tumor that can grow as large as 7 or 8 mm in diameter. It may remain contained in the tarsus or break through anteriorly beneath the skin or on the conjunctival side, possibly resulting in a fistula through which the granulation tissue protrudes. A marginal chalazion is a smaller granuloma involving the area of a meibomian gland near its marginal termination. Chalazia are more common on the upper lid, occur most often in adults, and are associated with seborrhea, chronic blepharitis, and acne rosacea.

THERAPY

Supportive. In general, most chalazia disappear in a few months without therapy. If the chalazion is small and causing no symptoms, treatment may not be required. A few seem to resolve with the use of hot packs. Systemic antibiotics are seldom indicated in the management of chalazion.

Ocular. Local injection of corticosteroids has been shown to be an effective, rapid form of treatment for chalazia. A volume of 0.5 to 2.0 ml of 5 mg/ml triamcinolone acetonide may be directly injected into the center of the chalazion. A second injection may be considered 2 to 7 days later if necessary.

Surgical. Surgical removal from the palpebral conjunctival side is preferred, unless a granuloma extends through skin or previous drainage has occurred externally and removal of the lesion is obviously easier by the external route. If secondarily infected, the chalazion should first be managed by heat, antibiotics, and, in selected cases, incision and drainage. A small chalazion may be treated by curettage and cauterization of the lining of the gland with phenol or trichloroacetic acid. A larger chalazion is more likely to be cured by surgical excision. Infiltration anesthesia and tarsal block are administered, and a chalazion clamp is applied. A vertical tarsal incision 2 to 3 mm from the lid margin is made. Identification and removal of the sac within its capsule are performed. Curettage and excision of the remaining tissue and sac are done carefully, being cautious not to remove normal tissue. However, in some cases, total removal of the tarsal plate within the area of the chalazion clamp without the need for curettage is the method of choice. Electrocautery may be used to prevent bleeding, although this is seldom necessary if pressure is applied for 4 to 5 minutes. A mild pressure bandage is applied for 4 hours.

If the external approach is used, a horizontal incision at least 3 mm from the lid margin is made in an existing crease, and the chalazion is removed. Normal lid tissue should not be sacrificed. Hemostasis is achieved with electrocautery. The wound is closed with 7-0 silk suture after the clamp is removed.

Occasionally, a chalazion involves both skin and conjunctiva; in such case, removal may be through both surfaces. A through-and-through hole should be avoided by offsetting the skin and conjunctival incisions.

Marginal chalazia that are improperly removed result in notching, trichiasis, and the loss of lashes. Most marginal chalazia are connected to another chalazion located farther from the lid margin. The contents may be expressed by rolling two cotton-tipped applicators toward the lid margin from both sides of the lid. If this is painful, a local anesthetic may be used. If the contents cannot be expressed, incision is made over the distal chalazion, and removal of the contents is by curettage. The marginal area of the eyelid is curetted, leaving a 3-mm bridge of normal tarsus nearest the lid margin to prevent notching. A pressure patch is then applied.

Ocular or Periocular Manifestations

Eyelids: Edema; granulation tissue; mass.
Other: Astigmatism.

PRECAUTIONS

Intralesional injection of corticosteroids is particularly suitable for a chalazion located near the lacrimal drainage apparatus because surgery in this area may lead to serious complications. Insoluble aqueous preparations are preferable to crystalline suspensions of corticosteroids to minimize complications of hypopigmentation and atrophy of the treated skin. A transconjunctival injection may also provide a further safeguard against these complications.

A lid incision should be made 2 to 3 mm from the lid margin to prevent notching. In general, normal lid tissue should not be sacrificed in attempting to completely remove a chalazion. A biopsy should be done on recurrent chalazia or those that seem unusual to rule out malignancy. If secondary infection exists, the pus should be evacuated, but no curettage should be performed.

COMMENTS

Conservative treatment is indicated, and in most cases, surgery should be performed only after a few weeks of hot packs. If multiple chalazia are present, they may be removed by careful dissection without fear of lid deformity, since this fibrous tissue heals without leaving gaps in the tarsal plate. Complete removal of the chalazion with the tarsal plate has not been reported to cause a lid deformity.

References

Dua HS, Nilawar DV: Nonsurgical therapy of chalazion. Am J Ophthalmol 94:424–425, 1982.

Duke-Elder S (ed): System of Ophthalmology. St. Louis, CV Mosby, 1965, Vol III, pp 242–247.

Epstein GA, Allen MP: Combined excision and drainage with intralesional corticosteroid injection in the treatment of chronic chalazia. Arch Ophthalmol 106:514–516, 1988.

Gershen HJ: Chalazion excision. Ophthalmic Surg 5:75–76, 1974.

King RA, Ellis PP: Treatment of chalazia with corticosteroid injections. Ophthal Surg 17:351–353, 1986.

Perry HD, Serniuk RA: Conservative treatment of chalazia. Ophthalmology 87:218–221, 1980.

Pizzarello LD, et al: Intralesional corticosteroid therapy of chalazia. Am J Ophthalmol 85:818–821, 1978.

Sloas HA Jr, et al: Treatment of chalazia with injectable triamcinolone. Ann Ophthalmol 15:78–80, 1983.

Soll DB, Winslow R: Surgery of the eyelids. In Duane TD (ed): Clinical Ophthalmology. Hagerstown, MD, Harper & Row, 1982, Vol V, pp 5:6–5:9.

Vidaurri LJ, Jacob P: Intralesional corticosteroid treatment of chalazia. Ann Ophthalmol 18:339–340, 1986.

DISTICHIASIS 743.63
(Districhiasis)

RICHARD L. ANDERSON, M.D., F.A.C.S.,
and JOHN B. HOLDS, M.D.

Salt Lake City, Utah

Congenital distichiasis—sometimes erroneously called "districhiasis"—is a rare condition in which an accessory row of eyelashes is present in or near the orifices of the meibomian glands. Cases have been reported with three (tristichiasis) and four (tetrastichiasis) rows of lashes. The accessory row (or rows) of lashes may consist of only a few cilia, or there may be a well-formed row. The extra cilia are generally smaller and less pigmented, although they may be as fully developed as the normal row in some cases. Abnormalities of the tarsal plate may result in slight eversion or marked ectropion of the eyelids.

Congenital distichiasis is frequently inherited as an autosomal dominant trait with high penetrance and variable expressivity. Distichiasis has also been reported in some forms of familial lymphedema (Meige's disease) in association with entropion, ptosis, vertebral anomalies, extradural cysts, webbed neck, yellow nails, and other systemic anomalies. It is also associated with trisomy 18, congenital heart defects, peripheral vascular anomalies, and congenital corneal hypesthesia. The significance of distichiasis lies in the chronic irritation of the cornea and conjunctiva caused by the aberrant cilia.

Acquired distichiasis is a term that has not been widely accepted, but describes a situation in which abnormal acquired lashes appear in the same location as those aberrant lashes in congenital distichiasis. The acquired distichiatic lashes tend to be short and wiry and cause more corneal irritation than in congenital distichiasis. Acquired distichiasis occurs in cases of Stevens-Johnson syndrome, toxic epidermal necrolysis, ocular pemphigoid, and chemical and physical injuries of the eyelids. Acquired distichiasis should be distinguished from trichiasis, which implies inturned or misdirected lashes that have a normal location in the anterior lamellae of the lid, because the anatomic location and treatment of the acquired distichiatic aberrant lashes differ.

In congenital distichiasis, a developmental anomaly occurs in which a complete pilosebaceous unit (with hair and glandular structures) is present in the posterior lamella. This probably represents a failure of the primary epithelial anlage to differentiate selectively into only a sebaceous gland. If this is the case, it would not represent a true metaplasia as some have suggested. An in utero injury leading to a metaplasia inducing congenital distichiasis seems unlikely.

In acquired distichiasis, certain stimuli (immunologic, chemical, or physical) provoke metaplastic change that results in the formation of a hair follicle within or adjacent to the sebaceous meibomian gland. The clinical evidence in many cases of Stevens-Johnson syndrome, pemphigoid, and chemical or physical injuries, as well as histologic studies, provide support for this hypothesis.

THERAPY

Ocular. No treatment is required in asymptomatic individuals. Lubricating agents should be used to protect the eye from irritation until definitive treatment is performed. Therapeutic soft contact lenses may also be employed as a temporary measure.

Surgical. Although many procedures have been described for the correction of distichiasis, none has gained general acceptance. These treatment modalities can be divided into the categories of epilation, electrolysis, surgical extirpation, and cryosurgery. Epilation is only a temporizing measure and results in the recurrence of cilia that are even more irritating. Electrolysis is complicated with many recurrences, scarring, and entropion. It is virtually impossible to isolate all the distichiatic cilia, and electrolysis is only applicable in cases with very limited involvement. Procedures of microscopic identification of the follicles through a trap-door-type of posterior tarsal incision or other tarsal dissection followed by their obliteration are time consuming and tedious and fraught with recurrence because of incomplete excision. Splitting of the eyelid at the gray line with excision of the marginal portion of the tarsus can lead to entropion and trichiasis. The use of nasal mucosal, tarsoconjunctival, or buccal grafts in an attempt to reconstruct the posterior lamella is time consuming and unpredictable and results in eyelid margin disfigurement.

Cryosurgery is the most effective method available for obliterating aberrant lashes of the eyelid. Temperatures of -15 to $-20°C$ result in permanent destruction of the lash follicle; temperatures of $-30°C$ and lower cause increased necrosis and scarring. With standard forms of cryosurgical treatment, not only the abnormal posterior lashes but also the normal anterior cilia are lost. Despite efforts to limit this loss with the use of thermocouple monitoring, optimal treatment criteria have not been established. Additionally, depigmentation of the skin occurs, which is especially disfiguring in pigmented individuals. Lid splitting and posterior lamellar cryotherapy are recommended; these procedures preserve the normal anterior lashes and avoid depigmentation while obliterating the aberrant cilia in the posterior lamella.

Lidocaine with epinephrine (1:100,000) is injected under the skin and conjunctiva of the eyelid. Topical 2.5 per cent phenylephrine is placed in the conjunctival cul-de-sac to provide added vasoconstriction. The eyelid is split at the gray line with a No. 11 scalpel blade. Magnification, by either operating microscope or loupes, is used to verify the gray line and to ensure that all aberrant lashes are included in the posterior lamella. The incision must be made perpendicular to the lid margin. The lid splitting is continued by blunt and sharp dissection with scissors, maintaining a plane on the anterior surface of the tarsal plate. Care is taken to avoid the normal anterior lash follicles, as trauma may result in the loss of normal lashes or trichiasis. The lid splitting is continued for a sufficient distance up the tarsus to ensure that the cryoprobe, when applied, will not inadvertently freeze the normal anterior cilia. Hemostasis is obtained by compression and bipolar cautery. Using the large beveled tip of the nitrous oxide eyelid cryoprobe (Cryomedics), the posterior lamella is frozen to −20 to −25°C. Temperature is monitored by a thermocouple. Once experience has been gained with the technique, it may be possible to omit the thermocouple. The surgeon attempts to obtain a rapid freeze and slow thaw to room temperature, followed by a second freeze and slow thaw. Care is taken not to freeze the anterior lamella of the eyelid during this procedure.

After all areas of the posterior lamella have been treated, the anterior lamella is recessed 2 mm from the lid margin by placing 6-0 chromic horizontal mattress sutures to position the recessed anterior lamella on the tarsus. Care is taken to direct the lashes in a slightly everted position, for any misdirected lashes may become trichiatic. The 2-mm anterior lamellar recession helps prevent the normal anterior lashes from misdirecting posteriorly and becoming trichiatic. Without this recession, the anterior lamella may override the posterior lamella. Within a month, the anterior lamella will have migrated toward the margin so that the anterior recession is unnoticed. Topical steroid-antibiotic ointment is placed in the eye and on the lid margin. No patch is applied for fear of misdirecting lashes.

Ocular or Periocular Manifestations

Conjunctiva: Conjunctivitis; scarring; symblepharon shrinkage.
Cornea: Erosions; keratitis; keratoconjunctivitis sicca; secondary vascularization and scarring.
Eyelids: Blepharoptosis; ectropion; entropion; reactive spasms and squeezing.

PRECAUTIONS

Considerable edema may be present postoperatively. If both upper and lower eyelids require surgery, the eyelids may be closed by the edema on the first postoperative day. Conjunctival shrinkage disorders may be aggravated by cryosurgery or other surgery. Recurrence of an isolated cilium, induction of trichiasis, or loss of normal lashes are possible. Slight thickening of the eyelid margin may occur.

COMMENTS

In congenital distichiasis the most common side effects experienced with cryosurgery are transient edema and slight thickening of the lid margin. Fewer complications occur in congenital than in acquired distichiasis for these eyelids react normally to cryosurgery and other surgery.

Acquired distichiasis is a much more difficult condition to treat than congenital distichiasis. Follow-up of patients with acquired distichiasis for a minimum of 2 years showed great improvement after lid splitting and posterior lamellar cryosurgery. Epilation of a trichiatic lash or isolated cryosurgical touch-up to a recurrent distichiatic or trichiatic lash may be required occasionally. It is difficult to determine if these cases represent treatment failure or continuation of the metaplastic process in the eyelids. Small areas of sparse to absent lashes along the lid margin were present in only a few eyelids. Conjunctival keratinization was markedly improved in most cases. The incidence of complications with cryosurgery or surgery is much higher in patients with the conjunctival shrinkage syndromes than in normal subjects. Considering the natural history and the extent of the disease processes in these patients followed (Stevens-Johnson syndrome and chemical injury), these results are very encouraging in these very difficult conditions. This technique gains the advantages of cryosurgery for the treatment of distichiasis while avoiding many of the disadvantages.

References

Anderson RL, Harvey JT: Lid splitting and posterior lamella cryosurgery for congenital and acquired distichiasis. Arch Ophthalmol 99:631–634, 1981.

Dortzbach RK, Butera RT: Excision of distichiasis eyelashes through a tarsoconjunctival trapdoor. Arch Ophthalmol 96:111–112, 1978.

Duke-Elder S (ed): System of Ophthalmology. St. Louis, CV Mosby, 1963, Vol III, pp 873–876.

Frueh BR: Treatment of distichiasis with cyrotherapy. Surv Ophthalmol 12:100–103, 1981.

Goldstein S, et al: Distichiasis, congenital heart defects and mixed peripheral vascular anomalies. Am J Med Genet 20:283–294, 1985.

Kremer I: Corneal hypoaesthesia in asymptomatic familial distichiasis. Br J Ophthalmol 70:132–134, 1986.

Mehta L, et al: Trisomy 18 in a 13 year old girl. J Med Genet 23:256–257, 1986.

Teillac D, et al: Toxic epidermal necrolysis in children (Lyell's syndrome). Apropos of 18 cases. Arch Fr Pediatr 44:583–587, 1987.

White JH: Correction of distichiasis by tarsal resection and mucous membrane grafting. Am J Ophthalmol 80:507–508, 1975.

Wolfley D: Excision of individual follicles for the

management of congenital distichiasis and localized trichiasis. J Pediatr Ophthalmol Strabismus 24:22–26, 1987.
Wood JR, Anderson RL: Complications of cryosurgery. Arch Ophthalmol 99:460–463, 1981.

ECTROPION 374.10

RICHARD D. LISMAN, M.D., F.A.C.S., *and* STEPHEN SOLL, M.D.

New York, New York

Ectropion is the outward turning of the eyelid margin that may involve the upper, lower, or both eyelids. It may vary from a mild eversion of a portion of the lid to a total eversion of the entire lid. In longstanding cases, the conjunctiva becomes hyperemic and then hypertrophic. As a result of the drying, it may become keratinized. Ectropion may be classified as congenital, atonic, cicatricial, allergic, or mechanical.

Congenital ectropion is usually due to a vertical deficiency and rarely to a horizontal deficiency of the skin and occasionally the underlying tissue. All of the eyelids may be involved; however, it occurs most often in the lateral one-third of the lower eyelids. Often, there are other associated ocular abnormalities, including blepharophimosis, telecanthus, epicanthus inversus, and ptosis.

Atonic ectropion includes an involutional (senile) and a paralytic type. The involutional type is characterized by excessive horizontal eyelid length associated with weakness of the pretarsal portion of the orbicularis muscle. Horizontal stretching of the tarsus and laxity of both the medial and lateral canthal tendons contribute to an increase in horizontal eyelid length. These patients are usually annoyed by epiphora secondary to an associated punctal ectropion of the lower lid. The constant wiping of their eyes additionally stretches the eyelid and draws the punctum away from the tear pool. Paralytic ectropion occurs with seventh nerve palsy and is often unilateral. Etiologies include Bell's palsy, trauma, cerebrovascular accident, or resection of tissue along the course of the peripheral nerve distal to the foramen lacerum. The atonic lower eyelid is susceptible to gravitational effects and, if not corrected, will become more prominent with the passage of time. Thus, treatment depends on the permanency of the involvement.

Cicatricial ectropion is the result of shortened anterior lamellae of the eyelid, usually secondary to scar contracture. Thermal, chemical, mechanical, or previous surgery can all be responsible for scar formation. The overzealous resection of skin during blepharoplasty is another cause of cicatricial ectropion.

Skin grafting is the only treatment for severe cicatricial ectropion.

Allergic ectropion is usually reversible and is most often due to contact dermatitis of the eyelids. The offending medication or cosmetic irritant should be discontinued. Treatment with the use of a bland skin ointment and massage should be attempted first. In longstanding cases, scarring may have set in, and management is similar to cicatricial ectropion.

Mechanical ectropion is caused by heavy eyelid tumors or the displacement of eyelid tissue secondary to unrepaired displaced orbital fractures. Removal of the underlying cause is usually sufficient treatment. Often, mechanical ectropion is due to fluid accumulation in the eyelid, and the patient should be evaluated for sinus, thyroid, renal and other medical problems.

Therapy

Ocular. Topical ophthalmic lubricating agents should be used to protect the globe from exposure. Applications of 0.5 to 1.0 per cent methylcellulose may be given at periodic intervals. If the patient has a poor Bell's phenomenon and lid malposition, even continuous application of artificial lubricants may be inadequate. Taping the lids closed or wearing a protective moist chamber plastic bubble may provide some temporary relief, but may excoriate the skin with long-term use. Bandage soft lenses are subject to desiccation just as is the corneal epithelium and may be ineffective. Pressure patches can be used for the temporary treatment of corneal epithelial defects.

The outward turning of an eyelid produces a keratinization of the lid margin, which predisposes the lid to crusting and the development of blepharitis. Eyelid hygiene and the short-term use of topical antibiotics are useful in the control of ocular infections. In most cases, the definitive treatment of ectropion is surgical.

Surgical. Preoperative diagnosis of the underlying ectropion pathology dictates which route of surgical correction is to be undertaken. A single or combination of procedures may be applied to correcting more than one type of ectropion. The history and complete ophthalmologic examination will reveal under which classification the ectropion falls.

Involutional (senile) lower lid ectropion may be corrected, as with all types of ectropion, in many different ways. Treatment with thermal cautery may be used in mild involutional ectropion. It is basically a destructive procedure and is rarely used. However, it is useful on nonsurgical candidates as it may be performed on an outpatient basis. A series of diathermy punctures are made through the conjunctiva and underlying tissue below the border of the tarsus. The skin is not penetrated. This procedure may be repeated if the initial cauterization is not successful. Another procedure useful with nonsurgical candidates is the use of sutures. The two-suture technique of Snellen involves passing two double-armed sutures, either 4-0 silk or chromic gut, in mattress fashion, first through the inferior border of tarsus and then emerging cutaneously at the level of the orbital rim and tied over with pledgets. Sutures are passed at the junction of the intermediate and medial one-third of the eyelid and at the lateral one-third of the eyelid. Silk sutures are removed after 7 to 10 days, and gut sutures may be left in or removed. Recurrence is the main complication with the above procedures. When it happens, another, more definitive type of ectropion operation should be performed, as described below.

Pentagonal resection of lower eyelid tissue is one of the most permanent methods of correcting involutional ectropion when caused solely by a horizontal lid laxity. The resection is taken in the area of greatest involvement, usually at the junction of the intermediate and lateral one-third of the lower eyelid. The standard horizontal shortening is performed by incising the eyelid through-and-through with a razor blade knife, overlapping the two free edges of the eyelid margin, and again incising the eyelid and resecting the portion easily overlapped. A wedge of eyelid in the shape of an upside-down pentagon is removed, and the eyelid is reconstructed by first aligning the lid margin. This alignment is done with three 6-0 silk sutures, each passed in a symmetric fashion on either side of the vertical eyelid incision. The first of these sutures is passed through the eyelash line, the second through the meibomian gland orifices, and the third through the gray line. These three sutures are left long, placed anteriorly away from the globe, and sutured down to the skin so as not to strike the cornea. The skin is closed in a routine manner, after one or two absorbable sutures are used to close the tarsus.

The Byron Smith modification of the Kuhnt-Szymanowski procedure is useful if there is a marked redundancy of lower lid skin. In this procedure, first a subciliary incision is performed, elevating a skin flap to the inferior orbital rim. An inverted pentagonal resection of the lateral third and medial two-thirds of the lower lid is then excised and reapproximated, as described above. The skin is then draped back into position, and any excess skin is excised. The skin is closed with 6-0 silk, as in a blepharoplasty.

When the eyelid is lengthened horizontally and the lower punctum is everted, correction is best applied with the Byron Smith "Lazy T" procedure. Four millimeters lateral to the lower punctum, a pentagonal lid resection is performed. Five millimeters inferior to the canaliculus, a horizontal incision through conjunctiva and submucosa is made, contiguous with the lid resection, which is closed with 6-0 plain sutures. Thus, both horizontal laxity and punctal eversion are corrected.

If laxity of the medial canthal tendon is present, tightening of the tendon may be performed. The medial canthal tendon is approached with a curvilinear vertical incision in the medial canthal region; the tendon is dissected and identified. Nonabsorbable synthetic sutures are used in a mattress fashion to plicate the medial canthal tendon or to detach it from its insertion and reattach it in a firmer position to the periosteum over the anterior lacrimal crest.

Lateral tarsal strip suspension may be used for moderate generalized or lateral involutional ectropion. A lateral canthotomy is performed, and the inferior portion of the lateral canthal tendon is severed. From the ends of the canthotomy incision, a skin incision is carried medially for several millimeters parallel to and inferior to the lash line. The skin is undermined. The lateral border of the severed eyelid is grasped, and the eyelid is positioned in apposition to the lateral orbital rim. If there is overlapping segment of tarsus, then it is excised where it is in contact with the lateral orbital rim. The freshened tarsal edge is sutured just superior to the lateral orbital tubercle and within the lateral orbital rim on to the periosteum. Tarsus is sutured to periosteum with Prolene, Supramid, Mersilene, or PDS.

Paralytic ectropion occurs with facial nerve paralysis and most often is unilateral. Treatment depends on the duration of involvement. If the paralysis is temporary, as may occur with Bell's palsy, then treatment may only be medical. Treatment consists of topical lubricating drops, ointments, and moist chambers. If necessary, eyelids may be taped at bedtime to prevent corneal exposure. If resolution of the facial palsy is incomplete after a 3- to 6-month period, the paralysis of the lower lid usually results in stretching of the canthal tendons and a horizontal lower lid laxity results. The surgical approach is similar in fashion to that previously mentioned. The medial canthal tendon may be plicated or the lower eyelid horizontally shortened. The most common protective surgical procedure for permanent facial paralysis is a medial and lateral tarsorrhaphy that involves permanently anastomosing the upper and lower eyelid margins at the medial and the lateral aspects of the eyelids. Insertion of spacer grafts between the lower tarsus and lower lid retractors aids in lower lid support. Spacer grafts include ear cartilage, sclera, fascia lata, and hard palate mucosal grafts. Fascia lata (autogenous or banked) sling may also be used in the correction of paralytic ectropion. The sling is sutured to the medial canthal tendon and adjacent periosteum and slung across the lower eyelid margin between the orbicularis muscle and the tarsus; it is then attached to the lateral canthal tendon and periosteum of the lateral orbital rim. Nonabsorbable 4-0 nylon or prolene sutures are used to anchor the fascia lata sling to adjacent sutures. Temporalis muscle transfer can be combined with other reconstructive facial surgery to produce better cosmesis and function on the involved side. The temporalis muscle is innervated by the motor division of the fifth cranial nerve and thus is not affected in seventh nerve paralysis. This operation gives dynamic function to both the upper and lower lids. Blink occurs each time the temporalis muscle is activated. Eyelid springs to reanimate the lid and correct ectropion are another method of repair; however, it is fraught with complications.

Cicatricial ectropion is corrected with a lengthening of the anterior lamella of the eyelid. V to Y plasties are important tools to be used in the lengthening of scarred eyelids. Excision of the cicatricial scar and moving a flap or filling the defect with a free graft are the most common methods of lengthening a vertically contracted eyelid. V to Y plasties are constructed by making a V-shaped incision and undermining the center skin flap, letting it retract, and resuturing the wound in the shape of a "Y." Z plasties are performed by making a Z-shaped incision, undermining the flaps, and transposing them to relieve tension in the direction desired. Transposition flaps may also be used and are most useful when the cicatricial ectropion involves the lateral one-third or one-half of the lower lid. In this procedure a donor flap from the upper eyelid is transposed laterally to the lower eyelid by a hinge.

When congenital ectropion is due to a vertical deficiency of skin and underlying tissue, the horizontal eyelid length usually is adequate, as are the tarsal and conjunctival tissues. Treatment for this type is with a transposition skin flap from an uninvolved to an involved eyelid or the use of a free full-thickness skin graft. A congenital ectropion, due to excessive horizontal eyelid length, should be managed by a wedge resection of the involved portion of the eyelid, as described under involutional ectropion.

Ocular or Periocular Manifestations

Conjunctiva: Chronic conjunctivitis; keratinization, thickening.
Cornea: Exposure keratitis; toxic keratitis.
Eyelids: Keratinization of the eyelid margins.
Lacrimal System: Increased tear osmolarity.

PRECAUTIONS

In the repair of any cicatricial ectropion, the basic principles of surgery should be followed. All progressive scarring should be ceased before surgery is performed. When surgery is performed, the removal of all scar tissue is crucial for its success.

In the treatment of facial palsy, temporary and permanent tarsorrhaphies are basic and

adequate treatment to allow corneal coverage in expectation of the resolution of the seventh nerve palsy.

COMMENTS

Many procedures have been described for the treatment of the classifications of ectropion. Before appropriate treatment can be instituted, the surgeon must diagnose accurately the cause and type of ectropion. Taping the lids in the corrected position before surgery is useful as a prognostic indicator of the surgical result. Simulating a tightened canthal tendon or the addition of skin will also help indicate the final result.

References

Beard C: Ptosis, 3rd ed. St. Louis, CV Mosby, 1981.
Bosniak S: Ectropion. *In* Smith B (ed): Ophthalmic Plastic and Reconstructive Surgery. St. Louis, CV Mosby, 1987.
Lisman, RD, Rees, T: Correction of ectropion—Round table discussion. Perspectives in Plastic Surgery. New York, Quality Medical Publishing, 1988.
Lisman RD, Rees T, Baker D, Smith B: Tarsal suspension as a factor in lower lid blepharoplasty. Plast Reconstr Surg 79:6, 1987.
Miller GR, Tenzel RR, Buffam, FV: Lid taping in the preoperative management of tearing or asthenopia. Arch Ophthalmol 94:1289–1290, 1976.
Smith B: The "Lazy-T" correction of ectropion of the lower punctum. Arch Ophthalmol 94:1149–1150, 1976.
Smith B, Cherubini TD: Oculoplastic Surgery: A Compendium of Principles and Techniques. St. Louis, CV Mosby, 1970.
Soll DB: Entropion and ectropion. *In* Soll DB (ed): Management of Complications in Ophthalmic Plastic Surgery. Birmingham, Aesculapius, 1976, pp 132–206.

ENTROPION 374.00
ROGER A. DAILEY, M.D.
Portland, Oregon

Entropion of the eyelids is defined as an inversion of the eyelid margin so that the margin itself, the cilia, and sometimes the external keratinizing squamous epithelium of the lid are brought into contact with the surface of the cornea, producing corneal irritation and abrasion. Entropion can occur in the upper lid and/or lower lid. It can be classified as congenital, cicatricial, spastic, or involutional. The choice of appropriate management is greatly dependent on establishing the correct diagnosis initially. Several other eyelid abnormalities can simulate entropion, such as epiblepharon, epicanthal folds, trichiasis, or distichiasis. A careful history and examination should allow the clinician to make the correct diagnosis.

Congenital entropion is a rare disorder, with a higher incidence in female infants. The diagnosis is based on an actual inturning of the eyelid margin. It can be confused with epiblepharon, which is an anomalous fold of the pretarsal skin that forces the eyelashes to orient inward toward the globe. Individuals who suffer from cicatricial entropion of either lid typically have a history of ocular inflammation, such as that occurring with trachoma, Stevens-Johnson syndrome, or ocular pemphigoid. Chemical or heat burns can cause a cicatricial entropion and shortening of the posterior lamella. Spastic entropion is typically found in individuals who have recently had intraocular surgery or an external ocular inflammation. Involutional or senile entropion is probably the most common type seen in the average clinician's office. It is rare to see this condition in the upper lid; in the lower lid, it occurs as a result of three factors: (1) the lower lid retractors lose control of the inferior margin of the tarsus, allowing it to rotate anteriorly and superiorly; (2) the preseptal muscle tends to override the pretarsal muscle; and (3) weakness of the inferior tarsal muscle of the capsulopalpebral head allows the anatomic rotation of the lid margin. Enophthalmos in the older age population also contributes to this problem. In years past, there has been some speculation as to the role of the muscle of Riolan in producing involutional entropion; however, Jones was careful to point out that the muscle of Riolan inserts medially and laterally into the superficial head of the pretarsal muscle, not the deep head. Therefore, it is mechanically impossible for the muscle of the Riolan to inwardly rotate the lid margin.

THERAPY

Ocular. It is important to remember that the entropion, whatever the cause, can affect the cornea, and significant problems may result. Temporary measures to deal with the entropion should be used until a more definitive procedure can be done. Artificial tears and petrolatum ointments can be used to protect the cornea. If there is evidence of external ocular infection, an appropriate antibiotic should be used to prevent infectious keratitis. Taping the lid margin to maintain an appropriate position relative to the cornea can also be helpful.

Surgical. The definitive treatment of this disorder is surgery. The surgical technique employed is dependent on the etiology of the entropion, which lid is involved, and, in some cases, the general healthy and disposition of the patient.

Congenital entropion is associated with spasm and hypertrophy of the pretarsal orbicularis muscle fibers and a relative deficiency of the tarsal plate. These anatomical findings are usually most prominent medially in the lower lid. However, the concept of orbicularis hypertrophy has been disputed, and a retractor disinsertion from the tarsus has been proposed as a cause of congenital entropion. Repair involves a small subciliary incision with dissection of an anterior skin flap to separate skin from the underlying orbicularis muscle. A small amount of preseptal muscle is then dissected out of this area, and the inferior retractors of the lower lid are identified. The inferior retractor attachment to the inferior border of the lower tarsus is reinforced with one to three interrupted 6-0 vicryl sutures, and the skin is closed with interrupted sutures of the surgeon's choice.

Spastic lower lid entropion tends to be a transient condition requiring treatment of the underlying condition that initially produced it, such as external ocular inflammation. In addition, the entropion produced must be relieved temporarily. The placement of Quickert sutures provides quick, safe, temporary relief of entropion. This can be done on an outpatient basis or at the patient's bedside with local infiltrative anesthetic. One needle of a double-armed suture of 5-0 chromic catgut or 5-0 Vicryl suture is placed deep in the conjunctival fornix and brought anteriorly and superiorly through the lid tissues so that it exits the skin near the lid margin, beneath the lash line. The second needle is then passed in a similar fashion 3 to 4 mm laterally. Two additional double-armed sutures are placed, one medially and one laterally, in a similar fashion. The sutures are tied, causing an eversion of the lid margin, and typically a small amount of overcorrection is desired. Good lid approximation to the globe is usually obtained within 1 to 2 weeks. If overcorrection persists, the sutures can be cut.

In discussing involution entropion, Lester Jones quoted an old medical axiom: "To cure disease surgically, you should not try to make the anatomy conform to your technique; you should make your technique conform to the anatomy." Many procedures have been described to treat senile entropion; however, the majority of them ignore the anatomic defects mentioned above that led to the development of the entropion. Ziegler cautery, the Fox and Bick procedures, and numerous other procedures involving surgical maneuvering of the protractor muscles are now mainly of historic interest. The preferred treatment of involutional entropion is a procedure described by Jones and Wobig (1976) involving debulking of the preseptal muscle and anatomic reattachment of the lower lid retractors to the inferior tarsal border.

This procedure can be performed using topical proparacaine anesthesia and local infiltrative anesthesia consisting of 2 per cent lidocaine with epinephrine 1: 100,000 with hyaluronidase. A subciliary incision is made from the puncta to the lateral canthus area. If a lower lid blepharoplasty is to be combined with this correction, this incision can be carried laterally in a "crow's foot." If horizontal laxity of the lower lid is present and a horizontal shortening procedure is indicated, the subciliary incision can be combined with a lateral cantholysis and tarsal tongue procedure, as described by Anderson (1982). This procedure should be done before the retractor repair. With the incisions completed, an anterior skin-muscle flap is developed that extends inferiorly approximately to the level of the infraorbital rim. A small to moderate amount of preseptal muscle is then resected. The septum is then incised its entire length horizontally. This procedure allows the surgeon to identify the lower lid fat pads, which are analogous to preaponeurotic fat in the upper lid. Superior to the fat pads, the surgeon will be able to identify the white glistening fibers of the inferior retractors of the lower lid, and typically there will be disinsertion from the inferior border of the lower lid tarsus or a dehiscence of the retractors. Any excess fat to be removed can be done at this point, using a cross-clamping technique with a hemostat followed by cautery of any hemorrhage sites. The inferior retractors are anatomically approximated to the inferior border of the tarsus with three interrupted 5-0 Vicryl sutures. The patient is asked to look superiorly and open the mouth widely, and the skin is unfolded and reapproximated to the superior margins of the wound. If an excess amount of skin is present, it can be removed with sharp dissection at this time. After the patient has been asked to relax, the skin edges are reapproximated with multiple interrupted 6-0 silk or plain fast-absorbing gut sutures. The key to this procedure is to restore the downward and backward motion provided by the inferior lid retractors.

Cicatricial entropion provides the surgeon with a difficult challenge. This disorder, if not corrected or treated appropriately, can result in significant impairment of vision. The entropion secondary to trachoma is one of the leading causes of blindness in the world today. The procedure selected by the surgeon depends on whether the upper or lower lid is affected and the severity of the disease.

Procedures designed to correct upper lid entropion must correct the posterior lamellar contraction and allow the eyelashes to rotate outward, away from the eye. For mild to moderate amounts of cicatricial upper lid entropion, a lid splitting procedure works well. After local infiltrative anesthesia, the gray line is identified and the lid incision is made at this point from lateral canthus to punctum to create an anterior and posterior lamella. The posterior lamella consists of conjunctiva and tarsus, and the anterior lamella consists of skin, orbicularis muscle, lashes, and tarsus. Hemostasis can be obtained with a hand-held thermal cautery unity or electrocautery. If

there is any significant distichiasis or trichiasis at the time, these areas can be treated with freeze-thaw-freeze-thaw cryoepilation. Monitoring tissue temperature with a thermocouple to −20°C is advised by some surgeons. Then the lid edges are reapproximated; however, the anterior lamella is recessed superiorly relative to the posterior lamella and sutured in place with several interrupted 5-0 or 6-0 vicryl rotational sutures. In moderate to severe cases, Baylis and Silkiss (1987) have suggested severing the attachments of Müller's muscle and conjunctiva from the superior border of the tarsus, in addition to the lid splitting and anterior lamella recession. This posterior defect is left open to re-epithelialize without contraction. One to two millimeters blepharoptosis may be present postoperatively.

A buccal mucosa graft can be laid between the edge of the posterior lamella and the anterior lamella and held in place with 6-0 vicryl or 6-0 plain fast-absorbing gut sutures. The mucosal graft is easily obtained from the buccal surface of the lower lip or cheek. After local infiltration, it is harvested freehand and then thinned as much as possible of its underlying subcutaneous tissue. The harvest graft bed is allowed to heal without any specific dressing or treatment. If the harvest is from the cheek area, one must be careful to avoid the opening of Stensen's duct from the parotid gland. It is usually opposite the second upper molar on either side.

In severe cases of upper lid entropion, it is often advisable to use a so-called spacer. This can be done using a composite graft of nasal septal cartilage with its overlying mucosa. It can be harvested either by an eye surgeon familiar with nasal anatomy or by an otorhinolarygologist. For cicatricial entropion, it is suggested that the cartilage not be thinned as it sometimes is for upper eyelid reconstruction. Thinning is thought to make the cartilage graft more vulnerable to warp during the healing process and to increase the chances of postoperative entropion. This procedure is started the same way as the upper lid splitting, although the incision should be somewhat posterior to the gray line at the mucocutaneous junction, rather than at the gray line. Once the anterior and posterior lamella have been separated adequately, any markedly diseased, warped tarsus is resected, and the nasal composite graft is contoured to fit in the remaining space between the patient's tarsus and the margin. It is then held in place with either 6-0 Vicryl sutures or a running 6-0 Prolene. The Prolene is removed about 10 days later. The mucosal surface is then approximated to the lid margin on the conjunctival surfaces so that there is a moist surface in contact with the cornea. The posterior lamella spacer then forces the eyelashes forward, away from the eye. For patients with Stevens-Johnson syndrome and ocular pemphigoid that have chronic epidermalization of the conjunctiva, McCord and Chen (1983) have described a technique that combines tarsal polishing to remove epidermalized conjunctiva with a smooth 3 mm dermabrading tip and a subsequent full-thickness buccal mucous membrane graft into the lid splitting and spacer procedures.

Lower lid entropion can be repaired using basically the same procedures as described for the upper lid entropion; in addition to using a nasal composite graft, auricular cartilage can be used in the lower lid to act as a spacer. Eye bank sclera has been used, but unfortunately, it is relatively unsatisfactory as it is not stiff enough to resist the postoperative healing forces that cause the entropion to recur. In cases of mild to moderate lower lid entropion, the Weiss procedure has been used. It involves a two-step transverse blepharotomy incision made through the skin, muscle (first step), and tarsus and conjunctiva (second step) 3 mm below the lid margin. Three or four double-armed mattress sutures of 5-0 silk are passed from the conjunctival fornix side of the incision into the wound, exiting the anterior surface of the proximal tarsus, and then into the superior portion of the wound and brought out through the skin near the eyelashes and tied to obtain the desired amount of overcorrection. This forces the eyelashes to rotate outward. This will usually resolve within 1 or 2 weeks. If the overcorrection is persistent and exposure keratitis is a problem, the sutures can be removed; removal typically results in some reduction of the overcorrection. This procedure can be performed for upper lid entropion, but the double-armed sutures must enter the cut edge of the tarsus, not the conjunctiva, to avoid abrading the cornea.

In cases where the entropion is clearly a vertical shortening of the posterior lamella, the hard palate mucosal graft is gaining popularity. This graft provides both structural support and mucosal surface.

Ocular or Periocular Manifestations

Conjunctiva: Chronic conjunctivitis; chemosis.
Cornea: Mechanical keratitis; corneal ulcer.
Eyelids: Swelling; erythema; trichiasis.
Lacrimal System: Epiphora.

PRECAUTIONS

The key to treatment of this disorder is accurate diagnosis and the subsequent choice of an appropriate surgical technique. In addition, the surgeon must have a thorough knowledge of the upper and lower eyelid anatomy and must try to make the surgical technique conform to that anatomy. A small amount of overcorrection postoperatively is usually desired to ensure that the entropion does not recur. If the overcorrection persists, it may require release of sutures or possibly a

second procedure. It is important to operate on patients who are not on any platelet inhibitors (e.g., aspirin or nonsteroidal anti-inflammatory agents) or anticoagulants, e.g., warfarin, or heparin. There is a small risk to the patient's vision with these procedures, especially in the lower lid, should they have a significant retrobulbar hemorrhage postoperatively. They should be cautioned about this complication and instructed to call the surgeon immediately if they develop significant periorbital swelling associated with pain. If swelling and pain do develop, the incision should be opened immediately, the hematoma evacuated, and the bleeding site identified and cauterized. The wound can then be reapproximated. One should be careful not to remove too much fat since enophthalmos is often one of the contributing factors in many cases of this disease, particularly involutional entropion.

COMMENTS

The conservative treatment of taping the lower lid into position typically does not work, as the skin gets moist from epiphora and the tape slips. However, it can be used as a prognostic indicator in patients who are skeptical about having surgery. The above procedures are typically performed in the operating room using local infiltrative anesthesia and topical proparacaine; however, some procedures, such as the Quickert-Rathbun sutures, can still be done easily in the office or at the bedside. Secondary ocular problems typically resolve quickly with the anatomic correction of the eyelid abnormalities; however, careful monitoring of the cornea throughout the postoperative period is a priority.

References

Anderson RL: The tarsal strip. *In* Transactions of the New Orleans Academy of Ophthalmology. St. Louis, CV Mosby, 1982, pp 352–363.

Bartley GB: Posterior lamella eyelid reconstruction with a hard palate mucosal graft. Am J Ophthalmol 107:609–612, 1989.

Baylis HI, Silkiss RZ: A structurally oriented approach to the repair of cicatrical entropion. Ophthalmic Plast Reconstr Surg 3:17–20, 1987.

Callahan A: Correction of entropion from Stevens-Johnson syndrome. Use of nasal septum and mucosa for severely cicatrized eyelid entropion. Arch Ophthalmol 94:1154–1155, 1976.

Jones LT, Wobig JL: Surgery of the Eyelids and Lacrimal System. Birmingham, Aesculapius, 1976, pp 123–131.

Jones LT, Reeh MJ, Wobig JL: Senile entropion. A new concept for correction. Am J Ophthalmol 74: 321–329, 1972.

McCord CD, Chen WP: Tarsal polishing and mucous membrane grafting for cicatricial entropion, trichiasis, and epidermalization. Ophthalmic Surg 14:1021–1025, 1983.

Quickert MH, Wilkes DI, Dryden RM: Non-incisional correction of epiblepharon and congenital entropion. Arch Ophthalmol *101*:778–781, 1981.

Tse DT, Anderson RL, Fratkin JD: Aponeurosis disinsertion in congenital entropion. Arch Ophthalmol *101*:436–440, 1983.

Weiss FA: Surgical treatment of entropion. J Int Coll Surg *21*:758–760, 1954.

EPICANTHUS 743.63

ROGER A. DAILEY, M.D.

Portland, Oregon

The term "epicanthus" refers to a relatively vertical fold of skin that is located between the medial canthus and the nose and may cover part or all of the inner canthus of the eye. Four separate types have been described. *Epicanthus supraciliaris* is a vertical fold of skin that extends from just below the brow to an area just over the infraorbital rim, usually obscuring the caruncle. In *epicanthus palpebralis*, the skin fold extends from the medial aspect of the upper lid to the medial aspect of the lower lid in a rather symmetric fashion and often obscures the caruncle. This is the most common configuration. *Epicanthus tarsalis* refers to a fold that begins laterally and extends over the entire lid, ending in the medial canthus. This is the typical Oriental upper lid configuration. Epiblepharon of the upper lids is distinguished from epicanthus tarsalis by its lack of a true superior palpebral fold and the presence of a fold of skin that overlaps the eyelid margin and presses the lashes against the cornea. Finally, *epicanthus inversus* is similar to epicanthus tarsalis, but involves the lower lid. It usually occurs as a part of Komoto's tetrad of blepharoptosis, blepharophimosis, telecanthus, and epicanthus inversus. Blepharophimosis refers to narrowing of the palpebral aperture in its horizontal dimension. Rarely, the tetrad can occur as a developmental anomaly, but more commonly it is transmitted as an autosomal dominant trait with 100 per cent penetrance. The blepharoptosis is usually associated with poor function.

THERAPY

Surgical. In patients with these disorders, it is important to avoid early operation if possible. Many forms of epicanthus that are present when a child is young will become less apparent as the child matures and growth of the dorsum of the nose occurs. The exception is epicanthus inversus, which typically shows little improvement with age. In these children, the skin tends to be very stiff early on and difficult to work with surgically, but becomes more amenable to intervention at a later age. No spinal abnormalities have ever been reported from patients who have had blepharoptosis for many years, and amblyopia is rare in these patients and is usually associated with other problems, such as anisometropia and astigmatism. Consideration should be given to doing surgery before the child enters school because of potential associated psychological problems with this perceived facial anomaly. Larger children tend to yield better surgical results.

Numerous surgical methods to correct epicanthus have been described. Most surgeons would agree that it is best to correct the epicanthus first, along with any associated telecanthus or blepharophimosis, and then at a later time correct the blepharoptosis either with a sling if the levator function is 4 mm or less or with a levator resection if the function is greater. Supramid suture slings can be performed on patients as a temporary measure if the surgery is done before 3 years of age, or banked fascia lata can be used as well. After the age of 3, the patient's own fascia lata can be harvested from the leg.

Several different techniques have been described to correct epicanthus: Spaeth's epicanthus operation, Verwey Y-to-V operation, double Z plasty, Mustarde's technique, the Y-to-W procedure, Roveda's technique, and, more recently, the five-flap procedure. Spaeth's technique, which involves excision of a portion of the fold of skin, is generally reserved for only mild cases of epicanthus inversus. The Verwey Y-to-V operation is more commonly used for epicanthus repair, especially epicanthus palpebralis.

Double opposing Z plasties work well for epicanthus supraciliaris or epicanthus tarsalis. This procedure is very similar to the Mustarde procedure. It is much easier to transpose the skin flaps of this double Z if all of the incisions are made medially to the epicanthal fold and the incisions are not extended onto the lids themselves. The Mustarde technique combines a Y-to-V with double opposing Z plasty. Some surgeons feel that the measurements to set this procedure up are unduly complex, and the flaps tend to be irregular and can be difficult to transpose. The basic Y-to-W and Roveda's technique are essentially the same procedure. Roveda's technique, again, involves larger irregularly shaped flaps that can be difficult to transpose.

Anderson and Nowinski (1989) recently described a procedure that they termed the five-flap technique, which is a modified Y-to-V procedure combined with a double Z plasty. It has the advantage of being simple to mark out on the lid, and the flaps are small and relatively easy to transpose.

No matter which of the above procedures are chosen for a patient with epicanthus, some features remain generally consistent throughout. Typically, the patients who are operated on are from 3 to 5 years of age. Since epicanthus invariably occurs bilaterally, both sides can be done at the same time. A general anesthetic is used, mainly because of the child's age. A local anesthetic with epinephrine helps control hemostasis. Once the flaps are raised, any excess orbicularsis muscle can be resected, and the medial canthal tendon is easily visualized. Since there is usually associated telecanthus, it can be repaired with a medial canthal tendon resection or, in severe cases, transnasal wiring. It is important to avoid injuring the canaliculus or lacrimal sac. Closure is performed with a suture of the surgeon's choice. Blepharophimosis can also be repaired at this time via a lateral canthoplasty.

Ocular or Periocular Manifestations

Conjunctiva: Hypoplasia of the caruncle and semilunar folds.
Eyelids: Blepharophimosis; blepharoptosis; telecanthus.
Lacrimal System: Punctal stenosis; lateral displacement of puncta.
Other: "Lop" ears; amblyopia; strabismus and double elevator palsy.

PRECAUTIONS

As always, accurate diagnosis is the key to a satisfactory result. Epiblepharon is essentially an exaggeration of epicanthus tarsalis. Although epicanthus is typically bilateral, epiblepharon can be unilateral. It can occur in either the upper or lower lid and usually regresses spontaneously without any surgery. Epicanthus is a cause of pseudostrabismus; therefore, it is important in these patients to check not only visual acuity but also to use a prism alternating cover test to rule out true strabismus.

Scarring in these patients can be quite exuberant in the initial postoperative weeks. It is important to reassure the parent that it will diminish with time. Topical steroid ointments can be measured into the area and are felt to be of some benefit. There is no evidence that vitamin E ointment is helpful beyond the benefit gained from massaging alone. Radiation to the scarred area should not be used.

COMMENTS

Epicanthus supraciliaris, palpebralis, and tarsalis tend to regress spontaneously with age and only occasionally require surgical correction. In some patients in whom the epicanthus is minimal and a ptosis repair is performed, the epicanthus is exaggerated. In this instance, a Y-to-V or simple single Z plasty often takes care of the epicanthus. Amblyopia is occasionally found in these patients with epicanthus and blepharoptosis. It is important to check the visual acuity and also to rule out significant refraction errors.

References

Anderson RL, Nowinski TS: The five-flap technique for blepharophimosis. Arch Ophthalmol 107:448–452, 1989.

Beard C: Ptosis. St. Louis, CV Mosby, 1976, pp 218–235.

Callahan A: Surgical correction of the blepharophimosis syndromes. Trans Am Acad Ophthalmol Otolaryngol 77:687–695, 1973.

Callahan MA, Callahan A: Ophthalmic Plastic and Orbital Surgery. Birmingham, Aesculapius, 1979, pp 36–41.

Crawford JS, Apt RK: Congenital anomalies. In Silver B (ed) Ophthalmic Plastic Surgery. Rochester, American Academy of Ophthalmology and Otolaryngology, 1977, pp 74–79.

Hughes WL: Surgical treatment of congenital palpebral phimosis. The Y-V operation. Arch Ophthalmol 54:586–590, 1955.

Johnson CC: Epicanthus. Am J Ophthalmol 66:939–946, 1968.

Johnson CC: Epicanthus and epiblepharon. Arch Ophthalmol 96:1030–1033, 1978.

Kohn R, Romano PE: Blepharoptosis, blepharophimosis, epicanthus inversus and telecanthus—A syndrome with no name. Am J Ophthalmol 72:625–632, 1971.

EYELID COLOBOMA 743.62

JOHN D. BULLOCK, M.D., M.S., F.A.C.S.,
Dayton, Ohio
and STUART H. GOLDBERG, M.D.
Hershey, Pennsylvania

A coloboma is a full-thickness defect of the eyelid. Colobomas may occur congenitally or as a result of accidental or surgical trauma (secondary to excision of eyelid tumors). Congenital colobomas are most commonly unilateral, lid-margin-based, triangular defects involving the medial third of the upper lid. However, a congenital eyelid coloboma may be bilateral, rectangular, or triangular; may be found on any aspect of the lid margin; and may occur on the lower or upper lid. Lower lid lesions usually are seen laterally. A benign dermoid tumor at the limbus or apex of the coloboma is encountered frequently. A congenital eyelid coloboma may be accompanied by a variety of other facial anomalies.

THERAPY

Ocular. Corneal protection is the primary therapeutic goal. Patients with small lid defects may be treated adequately with artificial tears and ophthalmic ointments. Commercially available optical bandages that provide an airtight moist chamber have been advocated. Patching at bedtime may be required in cases where significant corneal exposure occurs during sleep.

Surgical. Corneal protection and cosmesis are indications for surgical correction. Large congenital colobomas may necessitate immediate surgical intervention to prevent corneal compromise. Small defects that are well managed with topical lubricants may have surgical correction delayed until later in childhood.

Small colobomas can be corrected by direct closure. The edges of the colobomatous defect are freshened with sharp incisions, and precise anastomosis of the lid margin is performed. A meticulous two-layer approximation of the incised tarsal and skin margins achieves wound closure. Lateral cantholysis and placement of a near-far, far-near suture may be necessary to minimize horizontal tension along the wound margins.

A two-stage reconstruction may be required for lid defects exceeding 40 to 50 per cent. For large, lower lid colobomas, an upper lid tarsoconjunctival advancement flap with retroauricular skin graft to reconstitute the anterior lamella of the reconstructed lower lid (modified Hughes' procedure) has been recommended. Large upper lid colobomata can be reconstructed by advancement of full-thickness lower lid beneath a bridge of lower eyelid margin, with subsequent release of the flap in 8 to 12 weeks (Cutler-Beard procedure).

Alternative techniques of repairing large colobomas include use of a semicircular flap from the lateral canthal area and full-thickness lid rotational flaps.

Ocular or Periocular Manifestations

Choroid: Coloboma.
Conjunctiva: Symblepharon.
Cornea: Cicatrization; exposure keratopathy; opacities.
Eyelids: Trichiasis.
Lacrimal System: Obstruction.
Lens: Anterior polar cataract; subluxation.
Sclera: Epibulbar dermoid tumor.

PRECAUTIONS

Eyelid-sharing procedures should be used with caution in infants and young children due to the potential for occlusion amblyopia. The excision of associated limbal dermoid tumors must be undertaken with particular care. Pseudopterygium or symblepharon formation can result from attempts at simple excision. The use of lamellar grafts has been advocated.

COMMENTS

Lacrimal system obstruction is common in the setting of both upper and lower eyelid coloboma.

A complete ophthalmologic examination to rule out possible coexisting ocular anomalies should be performed at the time of surgery. Lower eyelid colobomas are characteristic of mandibulofacial dysostosis (Treacher Collins or Franceschetti syndrome); upper eyelid colobomas are commonly seen in oculoauricular dysplasia (Goldenhar's syndrome). Eyelid colobomas associated with corneal opacities and facial clefts are present in many patients with amniotic band syndrome.

References

Casey TA: Congenital colobomata of the eyelids. Trans Ophthalmol Soc UK 96:65–68, 1976.
Crawford JS: Congenital eyelid anomalies in children. J Pediatr Ophthalmol Strabismus 21:140–149, 1984.
Duke-Elder S: Normal and abnormal development. Congenital deformities. *In* Duke-Elder S (ed): System of Ophthalmology. St. Louis, CV Mosby, 1964, Vol 3, part 2, pp 836–840.
Guibor P: Surgical repair of congenital colobomas. Trans Am Acad Ophthalmol Otolaryngol 76:671–678, 1975.
Harley RD: Disorders of the lids. Pediatr Clin North Am 30:1145–1158, 1983.
Kidwell EDR, Tenzel RR: Repair of congenital colobomas of the lids. Arch Ophthalmol 97:1931–1932, 1979.
Miller MT, Deutsch TA, Cronin C, Key CL: Amniotic bands as a cause of ocular anomalies. Am J Ophthalmol 104:270–279, 1987.
Patipa M, Wilkins RB, Guelzow KW: Surgical management of congenital eyelid coloboma. Ophthalmol Surg 13:212–216, 1982.
Poswillo D: Pathogenesis of craniofacial syndromes exhibiting colobomata. Trans Ophthalmol Soc UK 96:69–72, 1976.

FLOPPY EYELID SYNDROME 374.9

LEE K. SCHWARTZ, M.D.,
and GARY L. AGUILAR, M.D.

San Francisco, California

The floppy eyelid syndrome is an uncommon and frequently unrecognized cause of chronic unilateral or bilateral papillary conjunctivitis. It is frequently associated with punctate epithelial keratitis. The syndrome is characterized by a triad of diffuse papillary conjunctivitis, a loose upper lid that readily everts by pulling it upward (positive lid eversion sign), and a soft rubbery tarsus that can be folded on itself. The lower lids may also be involved. Both sexes are affected, but males predominate. A frequent association with obesity has been observed. Reported cases range in age from between 12 and 65 years. The cause of tarsal laxity is unknown.

There is no definite association with systemic diseases of collagen or elastic tissue. Various associations have been reported with hyperglycinemia, keratoconus, keratotorus, psoriasis, blepharitis, and tear dysfunction. In addition, there have been associations with pachydermoperiostosis and obstructive sleep apnea.

The consequences of the floppy eyelid syndrome may be serious. *Staphylococcus aureus* corneal ulcer has been noted in association with the syndrome. Thus, routine cultures of the conjunctiva should be obtained. Bacterial conjunctivitis should be treated accordingly. In addition, bilateral corneal neovascularization has been reported as a rare but severe complication of the syndrome. Corneal scarring necessitates a penetrating keratoplasty for visual rehabilitation.

A study of 58 patients with chronic conjunctivitis of longer than 2 weeks' duration revealed that floppy eyelid syndrome was the cause of chronic conjunctivitis in 2 per cent of patients. In 31 per cent of patients, no specific cause was detected.

The mechanism of the chronic conjunctivitis is thought to be eyelid eversion during sleep with corneal-conjunctival-pillow contact. Not all cases, however, report nocturnal eyelid eversion. An alternative explanation is that there is a poor interface between the loose upper eyelid and the underlying bulbar conjunctiva. Both mechanisms, however, may be present to produce the symptoms, which probably explains why conservative treatment with eye shields and patching may not work. In addition, surgical eyelid tightening is usually curative.

Histopathologic investigations, including light and electron microscopy, have revealed chronic conjunctival inflammation with fibrosis and scarring. The appearance of tarsal collagen has been normal, with no abnormality of ultrastructure or distribution of the collagen and elastic fibers of the tarsus. One report indicated cystic degeneration and squamous metaplasia of the meibomian glands, along with abnormal keratinization and granuloma formation. This report suggested that meibomian gland dysfunction, along with the associated abnormalities of the tear film, may be partly responsible for the keratoconjunctivitis seen in the syndrome. Conjunctival scrapings reveal keratinized epithelial cells.

Symptoms include chronic ocular irritation or foreign body sensation, red eye, and mucous discharge. They are usually worse on awakening in the morning. Often, patients present with multiple ocular medications that have been prescribed by numerous ophthalmologists. Sometimes the syndrome may be masked by toxic medicamentosus from the numerous eye medications. The clinical findings are that of a papillary unilateral or bilateral conjunctivitis affecting the upper and/or lower lids, a superficial punctate keratitis, and corneal vascularization.

THERAPY

Supportive. Since the cause of the floppy eyelid and rubbery tarsus is unknown, therapy is aimed at preventing the probable nocturnal eyelid eversion. One method is to have the patient wear an eye shield while asleep. Not all symptoms are relieved by this treatment.

Surgical. A surgical remedy is often unavoidable. As the cause is simply one of excessive eyelid laxity, the cure involves an eyelid tightening procedure. A straightforward upper and lower pentagonal eyelid resection has been recommended as a remedy and is well within the surgical skills of most ophthalmologists. Other eyelid shortening procedures, such as the tarsal strip and Bick procedures, may also be used successfully to alleviate symptoms of patients with the floppy eyelid syndrome. An eyelid shortening procedure involving a full-thickness resection or a tarsal strip procedure must avoid injury to the secretory ductules of the lacrimal glands.

FULL-THICKNESS UPPER AND LOWER EYELID RESECTION. When performing the procedure on a patient with floppy eyelids, both the upper and the lower eyelids must undergo surgery to achieve symptomatic success. The principal caveat is to avoid injury to the lacrimal secretory ductules, which are approximately 5 mm above the lateral extreme of the upper tarsus. In addition, to avoid an unsightly buckling in the upper eyelid tarsus, the vertical excision must extend through the top of the tarsus.

UPPER AND LOWER LATERAL CANTHAL SUSPENSION PROCEDURE—THE TARSAL STRIP PROCEDURE. This procedure is an excellent technique for the repair of the floppy eyelid abnormality if used as described by Anderson (1979) on both upper and lower eyelids.

BICK PROCEDURE (MODIFIED). By applying the well-known principles of the Bick technique, with minor modifications, to upper and lower eyelids, one may use the technique successfully in the repair of the floppy eyelid. Floppy eyelids tend to require more eyelid excision than is needed when the Bick procedure is used for the repair of ectropion or entropion. Thus, it is preferable to place one clamp at a time, rather than both clamps simultaneously, as described by Bick. In performing a Bick-type upper eyelid excision, great care must be taken to avoid the secretory ductules of the lacrimal glands. They empty into the superior cul-de-sac approximately 5 mm above the lateral extreme of the tarsus.

Ocular or Periocular Manifestations

Conjunctiva: Papillary conjunctivitis with mucous discharge.
Cornea: Diffuse papillary epithelial keratitis.

Eyelids: Always involves upper lids; may also involve lower lids; soft rubbery tarsus; upper lid everts easily on itself by pulling upward.

PRECAUTIONS

In most cases, the accurate diagnosis is initially overlooked. Many patients are inappropriately treated with various topical or systemic medications. Some patients may exhibit toxic reactions to these chronically administered but ineffective antibiotics, artificial tears, or steroids. Surgical correction must avoid the ductules of the lacrimal glands.

COMMENTS

Early recognition of this clinical entity may spare a patient many unnecessary diagnostic procedures and treatment trials. By the time some patients are diagnosed appropriately, they may have a concurrent medicamentosa conjunctivitis. The duration of symptoms before diagnosis has ranged from 8 months to 14 years.

References

Anderson R, Gordy DD: The tarsal strip procedure. Arch Ophthalmol 97:2192–2196, 1979.

Bick MW: Surgical management of orbital tarsal disparity. Arch Ophthalmol 75:386, 1966.

Culbertson WW, Ostler HB: The floppy eyelid syndrome. Am J Ophthalmol 92:568–575, 1981.

Dutton JJ: Surgical management of floppy eyelid syndrome. Am J Ophthalmol 99:557–560, 1985.

Easterbrook M: Floppy eyelid syndrome. Can J Ophthalmol 20:264–265, 1985.

Fleishman JA, Hoffman RO: An unusual case of floppy eyelid syndrome. Ann Ophthalmol 20:468–469, 1988.

Gerner EW, Hughes SM: Floppy eyelid with hyperglycinemia. Am J Ophthalmol 98:614–616, 1984.

Goldberg R, et al: Floppy eyelid syndrome and blepharochalasis. Am J Ophthalmol 102:376–381, 1986.

Inbert P, Williamson W, Leger F, Gauthier L, Lagoutte F: Bilateral corneal neovascularization and floppy eyelid syndrome. A case report. J Fr Ophthalmol 13:223–225, 1990.

Moore MB, et al: Floppy eyelid syndrome management including surgery. Ophthalmology 93:184–188, 1986.

Parunovic A: Floppy eyelid syndrome. Br J Ophthalmol 67:264–266, 1983.

Schwartz LK, Gelender H, Forster RK: Chronic conjunctivitis associated with "floppy eyelids." Arch Ophthalmol 101:1884–1888, 1983.

HEMIFACIAL SPASM 351.8

JOHN R. SAMPLES, M.D.

Portland, Oregon

Hemifacial spasm is a facial movement disorder in which there is a sporadic synchronized contraction of many muscles on one side of the face. Unlike benign essential blepharospasm, which is a bilateral disease, hemifacial spasm is confined to one side of the face. Often, it begins with twitches in a single orbicularis muscle. The twitches last from seconds to minutes and are typically irregular and clonic. The spasm may start around the eye and spread to other muscles innervated by the seventh cranial nerve. Hemifacial spasm never spreads to muscles beyond those innervated by the facial nerve. Spasms are often precipitated or made worse by fatigue and stress.

Synkinesis is observed in hemifacial spasm, but not facial myokymia, from which hemifacial spasm must be differentiated. Facial myokymia is almost always a benign condition when it involves only a single muscle, such as the orbicularis oculi. However, in certain patients with multiple sclerosis or brainstem tumors, facial myokymia may be a presenting feature and may persist indefinitely. Symptomatic hemifacial spasm is caused by lesions compressing the facial nerve extraaxially, usually by aneurysm, arteriovenous malformation, or rarely a neoplasm involving the cerebellopontine angle. The majority of cases have been attributed to an aberrant blood vessel compressing the facial nerve.

Therapy

Systemic. Hemifacial spasm is usually refractory to medical therapy, although carbamazepine[‡] has been estimated to be of benefit in up to 30 per cent of patients with this disorder. Serum levels of this drug may be obtained and followed to achieve therapeutic levels.

Botulinum A toxin[†] may be injected locally to produce a reversible neuromuscular blockade that may be useful in relieving the spasms. Many patients feel that the toxin produces significant improvement. Complications of botulinum A toxin injection into the orbicularis and adjacent muscles include ptosis, ectropion, corneal exposure, and tearing. Tolerance to the toxin does not develop. Antibodies to botulinum A toxin do not develop with the dosage commonly used in facial spasm.

Surgical. Decompression of the facial nerve in symptomatic cases has been described as being effective. Operating on cryptogenic cases and decompressing the facial nerve from aberrant blood vessels have been recommended. However, this surgical approach requires a retromastoid craniectomy and microneurosurgical techniques.

Ocular or Periocular Manifestations

Eyelids: Intermittent clonic and tonic jerks confined to the muscles about the eyelid, coupled with an ipsilateral contracture of the facial musculature.

PRECAUTIONS

Carbamazepine produces potentially alarming side effects, including hematopoietic, cardiovascular, hepatic, and renal disturbances. Careful examination and close medical supervision are required with the use of this drug. Fatal aplastic anemia, agranulocytosis, thrombocytopenia, and purpura are among the hematologic complications associated with this drug. A complete blood count, including platelet, thrombin, and reticulocyte count with serum iron determination, should be performed before initiating carbamazepine therapy and frequently throughout.

Significant risks, including ipsilateral deafness and brainstem stroke, are involved in the operative management of this condition. These major complications must be weighed against the impairment of the patient and the expected benefit of surgery; the importance of selecting a qualified neurosurgeon to perform this procedure should be emphasized.

COMMENTS

Botulinum A toxin is a new and effective treatment for this disorder. A trial with botulinum A toxin injections is indicated before undertaking surgical therapy.

References

Elston JS: Botulinum toxin therapy for involuntary facial movement. Eye 2:12–15, 1988.
Gardner WJ: Concerning the mechanism of trigeminal neuralgia and hemifacial spasm. J Neurosurg 19:947–958, 1962.
Janetta PJ: Observations on the etiology of trigeminal neuralgia, hemifacial spasm, acoustic nerve dysfunction and glossopharyngeal neuralgia. Definitive microsurgical treatment and results in 117 patients. Neurochirugia 20:145–154, 1977.
Nielsen VK: Pathophysiology of hemifacial spasm. 1. Ephaptic transmission and ectopic excitation. Neurology 34:418–426, 1984.
Savino PJ, et al: Hemifacial spasm treated with botulinum A toxin injection. Arch Ophthalmol 103: 1305–1306, 1985.
Soso MJ, Nielsen VK: The lesion of hemifacial spasm is peripheral to the facial nucleus. Muscle Nerve 7:578, 1984.

HORDEOLUM 373.1
(Stye)

F. T. FRAUNFELDER, M.D.
Portland, Oregon

Hordeolum is a staphylococcal infection of the sebaceous glands of the eyelids. External hordeolum (stye) is caused by stasis with subsequent bacterial infection of the glands of Zeis or Moll. Internal hordeolum results from a secondary staphylococcal infection of a meibomian gland in the tarsal plate. Both internal and external hordeola are common sequelae of infectious blepharitis, and the most common infectious agent is *Staphylococcus aureus*. Hordeola usually begin with painful swelling and edema of the eyelid, which become localized. The purulent exudate of external hordeola often breaks through the skin near the eyelash line; however, the suppuration of the internal hordeolum occurs on the conjunctival side of the eyelid.

THERAPY

Ocular. Hordeola are usually self-limited and respond well to hot moist compresses. If applied early in the course of the infection, the hot compresses may prevent suppuration and abort the attack. To localize the infection, warm soaks administered four times daily for 15 minutes will increase the blood flow and tissue temperature so hydrolytic enzymes can break down tissue and form an abscess. Removal of the eyelashes in the affected area sometimes promotes better drainage of an external hordeolum.

After the hordeolum has started to drain or if there is a tendency to recur, topical ophthalmic antibiotics may be indicated. Tobramycin or gentamicin solution or ointment may be applied four times a day during the acute phase and continued twice daily for 1 week thereafter.

Topical ophthalmic corticosteroid therapy is rarely indicated and then only if inflammation is severe and threatening structural changes of the eyelid.

Systemic. If there are staphylococcal infections elsewhere or preauricular lymphadenopathy is present, systemic antibiotics may be necessary. Oral administration of 250 mg of erythromycin or 125 to 250 mg of dicloxacillin or cloxacillin may be given four times daily for up to 2 weeks. In chronic long-term prophylactic therapy, 250 mg of tetracycline, given orally twice daily 1 hour before meals, may be necessary for several months. Not infrequently, even antibiotic-sensitive staphylococcal organisms cannot be eradicated from the lids or nares. In these cases, lid hygiene, toxoids, a different course of systemic antibiotics, or such antiseptics as silver nitrate or gentian violet may be tried.

Surgical. After localization, these infections usually drain spontaneously, and the condition will subside. However, a stab incision in the area of the pointing abscess may occasionally be necessary. One must remember that there are frequently many pockets in large abscesses so multiple stab incisions may be necessary. If a local anesthetic is used, the injection is not given directly in the area of inflammation, but either above the upper border of the upper tarsus or below the lower border of the lower tarsus. A chalazion clamp is applied, and a horizontal incision is made over the pointing area if on the skin, or a vertical incision is made if conjunctival. The lash margins should be avoided so as not to injure lash roots. The wound edges are not resutured, but postoperative warm compresses and antibiotic ointment are used until closure occurs spontaneously.

Ocular or Periocular Manifestations

Conjunctiva: Cicatrization; exudates; hyperemia.
Eyelids: Cicatrization; destruction of follicles; distortion of lid margins; edema; erythema; madarosis.

PRECAUTIONS

Attempting to excise or curette all material in the presence of an acute inflammation can result in excision of an unnecessarily large amount of tarsal tissue. Systemic antibiotics are to be avoided, unless absolutely necessary. Tetracycline may act more by changing the lipoid content of the lid secretions than as an antibiotic in chronic long-term blepharitis.

As with all penicillins, one needs to consider the adverse effects. Immediate reactions that may occur within a matter of minutes or hours include urticaria, angioneurotic edema, and anaphylaxis, with a 10 per cent mortality rate. The accelerated reactions that may occur within the first 48 hours include urticaria, laryngeal edema, fever, rash, and erythema. The delayed reactions, which usually occur 2 to 10 years later, include a delayed urticaria, drug fever, rash, serum sickness, and diarrhea. Rarely does blood dyscrasia occur with this agent.

COMMENTS

The discharge from these infections is literally loaded with pathogenic staphylococci. Treatment following subsidence of the abscess should consist of measures to keep the staphylococci count on the eyelids at a minimum. Topical ophthalmic antibiotics may be effective and may aid in preventing recurrences. Hordeola are most frequent in debilitated patients, diabetics, and patients with chronic blepharitis.

References

Briner AM: Surgical treatment of a chalazion or hordeolum internum. Aust Fam Phys 16:834–835, 1987.
Briner AM: Treatment of common eyelid cyst. Aust Fam Phys 16:828–830, 1987.
Diegel JT: Eyelid problems. Blepharitis, hordeola, and chalazia. Postgrad Med 80:271–272, 1986.
Wilson LA: Bacterial conjunctivitis. In Duane TD (ed): Clinical Ophthalmology. Philadelphia, Harper & Row, 1979, Vol IV, pp 4:12–16.

LAGOPHTHALMOS 374.20
RICHARD P. JOBE, M.D.
Palo Alto, California

Lagophthalmos, the inability to close the eyelids fully, can result from excessive projection of the eye in the orbit, inadequate vertical dimensions of either lid, or malfunction of the orbicularis oculi. Appropriate therapy is dependent upon accurate diagnosis. Proptosis caused by congenital deformity, as in Crouzon's syndrome, requires craniofacial surgery for definitive cure. If proptosis is caused by tumor, orbital wall displacement secondary to trauma, or exophthalmos of hyperthyroidism, definitive treatment requires correction of the cause. In hyperthyroidism, surgical decompression of the orbit may perhaps be necessary if medical and radiologic treatment fail. Lid retraction caused by burns or the traumatic loss of eyelid tissue requires plastic surgical reconstruction of the lids to restore the capacity to cover the eye. Paralytic lagophthalmos secondary to decreased orbicularis oculi muscle tone is commonly seen in Bell's palsy.

The presence of lagophthalmos of any origin requires prompt efforts to protect the eye because of the loss of the natural hygienic properties of lid cover. Neglect of lagophthalmos results in painful dryness and, ultimately, keratitis or corneal ulceration. Conservative measures should begin as soon as it is evident that the lids will not close, before symptoms occur, and while the cause is being determined.

THERAPY

Ocular. Maintenance of a moist surface on the eye is critical to the management of lagophthalmos. This is the purpose of the lid suture or adhesion. Petrolatum ointment for longer action or artificial tears is a critical part of the armamentarium. The addition of occlusal techniques is also helpful. A moisture chamber made of a cone of x-ray film taped over the eye is often used. Prefabricated moisture chambers of clear plastics are also available. Thin polyethylene film can be taped over the eye, or a moisture chamber or wind screen can be attached to the frame of the spectacles. One should be particularly cautious in patching the eye in lagophthalmos, because the lids can open under the patch, causing corneal abrasion. Soft contact lenses occasionally can be useful in chronic irritative conditions caused by mild or partially corrected lagophthalmos.

When the condition is severe, lid suture or lid adhesion should be considered promptly. Lid suture is usually done in the central lids, using 5-0 monofilament plastic suture material. A stitch is placed beginning about 5 mm above the upper lid margin, passed out of the lid margin at the gray line, then into the lower lid at the gray line, and out through the skin about 5 mm below the margin. It is then passed in and out of the small piece of rubber or plastic that will serve as a bolster and returns about 6 mm away from the first pass by the opposite identical route through both lids. It is then tied snugly over another bolster. This can be done quickly under local anesthesia. The lid suture can be expected to be effective for several weeks if it is not tied too tightly to avoid cutting through the tissues. If an adhesion is needed for longer or permanent use, one merely removes the epithelium from the lid margins before placing the sutures, and the sutures may be left for 12 to 14 days.

Concurrent trigeminal defects with the loss of corneal reflex or sensation add greatly to the difficulty of management of lagophthalmos. This is particularly true in the paralytic lagophthalmos of facial paralysis if one attempts to balance protection and appearance. Cooperative patients with intact corneal sensation can often be managed by techniques that allow the ocular aperture to be preserved. Where a trigeminal defect coexists, permanent tarsorrhaphy is often necessary to protect the eye, to the detriment of the patient's appearance. The temporalis muscle and fascia dynamic sling into both lids can often achieve the necessary compromise between protection and appearance in this situation.

The management of paralytic lagophthalmos involves both lids. The lower lid must be gently held against the globe. This can be accomplished temporarily by placing tapes across the lower lid just below the cilia, drawing the lid laterally and superiorly along an upper lateral crow's foot line. Similarly, the upper lid can be stiffened and held down by the application of a crescent of stiff tape between the cilia and brow.

Surgical. In studying the laxity of the lower lid, its source must be identified. In long-standing paralytic lagophthalmos, often the tendinous structure between the medial lower tarsus (punctum) and the medial canthus is stretched, allowing the punctum and tarsus to fall out and laterally. When this condition is present, a medial canthoplasty is indicated as a part of the support system for the lower lid. The usual procedures for elevation of the lower lid are less effective if this medial laxity is present. The most common useful procedure for correction of mild paralytic lagophthalmos, particularly in younger individuals where orbicularis function is in part replaced by the elasticity of the eyelid skin, is the McLaughlin lateral canthoplasty. This procedure can be done in a few minutes under local anesthesia. It consists of closure of the lateral 4 to 5 mm of the lid aperture, overlapping the upper lid with the lower lid, and attaching the two tarsal plates together, supporting the lower lid and providing a touch of animation into the lower lid as the lower tarsus rises with the upper on levator contraction. In normal lids, the tarsal plates do not contact each other. The procedure is done by incising at the gray line from a point 5 mm medial to the lateral canthus of either lid around the conjunctivo-cutaneous junction of the canthus to the same point on the opposite lid. A triangle of conjunctiva is removed along the lid margin of the upper lid, and a triangle of skin with cilia is removed from the lid margin of the lower lid. A 5-0 monofilament suture is passed from a point 5 mm above the upper cilia through the upper tarsus and both triangular wounds and then through the lower tarsus and conjunctiva. It is passed back through both lids, wounds, and skin, and it is tied over a bolster for 10 days. This procedure is useful in permanent lagophthalmos, but should be avoided in patients whose condition may be temporary, as it is difficult to restore normal canthal anatomy on release of this tarsorrhaphy. A Kuhnt-Szymanowski procedure is occasionally useful if the dimensional anatomy permits it without additional deformity.

The best durable support for the lower lid that sacrifices nothing aesthetically is a fascia lata or palmaris longus tendon sling passed through the lower lid below the margin from the medial canthal tendon to a hole drilled above the lateral canthus in the orbital rim. It should be just tight enough to hold the lid on the globe against a gentle downward pull. Such a sling will hold up well with time and will relieve many symptoms. The sling is about 3 mm wide and is sutured to the medial canthal tendon and the orbital periosteum or itself laterally after passing in and out through a small hole drilled in the bone. A third incision below the cilia in the central lower lid is helpful in passing the sling. Unless the lower lid is against the globe, measures to assist the upper lid in lagophthalmos will fail.

The upper lid in most cases of lagophthalmos has a functioning levator muscle that keeps the lids open and is the cause of most of the problems resulting from lagophthalmos. Sometimes, iatrogenic lagophthalmos, intentional or unintentional, results from overaggressive correction of ptosis. If the overcorrected ptosis causes persistent problems, a release of the correction may be warranted.

The temporalis muscle and fascia transfer of Gillies is particularly useful in lagophthalmos of Hansen's disease and where the cornea is insensitive. In this situation, the closure is active and muscular. It is a complex operation and often causes paradoxical eye closure with chewing and, uniformly, a bulge over the lateral orbit where the muscle belly is transferred toward the eye. This procedure actively replaces the orbicularis in both lids.

Foreign material placed within the lids may counteract the levator action. The use of a stainless-steel spring between the brow and upper tarsus has a few advocates who, however, seem to employ it less frequently as they accumulate experience. A silicone rubber loop around both lids has also been used to hold the lids together. In addition, magnets made of an alloy of cobalt and platinum have been placed in both lids such that the force will close the lids. The least complicated procedure and therefore the most applicable one is lid loading. It is done by addition of a gold weight to the upper lid. (Gold lid loads are available in the United States only at MedDev Corporation (800) 543-2789.) Such weights are usually about 4.5 mm high, 1 mm thick, and as long as is necessary to achieve the desired weight. As a preliminary test, weights are glued to the lid with benzoin to determine the necessary force. If the facial palsy is long-standing, the weight should be about 0.2 gm greater than the ideal on testing as the levator will strengthen with the weight in place.

At surgery, the upper tarsus is exposed, and the weight is sutured in place to the orbital septum or levator aponeurosis sufficiently high in the lid that it is above the thin supraciliary lid. The orbicularis and skin are closed over the lid load, and the operation is completed in a few minutes. In the event of recovery of orbicularis function, the load can be easily removed without adverse effect.

Recent reports from Britain present an incidence of extrusion of gold lid loads of about 10 per cent. Both reports suggest that the loads were not sutured into position when placed. This discouraging information caused the author to arrange a survey of over 600 customers of MedDev Gold Lid Loads, of whom 167 replied, representing over 2000 procedures. An incidence of extrusion of 2.6 per cent was deduced from this informal survey of surgeons who are presumed to have placed a suture through the holes in the implant. These explanations were given for these failures: radiation, thin skin, a too-large implant, poor placement. etc. Therefore, it seems to be particularly desirable to suture the implant into position when it is placed. It will soon become well encapsulated, but it is beneficial to have it relatively immobile early on.

Ocular or Periocular Manifestations

Cornea: Epithelial defects; keratitis; opacity; perforation; ulcer; xerosis.
Eyelids: Blepharochalasis (upper lid); ectropion (lower lid).
Other: Epiphora; visual loss.

PRECAUTIONS

Although successful attempts at improving lid closure by weighting the upper lid or attaching springs have been reported, problems with these devices exist. Difficulties in the adjustment and tension maintenance of the stainless-steel spring may develop, and the likelihood that the spring will wear through the lid at some time necessitates the patient's continuous proximity to a surgeon familiar with the technique. Likewise, the elastic force of the silicone rubber loop may ultimately stretch the tissue through which it passes and will lose some tension. To have enough force to close the lids, the elasticity must also pull back against the eye, precluding the use of contact lenses. Although the use of magnet is a popular procedure in Germany where the magnets are made, problems have included extrusion, incorrect selection of magnets, and the weight of the lower magnet when the eye is open. The technique has been quite successful in the hands of those with experience, particularly if the magnets are placed in position before the levator muscle shortens due to myotonic contracture as a result of loss of opposing force.

COMMENTS

Although nerve anastomosis, muscle transfers, and other more exotic and definitive measures for correction of facial paralysis are often quite successful, they do not always achieve enough ocular protection to preclude the measures outlined here. Often, surgical ocular protection is wise in contemplation of either spontaneous or postoperative nerve regeneration.

The procedures that preserve appearance may provide somewhat less protection for the eye than tarsorrhaphy and should be used only in patients who can be reliably expected to use adequate protection to achieve comfort and safety. The constant exposure of the cornea results in excessive evaporation of the tear film, dryness of the cornea, and an exposure keratitis. These conditions may progress to infection, corneal ulceration, perforation of the globe, and blindness.

References

Barclay TL, Roberts AC: Restoration of movement to the upper eyelid in facial palsy. Br J Plast Surg 22:257–261, 1969.
Beard C: Diseases of the lids. *In* Dunlap EA (ed): Gordon's Medical Management of Ocular Dis-

ease, 2nd ed. Hagerstown, MD, Harper & Row, 1976, p 131.

Guy CL, Ransohoff J: The palpebral spring for paralysis of the upper eyelid in facial nerve paralysis: Technical note. J Neurosurg 29:431–433, 1968.

Jobe RP: A technique for lid loading in the management of the lagophthalmos of facial palsy. Plast Reconstr Surg 53:29–32, 1974.

Kelly SA, Sharpe DT: Gold eyelid weight in patients with facial palsy: A patient review. Plas Reconstr Surg. 89:3, 1992.

May M: Gold weight and wire spring implants as alternatives to tarsorrhaphy. Arch Otolaryngol Head Neck Surg 113:656–660, 1987.

Mühlbauer WD: 5 Jahre Erfahrung mit der Lidmagnetimplantation beim paretischen lagophthalmus. Klin Monatsbl Augenheilkd 171:938–945, 1977.

Pickford MA, Scamp T, Harrison DH: Morbidity after gold weight insertion into the upper eyelid in facial palsy. Br J Plast Surg 45:460–464, 1992.

Townsend DJ: Eyelid reanimation for the treatment of paralytic lagophthalmos: Historical perspectives and current applications of the gold weight implant. Ophthal Plast and Reconstr Surg 8:196–201, 1992.

Wood-Smith D: Experience with the Arion prosthesis. In Tessier P, et al: Plastic Surgery of the Orbit and Eyelids. New York, Masson, 1981.

LID MYOKYMIA 333.2

BYRON L. LAM, M.D.

Little Rock, Arkansas

Myokymia is the spontaneous fine fascicular contraction of muscle without muscular atrophy or weakness. Eyelid myokymia usually involves the orbicularis oculi of one of the lower eyelids, although occasionally the upper eyelids can be affected. These irregular contractions are usually intermittent and may persist for weeks to months. The disorder is generally not associated with any organic disease, although it is often attributed to stress and fatigue. Possible precipitating factors include overwork; lack of sleep; excessive coffee, alcohol, or smoking; and irritative corneal or conjunctival lesions. Patients may complain of eye jumping or even oscillopsia. These symptoms may decrease when the eyelid is pulled manually. Fine contractions of the eyelid are usually visible and often are more apparent to the patient than to the observer. Rarely, the contractions may be vigorous enough to cause movement of the globe, producing pseudonystagmus. The focus of irritation is most likely in the nerve fibers within the muscle.

THERAPY

Supportive. Eyelid myokymia is usually a self-limited condition. Reassurance and re-

duction in precipitating factors are appropriate for most patients.

Systemic. Treatment should be reserved only for severe cases. The efficacy of various modalities is difficult to evaluate because the condition usually resolves spontaneously. Oral antihistamines, such as promethazine[‡] 12.5 mg to 25 mg, up to three times daily, or tripelennamine[‡] 25 mg to 75 mg, four times daily, may be used in severe cases. Oral quinine 0.2 to 0.3 gm once to twice daily for 3 days may be used either alone or in combination with antihistamines. Quinine is contraindicated in pregnancy and should be discontinued if tinnitus or visual disturbance occur.

Ocular or Periocular Manifestations

Eyelids: Fine rippling contractions.
Other: Oscillopsia; pseudonystagmus.

PRECAUTIONS

Myokymia may be caused by topical ocular use of indirect parasympathomimetics, such as physostigmine. Persistent myokymia followed by spastic paretic facial contracture is an important, although uncommon sign of disease in the dorsal pons. It may be seen in multiple sclerosis, brainstem neoplasms (e.g., glioma, metastatic disease), trigeminal neuralgia, and myasthenia gravis.

COMMENTS

Eyelid myokymia is generally a benign self-limiting condition that requires no workup. Medical treatment is seldom necessary. Clinicians should be aware that eyelid myokymia may rarely present as a precursor or as part of facial myokymia, indicating brainstem disease.

References

Andermann F, et al: Facial myokymia in multiple sclerosis. Brain 84:31–44, 1961.

Givner I, Jaffe NS: Myokymia of the eyelids. A suggestion as to therapy: Preliminary report. Am J Ophthalmol 32:51–55, 1949.

Krohel GB, Rosenberg PN: Oscillopsia associated with eyelid myokymia. Am J Ophthalmol 102:662–663, 1986.

Lowe R: Facial twitching. Trans Ophthalmol Soc Aust 11:129–133, 1951.

Reinecke RD: Translated myokymia of the lower eyelid causing uniocular vertical pseudonystagmus. Am J Ophthalmol 75:150–151, 1973.

Rubin M, Root JD: Electrophysiologic investigation of benign eyelid twitching. Electromyogr Clin Neurophysiol 31:377–381, 1991.

Sogg RL, Hoyt WF, Boldrey E: Spastic paretic facial contracture: A rare sign of brainstem tumor. Neurology 13:607–612, 1963.

LID RETRACTION 374.41

J. TIMOTHY HEFFERNAN, M.D.,

Seattle, Washington

and RICHARD R. TENZEL, M.D.

North Miami Beach, Florida

Lid retraction is a disorder of eyelid position that can affect the upper lid, the lower lid, or both. The condition is characterized by the appearance of a band of white sclera between the limbus and the eyelid margin or margins when the eyes are in primary position.

The most common etiology of eyelid retraction is thyroid ophthalmopathy that may be present with or without exophthalmos. Other causes of upper eyelid retraction include overcorrection of ptosis repair, Marcus Gunn jaw-winking syndrome, and some lesions of the rostral midbrain. Those lesions produce a symmetric, bilateral retraction of the upper eyelids.

Lower eyelid retraction can result from thyroid eye disease or large recessions of the inferior rectus and be a complication of other surgeries in the lower lid, such as blepharoplasty and blow-out fracture repair. In this latter group of conditions, one typically finds significant scarring of the central lamella. The anatomic basis of lower lid retraction in inferior rectus recession involves anterior extensions of Tenon's capsule that surround the inferior rectus and the inferior oblique, thus forming Lockwood's ligament. Lockwood's ligament is the origin of the capsulopalpebral fascia that inserts on the lower tarsal border.

THERAPY

Surgical. Upper eyelid retraction can be corrected by recession of Müller's muscle and levator aponeurosis. This procedure is best done with local anesthesia on an awake and alert patient. Doing so allows the surgeon to lower the lid progressively while evaluating the response of the lid after each step. An incision is made through the skin at the lid crease. The orbital septum is identified and opened entirely across the lid. Protruding orbital fat can be removed as indicated. At this point, the patient is instructed to open the eyes, and the position of the lid is noted. This level is compared to the preoperative height. Any change in level is noted and if an elevation (common) or lowering (uncommon) has occurred, this amount of change is used to determine whether the lid position at the end of the procedure should be at, above, or below the desired final lid height. The levator is cut and disinserted from the tarsus. When Müller's muscle is reached, a Desmarre retractor is placed beneath the lid and the lid put on a stretch. A plane of dissection is created between the conjunctiva and Müller's

muscle, which allows Müller's muscle and the levator aponeurosis to be recessed en bloc. The recession is initially confined to the temporal two-thirds of the lid to prevent nasal overcorrection. During the dissection, the patient is repeatedly asked to open the eyes so the level of the lids can be evaluated. If more nasal correction is required, it is done in small segments. When the desired end point is reached, a 6-0 mersilene suture is placed partial thickness in the superior edge of the tarsus and brought through the lid retractors. This suture suspends the lid at the desired height and prevents further recession of the retractors. The lid crease is then formed at the desired height by attaching the orbicularis muscle to the tarsus with three nonabsorbable horizontal mattress sutures.

Lower eyelid retraction may be approached through a conjunctival incision at the lower edge of the tarsus. The conjunctiva is dissected from the posterior surface of the lower eyelid retractors beyond the reflection of the inferior conjunctival cul-de-sac, thus cutting the connections of the capsulopalpebral fascia to the fornix. Dissection then goes through the lid retractors at the lower edge of the tarsus and continues down the anterior face of the orbital septum. This allows the lower lid retractors to recess en bloc. The orbital septum can then be opened and fat removed. If scarring from previous surgery is present, it can be excised at this point. A strip of donor sclera 2.5 times the amount of desired recession is then placed between the retractors and the tarsus and sutured into position with a running absorbable or nonabsorbable suture. Traction sutures are taped over the brow for 24 hours. An initial postoperative overcorrection is desirable.

Alternatively, the hammock sling procedure may be used. A skin-muscle flap is made temporally using a blunt Stevens scissors. An incision is made through the lower eyelid retractors below the tarsal plate, and the conjunctiva is separated from the lid retractors beyond the reflection of the inferior fornix. The lower eyelid retractors are allowed to recess into the orbit. Without disturbing its medial and lateral attachments, the pretarsal orbicularis muscle is separated from the tarsus. The muscle is then rotated inferiorly and sutured between the inferior border of the tarsus and the superior border of the lid retractors, thus forming a hammock of pretarsal orbicularis muscle. A 2-mm horizontal lateral canthotomy is performed at the desired level of the new lateral canthus. The lid is overlapped, and redundant lid is excised. The cut edge of the tarsus is sutured to the medial cut edge of the lateral canthal tendon with interrupted sutures of 7-0 Vicryl. A skin graft may be used, if necessary.

When performing a large recession of the inferior rectus, one may avoid lid retraction by careful and complete dissection of Lockwood's ligament. If lid retraction occurs despite this procedure, a recession of the lid retractors as described earlier can be done. However, a scleral graft should not be necessary.

Ocular or Periocular Manifestations

Cornea: Exposure keratitis.
Eyelids: Lagophthalmos; ptosis.
Orbit: Exophthalmos.
Other: Chemosis; diplopia; incomitant strabismus.

PRECAUTIONS

In thyroid patients, all eyelid surgery should be postponed until the metabolic status and lid levels are stable for at least 6 months. Furthermore, if orbital decompression and strabismus repair are contemplated, these procedures should precede eyelid surgery.

Ideally, lid retraction caused by overcorrection of ptosis should be recognized and corrected in the first 10 to 14 days after the initial surgery. Doing so greatly facilitates the repair because healing has not yet occurred and one may simply reopen the wound and resuture the levator aponeurosis at the desired height.

Lids receiving scleral implants become thickened and edematous postoperatively, and the sclera resorbs in an unpredictable manner in many cases. Therefore, scleral grafts may end up less than cosmetically acceptable and require further surgery.

COMMENTS

Classically, upper eyelid retraction in thyroid eye disease was considered to be caused by increased innervation to Müller's muscle. It is now recognized, however, that many other forces are also at work, including inflammatory adhesions between the levator aponeurosis and adjacent tissues, thickening and loss of elasticity of the levator, and increased innervation of the superior rectus and levator muscle to compensate for a contracted inferior rectus. Retraction of the lids secondary to the conditions described here is amenable to correction, but each case must be evaluated individually. The patient must be warned that additional procedures may be necessary.

Lid retraction operations may be used not only to protect the cornea but also to make a cosmetically deforming exophthalmos less apparent or to avoid an orbital decompression procedure with its attendant complications.

References

Dryden RM, Soll DB: The use of scleral transplantation in cicatricial entropion and eyelid retraction. Trans Am Acad Ophthalmol Otolaryngol 83:669, 1971.
Heffernan JT, Tenzel RR: Correction of vertical retraction of the lower lid with an orbicularis hammock. Ophthalmic Plast Reconstr Surg 5:92–98, 1989.

MADAROSIS 374.55
(Loss of Eyelashes)

ALLEN M. PUTTERMAN, M.D.
Chicago, Illinois

Madarosis, the loss of eyelashes, can be an undesirable cosmetic deformity. It can be caused by systemic or topical infections and inflammations, hysteric plucking of hairs, surgery, and trauma. The hair loss may involve the entire lid, but frequently involves only a segment.

Systemic causes of madarosis include generalized disorders, such as alopecia areata (characterized by an area or areas of sharply defined baldness) and alopecia artefacta (baldness due to neurotic plucking of hairs or cilia). Other systemic causes of madarosis are lupus erythematosus, psoriasis, and seborrhea in which loss of eyelashes follows inflammation of the lids, as well as leprosy, syphilis, tuberculosis, sickle cell anemia, and endocrine disorders. Topical infections and inflammations, such as ulcerative and allergic blepharitis, frequently lead to loss of cilia that is usually segmental.

Madarosis is also a complication of eyelid surgery. Absent lashes frequently occur when full-thickness segments of the lids are excised in the treatment of eyelid carcinoma. In other eyelid surgery, especially that related to the treatment of ptosis and benign tumors, lashes can be lost because of the undermining of skin from orbicularis within 2 mm of the lid margin. Traumatic lid lacerations and avulsions are still other causes of madarosis.

THERAPY

Supportive. The treatment of absent cilia after surgery or trauma and the control of systemic and topical infections and inflammation are difficult. Certainly, the need for treatment varies, since many patients have a cosmetically acceptable appearance without lashes, especially if madarosis involves a small segment of the lid or even the entire lower lid. The easiest treatment is achieved with makeup. Eyelid liner, mascara, and false eyelashes can camouflage the defect and frequently produce a better cosmetic appearance than that achieved surgically. False eyelashes can be applied to a segment of the lid. In addition, makeup experts can attach false lashes to surrounding normal cilia by a weaving process.

Systemic. Therapy for madarosis is aimed at treating the specific illnesses that are causing it. Medical management of these systemic problems, including the emotional problems of alopecia artefacta, frequently leads to regrowth of the cilia. The treatment of topical causes of madarosis, such as ulcerative and allergic blepharitis, are discussed in other areas of this book. In general, lid hygiene, lid scrubs with baby shampoo, and application of topical antibiotics (such as erythromycin) to the lid margins will control seborrheic blepharitis and prevent further loss of lashes. Allergic blepharitis is treated by eliminating the offending antigens and the application of topical steroids.

Surgical. The most pleasing surgical results are achieved in patients who have had a segmental loss of lashes. The treatment consists of an eyelid excision of a full-thickness pentagon segment in the area without lashes. The surrounding normal lid segments are then connected together. Three 6-0 black silk double-armed sutures are placed through the lid margins. One suture is placed through the squared corners where conjunctiva meets tarsus entering through the posterior aspect of the tarsus. The second suture is placed through the gray line. The third suture is placed through the most posterior row of cilia. The suture enters and exits from similar areas on each edge of the wound to avoid lid notching postoperatively. Sutures are triple-tied, and the ends of the posterior two sutures are tied over the cilia suture, so that when all six ends are cut they point away from the cornea to avoid suture keratopathy. Two to three Vicryl double-armed sutures are then passed through the pretarsal fascia and the anterior aspect of the tarsus on each side of the wound below the lid margin. The skin is closed with a continuous 6-0 black silk suture.

If the normal lid segments connect together with too much tension, a lateral canthotomy and cantholysis with or without a semicircular temporal flap may be needed. This is especially important in the upper eyelid where a tight eyelid can cause ptosis. Also, it is possible to attach a segment of the lid with normal cilia to the lid segment that has a few absent cilia. Doing so decreases the area of madarosis, and a smaller area of absent lashes is usually acceptable. The lateral canthotomy and cantholysis and semicircular flap will leave the temporal lid segment without lashes. This too is more cosmetically acceptable than absent central lashes.

Transplantation of hairs from the eyebrow to the eyelid is another alternative treatment of madarosis. An incision is made at the junction of the skin-lid margin over the absent lash area. The direction of the brow hairs is studied, and the hairs pointing in the desired direction are chosen. A portion of the eyebrow that is equivalent in length and width to the lid with absent cilia and consisting of four rows of hairs is excised from the eyebrow. The correct depth of the graft is critical; it must include the hair follicles while avoiding too much subcutaneous tissue. The graft is sutured to surrounding skin and lid margin so that the hairs are pointing away from the cornea and correspond to the direction of the adjacent normal cilia. Usually, the outer two rows of hairs eventually slough off. This procedure commonly leads to loss of hairs over parts of the graft and usually unsatisfactory cosmetic results.

Still another alternative to lash transplantation is to remove a segment of the normal temporal lashes and place them, as described above, into the area of madarosis. Naugle (1982) has advocated this approach and claims good results. Again, the cost of losing temporal lashes to create central lashes is a cosmetically desirable trade. Good results have also been achieved with the placement of individual lash grafts into areas of madarosis.

Blepharopigmentation is a technique in which pigment is tattooed into the eyelids. It is chiefly advocated to simulate eyeliner or to enhance the eyelashes. However, it can also be used to simulate eyelashes and is especially effective if the eyelashes are sparse, rather than totally absent. Equipment and pigment are available through Dioptics and Cooper-Vision. Pigment is applied beneath the skin in the desired density with a rapidly pulsating needle that is covered with pigment.

PRECAUTIONS

The transplantation of eyebrow hairs into the eyelid must not be considered a cure for madarosis. The relatively high incidence of postoperative loss of transplanted brow hairs and the frequently conspicuous appearance of the brow hairs that remain should alert the surgeon to surgical failure. Blepharopigmentation was initially a popular technique, but now is used only occasionally. One of the main problems has been the difficulty of removing pigment in patients who do not like the density or areas to which it was applied.

COMMENTS

Madarosis (loss of eyelashes) has systemic, topical, hysteric, traumatic, and surgical causes. The first three categories can be treated medically. Makeup, horizontal lid shortening, and brow and lid grafts can be used to treat traumatic and surgical causes.

References
Naugle T: Cited by Caldwell D: Eyelash loss corrected by ciliary transplantation. Ophthalmol Times 7:52–53, 1982.

Putterman AM: Basic oculoplastic surgery. In Peyman GA, Sanders DR, Goldberg MF (eds): Principles and Practice of Ophthalmology. Philadelphia, WB Saunders, 1980, pp 2292–2295.

Putterman AM, Migliori ME: Elective excision of permanent eyeliner. Arch Ophthalmol *106*:1034, 1988.

MARCUS GUNN SYNDROME 742.8

(Jaw-Winking Syndrome, Trigemino-Ocular Motor Synkinesis)

ROGER A. DAILEY, M.D.,

Portland, Oregon

and AMY AIELLO, M.D.

Phoenix, Arizona

The jaw-winking syndrome, described by Marcus Gunn in 1883, is one type of congenital ptosis of a synkinetic nature that classically consists of ptosis of the upper eyelid associated with involuntary retraction of the lid during contraction of the ipsilateral pterygoid muscle. This syndrome accounts for 4 to 6 per cent of all congenital ptosis cases. It is usually noted shortly after birth. As the infant begins to nurse, the ptotic lid rhythmically jerks upward. The retraction is most commonly demonstrated by opening and closing the mouth or moving the jaw from side to side. It is rarely demonstrated by coughing, smiling, Valsalva maneuvers, swallowing, inspiration, or contraction of the platysma muscle. It seems from electromyographic studies that there is a synkinetic relationship between the external pterygoid muscle and the levator muscle. The lid elevates with jaw thrusting to the opposite side (ipsilateral external pterygoid) or with the jaw projecting forward or mouth opening (bilateral external pterygoid). The less common type is the internal pterygoid levator synkinetic group in which the lid elevates with the muscle closing or teeth clenching. The ptosis, as well as the retraction ("winking"), varies in severity from minimal to cosmetically unacceptable, and either component may dominate the clinical picture. The condition is usually sporadic, but familial cases have been reported. It is almost always unilateral and more severe in downgaze. The Marcus Gunn syndrome is persistent throughout life, although it may become less conspicuous with time as patients learn to control or mask its features. The explanation for the often bizarre manifestation of this syndrome is a congenital misdirection of part of the fifth cranial nerve to a branch of the third cranial nerve that supplies the levator muscle. Therefore, stimulation to the jaw sends impulses to the poorly innervated levator. Several series have reported significant associations with other ocular problems, including strabismus, anisometropia, amblyopia, and Duane's syndrome. The frequency of strabismus has been reported as high as 58 per cent and includes superior rectus palsies, double elevator palsies, and as horizontal deviations.

THERAPY

Supportive. Amblyopia if present needs to be treated vigorously, and anisometropia must be corrected if significant.

Surgical. As the patient with Marcus Gunn syndrome brings to the clinician two separate problems—ptosis and jaw-winking—the satisfactory elimination of both is often a challenging endeavor. In evaluating a patient, one must decide which component is more cosmetically intolerable; only then can the surgical plan be tailored accordingly and the best results obtained. A discussion with the patient and/or the parents is important to ensure that they have realistic expectations and are aware that a compromise may be necessary.

In patients with very mild ptosis (<2 mm) and mild jaw-wink (3-4 mm), one can perform a Müller's muscle conjunctival resection as described by Putterman or a levator resection; no treatment may even be acceptable. If the ptosis is moderate and the jaw-winking minimal, a levator resection is the treatment of choice. Undercorrection of the ptosis has been a complication of this approach, and it is recommended that the resection be greater (4-5 mm more) than in the usual case of congenital ptosis. Unfortunately, an exacerbation of the jaw-wink may then occur as this procedure strengthens the levator muscle and the eyelid excursion now begins at a higher level.

When the jaw-winking component is severe, a levator resection only exacerbates the wink. In this case one needs to obliterate the jaw-wink by release of the levator aponeurosis followed by a frontalis suspension. Dryden and co-workers (1982) described a reversible technique of suturing the levator aponeurosis to the arcus marginalis of the upper orbital rim to ensure its deactivation. Bilateral levator release with fascia lata suspension of both eyelids is the procedure of choice as it avoids the often marked asymmetry of unilateral surgery. Bilateral levator suspension combined with only unilateral levator excision of the affected eye is also advocated ("Cluchen-Beard" operation). If the patient or parents refuse bilateral surgery, the frontalis suspension may be performed on the affected eye with or without prior levator release.

To effect a levator release, a skin crease incision is made, and a small amount of preseptal orbicularis is resected. The underlying system is identified and incised nearly its entire length horizontally. This allows identification of the levator aponeurosis, which is released from the tarsus and attached to the arcus marginalis with multiple 5-0 Dacron sutures. Care should be taken to avoid the supraorbital neurovascular bundle. A frontalis sling of the surgeon's choice can then be performed. A double rhomboid as described by Beard (1981) is an excellent choice in the setting.

In cases in which the wink is not prominent and the levator does not need to be released, the authors prefer a transconjunctival frontalis suspension. Before age 3, use of a synthetic sling is suggested, such as 2-0 Proline. Banheal fascia can be used, but in the authors' experience, this material has not been satisfactory. After age 3, the child's own fascia lata has developed sufficiently to enable harvesting either from midthigh or the hip area.

A stab incision is made at the upper edge of the brow where elevation of the eyelid by the surgeon's finger gives the most pleasing cosmetic appearance. This incision need not be carried down to periosteum. A small amount of skin undermining will ensure good closure over the fascia knot later.

The eyelid is then everted over a Desmarres retractor and held in place with a forceps. A fascia lata strip measuring approximately 3 mm in width and 12 to 15 cm in length is loaded on a half-circle, reverse-cutting needle (Richard Allan No. 2164-4) and passed horizontally through the lid just anterior to the superior tarsal border. This horizontal limb should measure approximately 6 to 10 mm depending on the patient's size. An attempt is made to incorporate the tarsal plate.

The needle is then placed back in the lid where it has just exited and driven in a slightly posterior direction to an area immediately behind the superior orbital rim, "walked" anteriorly over the rim, and brought out through the brow incision. Before pulling this vertical fascia limb through, a small piece of 4-0 silk is placed as a marker suture at the junction of the horizontal and vertical limbs to facilitate removing the vertical portion, should repositioning of the fascia be necessary.

The needle is then reloaded with the opposite end of the fascia, brought through the entry site of the horizontal limb, and then directed superiorly to the brow incision in the same fashion. A small piece of silk is again placed at the junction. The result is a triangle-shaped sling with its base at the anterior-superior tarsal margin.

At this point, the two vertical limbs can be tied temporarily to check height, lid margin contour, and symmetry. If adjustments need to be made, the fascia can be removed in part or totally and replaced until the desired effect is achieved. The silk marker sutures are then removed, and the fascia is secured with a square knot. A 5-0 Dacron suture is tied in between throws of the fascia to help stabilize the knot. At this point, a good lid crease should be present, and the lid margin should be 1 to 2 mm above the desired postoperative level and in apposition with the globe. Infe-

rior pressure on the brow will relax suspension and should allow the eye to close.

Ocular or Periocular Manifestations

Extraocular Muscles: Double elevator palsy; superior rectus palsy.
Other: Amblyopia; anisometropia; Duane's syndrome.

PRECAUTIONS

An associated elevator palsy or superior rectus palsy with a hypertropia in the primary position should be treated before levator resection. Levator resection alone treats only the ptosis and often undercorrects it. It may also exaggerate the jaw-wink and be associated with cosmetically significant eyelid lag. Undercorrections are often the rule, even with frontalis suspension, and necessitate further surgery. It may be prudent to overcorrect purposefully by 1 to 2 mm at the time of surgery.

COMMENTS

Several modifications of the frontalis suspension have been advocated. The authors favor the transconjunctival suspension in cases where the levator has not been released. The advantages of this approach include a smaller chance of infection since it avoids low anterior skin incisions near the lash line, avoidance of visible traction lines below the skin, and facilitation of crease formation since the fascia is placed posteriorly to the orbital septum. In addition, normal attachments of the levator to the tarsus and skin are preserved so that, when the brow is elevated by the frontalis muscle, the lid is indirectly raised and normal lid margin contour and apposition to the globe are maintained. This procedure is also inherently safer as the needle used to pass the fascia lata is never directed toward the eyeball, therefore minimizing the chance of ocular penetration.

References

Beard C: Ptosis. 3rd ed. St. Louis, CV Mosby, 1981, pp 113–115, 208–210.
Beyer-Machule CK, Johnson CC, Pratt SG, Smith BR: The Marcus Gunn phenomenon. Orbit 4:15, 1985.
Bullock JD: Marcus Gunn jaw-winking ptosis: Classification and surgical management. J Pediatric Ophthalmol Strabismus 17:375, 1980.
Callahan A: Correction of unilateral blepharoptosis with bilateral eyelid suspension. Am J Ophthalmol 74:321–326, 1972.
Dailey RA, Wilson DJ, Wobig JL: Transconjunctival frontalis suspension (TCFS). Ophthalmol Plast Reconstr Surg 7(4), 1991.
Darcet TW, Crawford JS: The quantification, natural course, and surgical results in 57 eyes with Marcus Gunn (jaw-winking) syndrome. Am J Ophthalmol 92:702–707, 1981.
Dryden RM, Fleuringer JL, Quickert MH: Levator

transposition and frontalis sling procedure in severe unilateral ptosis and paradoxically innervated levator. Arch Ophthalmol *100*:462, 1982.

MELANOCYTIC LESIONS OF THE EYELIDS 172.1
(Melanoma, Nevi, Oculodermal Melanocytosis)

VITALIANO B. BERNARDINO, JR., M.D.,
WILLIAM C. LLOYD III, M.D., F.A.C.S.,
and MICHAEL A. NAIDOFF, M.D.

Philadelphia, Pennsylvania

Whenever a pigmented lesion of the eyelid or periorbital skin is discovered, it is important to determine whether the growth is benign, malignant melanoma, or a melanoma precursor. Historically, the reported incidence of eyelid malignant melanoma has been extraordinarily low—often quoted as 1 per cent of all eyelid neoplasms. However, recent data track the diagnosis of malignant melanoma as the fastest-rising cancer unrelated to smoking. Malignant melanoma is the most common potentially fatal skin neoplasm, yet overall survival is greatly improved with early diagnosis and treatment. For these reasons, all melanocytic eyelid lesions warrant careful examination. The examiner must be familiar with those clinical features that will help establish a correct diagnosis and affect an appropriate management plan.

Melanin is synthesized in the melanocyte and is the most common endogenous cutaneous pigment. Melanocytes reside both in the epidermis and dermis. Any workable classification of melanocytic lesions should distinguish those that involve the superficial (epidermal) melanocytes from those that arise in the deep set of melanocytes.

The majority of melanocytic lesions originate from epidermal melanocytes, including nevi, freckles, lentigines, melanomas, and melanoma precursors. Blue and cellular nevi, the nevus of ota (oculodermal melanocytosis), and some rare forms of melanoma are examples of lesions from the deep melanocytes. Because of their deeper location in the skin, deep melanocytes frequently impart a bluish discoloration to the lesion when viewed from the surface. The overwhelming majority are benign in nature. Lesions from epidermal melanocytes, on the contrary, demonstrate variations in the brown color of melanin. Most melanomas and melanoma precursors involve the superficial melanocytes.

Many nonmelanocytic lesions may be pigmented and confused with nevi and melanoma. The clinical challenge is to distinguish the melanocytic from the nonmelanocytic and the malignant from the benign conditions.

Proper management relies on diagnostic accuracy. A complete family history is essential. Patients should be examined under ideal lighting conditions. The slit lamp is particularly useful. The ophthalmologist should palpate, measure, and record all pertinent findings. Photographic documentation should be done. When the history is unclear, the patient or guardian should be instructed to bring past photographs, if available. Full body examination is indicated in the presence of any suspicious pigmented eyelid lesion.

Epidermal melanocytes produce three familiar, nonpalpable lesions. Freckles (ephelides) are small, sharply demarcated macules that appear in childhood and darken with sun exposure. The melanin is produced by reactive dendritic melanocytes. Freckled skin does not carry an increased number of melanocytes. Lentigo simplex clinically resembles a freckle; however, it is often darker and somewhat larger, and its color is unaffected by sunlight. Lentigo simplex is actually a monolayer of primitive nevus cells. Multiple facial lentigines may suggest Peutz-Jeghers syndrome, and the patient should be evaluated for the possibility of intestinal polyps and occult visceral tumors. The unrelated and misnamed lentigo senilis (also called solar lentigo, age spot) is observed in 90 per cent of elderly Caucasians, and it represents a noncancerous focal hyperpigmentation on sun-exposed skin. Lentigo senilis is a dark brown macule that usually measures 4 to 10 cm in diameter.

As mentioned earlier, the presence of melanocytes within the dermis imparts a more bluish appearance to the skin lesion. This finding is attributed to the scattering of light by these deeply situated pigmented cells (Tyndall phenomenon), and two familiar eyelid lesions are in this category. A blue nevus is a circumscribed papule 3 to 8 mm in diameter and is often located at the eyelid margin. Nevus of ota represents a more diffuse dermal melanocytosis observed in conjunction with ipsilateral ocular melanocytosis (melanosis oculi), leading to the characteristic slate-gray appearance of the globe. Patients with Nevus of ota are reported to have an increased risk of *uveal* melanoma, and routine ophthalmoscopic examinations are warranted.

Eyelid skin nevi can be congenital or acquired. Congenital nevi are visible from birth and carry an increased risk of becoming malignant melanoma in the first decade of life. Since most nevi appear at birth or in early childhood, it is not always possible to categorize accurately a pigmented lesion described as being present all the patient's life. Although congenital and acquired nevi share a common cytologic derivation, only congenital nevi are implicated in the development of malignant melanoma, whereas acquired nevi are no more likely to undergo malignant transformation than any other melanocyte in the body.

Common nevi are histopathologically classified based on their location within the skin layers. Junctional nevi are purely intraepithelial and reside immediately above the epidermal-dermal junction within the epidermal basal epithelium. Junctional nevi bear the most immature nevus cells, are often darkly pigmented, remain flat, and tend to enlarge over time. Intradermal nevi, on the other hand, are situated exclusively within the dermis. This deeper lesion is composed of aging, migrated nevus cells that have exhausted most of their capacity to make melanin. Consequently, the intradermal nevus usually forms an elevated mass with faint, if any, pigmentation. It carries the most benign overall prognosis. Because of its pale coloration, this elevated mass is often clinically confused with a verruca or papilloma. In addition, because these nests of nevus cells can extend deep into the dermis or tarsus, the microscopic appearance of an intradermal nevus may masquerade as an invasive cancer. Cilia are often found within intradermal nevi. It is the most frequently diagnosed nevus in the periorbital skin. Lastly, compound nevi are moderately pigmented and minimally elevated because the nevus cells occupy both epidermis and dermis. The compound nevus clinically and histopathologically exhibits morphologic characteristics between the extremes previously discussed in the junctional and intradermal varieties. Most congenital nevi are compound nevi, and it is the less mature junctional component of the compound nevus that poses a risk for melanoma. A striking example of a congenital nevus is the split or kissing nevus wherein the apposing skin margins and conjunctiva of the embryologically fused eyelids harbor this hyperpigmentation.

Several unusual variant conditions deserve mention. Balloon cell nevi appear during youth and are indistinguishable from a common acquired nevus; they rarely exceed 5 mm in diameter, and the diagnosis is based on its histology. The Spitz tumor (spindle-epithelioid nevus) is a weakly pigmented, benign, rapidly growing compound nevus seen in children and young adults. This pinkish-tan mass enlarges up to 10 mm in diameter over a period of months and then ceases further growth. Dysplastic nevi are present in 8 per cent of the normal population and behave differently than most nevi. They tend to be larger, with a diameter exceeding 4 mm, and identify themselves with haphazard patches of tan, brown, and pink color. They are, however, most frequently encountered in the skin of the trunk and back. The borders of dysplastic nevi are indistinct. Although dysplastic nevi are reported to have an increased risk of engendering malignant melanoma, the vast majority of these lesions never become cancerous. Therefore, close observation of dysplastic nevi, not prophylactic excision, is warranted. Dysplastic nevi can occur sporadically or follow a hereditary pattern (B-K mole syndrome). The latter group is at risk of developing multicentric cutaneous melanomas elsewhere on the body.

Nevi, as a group, pose several clinical problems. The larger and darker pigmented spots may be cosmetically unattractive. Some congenital eyelid nevi may enlarge sufficiently to result in mechanical ptosis and amblyopia. The hormonal influence of puberty can stimulate quiescent lesions and alarm the patient. Finally, patients may harbor fears of a malignant melanoma arising from an acquired nevus despite reassurances about the true rarity of such an occurrence. The chance of any single nevus transforming into melanoma is so extremely remote that it is felt to be inappropriate to excise nevi in hopes of eliminating a melanoma precursor lesion. The significance of a positive family history for malignant melanoma cannot be overemphasized, as it is these patients whose lesions most deserve careful scrutiny.

Despite the rarity of primary eyelid malignant melanoma, the diagnosis cannot be dismissed. Approximately 75 per cent of cutaneous malignant melanoma arises de novo from atypical melanocytes without any history of a pre-existent lesion. Lentigo maligna (Hutchinson's melanotic freckle) is a flat dark macule seen on the sun-exposed skin of elderly individuals. The canthal angles and lower eyelid are frequent sites. This slowly growing lesion has a prolonged horizontal (centrifugal) growth phase. Dermal invasion is encountered in approximately 30 per cent of cases, changing the diagnosis to lentigo malignant melanoma. Clinical signs of this change may not be visible. Five-year survival after complete excision exceeds 90 per cent.

The most frequently diagnosed eyelid melanoma is the superficial spreading melanoma. The lesion is encountered even among younger patients, and it can arise on all skin surfaces regardless of sun exposure. It is palpable early in its clinical course and exhibits varying color from brown to gray or rose. Its oval configuration is disrupted by protrusions and indentations. The presence of nodules signals vertical invasion. One recent study has shown that the most common form of eyelid melanoma was nodular melanoma (59 per cent), whereas superficial spreading melanoma and lentigo maligna melanoma represented 22 per cent and 19 per cent of cases, respectively. Microscopy reveals the pagetoid spread of uniformly atypical melanocytes in the epidermis, with basal nests of atypical cells. Superficial spreading melanoma carries a poorer prognosis than lentigo maligna melanoma. Nodular cutaneous malignant melanoma is a very rare eyelid lesion. Affected individuals present with a rapidly growing palpable mass with nonuniform pigmentation. It has a short horizontal growth phase, quickly becomes invasive, and, as expected, carries the poorest diagnosis.

A complete evaluation of melanocytic lid lesions must consider other benign and malignant diagnoses in addition to nevi and melanoma. Seborrheic keratosis is a benign papilloma that is usually darker than the adjoining skin due to chronic secondary pigmentation. Seborrheic keratoses have a greasy feel and a characteristic "stuck-on" appearance. Vascular lesions of the skin can produce elevated skin masses with very suspicious coloration. Common examples include angiokeratoma, venous lake, and thrombosed capillary aneurysms. Dermatofibroma is an outdated descriptive term for a benign fibrous histiocytoma. This ill-defined nodular skin growth can harbor dispersed melanin or, more often, brown hemosiderin from degenerated blood within the slowly enlarging proliferation of dermal fibroblasts. Cystic lesions, such as a hidrocystoma (sudoriferous cyst, sweat ductal cyst) can also contain blood breakdown products. Easily overlooked changes to eyelid skin include an infarcted acrochordon (skin tag) or skin tattooing from unrecognized foreign body particles. Finally, other skin cancers can also appear darker than the surrounding skin. Secondary pigmentation is a known phenomenon in actinic keratoses, basal cell carcinoma, and squamous cell carcinoma. Accordingly, all adults presenting with any newly acquired pigmented lid mass should be carefully considered for biopsy.

THERAPY

Supportive. Not all pigmented eyelid lesions require excision. For many patients a clear explanation is all that is necessary. Today, those patients seeking cosmetic improvement can select from a wide variety of nonirritating occlusive make-up products. Photodocumentation is vital in order for the surgeon to assess the clinical course objectively. All patients need to be thoroughly advised of the warning signs that may herald the onset of a premalignant or malignant condition: changes in size, coloration, or topography and the presence of satellite lesions, ulceration, or bleeding.

Surgical. Surgical excision remains the principal treatment of pigmented eyelid lesions. Indications include the clinical suspicion of malignant melanoma, documented change or atypical behavior in an existing lesion, and a patient's preference for removal of an unsightly mass. Certainly, when the nature of the lesion is in doubt, a simple biopsy should be performed. Eyelid lesions should not receive pretreatment with cryo, dermabrasion, cauterization, laser, or radiation before biopsy, as doing so serves only to confuse the pathologist. Frozen section techniques are discouraged for management of an initial biopsy; excisional biopsies are preferable. When complete excision will result in profound lid disfigurement, shave biopsies are often acceptable to establish an initial diagnosis; however, this technique may lead to recurrences, and specimens from repeat biopsies can mimic a more worrisome diagnosis. All excised tissue should be forwarded for pathologic processing. Patients should be counseled beforehand regarding the possible need for repeat excision. Specimen reports should include a pertinent clinical history, and a simple orientation sketch will greatly facilitate tissue interpretation. Tissue margins will be carefully studied for evidence of atypia. When considering the adequacy of excision for cutaneous melanoma, the ophthalmologist must weigh the likelihood of recurrence in a biopsy with clean margins versus the morbidity associated with radical eyelid excision. Specific recommendations for every situation are beyond the scope of this article.

COMMENTS

The overall prognosis for excised primary eyelid malignant melanoma is extremely favorable. Most of these melanomas are discovered and treated before local disease can spread. Tumors excised with clean margins that are less than 2 mm deep most likely have not released micrometastasis. In contrast, late cases of melanoma with frank preauricular and cervical adenopathy are candidates for palliative therapy.

Regardless of the specific diagnosis and whether surgery was performed, all patients presenting with pigmented eyelid lesions require routine follow-up examinations with appropriate photodocumentation.

References

Elder DE, Murphy GF: Melanocytic Tumors of the Skin. Washington, American Registry of Pathology, 1991, pp 1–15.

Folberg R, Bernardino VB Jr, Bernardino EA: Pigmented eyelid lesions. In Hornblass A (ed): Oculoplastic, Orbital and Reconstructive Surgery. Baltimore, Williams & Wilkins, 1988, pp 259–270.

Grossniklaus HE, McLean IW: Cutaneous melanoma of the eyelid: Clinicopathologic features. Ophthalmology 98:1867–1873, 1991.

Keeling JH III: Pigmentary problems. In Griffith DG, Salasche SJ, Clemons DE (eds): Cutaneous Abnormalities of the Eyelid and Face. New York, McGraw-Hill, 1987, pp 169–191.

Lever WF, Schaumburg-Lever G: Histopathology of the Skin. Philadelphia, JB Lippincott, 1990, pp 756–797.

Maize JC, Ackerman AB. Pigmented Lesions of the Skin. Philadelphia, Lea & Febiger, 1987, pp 225–320.

ORBITAL FAT HERNIATION 374.34

(Adipose Palpebral Bags, Baggy Eyelids)

ALLEN M. PUTTERMAN, M.D.

Chicago, Illinois

In addition to cardiorenal disease, apparent prolapses of skin around the eyes primarily represent a true herniation of encapsulated orbital fat through an opening between the rims of the orbital septum and levator aponeurosis in the upper lid or between the junction of the rim of the septum and the capsulopalpebral fascia in the lower lid. These areas are anatomically weak so that orbital fat can protrude through the junctions, producing a hernia of fat. Orbital fat herniation must be distinguished from but also may be associated with dermatochalasis, which is excessive skin. These conditions pose cosmetic problems, especially in females, and may require surgical correction.

THERAPY

Surgical. At present, the only satisfactory method of treatment is surgical excision of the protruding fat. An incision is made through the upper eyelid crease or about 2 mm below the lower eyelid margin, and a skin-orbicularis flap is dissected either superiorly or inferiorly. The orbital septum is then located and tagged with 4-0 black silk sutures. The hernial sac is incised, and the fat is excised and cauterized until gentle pressure applied to the globe fails to prolapse the fat. The detached septum is not reattached to the levator or capsulopalpebral fascia, but is left to reattach spontaneously. Excessive skin and orbicularis muscle are excised as necessary, and the skin-orbicularis flaps are resutured at the original site of incision.

An alternative technique is to remove the herniated orbital fat through an internal lower eyelid approach. An incision is made through conjunctiva, Müller's muscle, and capsulopebral fascia several millimeters above the inferior fornix. The lid margin is pulled downward and outward with a Desmarres retractor while the conjunctiva, Muller's muscle, and capsulopalpebral fascia at the inferior aspect of the wound are pulled upward and secured to the upper lid margin. Dissection along the capsulopalpebral fascia with cotton-tipped applicators allows identification of the orbital fat pads. The fat that prolapses with general pressure to the eyelids is removed from the temporal, central, and nasal fat areas, and then the conjunctiva is reapproximated with three 6-0 plain interrupted sutures.

PRECAUTIONS

Although most cases of baggy eyelids represent true herniation, treatment, as for hernias elsewhere in the body, does not at present provide good results. If the protruding sac of fat is pushed back into place and the detached septum reattached, the problem usually recurs. Recurrence may result from the use of absorbable rather than permanent sutures. It is also possible that the exposed herniated orbital fat becomes abnormal and therefore cannot be replaced.

Lid retraction and lagophthalmos are complications of baggy eyelid surgery, especially when performed via an external approach in the lower eyelid. Since the septum is a strong inelastic tissue, the position of its reattachment to the levator and capsulopalpebral fascia may explain these complications. Therefore, it is important that the septum is in a satisfactory position in relation to the levator and capsulopalpebral fascia before closing the wound. On the upper lid, the septum should be about 10 mm above the superior tarsal border; in the lower lid, it should be about 5 mm below the inferior tarsal border.

To avoid loss of cilia, the uppermost incision on the lower lid must not be made too close to the lid margin. The surgeon must identify the inferior oblique muscle to avoid its injury with internal blepharoplasty. Normally, the optimal position for the lower lid incision is 2 mm below the lashes. It is also important to differentiate baggy eyelids caused by herniation of orbital fat from eyelid edema secondary to metabolic problems. Pressing on the eye through the closed eyelids will lead to increased orbital fat herniation, whereas lid edema will remain unchanged.

COMMENTS

Surgical procedures for correcting baggy eyelids have been based on three different concepts regarding the pathogenesis of this condition: there is too much orbital fat, the orbital septum is absent, and the septum is thinned and degenerated with a direct herniation of the fat through it. Careful inspection shows that the condition does indeed represent a true herniation, but a thinned septum is not usually responsible for it. In most patients, the septum itself, though not its attachments, is found to be normal.

References

Putterman AM (ed): Cosmetic Oculoplastic Surgery. New York, Grune & Stratton, 1982.

Putterman AM: Upper eyelid blepharoplasty. *In* Hornblass A (ed): Ophthalmic and Orbital Plastic and Reconstructive Surgery. Baltimore, Williams & Wilkins, 1988, pp 474–484.

Putterman AM (ed). Cosmetic Oculoplastic Surgery, 2nd ed. Philadelphia, WB Saunders, 1993.

Putterman AM, Urist MJ: Baggy eyelids—A true hernia. Ann Ophthalmol 5:1029–1032, 1973.

Putterman AM, Urist MJ: Surgical anatomy of the orbital septum. Ann Ophthalmol 6:290–294, 1974.

Safian J: A late report on an early operation for

"baggy eyelids." Plast Reconstr Surg 48:347–348, 1971.

Sayoc BT: Pathogenesis and management of adipose palpebral bags. Philippine J Ophthalmol 5: 128–135, 1973.

Ptosis 374.30
(Blepharoptosis)

JOHN H. SULLIVAN, M.D.

San Francisco, California

The term "blepharoptosis" refers to the condition in which the upper eyelid margin is abnormally low. The upper lid may rest at any position between the superior pupillary border and upper limbus and be considered normal. It is difficult, therefore, to designate the exact height at which an eyelid should be defined as ptotic. The position of the fellow eyelid and the configuration of the upper face can mitigate the significance of a ptotic eyelid. A small amount of ptosis may be undetectable if it is bilateral and symmetric but may be quite apparent if unilateral, especially if the eyes are prominent.

Elevation of the lid is accomplished by the simultaneous contraction of the levator palpebrae superioralis and the upper tarsal (Müller's) muscle. The levator is a striated muscle under voluntary control and is similar in most respects to other extraocular muscles. On upgaze the normal lid rises 10 to 20 mm. Most of the movement is generated by the levator. Perhaps 3 to 4 mm of excursion is attributable to Müller's muscle. This involuntary muscle contains smooth fibers and is controlled by the autonomic nervous system. Its tone and the height of the lid vary according to the state of consciousness and the level of adrenergic discharge.

Beard (1978) revised his original classification of ptosis from congenital and acquired subtypes to reflect an etiologic taxonomy.

- Levator maldevelopment
  - Simple
  - With superior rectus weakness
- Other myogenic ptosis
  - Blepharophimosis syndrome
  - Chronic progressive external ophthalmoplegia
  - Oculopharyngeal syndrome
  - Progressive muscular dystrophy
  - Myasthenia gravis
  - Congenital fibrosis of the extraocular muscles
- Aponeurotic ptosis
  - Senile ptosis
  - Late-developing hereditary ptosis

- Stress or trauma to levator aponeurosis
  - After cataract surgery
  - After other local trauma
  - Blepharochalasis
  - Associated with pregnancy
  - After Graves' disease
- Neurogenic ptosis
  - Ptosis caused by lesions of the oculomotor nerve
  - Post-traumatic ophthalmoplegia
  - Misdirected third nerve ptosis
  - Marcus Gunn jaw-winking ptosis
  - Horner's syndrome
  - Ophthalmoplegic migraine
  - Multiple sclerosis
- Mechanical ptosis
- Apparent ptosis
  - Due to lack of posterior lid support
  - Due to hypotropia
  - Due to dermatochalasis

The designation "true congenital ptosis" is a specific *maldevelopment of the levator muscle*. Fibrous and fatty tissue replace the normal muscle fibers in proportion to the severity of ptosis. Müller's muscle is usually unaffected. These inelastic fibers inhibit the lid from fully elevating on contraction (decreased levator function) or lowering on relaxation (lid lag). Since these dystrophic changes are rarely found in other types of ptosis, the finding of lid lag is an important indicator of levator maldevelopment. The term "congenital ptosis" may be confusing. A newborn may present with an acquired myogenic or neurogenic ptosis that by definition is congenital but is not the result of levator maldevelopment.

Levator maldevelopment is an uncommon disorder and occurs most often as an isolated unilateral finding. It may be associated with other ocular abnormalities. The *superior rectus* may also be dystrophic. These patients are identified by their inability to elevate the ptotic eye fully on upgaze. Some patients display a bizarre synkinetic movement of the upper eyelid known as *Marcus Gunn jaw-winking*. When the jaw is opened widely or deviated to the contralateral side, the pterygoid muscles are stimulated, and an aberrant impulse is sent to the levator muscle. During the act of eating, the upper eyelid may repeatedly dart over the superior limbus. *Blepharophimosis* is another uncommon variation of levator maldevelopment. Ptosis is bilateral and severe with poor levator function. It is associated with telecanthus, epicanthus inversus, and cicatricial ectropion of the lower lids. *Amblyopia* is uncommonly associated with ptosis and is usually secondary to concomitant astigmatism or myopia. Deprivational amblyopia is rare unless the lid is completely closed such as in oculomotor nerve palsy.

Acquired ptosis is more common than congenital ptosis and usually is the result of aging, neuropathy, or trauma. The distinction between levator maldevelopment and acquired ptosis is important because much less surgery is required for the correction of acquired ptosis. Acquired ptosis may be myogenic, aponeurotic, neurogenic, or mechanical. It is frequently caused by the disinsertion or dehiscence of the levator aponeurosis. This is believed to be the mechanism of senile (involutional) ptosis, postcataract ptosis, and many instances of traumatic ptosis. Neurologic causes of acquired ptosis include Horner's syndrome, oculomotor nerve palsy, myasthenia gravis, and chronic progressive external ophthalmoplegia.

Horner's syndrome causes ptosis by paralysis of Müller's sympathetic muscle. Other features of the syndrome—miosis, elevation of the lower lid, and anhidrosis—may be absent or so subtle that the diagnosis can be established only by testing pupillary response to topical cocaine (inhibits dilation). Ptosis from Horner's syndrome is usually mild and associated with good levator function. Ptosis may be the only manifestation of myasthenia gravis. Fatigue of the lid is often a clue, but a test of intravenous edrophonium chloride may be necessary to make the diagnosis.

Pseudoptosis can be a source of confusion. The upper lid is low in an eye that is hypotropic. When the eye is in primary position the lid is normal. With advanced dermatochalasis, redundant skin may overhang the lid margin, giving the appearance of ptosis.

THERAPY

Surgical. Effective management requires familiarity with several surgical techniques. *Minimal ptosis* with good levator function regardless of etiology is most easily repaired by Müllerectomy or tarso-Müllerectomy. The Fasanella-Servat procedure remains the most popular of this type because of its simplicity and predictability. In this operation, the upper lid is everted; a clamp is placed over the upper tarsus, conjunctiva, and Müller's muscle; and these tissues are resected.

Moderate ptosis (2 to 3 mm) with fair function (5 to 7 mm) resulting from levator maldevelopment is most often treated by moderate to large levator resection. Levator resection has been the mainstay of surgery for levator maldevelopment. An internal (conjunctival) or external (cutaneous) approach can be used. The conjunctival approach has the advantage of adjustability in the event of overcorrection. The resected levator is secured to the tarsus by mattress sutures knotted on the skin surface. Their early removal combined with manipulation allows the lid to be lowered in the immediate postoperative period. The external approach provides additional exposure, which is necessary for a maximum resection (greater than 23 mm). Many surgeons now advocate aponeurosis advancement for levator maldevelopment.

The amount of levator to be resected may be determined by two methods. Predetermination can be made by Beard's guidelines of levator function and the severity of ptosis. Variations in technique, such as the magnitude of tarsal resection, placement of sutures, and effect of cutting the levator horns, influence the final lid position. Berke determines the amount of levator to be resected by the position of the lid during surgery. This method is predicated on the knowledge that the lid will elevate or drop postoperatively in proportion to levator function. The surgeon should be aware of both methods to predict the size of resection, confirm the choice during surgery, and anticipate postoperative changes.

Moderate or severe ptosis with good function, a high lid crease, and thin lid are indications of aponeurosis disinsertion. Exploration and repair of the aponeurosis through a lid fold incision are the procedures of choice. Under local anesthesia it is usually not difficult to identify the aponeurosis and to attach it to the tarsus. The lid is set slightly higher than the final desired result to compensate for stimulation of Müller's muscle. Because it is difficult to predict the postoperative lid position, over- and undercorrections are not uncommon after aponeurosis surgery.

Severe ptosis (4 mm or more) with poor levator function (4 mm or less) requires an auxiliary elevating force. The most useful technique is the suspension of the lid to the frontalis muscle. Elevation of the lid is then effected by raising the eyebrow. Autogenous fascia lata has been found to be superior to synthetic or other biologic materials for this purpose.

Ptosis associated with superior rectus weakness requires a larger than usual resection of levator. Ptosis with blepharophimosis almost always requires brow suspension because of poor levator function. Ptosis with Marcus Gunn syndrome is usually unilateral. If the normal action of the mandible in eating and speaking does not produce noticeable lid movement, surgery is limited to correction of the ptosis. Elimination of the aberrant lid movement requires excision of the levator muscle and brow suspension. Unilateral brow suspension, however, is rarely satisfactory because of insufficient stimulus to raise the affected brow. Bilateral suspension with excision of both levators produces the most symmetric result. Correction of ptosis caused by myasthenia and chronic progressive external ophthalmoplegia may be complicated by progressive deterioration and extraocular muscle weakness. To avoid exposure keratitis, undercorrection is advised.

PRECAUTIONS

The most frequent complication of ptosis surgery is undercorrection of congenital levator maldevelopment. Repair of undercorrection necessitates reoperation, whereas management of overcorrection is much easier. Early removal of sutures, massage, and stretching are sufficient for most cases of overcorrection. Levator tenotomy is used when conservative treatment fails. Lid lengthening by scleral graft is useful in the late repair of severe lagophthalmos. Eye bank sclera preserved in alcohol is used in the same manner as in correction of lid retraction from Graves' disease.

Entropion and lid contour abnormalities can be minimized by resection of no more than half the tarsal plate. Failure to remove skin from the upper lid after a large levator resection will produce a low lid fold and spoil the appearance of an otherwise excellent job. Damage to the superior rectus or superior oblique can occur during ptosis surgery and may result in diplopia. Caution should always be used in cutting the horns of the aponeurosis. Identification of the superior rectus can be facilitated by a bridal suture.

COMMENTS

The outcome of ptosis surgery in patients with less than good levator function is never perfect. Lid asymmetry will always be present in some position of gaze. The limitations of surgery are generally better accepted by patients with congenital defects than those whose problem has been recently acquired. In either setting, a discussion of realistic goals before surgery can prevent the problem of an unhappy patient despite the best possible result. The surgeon should be familiar with the intricate anatomy of the lid and be capable of using different procedures to manage various types of ptosis.

References

Anderson RL: Age of aponeurotic awareness. Ophthalmol Plast Reconstr Surg 1:69, 1985.
Beard C: Ptosis surgery past, present, future. Ophthalmol Plast Reconstr Surg 1:69, 1985.
Beard C, Sullivan JH: Ptosis—Current concepts. Int Ophthalmol Clin 18:53–73, 1978.
Buckman G, Jakobiec FA, Hyde K, Lisman RD, Hornblass A, Harrison W: Success of the Fasanella-Servat operation independent of Müller's smooth muscle excision. Ophthalmology 96:413–418, 1989.
Callahan MA, Beard C: Beard's Ptosis, 4th ed. Birmingham, Aesculapius, 1990.
Jones LT, Quickert MH, Wobig JL: The cure of ptosis by aponeurotic repair. Arch Ophthalmol 93:629–634, 1975.
Linberg JV, Vasquez RJ, Chao GM: Aponeurotic ptosis repair under local anesthesia. Prediction of results from operative lid height. Ophthalmology 95:1046, 1988.
Merriam WW, Ellis FD, Helveston EM: Congenital blepharoptosis, anisometropia, and amblyopia. Am J Ophthalmol 89:401–407, 1980.
Putterman AM, Urist MJ: Müller muscle-conjunctiva resection. Technique for treatment of blepharoptosis. Arch Ophthalmol 93:619–623, 1975.

SEBORRHEIC BLEPHARITIS 373.00

MICHAEL HALSTED, M.D., and JAMES P. McCULLEY, M.D.

Dallas, Texas

Chronic blepharitis is a disease that is commonly encountered by the practicing ophthalmologist. There is an updated classification of chronic blepharitis based on clinical signs and symptoms. This current classification subdivides chronic blepharitis into six categories: (1) staphylococcal blepharitis, (2) pure seborrheic blepharitis, (3) mixed staphylococcal/seborrheic blepharitis, (4) seborrheic blepharitis with meibomian seborrhea, (5) seborrheic blepharitis with secondary meibomianitis, and (6) meibomian keratoconjunctivitis or primary meibomianitis.

Seborrheic blepharitis commonly presents in an older age group (mean age, 50 years) and has a longer duration of symptoms than staphylococcal blepharitis. Symptoms of mattering, burning, and foreign body sensation, once present, are not associated with as frequent exacerbations as in patients with staphylococcal lid disease, but are chronic with minimal waxing and waning. The eyelids are frequently less inflamed, and the debris deposited on the eyelid margin has an oily and greasy consistency that is often called scurf. Mixed staphylococcal/seborrheic blepharitis is marked by more frequent exacerbations of symptoms and is discussed in detail in the next section.

Seborrheic blepharitis with associated meibomian seborrhea frequently presents with pronounced complaints of severe burning in the morning. Although patient symptoms are marked, the clinical signs are frequently less prominent. The foremost finding is engorged meibomian glands filled with retained secretions (meibum) that can be easily expressed on eyelid massage. The tear film has a foamy appearance that is most noticeable in the lateral canthal region.

Seborrheic blepharitis with a secondary meibomianitis presents with symptoms similar to those of seborrheic blepharitis alone, but with more significant periods of exacerbation of symptoms. The anterior/ciliary lid changes are also similar to those found in patients with seborrheic blepharitis, but examination of the posterior lid reveals patchy, scattered inflammation surrounding the meibomian glands. The affected glands are inflamed and dilated with retained solidified meibum. The involved gland orifices are blocked with inspissated secretions that are not easily expressible on massage.

Meibomian keratoconjunctivitis is distinguished from other seborrheic blepharitis by a shorter duration of symptoms at the time of presentation and a more pronounced inflammation of the eyelids. The anterior/ciliary aspect of the lids are frequently only minimally involved with deposition of an oily scurf. The prominent feature is diffuse inflammation around the meibomian glands, which are dilated with retained meibum that is not easily expressed. The orifices of the glands are obstructed and pout with inspissated secretions. There is a marked inflammation around the meibomian glands and the orifices. This constellation of findings gives an overall picture of thickened and inflamed eyelids.

In addition to the lid findings, an important associated condition found in these patients is keratoconjunctivitis sicca (KCS). The symptoms of KCS are similar to and may be masked in the complaints of patients whose predominant problem is related to blepharitis. However, patients with chronic blepharitis have been shown to have changes in the composition of meibum, which may lead to alterations in the tear film, thereby predisposing these patients to associated ocular surface problems related to an unstable tear film. Nonetheless, recent studies have documented the occurrence of concurrent KCS in patients with chronic blepharitis in 25 to 60 per cent of the patients. It is imperative to look for an accompanying dry eye state in these patients and to treat it when present.

Extensive culturing, both aerobic and anaerobic of normals and patients with each form of chronic blepharitis, has revealed a significantly greater incidence of colonization by Staphylococcus aureus species only in the staphylococcal and mixed staphylococcal/seborrheic subgroups. There was no significant difference in the incidence of coagulase-negative staphylococcus (C-NS), Propionibacterium acnes, or any other bacteria isolated in any of the various patient subgroups compared to normal controls. Cultures of meibum revealed no evidence to support its role as a reservoir for bacterial colonization in any form of chronic blepharitis.

The possible role of bacterial lipases in modifying the composition of meibum and differences in the biochemical composition of meibum in the various subgroups of chronic blepharitis have also been examined. Careful studies have shown that there is a higher percentage of C-NS species capable of de-esterifying fatty waxes and cholesteryl-esters in the types of chronic blepharitis with meibomian gland involvement. In addition, it has been demonstrated that the free fatty acid component of meibum in patients with meibomian gland involvement varies from that of normals. The exact role of bacterial lipases and variation in the biochemical components of meibum as factors in the pathophysiology of chronic blepharitis, as possible markers for diagnosis, or as new avenues for therapeutic intervention requires further elucidation.

THERAPY

Supportive. First and foremost in the treatment of chronic seborrheic blepharitis is the understanding by both patient and physician that the disease is chronic, occasionally marked by bothersome exacerbations of symptoms and signs, and one for which there is presently no definitive cure. The goals of therapy are to control the disease, maintain vision, and avoid secondary complications. There are characteristically two phases of therapy. The first is to bring the disease under control and then subsequently to taper the therapy to a minimum that will provide long-term control of the chronic disease process and prevent exacerbations.

Ocular. The mainstay of treatment for chronic blepharitis is lid hygiene. This must be carefully explained and demonstrated so that it will be performed properly by the patient. The aim is to remove eyelid debris adequately and restore normal meibum secretory flow.

A warm and moist compress, usually a facecloth run under a flow of water as warm as can be tolerated, should be applied to the closed eyelids for 5 to 10 minutes. As the compress cools, it should be rewarmed in a similar fashion. After the use of compresses, the tarsus containing the meibomian glands should be massaged against the globe in patients with meibomian gland involvement. This is best accomplished by rotating the tip of a finger placed just outside the lashes and applying enough pressure to the tarsus against the globe to express the contents of the glands onto the lid margin. In patients with meibomianitis, it is hoped that the warm compresses will raise the temperature of the lid sufficiently to surpass the melting point of the abnormal retained meibum. Debris is then scrubbed from the lid margin with a clean facecloth and a nonirritating baby shampoo or a commercially available eyelid scrub. The lids are then rinsed until free of shampoo. Initially, lid hygiene is required two to four times a day, but may then be tapered to once or twice a day, usually upon waking and at bedtime. The most important time to perform lid hygiene is in the morning, as the debris collects and builds up on the lids when closed during sleep.

The use of topical antibiotic is recommended in all patients except those with seborrheic blepharitis alone. The recommended topical antibiotic treatment is detailed in the next article on staphylococcal blepharitis.

Systemic. The use of systemic antibiotics in addition to local treatment is indicated in all patients with primary meibomianitis or patients with secondary meibomianitis unresponsive to local therapy. Initially, patients with meibomianitis require 250 mg of oral tetracycline four times a day to bring the inflammation under control. The mechanism of action is felt to be related to tetracycline-induced bacterial lipase inhibition and decreased free fatty acid production. In patients with secondary meibomianitis or meibomian keratoconjunctivitis without associated rosacea, the dose of tetracycline may frequently be tapered and discontinued over the course of 3 to 4 months. However, patients with meibomian keratoconjunctivitis in conjunction with rosacea frequently require a chronic low daily dose of 250 mg to control their symptoms.

In patients with seborrheic blepharitis, it is important also to look carefully for concurrent seborrheic dermatitis. The degree and distribution of involvement vary greatly from patient to patient. Involvement of the scalp, retroauricular, nasolabial, brow, and sternal regions has all been reported in patients presenting with seborrheic blepharitis. In patients who have an associated significant dermatitis, consultation with a dermatologist is prudent.

Ocular or Periocular Manifestations

Conjunctiva: Concretions; cystic changes; hyperemia; papillary hypertrophy.
Cornea: Marginal cicatrization; pannus formation; punctate epithelial erosions; punctate epithelial keratitis.
Eyelids: Chalazion; collarettes; debris; edema; erythema; hordeolum; madarosis; meibomian gland changes; poliosis; scaling.

PRECAUTIONS

In patients who require systemic tetracycline, appropriate precautions need to be taken. Tetracycline should be taken on an empty stomach, i.e., 1 hour before or 2 hours after meals. If associated gastrointestinal irritation presents as a side effect, 100 mg of doxycycline twice a day, which may be taken with food, can be substituted. Tetracycline or doxycycline should not be administered to children because of the effect on dental enamel. In addition, it is contraindicated in pregnant women and lactating mothers. When tetracycline is contraindicated, erythromycin is a suitable alternate.

COMMENTS

Although a chronic and bothersome disease, seborrheic blepharitis when correctly diagnosed and treated can usually be brought under control and the patient's symptoms reduced greatly. It is imperative that the chronic nature of the disease be explained to the patient so that false expectations may be put to rest at the onset. The close interrelationship between eyelid, tear film, and an intact and healthy ocular surface demands that careful attention to the tear film and ocular surface be paid when examining patients with blepharitis so that associated or underlying abnormalities do not go undiagnosed and untreated.

References

Bowman RW, Dougherty JM, McCulley JP: Chronic blepharitis and dry eyes. Int Ophthalmol Clin 27: 27–35, 1987.
Dougherty JM, McCulley JP: Analysis of free fatty acid component of meibomian secretions in chronic blepharitis. Invest Ophthalmol Vis Sci 27: 52–56, 1986.
Dougherty JM, McCulley JP: Bacterial lipases and chronic blepharitis. Invest Ophthalmol Vis Sci 27: 486–491, 1986.
Leibowitz HM, Capino D: Correspondence to the editor. Arch Ophthalmol 106:720, 1988.
McCulley JP: Blepharoconjunctivitis. Int Ophthalmol Clin 24:65–77, 1984.
McCulley JP: Blepharitis associated with acne rosacea and seborrheic dermatitis. Ann Ophthalmol 17:53–57, 1985.
McCulley JP, Dougherty JM: Bacterial aspects of chronic blepharitis. Trans Ophthalmol Soc UK 105:314–318, 1986.
McCulley JP, Sciallis GF: Meibomian keratoconjunctivitis. Am J Ophthalmol 84:778–793, 1977.
McCulley JP, Dougherty JM, Deneau DG: Classification of chronic blepharitis. Ophthalmology 189:1173–1180, 1983.
Pollack FM, Goodman DF: Correspondence to the editor. Arch Ophthalmol 106:719–720, 1988.

STAPHYLOCOCCAL AND MIXED STAPHYLOCOCCAL/ SEBORRHEIC BLEPHAROCONJUNCTIVITIS 372.20

DONNA D. BROWN, M.D.,
and JAMES P. McCULLEY, M.D.

Dallas, Texas

Blepharoconjunctivitis is one of the most commonly encountered diseases in ophthalmology. In 1982, a classification of chronic blepharitis was introduced that has served as a good framework on which to build our thinking about this disease. This classification scheme was based on careful ophthalmologic and dermatologic examinations, cultures of the lids and conjunctiva, and lipid studies. The categories described were (1) staphylococcal; (2) seborrheic-alone, mixed seborrheic/staphylococcal, seborrheic with meibomian seborrhea, and seborrheic with secondary meibomianitis; (3) primary meibomianitis; and (4) other, including atopic, psoriatic, fungal, etc.

Chronic staphylococcal blepharoconjunctivitis characteristically has a history of waxing and waning signs and symptoms that are usually of shorter duration than those of other types of blepharoconjunctivitis. These patients are usually younger, with a mean age of 42 compared with 51 years for other types of blepharitis. It is more common in females, with 80 per cent of cases occurring in females. Staphylococcal blepharitis is characterized by collarettes and less greasy debris than seborrheic blepharitis. The eyelids of patients with staphylococcal blepharitis alone or in association with seborrheic blepharitis are more inflamed than other subgroups. There is a lack of associated dermatologic abnormalities in the staphylococcal group. Results of aerobic and anaerobic cultures from lids and conjunctiva showed that the only blepharitis groups with a significant percentage of positive cultures for *Staphylococcus aureus* were the clinically defined groups of staphylococcal and mixed staphylococcal/seborrheic groups.

In the pure staphylococcal group, blepharitis is treatable and possibly curable, in contrast to other forms of the disease, which usually can only be controlled. Clinical features of staphylococcal blepharoconjunctivitis include inflamed eyelids with erythema and sometimes edema along the anterior ciliary portion of the lid and not uncommonly madarosis. The eyelid margin is frequently involved as well. There may be telangiectatic changes along the lid margin.

Crusting of the lashes occurs with collarettes surrounding individual cilia. Anterior or posterior hordeola occur intermittently. Fifteen per cent of patients develop bulbar and tarsal conjunctival changes, including injection and, when chronic, papillary hypertrophy of the tarsal conjunctiva. With acute exacerbation, a follicular response may develop over the inferior tarsal plate. A keratitis characterized by punctate epithelial erosions involving the inferior one-third of the cornea, which may be secondary to staphylococcal exotoxin, may occur. Other possible causes of this keratitis include an abnormal blink mechanism or destabilization of the tear film. A more severe keratitis leading to phlyctenular changes and corneal ulcers can occur. Infiltrates with a marginal keratitis may also occur. Fifty per cent of patients with staphylococcal blepharoconjunctivitis also have associated keratoconjunctivitis sicca that may have an associated corneal punctate epitheliopathy.

Forty-six per cent of eyelid cultures from patients with clinical staphylococcal blepharoconjunctivitis have been found to be positive for *S. aureus* and 92 per cent were positive for *S. epidermidis*. Conjunctival cultures were 23 per cent positive for *S. aureus*, and 85 per cent were positive for *S. epidermidis*. Other organisms that may be cultured are *Corynebacterium* species, *Propionibacterium acnes*, and other *Propionibacterium* species.

Mixed seborrheic/staphylococcal blepharoconjunctivitis exhibits signs of both types of blepharitis and an equal male/female distribution. The debris is characteristically an oily, greasy crusting on the anterior lid and collarettes on the lashes. Characteristically, these patients have a chronic history, with periods of significant exacerbation of the inflammatory process representing the chronic seborrheic component and exacerbation occurring when the bacterial component becomes active. They typically have more inflammation than in seborrheic blepharoconjunctivitis alone.

Approximately 35 per cent of patients with mixed seborrheic/staphylococcal blepharoconjunctivitis have associated keratoconjunctivitis sicca. Most of the patients in the seborrheic/staphylococcal group also have seborrheic dermatitis. Keratoconjunctivitis is common in mixed seborrheic/staphylococcal blepharoconjunctivitis with mild inferior tarsal conjunctival papillary hypertrophy, bulbar conjunctival injection, punctate epithelial erosions over the inferior third of the cornea, and rarely follicular hypertrophy over the inferior tarsal conjunctiva.

More than 80 per cent of patients in the mixed group have positive eyelid cultures for *S. aureus*, and 50 per cent have positive conjunctival cultures. Almost all patients have positive lid cultures for *S. epidermidis*, and more than 80 per cent have positive conjunctival cultures.

THERAPY

Ocular. Although treatment for most types of chronic blepharitis is aimed at control rather than cure, treatment for staphylococcal blepharitis may be curative. There may, however, be intermittent recurrences or exacerbation of the inflammatory process after the initial treatment has led to resolution. In such patients, a less intense maintenance regimen of treatment is required. Treatment usually requires 2 to 8 weeks of intense therapy, with lessening of treatment after the initial, more severe signs have resolved.

The most important component of the initial therapy is the use of warm compresses aimed at loosening debris and liquefying meibomian secretions, which are followed by eyelid scrubs. It is important to instruct patients carefully in the technique of applying hot compresses and performing eyelid scrubs. The first step is to soak a clean facecloth in water as warm as the eyelids can tolerate and to apply it to the eyelid. This should be done for 5 to 10 minutes, rewarming the wash cloth as often as is necessary to maintain the warm temperature. Applying the compress loosens the debris and liquefies sebaceous secretions, which may then be removed with the lid scrubs with an innocuous soap, such as one of the baby shampoos or commercial lid scrubs. Some advise using diluted baby shampoo, but full-strength shampoo is recommended. Again, a wet facecloth is used to which shampoo has been applied, with the patient scrubbing in a left-to-right motion. Both the upper and lower lids are scrubbed, as well as the eyebrows. Excess soap is rinsed away. A facecloth is preferred over a cotton-tipped applicator because frequently either the globe is traumatized with the cotton-tipped applicator or the patient does not adequately perform scrubs because of the fear of traumatizing the globe. The patient should realize that the purpose of the compresses and scrubs is to remove the debris from the lids and lashes. The soap scrubs also help lyse bacterial membranes and thus decrease the bacterial count.

With clinical evidence of infection, cultures of the eyelids and conjunctiva may be done, but are not required. Most staphylococcal species are sensitive to bacitracin, erythromycin, chloramphenicol, gentamicin, and tobramycin. In patients with clinical evidence of staphylococcal or mixed seborrheic/staphylococcal blepharoconjunctivitis, an antibiotic ointment may be used empirically after the lid scrubs. Bacitracin, which is highly effective against all staphylococci, is the first drug of choice. It is bactericidal and has a low incidence of associated allergic reactions. Erythromycin is the second drug of choice. The aminoglycosides are usually reserved for sight-threatening conditions and for treating resistant organisms.

The antibiotic ointment is rubbed into the eyelid along the lash margin after the warm compresses and scrubs have been done. One-fourth inch of ointment is also instilled into the inferior cul-de-sac at bedtime. With this approach, no ointment is instilled into the tear film during the day. If the infectious process is severe enough to raise concern about the potential for developing a corneal infection, an aminoglycoside is recommended because it is available in both ointment and drop form. This allows the use of only one antibiotic with the ointment being rubbed into the lids and lashes, as well as being instilled into the cul-de-sac at bedtime; the drops are applied to the ocular surface during the day. Tobramycin is recommended because of its broad spectrum of action and relative lesser toxicity.

After the initial inflammatory signs have resolved, the above regimen may be tapered to a frequency that keeps the condition stable. The compresses and lid scrubs are frequently required on a long-term basis and are most beneficial in the morning because during the night organisms and debris have accumulated on the lids. Occasionally, long-term antibiotic ointment is required, in which case the weekly alteration of antibiotic may decrease the risk of selection of resistant organisms.

Rarely, topical steroids are used when hypersensitivity infiltrates persist, but they are not recommended for routine use in acute or chronic blepharitis. Most often, eyelid hygiene and antibiotic therapy will clear hypersensitivity keratitis. The use of steroids is risky and especially so in dry-eyed patients as further suppression of the immune system may create an increased potential for infec-

tion. In any patient, severe bacterial or fungal infections may occur with long-term steroid use.

Occasionally, especially in children, systemic antibiotic therapy is necessary. Erythromycin, a cephalosporin, or a penicillinase-resistant penicillin may be used in these patients.

Sensitivity testing for *Staphylococcus* species has shown some strains to be resistant to sulfonamides. Therefore, based on current knowledge of mechanisms that lead to the development of staphylococcal blepharoconjunctivitis, sulfonamides are not recommended as an antimicrobial agent.

Not uncommonly, keratoconjunctivitis sicca (KCS) coexists with staphylococcal blepharitis. It is sometimes difficult to diagnose during an acute episode of staphylococcal blepharitis, but is later discovered after the blepharitis is under control. Topical preservative-free artificial tear therapy should be initiated when KCS coexists. Occasionally other measures, such as punctal occlusion, may be required. Patients appropriately treated for KCS may be less likely to develop recurrent bacterial blepharoconjunctivitis.

Treatment of mixed seborrheic/staphylococcal blepharoconjunctivitis is aimed at control and not cure. Warm compresses followed by application of either bacitracin or erythromycin ointment two to four times daily as described for the treatment of staphylococcal blepharoconjunctivitis should be done. It usually takes 2 to 8 weeks of intense therapy initially to control inflammation. After this time, tapering treatment to a frequency necessary to control inflammation is the goal. The regime typically consists of warm compresses and lid scrubs once or twice daily. Thirty to thirty-five per cent of patients also have KCS that requires therapy.

Ocular or Periocular Manifestations

Conjunctiva: Conjunctivitis; injection; mucous or mucopurulent discharge; phlyctenules.

Cornea: Epithelial erosions; marginal infiltrates; phlyctenules; ulceration; vascularization.

Eyelids: Chalazion; collarettes; debris; edema; erythema; hordeolum; madarosis; meibomian gland changes; poliosis; scaling.

Other: Seborrheic skin changes in mixed seborrheic/staphylococcal blepharoconjunctivitis.

Precautions

Medicamentosa conjunctivitis secondary to the topical treatment may occur, especially in patients with associated keratoconjunctivitis sicca. The patient may be reacting to the antibiotic or possibly to a preservative in a tear preparation. Preservative-free tear preparations are recommended. Discontinuation of all potentially toxic medication should result in significant improvement. Allergies to bacitracin and erythromycin are unusual but may occur, necessitating alternate therapy. Of course, patients may be allergic to a systemic antibiotic being used, especially penicillin, and a careful history to elicit this information is necessary. Chemicals present in the soaps may cause hypersensitivity and allergic reactions.

Occasionally, more severe keratitis, phlyctenular changes, and even corneal ulceration may occur that require more intensive therapy.

COMMENTS

Blepharoconjunctivitis is a condition that is commonly encountered by the ophthalmologist. Close observation of the specific eyelid, conjunctival, and corneal changes will help determine the type of blepharoconjunctivitis present, thus determining the type of treatment regimen best suited for the individual patient. Eyelid hygiene and topical antibiotics as described earlier cure or control staphylococcal blepharoconjunctivitis or mixed seborrheic/staphylococcal blepharoconjunctivitis. When these therapies fail, attention should be given to other possible diagnoses or additional underlying problems. Occasional discontinuation of all therapy and culturing or reculturing of the eyelids and conjunctiva will aid in the diagnosis and treatment.

References

Bowman RW, Dougherty JM, McCulley JP: Chronic blepharitis and dry eyes. Int Ophthalmol Clin 27: 27–35, 1987.

Bowman RW, Miller K, McCulley JP: Diagnosis and treatment of chronic blepharitis. *In* Focal Points: Clinical Modules for Ophthalmologists. American Academy of Ophthalmology, 1988.

Dougherty JM, McCulley JP: Comparative bacteriology of chronic blepharitis. Br J Ophthalmol *68*: 524–528, 1984.

McCulley JP: Blepharoconjunctivitis. Int Ophthalmol Clin 24:65–77, 1984.

McCulley JP, Sciallis GF: Meibomian keratoconjunctivitis. Am J Ophthalmol *84*:788–793, 1977.

McCulley JP, Dougherty J, Deneau DG: Classification of chronic blepharitis. Ophthalmology *89*: 1173–1180, 1982.

Smolin G, Okumoto MA: Staphylococcal blepharitis. Arch Ophthalmol *95*:812–816, 1977.

Thygeson P: Complications of staphylococcal blepharitis. Am J Ophthalmol *68*:446–449, 1969.

SYMBLEPHARON 372.63

DAVID W. VASTINE, M.D.,
and ROBERT L. STAMPER, M.D.

San Francisco, California

Symblepharon is an adhesion between the palpebral conjunctiva and the bulbar conjunctiva or cornea. It may be localized and of little clinical consequence or large enough to interfere with normal eyelid or extraocular muscle function. Although congenital symblepharon is a rare occurrence, symblepharon formation is usually a result of trauma, radiation, burns, severe inflammation, or infection. Chemical burns, Stevens-Johnson syndrome, and ocular cicatricial pemphigoid are some of the conditions that cause the more severe adhesions. If the cornea is directly involved or the symblepharon leads to exposure, vision may be impaired. The pathogenesis seems to be intimately related to the direct apposition of two denuded epithelial surfaces, conjunctival and/or corneal, which results in scarring, shrinkage, and adherence of the tissues. Disruption of a single epithelial surface rarely leads to the formation of symblepharon.

THERAPY

Ocular. Symblepharon is easier to prevent than to treat. The denuded surfaces must be separated until re-epithelialization has occurred. Classical prophylaxis and early treatment have been to break early symblepharon with a glass rod or, if none is available, with an ordinary glass thermometer (the opposite end of the bulb). Rectal thermometers are preferred (over oral) as they are thicker and less likely to break in the eye. This symblepharon lysis must be done at least twice a day to be effective. Often, this kind of regimen is inconvenient, if not impossible, to accomplish. In severe cases, the glass rod lysis technique cannot keep up with the formation of adhesions.

A variety of conformers and stents have been advocated to keep the raw surfaces separated. None of these devices is entirely satisfactory because they do not prevent subepithelial fibrosis, which may lead to extrusion. A methylmethacrylate conformer with a large central opening to allow clearance of the cornea during normal ocular movement is recommended. The denuded conjunctival surfaces are separated by the conformers or stents, and thus, healing can occur without the formation of adhesions. In children or uncooperative patients, sterilized Saran wrap, thin silicone sheeting, plastic surgical drape, or other similar thin, flexible, plastic material can be used to separate the conjunctival surfaces. The material must be sutured in place deep in the fornix so that it covers the affected conjunctival surface.

Conjunctival Z-plasty and other simple conjunctival manipulations may be helpful in the less severe cases once the disease process is quiescent. In the more severe cases, some form of mucous membrane grafting must be used. Any surgical repair should be delayed until the acute process or trauma has been controlled. Use of anti-inflammatory agents or immunosuppression is often required to control the acute disease. The mucous membrane graft replaces the denuded epithelium of at least one of the two surfaces. Although the mucous membrane of the mouth has been the most commonly used source, excellent results have been reported with autologous conjunctiva taken from the ipsilateral conjunctiva when the defect is small or from the contralateral conjunctiva when the defect is large. Use of autologous conjunctival grafts seems to limit subepithelial fibrosis and graft and submucosal shrinkage. This preferred approach provides more normal surface characteristics and tear function than buccal or labial mucosa. In those cases where foreshortening of the conjunctival fornices causes extrusion of a conformer, either conjunctival or mucous membrane grafting may be the only way to prevent serious lid deformity or extraocular muscle restriction.

Ocular or Periocular Manifestations

Cornea: Exposure keratitis; keratoconjunctivitis sicca; opacity.
Eyelids: Adhesions; deformity; distichiasis; entropion; lagophthalmos.
Lacrimal System: Epiphora; punctal occlusion.
Other: Blinding; diplopia; restriction of extraocular motility.

PRECAUTIONS

All attempts at therapy assume that the basic disease process is nonprogressive. If the process is progressive, almost all attempts at therapy will fail. The glass rod lysis technique should be used in the first 24 to 48 hours. In mild to moderate cases, the lysis should be continued until the opposing conjunctival surfaces have re-epithelialized as demonstrated by the lack of fluorescein staining of the conjunctival or corneal surface. If symblepharon continues to form despite lysis, a rigid donut-shaped conformer can be placed into the conjunctival fornices. Although normal eyes frequently do not tolerate a conformer, a soft bandage contact lens placed on the cornea before fitting may make the scleral shell tolerable. If the eye cannot tolerate the conformer or the newly forming symblepharon expels the conformer, a mucous membrane graft should be considered, once the situation has stabilized.

No therapeutic measures will work if there is extensive subconjunctival fibrosis or the fornices have been significantly shortened. All subconjunctival fibrosis should be carefully and completely resected before attempting any other type of treatment. If conjunctival grafts are used, only the mucosa should be transplanted, and care should be taken to leave at least 1 to 2 mm of normal conjunctiva at the limbus at the donor site. In cases of severe alkali burns when all normal cell transformation has been eliminated, a deliberate attempt to transfer the limbal conjunctiva and Palisades of Voyt is recommended to supply normal stem cells for proper corneal and conjunctival cell transformation and re-epithelialization. A partial-thickness mucous membrane graft from the mouth can be used, although this material is more likely to shrink and may be cosmetically and functionally less satisfactory than autologous conjunctiva.

In the late cicatricial stages, dry eye syndrome with severe irritation, distichiasis, trichiasis, and ankyloblepharon may occur. In addition, the puncta may scar over with resultant epiphora. Localized procedures, such as repeat punctal dilation, repair of associated ankyloblepharon, and conjunctival deformities, may be necessary.

COMMENTS

Symblepharon is one of the most frustrating eyelid problems. Progressive disease essentially prevents satisfactory therapy. Extensive scarring will hinder therapy unless it is totally removed. However, with diligence, attention to detail, and cooperation on the part of the patient, many cases previously consigned to blindness can be helped.

References

Belin MW, Hannush SB: Mucous membrane abnormalities. *In* Abbott RL (ed): Surgical Intervention in Corneal and External Diseases. Orlando, Grune & Stratton, 1987.

Duke-Elder S (ed): System of Ophthalmology. St. Louis, CV Mosby, 1965, Vol VIII, pp 6–8.

Kaufman HE, Thomas EL: Prevention and treatment of symblepharon. Am J Ophthalmol 88: 419–423, 1979.

Schwab IR, Stamper RL: Symblepharon lysis with a thermometer. Am J Ophthalmol 90:270–271, 1980.

Thoft RA: Keratoepithelioplasty. Am J Ophthalmol 97:1, 1984.

Vastine DW, Stewart WB, Schwat IR: Reconstruction of the periocular mucous membrane by autologous conjunctival transplantation. Ophthalmology 89:1072–1081, 1982.

TRICHIASIS 374.05

F. T. FRAUNFELDER, M.D.

Portland, Oregon

Trichiasis is a condition in which the eyelashes are directed toward the globe and irritate the cornea and the conjunctiva. The primary problem caused by trichiasis is secondary corneal abrasion or ulceration with or without infection, and it may well be one of the leading causes of corneal ulcers in the older age group. The condition most often occurs secondary to chronic blepharitis, but may also be associated with trachoma, cicatricial pemphigoid, alkaline burns, and eyelid injuries. One needs to differentiate trichiasis from entropion, since the latter condition is treated with a different surgical procedure.

THERAPY

Surgical. Epilation provides temporary relief of trichiasis. Since the normal growth cycle of an eyelash is 6 to 8 weeks, the abnormal eyelashes usually recur within a few weeks. In general, epilation is only a temporizing measure, and a more definitive procedure usually needs to be done.

Electrolysis can be effective; however, few ophthalmologists use electrolysis for more than a few lashes primarily because it takes a great deal of time to put an electrode down each individual hair follicle. In addition, scarring and secondary entropion may occur with this type of treatment. Various electrolysis instrumentations are available; some are satisfactory, whereas others, especially the battery-operated instruments, can be erratic in function.

Cryotherapy is rapidly gaining in popularity. If at least half or the whole lid needs to be treated, cryospray is preferred. The cryoprobe is satisfactory if less than half of the lid needs to be treated.

If over half of the lid margin is to be treated, equal parts of bupivacaine and lidocaine with epinephrine are injected along the base of the hair follicles, and a topical local anesthetic is applied to the eye. A thermocouple may be placed at the base of a few hair follicles, usually temporally if all the hair follicles in the lid are to be destroyed. The lid is partially everted so that the spray can be directed perpendicular to the lid margin. A Berke-Jaeger shield should be placed in the cul-de-sac to protect the eye. The area over the thermocouple is frozen to −15°C, and the size of the iceball to achieve this temperature is then used as a guide or template to freeze the areas away from the thermocouple. The iceball is extended along the lid margin by slowly advancing the nasal edge of the ice using an intermittent or "pulse" spray technique. The ice front (iceball on the skin) is advanced by moving the tip a little more nasally.

After a complete thaw, the freezing procedure is repeated. Cryosurgery in this manner is used only to treat extensive trichiasis. Once the physician has done a few of these procedures, the thermocouple is seldom used since one rapidly gets a "feel" for the amount of freeze which is necessary.

When treating lesions that involve less than half of the lid margin, anesthesia is rarely necessary. Under the slit lamp, a felt-tipped pen is used to mark the skin in the areas corresponding to the lashes to be destroyed. The lid is pulled away from the eye by grasping the skin with thumb and forefinger. The probe is placed on the lash line adjacent to the skin mark. The liquid nitrogen is started a second before touching the skin so the probe immediately "sticks" to the area to be frozen. Freezing is continued until a 3-mm diameter iceball (from the edge of the probe tip to the end of the ice front) forms. The area is allowed to thaw until the probe can be removed, or the ice front continues from the cryogen still in the probe, and the probe is "cracked" off the skin. The lid should be kept away from the eye to allow for a "slow" thaw. The tip of the probe is washed with sterile solution to warm the probe tip so that the tip will easily adhere or freeze to the lid on the second application. The procedure is repeated, and the involved lashes are removed manually. This procedure is repeated in multiple areas as needed.

Other cryogens, such as nitrous oxide, are satisfactory and in common usage. Greater areas of frozen tissue are necessary to obtain the results of liquid nitrogen.

Laser thermoablation of ciliary follicles and excision of individual follicles may be alternatives in the treatment of localized trichiasis. Argon laser treatment is performed with a spot-size beam of 50 to 200 μm, of 0.1- to 0.2-second duration, and 1,000 to 1,200 mW power under local anesthesia. Approximately 12 to 15 applications are necessary to destroy the follicles. This technique is suitable when a few fine cilia are involved. Excision of individual follicles is ideal for resecting the occasional aberrant eyelash that may appear at the edge of a wound after horizontal shortening of an eyelid or eyelid laceration; however, this technique is tedious and time consuming.

Ocular or Periocular Manifestations

Conjunctiva: Chemosis; hyperemia.
Cornea: Erosion; punctate keratopathy; ulcer.
Other: Foreign body sensation; lacrimation; photophobia.

PRECAUTIONS

When using any cryogen, measures must be taken to prevent damage to the cornea and adjacent skin from either runoff or direct contact with the probe. The use of a nonmetallic lid plate may be helpful. Edema of the lid and cheek may persist for as long as 1 week after treatment. Occasionally, patients may experience moderately severe pain beginning 5 to 6 hours after using the combination of a long- and short-acting local anesthetic. In general, aspirin alone is all that is necessary to control this pain. There is a loss of sensory nerves in this area within 18 to 24 hours, which may last for 6 to 12 weeks. Cutaneous depigmentation is an invariable sequela to cryotherapy, and repigmentation may take as long as 2 years to occur. Cryotherapy has not been used extensively in African-American patients because of the marked susceptibility of pigment cells to freezing and the subsequent problem of depigmentation. By applying the cryoprobe to the lid margin and conjunctival surface instead of to the skin, it is possible to limit the degree of depigmentation in highly pigmented lids. Thus, the complication of cosmetic blemish and the risk of actinic damage and its sequelae are decreased. However, because of the possible complications of chronic or permanent vitiligo, seldom should a darkly pigmented eyelid be treated with cryotherapy.

Lids that have been badly scarred from previous disease, prior surgery, or radiation should be treated with caution, as segmental necrosis or aggravation of an entropion may occur. In patients with sensory or motor deprivation of the lid, care should be taken when treating with cryosurgery, since there have been reported cases of lid necrosis.

If ocular pemphigoid is in an acute phase, it should not be treated because doing so may precipitate symblepharon. However, ocular pemphigoid may be treated if the disease is in a quiescent phase.

Caution should be used when treating young patients with cryotherapy because atrophic skin in the area treated is a potential complication. In some patients, thinning of the eyelid may occur. In addition, this thinning may, in rare instances, cause problems with the tear film, since the meibomian glands are destroyed. Yet, this complication is rarely found. The main problem with freezing large areas with cryosurgery is that, at each end of the areas that are not treated, there appears to be some constricte of the lid and an entropion-type process occurs, causing trichiasis to each side of the frozen area.

COMMENTS

If large segments of the lashes are to be treated, cryosurgery should be done with epinephrine in the local anesthetic, since it enhances the loss of lashes. The larger lashes seem to be more cryosensitive than the fine lanugo hairs. Individual lashes can be treated by isolated refreezing with a small probe.

Cryotherapy with the retina cryoprobe instrumentation using double-freeze thaws has

not been very successful. Although nitrous oxide units are satisfactory, liquid nitrogen is preferred because only one cryo unit is needed and a much smaller area of the lid is frozen, although much more intensely.

References

Awan KJ: Argon laser treatment of trichiasis. Ophthalmic Surg 17:858–660, 1986.
Delaney MR, Rogers PA: A simplified cryotherapy technique for trichiasis and distichiasis. Aust J Ophthalmol 12:163–166, 1984.
Johnson RLC, Collin JRO: Treatment of trichiasis with a lid cryoprobe. Br J Ophthalmol 69:267–270, 1985.
Majekodunmi S: Cryosurgery in treatment of trichiasis. Br J Ophthalmol 66:337–339, 1982.
Peart DA, Hill JC: Cryosurgery for trichiasis in black patients. Br J Ophthalmol 70:712–714, 1986.
Wolfley D: Excision of individual follicles for the management of congenital distichiasis and localized trichiasis. J Pediatr Ophthalmol Strabismus 24:22–26, 1987.

XANTHELASMA 374.51
(Xanthelasma Palpebrarum, Xanthoma Palpebrarum)

F. T. FRAUNFELDER, M.D.

Portland, Oregon

Xanthelasma is a form of cutaneous xanthomatosis that is characterized by the presence of rounded or oval, dull yellow, slightly elevated plaques in the skin of the eyelids. The lesions are usually located near the inner canthi and generally begin on the upper eyelid. Xanthelasma may first appear in early middle age, often in females. A minority of patients with xanthelasma have frank hyperlipidemia, although a tendency toward enhanced atherogenicity may be seen. However, these lesions commonly occur in patients with essential hyperlipidemia and in patients, such as diabetics, with secondary hyperlipidemia. Histologically, these lesions are composed of foamy histiocytes. Histochemical analysis of the lipid vacuoles in early lesions may closely resemble that of serum lipids, but the contents of older lesions differ from that of the serum lipids. In chronic lesions, there is an increase in the number of fibroblasts and long-spaced collagen.

THERAPY

Supportive. A serum lipid profile should be investigated to rule out hyperlipidemic syndromes and other associated diseases, such as cirrhosis, diabetes mellitus, and arteriosclerosis. Dietary treatment of hyperlipidemia may induce a regression in xanthelasma, although this response may be quite delayed.

Surgical. Cosmetic surgery on eyelids with xanthelasma can be performed. After removal of the xanthelasma from the eyelid, the defect is usually closed in a horizontal direction without causing a lid deformity. When the xanthelasma is large, a musculocutaneous flap may be used to close the defect.

An alternative method of treatment of xanthelasma is application of 75 per cent trichloroacetic acid or dichloroacetic acid. A local anesthetic is first applied beneath the lesion. Each end of a double-tipped cotton applicator is dipped into either the acidic or saturated sodium bicarbonate solution. Using the tip dipped in the acidic solution, this solution is applied in an ever-increasing circular pattern, starting from the center until the edges of the lesion are reached. After 5 to 10 seconds, the treated area turns white and bubbles. Using the tip dipped in the neutralizing solution, the treated area is sponged off with sodium bicarbonate. For 4 to 6 weeks, the treated area will form scabs, which often peel off; however, excellent cosmetic results will be attained with this method. Small areas can be retreated again, if necessary.

PRECAUTIONS

If a patient with hyperlipidemia has xanthelasma, treatment of hyperlipidemia may improve the systemic disease, but will not necessarily cause the xanthelasma to regress. However, patients treated with the cholesterol-lowering drug lovastatin have experienced a decrease in intensity and possible resolution of the xanthelasma.

Cosmetic revision of the lid lesions may need to be performed, especially with recurrences of xanthelasma. It is this type of problem that may result in a lid deformity, such as ectropion.

COMMENTS

Xanthelasma should be a signal to the physician that carbohydrate and lipid metabolism states require further investigation. Although 60 per cent of patients with xanthelasma have normal serum lipid profiles, more subtle changes in lipid composition might be found. In fact, several other abnormalities of plasma lipoproteins have been reported, which may indicate a tendency toward enhanced atherogenicity. Therefore, normolipidemic patients with xanthelasma may indeed possess a less obvious, yet potentially clinically significant disturbance of lipid metabolism.

References

Crawford JB: Neoplastic and inflammatory tumors of the eyelids. *In* Duane TD (ed): Clinical Ophthalmology. Philadelphia, Harper & Row, 1987, Vol IV, pp 3:10–12.

Depot MJ, et al: Bilateral and extensive xanthelasma palpebrarum in a young man. Ophthalmology *91*:522–527, 1984.

Hosokawa K, et al: Treatment of large xanthomas by the use of blepharoplasty island musculocutaneous flaps. Ann Plast Surg *18*:238–240, 1987.

Roederer GO, Bouthillier D, Davignon J: Xanthelasma palpebrum and corneal arcus in octogenarians. New Engl J Med *317*:1740, 1987.

Rouffy J, et al: Xanthelasma palpebrarum and dyslipoproteinaemia: Two retrospective studies. Ann Dermatol Venereol *109*:231–235, 1982.

Smith RE, Lee JS: The cornea in systemic disease. *In* Duane TD (ed): Clinical Ophthalmology. Philadelphia, Harper & Row, 1980, Vol IV, pp 15:15–17.

SECTION 24

GLOBE

ANOPHTHALMOS 743.00

DANIEL MARCHAC, M.D.

Paris, France

Anophthalmos with complete absence of ectodermal and mesodermal tissues of the eye is extremely rare. In fact, microphthalmos resulting from arrest of development of the eyeball at various stages of growth of the optic vesicle is usually observed; such malformation is sometimes sporadic or congenital (autosomal dominant or recessive). External influences during pregnancy, such as rubeola or toxoplasmosis, may also play a role in some cases.

The development of the orbital region is correlated with the outgrowth of the eyeball, as demonstrated by a reduction in the volume of the orbit up to 60 per cent of the normal size after removal of eyeballs in embryos.

In microphthalmos, the orbit does not usually develop properly, with resultant loss of projection of the adjunct frontal and malar areas, particularly a small bony cavity. This small bony cavity does not allow proper fitting of a prosthesis.

THERAPY

Ocular. Anophthalmos or microphthalmos is a pediatric ocular emergency. If started in the first months of life, the use of conformers can enlarge a small cavity and allow the orbit to attain almost normal proportions. A very careful follow-up with rapidly increasing sizes of conformers will generally produce a cavity adaptable to fitting a prosthesis and a good-sized orbit.

Surgical. In early stages, an inflatable expander is the preferable solution to enlarge the orbit if the conformers were not tolerated. The expansion is best done during the first year of life. The expander—a small empty silicone bag—is placed deep into the orbit and is linked by a tube passing through the lateral wall to a filling chamber placed in the temporal area. The expansion is carried out on a weekly basis by gradually filling the expander with saline solution. Many technical problems may be encountered, but excellent results can be achieved this way.

If enlargement with conformers or with expanders was not undertaken or was not successful, the orbit remains too small to fit a

prosthesis. The lateral orbital wall needs to be displaced medially, as it is located just where the lateral part of the cavity should be created. To create a cavity in front of the bone is a poor solution, that will not give enough depth for a suitable prosthesis to project the eyelids properly. The bony orbit generally has to be enlarged in three directions: laterally, superiorly, and inferiorly. This surgical orbital expansion can be obtained by an osteotomy, dividing the existing orbital rim in three parts in a step-like fashion that allows bony contact where expanded.

A limited intracranial approach is necessary when the orbital roof has to be elevated, which is not always the case. This operation is performed through a scalp bicoronal approach. The creation of a good-sized socket is done in a second stage. Final touch-up with skin and cartilage grafts are often necessary to lengthen the eyelids.

Ocular or Periocular Manifestations

Conjunctiva: Shallow lower fornix; small socket.

Extraocular Muscles: Absent.

Eyelids: Absent levator function; absent lid fold; orbicularis contraction; shortening in all directions.

Globe: Decreased or absent amount of tissue.

Lacrimal System: Absent ducts and glands.

Orbit: Medial deviation; reduced orbital rim; small optic foramen.

PRECAUTIONS

Results are often disappointing because of an immobile prosthesis, as well as such eyelid malformations as short and immobile eyelids. Early treatment is advocated for enlargement of eyelid structures.

COMMENTS

Surgical creation of a good-sized cavity and subsequent enlargement of eyelids are long and complicated processes. If the patient is more than a few years old, however, this reconstruction is the only choice. The psychologic benefit makes it worthwhile; it should deal first with the bony problems. Early treatment with conformers should certainly be ap-

604

plied whenever possible to try to avoid this surgical procedure.

References

Kennedy RE: The effect of early enucleation on the orbit in animals and humans. Am J Ophthalmol 60:277–306, 1965.

Marchac D, et al: Orbital expansion for anophthalmia and micro-orbitism. Plast Reconstr Surg 59: 486–491, 1977.

Mustardé JC: The orbital region. *In* Mustardé JC (ed): Plastic Surgery in Infancy and Childhood. Edinburgh, Livingstone, 1971, pp 232–237.

Mustardé JC: The orbital rim. *In* Mustardé JC, Jancsous IT (eds): Plastic Surgery in Infancy and Childhood. Edinburgh, Churchill Livingston, 1988, pp 150–155.

Rodallec A, et al: Anophtalmies congenitales. Contrôle de l'ostéogenèse par prosthèse expansive intraorbitaire. J Fr Ophtalmol 11:661–668, 1988.

BACTERIAL ENDOPHTHALMITIS 360.0

SID MANDELBAUM, M.D.,

New York, New York

and RICHARD K. FORSTER, M.D.

Miami, Florida

Bacterial endophthalmitis is inflammation of intraocular tissues resulting from bacterial infection. The most frequent cause is recent intraocular surgery during which the organisms apparently gain access to the interior of the eye. Bacterial endophthalmitis may also occur after penetrating ocular trauma; endogenously via blood-borne spread from a site of infection elsewhere in the body; or in eyes with filtering blebs, even years after surgery, presumably by penetration of the organisms through the bleb. Infectious endophthalmitis may result from any ocular penetration, no matter how innocuous it might seem; self-sealing traumatic or surgical corneal perforations, surgical posterior capsulotomies, and even cutting of deeply placed sutures after ocular surgery have all resulted in endophthalmitis. The vitreous is the intraocular site most involved by the well-developed infectious process; this is the case even when the injury or surgery is confined to the anterior segment or the patient is phakic. Therefore, the cornerstone of laboratory evaluation is to sample and culture the vitreous if infectious endophthalmitis is considered.

Infectious endophthalmitis should be suspected whenever inflammatory signs and symptoms after intraocular surgery or penetrating trauma are out of proportion to those anticipated in the particular clinical setting.

Bacterial endophthalmitis usually presents between 1 and 4 days after surgery or trauma. Pain is a prominent symptom, although it is not invariably present. Signs include lid and conjunctival edema, hyperemia, exudate, corneal edema, and especially anterior chamber reaction (often with hypopyon) and vitreitis. Less virulent bacteria, especially *Staphylococcus epidermidis*, may incite a lower-grade inflammatory reaction that may not become evident for a week or more postoperatively. *Propionibacterium acnes* particularly, but other less virulent bacteria as well, has been associated with a syndrome of painless, usually progressive intraocular inflammation that may not present for months after surgery; some of these cases presented only after Nd: YAG posterior capsulotomy. Organisms are thought to have been sequestered in the peripheral capsular bag and then liberated either spontaneously or by the laser capsulotomy. Endophthalmitis caused by fungi is also indolent, often with an apparent latent period of days to weeks after surgery or trauma before the inflammation becomes evident.

Patients with blebs either as a result of glaucoma filtration surgery or that are inadvertently created during cataract extraction are susceptible to bacterial endophthalmitis months or years after their surgical procedure. Potential sources of infection include normal conjunctival flora, episodes of bacterial conjunctivitis, use of contact lenses, and contaminated medicine dropper bottle tips. Many ophthalmologists are not sensitive to the possibility of bacterial endophthalmitis in these eyes; therefore, they are often treated with steroids for presumed idiopathic uveitis until an infectious etiology is considered.

The most common organism isolated from eyes with endophthalmitis in the postoperative period is *Staphylococcus epidermidis*. More virulent organisms that may be isolated include *S. aureus*, *Proteus*, and *Pseudomonas*. Organisms previously felt to be nonpathogens are increasingly being isolated, which suggests that under appropriate circumstances almost any organism is capable of causing endophthalmitis. *Bacillus cereus* has been associated with fulminant endophthalmitis after ocular trauma. In the group of patients with filtering blebs, streptococci seem to be responsible for the majority of cases; the most common gram-negative organism isolated has been *Hemophilus influenzae*, a very unusual cause of endophthalmitis in other circumstances.

The differential diagnosis of bacterial endophthalmitis includes the many entities that cause intraocular inflammation. Postoperatively, retained lens material, particularly nuclear fragments, incarceration of iris or vitreous in the wound, inflammation induced by intraocular lens or other foreign body, and exaggerated postoperative iridocyclitis are all causes of sterile inflammation. Blood in the vitreous may simulate inflammation. An unrecognized retained foreign body is a potential cause of posttraumatic inflammation. If there is suspicion that the eye is infected, however, it is safest to culture aqueous and vitreous and begin therapy as outlined below.

THERAPY

Ocular. Patients with suspected infected endophthalmitis require sampling and culture of at least vitreous (preferably also aqueous) and institution of broad-spectrum antibiotic therapy. It is generally agreed that since antibiotics appropriately administered directly into the vitreous cavity seem safe both experimentally and clinically and achieve the highest intravitreal antibiotic levels, this is the preferred route. Systemic, periocular, and topical antibiotics are usually also administered, although the beneficial effect of these additional routes of antibiotic delivery is uncertain.

Patients with presumed infectious endophthalmitis are usually given retrobulbar or general anesthesia; a beveled incision partially through peripheral clear cornea may then be made with a razor-blade knife under microscopic control. A 25-gauge needle attached to a tuberculin syringe is then used to enter the anterior chamber carefully through this incision, and 0.1 to 0.2 ml of aqueous is aspirated. The aqueous is immediately inoculated on fresh culture media. Vitreous is generally obtained through a separate pars plana sclerotomy site, 3.5 to 4.0 mm posterior to the limbus. It can be obtained by gentle aspiration using a 22-guage needle attached to a syringe, inserted through the sclerotomy into the midvitreous cavity; careful manipulation of the needle may be required to locate a pocket of liquid vitreous. In those cases where an adequate vitreous sample cannot be obtained by gentle aspiration, a mechanized vitreous cutter is inserted through the sclerotomy and a localized vitrectomy performed. The vitrectomy sample is reserved for culture. The remainder of the vitrectomy specimen, usually diluted with the infusion solution, is passed through a filter system to concentrate it, and the disposable filter paper is inoculated directly onto the culture media. All samples should be inoculated onto culture media as soon as possible, preferably in the operating room. Lid and conjunctival cultures should also be obtained either at or before surgery.

Once aqueous and vitreous samples have been obtained, the previously prepared antibiotics for intravitreal injection, each in a separate tuberculin syringe with a 25-gauge needle, are then slowly injected into the midvitreous, inserting each needle through the sclerotomy site. For initial therapy, 100 μg of gentamicin* in 0.1 ml (or 400 mg of amibacin in 0.1 ml) and 1.0 mg of vancomycin* in 0.1 ml are injected. The sclerotomy and keratotomy sites are closed by one suture.

In addition to intravitreal antibiotics, systemic, periocular, and topical antibiotics are usually given. The additive benefit of systemic antibiotics is uncertain, but they are commonly administered intravenously during hospitalization. The combination of an aminoglycoside (1 mg/kg every 8 hours) and cefazolin (1 gm every 6 hours) has been used although many strains of staphylococci have become resistant to cefazolin. If an aminoglycoside and vancomycin are administered systemically, caution must be used due to potential systemic toxicity. Subconjunctival injections of 40 mg of gentamicin*, 125 mg of cefazolin*, or 25 mg of vancomycin* may be repeated daily. Fortified eyedrops of gentamicin§ (9.1 mg/ml), cefazolin§ (50 mg/ml), or vancomycin§ (50 mg/ml) may be administered every hour or two. Topical cycloplegic agents should also be given. Adjustments in antibiotic therapy are made based on antibiotic sensitivities of the isolated organism and clinical response. In particular, the administration of toxic antibiotics should be discontinued if the isolated organism is sensitive to less toxic agents.

Steroids are helpful in reducing the inflammation caused by the infectious process. Although not universally recommended, intravitreal dexamethasone*, 400 μg in 0.1 cc, is administered by many experienced practitioners along with initial intravitreal antibiotics. Oral prednisone may be given in a daily dose of 40 to 80 mg with rapid tapering after 7 to 10 days, depending on the extent of intraocular inflammation and the patient's medical status. Topical corticosteroids should be administered after the initial diagnostic and therapeutic intervention to reduce anterior segment inflammation. Steroids should not be used at all if, based on the clinical picture, fungal infection is a consideration.

Surgical. The role of vitrectomy in the management of bacterial endophthalmitis remains uncertain. Vitrectomy may be a technically difficult procedure in infected eyes because of limited visualization of intraocular structures, uveal engorgement, and retinal edema. Nonetheless, it may offer advantages in terms of removal of infectious organisms and inflammatory debris and elimination of loculated pockets, thus improving fluid and antibiotic circulation in the vitreous cavity. It has been shown in an experimental model of endophthalmitis that the vitreous was sterilized more frequently in eyes with combined vitrectomy and antibiotic administration than in those given antibiotics alone. The risks of vitrectomy under these circumstances must be balanced against the potential benefits for each individual case. Initial vitrectomy is recommended in advanced infections at presentation. For less advanced inflammation, initial treatment with intravitreal and ancillary antibiotics (after diagnostic sampling) may be equally effective. If improvement is not apparent within 36 to 48 hours or if a virulent organism, such as *Pseudomonas*, is isolated, vitrectomy is then performed, taking care to avoid the friable retinal surface. Antibiotics are carefully injected at the completion of the vitrectomy. The role of vitrectomy is being evaluated in a NIH-sponsored multicenter study, the Endophthalmitis Vitrectomy Study.

PRECAUTIONS

Endophthalmitis is certainly a condition that is better prevented than treated. Careful preoperative attention to blepharitis, the lacrimal system, and infections elsewhere in the body is mandatory. Generally preoperative conjunctival cultures are not routinely performed. The use of preoperative topical antibiotics seems to decrease the incidence of endophthalmitis, but none of the studies performed to date has been definitive. The optimum dosing schedule and best antibiotic to use for preoperative prophylaxis, if selected, are uncertain. Preoperative instillation of 5 per cent povidone-iodine solution into the conjunctival sac with subsequent irrigation reduced the incidence of culture-positive endophthalmitis in one study; this finding awaits confirmation. Subconjunctival antibiotics are administered at the conclusion of surgery by most practitioners, although their use entails some risk and their benefit in preventing postoperative infection is still uncertain. Antibiotics cannot replace meticulous attention to sterility within the operating suite. In patients with filtering blebs, the use of contact lenses presents an additional hazard to be avoided, if at all possible. In cases of intraocular trauma, systemic and periocular antibiotics are recommended, although no firm data are available indicating their effectiveness in preventing endophthalmitis.

Clinically, the two major determinants of visual prognosis in bacterial endophthalmitis are the virulence of the infecting organism and the rapidity of institution of appropriate therapy. Most ophthalmologists are reluctant to make this diagnosis in their postoperative patients; precious time is often lost when a "wait-and-see" attitude is adopted. A hypopyon is not an invariable finding early in the course of endophthalmitis; too frequently, patients are followed with unexplained intraocular inflammation until they develop a hypopyon, at which time the diagnosis of endophthalmitis is first entertained. If infection is a possibility, the vitreous should be cultured. Aqueous cultures alone have repeatedly been shown to be inadequate; on the other hand, there are only very rare cases of positive aqueous cultures when the vitreous culture is negative. Empiric antibiotic therapy without vitreous cultures or in less than full doses is rarely appropriate. The response is likely to be incomplete, and further diagnostic studies and therapy are compromised. If the local environment does not provide sufficient experience or facilities to manage a case of endophthalmitis, it is in the best interest of both the patient and physician to make a prompt referral to a center where such facilities are available.

Care needs to be taken in the administration of intravitreal antibiotics; dilutions must be carefully done so that the final concentration is correct. Intravitreal antibiotics must be injected slowly to avoid retinal damage from the impact of the antibiotic solution. Doses of systemic cephalosporins and aminoglycosides must be reduced if renal function is compromised. Even if renal function is normal, the serum creatinine should be checked periodically when systemic aminoglycosides are administered.

COMMENTS

Although advances in the treatment of endophthalmitis in the form of more effective antibiotics, anti-inflammatory agents, and drug delivery systems may be anticipated, the greatest positive effect on the outcome of any individual case will almost certainly be that of earlier diagnosis and institution of therapy. In some respects, infectious endophthalmitis is similar to infectious meningitis; serious consideration of either diagnosis obligates the initiation of diagnostic and therapeutic measures. Although these measures are invasive, the risk:benefit ratio is such that their early application in cases of suspected endophthalmitis is a more prudent approach than observation until the diagnosis is certain.

References

Cottingham AJ Jr, Forster RK: Vitrectomy in endophthalmitis. Results of study using vitrectomy, intraocular antibiotics, or a combination of both. Arch Ophthalmol 94:2078–2081, 1976.

Diamond JG: Intraocular management of endophthalmitis. A systematic approach. Arch Ophthalmol 99:96–99, 1981.

Doft BH: The endophthalmitis vitrectomy study (Editorial). Arch Ophthalmol 109:487–488, 1991.

Driebe WT Jr, Mandelbaum S, Forster RK, et al: Pseudophakic endophthalmitis. Diagnosis and management. Ophthalmology 93:442–448, 1986.

Flynn HW Jr, Pflugfelder SG, Culbertson WW, Davis JL: Recognition, treatment and prevention of endophthalmitis. Sem Ophthalmol 4:69–83, 1989.

Forster RK: Endophthalmitis. In Duane TD (ed): Clinical Ophthalmology. Philadelphia, Harper & Row, 1987, Vol IV, pp 24:1–21.

Forster RK, Abbott RL, Gelender H: Management of infectious endophthalmitis. Ophthalmology 87:313–319, 1980.

Jeglum EL, Rosenberg SB, Benson WE: Preparation of intravitreal drug doses. Ophthalmic Surg 12:355–359, 1981.

Meisler DM, Mandelbaum S: Propionibacterium-associated endophthalmitis after extracapsular cataract extraction. Ophthalmology 96:54–61, 1989.

Menikoff JA, Speaker MG, Marmor M, Raskin EM. A case-control study of risk factors for postoperative endophthalmitis. Ophthalmology 98:1761–1768, 1991.

O'Day DM, et al: *Staphylococcus epidermidis* endophthalmitis. Visual outcome following noninvasive therapy. Ophthalmology 89:354–360, 1982.

Peyman GA, Vastine DW, Raichand M: Symposium: Postoperative endophthalmitis. Experimental aspects and their clinical application. Ophthalmology 85:374–385, 1978.

Speaker MG, Menikoff JA: Prophylaxis of endophthalmitis with topical povidone-iodine. Ophthalmology 98:1769–1775, 1991.

Speaker MG, Milch FA, Shah MK, et al: Role of external bacterial flora in the pathogenesis of acute postoperative endophthalmitis. Ophthalmology 98:639–650, 1991.

Starr MB: Prophylactic antibiotics for ophthalmic surgery. Surv Ophthalmol 27:353–373, 1983.

FUNGAL ENDOPHTHALMITIS 360.1

WOODFORD S. VAN METER, M.D.,
and JACK L. HOLLINS, M.D.

Lexington, Kentucky

Although fungi rank behind bacteria and viruses in overall incidence as a cause of ocular infection, they often produce greater structural and functional damage to the eye. Fungal endophthalmitis is slowly progressive, rather than fulminant, and complications of fungal endophthalmitis are exacerbated by the propensity of fungi to mimic other infections or neoplastic diseases thereby delaying diagnosis and treatment.

Fungal endophthalmitis can be exogenous, when the infection is associated with an external source, such as penetrating trauma, previous intraocular surgery, or inoculation of the eye through an infected cornea or sclera, or endogenous from the hematogenous spread of fungal infection to the eye from elsewhere in the body. Sources for endogenous fungal endophthalmitis are intravenous drug abuse, a compromised immune system, or an infected indwelling catheter, shunt, or prosthesis.

The time from intraocular inoculation to clinical endophthalmitis averages 10 to 14 days, although the time can be more or less depending on the size of the inoculum, the competency of the patient's immune defense mechanisms, and the concomitant administration of corticosteroids or antifungal agents during the infection period. Early symptoms of fungal endophthalmitis may include conjunctival injection with varying amounts of pain and decreased vision. Objective findings are caused by host inflammation due to fungal elements and include anterior chamber cells and flare, hypopyon, vitreous cells, vitreous clouds or veils, and white plaques on the pars plana, lens capsule, or intraocular lens. More fulminant infections may cause fibrinous membranes in the anterior chamber and vitreous veils, snowballs, or calcific plaques in the posterior segment. Endogenous fungal endophthalmitis may be associated with a white fluffy retinal infiltrate with or without retinal hemorrhage. There may be variable extension of a retinal infiltrate into the vitreous, depending on the stage of the infection and the capacity of the host immune response.

In suspected fungal endophthalmitis, aqueous and vitreous samples for smears and cultures are very important for identification of the infecting organism. A vitreous specimen cultured on multiple media should be considered the first stage in treatment of any case of fungal endophthalmitis. It is usually unwise to initiate broad-spectral antifungal therapy for suspected fungal endophthalmitis without first making every effort to identify the causative organism, because different fungal elements may respond differently to the various antifungal agents. Because resolution of infection can be slow and the patient's clinical condition can deteriorate even after appropriate therapy is instituted, it is advantageous to know that the infecting organism is sensitive to the treatment offered.

A careful history can often assist with identification of the causative organism. Septate filamentous fungi, such as aspergillus and *Fusarium*, are common after trauma. *Aspergillus* has a high frequency among grain farmers or poultry breeders. Infections due to *Candida*, a yeast, can be endogenous or exogenous, but *Candida* endophthalmitis is often associated with *Candida* infection elsewhere in the body. *Paecilomyces* can cause chronic low-grade endophthalmitis after cataract surgery, but is rare.

The importance of positive identification of the causative organism cannot be overemphasized. A vitreous tap or vitreous biopsy specimen filtered through a millipore filter or centrifuged and plated on a slide will concentrate any organisms present. Filtering or centrifugation improves the chances of positive identification over a vitreous tap that is immediately plated on a slide without an attempt to concentrate the organisms. In its middle to late stages fungal endophthalmitis can produce calcific plaques on the iris, capsular bag, intraocular lens, or pars plana. The incidence of positive cultures is greatly increased if biopsy or aspiration can be directed toward vitreous clouds or calcific plaques, rather than blindly aspirating clear vitreous specimens. Anterior chamber aspirates yield a reduced incidence of positive cultures compared to vitreous aspirates. A vitreous sample is therefore essential, whereas an anterior chamber aspirate may not be helpful.

Vitreous specimens should be inoculated onto blood agar, chocolate agar, liquid brain heart infusion (BHI), and thioglycollate broth at 37°C and at 25°C specimens should be inoculated for Sabouraud's agar, blood agar, and BHI with gentamicin. Cultures should always be held at least 2 weeks for observation. Some laboratories routinely discard cultures that have no growth after 48 hours. Cultures for suspected fungal endophthalmitis discarded before 14 days may be falsely read as negative.

THERAPY

Systemic. Initial therapy should include removal of any infecting exogenous agent and treatment of fungal keratitis, scleritis, or any systemic condition predisposing to fungal endophthalmitis. Every effort should be made to identify a specific organism, so that treatment can be directed more efficaciously toward the offending agent (see sections on endophthalmitis due to specific fungus).

Treatment of fungal endophthalmitis consists of topical, subconjunctival, intravenous, and intravitreal administration of antifungal agents. Because of the limited corneal penetration of most topical antifungal agents, because of local complications associated with subconjunctival injections* of antifungal drugs, and because of the systemic side effects of intravenous administration, vitrectomy to identify the affecting agent and remove the infected tissue combined with intravitreal injection* of antifungal drugs is the most efficacious treatment.

Drugs available for intravenous treatment for fungal endophthalmitis are amphotericin B and miconazole. Amphotericin B binds to cell membrane sterols, increasing cell membrane permeability and causing leakage of cell contents and cell death. Amphotericin B‡ is administered intravenously in dextrose and water because it precipitates in saline solution. Because of the undesirable systemic side effects of amphotericin B, a 1-mg test dose administered in 100 cc of D_5W over 1 hour is given first. If there is no severe reaction to the test dose, the test dosage can be followed with a therapeutic dose of 0.5 mg/ kg/day (30 to 40 mg average daily dose) given in four divided doses every 6 hours. If nausea or side effects are particularly troublesome, extending the infusion time to every 8 hours may be helpful. Premedication of the patient with aspirin, diphenhydramine, and/ or meperidine may reduce or eliminate uncomfortable side effects. Miconazole, a first-generation imidazole, binds to sterols in fungal cell membranes and is effective against a wide spectrum of fungi. Miconazole is usually administered intravenously with a total daily dosage of 0.6 to 1.8 gm/day given in three divided doses.

Oral antifungal agents are flucytosine, ketoconazole, and fluconazole. Flucytosine is effective against *Candida* and *Cryptococcus* species and is synergistic with amphotericin B. Flucytosine can be administered orally 100 mg/kg/day given in four divided doses.

However, drug resistance to flucytosine has been noted in up to 50 per cent of fungal isolates tested with this drug. Blood flucytosine levels should be measured and the dose of flucytosine adjusted if toxic levels (greater than 100 to 150 mc/ml) are obtained. Elevated liver enzymes and hepatomegaly occur in 50 per cent of patients on flucytosine, but resolve after the drug is stopped.

Ketaconazole is an effective oral antifungal agent with a broad spectrum of activity. Ketoconazole is supplied in 200-mg tablets and is administered orally in a single daily dose of 200 mg per day (400 mg for severe infection). Ketoconazole requires an acid pH in the stomach for absorption, and patients who are receiving antacids or histamine H_2 blockers may not be suitable candidates for this drug.

Fluconazole, a third-generation imidazole, is given orally in a single dose of 50 to 100 mg per day. Fluconazole has good antifungal antibody, but ingestion of this drug over several weeks can cause severe depression that is clinically significant and may necessitate its discontinuance.

Ocular. Ocular treatment consists of the topical and subconjunctival application* of antifungal agents. Topical ophthalmic antifungal agents do not provide useful intravitreal levels, but can be used to treat fungal keratitis or scleritis while the endophthalmitis is treated with vitrectomy and intravitreal injection. Natamycin 5 per cent ophthalmic suspension is available for the treatment of corneal ulcers. Natamycin is similar to amphotericin B in its activity, and if natamycin cannot be used, amphotericin B 0.2 per cent topical solution* can be used until natamycin is obtained. In cases of fungal keratitis refractory to natamycin or amphotericin B therapy, a miconazole* 1 per cent solution prepared from undiluted intravenous miconazole can be administered topically hourly. There is poor vitreous penetration of subconjunctival drugs, and the risk of local side effects from the subconjunctival injection of antifungal compounds makes subconjunctival administration questionably useful as an adjunctive therapy. Subconjunctival injections are not as efficacious as intravenous or intravitreal administration. Subconjunctival injection of amphotericin B* in a dosage of 0.75 to 4.0 mg in 1.0-mm aqueous suspension can be given, but is painful. Miconazole, 5 or 10 mg of undiluted intravenous preparation in 1 cc, can also be injected subconjunctivally.* The half-life of intraocular amphotericin B in patients who have not undergone vitrectomy is approximately 1 week, and repeat injection should be delayed until after the half-life period is ended. Patients who are aphakic and have undergone vitrectomy may have rapid clearing, and a second dose should be administered in 24 hours.

Miconazole can be injected intravitreally* 40 mg, but is not often used because of the good ocular penetration of oral ketoconazole.

Subconjunctival injections are not as efficacious as intravenous or intravitreal administration. Subconjunctival injection of amphotericin B* in a dosage of 0.75 to 4.0 mg in 1.0 mm aqueous suspension can be given, but is painful. Miconazole, 5 mg of undiluted intravenous preparation in 1 cc, can be injected subconjunctivally.*

Intraocular injection of amphotericin B or miconazole is the most efficacious means of drug delivery for fungal endophthalmitis, but should be deferred until sufficient cultures have been taken to identify the causative organism. The intravitreal dosage of amphotericin B is 5 mcg in 0.1 ml. The half-life of amphotericin B in patients who have not undergone vitrectomy is approximately 1 week, and repeat injection should be delayed until after the half-life period is ended. Patients who are aphakic and have undergone vitrectomy may have rapid clearing, and a second dose should be administered in 24 hours. Miconazole 40 mcg in 0.1 ml can be injected intravitreally.* For severe infections and/or if there is no known causative organism, amphotericin B and miconazole can be administered together.

Surgical. Vitrectomy is helpful in most cases of fungal endophthalmitis to facilitate culture of the causative organism, remove the bulk of the infective organisms, sterilize the vitreous cavity, and improve aqueous circulation into the vitreous to circulate therapeutic drug molecules and wash out offending fungal elements. In cases of recurrent infection or inflammation in patients with an intraocular lens, the intraocular lens implant and entire centrifugation or filtration of vitreous specimens can concentrate the organisms and improve the chances of a positive culture. The capsular bag should be removed for culture and to reduce potential scaffolding for infection. The efficacy of obtaining identifiable cultures from blind removal of clear vitreous is low, but aspiration of white clouds, calcific plaques, or opacified portions of residual capsule improves the chances of a positive culture of the offending organism. Chronic low-grade postoperative fungal endophthalmitis can be associated with multiple negative cultures unless specific identifiable vitreous plaques or opacities can be identified, removed, and cultured. Fungal elements can often be cultured from the capsular bag or from residual capsule elements when there is no specific vitreous pathology other than minimal cells in postoperative fungal endophthalmitis.

PRECAUTIONS

Amphotericin B has toxic systemic side effects, and patients should be carefully monitored for serum electrolytes and kidney function parameters. A small percentage of patients may develop a transient rise in liver enzymes with ketoconazole or flucytosine. Fluconazole can result in serous depression if treatment extends beyond several weeks, but it remits after the drug is stopped.

Decisions regarding the use of topical corticosteroids can be complex, but in general steroid therapy has no place in the management of fungal endophthalmitis unless the causative organism has been isolated and definitively identified and specific therapy to which the organism is sensitive has been instituted. Corticosteroids can inhibit the host response to the infecting organism, thereby promoting undesirable progression of the infectious process. Excessive inflammatory host responses can be highly destructive and produce undesirable permanent structural alterations in the eye. The careful use of topical or systemic corticosteroids may be indicated to mediate these inflammatory changes once the infection has been controlled.

COMMENTS

The essentials of current treatment of fungal endophthalmitis are identification of the causative organism from culture of vitrectomy or vitreous tap specimens and subsequent treatment with vitrectomy, intraocular amphotericin B or miconazole injection, or ketoconazole. When doing a vitreous tap or injecting intravitreal antifungal agents, care should be taken to avoid the crystalline lens and peripheral retina and to make certain that the dosage of antifungal agents is correct.

References

Bauman WC, D'Amico DJ: Surgical techniques in diagnosis and management of suspected endophthalmitis. J Int Ophthalmol Clin 32:113–128, 1992.

Brod RD, et al: Endogenous Candida endophthalmitis: Management without intravenous amphotericin B. Ophthalmology 97:666–674, 1990.

Cusumano A, et al: Mycotic infection of the capsular bag in post operative endophthalmitis. J Cat Refract Surg 17:503–505, 1991.

Forester RK, Abbott RL, Gelender H: Management of infectious endophthalmitis. Ophthalmology 87:313–319, 1980.

Foster CS: Miconazole therapy for keratomycosis. Am J Ophthalmol 91:622–629, 1981.

Foster CS, et al: Ocular toxicity of topical antifungal agents. Arch Ophthalmol 99:1081–1084, 1981.

Jones DB: Therapy of post surgical fungal endophthalmitis. Ophthalmology 85:357, 1978.

McGuire LW, et al: Fungal endophthalmitis: An experimental study with a review of seventeen human ocular cases. Arch Ophthalmol 109:1289–1296, 1991.

Plugfelder SC, et al: Exogenous fungal endophthalmitis. Ophthalmology 95:19, 1988.

NANOPHTHALMOS 743.10

ROBERT J. BROCKHURST, M.D.

Boston, Massachusetts

Nanophthalmos is a rare bilateral type of microphthalmos that usually shows an autosomal recessive hereditary pattern. In contrast to the more common form of microphthalmos, which is usually unilateral and associated with poor vision and other ocular defects, the nanophthalmic eye is essentially a small eye with microcornea and a crystalline lens of normal (or slightly larger) size. Vision in younger patients who have not yet developed complications is usually normal with a strong (+10 to +20 diopters) hyperopic correction. Patients can easily be recognized by the fact that they wear "cataract glasses," but are phakic.

Since these eyes have a short axial length and diameter (14 to 20 mm), they appear deeply set in the orbits, the palpebral fissures are narrow, and they are difficult to examine and operate on. Because the eyeball has an overall small volume and the lens is of normal size, there is an abnormally large lens/eye volume ratio (LEV ratio) of 10 to 30 per cent. In normal eyes, the LEV ratio is about 4 per cent. As a consequence of the large LEV ratio, the anterior chamber becomes compromised, and peripheral anterior synechiae develop, resulting in angle-closure glaucoma.

In all nanophthalmic eyes, the sclera is abnormally thick, shows larger collagen bundles than a normal eye, and contains an abnormally high quantity of proteoglycans or glycosaminoglycans. Nanophthalmos has been reported to occur in the mucopolysaccharidoses, which are characterized by excessive deposits of proteoglycans in the tissues. With aging, the thickened abnormal sclera becomes more sclerotic and causes increased resistance to venous outflow via the vortex veins, as well as the trans-scleral passage of fluids and proteins. These changes result in congestion of the choroidal vasculature and thickening of the choroid. Clinically, it can be recognized by the absence of the normal choroidal vascular pattern. Finally, the congestion becomes so severe that choroidal effusion develops, often anteriorly in a circumferential annular form. This phenomenon causes further embarrassment of the anterior chamber angle by rotating the iris root forward. Measurement of episcleral venous pressure shows normal values.

Thus, it seems that the glaucoma that complicates nanophthalmos is the result of a basic abnormality of the LEV ratio plus an unsuspected peripheral choroidal detachment secondary to resistance to vortex venous drainage. Ultrasound and magnetic resonance imaging studies have confirmed the existence of a peripheral, annular, choroidal detachment before the development of increased intraocular pressure.

Uveal effusion with choroidal and nonrheg-matogenous retinal detachment can occur spontaneously in advanced cases because of the increasing resistance to venous drainage via the vortex veins and the scleral resistance to passage of proteins and fluids from the eye. In patients with glaucoma and peripheral anterior choroidal detachment, surgical procedures that result in a sudden lowering of the intraocular pressure to zero, at the time of surgery, may produce a rapid severe effusion with total retinal detachment 1 to 4 days after the surgery.

THERAPY

Ocular. Medical therapy should be employed in early cases of chronic open-angle glaucoma. Timolol in 0.25 or 0.5 per cent concentration may be used twice a day, as well as other types of beta blockers.

Systemic. Carbonic anhydrase inhibitors, such as acetazolamide, may be used in doses of 250 mg four times a day if the intraocular pressure fails to respond to local therapy alone.

In general, medical treatment of uveal effusion with nonrhegmatogenous retinal detachment has been disappointing, but occasionally patients respond to systemic steroid treatment. A daily dose of 100 mg of prednisone for 1 week followed by 100 mg every other day for an additional 4 to 8 weeks, may result in subsidence of the detachment.

Surgical. Argon and YAG lasers are of value in chronic angle-closure glaucoma that cannot be controlled medically. Iridotomy can be used to relieve the pupillary block. Moreover, surface treatment of the iris results in flattening of the convex iris (gonioplasty), thereby opening the angle so that medical therapy may once again be successful.

Customary retinal detachment procedures for nonrhegmatogenous retinal detachment occurring in nanophthalmic eyes are ineffective. Treatment by scleral resection (to normalize the excessively thick sclera) and sclerotomies to drain suprachoroidal fluid are usually successful. Although Gass (1983) has shown that this procedure is effective if the vortex vein areas are avoided, the choroidal congestion is not relieved and the recurrence rate is significant. If the scleral resection is performed over the vortex veins to relieve the constricting effect of the thick abnormal sclera, the choroidal congestion is relieved and recurrence is rare. In some cases where the retina is very highly detached, the postoperative recovery period can be shortened by draining subretinal fluid at the time of vortex vein decompression.

Ocular or Periocular Manifestations

Anterior Chamber: Shallow; narrow angle; peripheral anterior synechiae.

Choroid: Thickening; choroidal vascular pattern not visible; peripheral choroidal detachment.

Cornea: Decreased diameter.

Eyeball: Small (less than 20 mm in axial length).

Eyelids: Narrow palpebral fissures.

Iris: Forward displacement; poor pupillary dilation.

Lens: Normal or slightly larger than normal.

Optic Nerve: Pallor; cupping.

Orbit: Deeply set eyes.

Refraction: Extremely hyperopic, >6 diopters.

Retina: Macular fold; nonrhegmatogenous detachment.

Sclera: Very thick (2 to 3 mm); high concentration of proteoglycans; larger and more interwoven collagen bundles.

PRECAUTIONS

Miotics may aggravate chronic open-angle glaucoma by increasing the degree of pupillary block. In addition, conventional glaucoma surgery should be avoided because of the significant risk of postoperative malignant glaucoma and retinal detachment. The sudden decompression of the globe aggravates the uveal effusion and may lead to severe retinal detachment. If filtering surgery is necessary, it should be preceded or accompanied by scleral resection, preferably over the vortex veins. Lens extraction may also be followed by retinal detachment; however this complication may be prevented by prior vortex vein decompression.

Peripheral iridectomy and filtering procedures may be followed by malignant glaucoma. Finally, choroidal detachment may be mistaken for malignant melanoma, and as a result unnecessary enucleation may be performed.

COMMENTS

A genetic predisposition causes the eye to fail to grow to proper dimensions, resulting in narrowing of the anterior chamber angle. With age, choroidal elevation in the periphery results in forward displacement of the iris and further embarrassment of the angle. It is possible that vortex vein decompression, which would decrease the peripheral choroidal detachment, might prevent some patients from developing chronic open-angle glaucoma.

References

Allen KM, Meyers SM, Zegarra H: Nanophthalmic uveal effusion. Retina 8:145, 1988.

Bill A: Movement of albumin and dextran through the sclera. Arch Ophthalmol 74:248, 1965.

Brockhurst RJ: Nanophthalmos with uveal effusion: A new clinical entity. Trans Am Ophthalmol Soc 72:371–403, 1974.

Brockhurst RJ: Vortex vein decompression for nanophthalmic uveal effusion. Arch Ophthalmol 98:1987–1990, 1980.

Brockhurst RJ: Cataract surgery in nanophthalmic eyes. Arch Ophthalmol 108:965–967, 1990.

Calhoun FP Jr: The management of glaucoma in nanophthalmos. Trans Am Ophthalmol Soc 73:97–122, 1975.

Gass JDM: Uveal effusion syndrome: A new hypothesis concerning pathogenesis and technique of surgical treatment. Retina 3:159–163, 1983.

Goldberg MF, Duke JR: Ocular histopathology in Hunter's syndrome. Arch Ophthalmol 77:503, 1967.

Good WV, Stern WH: Recurrent nanophthalmic uveal effusion syndrome following laser trabeculoplasty. Am J Ophthalmol 106:234, 1988.

Johnson MW, Gass JDM: Surgical management of the idiopathic uveal effusion syndrome. Ophthalmology 97:778, 1990.

Kimbrough RL, et al: Angle-closure glaucoma in nanophthalmos. Am J Ophthalmol 88:572–579, 1979.

Trelstad RL, Silbermann NN, Brockhurst RJ: Nanophthalmic sclera: Ultrastructural, histo-chemical and biochemical observations. Arch Ophthalmol 100:1935–1938, 1982.

Vine AK: Uveal effusion in Hunter's syndrome: Evidence that abnormal sclera is responsible for the uveal effusion syndrome. Retina 6:57, 1986.

Ward RC, et al: Abnormal scleral findings in uveal effusion syndrome. Am J Ophthalmol 106:139, 1988.

SECTION 25

INTRAOCULAR PRESSURE

APHAKIC AND PSEUDOPHAKIC PUPILLARY BLOCK 365.61

CLAUDIA U. RICHTER, M.D.,
and B. THOMAS HUTCHINSON, M.D.

Boston, Massachusetts

Pupillary block is the obstruction to aqueous humor outflow from the posterior chamber to the anterior chamber of the eye. It causes shallowing of the anterior chamber and, if untreated, the development of peripheral anterior synechiae and chronic angle-closure glaucoma. Treatment must be prompt and vigorous to prevent chronic angle-closure glaucoma. Although pupillary block may develop in the phakic and unoperated eye with iritis and posterior synechiae, it occurs more often after cataract surgery, with or without intraocular lens implantation. Pupillary block may occur after intracapsular and extracapsular cataract surgery; the implantation of anterior chamber, iris plane, and posterior chamber intraocular lenses; and with either peripheral or sector iridectomies.

Aphakic and pseudophakic pupillary block develop when the pupillary aperture and iridectomies are occluded by vitreous, inflammatory membranes, capsular or cortical remnants, and/or an intraocular lens. Inflammation causing iridovitreal, iridocapsular, or iridopseudophakic adhesions is the primary cause of aphakic and pseudophakic pupillary block. A wound leak may contribute to the development of pupillary block by allowing iridovitreal adhesions to develop. After intracapsular cataract extraction, vitreous alone may obstruct patent peripheral iridectomies and cause pupillary block if there is also obstruction to aqueous flow through the pupil, i.e., by vitreous or an intraocular lens.

Pupillary block frequently presents in the first few days to weeks after surgery, but also may appear months to years later. Aphakic pupillary block classically presents with a shallow or flat anterior chamber, elevated intraocular pressure, and vitreous occluding the pupillary aperture and iridectomies. Pseudophakic pupillary block with an anterior chamber intraocular lens presents with a deep central anterior chamber with pupillary iris held posterior to the lens, but a shallow peripheral anterior chamber with an iris bombe configuration. Pseudophakic pupillary block with a posterior chamber lens may have a deep central anterior chamber and peripheral iris bombe or a more uniform shallowing of the anterior chamber with anterior displacement of the intraocular lens. The gonioscopic picture may be quite variable; the filtration angle is usually completely closed, but incomplete or early pupillary block may only cause a narrowing or partial closure of the angle. The intraocular pressure may be low or normal in early pupillary block, due to a wound leak or decreased aqueous production from inflammation or a choroidal detachment.

The differential diagnosis of aphakic pupillary block includes wound leak, choroidal detachment (serous or hemorrhagic), and posterior aqueous entrapment (aphakic malignant glaucoma). A wound leak typically presents with a low intraocular pressure and a positive 2 per cent fluorescein test. A choroidal detachment may mimic pupillary block with shallowing or flattening of the anterior chamber, with or without angle closure, and with a low-to-normal pressure caused by decreased aqueous production. Ultrasonography may help detect peripheral choroidal effusions.

Posterior aqueous entrapment (malignant glaucoma) is similar to pupillary block in its development of a shallow or flat anterior chamber. This condition develops when aqueous humor flow is directed into or behind the vitreous because of increased resistance through the anterior vitreous. The resistance may occur at the level of the ciliary body and has been called "ciliovitreal block." The misdirection of aqueous humor pushes the iris forward, flattens the anterior chamber, and occludes the angle. Thus, both pupillary block and posterior aqueous entrapment have shallow or flat anterior chambers and variable intraocular pressures early in their course, but both ultimately have elevated pressures. The final distinction between these two disorders can only be made by the eye's response to medical and laser treatment or surgery.

The incidence of aphakic and pseudophakic pupillary block may be minimized by careful suture placement to prevent wound leaks and the use of topical steroids to decrease inflammation and minimize synechiae. Basal peripheral iridectomies performed during cataract surgery reduce the incidence of pupillary block.

THERAPY

Ocular. The goals of medical therapy are to break the pupillary block, deepen the an-

613

terior chamber, and prevent chronic angle-closure glaucoma. The first step has traditionally been to move the iris pharmacologically in order to break any adhesions. Cycloplegics (cyclopentolate or tropicamide) with the addition of 2.5 per cent phenylephrine as an active mydriatic are often successful. Alternating miotics and mydriatics may be helpful in breaking synechiae: 4 per cent pilocarpine every 10 minutes for six doses followed by 2.5 per cent phenylephrine and 1 per cent cyclopentolate every half-hour for three doses.

If the intraocular pressure is elevated, a topical beta-adrenergic antagonist (betaxolol, levobunolol, metipranolol, or timolol), apraclonidine, and a systemic carbonic anhydrase inhibitor (250 mg acetazolamide every 6 hours or 50 mg methazolamide every 8 hours) should be used unless systemically contraindicated. Osmotic agents are helpful if the intraocular pressure is quite high. A dosage of 1.5 gm/kg body weight of 45 per cent isosorbide may be given if the patient can tolerate oral therapy, or 1.5 gm/kg body weight of 20 per cent mannitol may be given intravenously. Lowering the intraocular pressure makes the iris more responsive to topical medications, decreases iris congestion, and reduces the "forcefulness" of closure between the iris and the trabecular meshwork. Corneal edema will begin to resolve as the intraocular pressure is reduced. In addition, the antiglaucomatous medications serve to protect both the recently operated wound and the optic nerve from significant compromise. Topical steroids should be used liberally to decrease the inflammatory response and inhibit synechiae formation.

Surgical. A laser iridectomy is usually successful in relieving pupillary block if medical therapy fails. Even if medical therapy relieves the pupillary block, a laser iridectomy should be performed to decrease the possibility of recurrence. Either the neodymium:YAG, argon, or diode laser may be used. However, the neodymium:YAG laser frequently allows more rapid iris penetration and, if available, is the laser of choice. If the cornea is edematous, topical glycerin frequently provides adequate clearing to allow a neodymium:YAG iridectomy. Two or three laser iridectomies are recommended because even neodymium: YAG iridectomies may be occluded by iris folds as a billowing iris returns to its normal position.

If several iridectomies fail to relieve the apparent pupillary block, and a wound leak and choroidal detachment have been eliminated as possible causes of the shallow anterior chamber, the diagnosis is posterior aqueous entrapment. The neodymium:YAG laser can be used to disrupt the anterior hyaloid face and relieve the posterior aqueous entrapment. It can be focused through a large peripheral iridectomy at the presumed peripheral hyaloid using low energy (1 to 2 millijoules) or through a positioning hole in the intraocular lens if one is present and visible. If a peripheral iridectomy is not present or inaccessible, the neodymium:YAG laser can be used to perform a posterior capsulotomy and then to disrupt the anterior hyaloid face centrally.

If ocular and laser therapy fail to relieve the pupillary block or posterior aqueous diversion, surgery is necessary. If the laser is unable to establish a patent peripheral iridectomy because of total flattening of the anterior chamber or severe corneal clouding that is unresponsive to medically lowered intraocular pressure and topical glycerin, a surgical peripheral iridectomy with chamber deepening is indicated. However, if one or more patent laser iridectomies in addition to photodisruption of the hyaloid face fail to relieve the block and deepen the anterior chamber, a surgical vitrectomy or vitreous tap is necessary to relieve the posterior aqueous entrapment.

Retrobulbar anesthesia* should be used cautiously, as these eyes frequently have a recent surgical wound and a congested orbit. The orbital congestion both decreases the effectiveness of retrobulbar anesthesia and increases the risk of retrobulbar hemorrhage. General anesthesia may be necessary for some of these eyes.

A surgical iridectomy should be preceded by deepening the anterior chamber. A paracentesis is performed first, employing a Wheeler or similar knife needle to produce a shelving tract through the peripheral cornea into the anterior chamber. The anterior chamber is reformed by injecting balanced salt solution through the paracentesis wound. Posterior sclerotomies, in one or two lower quadrants, are placed to drain any suprachoroidal fluid. The anterior chamber is again reformed if significant suprachoroidal fluid is found, and removal of fluid from the sclerotomies and injection into the anterior chamber are repeated as necessary to evacuate the suprachoroidal space. If no suprachoroidal fluid is present and the intraocular pressure is elevated, vitreous aspiration or removal may be necessary before the anterior chamber can be deepened.

If the anterior chamber remains deep after its reformation as above and communication exists between the anterior and posterior chambers with the iris in the normal aphakic position, one need not proceed further. If pupillary block persists, injection of aqueous humor into the anterior chamber will cause the iris to funnel posteriorly toward the optic nerve, but will be prevented from entering the posterior chamber by the same obstruction causing the pupillary block. Persistence of pupillary block, indicated by the funneling of the iris, is treated by performing a surgical peripheral iridectomy.

If the anterior chamber is not maintained and there is no flow of aqueous from the posterior chamber after a peripheral iridectomy or if patent laser iridectomies fail to deepen the anterior chamber, posterior aqueous entrapment may be present. A pars plana vitrectomy is performed to excise the central anterior vitreous gel and any vitreous behind the iridectomies to create a pathway for normal anterior flow of aqueous. Residual cortical lens material after extracapsular cataract surgery may cause an inflammatory reaction in the lens equatorial region and contribute to the obstruction to aqueous flow. In these eyes, a small area of zonules and capsule should be removed to ensure an anterior pathway for aqueous humor. In eyes with posterior chamber intraocular lenses, one should remove as few zonules as possible to prevent lens dislocation. If a vitrectomy instrument is not available and the eye is aphakic, discission of the anterior hyaloid through an air bubble into the vitreous gel may re-establish aqueous flow. If a vitrectomy instrument is not available and the eye is pseudophakic, vitreous may be aspirated with a 19-gauge needle.

After the relief of choroidal detachment, pupillary block, or posterior aqueous entrapment, one should check the original cataract incision for a wound leak that might have developed with the operative manipulation of the eye. Sterile 2 per cent fluorescein and slight pressure on the globe are recommended.

Postoperatively, cycloplegics, topical steroids, and topical broad-spectrum antibiotics are used.

Ocular or Periocular Manifestations

Anterior Chamber: Shallow or flat.
Conjunctiva: Variable inflammation.
Cornea: Epithelial and stromal edema; striae (if extensive iridocorneal, vitreocorneal, or pseudophakic-corneal contact or elevated intraocular pressure).
Iris: Bombe configuration; occluded iridectomies; peripheral anterior synechiae; posterior synechiae.
Vitreous: Anterior hyaloid or capsular-cortical remnants adherent to the borders of the pupil and all iridectomies.
Other: Choroidal detachment; elevated intraocular pressure; posterior aqueous pockets.

PRECAUTIONS

It is imperative that the surgeon not become overly aggressive in the use of medical therapy, which may have significant and even catastrophic side effects. Only cautious use of 2.5 per cent phenylephrine is appropriate as this medication may cause a systemic hypertensive crisis. In addition, contraindications to topical ophthalmic beta-adrenergic antagonists, systemic osmotics, or carbonic anhydrase inhibitors must be observed carefully.

Delay in the therapy of pupillary block should be avoided, as spontaneous resolution and reformation of the anterior chamber with an open angle are rare. Furthermore, it is important to remember that a serous choroidal detachment and pupillary block may exist concurrently; the surgeon should not be lulled into complacency by a low or normal intraocular pressure that remains low only as long as the choroidal detachment persists. Although the chamber may deepen slightly after the relief of choroidal detachment, an elevated pressure will invariably result when aqueous secretion returns to normal if the pupillary block has not been treated.

The relief of pupillary block by ocular therapy or laser or surgical iridectomy does not guarantee that the angle will reopen, but only that the chamber will deepen. Significant residual peripheral anterior synechiae may cause chronic angle-closure glaucoma. Gonioscopy should be repeated after resolution of pupillary block or posterior aqueous entrapment. If more than 60 to 90 degrees of the angle remains closed by synechiae, laser gonioplasty may open the angle by causing contraction of the iris stroma. If significant angle closure is unresponsive to laser gonioplasty, especially if the intraocular pressure is elevated, then operative goniosynechialysis may open the angle adequately to minimize or prevent angle-closure glaucoma.

COMMENTS

Visual loss from chronic angle-closure glaucoma following pupillary block can be minimized by efforts to decrease the incidence of pupillary block, prompt and vigorous treatment to ensure that the obstruction to aqueous flow is removed, gonioscopy to detect residual peripheral anterior synechiae, and laser or surgical therapy to break any synechiae. These careful and vigorous efforts will ensure that most patients who do develop aphakic or pseudophakic pupillary block will be left with a functioning trabecular meshwork.

References

Dickens CJ, Shaffer RN: The medical treatment of ciliary block glaucoma after extracapsular cataract extraction. Am J Ophthalmol 103:237, 1987.

Epstein DL, Steinert RF, Puliafito CA: Neodymium-YAG laser therapy to the anterior hyaloid in aphakic malignant (ciliovitreal block) glaucoma. Am J Ophthalmol 98:137–143, 1984.

Forman JS, et al: Pupillary block following posterior chamber lens implantation. Ophthalmic Laser Ther 2:85–97, 1987.

Lynch MG, et al: Surgical vitrectomy for pseudophakic malignant glaucoma. Am J Ophthalmol 102:149–153, 1986.

Mandelcorn MS, Maatanen H: Laser iridotomy in post-traumatic and post-surgical pupillary block: A report of five cases. Can J Ophthalmol 13:163–165, 1978.

Samples JR, et al: Pupillary block with posterior chamber intraocular lenses. Arch Ophthalmol 105:335–337, 1987.

Shrader EC, et al: Pupillary block and iridovitreal block in pseudophakic eyes. Ophthalmology 91:831–837, 1984.

Simmons RJ, et al: Laser gonioplasty for special

problems in angle closure glaucoma. *In* Symposium on Glaucoma. Transactions of the New Orleans Academy of Ophthalmology. St. Louis, CV Mosby, 1981, pp 220–235.

Tomey KF, Traverso CE: Neodymium-YAG laser posterior capsulotomy for the treatment of aphakic and pseudophakic pupillary block. Am J Ophthalmol *104*:502–507, 1987.

Van Buskirk EM: Pupillary block after intraocular lens implantation. Am J Ophthalmol *95*:55–59, 1983.

Werner D, Kaback M: Pseudophakic pupillary-block glaucoma. Br J Ophthalmol *61*:329–333, 1977.

CORTICOSTEROID-INDUCED GLAUCOMA 365.31

JOHN R. SAMPLES, M.D.

Portland, Oregon

Corticosteroids may cause elevated intraocular pressure through any route of administration, including oral, inhaled, topical, and periocular. Individuals vary a great deal in their sensitivity to corticosteroids. Approximately one-third of normal individuals will have some type of pressure elevation in response to the use of corticosteroids. Age seems to be an important factor in determining this; children may be particularly susceptible. Several cases of steroid-induced glaucoma in children have been reported, and in some instances, congenital glaucoma may actually be corticosteroid related.

In addition to the age of the patient, the magnitude of intraocular pressure elevation is determined by dose, route of administration, frequency, duration of treatment, and the predisposition of the individual to respond to corticosteroids. Almost every individual will have glaucomatous optic nerve changes and visual field loss if the duration of exposure is great enough. Since many individuals have a normal optic nerve, a patient with elevated intraocular pressure secondary to corticosteroid therapy may not have any glaucomatous damage. Patients who are already known to have open-angle glaucoma may become refractory to medical treatment.

THERAPY

Ocular. It is important to discontinue corticosteroids when a steroid-induced glaucoma is suspected if the underlying condition will permit. Whether the pressure falls will depend on the concurrent presence of uveitis or other causes that raise the intraocular pressure. Permanent alteration in the trabecular

cells and in the cellular events surrounding outflow may occur as a result of corticosteroid use. Patients with corticosteroid-induced pressure elevations respond to the usual antiglaucoma medications, including miotics, epinephrine, dipivefrin, beta-adrenergic antagonists, and carbonic anhydrase inhibitors. Corticosteroid glaucoma generally does not respond to laser trabeculoplasty.

If an ocular steroid is needed, it is sometimes useful to use a weaker synthetic steroid, such as fluoromethalone, which will cause less pressure elevation for a given amount of anti-inflammatory effect. Topical nonsteroidal anti-inflammatory agents that are potent enough to penetrate the eye and have significant anti-inflammatory action have recently become available. In select cases, they may prove to be useful substitutes for steroids. Topical diclofenac or keterolac may have significant potency as well as a useful anti-inflammatory effect when used four times a day.

The metabolism of steroids in systemic tissues, as well as the eye, seems to be a major determinant of steroid effects and side effects. A major part of the increased potency of steroids, such as dexamethasone systemically, is due to substitutions occurring on the cortisol molecule, some of which decrease degradation and others of which increase binding to steroid receptors. In direct contrast, steroids that are synthesized using progesterone rather than cortisol as the foundation molecule, such as fluoromethalone and medrysone, seem particularly susceptible to degradation. In the eye, both medrysone and fluoromethalone have a lower tendency to raise the intraocular pressure, but they are not considered as efficacious in treating ocular inflammation, probably because of the inactivation due to metabolism.

Surgical. Corticosteroid-induced glaucomas may require filtering surgery if they do not remit. Any decision to perform surgery must be based on the appearance of the visual field, as well as the optic nerve. Occasionally, corticosteroid-induced glaucomas are observed in the presence of a functioning filter or a seton procedure. Glaucomatologists vary in their opinion on whether or not steroid-induced pressure elevations can be a significant problem when an outflow procedure, such as trabeculectomy or a seton procedure, has been performed. It is suggested that a trial off corticosteroids or with a low-potency steroid, such as fluoromethalone, be undertaken. The diagnosis of steroid-induced pressure elevation after filtration should consider other etiologies of bleb failure, such as closure of the internal aspect of the filtering fistula and subconjunctival scarring.

Ocular or Periocular Manifestations

Eyelids: Slight ptosis.
Lens: Cataracts, particularly posterior subcapsular cataracts.

Optic   Nerves: Glaucomatous   optic neuropathy.

Other: Increased intraocular pressure; visual field loss.

PRECAUTIONS

Whenever a patient undergoes corticosteroid therapy, a baseline examination and close follow-up are mandatory. Patients who are given oral prednisone chronically may be particularly at risk and should have an eye examination to ascertain that they have not developed a steroid-induced glaucoma.

Although the side effects of corticosteroids are enumerated above, one should bear in mind that steroid injections can also cause problems because of the preservatives used and because of the direct toxicity of high steroid concentration on certain cell types. Periocular methylprednisone preparations may show steroid-related effects for longer than is generally appreciated.

COMMENTS

Many corticosteroid-induced glaucomas result from the inappropriate use of corticosteroids for minor conditions, such as eye irritation or contact lens discomfort. Also, it is not uncommon for patients who have been treated with oral steroids to have pressure elevations. The failure of a physician to recognize corticosteroid-induced glaucoma may lead to needless visual loss and difficult medical-legal problems.

References

Armaly MF: Effects of corticosteroids in intraocular pressure and fluid dynamics. I. The effect of dexamethasone in the normal eye. Arch Ophthalmol 74:82, 1963.

Armaly MF: Effects of corticosteroids on intraocular pressure and fluid dynamics. II. The effects of dexamethasone in the glaucomatous eye. Arch Ophthalmol 74:92, 1963.

Armaly MF: Statistical attributes of steroid hypertensive response in the clinically normal eye. Invest Ophthalmol Vis Sci 4:187, 1965.

Kass MA, Kolker AE, Becker B: Chronic topical corticosteroid use simulating congenital glaucoma. J Pediatr 81:1175, 1972.

Kwak HW, D'Amico DJ: Evaluation of retinal toxicity in pharmacokinetics of dexamethasone after intravitreal injection. Arch Ophthalmol 110:259–266, 1992.

Nabih M, Peyman GA, Tawakol ME, Naguib K: Toxicity of high dose intravitreal dexamethasone. Int Ophthalmol 15:223–235, 1991.

Ohji M, Knoshita S, Ohmi E, Kuwayama Y: Marked intraocular pressure response to instillation of corticosteroids in children. Am J Ophthalmol 112:450–454, 1991.

Polansky JR: Side effects of ophthalmic therapy with anti-inflammatory steroids. Curr Opin Ophthalmol 3:259–272, 1992.

Polansky JR, Alvarado JA: Isolation and evaluation of target cells in glaucoma research: Hormone receptors and drug responses. Curr Eye Res 4:267–279, 1985.

Smith R, Nozik RA: Uveitis: A Clinical Approach to Diagnosis and Management. Baltimore, Williams & Wilkins, 1982.

EXFOLIATION SYNDROME 365.52
(Capsular Glaucoma, Exfoliative Glaucoma, Pseudoexfoliation of the Lens Capsule)

AHTI TARKKANEN, M.D.

Helsinki, Finland

Exfoliation syndrome (ES) is characterized by grayish flakes that coat the surfaces of the anterior segment of the eye. The deposits can be found on the lens capsule, the ciliary processes, the zonules, and the pupillary margin. The pathologic deposits produce three different zones on the anterior lens capsule: a translucent central disc; a granular girdle around the periphery, called the peripheral band; and a clear zone separating these two areas. The central disc in the pupillary area may be quite faint and is easily missed without dilation of the pupil. Its border, however, is then seen and is more clearly outlined by a few dandruff-like deposits and a white-grayish ring at the edge. The central disc is not a constant feature of the exfoliation syndrome. The peripheral band, however, is always present and shows the characteristic granular appearance. The clear intermediate zone contains no deposits. Occasionally, however, one may see some loose flakes and a bridge extending from the peripheral band to the central disc. In addition, the flakes have been observed as precipitates on the posterior surface of the cornea, floating freely in the anterior chamber, on the anterior surface of the iris, in the pupillary border, and in aphakic eyes on the hyaloid. The pupillary border may appear atrophic with a characteristic moth-eaten appearance. Transillumination of the iris in the midperiphery is often seen. On gonioscopy, the pigmentation of the trabecular meshwork may extend anterior to the Schwalbe's line (Sampaolesi's line).

About 20 per cent of patients with ES show abnormalities of intraocular pressure. Glaucoma associated with ES is called capsular glaucoma. Capsular glaucoma is often far advanced when diagnosed, and the progression of visual field loss is more severe than in chronic simple glaucoma. However, no difference in the degree of damage is found when intraocular pressure has been equally controlled. Elevated intraocular pressure in capsular glaucoma is more resistant to medical therapy. Furthermore, by histopathologic studies it has been shown that absolute neovascular glaucoma is more common in capsular than chronic simple glaucoma in elderly individuals.

In large clinical series, ES has been found to be unilateral in approximately one-third of the patients, but it may progress to bilateral involvement with time. In Caucasians, it occurs more often in females in a ratio about 2.3:1. ES is known to be age dependent, and there is a clear increase with advancing age. The prevalence is low in individuals younger than 60 years, whereas there is an increase from 1 per cent in the age group 60 to 69 years to 4.8 per cent in the group 70 to 79 years. In individuals aged 80 years or more, the prevalence is over 8 per cent. There are exceptional populations though, in which ES seems to appear about 10 years earlier. Familiar occurrence of ES has been described by several authors. ES has now been described in practically all parts of the world, but recent data support the opinion that ES is not uniformly distributed in different countries.

THERAPY

Supportive. Patients with ES with normal intraocular pressure and normal optic discs require only regular follow-up examinations.

Ocular. In capsular glaucoma, beta-blocking agents, such as timolol, levobunolol, or betaxolol, are used to lower intraocular pressure. These agents may be used topically every 12 or 24 hours. They lower intraocular pressure by reducing the aqueous production. Epinephrine or dipivefrin may be instilled once or twice daily to decrease the production of aqueous humor and to increase the facility of outflow. Dipivefrin is a prodrug that is converted into epinephrine within the eye. One to 4 per cent pilocarpine solution can be applied two to four times daily to decrease intraocular pressure by increasing the facility of outflow. Alternatively, 0.75 to 3.0 per cent carbachol can be instilled two to three times daily.

Systemic. Carbonic anhydrase inhibitors may be added to the treatment with topical agents. Acetazolamide may be prescribed orally from 65 to 250 mg three to four times a day. A sustained-release preparation of acetazolamide may also be tried. As alternatives to acetazolamide, methazolamide or dichlorphenamide may be used. The common dosage of methazolamide varies from 50 to 100 mg, orally three times a day; the dose of dichlorphenamide ranges from 25 to 50 mg orally three to four times a day.

Surgical. Argon laser trabeculoplasty can be performed as treatment of capsular glaucoma before a filtering operation is considered. Fifty to 60 applications of 50-μm spots of the argon laser with 0.1-second duration are evenly spaced over 180 degrees of the trabecular meshwork. One may begin with an initial power setting of 300 mW and increase up to 1000 mW to produce blanching of trabecular pigment or minimal bubble formation. Eyes with capsular glaucoma show a pigmented trabecular meshwork, which is a prerequisite for a successful operation. The reduction of intraocular pressure is caused by increase of the outflow facility. Primary success rates of 80 per cent have been reported. The greater therapeutic reduction of intraocular pressure in capsular glaucoma as compared to chronic simple glaucoma may be due to a higher pretreatment intraocular pressure level. The secondary effects of laser trabeculoplasty in capsular glaucoma include an acute undesired intraocular pressure elevation immediately posttreatment. One has to remember that the primary success rate of 80 per cent may drop to 30 to 40 per cent in 4 years after treatment. Careful follow-up of patients with capsular glaucoma is mandatory, especially after a successful argon laser trabeculoplasty. With developing failure, another 180 degrees of the chamber angle can be treated.

Filtering surgery is more effective in lowering intraocular pressure than argon laser trabeculoplasty. The decision to operate should not be postponed until the late stage of the disease. The use of viscoelastic materials during surgery will prevent loss of anterior chamber and intraocular bleeding during operation and may prevent or lessen postoperative hypotony and cataract formation. Furthermore, a tight initial closure of the filtering bleb followed by daily suture cutting will ensure filtration without the well-known immediate complications of filtering surgery. The difficulties in the medical management of capsular glaucoma are illustrated by the fact that, among consecutive patients with chronic open-angle glaucoma who required filtering surgery, capsular glaucoma accounted for 62 per cent of the cases in one medical center.

Cataract surgery in eyes with ES may be linked to several problems. Eyes with ES may show spontaneous subluxation of the lens in 2 per cent of cases, which may go unnoticed because of the absence of iridodonesis. This condition may be due to increased iris rigidity caused by infiltration of the iris stroma by exfoliation material. There may be a strong bonding of the posterior surface of the iris to the pre-equatorial lens capsule, preventing good pupillary dilation. The zonular fibers are known to be weak in ES and the central posterior lens capsule very thin. These features make ES a major risk factor in extracapsular cataract surgery. In a series of unselected cataract operations, the incidence of vitreous loss was 1.6 per cent in cataracts without ES and 11.1 per cent in those with ES. When these complications are feared, sector iridotomy is performed, and the haptics of the intraocular lens should be placed into the ciliary sulcus. Anterior chamber intraocular lenses were previously not recommended in ES because it was feared that the haptics in the chamber angle may further decompensate aqueous outflow. The author's experience has shown that in the absence of capsular-zonular support the intraocular lens may be placed in the anterior chamber.

Cataract surgery in capsular glaucoma may present further problems. If the intraocular pressure has been controlled by medication, laser therapy, or previous filtering surgery, extracapsular cataract extraction and posterior chamber intraocular lens implantation are recommended. If, however, the intraocular pressure cannot be brought under control, cataract surgery may be followed by very high intraocular pressures, which usually do not respond to any treatment. Initial filtering surgery will control the intraocular pressure, and cataract surgery can be performed 4 to 6 months later. This approach is safe and can be recommended to patients who do not need immediate visual restoration and who show high intraocular pressures while on maximum tolerated medical therapy. In contrast, one should consider glaucoma triple procedure, trabeculectomy, extracapsular cataract surgery, and posterior chamber lens implantation in patients who need immediate visual restoration. Furthermore, this approach may be used to improve glaucoma control in borderline cases or in patients with advanced glaucomatous optic nerve damage. The visual results are satisfactory, and immediate elevated postoperative intraocular pressure can be avoided. The long-term effects of this operation to the intraocular pressure will be known later, but the patient has undergone only one operation. This procedure, however, is recommended only to experienced surgeons. The postoperative course may be complicated by fibrinoid reaction in the anterior chamber. One to five days postoperatively, fibrinoid deposits, threads, and grayish mass may appear in the anterior chamber as the result of the leaking iris capillaries. Eyes with ES or capsular glaucoma are at risk for this complication, which can be mistaken as postoperative purulent endophthalmitis.

Ocular or Periocular Manifestations

Anterior Chamber: Exfoliation material on trabecular meshwork; pigment cells on trabecular meshwork.
Cornea: Exfoliation material or pigment granules on the endothelium.
Iris or Ciliary Body: Exfoliation material on the pupillary margin and ciliary processes; depigmentation of the pigment layer of the iris; exfoliation material or pigment granules on the iris in the pupillary border.
Lens: Exfoliation material on the anterior lens capsule; peripheral band-central disc.
Optic Nerve: Glaucomatous cupping in capsular glaucoma.
Other: Elevated intraocular pressure.

PRECAUTIONS

The drugs used in the treatment of capsular glaucoma can cause undesirable side effects. Their toxic effect can be additive to systemic drugs prescribed to the patient by the family physician or internist. Timolol should be avoided in patients with a history of asthma or other lung or heart problems. Epinephrine may be associated with conjunctival irritation, allergic conjunctivitis, and even adrenochrome deposition in the conjunctiva, as well as heart arrhythmia and blood pressure elevation. Pilocarpine and carbachol may cause headache, accommodative spasm, and decreased visual activity. Carbonic anhydrase inhibitors may be associated with malaise, fatigue, unexplained weight loss, nausea, diarrhea, depression, and paresthesias. They may further exacerbate nephrolithiasis. To avoid systemic side effects of the topical drugs, the patient should be advised to occlude the tear duct after instilling the eyedrop or to keep the eyes closed without blinking for about 2 minutes after instillation of the drops.

COMMENTS

Exfoliation material has a fibrillar structure. The fibrils are 20 to 30 nm thick with 10-nm subunits and may be 800 to 900 nm long. Sometimes, they may show a banding periodicity of 50 nm. The material arises probably from the epithelium of the iris and the ciliary body, perhaps as the result of an unknown metabolic disorder. From these areas, the material enters the aqueous humor and is deposited on the anterior lens capsule, zonules, vitreous face, the iris, the trabecular meshwork, and the corneal endothelium. Histochemical studies have demonstrated the presence of glycosaminoglycans. Recent studies of lectin binding to the exfoliative material show that glycoconjugates present in the superficial zonular lamella, zonular fibers, and the nonpigmented epithelium of the ciliary body have a rather similar lectin-binding profile to that of exfoliative material. Of interest is that the lens capsule was essentially unreactive with all lectins used. About 20 per cent of the patients with ES show abnormalities of intraocular pressure. This data can lead to the conclusion that capsular glaucoma results from an overload of an already impaired drainage system by exfoliation material and by pigment granules. This combination is often followed by high intraocular pressures and rapid loss of visual field. Corticosteroid testing has indicated that primary open-angle glaucoma and capsular glaucoma are separate disease entities.

Exfoliation material has been shown to infiltrate even the juxtacanalicular connective tissue and to enter within the giant vacuoles of the endothelium of the Schlemm's canal. This infiltration may explain the poor response of capsular glaucoma to miotic therapy. Furthermore, the ciliary processes in eyes with ES show marked degenerative changes in addition to the exfoliative material. These changes may lead to hyposecretion of aqueous humor. Again, this phenomenon would explain why eyes with capsular glaucoma may be unresponsive to drugs that lower intraocular pressure by decreasing aqueous production.

References

Karjalainen K, Tarkkanen A, Merenmies L: Exfoliation syndrome in enucleated haemorrhagic and absolute glaucoma. Acta Ophthalmol 65:3, 1987.

Naumann GOH: Exfoliation syndrome as a risk factor for vitreous loss in extracapsular cataract surgery. Acta Ophthalmol 66(Suppl 184):129–131, 1988.

Ruotsalainen J, Tarkkanen A: Capsule thickness of cataractous lenses with and without exfoliation syndrome. Acta Ophthalmol 65:444–449, 1987.

Schönherr U, Küchle M, Händel A, Lang GK, Naumann GOH: Pseudoexfoliationssyndrom mit und ohne Glaukom als ernstzunehmender Risikofaktor bei der extrakapsulären Kataraktextraktion. Fortschr Ophthalmol 87:588–590, 1990.

Tarkkanen A, Forsius H (eds): Exfoliation syndrome. Acta Ophthalmol 66(Suppl 184):1–7, 1988.

Wålinder P-EK, Olivius EOP, Nordell SI, Thorburn WE: Fibrinoid reaction after extracapsular cataract extraction and relationship to exfoliation syndrome. J Cataract Refract Surg 15:526–530, 1989.

GHOST CELL GLAUCOMA 365.89

DAVID G. CAMPBELL, M.D.

Hanover, New Hampshire

Ghost cell glaucoma is a rare form of secondary glaucoma in which elevation of intraocular pressure may occur after vitreous hemorrhage and the development of a disruption in the anterior hyaloid face that allows the contents of the vitreous cavity to pass forward into the anterior chamber. Characteristically, the main component of the vitreous hemorrhage that passes forward into the anterior chamber is degenerated red blood cells— ghost cells. Extracellular hemoglobin debris tends to remain behind in the vitreous cavity, trapped within vitreous and/or fibrin strands. The cause of the glaucoma is obstruction of the intertrabecular spaces of the trabecular meshwork by the ghost cells, which are less pliable than fresh red blood cells. Macrophages and 1 *u* hemoglobin particles, Heinz bodies, are found occasionally in the anterior chamber as well, although ghost cells predominate overwhelmingly.

Ghost cell glaucoma characteristically occurs in association with vitreous hemorrhage after cataract extraction, after trauma with vitreous hemorrhage and disruption of the anterior hyaloid face, and after vitrectomy for vitreous hemorrhage.

THERAPY

Supportive. If the intraocular pressure is very high and there is pain secondary to this elevation, analgesics may be valuable in controlling discomfort. Oral doses of acetaminophen, 300 to 500 mg every 4 to 6 hours, may be given. Occasionally, narcotics are necessary.

Ocular. A topical beta blocker and/or dipivefrin, and/or a miotic, should be used initially to attempt to lower an elevated intraocular pressure due to ghost cell glaucoma. Solutions of 0.1 per cent dipivefrin or 0.25 to 0.50 per cent timolol may be used every 12 hours to complement miotics, such as 1 to 4 per cent pilocarpine instilled every 6 hours.

Systemic. If topical ocular medications do not sufficiently lower the intraocular pressure, systemic therapy is indicated. Carbonic anhydrase inhibitors are used in full adult dosage; either 250 mg of acetazolamide every 6 hours or 50 mg of methazolamide every 8 hours may be administered orally. If the intraocular pressure still remains high and there is severe pain or fear of damage to the optic nerve, osmotic agents are indicated to lower the intraocular pressure. One to 1.5 gm/kg of a 50 per cent solution of glycerin mixed with fruit juice on ice can effectively lower the intraocular pressure for a few hours. If necessary, intravenous infusion of 2 gm/kg of a 20 per cent solution of mannitol may be given over a 20-minute period. If osmotic agents are contraindicated for any reason, a paracentesis procedure should be substituted at this stage.

In many cases, medical therapy may suffice to control this transient elevation of intraocular pressure. Therapy may be required for a period of weeks to months, until the point is reached at which the supply of ghost cells from the vitreous cavity is exhausted and they no longer continue to pass into the anterior chamber.

Surgical. If medical therapy fails, the intraocular pressure remains elevated, and a painful eye results, surgical therapy then becomes necessary. The first treatment advised is a paracentesis, combined with a washout or irrigation of the contents of the anterior chamber. This is accomplished through a beveled paracentesis incision that begins in the clear cornea near the limbus laterally and extends toward the inferior angle. The incision is made wide enough so that easy escape of fluid out around a cannula can occur. Then, 15 ml of balanced salt solution is passed through a small cannula without a sharp point into the anterior chamber directed toward the inferior angle. The direction of the flow is regulated around the angle so that the accumulation of ghost cells on the trabecular meshwork and within the anterior chamber is dislodged. One washout should be performed and repeated, if necessary. At the time of irrigation, the contents of the anterior chamber should be aspirated and examined histologically under phase-contrast microscopy. This will allow proper histologic diagnosis of ghost cell glaucoma.

If two anterior chamber washouts are unsuccessful, a vitrectomy is indicated to irrigate and remove most, if not all, of the ghost cells and hemorrhagic debris within the vitreous cavity. If the greater portion of the ghost cells is removed, further entry into the anterior chamber will be prevented and the glaucoma will resolve. If this fails, cyclocryotherapy can be effective in lowering the intraocular pressure.

Ocular or Periocular Manifestations

Anterior Chamber: Flare; multitude of tiny, khaki-colored cells; occasional pseudohypopyon (khaki-colored, indicating ghost cell layer); open angle.
Cornea: Edema (when pressure is high).
Iris or Ciliary Body: Open trabecular meshwork (may be covered by pathognomonically khaki-colored layer of cells); signs of injury (if caused by trauma).
Optic Nerve: Atrophy without cupping (if pressure has been high for short periods of time); glaucomatous cupping (if pressure elevation is prolonged).
Vitreous: Hemorrhage (fresh or often characteristic khaki color).
Other: Elevation of intraocular pressure (moderate to marked); ocular pain (moderate to marked).

Precautions

Ghost cell glaucoma must not be misdiagnosed as glaucoma secondary to uveitis or to endophthalmitis. In uveitis, keratic precipitates can be pathognomonic. In addition, there is an absence of the characteristic khaki-colored cells in the anterior chamber and vitreous and of a history of hemorrhage within the vitreous. The pseudohypopyon that occurs with ghost cell glaucoma is pathognomonically khaki-colored. A white hypopyon suggests either uveitis or endophthalmitis.

Comments

Occasionally, ghost cell glaucoma must be differentiated from neovascular glaucoma. In the latter, neovascularization at the pupillary margin and in the angle accompanied by secondary synechial closure is pathognomonic of this condition, which is often associated with vitreous hemorrhage. In ghost cell glaucoma, the angle is open, and the anterior chamber is filled with tiny, khaki-colored cells. Clearing of an edematous cornea with topical glycerin may allow new vessels to be appreciated.

Ghost cell glaucoma is a temporary glaucoma; generally, the intraocular pressure will return to normal once the supply of ghost cells from the vitreous cavity is exhausted. Permanent open-angle glaucoma secondary to the effect of ghost cells within the trabecular meshwork has not been reported.

References

Campbell DG: Ghost cell glaucoma. *In* Ritch R, Shields MB (eds): The Secondary Glaucomas. St. Louis, CV Mosby, 1982, pp 320–327.
Campbell DG, Simmons RJ, Grant WM: Ghost cells as a cause of glaucoma. Am J Ophthalmol *81:* 441–450, 1976.
Fenton RH, Zimmerman LE: Hemolytic glaucoma. An unusual cause of acute open-angle secondary glaucoma. Arch Ophthalmol 70:236–239, 1963.
Phelps CD: Hemolytic glaucoma. *In* Fraunfelder FT, Roy FH: Current Ocular Therapy 2. Philadelphia, WB Saunders, 1980, pp 447–448.
Phelps CD, Watzke RC: Hemolytic glaucoma. Am J Ophthalmol *80:*690–695, 1975.

GLAUCOMA AFTER OCULAR CONTUSION 921.3
(Angle Recession 364.77)

JOHN C. MORRISON, M.D.

Portland, Oregon

Ocular contusion, usually the result of blunt ocular trauma, compresses the cornea posteriorly, forcing aqueous humor laterally and creating shearing forces between the anterior uvea and its attachments to the limbus. Such forces cause variable damage to the ciliary muscle, trabecular meshwork, and iris. Ciliary muscle and iris tears may rupture the ciliary vasculature, producing a hyphema, the most common presentation for ocular contusion.

After the hyphema resolves, several characteristic abnormalities may result, including iridodialysis, cyclodialysis, and angle recession. Although angle recession may present with a deepened anterior chamber, the diagnosis usually requires detailed gonioscopy of the injured eye and careful comparison with the uninjured fellow eye. Because the shearing forces can tear the face of the ciliary muscle fibers, a cleft may appear in the ciliary body band, making it appear several times wider than the trabecular meshwork and producing apparent "recession" of the iris root.

Sclera may occasionally appear in the depths of this cleft with an extensive tear of the ciliary muscle. Damage to the uveal meshwork may range from focal iris process tears to a complete stripping away from the scleral spur, rendering it unusually white and prominent. Actual tears in the corneoscleral meshwork may also be seen, but are much more subtle. Other signs of contusion include peripheral anterior synechiae, tearing of the iris root (iridodialysis), and separation of the ciliary body from the scleral spur (cyclodialysis). A single eye can present with one or more of these signs, involving variable amounts of the angle from a single clock hour to its entire circumference.

Glaucoma following ocular contusion is also highly variable. Although most eyes demonstrate elevated intraocular pressure within several weeks after the injury, some do not develop glaucoma until years later. Early elevations of intraocular pressure, which are often transient, may be caused by hyphema, traumatic iritis with inflammation of the trabecular meshwork, or lens dislocation with pupillary block. Alternatively, no obvious cause may be apparent. Other eyes have an initially normal or slightly low intraocular pressure, usually secondary to depressed aqueous humor formation from iridocyclitis, but occasionally from increased outflow via trabecular meshwork tears or a cyclodialysis cleft. With time, approximately 4 to 9 per cent of patients with angle recession involving more than 180 degrees of the angle circumference eventually develop glaucoma. Most cases of late glaucoma arise from gradual scarring of the trabecular meshwork. Other causes may include gradual closure of a cyclodialysis cleft or extension of endothelium over the chamber angle with deposition of a Descemet's-like membrane.

THERAPY

Ocular. If an early rise in intraocular pressure is felt to be caused by traumatic iritis, a trial of topical 1 per cent prednisolone acetate four times daily with a cycloplegic, such as scopolamine, may be beneficial. Otherwise, initial treatment of elevated intraocular pressure, either of early or late onset, should begin with a beta-blocking agent, 0.25 to 0.5 per cent timolol, 0.5 per cent levobunolol, or 0.5 per cent betaxolol, used once or twice daily. Twice-daily 1 per cent epinephrine and 0.1 per cent dipivefrin, 2 to 4 per cent pilocarpine four times daily, or acetylcholinesterase inhibitors (0.06 to 0.25 per cent echothiophate) twice daily may provide additional reduction of intraocular pressure. However, the effectiveness of these agents may be limited by extensive trabecular meshwork damage and disinsertion of the ciliary muscle.

Systemic. If topical medications fail to lower intraocular pressure satisfactorily, systemic carbonic anhydrase inhibitors may be necessary. These include 125 to 250 mg of oral acetazolamide four times daily or 50 to 100 mg of oral methazolamide twice daily.

Surgical. Surgery is necessary if maximally tolerated medical therapy does not lower intraocular pressure into a satisfactory range or if progressive visual field loss or disc atrophy is observed. Although generally not successful in angle-recession glaucoma, standard argon laser trabeculoplasty should precede filtering surgery if trabecular damage or peripheral anterior synechiae are not extensive. If the optic nerve is already severely damaged, premedication with a single drop of 1 per cent apraclonidine[†] may be used to reduce the likelihood of an abrupt rise in intraocular pressure following laser. If all of the above measures are unsuccessful, a filtering procedure (trabeculectomy) is indicated to control pressure and preserve vision. Adjunctive 5-Fluorouracil[‡] or mitomycin C[‡] are often indicated by the history of trauma and inflammation, along with the relatively young age of many patients with this form of glaucoma. Full-thickness operations, including trephination, sclerectomy, or thermal sclerostomy, are similarly effective, but have a higher rate of complications, such as flat chamber and choroidal effusions, and should not be performed with adjunctive antimetabolites.

Ocular or Periocular Manifestations

Anterior Chamber: Bare, white scleral spur; deep anterior chamber; peripheral anterior synechiae; trabecular meshwork tears.

Cornea: Blood staining.

Iris and Ciliary Body: Cyclodialysis; iridodialysis; irregular pigmentation of ciliary body band and trabecular meshwork; wide ciliary body band.

Lens: Cataract, ruptured zonules with vitreous herniation.

Optic Nerve: Glaucomatous cupping; pallor.

Retina: Commotio retinae (early); detached vitreous base; retinal holes; retinodialysis.

Other: Elevated intraocular pressure; hypotony, vitreous hemorrhages.

PRECAUTIONS

The efficacy of topical and systemic agents should always be balanced against their safety and the patient's tolerance of their side effects. In patients with reactive respiratory disease, beta-blockers should be limited to betaxolol, a relatively selective beta$_1$ antagonist, with the consent of the patient's internist and careful monitoring of pulmonary functions. Echothiophate should not be used in phakic patients as they have a cataractogenic potential. Systemic carbonic anhydrase inhibitors possess many, usually self-limited, side effects, including acidosis, paresthesia, loss of appetite, loss of libido, and fatigue. Renal stones may accompany the acidosis, and potassium depletion may result if carbonic anhydrase inhibitors are used with diuretics. Rare, life-threatening blood dyscrasias have also been associated with carbonic anhydrase inhibitors and regular blood counts, including platelets, have been advocated for patients using these drugs. Daily subconjunctival 5-Fluorouracil injections* for the first week after surgery and every other day for the second week may produce epithelial corneal erosions that heal slowly. Both 5-fluorouracil‡ and mitomycin C‡ (applied topically to the episclera immediately before creating the limbal fistula) can be associated with conjunctival wound leaks and spontaneous holes, as well as occasional severe hypotony, maculopathy, and the permanent loss of visual acuity.

COMMENTS

Over 90 per cent of ocular contusions severe enough to cause a traumatic hyphema have gonioscopically visible angle recession or other damage to the anterior chamber angle. Since nearly 10 per cent of eyes with more than 180 degrees of angle recession may ultimately develop glaucoma, these abnormalities should be considered evidence of concomitant injury to the trabecular meshwork. All eyes with traumatic hyphema should therefore be examined by careful gonioscopy for angle recession, iridodialysis, or cyclodialysis after the blood has completely cleared and a good view re-established. Although glaucoma is most likely to present during the first year after injury, patients with greater than 180 degrees of angle recession should have yearly tonometry and optic nerve evaluations for the remainder of their lives.

References

Epstein DL: Chandler and Grant's Glaucoma, 3rd ed. Philadelphia, Lea & Febiger, 1986, pp 296–310.
Howard GM, Hutchinson BT, Frederick AR: Hyphema resulting from blunt trauma. Gonioscopic, tonographic, and ophthalmoscopic observations following resolution of the hemorrhage. Trans Am Acad Ophthalmol Otolaryngol 69:294–306, 1965.
Kaufman JH, Tolpin DW: Glaucoma after traumatic angle recession. A ten-year prospective study. Am J Ophthalmol 78:648–654, 1974.
Shields MB: Textbook of Glaucoma, 2nd ed. Baltimore, Williams & Wilkins, 1987, pp 328–333.
Tonjum A: Gonioscopy in traumatic hyphema. Acta Ophthalmol 44:650–664, 1966.
Wolff SM, Zimmerman LE: Chronic secondary glaucoma. Associated with retrodisplacement of iris root and deepening of the anterior chamber angle secondary to contusion. Am J Ophthalmol 54:547–562, 1962.

GLAUCOMA ASSOCIATED WITH ANTERIOR UVEITIS 365.62

M. BRUCE SHIELDS, M.D.

Durham, North Carolina

Anterior uveitis influences intraocular pressure through effects on both aqueous humor production and resistance to aqueous outflow. Inflammation of the ciliary body usually leads to reduced aqueous production, and if this reduction outweighs a concomitant increase in resistance to outflow, the intraocular pressure will be reduced, which is typically the case in acute anterior uveitis. In other cases, inflammation-induced alterations in the aqueous outflow system may be sufficient to cause pressure elevation and secondary glaucoma.

The mechanisms by which anterior uveitis increase resistance to aqueous outflow are numerous and only partially understood. They may be associated with acute, subacute, or chronic iridocyclitis. Acute iridocyclitis is characterized by ciliary flush, slight miosis, variable degrees of aqueous flare and cell, and frequent keratic precipitates. Symptoms usually include mild to moderate ocular pain, photophobia, and blurred vision, unless marked secondary intraocular pressure elevation has developed with severe pain and corneal edema. Subacute iridocyclitis produces few or no symptoms, but can have serious consequences because its complications, including secondary glaucoma, may go undetected until advanced damage has occurred. Mechanisms of increased resistance to aqueous outflow with both acute and subacute forms of anterior uveitis are usually of the open-angle type and include obstruction of the trabecular meshwork by inflammatory cells or fibrin, swelling or dysfunction of the trabecular lamellae or endothelium, and inflammatory precipitates on the meshwork. Much less commonly, these forms of uveitis may be associated with secondary angle-closure glaucoma by forward rotation of the ciliary body or by lens-iris diaphragm displacement from an associated posterior uveitis.

Chronic anterior uveitis may follow either acute or subacute iridocyclitis, but is characterized by a protracted course of months to years, often with remissions and exacerbations, and is particularly prone to cause secondary glaucoma. The mechanisms of obstruction to aqueous outflow may be open angle, in which the meshwork is scarred or covered by a membrane, closed angle due to contracture of the membrane or inflammatory precipitates, or after posterior synechia formation with subsequent iris bombé. Another mechanism of secondary glaucoma to be considered during the treatment of any form of anterior uveitis is steroid-induced glaucoma.

THERAPY

The treatment should first be directed at the underlying etiology of the ocular inflammation, such as an infectious process, if this is apparent. In the vast majority of cases, however, a definite cause of the anterior uveitis is never clearly established, and most are presumed to represent an autoimmune mechanism. The treatment in these situations is nonspecific, with anti-inflammatory agents usually constituting the first approach in the treatment plan. In many cases, resolution of the inflammatory process is sufficient to control the intraocular pressure, although other cases require medical and even surgical management of the secondary glaucoma.

Ocular. Corticosteroids constitute the first line defense in most cases of anterior uveitis. Topical administration is usually preferred, and commonly used corticosteroids include prednisolone 1.0 per cent or dexamethasone 0.1 per cent. A typical maintenance dose is one drop four times daily, although more frequent instillation, such as every hour, may be required initially or in severe cases. In a rabbit model of keratitis, instillation every 15 minutes or five doses at 1-minute intervals each hour was more effective than an hourly regimen. If topical administration is inadequate, periocular injections* (e.g., dexamethasone phosphate, prednisolone succinate, or methylprednisolone acetate) or systemic administration (e.g., prednisone) may be required.

Nonsteroidal anti-inflammatory agents may be needed when corticosteroids are inadequate or contraindicated. These include prostaglandin synthetase inhibitors (e.g., aspirin[‡], indomethacin[‡], imidazole[‡], indoxole[†], or dipyridamole[‡]) and immunosuppressive agents (e.g., methotrexate[‡], azathioprine[‡], or chlorambucil[‡]). One regimen that is reported to be effective in cases of severe chronic uveitis, which have been poorly responsive or unresponsive to corticosteroid therapy, is long-term daily administration of prednisone 10 to 15 mg combined with azothioprine 2.0 to 2.5 mg or chlorambucil 6 to 8 mg.

In conjunction with anti-inflammatory agents, a mydriatic-cycloplegic (e.g., atropine 1 per cent, homatropine 1 to 5 per cent, or cyclopentolate 0.5 to 1 per cent) is usually indicated to avoid the formation of posterior synechiae and to relieve the discomfort of ciliary muscle spasm.

Antiglaucoma medication should be added to the treatment plan if the magnitude of the intraocular pressure elevation poses an immediate threat to vision or if the pressure does not respond adequately to anti-inflammatory therapy alone. Miotics are generally contraindicated in the inflamed eye, because they may aggravate the inflammation, increase the chances of posterior synechiae formation, and worsen the discomfort from ciliary muscle spasm. Therefore, topical beta blockers (timolol 0.25 or 0.5 per cent, betaxo-

lol 0.25 or 0.5 per cent, levobunolol 0.25 or 0.5 per cent, metipranolol 0.3 per cent, or carteolol 1.0 per cent), epinephrine 0.5 to 2 per cent, or dipivalyl epinephrine 0.1 per cent, twice daily are usually the initial drugs of choice. When further pressure reduction is needed, a carbonic anhydrase inhibitor (e.g., methazolamide 15 to 50 mg twice daily or acetazolamide 250 mg four times daily or 500-mg sustained-release capsules, twice daily) may be added. Hyperosmotic agents (e.g., oral glycerol or isosorbide or intravenous mannitol) and topical apraclonidine 1.0 per cent may also be used for short-term, emergency control of secondary glaucoma.

Surgical. It is a general rule that surgery should be avoided when possible in the inflamed eye. When surgical intervention is needed for intraocular pressure control, however, it is best to select the procedure with the least amount of intraocular involvement. For example, a laser iridotomy is preferable to a surgical iridectomy when a pupillary block mechanism is believed to be present. For open-angle cases that are uncontrolled by maximum medical therapy, a filtering procedure is usually indicated. An alternative approach, called trabeculodialysis, has been described in which a goniotomy knife is used to incise above the trabecular meshwork and then peel the meshwork downward. Laser trabeculoplasty should be avoided when active inflammation is present, since it can lead to a significant postoperative intraocular pressure rise.

Ocular or Periocular Manifestations

Anterior Chamber: Aqueous cells and flare.
Anterior Chamber Angle: Inflammatory precipitates; peripheral anterior synechiae.
Conjunctiva: Ciliary flush.
Cornea: Keratic precipitates; edema.
Other: Glaucoma.

PRECAUTIONS

Prompt, aggressive treatment of anterior uveitis is necessary to avoid serious sequelae, including complicated cataracts and chronic secondary glaucoma. However, the medications required in the treatment plan have a significant potential for adverse reactions and must be used with extreme caution. The risk of steroid-induced glaucoma exists with the use of either topical or periocular corticosteroids and, to a lesser extent, with systemic steroids. The newer progesterone-like steroids (medrysone and fluorometholone) have a lower potential for induced pressure elevation, but are not completely devoid of this property. Care must also be taken to rule out viral or fungal infections when steroids are to be prescribed. When using nonsteroidal anti-inflammatory agents, the risk of gastrointestinal irritation must be considered with most prostaglandin synthetase inhibitors, whereas the possibility of hematologic disorders requires constant monitoring during the use of immunosuppressive agents.

The potential for angle-closure glaucoma must be assessed before prescribing a mydriatic-cycloplegic or epinephrine compounds. With topical beta blockers, the most serious potential consequences are related to systemic side effects and include reduced pulse rate, weakened myocardial contractility, bronchospasm, and central nervous system disorders. The most significant risks of treatment with carbonic anhydrase inhibitors are electrolyte imbalance, systemic acidosis, gastrointestinal distress, genitourinary disorders including renal calculi, and blood dyscrasias. With hyperosmotic therapy, nausea and vomiting may occur with the oral preparations, which may lead to loss of any therapeutic effect, whereas cardiovascular overload may be a problem with intravenous mannitol, particularly if there is a history of congestive heart failure.

When surgical intervention is required in the inflamed eye, a major cause of failure is excessive postoperative iridocyclitis, necessitating the use of aggressive steroid therapy during this period. In addition, the adjunctive use of pharmacologic agents to modulate wound healing, such as 5-fluorouracil and mitomycin-C, may significantly improve the success rate of filtering surgery in these patients.

References

Andrasch RH, Pirofsky B, Burns RP: Immunosuppressive therapy for severe chronic uveitis. Arch Ophthalmol 96:247–251, 1978.

Bolliger GA, Kupferman A, Leibowitz HM: Quantitation of anterior chamber inflammation and its response to therapy. Arch Ophthalmol 98:1110–1114, 1980.

Epstein DL, Hashimoto JM, Grant WM: Serum obstruction of aqueous outflow in enucleated eyes. Am J Ophthalmol 86:101–105, 1978.

Jampel HD, Jabs DA, Quigley HA: Trabeculectomy with 5-fluorouracil for adult inflammatory glaucoma. Am J Ophthalmol 109:168–173, 1990.

Kanski JJ, McAllister JA: Trabeculodialysis for inflammatory glaucoma in children and young adults. Ophthalmology 92:927–930, 1985.

Leibowitz HM, Kupferman A: Optimal frequency of topical prednisolone administration. Arch Ophthalmol 97:2154–2156, 1979.

Panek WC, Holland GN, Lee DA, Christensen RE: Glaucoma in patients with uveitis. Br J Ophthalmol 74:223–227, 1990.

Spinelli HM, Krohn DL: Inhibition of prostaglandin-induced iritis. Topical indoxole versus indomethacin therapy. Arch Ophthalmol 98:1106–1109, 1980.

GLAUCOMA ASSOCIATED WITH ELEVATED VENOUS PRESSURE 365.82

JOHN R. SAMPLES, M.D.

Portland, Oregon

Systemic disorders that raise the episcleral venous pressure can cause glaucoma as the increased pressure creates resistance to outflow in Schlemm's canal. Schlemm's canal is connected to the episcleral and conjunctival veins by a complicated system of vessels. Most vessels carrying aqueous humor from Schlemm's canal are directed posteriorly, with the vast majority draining into episcleral veins. A few cross the subconjunctival tissue and drain into conjunctival veins. Episcleral veins drain into the cavernous sinus via the anterior ciliary and superior ophthalmic veins, whereas the conjunctival veins drain into the superior ophthalmic or facial veins via the palpebral and angular veins. The normal episcleral venous pressure ranges between 8 and 10 mm Hg. Patients with primary open-angle glaucoma do not appear to have episcleral venous pressure elevations. In fact, there seems to be a negative correlation, with ocular hypertensive patients having significantly lower episcleral venous pressure.

Elevated venous pressure is one means by which patients with thyroid eye disease may have elevated intraocular pressure. Elevated venous pressure may occur in association with a carotid cavernous fistula. The most consistent finding in patients with an elevated episcleral venous pressure is tortuous and dilated episcleral and bulbar conjunctival vessels. When the meshwork is open, one may observe blood reflux into Schlemm's canal. Noteworthy, however, is at least one study's suggestion that elevated venous pressure may be associated with increased outflow caused by widening of Schlemm's canal. Prolonged elevation of episcleral venous pressure seems likely to lead to a reduction in outflow.

There are four categories of patients with elevated episcleral venous pressure. The first have venous obstruction. In patients with thyroid eye disease, contracture of extraocular muscles and the infiltration of plasma cells and lymphocytes into the orbit may lead to an elevated venous pressure. It must be kept in mind that thyroid dysfunction may be associated with abnormal scleral rigidity. Retroorbital tumors, cavernous sinus thrombosis, and lesions that obstruct venous return from the head may also cause venous obstruction and elevated venous pressure.

Persons with carotid cavernous fistulas comprise the second category of patients with elevated venous pressure. The typical carotid cavernous fistula occurs as a result of severe head injury; a large fistula is created between the internal carotid artery and the surrounding cavernous sinus venous plexus. The condition is characterized by pulsating exophthalmos, a bruit over the globe, conjunctival chemosis, engorgement of episcleral venous veins, and restriction of motility with evidence of ocular ischemia. The shunting of the internal carotid cavernous fistula causes high flow and high pressure. A more recently appreciated form of carotid cavernous fistula is the "low-flow" shunt. These small fistulas may occur without a history of trauma. In these cases, the shunt is fed by a meningeal branch of the intracavernous internal carotid artery or external carotid artery that empties directly into the cavernous sinus or adjacent dural vein that connects with the cavernous sinus. Whether the patient has a high-flow or low-flow shunt, elevated pressure occurs. Venous back pressure may increase the episcleral venous pressure, which is the most common cause of intraocular pressure rise with the fistula. Angle-closure glaucoma has also been reported in association with carotid cavernous fistula.

A third condition that can lead to elevation of episcleral venous pressure is Sturge-Weber syndrome where a hamartoma arises from the vascular tissue and produces a characteristic port-wine stain hemiangioma of the skin in a trigeminal distribution. Several mechanisms of glaucoma are possible in these patients, but at least some patients seem to have an open anterior chamber angle with small arteriovenous fistulas in the episcleral venous pressure. Orbital varices have not been associated with glaucoma, perhaps because intraocular pressure is likely to be normal between episodes. When orbital varices are present, elevated episcleral venous pressure is usually associated with stooping over or the Valsalva maneuver.

Finally, idiopathic cases of elevated episcleral venous pressure have been reported. These patients are elderly with no family history of the condition. The cause of the elevated venous pressure is unknown, and the associated glaucoma may be severe.

THERAPY

Ocular. The treatment for glaucoma associated with elevated venous pressure is no different than for other forms of glaucoma, so long as the angle is open. In cases where carotid cavernous fistula or low-flow shunt is present, pharmacologic glaucoma control should be considered before surgical intervention is contemplated when the glaucoma is the only condition prompting consideration of surgery. In some instances, angiography alone is sufficient to prompt low-flow fistulas to close spontaneously.

Surgical. If surgical intervention is necessary, a filtering procedure should be employed. There is no doubt that these patients are at substantially increased risk for uveal effusion and expulsive hemorrhage. It has been recommended that drainage of the suprachoroid be routinely performed at the time of surgery. Prophylactic sclerotomies should routinely be performed when the filtering procedure is performed.

Ocular or Periocular Manifestations

Ciliary Body: Ciliary congestion; detachment.
Conjunctiva: Dilated, tortuous bulbar conjunctival vessels.
Optic Nerve: Glaucomatous cupping.
Sclera: Dilated, tortuous episcleral veins.
Other: Increased intraocular pressure.

PRECAUTIONS

Repair of carotid cavernous fistulas may be hazardous and is at present a controversial area in neurosurgery. If glaucoma is the sole cause for intervention, one should be certain that it is significant, difficult to treat, and visual field progression is present.

COMMENTS

Elevated episcleral venous pressure as a cause of glaucoma is often overlooked. Because these patients do have increased complications at the time of filtering surgery, careful consideration of episcleral and conjunctival vessels before filtration is always indicated.

References

Barany EH: The influence of extraocular venous pressure on outflow facility in Cercopithecus ethiops Macacafascicularis. Invest Ophthalmol Vis Sci 17:711–717, 1978.

Bellows AR, et al: Choroidal effusion during glaucoma surgery in patients with prominent episcleral vessels. Arch Ophthalmol 97:493–497, 1979.

Harris GJ, Rice PR: Angle closure and carotid cavernous fistula. Ophthalmology 86:1521–1529, 1979.

Henderson JW, Schneider C: The ocular findings in carotid cavernous fistula in a series of 17 cases. Am J Ophthalmol 48:585–597, 1959.

McLenachan J, Davies DM: Glaucoma and the thyroid. Br J Ophthalmol 49:441–444, 1965.

Palestine AG, Young BR, Pipegras DG: Visual prognosis and carotid cavernous fistula. Arch Ophthalmol 99:1600–1603, 1981.

Phelps CD: The pathogenesis of glaucoma in Sturge-Weber syndrome. Ophthalmology 85: 276–286, 1978.

Phelps CD, Thompson HS, Ossoinig KC: The diagnosis and prognosis of atypical carotid cavernous fistulas (Red-eyed shunt syndrome). Am J Ophthalmol 93:423–436, 1982.

Podos SM, Minas TF, MacRif J: A new instrument to measure episcleral venous pressure. Comparison of normal eyes and eyes with primary open angle glaucoma. Arch Ophthalmol 80:209–213, 1968.

Radius RL, Maumenee AE: Dilated episcleral venous vessels and open-angle glaucoma. Am J Ophthalmol 86:31–35, 1978.

Sanders MD, Hoyt WF: Hypoxic ocular sequelae of carotid cavernous fistula. The study of causes of visual failure before and after neurosurgical treatment in a series of 25 cases. Br J Ophthalmol 53:82–97, 1969.

Talusan ED, Schwartz B: Episcleral venous pressure—Differences between normal ocular hypertensive and primary open-angle glaucoma. Arch Ophthalmol 99:824–828, 1981.

GLAUCOMA ASSOCIATED WITH INTRAOCULAR LENSES 365.59

GEORGE A. CIOFFI, M.D.,
and E. MICHAEL VAN BUSKIRK, M.D.

Portland, Oregon

Recent developments in the design and implantation of intraocular lenses have permitted their use in almost all patients undergoing cataract extraction. Intraocular lenses have afforded a closer approximation of phakic vision, which has been welcomed by both cataract patients and surgeons alike. Along with the increased incidence of lens implantation from this burgeoning technology, virtually all varieties of intraocular lenses have been associated with a variety of types of glaucoma. After lens implantation both permanent and transient intraocular pressure rises have been noted. Although both posterior chamber and anterior chamber lenses have been associated with these complications, it is the authors' experience that anterior chamber lenses are much more likely to be associated with elevations of intraocular pressure than are posterior chamber intraocular lenses. This may be related to the fact that anterior chamber lenses are often placed in eyes that have developed complications during cataract surgery, such as a rupture of the posterior capsule and/or vitreous loss. These eyes are more prone to chronic inflammation, as well as peripheral anterior synechiae. Pressure elevations also occur in greater frequency after placement of anterior chamber lenses, even in the absence of other complications. With the advent of ciliary sulcus-fixated posterior chamber intraocular lenses, new questions arise concerning their long-term effect on the eye and the stability of their placement.

Glaucoma in the aphakic or pseudophakic eye may occur both in an open- or closed-angle form. The etiology of pressure elevations in an eye with an open angle may be secondary to a variety of postoperative conditions. Postoperative inflammation after intraocular lens placement is among the most common presumptive etiology of acute intraocular pressure elevation after surgery. Intracameral manipulation leads to a partial breakdown of the blood aqueous barrier after the surgery. Intraocular lenses themselves must also be suspected in cases of chronic postoperative inflammation. However, inflammation can be seen in the absence of an intraocular lens. Patients with postoperative inflammation characteristically have a mild cellular reaction in the anterior chamber, with a muddy "spattering" of inflammatory debris in the trabecular meshwork. It is hypothesized that this trabecular inflammation decreases outflow, resulting in the elevation in intraocular pressure. Past experience with iris fixation anterior chamber lenses has shown a high incidence of postoperative inflammation and increased intraocular pressure. Chafing of the posterior iris surface by the lens haptics may lead to increased inflammation with a posterior chamber intraocular lens.

Improperly sized anterior chamber lenses or the placement of a rigid anterior chamber lens may erode into the peripheral iris, trabecular meshwork, and even peripheral cornea. This may lead to chronic inflammation, as well as bleeding and glaucoma (the so-called UGH syndrome). By the same token, lens haptics in the posterior chamber, especially when fixed in the ciliary sulcus, may cause iris pressure necrosis of the ciliary body, ischemia, and associated inflammation.

With both posterior chamber and anterior chamber lenses, hyphema may result from erosion of the haptics into a blood vessel. A hyphema may also result from bridging vessels over the cataract wound closure that can bleed intermittently, even years after the surgery. Red blood cells alone can overwhelm the trabecular outflow system and cause elevations in intraocular pressure. In hemolytic glaucoma, hemosiderin-laden macrophages occlude the trabecular meshwork. As well, ghost cell glaucoma may result when the normal erythrocyte degenerates into a less pliable, spherical cell. The classic description is that of khaki-colored cells in the anterior chamber (liberated from the vitreous) that obstruct the outflow angle; these cells have an increased difficulty exiting through the trabecular meshwork and obstruct outflow.

Vitreous loss at the time of surgery can be associated with both an increase in intraocular inflammation and possible vitreous extending into the anterior chamber and obstructing trabecular meshwork. Other forms of trabecular meshwork damage from either an anterior chamber intraocular lens haptic or intraocular manipulation may occur. Depending on the style of cataract incision, the anterior chamber can be entered through the trabecular meshwork. In a patient with decreased facility of outflow before surgery, further intraoperative damage to the trabecular meshwork may result in postoperative problems.

Intraocular pressure elevations may result from various intracameral agents used at the time of surgery. All the viscoelastic agents, such as Healon, Amvisc, or Occucoat, if left in the eye at the completion of surgery, have been associated with at least transiently elevated intraocular pressures. The use of alpha-chymotrypsin during intracapsular cataract extraction may cause marked elevations of intraocular pressures usually 2 to 5 days after surgery. This elevation is probably due to a combination of both zonular debris and direct effects of alpha-chymotrypsin on the trabecular meshwork. Retained lens cortical material may also temporarily obstruct the trabecular outflow, as well as incite increased postoperative inflammation. Campbell and associates (1980) have presented convincing evidence to support the hypothesis that rubbing of the peripheral iris by the lens zonules may lead to pigmentary dispersion syndrome in phakic eyes. A similar mechanism may be implicated in pseudophakic eyes. Posterior chamber intraocular lenses rub on the posterior surface of the iris, creating pigment dispersion. These patients have transillumination defects at the site of the supporting lens haptics. Pigment granules are seen in the anterior chamber, as well as on the anterior surface of the iris, intraocular lens, and in the trabecular meshwork.

Intraocular pressure elevation secondary to steroid response is often a concern of surgeons during the postoperative period. It has been the authors' experience that residual intraocular inflammation is a much more common cause of intraocular pressure elevation than is steroid response. Inadequately treated inflammation with decreasing doses of topical steroids may masquerade as a steroid response. Intraocular pressure elevations secondary to previously undiagnosed ocular inflammatory syndromes may also be confused with a response to the steroids when in fact inflammatory trabeculitis is the etiology of the pressure elevation.

Finally, among the open-angle varieties of glaucoma, preexisting primary open-angle glaucoma must be considered. Patients may exhibit normal preoperative intraocular pressures on screening exams, but the decreased ability to examine the posterior pole because of the cataract may impair a full glaucoma evaluation. These patients may be identified in the frequent postoperative examinations after cataract surgery, and the pressure elevations may be unrelated to the surgery itself.

Patients also exhibit closed-angle varieties of glaucoma after cataract surgery that are associated with peripheral anterior synechiae. Most common in this group is pupillary block from either an anterior or posterior chamber intraocular lenses. This complication is much less frequent with a posterior chamber intraocular lens. Patients with diabetes mellitus or with small, hyperopic eyes, which are prone to angle closure, may benefit from a peripheral iridectomy at the time of surgery. Other forms of pupillary block, with the vitreous face or posterior capsule in the absence of an intraocular lens occluding the pupil, also result in angle-closure glaucoma. Seclusio pupillae results when prolonged inflammation causes posterior synechiae of the iris to the anterior surface of a posterior chamber intraocular lens. It may also occur if the anterior surface of the iris fixes to the posterior face of an anterior chamber intraocular lens. This results in an iris bombé configuration and total angle closure.

A particularly difficult form of postoperative angle-closure glaucoma is aqueous misdirection syndrome or malignant glaucoma. All forms of intraocular lenses have been associated with this type of glaucoma. Posterior diversion of the aqueous humor produces a forward shift of the lens and iris, resulting in angle-closure glaucoma even in the presence of an iridectomy. Before surgery, these eyes often exhibit a shallow anterior chamber, poorly controlled angle-closure glaucoma, peripheral anterior synechiae, or even a history of phakic malignant glaucoma. After surgery, a shallow anterior chamber with the iris, implant, and posterior capsule appearing to bulge forward toward the cornea is found, even in the presence of a patent iridectomy. Vitreous may be compacted against the posterior capsule with a relatively clear, aqueous-containing space deep within the posterior segment. Ultrasonography can sometimes identify an echolucent, aqueous pocket in the vitreous.

Angle-closure glaucoma in the absence of pupillary block also occurs after lens implantation. A flat anterior chamber secondary to a wound leak or inadvertent filtering bleb at the site of the cataract incision should be suspected. Chronic inflammation with late-onset, progressive, peripheral anterior synechiae are occasionally found after otherwise uneventful implantations of posterior chamber lenses. These patients first exhibit peripheral anterior synechiae localized over the lens haptics, which progress over time to total angle closure. Another form of angle-closure glaucoma to be considered is neovascularization of the iris and of the angle structures. Epithelial downgrowth or fibrous ingrowth may occur after cataract surgery and lead to progressive angle-closure glaucoma.

THERAPY

Ocular. The management of elevations in intraocular pressure after intraocular lens placement should be directed toward the specific pathogenesis of the pressure rise. Increased intraocular pressure that results from prolonged inflammation usually responds well to topical corticosteroids, such as 1 per cent prednisolone acetate, which are administrated every 1 to 4 hours until the anterior chamber inflammation and the intraocular elevated pressure resolve. Depending on the state of the optic nerve and the height of the intraocular pressure elevation, aqueous formation inhibitors, such as beta-adrenergic antagonists, may be used to suppress aqueous humor formation. Topical cycloplegic agents, such as 5 per cent homatropine, are useful to produce ciliary muscle relaxation and prevent other complications, such as pupillary block. In general, epinephrine preparations are avoided because of their association with cystoid macular edema and a possible contribution to chronic inflammation. Uveitis glaucoma does not generally respond well to miotics. In fact, miotics may increase the inflammation by disrupting the blood-aqueous barrier. However, if intraocular pressure remains elevated after other ocular hypotensive agents have been employed and inflammation has subsided, a therapeutic trial of miotics, such as 4 per cent pilocarpine four times daily or 3 per cent carbachol three times daily, may be tried in the presence of a patent iridectomy and no evidence of pupillary block.

Pseudophakic pigment dispersion syndrome often responds to conventional ocular hypotensive agents, including miotics, beta-adrenergic blockers, and adrenergic agonists. As with phakic pigment dispersion syndrome, these eyes often do well with low-dose miotics that fix the pupil and prevent iris chafing. The addition of aqueous suppressant agents, such as beta-adrenergic blockers, is also effective in controlling intraocular pressure.

Systemic. Systemic carbonic anhydrase inhibitors may be prescribed either on a short-term or chronic basis for any of the conditions in which intraocular pressure is unacceptably high for the health of the optic nerve. Such osmotic agents as glycerin, mannitol, or isosorbide are often used for breaking attacks of pupillary block and as a temporary measure for patients awaiting surgery.

Surgical. Glaucoma resulting from a mechanical distortion or damage of the anterior chamber angle often requires surgical management. The surgeon should be sure that the inflammatory component has been suppressed before undertaking surgical intervention. Pupillary block glaucoma invariably requires the placement of an iridotomy or iridectomy. A surgical peripheral iridectomy is always indicated at the time of anterior chamber intraocular lens placement. Iridotomies can typically be placed using a laser; however, an edematous cornea may preclude the placement of an iridotomy, and a surgical iridectomy may need to be performed. If at all possible pupillary block should be broken medically with topical and/or oral agents before surgical intervention. Topical mydriatic/cycloplegics can be used to dilate the pupil and displace the iris diaphragm posteriorly. Short-acting mydriatics are preferred because

their action can be easily reversed if the pupil becomes too dilated to place a laser iridotomy.

For cases of glaucoma secondary to chronic inflammation, mechanical distortion of the anterior chamber, or pigmentary dispersion, the primary surgical decision is whether or not to remove the intraocular lens. In many cases the same factors that lead to the insertion of the intraocular lens initially make the surgeon reluctant to remove it. Most often it is difficult to attribute the intraocular inflammation to the presence of the intraocular lens; therefore, the inflammation is treated medically and the lens is left in place. However, if progressive peripheral anterior synechiae or extensive adhesions between the iris and the intraocular lens itself are developing, it is preferable to remove the lens before it becomes technically dangerous to do so. These adverse outcomes are more often seen with anterior chamber intraocular lens, but may occur with posterior chamber lenses as well.

Laser trabeculoplasty in aphakic or pseudophakic eyes may have more limited success than in eyes that have not had cataract surgery. This is especially true in aphakic eyes where vitreous extends into the anterior chamber. However, recent reports have found significant intraocular pressure lowering after argon laser trabeculoplasty in pseudophakic eyes, some of which have previously undergone filtering surgery. In patients with postoperative open-angle glaucoma, laser trabeculectomy is a therapeutic option. In the presence of active intraocular inflammation, laser trabeculoplasty should be avoided.

Cyclodestructive procedures, such as transcleral nd:YAG laser cycloablation or cyclocryotherapy, are generally reserved for eyes with poor visual potential. These procedures are generally felt to be less invasive than complex surgical protocols and may be appropriate in eyes that have undergone multiple complications after cataract surgery. Cyclodestructive procedures require at least a partially functioning trabecular outflow system because a total obstruction of the trabeculectomy meshwork would require total aqueous suppression, resulting in hypotony. The authors generally reserve cyclodestructive procedures as palliation only after other medical and surgical alternatives have been exhausted.

In the absence of extensive inflammation and conjunctival scarring, conventional trabeculectomy surgery may be used in pseudophakic eyes. The presence of an intact posterior capsule and the absence of vitreous in the anterior chamber greatly increase the success of such surgery. Adjunctive antimetabolite therapy, such as mitomycin-C and 5-fluorouracil, has been shown to increase the success rate of trabeculectomy in such eyes. In eyes with extensive conjunctival scarring of both superior quadrants, seton procedures, such as Baerveldt or Molteno implants, may be considered.

PRECAUTIONS

Pupillary block glaucoma may occur immediately after surgery, as well as years after intraocular lens implantation. All patients with anterior chamber intraocular lenses require long-term, careful observation and should be warned to consult their ophthalmologist promptly if symptoms of angle-closure glaucoma occur. Patients may have extensive, permanent angle closure when the first symptoms of pupillary block glaucoma are observed. The surgeon must be prepared to perform filtration surgery if an insufficient open angle exists after placement of an iridotomy. Patients with pupillary block occurring acutely after surgery should be evaluated for a possible wound leak.

An ocular hypertensive response may occur after capsulotomy with a nd:YAG laser in the pseudophakic eye. The mechanism of this glaucoma is not well understood, and the pressure elevation is typically self-limited. Anti-inflammatory agents are typically used postoperatively, and the use of perioperative apraclonidine has diminished the incidence of this complication.

COMMENTS

Implantation of intraocular lenses has become a standard protocol after cataract extraction during the past several decades. New varieties of pseudophakic glaucoma continue to be described with virtually all types of intraocular lenses. The ophthalmologist performing cataract surgery with intraocular lens implantation must be prepared to deal with such sequelae as they develop. With improved technical development of flexible anterior chamber lenses, the high rate of complications seen after implantation of the rigid varieties of these lenses may decrease. The association of rigid anterior chamber lenses, especially those with closed loop haptics, with bleeding, chronic uveitis, and pseudophakic bullous keratopathy may also decrease with these newer lenses. With the advent of foldable posterior chamber intraocular lenses, smaller wound sizes, and less intracameral manipulation, the incidence of glaucoma after cataract surgery may decrease. It is too early to predict the impact of foldable lenses at this time. Because intraocular pressure may increase, even after uncomplicated cataract surgery, patients, especially those with pre-existing open-angle glaucoma, must be followed closely during the postoperative period. Maximizing intraocular pressure control by promptly eliminating contributing factors may prevent further compromise of the optic nerve.

References

Apple DJ, et al: Complications of intraocular lenses. A historical and histopathological review. Surv Ophthalmol 29:1, 1984.

Campbell DG: Pigmentary dispersion and glaucoma. A new theory. Arch Ophthalmol 97:1667–1672, 1980.
De Heer LJ: Glaucoma as a problem in intraocular lens implantation. Doc Ophthalmol 49:337–346, 1980.
Ellingson FT: The uveitis-glaucoma-hyphema syndrome associated with the Mark VIII anterior chamber lens implant. J Am Intraocular Implant Soc 4:50–53, 1978.
Kielar RA, Stambaugh JL: Pupillary block glaucoma following intraocular lens implantation. Ophthalmol Surg 13:647–650, 1982.
Robin AL, Pollack IP: Argon laser trabeculoplasty in secondary forms of open-angle glaucoma. Arch Ophthalmol 101:382–384, 1983.
Rowsey JJ, Gaylor JR: Intraocular lens disasters. Peripheral anterior synechia. Ophthalmology 87:646–664, 1980.
Samples JR, Van Buskirk EM: Pigmentary glaucoma associated with posterior chamber intraocular lenses. Am J Ophthalmol 100:385–388, 1985.
Samples JR, et al: Pupillary block with posterior chamber intraocular lenses. Arch Ophthalmol 105:335–337, 1987.
Tomey KF, Traverso CE: The glaucoma in aphakia and pseudophakia. Surv Ophthalmol 36:79–112, 1991.
Van Buskirk EM: Pupillary block after intraocular lens implantation. Am J Ophthalmol 95:55–59, 1983.
Van Buskirk EM: Pseudophakic glaucoma. In Weinstein GW (ed): Open Angle Glaucoma. Contemporary Issues in Ophthalmology. New York, Livingstone, 1986, Vol 3, pp 133–154.
Van Buskirk EM: Late onset, progressive, peripheral anterior synechiae with posterior chamber intraocular lenses. Ophthalmic Surg 18:115–117, 1987.

GLAUCOMA ASSOCIATED WITH INTRAOCULAR TUMORS 365.64

CAROL L. SHIELDS, M.D., and JERRY A. SHIELDS, M.D.

Philadelphia, Pennsylvania

A number of intraocular tumors can produce ipsilateral elevation of the intraocular pressure. In such instances, there may be a delay in clinical recognition of the underlying neoplasm while the patient is treated for the secondary glaucoma. In cases of malignant tumors, this delay in diagnosis can have serious consequences.

In contrast to the primary glaucomas, which are generally bilateral, tumor-induced secondary glaucomas are almost always unilateral. The mechanism of the secondary glaucomas varies with the location, size, and type of tumor. Malignant tumors in the iris and ciliary body are more likely to obstruct aqueous outflow by directly infiltrating the trabecular meshwork. More posteriorly located intraocular neoplasms can produce anterior displacement of the lens-iris diaphragm causing angle closure, they may induce iris and angle neovascularization causing neovascular glaucoma, or they may liberate tumor cells in the anterior chamber angle, blocking aqueous outflow.

Primary Tumors of the Uvea

Uveal nevi are benign lesions that rarely produce secondary glaucoma. Occasionally, however, localized or diffuse uveal nevi can lead to secondary glaucoma. This occurs most often with a melanocytoma or with a diffuse nevus of the iris. Melanocytoma is a specific variant of nevus that usually occurs in the optic disc, but which can arise anywhere in the uveal tract. Those located in the optic disc or choroid rarely produce secondary glaucoma, whereas those that occur in the ciliary body or iris are more likely to produce secondary glaucoma. This tumor has an unusual tendency to undergo necrosis and fragmentation, liberating pigment into the anterior chamber and trabecular meshwork.

With regard to iris melanoma, the most common mechanism of glaucoma is direct invasion of the trabecular meshwork by tumor tissue. Occasionally it may bleed spontaneously, leading to hyphema and increased intraocular pressure. The diffuse iris melanoma produces a classic syndrome of acquired hyperchromic heterochromia and ipsilateral glaucoma.

In contrast to iris melanoma, ciliary body melanoma tends to attain a fairly large size before diagnosis. Ciliary body melanomas can produce secondary glaucoma by causing anterior displacement of the iris with secondary angle closure or by growing anteriorly into the trabecular meshwork and obstructing aqueous outflow. Less commonly, they can produce a hyphema, undergo necrosis, or cause iris neovascularization, all of which can lead to secondary glaucoma.

In the authors' series of 1913 eyes with choroidal melanoma, only 32 (2 per cent) had secondary glaucoma. In most prior series, the incidence of secondary glaucoma has been higher. This trend reflects the earlier clinical recognition and treatment of choroidal melanomas in recent years.

When secondary glaucoma occurs due to a choroidal melanoma, its cause is iris and angle neovascularization (56 per cent) or anterior displacement of the lens-iris diaphragm and secondary angle closure (44 per cent). Large necrotic choroidal melanomas can occasionally produce intraocular inflammation or hemorrhage, which can further contribute to secondary glaucoma.

Other rare uveal tumors, such as neurilemomas, leiomyomas, and neurofibromas, can produce secondary glaucoma by the same mechanisms.

Metastatic Tumors to the Uvea

Malignant tumors from distant primary sites metastasize via hematogenous routes to the uveal tract and rarely to the retina or optic nerve. Choroidal metastases only produce secondary glaucoma when they attain a large size, whereas iris and ciliary body metastases frequently produce secondary glaucoma because of their tendency to be friable and also to involve the angle structures. In the authors' series of patients with uveal metastases, secondary glaucoma was found in 64 per cent of iris metastasis, 67 per cent of ciliary body metastasis, and 2 per cent of choroidal metastasis. Metastatic tumors to the intraocular structures most commonly occur from primary sites in the breast and lung and less often from the gastrointestinal tract and kidney.

Iris and ciliary body metastases usually produce secondary glaucoma by seeding into the anterior chamber angle and trabecular meshwork, mechanically blocking aqueous outflow. In some cases, a solid growth of tumor cells can assume a ring-type infiltration of the trabecular meshwork, resulting in intractable glaucoma.

Metastatic tumors to the choroid appear as single or multiple elevated or diffuse lesions and often associated with a secondary nonrhegmatogenous retinal detachment. The most common mechanism of glaucoma with choroidal metastases is angle closure due to anterior displacement of the lens-iris diaphragm secondary to total retinal detachment. Neovascular glaucoma can occur in advanced cases with total retinal detachment.

In general, eyes with choroidal metastases are best managed by external beam radiotherapy to the involved eye, combined with any chemotherapy that the patient may be receiving for associated systemic metastasis. Such treatment may control associated secondary glaucoma, but supplemental medical treatment of the glaucoma may be necessary. In rare instances, the associated glaucoma can produce such severe pain that palliative enucleation is necessary.

Primary Tumors of the Retina

The most important tumors of the sensory retina include retinoblastoma, vascular tumors, and glial tumors. Retinoblastoma, the most important retinal tumor, frequently produces secondary glaucoma. In rare instances, advanced retinal capillary hemangiomas can produce secondary glaucoma in association with a total retinal detachment.

In the authors' series of 248 patients with retinoblastoma, about 17 per cent of 303 affected eyes had secondary glaucoma. The secondary glaucoma was due to iris neovascularization in 72 per cent of cases, to angle closure secondary to anterior displacement of the lens-iris diaphragm in 26 per cent of cases, and to tumor seeding into the anterior chamber in 2 per cent of cases. In cases with iris neovascularization, secondary hyphema sometimes contributed to the mechanism of glaucoma.

Tumors of the Nonpigmented and Pigmented Epithelium

Tumors of the nonpigmented epithelium of the ciliary body include medulloepithelioma, adenoma, and adenocarcinoma. The medulloepithelioma (previously called diktyoma) is an embryonic ciliary body tumor that becomes clinically apparent in the first few years of life. It can be benign or malignant, but the malignancy is low grade and the systemic prognosis is generally excellent. In the five cases of this rare tumor that the authors have managed, three patients had secondary glaucoma. In a large series from the Armed Forces Institute of Pathology, glaucoma occurred in 46 per cent of cases. In these cases, glaucoma can occur secondary to iris neovascularization or from direct invasion of the anterior chamber angle structures by the tumor. In some instances, hyphema or cysts in the anterior chamber may also contribute to obstruction of aqueous outflow.

Acquired tumors of the nonpigmented ciliary epithelium are rare, slow-growing, benign or lowly malignant lesions, and they rarely produce secondary glaucoma. Primary tumors of the pigmented epithelium (adenoma and adenocarcinoma) of the iris, ciliary body, and retina are rare. The mechanisms of glaucoma are the same as those of malignant melanoma.

Lymphoid Tumors and Leukemias

Lymphoid tumors and leukemias are grouped together here because they can produce a similar infiltration of the uveal tract and retina. The most important lymphoid tumors of the intraocular structures include benign reactive lymphoid hyperplasia (BRLH) of the uvea and malignant lymphoma, particularly large-cell lymphoma (histiocytic lymphoma, reticulum cell sarcoma). Secondary glaucoma most often occurs from direct infiltration of the anterior chamber angle and thickening of the iris and ciliary body by tumor cells. These actions result in blockage of aqueous outflow and secondary elevation of intraocular pressure.

Systemic Hamartomatoses (Phakomatoses)

The classic phakomatoses include encephalofacial hemangiomatosis (Sturge-Weber syndrome) neurofibromatosis, retinocerebellar capillary hemangiomatosis (von Hippel-Lindau syndrome), and tuberous sclerosis. The two conditions that are more likely to be associated with either infantile or juvenile glaucoma are encephalofacial hemangiomatosis and neurofibromatosis.

THERAPY

Ocular. The management of glaucoma secondary to intraocular tumors should depend on the type of tumor. In cases of benign tumors, it is often appropriate to first treat the glaucoma medically. In cases of malignant tumors, it may be appropriate to first treat the tumor in hopes of relieving the glaucoma. In cases of uveal melanoma, melanocytoma, metastasis, and lymphoid infiltration, the glaucoma may resolve with the primary treatment of the tumor either by surgical resection or radiotherapy. If the glaucoma persists despite effective therapy, then medical management of the secondary glaucoma is warranted. Generally, antiglaucoma eyedrops and systemic carbonic anhydrase inhibitors are instituted as necessary.

Surgical. Most melanocytic iris tumors should be managed initially by periodic observation, and any associated glaucoma should be managed medically. If the tumor shows evidence of growth or if the secondary glaucoma cannot be controlled, then surgical intervention should be considered. In cases of circumscribed tumors, excision of the tumor by a partial iridectomy, sometimes with laser or surgical trabeculectomy to control the glaucoma, can be undertaken. In the case of a diffuse iris melanoma with secondary glaucoma, enucleation is generally necessary. Fine-needle aspiration biopsy is indicated to differentiate melanoma from melanocytoma or nevus. The authors have found that open biopsy of the iris tumor or surgery to control the glaucoma in cases of diffuse iris melanoma can predispose to extrascleral extension of the tumor. In the case of iris melanocytoma, the liberated pigment in the trabecular meshwork may gradually disappear following complete excision of the main tumor by iridectomy or iridocyclectomy.

Before initiating treatment, small ciliary body melanomas can be managed by simple periodic observation until growth is documented. Somewhat larger tumors can be managed by local resection or episcleral plaque radiotherapy. Most tumors that are large or infiltrative enough to produce secondary glaucoma are generally best managed by enucleation of the affected eye. Careful medical evaluation and follow-up are warranted because of the relatively high risk of metastatic disease in cases of ciliary body melanomas with secondary glaucoma. In the authors' series of patients with ciliary body melanomas, 50 per cent of patients with secondary glaucoma died from metastatic melanoma within 2 years of the diagnosis.

The options in management of choroidal melanomas are well outlined in the literature and include simple observation, photocoagulation, radiotherapy, local resection, enucleation, and even orbital exenteration. Unfortunately, choroidal melanomas that have produced secondary glaucoma are generally so large that enucleation is necessary.

In some cases of uveal metastases associated with secondary glaucoma, the glaucoma may ultimately require laser or surgical trabeculectomy, cyclocryotherapy, retrobulbar alcohol injection, or even enucleation. Since most affected patients have a poor systemic prognosis, enucleation should be avoided if possible and the goal should be to make the patient comfortable.

The selected management of retinoblastoma should depend on the overall clinical findings and can include enucleation, radiotherapy, cryotherapy, and photocoagulation. In cases with secondary glaucoma, the tumor is usually quite advanced, and enucleation is considered the treatment of choice. In most cases of retinoblastoma associated with secondary glaucoma, the optic disc cannot be visualized ophthalmoscopically because of the large tumor within the eye. Therefore, it is particularly important in these cases to obtain a long section of optic nerve stump along with the globe at the time of enucleation, since the most important route of extraocular extension of this tumor is through the optic nerve to the central nervous system.

Management of small intraocular medulloepitheliomas consists of an attempt at local resection by a cyclectomy because the tumor is usually benign. Unfortunately, it is extremely difficult to remove such tumors completely, and recurrence is common, eventually requiring enucleation. In cases with glaucoma, enucleation is usually necessary because of pain or because malignancy cannot be excluded clinically.

Irradiation and Chemotherapy. The management of iris and ciliary body metastases should be systemic chemotherapy or other management that the patient is receiving for the systemic cancer. If the ocular tumor continues to proliferate, then external beam radiotherapy to the eye, giving 3500–4000 cGy to the affected eye in divided doses over a 4-week period, should be initiated. If the uveal metastasis is the patient's only active metastatic focus, then local plaque radiotherapy is certainly justified. This form of radiotherapy takes approximately 4 days and spares the uninvolved remainder of the eye and orbit. If any associated secondary glaucoma does not resolve after chemotherapy and radiotherapy, acetazolamide, timolol, or other medications should be continued to control the intraocular pressure and to keep the patient comfortable. In many instances, the glaucoma will progress relentlessly, and laser or filtering surgery can

be attempted. This decision should be made in light of the patient's prognosis, and enucleation should be avoided if the systemic prognosis is dismal.

The appropriate management of intraocular lymphoid tumors and leukemias is ocular radiotherapy combined with the chemotherapy that the patient may be receiving for the systemic disease. In the case of BRLH, about 2000 cGy is generally sufficient, whereas in the case of malignant lymphoma about 3000 to 4000 cGy may be necessary to bring about good resolution of the tumor. In some cases, the glaucoma resolves with the radiotherapy or chemotherapy, but in cases with severe glaucoma, this treatment may not help and enucleation of the eye, if it is blind and painful, may be necessary.

Ocular or Periocular Manifestations

Anterior Chamber: Hyphema; hypopyon; tumor seeds in aqueous or angle.
Choroid: Tumor.
Ciliary Body: Tumor.
Conjunctiva: Injection.
Cornea: Tumor clumps on endothelium.
Episclera: Tumor sentinel vessels over ciliary body tumor.
Eyelids: Edema.
Iris: Nodules; diffuse thickening; heterochromia; neovascularization.
Lens: Subluxed lens or cataract from ciliary body tumor compression or from chronic large bullous retinal detachment.
Optic Nerve: Glaucomatous cupping; engorgement.
Retina: Nonrhegmatogenous retinal detachment; endophytic or exophytic retinoblastoma.
Vitreous: Tumor seeds from retinoblastoma, melanoma, or lymphoma; hemorrhage.

PRECAUTIONS

A patient who presents with unexplained unilateral glaucoma could be harboring an unsuspected intraocular malignant tumor. Laser surgery or filtering procedures are contraindicated until a complete ophthalmologic examination, including careful indirect ophthalmoscopy, is performed to exclude the possibility of tumor. In cases where the posterior pole or ciliary body cannot be viewed because of opaque media, ultrasonography, transillumination, or other procedures are necessary to rule out a tumor. It is particularly important not to perform glaucoma surgery or vitrectomy on a child with vitreous cells and unilateral glaucoma until the possibility of retinoblastoma is excluded.

COMMENTS

The management of tumor-induced glaucoma usually consists of enucleation because most cases are due to advanced uveal melanoma or retinoblastoma. In cases of benign tumors, medical therapy can be attempted first, followed by laser or surgical therapy. It should be emphasized that the management of glaucoma secondary to iris tumors is a very difficult problem, because many such tumors are relatively benign histopathologically and all efforts are made to control the glaucoma by medical or laser treatment before surgical intervention. Trabeculectomy is controversial in the management of iris melanomas because of the possibility of tumor spread into the filtering bleb and episcleral tissues.

References

Broughton WL, Zimmerman LE: A clinicopathologic study of 56 cases of intraocular medulloepitheliomas. Am J Ophthalmol 85:407–418, 1978.
Shields JA, Annesley WH, Spaeth GL: Necrotic melanocytoma of iris with secondary glaucoma. Am J Ophthalmol 84:826–829, 1977.
Shields JA, Shields CL: Intraocular Tumors: A Text and Atlas. Philadelphia, WB Saunders, 1992.
Shields JA, Shields CL, Donoso LA: Management of posterior uveal melanoma. Surv Ophthalmol 36:161–195, 1991.
Shields JA, Shields CL, Donoso LA, Lieb WE: Changing concepts in the management of retinoblastoma. Ophthalmic Surg 21:72–76, 1990.
Shields CL, Shields JA, Shields MB, Augsburger JJ: Prevalence and mechanisms of secondary intraocular pressure elevation in eyes with intraocular tumors. Ophthalmology 94:839–846, 1987.

GLAUCOMA FOLLOWING BLEB FAILURE 365.89

DAVID A. LEE, M.D., M.S., F.A.C.S., and MANOLITO R. REYES, M.D.

Los Angeles, California

The basic mechanism of glaucoma filtration surgery is the creation of a fistula in the area of the corneoscleral limbus so as to form a bleb by channeling the aqueous humor from the anterior chamber into the subconjunctival space. This process circumvents the pathologically obstructed outflow system in the glaucomatous eye. A good bleb appears as a localized or diffuse area of conjunctival elevation that has a thin, transparent wall with microcystic changes on the surface and few blood vessels. Blebs may fail to function soon after surgery (within the first 2 weeks) or later in the postoperative period.

Early-onset bleb failures may be due to obstruction of the sclerostomy site by Descemet's membrane, iris, vitreous, ciliary process, lens, or blood clot. These causes are suspected

when there is elevated intraocular pressure with a deep anterior chamber and a low or absent bleb. If viscoelastic material is used to maintain the anterior chamber during and after surgery or to prevent hypotony, it may obstruct the flow of aqueous through the sclerostomy. Oversuturing of the scleral trabeculectomy flaps may be the most common cause of early bleb failure. In this case, there may be too many sutures, or the sutures may be too tightly tied.

A flat anterior chamber with a patent iridectomy and elevated intraocular pressure following a filtering procedure in a small eye may be due to malignant glaucoma. Pupillary block must first be ruled out by confirming the patency of the iridectomy.

Late-onset bleb failure may occur during the second postoperative week or later as the result of an encapsulated or encysted bleb. Such a bleb is highly elevated and frequently injected, smooth domed, thick walled, localized, and without surface microcystic changes. It is lined with a layer of fibrous tissue that prevents the passage of aqueous humor through the bleb wall.

Progressive scarring of the filtering bleb may occur within the first month after surgery or later. The wound healing process starts when damaged tissues release vascular components and inflammatory mediators into the extravascular space. Epithelialization then ensues by the movement of epithelial cells into the wound. Neutrophils, macrophages, and fibroblasts enter the wound, and each plays a significant role as the wound healing process continues. Neutrophils have antibacterial and chemotactic properties, macrophages are involved in the phagocytosis of cellular debris, and fibroblasts are responsible for the synthesis and secretion of collagen and other extracellular matrix proteins that fill the wound. Proliferation of episcleral and subconjunctival Tenon's fibroblasts creates excessive scar tissue that obstructs the sclerostomy externally, resulting in a flat, scarred conjunctival bleb and increased intraocular pressure. Control of this wound healing process may prevent bleb failure after glaucoma filtering surgery.

THERAPY

Ocular. Digital massage should be used initially in attempting to save marginally filtering blebs. The purpose of this massage is to open the sclerostomy wound by applying pressure either adjacent to the scleral trabeculectomy flap or on the lower lid against the inferior part of the globe while the patient is looking superiorly. Digital massage can be performed repeatedly by the physician in the office or by the patient at home. The efficacy of the massage should be established by measuring intraocular pressure before and after its performance in the office before it is performed on an ongoing basis. If the patient will be doing the massage, careful instruction is necessary to avoid any complications. Topical antiglaucoma therapy, such as beta blockers, or systemic medication, such as carbonic anhydrase inhibitors, may be administered to patients who have persistently elevated intraocular pressure in spite of digital massage.

Surgical. In cases of early-onset bleb failure due to a sclerostomy site obstructed by Descemet's membrane, iris, vitreous, ciliary process, lens, or blood clot, an argon or Nd:YAG laser can be of benefit in removing the obstructing material. If this procedure is not successful, a surgical revision of the filtering bleb to remove the obstruction may be necessary. Oversuturing of the scleral trabeculectomy flap can be relieved by cutting the sutures with an argon laser using a Hoskins or Zeiss lens pressed on the conjunctiva overlying the sutures in order to visualize the sutures more clearly.

Failure to create and maintain a patent peripheral iridectomy after filtering surgery may result in pupillary block glaucoma. The definitive treatment for this complication is laser or surgical peripheral iridectomy. Ciliary block glaucoma requires aggressive medical treatment with cycloplegics (atropine), beta blockers, carbonic anhydrase inhibitors, and hyperosmotic agents. If medical therapy proves unsuccessful in relieving the block, Nd:YAG laser disruption of the anterior hyaloid face or argon laser photocoagulation of the visible ciliary processes through the patent iridectomy may allow the entrapped aqueous humor in the vitreous cavity to escape and reform the anterior chamber. If laser therapy is not possible or is ineffective, a pars plana anterior vitrectomy and hyaloidectomy may be curative.

An encapsulated bleb can initially be managed conservatively with beta blockers and/or carbonic anhydrase inhibitors because the capsule of the bleb frequently becomes more permeable to aqueous humor with time. Other methods of digital massage directly compressing the bleb may be performed. After topical anesthetization of the conjunctiva, a moistened cotton applicator can be pressed onto the dome of the encapsulated bleb. Alternatively, digital pressure can be applied through the eyelid overlying the bleb as the patient looks downward. The direct pressure compresses the bleb and closes the trabeculectomy scleral flap, forcing the entrapped aqueous humor through the encapsulated wall into the adjacent subconjunctival space. Either of these procedures can be repeated several times to enlarge the bleb.

Two surgical techniques may be useful in managing encapsulated blebs if time, medical therapy, and massage fail to resolve the condition. The first is needling of the encapsulated bleb, a relatively simple technique in which a 30-gauge needle is passed subconjunctivally to the encapsulated bleb and holes are pierced in the capsule. The second approach is to reopen the conjunctival incision carefully and partially or completely excise the encapsulated wall. An antimetabolite drug, such as 5-fluorouracil (5-FU), may be used as an adjunct to these techniques to prevent reformation of the bleb capsule.

Antineoplastic agents, which exert their cytotoxic effect by interfering with DNA or RNA replication, protein synthesis, or cell division, directly affect fibroblast migration and proliferation and collagen synthesis. The most commonly used clinical agents are 5-FU and mitomycin. 5-FU is usually given as a subconjunctival injection* after glaucoma filtering surgery at a dose of 5 mg in 0.5 ml, as frequently as twice a day during the first postoperative week, and then once a day during the second postoperative week. Mitomycin* is usually applied intraoperatively during glaucoma filtering surgery using a Weck cell sponge saturated with a solution of 0.3 to 0.4 mg per ml of mitomycin. These regimens for 5-FU and mitomycin can be modified according to clinical response and toxic reactions.

Ocular or Periocular Manifestations

Anterior Chamber: Deep in cases of blocked sclerostomy; shallow in cases of malignant and pupillary block glaucoma.

Conjunctiva: Conjunctival injection; flat bleb; encapsulated bleb.

Cornea: Epithelial edema associated with elevated intraocular pressure.

Optic Nerve: Glaucomatous cupping.

Other: Increased intraocular pressure; glaucomatous visual field defect.

PRECAUTIONS

Glaucoma filtering surgery should be performed carefully so as to minimize trauma to the conjunctiva and sclera and thus reduce inflammation and fibrosis. Gentle manipulation of the conjunctiva with smooth forceps to avoid buttonholes and mild cautery to prevent excessive inflammation and charring when controlling bleeding are important. Conjunctival wound closure is critical so as to avoid wound leaks and flat anterior chambers in the immediate postoperative period. Postoperative medical management includes topical steroids, cycloplegics, and antibiotics. Steroids are known to inhibit prostaglandin synthesis, thus reducing the amount of inflammation. Steroids can be given initially at the conclusion of surgery as a subconjunctival injection* and then maintained as topical applications for several weeks. Cycloplegics, such as atropine, relieve ciliary body spasm, dilate the pupil, and deepen the anterior chamber by pulling the lens-iris diaphragm posteriorly. Prophylactic topical antibiotics can prevent postoperative infection. Usually eyes with very thin blebs require close observation for signs of infection. Infections of the bleb usually impair or prevent the bleb from functioning and cause endophthalmitis. Smears and cultures of the bleb, conjunctiva, aqueous humor, and vitreous should be taken before initiating aggressive systemic and topical antibiotic therapy.

Digital massage should be used cautiously and under careful supervision. Improper massage can injure the bleb, create a corneal abrasion, or result in excessive hypotony. Laser sclerostomy revision carries a risk of transient increases in intraocular pressure, uveitis, and damage to the cornea, iris, lens, conjunctiva, and retina. Laser suture lysis of trabeculectomy flap sutures entails the danger of bleb leaks and hypotony. Bleb needling procedures carry the risks of bleb leaks, infection, and inadvertent intraocular penetration. Surgical bleb revision has the same risk as the original filtering surgery, as well as the risk of recurrence of scar tissue formation and bleb failure. Complications stemming from the use of the antimetabolites—5-FU and mitomycin—include corneal and conjunctival epithelial defects, superficial punctate keratitis, corneal edema and ulceration, and bleb ruptures. Awareness of early signs of toxicity and prompt treatment can prevent or minimize severe complications. Therapy should be discontinued temporarily if mild complications occur and curtailed if severe complications arise.

COMMENTS

The failing filtering bleb presents the ophthalmic surgeon with a challenging management problem. It is best to minimize the chances of its occurrence through the practice of meticulous and careful surgical technique. Medications that decrease inflammation and scar tissue formation will improve the chance of success. Standard methods for managing early bleb failure include digital massage, laser suture lysis, and bleb needling. New techniques are being developed to revive failing blebs. The Nd:YAG laser can be used in a transconjunctival approach to disrupt an encapsulated bleb wall. Alternatively, high-intensity focal therapeutic ultrasound can be applied to the area of a failed or failing bleb to improve the drainage of aqueous humor, probably by increasing scleral permeability. By far the most common cause of glaucoma filtering bleb failure is the excessive wound healing response. New drugs and drug delivery systems are being investigated to directly address this issue so as to control the intraocular pressure and preserve vision and optic nerve function in glaucoma patients.

References

Addicks EM, Quigley HA, Green WR, Robin AL: Histologic characteristics of filtering blebs in glaucomatous eye. Arch Ophthalmol 101:795–798, 1983.
Ewing RH, Stamper RL: Needle revision with and without 5-fluorouracil for the treatment of failed filtering bleb. Am J Ophthalmol 110:254–259, 1989.
The Fluorouracil Filtering Surgery Study Group: Fluorouracil Filtering Surgery Study one-year follow-up. Am J Ophthalmol 108:625–635, 1989.
Hoskins HD, Kass MA: Complications and failure of filtering surgery. In Hoskins HD, Kass MA (eds): Becker-Shaffer's Diagnosis and Therapy of the Glaucomas, 6th ed. St. Louis, CV Mosby, 1989, pp 583–604.
Rankin GA, Latina MA: Transconjunctival ND: YAG laser revision of failing trabeculectomy. Ophthalmic Surg 21:365–367, 1980.
Shields MB: Filtering surgery. In Shields MB: Textbook of Glaucoma, 3rd ed. Baltimore, Williams & Wilkins, 1992, pp 577–611.
Skuta GL, Beeson CC, Higginbotham ES, Lichter PR, Musch DC, Bergstrom TJ, Klein TB, Falck FY: Intraoperative mitomycin versus postoperative 5-fluorouracil in high-risk glaucoma filtering surgery. Ophthalmology 99: 438–444, 1992.
Tahery MM, Lee DA: Review: Pharmacologic control of wound healing in glaucoma filtration surgery. J Ocular Pharmacol 5:155–169, 1989.
Van Buskirk EM: Assessment and management of filtering blebs. In Mills RP, Weinreb RN (eds): Glaucoma Surgical Techniques. San Francisco, American Academy of Ophthalmology, 1991, pp 99–116.
Yablonski M, Masonson HM, El-Sayyad F, Dennis PH, Hargrave S, Coleman DJ: Use of therapeutic ultrasound to restore failed trabeculectomies. Am J Ophthalmol 103:492–496, 1987.

THE GLAUCOMA SUSPECT 365.00

JOHN C. MORRISON, M.D.

Portland, Oregon

Glaucoma is a lifelong disease that requires chronic medical therapy and, occasionally, intraocular surgery. Because of the expense and potential for adverse ocular and systemic side effects, diagnosing glaucoma and instituting therapy are important medical decisions with lasting consequences.

Because nearly all glaucoma therapy is intended to lower intraocular pressure (IOP), the diagnosis of glaucoma requires recognizing the characteristic features of glaucomatous optic nerve damage and making a clinical judgment that the patient's current IOP will cause progressive deterioration. This judgment is obvious in patients with markedly elevated IOP and extensive optic nerve damage. However, many patients with optic nerves suggestive of glaucoma do not have elevated IOP, and the risks of antiglaucoma therapy cannot be immediately justified. Such patients are considered glaucoma suspects and warrant close observation.

Recognition of the glaucoma suspect hinges on the appearance of the optic nerve. Asymmetric cupping between the right and left eyes and focal erosions of the neuroretinal rim aid in differentiating glaucomatous discs from those with large, "physiologic" cups. Glaucoma often preferentially damages the superior and inferior neuroretinal rims, producing "vertical" elongation of the cup. Studies of normal optic nerves suggest that the inferior neuroretinal rim is usually thicker than the superior. A reversal of this relationship may be a subtle sign of inferior disc damage.

Accurate assessment of the optic disc depends on determining the contour of the disc surface. This requires routine use of three-dimensional techniques, such as stereo biomicroscopic funduscopy with a contact lens, Hruby lens, or a 90 diopter lens. Two-dimensional viewing with the direct ophthalmoscope requires accurate determination of surface detail and frequent corroboration with stereo techniques. Poor visibility due to patient movement may require stereo fundus photography for a permanent record that can be studied at leisure and used for future comparisons.

THERAPY

Ocular. Treatment of the glaucoma suspect involves close monitoring of IOP and careful examination for early manifestations of progressive loss of visual function. Because diurnal IOP fluctuation is accentuated in glaucoma, all-day pressure curves or random pressures taken at different times of the day may reveal higher pressures than those seen on initial examination. Tonography, although cumbersome, may identify patients who have low outflow facility and are likely to have wider pressure variations. Determining IOP before and after instilling a cycloplegic is more practical and can be easily incorporated into the standard office practice.

Recent advances in optic nerve head analysis and automated, quantitative perimetry now allow careful appraisal of the appearance and function of the optic nerve over time. Stereo disc photography provides a permanent record for future comparisons, although the angle of separation must be kept constant and the apparent cupping may differ from that seen by direct examination. Automated disc analyzers using standard photography with software for longitudinal comparisons of disc contour and nerve fiber layer thickness have found limited usefulness. However, similar instruments based on the scanning laser ophthalmoscope are relatively independent of pupil size and media opacities, two frequently encountered problems in the elderly population.

The nerve fiber layer appearance should be used to corroborate the optic disc appearance. Best viewed temporally with red-free light approximately 1 disc diameter from the nerve head, its distinct striations are thickest in the arcuate bundles and thinner in between, producing a characteristic "light-dark-light" appearance. Departure from this pattern, with either focal or generalized thinning, is usually reflected in the disc contour. However, pathologic nerve fiber layer thinning without significant cupping occasionally occurs in patients with small optic nerve heads, such as hyperopes with intermittent angle-closure glaucoma.

Longitudinal analysis of the nerve fiber layer over time using red-free photography has proven too subjective for routine use. However, the scanning laser ophthalmoscope can provide detailed maps of nerve fiber layer thickness that may be useful for detecting progressive tissue loss.

Typically, changes in the disc and nerve fiber layer precede visual field defects. However, automated visual field analysis can help in monitoring the glaucoma suspect, particularly if equivocal or borderline changes are present. Hemifield and change analysis programs provide quantitative, reliable measurements of visual field sensitivity for detecting progressive optic nerve damage.

Ocular or Periocular Manifestations

Nerve Fiber Layer: Diffuse thinning; focal, wedge defects.

Optic nerve: Increased cupping with vertical elongation; focal neuroretinal rim erosion, especially superior and inferior.

Visual Fields: Generalized depression; focal sensitivity loss; nasal "steps."

PRECAUTIONS

The detection of glaucomatous optic nerve damage relies heavily on the contour of the optic nerve head, with less emphasis on pallor. Disc pallor that involves the neuroretinal rim is atypical for glaucoma and suggests an intracranial process or neurogenic problem. In such cases, neuro-ophthalmic evaluation and possibly MRI studies are indicated.

Other conditions that mimic glaucomatous optic nerve damage include optic nerve colobomas, the morning glory syndrome, and optic nerve pits. These can be recognized by their characteristic associated findings. Large "physiologic" cups, although not glaucomatous, are often associated with myopia. Because myopia is a risk factor for glaucoma with potentially increased optic nerve susceptibility to IOP, such patients should have routine examinations, particularly if other risk factors are present, including black race, family history, and vascular disease.

COMMENTS

Once identified, the glaucoma suspect is unlikely to undergo rapid, progressive optic nerve damage. Therefore, the decision to start therapy need not be made on the basis of a single examination. Once unacceptable IOP is documented or progressive deterioration in the optic nerve head appearance or visual function occurs, treatment with standard glaucoma therapy is indicated. Similar principles apply to altering therapy in established glaucoma patients, particularly when surgery seems indicated.

References

Jonas JB, Zach FM, Gusek GC, Naumann GOH: Pseudo-glaucomatous physiologic large cups. Am J Ophthalmol 107:137–144, 1989.
Miller JM, Caprioli J: An optimal reference plane to detect glaucomatous nerve fiber layer abnormalities with computerized image analysis. Graefe's Arch Ophthalmol 230:124–128, 1992.
Quigley HA, Green WR: The histology of human glaucoma cupping and optic nerve damage: Clinic pathologic correlation in 21 eyes. Ophthalmology 86:1803, 1979.
Sommer A, D'Anna SA, Kues HA, George T: High-resolution photography of the retinal nerve fiber layer. Am J Ophthalmol 96:535, 1983.
Sommer A, Quigley HA, Robin AL, Miller NR, Katz J, Arkell S: Evaluation of nerve fiber layer assessment. Arch Ophthalmol 102:1766, 1984.
Trobe, Glaser JD, Cassady JS, Herschler J, Anderson DR: Non-glaucomatous excavation of the optic disc. Arch Ophthalmol 98:1046, 1980.

GLAUCOMATOCYCLITIC CRISIS 364.22
(Posner-Schlossman Syndrome)

ABRAHAM SCHLOSSMAN, M.D., F.A.C.S.

New York, New York

Glaucomatocyclitic crisis is unilateral glaucoma characterized by recurrent attacks of glaucoma that are usually associated with signs of mild cyclitis. The disease generally occurs in patients between 20 to 50 years of age, with individual attacks of ocular hypertension lasting from a few hours to 1 month, but very rarely over 2 weeks. The onset of symptoms is acute with minimal ocular discomfort, blurred vision, and colored halos around lights. The intraocular pressure fluctuates, but initially is usually between 40 and 60 mm Hg. A few keratic precipitates are present, and the pupil of the affected eye is larger than that of the other. Synechiae generally do not develop. The prognosis is excellent, with no permanent changes detectable in the visual fields after an attack.

Knox (1988) has stressed multifactorial etiologies in relation to the Posner-Schlossman syndrome. Of 32 patients suffering from this condition, 68 per cent of the male and 38 per cent of the female patients demonstrated symptoms of peptic ulcer. The relationship to allergy has been emphasized by Demailly and co-workers (1985), who described allergic aspects of 13 patients with the syndrome.

THERAPY

Ocular. Treatment of the ocular hypertension should be limited to the attack and should consist of the use of mild miotics, such as 0.5 to 2.0 per cent pilocarpine or 0.25 to 0.50 per cent timolol. Topical ocular corticosteroids are used one to four times daily to control inflammation and are especially helpful during the acute phase. Occasional pupillary dilation with 10 per cent phenylephrine usually confirms that no synechiae are forming.

Supportive. Analgesics or tranquilizers may be helpful during attacks to control pain and apprehension. Follow-up examinations are important to monitor inflammation or pressure elevation.

Ocular or Periocular Manifestations

Anterior Chamber: Cells and flare.
Cornea: Epithelial edema; keratic precipitates.
Iris: Anterior and posterior synechiae (rare); ciliary flush; hypochromic heterochromia.
Optic Nerve: Glaucomatous cupping (rare).
Other: Decreased visual acuity (temporary); increased intraocular pressure; mydriasis.

PRECAUTIONS

Strong miotics and, perhaps, strong mydriatics tend to aggravate the symptoms by producing pain, congestion, and spasm of the ciliary muscle.

In view of the ineffectiveness of surgical measures and the benign and self-limited nature of the disease, there exists no indication for any surgical intervention in this syndrome. Medical therapy between attacks is not indicated.

Topical corticosteroids give good results by allaying ciliary irritability. However, corticosteroid-induced glaucoma may occur if such treatment is prolonged.

COMMENTS

The value of recognizing this syndrome lies in the fact that surgical procedures not only are unnecessary but are definitely contraindicated in this condition. Glaucomatocyclitic crises differ from acute narrow-angle glaucoma and glaucoma secondary to uveitis in that the angle of the anterior chamber is open, even at the height of an attack, and the eye is white with minimal pain during attacks. Also, facility of outflow is normal between attacks, and provocative tests give normal responses.

References

Demailly P, Zaegel R, Blamanthier J, et al: Syndrome de Posner Schlossman et allergie. J Fr Ophthalmol 8:773–777, 1985.

de Roeth A Jr: Glaucomatocyclitic crisis. Am J Ophthalmol 69:370–371, 1970.

Hollwich F: Zur Klinik und Therapie des Posner-Schlossman Syndroms. Klin Monatsbl Augenheilkd 172:736–744, 1978.

Knox DL: Glaucomatocyclitic crises and systemic disease: Peptic ulcer, other gastrointestinal disorders, allergy and stress. Trans Am Ophthalmol Soc 86: 473–495, 1988.

Posner A, Schlossman A: Syndrome of unilateral attacks of glaucoma with cyclitic symptoms. Arch Ophthalmol 39:517–535, 1948.

Posner A, Schlossman A: Further observations on the syndrome of glaucomatocyclitic crises. Trans Am Acad Ophthalmol Otolaryngol 57:531–536, 1953.

Reibaldi A, Avitabile T: Topical indomethacin in Posner and Schlossman's syndrome. J Ocular Ther Surg 4:28–31, 1985.

Theodore FH: Observations on glaucomatocyclitic crises (Posner-Schlossman syndrome). Br J Ophthalmol 36:207–210, 1952.

Varma R, Katz LJ, Spaeth GL: Surgical treatment of acute glaucomatocyclitic crisis in a patient with primary open-angle glaucoma. Am J Ophthalmol 105:99–100, 1988.

INFANTILE GLAUCOMA 743.20
(Primary Congenital Open-Angle Glaucoma)

DAVID S. WALTON, M.D.

Boston, Massachusetts

Infantile glaucoma is a specific type of childhood glaucoma and the most common cause of glaucoma in early childhood. It is caused by polygenic inheritance and is usually bilateral. The elevation of intraocular pressure is caused by a defect of the internal surface of the filtration angle. The severity of the disease is quite variable, and there is a marked difference between patients with respect to the severity of symptoms and corneal signs and, subsequently, the age of diagnosis. Most patients are symptomatic before 3 months of age and diagnosed before 9 months of age. They usually possess significant light sensitivity, corneal stigmata of increased eye pressure (including defects in Descemet's membrane), and variable amounts of optic nerve cupping.

THERAPY

Surgical. The treatment of infantile glaucoma is surgical. Internal goniotomy or trabeculotomy is indicated. Surgery should be performed by surgeons experienced with these procedures and in the care of children with glaucoma. If control is not attained after repeating these procedures, other surgery must be considered. Trabeculectomy is not as successful during the first year of life compared to later in childhood. It is, however, the next surgical procedure of choice if the glaucoma cannot be controlled medically after goniosurgery with the use of carbonic anhydrase inhibitors and other glaucoma medications. Trabeculectomy surgery combined with the use of topically applied mitomycin-C* at surgery should be considered. Drainage devices, such as a Molteno implant, should next be considered, followed by cycloablative procedures.

Ocular. Miotics rarely are helpful for this type of glaucoma. In young children, timolol has also not proven to be a useful agent. Carbonic anhydrase inhibitors lower the eye pressure significantly in young children, but acetazolamide infrequently normalizes the pressure in infantile glaucoma. However, these agents are useful to achieve some clearing of the corneal edema and to lower the pressure before surgery is performed or to enhance pressure control after surgery.

Ocular or Periocular Manifestations

Anterior Chamber: Deep, flat iris.

Ciliary Body: Poorly defined and occasionally narrow ciliary body band; poorly defined or absent scleral spur.

Cornea: Breaks in Descemet's membrane; enlargement; epithelial edema; limbal thinning; stromal edema.

Iris: Easily visible peripheral iris blood vessels and posterior pigmented epithelium.

Optic Nerve: Atrophy; glaucomatous cupping.

Other: Amblyopia; epiphora; myopia.

PRECAUTIONS

There are many causes of glaucoma in infancy and early childhood. Both primary childhood glaucomas and secondary causes of glaucoma must be considered. Careful examination of the patient with childhood glaucoma must be performed to rule out the presence of systemic or related ocular abnormalities before the diagnosis of primary congenital open-angle glaucoma can be made with confidence.

COMMENTS

The infant's eye is quickly damaged by increased intraocular pressure. The earlier the diagnosis of glaucoma is made and the more effectively pressure is brought under control, the less likely will be the occurrence of secondary glaucomatous changes, such as tears in Descemet's membrane, increase in corneal size, corneal edema, damage to the optic discs, and visual field defects.

However, one must remember that vision, not pressure control alone, must be the goal of the ophthalmic surgeon. All children with infantile glaucoma should be examined regularly. Refraction should be part of the routine periodic examination of these children. If a child develops a deviation or a significant degree of anisometropia, treatment to prevent amblyopia should be begun promptly. Finally, the patient must have continuing examination for life to avoid the tragic loss of vision that can accompany later undetected increases in intraocular pressure.

References

Anderson DR: The development of the trabecular meshwork and its abnormality in primary infantile glaucoma. Trans Am Ophthalmol Soc 79:458–485, 1981.

DeLuise VP, Anderson DR: Review: Primary infantile glaucoma. Surv Ophthalmol 28:1–19, 1983.

Shaffer TN, Weiss DI: Congenital and Pediatric Glaucomas. St. Louis, CV Mosby, 1970, pp 37–59.

Walton DS: Primary congenital open-angle glaucoma. A study of the anterior segment abnormalities. Trans Am Ophthalmol Soc 77:746–768, 1979.

Walton DS: Primary congenital open-angle glaucoma. In Chandler PA, Grant WM (eds): Glaucoma, 2nd ed. Philadelphia, Lea & Febiger, 1979, pp 329–343.

JUVENILE GLAUCOMA
365.14

MARIANNE E. FEITL, M.D.,

Danville, Pennsylvania

and THEODORE KRUPIN, M.D.

Chicago, Illinois

Juvenile glaucoma is not a single disease entity; rather, it is a heterogeneous grouping of glaucomas defined by an onset in older children and young adults. Age limits for this grouping are arbitrarily set at between 3 to 5 and 30 to 35 years of age, which is after the onset of most cases of infantile glaucoma and before the manifestation of most adult primary glaucomas. In a large series of glaucoma patients, only a small number, approximately 0.02 per cent, were diagnosed within this age interval. Unfortunately, because of a low index of suspicion on the part of the physician, the diagnosis of glaucoma within this age group is easily overlooked.

Milder cases of primary congenital glaucoma may go unrecognized until later in childhood. These children show no sign of ocular discomfort and have perfectly clear corneas with only mild corneal enlargement or breaks in Descemet's membrane (Haab's striae). Progressive myopia and corneal enlargement may rarely occur in glaucoma in children over the age of 3 years, although severe buphthalmos does not generally occur. Juvenile-onset glaucoma can occur in other conditions associated with abnormal iridocorneal angles: aniridia, iridocorneal dysgenesis (Axenfeld's or Rieger's syndrome), Stürge-Weber syndrome, neurofibromatosis, and Lowe's syndrome.

Glaucoma secondary to traumatic angle recession, hyphema, glaucomatocyclitic crisis, and rubeosis iridis may occur in this age group. Neoplasia, including the phakomatoses, retinoblastoma, acute leukemia, juvenile xanthogranuloma, and medulloepithelioma, may also cause secondary glaucoma. An important cause of secondary glaucoma is previous surgery for congenital cataract. Glaucoma may also be found in patients with congenital rubella. Glaucoma in ocular rubella may be caused by iridocyclitis, angle anomalies resembling primary congenital glaucoma or mesodermal dysgenesis, an intumescent lens, or pupillary block after cataract extraction. Although the ocular abnormalities are usually noted in the neonatal period, the glaucoma may have its onset in later childhood or young adulthood. These late-onset glaucomas are most often found in eyes with microphthalmia and cataracts.

Patients with juvenile rheumatoid arthritis (JRA) have a significant incidence (8 to 24 per cent) of uveitis that may lead to glaucoma. Female patients and patients with mono- or pauciarticular JRA have a higher incidence of iridocyclitis than those with the polyarticular form. Since patients are often asymptomatic, they must be examined frequently for ocular involvement. Of note, no parallel has been found between the activity of the iridocyclitis and the joint disease. The iritis may first develop in patients over the age of 16, although an earlier onset is more common. Appropriate treatment with cyclopegics and steroids should be instituted to prevent peripheral anterior synechiae or neovascular membranes. In addition, topical cycloplegics increase uveoscleral outflow, which may reduce intraocular pressure. Antiglaucoma therapy should be instituted if necessary. Topical miotics are avoided since these agents can increase intraocular inflammation and decrease uveoscleral outflow resulting in a paradoxical rise in intraocular pressure. Other important causes of uveitis include sarcoidosis, ankylosing spondylitis, herpes zoster, syphilis, and possibly tuberculosis.

Some cases of juvenile-onset glaucoma resemble primary open-angle glaucoma of the adult type. The possibility of secondary open-angle glaucoma related to topically applied corticosteroids, especially in contact lens wearers, must be eliminated by a careful history. In contrast to primary open-angle glaucoma, which characteristically occurs after the age of 40 years, there is a preponderance of male patients and of myopia in juvenile-onset glaucoma.

In addition, pigmentary glaucoma may have its onset during this age interval. These patients characteristically show mid-peripheral iris transillumination defects and pigment deposition on the corneal endothelium (Krukenberg's spindle), trabecular meshwork, iris, and lens. Pigmentary glaucoma seems to become less severe in some patients with advancing age. This decrease in severity may be due to an increase in the axial length of the lens, which elevates the peripheral iris above the lens zonules and decreases pigment liberation. Intraocular pressure in pigmentary glaucoma is subject to large spontaneous fluctuations, which must be considered in evaluating the response to medical treatment. These patients occasionally manifest the classic symptoms of an acute intraocular pressure rise, particularly after an iris pigment "shower" from mydriasis or physical exercise.

Primary angle-closure glaucoma is extremely rare in young people. When present, it is usually of the plateau iris type. Angle-closure glaucoma in children as a result of pupillary block is usually secondary to other ocular disorders, including anterior uveitis, microcornea, spherophakia (Marchesani's syndrome), a dislocated lens (Marfan's syndrome or homocystinuria), retrolental fibroplasia, or intraocular surgery, particularly for congenital cataracts.

THERAPY

Ocular. Most patients with juvenile open-angle glaucoma should be given a thorough trial with medical therapy. Treatment is tempered by the same considerations as with the adult glaucomas. Children are less likely than adults to complain of drug side effects and thus must be watched and questioned more carefully. The beta-adrenergic blocking drugs should be used with caution in children. Although these agents can be effective, nonselective beta blockers should be avoided in patients with asthma because of their bronchospastic effects. Betaxolol (Betoptic), a se-

lective β_1-antagonist, may be tolerated in patients with pulmonary disease. Beta blockers also should be used cautiously in patients with heart problems, including congestive heart failure. Topical epinephrine or its prodrug dipivefrin administered twice daily is an excellent hypotensive agent in juvenile patients and may be used alone or in combination with miotics or other agents. Maculopathy that is reversible on stopping the topical medication can occur in aphakic eyes with either epinephrine or dipivefrin.

Oral carbonic anhydrase inhibitors are often useful and better tolerated than miotics in young glaucoma patients. Acetazolamide in daily oral doses of 15 to 30 mg/kg is administered in divided doses. Methazolamide may cause fewer side effects than acetazolamide. The possibility of renal calculi should be borne in mind and indicated to the parents. In addition, there may be a possible association of the carbonic anhydrase inhibitors with bone marrow depression and aplastic anemia. Future clinical availability of a topical carbonic anhydrase inhibitor may provide better tolerance and reduced side effects.

Topical pilocarpine is an effective ocular hypotensive agent, particularly in children with open iridocorneal angles. However, despite this drug's efficacy the induced miosis and myopia may cause sufficiently disabling symptoms to prevent its use. Occasionally, bedtime administration of pilocarpine gel is better tolerated than pilocarpine drops. Membrane-controlled pilocarpine delivery systems (Ocuserts) offer the advantages of less miosis, less induced myopia, and theoretically better diurnal intraocular pressure control. However, some patients have difficulty retaining these membranes in the cul-de-sac. Carbachol is also an excellent replacement or alternate drug for pilocarpine when resistance has developed.

Young patients should be examined frequently until maintenance of a satisfactory intraocular pressure level is achieved. In the absence of reliable visual fields, one must rely more heavily on correlation of intraocular pressure level and the stability of optic disc damage.

Surgical. Medical therapy is usually less effective in juvenile than adult-onset primary glaucoma, and surgical intervention is often necessary. Iridectomy is the procedure of choice in primary or secondary angle closure. Mechanical and technical incompatibilities of the slit-lamp-based laser and the need for general anesthesia may dictate a surgical iridectomy, rather than a laser iridotomy.

Goniotomy or ab externo trabeculotomy is indicated as the initial surgery in eyes with congenital glaucoma. Gonioscopically, the iridocorneal angle has a thick, spongy, and ground-glass uveotrabecular meshwork with poorly defined normal landmarks. The surgeon should attempt to include as many clock hours of the circumference as possible during the goniotomy incision. The same consideration applies for trabeculotomy, which functions similarly to goniotomy. Trabeculotomy is currently the preferred procedure by most surgeons and is the procedure of choice when corneal clouding prevents visualization of angle structures. Surgical results in congenital glaucoma are similar after either procedure. In addition, excellent results are claimed after trabeculotomy in infantile and juvenile glaucoma.

Filtration surgery, full or partial thickness (trabeculectomy), is less likely to be successful in juvenile than in adult glaucoma. The lower success rate in younger patients may relate both to increased postoperative scarring and to the types of glaucomas that tend to occur in this age group. Postoperative bleb encapsulation is more common in juvenile glaucoma patients. Trabeculectomy in eyes with previous surgery or secondary glaucoma, particularly neovascular glaucoma, has a poor prognosis. Age as an isolated factor may have its greatest influence on surgical outcome in patients under 30 years of age. In one series, trabeculectomy for primary glaucoma was successful in 25 of 30 (83 per cent) patients aged 30 to 49 years, but only in 4 of 9 (44 per cent) patients under 30 years of age. In youth, Tenon's tissue is more extensive, postoperative hypotony may be prolonged, wound healing may be more vigorous, and postoperative examination is often less than ideal. Because limbal surgical landmarks can be obscure, transillumination at the time of surgery is recommended to avoid placing the sclerostomy incision too posterior. A lamellar scleral flap helps identify the limbal surgical anatomy, in particular the scleral spur. It aids proper surgical entry into the anterior chamber. In addition, the scleral flap lowers the incidence of a postoperative flat anterior chamber and results in a thicker, more diffuse filtration bleb. However, the surgeon should remember that the sclera may be thinner in the juvenile eye, making scleral flap dissection more difficult. Corticosteroids should be used after filtration surgery to diminish postoperative inflammation and scarring of the bleb. A sub-Tenon's injection of a short-acting corticosteroid, such as dexamethasone* or triamcinolone*, at the completion of surgery and the use of topical corticosteroid drops or ointment after surgery are recommended.

Adjunctive antimetabolites should be used to slow wound healing and scar formation and increase the success rate of trabeculectomy in this patient population. Postoperative subconjunctival injections* of 5-fluorouracil are usually impossible in very young patients. Intraoperative application of mitomycin-C[‡] is an option in these patients. Both 5-fluorouracil[‡] and mitomycin-C are associated with thinner, more cystic blebs and may carry a higher rate of complications, such as wound leaks, chronic hypotony, and possibly late endophthalmitis. Releasable scleral flap sutures may be used at the time of surgery in young patients to control postoperative bleb function and reduce the occurrence of early postoperative hypotony. These sutures are removed at the time of examination under anesthesia.

Cyclocryotherapy has several useful applications in the management of juvenile glaucoma. It may be effective in aphakic patients with an open or partially open anterior chamber angle. It may also be used to provide intraocular pressure control in circumstances where filtration surgery is likely to fail. This procedure has a high complication rate (e.g., phthisis bulbi and loss of vision) when used in the therapy of neovascular glaucoma. New types of cyclodestructive procedures, such as Nd:YAG transcleral laser and therapeutic ultrasound, have limited experience in juvenile glaucoma. Their potential complications are not fully known in the young patient.

Seton devices have been used in juvenile-onset glaucoma eyes that have failed routine filtrating surgery. Encouraging results have been reported using various posterior tube shunt implant devices. These devices place an open plastic tube into the anterior chamber that is attached to an equatorial episcleral plate, resulting in a posterior bleb over the area of the encapsulated explant.

PRECAUTIONS

Perhaps the saddest error in dealing with these patients is the failure to recognize the condition early. The fellow eye of patients with apparent uniocular congenital glaucoma should be followed very carefully for possible late-onset congenital glaucoma. Young patients with advancing high myopia should be regarded as potential candidates for glaucoma. Applanation tonometry is preferable to Schiötz tonometry in these patients because of their low ocular rigidity. A positive family history of glaucoma in children should suggest examination of the patient's relatives and siblings.

COMMENTS

With the availability of hand-held portable applanation tonometers, office measurement of intraocular pressure can usually be performed on most children. It should be considered part of the complete pediatric ophthalmologic examination whenever glaucoma is suspected and should be performed in all patients who can cooperate. Gonioscopy may be performed successfully in many children, often with surprising ease. Reliable visual fields are difficult to obtain in young children, placing more responsibility on the ophthalmologist for accurate assessment and recording of optic disc appearance. Routine examination of the optic disc should be done in all patients. In children on whom tonometry cannot be performed, the optic disc examination may reveal suspected or definite damage from elevated intraocular pressure. In those patients, further examination under anesthesis is warranted. If possible, the optic disc should be photographed in individuals with suspected or proven juvenile-onset glaucoma. Rapid increase and reversal of cupping are seen much more frequently in children with glaucoma than in adults.

References

Barsoum-Homsy M, Chevrette L: Incidence and prognosis of childhood glaucoma. Ophthalmology 93:1323–1327, 1986.
Boger WP III, Walton DA: Timolol in uncontrolled childhood glaucomas. Ophthalmology 88:253–258, 1981.
Chew E, Morin JD: Glaucoma in children. Pediatr Clin North Am 30:1043–1061, 1983.
Chopra H, Goldenfeld M, Krupin T, Rosenberg LF: Early postoperative titration of bleb function: Argon laser suture lysis and removable sutures in trabeculectomy. J. Glaucoma 1:54–57, 1992.
Dicken JC, Hoskins HD Jr: Diagnosis and treatment of congenital glaucoma. In Ritch R, Shields MB, Krupin T (eds): The Glaucomas. St. Louis, CV Mosby, 1989, Vol II, pp 773–785.
Falck FY Jr, Skuta GL, Klein TB: Mitomycin versus 5-fluorouracil antimetabolite therapy for glaucoma filtration surgery. Sem Ophthalmol 7:97–109, 1992.
Gressel MG, Meuer DK, Parrish RK II: Trabeculectomy in young patients. Ophthalmology 91:1242–1246, 1984.
Hoskins HD Jr, Hetherington J Jr, Magee SD, Naykhin R, Magliazzo CV: Clinical experience with timolol in childhood glaucoma. Arch Ophthalmol 103:1163–1166, 1985.
Kass MA, Kolker AE, Gordon M, Goldberg I, Krupin T, Becker B: Acetazolamide and urolithiasis. Ophthalmology 88:261–265, 1981.
Krupin T. Surgical treatment of glaucoma with the Krupin-Denver valve. In Cairns JE (ed): Glaucoma. London, Grune & Stratton, 1986, Vol I, pp 239–245.
Molteno ACB: Use of Molteno implants to treat secondary glaucoma. In Cairns JE (ed): Glaucoma. London, Grune & Stratton, 1986, Vol I, pp 211–238.
Richter CU, Shingleton BJ, Bellows AR, Hutchinson BT, O'Connor T, Brill I: The development of encapsulated filtering blebs. Ophthalmology 95:1163–1168, 1988.
Ritch RP: Pigmentary glaucoma—A self-limited entity. Ann Ophthalmol 15:115–116, 1983.
Walton DS: Juvenile open-angle glaucoma. In Chandler PA, Grant WM (eds): Glaucoma, 3rd ed. Philadelphia, Lea & Febiger, 1986, pp 528–529.
Whiteside-Michel J, Liebmann JM, Ritch R: Initial 5-fluorouracil trabeculectomy in young patients. Ophthalmology 99:7–13, 1992.

LENS-INDUCED GLAUCOMA 365.51
(Phacolytic Glaucoma)

DAVID L. EPSTEIN, M.D.

Durham, North Carolina

Phacolytic glaucoma classically refers to a secondary open-angle glaucoma of rapid onset associated with a leaking hypermature or mature cataract. Although obstruction of the trabecular meshwork by lens-protein-engorged macrophages has been postulated to be a mechanism for such glaucoma, recent studies have indicated that direct obstruction of the outflow pathways by the leaking lens proteins themselves may be an important factor.

Patients with phacolytic glaucoma present with an acute elevation of intraocular pressure, frequently to very high levels. Corneal epithelial edema is usual. The angle is open. Slit-lamp examination of the anterior chamber usually reveals heavy flare, but a variable cellular content. Often, chunky white particles, larger than cells, can be seen floating in the aqueous. Cellular reaction may be minimal. Although the condition is usually associated with a mature or hypermature cataract, rare cases can occur with immature cataracts, which may leak posteriorly. Patches of white material that are probably macrophages can often be seen on the lens capsule.

THERAPY

Ocular. Most often, eyes with phacolytic glaucoma show minimal response to topical ophthalmic antiglaucoma or anti-inflammatory therapy. However, other types of glaucoma caused by retained lens cortex after extracapsular cataract surgery or lens injury may respond to medical therapy. The latter type of glaucoma is probably caused by direct obstruction of the outflow channels by the liberated particulate lens material or possibly by the inflammatory reaction to such lens material. In such cases, if not too much free lens material is present, medical therapy consisting of cycloplegics, apraclonidine, beta blockers, carbonic anhydrase inhibitors, and possibly corticosteroids may control the intraocular pressure until the lens material is spontaneously absorbed. If the glaucoma is severe, the residual lens material must be removed surgically.

The eye pressure in phacolytic glaucoma (leaking hypermature cataract) will usually rise progressively and may be temporarily reduced by topical beta blockers, apraclonidine, systemic carbonic anhydrase inhibitors, and osmotic therapy. Initially, topical 0.5 per cent timolol, levobunolol, betaxolol, or other beta blockers may be used every 12 hours to lower the pressure temporarily. One per cent apraclonidine may be administered every 12 hours, and 250 mg of acetazolamide may be given intravenously. This may be repeated in 30 to 60 minutes and then every 6 hours. A 50 per cent solution of glycerin in fruit juice or cola drink may be given orally in doses of 1.5 gm/kg (0.7 ml/kg), or an intravenous solution of 1 to 2 gm/kg of mannitol may be necessary in patients who are vomiting.

Pain medication is frequently necessary, and 50 mg of intramuscular meperidine may be of value.

Surgical. The intraocular pressure should be followed closely, and emergency cataract extraction may be required. It is not certain whether extra- or intracapsular surgery is best. The benefits of extracapsular techniques in routine cataract surgery are clear. However, vitreous loss in phacolytic eyes can be especially disastrous. Residual lens material even without vitreous loss can cause uveitic complications. Because of the fragile nature of the leaking lens capsule, chymotrypsin should be used in intracapsular surgery. A planned or unplanned extracapsular extraction, in which hypermature lens material is left in the eye, may be very deleterious postoperatively. An intact senile nucleus should never be allowed to remain in the eye after extracapsular surgery, since it will invariably cause a severe lens reaction. Phacoanaphylaxis may result when lens material is sequestered in the eye, especially in the vitreous. When vitreous loss occurs during an extracapsular extraction, as much lens material as possible should be removed, primarily at the time of the surgery.

A recent report documents that planned extracapsular cataract surgery with a posterior chamber intraocular lens following thorough removal of lens material can be safe and effective in phacolytic glaucoma.

After uncomplicated cataract surgery, the intraocular pressure returns to normal within a few days.

PRECAUTIONS

In the differential diagnosis of phacolytic glaucoma, one must consider that a swollen cataractous lens can induce angle-closure glaucoma.

Secondary open-angle glaucoma caused by non-lens-related primary uveitis can certainly occur in patients with cataracts. Characteristic of phacolytic glaucoma is the eventual failure of response to topical ophthalmic therapy. When in doubt as to whether glaucoma is caused by phacolysis or primary uveitis, such as in the case of an immature cataract, standard medical therapy for uveitis should be tried first. Diagnostic paracentesis can establish the correct diagnosis by the presence of macrophages.

In cases of phacolytic glaucoma with lenses that are dislocated into the vitreous, the presentation may be more subacute and the ocular signs more subtle. Differential diagnosis includes traumatic angle-recession glaucoma, primary open-angle glaucoma, and an idiopathic type of chronic open-angle glaucoma that is apparently not related to obvious angle recession or lens reaction.

COMMENTS

Phacolytic glaucoma usually occurs unilaterally. The preoperative vision is not indicative of the vision to be obtained postoperatively, since the postoperative results are surprisingly good if the intraocular pressure has not been elevated for significant periods of time. This is true even in patients with questionable light perception and projection preoperatively. In one series, at least 25 per cent of the eyes with phacolytic glaucoma had angle recession. The cause of this condition is unknown, although it may indicate that many of these eyes had trauma that led to cataract formation.

References

Epstein DL: Lens-induced glaucoma. In Epstein DL (ed): Chandler and Grant's Glaucoma, 3rd ed. Philadelphia, Lea & Febiger, 1986, pp 320–331.

Epstein DL, Jedziniak JA, Grant WM: Identification of heavy-molecular-weight soluble protein in aqueous humor in human phacolytic glaucoma. Invest Ophthalmol Vis Sci 17:398–402, 1978.

Epstein DL, Jedziniak JA, Grant WM: Obstruction of aqueous outflow by lens particles and by heavy-molecular weight soluble lens proteins. Invest Ophthalmol Vis Sci 17:272–277, 1978.

Lane SS, Kopietz LA, Lindquist TD, Leavenworth N: Treatment of phacolytic glaucoma with extracapsular cataract extraction. Ophthalmology 95:749–753, 1988.

Lazzaro, EC: Phakolytic glaucoma: Case presentation. Ann Ophthalmol 4:773–776, 1972.

Pollard ZF: Phacolytic glaucoma secondary to ectopia lentis. Ann Ophthalmol 7:999–1001, 1975.

Rosenbaum JT, Samples JR, Seymour B, Langlois L, David L: Chemotactic activity of lens proteins and the pathogenesis of phacolytic glaucoma. Arch Ophthalmol 105:1582–1584, 1987.

Uemura A, Sameshima M, Nakao K: Complications of hypermature cataract: Spontaneous absorption of lens material and phacolytic glaucoma-associated retinal perivasculitis. Jpn J Ophthalmol 32:35–40, 1988.

LOW-TENSION GLAUCOMA 365.12

STEPHEN M. DRANCE, M.D.

Vancouver, British Columbia, Canada

Low-tension glaucoma is a form of open-angle glaucoma in which damage to the optic nerve and visual field occurs with intraocular pressures that are always within normal limits. It is usually bilateral and typically occurs in older individuals. Low-tension glaucoma is probably caused by a deficiency of blood supply to the optic nerve as a result of many interacting factors, such as arteriosclerosis, hemodynamic crisis, low blood pressure, carotid disease, intermittent cardiac arrhythmias, and diabetes. Some of these entities cause a transient, others a permanent, imbalance in the intraocular pressure and the optic nerve perfusion pressure, resulting in damage to neurons. In the presence of these factors, poor perfusion of the optic nerve may occur, even with normal intraocular pressure. Forty-seven per cent of low-tension glaucoma patients have been found to suffer from migraine headaches. In the future, many other factors that contribute to the circulation difficulty may be discovered. It has recently been found that there may be two glaucoma populations, the first being predominantly vasospastic to cold and sensitive to all levels of intraocular pressure, whereas the second is a nonvasospastic group predominantly with markers for small vessel disease and who may not be as responsive to intraocular pressure. These two groupings occur in both open-angle glaucoma and normal-tension glaucoma. Some cases of low-tension glaucoma are falsely diagnosed because of low coefficients of ocular rigidity in which the actual pressure in the eye is higher than that recorded with an indentation tonometer. In others, large diurnal intraocular pressure fluctuations are missed when the pressure is recorded only during the day. Other causes of cupping of the optic disc, atrophy of the nerve fiber bundle type, and visual field loss must always be ruled out.

THERAPY

Ocular. Attempts should be made to reduce the level of intraocular pressure to the lowest possible level, particularly in those patients who are vasospastic to cold. Such pressure reduction may arrest the progression of the disease in some individuals. However, it is not clear whether this pressure reduction is in fact successful and under what circumstances. A 6-year collaborative study is currently underway to test the hypothesis that a 30 per cent pressure reduction in normal tension glaucoma patients is of benefit. Pilocarpine in 1 or 2 per cent concentration four times a day is probably the first agent. It has been shown that when used in conjunction with laser trabeculoplasty it is capable of reducing intraocular pressure by 30 per cent in approximately 60 per cent of patients with normal tension glaucoma. If pilocarpine is not effective in conjunction with the laser, 0.5 to 2 per cent epinephrine twice daily can be added to this regimen. Acetazolamide is often the most useful drug for good pressure reduction at low intraocular pressure levels. In

patients who are vasospastic, the nonspecific beta-blockers should probably not be used because of their potential vasospastic properties. In patients who have small vessel disease, low doses of aspirin may be helpful, and calcium channel blockers should be tried in patients who are vasospastic but whose blood pressure is not too low so as to be contraindicated.

Supportive. Medical and neurologic evaluation at repeated intervals is indicated. Hypertension should be controlled, but precipitous episodes of iatrogenic or spontaneous hypotension may aggravate the condition. Any disease that can cause an intermittent or constant decrease in the blood supply to the optic nerve should be treated.

Surgical. The majority of patients with normal-tension glaucoma will not become completely blind during their lifetime. When the disease is progressing and threatening fixation, particularly in younger individuals, filtering surgery may be necessary to lower the pressure as much as possible. Under such circumstances, a full-thickness sclerectomy may be considered, or a trabeculectomy with the use of an antifibrosis regimen has shown promise. If patients continue to progress in spite of this pressure reduction, an optic nerve sheath decompression may be considered. Sporadic cases of improvement with this procedure have been reported, but no definitive recommendations can be made at this time.

Ocular or Periocular Manifestations

Optic Nerve: Atrophy; cupping; hemorrhage.
Other: Scotoma or other visual field defects.

PRECAUTIONS

Flame-shaped hemorrhages on the optic disc may indicate ischemia and the site of potential optic nerve head damage. Without treatment, the disease may progress similarly to primary open-angle glaucoma. Moderate-to-heavy antiglaucoma medications may reduce ocular pressure. However, even the most intensive medical treatment often produces little reduction of intraocular pressure. Even when pressure is reduced, the disease may still continue to progress.

COMMENTS

Low-tension glaucoma is not a rare entity. There are probably four patients with chronic open-angle glaucoma for every one patient with low-tension glaucoma. One has to rule out elevations of intraocular pressure by recording pressure at frequent intervals around the clock. Such diurnal tension curves are not always readily obtainable, but in this condition are very valuable. Tonography is not a good substitute, although eyes with unstable intraocular pressures generally seem to have lower coefficients of outflow facility. The presence of low coefficients of outflow facility makes it more likely that the intraocular pressure may have higher peaks of abnormal pressure than those recorded during the day, but it may also indicate that the individual had previously high intraocular pressures ("burnt-out" chronic open-angle glaucoma).

References

Chumbley LC, Brubaker RF: Low-tension glaucoma. Am J Ophthalmol 81:761–767, 1976.

Drance SM: Some factors in the production of low-tension glaucoma. Br J Ophthalmol 56:229–242, 1972.

Drance SM, et al: Studies of factors involved in the production of low-tension glaucoma. Arch Ophthalmol 89:457–465, 1973.

Levene RZ: Low-tension glaucoma: A critical review and new material. Surv Ophthalmol 24:621–664, 1980.

Phelps CD, Corbett JJ: Migraine and low-tension glaucoma. Invest Ophthalmol Vis Sci 26:1105, 1985.

Schulzer M, Drance SM, Carter CJ, Brooks DK, Douglas GR: Biostatistical evidence for two distinct chronic open-angle glaucoma populations. Br J Ophthalmol 74:195–200, 1990.

Simmons RJ, Singh OS: Shell tamponade in glaucoma surgery. In Symposium on Glaucoma. New Orleans Academy of Ophthalmology. St. Louis, CV Mosby, 1981, pp 242–252.

Spaeth GL: Tonography and tonometry. In Duane TD (ed). Clinical Ophthalmology. Hagerstown, MD, Harper & Row, 1982, Vol III, pp 47:22–23.

MALIGNANT GLAUCOMA 365.20

(Ciliary Block, Iridovitreal Block, Posterior Aqueous Diversion, Vitreolenticular Ciliary Block)

JOHN C. MORRISON, M.D.

Portland, Oregon

Malignant glaucoma, thought to occur through misdirection of aqueous humor into the vitreous body, should be considered in cases of elevated intraocular pressure with a shallow or flat anterior chamber that persists despite a peripheral iridectomy. Classically described after either filtering surgery or surgical peripheral iridectomy for pupillary block in phakic eyes, this condition can also occur in aphakia and without prior surgery. Malignant glaucoma is being increasingly reported in eyes with posterior chamber intraocular lenses, although the pathogenesis and response to treatment may be different than in the phakic eye.

In phakic eyes, malignant glaucoma apparently results from conditions that shift the lens-iris diaphragm anteriorly, such as glaucoma surgery, trauma, inflammation, miotics, and the discontinuation of postoperative cycloplegics. In addition to axial shallowing of the anterior chamber, the ciliary processes may appear unusually prominent and compressed against the lens equator. When visible, the anterior vitreous face may have a glassy, thickened texture, with clear spaces in the anterior vitreous. Although nearly half of these cases respond to medical therapy, the glaucoma often is not relieved until the anterior vitreous face is incised or ruptured. These observations suggest that, in malignant glaucoma, aqueous humor is diverted into the vitreous body (aqueous misdirection) possibly secondary to obstruction of anterior aqueous flow by ciliary-process-lens apposition (ciliary block, ciliolenticular block). An abnormally impervious vitreous face prevents anterior flow of the aqueous humor into the posterior chamber, resulting in forward movement of the vitreous face, lens, and iris to produce angle closure that cannot be reversed with either surgical or laser peripheral iridectomy.

Currently, malignant glaucoma is most commonly seen after extracapsular cataract surgery with posterior chamber lens implantation, often in eyes without pre-existing angle closure or anatomically narrow angles. This finding suggests that the mechanism of aqueous diversion in pseudophakia is unique and is possibly caused by the presence of cortical remnants and retention of the posterior capsule. In aphakia, posterior diversion of aqueous humor is thought to result from adherence of vitreous to the ciliary processes or blockage of the pupil an peripheral iridectomy by the vitreous face (iridovitreal block).

THERAPY

Ocular. Medical therapy is directed toward suppressing aqueous humor formation, dehydrating the vitreous body, and shifting the lens-iris diaphragm posteriorly. Aqueous humor formation can be reduced with a topical beta-blocking agent, such as 0.5 per cent timolol or levobunolol, used twice daily. Intensive cycloplegia and mydriasis with 1 per cent atropine and 2.5 per cent phenylephrine three to four times daily will reverse the forward movement of the ciliary body and pull the lens posteriorly against the vitreous face to help deepen the anterior chamber and possibly relieve ciliary block. Miotics are contraindicated, since they cause anterior movement of the lens-iris diaphragm and can aggravate angle closure.

Systemic. Carbonic anhydrase inhibitors, such as oral acetazolamide 125 to 250 mg four times daily or methazolamide 50 to 100 mg twice daily after an oral or intravenous loading dose (1 gm acetazolamide), help lower intraocular pressure by decreasing aqueous humor production. Hyperosmotics have a specific role in the treatment of malignant glaucoma. They dehydrate the vitreous, decreasing the anterior pressure of the vitreous face and aiding cycloplegics in deepening the anterior chamber. Oral glycerin or isosorbide, 1 to 2 gm/kg of a 50 per cent solution, can be given every 12 hours as tolerated. Isosorbide is preferred in diabetic patients, since the metabolism of glycerin may cause hyperglycemia. If nausea and vomiting prevent oral therapy, 20 per cent intravenous mannitol in a dose of 2 gm/kg given over 30 minutes is equally effective.

In phakic eyes, the above medical regimen should be continued for 4 to 5 days, by which time intraocular pressure in approximately half of the patients will be controlled. After this, medical therapy can be withdrawn gradually, beginning with the hyperosmotics and carbonic anhydrase inhibitors, followed by the beta blockers and mydriatics. Cycloplegics should probably be continued indefinitely, as malignant glaucoma unresponsive to medical therapy may occur if they are stopped.

Aphakic and pseudophakic eyes should also receive a trial of the same medical regimen. However, response of these eyes to medical therapy is generally poor, probably because they lack a normal crystalline lens and cycloplegics can no longer effectively counteract anterior movement of the vitreous face. If rapid improvement does not occur, one should proceed to surgical treatment.

Surgical. Definitive surgery for malignant glaucoma involves opening the anterior vitreous face to give diverted aqueous humor direct access to the posterior and anterior chamber. This can be accomplished with the neodymium:YAG laser using single 2- to 5-mJ pulses in aphakic and pseudophakic eyes, either through the pupil or through the peripheral iridectomy if the vitreous face can be seen between the ciliary processes. Neodymium:YAG laser treatment is less successful in phakic eyes, which generally require a mechanical anterior vitrectomy.

If Neodymium:YAG laser treatment to the anterior vitreous face is unsuccessful, direct argon laser photocoagulation of visible ciliary processes through the peripheral iridectomy, combined with conventional medical therapy, may occasionally eliminate the need for more invasive surgery.

If neither medical nor laser treatments are successful in relieving malignant glaucoma, surgical incision of the anterior and, if possible, the posterior face of the vitreous should be attempted. An ultrasound should first be done to check for suprachoroidal hemorrhage. If it is negative and a sufficient view of the posterior pole exists, the surgeon should perform a mechanical subtotal anterior vitrectomy through the pars plana.

If the view of the posterior pole is not adequate for vitrectomy, the vitreous aspiration

as described by Chandler (1968) is indicated. In phakic eyes, a sclerotomy is made 3 to 3.5 mm posterior to the limbus and treated with diathermy to prevent bleeding of the underlying pars plana. An 18- to 20-gauge sharp needle is then passed 12 mm into the globe toward the optic nerve, and fluid is allowed to escape spontaneously. An additional 1 to 1.5 ml of fluid is then aspirated and the anterior chamber partially reformed by injecting balanced salt solution through a preplaced paracentesis. Air is injected to deepen the anterior chamber to myopic depth, but still leaving the eye soft. Atropine should be used for an indefinite period after the operation. Occasionally, this procedure may have to be repeated to control the attack finally.

In aphakic eyes, Neodymium:YAG disruption of the anterior vitreous face often dramatically deepens the anterior chamber with lowering of intraocular pressure. If not, mechanical vitrectomy or vitreous aspiration can be performed via the limbus and through the pupil. If a posterior chamber lens is present, a pars plana anterior vitrectomy is required, with particular attention to eliminating lens capsule and cortical remnants immediately behind an otherwise patent peripheral iridectomy.

Ocular or Periocular Manifestations

Anterior Chamber: Angle closure; shallow or flat centrally.
Ciliary Body: Ciliary process apposition or overlapping of the lens equator.
Cornea: Edema (from high intraocular pressure of lenticular touch).
Lens: Anterior shift of lens; cataract (from corneal touch).
Optic Nerve: Glaucomatous cupping; pallor.
Other: Clear spaces in vitreous; elevated intraocular pressure; thickened, glassy appearance of anterior vitreous face.

PRECAUTIONS

Patients receiving the medical regimen outlined earlier should be carefully monitored for adverse, life-threatening side effects. Hyperosmotic agents produce an osmotic diuresis with depletion of fluids and electrolytes. However, these same drugs can precipitate pulmonary edema in patients with poor cardiac or renal function. Carbonic anhydrase inhibitors can cause hypokalemia if used with diuretics and metabolic acidosis in patients with pulmonary insufficiency. Rare, life-threatening blood dyscrasias have been reported. Blood pressure should be monitored because topical 2.5 per cent phenylephrine may exacerbate pre-existing hypertension. In patients with reactive airway disease, beta blockers should be limited to betaxolol with the consent of the patient's internist and close monitoring of pulmonary function.

If vitreous aspiration is required, the needle should be clamped 12 mm from its tip with a hemostat, which will thus prevent it from being inserted too far into the eye and traumatizing the retina or optic nerve head. The insertion site of the needle should be placed carefully between 3 to 3.5 mm from the limbus, since a more posterior insertion will enter through the vitreous base and not successfully incise the anterior vitreous face. A more anterior insertion may damage the lens. The eye should be moderately hypotonic at the end of the operation, since overfilling the anterior chamber may divert more fluid or air into the vitreous and the anterior chamber will once again flatten.

COMMENTS

Malignant glaucoma occurs in only 1 to 4 per cent of patients requiring surgery for pupillary block. However, this condition may also develop in apparently normal eyes after cataract extraction and posterior chamber lens implantation and should be considered whenever a shallow anterior chamber and elevated intraocular pressure coexist.

Elevated intraocular pressure with a shallow anterior chamber may also result from pupillary block, a swollen or dislocated lens, ciliochoroidal effusion, and suprachoroidal hemorrhage. Before diagnosing malignant glaucoma, one should check first for a patent iridectomy. Asymmetric or extreme shallowing of the central anterior chamber also differentiates malignant glaucoma from pupillary block, since the lens is not forced anteriorly in the latter. In pseudophakia, many cases of "pupillary block" may in fact be malignant glaucoma. The appearance of vitreous bulging around the posterior chamber lens optic or through the peripheral iridectomy can clarify the diagnosis. Furthermore, an ultrasound may demonstrate a compressed anterior vitreous face and clear spaces posteriorly that presumably are filled with aqueous humor.

Although ciliochoroidal effusions are usually associated with hypotony, ciliary detachment may occasionally mechanically obstruct the chamber angle and elevate eye pressure. If the fundus is not easily seen or the red reflex is absent, ultrasound may help diagnose choroidal effusions, as well as suprachoroidal hemorrhage, which usually causes sudden, severe pain.

Patients with malignant glaucoma in one eye have a significant chance of developing the same condition in the other eye if an angle-closure attack required subsequent surgery. Prophylactic laser iridotomy should therefore be done as soon as possible in all fellow eyes. If surgery is required, cycloplegics should be used postoperatively.

References

Chandler PA, Simmons RJ, Grant WM: Malignant glaucoma. Medical and surgical treatment. Am J Ophthalmol 66:495–502, 1968.
Epstein DL, Steinert RF, Puliafito CA: Neodymium-YAG laser therapy to the anterior hyaloid in aphakic malignant (ciliovitreal block) glaucoma. Am J Ophthalmol 98:137–143, 1984.
Hershler J: Laser shrinkage of the ciliary processes. A treatment for malignant (ciliary block) glaucoma. Ophthalmology 87:1155–1159, 1980.
Lynch MG, et al: Surgical vitrectomy of pseudophakic malignant glaucoma. Am J Ophthalmol 102:149–153, 1986.
Rieser JC, Schwartz B: Miotic-induced malignant glaucoma. Arch Ophthalmol 87:706–712, 1986.
Shaffer RN: The role of vitreous detachment in aphakic and malignant glaucoma. Trans Am Acad Ophthalmol Otolaryngol 58:217–231, 1954.
Shields MB: Textbook of Glaucoma, 2nd ed. Baltimore, Williams & Wilkins, 1987, pp 334–339.
Shrader CE, et al: Pupillary and iridovitreal block in pseudophakic eyes. Ophthalmology 91:831–837, 1984.
Simmons RJ: Malignant glaucoma. Br J Ophthalmol 56:263–272, 1972.
Weiss DJ, Shaffer RN: Ciliary block (malignant) glaucoma. Trans Am Acad Ophthalmol Otolaryngol 76:450–460, 1972.

OCULAR HYPERTENSION 365.04

JEFFREY M. LIEBMANN, M.D.,
JANET B. SERLE, M.D.,
STEVEN M. PODOS, M.D.,
and ROBERT RITCH, M.D.

New York, New York

Glaucoma is a progressive optic neuropathy characterized by a specific pattern of optic nerve head damage and visual field loss. The most important risk factor for the development of glaucomatous damage is elevated intraocular pressure (IOP). Other risk factors include a family history of glaucoma, myopia, black race, diabetes mellitus, and ophthalmic conditions that lead to secondary forms of glaucoma.

Ocular hypertension is not a specific disease, but a descriptive term used to define the status of an eye that has an "abnormally high" IOP but shows no clinically detectable glaucomatous damage. Large population studies performed a generation ago suggest that mean IOP is 15 to 17 mm Hg. Elevated IOP is then arbitrarily defined as being two standard deviations or more above the mean. As a result, IOP greater than 21 mm Hg has been considered abnormal. The distribution of IOP within the population approximates a Gaussian curve but, rather than being symmetric about the mean, is skewed to the right.

A skewed frequency distribution indicates that 95 per cent of the area under the distribution curve does not lie within two standard deviations of the mean. Therefore, the upper limit of "normal" IOP is not necessarily 21 mm Hg, nor is an eye with a "normal" IOP immune to glaucomatous damage. Consequently, the concept of a specific maximum "normal" IOP is both misleading and deleterious to optimal patient management.

An IOP of 22 mm Hg or greater, in the absence of visual field loss or glaucomatous cupping, has conventionally been used to discriminate between normal IOP and ocular hypertension. Included in this category are (1) eyes with an IOP that may be abnormal with regard to the mean but that may be "normal" for those particular eyes, (2) eyes defined as having elevated IOP but that may never (during the patients' lifetimes) develop glaucomatous damage because of the ability of the optic nerve head to withstand that particular pressure, and (3) eyes that are destined to develop damage but that have not yet done so. Given the much larger segment of the general population with an IOP less than 22 mm Hg, a significant portion of the glaucoma population has a statistically normal IOP, despite the lower incidence of the disease in the normal group.

Estimates of the prevalence of definite open-angle glaucoma in a number of population studies vary between 0.25 and 0.75 per cent, whereas the prevalence of ocular hypertension is approximately 2 per cent of the population between the ages of 40 and 50 and as high as 8 per cent of those between 70 and 80. The prevalence of glaucoma increases with age from about 0.2 per cent of those aged 50 to 54 years to about 2.0 per cent of those aged 70 to 74 years. A number of studies have demonstrated that the higher the IOP, the greater the chance of developing glaucomatous damage over a period of time. Nevertheless, the great majority of patients with IOPs greater than 21 mm Hg will not develop glaucomatous damage. Most long-term studies of untreated ocular hypertensives with an IOP less than 30 mm Hg indicate that about 1 per cent per year will develop glaucomatous damage. This incidence is actually lower than the mortality rate for these patients. Thus, IOP alone is not necessarily a sufficient criterion upon which to base the decision to institute treatment.

Until recently, the presence or absence of glaucomatous damage was determined on the basis of the appearance of the optic nerve head and visual field. The advent of more accurate and sensitive photographic methods and psychophysical testing may enable the detection of earlier glaucomatous changes, and it now becomes necessary to consider both what is meant by the term "ocular hypertension" and what criteria should be used to place a patient on antiglaucoma medications. How useful is the concept of ocular hypertension if its meaning changes with the increasing refinement of tests? The long-term goal in treating the patient is to prevent functional visual loss. At present, no repeatable, reliable prognostic test exists to determine which patients with elevated IOP will go on to develop glaucomatous damage.

THERAPY

Ocular. Drug treatment is the same as for primary open-angle glaucoma. The crucial difference lies in the decision as to which patients to treat and which to observe.

Certain factors have been implicated as predisposing an "ocular hypertensive" eye to glaucomatous damage. Among these are glaucomatous damage in the contralateral eye, elevated IOP, recent onset of elevated IOP, myopia, congenitally large cup-to-disc ratio, family history of glaucoma, diabetes mellitus, circulatory disorders, and anemia. African-Americans are more likely to develop both elevated IOP and glaucomatous damage at any given level of IOP than whites. A cup:disc ratio asymmetry of 0.2 or greater between the two eyes, evidence of nerve fiber layer damage, or focal damage to the neural rim is highly suspicious. The absolute numerical value of the IOP that the ophthalmologist feels safe not treating is also important. In the absence of other risk factors, it is recommended to institute treatment for one or both eyes at a pressure range of about 25 to 30 mm Hg, depending on the effectiveness of medications, side effects, and the age and wishes of the patient.

Observation is the simplest form of follow-up. The frequency of observation should vary directly with the level of IOP and the number of risk factors. Since glaucomatous visual field loss is not present in patients with ocular hypertension, serial tonometry and disc evaluation are important parameters to follow. Helpful adjuncts are periodic stereophotography of the discs, red-free photographs of the nerve fiber layer, and office determination of the diurnal curve to determine the time of peak pressure. In ocular hypertensive patients, office determination of IOP between 8 A.M. and 5 P.M. is usually sufficient.

PRECAUTIONS

Once the decision to treat in the absence of detectable glaucomatous damage has been made, one should choose a drug that lowers IOP effectively with the least amount of discomfort to the patient. A uniocular therapeutic trial should be performed when instituting therapy to ensure that it is actually the drug that is lowering IOP, rather than fluctuation due to diurnal or other variations. If a patient with symmetric elevation of IOP achieves a significant lowering of pressure in the treated eye, one may then elect to treat both eyes or to continue to treat one eye and observe the other. One is treating a patient, not a number, and one should not become obsessed with lowering the pressure to the "normal" range. A drop from 35 to 25 mm Hg may be quite sufficient to protect the patient from the future development of glaucomatous damage. Systemic carbonic anhydrase inhibitors have significant side effects and should be reserved for ocular hypertensive patients with high IOPs and multiple risk factors who have not responded sufficiently to topical therapy. Laser trabeculoplasty may be useful in recalcitrant cases.

Certain patients merit more aggressive treatment. These include patients who are monocular patients, who have developed a branch or central retinal vein occlusion in either eye, or who have systemic arterial occlusive disease. In addition, higher myopia predisposes to glaucomatous optic nerve injury at lower pressures than lesser amounts of myopia, emmetropia, or hyperopia.

COMMENTS

The fact that one is dealing with a physical sign and not a rigidly definable disease entity should encourage the ophthalmologist to take into account the other contributory factors mentioned in the individualization of treatment for any particular patient. It would be better to call the patient a "glaucoma suspect." In addition to being more flexible and less compartmentalizing a term than "ocular hypertension," it allows inclusion of those patients who may be suspected of having early glaucoma in the absence of elevated IOP, such as those with large or asymmetric cup-to-disc ratios.

References

Chandler PA, Grant WM: "Ocular hypertension" vs. open-angle glaucoma. Arch Ophthalmol 95: 585–586, 1977.

Chauhan BC, Drance SM, Douglas GR: The time-course of intraocular pressure in timolol-treated and untreated glaucoma suspects. Am J Ophthalmol 107:471–475, 1989.

Colton T, Ederer F: The distribution of intraocular pressures in the general population. Surv Ophthalmol 25:123–129, 1980.

Epstein DL, Krug JH Jr, Hertzmark E, Remis LL, Edelstein DJ: A long-term clinical trial of timolol therapy versus no treatment in the management of glaucoma suspects. Ophthalmology 96:1460–1467, 1989.

Graham P: Epidemiology of chronic glaucoma. In Heilmann K, Richardson KT (eds): Glaucoma. Conceptions of a Disease. Philadelphia, WB Saunders, 1978, pp 7–17.

Hoskins HD Jr: Definition, classification and management of the glaucoma suspect. In Symposium on Glaucoma. Transactions of the New Orleans Academy of Ophthalmology. St. Louis, CV Mosby, 1981, pp 19–29.

Hovding G, Aasved H: Prognostic factors in the development of manifest open-angle glaucoma.

A long-term follow-up study of hypertensive and normotensive eyes. Acta Ophthalmol 64: 601–608, 1986.

Kass MA, Gordon MO, Hoff MR, Parkinson JM, Kolder AE, Hart WM Jr, Becker B: Topical timolol administration reduces the incidence of glaucomatous damage in ocular hypertensive individuals. A randomized, double-marked long-term clinical trial. Arch Ophthalmol 107:1590–1598, 1989.

Kass MA, et al: Risk factors favoring the development of glaucomatous visual field loss in ocular hypertension. Surv Ophthalmol 25:155–162, 1980.

Kolker AE, Becker B: "Ocular hypertension" vs. open-angle glaucoma: A different view. Arch Ophthalmol 95:586–587, 1977.

Krupin T, Podos SM: The glaucomas: Classification and synthesis. In Heilmann K, Richardson KT (eds): Glaucoma. Conceptions of a Disease. Philadelphia, WB Saunders, 1978, pp 348–369.

Phelps CD: Ocular hypertension: To treat or not to treat? Arch Ophthalmol 95:588–589, 1977.

Schwartz B: Roundtable discussion. Management of ocular hypertension. Surv Ophthalmol 25: 215–221, 1980.

Shaffer R: "Glaucoma suspect" or "ocular hypertension?" Arch Ophthalmol 95:588, 1977.

Somner A: Intraocular pressure and glaucoma. Am J Ophthalmol 107:186–188, 1989.

Spaeth GL: Ocular hypertension: Reasons for abandonment of the term. Int Ophthalmol 19:37–49, 1979.

Tielsch JM, Sommer A, Katz J, Royall RM, Quigley HA, Javitt J: Racial variations in the prevalence of primary open angle glaucoma. The Baltimore Eye Survey. JAMA 266:369–374, 1991.

Wilson MR, et al: A case-control study of risk factors in open-angle glaucoma. Arch Ophthalmol 105:1066–1071, 1987.

OCULAR HYPOTONY 360.3

DAVID J. WILSON, M.D.

Portland, Oregon

Ocular hypotony lacks a specific definition, but is generally considered to be present when low intraocular pressure results in demonstrable effects on the eye. The intraocular pressure at which clinical effects become apparent is variable and depends on the speed of onset and the underlying cause for the decreased intraocular pressure. Generally, no ocular effects is noted until the intraocular pressure is below 6.5 mm Hg, and usually the intraocular pressure must fall to 0 to 4 mm Hg before deleterious effects become apparent. Hypotony of this degree is usually caused by wound leaks resulting from trauma or surgery, cyclodialysis, iridocyclitis, retinal detachment, or ciliochoroidal detachment. Other less common causes of hypotony include vascular occlusive disease (carotid artery occlusive disease, temporal arteritis, and central retinal artery or vein occlusion), osmotic hypotony (dehydration, diabetic coma, and uremia), myotonic dystrophy, after glaucoma filtration surgery, and pre-phthisis bulbi.

THERAPY

Ocular. The most important factor in treating ocular hypotony is recognition of the underlying cause of the low intraocular pressure. In the setting of trauma or postoperatively, it is essential to assess for the possibility of a wound leak. Seidel's test should be performed under topical anesthesia to evaluate for the presence or absence of a wound leak. In this test, the lids are held in a separated position, and a fluorescein-impregnated paper is used to apply fluorescein to the area of the suspected leak. It is important to apply the fluorescein in a highly concentrated form; otherwise, small leaks may go undetected. If a leak is not detected, gentle digital pressure should be applied to the eye to see if one becomes evident. The management of postoperative wound leaks is discussed in the article of postoperative flat anterior chamber, and the repair of penetrated globes is covered under indirect global ruptures and sharp scleral injuries.

With persistent hypotony after trauma or surgery in the absence of a wound leak, a cycloidialysis should be suspected. This diagnosis may be substantiated by gonioscopy. If a cyclodialysis is identified, surgical repair may be undertaken if the hypotony is clinically significant, i.e., if it is resulting in pain or decreased vision that warrants the risks of surgical repair. Closure of cyclodialyses has been described using diathermy, cryotherapy, suturing of the ciliary body, external plombage, and argon laser photocoagulation.

Rhegmatogenous retinal detachment is frequently associated with mild hypotony, but marked hypotony may occur. The recognition and treatment of retinal detachment are covered in a separate section.

Iridocyclitis may cause mild hypotony and may be associated with any of the above conditions. Before attributing hypotony solely to iridocyclitis, other possibilities should be excluded. Likewise, if surgical intervention for cyclodialysis is contemplated and iridocyclitis is also present, a trial of topical steroids is warranted to determine if eradicating the iridocyclitis will relieve the hypotony.

Ciliochoroidal detachment or effusion is commonly associated with hypotony, but its pathogenetic role in hypotony is unclear. Pederson has demonstrated that detachment of the ciliary body with silicone oil in the monkey does not result in hypotony. However, ciliochoroidal detachment is a common accompaniment of hypotony in humans, and drainage of suprachoroidal and supraciliary fluid in some cases resolves the ocular hypotony. The indications and procedure for drainage of ciliochoroidal detachments are discussed in a separate section.

Ocular hypotony is an infrequent occurrence after standard glaucoma filtration surgery. However, with the use of antimetabolites in conjunction with glaucoma filtration surgery, ocular hypotony is being seen with increasing frequency. The visual loss and chorioretinal folds present in these patients do not always respond to measures to increase the intraocular pressure. These measures generally include treating the filtering bleb with various agents to decrease filtration.

Ocular or Periocular Manifestations

Anterior Chamber: Shallow.
Ciliary Body: Ciliary congestion; cyclodialysis; detachment.
Cornea: Folds in Bowman's and Descemet's membrane.
Iris: Anterior synechia; anterior uveitis.
Retina: Detachment; folds; macular edema.
Other: Cataract; decreased vision; ocular pain; optic nerve head edema.

PRECAUTIONS

Successful treatment of ocular hypotony requires recognition of its cause. A careful eye examination, including Seidel's test for wound leaks, gonioscopy for cyclodialysis, and fundus examination to evaluate for choroidal or retinal detachment, should be conducted.

COMMENTS

In the absence of a wound leak, treatment of asymptomatic ocular hypotony may not be necessary. Therapeutic intervention in ocular hypotony should be attempted only after the physician and patient have weighed the relative risks and benefits of the planned intervention.

References

Barasch K, Galin MA, Baras I: Postcyclodialysis hypotony. Am J Ophthalmol 68:644–645, 1969.

Brubaker RF, Pederson JE: Ciliochoroidal detachment. Surv Ophthalmol 27:281–289, 1983.

Demeler U: Refixation of the ciliary body after traumatic cyclodialysis. Dev Ophthalmol 14:199–201, 1987.

Harbin, TS Jr: Treatment of cyclodialysis clefts with argon laser photocoagulation. Ophthalmology 89:1082–1083, 1982.

Jampel HD, Pasquale LR, Dibernardo C: Hypotony maculopathy following trabeculectomy with mitomycin C. Arch Ophthalmol 110:1049–1050, 1992.

Joondeph HC: Management of postoperatiave and posttraumatic cyclodialysis clefts with argon laser photocoagulation. Ophthalmic Surg 11:186–188, 1980.

Maumenee AE, Stark WJ: Management of persistent hypotony after planned or inadvertent cyclo-dialysis. Am J Ophthalmol 71:320–327, 1971.

Pederson JE: Hypotony. *In* Duane TD (ed): Clinical Ophthalmology. Philadelphia, Harper & Row, 1984, Vol 3, pp 58:1–8.

Pederson JE: Ocular hypotony. Trans Ophthalmol Soc UK 105:220–226, 1986.

Pederson JE, Gaasterland, DE, MacLellan HM: Experimental ciliochoroidal detachment: Effect on intraocular pressure and aqueous humor flow. Arch Ophthalmol 97:536–541, 1979.

Portney GL, Purcell TW: Surgical repair of cyclo-dialysis induced hypotony. Ophthalmic Surg 5: 30–32, 1974.

OPEN-ANGLE GLAUCOMA 365.10

MARTIN WAND, M.D.,

Hartford, Connecticut

and ROBERT N. SHAFFER, M.D., F.A.C.S.

San Francisco, California

Open-angle glaucoma (OAG) is usually a bilateral chronic disease characterized by glaucomatous optic nerve changes and/or glaucomatous visual field (VF) changes. By definition, the iridocorneal angle is open; it typically occurs in adults, and there is no other etiology responsible for the optic nerve or VF changes. Glaucomatous optic nerve changes include progressive optic nerve cupping or thinning of the optic nerve rim and loss of nerve fiber layer as noted on red-free illumination. Glaucomatous VF changes include a nasal step, paracentral scotoma, or arcuate scotoma extending from the blind spot.

The intraocular pressure (IOP) is usually elevated, but this is not a prerequisite for an eye to develop glaucomatous optic nerve changes or VF loss. In the past, an elevated IOP has always been assumed to be the cause of OAG and thus was always an integral part of the definition. However, over the past decade, our concept of OAG has undergone a fundamental change, based on previously inexplicable clinical findings. Up to 30 per cent of patients can have typical glaucomatous optic nerve and/or VF changes with "normal" IOPs (≦ 21 mm Hg), and up to 20 per cent of patients can continue to have progressive optic nerve and/or VF changes despite a lowering of the IOP to "normal" levels. The current feeling is that OAG is an optic neuropathy and that high IOP is not the only cause of glaucomatous nerve damage or VF loss. For each optic nerve, there is a range of IOPs above which progressive nerve damage and VF loss will occur and below which loss will not occur. The upper limit of normal was generally assumed to be approximately 21

mm Hg for everyone, but it is now realized that the susceptibility to optic nerve damage is different for different people and may vary in the same individual at different times in the course of the disease. Although elevated IOP is not a necessary component of OAG, it remains the major known causative factor in glaucomatous optic nerve damage and VF loss and the main element that can be controlled. Other risk factors include large optic nerve cup, older age, positive family history, African-American race, high myopia, diabetes mellitus, and systemic hypertension.

Over one million Americans have been diagnosed with OAG, and it is estimated that at least another one million Americans have undiagnosed OAG. After age-related macular degeneration, it is the second most common cause of blindness in the United States, and among African-Americans, it is the leading cause of blindness. The American Academy of Ophthalmology (AAO) estimates that there are over three million office visits per year for the diagnosis and treatment of OAG, making it one of the major ocular and public health problems in this country. Unfortunately, present screening based on IOP measurements has not proved satisfactory in identifying the individual at risk of glaucomatous optic nerve damage and VF loss. As already mentioned, up to 30 per cent of patients with OAG may have a "normal" IOP, and up to 50 per cent of individuals with OAG may have a "normal" IOP at any single IOP measurement. Using IOP screening alone, many individuals at risk would be missed. Ideally, IOP measurement must be combined with optic nerve and VF evaluation. The AAO Preferred Practice Pattern guidelines for quality eye care, state that a periodic comprehensive ocular examination is the best way to identify the patient at righ risk of developing OAG. All asymptomatic patients over 65 years should have a comprehensive ocular examination every 1 to 2 years; all African-Americans over the age of 20 should have one every 3 to 5 years, and those over the age of 40 should have one every 2 to 4 years.

Because many studies have shown the beneficial effects of lowering the IOP and because at the present time IOP is the only risk factor amenable to therapeutic intervention, all current treatment modalities are aimed at lowering the IOP.

THERAPY

The therapeutic goal in OAG is to prevent further optic nerve damage and further VF loss using modalities with minimal and acceptable side effects. In attempting to lower the IOP, the end point or "target" pressure will vary depending on many factors. In general, the more damage there is to an optic nerve, the lower the IOP necessary to prevent further damage. The rapidity in development of the present damage, the extent of damage in the fellow eye, positive family and racial history, and systemic risk factors all dictate a lower target IOP. Also as a general rule, when the IOP is high, the target IOP should be below 21 mm Hg, and when the IOP is initially in the "normal" range, the target IOP should be at least one-third lower than the initial IOP. Unfortunately, there is no way at the present time of knowing whether any target IOP is indeed a "safe" IOP for any individual eye. Periodic reassessment of the optic nerve and VF is necessary to determine if further damage has occurred. If so, reassessment of the therapy is necessary with a new and lower target IOP.

OCULAR

Beta Blockers. The mainstay of medical therapy is topical beta blockers. Nonselective $beta_1$ and $beta_2$ blockers—timolol, levobunolol, carteolol, and metipranolol—and the selective $beta_1$ blocker, betaxolol, are currently available. They act by decreasing aqueous production by approximately 30 per cent. Except for slight topical anesthesia, the ocular and visual side effects are minimal. Because blockage of $beta_1$ fibers decreases cardiac muscle contraction and blockage of $beta_2$ fibers increases pulmonary smooth muscle contraction, topical beta blockers can cause bradycardia, decreased cardiac output, and difficulty in breathing, resulting in congestive heart failure and asthma. Depression, general mood changes, and confusion may also result, and in men, impotence is a reported complication of treatment. Selective $beta_1$ blockers have a lesser ocular hypertensive effect, but also have a lower incidence of pulmonary and central nervous system side effects.

Dose-response studies of these drugs suggest that a 0.25 per cent solution daily is sufficient in most patients, but practically speaking, most patients receive 0.5 per cent solutions twice a day.

Parasympathomimetic Agents. The direct-acting parasympathomimetic drug, pilocarpine has been employed for over one century and was the initial drug of choice for OAG before the introduction of the beta blockers. Pilocarpine causes contraction of the iris sphincter and ciliary muscles. The resulting traction on the scleral spur opens the trabecular meshwork, increases the facility of outflow, and decreases the IOP up to 20 per cent. However, the ciliary muscle spasm is painful and produces a fluctuating myopia that is often intolerable to younger patients. The miotic pupil decreases night vision and is especially annoying in elderly patients because of the frequent coexistence of cataracts. Because of these significant side effects, pilocarpine has been relegated to a second-line drug after the beta blockers. Its ocular hypotensive effect is additive to the beta blockers,

and recent studies suggest that a combination solution of beta blocker and pilocarpine in twice-daily dosage may minimize the ocular side effects without a corresponding loss of therapeutic efficacy. Starting dosages may be as low as 1 per cent twice a day. The generally accepted maximal treatment schedule is 4 per cent four times a day. The initial use of pilocarpine may result in pain from the ciliary spasm, but this usually lessens with time. Frequently, it is more tolerable to start the patient at a lower dosage and frequency. Sometimes, the ocular and visual side effects may be minimized with the use of topical pilocarpine gel at bedtime or an Ocusert slow-release system in the ocular fornices once per week. Other rare side effects of topical pilocarpine include tear duct occlusions, ocular pseudopemphigoid, and an increased incidence of retinal detachment. Although infrequent and therefore overlooked by ophthalmologists and primary care physicians, the cholinergic side effects of pilocarpine may cause gastrointestinal activity resulting in nausea, vomiting, and diarrhea, and, more important, increased pulmonary secretions resulting in pulmonary congestion.

Carbachol, another direct- and indirect-acting parasympathomimetic agent, may be tried in case of allergy or intolerance to pilocarpine. The dosage is 0.25 to 3.0 per cent two to four times a day.

Phospholine Iodide (echothiophate) is an indirect-acting parasympathomimetic agent that acts through the inhibition of acetylcholinesterase. It is available in strengths of 0.0625, 0.125, and 0.25 per cent, with 0.125 per cent equivalent in action to 4 per cent pilocarpine. The usual dosage is twice a day. The ocular and systemic side effects are similar to pilocarpine. It is infrequently used now, which is unfortunate, because it can have a significant ocular hypotensive effect in aphakic and pseudophakic patients. Furthermore, in older patients, the visual side effects of a miotic are not major problems. Because it depletes the body of acetycholinesterase and pseudocholinesterase, if the muscle relaxant, succinylcholine, is used in general anesthesia, prolonged respiratory paralysis can occur. Anesthesiologists must be warned that the patient is using Phospholine Iodide.

Sympathomimetic Agonists. The epinephrine family of drugs exerts its hypotensive effects through a combination of decreased aqueous production and increased facility of outflow. The exact mechanisms of how these drugs work are still unclear. Their ocular hypotensive effect does not seem to be additive to the nonselective beta blockers, but is somewhat additive to the selective $beta_1$ blockers so that the total ocular hypotensive effect with this combination is of the same magnitude as using a nonselective beta blocker alone. The epinephrine compounds are available in different salt forms and in strengths of 0.25, 0.5, 1 and 2 per cent. The borate formulation with a pH of 7.0 is more comfortable than the bitartrate formulation, which has a pH of 3.5. Ocular side effects include transient stinging, black pigment (adrenochrome) deposits in the conjunctiva from chronic use, and a high incidence of localized allergic reaction necessitating discontinuation. Epinephrine should not be used in narrow-angle eyes as the resulting pupillary dilation might cause angle closure. An infrequent but significant ocular complication is cystoid macular edema in the aphakic and pseudophakic eye. This complication is usually reversible upon discontinuing the medication. Systemic side effects from adrenergic stimulation include tachycardia, systemic hypertension, and anxiety.

In an attempt to lower its local and systemic side effects, the pro drug dipivefrin was developed. It is lipophilic and penetrates through the cornea into the anterior chamber about 15 times more readily than epinephrine, which is hydrophilic. Thus, a 0.1 per cent concentration of dipivefrin is pharmacologically equivalent to 2 per cent epinephrine, but causes a significantly decreased incidence of ocular and systemic side effects. Allergy requiring discontinuation, however, still occurs in approximately 20 per cent of the patients.

An alpha$_1$ agonist, apraclonidine, is now available for short-term use as a hypotensive agent. It seems to act by increasing uveoscleral outflow and can decrease IOP up to 40 per cent. It seems to be additive to the beta blockers and has proven to be effective in aborting or blunting the IOP spikes commonly seen after argon laser trabeculoplasty, Nd:YAG laser posterior capsulotomy, and cataract extraction. Currently, it is available only as a 1 per cent solution in droppettes containing only two or three drops for one-time use. Its role in the chronic treatment of OAG has not yet been defined, but phase III studies are currently underway, and availability as a 0.5 per cent solution in 5-ml bottles for long-term twice a day use is anticipated in the next few years.

Systemic. Carbonic anhydrase inhibitors (CAI) lower IOP by decreasing aqueous production. At therapeutic levels, aqueous production can be decreased by 30 per cent. Their effect is additive to the beta blockers and the miotics. Systemic administration by oral, intramuscular, and intravenous modes is currently available. Topical CAIs should be clinically available within the next few years.

Many systemic side effects are experienced with this group of drugs. Paresthesias of the extremities are common, as are generalized malaise; lethargy; mood changes, especially depression; gastrointestinal symptoms of nausea and vomiting, dyspepsia, and diarrhea; and the loss of libido in men. Kidney stones are a potential complication, but seem to be less frequent with methazolamide than the other CAIs. All CAIs can decrease serum potassium levels, but generally this is not a problem unless a patient is already on another diuretic. Because all CAIs are sulfa compounds, anyone with an allergy to sulfa should not take this medication. Idiosyncratic blood dyscrasias may occur, including life-threatening aplastic anemia. These are extremely rare, and there is no blood test that can reliably predict who is susceptible to this complication.

Acetazolamide is available in 125-mg and 250-mg tablets and in 500-mg sustained-release (sequel) capsules; the dosage ranges from 125 mg twice a day to 250 mg four times a day. The 500-mg sequels twice a day seem to be associated with less side effects than 250 mg four times a day. Methazolamide is usually given 25 to 50 mg three times a day and also seems to have less systemic side effects than comparable doses of acetazolamide. Dichlorphenamide is another CAI that is used in dosages of 25 to 100 mg two to four times a day.

Laser. Argon laser treatment of the trabecular meshwork (argon laser trabeculoplasty or ALT) is successful in lowering the IOP in up to 90 per cent of treated eyes with adult-onset OAG. This figure, however, includes eyes with a pressure lowering of only a few mm Hg, which may not achieve the "target" pressure for that eye. The average decrease in IOP is 4 to 8 mm Hg, with a range of 1 to 15 mm Hg. In general, the higher the initial IOP, the greater the absolute and percentage decrease in IOP. Studies have shown that up to 55 per cent of the treated eyes are still under control at the end of 5 years. Retreatment may be performed, but the reported success in lowering the IOP rate is from 30 to 70 per cent and is probably close to 50 per cent or lower. In addition, the magnitude of the IOP lowering with retreatment is not as great and does not last as long as after initial therapy. Treatment over 180° seems to produce as good IOP control in most eyes as an initial 360° of treatment and is associated with less side effects. If need be, the other 180° can be treated at a later time. Forty to fifty spots, 50 μm in size, are applied evenly over 180° of the anterior trabecular meshwork. Most patients will develop some iritis after the treatment, but it is easily controlled with topical steroids for a few days. Some patients can spike a high IOP within hours after treatment. In an eye with a compromised optic nerve, this spike can be potentially sight-threatening. Therefore, all patients undergoing ALT should have the IOP checked within 1 hour after treatment, and if the IOP is elevated, appropriate therapy should be instituted. Some physicians prefer to pretreat patients with apraclonidine to prevent or at least blunt the posttreatment IOP spikes.

SURGICAL

Filtration Surgery. Filtration surgery has traditionally been reserved as the treatment of last resort. Before many of the newer medications and ALT became available, surgical intervention occurred much earlier than it does currently. The success rate in eyes with primary OAG that have not had any previous surgery is at least 75 per cent. The success rate is significantly lower if previous cataract or filtration surgery has been performed. The success rate is also significantly lower for African-Americans and in younger patients, probably on the basis of their more rapid healing process.

The two major groups of filtration procedures are guarded and unguarded procedures. The guarded procedures include various forms of trabeculectomy. The unguarded procedures include trephine, posterior lip sclerectomy, and cautery sclerostomy. In general, the unguarded procedures result in a lower IOP and longer IOP control than the guarded procedures, but the guarded procedures are associated with a lower postoperative complication rate and seem to be associated with a lower incidence of late endophthalmitis. As with any surgical procedure, hemorrhage and infections, although rare, are always potential postoperative complications. In addition, specific to filtration procedures, progression of cataract, flat anterior chamber, choroidal effusion, and suprachoroidal hemorrhage may develop in the immediate postoperative period, and further surgical intervention may be necessary. Failure of adequate filtration remains the major setback of surgery, but newer techniques are increasing the chances of successful filtration. The intraoperative use of mitomycin-C[‡] and the postoperative use of 5-fluorouracil[‡] have significantly increased the chances of successful filtration, especially in eyes with low chances of success—those with previous ocular surgery and complicated glaucomas with iritis or rubeosis iridis, or in African-Americans and young patients. This gain in successful filtration is offset by slightly increased incidence of persistent hypotensive maculopathy and late-onset endophthalmitis. Long-term prospective studies will determine the ultimate role of antimetabolites in filtration surgery. In addition, newer filtration techniques involving mechanical trephines and lasers to produce sclerostomies are in clinical trials, and their place in the surgical armamentarium for OAG will be determined in the future.

Seton Procedures. If there is a great deal of conjunctival scarring present to prevent the successful completion of a standard filtration procedure, various implants (setons) have been developed to drain aqueous from the anterior chamber to a mechanically maintained subconjunctival space in the peri-equitorial region of the eye. These devices include the Molteno, Baerveldt, Krupin-Denver, Schocket, and White implants. All of them share common problems of blockage of the internal and external osteum, erosion of the implant, hypotony, and failure to function. All attempts at standard filtration surgery with and without antimetabolites should be tried before using these devices.

Cyclodestructive Surgery. When all attempts at filtration surgery have failed and the IOP is still too high, then a cyclodestructive procedure should be considered. Either through cryotherapy or Nd:YAG laser photodisruption of the ciliary processes, the source of aqueous production is ablated permanently. The major complication of this procedure is that it is a nonreversible destructive procedure and permanent hypotony with phthisis may result. Posttreatment inflammation and pain may also occur. Nd:YAG laser cyclophotocoagulation is associated with less posttreatment discomfort and phthisis than cyclocryotherapy and seems to be the treatment of choice at the present time. Recent reports of sympathetic ophthalmia after Nd:YAG cyclophotocoagulation need to be evaluated. These procedures are performed only as a last resort.

PRECAUTIONS

There are several problems unique to OAG. It is a chronic disease for which there is no cure; lifetime follow-up and treatment are necessary. Until the end stages of the disease, there are no symptoms. It is therefore understandable that the nickname for OAG is the "silent thief." Yet, the medications to treat this disease are expensive and can cause a great deal of ocular and systemic side effects, which are sometimes life threatening, and must be taken on an around-the-clock schedule. Successful treatment, by medications, lasers, or surgery does not result in any tangible benefit obvious to the patient. The patient has to accept on faith alone that there is control of the OAG. In accepting surgery, the patient has to subject an apparently normal eye to pain, discomfort, transient and sometimes permanent decrease in vision, as well as the remote possibility of losing the eye. Even if the surgery is successful, the eye does not see any better, and there is now a "bump" under the eyelid, sometimes associated with epiphora; the only comfort is the assurance from the physician that everything is "great." Compliance with any medical therapy is difficult, but it is easy to see why it is a major problem in OAG. Studies have shown that up to 50 per cent of patients do not take their eye medications conscientiously. Failure to achieve a target IOP or failure to prevent progressive optic nerve damage despite achieving a target IOP is often due to lack of patient compliance.

Education of the patient and the family is therefore of paramount importance with OAG. Prescribing the appropriate treatment is only half of the physician's responsibility to the patient. Without proper education so that the patient appreciates the magnitude of the problem and the importance of adhering to the treatment regimen and scheduled follow-up examination, even the most efficacious medications and surgical procedures will fail.

Some of the major complications of medications used in the treatment of glaucoma have already been mentioned. It goes without saying that patients should be informed of these potential side effects and urged to call the physician with any new or unexplained symptoms after the institution of a new antiglaucoma medication. Also, it is important that patients be told to inform their primary care physicians of all new antiglaucoma medications. Finally, patients should be instructed either to close the lids or occlude the punctum after eyedrops to minimize systemic absorption and side effects.

COMMENTS

The traditional approach to the treatment of OAG has been to initiate therapy with medications. When maximal tolerable medical therapy failed, ALT was performed. When that failed, surgery was the last resort. Recently, papers have been published questioning this approach. Should laser or even surgery be the initial treatment of choice in a newly diagnosed case of OAG? These are valid questions to ask, and there should be no dogma in the treatment of this difficult disease. The side effects of medical therapy are common and serious. These side effects can drastically alter the patient's quality of life and even threaten the patient's survival. The compliance problem must be factored into the treatment equation. Furthermore, the high cost of medications and a patient's inability to keep regular follow-up appointments may all justify earlier or even initial laser therapy. Strong family and/or racial history, history of glaucomatous loss in a fellow eye, advanced optic nerve cupping and VF loss on the initial examination, and older age may all justify early or even initial surgical intervention. Studies are underway to help answer these important questions. Yet, regardless of the results of these studies, the most important fact to remember is that the patient with OAG is a unique individual and requires the individualized supervision of a caring eye physician.

References

American Academy of Ophthalmology: Comprehensive Adult Eye Evaluation, Preferred Practice Pattern. San Francisco, American Academy of Ophthalmology, 1992.

American Academy of Ophthalmology: Primary Open Angle Glaucoma, Preferred Practice Pattern. San Francisco, American Academy of Ophthalmology, 1992.

Epstein DL (ed): Chandler-Grant's Glaucoma, 3rd ed. Philadelphia, Lea & Febiger, 1986.

Hoskins HD Jr, Kass MA: Becker-Shaffer's Diagnosis and Therapy of the Glaucomas, 6th ed. St. Louis, CV Mosby, 1989.

Shields MB, Ritch R, Krupin T: The Glaucomas. St. Louis, CV Mosby, 1990.

PEDIATRIC APHAKIC GLAUCOMA 365.14

JOHN R. SAMPLES, M.D.

Portland, Oregon

Pediatric aphakic glaucoma is generally underappreciated due to the difficulty clinicians encounter in examining infants and children and obtaining an accurate assessment of intraocular pressures and the optic nerve. Many of the causes of aphakic glaucoma in children are similar to those seen in adults. For instance, children may also have aphakic pupillary block, particularly when there has been inadequate removal of anterior vitreous at the time of lensectomy surgery. Aphakic glaucomas in children, including open-angle glaucoma, may be related to inflammation of the trabecular meshwork that leads to angle-closure glaucoma secondary to development of synechia. The aphakic small eye may be particularly susceptible to angle closure. As a result, monitoring of intraocular pressure, corneal diameter, refractive changes, and the appearance of the optic nerve in pediatric patients who have undergone cataract extraction is advisable.

The diagnosis of pediatric aphakic glaucoma depends upon assessment of the eye. In children over the age of 3, it is often possible to measure intraocular pressure with a Perkins hand-held applanation tonometer or a Tonopen. Any tonometric measurement needs to take into account the status of the cornea (astigmatism, corneal compliance, and hydration) and the method of measurement. If cooperation is not possible, then an examination with chloral hydrate sedation or under general anesthesia may be undertaken. Some type of pressure measurement should be obtained 3 and 6 months after surgery and yearly thereafter in all aphakes. Gonioscopy is particularly important and allows one to gain valuable information about the etiology of the glaucoma that is present. An open-angle glaucoma with a dysfunctional trabecular meshwork, similar to primary congenital glaucoma, may become manifest at any age. Whether or not such glaucomas may be particularly associated with cataract, yet be independent of cataract removal, is not clear. Angle-closure glaucoma is most often seen in pediatric aphakic patients when residual cortical material has remained in the eye and provoked inflammation. It is also seen in patients who have sustained pupillary block, often through mechanisms related to forward displacement of the vitreous. The later mechanism is occasionally seen after lensectomy in children with retinopathy of prematurity.

With time and patience, many older pediatric patients may successfully complete visual field testing. Often, it is helpful to test only one eye at a time, giving the child frequent breaks and substantial encouragement.

Some children perform well on automated perimetry examinations using the Humphrey automated perimeter. New, fast perimetry strategies, such as the Humphrey Fastpac, may be especially useful for pediatric patients.

Particularly in pediatric patients, the diagnosis of glaucoma should never rest on the measurement of a single elevated intraocular pressure. Children who are squeezing their eyelids may raise their intraocular pressure. Intraocular pressures vary substantially over the course of the day, and an increase in diurnal variation of intraocular pressure is characteristic of glaucoma. Any history of corticosteroid treatment should be taken into account before making the diagnosis of pediatric aphakic glaucoma. Like adults, children may sustain elevated intraocular pressure when exposed to corticosteroids. Elevated intraocular pressures have been observed with the use of topical systemic and dermatologic routes of administration of corticosteroids.

THERAPY

Ocular. All antiglaucoma medications have significant side effects, and for this reason, a decision to treat needs to be weighed carefully against the potential for medications to have adverse effects. This is more true in the pediatric population than in others where very high blood levels of some agents, such as beta blockers, may be achieved. Pediatric aphakic glaucoma patients are often treated with medications on a chronic basis, not because medications are a desirable therapeutic alternative but because complications associated with the surgical treatments are high. The prevailing wisdom among glaucomatologists is that children will not do well with trabeculectomy procedures, although trabeculectomies with antimetabolite therapy have been reported to succeed in younger children. Long term follow-up data on such patients are lacking. Toxicity concerns related to the use of 5-fluorouracil and mitomycin-C after filtration procedures in young children are significant and have not yet been addressed fully.

Beta blockers may be used in children with good results. However, it is important to monitor children carefully for toxicity. Extreme caution is required in children under 1 year of age. Parents should use punctal occlusion to limit the systemic absorption of these medications. Further, it should be borne in mind that these medications do not have FDA approval for pediatric use. A child's pediatrician should be notified that a beta blocker is being used. The parents should be cautioned to observe the child for unexplained cough, a decrease in exercise tolerance, hair loss, palpitations, and other related side effects. Beta blockers should not be used in children who have been diagnosed as having reactive airway disease or any disease of the central nervous system. Because side effects may be fewer, a cardioselective beta blocker, such as betaxolol, offers some advantage in pediatric use.

Miotics, such as pilocarpine and carbachol, are generally tolerated by children. However, parents may have a difficult time complying with a four time a day regimen for pilocarpine. There is no published experience using pilocarpine as a gel vehicle (Pilogel, Alcon). However, such medication is traditionally used after goniotomy and may be of value in lowering pressure in some individuals. Phospholine iodide may be used twice daily, but can cause many complications.

Carbonic anhydrase inhibitors successfully lower pressure in children. Oral agents may be useful on a short-term basis, but the use of oral agents should not be continued over 3 months except in unusual circumstances. A topical carbonic anhydrase inhibitor, which may be released by the time this book is published, may be quite useful in children. Parents need to be informed about the potential side effects, including kidney stones and potentially life-threatening bone marrow aplasia. These drugs should not be used if there is a history of sulfa allergy. A complete blood count before their use, at 2-month intervals after they are initiated, and 6 months after they are initiated is advised in pediatric patients. Recommendations regarding a CBC in adults are controversial since clinical symptoms may often seem to indicate toxicity and since periodic CBCs may not be an efficient method for detection of a bone marrow problem. However, such blood tests seem especially logical in children where there may be more difficulty in obtaining an accurate history.

Surgical. Laser trabeculoplasty has no place in the management of pediatric aphakic glaucomas. The trabecular meshwork has often been inflamed, and trabeculoplasty may worsen the problems associated with treatment. Cyclocryotherapy has been a traditional treatment for intractable pediatric aphakic glaucoma, but it carries a significant risk of phthisis and pain. Laser cyclophotocoagulation using either a contact or noncontact method seems to be less painful for patients and carries less risk of phthisis, but may require more repeat treatments. Traditional filtering surgery has not been successful in pediatric patients. However, as noted above, 5-fluorouracil and mitomycin-C used adjunctively may improve its effectiveness. Seton procedures, such as the implanting of the Molteno seton and the Baerveldt seton or one of a number of newly introduced devices, may be very effective in pediatric patients. Such procedures are fraught with complications, but the potential rewards of long-term pressure control are great. An ophthalmologist electing to perform these procedures should have significant experience using them in adults before employing them in children.

Ocular or Periocular Manifestations

Cornea: Corneal edema.
Optic Nerve: Significant optic nerve cupping.
Other: Visual disturbance and visual loss.

PRECAUTIONS

Surveillance for pressure elevation is the key to effective detection of these disorders. Treatment of these patients should not neglect amblyopia management.

COMMENTS

Tube implants and valves for the patient that is actually sustaining optic nerve damage may represent the best alternative for therapy. However, monitoring children after the implantation of such devices may be particularly difficult. Extrusion of setons, as well as adjustments in the location of a tube because of minor trauma, growth, or incarceration of the iris, may occur.

References

Kwitko ML: Glaucomas in Infants and Children. New York, Appleton Century Crofts, 1973.
Passo M, Palmer EA, Van Buskirk EM: Plasma timolol in glaucoma patients. Ophthalmology 11: 1361–1363, 1984.

PHACOANAPHYLACTIC ENDOPHTHALMITIS
360.19
(Endophthalmitis Phacoanaphylactica, Phacoanaphylactic Uveitis, Phacoantigenic Uveitis)

BARTON L. HODES, M.D.

Tucson, Arizona

Phacoanaphylactic endophthalmitis historically has been viewed as an inflammatory disease of the eye that results from immunologic sensitization of a patient to lens protein that is released from its sequestered capsular bag by a lens injury, whether surgical, traumatic, or spontaneous. The fact that the liberation of lens protein only rarely causes an immune response has led investigators to conclude that an alteration in the natural tolerance of the body to lens protein is essential

for liberated lens protein to become antigenic; this process seems to be T-cell mediated.

Clinically, phacoanaphylactic endophthalmitis (PE) may present with a spectrum that ranges from a mild anterior uveitis to a severe hypopyon uveitis resembling infectious endophthalmitis. The onset of the inflammation may be as early as 24 hours, although this is more consistent with an infectious etiology, or as late as 2 weeks after lens injury. It typically presents 3 to 5 days after injury in patients already sensitized to lens protein, whereas 10 to 14 days is more common after initial lens injury. Lid edema, chemosis, mutton-fat keratic precipitates, and formation of dense posterior synechiae may occur. Secondary glaucoma and cyclitic membrane formation are not uncommon.

The differential diagnosis includes toxic, mechanical, and infectious etiologies. PE should always be included in this differential diagnosis. In the presence of hazy media, diagnostic ultrasonography is helpful in identifying retained intravitreal lens material; its dissolution over time with therapy can also be monitored ultrasonographically. Ultrasonography may also identify early vitreous organization and indicate the need for prompt therapeutic vitrectomy and possible intravitreal corticosteroids.

THERAPY

Aggressive treatment directed at the most likely etiology is essential. Depending upon the severity of the inflammation, a diagnostic vitrectomy to attempt to isolate microorganism(s) may be essential. Prompt suppression of inflammation to prevent the destruction of ocular tissues by the inflammatory process is the hallmark of therapy; whenever possible, this may be facilitated by the removal of retained lens material.

Ocular. Vigorous anti-inflammatory therapy consistent with the severity of inflammation should be initiated without delay. High-dose systemic corticosteroids (80 mg to 120 mg prednisone daily) with as rapid tapering as possible, frequent topical corticosteroids (prednisolone acetate 1 per cent every hour), and sub-Tenon's injections* of corticosteroids (preferably aqueous, not depot) accompanied by cycloplegics/mydriatics constitute the therapeutic armamentarium.

Ocular or Periocular Manifestations

Anterior Chamber: Cells and flare; hypopyon; mutton-fat keratic precipitates.
Conjunctiva: Chemosis; hyperemia; scant to no discharge.
Cornea: Edema; striae in Descemet's membrane.
Globe: Vitreous membranes; pupillary membranes; retinal detachments; decreased

vision; eyelid edema; synechiae, posterior and anterior; pupillary seclusion; secondary glaucoma.

PRECAUTIONS

PE is easily confused with infectious endophthalmitis; in both, early etiologic diagnosis is vital to preserve visual function as prolongation of either leads to irreversible damage to ocular structures. Although intensive antibiotics (systematic and intravitreal) are essential to salvage an eye with infection, they are of no value in management of PE.

COMMENTS

PE may occur after penetrating ocular trauma involving the lens, "uncomplicated" extracapsular cataract surgery, or cataract surgery that is complicated by posterior luxation of lens material.

References

Hodes BL, Stern G: Phacoanaphylactic endophthalmitis: Echographic diagnosis of phacoanaphylactic endophthalmitis. Ophthalmic Surg 7:60–64, 1976.
Marak G: Phacoanaphylactic endophthalmitis. Surv Ophthalmol 36:325–339, 1992.
Smith RE, Weiner P: Unusual presentation of phacoanaphylactic endophthalmitis following phacoemulsification. Ophthalmic Surg 7:65–68, 1976.

PIGMENTARY GLAUCOMA 365.13
(Pigment Dispersion Syndrome)

DAVID G. CAMPBELL, M.D.

Hanover, New Hampshire

Pigmentary glaucoma is a form of glaucoma in which there is usually bilateral elevation of intraocular pressure, open angles, and a heavy accumulation of pigment within the trabecular meshwork. The disease most characteristically occurs in relatively young, male Caucasian myopes. Initially, symptoms are usually absent due to slow and quiet elevation of intraocular pressure. Haloes due to corneal edema resulting from rapid elevation of pressure may occasionally occur, particularly after exercise. Primary findings are characteristic radial defects in the pigment epithelium in the outer periphery of the iris, seen by iris transillumination. These defects constitute the source of pigment that is dispersed throughout the posterior and anterior segments of the eye and within the trabecular

meshwork. This pigmentary dispersion is noted on the posterior surface of the cornea in the form of a Krukenberg spindle, on and within the trabecular meshwork, on the anterior surface of the iris, occasionally upon the zonular fibers, characteristically as a ring on the posterior peripheral surface of the lens, and occasionally as free pigment particles within the aqueous itself. In untreated eyes, there is a characteristic posterior bowing of the peripheral iris early in the course of the disease. The cause of the syndrome seems to be due to mechanical rubbing between the bowed posterior surface of the iris and packets of anterior zonules in predisposed eyes. If untreated, pigmentary glaucoma can lead to optic nerve damage, visual field loss, and blindness. In some cases, however, pigmentary glaucoma can resolve spontaneously. This resolution seems to be due to forward movement of the peripheral iris off of the zonules secondary to increasing lens size and increasing relative pupillary block due to age.

THERAPY

Ocular. In these generally young patients, either a beta blocker or dipivefrin may be used as initial therapy to lower the intraocular pressure. Timolol, 0.25 or 0.5 per cent, or Betoptic-S may be administered in each eye twice a day. One per cent dipivefrin may also be used twice a day.

One to 4 per cent pilocarpine may be applied every 6 hours to decrease the intraocular pressure by increasing aqueous outflow facility. An alternative to pilocarpine can be 0.75 to 3.0 per cent carbachol instilled in each eye every 8 hours. If pigmentary glaucoma worsens and optic nerve damage results, pilocarpine should be administered to the eye with the highest intraocular pressure, even in those patients in whom pilocarpine is not tolerated bilaterally because of accommodative blurring. An increase in the number of iris transillumination defects, the dispersion of pigment in the anterior segment or the degree of darkness of pigment in the trabecular meshwork, and a decrease in the facility of outflow with increased intraocular pressure are signs of worsening of pigmentary dispersion. Studies indicate that the flattening of the iris associated with chronic pilocarpine usage may lift the peripheral iris off the zonules, stop the abrasion to the posterior surface of the iris, and stop the alluvial flow of pigment to the trabecular meshwork, and, in some cases, allow the trabecular meshwork to begin to recover. This recovery becomes manifest as an increase in the facility of outflow and a decrease in the untreated intraocular pressure.

Systemic. When topical therapy is unsuccessful, carbonic anhydrase inhibitors may be instituted. Oral administration of 125 to 250 mg of acetazolamide may be given four times daily in adults; children may be given 5 mg/

kg every 6 hours. Acetazolamide sequels, 500 mg every 12 hours, are better tolerated than the tablets. Methazolamide, 50 mg orally every 8 hours, may be used instead of acetazolamide, and even lower doses, 25 mg twice daily, should be tried initially. The incidence of unwanted kidney stones may be less with methazolamide.

Surgical. If maximum tolerated medical therapy fails and cupping of the optic disc or visual field defects progress, surgical therapy is indicated. Laser trabeculoplasty is the treatment of choice if there is progressive disc and field damage or the intraocular pressure level is considered unsafe for a particular eye.

An effective laser treatment may be 80 applications spaced evenly over the circumference of the trabecular meshwork for 360°, of 0.1-second duration, and 50-micron spot size, with just enough power to cause a white blanched spot or tiny bubble formation within the mid- to upper trabecular meshwork. Because it is easy to overtreat these heavily pigmented meshworks and to obtain no pressure lowering or even unwanted permanent elevation, the power setting should be reduced to approximately half of the normal setting. Temporary pressure rise after laser treatment should be watched for and treated with a topical or systemic glaucoma medication, if necessary.

The creation of an iridotomy into a posteriorly bowed iris will cause the iris to flatten immediately and permanently. It may therefore be possible to prevent the conversion from the pigmentary dispersion syndrome (characteristic findings, but without an abnormal elevation of intraocular pressure) to pigmentary glaucoma (characteristic findings with an elevation of intraocular pressure), and it may be possible to halt the progression of and/or to reverse established pigmentary glaucoma. The flattening of the iris will prevent any further loss of pigment from the iris by zonular abrasion. In established pigmentary glaucoma, if the trabecular meshwork has not been irreversibly damaged by pigment, the interruption of further pigment flow to the meshwork may allow a degree of recovery, increasing the facility of outflow and lowering the baseline or the untreated intraocular pressure. Prospective studies will determine the overall effectiveness of this form of therapy and who should receive it. At the present time, an iridotomy should be considered for a rapidly worsening case of pigmentary glaucoma. Certainly, patients destined to develop only the pigmentary dispersion syndrome (and no glaucoma) should not have an iridotomy performed.

If laser trabeculoplasty fails, filtering surgery is the treatment of choice for progressive disc and field damage. Either a guarded filtration procedure, such as a trabeculectomy, or a filtration procedure, such as a trephine or thermal sclerotomy, can be effective. Goniotomy and cyclodialysis are of low effectiveness.

Ocular or Periocular Manifestations

Anterior Chamber: Free pigment particles in aqueous, particularly after dilatation or exercise.

Cornea: Pigmentary endothelial deposits (Krukenberg spindles).

Iris: Characteristic and pathognomonic peripheral radial slit-like transillumination defects; pigment on surface of iris.

Lens: Circular pigmentary deposit on posterior peripheral lens surface; heavy pigment deposition on zonules (occasional).

Optic Nerve: Glaucomatous cupping with characteristic glaucomatous visual field loss.

Other: Increased intraocular pressure; myopia.

PRECAUTIONS

Cycloplegic therapy can cause a pressure rise in these patients, just as in most open-angle glaucomas. This is due to decreased aqueous outflow facility secondary to the loss of the normal ciliary muscle tone exerted upon the scleral spur in these predisposed eyes. If a patient has bilateral pigmentary glaucoma that is worsening in both eyes, bilateral chronic miotic therapy is recommended for the reasons given above. If the patient is young, the accommodative blurring of vision that follows parasympathomimetic therapy is often so disabling that the patient cannot maintain a normal pattern of life. This causes decreased compliance, which must be watched for. If the patient cannot use bilateral therapy, at least unilateral therapy should be encouraged for the eye with the highest pressure. Before the institution of miotic therapy in these myopic eyes, a peripheral retinal examination should be performed, and any areas of retinal weakness should be treated to avoid induced rhegmatogenous retinal detachment.

If it is determined that the glaucoma has stabilized or perhaps begun to improve, as can happen in some cases, an occasional discontinuation of medication is in order to be certain that the medications being used are needed.

The usual precautions in regard to glaucoma medications, as described in the section on open-angle glaucoma, should be observed.

COMMENTS

Some patients with pigmentary glaucoma can develop an acute pressure rise following vigorous exercise, an increase which is due to a transient influx of released pigment to the trabecular meshwork. This pressure rise generally does not last more than a few hours but may lead to very high pressures that can damage the optic nerve. Therefore, patients should be checked after vigorous exercise; if an acute intraocular pressure rise occurs, that form of exercise should either be discontinued or topical pressure-lowering medications should be used whenever possible during and after exercise to avoid this increased pressure.

The prognosis for patients with pigmentary glaucoma can vary. The disease may become rapidly worse and require maximum medical or surgical therapy, or it can reach a plateau stage in which progression stops and, in some cases, spontaneous improvement follows.

References

Campbell DG: Pigmentary dispersion and glaucoma. A new theory. Arch Ophthalmol 97:1667–1672, 1979.

Epstein DL: Pigment dispersion and pigmentary glaucoma. *In* Chandler PA, Grant WM (eds): Glaucoma. 2nd ed. Philadelphia, Lea & Febiger, 1979, pp 122–129.

Lichter PR: Pigmentary glaucoma—Current concepts. Trans Am Acad Ophthalmol Otolaryngol 78:309–313, 1974.

Lichter PR: Pigmentary glaucoma. Fraunfelder FT, Roy FH: Current Ocular Therapy 2. Philadelphia, WB Saunders, 1980, pp 465–466.

Sugar HS, Barbour FA: Pigmentary glaucoma. A rare clinical entity. Am J Ophthalmol 32:90–92, 1949.

PLATEAU IRIS 743.8

ROBERT RITCH, M.D.,
and STEVEN M. PODOS, M.D.

New York, New York

Plateau iris refers to an anatomic configuration in which the iris is inserted anteriorly on the ciliary body face and the iris root angulates forward and then centrally. The result is somewhat akin to a bird's-eye view of a mesa (hence the name): The iris surface appears flat and the anterior chamber deep on slit-lamp examination, but the angle is narrow on gonioscopy, with a sharp drop-off of the peripheral iris. By contrast, in primary angle-closure glaucoma, the most common form of angle closure, the anterior chamber is shallow and the iris surface rounded (iris bombé).

Patients with plateau iris who develop angle-closure glaucoma tend to be younger than those with primary angle closure. The younger the patient, the greater the chance that the angle closure is due purely to angle crowding without pupillary block. Most patients, however, have some element of relative pupillary block superimposed upon a plateau iris configuration, but the degree of block necessary to induce angle closure is less than in primary angle-closure glaucoma. This seems to account for the deeper anterior chamber and flatter iris surface in eyes with plateau iris that develop angle closure.

Because of the pupillary block component, angle closure in most patients with plateau iris is successfully relieved by laser iridotomy. A minority, however, are subject to repeated attacks of angle closure despite a patent iridotomy, usually after pharmacologic dilation of the pupil but sometimes spontaneously. The term "plateau iris syndrome" has been used to describe these patients, and it is a relatively rare entity.

It has recently been recognized, however, that these patients, defined as having "complete" plateau iris syndrome comprise only a small proportion of patients with plateau iris who are capable of some degree of angle closure after iridotomy. Far more common are those capable of appositional closure, either spontaneously or after pupillary dilation, without a concomitant rise in intraocular pressure. These patients are defined as having "incomplete" plateau iris syndrome.

The important difference between the complete and incomplete syndromes is the level of the iris stroma with respect to the angle structures or the "height" to which the plateau rises. If the angle closes to the upper trabecular meshwork or Schwalbe's line, intraocular pressure rises, whereas if the angle closes only the lower portion of the angle, the pressure remains unchanged.

The peripheral iris configuration is consistent with abnormally large or anteriorly positioned ciliary processes pushing the peripheral iris anteriorly. In primary angle closure due to relative pupillary block, indentation gonioscopy pushes the iris root posteriorly, opening the angle. In plateau iris, the deepest point of indentation is not at the iris periphery, but approximately two-thirds of the distance between the center of the pupil and the iris root. The peripheral iris then rises again to conform to the hump created by the ciliary processes. This has been confirmed by high-resolution anterior segment ultrasonic biometry.

THERAPY

Surgical. The initial treatment of choice for an angle-closure glaucoma with plateau iris configuration is laser iridotomy. If, in the presence of a patent iridotomy, the angle remains spontaneously appositionally closed and intraocular pressure either normal or elevated, there are two choices. Low-dose pilocarpine may open the angle and, if tolerated well by the patient, may be used for maintenance. In these cases, one per cent pilocarpine twice daily is usually sufficient. The alternate choice is to perform argon laser peripheral iridoplasty. This procedure alters the configuration of the plateau iris periphery to remove the sharp angulation. Laser settings of 500-

μm spot size, with an exposure time of 0.5 second, and an intensity of 200 to 300 mW achieve sustained contraction of the peripheral iris. If miotics are needed for control of intraocular pressure after iridotomy, then iridoplasty is indicated only if the angle remains spontaneously appositionally closed on miotics.

If the angle is open after iridotomy but closes appositionally with pupillary dilation, treatment is indicated if intraocular pressure rises with closure. If closure is incomplete, observation for the development of future spontaneous closure is indicated.

PRECAUTIONS

If plateau iris configuration is diagnosed incidentally in an eye with an open angle, caution should be exercised in dilation and the patient followed gonioscopically at routine intervals for signs of progressive angle closure. If the patient presents with elevated intraocular pressure, careful indentation gonioscopy should be performed as in all cases of glaucoma, so that the condition is not confused with open-angle glaucoma because of the normal depth of the anterior chamber and relatively flat iris surface on direct examination.

COMMENTS

The most common cause of differential diagnostic confusion on routine examination is a prominent peripheral iris roll. With this iris picture, however, the peripheral iris does not occlude the angle on dilation, and it does not predispose to angle-closure glaucoma.

If the condition was not diagnosed before iridotomy and intraocular pressure is elevated postoperatively, careful gonioscopy should be performed. If the angle is open, such diagnoses as secondary damage to the trabecular meshwork should be considered. If the angle is closed, the differential diagnosis should include ciliary block or malignant glaucoma, in which the anterior chamber is flat or extremely shallow; peripheral anterior synechiae, which can be ruled out by indentation gonioscopy; or incomplete iridotomy.

Although plateau iris syndrome usually occurs in the postoperative period, it may occur up to years later, and patients with plateau iris configuration should not be assumed to be permanently cured if plateau iris syndrome does not develop immediately.

References

Epstein DL: Chandler and Grant's Glaucoma, 3d ed. Philadelphia, Lea & Febiger, Philadelphia, 1986.
Kolker AE, Hetherington J Jr: Becker-Shaffer's Diagnosis and Therapy of the Glaucomas, 5th ed. St. Louis, CV Mosby, 1983.
Lowe RF: Primary angle-closure glaucoma: A review of ocular biometry. Aust J Ophthalmol 5:9–17, 1977.
Lowe RF, Ritch R: Angle-closure glaucoma—Clinical Types. In Ritch R, Shields MB, Krupin T (eds): The Glaucomas. St. Louis, CV Mosby, 1989.
Pavlin CJ, Ritch R, Foster FS: Ultrasound biomicroscopy in plateau iris syndrome. Am J Ophthalmol 113:390–395, 1992.
Ritch R: Plateau iris is caused by abnormally positioned ciliary processes. J Glaucoma 1:23–26, 1992.
Ritch R: Argon laser peripheral iridoplasty: An overview. J Glaucoma (in press).
Ritch R, Solomon IS: Glaucoma surgery. In L'Esperance FA Jr (ed): Ophthalmic Lasers, 3rd ed. St. Louis, CV Mosby, 1993.
Törnquist R: Angle-closure glaucoma in an eye with a plateau type of iris. Acta Ophthalmol 36: 419–423, 1958.
Wand M, et al: Plateau iris syndrome. Trans Am Acad Ophthalmol Otolaryngol 83:122–130, 1977.

PRIMARY ANGLE-CLOSURE GLAUCOMA 365.20
(Primary Closed-Angle Glaucoma, Primary Narrow-Angle Glaucoma)

YOSHIAKI KITAZAWA, M.D. Ph.D.

Gifu, Japan

Primary angle-closure glaucoma is caused by increased intraocular pressure and obstruction of aqueous humor outflow resulting from the closure of the angle by the peripheral root of iris. It is a bilateral disease and affects those who are born with a narrow angle. The outflow channels of aqueous, including the trabecular meshwork, are normal before the closure of angle takes place.

In its early stage, the closure of the angle is nothing more than the contact between the trabecular meshwork and the root of the iris and is reversible once pupillary block is eliminated. However, as time goes by, the root of the iris becomes adherent to the trabeculum, forming peripheral anterior synechiae that cannot be relieved by breaking pupillary block.

Although the mechanism of pressure rise is identical, symptoms vary markedly depending on the magnitude and the speed of the intraocular pressure rise. With prodromal or intermittent angle-closure glaucoma, symptoms are caused by the rapid elevations and decreases of intraocular pressure. A steaminess of the cornea is caused by the abrupt rise of pressure as a result of sudden angle occlusion. Symptoms may consist of foggy or hazy vision with rainbow-colored halos around lights. Ocular congestion or discomfort may occur. Symptoms spontaneously subside in a few hours if the pupillary block is relieved by the miosis. The miosis may occur when the patient goes to a brighter environment or to sleep.

In the acute attack of primary angle-closure glaucoma, the symptoms are precipitated by pupillary dilation resulting from mydriatic drops, dim light, or emotional upset. Once angle closure is established, the symptoms of the intermittent or prodromal attack become more severe and permanent; they include blurred, foggy vision with colored halos around lights, ocular congestion, and pain. Also, nausea and vomiting may occur and are due to autonomic stimulation.

In chronic primary angle-closure glaucoma, the pressure rises insidiously as the closed area of the angle gradually increases, and patients may be totally free from symptoms or may experience some ocular discomfort and halos. Chronic primary angle-closure glaucoma cannot be differentiated from primary open-angle glaucoma on the basis of symptoms. Visual field defects and optic disc changes are also very similar in these two different glaucomas.

THERAPY

Supportive. The patient with acute primary angle-closure glaucoma should be admitted to the hospital to initiate intensive medical therapy that is usually a prelude to surgery. Analgesics may be used to control pain and apprehension. Administration of 300 to 600 mg of aspirin every 6 to 8 hours is usually adequate; if not, 50 to 100 mg of meperidine may be used.

In chronic primary angle-closure glaucoma, medical therapy can be less intensive than in an acute attack. Since there is no pain, analgesics are not necessary, and patients may be treated as outpatients.

Ocular. Cholinergic agents are used to pull the iris away from the angle. In acute primary angle-closure glaucoma, one or two drops of 1 to 3 per cent pilocarpine or 0.75 to 1.5 per cent carbachol should be instilled every 5 minutes for four times, then three or four times every half-hour, and thereafter every 1 to 2 hours. Moxisylyte,[+] an alpha-adrenergic blocking agent, may be effective in breaking attacks of acute closure. Instilled topically every 10 to 15 minutes in a 0.5 per cent solution, it inhibits contraction of the dilator muscle of the iris. As a result, pilocarpine constricts the pupil more effectively when applied with moxisylyte. Twice-daily administration of 0.25 or 0.50 per cent timolol may be added to miotics. Corticosteroids are useful in controlling inflammation. One to two drops of 0.1 per cent dexamethasone are given three to four times a day. To obtain a prompt normalization of pressure, topical drops should be used in conjunction with systemic medications.

In chronic angle-closure glaucoma, 1 to 3 per cent pilocarpine should be instilled every 4 to 6 hours. Twice-daily administration of 0.25 or 0.5 per cent timolol may be a supplement to pilocarpine.

Systemic. To break an acute attack, hyperosmotic agents are used that reduce intraocular pressure promptly. Oral glycerin may be administered in a 50 per cent solution in a dosage of 2 to 3 ml/kg. Oral isosorbide is an alternative to oral glycerin. It is administered in doses of 1 to 2 gm/kg and is preferred in diabetics as a metabolically inactive agent. Isosorbide is usually better tolerated than glycerin. If the patient is nauseated or oral glycerin has failed to be effective, 20 per cent mannitol may be given intravenously in a dose of 1 to 2 gm/kg, or 30 per cent urea may be given intravenously in a dose of 1.0 to 1.5 gm/kg. Carbonic anhydrase inhibitors, such as acetazolamide, are given by mouth in a dose of 250 mg four times daily. If the patient cannot take oral medication because of nausea, 500 mg of acetazolamide should be injected intravenously.

With chronic primary angle-closure glaucoma, hyperosmotic agents are of less value and are employed as a preoperative measure. Carbonic anhydrase inhibitors are used as for primary open-angle glaucoma; 250 mg of acetazolamide four times daily or 50 mg of methazolamide three times daily may be administered.

Surgical. Treatment of primary angle-closure glaucoma consists of peripheral iridectomy or laser iridotomy after the intraocular pressure has been normalized. In acute angle-closure glaucoma, the eye should be operated on promptly unless most of the angle has been confirmed to be open after the attack has been completely broken with medical measures. Iridectomy may be done surgically, or argon, Q-switched Nd:YAG, and diode laser may be used to create an iridotomy (laser iridotomy). If the acute attack of angle closure does not respond to intensive medical therapy, filtration surgery may be considered.

In chronic primary angle-closure glaucoma, laser iridotomy or surgical iridectomy is the operation of choice. It should be done even though intraocular pressure is normalized with medical therapy to avoid the progress of the synechial closure of the angle. Filtration surgery should not be performed unless iridectomy has failed to normalize intraocular pressure.

Ocular or Periocular Manifestations

(A) refers to acute angle-closure glaucoma; (C) indicates chronic angle-closure glaucoma.

Anterior Chamber: Closed angle (A, C).
Conjunctiva: Chemosis (A); hyperemia (A).
Cornea: Epithelial edema (A); folds in Descemet's membrane (A); hypesthesia (A); pigment on posterior surface (A).

Iris: Convex (C); forward displacement (A); peripheral anterior synechiae; posterior synechiae (A); sector atrophy, usually in the upper half (A).

Lens: Glaukomflecken or cataracta disseminata subcapsularis glaukomatosa (A).

Pupil: Dilatation, vertically oval, mid-dilated, and fixed (A).

Other: Increased intraocular pressure (A, C); visual field defects (A, C).

PRECAUTIONS

Intravenous hyperosmotic agents cause headache, dizziness, nausea, and vomiting; oral glycerin particularly tends to induce nausea. Urinary retention may be brought about by intense diuresis. Pulmonary edema and congestive heart failure may be precipitated in elderly patients with borderline cardiac and renal function; this is especially true of mannitol, which greatly increases blood volume. Cellular dehydration, including cerebral dehydration, may occur more often with mannitol and results in mental disorientation. Urea can cause skin slough and phlebitis, if it extravasates. Rebound elevation of intraocular pressure is common with urea.

Systemic toxicity following multiple topical applications of cholinergic drops may occur. Potent anticholinesterase inhibitors, such as echothiophate and demecarium, should not be used because of their tendency to precipitate angle closure as a result of aggravation of pupillary block and vascular congestion.

Epinephrine is contraindicated as it induces pupillary dilation. Adrenergic beta-blocking agents, including timolol, are considered to be supplementary to miotics as they possess no miotic effect.

COMMENTS

Acute primary angle-closure glaucoma is an ophthalmic emergency and requires immediate medical therapy. All medical measures should be used simultaneously to normalize elevated intraocular pressure. Once the pressure is brought under control, pressure gonioscopy with a Zeiss four-mirrored lens or Kitazawa's goniolens for this purpose is necessary to confirm the diagnosis and to evaluate the extent of peripheral anterior sy-

nechiae. If the angle is open at least one-quarter of the entire circumference, a peripheral iridectomy or laser iridotomy may be postponed until the eye becomes less irritated. If the angle is closed with peripheral anterior synechiae more than three-quarters in its circumference or the intraocular pressure responds poorly to maximum medical therapy, an immediate peripheral iridectomy or laser iridotomy should be performed. If the angle is open as much as half of the entire circumference, iridectomy is likely to normalize intraocular pressure without medication postoperatively. The more extensive the peripheral anterior synechiae, the more likely antiglaucoma medications will be needed to maintain a normal intraocular pressure after surgery. The fellow eye should also be treated with topical miotics in order to avoid an acute attack. Prophylactic laser iridotomy may be preferred to surgical iridectomy because of its safety and convenience.

Chronic primary angle-closure glaucoma should be treated surgically even when the intraocular pressure is normalized with medication. Since pupillary block cannot be eliminated by medical therapy, peripheral anterior synechiae always increase in width and height, regardless of the level of intraocular pressure.

References

Forbes M: Gonioscopy with corneal indentation. A method for distinguishing between appositional closure and synechial closure. Arch Ophthalmol 76:488–492, 1966.

Halasa AH, Rutkowski PC: Thymoxamine therapy for angle-closure glaucoma. Arch Ophthalmol 90:177–179, 1973.

Lowe RF: Primary angle-closure glaucoma: Biometry and the clinician. *In* Etienne R, Paterson GD (eds): International Glaucoma Symposium. (XXII International Congress of Ophthalmology, Albi, France, 1974). Marseille, Diffusion Generale de Librarie, 1975, pp 247–272.

Nakamura Y, Kitazawa Y: A new goniolens for corneal indentation gonioscopy. Acta Ophthalmol 49:964–970, 1971.

Pollack IP: Laser iridotomy: Current concepts in technique and safety. Int Ophthalmol Clin 21:137–144, 1980.

Sugar HS: Surgical decision, technique and complications of peripheral iridectomy for angle-closure glaucoma. Ann Ophthalmol 7:1237–1241, 1975.

IRIS AND CILIARY BODY

ACCOMMODATIVE SPASM
367.53

WILLIAM E. SCOTT, M.D.

Iowa City, Iowa

Accommodative spasm (spasm of the near reflex) is an overactivity of accommodation wherein the refractive power of the eye is increased and the patient has an induced myopia. The tone of the ciliary muscle is increased, and a constant accommodative effort is expended by the parasympathetic nervous system to bring both the far point and near point closer. It is an involuntary action that may be constant or intermittent. Spasm of accommodation may be associated with headaches, photophobia, eyestrain, defective vision for near and distance, inability to concentrate, and intermittent homonymous diplopia. The distant vision may be blurred because of the pseudomyopia. Macropsia may also occur, as well as browache, ocular fatigue, and inability to maintain visual or mental concentration. These patients also present with limitations of abduction, which may result in the misdiagnosis of a sixth cranial nerve palsy. The differential diagnosis consists of abducens palsy, thyroid eye disease with secondary involvement of the medial recti, myasthenia gravis, convergent strabismus, divergence insufficiency, or ocular motor apraxia.

The etiology of accommodative spasm usually has a functional basis, but it may be associated with organic disease. Raymond and Compton (1990) reported a case of a patient with a progressive 11-year history of spasm of the near reflex associated with cerebral vascular accidents. Spasm of the near reflex has been reported in association with head injury and may resolve in 1 to 2 years. Moster and Hoenig (1989) described a transient occurrence of spasm of the near reflex in a patient with an adenocarcinoma of the gall bladder and an encephalopathy associated with sepsis and with renal and hepatic failure. Spasm of accommodation occurs in patients usually under the age of 40 when it is functional in origin. In cases associated with organic disease, the onset may be in the later years of life.

THERAPY

Ocular. Treatment of accommodative spasm is difficult and is largely based on relief of symptoms. In patients with blurred distance vision, one should not hesitate to prescribe a minus power lens, even though it is for pseudo-and not true myopia. The use of a minus lens will not influence the basic refractive error. As the patient becomes older and accommodation lessens, the spastic state will disappear, as well as the pseudomyopia. The glasses should be worn as needed.

When the complaint is blurred near vision, one should correct for near vision and inform the patient to expect distant vision to be blurred. If close work tends to cause further relapses, stronger lenses for this work may bring relief. The recommendation should be made that the glasses be worn only for prolonged near use.

A careful explanation to the patient of the condition will avoid unnecessary anxiety and constant lens corrections. Occasionally, a concurrent regimen of an antispasmodic, such as belladonna, and a mild sedative may be helpful to these patients.

PRECAUTIONS

Cycloplegics, such as atropine and homatropine, have been advocated for the treatment of accommodative spasm. However, the spasm is broken only during the use of the cycloplegic and generally recurs when it is discontinued. In addition, temporary reading glasses are usually needed. Such glasses are not tolerated by most patients, and it has never been shown that the spasm is influenced by them.

Accommodative spasm may be caused by miotic drugs, such as pilocarpine, physostigmine, echothiophate, neostigmine, and isoflurophate. This condition may be quite distressing to a patient beginning miotic therapy for glaucoma. Accommodative spasm may also be associated with overdosage of such drugs as morphine, alcohol, or digitalis.

COMMENTS

A tonic accommodation is a rare phenomenon in which an accommodative posture is prolonged so that the change in focus from distant to near objects or vice versa is delayed. The patient may need bifocal lenses if the defect is great. The site of the casual lesion is unknown, but has occasionally been associated with syphilis, measles, diabetes, alcoholism, Graves' disease, and trauma.

References

Dagi LR, Chrousos GA, Cogan DC: Spasm of the near reflex associated with organic disease. Am J Ophthalmol 103:582–585, 1987.

Herman P: Convergence spasm. Mt Sinai J Med 44: 501–509, 1977.

Manor RS: Use of special glasses in treatment of spasm of near reflex. Ann Ophthalmol 11:903–905, 1979.

Moore S, Stockbridge L: Another approach to the treatment of accommodative spasm. Am Orthopt J 23:71–72, 1973.

Moster ML, Hoenig EM: Spasm of the near reflex associated with metabolic encephalopathy. Neurology 38:150, 1989.

Nirankari VS, Hameroff SB: Spasm of the near reflex. Ann Ophthalmol 12:1050–1051, 1980.

Raymond GL, Compton JL: Spasm of the near reflex associated with cerebrovascular accident. Aust NZ J Ophthalmol 18:407–410, 1990.

Sloane AE, Kraut JA: Spasm of accommodation. Doc Ophthalmol 34:365–369, 1973.

ANIRIDIA 743.45

DAVID S. WALTON, M.D.

Boston, Massachusetts

Aniridia is a genetically determined condition with multiple congenital ocular anomalies and in which dystrophic changes progress from early childhood. Externally, there appears to be a total absence of the iris, although gonioscopy reveals some iris in all eyes. Approximately 50 per cent of patients with aniridia develop progressive glaucoma. Nearly all have visual problems. The visual acuity is usually markedly decreased (20/100 to 20/400) because of an associated foveal hypoplasia. In rare cases, the visual acuity can be as good as 20/50. The glaucoma in aniridia characteristically develops in late childhood and often seems to depend on the extent of the attachment of the iris stump to the trabecular meshwork. The iris deformity is always bilateral, but can show marked asymmetry. Approximately two-thirds of patients with congenital aniridia have a positive family history of the autosomal dominant inheritance, whereas the remainder of cases are sporadic. There is a significant association with Wilms' tumor, other genitourinary defects, retardation, and aniridia in certain sporadic cases that also possess a deletion of short arm of the eleventh chromosome. In glaucoma associated with aniridia, the cornea is rarely enlarged, and breaks in Descemet's membrane almost never occur, unless the glaucoma occurs in infancy, which is uncommon.

THERAPY

Ocular. Miotics are used to improve outflow facility and thus lower the intraocular pressure. Beta-adrenergic blockers have also been of inconsistent value.

Systemic. Carbonic anhydrase inhibitors are used to lower intraocular pressure by suppressing secretion of aqueous humor, if topical ocular miotics prove inadequate alone. The usual oral daily adult dosage of acetazolamide is 125 to 250 mg every 6 hours or 500-mg Sequels every 12 to 24 hours. Alternatively, methazolamide in doses of 25 to 100 mg every 8 to 12 hours may be used, with apparently less risk of kidney stone formation. For children, a daily dose of 3 mg/kg of methazolamide or 15 mg/kg of acetazolamide is used daily.

Surgical. In the majority of patients, medical therapy is helpful, but may eventually prove inadequate, and antiglaucoma surgery becomes indicated. If the glaucoma has become poorly controlled in spite of medical treatment, goniosurgery to dissect the iris stump from the trabecular meshwork may be temporarily effective in increasing the response to medical therapy, but it rarely has a lasting beneficial effect. In contrast, early prophylactic goniotomy in aniridia cases in which the iris stump is just beginning to develop synechiae to the trabecular meshwork may prove valuable in both the prevention of glaucoma and the treatment of early glaucoma. Trabeculectomy may be useful in some patients. Full-thickness filtration surgery also may be successful, but the risks of postoperative flat chamber and secondary corneal injury by the lens make this procedure more risky than trabeculectomy. For advanced aniridia glaucoma unresponsive to other treatment, cycloablative procedures are of value.

Cataract surgery is often necessary in time. Aspiration cataract extraction is used in the young patient, and extracapsular cataract extraction is used in older patients for removal of the opacified lens.

A peculiar corneal epithelial dystrophy usually develops, starting at the limbus and progressing centrally, but it rarely requires treatment. Penetrating keratoplasty for complete corneal opacification has been disappointing. Prolonged patching may be necessary for chronic epithelial breakdown in such cases.

Ocular or Periocular Manifestations

Conjunctiva: Hyperemia.
Cornea: Circumferential epithelial dystrophy with pannus; degeneration and progressive opacity.
Iris: Iris blockage of the trabecular meshwork; narrow peripheral rim only.
Lens: Displacement (superior); progressive opacification.

Optic Nerve: Atrophy; cupping; disc hypoplasia.
  Pupil: Enlarged.
  Retina: Absence of foveal reflex; foveal hypoplasia; white dots at the ora serrata.
  Other: Glaucoma; nystagmus.

PRECAUTIONS

The risk of aniridic glaucoma dictates careful attention to these patients since there may be a gradual increase in intraocular pressure over a number of years. Goniosurgery is effective in some patients and is apparently best performed earlier, but the absence of iris increases the risk to the lens during the procedure. Accordingly, goniosurgery is best done by surgeons experienced in goniotomy-type surgery and thoroughly familiar with abnormalities of the angle in aniridia glaucoma.

The risks that miotics will promote lens opacities and that epinephrine will affect the macula in aniridia are unknown. Aniridic eyes nearly always undergo breakage of some of the lens zonules below, with upward displacement of the lens. These eyes also frequently develop cataracts. Miotics may cause shallowing of the anterior chamber and blockage of the angle secondary to anterior rotation of the iris leaf circumferentially.

COMMENTS

Recognition of aniridia by pediatricians and parents often occurs in infancy. This is important, not only because of the high risk of glaucoma but also because of the risk of associated Wilms' tumor in certain sporadic cases of aniridia. Chromosomal examination is indicated in the evaluation of all patients with aniridia and is mandatory in sporadic cases under 10 years of age. In the presence of a deletion of the short arm of the eleventh chromosome, the risk of Wilms' tumor is significantly increased. Familial cases seem to be at no increased risk for Wilms' tumor. The average age for development of Wilms' tumor is somewhat younger in patients with aniridia (mean average, 3.6 years). These tumors are grossly and microscopically identical to those that appear in otherwise normal individuals. Early diagnosis and treatment of the tumor can be life saving.

The pediatrician should be alerted to the risk that Wilms' tumor might develop. These children must have a careful physical examination, and blood pressure should be measured regularly. In addition to chromosomal studies, developmental evaluation and examination for other congenital anomalies should be a part of the care of these children. Renal ultrasonography is indicated every 3 months for patients with a chromosomal deletion and at least every 6 months for sporadic cases without a detectable chromosome defect.

At 6- to 12-month intervals, an ophthalmic examination, including tonometry and gonioscopy, should be performed. If necessary, these procedures should be done under anesthesia. In some infants, it is possible to do Perkins' applanation tonometry and gonioscopy without general anesthesia while the baby is being fed.

References

Elsas FJ, et al: Familial aniridia with preserved ocular function. Am J Ophthalmol 83:718–724, 1977.
Francois J, Coucke D, Coppieters R: Aniridia-Wilms' tumour syndrome. Ophthalmologica 174: 35–39, 1977.
Friedman AL: Wilms' tumor detection in patients with sporadic aniridia: Successful use of ultrasound. Am J Dis Child 140:173–174, 1986.
Grant WM, Walton DS: Progressive changes in the angle in congenital aniridia, with development of glaucoma. Am J Ophthalmol 78:842–847, 1974.
Pilling GP IV: Wilms' tumor in seven children with congenital aniridia. J Pediatr Surg 10:87–96, 1975.
Riccardi VM, et al: Chromosomal imbalance in the aniridia-Wilms' tumor association: 11p interstitial deletion. Pediatrics 61:604–610, 1978.
Walton DS: Aniridic glaucoma: The results of gonioscopy to prevent and treat this problem. Trans Am Ophthalmol Soc 84:59–70, 1986.

FUCHS' HETEROCHROMIC IRIDOCYCLITIS 364.21

THOMAS J. LIESEGANG, M.D.

Jacksonville, Florida

Fuchs' heterochromic iridocyclitis is readily recognized when it presents with its classic clinical appearance. These findings include heterochromia of the irides (usually the lighter iris is present in the involved eye), absence of conjunctival infection, specific atrophic changes on the iris surface, minimal cell and flare, widely scattered small nonconfluent keratic precipitates, vitreous cells, absence of posterior synechiae, a complicated cataract, and occasional glaucoma. It can occur at all ages in both sexes. It may present as an asymptomatic finding early in its course with minimal ocular symptoms of floaters or in some patients only after the development of a cataract. The disease is recognized in about 5 per cent of patients presenting with uveitis. In about 10 per cent of cases the disease is bilateral, and this may require an astute clinician to make the diagnosis. If the disease is unilateral at presentation, it usually remains a unilateral disease.

Fuchs' heterochromic iridocyclitis is frequently misdiagnosed by the ophthalmologist who does not see a large number of uveitis patients because of the unrecognized atypical variants of the syndrome. The presentation, progression, and prognosis of this disease vary widely. There is a variable degree and progression of iris atrophy involving both the anterior portion of the iris and the posterior pigmented layer. This atrophy is evident as a generalized blunting, flattening, or blurring of the surface markings of the iris crypts or rugae, especially when compared with the other eye. The whole iris tissue demonstrates rarefaction and transparency, with a moth-eaten appearance and defects in the posterior pigmented layer and anterior stromal thinning with sphincter muscle atrophy. The pupil is sometimes irregular or larger because of sphincter atrophy. Transillumination defects are best seen with retroillumination. In a brown-eyed individual, it may be difficult to detect the iris atrophy because both layers of the iris are of the same color and texture (no heterochromia). In some individuals there is more atrophy of the anterior layer such that the iris can appear darker in the affected eye (reversed heterochromia). Daylight examination is the best for detecting subtle heterochromia. Gaps or absence of the pupillary ruff is frequently seen. Gelatinous nodules (probably plasma cells) are occasionally seen at the pupillary margin or on the iris surface. The iris atrophy tends to be more prominent around the pupillary area. The absence of posterior synechiae is a constant feature of the disease, although there may be small residual pigment deposits on the anterior lens capsule from previous Koeppe nodules.

With iris atrophy, vessels within the iris stroma become more noticeable, and as the disease progresses, they become straighter and narrower. Fluorescein angiography of the iris in patients with Fuchs' iridocyclitis has demonstrated an ischemic vasculopathy and infarction along with increased permeability of vessels on the iris surface, limbus, and the ciliary body. Over time, this ischemia evolves to a fine rubeosis involving the iris surface, angle, and possibly the ciliary body. This iris ischemia is probably an initiating cause of the iris atrophy. The fragile blood vessels in the angle are susceptible to bleeding either spontaneously or in association with a sudden reduction of pressure in the anterior chamber. The filiform hemorrhage seen in the chamber angle or on the peripheral iris after paracentesis, glaucoma, or cataract surgery is known as Amsler's sign and is characteristic of the disease. Small peripheral anterior synechiae are occasionally seen in areas of fine rubeosis; they may be transient. In some patients a felt-like membrane develops within the angle in areas of previous fine rubeosis either with or without glaucoma. In rare cases, blood-containing cysts of the ciliary body are seen and may proceed to vitreous hemorrhages upon rupture.

The cell and flare in the anterior chamber and the anterior vitreous are usually very mild. The keratic precipitates are extremely characteristic, although they are evanescent in some patients. They are small, widely scattered, round, gray-white precipitates that have a tendency to involve the whole back surface of the cornea. This is one of the only diseases in which the keratic precipitates may involve the superior part of the cornea, occasionally selectively. Between the precipitates are fine, wispy cotton-like filaments that are even more evanescent. The keratic precipitates of this disorder are never confluent, large, or greasy. Within the vitreous there may also be heavy stringy or dust-like particles adherent to a degenerative vitreous framework. After cataract surgery or occasionally spontaneously, dense vitreous veils may form, possibly related to bleeding in the ciliary body area. These veils may preclude vision or lead to further intraocular inflammation. The eyes with Fuchs' heterochromia iridocyclitis are usually white and quiet externally, but can be inflamed on occasion, especially in association with vitreous hemorrhage or glaucoma.

Glaucoma is a common finding in patients with long-term or more severe progression of the disease (up to 60 per cent). It is also the primary reason for permanent loss of vision with this condition. It is felt to be caused by sclerosis of the trabecular meshwork or collapse of the canal of Schlemm, but the findings of peripheral anterior synechiae, felt-like membrane in the angle, and trabecular spaces filled with plasma cells are alternate mechanisms of disease. The iris and angle fine rubeosis does not lead to synechial closure. Elevated intraocular pressure may be intermittent initially and may respond to topical steroids (an inflammatory glaucoma), but in many cases, it becomes recalcitrant to steroids, as well as antiglaucoma medications. Patients with this disorder are poor candidates for successful argon laser trabeculoplasty. Filtering surgery is frequently required and has a variable success rate.

Cataract is a consistent feature of Fuchs' iridocyclitis. It begins as a posterior subcapsular cataract and has a tendency to progress to hypermaturity. Occasionally, the iris heterochromia becomes more obvious when the cataract matures. Patients with milder forms of the disease do well with extracapsular surgery (with or without an intraocular lens), but patients with more severe disease very frequently have anterior chamber or vitreous hemorrhage, severe glaucoma, pupillary or vitreous membranes, or corneal edema in the aftermath of intraocular surgery.

The cornea in most patients with this disorder is probably normal, although patients have been noted with guttata in only the affected eye or a reduced endothelial cell count. Areas of darkness spanning several endothelial cells or intercellular blebs have been seen on specular microscopy. Some patients have demonstrated central or peripheral corneal decompensation after intraocular surgery, suggesting poor endothelial tolerance. This may correlate with hypoprofusion of the iris.

Chorioretinal lesions with the distinctive appearance of focal atrophy with a hyperpigmented border have been described in several patients with Fuchs' uveitis. Many but not all have a positive serologic test for toxoplasmosis. A few patients have been described with a retinal vasculitis. In many instances, the fundus cannot be viewed because of the cataract.

The pathogenesis of the condition is unknown, although for many years it was felt to be a degenerative or trophic condition, specifically of the nervous system or perhaps a vascular insufficiency. Genetic studies have not been revealing. Taking all present pathologic and clinical information into account, there is significant evidence to suggest that the disease is an occlusive vasculitis as a result of a localized immunologic reaction. Large numbers of plasma cells, immunoglobins, and immune complexes are found locally within several ocular tissues without evidence of systemic immune disease. Cellular and humoral immunity to corneal antigens can be present, but it is not clear whether these are epiphenomena. Vascular occlusion causes hypoxia, neovascularization, and subsequent hemorrhages. It is conceivable that certain processes, such as toxoplasmosis, may initiate the process in some patients so that this single clinical entity may have different etiologies. Early glaucoma is probably related to the obstruction of the trabecular spaces by plasma cells, but later in the course, trabecular sclerosis or vascular ischemia and rubeosis may play a more prominent role.

THERAPY

Ocular. The majority of patients with Fuchs' heterochromic iridocyclitis have few symptoms and do not require treatment other than periodic observation. Steroid drops can reduce the anterior chamber reaction and the symptoms of floaters and can occasionally lower the intraocular pressure during intermittent attacks of glaucoma. The use of topical steroids, however, is generally not indicated. Glaucoma is the most significant therapeutic problem. It may respond initially to topical steroids, but later becomes refractory to steroids. Milder cases may respond to topical or systemic antiglaucoma medications, but more severe cases will be refractory. Cycloplegics are not helpful.

Surgical. Argon laser trabeculoplasty is usually not successful and probably should be avoided if there are significant peripheral anterior synechiae, fine vessels in the angle, or a felt-like membrane. Filtration surgery is frequently indicated, but anterior chamber and vitreous hemorrhage and intraocular inflammation preclude success in many cases. Light cyclocryotherapy before filtration surgery may reduce the complications that apparently are caused by neovascularization.

With milder forms of the disease, cataract surgery (even with an intraocular lens) has a good success rate. Extracapsular cataract extraction is preferred over an intracapsular cataract operation. In more severe forms of the disease, glaucoma, intraocular bleeding, and inflammation frequently preclude successful cataract surgery. Corneal transplantation has been required in only a limited number of these patients, but has met with poor success because of peripheral anterior synechiae and glaucoma in these selected patients.

Ocular or Periocular Manifestations

Angle: Felt-like membrane; fine peripheral anterior synechiae (PAS); fine rubeosis; hyphema (occasional).

Conjunctiva: Ciliary flush (occasional); quiescent (usually).

Cornea: Central or peripheral corneal edema after intraocular surgery; dark areas on specular microscopy; guttata (occasional); lower endothelial cell count.

Fundus: Focal, atrophic chorioretinal scars with pigmented borders.

Intraocular Pressure: Increased.

Lens: Posterior subcapsular cataract with tendency to progression.

Uvea: Anterior stromal and posterior pigment iris atrophy, especially in the pupillary zone; lack of crisp iris detail; gaps in the pupillary ruff around the pupil with transillumination iris defects; heterochromia frequently reversed or subtle; iris vessel straight, narrow, and more evident; rubeosis; small, round, nonconfluent keratic precipitates, especially on the superior cornea; fine filaments between keratic precipitates; mild cell and flare.

Vitreous: Cells adherent to vitreous framework, condensed vitreous veils (occasional).

PRECAUTIONS

The diagnosis is frequently missed because the wide spectrum of the disease is not appreciated. The term "heterochromia" is probably inappropriate because it is frequently absent. Once the disease is confirmed, further medical work-up for uveitis is not needed. If the disease is unilateral at presentation, it usually remains unilateral. Rarely, the disease is present in other family members; some patients report heterochromia since childhood. Steroid therapy is usually not successful or indicated. These patients must be followed periodically to monitor for glaucoma, cataracts, or corneal disease.

COMMENTS

The prognosis varies with the progression and severity of the clinical findings, especially with regard to iris stromal atrophy and rubeosis. The significance of toxoplasmosis-like scars is not known. In milder cases, intraocular surgery is usually successful. In more advanced cases (for example, in patients with severe glaucoma), both cataract and glaucoma surgery have a significant incidence of complications.

References

Berger BB, Tessler HH, Kottow MH: Anterior segment ischemia in Fuchs' heterochromic cyclitis. Arch Ophthalmol 98:499, 1980.

Brooks AM, et al: Progressive corneal endothelial cell changes in anterior segment disease. Aust NZ J Ophthalmol 15:71–78, 1987.

Jones NP: Extracapsular cataract surgery with and without intraocular lens implantation in Fuchs' heterochromic uveitis. Eye 4:145–150, 1990.

La Hey E, Mooy CM, Baarsma GS, et al: Immune deposits in iris biopsy specimens from patients with Fuchs' heterochromic iridocyclitis. Am J Ophthalmol 113:75–80, 1992.

La Hey E, Rothova A, Baarsma GS, et al: Fuchs' heterochromic iridocyclitis is not associated with ocular toxoplasmosis. Arch Ophthalmol 110:806–811, 1992.

Liesegang TJ: Clinical features and prognosis in Fuchs' uveitis syndrome. Arch Ophthalmol 100:1622–1626, 1982.

O'Connor GR: Heterochromic iridocyclitis. Trans Ophthalmol Soc UK 104:219–231, 1985.

Schwab IR: The epidemiologic association of Fuchs' heterochromic iridocyclitis and ocular toxoplasmosis. Am J Ophthalmol 111: 356–362, 1991.

Tabbut BR, Tessler HH, Williams D: Fuchs' heterochromic iridocyclitis in blacks. Arch Ophthalmol 106:1688–1690, 1988.

IRIDOCORNEAL ENDOTHELIAL SYNDROME 364.51

(Chandler's Syndrome, Cogan-Reese Syndrome, ICE Syndrome, Progressive "Essential" Iris Atrophy)

M. BRUCE SHIELDS, M.D.

Durham, North Carolina

The iridocorneal endothelial (ICE) syndrome is a spectrum of disease that includes Chandler's syndrome, progressive iris atrophy, and the Cogan-Reese syndrome. Common to each condition is an alteration of the corneal endothelium, which has a fine, hammered silver appearance by slit-lamp biomicroscopy and typical changes by specular microscopy. In many cases, the endothelial disorder gives rise to corneal edema of variable degree. Ultrastructural studies of advanced cases reveal a multilayered Desce-

met's membrane lined by scant, abnormal cells.

Also common throughout this spectrum of disease is peripheral anterior synechiae, which often extend to or beyond Schwalbe's line. These synechiae typically spread circumferentially around the anterior chamber angle, eventually leading to secondary glaucoma in a high percentage of cases. A third feature, and that for which the clinical variations are most easily distinguished, is changes in the iris. In Chandler's syndrome, iris abnormalities are either absent or limited to mild pupillary distortion and stromal atrophy, whereas progressive iris atrophy is characterized by marked corectopia, ectropion uvea, and atrophy with hole formation. The Cogan-Reese syndrome may have any degree of iris changes, but has the additional feature of nodules on the stromal surface of the iris. According to the membrane theory of Campbell (1978), an endothelial membrane from the abnormal corneal endothelium grows across the anterior chamber angle and onto the iris and subsequently undergoes contraction, leading to the aforementioned changes of both structures. A clinical comparison suggests that corneal edema is more common with Chandler's syndrome, whereas secondary glaucoma is seen more often with the other two subsets.

The ICE syndrome is almost always unilateral and typically becomes apparent during young adulthood, with a predilection for females. There is usually no family history of the disease or associated systemic diseases. Typical presenting complaints include visual disturbance, ranging from a mild blur in the morning hours to marked, persistent reduction, and alterations in the pupil or iris.

THERAPY

Managing patients with the ICE syndrome often involves treatment of the corneal edema, the secondary glaucoma, or both. Medical therapy may suffice for either problem, although a high percentage of patients eventually require surgical intervention.

Ocular. The corneal edema is dependent to a degree on the level of intraocular pressure, although it may occur with normal pressures. Control of both corneal edema and secondary glaucoma, therefore, may be accomplished in some cases with antiglaucoma medications. Due to the obstruction of the trabecular meshwork by the membrane or synechia, drugs that reduce aqueous production, such as topical beta blockers (timolol 0.25 or 0.5 per cent, betaxolol 0.25 or 0.5 per cent, levobunolol 0.25 or 0.5 per cent, metipranolol 0.3 per cent, or carteolol 1.0 per cent twice daily) or carbonic anhydrase inhibitors (e.g., methazolamide 25 to 50 mg twice daily or acetazolamide 500-mg sustained-release capsules twice daily or 250 mg four times daily) are usually the most efficacious. However, pilocarpine or epinephrine may also be effective, especially in the early stages of the disease. In some cases, additional measures may be required for the corneal edema, such as topical hypertonic saline solutions or a soft contact lens.

Surgical. The corneal edema in some patients eventually becomes intractable to all nonsurgical measures. Glaucoma filtering surgery has been used to control the edema by further intraocular pressure reduction. However, the edema may persist despite pressures in the subteens, and penetrating keratoplasty is the preferred surgical technique for management of the corneal edema when the intraocular pressure is controlled at a level sufficient to prevent progressive glaucomatous optic atrophy. When the secondary glaucoma is uncontrolled medically, filtering surgery is the procedure of choice. Laser trabeculoplasty is not effective in these cases.

Ocular or Periocular Manifestations

Anterior Chamber Angle: Peripheral anterior synechiae.
Cornea: Endothelial alteration; edema.
Iris: Chandler's syndrome: mild atrophy and pupillary distortion; progressive Iris Atrophy: advanced atrophy with holes, corectopia, and ectropion uvea; Cogan-Reese syndrome: any degree of atrophy with nodules on the iris stroma.
Other: Secondary glaucoma.

PRECAUTIONS

Potential adverse reactions with beta blockers include bradycardia, weakened myocardial contractility, bronchospasm, and central nervous system alterations. Serious side effects of carbonic anhydrase inhibitors include serum electrolyte imbalance, systemic acidosis, gastrointestinal distress, genitourinary problems, including renal calculi, and blood dyscrasias. The ICE syndrome may be confused with other disorders, which can lead to incorrect therapy. The corneal changes must be distinguished from those of Fuchs' endothelial dystrophy and posterior polymorphous dystrophy. The iris dissolution may resemble the changes in the Axenfeld-Rieger syndrome, whereas the iris nodules may be confused with the iris nevus syndrome, neurofibromatosis, nodular iritis, or malignant melanoma, the latter having mistakenly led to enucleation.

COMMENTS

The subtle changes of Chandler's syndrome are often missed, making it a frequently overlooked cause of unilateral glaucoma. This misdiagnosis is best avoided by careful slit-lamp inspection of the posterior cornea for the

typical fine, hammered silver appearance, as so clearly described by Chandler.

References

Campbell DG, Shields MB, Smith TR: The corneal endothelium and the spectrum of essential iris atrophy. Am J Ophthalmol 86:317–324, 1978.
Chandler PA: Atrophy of the stroma of the iris. Endothelial dystrophy, corneal edema, and glaucoma. Am J Ophthalmol 41:607–615, 1956.
Cogan DG, Reese AB: A syndrome of iris nodules, ectopic Descemet's membrane, and unilateral glaucoma. Doc Ophthalmol 26:424–433, 1969.
Hirst LW, Quigley HA, Stark WJ, Shields MB: Specular microscopy of iridocorneal endothelial syndrome. Am J Ophthalmol 89:1–21, 1980.
Lichter PR: The spectrum of Chandler's syndrome: An often overlooked cause of unilateral glaucoma. Ophthalmology 85:245–251, 1978.
Richardson TM: Corneal decompensation in Chandler's syndrome. A scanning and transmission electron microscopic study. Arch Ophthalmol 97:2112–2119, 1979.
Shields MB, Campbell DG, Simmons RJ, Hutchinson BT: Iris nodules in essential iris atrophy. Arch Ophthalmol 94:406–410, 1976.
Shields MB, Campbell DG, Simmons RJ: The essential iris atrophies. Am J Ophthalmol 85:749–759, 1978.
Shields MB, McCracken JS, Klintworth GK, Campbell DG: Corneal edema in essential iris atrophy. Ophthalmol 86:1533–1548, 1979.
Wilson MC, Shields MB: A comparison of the clinical variations of the iridocorneal endothelial syndrome. Arch Ophthalmol 107:1465–1468, 1989.

IRIS BOMBÉ 364.74
LEONARD CHRISTENSEN, M.D.
Portland, Oregon

Iris bombé is a pathologic extension of pupillary block whereby the iris is bound to the lens at the pupillary border by firm fibrotic adhesions. These adhesions form most frequently, but not invariably, from chronic iridocyclitis of diverse etiology. When the adhesion is sufficiently firm and complete (seclusio or occlusio pupillae), the flow of aqueous from the posterior chamber is impeded to the extent that the pressure required to drive aqueous into the anterior chamber exceeds the pressure required to drive it out. At that level, the peripheral leaf of the iris bows forward. If the blockage is of sufficient magnitude, the iris is displaced firmly against the trabecula. In turn, the aqueous outflow from the anterior chamber is blocked, creating an acute or subacute angle-closure glaucoma. Iridolenticular adhesions are almost always related to inflammation of the iris. Initially, there is an outpouring of fibrin from the iris, creating soft adhesions to the adjacent lens. If not interrupted, this outpouring is followed by fibrocytic proliferation from the iris stroma, with consequent formation of firm, medically irreversible adhesions.

THERAPY

Ocular. Prophylaxis is most important. Initially, the iris adhesions are uniform and susceptible to medical management by mobilization of the pupil. In active iritis, the pupil should be maximally dilated to prevent iridolenticular adhesions. By alternately employing miotics occasionally, mobilization of the iris may be retained. This will further ensure against formation of adhesions.

Once formed, the fibrocytic adhesions are almost impossible to disrupt by medical means. Dilating agents, including combinations of cycloplegics and mydriatics, such as 2.5 or 10 per cent phenylephrine with 1 per cent atropine, 1 per cent cyclopentolate, or 5 per cent homatropine, may be tried. However, if the intraocular pressure is significantly high, surgical intervention should be employed as soon as possible.

Systemic. Systemic control of glaucoma may be temporarily gained by employment of osmotic agents or carbonic anhydrase inhibitors, but invariably surgery must be performed. Of the osmotic agents, 20 per cent intravenous mannitol is most effective, although oral administration of 0.75 to 1.5 gm/kg of glycerin may be sufficient temporarily.

Surgical. The aim of treatment is to re-establish communication between the posterior and anterior chamber. This may be accomplished by surgical transfixation of the iris or surgical iridectomy. The most recent innovation is iridectomy by argon or YAG laser. If the iris is in contact with the cornea at the site of perforation, heat injury to the cornea might occur. However, this injury should be discrete and at the periphery.

Surgical management consists of establishing the free flow of aqueous from the posterior chamber to the anterior chamber, thus relieving the pressure against the iris. This permits the iris to fall back from the cornea and opens the angle and escape channels. However, sometimes the iris does not fall back spontaneously. Once the anterior chamber is entered, active displacement of the iris by instrumentation is then required.

Transfixion of the iris is mentioned in the older literature. It is achieved by inserting a Graefe (or Wheeler) knife through the cornea, the iris both peripherally and centrally, and the cornea of the opposite side. Although effective, the incisions may close off because of their small size. Damage to the lens can also occur.

A peripheral irridectomy through an ab externo incision is very effective, simple, and safe. In addition, an iris spatula can be inserted between the iris and lens at the pupillary border, thus freeing up the adhesions; however, care must be taken to avoid injury to the lens. Also, the iris spatula can be employed to displace the iris from the posterior corneal surface if necessary. If recurrence is a threat, the peripheral iridectomy can be converted to a sector iridectomy, ensuring against such an event.

Ocular or Periocular Manifestations

Anterior Chamber: Cloudy aqueous.
Cornea: Keratic precipitates; thickened.
Iris: Anterior synechiae; dilated blood vessels; iridolenticular adhesions; posterior synechiae.
Lens: Anterior subcapsular opacity.
Other: Glaucoma.

PRECAUTIONS

Repeated instillation of 10 per cent phenylephrine may produce a systemic vasopressor response, particularly in very young or debilitated patients. Intravenous injections of mannitol may produce mental confusion, particularly in aged or debilitated patients. Although quite safe, this latter agent should be used with caution.

If transfixion is to be employed, care should be taken to avoid the lens, and the surgeon must appreciate that the communication can readily be closed in the face of active inflammation. With iridectomy, suction applied at the opening of the incision delivers the iris to the external surface, and the iris can be readily grasped for an iridectomy. This avoids any chance of lens injury that might occur with insertion of forceps to grasp the iris.

COMMENTS

Iris bombé is essentially the aftermath of iridocyclitis. It may be prevented by maximal pupillary dilation and active mobilization of the pupil early in the disease. Once established, it is almost always a surgical problem best resolved by peripheral or sector iridectomy.

References

Abraham RK, Miller GL: Outpatient argon laser iridectomy for angle closure glaucoma: A two-year study. Trans Am Acad Ophthalmol Otolaryngol 79:529–538, 1975.

Duke-Elder S (ed): System of Ophthalmology. St. Louis, CV Mosby, 1966, Vol IX, p 178.

Shin DH: Argon laser iris photocoagulation to relieve acute angle-closure glaucoma. Am J Ophthalmol 93:348–350, 1982.

Tomey KF, Traverso CE, Shammas IV: Neodymium-YAG laser iridotomy in the treatment and prevention of angle closure glaucoma. A review of 373 eyes. Arch Ophthalmol 105:476–481, 1987.

IRIS CYSTS 364.6

(Epithelial Cysts, Epithelial Implantation Cysts, Spontaneous Congenital Iris Cysts)

KENNETH C. SWAN, M.D.

Portland, Oregon

Iris cysts are of two general types: cysts that originate within the intraepithelium or stroma and implantation cysts from intraocular surgery or trauma. Intraepithelial cysts represent an incomplete obliteration or reestablishment of the space between the two layers of the secondary optic vessel. The outer layer is composed of pigment epithelium and presents as a black globular mass behind the iris, which does not transilluminate. Peripherally, the cysts may present as globular protrusions as the overlying iris stroma is pushed anteriorly. They may extend through the iris into the anterior chamber. Iris cysts may be concealed, unless the pupil is dilated. More than one cyst may be noted in the same eye or in the other eye. Iris nodules and cysts also may occur as a proliferative response to miotic therapy for glaucoma or accommodative esotropia.

Stromal cysts typically are nonpigmented and semitransparent because they are lined by an external type of epithelium that may have goblet cells. They may be congenital or caused by implantation of corneal or conjunctival epithelium from surgery or trauma. Clinical findings may include pupillary distortion, iridocyclitis, and glaucoma. Cysts may enlarge and eventually fill the anterior chamber, with potential loss of the eye. The rate of growth of these cysts is quite variable.

THERAPY

Ocular. Iris cysts induced by miotic therapy partially recede when miotics are discontinued. In the management of accommodative esotropia, these cysts reportedly can be minimized by the concomitant use of 2.5 per cent phenylephrine given intermittently.

Surgical. The management of implantation or embryonal epithelial cysts of the iris is in a large part dependent on their growth pattern. Some small cysts will remain stationary and asymptomatic; these should only be observed. Those with evidence of growth require therapy.

For cysts that involve the corneal or limbal stroma, chemical cauterization is indicated. Retrobulbar anesthesia* is used for adults and general anesthesia for children. High magnification with the surgical microscope is essential. A discission knife is used to make a track into the cyst. The knife is withdrawn, and a short, blunt-tipped 30-gauge needle attached to a 2 ml syringe containing 0.5 ml of 20 per cent trichloroacetic acid is introduced. The cyst is aspirated, and then, without withdrawal of the needle, the mixture of cyst fluid and trichloroacetic acid is carefully injected.

The clear walls of the cyst and the protein in the cyst fluid immediately turn white. The cyst contents are aspirated to collapse the cyst completely before the needle is withdrawn. Suction is maintained as the needle is withdrawn to avoid spread of the acid into the stromal tissue. Only a minimal coagulation of the conjunctiva occurs at the puncture site. Iris cysts not in contact with the wall of the eye cannot be injected safely, but simple surgical excision, performed the same way as an iridectomy, is curative.

Epithelial cysts may also be treated with xenon arc photocoagulation. Other methods advocated include extensive surgical procedures with iridocyclectomy and corneal or corneoscleral transplants, diathermy, electrolysis, cryotherapy, and argon laser coagulation of corneal cysts. X-ray irradiation has largely been abandoned.

Ocular or Periocular Manifestations

Lens: Cataract; subluxation (with pressure).
Pupil: Distortion; pigmented nodules.
Other: Corneal edema; decreased visual acuity; glaucoma; uveitis.

PRECAUTIONS

Therapy is not always indicated in the management of epithelial cysts of external origin; however, if one elects to observe these lesions, they must be seen at regular 6-month intervals because they may enlarge dramatically after a dormant period. After the decision to treat is made, one must treat aggressively and effectively. Incomplete management and disruption of the cyst wall can convert a localized epithelial cyst into a diffuse epithelial growth.

When injecting sclerosing fluids, such as 20 per cent trichloroacetic acid, one must take great care to inject only into the cyst and not into the cornea or conjunctiva, or an opacity and severe iritis will result. Inadvertent injection of trichloroacetic acid into the anterior chamber can cause irreversible corneal, iris, and lens damage. There are usually no adverse reactions after an initial 10-day period of mild iritis. In occasional instances, a second injection has been required 1 to 6 months later.

Photocoagulation also requires great care. Inadvertent "explosions" can rupture the cyst wall, converting the cyst into an epithelial downgrowth. Cataracts or corneal and iris changes may occur with improper use of this technique. Excessive treatment may require hospitalization because postoperatively a moderately severe plastic iritis may develop, sometimes with secondary glaucoma. Photocoagulation does cause shrinkage of the iris, resulting in a slightly updrawn pupil.

It should be explained to the patient before

initiating any form of therapy that multiple treatments may be necessary. These cysts may even reappear years after surgery, chemical cautery, or photocoagulation. Therefore, long-term follow-up is necessary.

COMMENTS

With renewed interest in extracapsular cataract extraction, an increased incidence of epithelial implantation or even downgrowths can be expected to result from accidental incarceration of the lens capsule in the limbal or corneal wound.

References

Duke-Elder S (ed): System of Ophthalmology. St. Louis, CV Mosby, 1964, Vol III, pp 603–606; 1966, Vol IX, pp 769–775.

Neumann GO, Rummelt V: Block excision of cystic and diffuse epithelial ingrowth of the anterior chamber. Arch Ophthalmol 110:223–227, 1992.

Rosenquist RC, Fraunfelder FT, Swan KC: Treatment of conjunctival epithelial cysts with trichloracetic acid. J Ocul Ther Surg 4:51–55, 1985.

Scholtz RT, Kelley JS: Argon laser photocoagulation treatment of iris cysts following penetrating keratoplasty. Arch Ophthalmol 100:926–927, 1982.

Swan KC: Iris pigment nodules complicating miotic therapy. Am J Ophthalmol 37:886–889, 1954.

Swan KC: Epithelial cell cysts of the anterior chamber treated by acid injections. Doc Ophthalmol 18:363–370, 1979.

IRIS MELANOMA 190.0

H. JOHN SHAMMAS, M.D.

Los Angeles, California

It is generally agreed that iris melanomas are relatively benign. However, when a pigmented iris lesion is noted on slit-lamp examination, it should be documented with photographs and observed at regular intervals for evidence of growth. Signs of active growth include an increase in size, new vessel formation, implantation growths, pupil distortion, and ectropion uvea. Spontaneous hyphema and secondary glaucoma occasionally complicate the course of highly vascularized melanomas. Iris melanomas grow either into the anterior chamber or along the iris surface, ultimately invading the angle and ciliary body. The iris pigment epithelium seems to be a barrier to the invasion of the posterior chamber. Diffuse iris melanomas are the result of widely scattered areas of neoplasia.

Extension of the iris melanoma into the ciliary body carries a more severe prognosis. The extension is usually not recognized early, and as a consequence, the ciliary body tumor may become quite large before it is diagnosed. The tumor's thickness can be accurately measured by ultrasonography using standardized A-scan techniques.

THERAPY

Supportive. A conservative approach is recommended at the time of initial diagnosis until definite evidence of growth is established. Iris melanomas can be followed for long periods of time because of their benign nature. Small pigmented iris tumors are initially checked every 3 months, and if there is no evidence of growth after a year, the interval can be extended to 4 or 6 months. Large iris tumors are followed at a much shorter interval, especially if they are complicated by iris neovascularization and/or secondary glaucoma.

Surgical. The surgical therapy includes iridectomy, iridocyclectomy, and enucleation depending on the tumor's size and location. Surgery should only be considered when active signs of growth are documented over short follow-up periods.

An excisional iridectomy is indicated for melanomas localized to the iris. The specimen should be pinned to a flat surface and the borders identified so that the limits of the lesion can be determined. Measures should be taken to prevent the tissue from curling and wrinkling, which may distort the histologic findings. If there is residual tumor, it would seem safe to leave the eye alone until regrowth is evident, especially if the tumor is histologically benign.

If an iris melanoma has extended into the ciliary body, an iridocyclectomy can be performed. Good results can be expected because iris melanomas are relatively benign. There are many ways of accomplishing an iridocyclectomy; however, an en bloc excision with preservation of the outer scleral layers seems to be the safest.

Enucleation is recommended for diffuse iris and ciliary body melanomas that cannot be managed by local excision and for incompletely excised tumors that are histologically malignant.

Ocular or Periocular Manifestations

Anterior Chamber: Depth variations; hyphema.

Iris: Chronic uveitis; ectropion uvea; freckles; heterochromia; pigmented mass.

Other: Decreased visual acuity, glaucoma; hypotension; prominent episcleral vessels; pupillary distortion; refractive disorders.

PRECAUTIONS

Melanomas have to be differentiated from benign iris lesions, such as nevi, freckles, or melanocytomas. When making the final diagnosis, one must remember that melanomas are rare in children and non-Caucasians. A complete physical examination and laboratory studies, such as blood counts, liver function tests, and radiologic studies, should be performed to make sure that the tumor is not a metastatic lesion to the iris.

Surgical therapy is not without its risks. Most iris melanocytic lesions do not enlarge and can be observed safely. If the lesion shows only slight growth on follow-up examinations, careful observation may be recommended, but if the lesion shows more pronounced and progressive growth, then complete excision is warranted. Complications of iridectomy include hyphema, cataract, wound dehiscence, and episcleral seeding of the tumor. Complications of iridocyclectomy include vitreous loss, cataract, high astigmatism, and incomplete excision.

Radiotherapy has no place in the treatment of iris melanomas. The cytology makes it unlikely that radiation would be effective. One case of successful laser treatment of a recurrent tapioca melanoma of the iris and ciliary body has been reported. Metastatic lesions from an iris melanoma are extremely rare. One case of hepatic metastasis has been reported to occur 17 years after enucleation of an eye harboring a diffuse iris melanoma.

COMMENTS

An accurate diagnosis and evidence of active growth should be established before any therapy is considered.

References

Arentsen JJ, Green WR: Melanoma of the iris: Report of 72 cases treated surgically. Ophthalmic Surg 6:23–37, 1975.
Dart JK, Marsh RJ, Garner A, Cooling RJ: Fluorescein angiography of anterior uveal melanocytic tumors. Br J Ophthalmol 72:326–336, 1988.
Demeler U: Fluorescence angiographical studies in the diagnosis and follow-up of tumors of the iris and ciliary body. Adv Ophthalmol 42:1–17, 1981.
Kersten RC, Tse DJ, Anderson R: Iris melanoma. Nevus or malignancy? Surv Ophthalmol 29:423–433, 1985.
Makley TA Jr: Management of melanomas of the anterior segment. Surv Ophthalmol 19:135–153, 1974.
Memmen JE, McLean IW: The long-term outcome of patients undergoing iridocyclectomy. Ophthalmology 93:429–432, 1990.
Rones B, Zimmerman LE: The prognosis factors in choroidal and ciliary body melanomas. Arch Ophthalmol 95:63–69, 1977.
Shields JA, Sanborn GE, Augsburger JJ: The differential diagnosis of malignant melanoma of the iris: A clinical study of 200 patients. Ophthalmology 90:716–720, 1983.
Shields JA, Shields CL: Hepatic metastases of diffuse iris melanoma 17 years after enucleation. Am J Ophthalmol 106:749–750, 1988.
Shields MB, Proia AD: Neovascular glaucoma associated with an iris melanoma. A clinicopathologic report. Arch Ophthalmol 105:672–674, 1987.
Sunba MSN, Rahi AHS, Morgan G: Tumors of the anterior uvea. I. Metastasizing malignant melanoma of the iris. Arch Ophthalmol 98:82–85, 1980.
Territo C, Shields CL, Shields JA, Augsburger JJ, Schroeder RP: Natural course of melanocytic tumors of the iris. Ophthalmology 95:1251–1255, 1988.
Wilson RS, Fraunfelder FT, Hanna C: Recurrent tapioca melanoma of the iris and ciliary body treated with the argon laser. Am J Ophthalmol 82:213–217, 1976.

IRIS PROLAPSE 364.8

DAVID LITOFF, M.D.

Greenwich, Connecticut

Iris prolapse is an uncommon complication of cataract surgery. It can also occur after glaucoma surgery or corneal transplantation or as a result of an acute degenerative process, infection, or injury. With placoemulsification and small incision cataract surgery, iris prolapse is becoming increasingly rare.

Iris prolapse is usually a manifestation of wound failure. Most commonly it occurs in the immediate postoperative period; however, a delayed form can occur weeks or months after surgery. The delayed form of iris prolapse is often incomplete, with the iris becoming incarcerated in the wound. In both forms, the pupil becomes distorted in a teardrop fashion with the point toward the site of iris prolapse. Usually, the prolapsed iris fills the wound gap and maintains a watertight seal; however, occasionally a filtering bleb or even a flat chamber can accompany iris prolapse.

The etiology of iris prolapse can be divided into two categories. The first form is due to inadequate wound closure with poor wound architecture or an insufficient number of sutures. The second form is due to a sudden rise in intraocular pressure resulting in a wound dehiscence and iris prolapse. This pressure increase can be caused by eye rubbing, coughing, vomiting, wheezing, or pupillary block. Iris prolapse is a serious complication and can cause endophthalmitis, hypotony, cystoid macular edema, epithelial downgrowth, fibrous downgrowth, uveitis, and increased against-the-rule astigmatism. To prevent iris prolapse, careful attention to wound closure is extremely important. Postoperatively, an eye shield can prevent inadvertent trauma in the early postoperative period.

THERAPY

Ocular. The treatment of iris prolapse depends on its etiology, size, and duration. In the immediate postoperative period, a small iris prolapse can be treated with maximal ocular hypotension with a strong miotic. Although this is rarely successful, it should be attempted because it can avoid a return to the operating room.

Surgical. If medical treatment is unsuccessful, surgery is needed to reposit the iris. If the eye is very inflamed, general anesthesia is preferable. A stab incision can be made 45 degrees from the edge of the prolapse at the limbus. After injection of a small amount of a viscoelastic, acetylcholine is injected into the anterior chamber. Next, a cyclodialysis spatula can be used to sweep the iris back into position. An alternative method involves pushing the iris directly back into the wound with an iris spatula. If no peripheral iridectomy is present, one should be considered. The viscoelastic should be removed from the eye and the wound then closed with additional sutures. If the iris prolapse is large and over 96 hours old, it is better to excise the prolapsed iris. The late occurrence of an iris prolapse that is small and covered with conjunctiva can often be observed without treatment.

Other methods that have been reported for the treatment of iris prolapse include photocoagulation, cryotherapy, and cauterization with trichloroacetic acid or silver nitrate. These methods do not yield consistently good results and may create more inflammation or worsening of the iris prolapse.

References

Duke-Elder S (ed): System of Ophthalmology. St. Louis, CV Mosby, 1965, Vol VIII, pp 635–636.

Jaffe NS, Jaffe MS, Jaffe GF: Cataract Surgery and Its Complications. 5th ed. St. Louis, CV Mosby, 1990, pp 577–581.

Wand M, Olive GM, Mangiaracine AB: Corneal perforation and iris prolapse due to mima polymorpha. Arch Ophthalmol 93:239–241, 1975.

PARS PLANITIS 363.21

(Angiohyalitis, Chronic Cyclitis, Cyclitis, Peripheral Uveitis, Peripheral Uveoretinitis, Vitreitis)

DANIEL H. SPITZBERG, M.D., F.A.C.S.

Indianapolis, Indiana

Pars planitis is a common inflammation seen in young adults. Most cases last for decades and are usually bilateral. The minimum criterion for diagnosis is the presence of a snowbank or at least a few snowballs in the peripheral inferior retina. The cause of pars planitis is unknown. The most important guide for therapy is the degree of cystoid macular edema, and the most important feature for diagnosis is the snowbank. Pars planitis is the most commonly overdiagnosed uveitis syndrome. Ophthalmologists often make the diagnosis apparently because of cystoid macular edema; however, such macular edema is common in many different types of uveitis and is of therapeutic but not diagnostic interest.

THERAPY

Ocular. The goal of therapy is not to eradicate all signs and symptoms but to reduce the inflammation so that hypotony, cystoid macular degeneration, vitreous traction, retinal detachment, and cyclitis membrane formation will not significantly reduce visual acuity. If the disease is unilateral or asymmetric or if the patient does not tolerate systemic corticosteroids, periocular injections of methylprednisolone* may be necessary. A topical local anesthetic should be applied at least five times over the area to be injected. The head should be tilted so that gravity will pull the anesthetic into the cul-de-sac. An injectable anesthetic is neither necessary nor advisable. A 2-ml syringe is used to inject 0.5 ml of the 80 mg/ml concentration of methylprednisolone. The easiest place to make the injection is inferotemporally. The point of the needle should be placed 3 to 4 mm in front of the cul-de-sac and between blood vessels. It should be pushed into the hilt, *following the curve* of the sclera by the use of lateral motion of the needle over an area of 5 mm. This is a most valuable maneuver, since it allows one to hug the sclera as the needle goes in. The barrel of the syringe must be moved a large distance as one goes around the eyeball in order to keep the needle point near the eye. Keeping the needle near the eye with the aperture facing the sclera reduces the patient's discomfort and increases the penetration of the steroid because it keeps the medication closer to the sclera and not out in the orbital tissues. This lateral motion also avoids impaling the eyeball, since the ophthalmologist will immediately be aware that the sclera has been engaged if such a movement is used. By putting the injection far back, the side effects of chemosis and ptosis are decreased and the white material is not visible. If repeated injections are necessary, the superotemporal quadrant is usually varied with the inferotemporal. If a patient develops an allergy to methylprednisolone, the diagnosis should be confirmed by 0.01 ml injected intradermally and read at 2 days, and the patient should be switched to another agent, such as triamcinolone (40 mg/ml).

These periocular injections may be given

from every 2 to 16 weeks, depending on the patient's needs. At the beginning of treatment they should be given every 2 weeks until the patient's vision reaches a maximum level, and then they should be tapered to the minimal amount necessary to maintain the vision at the desired level. Since the disease lasts for decades, one should hesitate to stop medication completely, unless one can taper down to nothing without a relapse in vision. Additional topical corticosteroids or a mydriatic may not be necessary because the anterior chamber reaction is usually mild.

Systemic. Since the disease is usually bilateral and the process is extremely chronic, the systemic use of corticosteroids on an alternate-day regimen is recommended. Fifty to 100 mg of prednisone may be given every other day after breakfast, and the dosage should be adjusted depending on the therapeutic response, as well as the ocular and systemic complications of such therapy. Steroid treatment should be continued as long as ocular and systemic complications are not serious, and alternate-day administration can be continued for decades in some patients. Stopping medication will cause the cystoid changes in the macula to return and the vision to decrease. The ophthalmologist should monitor the patient's vision and should document the degree of cystoid macular edema by fluorescein angiography.

When corticosteroids are not adequate, some authorities use immunosuppressive agents. Although immunosuppressive agents are effective, they are life threatening and should not be used for mild or unilateral cases.

Surgical. Another alternative if corticosteroids are ineffective is cryotherapy. Utilizing indirect ophthalmoscopy, cryotherapy should be administered using a nitrous oxide or carbon dioxide retinal probe over the uninvolved and surrounding areas. An iceball should cover the exudative focus and then be allowed to thaw. It is then immediately refrozen to the same extent. Uninvolved ciliary body and retina are treated one probe width beyond the recognizable inflammatory reaction. A single depot injection of corticosteroids* is given to minimize the inflammatory effects of the cryotherapy. Cryotherapy may need to be repeated in 3 to 4 months.

PRECAUTIONS

Immunosuppressive agents should be supervised by an oncologist, rheumatologist, hematologist, or any other expert in their use. They have an additive effect when used with corticosteroids and have the advantage of not causing glaucoma or posterior subcapsular cataracts.

COMMENTS

About 80 per cent of cases of pars planitis do not need treatment. The patient should be treated only for a definite decrease in vision caused by cystoid macular edema and should not be treated for floaters. The level at which therapy is begun varies from a vision of 20/25 to 20/40. Evidence of the deleterious effects of smoking and pars planitis has been shown, and it is recommended that smoking be discontinued.

References

Aaberg TM, Cesarz TJ, Flickinger RR Jr: Treatment of peripheral uveoretinitis by cryotherapy. Am J Ophthalmol 75:685–688, 1973.

Aaberg TM, Cesarz TJ, Flickinger RR Jr: Treatment of pars planitis. I. Cryotherapy. Surv Ophthalmol 22:120–125, 1977.

Buckley CE III, Gills JP Jr: Cyclophosphamide therapy of peripheral uveitis. Arch Intern Med 124:29–35, 1969.

Giles CL: The use of methotrexate in the treatment of uveitis. Univ Mich Med Cent J 35:30–31, 1969.

Henderly DE, Genstler AJ, Rao NA, Smith RE: Pars planitis. Trans Ophthalmol Soc UK 105:227–232, 1986.

Henderly DE, Haymond RS, Rao NA, Smith RE: The significance of the pars plana exudate in pars planitis. Am J Ophthalmol 103:669–671, 1987.

Lazar M, Weiner MJ, Leopold IH: Treatment of uveitis with methotrexate. Am J Ophthalmol 67:383–387, 1969.

Nussenblatt RB, Palestine AG, Chan CC: Cyclosporine therapy for uveitis: Long-term follow-up. J Ocul Pharmacol 1:369–382, 1985.

Schlaegel TF Jr: Recent advances in uveitis. Ann Ophthalmol 4:525–552, 1972.

Schlaegel TF Jr: Peripheral uveitis. JAMA 223:696, 1973.

Schlaegel TF Jr, Weber JC: Treatment for pars planitis. II. Corticosteroids. Surv Ophthalmol 22:120–130, 1977.

Wakefield D, Dunlop I, McCluskey PJ, Penny R: Uveitis: Aetiology and disease associations in an Australian population. Aust NZ J Ophthalmol 14:181–187, 1986.

Wong VG, Hersh EM: Methotrexate in the therapy of cyclitis. Trans Am Acad Ophthalmol Otolaryngol 69:279–293, 1965.

RUBEOSIS IRIDIS 364.42
(Neovascular Glaucoma)

JOHN R. SAMPLES, M.D.

Portland, Oregon

Rubeosis iridis is a condition in which the iris develops neovascularization, often starting along the pupillary margin and progressing across the root of the iris into the trabecular meshwork. It occurs as a complication of diseases in which there is retinal ischemia and is frequently associated with a severe form of secondary glaucoma, which has been termed neovascular glaucoma or rubeotic glaucoma.

The growth of new blood vessels is associated with a fibrovascular membrane growing on the anterior surface of the iris and into the anterior chamber angle. These vessels can spread rapidly to cover the iris and trabecular meshwork, ultimately leading to the development of peripheral and anterior synechiae and to closure of the anterior chamber angle. The peripheral anterior synechiae gradually coalesce to close the angle in a zipper-like fashion.

About one-third of patients with rubeosis iridis have diabetic retinopathy. Central retinal vein occlusion accounts for about 28 per cent of all cases of rubeosis iridis. Other causes include retinal detachment that may be chronic and may be associated with malignant melanoma. Uveitis can also cause the development of rubeosis iridis. End-stage glaucoma may result in rubeosis iridis, probably because of persistent elevated pressures leading to a central vein occlusion and its consequences. Carotid artery obstructive disease, retrolental fibroplasia, sickle cell anemia, intraocular tumors, and carotid cavernous fistulas may lead to the development of neovascular glaucoma.

Many of the conditions that cause rubeosis share an underlying development of retinal hypoxia. It seems likely that this hypoxia leads to a "cell signal" that stimulates the angiogenesis and proliferation of new blood vessels. Similar signals may be present in uveitis, and the generation of a neovascular stimulus through a peptide signal thus seems likely. If such a peptide signal does emanate from hypoxic retina, it would be expected that removal of either vitreous or lens would increase rubeosis iridis in eyes with diabetic retinopathy. This has proven to be the case and is evidence for a diffusable angiogenic factor.

There are several stages in the development of rubeosis. At first, the intraocular pressure is normal, unless other underlying or associated abnormalities of the trabecular meshwork are present. Slit-lamp biomicroscopy using high-level magnification reveals small dilated tufts of capillaries with randomly oriented vessels on the surface of the iris near the pupillary margin. These new vessels characteristically leak fluorescein. Neovascularization progresses from the pupillary margin toward the root of the iris. Initially, gonioscopy shows a normal, open anterior chamber angle, and later single vascular trunks are seen crossing and arborizing into the trabecular meshwork. In a subsequent phase, the rubeosis becomes more florid, and a fibrovascular membrane that covers the anterior chamber angle and anterior surface of the iris is appreciated. As the membrane contracts, iris pigment epithelium is everted through the pupil onto the surface of the iris, leading to ectropion uvea. Glaucoma occurs as a result of inflammatory reactions that take place in the eye, the development of subsequent hyphema, the covering of the fibrovascular membrane over the trabecular meshwork, and the development of peripheral anterior synechiae. It is important to distinguish between an open angle and an angle that is covered with synechiae; if the angle is open, there is still hope for achieving some regression of the vessels in the angle when panretinal photocoagulation is performed. In the final phase as the angle becomes completely closed, the glaucoma is quite severe, and surgical intervention is required to alleviate the pressure.

THERAPY

Ocular. The intraocular pressure should be lowered through the use of topical and systemic medications. It may be prudent to avoid miotics in these cases, since they may produce a forward shift of the lens-iris diaphragm. Initial therapy should include a topical ophthalmic beta blocker twice daily or 1 per cent epinephrine twice daily. The use of an adjunctive oral carbonic anhydrase inhibitor, such as acetazolamide, may be useful. Long-acting cycloplegics, such as 1 per cent atropine twice daily, as well as the use of the more potent topical ophthalmic steroids, are helpful in reducing pain and controlling the inflammatory response that is evident in the eye. Neovascular eyes that have reached an end stage and that are not candidates for surgical therapy require the use of chronic cycloplegics and steroids. Glycerol and mannitol, osmotic agents, can be used temporarily before surgery. Some workers have advocated radiation management in neovascular glaucoma, both for analgesia and to treat the underlying cause. Direct radiation is used, and the mechanism of action is unclear. This treatment is controversial.

Surgical. Surgical management depends on the phase at which the rubeosis is encountered. Eyes in the early phase of development of rubeosis do best with panretinal photocoagulation and carefully timed medical treatment of the glaucoma. In many instances, regression of vessels in the angle is observed after panretinal photocoagulation, and it is possible to forestall glaucoma surgery. In other instances when the pressure is quite elevated and the acuity of the eye remains at a level sufficient to retain vision, it is best to proceed with filtering surgery soon after panretinal photocoagulation. Panretinal photocoagulation inhibits the growth of rubeosis and permits the involution of active rubeosis, with subsequent improvement in outflow facility in the anterior segment. Panretinal photocoagulation is most effective when it is used prophylactically, as, for example, in a central retinal vein occlusion in which rubeosis is significantly correlated with the extent of retinal capillary nonperfusion. Fundus fluorescein angiography should be obtained whenever possible after a vein occlusion. When extensive retinal capillary nonperfusion is documented, prophylactic treatment is indicated. Because vitrectomy and lensectomy are frequently followed by the development of rubeosis, prophylactic panretinal photocoagulation after these procedures is indicated, particularly when peripupillary fluorescein leakage has been detected. In selected cases, panretinal photocoagulation may reverse intraocular pressure elevation in the early open-angle glaucoma stage of rubeosis iridis.

Goniophotocoagulation is the application of direct photocoagulation to angle vessels. It seems to be most effective for rubeosis in its earliest stages. When used and directed at the trunk vessels crossing the angle, it can provide an effective adjunct to the eventual development of intractable neovascular glaucoma. This procedure does not have any effect upon the subsequent development of rubeosis and is best regarded only as a supplement and not a replacement for a retinal ablative procedure.

Once extensive panretinal peripheral anterior synechiae or the development of a fibrovascular membrane has occurred in the angle, it is unlikely that goniophotocoagulation will have any beneficial effect upon intraocular pressure. Traditionally, filtering surgery in eyes with neovascular glaucoma has been regarded as rarely successful both because of a high risk of intraoperative bleeding and the postoperative progression of the fibrovascular membrane. However, when panretinal photocoagulation possibly combined with goniophotocoagulation is undertaken before filtration, a much more successful result may be obtained. Panretinal photocoagulation, topical steroids, cycloplegics, and the time for these measures to have an effect are important preoperative adjuncts to filtering surgery. In one report, adequate control was obtained in 67 per cent (16 of 24 eyes) after filtration surgery. In eyes that have not previously had conjunctival surgery, a trabeculectomy works well. The excised limbal block should be so anterior that one can perform a careful dissection of corneoscleral tissue away from peripheral anterior synechiae. The iris may then be inspected and surface vessels may be coagulated with a bipolar cautery as described by Herschler (1979). Krupin (1983) has reported good results with neovascular glaucoma patients with the implantation of setons. Preliminary results have been promising with the implantation of tubes and with the Molteno seton.

The adjunctive use of fluorouracil has substantially increased the chances of success in patients undergoing routine trabecular filtering surgery for neovascular glaucoma. A variety of treatment protocols have been proposed. Optimal parameters for the treatment with fluorouracil remain to be settled. At present 0.1 ml of a solution containing 50 mg/ml of fluorouracil* is recommended for subconjunctival injection at a variety of sites,

none of which is in the immediate vicinity of the filtering bleb.

A variety of cyclodestructive procedures have been advocated for some cases of neovascular glaucoma. They are usually more palliative than vision-maintaining. In addition to cyclocryotherapy, the use of both therapeutic ultrasound and of a YAG laser cyclodestructive procedure has been advocated. Since eyes with advanced rubeosis have minimal outflow, one must obliterate nearly the entire ciliary body in order to control intraocular pressure. Often, a cycloablative procedure will enable maintenance of a useful eye, staving off the need for enucleation. At present, such eyes treated with 180° of cyclocryotherapy use a 1-minute freeze at −80°C directly over the ciliary body, with a total of six applications throughout the 180°. If these fail to lower the pressure, treatment is repeated embracing 90° of previously treated ciliary body and 90° new areas.

Ocular or Periocular Manifestations

Iris: Neovascularization.
Trabecular Meshwork: Neovascularization; peripheral anterior synechiae; angle closure.

PRECAUTIONS

Rubeosis iridis and neovascular glaucoma develop rapidly after central retinal vein occlusion and vitrectomy. Vigilance is needed to detect these conditions early, since treatment and outcome are far better with earlier detection. Prophylactic treatment is a consideration when nonperfused ischemic areas of retina are detected on fluorescein angiogram.

COMMENTS

Diabetic eyes that develop neovascular glaucoma have often previously undergone vitrectomy and lensectomy, making them poor candidates for limbal filtration surgery. In some instances, a Molteno implant may be useful. Alternatively, cyclodestructive procedures should be considered. When the media are too hazy and a retinal photoablative procedure is needed, a panretinal cryoablation should be considered. Neovascular glaucoma associated with retinal detachment has been reported to be associated with the development of intravitreal neovascularization from ciliary body after cyclocryotherapy.

References

Allen RC, et al: Filtration surgery in the treatment of neovascular glaucoma. Ophthalmology 89: 1181–1187, 1982.

Ancker E, Molteno ACB: Molteno drainage implant for neovascular glaucoma. Trans Ophthalmol Soc UK 102:122–124, 1982.

Ehrenberg M, et al: Rubeosis iridis: Preoperative

iris fluorescein angiography and periocular steroids. Ophthalmology 91:321–325, 1984.

Goldberg MF, Erickson ES: Intravitreal ciliary body neovascularization. Ophthalmic Surg 8:62–70, 1977.

Herschler J, Agness D: A modified filtering procedure for neovascular glaucoma. Arch Ophthalmol 97:2339–2341, 1979.

Heuer DK, et al: 5-fluorouracil in glaucoma filtering surgery. Ophthalmology 91:384–393, 1984.

Krupin T, et al: Long-term results of valve implants in filtering surgery for eyes with neovascular glaucoma. Am J Ophthamol 95:775–782, 1983.

Priluch IA, Robertson DN, Hollinhorst RW: Long-term follow-up of occlusion in central retinal vein in young adults. Am J Ophthalmol 90:190–202, 1980.

Simmons RJ, Depperman SR, Dueker DK: The role of gonio-photocoagulation neovascularization of the anterior chamber angle. Ophthalmology 87:79–82, 1980.

Zegarra H, Gutman FA, Conforto J: The natural course of central retinal vein occlusion. Ophthalmology 86:1931–1939, 1979.

UVEITIS 364.3

JAMES T. ROSENBAUM, M.D.

Portland, Oregon

Many different processes, including infection, malignancy, and immune-mediated diseases, can result in inflammation of the uveal tract. These diseases can be categorized on the basis of the portion of the uveal tract that is affected. The size and distribution of keratic precipitates, the suddenness of onset, the duration of inflammation, and the association with various complications can also be helpful in categorizing uveal inflammation. The treatment of uveitis depends on the specific diagnosis (e.g., herpes simplex keratouveitis is obviously approached differently from phacolytic glaucoma), the duration and severity of the inflammation, the location of the inflammation, and the presence of potential complications.

In designing therapy for a patient with uveitis, one must first exclude an underlying infection or malignancy. Syphilis has protean ocular manifestations and must be excluded by an appropriate serologic study, such as a fluorescent treponemal antibody absorption test. Such diagnostic entities as toxoplasmosis, herpes zoster ophthalmicus, herpes simplex keratouveitis, toxocariasis, acute retinal necrosis (which is caused by viruses from the herpes family), and infection in the immunocompromised host must be recognized and treated with specific antimicrobial therapy. Malignancies, including melanoma, lymphoma, leukemia, and retinoblastoma, may masquerade as uveitis and fail to respond to anti-inflammatory drugs.

The systemic illnesses associated with uveitis include sarcoidosis, ankylosing spondylitis, Reiter's syndrome, juvenile-onset rheumatoid arthritis, inflammatory bowel disease, interstitial nephritis, Behçet's disease, Vogt-Koyanagi-Harada syndrome, Sjögren's syndrome, and multiple sclerosis. In most cases, a careful history should lead one to suspect a related systemic disease if it is present. Of course, some of the therapeutic options for the systemic illnesses (e.g., corticosteroids for sarcoidosis or surgery for refractory inflammatory bowel disease) influence the course of the eye disease.

THERAPY

Ocular. Therapy for an acute iritis or iridocyclitis should include both a topical corticosteroid and a mydriatic or cycloplegic. By relieving spasm of the ciliary muscles, a dilating drop reduces pain. In addition, it should prevent the complication of posterior synechiae. Choices include scopolamine (0.25 to 0.5 per cent), homatropine (2 to 5 per cent), cyclopentolate (0.5 to 2.0 per cent), and atropine (0.5 to 2 per cent). Tropicamide (1 per cent) is an alternative if the inflammation is mild. The dose of the dilating drop should be adequate to reduce pain and to produce dilation without maintaining the pupil constantly in a fully dilated position.

Topical corticosteroids include dexamethasone, hydrocortisone, prednisolone, and progesterone-like compounds, including fluorometholone and medrysone. One of these should be started as soon after the onset of inflammation as possible. Often, patients with recurrent iritis experience a prodromal illness before cell and flare are detected in the anterior chamber. The initiation of topical corticosteroids at this time is optimal. Generally, the drops are given as frequently as every hour until improvement begins. Dexamethasone ointment may be added at night. Although topical steroids do vary in their tendency to elevate intraocular pressure, the rise in pressure probably correlates with the potency of the anti-inflammatory effects. Thus, the progesterone-like compounds are less likely to elevate pressure, but are also less potent in controlling inflammation.

If topical therapy is not adequate, a periocular injection of corticosteroids is an alternative. Periocular injections are an excellent choice for therapy if the disease is unilateral or posterior to the lens or both. One study has suggested that a superior, posterior, sub-Tenon's capsule approach may be more effective than an inferior approach. Corticosteroid preparations available for periocular injection include dexamethasone*, methylprednisolone*, triamcinolone*, and betamethasone*. An injection of 1.0 ml of most commercial preparations can be repeated every 2 to 6 weeks in an effort to control inflammation.

The author's practice is to repeat the injection on at least one occasion before concluding that it is not effective because therapeutic benefit may vary depending on placement of the medication.

Systemic. Oral corticosteroids are indicated for intraocular inflammation that has not responded to topical or periocular medications and that is not secondary to infection or malignancy. The goal of therapy is usually not to eliminate inflammation but to reduce it to a level acceptable to the patient while using the lowest possible dose of potentially toxic medication. An amount comparable to 60 mg of prednisone taken in the morning as a single oral dose is frequently used to initiate therapy. Alternate-day therapy with corticosteroids is both less toxic and less efficacious. Dividing the daily dose is likely to increase benefit, but also to increase toxicity. The dose of corticosteroids should be adjusted based on the activity of the inflammation. The benefits of corticosteroids are balanced by their risks, which are proportionate to the dosage and duration of therapy.

Four weeks of moderately high doses of corticosteroids equivalent to 40 to 60 mg of prednisone daily are generally sufficient to determine if the medication is beneficial. Oral corticosteroids should not be discontinued abruptly. A tapering schedule should be used to discontinue corticosteroids, especially if the duration of therapy has been longer than 4 weeks. Pulse therapy with corticosteroids (as much as 1 gm of methylprednisolone daily, intravenously for 3 consecutive days) has been reported to benefit a limited number of patients who do not respond adequately to oral regimens.

Guidelines for the use of systemic immunosuppressive therapy have been suggested by the International Uveitis Study Group. These guidelines include bilateral disease, best corrected vision no better than 20/50, and failure either to respond or to tolerate oral corticosteroids. Drugs within this category include cyclosporine[‡] and cytotoxic medications, such as azathioprine[‡], chlorambucil[‡], cyclophosphamide[‡], and methotrexate[‡]. Cyclosporine at a daily dose of 2.5 to 10 mg/kg orally has resulted in improved visual acuity in many patients who have not improved with corticosteroids. However, this dose is frequently associated with nephrotoxicity. Other problems associated with cyclosporine include hepatotoxicity, hirsutism, hypertension, gingivitis, malaise, and lymphoid malignancy. The cytotoxic drugs are all associated with cytopenias. All of these immunosuppressive agents predispose to the development of opportunistic infections.

The benefit of either oral or topical nonsteroidal anti-inflammatory drugs, such as indomethacin[‡] or flurbiprofen[‡], has not been established in uveitis. Since multiple mediators undoubtedly contribute to the process of inflammation, future pharmacologic modalities may inhibit such phlogistic substances as oxygen radicals, platelet-activating factor, interleukin-1, or neuropeptides.

PRECAUTIONS

Ocular toxicity from oral, periocular, or topical corticosteroids includes posterior subcapsular cataract, raised intraocular pressure, and reduced response to infection.

An inadvertent intraocular injection of corticosteroids will normally result in permanent visual loss. Other potential hazards of periocular injections include pain or discomfort, ptosis, hemorrhage, infection, fat atrophy, and an allergic reaction to the drug vehicle. Depot injections of corticosteroids may occasionally need to be removed in order to control intraocular pressure.

The adverse reactions from oral corticosteroids include personality changes, such as mania, psychosis, or sleep disturbance; weight gain and fat redistribution; adrenal suppression; acne; osteoporosis; avascular necrosis; immunosuppression, including reduced fever and pain from an infection, such as appendicitis; diabetes; easy bruisability; poor healing; menstrual irregularity; peptic ulcer disease; and reactivation of latent infection.

COMMENTS

The complications from uveitis may include cystoid macular edema, synechiae, band keratopathy, cataract, glaucoma, neovascularization, and retinal detachment. If therapy for the underlying inflammation cannot control or prevent a complication, the complication must obviously be addressed separately if appropriate. Band keratopathy, for example, may require chelation therapy or even corneal transplantation. Vitrectomy is an option for severe vitreous opacification that has failed anti-inflammatory therapy. Vitrectomy, however, may worsen underlying cystoid macular edema if present. Cryotherapy is sometimes used for localized therapy of pars plana exudates. It may, however, increase the risk of retinal detachment. Cataract surgery should optimally be performed in an eye with minimal active inflammation.

References

Andrasch RH, Pirofsky B, Burns RP: Immunosuppressive therapy for severe chronic uveitis. Arch Ophthalmol 96:247–251, 1978.

Nussenblatt RB, Palestine AG, Chan CC: Cyclosporin A therapy in treatment of intraocular inflammatory disease resistant to systemic corticosteroids and cytotoxic agents. Am J Ophthalmol 96P:275–282, 1983

Nussenblatt RB, Palestine AG, Chan CC, et al: Randomized, double-masked study of cyclosporine compared to prednisolone in the treatment of endogenous uveitis. Am J Ophthalmol 112:1348, 1991.

Rosenbaum JT: Immunosuppressive therapy of uveitis. Ophthalmol Clin North Am (in press).

Rubin RM, Samples JR, Rosenbaum JT: Prostaglandin-independent inhibition of ocular vascular permeability by a platelet-activating factor antagonist. Arch Ophthalmol 106:1116–1120, 1988.

Smith RE, Nozik RA: The nonspecific treatment of uveitis. In Uveitis. A Clinical Approach to Diagnosis and Management. Baltimore, Williams & Wilkins, 1989, pp 51–76.

SECTION 27

LACRIMAL SYSTEM

ALACRIMA 375.5

DAVID E. COWEN, M.D.,
and JEFFREY J. HURWITZ, M.D.,
F.R.C.S.(C)

Toronto, Ontario, Canada

Alacrima refers to a spectrum of congenital lacrimal secretory disorders ranging from complete absence of tears to hyposecretion to a rare condition wherein there is a selective absence of tearing in response to emotional stimulation with a normal secretory response to mechanical stimulation. Suggested etiologic mechanisms have included; nuclear aplasia, failure of central nervous system connections, aplasia or hypoplasia of the lacrimal gland and disturbance or failure of peripheral neural connections.

Systemic associations of alacrima are well known and described. The Riley-Day Syndrome (RDS, familial dysautonomia), anhidrotic ectodermal dysplasia (AED), Sjögren's syndrome, and Allgrove's or the Triple A syndrome (3A syndrome) consisting of achalasia, alacrima and ACTH insensitivity and its variants, all have a component of alacrima. It is known to occur in association with other congenital abnormalities including palsies of the fifth, sixth, seventh, eighth, or twelfth cranial nerves. Inheritance patterns of autosomal recessive and dominant have been recorded.

Isolated congenital alacrima is exceedingly rare although at least two case reports have been recorded. The inheritance pattern appears to be autosomal dominant in these cases. Distinguishing isolated inherited congenital alacrima requires knowledge of the other systemic processes in which it might be found as well as the pattern of inheritance in the family of the patient. AED can be ruled out by the absence of the following: absent or decreased sweating and salivation, intolerance to heat, hypotrichosis, total or partial anodontia, prematurely aged skin, and sex-linked recessive inheritance. RDS can be eliminated by its autosomal recessive inheritance and almost exclusive restriction to people of Jewish descent. Furthermore, tear production in response to systemic administration of neostigmine bromide and edrophonium chloride is not evident in inherited congenital alacrima. Sjögren's syndrome rarely has an hereditary component and is associated with xerostomia, salivary gland enlargement, and collagen diseases, findings which are not seen in isolated alacrima.

Characteristically, these children have a history of absent tears when crying. It is not uncommon for children with alacrima to be asymptomatic and comfortable. Conversely, irritative symptoms with photophobia, foreign body sensation and hyperemia may be present. Patients with these symptoms may have a very low to absent Schirmer's test, evidence of superficial punctate epithelial defects (SPK) with fluorescein staining on slit lamp exam, and a thick mucoid discharge. Normal lacrimation with its attendant dilutional and antimicrobial activity is decreased resulting in frequent blepharoconjunctivitis. Histopathologic examination reveals hydropic degeneration of the conjunctival epithelium similar to keratoconjunctivitis sicca. Most cases are bilateral although a unilateral case associated with facial hypoplasia has been reported.

THERAPY

Ocular. Symptomatic cases may be managed with artificial tears used as frequently as necessary to relieve ocular irritation. Petrolatum ointment (Lacrilube etc.) may be used at night. Attention should be paid to possible allergic responses to preservatives. More severe cases may be treated with more viscous methylcellulose preparations. Progressive symptoms may require the use of sustained release ocular inserts.

Blepharoconjunctivitis may be treated with hot compresses and the addition of antibiotic drops and/or ointments.

Selected cases of keratoconjunctivitis sicca, especially with recurrent corneal erosion or ulceration, may be helped by the use of therapeutic contact lenses with aggressive topical lubrication and antibiotics as indicated. Moisture chambers at night may be attempted although compliance in children is poor. A trial of temporary punctal plugs should be attempted when conservative, topical therapy does not relieve the symptoms. If symptoms improve, surgical options should be considered.

Surgical. In severe cases, not relieved by conservative measures, punctal occlusion should be attempted. Inferior puncta followed by superior puncta, if indicated, may be occluded by thermal, electrical or laser methods.

Continued symptoms and evidence of corneal compromise should then be addressed by permanent tarsorrhaphy.

Systemic. Cases of autonomic dysfunction have been treated with subcutaneous injections of 0.25 mg of neostigmine or 3.0 mg of methacholine. Neurologic consultation should accompany such treatment.

Ocular or Periocular Manifestations

Conjunctiva: Hyperemia, thick mucoid discharge.

Cornea: Hypesthesia (associated with RDS); interstitial keratitis; pannus, subepithelial opacity; superficial punctate keratoconjunctivitis; ulcer.

Extraocular Muscles: Paralysis of V, VI, or VII cranial nerves.

Eyelids: Chronic or recurrent blepharoconjunctivitis.

Other: Decreased tear secretion; decreased vision; irritation; photophobia; foreign body sensation.

PRECAUTIONS

Sensitization to any of the commercially available ocular lubricants or inserts may occur. In addition, ocular inserts may cause blurring of vision during the last few hours of effectiveness. Close observation of the status of the cornea monitoring for development of corneal ulceration.

COMMENTS

Alacrima should be considered in the differential diagnosis of red irritable eyes in young children, even without a definite history by the parents. Knowledge of other possible systemic findings may aid in diagnosis and possible treatment (RDS, AED, Sjögren's)

Long-term follow-up is necessary even in asymptomatic cases in light of the possibility of the development of keratoconjunctivitis sicca.

References

Beard C: Abnormalities of eyelids, lacrimal system, and orbit. *In* Congenital Anomalies of the Eye. Transactions of the New Orleans Academy of Ophthalmology, St. Louis, CV Mosby, 1968, p 411.

Coverdale H: Some unusual cases of Sjögren's syndrome. Br J Ophthalmol 32:669, 1948.

Davidoff E, Friedman AH: Congenital alacrima. Surv Ophthalmol 22:113, 1977.

Duke-Elder S (ed): System of Ophthalmology. St. Louis, CV Mosby, 1963, Vol. III, pp 913–917.

Kruger KE: Congenital absence of lacrimation in a family. Klin Monatsbl Augenheilk 124: 711, 1954.

Lisch K: Uber hereditares vorkommen des mit keratoconjunctivitis sicca verbunden Sjögren schen sumptomen komplexes. Arch Augenheilkd 110: 357, 1937.

Mondino BJ, Brown SI: Hereditary congenital alacrima. Arch Ophthalmol 94:1478, 1976.

Riley CM: Familial autonomic dysfunction. JAMA 149:1532, 1952.

Sjögren H, Eriksen A: Alacrimia congenita. Br J Ophthal 34:691, 1950.

Thurnam J: Two cases in which the skin, hair and teeth were very imperfectly developed. Med Chir Trans 31:71, 1848.

CONGENITAL ANOMALIES OF THE LACRIMAL SYSTEM 743.65
(Anlage Duct, Closed Nasolacrimal Duct)

JOHN L. WOBIG, M.D.

Portland, Oregon

Congenital anomalies of the lacrimal system may include an absence of one or more canaliculi, multiple puncta, or anomalies of the nasolacrimal duct. The duct that ends at or near the vault of the inferior meatus and fails to perforate the nasal mucosa is by far the most common variation; however, there are large varieties of obstructions and abnormalities of the nasolacrimal outflow system. Congenital anomalies of the motor mechanism occasionally occur even when the lacrimal passages are normal. There may be paralysis of the entire orbicularis oculi muscle or only of the medial ends of the pretarsal and preseptal muscle fibers. Congenital dacryocystocele, also known as congenital mucocele or amniotocele, is identified by a blue-gray cystic swelling below the medial canthus. Associated with a dacryocystocele can be a cystic nasal distention of the nasolacrimal duct. The infant can have respiratory distress and will need probing and puncture of the nasolacrimal cyst. The lacrimal anlage duct anomaly occurs when the rod of cells that extends from the posterior surface of the anlage to the deeper part of the lacrimal fossa to become the origin of the tear sac proliferates and canalizes instead of degenerating. It may occur bilaterally and be inherited as an autosomal dominant trait.

THERAPY

Ocular. If inflammation is present, systemic and topical ophthalmic antibiotics may be indicated. In addition, a decongestant medication in an aqueous vehicle should be prescribed for local conjunctival use. If the inflammation is not acute, the parents should be taught to exert pressure over the top of the tear sac four or more times a day for 1 to 2 weeks.

Surgical. Unless the epiphora has subsided completely within 2 weeks, probing under local anesthesia should be considered for children under 6 months of age. A probe that will slide through the canaliculus without resistance must be chosen. A dark line should be marked at 12 mm and another at 20 mm from the tip of the silver probe by applying tincture of iodine with a toothpick. The probe should then be passed vertically through the lower punctum and then horizontally through the canaliculus, with the convex side of the curve inferiorly. As soon as the sac is entered, the probe should again be held vertically, with the convexity turned medially. If the probe stops at the 12 mm mark and on manipulation no passage beyond is found, probing should stop there. Probably there is no nasolacrimal canal and therefore no duct. These patients should have a dacryocystorhinostomy between 6 and 12 months of age, depending on the severity of the discharge and infection. If the probe passes down to the 20-mm mark, the probe is at the level of the inferior meatus. The probe should then be passed to the obstructed end of the duct and turned, with the convex side laterally. The probe, which should be against the mucosal side of the wall, should be given a quick, sharp push. Before withdrawing the probe, a metal instrument, such as another probe, should be passed into the inferior meatus of the nose so that a "metal-to-metal" touch will prove that the tip of the first probe is in the nasal cavity.

Inferior turbinotomy under general anesthesia should be performed on all recurrent cases. When probing fails to penetrate the nasal mucosa, the surgeon should try to impale the probe between the bone and the tip of a Freer elevator, which is passed into the inferior meatus with the curved edge toward the lateral wall about 20 mm from the entrance of the nares. The sharp edge of the elevator is then moved up and down the probe, cutting and scraping through the overlying mucosa until metallic contact is made. If it does not locate the probe laterally, the elevator should be turned over and a search made for the probe on the wall of the inferior turbinate. If the mucosa of the inferior turbinate cannot be opened over the probe, a turbinate punch should be used to remove that part of the obstructing tissue. The turbinate is then infractured.

Lacrimal amniotoceles may be treated conservatively as long as there is no sign of infection. If necessary, the nasolacrimal duct may be probed and opened.

The technique for excision of the anlage duct, performed under local anesthesia, should include an injection of two or three drops of 2 per cent methylene blue into the duct. A probe should be passed in far enough to give the direction of the duct. An incision should be made only through the skin in line with the duct. The duct is then freed by blunt dissection, keeping the probe in place. When the medial canthal tendon is reached, the duct should be ligated and excised and the skin closed with interrupted sutures.

Ocular or Periocular Manifestations

Lacrimal System: Atresia; dacryoadenitis; dacryocystitis; displacement of punctum; ectasia of lacrimal passage; ectropion of punctum; epiphora; fistula; occlusion of nasolacrimal duct or canaliculi; supernumerary puncti.
Other: Paralysis of seventh nerve.

PRECAUTIONS

With the possible exception of newborn infants, there seems to be no age limit for the treatment of these anomalies. The canalicular epithelium should always be handled carefully to produce minimal trauma during manipulations. Except at the point of obstruction in the inferior meatus of the nose, the use of force during probing is contraindicated.

The earlier the obstruction is removed, the higher is the incidence of cure. This is because the vigor and growth of the lacrimal epithelium are probably greatest at birth. The more chronic the infection and the greater the fibrotic and inflammatory changes, the more difficult it is to prevent recurrence. Dilation of the punctum should not be done with a Ziegler-type dilator, as it often causes a tear.

COMMENTS

Anomalies involving the excretory lacrimal system are much more common congenitally than are secretory anomalies. Rarely, an anomalous lacrimal secretory duct is found opening on the cutaneous surface of the upper eyelid. A secretory duct is sometimes diverted into a bulbar conjunctival nevus or dermoid. Although fistulas of the lacrimal ducts are usually acquired, they may also develop congenitally and can be excised.

In about 30 per cent of newborn infants, the duct is still closed. Apparently, the last barrier to canalization is the fibrous layer of the nasal mucoperiosteum. This should be considered a normal event, unless it fails to open within the first 2 or 3 postpartum weeks.

References

Beard C: Congenital and hereditary abnormalities of the eyelids, lacrimal system, and orbit. *In* Beard C, et al (eds): Symposium on Surgical and Medical Management of Congenital Anomalies of the Eye. St. Louis, CV Mosby, 1968, pp 411–415.

Caputo AR, et al: Definitive treatment of congenital lacrimal sac fistula. Arch Ophthalmol *96*:1443–1444, 1978.

Frankel CA: The treatment of dacryostenosis (Letter). JAMA *260*:2666, 1988.

Jones LT, Wobig JL: Surgery of the Eyelids and Lacrimal System. Birmingham, Aesculapius, 1976, pp 157–173.

Lipton J, Jacobs N, Rosen ES: Bilateral acute dacryocystitis in an infant. Br J Hosp Med 38:251, 1987.

DACRYOADENITIS 375.00

JOHN L. WOBIG, M.D.

Portland, Oregon

Dacryoadenitis is an inflammatory enlargement of the lacrimal gland caused by infection, granulomatous disease of unknown cause, or a benign lymphoepithelial lesion. Acute dacryoadenitis may affect either the palpebral or orbital lobe of the gland separately or together. Acute palpebral dacryoadenitis usually presents as orbital pain followed by edema of the upper lid, which results in an S-shaped curved lid deformity and a preauricular lymph node. Palpation of the lid shows a tender nut-shaped swelling continuous with neither the orbit nor the ciliary margin. The conjunctiva may be injected and chemotic, sometimes with mucus discharge. The disease may run a brief course and then resolve, or it may progress to suppuration. Acute orbital dacryoadenitis is rarer than the palpebral form and presents with the same, although accentuated, symptoms. In addition, there is usually some proptosis as a result of the swelling extending under the orbital rim. There may be some limitation of ocular mobility with diplopia, and sometimes there is a convergent squint. Chronic dacryoadenitis usually presents as a painless swelling in the upper and outer part of the lid, accompanied by ptosis. A hard mass is palpable under the upper and outer rim of the orbit. Displacement of the globe downward and inward occurs with diplopia on looking up and out, but proptosis is rare.

THERAPY

Supportive. The therapy of dacryoadenitis is determined by the etiology. For dacryoadenitis that is a complication of systemic disease, therapy should be directed toward the overall treatment of the generalized disorder. Dacryoadenitis that is a complication of a viral disease (most commonly mumps) should be treated symptomatically. Local application of heat or cold offers some relief. Bedrest and salicylates are suggested. Dacryoadenitis secondary to sarcoidosis should be treated by systemic corticosteroids.

If the causative organism can be identified in a bacterial infection of the lacrimal gland, appropriate antibiotic therapy should be given. Hot packs followed by symptomatic therapy may give some relief.

Ocular. If discharge is present, lavage of the conjunctival sac is indicated. If lacrimal function is not adequate, replacement therapy with tear substitutes should be instituted.

Surgical. If suppuration occurs, early incision is indicated. This should be done through the conjunctiva if the palpebral lobe is involved or through the skin if the orbital lobe is affected.

Ocular or Periocular Manifestations

Conjunctiva: Chemosis; fistula; hyperemia; mucous discharge.
Eyelids: Edema; erythema; ptosis.
Globe: Proptosis.
Lacrimal System: Edema; inflammation; suppuration.
Other: Convergent squint; diplopia; ocular pain; preauricular lymphadenopathy.

PRECAUTIONS

An acute palpebral dacryoadenitis may suggest a chalazion or hordeolum. Eversion of the lid will rule out these diagnoses. Tenderness and swelling of the gland and localized chemosis are also characteristic features. Acute orbital dacryoadenitis may present a general picture suggesting orbital cellulitis.

COMMENTS

It is generally believed that lacrimal gland enlargements are caused by tumors or inflammations, with inflammations representing the more frequent cause. Among granulomatous diseases resulting in lacrimal gland inflammation, sarcoidosis and Sjögren's syndrome are the most prominent. The lacrimal gland may also experience chronic inflammation and ultimately fibrosis as sequelae to radiation or loss of innervation. However, lacrimal gland enlargement may be due to causes other than inflammation. Nutritional deficiencies, alcoholism, diabetes, tumors, and use of certain drugs may cause enlargement of the lacrimal gland. The infrequency of reported cases of dacryoadenitis reflects the fact that the lacrimal gland is housed in a bony cavity that is not regularly palpated and can conceal moderate enlargement.

References

Duke-Elder S (ed): System of Ophthalmology. St. Louis, CV Mosby, 1974, Vol VIII, pp 601–622.

Jakobiec FA, Jones IS: Orbital inflammations. In Duane TD (ed): Clinical Ophthalmology. Hagerstown, MD, Harper & Row, 1982, Vol II, 35: pp 64–69.

Jakobiec FA, Gess L, Zimmerman LE: Granulomatous dacryoadenitis caused by Schistosoma haematobium. Arch Ophthalmol 95:278–280, 1977.

DACRYOCYSTITIS 375.30

ROGER A. DAILEY, M.D.

Portland, Oregon

Dacryocystitis refers to an inflammation of the lacrimal sac. It occurs primarily because of nasolacrimal duct obstruction that was either present at birth (congenital) or acquired. Secondary dacryocystitis can be caused by the spread of infection from the nose or paranasal sinuses, trauma, or in association with some systemic disorder, such as tuberculosis, syphilis, or Hansen's disease (leprosy).

The incidence of congenital obstruction of the nasolacrimal duct in newborn infants is approximately 2 to 6 per cent. It occurs bilaterally in one-third of these cases. The formation of the lacrimal outflow system relies on canalization of an epithelial cord formed by invagination of surface ectoderm over the naso-optic fissure. Canalization occurs in a segmented fashion, which is normally completed by the time of birth or shortly thereafter. Although this canalization may fail at any point, it usually does so at the lower end, leaving an imperforate membrane where the ostium of the duct into the inferior meatus of the nose should be. Bony obstruction of the nasolacrimal duct can also occur.

Rarely, an infant will be born with an amniotocele. This markedly distended lacrimal sac appears as a bluish swelling below the medial canthal tendon and can be mistaken for a hemangioma. Alleyways are sterile initially but, if unresolved, can develop a secondary dacryocystitis.

Typically, infants with obstruction of the nasolacrimal duct have a history of epiphora and chronic blepharoconjunctivitis. The sac will swell if it is unable to decompress either spontaneously or with external massage.

The majority of cases of dacryocystitis are acquired, and the infection begins in the lacrimal system. Despite a protective mucosal barrier of stratified columnar epithelium and the bacteriostatic action of tear lysozymes, any stasis with accumulation of tear-sac products because of partial or complete obstruction of the nasolacrimal duct will predispose the lacrimal system to infection. Idiopathic acquired closure usually occurs in middle-aged adults with a 3:1 preponderance among females. It is rare among African-Americans. A heredofamilial tendency has been noted in some cases.

There are many known causes of acquired nasolacrimal duct obstruction. Intermittent or partial obstruction can be caused by dacryolith in 15 per cent of cases. Obstruction can occur in association with mycotic infections with fungi, such as *Actinomyces israelii*. Many types of tumors can occur in the nasolacrimal duct or lacrimal sac. Most of these are primary tumors of epithelial origin, such as papillomas, adenomas, and carcinomas. Secondary tumors from the sinus, nose, and orbit have been reported. Metastatic disease is very rare. Both dacryoliths and tumors can be associated with bloody tears. Patients with a tumor typically have a dacryocystitis associated with irreducible mass. Jones testing reveals a partial obstruction with an excretory system that is patent to irrigation.

THERAPY

Ocular. During the first few weeks of life, the majority of cases of nasolacrimal duct obstruction resolve spontaneously. In the absence of spontaneous resolution, the parents are instructed to massage over the lacrimal sac in such a way as to obstruct the canaliculi and increase the hydrostatic pressure in the lacrimal sac. Occasionally, parents will report a "popping" sensation, which is followed by resolution of the epiphora. In those patients with mucopurulent discharge, parents are instructed to use an antibiotic solution. In some series, over 90 per cent of infants cleared by 1 year of age.

Acquired dacryocystitis is initially treated with topical antibiotic or antibiotic-steroid solutions for 2 weeks. Warm compresses over the lacrimal sac are also helpful. Probing and irrigation of the canaliculi and lacrimal excretory system in the office can help, but it is not definitive treatment.

Acute dacryocystitis is exquisitely painful for the patient. An attempt should be made to decompress the sac when the patient is first seen to relieve the pressure. This technique is discussed below. After decompression, the patient is given a topical antibiotic (with or without steroid) solution. Systemic therapy in the form of 1 gm of oral dicloxacillin administered in divided doses is instituted for 10 to 14 days. Warm compresses may resolve the cellulitis, if present, but they increase the chance of formation of a dacryocutaneous fistula, if one was not iatrogenically created to drain the sac. If the sac has been decompressed, the excretory system should be irrigated with a suitable topical antibiotic (with or without steroid).

Surgical. Probing is indicated any time after 2 months of age, either because of parental request or the surgeon's philosophy. The technique is described in congenital anomalies of the lacrimal system (see p. 684). It can be done in the office in infants younger than age 6 months. Probing in the office or hospital in experienced hands is associated with very little morbidity. Past the age of 6 months, a short general anesthetic is recommended for most cases. If the dacryocystitis is allowed to persist beyond 13 months of age, the number of patients requiring a dacryocystorhinostomy at a later date increases.

If the initial office probing fails, the child is brought to the hospital operating room and probed again. If the inferior meatus is at all tight, the inferior turbinate is fractured medially with a Freer elevator or straight hemostat. The excretory system is then intubated with silicone that has been glued on the ends of Quickert probes. A square knot is tied in the silicone, and it is allowed to retract into the inferior meatus. The puncta should be checked to be sure the silicone tension is not excessive. The tube is left in place for 6 weeks and then removed either through the nose or upper canalicular system.

When a patient is seen initially for an acute dacryocystitis, as mentioned above, an attempt should be made to decompress the swollen, tender sac. Massage of the area typically meets with significant resistance from the patient because of pain. Topical proparacaine is applied to the ocular surface, and then 4 per cent cocaine solution is used topically to numb the puncta, and the canaliculi may be irrigated with the 4 per cent cocaine solution. At this time, the punctum is dilated with a 1 or 2 Jones punctal dilator. The upper or lower canaliculus is probed gently with a Bowman 1 or 2 probe. Once the tip of the probe comes into contact with the common canalicular area, the probe is gently advanced past the swollen valve of Rosenmuller into the sac. It is important at this stage not to use excessive pressure and create a false passage. Often, if the probe can be placed into the lacrimal sac, the contents will drain around the probe and through the opposite canaliculus and puncta, allowing for sac decompression. If this does not happen, the probe can be removed and the sac irrigated again with the 4 per cent cocaine solution. An attempt is then made to place the probe into the sac, and at this time the probe is turned 90° cephalad with the convexity of the curve in the probe against the nose. The probe is then passed toward the nasolacrimal duct. The probe is gently advanced through the duct into the nose and removed. With a small amount of pressure externally, the sac can be decompressed into the nose and oropharynx. If this is achieved, irrigation with an antibiotic-steroid solution is helpful in resolving the acute episode of dacryocystitis.

If decompression cannot be achieved by probing, a dacryocutaneous fistula can be created by lancing the swollen sac through the overlying skin with a Number 11 Bard-Parker blade.

Dacryocystorhinostomy is performed early on infants with amniotoceles or acute dacryocystitis. It is also performed when the more conservative measures discussed above fail. It is best to wait until the child is at least 1 year of age. The technique is essentially the same as that used in adults with minor variations. A general anesthetic is always used, and silicone intubation is always performed. The silicone used has an outside diameter of 0.032 mm.

Dacryocystorhinostomy in an adult can be done under general anesthesia or monitored anesthesia care (MAC) with intravenous sedation. Hemostasis is not as satisfactory with general anesthesia, unless hypotensive anesthesia is used. The patient is placed in a supine position on the operating table with a slight reverse Trendelenburg orientation to the table. If the dacryocystitis involves both lacrimal sacs, surgery can be performed bilaterally. A dacryocystorhinostomy can be performed either by external skin approach or intranasal approach. The following describes a standard external skin approach to dacryocystorhinostomy.

The local anesthetic, consisting of 2 per cent lidocaine with epinephrine 1:100,000 with hyaluronidase, is injected into the area where the skin incision will be made and also around the upper and lower canaliculus. Regional block injections of the supratrochlear nerve and the infraorbital nerve can also be used. In children, the preferred local anesthetic is 1 per cent lidocaine with epinephrine 1:200,000 and hyaluronidase. A standard facial prep with povidone-iodine solution is performed, and the patient is draped so that the nose remains out for easy access during the case. A nasal packing consisting of one-half-inch packing gauze soaked first in epinephrine 1:1000 and then 10 per cent cocaine solution is placed in the nose area of the anterior rip of the middle turbinate. The skin incision is initiated 11 mm medial to the medial canthus and slightly above the insertion of the medial canthal tendon and extended approximately 18 mm inferolaterally toward the nasolabial fold. The subcutaneous tissue is opened with sharp dissection, and the orbicularis muscle fibers are separated with blunt dissection down to the periosteum over the frontal process of the maxillary bone medial to the anterior lacrimal crest. Care is taken to avoid the angular vein. The periosteum is incised vertically and spread laterally and medially until the anterior lacrimal crest can be identified. The sac is elevated out of the lacrimal fossa somewhat so that the opening of the nasolacrimal duct can be identified. It is important, at this time, to have identified the medial canthal tendon, as it is an important landmark superiorly. In general, the medial canthal tendon should not be removed from its insertion on the nose. Local anesthetic is injected into the sac at this point, and a cotton pledget, soaked first in the epinephrine and cocaine solutions, is placed into the lacrimal fossa between the lacrimal bone and the sac to allow for increased anesthesia and hemostasis. The nasal packing is removed. The bony ostium is then created medial to the anterior lacrimal crest, using a power drill and dental burr. Care is taken to avoid the nasal mucosa. The bridge of bone between the ostium and lacrimal sac can be removed with a rongeur and Kerrison punch after the cotton pledget is removed. The self-retaining retractors are relaxed, and the upper canaliculus is probed with a Bowman 1 or 2 probe; once in the sac, it is used to tent the sac medially where it can be opened with sharp dissection, creating an anterior and posterior flap. The nasal mucosa is incised as well to create an anterior and posterior flap. These posterior flaps, both from the lacrimal sac and from the nasal mucosa, are excised and not closed surgically. Once the nasal mucosa has been violated, the patient's airway is no longer protected from hemorrhage. Suction is used to avoid airway obstruction. If there is a fair amount of bleeding, an absorbable, hemostatic collagen or oxidized cellulose can be placed in the area of the posterior flaps. The appropriate size of silicone, glued on the Quickert probes, is then passed through the upper and lower canaliculi, one at a time, into the nose posterior to the anterior flaps. The probe can be brought through the external nares using a straight hemostat. The Quickert probes are removed, and the silicone is tied at the end of the case. The anterior flaps are then closed with two or three interrupted 5-0 Dacron sutures. The hemostatic collagen can be left in place, as it will be absorbed. After closure of the anterior flaps, the periosteum and deep muscular layers can be closed with interrupted or running 6-0 vicryl sutures, and the skin is closed with a stitch and suture of the surgeon's choice. The silicone is then tied in place with a square knot and cut, and the knot is allowed to retract into the inferior meatus. It is important to check the puncta and make sure that there is no tension on the silicone that could cause a cheese-wiring of the silicone through the canaliculi.

In the past two years, intranasal dacryocystorhinostomy has experienced renewed interest with the use of nasal endoscopy and KPT: YAG and Holmium: YAG lasers. Transcanalicular laser dacryocystorhinostomy has also shown some promise. Unfortunately, follow-up reports are showing a much higher failure rate than is seen with conventional dacryocystorhinostomy surgery. The absence of an external scar and less ecchymosis and swelling are its principal advantages.

Ocular or Periocular Manifestations

Conjunctiva: Conjunctivitis.
Cornea: Keratitis; ulceration.
Lacrimal System: Canalicular discharge; pain, swelling, and tenderness over the lacrimal sac (especially with digital pressure); epiphora.
Orbit: Cellulitis.
Other: Periorbital edema and periorbital hyperemia; panophthalmitis; sinusitis; meningitis.

PRECAUTIONS

When probing the canalicular system in either the infant or adult, the surgeon must be careful to avoid creating a false passage. This can best be avoided by maintaining good lateral pressure on the lid to avoid an accordion effect of the canaliculus as the probe is advanced. In addition to this pressure, only gentle pressure should be used with the probe, never forcing it where it will not advance easily.

It is extremely important that the silicone in the puncta is checked to ensure that canalicular erosion does not occur because of excessive tension. When removing the silicone in adults after 6 weeks, it is best to take it out through the nose with a hemostat, after cutting the loop between the two puncta. Often, this is difficult or impossible to do in the child, so the knot can be rotated and brought out through the upper canaliculus, which is preferred over the lower canaliculus because of the potential for cicatricial closure. The inferior canaliculus, which is thought to be the canaliculus that is responsible for the majority of tear removal, is thus spared any possible trauma.

Dacryocystorhinostomy is 90 to 95 per cent successful; however, failures can occur. The failures are typically a result of membrane formation over the internal ostium of the surgically created fistula into the nose. This membrane can be identified by placing a 1 or 2 Bowman probe through a canaliculus into the fistular area, tenting the newly formed cicatricial membrane into the nose, and observing it through the external nares using a nasal speculum. The probe can be advanced through the membrane and identified in the nose. The membrane around the probe can then be excised and the patient reintubated with silicone. In most cases, this procedure will resolve the continued epiphora. In cases where the anterior tip of the middle turbinate is obstructing the ostium, it can be removed with a universal turbinate punch.

Postoperative complications include periorbital ecchymosis and swelling. There will be formation of a scar on the face, which is usually barely visible after 4 to 6 months. Silicone erosion of the canaliculus can occur if the tension on the silicone is too great. Pyogenic granulomas can form around the silicone at the puncta and in the nose; these are easily excised and the base cauterized. The silicone tube can occasionally be caught by the patient and retracted from the puncta, leaving an externalized loop. Patients are instructed postoperatively to tape this over onto the nose, should it occur. When they are seen in the office, the tube is either repositioned or removed. Cerebrospinal fluid leaks have been reported, but with careful attention to anatomy and technique, these leaks can be avoided. They typically result from bony fracture of the floor of the anterior cranial fossa and/or the cribriform plate as a result of rotational force used when removing bone with the rongeur or fracturing an ethmoid air cell. Orbital hemorrhage with proptosis has also been reported. It is a very rare complication of this surgery.

COMMENTS

As always, the appropriate management of any disease entity relies on accurate clinical diagnosis. A history of tearing with muco-purulent regurgitation from the puncta or acute inflammation in the area of the lacrimal sac, combined with Jones tests that would suggest blockage of the nasolacrimal duct, allows the surgeon to feel comfortable proceeding with probing and silicone intubation in a child or dacryocystorhinostomy in an adult.

Many authorities in this field suggest using dacryocystography in the preoperative evaluation. It is felt that doing so better delineates certain problems, such as dacryoliths and tumors, and the exact location of obstruction in some cases. Scintiscanning has also been used in the preoperative evaluation, but it is mainly confined to experimental evaluation and is rarely of clinical necessity. Collagen absorbable hemostat (Instat-Johnson and Johnson) is not only helpful intraoperatively to control hemorrhage but also makes a postoperative Vaseline gauze packing unnecessary. In addition, first-day postoperative hemorrhage is rare. No significant complications have been encountered with collagen use.

References

Dailey RA, Wobig JL: Use of collagen absorbable hemostat in dacryocystorhinostomy. Am J Ophthalmol 106:109–110, 1988.

Font RL: Lacrimal drainage system. In Spencer WH (ed): Philadelphia, WB Saunders, 1986, pp 2312 2336.

Gonnering RS, Lyon DB, Fisher JC: Endoscopic laser assisted lacrimal surgery. Am J Ophthalmol 108:1172, 1990.

Hurwitz JL, Victor WH: The role of sophisticated radiologic testing in the assessment and management of epiphora. Ophthalmology 92:407–413, 1985.

Jones LT, Wobig JL: Surgery of the Eyelids and Lacrimal System. Birmingham, Aesculapius, 1976, pp 163–167.

Kushner BJ: Congenital nasolacrimal system obstruction. Arch Ophthalmol 100:597–600, 1982.

Milder B, Demorest BH, Wobig JL: The lacrimal system. In Silver B (ed): Ophthalmic Plastic Surgery. Rochester, American Academy of Ophthalmology and Otolaryngology, 1977, pp 161–189.

Neuhaus RW, Baylis HI: Cerebrospinal fluid leakage after dacryocystorhinostomy. Ophthalmology 90:1091–1095, 1983.

Paul TO: Medical management of congenital nasolacrimal duct obstruction. J Pediatr Ophthalmol Strabismus 22:68–70, 1985.

Slonim CB, Older JJ, Jones PL: Orbital hemorrhage with proptosis following a dacryocystorhinostomy. Ophthalmic Surg 15:774–775, 1984.

Wesley RE: Inferior turbinate fracture in the treatment of congenital nasolacrimal duct obstruction and congenital nasolacrimal duct anomaly. Ophthalmic Surg 16:368–371, 1985.

DACRYOLITH 375.57

BENJAMIN MILDER, M.D.
Saint Louis, Missouri

A dacryolith is a concretion or stone in the lacrimal canaliculus or sac. Dacryoliths are generally caused by mycotic infections and appear as doughy or granular masses made up of degenerated cells, fungi, and amorphous debris. They are noncalcific and therefore not usually visible by x-ray. *Candida, Aspergillus, Nocardia,* and *Actinomyces* have been identified in canalicular dacryoliths. The canalicular dacryolith is usually a part of the picture of mycotic canaliculitis. The incidence of canaliculitis varies with climate and geography; it is found more commonly in the farming areas of the Midwest than in the coastal regions of the United States.

Infrequently, a foreign body within the canaliculus may form a nidus for a stone, building up strata of fibrin, necrotic cells, inspissated mucus, and, occasionally, calcium salts. Ordinarily, the disease is unilateral, and only one canaliculus is involved. The clinical picture is characterized by a fullness in the nasal one-third of the affected eyelid, often with angular conjunctivitis, and creamy white pus that exudes from a patulous punctum or that can be expressed by light pressure. The pus may contain sulfur granules. Canaliculitis, with or without a dacryolith, should be suspected in any unilateral nasal angle conjunctivitis that persists despite treatment.

The dacryolith in the lacrimal sac or nasolacrimal duct is an indication of stasis. In most instances, the excretory system is patent, but nonfunctioning (functional block). There is usually a history of one or more bouts of acute dacryocystitis. In about 20 per cent of cases of chronic dacryocystitis with a patent outflow system, a dacryolith will be found at surgery. Foreign matter and mycotic infection have been implicated in the formation of lacrimal sac "stones," but studies have rarely confirmed such etiologic agents.

Dacryoliths are noncalcific and therefore radiolucent. Although calcium salts may be present, they are rarely sufficient to produce an identifiable radiographic shadow. No systemic calcium abnormality nor hypersecretion of calcium in the tears has been found in association with dacryoliths. Since the stone cannot be identified by palpation, contrast dacryocystography is necessary to confirm the diagnosis before surgical intervention. The dacryocystogram reveals the patent system, stasis in the sac, and a characteristic radiolucent central area in the sac or duct. Clinically, there is chronic dacryocystitis, epiphora, mild deep tenderness, and, occasionally, dilation of the lacrimal sac.

THERAPY

Systemic. If the canaliculitis is an isolated infection that is unrelated to a more widespread disease, local treatment will prove more effective than systemic therapy. When systemic therapy is indicated and the infectious agent is *Actinomyces*, penicillin G (250,000 units every 4 hours for adults) or minocycline (100 mg every 12 hours) is indicated. For *Nocardia* infection, Bactrim (trimethoprim and sulfamethoxazole) is the preferred systemic agent. For *Candida* and other yeast forms, mycostatin is the drug of choice.

The systemic treatment of fungus canaliculitis with dacryoliths has been disappointing. If topical therapeutic agents are not effective after a period of 2 or 3 weeks, surgical intervention is necessary.

Ocular. *Candida, Nocardia,* and *Aspergillus* can be diagnosed by the finding of septate hyphae in a microscopic examination of the pus, using a KOH hanging drop preparation (a single drop of 10 per cent KOH on a glass slide). The fungal agents can be cultured in thioglycollate broth. For topical therapy, a suspension of 20,000 units/ml of nystatin* may be employed, using one drop four times a day and irrigating the suspension into the infected canaliculus every second or third day. Nystatin is nontoxic to the cornea and conjunctiva. For treatment of *Actinomyces*, penicillin G*, in a concentration of 50,000/ml, may be employed in the same manner.

Surgical. Surgical intervention is necessary for removal of concretions in the canaliculus. The horizontal limb of the canaliculus should be split open on the conjunctival aspect of the lid with a lacrimal probe in place. The concretions and infected mucosa are curetted. The remaining mucosal lining is destroyed with tincture of iodine. It is not necessary to suture the canaliculus, although patency should be confirmed after the infection has subsided. Dacryoliths within the lacrimal sac present a different problem. They are a sign of lacrimal sac disease, and the removal of the dacryolith must be combined with dacryocystorhinostomy. Simple removal of the stone is not sufficient. The loss of lacrimal excretory function is remedied by the dacryocystorhinostomy.

Ocular or Periocular Manifestations

Conjunctiva: Nasal angle conjunctivitis.
Lacrimal System: Canaliculitis; dacryocystitis; distention of the sac; epiphora; moderate deep tenderness; patulous punctum; purulent discharge; "sulfur granules."

COMMENTS

The excretory system is usually patent in the presence of a dacryolith in the lacrimal sac because the dacryolith is a result of nonfunction and resulting stasis. The diagnosis can be made preoperatively by contrast dacryocystography and the calculus identified by the radiolucent area in the lacrimal sac or naso-

lacrimal duct shadow. Dacryoscintillography identifies the patency and functional impairment, but does not outline the dacryolith as precisely as contrast dacryocystography.

References

Bohigian GM: Handbook of External Diseases of the Eye. Fort Worth, Alcon, 1980, p 163.
Bradbury JA, Rennie IG, Parsons MA: Adrenaline dacryolith: Detection by ultrasound examination of the nasolacrimal duct. Br J Ophthalmol 72: 935–937, 1988.
Duke-Elder S (ed): System of Ophthalmology. St. Louis, CV Mosby, 1974, Vol XIII, pp 768–770; 1972, Vol XIV, pp 652–655.
Hawes MJ: The dacryolithiasis syndrome. Ophthalmol Plast Reconstr Surg 4:87–90, 1988.
Herzig S, Hurwitz JJ: Lacrimal gland calculi. Can J Ophthalmol 14:17–20, 1979.
Hurwitz JJ, Welham RAN, Maisey MN: Intubation macrodacryocystography and quantitative scintillography: The "complete" lacrimal assessment. Trans Am Acad Ophthalmol Otolaryngol 81:575–582, 1976.
Jay JL, Lee WR: Dacryolith formation around an eyelash retained in the lacrimal sac. Br J Ophthalmol 60:722–725, 1976.
McCord CD Jr: The lacrimal drainage system. In Duane TD (ed): Clinical Ophthalmology. Hagerstown, MD, Harper & Row, 1982, Vol IV, p 13: 14.
Milder B, Weil BA: The Lacrimal System. Norwalk, CT, Appleton-Century-Crofts, 1983, pp 127–129.

EPIPHORA 375.20
JOHN L. WOBIG, M.D.
Portland, Oregon

Epiphora is the result of hypersecretion or failure of the lacrimal excretory system to function. Many conditions cause epiphora. Stimulation of the fifth cranial nerve due to any pathologic conditions, such as corneal foreign body, corneal ulcer, or nasal pathology, will cause a reflex hypersecretion. Abnormalities of the distributional system, such as entropion or ectropion, as well as constriction or complete closure of the puncta, canaliculi, tear sac, or tear duct, may also result in epiphora.

THERAPY

Ocular. Local disorders of the eye, such as corneal ulcers, intraocular disease, allergies, and nasal pathology, are treated conservatively. The treatment is initially directed toward the cause and, when unsuccessful, toward reducing hypersecretion.

Conservative treatment of the congenitally closed nasolacrimal duct should be attempted initially. Massage of the tear sac for several weeks and instillation of antibiotic drops for infections are recommended for as long as they are effective. Canaliculitis responds temporarily to eyedrops of 10 per cent potassium iodide*, but the disease usually follows a course of remissions and exacerbations until surgical intervention prevails. Acute and chronic forms of dacryocystitis are initially managed by topical ophthalmic and systemic antibiotics. This condition also goes through periods of remission and exacerbations until resolved by a dacryocystorhinostomy.

Surgical. Hypersecretion that cannot be diagnosed or treated conservatively may be helped by a conjunctival dacryocystorhinostomy. This procedure is preferable to removal of the accessory lacrimal lobe or cautery to the ducts of the lacrimal gland. Surgery to the distributional system is generally done to correct entropion or ectropion. In order for the lacrimal pump to work, the lids must be in proper apposition to the globe. Ectropion is usually corrected by horizontal lid-shortening procedures, and entropion is repaired by reattaching the retractors of the lower eyelid to the tarsus.

Several surgical procedures are employed to correct the obstruction. The punctum can be opened with a Habb needle knife under the microscope. Spastic closure of the punctum is opened by a one-snip procedure. The posterior portion of the punctum is cut vertically for approximately 2 mm. This must be dilated several times after the one-snip procedure to correct the spastic closure. If this fails, a silicone tube can be intubated through the lacrimal system. Mild eversion of the punctum is best handled by a one-snip procedure, with removal of a diamond-shaped wedge of conjunctival tissue just inferior to the punctum.

The canaliculus occludes because of flaccidity, lacerations, and cicatrization secondary to chronic use of some eyedrops and infection. The lacerations and narrowing of the canaliculus are best treated by silicone intubation. This technique is performed as described by Quickert and Dryden and gives the best anatomic repair, as well as allows the stent to remain in the canaliculus for a longer period of time than any other previously used stents. A one-snip is done on both the upper and lower punctum. Silicone wedged on a probe, such as the Quickert probe, is placed alternately through the upper and lower canaliculus, tear sac, and nasolacrimal duct. The probe is visualized in the inferior meatus and pulled out of the nose by either a grooved director or a hemostat. The probes are removed from the silicone, and the silicone is tied in a square knot and allowed to retract into the nose. Complete absence or obliteration of the canaliculus is repaired by the Jones' method of a conjunctival dacryocystorhinostomy. Concretions of the canaliculus can be removed by a small ring ear curette. If

this is unsuccessful, then the canaliculus is slit open, and the concretions are removed under direct visualization. No stent is needeed after removing the concretions, since the canaliculus can be primarily closed.

The tear sac obliteration can be caused by infection, dacryoliths, and, rarely, tumors. Acute and chronic dacryocystitis are best treated by dacryocystorhinostomy. Dacryocystectomy should be reserved for malignancy of the tear sac only. Dacryoliths are removed via a dacryocystorhinostomy, since there is usually an anatomic malfunction of the sac or duct that causes the stones to develop.

The nasolacrimal duct can be occluded on a congenital basis and responds best to probing. Early probing of the nasolacrimal duct with a number 0 or 00 probe before 6 months of age has an excellent cure rate. If the infant is over 1 year of age, an infracture of the turbinates should be combined with probing. Stenosis of the nasolacrimal duct in adults is treated by a dacryocystorhinostomy.

PRECAUTIONS

Probing for therapeutic purposes should be confined to infants, whereas probing in adults should be limited to diagnostic tests. Dacryocystorhinostomy is the preferred treatment for most cases of epiphora, and a dacryocystectomy should be avoided. Lacrimal surgery necessitates a thorough knowledge of the lateral wall of the nose.

COMMENTS

A lacrimal evaluation should include inspection, palpation, and the proper diagnostic tests. The lacrimal distributional, secretory, and excretory systems should all be evaluated to diagnose properly the underlying cause of epiphora.

References

Cassady JV: Developmental anatomy of nasolacrimal duct. Arch Ophthalmol 47:141–158, 1952.

Jones LT: Epiphora: Its causes and new surgical procedures for its cure: Preliminary report. Am J Ophthalmol 38:824–831, 1954.

Jones LT, Wobig JL: Surgery of the Eyelids and Lacrimal System. Birmingham, Aesculapius, 1976.

Tenzel RR: Canaliculo-dacryocystorhinostomy. Arch Ophthalmol 84:765, 1970.

Veirs ER: Lacrimal Disorders: Diagnosis and Treatment. St. Louis, CV Mosby, 1976.

Wobig JL: The office management of the lacrimal excretory system. JCE Ophthalmol December, 1978, pp 13–24.

Wobig JL: Lacerations of the Lacrimal Excretory System. Ocular Trauma. New York, Prentice Hall, 1979.

Wobig JL: Epiphora. Causes and treatment. Perspect Ophthalmol 5:177–181, 1981.

LACRIMAL GLAND TUMORS 224.2

(Adenoid Cystic Carcinoma, Benign
Epithelial Tumors, Benign Mixed Tumors,
Inflammatory or Lymphoid Tumors,
Malignant Epithelial Tumors, Malignant
Mixed Tumors)

RICHARD D. CUNNINGHAM, M.D., M.S.

Temple, Texas

The lacrimal gland lies in the superolateral portion of the orbit. It consists of a palpebral lobe located in the temporal portion of the upper eyelid and a larger orbital lobe that lies in the lacrimal fossa, just behind the orbital rim. Tumors of the lacrimal gland account for approximately 10 to 12 per cent of orbital masses undergoing biopsy. They are generally classified into those originating from epithelial elements of the lacrimal gland (benign and malignant epithelial tumors) and those originating from the nonepithelial elements (acute and chronic inflammation and benign and malignant lymphoid tumors). It is now generally accepted that the majority of lacrimal gland lesions consist of nonepithelial elements (70 to 80 per cent) and the remainder (20 to 30 per cent) of benign and malignant epithelial lesions. Malignant epithelial tumors of the lacrimal gland are considerably less common than previously believed.

Several important factors must be considered in the clinical evaluation of a patient with a lacrimal gland tumor: (1) the clinical history, especially the type and duration of symptoms; (2) the presence or absence of radiographically demonstrable bone changes contiguous to the lacrimal gland lesion; and (3) the configuration of the soft tissue portion of the lesion.

Benign mixed tumors (pleomorphic adenomas) account for the majority of epithelial lesions of the lacrimal gland. These are slow-growing tumors originating from ductular elements of the lacrimal gland. They are surrounded by an imperfect pseudocapsule that is transversed by fingers of tumor cells. Histologically the tumor consists of unusual mesenchymal elements (myxoid, chondroid, and osteoid) and tubular epithelial units. The typical presentation of a benign mixed tumor is that of a painless, slowly enlarging mass in the temporal aspect of the upper orbit without clinical signs of inflammation. The mass effect causes inferonasal displacement of the globe and moderate proptosis. Patients tolerate the displacement of the globe very well and rarely report diplopia or visual loss, in fact, many such tumors are present several years before causing severe symptoms. Conventional x-ray studies usually reveal expansion of the lacrimal fossa without bone destruction. Computed tomography or MRI of the orbit reveals a rounded or globular soft tissue mass and confirms the absence of contiguous destruction.

Adenoid cystic carcinoma is the most common malignant epithelial tumor of the lacrimal gland. The tumor is composed of aggregates of basaloid cells that proliferate around circular acellular spaces, giving the tumor a "Swiss cheese" appearance. These highly malignant tumors also cause inferior and nasal displacement of the globe, but these patients frequently complain of pain, numbness, diplopia, and visual disturbances. Symptoms develop quickly—usually within 6 months and almost always within 1 year. CT or MRI of the orbit reveals a circumscribed tumor that frequently extends medially and posteriorly into the orbit and usually shows contiguous bony changes with ragged infiltrating edges projecting from the main mass. The commonly experienced symptom of pain results from periorbital and/or perineural invasion by the tumor. Multiple recurrences and a high mortality rate, approaching 90 per cent at 15 years, are the result of bone, soft tissue, and perineural extension within the orbit and cranium. The tumor does not metastasize early, but eventually will disseminate hematogenously to the lungs and lymphogenously to regional nodes.

Malignant mixed tumor (pleomorphic adenocarcinoma) represents a malignant degeneration of a benign pleomorphic adenoma. Patients with malignant mixed tumor tend to be older (50 to 60 years of age) when compared to those harboring benign mixed tumors or adenoid cystic carcinoma (30 to 40 years of age). There are three types of presentation of malignant mixed tumors. The first is that of a benign mixed tumor that has been incompletely excised. After several benign recurrences, the tumor ultimately degenerates into a malignant mixed tumor. The benign recurrences tend to occur over 3- to 5-year intervals, but when a malignant transformation occurs the patient will become symptomatic over a much shorter period of time (3 to 6 months). The second mode of presentation is that of a patient who has the typical history of a benign mixed tumor (painless, slow-growing, lacrimal mass without symptoms for longer than 1 year) and then suddenly over a 3- to 6-month period notices an exacerbation with more rapid growth or symptoms. The third presentation is that of a patient who has the same clinical course as patients with de novo malignancies.

Nonepithelial lesions of the lacrimal gland account for approximately 75 per cent of lesions undergoing biopsy. Of these, approximately 4/5 are inflammatory and 1/5 are lymphoid tumors. Classification of these lymphoid lesions is still somewhat controversial. The majority are considered to be benign reactive lymphoid hyperplasia. Atypical lymphoid hyperplasia, true malignant lymphoma, and plasmacytoma account for the remainder of the tumors. These tumors tend to occur in older patients and present insidiously without signs of overt inflammation or pain. Computed tomography or MRI of the orbit in inflammatory swelling or lymphoid tumors show a more diffuse flattened enlargement of the gland in contrast to the globular rounded appearance of epithelial lesions.

THERAPY

Systemic. Proper treatment of patients with lacrimal gland tumors is dependent on accurate categorization, which is based on the clinical course, examination, and radiographs made before treatment. Patients with a very short history of lacrimal gland enlargement (less than 3 months) associated with inflammatory signs and without x-ray abnormalities can be treated depending on the clinical diagnosis. Systemic antibiotics are indicated in suppurative dacryoadenitis; systemic corticosteroids are recommended in the treatment of inflammatory pseudotumor. There should be a progressive decrease in mass size over the next 2 to 3 weeks with eventual complete resolution. If any mass remains, the patient should then have an incisional biopsy either through an anterior transseptal approach or transconjunctival approach to rule out a malignant epithelial tumor. Care should be taken during this biopsy not to violate the periorbita, as doing so could allow the potential extraperiosteal spread of malignant cells.

Surgical. Patients thought to have a benign mixed tumor based on the clinical course and typical radiographic findings (slowly progressive, noninflammatory mass lesion present for over 1 year) should not have a biopsy. Incomplete excision of a benign mixed tumor dooms the patient to multiple recurrences and the risk of malignant degeneration. The tumor should be excised in toto by a lateral orbitotomy, without disruption of its capsule, along with all surrounding tissues (lacrimal gland, conjunctiva, levator aponeurosis, and overlying periorbita). Since irradiation of benign mixed tumors has been suggested to increase the incidence of malignant change, no benign mixed tumor, either primary or recurrent, should be irradiated.

Patients with a noninflammatory lacrimal gland mass of less than 1 year's duration should be suspected of having a malignant epithelial tumor. These patients often have pain, diplopia, vision deficit, and characteristic x-ray findings. An incisional biopsy through an anterior transseptal or transconjunctival incision (not violating the periorbita) should be performed to establish the diagnosis based on permanent histologic sections. Once the diagnosis of a malignant epithelial tumor (adenoid cystic carcinoma, malignant mixed tumor, or another epithelial malignancy) is established, the patient should be thoroughly evaluated to rule out intracranial invasion or systemic metastasis. If neither of these is present, an attempt at a "curative" radical resection is performed. It should include the en bloc resection of the periorbital skin, eyelids, orbital contents, a portion of the bony lateral wall, and the roof of the orbit up to the midline. This is a major surgical undertaking and requires a neurosurgeon in addition to an orbital surgeon. Postoperative radiotherapy of 6000 rads delivered over 6 weeks is recommended.

Radiotherapy alone in inoperable cases can offer palliation, but not a cure. In general, the response of malignant tumors to radiation therapy is related to the histology, the extent of initial therapy, and the dose of radiation. Radical exenteration is a cosmetically disfiguring procedure, and the patient should be advised of this matter preoperatively. To date, there are too few patients who have been treated by this procedure to know if long-term survival will in fact be enhanced. Prognosis for these patients is very poor. If incisional biopsy indicates a diagnosis other than malignant epithelial tumor (e.g., lymphoma, inflammatory cellular infiltration etc.), appropriate anti-inflammatory or radiation therapy is initiated. Radiation therapy to the orbit including the conjunctiva to a tumor dose of 3000 to 4000 rads offers a good chance of local tumor control for lymphatic lesions.

Patients who are suspected clinically of having a malignancy in a recurrent benign mixed tumor should have an anterior transseptal or transconjunctival biopsy done on the recurrent tissue, and once malignant tissue has been discovered, radical surgery should be performed as mentioned above. The patient, of course, should first be studied for possible regional or distant metastasis. Patients who have never been treated before but present with a 2- to 3-year history of a slow-growing mass followed by a rapid acceleration of symptoms should have a biopsy through the lid or conjunctiva followed by radical surgery if the diagnosis of malignancy has been confirmed.

PRECAUTIONS

A working diagnosis must be formulated before treatment of any mass lesion of the lacrimal gland. Inflammatory lesions of the lacrimal gland usually present with rather rapid onset of tenderness and erythema of the overlying eyelid and a painful mass without bone destruction. A biopsy must be done on any lacrimal gland mass originally thought to be inflammatory that does not completely resolve through an anterior (eyelid) incision; however, biopsies should not be performed on suspected benign mixed tumors.

COMMENTS

Approximately 10 to 15 per cent of epithelial tumors of the lacrimal gland represent types of carcinoma other than malignant mixed tumors or adenoid cystic carcinomas. These cases are either de novo adenocarcinomas, squamous cell carcinomas, undifferentiated carcinomas, or mucoepidermoid carcinomas. Except for the last type, these tumors have the poorest prognosis for survival of all lacrimal malignancies. They tend to occur in older patients (50 to 70 years of age). The clinical presentation is usually similar to an adenoid cystic carcinoma. These tumors should be managed surgically as previously outlined. Additionally, one could entertain the possibility of performing preauricular and cervical lymph node dissections because these lesions tend to metastasize early to regional lymph nodes. The same proposal for regional lymph node dissections can be made for adenocarcinomas arising in benign mixed tumors. There is no chemotherapeutic protocol reported to be effective for treatment of primary or metastatic lacrimal gland tumors.

References

Brada M, Henk JM: Radiotherapy for lacrimal gland tumors. Radiother Oncol 9:175–183, 1987.

Byers RM, et al: Combined therapeutic approach to malignant lacrimal gland tumors. Am J Ophthalmol 79:53–55, 1975.

Font RL, Gamel JW: Epithelial tumors of the lacrimal gland: An analysis of 265 cases. In Jakobiec FA (ed): Ocular and Adnexal Tumors. Birmingham, Aesculapius, 1978, pp 787–805.

Font RL, Patipa M, et al: Correlation of computed tomographic and histopathologic features in malignant transformation of benign mixed tumor of the lacrimal gland. Surv Ophthalmol 34:449–452, 1990.

Henderson JW: Orbital Tumors, 2nd ed. New York, Brian C Decker, 1980, pp 394–423.

Jones IS: Surgical considerations in the management of lacrimal gland tumors. Clin Plast Surg 5:561–569, 1978.

Krohel GB, Steward WB, Chavis RM: Orbital Disease, A Practical Approach. New York, Grune & Stratton, 1981, pp 129–132.

Marsh JL, et al: Lacrimal gland adenoid cystic carcinoma: Intracranial and extracranial en bloc resection. Plast Reconstr Surg 68:577–585, 1981.

Mauriello JA, Flanagan JC: Management of Orbital and Ocular Adnexal Tumors and Inflammations. New York, Field & Wood, 1990.

Shields CL, Shields JA: Review of lacrimal gland lesions. Trans PA Acad Ophthalmol 42:925–930, 1990.

Spencer WH: Ophthalmic Pathology, 3rd ed. Philadelphia, WB Saunders, 1986.

Wright JE, Steward WN, Krohel GB: Clinical presentation and management of lacrimal gland tumors. Br J Ophthalmol 63:600–606, 1979.

LACRIMAL HYPERSECRETION 375.20

MICHAEL A. LEMP, M.D.,
and PAUL C. KEENAN, M.D.
Washington, District of Columbia

Lacrimal hypersecretion is excessive tearing caused by increased secretion from the lacrimal glands. It must be distinguished from epiphora, which is excessive tearing caused by a blockage of the tear drainage system. High Schirmer's test values in the presence of a patent drainage system indicate lacrimal hypersecretion. Lacrimal hypersecretion is usually an intermittent paroxysm without any ill effects other than social or cosmetic embarrassment. It can be divided into primary or secondary hypersecretion.

Primary lacrimal hypersecretion is very rare and is caused by a direct disturbance of the lacrimal gland. It can be initiated by strong parasympathomimetics, such as pilocarpine, or seen in early cases of lacrimal gland tumors or inflammation; it may also occur with hyperthyroidism, hypothyroidism, and in patients taking birth control pills. Cases of lacrimal gland fistulas have been reported with symptomatic lacrimal hypersecretion.

Secondary lacrimal hypersecretion is more common and is either central, psychic, or neurogenic. Central or psychic hypersecretion occurs in emotional states only after the first few months of life or at times of physical pain, or it can be hysterical in nature. Neurogenic lacrimal hypersecretion has many different causes, of which reflex trigeminal irritation is the most common. Reflex irritation in the area of distribution of any of the three branches can cause lacrimation. Such external irritants as smog, fog, or pollutants; local inflammation; entropion; ectropion; foreign bodies; and accommodative strain all can cause lacrimation. Reflex visual irritation by bright lights causes lacrimation as well. Facial nerve or sphenopalatine ganglion irritation can cause excessive lacrimation. Paradoxical gustatory lacrimal reflexes—that is, crocodile tears—occur after aberrant regeneration of the facial nerve. Reflex lacrimation also accompanies such physiologic acts as yawning, laughing, or vomiting.

THERAPY

Supportive. The first step in treatment is to establish the etiology of lacrimal hypersecretion. Doing so requires a complete ophthalmologic examination and probably an ear, nose, and throat evaluation. Treatment should be directed to the cause, especially in local reflex irritation. When a cause cannot be determined or eliminated, mild cases might be managed by topical astringent vasoconstrictive drops.

Surgical. Partial or total extirpation of the lacrimal glands is to be considered only in the most annoying cases, as there is a real and serious possibility of developing a dry eye. A surgical approach might involve removal of the palpebral lobe, which also leads to destruction of the ductules of the orbital lobe, or only the selective excision of excretory ductules subconjunctivally. In cases of lacrimal fistula, surgical redirection is performed. The sphenopalatine ganglion may also be blocked temporarily with local anesthetic injections; if it is useful, an alcohol block may be done. This is especially helpful in cases where there is nasal pathology or paradoxical weeping.

PRECAUTIONS

Surgical removal of part or all of the main lacrimal gland carries the risk of inducing a dry eye. The total mass of the acceessory lacrimal glands is variable; the amount of functional lacrimal tissue remaining after surgery probably determines the adequacy of tear production. Extreme caution should be exercised in deciding to remove the main lacrimal gland.

COMMENTS

Hypersecretion of tears, which is rare, should be distinguished from epiphora caused by obstruction of the lacrimal outflow pathway. The latter condition is much more common, and drainage studies should yield a positive diagnosis. Other causes, such as inflammatory disease and senile ectropion, should be suspected and treated vigorously, if present.

References

Clark WN: Lacrimal hypersecretion in children. J Pediatric Ophthalmol Strabismus 24:204, 1987.

Duke-Elder S (ed): System of Ophthalmology. St. Louis, CV Mosby, 1971, Vol XII, pp 959–965; 1974, Vol XIII, pp 597–599.

Gillette TE, et al: Histologic and immunohistologic comparison of main and accessory lacrimal tissue. Am J Ophthalmol 89:724–730, 1980.

Jones I, Jacobiec F, Nolan B: Patient examination and introduction to orbital disease. In Tasman W, Jaeger EA (eds): Duane's Clinical Ophthalmology, rev. ed. Philadelphia, Harper & Row, 1991, Vol 2.

O'Connor MA: Congenital fistula of the lacrimal gland. Br J Ophthalmol 69:711–713, 1985.

Scherz W, Dohlman CH: Is the lacrimal gland dispensable? Keratoconjunctivitis sicca after lacrimal gland removal. Arch Ophthalmol 93:281–283, 1975.

LACRIMAL HYPOSECRETION 375.15

MICHAEL A. LEMP, M.D.,
and PAUL C. KEENAN, M.D.

Washington, District of Columbia

Recent evidence suggests that all aqueous tear production by both the main and accessory lacrimal glands occurs as a result of reflex stimulation. Stimulation may be minimal, such as by normal indoor air currents, or considerable, such as by a surface foreign body. The previous distinction between reflex and "basal" tearing has been largely abandoned.

The tear film is composed of three components: lipid derived from the meibomian glands, mucus derived from conjunctival goblet cells, and aqueous tears produced by the main and accessory lacrimal glands. Mucus that renders the ocular surface wettable is reduced in conditions resulting in conjunctival scarring, such as erythema multiforme (Stevens-Johnson syndrome), ocular pemphigoid, chemical burns, and trachoma. Lipid production is reduced in ectodermal dysplasia. By far, the vast majority of cases of lacrimal hyposecretion, however, involve the aqueous component of tears. Decreased aqueous tear production occurs gradually with advancing age. It occurs more frequently in females and in the menopausal and postmenopausal years.

Keratoconjunctivitis sicca, the result of decreased aqueous tear production, can be seen in association with generalized collagen vascular disorders and the triad of dry eyes, dry mouth, and arthritis referred to as Sjögren's syndrome. Less frequently, keratoconjunctivitis can be seen as a result of familial dysautonomia (Riley-Day syndrome). Moreover, drugs with anticholinergic side effects can also cause a decrease in aqueous tear production.

THERAPY

Ocular. Artificial tears can be used to supplement deficient tear production. In general, nonviscous tears containing polyvinyl alcohol or adsorptive polymers form the mainstay of treatment. The frequency of dosage depends on the severity of the condition; relatively mild conditions respond well to the use of one drop of tears two to four times a day, whereas more severe conditions require more frequent instillation. A major advance in the use of tear substitutes has been the introduction of preservative-free ocular lubricants. Preservatives are toxic to the ocular surface and can lead to a worsening of surface disease with frequent applications. Unit-dose package solutions without preservatives, although costly, can be useful for many patients. In more advanced conditions, the use of a sustained-release polymeric rod containing hydroxypropyl cellulose inserted in the inferior cul-de-sac provides relief for from 6 to 12 hours. In many patients, however, this polymeric rod must be used in conjunction with artificial tears. In addition, the use of a bland lubricating ointment on retiring at night can be quite helpful.

Keratoconjunctivitis sicca tends to be associated with increased tear film viscosity as mucin, deprived of its normal aqueous solvent, becomes more viscous. The use of a 10 or 20 per cent acetylcysteine* solution helps reduce this viscosity.

In severe cases of keratoconjunctivitis sicca, particularly those with filamentary keratitis, a bandage soft contact lens can be particularly useful. These lenses, however, must be used in conjunction with artificial tears, and their use carries a certain risk of infection. Many clinicians prefer to use a prophylactic antibiotic drop along with these lenses. These lenses can provide a remarkable degree of comfort and can melt away filaments in a very short period of time.

Systemic. In general, corticosteroids and antimetabolites are not useful in the treatment of keratoconjunctivitis sicca. In certain other severe inflammatory processes associated with ocular drying, such as ocular pemphigoid and Stevens-Johnson syndrome, however, they can be effective. Their use carries significant hazards; caution and close systemic monitoring are required.

In some menopausal and postmenopausal females with marked ocular surface disease associated with keratoconjunctivitis sicca, the use of systemic estrogen‡ replacement therapy can be useful. It must be done in conjunction with gynecologic monitoring.

Topical. Recently, a retinoid topical ointment‡ has been reported to be useful in reversing conjunctival squamous cell metaplasia seen in association with dry eye conditions. Its use, however, remains experimental.

Surgical. Punctal occlusion by cautery is useful in severe cases of keratoconjunctivitis sicca, but should be used with caution because of the fluctuating nature of the condition. In general, repeated Schirmer tests of 1 mm or less or persistent ocular surface disease or both are necessary before the decision to cauterize the puncta is necessary. Too casual use of punctal cautery can cause epiphora.

A lateral tarsorrhaphy, which decreases the exposed area of the ocular surface, brings the conjunctival capillaries in constant apposition with the ocular surface, and lessens the shearing forces of the lid on the ocular surface, can be dramatically effective in reversing the ocular surface disease associated with several dry eye states.

Ocular or Periocular Manifestations

Cornea: Superficial punctate erosions; persistent epithelial defects; ulcer (rare).

Lacrimal System: Atrophy of the main and accessory lacrimal glands.

PRECAUTIONS

The ocular surface defense system is compromised in cases of keratoconjunctivitis sicca. These patients are therefore more prone to infections, particularly blepharitis and conjunctivitis. Exacerbations of symptoms may not be caused by a further decrease in tear production, but rather by concomitant blepharitis. Attention should be directed to the treatment of these infections when they occur.

COMMENTS

The management of a patient with moderate to severe lacrimal hyposecretion demands interest and perseverance on the part of the physician. These patients require long-term supportive help in an attempt to find which combination of treatments will provide satisfactory comfort. They should also be reassured that in the vast majority of cases this condition does not seriously affect vision.

References

Holly FJ, Lemp MA: Tear physiology and dry eyes. Surv Ophthalmol 22:69–87, 1977.
Jordan A, Baum J: Basic tear flow. Does it exist? Ophthalmology 87:920–930, 1980.
Lemp MA: Recent developments in dry eye management. Ophthalmology 94:1299–1304, 1987.
Lemp MA, Blackman JH: Ocular surface defense mechanisms. Ann Ophthalmol 13:61–63, 1981.

MIKULICZ'S SYNDROME 710.2
(Dacryosialoadenopathy, Mikulicz-Radecki Syndrome, Mikulicz-Sjögren Syndrome)

F. HAMPTON ROY, M.D., F.A.C.S.

Little Rock, Arkansas

Mikulicz's syndrome is a symptom complex caused by a variety of systemic diseases with secondary involvement of the salivary glands with or without lacrimal gland involvement. Marked salivary gland involvement may interfere with eating and speaking. This symmetric swelling of the lacrimal gland is slow and usually painless. The swelling causes gradual difficulty in opening the eye, slight edema of the lids, and minimal congestion of the conjunctiva. Pseudoptosis may occur from narrowing of the lid of the palpebral fissures and difficulty in raising the upper lid. The enlarged lacrimal gland may cause exophthalmos with medial displacement. The primary systemic diseases implicated in this syndrome are leukemia, lymphosarcoma, tuberculosis, syphilis, sarcoidosis, mumps, and Waldenstrom's macroglobulinemia. The course of Mikulicz's syndrome is related to the systemic disorder. It occurs most commonly during the fifth and sixth decades and affects females more often than males.

THERAPY

Systemic. Systemic corticotropin and corticosteroids may decrease the lacrimal and parotid gland enlargement in Mikulicz's syndrome. Prednisone in a daily dose of 5 to 20 mg or more should be given orally to control inflammation.

Chemotherapy may be helpful in cases of malignant lymphoma. Mechlorethamine in a dose of 0.4 mg/kg should be given intravenously as a single dose or divided over 2 separate days. The total dosage for patients who have had prior radiation or chemotherapy should be limited to 0.2 to 0.3 mg/kg.

Ocular. Topical corticosteroids and cycloplegics usually control the uveitis. When there is deficient lacrimal secretion, artificial tears should also be applied several times a day. A therapeutic contact lens may also be tried with some success.

Surgical. With a proven carcinoma or a malignant mixed tumor of the lacrimal gland, exenteration is usually the treatment of choice. The bony orbital wall of the lacrimal gland fossa surrounding the orbit should be resected, even if no gross involvement can be demonstrated by x-ray. Recurrent disease is likely beyond the region of the lacrimal gland fossa, which may require a more extensive resection. In the case of a benign mixed tumor, exposure at the time of operation should be adequate to enable inspection of the contiguous bone and resection of any of the involved areas. If a dermoid cyst or cholesteatoma is present, excision or drainage with ablation is indicated.

Ocular or Periocular Manifestations

Conjunctiva: Chemosis; follicular conjunctivitis; nodules; phlyctenules.

Cornea: Infiltration; keratoconjunctivitis sicca.

Eyelids: Edema; nodules; ptosis.

Iris: Anterior uveitis; granuloma; posterior synechiae.

Lacrimal System: Dacryoadenitis; decreased tear secretion; hypertrophy of lacrimal gland.

Optic Nerve: Atrophy; optic neuritis.

Retina: Candlewax spots; periphlebitis.

PRECAUTIONS

Overgrowth of bacteria, fungi, yeast, and viruses can occur with the indiscriminate use of corticosteroids. Frequent blood counts, including platelets, should be done whenever the patient is on mechlorethamine.

COMMENTS

Bilateral or unilateral enlargement of the lacrimal gland, with or without enlargement of one or more of the salivary glands, is often associated with Sjögren's syndrome, keratoconjunctivitis sicca, xerostomia, or rheumatoid arthritis. The prognosis for benign mixed tumors in Mikulicz's syndrome is good; however, the prognosis for all malignant tumors is poor.

References

Meyer D, Yanoff M, Hanno H: Differential diagnosis in Mikulicz's syndrome. Mikulicz's disease, and similar disease entities. Am J Ophthalmol 71:516–524, 1971.

Penfold DN: Mikulicz's syndrome. J Oral Maxillofac Surg 43:900–905, 1985.

Smith FB: Benign lymphoepithelial lesion and lymphoepithelial cyst of the parotid gland in HIV infection. Prog Aids Pathol 2:61–72, 1990.

Som PM, et al: Manifestations of parotid gland enlargement: Radiographic, pathologic, and clinical correlations. Part II: The disease of Mikulicz's syndrome. Radiology 141:421–426, 1981.

UVEOPAROTID FEVER 135
(Heerfordt's Syndrome, Uveoparotitis)

R. PITTS CRICK, F.R.C.S. (Eng), F.R.C.Ophth.,

London, England

and AIDAN MURRAY, F.R.C.S.

Cork, Ireland

Uveoparotid fever is a rare form of sarcoidosis that is characterized by uveitis, enlargement of the parotid and other salivary glands, and facial nerve paresis. However, the signs of the syndrome may be incomplete, and they may be associated with many other ophthalmic and general manifestations. There is an increased liability to florid forms of sarcoidosis in the African-American population, and when sarcoid uveitis is severe, it is particularly likely to be associated with raised intraocular pressure during the active stage. Broad adhesions across the drainage angle resulting from the fibrosis of iris nodules may later lead to chronic closed-angle glaucoma. As in any case of uveitis, secondary cataracts may form. Posterior uveitis frequently accompanies the anterior uveitis, but may appear to be present alone with snowball vitreous opacities and haze and whitish fundus lesions. Retinal vasculitis affecting the veins may be a prominent feature in some cases, but fluorescein angiography reveals that it is much more frequent than would be suspected on routine ophthalmoscopy. Only rarely are the lacrimal glands swollen, but they are frequently affected, and 65 per cent of sarcoid patients show evidence of tear deficiency, in contrast to 6 per cent of control patients. Tear deficiency tends to be severe in uveoparotid fever and may cause hyaline degeneration of the epithelial cells of the exposed conjunctiva and cornea. Conjunctival follicles with sarcoid histology are commonly present in the lower fornix and are a valuable source of biopsy material. Both the cornea and the conjunctiva may be involved in the deposits of calcium salts in exposed areas when sarcoidosis is complicated by hypercalcemia. In the cornea, this appears as a band opacity and may be associated with redness and discomfort. Such patients may become uremic from renal calcinosis. In addition to the facial palsy, in which the nerve may be involved above or below the level at which it is joined by the chorda tympani, sarcoid deposits at the base of the brain may cause other cranial nerve palsies. The optic nerve itself may be affected, with visual loss being associated with papilledema or optic atrophy. Diabetes insipidus from hypothalamic lesions may also occur. The skin of the eyelids may be affected by disfiguring sarcoid papules.

THERAPY

Systemic. Systemic treatment with corticosteroids is essential for all patients with uveoparotid fever. It will usually control the uveitis and retinal vasculitis, lead to resolution of the swollen parotid glands, improve the keratoconjunctivitis sicca by resolving lacrimal gland lesions, and restore a normal blood calcium level by increasing urinary excretion and decreasing intestinal absorption of calcium. In general, the dosage of corticosteroids is kept as low as possible to produce the desired response. Initially, daily oral administration of 40 to 60 mg of prednisone in conjunction with topical ophthalmic prednisolone, hydrocortisone, betamethasone, or dexamethasone may be necessary to control uveitis. This dosage may be slowly reduced over a period of some months, but must never be abruptly withdrawn. Central nervous system lesions usually resist treatment and may occasionally present grave therapeutic problems, especially if a large dosage is required for a long period.

Skin lesions are usually resistant to corticosteroid treatment and may be disfiguring. To avoid higher corticosteroid dosages, 200 mg of chloroquine[‡] may be given twice daily, although the cornea and retinal function must be reviewed regularly during treatment for signs of toxicity.

Ocular. The usual topical ophthalmic treatment for uveitis is mydriatic and cyclo-plegic medication. One per cent atropine in solution or ointment may be instilled several times daily, or 0.25 per cent scopolamine, 1 per cent cyclopentolate, or 1 per cent tropicamide may be substituted. All these parasympatholytic drugs may be aided by 10 per cent phenylephrine, which causes contraction of the sympathetically innervated dilator pupillae. In addition, local treatment with 0.1 per cent dexamethasone suspension, 0.5 per cent prednisolone solution, or 0.5 per cent hydrocortisone suspension or ointment may be used in a frequency of up to twice hourly and reduced gradually. Subconjunctival injections[*] are very useful in the initial treatment of severe cases. These injections may contain a long-acting corticosteroid, such as 20 mg of methylprednisolone in 0.5 ml, combined with 0.5 ml of a mixture containing 0.12 ml of a 1 : 1000 epinephrine solution, 1 mg of atropine, and 6 mg of procaine.

In most patients, keratoconjunctivitis sicca is not severe and requires little more than the use of methylcellulose solution every 2 to 4 hours. Only rarely is a filamentary keratitis encountered; it may require the addition of a mucolytic agent, such as 5 or 10 per cent acetylcysteine,[*] at intervals.

Acute corneal bland opacity usually responds to a rapid reduction of the serum calcium to normal levels by the use of corticosteroids and a low calcium diet, which will lead to early resolution. It may be necessary to remove a chronic band opacity surgically after the application of a chelating agent, such as edetate disodium,[*] which converts it to a mush that can be wiped away. The epithelium will then regenerate and cover the denuded area. In some cases, a corneal graft is required. The argon fluoride excimer laser, which produces an ultraviolet wavelength readily absorbed by all tissues and only penetrating by a few micrometers, causes photoablation in which the tissues are vaporized, it can be used to remove deposits of calcium salts in corneal band opacity.

Ocular or Periocular Manifestations

Conjunctiva: Follicles, hyperemia.
Cornea: Band keratopathy; keratoconjunctivitis sicca.
Eyelids: Sarcoid nodules.
Iris, Ciliary Body, or Choroid: Sarcoid nodules; uveitis.
Lacrimal System: Decreased tear secretion; infiltration of lacrimal gland.
Optic Nerve: Atrophy; papilledema.
Retina: Vasculitis.
Sclera: Episcleral nodules; episcleritis.
Vitreous: Haze; snowball opacities.
Other: Diplopia; paralysis of seventh nerve; proptosis; secondary cataract; secondary glaucoma; visual loss.

PRECAUTIONS

Topical and systemic corticosteroid therapy is usually essential, but the possibility of corticosteroid-induced cataracts or glaucoma should always be borne in mind. Care must be taken to exclude other diseases, such as diabetes, tuberculosis, or peptic ulcer, before corticosteroid therapy is instituted because the usual therapy may require modification.

COMMENTS

Uveoparotid fever must be regarded as a potentially severe form of sarcoidosis requiring prolonged energetic systemic corticosteroid therapy and close supervision. Its duration will depend on the progress of the disease. A delicate balance has to be preserved between tissue damage by sarcoidosis and the complications of corticosteroid treatment. Local therapy with mydriatics and corticosteroids alone is unlikely to control the uveitis of uveoparotid fever. However, these medications help raise intraocular concentrations even when systemic treatment is being given and may be used for local ocular defense over a long period when it is considered safe or desirable to withdraw systemic corticosteroids for the treatment of ocular or other lesions. Such patients should always be watched for signs of corticosteroid-induced glaucoma, which is more likely to be caused by local than by systemic treatment.

It is sometimes difficult to decide whether secondary glaucoma is caused by uveitis or corticosteroids. In either case, it is usually best to continue therapy and treat the raised intraocular pressure with oral acetazolamide or topical ophthalmic timolol solution, which both reduce aqueous production. Corticosteroid-induced cataracts may have to be accepted as a therapeutic risk in severe cases and should be subsequently treated with cataract extraction, although this procedure may present a difficult problem.

References

Bruins Slot WJ: Besnier-Boeck's disease and uveoparotid fever (Heerfordt). Ned Tijdschr Geneeskd 80:2859–2863, 1936.

Crick RP, Hoyle C, Smellie H: The eyes in sarcoidosis. Br J Ophthalmol 45:461–481, 1961.

Gartry G, Kerr Muir M, Marshall J: Excimer laser treatment of corneal surface pathology: A laboratory and clinical study. Br J Ophthalmol 75:258–269, 1991.

Heerfordt CF: Ueber eine Febris uveo-parotidea subchronica an der Glandula parotis und der Uvea des Auges lokalisiert und häufig mit Paresen cerebrospindler Nerven Kompliziert. Arch f Ophthalmol (Leipz) 70:254–273, 1909.

James DG, et al: Ocular sarcoidosis. Br J Ophthalmol 48:461–470, 1964.

Longscope WR, Freiman DG: A study of sarcoidosis based on a combined investigation of 160 cases including 30 autopsies from the Johns Hopkins Hospital and Massachusetts General Hospital. Medicine 31:1–132, 1952.

Scadding JG: Sarcoidosis. London, Eyre & Spottiswoode, 1967.

Smellie H, Hoyle C: The natural history of pulmonary sarcoidosis. Q J Med 29:539–558, 1960.

SECTION 28

LENS

ADULT CATARACTS
366.10

ROBERT C. DREWS, M.D., F.R.C.Ophth.

Clayton, Missouri

Adult cataract is not a single entity, and its different types display a wide variety of natural histories. The cataract that occurs in some alcoholics begins posterior subcapsularly and may become mature in 6 months or less. The specific cataract of diabetes mellitus consists of cortical flakes. These flakes may sometimes be seen in patients who have no diabetes themselves but only have a family history of the disease. Unless coupled with ordinary senile cataract, these flakes are slowly progressive and seldom coalesce sufficiently to obscure vision. Diabetes mellitus, however, may hasten the progression of senile cataract. Brunescent nuclear cataract is usually a very slowly progressive condition, and good visual acuity may persist for years, even after the nucleus becomes so dense that ophthalmoscopic examination of the retina is impossible. Since many adult cataracts are of this type, treatment with medications can seem to delay significantly the need for cataract surgery. Cortical cataracts (spokes and wedges) develop more rapidly than nuclear cataracts. Their course varies enough to make prediction hazardous.

THERAPY

Surgical. At the present time, cataract remains a surgical disease. There is no medical therapy of proven efficacy. Cataract surgery is almost always elective. When a patient's vision is no longer sufficient to meet his or her visual needs, that individual may decide on cataract surgery. Further decisions as to intracapsular or extracapsular surgery and postoperative optical correction with glasses, contact lenses, or an intraocular lens implant depend again upon the patient's needs and the surgeon's prejudices and skills. The majority of patients in the United States now receive extracapsular surgery and a posterior chamber lens implant.

Fortunately, cataract surgery has made stunning advances so that cataract is no longer the chief cause of blindness in the United States as it was not too many years ago. When surgery is needed, rapid, full visual rehabilitation is now available for the vast majority of patients with cataract.

Cataract surgery is occasionally needed to provide a view of the fundus to the eye, especially if there is an unresolvable question of tumor or if ablative retinal surgery is needed. Cataract surgery may be urgent or even become an emergency in cases in which the cataract has been neglected and has become hypermature with secondary uveitis or acute glaucoma. Acute glaucoma can be produced either by (1) swelling of the hypermature cataract with mechanical blockage of the chamber angle as the cataract pushes forward or (2) by leakage of cataract protein with a severe inflammatory response and clogging of the trabecular meshwork with macrophages filled with lens protein.

Ocular. Fifty years ago, a number of nostrums were used in the medical therapy of cataract, and even today a variety of drops are sold in most other countries with the claim that they will slow the progress of senile cataract. The public is willing to buy hope, and clinical impression is easily misled when harmless remedies are used against a disease, the natural history of which is only intermittently progressive.

There is a great deal of scientific interest today in the treatment of galactose cataract, since a specific metabolic defect is known. There is little evidence, however, that this defect plays any part in adult cataract; there is only hope that similar treatable enzyme deficiencies might be found. There is little immediate promise of any efficacious solution, however.

Chronic high-dose aspirin therapy (for arthritis) was thought to be associated with a diminished incidence of senile cataract, but this association has gone unsubstantiated. However, the possible relationship to tryptophan metabolism is of fundamental importance; it is only through an understanding of the biochemical mechanisms of cataract formation that an efficacious therapy can be found. Likewise, there has been a recent interest in the biochemical properties of vitamin E, but this too has gone the way of other treatment fads.

COMMENTS

Proving the efficacy of any therapy for adult cataract may be all but impossible. Valid

701

proof would require hundreds of patients using a treatment for a minimum of 5 to 10 years, with separate bottles of eyedrops for the right and left eye (one eye serving as a control) so that neither the patient nor the physician would know which bottle of drops contained the active ingredient. Thereafter, the code could be broken and the results analyzed to see if a difference in the progression rate of cataract could be demonstrated. Unfortunately, the original population would become statistically meaningless because of its hopeless decimation by death, loss to follow-up, and noncompliance. Noncompliance alone would make the study meaningless, especially when one combines informed consent with the necessity for religious usage of drops forever kept separate over a test period of several years. The alternate possibility of using the drops on randomly chosen patients would not change the death or dropout rate and would insufficiently increase compliance to make up for the loss of matched controls.

Vision in patients with cataracts is usually managed with changing glasses. When this is no longer adequate, surgery has to be considered.

References

Bettman JW: General surgical concepts: Patient selection. *In* Drews RC, Steele A (eds): Modern Trends in Cataract Surgery. West Yarmouth, MA, Butterworth, 1984.
Jaffe NS: Cataract Surgery and Its Complications. St. Louis, CV Mosby, 1990.

AFTER-CATARACTS
366.50

DAVID J. McINTYRE, M.D., F.A.C.S.

Bellevue, Washington

After-cataract is a poorly defined term referring to the residual lens remnants from trauma (or incomplete surgical extraction), as well as alterations in the tissues left behind in extracapsular cataract technique, and the results of their proliferation. In the instance of trauma or incomplete surgery, the eye may undergo a period of striking inflammation. Hemorrhagic, pigmentary, and fibrotic elements may enter the field, producing multiple synechiae, distortions of the pupil, and, occasionally, glaucoma or vitreous involvement with the risk of retinal detachment. Severe inflammation from this origin may result in phthisis bulbi. In the eye that is fortunate enough to avoid the inflammatory response, residual lens material may be isolated by sealing of the anterior and posterior capsular fragments. The Soemmering's ring and all of its variations result from this process. There is likely to be continued growth of new lens cortex, resulting in a slight enlargement of the Soemmering's ring over a period of years.

Currently, the greatest concern is with the after-cataract that develops after extracapsular cataract extraction. The pseudofibrotic changes in residual lens epithelial cells and the occasional growth of fibrous tissue from adhesions with the iris may ultimately result in a very heavy leathery membrane, which is a challenge in treatment.

In addition to changes in the material present at surgery, the long-term growth of secondary cortical fibers is also a problem. These fibers tend to grow across the posterior capsule in an irregular sheet or as nodular structures, classically known as Elschnig's pearls.

Severe inflammatory responses are readily apparent during the early course after trauma or surgery. In addition, those cases producing synechiae and distortion of the pupil are clearly visible at routine slit-lamp examination. After-cataract is not appropriately treated unless a visual disturbance or other complication arises. The visual effect is by far the most common indication for intervention.

Early visual disturbance may result from the presence of fibrous pseudometaplasia of cortical remnants on the central posterior capsule. It may also be greatly accelerated by a fibrinous exudation during the immediate postinjury period. Wrinkling and proliferation of an irregular layer of secondary cortex may result in late changes that occur gradually over a period of several years. The incidence of clinically significant after-cataract is often reported at 40 to 50 per cent.

A recent debate has arisen regarding the effect of the posterior chamber artificial lens implant. Numerous investigators have reported that the growth of secondary cortex and the development of Elschnig's pearls are at least retarded by the contact of an artificial lens with the posterior capsule. In this author's experience with in-the-bag placement of a posterior chamber lens with its convex surface against the posterior capsule, an 11 per cent posterior capsulotomy rate at the fourth postoperative year has been found.

THERAPY

Supportive. The great majority of fibrotic after-cataracts that result from inflammation can be prevented by currently available techniques of "clean" surgery. It is now commonly taught that trauma with lens involvement should be cleaned up thoroughly at initial repair. Modern techniques for managing both lens and vitreous have greatly enhanced the outlook after trauma. Modern techniques of extracapsular cataract extraction have also sharply reduced the occurrence of postoperative inflammation. The eye without residual cortex is generally white and quiet at the first dressing.

Metaplasia and continuing growth of the lens epithelial cells do occur, and long-term clouding of vision is a potential disadvantage to the patient with extracapsular cataract surgery. In addition to an attempt to attain "clean" cataract surgery, other approaches have been made to prevent the growth of secondary cortex. Three directions of concurrent investigations have generated enthusiasm. In early clinical trials with cryotherapy, the lens epithelial cells at the midperiphery of the anterior and posterior capsule are damaged by a series of freeze-thaw cycles. This is being evaluated with the use of a modified cryoprobe and careful technique that minimizes potential damage to adjacent tissues. In a second study, antimetabolites have been placed in the anterior chamber at the conclusion of surgery to destroy the lens epithelial cells chemically. In the human, these cells are actively dividing and therefore sensitive to damage by methotrexate* during their mitotic phase. The third investigation involves an antimetabolite bound to a monoclonal antibody† to the lens epithelial cells. None of these techniques is currently available for widespread use, but all suggest that a preventive approach to the growth of secondary cortex will soon be possible.

Surgical. As with any intraocular procedure, it must be recognized that there are certain risks inherent in intervention directed at after-cataract. The patient must be properly informed that endophthalmitis, retinal detachment, cystoid macular edema, and intraocular hemorrhage are among the potential risks. If a surgical procedure is performed, it must be done with appropriate aseptic preparation and with the pupil dilated as needed. At the present time, the treatment of after-cataract is divided into three categories: reaspiration, discission, and excision.

Reaspiration of secondary cortical growth or "polishing" of the posterior capsule is suggested as a conservative approach to the treatment of after-cataract. It is applicable only to those cases without significant fibrosis. Those patients considered to have an unusually high risk of retinal complication may be offered reaspiration, leaving the posterior capsule intact, on the basis of intuitive logic that suggests that the capsule may then continue to protect the posterior segment.

In many cases, reaspiration is technically very similar to the aspiration of residual cortex at the time of primary extracapsular surgery. The newly grown material may be stripped from the periphery and aspirated from the eye in the usual fashion. Maintenance of the anterior chamber volume with a viscoelastic substance is an important means of protecting the corneal endothelium during such an anterior segment procedure. The surgeon may choose instrumentation from among the modifications of the Kratz

scratcher, various curettes, the coaxial cannula, or any of a variety of other aspirating devices.

The classical *surgical discission* is done with various modifications of the Ziegler knife. Alternatively, a sharp hook on the tip of a fine disposable hypodermic needle may be used to incise or tear the thin posterior capsule. If fibrotic changes have produced an irregular tough membrane, the procedure may be significantly more difficult.

Recently, the Neodymium: YAG laser has become the most common instrument for posterior capsulotomy in the United States. Its astonishingly brief infrared energy creates a minute explosion in the transparent medium, thus causing a disruption of the capsular membrane. Lacking an incision, bacterial endophthalmitis is not a possible complication. However, early posttreatment secondary glaucoma is widely reported, along with cystoid macular edema, various maculopathies, and retinal detachment.

Occasionally, the after-cataract membrane may be so heavy and tough as to require *excision* with a vitreous suction/cutter. Such heavy scarring is usually associated with severe postoperative inflammation and extensive posterior synechiae formation. The individual case will dictate whether the procedure should be carried out via limbal or pars plana route.

PRECAUTIONS

As previously noted, the risks of preventive techniques in current evaluation are as yet unknown. On the other hand, the risks of active surgical therapy are quite well understood. All methods of posterior capsulotomy share the risks of cystoid macular edema, retinal detachment, and accelerated macular degeneration, etc.

Endophthalmitis is a very uncommon complication of surgical discission; proper aseptic technique and close postoperative observation must be exercised. As previously noted, endophthalmitis is not a risk with laser posterior capsulotomy. A far more frequent complication is cystoid macular edema. In the past several years, it has been demonstrated that the frequency of cystoid macular edema declines as the time increases between primary cataract surgery and the posterior capsulotomy. According to some reports, discission done at the time of surgery or up until 2 months postoperatively produces a cystoid macular edema rate approximately equal to intracapsular cataract surgery. On the other hand, discission performed 12 months after the initial procedure seems to have much less effect on the macula. Therefore, to minimize cystoid macular edema the surgeon should wait as long as possible after the initial cataract operation before doing a posterior capsulotomy by any method.

In addition to cystoid macular edema, progressive macular degeneration, retinal tears, and retinal detachment occur as complications of the posterior capsulotomy. The relationship to postcataract timing is not as yet well documented. There is a suggestion that some of these risks may be greater with laser than with surgical technique.

COMMENTS

The need for management of after-cataract will probably decrease strikingly in the next several years. Techniques are available for the management of trauma, inflammation, and residual lens material with minimum risk. Similarly, currently taught techniques of extracapsular cataract extraction include very effective removal of residual cortex and, when combined with the posterior chamber artificial lens implantation, may actually retard the growth of secondary cortex.

Either chemical or cryoepithelialysis may prove so effective that management of after-cataract will become a rare task indeed. In the meanwhile, either surgical or laser posterior capsulotomy is safe and effective for the treatment of visual impairment caused by after-cataract.

References

Aron-Rosa D: Pulse Yag Laser Surgery. Thorofare, NJ, CB Slack, 1981.

Chan R, Emery JM: Mitotic inhibitors in preventing posterior capsule opacification: 2½ years follow-up. In Caldwell D: Cryotherapy of the Posterior Capsule. Current Concepts in Cataract Surgery: Selected Proceedings of the 8th Biennial Cataract Surgical Congress, 1985.

Emery JM, McIntyre DJ: Extracapsular Cataract Surgery. St. Louis, CV Mosby, 1982.

Jaffe NS: Cataract Surgery and Its Complications, 2nd ed. St. Louis, CV Mosby, 1976, pp 380–388.

CONGENITAL AND INFANTILE CATARACTS 743.30

DAVID A. HILES, M.D.,
and C. SCOTT ATKINSON, M.D.

Pittsburgh, Pennsylvania

Congenital or infantile cataracts are being discovered more frequently early in the neonatal period or within the first few months of life by observant nonophthalmologic physicians or by parents. Juvenile- or adolescent-onset cataracts may not be diagnosed until later in childhood when progressive visual deficits or strabismus intervenes. Lens opacities may be unilateral or bilateral, involve part or all of the lens, and be stationary or progressive in nature. Cataracts without an identifiable etiology comprise about one-third of patients, whereas an additional 8 to 25 per cent have new autosomal dominant mutations. Cataracts are often associated with additional ocular defects, as well as with systemic, chromosomal, genetic, or syndrome-related anomalies. Syndromes with infantile cataracts include a variety of craniofacial, mandibulofacial, skeletal, apical, central nervous system, muscular, dermatologic, audiologic, metabolic, and renal entities. Cataracts also occur in association with such chromosomal anomalies as Down, Turner, Patau, Edward, Wolf-Hirschorn, cri-du-chat and trisomy 20p syndromes. Embryopathies, or nongenetic diseases, may affect the fetus and produce cataracts. These include the TORCH series with the rubella syndrome being most common, but other less common viral, bacterial, or protozoal infections also may induce lens opacification. Metabolic disturbances may induce a host of defects within enzyme systems that then induce cataracts related to diabetes, galactosemia, hypoparathyroidism, homocystinuria, mannosidosis, and Wilson, Fabry, and Refsum diseases, among others. Lens opacification may also occur in association with retinopathy of prematurity, infantile glaucoma, retinoblastoma, microphthalmos, anterior chamber cleavage syndromes, colobomas, aniridia, ectopia lentis, persistent hyperplastic primary vitreous (PHPV), retinal dysplasia, retinitis pigmentosa syndromes, retinoschisis, and retinal detachment. Ocular trauma in children frequently causes cataract formation, either at the time of the original injury or slowly evolving to more increased opacification with visual loss. Some opacities remain stationary without causing visual deficits. Ionizing radiation produces slowly progressive lens opacification that may occur many years after exposure. The effects of maternal drug, alcohol, and tobacco usage during pregnancy must be considered when investigating the etiology of cataracts in infants.

Infantile cataracts are also morphologically categorized according to the position of the opacity within the lens. Partial opacities may be located in the capsular or subcapsular regions of the anterior or posterior poles that include lenticonus and PHPV; arise in lamellar layers within the cortex; be located in the axial or embryonal, fetal or juvenile nuclear regions; or be membranous after the absorption of cortical and nuclear lens elements. Complete cataracts are those in which no fundus reflex is visible through widely dilated pupils.

THERAPY

Supportive. Many children with partial lens opacification are able to achieve high levels of visual development, but frequent monitoring with optical or amblyopia occlusion therapy is indicated to ensure this goal. Refraction with prescription of appropriate glasses helps prevent visual loss secondary to anisometropic amblyopia. Occlusion of the fellow eye may be necessary to prevent both anisometropic and deprivation amblyopia. Pupillary dilation with daily atropine drops is useful to enhance vision in patients with axial opacities; tinted glasses with bifocals are required to achieve optimal vision. If lens opacification increases in density or size with age, surgery is required. The visual prognosis for these older children with partial late-onset cataracts is enhanced as they have had a greater opportunity for phakic visual development with intact accommodation. Children with complete unilateral lens opacities discovered in the neonatal or early childhood periods frequently develop severe, often irreversible deprivation amblyopia that may be further complicated by the presence of microphthalmos. Patients with complete bilateral cataracts may develop deprivation amblyopia, microphthalmic eyes, syndrome-related defects, and nystagmus, all of which may further depress visual results.

Surgical.

BILATERAL CATARACTS. Patients with complete or dense axial cataracts 3 mm in diameter or larger that are discovered in the neonatal period require immediate cataract surgery to prevent deprivation amblyopia. The second eye is operated within a week of the first, providing there is minimal residual inflammation present in the first eye. Rarely are the two cataracts removed at the same operation. Incomplete cataracts arising within the same age group are removed when the visual fixation reflex is diminished, fundus details are obscured, or strabismus intervenes.

Patients up to about 8 years of age with similar complete or dense axial lens opacities require surgery when their fixation reflexes are decreased, corrected vision falls below 20/70, their visual behavior pattern or school performance deteriorates, fundus details are not observed, or strabismus occurs. Patients with an asymmetric onset of visually significant lens opacification may require surgery in the eye with the poorer vision and then only require surgery in the fellow eye many years later. Amblyopia arising in the aphakic eye must be monitored and treated with appropriate optical and occlusion therapy. If strabismus develops, surgery is indicated when central fixation is obtained in the deviating eye and the angle of strabismus remains stable.

UNILATERAL CATARACTS. Infants with unilateral infantile cataracts present a challenge to both physicians and parents seeking to obtain useful vision for the child. Recent evidence indicates that the optic axis must be cleared of opacities, appropriate optical correction placed, and occlusion therapy initiated before 17 weeks of age to achieve visual acuities in the aphakic eye of 20/40 or better. Perhaps occlusion of both eyes of a newborn infant with a unilateral cataract before surgery might enhance binocularity and prevent strabismus. Older children with unilateral cataracts require surgery when corrected vision falls below 20/70, central fixation is diminished, fundus details are obscured, or strabismus intervenes. Children with incomplete neonatal-, infantile-, or juvenile-onset cataracts require surgery when the same signs occur. These indications also apply to children with traumatic cataracts. Lens extraction may be performed at the time of primary repair of the globe if the lens capsule is lacerated or, more appropriately, at a second operation if the lens capsular opening is questionable or when the opacification develops more slowly.

CATARACT SURGERY. The cataract extraction technique for removal of both bilateral and unilateral cataracts is based upon the mode of aphakic optical correction selected as that mode determines the need to preserve the posterior capsule. For children younger than 1 year of age, the suggested procedure is a lensectomy combined with a large central anterior and posterior capsulectomy and an anterior vitrectomy. This operation may be accomplished through one or two small limbal incisions or through a pars plana incision. Both techniques use mechanical suction cutting devices that fragment and aspirate the lens elements in a one-stage operation. This procedure is designed to clear the visual axis of all obstruction and to prevent the occurrence of secondary membranes, thus reducing the need for secondary surgeries and decreasing the risk of amblyopia.

Aphakic rehabilitation is accomplished in infants younger than 1 year of age with unilateral and bilateral cataracts with contact lenses or aphakic spectacles. If these infants fail to wear these optical modalities successfully after 1 year of age, secondary intraocular lens or epikeratophakic grafts may be offered. These latter modalities are not offered to infants younger than 1 year of age because of the relative microphthalmos of the neonatal eye and the rapid myopic power shift that occurs during the first year of life.

Children older than 1 year of age may have either unilateral or bilateral cataracts removed by lensectomy-anterior/posterior capsulectomy-anterior vitrectomy operations as described and receive contact lenses or glasses for their aphakic optical correction. Epikeratophakic grafts may be applied at the time of cataract surgery, or as a secondary procedure, for the myopic power shift tendency has diminished and the graft powers will remain appropriate and stable. A posterior chamber intraocular lens may be implanted at the time of cataract extraction if the cataract surgery is limited to an anterior capsulectomy-lensectomy with mechanical suction cutting devices and the posterior capsule is preserved. This procedure requires that a secondary Nd:YAG laser posterior capsulotomy be accomplished 2 weeks after the lens is implanted, which may be repeated if the membrane reforms.

APHAKIC OPTICAL CORRECTIONS. Aphakic spectacles with a bifocal addition may be prescribed for all children with bilateral cataracts in whom contact lens compliance is inadequate, the parents are unable or reluctant to participate in their use, or other social or economic factors are present that render contact lens wear unsuccessful. Although glasses are expensive, they remain a noncontact, easily modified, reliable modality for aphakic optical correction for children. To reduce the weight of spectacles with very high refractive errors, a 20 diopter Fresnel press-on power prism may be applied to a carrier spectacle lens in which the residual sphere, cylinder, and bifocal are incorporated. Older children who object to thick unsightly aphakic glasses may be offered secondary epikeratophakic grafts or secondary intraocular lens implantation. However, children with unilateral aphakia do not readily wear or achieve visual success from glasses due to the unequal weight of the lenses, induced prism powers, and the large amounts of anisometropia and aniseikonia that lead to increased suppression and amblyopia formation.

Aphakic contact lenses are fitted within the first postoperative week or as soon as the surgical inflammatory response subsides. The initial K readings and trial lens fittings are accomplished under the same general anesthesia as the cataract operation. Lens powers are based upon a postoperative refraction plus the addition of two or three diopters for children younger than 2 to 3 years of age to compensate for their near visual world. Postoperative amblyopia therapy with light-tight occlusion of 75 to 95 per cent of the child's waking hours is undertaken as soon as the contact lens is worn. Frequent follow-up examinations with refraction and reduction of lens powers with growth of the eye are required during the first year of life. Older children require less frequent modifications of their lenses, but do require frequent monitoring of their visual development and amblyopia treatment schedules. The powers of the contact lenses are based upon accurate distance corrections while near vision is corrected with +2.50 bifocal additions in spectacles; this may be increased if a low-vision aid is needed.

Epikeratophakia refractive surgery consists of the application of a corneal onlay graft manufactured from human eyebank cornea lathed to a prescribed power and sutured into a peripheral groove in the host's epithelium-denuded cornea. Epigrafts are offered to children 1 year of age and older with unilateral or bilateral infantile or traumatic cataracts either during the primary cataract operation or at a secondary operation. Although graft failure rates approach 10 per cent, regrafting salvages 90 per cent of failed grafts. Visual acuities achieved by these children approximate those of other aphakic optical modalities. Epikeratophakic grafts, although still applied in selected cases, have not been approved by the FDA. Allergan Medical Optics, their commercial manufacturing company, has ceased promoting the product and training physicians in its use.

The use of intraocular lens implantation in children is increasing as most residents trained in current ophthalmology programs become proficient in this procedure for adults. Advantages to this mode of aphakic correction are constantly applied optics and reduction of anisometropia and aniseikonia. The lack of child and parental contact lens manipulation and its associated stress leads to an enhanced tolerance of amblyopia occlusion therapy as it remains the only therapy applied to the child other than bifocals for near vision.

Intraocular lenses are indicated for children 1 year of age and older who have corneal diameters greater than 9 mm; normal endothelial cell counts, angles, retinas, and optic nerves; and no chronic intraocular inflammation. If selected by the patients or parents after proper and adequate informed consent, intraocular lenses may be implanted as primary implants at the time of cataract surgery or as a secondary implant if the child fails to wear glasses or contact lenses.

Posterior chamber lenses are selected for primary implantation and in those secondary implant patients where a capsular support system exists or where the lens may be secured with transscleral sutures. The powers of the lens may be calculated from A-scan axial lengths, keratometry, and refraction or be empirically selected as an adult power that permits the child to grow toward emmetropia. Residual power, sphere, and bifocal additions are placed in glasses. All children opacify their posterior capsules due to proliferation of anterior capsular epithelial cells. A Nd:Yag laser capsulotomy is routinely scheduled 2 to 3 weeks after the lens is implanted in younger children or as needed in older children as they opacify their posterior capsules. Laser treatment is undertaken in young, uncooperative, or anxious children in a reclining position under general endotracheal anesthesia in the operating room.

Flexible open-looped anterior chamber lenses are occasionally implanted in children 2 to 3 years of age and older who lack a support system for a posterior chamber lens. The lens must be sized and configured accurately and be placed in the chamber angle under gonioscopic observation to avoid iris and corneal endothelial chafing or touch.

PRECAUTIONS

All neonates should have an examination of their eyes, with pupils dilated if necessary, and the clarity of the lens should be specifically noted before discharge from the newborn nursery. Children with unilateral cataracts that occlude the visual axis must be operated and optically corrected before 17 weeks of age to achieve maximum visual acuities. Occlusion of both eyes before surgery might prove beneficial to enhance binocular visual development by inhibiting stimulation of either eye before both eyes are capable of forming vision. Other children with significant bilateral cataracts discovered in the neonatal period often develop nystagmus on a visual deprivation or familial basis. It is thought that nystagmus might be prevented if the visual axes are cleared and optical correction is placed before its onset. Once nystagmus has become manifest, it will remain throughout life, creating its own visual deficit.

Spectacles prescribed for unilateral aphakia rarely are a successful method of optical correction leading to useful vision and the use of contact lenses. Therefore, epigrafts or intraocular lenses are considered. Contact lenses are widely used for aphakic children under 1 year of age, but the lens wear failure rate increases as the children increase in age. Smaller, hard lenses are useful for infants because of their ease of insertion and removal. Silicone lenses, either daily or extended wear, are worn comfortably by most babies, but the buildup of proteinaceous matter on the lens surface may occlude vision. Larger, soft lenses are also comfortable to wear with low loss rates, but frequent insertion and removal may graze or break these lenses. Extended-wear lenses are discouraged because of the complications of corneal ulcer formation. The importance of careful lens hygiene must be reinforced to the lens caretaker to reduce complications of breakage, loss, and infection.

Epikeratophakia grafts are considered in children older than 1 year of age who fail to wear contact lenses. Failure to obtain FDA approval for the manufacture of the lenticules and a lack of training programs by the manufacturing company have resulted in a marked decrease in their application. Epigraft infection, other failures necessitating removal and replacement, and power loss are the major complications of this procedure.

Posterior chamber intraocular lenses are implanted with greater frequency in younger children and in children with bilateral cataracts as more ophthalmologists become familiar with the operation. Careful selection of eyes to receive implants and the understanding and cooperative family caretakers enhance the success of the procedure. In addition, secondary Nd:YAG laser posterior capsulotomies performed on children who are reclining in the operating room under general endotracheal anesthesia is fundamental to the success of this program. Creation of apertures in thin capsules requires minimal laser energy. As the capsule thickens, higher levels of laser energy are required to disrupt them, which has led to an increased incidence of retinal detachments in adults.

Amblyopia occlusion therapy is mandatory for visual rehabilitation for children with unilateral aphakia, but the amount of occlusion time of the normal fixing eye still remains controversial. Up to 75 to 95 per cent of waking hours seems optimal, but lesser hours of occlusion might promote greater binocularity and less detrimental effects upon the fellow or occluded eye.

COMMENTS

Determination of the etiology of infantile cataracts and of associated ocular and systemic diseases requires a complete physical and ocular examination combined with appropriate laboratory, radiographic, audiologic, genetic, and other medical, educational, and social consultations as indicated. The ophthalmologist and the parents of the child are able to gain enhanced insight into the prognosis for visual recovery if these factors are known. Additional medical conditions might be prevented or treated in a more timely manner, and genetic counseling might suggest guidelines for future progeny if inherited defects are uncovered.

Unilateral cataracts in infants and children up to approximately 8 years of age often produce disappointing visual results due to deprivation amblyopia, microphthalmos, and strabismus; this poor result occurs in children with traumatic cataracts as well. Emphasis should be placed upon lens removal and optical correction of neonatal cataracts by 17 weeks of age to achieve optimum visual results. Light-tight occlusion therapy is instituted and monitored frequently, and if contact lenses are worn, repeated refractions with lens modifications are made as the lens powers decrease with increased axial length of the eye. The effect upon the fellow or occluded eye and upon optimum binocular development remains under investigation. Strabismus, a frequent coexistent finding, may require surgical management as visual improvement occurs, the angle of strabismus is constant, or when the child finds it leads to a poor self-image.

Ocular trauma-induced cataracts may require removal of the lens at the time of the repair of the original injury to the globe if the lens capsule is ruptured. The entry wound into the globe is closed, and a separate cataract incision is made so that the lens is removed during a well-rehearsed familiar operation. An intraocular lens may be placed into the eye if all of the parameters for implantation are present and the wound is not grossly contaminated. If lens capsular rupture is not well identified, it is prudent to close the original wound and observe the response of the eye to the trauma. When blood has cleared, the pressure is normal, and inflammation has subsided, a later cataract extraction may be performed under normal surgical conditions with or without lens implantation.

Amblyopia occlusion therapy and strabismus management may be required as the need arises.

Some children with bilateral cataracts may require surgery on both eyes within a few days or weeks of each other, whereas others may have an asymmetric onset of the lens opacification and require cataract surgery at times remote from each other. Careful monitoring of both eyes is required to correct amblyopia secondary to aphakia in the operated eye or deprivation amblyopia in the phakic eye as the cataract density increases. Children with bilateral cataracts, particularly if genetically incited or syndrome related, may have associated microphthalmos and nystagmus that further compromise visual results. Strabismus may intervene, and surgical correction may be required when fixation is central and the alignment is stable.

Children with unoperated cataracts being observed or others with aphakia may require support systems within the home and school if visual handicaps are present. Emotional and material support, counseling, and guidance often help the parents cope with the long-term care required for these patients and their disabilities. Special schools, homes, or institutions may be required for some patients with special needs. Information and appropriate referrals to these support groups should be presented to the families by the ophthalmologist.

Education of nonophthalmic physicians and other medical, social, and educational professionals must be emphasized by the ophthalmologic profession to ensure the timely referral of patients with cataracts so that optimal visual results for each child are obtained.

References

Cheng KP, Hiles DA, Biglan AW, Pettapiece MC: Visual results after early surgical treatment of unilateral congenital cataracts. Ophthalmology 98:903, 1991.

Drummond GT, Scott WE, Keech RV: Management of monocular congenital cataracts. Arch Ophthalmol 107:45, 1989.

Gregg FM, Parks MM: Stereopsis after congenital monocular cataract extraction. Am J Ophthalmol 114:314, 1992.

Hiles DA, Kilty LA: The newborn eye—Disorders of the first year of life. In Eisenberg SJ (ed): The Eye in Infancy, 2nd ed. Chicago, Year Book Medical Publishers, 1992.

Javitt JC, Tielsch JM, Canner JK, Steinberg EP: Increased risk of retinal complications associated with Nd:YAG laser capsulotomy. Ophthalmology 99:1487, 1992.

Lewis TL, Maurer D, Tytla ME, Bowering ER, Brent HP: Vision in the "good" eye of children treated with unilateral congenital cataract. Ophthalmology 99:1013, 1992.

Robb RM, Petersen PA: Outcome of treatment for bilateral congenital cataracts. Ophthalmic Surg 23:650, 1992.

DISLOCATION OF THE LENS 379.32
(Ectopia Lentis, Luxation of the Lens, Subluxation of the Lens)

BAILEY L. LEE, M.D.,
and PAUL STERNBERG, JR., M.D.

Atlanta, Georgia

The crystalline lens normally lies behind the iris and in front of the vitreous, held in position by the zonules. A dislocated lens, or ectopia lentis, occurs when the lens is not in its normal position. When a lens is decentered but remains in the pupillary area, it is subluxated. It is estimated that greater than 25 per cent of the zonular fibers must be disrupted for subluxation to occur. A luxated lens is completely displaced from the pupillary aperture, implying complete disruption of zonular fibers. The lens may be dislocated forward into the anterior chamber or posteriorly into the vitreous. Progressive dislocation of the lens may occur with a subluxated lens becoming totally luxated into the vitreous cavity. In addition to decreased vision, patients may complain of monocular diplopia because of the decentered lens. Exam may show iridodonesis or phakodonesis, as well as the displaced lens vitreous in the anterior chamber, pupillary block, progressive myopia, or marked astigmatism.

Trauma is the most common cause of lens dislocation, accounting for over half of the cases in most series. One needs to rule out predisposing conditions, such as syphilis. Traumatic dislocation of the lens is often accompanied by other evidence of contusive injury to the globe, including scleral rupture, hyphema, angle recession, glaucoma, iridodialysis, sphincter tears, cyclodialysis, iritis, cataract, vitreous hemorrhage, choroidal rupture, hemorrhagic choroidal detachment, retinal dialysis, retinal tears, commotio retinae, retinal detachment, and optic neuropathy.

Ectopia lentis is also a feature of a variety of systemic disorders, including Marfan's syndrome, homocystinuria, and Weill-Marchesani syndrome. The lens dislocation in Marfan's syndrome is usually superiorly and temporally, and is inferiorly and nasally with homocystinuria. Microspherophakia is typically seen in patients with Weill-Marchesani syndrome.

Since patients with Marfan's syndrome may have dilation or dissection of the aorta and cardiac valvular disease, and those with homocystinuria have a tendency to thromboembolism, it is important that the diagnosis be established before any surgical maneuvers are made that could precipitate vascular complications.

Other less common systemic disorders associated with ectopia lentis include sulfite oxidase deficiency, hyperlysinemia, focal dermal hypoplasia, Ehlers-Danlos syndrome, and mandibulofacial dysostosis. Ectopia lentis has been reported as an isolated autosomal dominant entity that may be expressed in the first few years of life in one form and during adulthood in the other (genetic spontaneous late subluxation of the lens). Ectopia lentis et pupillae is an autosomal recessive condition associated with corectopia. Other ocular disorders associated with ectopia lentis include congenital glaucoma, aniridia, and exfoliation syndrome. Since some of these conditions are heritable, genetic counseling should be encouraged in patients with a dislocated lens.

THERAPY

Supportive. The presence of a lens displaced from its normal position does not always mandate surgical intervention. In general, dislocated lenses with intact capsules can be tolerated well for long periods of time. If the subluxated lens is clear, refraction usually can be accomplished satisfactorily. Dilation of the pupil or pupilloplasty may be useful in some cases. If the lens is luxated into the vitreous cavity, an aphakic correction may be used. Pupillary block glaucoma from lens dislocation may respond to mydriatics. If this treatment is not successful, laser or surgical peripheral iridectomy should be attempted before lens removal. Topical cycloplegics and corticosteroids are often employed to control ocular inflammation associated with lens dislocation, particularly that caused by trauma.

Surgical. Surgical intervention is indicated when the dislocated lens becomes cataractous, either causing decreased visual function or preventing adequate retinoscopy in a child. Lens extraction may also be necessary with a clear lens where the edge is in the pupillary axis precluding suitable phakic or aphakic correction. Other indications include a dislocated lens leaking lens protein leading to a lens-induced uveitis or glaucoma, and irreversible luxation of the lens into the anterior chamber with pupillary block.

When planning surgery for a dislocated lens, the surgeon must remember that successful surgery depends on how well the vitreous is managed, since vitreous loss is likely because of ruptured zonules. A pars plana approach using vitreoretinal instrumentation decreases the risk of pulling on the vitreous with an aspiration needle, irrigation/aspiration handpiece, or cryoprobe, thereby reducing the likelihood of retinal tears and detachment. Also, a pars plana approach eliminates the chance of vitreous incarceration into the limbal wound.

The lens can be removed with a vitrectomy instrument or by phacofragmentation. The vitreous surrounding the lens should be managed with the cutting mode of the vitrectomy instrument to relieve any traction that may be transmitted to the peripheral retina. Lens fragments that have fallen posteriorly can be removed using standard three-port vitrectomy technique, and residual peripheral lens materials can be removed by performing gentle scleral depression to bring the pars plicata area into view.

In older patients, the lens may prove to be too hard for removal either with the vitrectomy instrument or phacofragmentation probe. In these instances, the lens may be removed by cryoextraction. It is important to avoid freezing the vitreous to prevent traction being transmitted to the peripheral retina as the lens is extracted. More recently, perfluorocarbon liquids have been used to support hard lenses, permitting removal anteriorly through the limbus by extracapsular techniques.

In some patients, the lens may become luxated into the anterior chamber, causing secondary glaucoma and corneal edema. In these cases, efforts may be made to displace the lens into the vitreous cavity. Often this displacement is unsuccessful, or if successful, luxation recurs shortly thereafter. Although pars plana surgery may be used for these lenses, intracapsular extraction through a limbal incision may be easier, particularly in the presence of corneal edema. The surgeon must anticipate the loss of vitreous and be prepared to perform an anterior vitrectomy. Preoperative placement of a Flieringa ring may prevent collapse of the globe.

PRECAUTIONS

If a retinal detachment is present in conjunction with a dislocated lens, removal of the lens should only be attempted if it precludes the surgeon's ability to visualize the retina. If it is necessary to remove the lens, pars plana surgery is preferred because of the smaller incisions and better immediate visualization of the fundus. The removal of a dislocated lens in the presence of a detached retina is hazardous; the lens must be aspirated into the vitrectomy or phacofragmentation probe and brought into the anterior vitreous away from the detached retina before attempting to cut or fragment the lens.

COMMENTS

Occasionally, lens cortex or the lens nucleus may become displaced into the vitreous as a complication of extracapsular cataract extraction or phacoemulsification. In some cases this complication can be well tolerated, but often it leads to uveitis, secondary glaucoma, and corneal edema. These lens fragments can be satisfactorily removed with pars plana vitrectomy techniques.

Extracapsular cataract surgery with intraocular lens implantation also may be complicated by early or late dislocation of the pseudophakos, usually as a consequence of inadequate capsular support. Partial dislocation may not require surgical intervention.

However, dislocation into the vitreous cavity can be managed successfully by pars plana vitrectomy and repositioning of the intraocular lens implant. In cases without adequate capsular support, the lens haptics can be sutured to the iris or sclera to prevent dislocation.

References

Chan CK: An improved technique for management of dislocated posterior chamber implants. Ophthalmology 99:51–57, 1992.

Chandler PA: Choice of treatment in dislocation of the lens. Arch Ophthalmol 71:765–786, 1964.

Fastenberg DM, Schwartz PL, Shakin JL, Golub BM: Management of dislocated nuclear fragments after phacoemulsification. Am J Ophthalmol 112:535–539, 1967.

Jarrett WH II: Dislocation of the lens. A study of 166 hospitalized cases. Arch Ophthalmol 78:289–296, 1967.

Maguire AM, Blumenkranz MS, Ward TG, Winkleman JZ: Scleral loop fixation for posteriorly dislocated intraocular lenses. Operative technique and long term results. Arch Ophthalmol 109:1754-1758, 1991.

Malbran ES, Croxatto JO, D'Alessandro C, Charles DE: Genetic spontaneous late subluxation of the lens. A study of two families. Ophthalmology 96:223–229, 1989.

Michels RG, Shacklett DE: Vitrectomy technique for removal of retained lens material. Arch Ophthalmol 95:1767–1773, 1977.

Nelson LB, Maumenee IH: Ectopia lentis. Surv Ophthalmol 27:143–160, 1982.

Plager DA, Parks MM, Helveston EM, Ellis FD: Surgical treatment of subluxated lenses in children. Ophthalmology 99:1018–1021, 1992.

Shapiro MJ, Resnick KI, Kim SH, Weinberg A: Management of the dislocated crystalline lens with a perfluorocarbon liquid. Am J Ophthalmol 112:401–405, 1991.

Sternberg P Jr, Michels RG: Treatment of dislocated posterior chamber intraocular lenses. Arch Ophthalmol 104:1391–1393, 1986.

Treister G, Machemer R: Pars plana surgical approach for various anterior segment problems. Arch Ophthalmol 97:909–911, 1979.

This work was supported in part by Research to Prevent Blindness, Inc., New York, New York.

LENTICONUS AND LENTIGLOBUS 743.36

MARSHALL M. PARKS, M.D.

Washington, District of Columbia

Lenticonus and lentiglobus are deformities of the anterior or posterior lens surfaces. The lens surface bows in the axial region 2 to 3 mm either forward into the anterior chamber or posteriorly into the vitreous. Lenticonus implies that the lens surface protuberance is conical; lentiglobus signifies that the lens surface is globular. The majority of cases are posterior lentiglobus. The etiology of posterior lentiglobus is unknown, but in many cases, the remnant of the hyaloid artery lies within the lentiglobus-involved portion of the posterior lens capsule. Persistent hyperplastic primary vitreous may also be associated with posterior lentiglobus. The posterior lentiglobus is presumed to result from a lens capsule weakness in the axial region that bulges increasingly with age under the intralenticular pressure. The anterior lens surface defects occur rarely and are usually bilateral, whereas the posterior lens surface defects are more common and often unilateral. Anterior lenticonus has been associated with spina bifida and Alport's and Waardenburg's syndromes.

Before cataract formation, the lentiglobus may appear as a 2- to 4-mm axial refractive defect by skiascopy that may be 6 to 15 diopters myopic compared to the slightly hypermetropic surrounding lens. The diagnosis is proven by slit-lamp biomicroscopy. Once the diagnosis is made, the progressively deteriorating character of the defect can be documented. The disrupted lens fiber lamellae become cataractous, which at first appear as a posterior axial opacity and eventually become a more diffuse cataract. Examination in the later stage precludes diagnosis. At least 90 per cent of cases are unilateral, being the most prevalent unilateral cataract in a normal-sized eye. Persistent hyperplastic primary vitreous (PHPV) cataracts, anterior polar cataracts, and congenital nuclear cataracts occur in microphthalmic eyes with corneas of 10 mm or less. Furthermore, the vast majority of posterior lentiglobus cases are acquired after the fixation reflex is developed, whereas PHPV and nuclear cataracts are congenital and deprive the patient of the opportunity to develop the fixation reflex in the involved eye.

THERAPY

Surgical. If visual acuity deteriorates, phacoemulsification with aspiration of the cataract associated with lenticonus and lentiglobus may be necessary. As the cataract is aspirated at surgery, the exposed diaphanous weak posterior lens capsule in the lentiglobus portion may become evident. Infusion of the irrigating solution into the anterior chamber bows the inherently defective portion of the lens capsule back into the vitreous cavity. Lowering the infusion bottle to near the level of the anterior chamber causes the lens capsule defect to bow forward toward the corneal endothelium. The lentiglobus portion of the posterior capsule often has calcium deposits within it. Usually, the diaphanous lentiglobus capsular defect tears before the lens cortex aspiration is completed, and vitreous may enter the anterior chamber.

PRECAUTIONS

Although lentiglobus usually is not detected at birth, the defect may be far advanced with rather diffuse cataracts already present. In contrast, some early diagnosed cases without significant cataract change and with essentially clear lenses may be followed for up to 10 years. However, the majority of the cases deteriorate and require surgery.

Glaucoma occurring 5 years or later after surgery is the most common serious complication of cataract surgery in children. However, its occurrence is rare in eyes with normal-sized corneas compared to small cornea eyes having nuclear cataracts and PHPV. Of the 72 eyes with small corneal diameters, 32 per cent developed open-angle glaucoma at a mean of 5.3 years from surgery, whereas only 1 of 18 posterior lentiglobus eyes developed aphakic glaucoma.

COMMENTS

Because cataractous changes often develop during the amblyogenic age (birth to 8 years), amblyopia is probably the most serious feature associated with this disorder. Another common problem encountered in unilateral posterior lentiglobus is the mistaken impression that the poor vision associated with the unilateral cataract is unimprovable; however, because poor vision may be recent, the prognosis for attaining nearly normal visual rehabilitation is good, if the surgery is performed early after onset.

A good rule to follow is that, if the axial refractive defect by skiascopy is 3 mm or larger and the infant or young child is too young to test visual acuity subjectively, amblyopia should be considered inevitable. Visual rehabilitation with lens surgery, contact lens, and occlusion therapy (if unilateral) of the good eye should be considered. In two recently published series, in the first group 49 per cent had 20/20 to 20/40 final visual acuities, and in the second 75 per cent of 18 patients obtained 20/40 or better.

References

Arnott EJ, Crawford MD'A, Toghill PJ: Anterior lenticonus and Alport's syndrome. Br J Ophthalmol 50:390–403, 1966.

Cheng KP, Hiles DA, Biglan AW, Pettapiece MC: Management of posterior lentiglobus. Pediatr Ophthalmol 28:143–149, 1991.

Crouch ER Jr, Parks MM: Management of posterior lenticonus complicated by unilateral cataract. Am J Ophthalmol 85:503–508, 1978.

Howitt D, Hornblass A: Posterior lenticonus. Am J Ophthalmol 66:1133–1136. 1968.

Johnson DA, Parks, MM: Cataracts in childhood: Prognosis and complications. Sem Ophthalmol 6: 201–211, 1991.

Parks MM: Visual results in aphakic children. Am J Ophthalmol 94:441–449, 1982.

Parks MM, Johnson DA, Reed GW: Long-term visual results and complications in aphakic chil-

dren: A function of cataract types. Ophthalmology (in press).

Stafford WR: Anterior lenticonus. Posterior lentiglobus. Report of cases and review of the literature. Am J Ophthalmol 56:654–658, 1963.

Tipshus AF: Posterior traumatic lenticonus. Arch Ophthalmol 82:548–549, 1969.

MICROSPHEROPHAKIA 743.36

HAROLD E. CROSS, M.D., Ph.D.

Tucson, Arizona

Microspherophakia is a rare condition in which the lens is small in equatorial diameter and slightly increased in anteroposterior dimensions, resulting in a small spherical lens. The entire lens equator is usually visible through a dilated pupil, and the ciliary zonules are elongated and irregular. Microspherophakia is usually bilateral, and subluxation of the lens is most frequently inferior, although it can dislocate or rotate anteriorly. Cataracts are also common. Myopia is consistently high with -5.00 to -20.00 diopters. Secondary glaucoma caused by pupillary block with progressive shallowing of the anterior chamber is the most serious complication.

Ultrastructural studies reveal abnormalities in both the lens and its suspensory zonules. Cortical lens fibers in cross-section are reduced to 20 per cent of normal. Zonules on the posterior lens surface are abnormally large with no evidence of prior attachment to ciliary processes. As yet, the causes of abnormal lens-zonule development remain obscure.

THERAPY

Ocular. Intraocular pressure control is of primary concern. Mydriatics and cycloplegics, such as cyclopentolate or tropicamide, may be of value in preventing pupillary block glaucoma, but prolonged mydriasis may allow the lens to migrate into the anterior chamber. Contact lenses should be considered in patients with high myopia.

Surgical. If the glaucoma is detected before peripheral anterior synechiae have formed, a peripheral iridectomy may be effective. If the peripheral anterior synechiae are severe, a filtration procedure may prove necessary.

Lens extraction for cataract or severe anterior displacement with intractable increased intraocular pressure may also be necessary.

Laser iridotomy may be preferable to the usual surgical approach to minimize complications. Postoperative miosis may reduce the risk of further lens dislocation, but this effect remains to be documented.

Supportive. Many ocular conditions that cause microspherophakia are hereditary. Therefore, whenever a sibling with microspherophakia is found, all other siblings in that family need to be examined, since a high frequency of visual loss occurs before diagnosis and management of unsuspected glaucoma.

Ocular or Periocular Manifestations

Lens: Anterior displacement; cataract; ectopia; inferior displacement.

Other: Decreased visual acuity; myopia; secondary glaucoma.

PRECAUTIONS

The visual prognosis for patients with microspherophakia is generally poor unless the diagnosis is made early and appropriate therapy instituted. Repeated episodes of elevated pressure lead to angle and optic nerve damage often in the first or second decades of life. It is therefore essential that all members of affected sibships be examined as early as possible. If the lens is clear, laser iridotomy is indicated prophylactically.

However, ectopia lentis and/or cataractous changes are often present as well. In such cases, serious consideration should be given to complete removal of the lens also as the primary treatment in the prevention of eventual glaucomatous nerve damage.

COMMENTS

Isolated microspherophakia is likely inherited only as an autosomal recessive disorder. Reports of other patterns of inheritance usually list other anomalies as well. This lens anomaly has been found in metabolic disorders, such as homocystinuria and Lowe's syndrome. It is also found in a variety of skeletal disorders, such as Marfan's syndrome, mandibulofacial dysostosis, Weill-Marchesani syndrome, chondrodysplasia punctata, and metaphyseal dysplasia.

References

Eustis HS, Yaplee SM, Kogutt M, Ginsberg HG: Microspherophakia in association with the rhizomelic form of chondrodysplasia punctata. J Pediatr Ophthalmol Strabismus 27:237–241, 1990.

Farnsworth PA, et al: Ultrastructural abnormalities in a microspherical ectopic lens. Exp Eye Res 27: 399–408, 1978.

Fujiwara H, Takigama Y, Ueno S, Okuda K: Histology of the lens in the Weill-Marchesani syndrome. Br J Ophthalmol 74:631–634, 1990.

Jensen AD, Cross HE, Paton D: Ocular complications in the Weill-Marchesani syndrome. Am J Ophthalmol 77:261–269, 1974.

Johnson VP, Grayson M, Christian JC: Dominant microspherophakia. Arch Ophthalmol 85:534–537, 1971.

Kemmetmueller H: Correction of bilateral severe myopia due to spherophakia with contact lenses. A case report. Contact Lens Med Bull 3:28–29, 1970.

Ritch R, Wand M: Treatment of the Weill-Marchesani syndrome. Ann Ophthalmol 13:665–667, 1981.

Sellyei LF Jr, Barraquer J: Surgery of the ectopic lens. Ann Ophthalmol 5:1127–1133, 1973.

Verboes A, Maldergem LV, Marneffe P, Dufier J-L, Maroteaux M: Microspherophakia-metaphyseal dysplasia: A "new" dominantly inherited bone dysplasia with severe eye involvement. J Med Genet 27:467–471, 1990.

SECTION 29

MACULA

AGE-RELATED MACULAR DEGENERATION 363.31

MICHAEL L. KLEIN, M.D.

Portland, Oregon

Age-related macular degeneration (AMD) is the leading cause of severe, irreversible loss of vision in older Americans. The underlying pathologic changes occur primarily at the level of the retinal pigment epithelium, Bruch's membrane, and choriocapillaris in the macular region. The earliest clinical manifestations of AMD are drusen, which appear as yellow deposits beneath the pigment epithelium; they are present throughout the fundus, but are especially prominent in the macula. Drusen occur commonly in older patients, are generally not associated with visual symptoms, and are considered by some to be precursors rather than an integral component of AMD.

Some patients with drusen do develop AMD with varying degrees of visual impairment. Most develop the dry or atrophic form, which is characterized by atrophic pigment epithelial changes and is usually associated with slowly progressive, mild visual loss. A smaller number develop the wet or exudative form that results in a more rapidly progressive and severe loss of vision. These patients comprise the vast majority of those with severe visual impairment from AMD, and the most common underlying feature of their disease is the presence of subretinal neovascularization (SRN). The resulting leakage, hemorrhage, and fibrovascular scar formation produce significant loss of central vision. In occasional cases, vitreous hemorrhage may occur and produce more profound impairment of vision. Another manifestation of exudative AMD is retinal pigment epithelial detachment, which may occur independently or in association with SRN.

THERAPY

Ocular. No medical treatment has been proven to be effective in preventing the development or altering the natural course of AMD. Certain nutritional supplements, including zinc,[‡] selenium,[‡] and vitamins C,[‡] E,[‡] and beta carotene,[‡] have been advocated as being of possible value. However, there is no conclusive evidence of their efficacy at this time. Long-term exposure to sunlight has been proposed as a contributing factor in the development of AMD. One epidemiologic study implicates exposure to shorter wavelengths of light in adult life, suggesting that tinted glasses that reduce ultraviolet and blue light might be beneficial. As of yet, however, there is no firm evidence to demonstrate a protective effect from the routine use of any type of tinted glasses. A pilot study of α-interferon indicated a possible benefit in retarding the growth of SRN in some patients. Favorable results have not yet been duplicated, and clinical trials are currently being carried out.

Surgical. Laser photocoagulation has been proven to be beneficial in reducing the incidence of severe visual loss in certain patients with SRN secondary to AMD. The Macular Photocoagulation Study reported favorable results using argon laser photocoagulation for extrafoveal SRN (200 μm or more from the center of the foveal avascular zone), krypton red laser photocoagulation for juxtafoveal SRN (0 to 200 μm from the center), and argon or krypton laser photocoagulation for subfoveal membranes (extending through the center of the foveal avascular zone). Principles of treatment in that trial included the use of a recent fluorescein angiogram; heavy, confluent burns covering the entire neovascular membrane; and the use of retrobulbar anesthesia*, except for subfoveal membranes.

With regard to wavelengths of laser, argon green laser is the most readily available and most commonly used modality in treating patients with SRN. When using the argon laser, the blue component should be avoided because of uptake by xanthophyll in the macula. The use of longer wavelengths, such as those produced by krypton red or dye red laser, may provide some advantage when treating SRN covered in part by blood, eyes with media opacities, such as cataract, and eyes with lesions occupying very large portions of the papillomacular bundle. However, certain complications are more common when using these wavelengths (see Precautions). The yellow wavelength of the dye laser provides certain theoretical advantages, including excellent absorption by subretinal blood vessels and maximum transmission through macular xanthophyll pigment. However, clinical advantages over other more accessible wavelengths have not been demonstrated. Limited

713

experience with the diode laser has demonstrated that it has the capability of closing SRN, either alone or accompanied by injection of indocyanine green dye to enhance its absorption. The relative value of any given wavelength over another in the treatment of SRN has yet to be demonstrated clinically. In the only two large randomized trials comparing the efficacy of different wavelengths, no significant differences were found between the argon green and krypton red lasers.

With regard to pigment epithelial detachments, the value of photocoagulation is uncertain. If accompanying SRN is identified, its treatment should be considered.

Vitreous hemorrhage usually clears spontaneously, but may persist for months or more. In some instances, vitrectomy may be indicated. Subretinal surgery employing vitrectomy techniques is currently under investigation for use in certain patients with SRN and its sequelae. It has been employed to evacuate large subretinal hemorrhage and to remove subfoveal neovascular membranes.

Ocular or Periocular Manifestations

Retina: Drusen; pigment epithelial atrophy; pigment epithelial detachment; subretinal exudate; subretinal fibrovascular scar; subretinal fluids, subretinal hemorrhage; subretinal neovascular membrane.

Precautions

Complications of photocoagulation include the following: (1) inadvertent foveal photocoagulation (the likelihood is lessened by using retrobulbar anesthesia and maintaining a constant awareness of foveal location by referring to the projected fluorescein angiogram during treatment); (2) macular pucker, especially with the argon laser, but it is seldom of visual significance; (3) hemorrhage from the choroid or the new blood vessel membrane (the likelihood is lessened by using longer-duration burns and avoiding the use of small spot sizes); and (4) retinal pigment epithelial tears. The last two complications are most likely to occur when using the red wavelengths.

When treating subfoveal membranes, immediate vision loss can be expectd, especially if initial vision is better than 20/200. Long-term benefits are most likely for lesions less than 2 disc areas in size.

Persistence and recurrence of SRN are unfortunately very common, occurring in over 50 per cent of treated eyes. Most recurrences develop within a year of treatment. Accordingly, careful postoperative follow-up is indicated to detect recurrences early, thereby allowing an opportunity for further treatment. The patient should be informed of the importance of daily monitoring of the vision in the treated eye. The use of an Amsler grid is help-ful for this purpose. Frequent postoperative examinations should be carried out, using clinical signs (history of decreased vision or Amsler grid changes or the appearance of subretinal fluid or blood on clinical examination) and fluorescein angiography to detect recurrences at the earliest possible time.

Comments

Patients with macular degeneration who have lost central vision in both eyes should be informed of the visual rehabilitation resources available to them. Low-vision optical aids and other devices along with a multitude of special services are available and can improve significantly the quality of life of many of these patients.

References

Gass JDM: Stereoscopic Atlas of Macular Diseases—Diagnosis and Treatment. St. Louis, CV Mosby, 1987, pp 60–97.
Hampton RG, Nelsen PT (eds): Age-Related Macular Degeneration—Principles and Practice. New York, Raven Press, 1992.
Macular Photocoagulation Study Group: Laser photocoagulation of subfoveal neovascular lesions in age-related macular degeneration—Results of a randomized clinical trial. Arch Ophthalmol 109:1220–1231, 1991.

CYSTOID MACULAR EDEMA 362.53
(CME, Cystoid Maculopathy, Irvine-Gass Syndrome)

WAYNE E. FUNG, M.D.

San Francisco, California

Cystoid macular edema (CME) has become a term that is used everyday by clinical ophthalmologists. Yet, the condition was not discovered until 1966, when Gass and Norton studied the so-called Irvine syndrome with intravenous fluorescein. This test clearly demonstrated that the cause of decreased central vision in these aphakic eyes was fluid accumulation in intraretinal spaces within the macular region. Since then, this same alteration of macular anatomy has been recognized in many seemingly diverse clinical situations (see Table 1). Cystoid macular edema is advanced as the reason for decreased central vision in all cases in which it can be proven, and yet our understanding of the pathologic process underlying its production is still very incomplete.

By far, the most common condition associated with cystoid macular edema is cataract surgery. Various investigators have determined the incidence following intracapsular cataract extractions to be between 40 and 60 per cent, whereas the incidence after planned extracapsular procedures of one type or another is around 10 per cent. The role played by the presence or absence of an intraocular lens and the style of intraocular lens, combined with an intra- or extracapsular procedure, has also been the subject of investigation. It has now been well established that lenses suspended in the pupil have the worst prognosis. The next worse are anterior chamber lenses, and the lens style with the lowest incidence of CME is the posterior chamber lens implanted "in the bag." Fortunately, in the great majority of these cases, the condition resolves spontaneously within 3 to 6 months. However, if the anterior hyaloid face is disrupted or formed vitreous is incarcerated into some portion of the corneoscleral wound, the condition may become chronic.

Diabetic retinopathy is the second most common condition associated with this change. It is largely seen in adults who became diabetics after the age of 30 years and who have had the condition for more than 10 years. Concomitant hypertension or arteriosclerosis makes the presence of this condition more likely. Other conditions known to be complicated by cystoid macular edema include exudative senile maculopathy with serous detachments of the macula, vasculopathies (tributary or central vein occlusions), postscleral buckling procedures, chronic uveitis, collagen vascular disease, aphakia with topical antiglaucoma epinephrine compounds, tumors of the choroid (melanomas and capillary hemangiomas), diabetic traction detachments, retinitis pigmentosa, nicotinic acid intoxication, and perifoveal retinal telangectasia.

TABLE 1. Conditions Having the Potential to Produce Cystoid Macular Edema

Pathophysiology	Clinical Examples
Chronic inflammation	After cataract surgery or scleral buckling; chronic uveitis
Vascular transudations	Retinal vascular occlusions; diabetes mellitus; Perifoveal, retinal telangiectasis
Hypoxia	Choroidal tumors and age-related macular degeneration
Structural alterations	Serous detachments from age-related macular degeneration; traction retinal detachment; epiretinal membranes
Disruption of RPE-pumping action	Retinitis pigmentosa
Toxic conditions	Nicotinic acid overdose

Based upon information produced within the past decade, the entity of cystoid macular edema may have two possible explanations: inflammation and anoxia. The inflammatory theory, proposed by Miyake (1977), suggests that the trauma of surgery to the anterior segment during a cataract extraction either stimulates the production of prostaglandins or creates a situation that retards their reabsorption within the eye. Whichever the case, prostaglandins presumably diffuse from the anterior segment to the posterior fundus and produce increased permeability of the perifoveal capillaries. In an independent report by Martin et al. (1977), round cells (lymphocytes and histiocytes) were found around the small vessels in the ciliary body and the perifoveal capillaries in eyes with chronic aphakic cystoid macular edema (Irvine-Gass syndrome). In other words, abnormal uveovitreal relationships in the anterior segment can definitely influence the integrity of the perifoveal capillaries. The inflammatory theory could account for the following situations: aphakic cystoid macular edema, early and late; chronic uveitis, including pars planitis; and postscleral buckling procedures.

The vascular occlusion theory readily explains the conditions seen with obvious retinal vascular disease and detachments of the retina when one considers that the outer third of the retina derives its nourishment from the choriocapillaris. Likewise, retinitis pigmentosa seems to be a disease of the retinal pigment epithelium and the retinal arterioles, and perifoveal telangiectasia produces shunts of the retinal circulation around the macula. The exact mechanism of cystoid macular edema with choroidal tumors, however, would seem obtuse were it not for the fact that Fine and Brucker's (1981) first case was precisely of this sort. Their electron microscopic examination of the retina in a nondiabetic eye containing a choroidal melanoma in the equatorial region demonstrated capillaries in the posterior pole with lumen reduced to a fine slit, secondary to swollen endothelial cells. This work conclusively showed that the macular cells most altered in these cases were the Müller cells of the central retina and that these alterations were most likely caused by occlusion of the retinal capillaries secondary to endothelial cell hypertrophy or edema. The Müller cells in Henle's layer were initially markedly swollen and later degenerated. Early in the process, the photoreceptor cells remain normal, and cystoid spaces in the retina are absent. As the condition persists, however, disruption of the Müller cells produces cystoid spaces in Henle's layer, and alteration of the microanatomy of the photoreceptors follows thereafter.

Recently, the above-mentioned intracellular theory of the origin of the (Müller cell) cysts has been challenged by Gass, Anderson, and Davis (1985). They hold that the cysts arise from expansion of the extracellular spaces of the retina by serous exudates within the inner plexiform and inner nuclear layers. This theory is based on electron microscopic examination of an eye from a 67-year-old woman; this eye contained a malignant melanoma of the choroid, just posterior to the ora along the 6 o'clock meridian. The tumor had been treated with a cobalt[60] episcleral plaque (10,000 rads) 3 years before enucleation. Immediately after enucleation, the eye was sectioned horizontally and immersed in cold 5 per cent gluteraldehyde, thus preserving the ultrastructure of the eye as pristinely as possible. These authors advance the following facts to support their hypothesis: (1) their electron microscopic observations; (2) the highly reversible function of an aphakic CME eye, arguing against cellular death and disruption; (3) the visible lack of occluded capillaries in the macula, arguing against the presence of anoxia; (4) the orderly arrangement of the cystic spaces, as seen on fluorescein angiography, arguing for fluid being incarcerated in extracellular spaces; and (5) the absence of visibly turbid fluid in the macula of an aphakic CME eye, arguing against an increased content of lipids and proteins in the cystic spaces. They suggest that the difference in the two observations (intracellular versus extracellular) most likely is the result of slower tissue fixation in the former eyes. Indeed, two of the eyes upon which the intracellular theory is based had been fixed in formalin before being refixed in gluteraldehyde.

THERAPY

Ocular. Since the pathophysiology of this condition is still in its formative stages, the patient must understand that only an approximate risk-benefit ratio can be estimated at this time with any of the modalities.

Prophylactic treatment of cataract patients with antiprostaglandin agents seems to reduce the high incidence of transient cystoid macular edema after an intracapsular procedure. Topical ophthalmic 1 per cent indomethacin* dissolved in sesame oil or water may be administered 1 day preoperatively and three or four times daily for 4 to 6 weeks. A clinical trial of 0.5 per cent topical ophthalmic suprofen[†] is also in progress.

Favorable responses may also be seen with oral antiprostaglandin agents. Fenoprofen[†] may be administered in doses of 60 mg three times daily, or 400 mg of ibuprofen[†] may be given three or four times daily. Doses may be gradually reduced after 2 weeks until an effective therapeutic level is found. More recently, an encouraging report using ketorolac trimethamine[†] in chronic cases (6 to 24 months of aphakic and pseudophakic cystoid macular edema) has appeared. The prospective protocol called for 30 patients to apply 0.5 per cent ketorolac or placebo drops four times daily for 60 days in a double-blind randomized study. The drug group demonstrated a significant (P = 0.005) improvement in vision.

Corticosteroids are still the mainstay of anti-inflammatory therapy. Topical prednisolone acetate may be administered in a concentration of one drop of 1 per cent four times a day, or five drops of 0.12 per cent every 4 hours while awake. Many patients show improvement of visual acuity within 1 to 2 weeks of the initiation of intensive corticosteroid therapy. It is very important to instruct the patient to keep the lids closed for 10 to 15 seconds after the successful instillation of a drop. Pressure over the inner canthus will trap the active medication in the ocular region and prevent the escape of the medication into the nasopharynx.

Oral therapy can also be employed. A dose of 20 mg of oral prednisone three to four times daily should be maintained for 1 week with gradual tapering to 40 mg per week over the next 2 weeks followed by 20 mg per week for another 2 to 3 weeks. Subtenon injection of 40 mg of triamcinolone* may also be delivered with a 27-gauge needle under topical anesthesia.

The recent introduction of cyclo-oxygenase inhibitors seems to be a very logical adjunct to the use of steroids. Acetazolamide (Diamox) has been shown experimentally to facilitate the transport of water across the retinal pigment epithelium from the subretinal space to the choroid. This was tested in a five-cycle cross-over regimen of treatment/no treatment. It is certainly a therapeutic tool to keep in mind.

The persistence of the cystic spaces within the retina very likely is caused by extravasation of serous fluid through damaged junctional complexes between endothelial cells of capillaries within the macula. Certainly, one sees the fluorescein accumulating in the intraretinal spaces during angiography, and it would not be difficult to believe that some, if not all, of the fluid leaks from capillaries with damaged junctional complexes.

At least two groups of investigators have reported dramatic improvement of chronic CME after treatment with hyperbaric oxygen. Ogura and colleagues (1987) reported two cases of branch vein occlusion that failed to respond to scattered laser treatment over periods ranging from 14 to 27 months, respectively. After 1 hour, twice-daily exposures to 2 atmospheres of oxygen from 4 to 14 days, retinal edema largely subsided and acuity improved from 20/70 to 20/20 and 20/25, respectively. In a randomized controlled series of eight cases of surgically aphakic eyes, all from 7 to 11 months postoperative, Ploff and Thom (1987) reported dramatic improvement in all patients receiving 2.2 atmospheres of oxygen for 1.5 hours twice daily for 7 days and then 2 hours daily for 14 days. They theorize that the beneficial effect occurs because hyperbaric oxygen may help heal the injured junctional complexes by causing constriction of the macular capillaries, along with stimulating collagen formation, which seals these spaces.

Laser. Laser therapy of the retina should be considered for diabetic maculopathy, branch vein occlusion, and some cases of central retinal vein occlusion. The parameters to consider consist of a patient's visual acuity and the fluorescein angiographic findings. For example, in the case of diabetic maculopathy and branch vein occlusion one criterion for treatment is that central vision should fall to at least 20/50 in the presence of cystoid macular edema. The other criterion would consist of angiographic evidence that the CME is actually due to the progression of intraretinal edema from vascular leaking sites to the central macula. The target of treatment should be the sites of leakage.

For central retinal vein occlusion, panretinal photocoagulation should be considered under two circumstances: (1) if neovascularization is developing on the disc or on other parts of the retina and (2) there is angiographic evidence of "nonperfusion" in the peripheral retina. If CME is present with a central retinal vein occlusion, and neovascularization of the disc and elsewhere is absent, a grid pattern of laser therapy across the central macula could be considered if the visual acuity has fallen to the 20/50 level.

Surgical. Anterior vitrectomy through either the limbal or pars plana approach in aphakic eyes with vitreous to the wound but *without* the presence of an intraocular lens has been found to be effective in improving the patient's condition in 75 per cent of the cases. All patients had angiographically proved cystoid macular edema for 6 months or longer. The goal of surgery was to restore microsurgically the anterior segment anatomy to normal by removing all abnormal visible vitreous connections. Because significant surgical complications can and have occurred with this procedure, it is recommended that this modality be held in reserve until medical treatment fails. In cases of an uncomplicated extra capsular procedure with an "in-the-bag" posterior chamber lens, pars plana vitrectomy has proven ineffective in a handful of chronic cases. Therefore, there is no evidence that surgery is at all indicated when there is no anterior segment distortion by vitreous or when vitreous traction on the macula is absent.

Finally, pars plana vitrectomy for pars planitis or chronic uveitis should only be considered after less invasive approaches have failed. Specifically, in the case of pars planitis, cryotherapy as described by Aaberg should be executed first before a vitrectomy is considered. Similarly, in the case of chronic uveitis, systemic and subtenon injections should be given a thorough trial before a vitrectomy is considered. The reason for caution in these two clinical situations is the fact that side effects, such as retinal tears, retinal detachment, and rubeosis iridis, are significant.

Finally, cystoid macular edema should be thought of as more of a medical problem than a surgical problem. The medical armamentarium has increased significantly over the past few years. It is only after medical treatment has failed and the proper indications for surgical approach are present that invasive procedures should be considered.

PRECAUTIONS

The most common adverse reactions to fenoprofen or ibuprofen that patients experience are related to the gastrointestinal tract (dyspepsia, constipation, nausea, vomiting, anorexia, and flatulence). Additional adverse reactions may include headaches, somnolence, dizziness, tremor, pruritus, tinnitus, and palpitations. To minimize side effects and facilitate absorption into the serum, these drugs should be ingested 30 minutes before each meal.

Oral corticosteroids should not be given to patients with a history of peptic ulcers or osteoporosis. Before subtenon injection of corticosteroids, the patient should first be tested for possible adverse response (elevated intraocular pressure) to steroids by topical applications because the periocular injection route most likely delivers the active ingredient to the eye for 1 month.

COMMENTS

Cystoid macular edema should be considered a *sign* of an underlying ocular disease process and not an entity in and of itself. Current investigation is aimed at testing the various hypotheses outlined earlier. Final conclusions should be forthcoming in the near future.

The role of light toxicity in causing cystoid macular edema has been considered by many clinicians. Light delivered to the retina via intravitreal fiberoptic devices has definitely been shown to be toxic to the retina, but it is unknown what role it plays in postoperative posterior vitrectomy cases with cystoid macular edema. The coaxial light of an operating microscope delivered to the posterior segment of an aphakic eye is responsible for producing a pink scotoma during the first postoperative week. Could light from the operating microscope be a cause of aphakic CME? In a prospective study by Kraff and associates (1985) no evidence could be found to substantiate this suspicion.

References

Bresnick, GH: Diabetic macular edema: A review. Ophthalmology 93:989–997, 1986.

Cox SN, Haye F, Bird AC: Treatment of chronic macular edema with acetazolamide. Arch Ophthalmol 106:1190–1195, 1988.

Fine BS, Brucker AJ: Macular edema and cystoid macular edema. Am J Ophthalmol 92:466–481, 1981.

Flach AJ: Cyclo-oxygenase inhibitors in ophthalmology. Therapeutic review. Surv Ophthalmol 36:259–284, 1992.

Flach AJ, Dolan BJ, Irvine AR: Effectiveness of ketorolac tromethamine 0.5% ophthalmic solution for chronic aphakic and pseudophakic cystoid macular edema. Am J Ophthalmol 104:301–302, 1987.

Fung WE, Vitrectomy-ACME Study Group: Vitrectomy for chronic aphakic cystoid macular edema: Results of a national, collaborative, prospective, randomized investigation. Ophthalmology 92:1102–1111, 1985.

Gas JDM, Anderson DR, Davis EB: A clinical, fluorescein angiographic, and electron microscopic correlation of cystoid macular edema. Am J Ophthalmol 100:82–86, 1985.

Kraff MC, et al: Factors affecting pseudophakic CME, Five randomized trials. Am Intraocular Implant Soc J 11:380–385, 1985.

Martin NF, Green WR, Martin LW: Retinal phlebitis in the Irvine-Gass syndrome. Am J Ophthalmol 83:377–386, 1977.

Miyake K: Prevention of cystoid macular edema after lens extraction by topical indomethacin (1). A preliminary report. Allbrecht von Graefes Arch Klin Ophthalmol 203:81–88, 1977.

Ogura Y, et al: Hyperbaric oxygen treatment for chronic CME after branch retinal vein occlusion. Am J Ophthalmol 104:301–302, 1987.

Ploff DS, Thom SR: Preliminary report on the effect of hyperbaric oxygen of CME. J Cataract Refract Surg 13:136–140, 1987.

EPIMACULAR PROLIFERATION 362.56
(Cellophane Maculopathy, Macular Pucker, Preretinal Macular Fibrosis, Surface Wrinkling Retinopathy)

JOSEPH E. ROBERTSON, Jr., M.D.

Portland, Oregon

Epimacular proliferation is a descriptive term used to characterize the condition in which the macular region is distorted by contraction of a fibrocellular membrane that has grown across the inner surface of the retina. These membranes are caused by proliferation of one or more of the following cell types: mononuclear inflammatory cells, astrocytes, fibrocytes, and retinal pigment epithelium cells. Many membranes contain numerous cell types. Stimuli that may induce such proliferation include inflammation, retinal tears, trauma, breaks in the internal limiting membrane from partial vitreous detachment, injury, retinal vascular disease, vitreous hemorrhage, surgery including cryotherapy and photocoagulation, and idiopathic causes.

The clinical appearance of these membranes may vary tremendously. They may be so thin as to be nearly transparent or so thick and opaque that visualization of the underlying retina becomes impossible. Most of these membranes have a matlike rather than shiny appearance when carefully observed. Such membranes may contain pigment, and many give a mottling or clumping appearance to the retinal pigment epithelium secondary to the tractional forces produced on the retina. Proper examination of these membranes requires high-power biomicroscopy, preferably with a fundus contact lens. The use of red free light is recommended by some examiners since its shorter wavelength is reflected more completely from the retinal surface.

Although the semi-opaque properties of these membranes may contribute to visual loss, most symptoms are probably due to distortion or localized detachment of the macula. Distortion of the retinal vessels may also increase vascular permeability and result in localized retinal edema. Significant leakage of dye into the extravascular retina is noted in approximately 20 per cent of cases when fluorescein angiography is used to evaluate these patients. Several clinical features of these membranes merit specific observation when surgical intervention is considered. Vessels that underlie the membrane are usually distorted in a wrinkled, twisted, and irregular manner, whereas vessels peripheral to the membrane generally appear straightened and even narrowed as they are pulled toward the epicenter, or point of maximal contraction. At least one edge of the membrane is often slightly elevated, and this should be noted since the edge is often the best location to initiate peeling of the membrane during surgery. However, failure to find such an edge during the preoperative examination does not preclude the patient from being an appropriate surgical candidate.

The prevalence of epimacular proliferation varies according to the clinical classification used. Most membranes show few signs of progression after their original detection, and the majority of patients are either asymptomatic or have minimal visual complaints. Autopsy studies have demonstrated an incidence of 2 to 4 per cent of eyes and 6 to 7 per cent of patients. The incidence does increase with advancing age. The increased incidence noted with advancing age may correlate with an increased incidence of posterior vitreous detachment (PVD). A PVD may cause breaks in either the internal limiting membrane or the retina, allowing the subsequent proliferation of fibrous astrocytes and/or retinal pigment epithelial cells. The rupture of the internal limiting membrane may actually represent the etiology of many cases of epimacular proliferation previously considered idiopathic.

THERAPY

Ocular. There is no current medical therapy for epimacular proliferation. Associated conditions, such as uveitis, may require topical or systemic treatment, but once contraction of this fibrocellar sheet has physically distorted the retina, there is no medical means of reversing the structural changes. Spontaneous separation of these membranes is well documented, but such an occurrence is exceedingly rare and only a handful of cases are described in the scientific literature. Photocoagulation is contraindicated in these individuals as the laser energy employed in such treatment has the potential to cause further shrinkage and contraction of the epiretinal membrane.

Surgical. Surgical removal of these membranes is accomplished using vitreoretinal microsurgical techniques and instrumentation. The results are good, with significant improvement in visual function now expected in over 90 per cent of cases. The best results are obtained in those cases with lesser degrees of preoperative retinal distortion and better preoperative visual acuities. Although prediction of the visual result is impossible in a given case, the "average" patient's visual function improves by approximately 50 per cent when tested by Snellen acuities. Although the Snellen acuity does improve significantly, most patients observe residual distortion of their central visual field, and the likely persistence of the symptoms does need to be discussed with surgical candidates during their preoperative evaluation.

Several methods for the surgical treatment of these membranes have been described. Common features of the various surgical approaches include a closed system, standard three-port vitrectomy set-up, and the use of 20-gauge picks, forceps, or scissors for the actual membrane removal. Delamination and peeling have their own advantages, and either is actually effective so long as the surgeon is conscientious in avoiding unnecessary trauma. Actual removal of vitreous is not essential to this procedure, but is advocated by many surgeons in the belief that the relative absence of vitreous facilitates the treatment of postoperative retinal detachment by injection of inert gas into the vitreous cavity. Late retinal detachment does occur in 4 to 8 per cent of cases. Reproliferation of the surface membrane is relatively rare, with recurrence noted only in 2 to 4 per cent of cases.

Ocular or Periocular Manifestations

Retina: Cystoid macular edema; distortion of posterior retina and retinal vessels; gray epiretinal membrane.

Vitreous: Pigment debris (associated retinal breaks); posterior detachment.

Other: Visual loss.

PRECAUTIONS

One must remember that, although epiretinal membranes are common, few patients ac-

tually require surgery for this condition. Most membranes cause only minimal symptoms. In one study, vision actually remained at 20/30 or better in 56 per cent of eyes and 20/50 or better in 78 per cent of affected eyes. Once symptoms are sufficient that the patient seeks evaluation, few membranes cause additional distortion. Most membranes are remarkably stable over long periods of observation. Thus, prophylactic removal is not indicated, and the decision regarding surgery should be made based on the patient's symptoms at the time of evaluation.

An increased degree of postoperative nuclear sclerosis is noted in a significant number of patients who undergo vitrectomy for this condition. Although considerable debate exists about the etiology for this change, increased macular sclerosis is probably functionally significant in one-third of surgically treated individuals. This issue should also be addressed with the patient preoperatively.

COMMENTS

Some ophthalmologists erroneously believe that an edge of the membrane must be visible before a patient can be considered a candidate for surgery. Access for removal (on iatrogenic edges) can always be created with the microsurgical blades now available. Improved surgical techniques and the observation that the best postoperative results are obtained in patients with better preoperative acuities have resulted in the more liberal use of vitrectomy for this condition. Although some vitreous surgeons would still limit surgical treatment to those eyes with 20/100 acuity or worse, many surgeons would now consider 20/60 a suitable threshold for surgical treatment. In very selected cases, compelling vocational needs may demand consideration of surgery in patients with even better visual function. The potential risks of any intraocular surgery, as well as the specific risk of retinal detachment and increasing nuclear sclerosis, must be considered carefully and discussed with all patients considering membrane removal.

References

Charles S: Vitreous Microsurgery, 2nd ed. Baltimore, Williams & Wilkins, 1987, pp 153–157.

deBustros S, Rice TA, Michels RG, Thompson JR, et al: Vitrectomy for macular pucker. Use after treatment of retinal tears or retinal detachment. Arch Ophthalmol 106:758–760, 1988.

deBustros S, Thompson JR, Michels RG, Rice TA, Glaser BM: Vitrectomy for idiopathic epiretinal membranes causing macular pucker. Br J Ophthalmol 72:692–695, 1988.

Gass JDM: Stereoscopic Atlas of Macular Diseases: Diagnosis and Treatment, 3rd ed. St. Louis, CV Mosby, 1987, pp 694–701.

Kampik A, et al: Epiretinal and vitreous membranes. Comparative study of 56 cases. Arch Ophthalmol 99:1445–1454, 1981.

Margherio RR, et al: The surgical management of epiretinal membranes. Ophthalmology *88*(Suppl):82, 1981.

Messner KH: Spontaneous separation of preretinal macular fibrosis. Am J Ophthalmol *83*:9–11, 1977.

Michels RG: Vitreous surgery for macular pucker. Am J Ophthalmol *92*:628–639, 1981.

Michels RG: Vitrectomy for macular pucker. Ophthalmology *91*:1384–1388, 1984.

Robertson DM, Buettner H: Pigmented preretinal membranes. Am J Ophthalmol *83*:824–829, 1977.

Sivalingam A, Eagle RC Jr, Duker JS, Brown GC, et al: Visual prognosis correlated with the presence of internal-limiting membrane in histopathologic specimens obtained from epiretinal membrane surgery. Ophthalmology *97*:1549–1552, 1990.

Trese M, Chandler DB, Machemer R: Macular Pucker. I. Prognostic criteria. II. Ultrastructure. Graefes Arch Clin Exp Ophthalmol *221*:12–15, 16–26, 1983.

Wise GN: Clinical features of idiopathic preretinal macular fibrosis. Am J Ophthalmol *79*:349–357, 1975.

MACULAR HOLE 362.54

MARK A. BRONSTEIN, M.D.,

Newport Beach, California

and GREGORY L. COHEN, B. S.

Tarrytown, New York

A macular hole is a loss of a circular or slightly oval area of retinal tissue in the macula. Typically, there is a marginal elevation of the retina around the hole that produces a gray halo or cuff, giving it the punched-out appearance of a doughnut. The hole and its halo rarely reach one disc diameter in size. Yellow clumps on the surface of the pigment epithelium may be seen in the depths of the hole. Frequently, inner and external layers of the retina are absent, causing a full-thickness macular hole.

The pathogenesis of macular holes is now thought to be vitreomacular traction occurring before a posterior vitreous detachment. Macular cyst formation, previously thought to be due to the loss of inner layer tissue, is now thought to be secondary to detachment of the macula as it is drawn anteriorly by contraction of the premacular vitreous. If the inner layer of the macula is gone but the external layer is intact, a lamellar hole exists. Biomicroscopy with a contact lens and fluorescein angiography are helpful in making these distinctions.

The vast majority of macular holes occur spontaneously in otherwise healthy elderly patients who are usually older than age 50. They are more common in females. Most macular holes are unilateral, and central visual loss is variable.

Macular holes can also occur secondary to blunt trauma. These macular holes may be round or oval and may also have irregular edges. They vary in size and occasionally may be larger than one disc diameter. These holes may be seen on early examination or later with the resolution of retinal edema.

A major complication of cystoid macular edema is a spontaneous rupture at the inner wall of the large cystoid space, which leads to the formation of a lamellar hole. A round or oval one-third disc diameter defect in the center of the macula occurs. The old deposits within the hole and the gray halo of marginal retinal elevation, which is typical of the full-thickness macular hole, are not present.

Infrequently, contraction of epiretinal membranes after a posterior vitreous detachment is a cause of macular hole formation. An operculum or tractional deformity of the adjacent retina should be present to make this diagnosis. The holes are oval or irregular in shape. They may resemble pseudoholes that involve epiretinal membranes alone. Fluorescein angiography differentiates between the two conditions.

Progressive myopia may also be associated with hole formation. The hole is usually quite small and round and is located in the paramacular region.

THERAPY

Ocular. Many patients with macular holes without a serous retinal detachment who are monocular or have decreased bilateral vision may benefit from low-vision aids, microscopes for reading vision, and telescopes for distance vision. As always, a comprehensive ocular examination including central visual field testing helps in the determination and design of the needed devices.

Surgical.

WHEN THE RETINA IS ATTACHED. There has been a recent interest in the surgical treatment of macular holes without a serous retinal detachment. Histopathologic specimens have shown the presence of epiretinal membranes along the edges and within the macular hole. Pars plana vitrectomy and suctioning techniques have been used to remove cortical vitreous and epiretinal membranes. This procedure is followed by an air fluid exchange. The surgical success rate for closing the hole is about 60 per cent. The overall success rate for improvement of visual acuity is about 40 per cent.

WHEN THE RETINA IS DETACHED. Surgery is indicated for serous retinal detachment caused by a macular hole. These detachments are slowly progressive, dependent in position to the hole, and do not reach the ora serrata. If these characteristics are not met, a diagnosis of peripheral break is more likely.

Internal surgical treatment is the procedure of choice. If no vitreous traction is present, as with a total posterior vitreous detachment, a paracentesis of the anterior chamber can be done followed by SF6 and C3F8 injection at the pars plana 4 mm behind the limbus. An alternative method is drainage of subretinal fluid externally and the injection of gas. The patient is then placed in a prone position for 5 to 24 hours. In many cases, this treatment effects a cure. If the retina redetaches, the above procedure can be repeated, followed by photocoagulation or cryopexy of the macular hole when the retina is flat.

If vitreous traction is present, as with an attached or partially attached vitreous, pars plana vitrectomy is indicated. It relieves the traction on the macular hole and provides a fluid space for use of an intraocular gas bubble. The subretinal fluid can be evacuated by internal drainage. Argon laser endophotocoagulation may be used to treat the macular hole.

In severe myopia with a marked staphyloma, the above surgical procedure may fail. A lensectomy and total liquid-silicone oil exchange may be done, followed by argon endophotocoagulation.

COMMENTS

The surgical treatment of macular holes without a serous retinal detachment is presently under study. Preselection must be done carefully. In approximately 90 per cent of patients with a macular hole, the fellow eye is not involved. Patients are usually elderly and should only be operated on if surgery could improve vision so that the quality of life improves. The rare patient who has bilateral macular holes may be an ideal candidate. Surgical trials are also underway for patients with impending macular holes. Because some patients with impending macular holes may improve with the spontaneous release of vitreomacular traction, this procedure is controversial and needs further study.

Retinal detachments caused by macular holes are extremely rare. If a retinal detachment has both a macular hole and a peripheral retinal break, the macular hole need not be closed. A rare exception could be a high myopic eye with staphyloma. Cystoid macular edema has a great propensity for spontaneous recovery unless there is a lamellar hole. If ocular inflammatory disease is present, treatment with cycloplegics, antiprostaglandins, and cortical steroids may be indicated. However, no evidence exists that pharmacologic agents can prevent or treat macular holes.

Knowledge of the different causes of and appearances of macular holes is essential. Biomicroscopy and fluorescein angiography are useful in determining which entity is present. Although macular holes are usually unilateral, the fellow eye must be examined for signs of macular change on initial and follow-up visits. If vision is impaired in both eyes, low-vision aids may be valuable.

References

Aaberg TM: Macular holes: A review. Surv Ophthalmol 15:139–162, 1970.

Aaberg TM, Blair CJ, Gass JDM: Macular holes. Am J Ophthalmol 69:555–562, 1970.

Benson WE: Retinal Detachment: Diagnosis and Management, 2nd ed. Philadelphia, JB Lippincott, 1988, pp 157–160.

Bronstein MA, Trempe CL, Freeman HM: Fellow eyes of eyes with macular holes. Am J Ophthalmol 92:757–761, 1981.

deBustros S, Wendel RT: Vitrectomy for impending and full thickness macular holes. Int Ophthalmol Clin 32:139–152, 1992.

Faye EE: Low-vision aids. In Duane TD (ed): Clinical Ophthalmology. Hagerstown, MD, Harper & Row, 1982, Vol 1, pp 46:5–14.

Gass JDM: Idiopathic senile macular hole: Its early stages and pathogenesis. Arch Ophthamol 106:629–639, 1988.

Kelly NE, Wendel RT: Vitreous surgery for idiopathic macular holes. Arch Ophthalmol 109:654–659, 1991.

Michaels RG, Wilkinson CP, Rice TA: Retinal Detachment. St. Louis, CV Mosby, 1990, pp 629–638.

Wiznia RA: Reversibility of the early stages of idiopathic macular holes. Am J Ophthalmol 107:241–245, 1989.

SOLAR RETINOPATHY 363.31

(Eclipse Burn, Foveomacular Retinitis, Photoretinitis, Solar Burn, Solar Retinitis, Sun Blindness)

ROGER A. EWALD, M.D.

Urbana, Illinois

Solar retinopathy is a pigmentary disturbance of the macula secondary to sun gazing. It is characterized by central and parafoveal depigmentation with perifoveal hyperpigmentation. The effects vary from a prolonged persistence of the negative afterimage of the sun or the appearance of scotoma to the permanent loss of central vision with objective signs of a retinal burn. In most cases of solar retinopathy, nothing abnormal is noticed immediately, except the dazzling sensation. However, shortly thereafter, a diffuse cloud floats with irregular undulations before the eyes and is usually associated with an irritating afterimage, photophobia, and occasionally photopsia and chromatopsia. Metamorphopsia, which is initially caused by displacement of the retinal elements with edema and eventually degenerative changes, may also appear in the central field. In mild cases, the macula becomes darker than usual, probably as a result of choroidal congestion. In the most severe cases, the central area may be raised and edematous, having a gray appearance and showing a dark central spot surrounded by perifoveal edema. The most striking characteristic of this disease is the development of a yellow foveal exudate. The exudate resolves in 10 to 14 days with the appearance of a reddish, foveal, "hole-like" lesion surrounded by a pale gray cuff of fine granular pigment within a larger ring of coarse pigment aggregation. Repeated sun gazing results in a mottled honeycomb pigmentary change in the macula with a dispersed light reflection.

Many investigators now believe that solar retinopathy is caused primarily by the photochemical effects of the short wavelengths in the visible spectrum of the sun, with some thermal enhancement from the longer wavelengths in the visible and near infrared. This would help explain those cases that cannot be accounted for solely on the basis of an acute thermal burn. The susceptibility of the retina to photic injury probably varies greatly among individuals.

THERAPY

Supportive. Aggressive public education about the danger of sun gazing may decrease the incidence of solar retinopathy. Emphasis should be placed on the risk inherent in gazing at the sun or other sources of bright light, particularly at the time of an eclipse. The safest advice for the public, and especially schoolchildren, is that under no circumstances should the sun be looked at directly using any type of filter whatsoever. Observing a solar eclipse through polarizing sunglasses or with photographic or x-ray film induces a false sense of security, prolongs exposure time, and results in retinal damage. Solar phenomena may be safely examined in an *indirect* manner, using a pinhole projection method with the observer's back to the sun.

Since extraction of the lens exposes the retina to near ultraviolet and short wavelength visible radiation, ophthalmic surgeons should be aware that the aphakic and pseudophakic eye is more susceptible to retinal damage from intense light sources than the phakic eye. This potential for retinal injury is clinically manifested by the complaint of erythropsia ("red vision") among aphakic and pseudophakic patients exposed to bright sunlight reflected from freshly fallen show. Possible retinal damage can be prevented by lenses (spectacle, contact, or intraocular) with filters that absorb wavelengths shorter than 450 to 500 nm. The sensitivity of the retina to short wavelengths of light may also have clinical significance for some retinal disorders,

such as senile macular degeneration and retinitis pigmentosa.

Solar retinopathy has resulted from minimal exposure, and initially, the patient may be totally unaware of the damage. Aphakic and pseudophakic patients, as well as the general public, should be encouraged to wear photoprotective lenses when engaged in such recreational activities as boating, sunbathing on bright sandy beaches, skiing, or hiking at high altitudes.

Systemic. The most useful measure after a sun gazing episode is the administration of systemic corticosteroids within 72 hours of exposure. A daily oral dosage of 60 mg of prednisone should be given and tapered over a 5-week period. A trial of systemic corticosteriods may decrease the retinal inflammatory reaction and improve the final visual result.

Ocular. In the acute stage, 20 mg of methylprednisolone* or 3 mg betamethasone* may be given by retrobulbar injection to minimize the chorioretinal reaction.

Ocular or Periocular Manifestations

Choroid: Congestion.
Retina: Absent foveal reflex; depigmentation and hyperpigmentation; foveal exudates and cyst; hyperemia; macular edema.
Other: Central scotoma; chromatopsia; frontal and temporal headaches; metamorphopsia; ocular and orbital pain; photophobia; photopsia; visual loss.

PRECAUTIONS

Cases of solar burns have occurred as a result of misconceived therapeutic measures to strengthen the eyes, as part of religious rituals, and while under the influence of psychotropic or hallucinogenic drugs. The deliberate observation of the sun with the intention of producing blindness as a means of self-mutilation has also been noted in individuals with a background of mental illness. Numerous cases of premeditated self-inflicted solar burns for secondary gain (limited duty, noncombat status, medical discharge) have been documented in military personnel). Solar retinitis associated with drug abuse should be considered in young patients who present with blurred vision, metamorphopsia, and central scotomas.

COMMENTS

In solar retinopathy, the visual prognosis is good if the central scotoma subsides or is markedly reduced during the first 4 weeks. Patients who have a final visual recovery of 20/30 or better usually achieve that within 6 weeks of onset. Nevertheless, some patients show gradual visual improvement for periods of as long as 1 year. Approximately 75 per cent of patients with eclipse burns or minimal solar exposure have a final visual acuity of 20/30 or better, but many have metamorphopsia or permanent central or paracentral scotoma or both. Cases of self-inflicted solar retinopathy with a background of mental illness, drug abuse, or malingering usually have more severe retinal damage, with only 35 to 50 per cent attaining a final vision of 20/30 or better.

References

Ewald RA: Sun gazing associated with the use of LSD. Ann Ophthalmol 3:15–17, 1971.

Ewald RA, Ritchey CL: Sun gazing as the cause of foveomacular retinitis. Am J Ophthalmol 70:491–497, 1970.

Gladstone GJ, Tasman W: Solar retinitis after minimal exposure. Arch Ophthalmol 96:1368–1369, 1978.

Mainster MA: Spectral transmittance of intraocular lenses and retinal damage from intense light sources. Am J Ophthalmol 85:167–170, 1978.

Penner R, McNair JN: Eclipse blindness. Report of an epidemic in the military population of Hawaii. Am J Ophthalmol 61:1452–1457, 1966.

Sadun AC, Sadun AA, Sadun LA: Solar retinopathy. A biophysical analysis. Arch Ophthalmol 102:1510–1512, 1984.

Taylor HR, et al: The long-term effects of visible light on the eye. Arch Ophthalmol 110:99–104, 1992.

Young RW: Solar radiation and age-related macular degeneration. Surv Ophthalmol 32:252–269, 1988.

Zigman S: Photohazards of intraocular lens implants in aphakia. Am J Ophthalmol 90:114–115, 1980.

SECTION 30

OPTIC NERVE

COMPRESSIVE OPTIC NEUROPATHIES 377.49

JOHN G. McHENRY, M.D.,
and THOMAS C. SPOOR, M.D., M.S.,
F.A.C.S.

Detroit, Michigan

Compressive optic neuropathies can occur secondary to intrinsic optic nerve sheath meningiomas or masses extrinsic to the intracranial or intraorbital optic nerve. Orbital masses can be intraconal or extraconal. Lacrimal tumors, mucoceles, and invasive sinus tumors are extraconal. Cavernous hemangiomas, schwannomas, and neurofibromas often occur within the muscle cone. Rhabdomyosarcomas, lymphomas, neuroblastomas, and metastases can occur either intraconally or extraconally. Dysthyroid optic neuropathy affects the extraocular muscles themselves, compromising the optic nerve at the orbital apex. Metastatic prostate carcinoma, fibrous dysplasia, Paget's disease of bone, osteopetrosis, and the hyperostoses associated with meningiomas affect the intracanalicular optic nerve. Intracranially, the optic nerve may be compressed by aneurysms and tumors. Intracranial tumors affecting the optic nerve include meningiomas, adenomas, metastatic tumors, and invasive sinus and nasopharyngeal carcinomas.

Compressive optic neuropathies usually manifest as slowly progressive visual loss. However, rapid growth or acute hemorrhage into an intraorbital or intracranial tumor may present with acute visual loss and mimic an acute optic neuropathy. Hemorrhage into a pituitary tumor may present as acute bilateral visual loss.

Computed tomography with contrast enhancement and magnetic resonance imaging with surface coils, gadolinium enhancement, and fat suppression techniques are essential for diagnosis and appropriate treatment.

THERAPY

Surgical. The location of a mass and its radiographic appearance are essential in determining whether the mass will be excised entirely, undergo biopsy, or be debulked. Encapsulated orbital masses may be removed entirely. Irregular orbital masses may undergo biopsy, be debulked, and treated with chemotherapy or radiation therapy. Optic nerve sheath meningiomas are difficult to excise without visual loss. They are usually slowly progressive and do not need to be excised unless they are extending intracranially. Excision then requires a combined orbital-intracranial approach. When there is optic canal compression by a meningioma, fibrous dysplasia, or metastatic prostate carcinoma, the optic canal can be decompressed extracranially through an external ethmoidectomy. The same approach can be used for dysthyroid optic neuropathy. The decompression is completed at the annulus of the optic canal since compression is occurring at the orbital apex. Dysthyroid optic neuropathy unresponsive to external ethmoidectomy and medial orbital decompression can be treated with 2000 rads of radiation of systemic corticosteroids.

PRECAUTIONS

All orbital surgeries are fraught with the possibility of iatrogenic damage to the optic nerve. The surgical field must have complete hemostasis at the conclusion of the operation. Bleeding into the closed orbital space can also cause a compressive optic neuropathy. Significant swelling occurs after any orbital surgery. Patients are routinely placed on 125 mg of intravenous methylprednisolone every 6 hours during the perioperative period to decrease orbital swelling. Because of the associated risk of erosive gastritis, they are also started on 150 mg of ranitidine[§] two times a day.

Extracranial optic canal decompression can be complicated by meningitis, cerebrospinal fluid leaks, pneumocephalus, sinusitis, esotropia, and symptomatic diplopia. The most feared complication is carotid bleeding. If attention is paid to the anatomic landmarks in the sphenoid sinus, the internal carotid artery may be avoided.

COMMENTS

Compressive optic neuropathies should be suspected in any patient with an afferent pupillary defect and optic atrophy, or in patients with a relative afferent pupillary defect (RAPD) and proptosis, injection, or ophthalmoplegia. These patients require a careful visual acuity, examination of the optic nerve head with a 78- or 60-diopter lens, and computerized perimetry with attention to mean deviation. Patients may or may not have optic atrophy, disc swelling, shunt vessels, ophthalmoplegia, injection, chemosis, strabismus, proptosis, pain, resistance to retropulsion, bruits, and periorbital changes. If patients are suspected of having a compressive optic neuropathy, they must undergo a CT scan of the head and orbits with at least 2 mm cuts and axial and coronal views with contrast. Depending on the findings of the CT scan, an MRI may or may not be necessary. Patients with optic atrophy should also have an FTA-ABS and VDRL. Careful attention must be paid to the visual field of the contralateral eye for superotemporal quadrant field defects that are suggestive of a junctional scotoma and an anterior chiasmal mass.

Patients with dysthyroid optic neuropathy will also respond to steroids, which are extremely useful in inflamed orbits. In patients with active hyperthyroidism, it is preferable to control the thyroid disease medically before surgery is attempted. If vision is threatened, the patient can be treated with radiation therapy with concomitant corticosteroids.

After treatment, all patients with compressive optic neuropathies should be followed with visual acuity and computerized perimetry, with attention to the mean deviation of the visual field. Afferent pupillary defects are followed with neutral density filters.

References

Joseph M: Extracranial decompression of the optic canal for frontobasal meningiomas. *In* Schmidek G (ed): Meningiomas and their Surgical Management. Philadelphia, WB Saunders 1991, pp 260–265.

Maniglia DS, Kronberg FG, Culbertson W: Visual loss associated with orbital and sinus diseases. Laryngoscope 94:1050–1059, 1984.

Maroon JL, Kennerdell JS: Surgical approaches to the orbit. J Neurosurg 60:1226–1235, 1984.

Stoll W, Busse H, Kroll P: Decompression of the orbit and the optic nerve in different diseases. J Cranio Maxillo Fac Surg 16:308–311, 1989.

CONGENITAL PIT OF THE OPTIC NERVE 377.4

P. K. MUKHERJEE, M.S.

Raipur, India

A congenital pit is a common anomaly of the development of the optic nerve. However, its presence is not appreciated until it produces defective vision. The frequency of congenital pit of the optic nerve is 1 in 10,000 live births. One-third of individuals with a congenital pit develop defective vision. Clinical features become obvious in the second and third decade, although it has been reported in a child aged 6 years; the oldest reported case was in an individual aged 62. It has no predilection for sex. In 15 to 20 per cent of cases, it is bilateral. Optic nerves with a congenital pit are generally larger than normal.

The color, position, number, and extent of congenital pit of the optic nerve vary. Seventy per cent are seen on the temporal side. This location is most apt to produce retinal pigment epithelium detachment and edema of the macula, which are often initially mistaken as idiopathic central serous retinopathy. Central pits are least likely to produce symptoms.

The number of pits varies from single to multiple. However, it is not the number but the position of the pit that influences the clinical picture. The color of the pit is generally translucent blue, similar to holes in normal lamina cribrosa. However, it may be gray, green, tan, or black. It is suggested that a dark color may not be the real color of the pit, but is due to the inability of light to reach the depth of the pit, which has steep walls. The presence of pigment in the pit may mimic melanocyte of the optic nerve.

The size of the pit may vary from pinhead sized to as large as the cup itself. Sometimes, the pit is covered by glial tissue revealing only a small pit, producing an occult hole. The pit may assume a slit-like or triangular shape. The glial tissue cover may pulsate with underlying retinal vessels. Retinal vessels may emerge or descend in a large pit that may involve about one-third of the disc. Papulomacular vessels are more common in eyes with a congenital pit of the optic nerve.

The exact genesis of a congenital pit of the optic nerve pit is not known. The most accepted view is that it is produced by the improper closure of fetal fissure. The exact mode of inheritance is also not established. Occurrence in siblings is known. The association of coloboma of the optic nerve with a congenital pit has been debated without any definite answer. Peripapillary scleral staphyloma has also been reported with congenital pit of the optic nerve.

Histologically, an optic pit consists of the herniation of dysplastic retina into the collagen-lined pocket extending posteriorly through a defect in the lamina cribrosa to the subarachnoid space. To produce visual symptoms, the pit, which is in fact a narrow channel, must communicate with the subarachnoid space of the optic nerve.

The pit of optic nerve may remain symptom free for a long time. It is most likely to produce a visual defect by the second and third decade. Field defects produced by these pits vary from enlargement of the blind spot to various papulomacular defects in the form of arcuate, paracentral, or centrocecal scotomas.

The most important complication that draws attention to its presence is the development of serous detachment of the sensory retina over the macular region, which may assume a circular form. The most common appearance is a tear-drop detachment with the apex on the lateral wall of the disc. It gradually expands to a rounded shape on the temporal aspect several discs in diameter between the superior and inferior temporal vessels.

Loss of vision with a pit of the optic nerve is more pronounced than that occurring with idiopathic serous detachment of the macula. It may produce metamorphopsia or relative scotoma. The exact nature of the detachment is not clear. The origin of fluid is still a matter of debate, but attention is now focused on two possibilities: vitreous and cerebrospinal fluid. Vascular leak from choroidal and retinal vessels has been excluded by fluorescein fundus angiography. Radio-isotope cisternography has failed to demonstrate any evidence of direct communication between the subarachnoid space and subretinal space.

In some eyes, cloudy precipitates may occur on the posterior surface of the detached retina, giving a false notion of solid detachment. With the passage of time, depigmentation of the detached retina occurs. Cystic retinal degeneration, marked thinning, and macular formation are common. The macular hole may be lamellar or full thickness. Subretinal neovascularization has often been reported in longstanding cases; neovascularization starts from the disc.

Fluorescein angiography has failed to show any leak from either the retinal or choroidal vascular system, which is the rule in idiopathic central serous retinopathy. However, in longstanding cases where subretinal neovascularization has taken place, new vessels may stand out prominently. In the early phase of fluorescein angiography, the pit is hypofluorescent, but in the late phase, it may show positive staining. Staining is more common with a retinal pigment epithelium detachment.

Spontaneous reattachment of the macula occurs in 25 per cent of cases. Reattachment may take place months or years after detachment, even without treatment. Reattachment is always associated with degenerative changes; hence, visual improvement is not possible.

Posterior vitreous detachment and vitreous bands have been reported. These bands when attached to the detachment have a poor prognosis.

THERAPY

Ocular. Treatment of a congenital pit of the optic nerve is always a disappointment due to the lack of precise knowledge of its exact mechanism and natural course. Attempts have been made to close the narrow neck of detachment at the optic nerve by various methods including photocoagulation. Photocoagulation of the pit itself has also been tried without much improvement. However, photocoagulation may enhance settlement of the detachment in a shorter period.

Surgical. If the macular detachment is associated with vitreous traction, a vitrectomy is attempted. A combination of vitrectomy, intravitreal gas, and photocoagulation may bring about reattachment, but visual improvement is not possible due to degenerative changes already present.

Ocular or Periocular Manifestations

Macula: Partial or full-thickness holes; subretinal neovascularization.

Optic Nerve: Coloboma of the disc; papulomacular vessel.

Retina: Cloudy precipitates on the back of a detached retina; depigmentation of the detached retina; cystic, retinal degeneration; serous detachment of retinal pigment epithelium.

Vitreous: Posterior vitreous detachment; traction bands.

PRECAUTIONS

The efficacy of photocoagulation should always be balanced against its possible damage to the papulomacular nerve fibers of the retina, which are likely to be damaged permanently.

COMMENTS

In all cases of central serous retinopathy, the optic nerve should be scanned carefully for the presence of pits. A case of central serous retinopathy that fails to reveal any vascular leak should always arouse suspicion of an optic pit. In unilateral cases, the other eye should be examined, and the patient should be warned about the possibility of occult holes. Even the siblings should be screened for the possibility of optic pits.

References

Alexander TA, Billson FA: Vitrectomy and photocoagulation in the management of serous detachment associated with optic disc pits. Aust J Ophthalmol 12:139, 1984.

Brockhurst RJ: Optic pits and posterior retinal detachment. Trans Am Ophthalmol Soc 73:264, 1975.

Gass JDM: Serous detachment of macula secondary to congenital pit of optic nerve head. Am J Ophthalmol 67:821, 1969.

Gordon R, Chatfield RK: Pits in optic disc associated with macular degeneration. Br J Ophthalmol 53:481, 1969.

Jack MK: Central serous retinopathy with optic pit treated with photocoagulation. Am J Ophthalmol 67:519, 1969.

Jay WM, Pope J Jr, Riffle JF: Juxtapapillary subretinal neovascularization associated with congenital pit of the optic nerve. Am J Ophthalmol 97: 655, 1984.

Sadun AA: Optic disc pits and associated serous macular detachment. Retina 799:805, 1989.

Sugar HS: Congenital pits in the optic disc and their equivalents associated with submacular fluids. Am J Ophthalmol 63:298, 1967.

DRUG-INDUCED OPTIC ATROPHY 377.34

ROBERTO GUERRA, M.D.

Modena, Italy

Several drugs are considered potential causes of optic atrophy. Those known agents that may cause optic atrophy include amiodarone, barbiturates, chloramphenicol, chloroquine, cisplatin, corticosteroids, digoxin, disulfiram, ergotamine, ethambutol, halogenated 8-hydroxyquinolines, hexachlorophene, hexamethonium, iodide compounds, isoniazid, lithium carbonate, monoamine oxidase inhibitors, nitroso ureas, oral contraceptives, penicillamine, perhexiline, phenothiazines, streptomycin, tryparsamide, and vincristine. Metronidazole, 2',3'-dideoxyinosine (ddI), ciprofloxacin and ofloxacin have been recently added to the suspect list. Optic neuropathy has been described as a rare complication with the use of several vaccines, including rabies, small pox, trivalent measles, mumps and rubella, diphtheria, and BCG. The cocaine-exposed newborn may have optic nerve abnormalities and delayed visual maturation.

Renal or hepatic failure, diabetes, arteriosclerosis, and alcoholism may enhance the neuropathic effect of the drugs. Optic atrophy is often associated with deficiencies of vitamin B_{12}, amino acids, and zinc.

A high incidence of optic neuropathies is caused by antitubercular agents. Ethambutol-induced optic neuropathy is rare with daily doses not exceeding 25 mg/kg. However, visual pattern-evoked potentials may reveal a high percentage of subclinical optic neuropathies during treatment. Spontaneous resolution usually occurs within 3 months of ethambutol withdrawal, although not always, and the loss of central vision may be permanent.

THERAPY

Ocular. Discontinuation of the suspected drug at the first sign of optic nerve dysfunction remains the most efficient treatment. If a chelating zinc agent, ethambutol, isoniazid, penicillamine, or quinolines are suspected, 100 to 250 mg of oral zinc sulfate[‡] three times daily may be given. Zinc does not seem to be of value if optic atrophy is far advanced. When vision does not improve within 10 to 15 weeks after ethambutol discontinuation, the only seemingly successful treatment reported is the parenteral administration of 40 mg of hydroxocobalamin.[§] This dose should be given for 10 to 28 weeks. Most patients treated this way usually recover full vision. Low serum levels of vitamin B_{12} and zinc have been found in patients with tobacco-alcohol amblyopia, and 20 mg of daily intramuscular hydroxocobalamin[§] for 4 weeks may be more effective than the usual 1-mg dose. Optic neuropathy induced by a ketogenic diet can be reversed by oral thiamine[‡], 50 mg daily for 6 to 12 weeks.

Ocular or Periocular Manifestations

Optic Nerve: Atrophy; pallor, papilledema.
Other: Blindness; central scotoma; constriction of visual fields; blue-yellow/red-green dyschromatopsia; hemianopsia.

PRECAUTIONS

The protracted administration of large doses of parenteral hydroxocobalamin did not cause adverse reactions in one series of 22 cases of ethambutol optic neuropathy. Zinc therapy seems to be theoretically sound because inherited or acquired zinc deficiency causes visual impairment and optic atrophy. Although its ability to restore some visual function has not been ascertained, oral zinc administration seems to be of value in correcting many general manifestations of zinc deficiencies. Because oral supplementary zinc sulfate may cause gastrointestinal irritation, zinc gluconate may be preferred. The amount of zinc administered depends on individual tolerance.

COMMENTS

Zinc serum levels should be checked in all optic neuropathies because a close correlation exists with the clinical course of the disease. Unfortunately, oral supplementary zinc did not prove effective in restoring vision, except in tobacco-alcohol amblyopia. More clinical work is needed to establish whether different zinc compounds, doses, and routes of administration will prove more effective. Hydroxocobalamin effectiveness is based on a still small number of observations and should be confirmed by more extensive studies. A prospective approach could be offered by gangliosides and glycosphingolipids, which have been reported to play a role in activating neuronal membrane enzymes. The number of toxic optic neuropathies treated with gangliosides is still too small to evaluate.

References

Bechetoille A, et al: Therapeutic effects of zinc sulfate on central scotoma due to optic neuropathy in men exhibiting excessive smoking and drinking habits. J Fr Ophthalmol 6:237–242, 1983 (Cited in Surv Ophthalmol 28:420, 1984).

Dette TM, et al: Visuell Evozierte Kortikale Potentiale zur Fruherkennung der Neuritis nervi optici unter Ethambutol therapie. Forschr Ophthalmol 88:546–548, 1991.

Good WV, et al: Abnormalities of the visual system in infants exposed to cocaine. Ophthalmology 99:341–346, 1992.

Guerra R, Casu L: Hydroxocobalamin for ethambutol-induced optic neuropathy. Lancet 2:1176, 1981.

Karcioglu ZA: Zinc in the eye. Surv Ophthalmol 27:114–122, 1982.

Lafeuillade A, et al: Optic neuritis associated with dideoxyinosine. Lancet 337:615–616, 1991.

Motolese E, et al: Neuropatia ottica tossica dopo somministrazione di chinolonici. Boll Ocul 69: 1011–1013, 1990.

Putnam D, et al: Metronidazole and optic neuritis. Am J Ophthalmol 112:737, 1991.

Vrabec TR, et al: Reversible visual loss in a patient receiving high-dose ciprofloxacin hydrochloride (Cipro). Ophthalmology 97:707–710, 1990.

Yen MY, Liu JH: Bilateral optic neuritis following Bacille Calmette-Guerin (BCG) vaccination. J Clin Neuro-Ophthalmol 11:246–249, 1991.

INFLAMMATORY OPTIC NEUROPATHIES 377.39

JOHN G. McHENRY, M.D.,
and THOMAS C. SPOOR, M.D., M.S., F.A.C.S.

Detroit, Michigan

Inflammatory optic neuropathies can be separated into those in which the inflammation occurs intradurally and those in which the inflammation occurs within the orbit and secondarily affects the optic nerve. These diseases can all be treated with corticosteroids. Their response to corticosteroids differentiates them from infectious optic neuropathies, which also have an inflammatory component but may be worsened by corticosteroids.

Inflammation within the optic nerve sheath can cause either an optic neuritis or an adhesive arachnoiditis. Inflammatory optic neuritides, such as systemic lupus erythematosis and sarcoidosis, may be associated with distended optic nerve sheaths and subarachnoid fluid surrounding the optic nerve, but intracranial pressure is not raised.

The diagnosis of optic neuritis is clinical. Patients are typically between the ages of 20 and 50 (mean, 30 to 35). Slightly more females are affected than males. The major symptom is visual loss. Visual function gradually decreases over several hours to several days. Rarely vision may decline over several weeks. Visual acuity varies from 20/25 to NLP. Color vision is reduced. Patients may complain of prodromal pain behind or above the eye. Some investigators feel that the pain is related to the inflammation of small terminal branches of the trigeminal nerve of the optic nerve sheath. Others feel that the pain is initiated by inflammation of the attachments of the ocular muscles to the optic nerve sheath. Occasionally the patients experience phosphenes.

Visual field defects are variable. Although the classical visual field defect is a central or centrocecal scotoma, any defect is possible. An afferent pupillary defect is almost always present. Other tests of optic nerve function include contrast sensitivity and visually evoked response tests. As the diagnosis is clinical, these tests are often superfluous.

Twenty to 40 per cent of patients with optic neuritis have some degree of optic disc swelling. Some patients have peripapillary flame-shaped hemorrhages, and some have vitreous cells. If there is extensive intraocular inflammation, a systemic disease should be suspected. Sheathing of the retinal veins can occur with anterior optic neuritis. When vitreous cells and venous sheathing is present, sarcoidosis or multiple sclerosis should be suspected.

Fifty per cent of patients will recover vision to 20/30 or better in 1 month. Seventy-five per cent recover to 20/30 or better within 6 months. Only 8 per cent will have vision worse than 20/200 after 6 months. The final outcome is unrelated to optic disc appearance. If visual acuity is going to improve, it usually will return rapidly over several days to weeks. Further recovery occurs slowly. However, even when visual acuity is 20/20 after recovery, there are abnormalities in contrast sensitivity and visual field.

Following optic neuritis, some patients describe transient visual blurring during exercise, a hot bath, or emotional stress (Uthoff's sign). It is most common in patients with multiple sclerosis, but it is also experienced in patients after idiopathic optic neuritis or Leber's optic neuropathy.

The evaluation of optic neuritis begins with a complete history and neuro-ophthalmic examination. In a patient under 45 years of age with pain on eye movement, visual acuity and field deficits, and optic disc swelling, the diagnosis is fairly straightforward. On examination, attention is paid to visual acuity. Afferent pupillary defects are graded with neutral density fibers. Computerized perimetry is performed, and attention is paid to mean deviation and corrected pattern standard deviation. Stereo disc photos are also obtained.

Optic neuritis in children presents differently and has a better prognosis than optic neuritis in adults. Disc swelling is found in more than 70 per cent of children. Fifty per cent have bilateral involvement. The majority of children have central scotomas. Visual acuity is usually less than 20/200. In spite of such poor vision on presentation, however, the visual prognosis is quite good. Complete recovery is typical, and recurrences are not as frequent as in adults. Neuroretinitis with disc swelling, peripapillary exudates, exudative retinal detachments, and macular stars are common. Fifty per cent of the patients with neuroretinitis have a history of a mild upper respiratory tract infection 1 to 2 weeks before the onset of visual symptoms. Unlike adults, children with optic neuritis rarely develop multiple sclerosis.

Optic neuritis may occur at any time during the course of multiple sclerosis. In one series in which patients were followed for 7 years, 20 per cent developed definite multiple sclerosis. Forty-five per cent of women and 11 per cent of men developed multiple sclerosis. The highest risk (51 per cent) occurred in the third decade. In another series with a mean follow-up of 7.6 years, 51 per cent of patients developed multiple sclerosis. A recent prospective study found that 74 per cent of women and 34 per cent of men presenting with mono-symptomatic optic neuritis developed multiple sclerosis over a 15-year period. Patients with pain or bilateral involvement are not more likely to develop multiple sclerosis, although recurrent attacks are more often associated with its development. Visual outcome has no bearing on whether optic neuritis will develop into multiple sclerosis. In a series of United States service men, neither race nor birth place was found to be significant.

Some patients with optic nerve inflammation do not manifest visual loss. These patients have perineuritis. Pathological specimens demonstrate polymorphonuclear optic nerve sheath arachnoid infiltration. The diagnosis is made after a lumbar puncture reveals normal intracranial pressure (ICP). A vascular etiology may underlie the disc swelling of some of these patients. Rickettsial inflammation of the blood vessels of the optic nerve may lead to disc swelling with normal ICP and normal vision.

Orbital inflammatory processes can secondarily involve the optic nerve. Patients with orbital inflammation present with variable pain, swelling, chemosis, proptosis, injection, warmth, and erythema that may be unilateral or bilateral. CT scanning is essential. Idiopathic orbital inflammation may present as an irregular mass, sinus disease, lacrimal gland enlargement, or an enlargement of the extraocular muscles without sparing of the tendons.

THERAPY

Ocular. The patient with optic neuritis is offered admission to the hospital. Neuroimaging (magnetic resonance with gadolinium enhancement) and lumbar puncture are performed before starting the patient on 500 mg IV methylprednisolone every 6 hours for 3 days. The drug is then tapered rapidly. Exquisitely steroid-responsive optic neuropathies that worsen upon tapering steroids

should suggest the possibility of an occult malignancy. Optic neuritis associated with collagen vascular diseases, such as systemic lupus erythematosis and sarcoidosis, may have poor responses and require extended therapy. The same regime may be used in patients with multiple sclerosis. Devic's disease is also responsive to steroids; however, extended therapy may be necessary. As there is no visual loss in perineuritis, the patient is followed with visual fields, photos, and visual acuity. If a patient is suspected of having orbital inflammation, treatment with 80 mg of prednisone daily and 150 mg of ranitidine two times a day for 2 weeks should be started. The patient is then re-examined. If there is improvement, steroid treatment is continued for 2 weeks and then gradually tapered by 20 mg/week until the patient is taking 20 mg/day. The patient is again re-examined. Recurrences are frequent, and steroids may be required at a higher level. Eventually steroids are tapered and discontinued. Patients who are unresponsive to treatment or recur after appropriate treatment undergo biopsy.

PRECAUTIONS

Patients treated with corticosteroids are also started on 150 mg of raniditine two times a day to prevent erosive gastritis and upper GI hemorrhage. The complications of steroid use are infrequent in patients under 60 years of age. Inflammatory optic neuropathies are unusual in patients over 45 years of age except for recurrent episodes of optic neuritis in patients with multiple sclerosis. Optic neuritis of the elderly may mimic nonarteritic anterior ischemic optic neuropathy; however, visual function often improves spontaneously and is usually diagnosed after the patient has recovered. A 45- to 60-year-old individual who is treated with intravenous corticosteroids and recovers visual function would most likely have optic neuritis. The use of intravenous megadose corticosteroids in patients older than 60 is associated with a high rate of arrhythmias, hypervolemia, myocardial infarction, and stroke. When steroids are used, they should be tapered rapidly, and the patient should be monitored for these problems.

COMMENTS

The optic neuritis treatment trial showed no significant difference in visual acuity ($P = 0.6$) after 6 months in patients treated with intravenous methylprednisolone and patients who were observed. However, visual field mean deviation did improve ($P = .056$). There was also significant improvement in color vision and contrast sensitivity. *Treatment solely with oral prednisone actually increased the risk of recurrence within 6 months of the initial episode and consequently is contraindicated.*

Fifty to eighty per cent of patients with optic neuritis develop some degree of optic disc pallor. The pallor is usually temporal, but may be generalized.

Since approximately 40 per cent of patients may have recurrent episodes, it is reasonable to treat optic neuritis aggressively with intravenous corticosteroids. If more of the optic nerve can initially be saved, more functioning axons are available if there is a recurrence.

References

Beck RW: Optic neuritis or anterior ischemic optic neuropathy? Arch Ophthalmol 110:1357, 1992.

Beck RW, Cleary PA, Anderson MM Jr, Keltner JL, Shults WT, Kaufman DI, Buckley EG, Corbett JJ, Kupersmith MJ, Miller NR, et al: A randomized controlled trial of corticosteroids in the treatment of acute optic neuritis. The Optic Neuritis Study Group. N Engl J Med 326:581–588, 1992.

Glaser JS: Optic neuritis and ischemic neuropathy. What we thought we already knew (Editorial; comment). Arch Ophthalmol 109:1666–1667, 1991.

Optic Neuritis Study Group: The clinical profile of optic neuritis: Experience of the Optic Neuritis Treatment Trial. Arch Ophthalmol 109:1673–1678, 1991.

Rizzo JF, Lessell S: Risk of developing multiple sclerosis after uncomplicated optic neuritis: A long-term prospective study. Neurology 38:185–190, 1988.

Spoor TC, Rockwell DL: Treatment of optic neuritis with intravenous megadose corticosteroids: A consecutive series. Ophthalmology 95:131–134, 1988.

ISCHEMIC OPTIC NEUROPATHY 377.41

SOHAN SINGH HAYREH, M.D., Ph.D., D.Sc., F.R.C.S.

Iowa City, Iowa

Ischemic optic neuropathy (ION) is a severe disease that causes blindness of sudden onset. The disorder comprises two distinct entities: anterior (AION) and posterior (PION) ischemic optic neuropathy. The former is an ischemic disorder involving the optic nerve head (supplied by the posterior ciliary artery circulation), whereas the latter is caused by occlusion of one or more nutrient arteries to the rest of the optic nerve. ION is multifactorial in origin, with usually many contributory risk factors. The common risk factors include atherosclerosis, arteriosclerosis, local microvascular disorders, diabetes mellitus, and arterial hypertension. Nocturnal hypotension is an important precipitating factor in AION in vulnerable persons with other vascular risk factors. However, the most important cause, particularly for posterior ciliary artery occlusion, is giant cell (temporal or cranial) arteritis,

which usually affects individuals in their sixties or older. Other less common causes include collagen vascular diseases, embolism, and massive systemic hemorrhages. Thus, AION can be subdivided into (1) arteritic (due to giant cell arteritis) and (2) nonarteritic (due to other causes) types.

Anterior ischemic optic neuropathy is a common blinding disorder in middle-aged and older persons, although no age is immune from it. The erroneous impression that it is a rare disease seen only in the elderly is based on lack of adequate knowledge and, sadly, results in frequent misdiagnosis.

The onset of AION is usually characterized by a sudden, painless, unilateral visual loss, mostly sectoral, although it is frequently total in giant cell arteritis. Occasionally, it may be progressive initially. Visual acuity may vary from no perception of light to perfectly normal central vision. The most important finding is the visual field defect, and the most common field defects in AION are inferior nasal, inferior altitudinal, and central scotoma. Other optic-disc-related visual field defects may include segmental, superior altitudinal, nerve fiber, or vertical defects and peripheral constriction. In AION, the optic disc initially shows on ophthalmoscopy a pink or pale-pink edema with frequent flame-shaped hemorrhages at the disc margin or adjacent retina. In half of the eyes with arteritic AION, the disc shows a characteristic chalky-white swelling with only a rare hemorrhage. In diabetics, the disc may be covered with a network of prominent fine vessels, mimicking neovascularization and thus leading to a mistaken diagnosis of proliferative diabetic retinopathy. The optic disc edema usually starts to subside in a couple of weeks, completely disappears in a couple of months, and leaves pallor of the disc that often has little correlation to the visual acuity or location of the visual field defects.

Once a diagnosis of AION is made, the most important first step is to differentiate arteritic from nonarteritic AION because blindness from giant cell arteritis is almost entirely preventable if diagnosed early and treated promptly. The differentiation can be made by the combined information applied by the following parameters: (1) systemic symptoms of giant cell arteritis; (2) amaurosis fugax episodes preceding the development of AION or in patients diagnosed to have giant cell arteritis; (3) elevated erythrocyte sedimentation rate (ESR) and C-reactive protein (CRP); (4) early massive visual loss varying from hand motion to no light perception; (5) chalky-white optic disc swelling; (6) evidence of posterior ciliary artery occlusion on fluorescein angiography, i.e. massive filling defect of the choroid, and (7) temporal artery biopsy. The author has found that combined information from these seven parameters can almost always help differentiate arteritic from nonarteritic AION, although no one of them is seen in every single case of giant cell arteritis.

AION is potentially a bilaterally crippling disease. The estimated 25th-percentile time to development of bilateral AION is much shorter in patients with arteritic AION (0.4 months) than in those with nonarteritic AION (32.4 months). In the author's series of cases of arteritic AION, AION (unilateral or bilateral) had almost invariably developed before systemic steroid therapy was started and did not develop after, indicating that this therapy is effective in preventing the development of AION in giant cell arteritis. Young diabetic males had the highest risk of developing bilateral AION.

Posterior ischemic optic neuropathy is much less common than AION. Its two most common causes are giant cell arteritis and collagen vascular diseases. There is a sudden visual loss and optic-nerve-related visual field defects. The visual acuity may vary from normal to no light perception. The fundus shows no abnormality (on ophthalmoscopy or fluorescein fundus angiography) at onset of the disease nor for about a month thereafter, but after about 5 to 6 weeks the optic disc develops pallor.

THERAPY

Supportive. Giant cell arteritis, with or without ION, is an ocular emergency. Since arteritic ION is a blinding disease with poor prognosis for recovery of vision and with a high risk of the second eye being involved soon after the first, the most important prophylactic measures are early and correct diagnosis of giant cell arteritis and prompt institution of aggressive systemic corticosteroid therapy.

Systemic. When in doubt, AION in persons over the age of 60 years should be regarded as caused by giant cell arteritis, particularly if a patient suddenly develops complete blindness in an eye, which sometimes may be preceded by attacks of transient amaurosis. The treatment is to institute anti-inflammatory therapy immediately with oral systemic corticosteroids in sufficiently high doses: 80 to 120 mg or even more of prednisone daily. In some patients, even megadose (equivalent to 1 gm) intravenous prednisone therapy at 6- to 8-hour intervals over 24 to 48 hours may be required before switching to the oral regimen. The object of the transient is to prevent the loss of vision in the second eye; it rarely produces any worthwhile visual recovery. The duration of high-dose therapy is guided by the response of ESR and CRP levels to treatment—a high dose is maintained until the levels of ESR and CRP reach the lowest stable stage (usually in 2 to 3 weeks). After that, prednisone is very gradually tapered down, maintaining the lowest levels of ESR and CRP. All these patients require a main-

tenance dose of prednisone to keep the disease under suppression, and determination of maintenance dose is a very slow and laborious process. The guiding principle in the reduction of prednisone and the determination of a maintenance dose is to titrate the dose of prednisone to keep the ESR and CRP at levels as low as possible. There is no other satisfactory standard for regulating corticosteroid therapy in these patients, and every patient reacts differently, so that no generalization is possible. These patients require prolonged corticosteroid therapy, usually for years, if not for the rest of their lives, and suddenly reducing or stopping the drug prematurely may produce visual loss.

Patients presenting with AION or PION caused by collagen vascular disease should be treated with high doses of systemic corticosteroids during the initial stages of the disease, before the onset of optic disc pallor. The treatment regimen is a starting dose of at least 80 mg of oral prednisone daily, continuing on this dosage for 2 weeks, and then slowly tapering to a maintenance dose of not less than 40 mg daily so long as the disc shows edema, which lasts for a maximum of 4 to 8 weeks from its onset. There may be a significant recovery of visual function in some of these patients after very early and adequate corticosteroid therapy.

There is no well-established treatment available for nonarteritic AION; however, in the author's series, a proportion of cases have achieved significant visual recovery in response to treatment with high doses of systemic corticosteroids when administered during the initial stages of the disease while the disc is edematous; this excellent response was found particularly in diabetics. Because the corticosteroids aggravate the diabetes, these patients require very stringent control of their diabetes by a diabetes specialist during corticosteroid therapy. Without such strict control, it may not be safe to give corticosteroid therapy to these patients.

Surgical. Some authorities advocate optic nerve sheath decompression in the treatment of nonarteritic AION, particularly in patients with progressive visual loss. This is a highly controversial treatment. The author, after extensive studies of the subject, finds that this procedure has no known scientific basis at all in the management of non-arteritic AION and could be dangerous.

PRECAUTIONS

In nonarteritic individuals, particularly those with a past history of AION in one eye, a sudden fall in systemic arterial blood pressure or an increase in intraocular pressure (after cataract extraction) should be prevented. The author's studies suggest that nocturnal hypotension is an important risk factor in the development of AION, which is further suggested by the most frequent occurrence of visual loss in AION during sleep. There is evidence that excessive systemic arterial hypotensive medication (especially when taken at bedtime) aggravates nocturnal hypotension, which is a risk factor in these cases. Cataract extraction in the same or fellow normal eye of these patients should be undertaken very cautiously because of the high risk of precipitating AION. All patients with unilateral ION should be warned to contact their physician immediately if there is any visual disturbance in the fellow eye. This measure will promote early diagnosis and the institution of adequate and appropriate therapy.

COMMENTS

Patients with ION caused by giant cell arteritis or collagen vascular disease benefit from corticosteroid treatment because of its anti-inflammatory property. In nonarteritic AION with diabetes mellitus or due to causes other than vasculitis, the rationale for corticosteroid treatment may be seriously questioned. Corticosteroids have many other properties as well as their anti-inflammatory one; one of them is to reduce capillary permeability. Administration of large doses of systemic corticosteroids is a standard and well-established treatment for cerebral edema of any etiology. Anoxia in ION most probably leads to increased vascular permeability of the optic nerve head capillaries, contributing partly at least to edema of the optic disc. The edema is an important factor in the production of visual loss, impeding further capillary circulation in the optic nerve head. This finding indicates that optic disc edema precedes visual loss. Corticosteroids probably reduce edema in ION by lowering capillary permeability and helping restore the circulation and function of the still surviving, although nonfunctioning, nerve fibers.

If systemic corticosteroid therapy is to show beneficial effects in ION caused by collagen vascular diseases, diabetes mellitus, or causes other than vasculitis, the treatment must be instituted at the earliest possible time while the optic disc still shows a fair amount of edema and recovery of axons is still possible. The chances of visual recovery are much greater if the treatment is started within 2 weeks after the onset of AION. Once the disc has become atrophic, no treatment is worthwhile, and it is pointless to use corticosteroids. The degree of recovery depends upon the amount of ischemic damage already inflicted, as well as upon the time lapse between the onset of AION and the start of treatment.

By no means do all cases show improvement, even if treatment is started promptly and vigorously; some even show further deterioration while on treatment. Since the treatment is given for no more than 4 to 6 weeks at the maximum, none of the serious side effects associated with long-term corticosteroid therapy is seen in most cases, except those with diabetes mellitus.

In addition to corticosteroid therapy, every attempt should be made to reduce the intraocular pressure to as low a level as possible in patients with AION, with a view to improving perfusion pressure in the optic disc vessels. (Perfusion pressure is equal to the mean blood pressure minus the intraocular pressure.) Any risk of marked nocturnal arterial hypotension should also be minimized.

References

Beri M, Klugman MR, Kohler JA, Hayreh SS: Anterior ischemic optic neuropathy. VII. Incidence of bilaterality and various influencing factors. Ophthalmology 94:1020–1028, 1987.

Hayreh SS: Anterior ischaemic optic neuropathy. III. Treatment, prophylaxis, and differential diagnosis. Br J Ophthalmol 58:981–989, 1974.

Hayreh SS: Anterior Ischemic Optic Neuropathy. New York, Springer-Verlag, 1975.

Hayreh SS: Anterior ischemic optic neuropathy. IV. Occurrence after cataract extraction. Arch Ophthalmol 98:1410–1416, 1980.

Hayreh SS: Anterior ischemic optic neuropathy. Arch Neurol 38:675–678, 1981.

Hayreh SS: Anterior ischemic optic neuropathy. V. Optic disc edema an early sign. Arch Ophthalmol 99:1030–1040, 1981.

Hayreh SS: Posterior ischemic optic neuropathy. Ophthalmologica 182:29–41, 1981.

Hayreh SS: Anterior ischemic optic neuropathy. VII. Clinical features and pathogenesis of posthemorrhage amaurosis. Ophthalmology 94:1488–1502, 1987.

Hayreh SS: Anterior ischaemic optic neuropathy: Differentiation of arteritic from nonarteritic type and its management. Eye 4:25–41, 1990.

Hayreh SS: The role of optic nerve sheath fenestration in management of anterior ischemic optic neuropathy. Arch Ophthalmol 108:1063–1064, 1990.

Hayreh SS: Ophthalmic features of giant cell arteritis. Clin Rheumatol 5:431–459, 1991.

Hayreh SS, Podhajsky P: Visual field defects in anterior ischemic optic neuropathy. In Greve EL (ed): Third International Visual Field Symposium. The Hague, Junk, 1979, pp 347–365.

Hayreh SS, Zahoruk RM: Anterior ischemic optic neuropathy. VI. In juvenile diabetics. Ophthalmologica 182:13–28, 1981.

Sergott RC, Cohen MS, Bosley TM, Savino PJ: Optic nerve decompression may improve the progressive form of nonarteritic ischemic optic neuropathy. Arch Ophthalmol 107:1743–1754, 1989.

OPTIC NEURITIS 377.30
(Papillitis, Retrobulbar Neuritis)

THOMAS C. SPOOR, M.D., M.S., F.A.C.S.,
Detroit, Michigan
and JOHN M. RAMOCKI, M.D.
Bloomfield Hills, Michigan

Optic neuritis is an inflammatory process affecting the optic nerve that may be secondary to viral, demyelinating, or autoimmune disease. The typical clinical picture occurs between 15 and 45 years of age and includes acute monocular loss of vision associated with retrobulbar pain, tenderness, and pain on ocular movement. These symptoms may be less severe when seen with acute retrobulbar neuritis. Examination reveals a relative afferent pupillary defect, dyschromatopsia, and a visual field defect, usually in the form of a central or cecocentral scotoma, but any visual field defect may be present. The majority of patients have retrobulbar neuritis and a normal-appearing optic disc during the acute episode. The patients sees nothing and the doctor sees nothing unless a relative afferent pupillary defect was elicited before dilating the pupils. In patients with papillitis, the optic nervehead is swollen with edema and hemorrhage present in the peripapillary nerve fiber layer.

Papillitis after viral respiratory infection tends to resolve and has a benign visual and neurologic prognosis without treatment. Optic neuropathies secondary to intrinsic demyelination (multiple sclerosis) result in recovery of good vision, with 75 to 90 per cent of patients achieving a visual acuity of 20/30 after 6 months. Visual recovery usually starts after 7 days, and full recovery may take weeks to months. However, studies have shown that 50 to 80 per cent of patients experience some degree of optic atrophy, and all patients reportedly develop a detectable nerve fiber layer defect after an episode of acute optic neuritis. Those patients with optic neuritis secondary to autoimmune disease, although clinically demonstrating a similar clinical picture to those described above, tend to manifest an atypical clinical course and suffer irreversible visual loss.

The initial diagnostic evaluation should include complete blood count, erythrocyte sedimentation rate, antinuclear antibody test, complement (C_3, C_4), serologic test for syphilis (FTA-ABS, VDRL), chest x-ray to detect specifically treatable entities, and formal visual fields to document baseline visual function. Data derived from the Optic Neuritis Treatment Trial (ONTT) indicate that extensive laboratory and radiologic testing is unproductive in patients with typical optic neuritis.

THERAPY

Systemic. The use of systemic corticosteroids in the treatment of optic neuritis is now less controversial than in the past. Earlier controlled studies failed to demonstrate any difference in the long-term outcome of patients with optic neuritis treated with pharmacologic doses of systemic corticosteroids. However, corticosteroids have been shown to shorten the duration of the acute attack in patients, presumably by decreasing the perineural inflammation, lessening axoplasmic stagnation, and reducing neuronal death.

Recent studies have shown that the clinical response to treatment with high-dose systemic corticosteroids may differ from the untreated natural course or from the clinical course of optic neuritis altered with pharmacologic doses of steroids. Visual acuity and visual fields seem to improve more rapidly (days versus weeks) in patients treated with high-dose corticosteroids. Additionally, progressive visual deterioration has not only been shown to be arrested but even reversed in some cases.

The recently completed Optic Neuritis Treatment Trial (ONTT) demonstrated that patients treated with intravenous methylprednisolone, 250 mg every 6 hours for 3 days, followed by 11 days of oral prednisone, had a more rapid recovery of vision and better visual function at 6 months follow-up than the placebo-treated control group. There were few significant side effects. Patients treated with oral prednisone alone had an increased incidence of repeat attacks of optic neuritis in the affected and the fellow eye. Subsequently, the use of oral prednisone alone is *not effective* treatment for optic neuritis and seems to increase the incidence of repeat attacks of optic neuritis. Treatment of typical optic neuritis with oral prednisone should be discouraged. Patients presenting with visual acuity worse than 20/40 or a marked loss of visual field should be treated immediately with high-dose intravenous methylprednisolone as described above.

Although the ONTT demonstrated that laboratory and neuroradiologic imaging was unproductive in patients with *typical* optic neuritis, the authors do obtain appropriate neuroimaging (CT or MR) and serologies in all patients with *atypical* optic neuritis.

The authors' present approach to management of patients with optic neuritis is predicted upon the initial visual function. Patients with visual acuity of 20/40 or better and mild visual field defects are observed for 7 to 14 days. If visual acuity or visual field deteriorates, they are treated with 250 to 500 mg intravenous methylprednisolone every 6 hours for 3 days, followed by a tapering course of oral prednisone 80 mg daily × 3 days, 60 mg daily × 3 days, 40 mg daily × 3 days, 20 mg daily × 3 days, and 10 mg daily × 3 days. Patients presenting with visual acuity worse than 20/40 or markedly compromised visual fields are offered treatment with the above regimen.

After treatment, visual acuity and fields are

followed weekly for 1 month, monthly for 3 months, and then every 6 months. These follow-up intervals are arbitrary. The true natural course of untreated optic neuritis, as well as that treated with megadose corticosteroids, is presently being studied in the cohort of patients enrolled in the ONTT.

Ocular. Periocular,* transeptal,* and retrobulbar* corticosteroids may also be given. Although these modes of steroid therapy may accelerate the recovery period, they offer no significant long-term benefit over untreated controls. Additionally, the potential risks of such treatment—namely, penetration of the globe or optic nerve—make local therapy less desirable than a short course of high-dose corticosteroids.

Ocular or Periocular Manifestations

Optic Nerve: Disc edema; disc hyperemia, late disc pallor; late nerve fiber layer dropout; nerve fiber layer exudates; splinter hemorrhages.
Pupil: Diminished light response; relative afferent pupillary defect.
Retina: Circinate maculopathy; exudates; hemorrhage; nerve fiber layer edema (peripapillary).
Uvea: Inflammatory cells in posterior segment.
Visual Fields: Arcuate defects; dyschromatopsia; photophobia; retrobulbar pain that increases with eye movement.

PRECAUTIONS

Since any entity that compresses the optic nerve (i.e., aneurysms, tumors, inflammatory masses) may mimic the clinical picture seen with optic neuritis, it is important to rule these conditions out, especially because they too may respond initially to systemic high-dose corticosteroids. Additionally, steroid therapy is not innocuous. Adverse reactions to systemic corticosteroids have been reported in 16.9 per cent of consecutively monitored hospitalized patients. Daily systemic corticosteroid treatment may be complicated by multiple, potentially serious side effects, including cataract formation, superinfection, electrolyte imbalance, leukocytosis, gastrointestinal bleeding, acute psychosis, aseptic necrosis of bone, hypertension, and hyperglycemia. These side effects may produce considerable morbidity and even mortality. The authors routinely administer H$_2$ blockers—ranitidine (Zantac) 150 mg by mouth twice daily—to patients treated with systemic corticosteroids. To minimize treatment complications, it is suggested that a thorough examination be conducted before treatment is begun, including a CT scan to detect a subtle sinusitis or mass lesion, a cerebrospinal fluid examination to detect subclinical infection, a neurologic evaluation to document mental status and detect subtle neurologic defects, and a general medical evaluation to detect electrolyte abnormalities, renal dysfunction, or diabetes. Additionally, visual function, mental status, and levels of serum glucose, blood urea-nitrogen, creatinine, and electrolytes are determined daily once therapy is started.

COMMENTS

The ONTT confirmed previous studies demonstrating that patients treated with high-dose intravenous corticosteroids improved more rapidly and had better visual function than those treated with placebo oral prednisone. Since it has been shown that 50 to 80 per cent of patients have some degree of optic atrophy after an acute attack of optic neuritis and therefore have some degree of visual deficit, it seems reasonable that reducing the amount of time that the optic nerve is exposed to compressive inflammatory forces should decrease damage to intraneuronal structures. High-dose systemic corticosteroids might accomplish this purpose.

References

Barnes MP, et al: Intravenous methylprednisolone infusion in multiple sclerosis. Neurology 30:702–708, 1980.
Beck RW: The optic neuritis treatment trial. Arch Ophthalmol 106:1051–1053, 1988.
Beck RW: The optic neuritis treatment trial. Implications for clinical practice. Arch Ophthalmol 110:331–332, 1992.
Beck RW, et al: A randomized, controlled trial of corticosteroids in the treatment of acute optic neuritis. N Engl J Med 326:581–588, 1992.
Bird AC: Is there a place for corticosteroids in the treatment of optic neuritis? *In* Brockhurst RJ, et al (eds): Controversy in Ophthalmology. Philadelphia, WB Saunders, 1977, pp 822–829.
Boston Collaborative Drug Surveillance Program: Acute adverse reactions to prednisone in relation to dosage. Clin Pharmacol Ther 13:694–698, 1972.
Bradley WG, Whitty CWM: Acute optic neuritis: Its clinical features and their relation to prognosis for recovery of vision. J Neurol Neurosurg Psychiatr 30:531–538, 1962.
Cohen MM, Lessell S, Wolf PA: A prospective study of the risk of developing multiple sclerosis in uncomplicated optic neuritis. Neurology 29:208–213, 1979.
Lessell S: Corticosteroid treatment of acute optic neuritis. N Engl J Med 326:634–635, 1992.
Rizzo JF, Lessell S: Risks of developing multiple sclerosis after uncomplicated optic neuritis: A long-term prospective study. Neurology 38:185–190, 1988.
Spoor TC: Treatment of optic neuritis with intravenous megadose corticosteroids. Ophthalmology 95:131–134, 1988.
Wakefield D, McCluskey P, Penny R: Intravenous pulse methylprednisolone therapy in severe inflammatory eye disease. Arch Ophthalmol 104:847–851, 1986.

PAPILLEDEMA 377.00
(Choked Disc)

THOMAS J. WALSH, M.D.

New Haven, Connecticut

Papilledema is noninflammatory congestion of the optic discs brought about by increased intracranial pressure. The most common cause of increased intracranial pressure is a space-occupying lesion, either a primary or metastatic tumor. If no mass or obstruction of cerebrospinal fluid is identified, pseudotumor cerebri should be considered. Since the literature is revealing more and more visual defects with benign intracranial hypertension, the name seems inappropriate. The term "idiopathic intracranial hypertension" is perhaps better, particularly if no specific cause can be identified. There are other nontumor causes of increased intracranial pressure as well. Tumors of the spinal cord and Guillain-Barre disease discharge proteins and other substances into the cerebrospinal fluid that block the absorbing channels of the cerebrospinal fluid and cause increased intracranial pressure. In addition, these substances may also be irritative or toxic and cause an arachnoiditis, which interferes with cerebrospinal fluid absorption, as well as producing an inflammatory reaction around the optic nerves that causes a decrease in vision. Certain disease states, such as nephritis, in combination with or as steroids are discontinued may cause idiopathic intracranial hypertension. It is also associated with such other entities as vitamin A intoxication, birth control pills, and tetracycline. It is therefore important not only to make the diagnosis of idiopathic intracranial hypertension but also to try and establish the cause of it or similar nonspatial-occupying lesions.

Unless careful and repeated evaluations of these patients are made, other causes of increased intracranial pressure may go undiagnosed. These may include gliomas that are isodense on CT, intracranial malignancies, and systemic malignancies that seed the subarachnoid space, such as lymphoma. Cord tumors, such as neurofibromatoses, can cause increased intracranial pressure without hydrocephalus and large ventricles. Infectious disease is always a consideration and may be low grade without the usual cerebral signs or symptoms of fever.

Whatever the cause, increased pressure on the visual systems will sooner or later cause a permanent loss of vision. Johnston and Paterson (1974) performed intraventricular monitoring in 20 patients. The commonest waves were of low amplitude (10 to 20 mm Hg). In eight of the cases plateau waves of 50 to 80 mm Hg lasting from 5 to 20 minutes were superimposed on the basic wave and were separated in time from 60 to 120 minutes. Therefore, a normal or abnormal spinal tap reading of intracranial pressure could be obtained de-

pending on what part of the curve was in place at the time of the tap. Cisternograms revealed a marked delay in the circulation time of cerebral spinal fluid, mostly in the subarachnoid space. The gradual rise in pressure and then its precipitous fall suggest a pressure gradient that is overcome by the rise in pressure at least temporarily. Other authors suggest multiple contributing factors, such as hypertension, to mention only one. Idiopathic intracranial hypertension may not be one disease and therefore may have more than one mechanism.

Corbett (1982) in a series of 57 patients and 114 eyes found vision or field defects in 49 per cent. Severe visual loss occurred in 14 patients, 13 of whom were hypertensive, which was considered a risk factor in idiopathic intracranial hypertension. The eight patients who were blind in that series were in the hypertensive group. Orcutt also demonstrated deficits on a tangent screen in 49 per cent of his cases, a finding that is comparable to Corbett's series. Wall (1987, 1991) in one series of 20 patients demonstrated visual defects in 75 per cent of the patients and in a later series of 50 patients the deficits were in the 96 percentile.

A common misperception about intracranial hypertension is that children with the diagnosis are more resistant to visual loss than adults. Lessell (1986) reported five such cases with visual loss, refuting the previous clinical impressions. However, vision tends to be preserved for a long period of time in the majority of patients with pseudotumor cerebri. This is not true of all cases and cannot be accurately predicted. The physician must follow these cases very carefully, since there is a fine line between judicious observation and neglect.

It is not known why vision tends to do better with increased intracranial pressure caused by pseudotumor cerebri than with other forms of prolonged increased intracranial pressure. One theory is that the fluctuation of increased intracranial pressure from abnormal to normal, which is common in idiopathic intracranial hypertension, may give the visual system a rest between significant rises in intracranial pressure. The periods of decrease in pressure do not last long enough, however, to clear the disc of edema.

The most common sign of idiopathic intracranial hypertension is papilledema. The clinical measurement of papilledema is the increase in the blind spot on perimetry. The usual explanations for this condition have involved displacement of the percipient elements of the retina away from the disc. It is seen on ophthalmoscopy by the concentric folds seen particularly on the temporal side of the disc called Paton's lines. They account for the absolute part of the scotoma. There is also a relative part to the scotoma as demonstrated by the size of the blind spot to different-sized targets. This may be a result of the elevation of the retina away from the choriocapillaris by edema, causing a relative ischemia to the percipient elements or the Stiles-Crawford effect. A more recent report by Corbett and co-workers (1988) suggests a refractive etiology for the relative deficit. In their case they theorized that an elevated peripapillary retina creates a hypermetropia, which produces the relative scotoma. The use of increasing plus lenses when performing the field reduces the relative scotoma. They felt that the blind spot would be reduced to almost normal size by this method. However, their report is of only one case. Just as the mechanism and causes of increased intracranial pressure are many, so may be the multiple factors that create the enlarged blind spot. Another report by Young, Knox and Walsh lends credence to refractive errors as a cause of field defects related to disc pathology. They found a similar correction for bitemporal hemianopias associated with tilted discs by using myopic lenses.

Another factor in the enlargement of the blind spot may be choroidal folds. The first report was by Nettleship in 1884. Bird and Sanders (1973) revived the idea with their report of eight such cases. Increased intracranial pressure is transmitted to the perineural optic nerve space and may then be transmitted to the globe. Two of their cases had acquired hypermetropia as is in keeping with Corbett's views. Pathologic study of the nerves in patients with papilledema reveal a distention of the sheath next to the insertion at the disc. This distention may press on the globe not only in the area of the disc causing the hypermetropia but may also cause horizontal striae. This transmitted pressure around the disc may also interfere with the peripapillary blood supply, which is a low-pressure system that is more easily affected than the retinal artery circulation. This interference is confirmed by a delay in fluorescein circulation time in the peripapillary area.

Transient visual obscurations, which are a unilateral or more commonly bilateral loss of vision lasting 5 to 20 seconds, have traditionally been considered a sign of increased intracranial pressure. Sadun, Currie, and Lessell (1984) report four patients with disc edema and no increased intracranial pressure with such visual symptoms. They felt that, if there is a common cause between their cases and those of increased intracranial pressure, increased tissue pressure in that retrolaminar area of lower vascular pressure is the likely etiology. The common denominator of all these cases is a disturbance of axoplasmic flow, which crowds the optic nerve in its sheath. Even slight variations in tissue pressure may affect the arterial flow in this low-pressure retrolaminar system and cause ischemia to the nerve. Cerebral autoregulation does compensate for pressure effects on the cerebral blood flow, but this occurs in the time frame of seconds. The low-pressure retrolaminar arterial system must be in such a delicate state of balance that momentary small tissue

pressure changes can have transient but profound changes in our optic nerve function.

THERAPY

Supportive. In any disease, it is important to identify the specific cause so that more appropriate and effective therapy can be administered. In the case of a tumor, the treatment is either surgical removal of the tumor, a shunting procedure to reduce the intracranial pressure, or radiation. Idiopathic intracranial hypertension is usually treated with well-established methods of supportive therapy, rather than the direct specific treatment. However, this may not always be the proper approach. A careful history may reveal the intake of certain substances, such as tetracycline and vitamin A, which can cause idiopathic intracranial hypertension. Obviously, discontinuance of these substances will result in a cure.

Systemic. The treatment of increased intracranial pressure depends on the specific cause. There are several therapeutic approaches to prolonged increased intracranial pressure with severe consequences to the visual system as is seen in idiopathic intracranial hypertension.

Many patients who have mild symptoms do not require treatment. However, they need to be followed just as closely as those who have severe complaints because of possible visual system deficits. Repeated spinal fluid taps have been advocated, but are not very pleasant for the patient. Since the spinal fluid pressure usually is restored to the previous level in about 2 hours, the rationale for the use of repeated spinal taps in a chronic disease is unclear. There is also the risk of infection with multiple taps. Repeated taps may cause tears in the dura, with chronic leaking of spinal fluid and perhaps worsening of the headache.

The use of carbonic anhydrase inhibitors, such as acetazolamide, decreases the production of cerebrospinal fluid, just as it reduces aqueous production in the eye. The usual dosage of acetazolamide that has been shown to be effective in reducing intracranial pressure has been projected at 4 gm daily. Side effects at this dosage level or even lower include gastrointestinal symptoms, disturbances in acid-base balance, and perioral and digital paresthesias. However, in the carbonic anhydrase inhibitor group, methazolamide theoretically may be a better choice, since it is known to cross the blood-brain barrier better than acetazolamide. No studies as yet have been performed to compare the two drugs. Diuretics in classes other than carbonic anhydrase inhibitors do not work as well.

Steroids[‡] are another therapeutic possibility. Steroids in themselves have serious side effects and have been implicated in causing idiopathic intracranial hypertension independently or in conjunction with the nephrotic syndrome. Most physicians treating idiopathic intracranial hypertension recommend steroid use for only a short course of treatment, such as several weeks.

Oral glycerin can also be used in doses of 75 ml two to three times a day to lower intracranial pressure. However, glycerin is not always tolerated well, particularly if there is any nausea; it should be chilled and mixed with some lime juice to make it more palatable. Although it is not the first choice of an oral medication, it is an alternative therapy.

Surgical. If the disease process does not abate and the medical treatment is not effective in stopping visual loss, then surgical intervention must be considered. There are two approaches in surgical treatment. The first is the lumboperitoneal shunt initially reported by Vander Ark in 1971. It has the advantage of normalizing the intracranial pressure rapidly and reducing the papilledema. Although any competent neurosurgeon can do this surgery, the operation is not perfect, and increased intracranial pressure may recur. At the other extreme, the shunt may filter excessively and lead to increased headache because of the shifting of intracranial contents and stretching of nerves.

Sergott's (1989) report on the Wills Hospital experience with lumboperitoneal shunts is not very encouraging. Their patients averaged five revisions.

The second surgical approach is an optic nerve decompression, which was first described by De Wecker in 1872. Davidson (1969) in England renewed interest in the procedure. Spoor and co-workers (1991) reported a series of 53 patients and 100 eyes operated on using optic nerve decompression. In their cases of acute papilledema 69 eyes had improved vision. In 32 cases of chronic papilledema, only 10 improved. Thirteen eyes had failed decompressions and required secondary and tertiary operations. The mechanism that makes this a rational treatment is not clear. Keltner (1988) suggested that optic nerve decompression serves as a filter for cerebral spinal fluid. The fact that the intracranial pressure remains high after optic nerve decompression in the majority of cases does not preclude a filtering mechanism. In some cases, the pressure, as well as the optic disc edema, was relieved. It has also been reported that unilateral decompression can produce bilateral optic nerve improvement in edema. This finding also supports the drainage theory. Sergott (1989) reported on 17 unilateral operated cases with bilateral improvement in 12. Corbett reported 16 such unilateral cases with bilateral improvement.

Optic nerve decompression has been effective in reversing visual loss from increased intracranial pressure, although the exact mechanism by which this is accomplished is not well understood. Kaye and his co-workers (1981) presented a 51-year-old female with a 14-month history of papilledema and pseudotumor cerebri. Because of worsening symptoms, increasing papilledema, and increasing transient obscurations, bilateral optic nerve sheath decompression was performed. Intracranial pressure was measured continuously postoperatively, and no significant lowering of intracranial pressure was recorded. However, the papilledema and symptoms decreased, and the patient was normal 2 months postoperatively. Therefore, optic nerve sheath decompression preserves optic nerve function, but apparently does not treat the underlying cause of increased intracranial pressure.

Ocular or Periocular Manifestations

Optic Nerve: Blurring of disc margins (initially nasal border); hemorrhages and exudates; obscuration and displacement of vessels; subtle vertical striae on temporal side.

Retina: Absence of spontaneous venous pulse; edema; hemorrhages and exudates.

Other: Enlarged blind spot; increased intracranial pressure; permanent visual loss; visual field loss (usually the inferior nasal quadrant initially with concentric contraction later).

PRECAUTIONS

Surgical therapy for any disease always has its hazards. However, being timid and waiting until the need for surgery is obvious may still produce a visual disaster. The optimal moment to abandon medical therapy and do a surgical procedure is impossible to determine accurately. Close and careful evaluation of vision and fields is all one can do in order to time surgical intervention properly.

The criteria for surgical intervention laid down by Dandy are still valid today. They are decreasing visual acuity, progressive concentric contraction of the field, increasing transient obscurations, and gliosis of the disc. Any or all of these are signs of a nerve that is beginning to decompensate and should be viewed as ominous indications for vision. Whether one chooses optic nerve decompression or a shunting procedure depends on the surgical expertise available. It is just as important to follow the fields once therapy or some definitive surgical procedure has been performed. The size of the blind spot should be measured both vertically and horizontally. The relative scotoma around and enlarging the blind spot may improve before there is visible evidence of a reduction in size of the blind spot. These improvements should be significant and not just 3 to 5 degrees, which could easily be a variation caused by the patient's varying level of alertness and general response to repeated testing.

COMMENTS

To suggest that the first decision in observing a disc is to decide whether there is true edema may seem presumptuous. However, this decision is not always easy. Even the presence of drusen of the optic nerve head does not preclude the patient from also having disc edema from any cause, including increased intracranial pressure. Once one decides that true disc edema is present, a decision whether it is papilledema due to increased intracranial pressure or to one of the other causes needs to be made so the proper ancillary tests and treatment can be instituted promptly. An improper workup can be worse than no workup at all, with this delay adding to the patient's visual deficit. A physician should constantly hone his or her clinical acumen, so that when the diagnosis of papilledema due to increased intracranial pressure is made, a proper program for patient management can be instituted promptly. The physician must walk that narrow path between reckless aggressiveness and bridled timidity.

References

Bird AC, Sander MD: Choroidal folds in association with papilledema. Br J Ophthalmol 57:89–97, 1973.

Buckell M, Walsh L: Effect of glycerol by mouth on raised intracranial pressure in man. Lancet 2:1151–1152, 1964.

Corbett JJ: Problems in the diagnosis and treatment of pseudotumor cerebri. J Can Sci Neurol 10:221–229, 1983.

Corbett JJ, Thompson S: The rational management of idiopathic intracranial hypertension. Arch Neurol 46:1049 1051, 1989.

Corbett JJ, et al: Visual loss in pseudotumor cerebri. Arch Neurol 39:461–479, 1982.

Corbett JJ, et al: Enlargement of the blind spot caused by papilledema. Am J Ophthalmol 105:261–265, 1988.

Davidson ST: A surgical approach to plesocephalic disc oedema. Trans Ophthalmol Soc UK 89:669–690, 1969.

De Wecker L: On incision of the optic nerve in cases of neuroretinitis. Int Ophthalmol Congr Rep 4:11–14, 1872.

Galbraith JEK, Sullivan JH: Decompression of the perioptic meningioma for relief of papilledema. Am J Ophthalmol 76:687–692, 1973.

Gucer G, Vierenstein L: Long-term intracranial pressure recording in management of pseudotumor cerebri. J Neurosurg 49:256–263, 1978.

Johnston I, Paterson A: Benign intracranial hypertension. II. CSF pressure and circulation. Brain 97:302–312, 1974.

Kaye AH, Galbraith JEK, King J: Intracranial pressure following optic nerve decompression for benign intracranial hypertension. Case report. J Neurosurg 55:453–456, 1981.

Kelman SE: Modified optic nerve decompression in patients with functioning lumboperitoneal shunts and progressive visual loss. Ophthalmology 98:1449–1453, 1991.

Keltner JL: Optic nerve sheath decompression. How does it Work? Has its time come? Arch Ophthalmol 106:1365–1369, 1988.

Lessell S, Rosman P: Permanent visual impairment in childhood: Pseudotumor cerebri. Arch Neurol 43:801–804, 1986.

Levin BE: The clinical significance of spontaneous pulsations of the retinal vein. Arch Neurol 35:37–40, 1978.

Maren TH: Carbonic anhydrase chemistry, physiology and inhibition. Physiol Rev 47:595–782. 1967.

Maren TH, et al: The pharmacology of methazolamide in relation to the treatment of glaucoma. Invest Ophthalmol 16:730–742, 1977.

Rabinowicz IM, Ben-Sira I, Zauberman H: Preservation of visual function in papilloedema. Observed for 3 to 6 years in cases of benign intracranial hypertension. Br J Ophthalmol 52:236–241, 1968.

Sadun AA, et al: Transient visual obscurations with elevated optic discs. Ann Neurol 16:489–494, 1984.

Sergott RC: Optic nerve sheath decompression. Curr Ther Ophthalmol Surg 8:302–306, 1989.

Spencer JD, et al: Benign intracranial hypertension without papilledema. Role of 24-hour CSF pressure monitoring in diagnosis and management. Neurosurgery 7:326–332, 1980.

Spoor TC, et al: Treatment of pseudotumor cerebri by primary and secondary optic nerve sheath decompression. Am J Ophthalmol 112:177–185, 1991.

Van Dyk HJL: Optic nerve sheath decompression: The ophthalmic surgeon approaches papilledema. In Burde RM, et al (eds): Symposium on Neuro-Ophthalmology. St. Louis, CV Mosby, 1976, pp 74–78.

Van Uitert RL, Eisenstadt ML: Venous pulsations not always indicative of normal intracranial pressure. Arch Neurol 35:550, 1978.

Walker AE, Adamkiewicz JS: Pseudotumor cerebri associated with prolonged corticosteroid therapy. Reports of four cases. JAMA 188:779–784, 1964.

Wall M, George D: Visual loss in pseudotumor cerebri. Arch Neurol 44:170 175, 1987.

Wall M, George D: Idiopathic intracranial hypertension. Brain 114:155–180, 1991.

TRAUMATIC OPTIC NEUROPATHY 377.49

JOHN G. McHENRY, M.D.,
and THOMAS C. SPOOR, M.D., M.S., F.A.C.S.

Detroit, Michigan

Midfacial and orbital fractures, as well as closed head injuries, can cause traumatic optic neuropathies (TON). The optic nerve can be impinged by broken bones within the optic canal, damaged by a compression-decompression injury, or compressed by a static force on the frontal bone. The exact mechanisms for traumatic optic neuropathies are controversial and are thought to result from a combination of compression and ischemia.

Many patients with traumatic optic neuropathies present to the emergency room unconscious or with severe associated injuries. Although it is impossible to obtain a visual acuity and visual field in an unconscious patient, it is often possible to diagnose a traumatic optic neuropathy. The pupils should be tested for a relative afferent pupillary defect (RAPD) A RAPD in a patient with orbital or midfacial trauma or closed head injury without associated ocular injuries is a sign of a traumatic optic neuropathy.

Retrobulbar and subperiosteal hemorrhages can compress the optic nerve, as can intraorbital air under pressure. Severe orbital emphysema can occur after a sinus injury. Some of the nasoethmoidal fractures create a ball-valve effect into the orbit. Each breath can force air into the orbit, further compressing the optic nerve. These are immediately treatable, readily reversible causes of TON.

Optic nerve avulsion can occur with penetrating injuries, as well as severe compression-decompression injuries. The fundus appearance is distinctive, with hemorrhages appearing at the site of the optic disc. Rarely, patients with optic nerve trauma can present with disc edema and hemorrhage. Some of these patients may have hemorrhage within the optic nerve.

THERAPY

Ocular. Patients with traumatic optic neuropathies are started immediately on 2 gm of intravenous methylprednisolone. A CT scan of the head and orbits is performed. If direct coronal scans cannot be obtained, reconstructed coronal images should be ordered. After the loading dose, the patient is begun in 2 hours on a course of 1 gm of intravenous methylprednisolone every 6 hours for 24 to 48 hours, at which point steroids are tapered. If there is no improvement in afferent pupillary defect, visual acuity, or visual field mean deviation, extracranial optic canal decompression may be considered. It is also considered if visual parameters deteriorate as the steroids are tapered.

Surgical. If a patient is to undergo extracranial optic canal decompression, steroids are increased in the perioperative period. The authors favor the transethmoidal approach via an external ethmoidectomy.

Retrobulbar hemorrhages are treated by canthotomy and cantholysis, along with intravenous megadose corticosteroids. If these procedures are unsuccessful, orbital decompression may be necessary. Although canthotomy and cantholysis can relieve some cases of compressive orbital emphysema, those patients with a sino-orbital ball valve need orbito-ethmoidal decompression.

There is no treatment for avulsion of the optic nerve. The rare patient with an optic nerve sheath hemorrhage may be helped by optic nerve sheath decompression.

PRECAUTIONS

All patients who are started on intravenous megadose corticosteroids are also started on ranitidine, 150 mg twice daily, to decrease the possibility of erosive gastritis or an upper GI hemorrhage. Steroids should be tapered quickly to avoid systemic complications, such as adrenal suppression or immunosuppression. Intravenous megadose corticosteroids can be used safely in patients under the age of 60. Older patients are subject to the mineralocorticoid effects of methylprednisolone, which can lead to hypervolemia, arrythmias, and myocardial infarction.

Extracranial optic canal decompression can be complicated by cerebrospinal fluid leaks, meningitis, pneumoencephalus, esotropia, and symptomatic epiphora. Although surgery within the sphenoid sinus occurs close to the carotid artery, if one stays superior and carefully burrs away the bony canal from lateral to medial and inferior to superior under direct visualization through an external ethmoidectomy with complete removal of the medial wall of the orbit, the probability of violating the carotid artery is minimized.

COMMENTS

Many patients with severe ocular injuries also have traumatic optic neuropathies. It is sometimes difficult to decide whether an afferent pupillary defect is secondary to optic nerve injury of an associated media opacity, such as hyphema or vitreous hemorrhage. Opacities can act as neutral density filters. If the diagnosis is in doubt, one can either err on the side of treatment, or one can perform an iopamidol CT myelogram looking for blockage of CSF flow through the optic canal. Those with blockage can be treated first with steroids and, if unsuccessful, with optic canal decompression.

References

Anderson RL, Panje RL, Gross LE: Optic nerve blindness following blunt forehead trauma. Ophthalmology 89:445–455, 1982.

Frenkel RP, Spoor TC: Diagnosis and management of traumatic optic neuropathies. Adv Ophthalmol Plast Reconstr Surg 6:71–90, 1987.

Joseph P, Lessell S, Rizzo J, Momose KJ: Extracranial optic nerve decompression for traumatic optic neuropathy. Arch Ophthalmol 108:1091–1093, 1990.

Lessell S: Indirect optic nerve trauma. Arch Ophthalmol 107:382–386, 1989.

Spoor TC, Hartel R: Treatment of traumatic optic neuropathy with corticosteroids. Am J Ophthalmol 110:665–669, 1990.

Spoor TC, Mathog RL: Restoration of vision after optic canal decompression. Arch Ophthalmol 104:804–805, 1986.

Wolin MJ, Lavin PJ: Spontaneous visual recovery from traumatic optic neuropathy after blunt head injury. Am J Ophthalmol 190:430–435, 1990.

VASCULOPATHIC OPTIC NEUROPATHIES 377.39

JOHN G. McHENRY, M.D.,
and THOMAS C. SPOOR, M.D., M.S.,
F.A.C.S.

Detroit, Michigan

The vasculopathic optic neuropathies cause optic nerve damage by ischemia, leading to axonal stasis, fluid transudation into the subarachnoid space, compression of already damaged axons, death of axons, and the further compromise of visual function. Vasculopathic optic neuropathies include both anterior ischemic optic neuropathy (AION) and posterior ischemic optic neuropathy (PION). Patients with ischemic optic neuropathies present with sudden visual loss, often noticed upon awakening. Visual function is compromised, and a relative afferent pupillary defect is present. Patients with AION manifest optic disc hemorrhages, edema, and pallor, whereas patients with PION have normal to atrophic discs.

Anterior ischemic optic neuropathies include both an arteritic form, associated with giant cell inflammation, and a more common nonarteritic form. Nonarteritic anterior ischemic optic neuropathy (NAION) occurs in a static and a progressive form, as well as a prodromal form of optic disc swelling with minimal visual loss that may resolve spontaneously. Static NAION may occur secondary to sectoral hypoperfusion of the optic nerve. Visual acuity may range from counting fingers to 20/20. Visual loss is stable. Static NAION can also occur after massive hypoperfusion of the optic nerve secondary to systemic hypotension or massive blood loss. In these cases, vision ranges from NLP to counting fingers. Patients with progressive NAION have a progressive deterioration in visual function after the initial episode of visual loss.

The workup for disc swelling and hemorrhage in a patient older than 45 with visual loss begins with a complete history. The review of systems focuses on visual loss, temporal pain, headaches, jaw claudication, tongue pain, and proximal muscle weakness. Visual acuity and the presence of a relative afferent pupillary defect or light-near dissociation are recorded. Pupillary defects are graded with neutral density filters. Computerized perimetry with calculation of mean deviation and corrected pattern standard deviation is performed. Slit-lamp biomicroscopy of the optic nerve head using a 78- or 60-diopter lens is helpful. Stereo disc photos are obtained, as is a 30° A-scan, looking for fluid within the optic nerve sheath. Finally, an erythrocyte sedimentation rate (ESR) is drawn.

The risk of giant cell arteritis (GCA) increases with age. It is extremely uncommon in patients under 50 years of age and increases dramatically above 80 years of age. It is also more common in females than males. Whites are much more commonly affected that African-Americans or Orientals. Clinical suspicions guide the evaluation.

Statistically, 45- to 75-year-old patients will be more likely to have NAION than giant cell arteritis. Appropriate laboratory evaluation includes CBC, platelets, ANA, RF, ESR, and anticardiolipin antibody. If the anticardiolipin antibodies are positive, antiphospholipid antibodies should be ordered.

Young patients with diabetes mellitis, sickle cell anemia, or hypertension may present with sectoral or diffuse optic disc swelling with visual loss. There have also been reports of patients taking oral contraceptives who have developed ischemic optic neuropathy. Sickle cell anemia should be excluded in young African-American patients with disc swelling and visual loss by performing a hemoglobin electrophoresis.

PION can occur secondary to intracranial artery or internal carotid ophthalmic artery atherosclerosis. It may also present with a tumor that disrupts the blood supply to the optic nerve. Trauma can disrupt the pial vessels within the optic canal that supplies the optic nerve, resulting in PION. The ophthalmic artery may also be disrupted by penetrating injuries or iatrogenically during paranasal sinus surgery. The fundus will then show a cherry-red spot with massive pallid edema of the optic nerve. Optic nerve vascular damage has also been implicated in radiation-induced optic neuropathy. The exact mechanism of visual loss is very complex and includes cytopathic, chromosomal, and immunologic factors, as well as vascular compromise. The common denominator of all of these posterior ischemic optic neuropathies is optic atrophy without antecedent disc swelling. PION is a diagnosis of exclusion.

THERAPY

Systemic. The treatment for giant cell arteritis is systemic corticosteroids. The authors evaluate and treat an elderly patient with profound visual loss, pallid edema, temporal pain, and tenderness in the following manner: an IV is started immediately, and the patient is given 500 mg of intravenous methylprednisolone. The patient is then given 150 mg of ranitidine or a comparable H_2 blocker and admitted to the hospital; 120 mg of oral prednisone is started concurrently. Laboratory requests include an erythrocyte sedimentation rate by the Westergren method, CBC, platelet, PLT, PT, PTT, anticardiolipin antibodies, ANA, FTA-ABS, VDRL, lytes, BUN, and creatinine. The ESR is but one piece of information that can lead to the diagnosis of GCA. Its specificity is extremely poor. Malignancies, infection, and collagen vascular diseases all may raise the ESR. It is said that if the ESR is half the age plus 10 for a woman, it is abnormal (half the age for a man). This is only a rough estimate.

If there is a greater than 10 per cent fluid shift on 30° A-scan, the patient is informed that they have an anterior ischemic optic neuropathy that may be progressing and that they should strongly consider combined temporal artery biopsy with optic nerve sheath decompression (ONSD) under retrobulbar anesthesia. This procedure should be performed as soon as possible.

Two hours after the first dose of methylprednisolone, the patient is started on a course of 250 mg of IV methylprednisolone every 6 hours for 48 hours and is continued on 120 mg of oral prednisone and 150 mg two times a day of ranitidine. If the temporal artery biopsy is positive, the patient is discharged on 120 mg of prednisone a day along with ranitidine. Steroids are slowly tapered over 6 to 12 months. This treatment is performed in conjunction with an internal medicine colleague or a rheumatologist. A systemic workup is essential. Serial ESRs guide the tapering of steroids.

If the biopsy is negative, then steroids are rapidly tapered over the ensuing week. If an optic nerve sheath decompression (ONSD) was not performed, the patient is seen in 24 to 48 hours for progressive visual loss. Visual loss occurs in 30 to 40 per cent of patients with nonarteritic anterior ischemic optic neuropathy. Visual acuity, computerized perimetry, and 30-degree A-scans for intranerve sheath fluid are performed. Patients are then followed at 1 week, 2 weeks, 1 month, 2 months, 3 months, and 6 months.

Patients with a lower clinical probability of GCA are started on 80 mg of prednisone with ranitidine, and a temporal artery biopsy is scheduled in the next several days. Patients with a higher probability of GCA are admitted, started on IV steroids and ranitidine, and scheduled for a temporal artery biopsy expeditiously.

Surgical. The treatment for NAION depends on whether the visual loss is progressive. If the patient gives a strong history of progression and there is significant fluid within the optic nerve sheath, ONSD is performed within 24 hours. If there is no history of progression or fluid within the optic nerve sheath, then the patient is examined again in 48 to 72 hours and the tests are repeated, looking for progression or fluid accumulation. If there is progression or fluid accumulation, the patient is offered ONSD. If progression has not occurred, the patient is seen again in 1 week, 2 weeks, 1 month, 2 months, and then monthly for 6 months.

There is presently no effective treatment for visual loss due to static NAION. Although optic nerve sheath decompression and intravenous megadose corticosteroids have been used to treat the AION of hypoperfusion and hypotension, the visual results are extremely discouraging. Similarly, there is no effective treatment for PION. Some patients with low-tension glaucoma may have the atherosclerotic form of PION.

PRECAUTIONS

Patients treated with systemic corticosteroids must be placed on H_2 blockers to decrease the risk of erosive gastritis, ulceration, and upper GI hemorrhages. The long-term use of corticosteroids can result in steroid myopathy, weakness, wasting, aseptic necrosis, immunosuppression, and adrenal suppression. After long-term use, tapering must proceed slowly. These patients are best followed in conjunction with an internist.

COMMENTS

Optic nerve sheath decompression for AION may improve visual acuity and visual field, but the patient is still left with a severe visual deficit. Patients with hypertension and diabetes are at highest risk for AION. There is a 40 per cent incidence of a second event in the fellow eye. Eyes with small cup:disc ratios are at particular risk. Rarely a patient will have a second event in the same eye. Patients may awake from major surgery bilaterally blind. It is important to differentiate blindness secondary to occipital infarction from blindness secondary to optic nerve infarcts. Immediately, there may be no sign other than minimal optic disc swelling. However, if optic nerve infarction has occurred, pallid edema will ensue over the next 24 hours. If a patient has some vision after the initial event and progressive visual loss can be documented, it may be reasonable to consider ONSD. The prognosis is very poor.

A prospective randomized clinical trial comparing observation to ONSD for NAION is currently underway. It will not, however, compare the efficacy of ONSD for static and progressive NAION. Previous studies have not shown ONSD to be effective in patients without progressive visual loss. This ineffectiveness may be related to the accumulation of subarachnoid fluid that occurs in some patients after an initial ischemic event. A cycle of ischemia, transudation, compression, and further ischemia ensues, leading to progressive visual loss. ONSD relieves the compression and breaks the cycle. Visual function is allowed to return to the level it was after the initial ischemic event.

References

Bogen DR, Glaser JS: Ischaemic optic neuropathy. The clinical profile and history. Brain 98:689–708, 1975.

Borchert M, Lessell S: Progressive and recurrent nonarteritic anterior ischemic optic neuropathy. Am J Ophthalmol 106:443–449, 1988.

Clearkin L, Caballero J: Recovery of visual function in anterior ischemic optic neuropathy due to giant cell arteritis. Am J Med 92:703–704, 1992.

Keltner JL: Giant-cell arteritis. Signs and symptoms. Ophthalmology *89*:1101–1110, 1982.

Repka MX, Savino PJ, Schatz NJ, Sergott RC: Clinical profile and long-term implications of anterior ischemic optic neuropathy. Am J Ophthalmol *96*:478–483, 1983.

Rizzo JF III, Lessell S: Posterior ischemic optic neuropathy during general surgery. Am J Ophthalmol *103*:808–811, 1987.

Sergott RC, Cohen MS, Bosley TM, Savino PJ: Optic nerve sheath decompression may improve the progressive form of NAION. Arch Ophthalmol *107*:1743–1754, 1989.

Spoor TC, Wilkinson MJ, Ramocki JM: Treatment of nonarteritic ischemic optic neuropathy with optic nerve sheath decompression. Am J Ophthalmol *111*:724, 1991.

Spoor TC, McHenry JG: Treatment of nonarteritic ischemic optic neuropathy with optic nerve sheath decomposition. Ophthalmology (in press).

SECTION 31

ORBIT

ENOPHTHALMOS 376.50

DAVID B. SOLL, M.D., F.A.C.S.

Philadelphia, Pennsylvania

Enophthalmos is a retrodisplacement of the eyeball into the orbit. It occurs in a variety of conditions when there is a disparity between the volume of the bony orbit and its contents. The most frequent cause is surgical anophthalmos. Other causes include congenital anophthalmos or microphthalmos. There is always some type of ocular remnant present in a socket even when it is classified as congenitally anophthalmic. Phthisis of the globe secondary to trauma or disease is also usually associated with orbital fat atrophy, and the amount of enophthalmos is thus accentuated. Orbital fractures, especially unrepaired or poorly repaired blow-out and naso-orbital fractures, are major causes of clinical enophthalmos. Sympathetic paresis, such as occurs in Horner's syndrome, often gives the appearance of enophthalmos; however, it is a pseudoenophthalmos and is secondary to a ptosis of the upper eyelid that is due to paralysis of Müeller's muscle, which is innervated by the sympathetic system.

Accompanying all forms of enophthalmos are usually a deep, superior eyelid sulcus and ptosis of the upper eyelid; the latter condition is secondary to inadequate support of the adnexal tissues by the globe. In many cases of orbital fracture, diplopia is also present secondary to the entrapment of extraocular muscles or tissue contiguous with the extraocular muscles, especially the inferior rectus-inferior oblique complex.

Enophthalmos of a prosthetic eye may be a particular problem after enucleation of the globe and may be accompanied by downward displacement of the prosthesis caused by relaxation of the lower eyelid. After enucleation of the globe, many physiologic and functional changes occur in the orbit. The anatomic position of the levator muscle complex is changed, and some atrophy of orbital fat occurs after all enucleation procedures.

THERAPY

Surgical. In patients with anophthalmic enophthalmos after enucleation, a modification of the prosthesis should be tried first. If this proves to be ineffective, a secondary implant may be inserted. Likewise, if an implant was not used during the initial enucleation procedure or an intraorbital implant has extruded, the secondary implant is best inserted posterior to all layers of Tenon's capsule, directly within the muscle cone. The surgical procedure consists of making a horizontal conjunctival incision in the center of the posterior wall of the socket. A central vertical incision through Tenon's capsule is then made, exposing the fat of the muscle cone. A spherical implant that has been encased in a scleral shell is inserted directly into the fatty tissue of the muscle cone. The implant should fit comfortably in the orbit. Usually a size 16- to 18-mm sphere is satisfactory; however, the size depends on the age of the patient and the volume of the orbit. Because of the problem of AIDS, fascia, either temporalis or fascia lata, has become a popular substitute for sclera. It is also possible to use an uncovered silicone or hydroxyapatite ball implant. Sutures may be directly inserted into the substance of a silicone ball. A 5–0 vicryl suture is placed at the apex of the implant through either the sclera or fascia. If a silicone ball has been used and it is not encased in sclera or fascia, the sutures are placed directly into the substance of the silicone ball. Two additional double-armed vicryl sutures are placed medially and laterally in positions where the medial and lateral rectus muscles would insert if the implant were a small globe. The preplaced medial and lateral sutures are brought through Tenon's capsule and conjunctiva and tied in the medial and lateral fornices, respectively. The apical double-armed suture is used to imbricate the central portion of Tenon's capsule. Any additional defects in Tenon's capsule are closed with interrupted 5–0 vicryl sutures. The conjunctiva is then undermined and closed with interrupted 6–0 plain gut sutures.

During the past few years, hydroxyapatite implants, which are manufactured from a coral derivative, have been used as orbital implants along with methylmethacrylate and silicone implants. These hydroxyapatite implants are invaded by blood vessels and become an integral part of the body. If a hydroxyapatite implant is used, it is ideally covered with sclera or fascia, leaving the posterior portion open. It is also possible to place an uncovered hydroxyapatite implant into the orbit. The author has not found it useful or necessary to dissect the retracted extraocular muscles when performing secondary implantations. If these muscles are readily visible and can easily be dissected, they will be used. If they are used, a window should be cut in the sclera or fascia where the muscle's normal position would be and the muscle is sutured into this window. Blood vessels will then invade the hydroxyapatite implant through this window, as well as through the posterior area. It is important to remember that if an extraocular muscle is sutured to the implant, its opposing muscle should also be sutured to the implant to avoid excessive implant rotation to one side or the other, or up or down. The author's experience has been that, even if the muscles are not sutured to the implant, if they are functional, the muscle pull on tissue that attaches to the implant will cause rotation of the implant. Blind dissection to retrieve an extraocular muscle will cause unnecessary trauma and subsequent tissue atrophy.

To achieve good motility of the implant, it is extremely important to ensure that the fornices are deep. If the fornices are shallow, the conjunctiva should be undermined deeply inferiorly, medially, and laterally. Conjunctival undermining superiorly has to be performed with a great deal of care to avoid injury to the levator muscle complex. If the fornices are shallow, the conjunctival undermining should be performed before the insertion of the secondary implant.

The use of de-epithelialized dermal grafts as a secondary implant also works very well. The implant is obtained from the lateral buttock area. The epithelium is removed, and the dermal part of the implant can then be sutured into the socket tissue with the fatty layer posteriorly. Another alternative is to encase the fatty layer of the de-epithelialized implant within the dermal layer; in other words, making the dermis the outer covering of a ball. It has been postulated that there is less tissue atrophy of the transplant when this technique is used. This de-epithelialized buttock fat ball implant is then inserted as either a secondary implant or as a primary implant. Their use is very valuable, especially in small orbits and in orbits where extrusion has occurred several times. Experience so far with these de-epithelialized dermal fat grafts has been very positive.

Another technique that is very useful for correcting enophthalmos and superior eyelid sulcus defects in the anophthalmic orbit is the subperiosteal insertion of room-temperature vulcanizing (RTV) Silastic. This material is used if an intraorbital implant is already present. It is injected subperiosteally into the orbit, usually under the inferior lateral orbital floor periosteum. The material is injected in a semi-isolid state. The rate of vulcanization depends upon the amount of catalyst mixed with the RTV silicone. Once solid, the material stays in position. The surgical approach is essentially the same as that for a blow-out orbital fracture. The orbital floor periosteum is dissected free of the underlying bone with a periosteal elevator, and a ribbon retractor is used to elevate orbital contents while the Silastic material is injected. It is important that none of this Silastic material extends anteriorly to the anterior orbital bony rim. The long-term results of using room-temperature vulcanizing Silastic material when correcting the enophthalmos in an anophthalmic orbit are very gratifying.

Because superior eyelid sulcus defects are so common in anophthalmic enophthalmic orbits, implants of de-epithelialized dermal fat placed subconjunctivally between the conjunctiva and the levator muscle, with the dermal side of the graft adjacent to the subconjunctival surface, have proven to be satisfactory in minimizing this defect. After the use of a de-epithelialized dermal fat graft under the upper eyelid, a smaller prosthesis is frequently required and eyelid motion is better. When enophthalmos occurs in an orbit with a seeing eye, it is much more difficult to correct. It is much easier to elevate an eye than it is to bring it forward. If there is an obvious orbital floor fracture with displacement of fragments or herniation of orbital contents into one of the sinuses, the orbital contents can be replaced in the orbit, the defect covered, and the contents supported with Supramid, silicone, Teflon, or autogenous bone floor implants. A 0.6-mm Supramid implant tailored to be just slightly larger than the size of the defect has been found to be ideal for supporting orbital contents.

During recent years, craniofacial surgeons have devised techniques to reconstruct defective bony areas, reposition orbital structures, and cosmetically repair cases of enophthalmos that were previously not treatable. During these procedures, the combined efforts of the ophthalmologist and the craniofacial surgeon are valuable.

Ocular or Periocular Manifestations

Eyelids: Dropped socket appearance; inability to close eyelids; ptosis; superior eyelid sulcus defects.

PRECAUTIONS

If the enophthalmos is not severe, various camouflages can be used. In an anophthalmic socket, tightening of a lax lower eyelid will often give better support to the prosthesis and help correct an apparent ptosis. If the ptosis is severe, it can usually be improved by modification of the prosthesis combined with a ptosis procedure, either a sling or a form of levator resection. The appearance of a superior lid sulcus defect can be made less obvious by a de-epithelialized fat graft on the internal surface of the upper lid. If the defect is still obvious, then a contralateral upper eyelid symmetrizing blepharoplasty can be considered. If this is done and if fat is removed from the contralateral upper eyelid in a monocular patient, only the lateral preaponeurotic fat should be excised. The ophthalmologist and patient should be aware of all risks when doing surgery on the lids or orbit of a monocular patient.

Camouflage procedures are very useful in the treatment of both patients with an anophthalmic socket and those who have enophthalmic enophthalmos in the presence of a seeing eye.

COMMENTS

Enophthalmos often develops late after unrepaired fractures and is a frequent complication of enucleation surgery. In the presence of a seeing eye, it is very difficult to correct the enophthalmos fully. Nothing should be done that will compromise vision. Craniofacial procedures work because the surgery is extraperiosteal and the orbital contents are not disturbed. However, complications can still occur. For this reason, the camouflage procedures already mentioned are extremely useful.

References

Aguilar EA: A re-evaluation of the indications for orbital rim fixation and orbital floor exploration in zygomatic complex fractures. Arch Otolaryngol Head Neck Surg 115:1025, 1989.

Arthurs B, Silverstone P, Della Rocca RC: Medial wall fractures. Adv Ophthalmol Plast Reconstr Surg 6:393–401, 1987.

Bite U, Jackson IT, et al: Orbital volume measurements in enophthalmos using three-dimensional CT imaging. Plast Reconstr Surg 75:502, 1985.

Bullock JD: Autogenous dermis-fat "baseball" orbital implant. Ophthalmic Surg 18:30, 1987.

Clinics in Plastic Surgery: Advances in Craniomaxillofacial Fracture Management. Philadelphia, WB Saunders, 1992.

Crockett DM, Funk GF: Management of complicated fractures involving the orbits and nasoethmoid complex in young children. Otolaryngol Clin North Am 24:119–137, 1991.

Dufresne CR, Manson PN, Iliff NT: Early and late complications of orbital fractures. Clin Plast Surg 15:239–253, 1988.

Gruss JS, Van Wyck L, Phillips JH, Antonyshyn O: The importance of the zygomatic arch in complex midfacial fracture repair and correction of posttraumatic orbitozygomatic deformities. Plast Reconstr Surg 85:878–890, 1990.

Hes J, deMan K: Use of blocks of hydroxyapatite for secondary reconstruction of the orbital floor. Int J Oral Maxillofac Surg 19:275–278, 1990.

Iverson RE, Vistnes LM, Siegel RJ: Correction of enophthalmos in the anophthalmic orbit. Plast Reconstr Surg 51:545–554, 1973.

Koornneef L: Eyelid and orbital fascial attachments and their clinical significance. Eye 1:130–134, 1988.

Nunery WR: Lateral canthal approach to repair of trimalar fractures of the zygoma. Ophthalmol Plast Reconstr Surg 1:175–183, 1985.

Nunery WR, Hetzler K: Dermal-fat graft as a primary enucleation technique. Ophthalmology 92:

1256, 1985 (see also Ophthalmology 93:418, 1986).

Pasket JP, Manson PN, Iliff NT: Nasoethmoidal and orbital fractures. Clin Plast Surg 15:209–223, 1988.

Raflo GT: Blow-in and blow-out fractures of the orbit: Clinical correlations and proposed mechanisms. Ophthalmic Surg 15:114–119, 1984.

Segrest DR, Dortzbach RK: Medial orbital wall fractures: Complications and management. Ophthalmol Plast Reconstr Surg 5:75–80, 1989.

Sergott TJ, Visnes LM: Correction of enophthalmos and superior sulcus depression in the anophthalmic orbit: A longterm follow-up. Plast Reconstr Surg 79:331, 1987.

Shore JW, et al: Management of complications following dermis-fat grafting for anophthalmic socket reconstruction. Ophthalmology 92:1342, 1985.

Smith B, Bosniak SL, Lisman RD: An autogenous kinetic dermis-fat orbital implant: An updated technique. Ophthalmology 89:1067–1071, 1982.

Soll DB: Insertion of secondary intraorbital implants. Arch Ophthalmol 89:214–216, 1973.

Soll DB: The anophthalmic socket. In Soll DB, Asbell RL (eds): Management of Complications in Ophthalmic Plastic Surgery. Birmingham, Aesculapius, 1976, pp 295–344.

Soll DB: The anophthalmic socket. Ophthalmology 89:407–423, 1982.

Soll DB: Evolution and current concepts in the surgical treatment of the anophthalmic orbit. Ophthalmol Plast Reconstr Surg 2:163, 1986.

Stanley RB, Mathog RH: Evaluation and correction of combined orbital trauma syndrome. Laryngoscope 93:856–865, 1983.

Waite PD, Carr DD: The transconjunctival approach for treating orbital trauma. J Oral Maxillofac Surg 49:499–503, 1991.

Whitaker LA: Aesthetic augmentation of the malar midface structures. Plast Reconstr Surg 80:337, 1987.

NONSPECIFIC ORBITAL INFLAMMATORY SYNDROMES 376.11

(Orbital Pseudotumors)

PETER J. DOLMAN, M.D., F.R.C.S.(C), and JACK ROOTMAN, M.D., F.R.C.S.(C)

Vancouver, British Columbia, Canada

Nonspecific orbital inflammatory syndromes (NSOIS) are a heterogeneous group defined by clinical and histologic signs of orbital soft tissue inflammation that cannot be attributed to local injury or infection nor to a specific entity, such as Graves' orbitopathy, Wegener's granulomatosis, or sarcoidosis.

Traditionally these syndromes were clumped under the generic term "pseudotumor," defined loosely as a non-neoplastic orbital inflammatory mass. Included in this broad group were lymphoid proliferations that currently are considered a separate disease spectrum ranging from benign lymphoid hyperplasia to lymphoma.

NSOIS account for 5 to 10 per cent of cases of orbital disease. Their cause is unknown, but they are probably immune disorders. There is no age, sex, or race predilection. They can be divided into three categories: acute/subacute NSOIS, sclerosing NSOIS, and granulomatous NSOIS.

Acute/subacute NSOIS develop over several days to weeks with pain, redness, edema, and local dysfunction. They are subdivided clinically on the basis of the primary orbital tissue involved: anterior (globe and surrounding orbit), myositis (extraocular muscle), dacryoadenitis (lacrimal gland), apical (orbital apex and cavernous sinus), and diffuse (entire orbital involvement). CT scans localize the involved areas with characteristic irregular margins surrounding the primary focus. Histologically, the affected tissues are infiltrated with a mixed population of neutrophils, plasma cells, histiocytes, macrophages, and lymphocytes.

Sclerosing NSOIS develop more insidiously and lead to orbital dysfunction as a result of progressive scarring and inflammation. Several authors recently have related this group of NSOIS to multifocal fibrosclerosis, which also includes retroperitoneal fibrosis, Riedel's sclerosing thyroiditis, and sclerosing cholangitis. They appear as homogeneous, dense lesions on CT scan incorporating both fat and surrounding structures. Histologically, the dominant feature is collagen deposition with a relatively scant, polymorphous inflammatory infiltrate.

Granulomatous NSOIS develop subacutely to chronically with minimal inflammatory signs around a palpable mass. Histologically they consist of granulomatous inflammation without an identifiable local or systemic cause.

THERAPY

Systemic. Oral corticosteroids are the first-line treatment for most nonspecific orbital inflammatory syndromes. Acute/subacute NSOIS typically respond dramatically to this therapy, with pain relief reported within hours. Idiopathic myositis and dacryoadenitis often can be controlled with lower doses (40 to 60 mg/day) tapered over 4 to 8 weeks. Anterior, diffuse, and apical inflammation require higher initial doses (prednisone, 60 to 100 mg/day) and a longer treatment course, with the drug tapered by 5 mg/week over 8 to 12 weeks. Re-exacerbations may occur and require the medicine to be increased to a level that controls the inflammation. Sclerosing NSOIS may initially respond to oral corticosteroids, but often become refractory and require additional therapy including chemotherapy or radiation. The initial recom-

mended dose is prednisone, 60 to 100 mg/day for 1 to 2 weeks; a successful response allows tapering over an 8- to 12-week period. Granulomatous NSOIS usually respond well to oral corticosteroids with a dosing and tapering schedule similar to that followed for idiopathic myositis and dacryoadenitis.

Oral corticosteroids should be used with caution in diabetics, hypertensives, and those with previous tuberculosis. Acutely, prednisone may cause hyperglycemia, hypertension, peptic ulcers, weight gain, and mood swings, including euphoria or psychosis. Prolonged therapy may cause cataracts, glaucoma, osteoporosis, acne, adrenocortical insufficiency, and aseptic necrosis of the femoral head.

Intralesional steroids have been used for localized NSOIS, including sclerotenonitis (anterior acute NSOIS), acute nonspecific dacryoadenitis, and granulomatous inflammatory masses. Triamcinolone acetonide (20 to 40 mg) and/or betamethasone (6 mg) may be injected* primarily or in cases refractory to or intolerant of systemic steroids. Secondary infections, atrophy of the overlying skin, globe perforations, and embolic occlusion of the central retinal artery leading to unilateral or bilateral blindness have been reported after the use of intralesional steroids.

Pulse-dose corticosteroids are being used increasingly for serious immune diseases. Methylprednisolone 1 gm/day can be administered intravenously on alternate days for three doses and is thought to destroy lymphocytes at these levels. It may be useful in more serious acute diffuse NSOIS with vision loss or in sclerosing NSOIS. Rare cases of arrhythmia and sudden death have been reported with pulse-dose steroids, but such treatment may avoid chronic steroid use with its many potential complications.

Nonsteroidal anti-inflammatory drugs may be used with steroids to allow a more rapid tapering regimen or alone in some patients with acute NSOIS who cannot tolerate steroids. Slow-release indomethacin 75 mg twice daily or ibuprofen 400 mg three times daily is typically administered for 1 to 2 weeks and then tapered over a 4-week period. Gastrointestinal distress, including peptic ulcers and bleeding, is the most frequent complication.

Cyclophosphamide is a potent, alkylating antineoplastic that may be helpful for NSOIS refractory to steroids or that recur repeatedly on attempted steroid-taper. It has been used most frequently in sclerosing NSOIS when steroids and irradiation have been unable to control disease progression. The daily dose is 1 to 4 mg/kg. It should not be used in patients with blood dyscrasias or hepatorenal dysfunction. Adverse effects include leukopenia, thrombocytopenia, sterile hemorrhagic cystitis, sterility, and carcinogenesis. Because of these serious side effects, a hematologist or oncologist should manage the treatment and provide appropriate monitoring.

Methotrexate is an antimetabolite that inhibits the reduction of folic acid and so interferes with tissue-cell reproduction. It may be used in recalcitrant cases of sclerosing NSOIS alone or in combination with steroids and cyclophosphamide. The dose is 5 to 15 mg weekly, with the minimal possible dose used to control the disease. This drug has serious toxicity, including ulcerative stomatitis, leukopenia, abdominal distress, hepatic and renal damage, and adverse interactions with steroids and nonsteroidal anti-inflammatory drugs. It must be administered under the direction of an oncologist or hematologist, and routine hemogram and liver and renal function tests are mandatory.

Azathioprine is a T-cell suppressant currently used in patients undergoing renal transplants or with severe rheumatoid arthritis. Although not described in the literature, it may be considered in cases of sclerosing NSOIS recalcitrant to steroids and radiotherapy. It has been used with steroids, but is contraindicated with or after cyclophosphamide therapy because of potential mutagenesis. The initial dose is 1 mg/kg/day, with therapeutic response expected at 6 to 8 weeks. Adverse effects include leukopenia and thrombocytopenia, gastrointestinal upset, hepatotoxicity, and carcinogenesis. Close monitoring of blood counts and liver function by an internist is required, with immediate withdrawal of the drug at the first sign of bone marrow depression or liver dysfunction.

Cyclosporine is a potent immunosuppressant that has been used in low doses (2 mg/kg/day) to control granulomatous orbital inflammatory disease where steroids, azathioprine, and cyclophosphamide were intolerable. Because of variable oral absorption, serum trough levels must be measured to reduce the risk of liver or kidney toxicity.

Surgical. Most cases of acute/subacute NSOIS with characteristic clinical and radiographic features may be treated with a therapeutic trial of steroids without obtaining biopsy. CT scans should show no sinus opacification nor orbital bone erosion. In some cases, doing a biopsy on acute NSOIS may actually exacerbate the inflammation. Steroid response should be dramatic and occur within several days; otherwise, prompt biopsy is indicated. Lesions of the lacrimal gland should all undergo biopsy before steroid therapy, since nonspecific inflammations are easily confused clinically and radiographically with lymphoid proliferations, specific systemic inflammations (sarcoid or Sjögren's) or epithelial neoplasia. Tissue diagnosis should also be made for insidious or sclerosing NSOIS and for orbital apex lesions to rule out cicatricial malignancies, lymphoid proliferations, or specific granulomatoses.

Excision (either in part or whole) of an inflammatory mass may be helpful in certain granulomatous or sclerosing NSOIS if the lesions are well localized and can be removed with little risk of functional damage.

Exenteration may be indicated ultimately for very aggressive sclerosing inflammations that have progressed relentlessly to cause blindness, an unsightly contracted orbit, and intractable pain, in spite of maximal medical and x-ray therapy.

Low-dose external beam gamma-radiotherapy (2,000 to 3,000 Rads divided into ten fractions) has proved effective for cases of sclerosing and acute NSOIS resistant to medical therapy. Early combined therapy should be considered for sclerosing lesions to limit functional loss. Apical lesions can be treated through a lateral port causing minimal globe exposure; anterior lesions are treated from the front with shielding of the cornea and lens. Radiotherapy should be avoided in diabetics because of reports of exacerbation of proliferative retinopathy. There have been no reports of secondary malignancies induced in the orbit at these low doses.

Ocular or Periocular Manifestations

Acute/subacute NSOIS:

Anterior: Lid injection and edema; chemosis; visual impairment; uveitis; limitation of movement; retinal detachment.

Apical: Impaired vision and ocular movement; orbital pain; minimal proptosis or chemosis.

Dacryoadenitis: S-shaped deformity of lid with lateral swelling; chemosis; tenderness; pouting of lacrimal ductules.

Diffuse: Same features with more severe involvement.

Myositis: Impaired, painful ocular movements; orbital pain; minimal proptosis or chemosis.

Granulomatous: Palpable orbital mass; minimal inflammatory signs around mass.

Sclerosing NSOIS: Insidious onset of proptosis; restricted ocular movement; orbital pain; vision loss.

PRECAUTIONS

Other diagnostic possibilities should be considered and ruled out before initiating therapy for nonspecific orbital inflammations. Orbital cellulitis may be confused with an acute anterior or diffuse NSOIS. Most cases of cellulitis arise from infected sinuses, which should be identified easily on CT scan. Uncertain cases should be biopsied for culture and histology before treating with antibiotics or anti-inflammatory agents. A rhabdomyosarcoma may cause sudden inflammatory signs in affected children, but CT evidence of orbital bony changes and the features of the primary lesion help distinguish this condition from NSOIS. Graves' orbitopathy occasionally may mimic a nonspecific myositis; the former usually develops more insidiously, has little pain with ocular movements, and rarely has

CT evidence of inflammation involving the tendons or surrounding soft tissues. Cicatricial malignancies may be confused for a sclerosing NSOIS or a discrete neoplasm for a chronic granulomatous NSOIS; tissue diagnosis is advised.

A biopsy should be performed for all lacrimal gland lesions, lesions refractory to steroids, insidious or sclerosing inflammations, and any acute orbital inflammation where the above differential diagnoses cannot be ruled out by clinical and radiologic findings.

An internist may help rule out systemic inflammatory syndromes in cases of granulomatous disease and also monitor side effects from long-term corticosteroids or other chemotherapeutic agents.

COMMENTS

Acute and subacute NSOIS are usually easily recognized by their characteristic clinical and radiologic features and their rapid response to corticosteroids with or without adjunctive nonsteroidal anti-inflammatory agents. A typical course of treatment is 6 to 8 weeks. Poorly responsive lesions should undergo biopsy before initiating other anti-inflammatory or x-ray therapy to rule out lymphoproliferative disorders or systemic inflammatory syndromes.

Sclerosing NSOIS undergo biopsy early, and the patient is examined systemically to rule out other sites of multifocal fibrosclerosis. Pulse-dose steroids, cyclophosphamide, or other chemotherapeutic agents described above, as well as radiotherapy alone or in combination, should be considered early to control the disease before permanent scarring and functional deficits occur. Local excision may help control the inflammatory mass; in relentless cases, exenteration may be the ultimate therapy.

Patients identified by biopsy as having granulomatous NSOIS should be screened by an internist for systemic entities, such as sarcoid or Wegener's granulomatosis, and treated appropriately. True nonspecific granulomatous inflammations often respond well to a brief course of systemic steroids, an intralesional steroid injection, or simple excision of the inflammatory mass.

References

Diaz-Llopis M, Menezo JL: Idiopathic inflammatory orbital pseudotumor and low-dose cyclosporine. Am J Ophthalmol 104:547–548, 1989.

Flanders AE, Mafee MF, Rao VM, Choi KH: CT characteristics of orbital pseudotumors and other orbital inflammatory processes. J Comp Assist Tomogr 13:40–47, 1989.

Kennerdell JS: Management of nonspecific inflammatory and lymphoid orbital lesions. Int Ophthalmol Clin 31:7–15, 1991.

Kennerdell JS: The management of sclerosing nonspecific orbital inflammation. Surv Ophthalmol 22:512–518, 1991.

Krohel GB, Carr EM, Webb RM: Intralesional corticosteroids for inflammatory lesions of the orbit. Am J Ophthalmol 101:121–123, 1986.

Leone CR, Lloyd WC: Treatment protocol for orbital inflammatory disease. Ophthalmology 92: 1325–1331, 1985.

Mauriello JA, Flanagan JC: Pseudotumor and lymphoid tumor: Distinct clinicopathologic entities. Surv Ophthalmol 34:142–148, 1989.

Rootman J, Nugent F: The classification and management of acute orbital pseudotumors. Ophthalmology 89:1040–1048, 1982.

Satorre J, Antle CM, O'Sullivan R, White VA, Nugent RA, Rootman J: Orbital lesions with granulomatous inflammation. Can J Ophthalmol 26: 174–195, 1991.

Weissler MC, Miller E, Fortune MA: Sclerosing orbital pseudotumor: A unique clinicopathologic entity. Ann Otol Rhinol Laryngol 98:496–501, 1989.

ORBITAL CELLULITIS AND ABSCESS 376.01

GEORGE O. STASIOR, M.D.,
and GREGORY B. KROHEL, M.D.

Albany, New York

Orbital cellulitis and abscesses are potentially lethal diseases of adults, children, and immunosuppressed patients. In the preantibiotic area, orbital cellulitis resulted in a 19 per cent death rate, blindness in 20 per cent of the affected eyes, and residual visual loss in another 13 per cent. It is a severe illness that must be managed with emergency hospitalization, blood and wound cultures, complete physical examination, orbital/sinus imaging, and aggressive intravenous antibiotic therapy. During the acute 48 to 72-hour period, antibiotic adjustment guided by positive cultures and drug-sensitivity testing will decrease morbidity and mortality. The complications of failed antibiotic treatment often require surgical intervention and may be life threatening.

The clinical presentation of orbital cellulitis is characterized by an acute febrile illness, leukocytosis, eyelid swelling and erythema, orbital pain, external ophthalmoplegia, proptosis, and potential visual loss. Acute orbital cellulitis can progress and cause severe complications if proper treatment is not initiated quickly. In children and immunosuppressed patients, preseptal cellulitis may progress rapidly to severe orbital cellulitis. Chronic orbital cellulitis, however, presents with a less fulminant course and is usually caused by inadequate antimicrobial treatment or retained foreign bodies.

Orbital cellulitis may be caused by either bacterial, fungal, or parasitic infections. Both acute and chronic orbital cellulitis can develop from direct inoculation, hematologic seeding, and spread from adjacent orbital structures. Direct bacterial inoculation of periorbital tissues results from both surgery and trauma. Special treatment considerations must be made for cases involving intraorbital foreign bodies and animal bites.

Hematologic seeding can result from systemic diseases that include subacute bacterial endocarditis, influenza, scarlet fever, vaccine, herpes simplex, and herpes zoster. Orbital cellulitis can also be spread from adjacent structures that include the eyelids, teeth, sinuses, tear sac (dacryocystitis), or middle ear. In children, the spread of infection from adjacent sinuses (especially the ethmoidal air cells) accounts for 84 per cent of postseptal cellulitis cases.

Fungal orbital cellulitis (aspergillosis or mucormycosis), although rare, can be fatal. The less acute aspergillosis cellulitis usually occurs in healthy patients and is often combined with optic neuropathy. Untreated cases of aspergillosis have a mortality rate as high as 80 per cent. Cases of mucormycosis orbital cellulitis can be fatal by causing vascular necrosis that extends into the brain. Predisposing factors of fungal orbital cellulitis include systemic steroid treatment, fluid/electrolyte imbalance, metabolic acidosis, and radiation. Mucormycosis classically presents in diabetic patients with metabolic acidosis. Characteristic gangrenous, well-circumcised lesions are often found on the nasal mucosa and palate. Fungal orbital cellulitis can progress rapidly to an orbital apex syndrome, presenting with headaches, proptosis, internal and external ophthalmoplegia, loss of vision, and second, third, fourth, and sixth cranial nerve palsies.

The complications of bacterial orbital cellulitis include subperiosteal abscess (7 per cent), meningitis (2 per cent), cavernous sinus thrombosis (1 per cent), visual loss (1 per cent), intracranial abscesses (1 per cent), and osteomyelitis of the facial bones (< 1 per cent). Subperiosteal abscesses are often caused by inadequate intravenous antibiotic treatment, which can result from treatment delay, polymicrobial infection, antibiotic-resistant organisms, or the inability of antibiotics to reach the abscess.

Cavernous sinus thrombosis is another severe complication of orbital cellulitis. It presents with the clinical signs of severe orbital cellulitis combined with intracranial symptoms of nausea, vomiting, headaches, and disorientation. Other symptoms include contralateral eyelid edema or proptosis, decreased sensation of the first and second divisions of the trigeminal nerve, and venous engorgement of the episcleral or retinal circulation. Mechanisms of visual loss in complicated orbital cellulitis include corneal exposure, inflammatory or neovascular glaucoma, exudative retinal detachment, optic neuritis, and central retinal vein or artery occlusion.

Orbital cellulitis is the most common cause of infectious proptosis. The differential diagnosis of inflammatory proptosis includes orbital cellulitis, neoplasms, thyroid-related ophthalmopathy, and idiopathic inflammation. Idiopathic orbital inflammations include orbital "pseudotumor," orbital myositis, and Wegener's granulomatosis. Thyroid-related ophthalmopathy or Graves' disease is the most common endocrine-related autoimmune orbitopathy. Graves' diseases can be differentiated from orbital cellulitis by its clinical signs and symptoms. Common neoplastic causes of inflammatory proptosis include lymphoma (both primary and systemic) and metastatic carcinoma, i.e., lung, breast, and prostate. Rhabdomyosarcoma, leukemia, and retinoblastoma should also be considered in the child. Arteriovenous malformations and carotid-cavernous fistulas are noninflammatory causes of congestive orbital proptosis that must be included in the differential diagnosis of orbital cellulitis.

THERAPY

Systemic. Treatment of orbital infections must be instituted rapidly. High-dose intravenous antibiotics are used after cultures are obtained and before the responsible organisms have been isolated. Orbital imaging studies, preferably CT scanning, are used to rule out the formation of subperiosteal and orbital abscesses, as well as the involvement of adjacent periorbital structures.

The most common bacterial pathogen in children is *Haemophilus influenzae*, which can be highly ampicillin resistant. Over 75 per cent of childhood orbital cellulitis includes *H. influenzae*, *Streptococcus pneumonia*, and *Staphylococcus aureus*. The recent use of *H. influenzae* vaccination may change the future epidemiology of cellulitis in children under 5 years old.

Infants with preseptal or orbital cellulitis are hospitalized and treated with intravenous ceftriaxone. The infant dose of ceftriaxone is intravenous 50 mg/kg every 12 to 24 hours, not to exceed 4 gm/day. In children, a combination of antibiotics is used. Nafcillin or oxacillin, 12.5 mg/kg, intravenously every 6 hours, is combined with cefuroxime, 25–33 mg/kg intravenously, every 8 hours not to exceed 4.5 gm/day. In children with severe cephalosporin or penicillin allergies, chloramphenicol 12.5–25 mg/kg intravenously every 6 hours may be given with hematologic monitoring. Upon discharge, children are treated with oral cefaclor for 5 to 7 days after the child is afebrile. Any signs of relapse on oral therapy warrant immediate rehospitalization and reinstitution of intravenous antibiotics.

In adults, the most common bacterial organisms include *Streptococcus pneumonia* and other streptococci, *S. aureus*, gram-negative aerobes, and non-spore-forming anaerobes. Common anaerobes include *Peptostreptococ-*

cus, Bacteroides, Clostridium, and *Fusobacterium.* Polymicrobial infections are common and often are not adequately covered with a single antibiotic.

Comprehensive coverage in the adult combines nafcillin or oxacillin 1.5 gm intravenously every 4 hours with penicillin G, 1 million units intravenously every 4 hours. Alternatives to penicillin include cefazolin 1–1.5 gm intravenously every 6 hours or cephalothin, 2 gm intravenously every 6 hours. In patients with severe cephalosporin or penicillin allergy, vancomycin 500 mg intravenously every 6 hours or ciprofloxacin 400 mg intravenously every 12 hours may be given. Vancomycin is also useful in treating methicillin-resistant *S. aureus* infections and may be used with gentamicin or rifampin for synergy.

In the presence of chronic sinusitis, anaerobic organisms must be considered, and clindamycin, 600 mg intravenously every 8 hours, may be added to the routine combination therapy. Metronidazole and chloramphenicol also have good anaerobic coverage. In cases of posttraumatic orbital cellulitis or where there is the suspicion of gram-negative organisms, intravenous aminoglycoside or fluoroquinilone should be added to the antibiotic regimen. Intravenous antibiotic therapy should be instituted for 7 to 10 days, followed by an additional 5 to 7 days of coverage by an appropriate oral antibiotic. Oral antibiotics are given if the patient is afebrile for at least 48 hours and shows clinical resolution of orbital cellulitis. Current oral discharge antibiotics include amoxicillin/clavulanate potassium, oral cephalexin, cefuroxime, or dicloxicillin. Antibiotic choice depends on availability, cost, and previous culture results and drug sensitivities.

The treatment of fungal orbital cellulitis is difficult and involves the correction of predisposing risk factors, high-dose intravenous amphotericin B, and surgical debridement. Since fungal cultures are often negative, tissue biopsies may be necessary to prove the presence of diagnostic hyphae.

Surgical. Surgery should be considered if aggressive intravenous antibiotic treatment begins to fail. Subperiosteal or orbital abscesses often require surgical drainage. Periorbital sinusitis and dental abscesses may also need to be drained to cure the adjacent orbital cellulitis. Adequate abscess drainage should be maintained for several days postoperatively. In cases of orbital trauma, it is important to explore the wound meticulously and to remove all foreign bodies.

Supportive. Antipyretics, such as aspirin and acetaminophen, should be used judiciously because they may mask the patient's febrile status. Other analgesics and sedatives may be used to help improve patient comfort. Corneal exposure should be treated with lubricating medication as necessary. Ocular hypertension can be treated topically, but may require systemic diuretics if the intraocular pressure rises higher than 30 mm Hg. Concomitant sinus infections may require topical nasal decongestion (phenylephrine 0.125 per cent for children and oxymetazoline hydrochloride 0.05 per cent for adults) and systemic antihistamines.

Ocular or Periocular Manifestations

Conjunctiva: Hyperemia; chemosis; vascular engorgement.

Eyelids: Erythema; edema; fluctuant abscess.

Globe: Choroidal folds; exposure keratitis; visual loss.

Optic Nerve: Edema; ischemia; atrophy.

Orbit: Periorbital inflammation; fullness to retropulsion; diplopia; painful external ophthalmoplegia; proptosis; subperiosteal abscess; orbital abscess.

Other: Anesthesia of dermatome supplied by the first and second division of the trigeminal nerve; osteomyelitis; subdermal crepitus.

PRECAUTIONS

Blood and wound cultures are mandatory in every patient suspected of having orbital cellulitis. At the time of initial presentation, cultures of the throat, nasal cavity, and conjunctiva may also be helpful. These cultures and their gram stain, when possible, are the appropriate guide for antibiotic therapy. It is important to obtain both gram stains and aerobic, anaerobic, and fungal cultures at the time of surgical drainage.

Orbital imaging should be obtained in all cases of suspected orbital abscesses, when a patient fails to respond to appropriate high-dose intravenous antibiotics, or when recurrence occurs on oral therapy. Orbital imaging includes sinus x-rays, orbital ultrasound, CT scans, and MR imaging. Orbital sinus x-rays are a cost-effective way to rule out adjacent sinus disease. CT scanning and orbital ultrasound can best define subperiosteal or orbital abscess formation. CT scanning best visualizes the presence of osteomyelitis. MR imaging with intravenous gadolinium is useful in following the progression of orbital inflammation and in ruling out organic foreign bodies.

In acute orbital cellulitis, an ophthalmic examination should be done every 4 to 6 hours to limit serious complications. The maximum allowable antibiotic doses should be administered in cases of severe orbital cellulitis with visual loss, subperiosteal or orbital abscesses, and cavernous sinus thrombosis. Triple intravenous antibiotics should completely cover gram-positive, gram-negative, and anaerobic bacteria. If improvement does not occur within 48 to 72 hours, surgical intervention may be necessary. In patients with cavernous sinus thrombosis or CT scan evidence of periorbital or sphenoid sinus involvement, prompt surgical drainage is indicated.

Special consideration should be given to cellulitis resulting from periorbital animal bites. It is important to document a history of previous splenectomy in patients with orbital cellulitis after a dog bite. Dog bites can inoculate the periorbital tissues with DF-2 (dysgonic fermenter-2). Cellulitis, vasculitis, sepsis and even death may develop in postsplenectomy patients. Intravenous penicillin or its derivatives are the recommended treatment of choice. In cases of periorbital cat bites, antibiotics should cover *Pasteurella*. Cellulitis can be treated with oral tetracycline.

Subdermal crepitus or orbital emphysema may be found in cases of traumatic orbital cellulitis. The possibility of an orbital fracture with air in the orbital tissues should be differentiated from crepitus secondary to anaerobic bacterial infection, i.e. clostridia. Antibiotic treatment of traumatic orbital cellulitis and "dirty" wounds should include coverage for anaerobes, and especially *Bacteroides fragilis*.

The side effects of different high-dose antibiotics must be taken into consideration when treating orbital cellulitis. Care should be taken when using chloramphenicol because of bone marrow suppression and aplastic anemia. When using clindamycin, one should be aware of *C. difficile* superinfection of the intestine, which may develop into pseudomembranous colitis. When treating severe cases of orbital cellulitis in children, immunosuppressed patients, and recurrences, an infectious disease consultation may be helpful.

COMMENTS

In general, improvement of orbital cellulitis is seen within 48 hours of aggressive intravenous antibiotic therapy. In 72 hours, eyelid edema and motility should be resolving. Complete resolution of proptosis and restoration of orbital motility should be seen in 10 to 14 days. Immunosuppressed patients must be followed more closely. In children or immunosuppressed patients, metastatic infection may develop after septicemia and may recur months after the original infection. Patients with immunosuppression, adjacent periorbital infections, metabolic imbalances, recurrence of orbital cellulitis, or systemic seeding may require a longer treatment duration and benefit from a team approach.

The team approach is useful in patients with severe orbital cellulitis. Treatment of the immunosuppressed or recurrent orbital cellulitis patient may require an infectious disease consultation. Pediatric consultation is helpful in correcting fluid/electrolyte imbalances during the acute febrile stage and with the administration of high-dose intravenous antibiotics to the child. Adjacent periorbital sinus infection or venous sinus thrombosis requires an otolaryngology surgery consultation. Signs of meningitis may require the

assistance of a neurologist concerning diagnosis and management. The team approach to severe orbital cellulitis may decrease complications and improve the patient's prognosis.

References

Abramowicz M (ed): The Medical Letter Handbook of Antimicrobial Therapy, New York, Medical Letter Co., 1992.

Bruce O: Infections of the eyelids and orbital cellulitis. *In* Hoeprich P, Jordan M (eds): Infectious Diseases. Philadelphia, JB Lippincott, 1989, pp 1124–1132, 1434–1438.

Freeman N, Green WR: Periocular infections. *In* Principles and Practice of Infectious Disease, New York, Harper & Row, 1990, pp 995–1001.

Handler LC, et al: The acute orbit: Differentiation of orbital cellulitis from subperiostial abscess by computerized tomography. Neuroradiology 33: 15–18, 1991.

Harris G: Subperiostial inflammation of the orbit: A bacteriological analysis of 17 cases. Arch Ophthalmol 106:947–952, 1988.

Jones D, Steinkuller P: Strategies for the initial management of acute preseptal and orbital cellulitis. Trans Am Ophthalmol Soc 86:99–112, 1988.

Steinkuller P, Jones D: Preseptal and orbital cellulitis and orbital abscesses. *In* Linberg JV (ed): Oculoplastic and Orbital Emergencies. New York, Appleton & Lange, 1990, pp 51–66.

Steinkuller P, Krohel G, Noel L: Focal Points: Orbital Cellulitis. Clinical Modules for Ophthalmologists, 1991, Vol IX, Module 11.

ORBITAL GRAVES' DISEASE 376.2
(Dysthyroid Orbitopathy, Endocrine Ophthalmopathy, Thyroid-Associated Eye Disease)

J. SCOTT KORTVELESY, M.D.,

Honolulu, Hawaii

and JOHN S. KENNERDELL, M.D.

Pittsburgh, Pennsylvania

The spectrum of disease in Graves' orbitopathy may range from mild symptoms to severe disfigurement and blindness. The diagnosis is made on clinical grounds, which may be supported by laboratory and other noninvasive testing. Typically, the patient is a female between the age of 30 and 50; however, Graves' orbitopathy can occur at any age. The overall female/male ratio is 3:1.

Thyroid-associated eye disease is a chronic orbital inflammation. Symptoms typically are insidious in onset, although acute cases may rarely be seen. Early symptoms and signs include foreign body sensation, dry eyes, and fullness to the lids. Upper eyelid retraction, diplopia, proptosis, and visual loss from optic neuropathy are other manifestations. These signs and symptoms do not occur in any particular order or progression. For example, a patient may present with Graves' optic neuropathy and little or no soft tissue signs, proptosis, diplopia, or lid retraction. This makes it difficult to predict the clinical course of a particular patient. Prophylactic treatments designed to prevent the onset of the various manifestations generally are not available. Therapies are therefore directed at the particular problems when they occur. The inflammatory process usually becomes quiescent in 6 months to 3 years; however, the changes caused by fibrosis are permanent.

Workup of the Graves' patient should include testing of visual acuity, color vision, pupillary examination, extraocular movements, motility measurements, lid evaluation, exophthalmometry readings, anterior segment examination (with attention to conjunctival injection and chemosis, plus corneal staining) and ophthalmoscopy. Intraocular pressure that increases on eccentric gaze suggests extraocular muscle involvement. Any indication of optic neuropathy (diminished acuity/color vision, afferent pupillary defect, or optic disc pallor/swelling) should be followed up with automated threshold visual field testing. Visual evoked response testing may occasionally be useful.

Additional testing, such as forced ductions, orbital ultrasonography, or CT or MRI scanning, may facilitate the diagnosis. All patients with a clinical diagnosis of Graves' orbitopathy should undergo a complete endocrine evaluation for thyroid disease. It typically begins with measurements of FT_4 (free thyroxine) and a sensitive TSH (thyroid-stimulating hormone). Other useful tests include T_3 uptake (a measure of the relative saturation of thyroid-binding globulin or TBG), T_3 (triiodothyronine), and radioactive iodine uptake (for differentiating forms of hyperthyroidism and planning therapy). Tests for microsomal antibodies (MSA) and thyroid-stimulating immunoglobulin (TSI) are useful markers for autoimmune thyroid disease when other tests are negative. Finally, the TRH stimulation test (thyrotropin) can be very valuable in detecting euthyroid Graves' disease. In general, the ophthalmologist should begin by ordering FT_4 and sensitive TSH levels. Further workup may be done with the assistance of an endocrinologist.

THERAPY

Patients with Graves' orbitopathy are managed on an individualized basis according to the predominant clinical findings, which may include one or more of the following: (1) congestion (soft tissue signs), (2) myopathy (diplopia), (3) lid retraction, (4) proptosis, and/or (5) optic neuropathy. Corneal involvement is secondary to lid retraction or proptosis. Man-

agement is then directed at the specific problem(s).

Systemic. The treatment of hyperthyroidism is best managed by an internist or endocrinologist. Propylthiouracil and methimazole inhibit the synthesis of thyroid hormones within the gland itself. Radioactive iodine (iodine [131]) accumulates in the thyroid gland and emits ionizing beta irradiation that destroys functioning thyroid cells. Propranolol[‡] suppresses some of the symptoms of hyperthyroidism, including tachycardia, palpitations, tremors, nervousness, hyperhidrosis, and spasticity.

Treatment of the orbitopathy is the domain of the ophthalmologist. Systemic corticosteroids are the mainstay of treatment for congestive symptoms and signs. Prednisone in doses of 60 to 100 mg per day may be useful for patients with lid edema, conjunctival chemosis and injection, tearing, and some cases of myopathy, proptosis, or optic neuropathy associated with congestion. Concomitant use of a diuretic, such as hydrocholorothiazide 50 mg a day, may help reduce orbital edema. In general, steroids should demonstrate an effect within 2 weeks if they are going to be useful; otherwise, they should be tapered and discontinued.

Other immunosuppressive agents (cyclophosphamide[‡], azathioprine[‡], and cyclosporine[‡]) as well as plasmapheresis, have also been used with varying success.

Ocular. Patients with Graves' orbitopathy frequently complain of grittiness and burning. Frequent lubrication of the ocular surface with artificial tears during the day and an ointment at night helps alleviate most of these symptoms. Topical vasoconstrictors (e.g., naphazoline) are of limited benefit for conjunctival chemosis and injection. Topical corticosteroids are generally not useful because of the protracted course of the disease. Most patients with Graves' orbitopathy and elevated intraocular pressure with eccentric gaze do not develop progressive optic nerve cupping. They have a pseudoglaucoma caused by a restrictive myopathy that exerts external pressure on the globe. Therefore, antiglaucoma medications are usually unnecessary. Sympatholytics, such as guanethidine[*], moxisylyte[†], and bethanidine[†], have been administered topically in cases of eyelid retraction. Despite their documented effectiveness, these agents suffer from significant ocular surface toxicity and limited availability in the United States.

In addition to topical therapy, a variety of other approaches can help improve patient comfort. Moisture chambers and swimmers' goggles help reduce corneal exposure, but have cosmetic limitations. Sunglasses reduce photophobia and tearing. Taping or patching the eyelids at night affords excellent protection in patients with lagophthalmos.

Retrobulbar corticosteroids[*] have been used in patients with contraindications for systemic administration; however, their effectiveness is unproven.

Small-angle tropias caused by restrictive myopathy can sometimes be treated with prisms. These prisms are prescribed to give fusion in primary and reading positions. Patients with large-angle or highly incomitant deviations frequently do not tolerate prism correction.

In selected cases of strabismus, botulinum toxin injections into the extraocular muscles may be of temporary benefit (2 to 3 months) before the advanced fibrotic changes occur.

Supportive. Home humidifiers may be helpful for patients with lagophthalmos or lid retraction with corneal exposure. Elevation of the head of the bed may reduce periorbital edema in patients with congestion.

Patients with dysthyroid orbitopathy are often quite distraught. They are beset with symptoms that may be annoying (tearing, foreign body sensation, photophobia), embarrassing (proptosis, lid retraction), or disabling (diplopia, visual loss). Usually, a careful discussion of the disease process, including reassurance that it is self-limiting, often allays many of the patient's fears. An explanation of the various medical and surgical options usually instills hope in even the most anxious patients. Careful follow-up should be emphasized to monitor progress and reinforce counseling.

Surgical. About 10 per cent of patients with clinical Graves' disease will need surgery for myopathy, lid retraction, proptosis, or optic neuropathy.

Orbital decompression is most beneficial in patients with lid retraction when their proptosis measures greater than 25 mm or they have compressive optic neuropathy. Coronal CT and MRI scans identify the largest muscles and help direct the ophthalmologist in planning the surgical strategy. When a decompression is performed to reduce proptosis, typically the medial or inferior walls are removed first. This removal may be augmented, if necessary, by lateral wall decompression; in exceptional cases, even the orbital roof can be safely decompressed. One wall results in decompression of 0 to 4 mm; two wall, decompression of 3 to 6 mm; three wall, decompression of 6 to 10 mm; and four wall, decompression of 10 to 17 mm. In patients undergoing decompression for compressive optic neuropathy with or without proptosis, the medial wall of the orbital apex is the most important area to be decompressed. Surgical approaches to decompression of the orbit include the lateral (modified Kronlein), medial (Lynch), transcranial (Naffziger), antralethmoidal (translid, fornix, or Ogura), or four-wall (Kennerdell-Maroon) procedures. A variety of combinations and modifications of these techniques have also been described.

In patients with proptosis less than 25 mm that is associated with lid retraction but without optic neuropathy, orbital decompression

is rarely necessary. Instead, surgery on the eyelid is usually sufficient to alleviate the corneal exposure and to mask disfiguring proptosis. For upper eyelid retraction of up to 2 mm, excision of Müllers muscle is adequate to correct the problem. For larger amounts of upper eyelid retraction, levator surgery becomes necessary. A variety of procedures have been described, including levator stripping, levator marginal myotomy, recession of the levator aponeurosis, or placement of a spacer (e.g., sclera, dura) between the aponeurosis and the upper tarsal border. Lower eyelid retraction is approached in a similar fashion. Disinsertion or extirpation of the lower lid retractors has been used with varying success. The most popular approach, however, is placement of a spacer between the disinserted capsulopalpebral fascia and the lower border of the tarsus. Sclera, cartilage, fascia, or a tarsal transplant from the upper lid have all been used successfully as spacers.

When the restrictive myopathy of Graves' orbitopathy induces a tropia that has been stable by prism measurement for 6 months or longer (off of steroids), eye muscle surgery can help restore ocular alignment. The goal is to create fusion in the primary and reading positions. Adjustable suture techniques are preferable in these patients to ensure a favorable postoperative alignment. Recessions are preferred over resections because of muscle restriction and the tendency for scar formation in the orbit of patients with Graves' disease. Overcorrection is preferred because postoperative adjustment is easier when tightening the sutures, i.e., reducing the recession.

The pathologic process of dysthyroid orbitopathy frequently leads to presenile prolapse of orbital fat in the upper and lower eyelid. This prolapse is caused by a combination of factors, including orbital congestion and inflammation, weakening of the orbital septum, and an increase in the volume of orbital fat. Cosmetic blepharoplasty should be approached with this in mind, concentrating on a more aggressive approach to fat removal while being conservative with skin excision.

When indicated, orbital decompression should be undertaken before strabismus or eyelid surgery because the decompression may alter the ocular alignment and eyelid position. Similarly, eye muscle surgery, especially inferior rectus recession, will affect the position of the eyelids. Accordingly, when eye muscle surgery is indicated, it is usually done before any contemplated eyelid surgery. Cosmetic blepharoplasty is best reserved for last when Graves' patients require more than one ophthalmic surgical procedure.

Irradiation. Radiation therapy has an important role in the management of the Graves' patient. The primary indication is in patients with disabling congestive symptoms, including conjunctival chemosis, prolapse, and injection, as well as rapidly progressive proptosis or optic neuropathy. Rare cases of diplopia caused by acute congestion may also benefit from radiation. Generally, congestive symptoms are first treated with corticosteroids. Radiation is reserved for patients with contraindications to steroid therapy or those who are dependent on them but suffer from side effects. External beam radiation in doses of 20 Gy are delivered to the orbit in ten fractions. Steroid therapy is best continued for 4 to 6 weeks after completion of the radiation, since it usually takes this long for radiotherapy to be effective. Radiation will commonly induce an exacerbation of inflammatory and congestive symptoms lasting 2 to 3 weeks. In fact, it is sometimes necessary to increase the steroid dose temporarily during the radiation treatments. As a rule, patients who do not respond to steroids or who are in the fibrotic, noncongestive stage of the disease process will not respond to radiation.

Ocular or Periocular Manifestations

Graves' disease is an orbitopathy and, as such, can affect virtually any structure of the orbit, ocular surface, or ocular adnexa. The eyeball itself is generally spared, except as a secondary effect, e.g., corneal exposure.

Conjunctiva: Chemosis; hyperemia; prolapse.

Cornea: Ulcerative keratitis; exposure keratopathy; perforation.

Extraocular Muscles: Infiltration and fibrosis of some or all muscles (most often inferior rectus, medial rectus, superior rectus); may range from mild limitation of gaze to immobility of the globe causing diplopia or head posturing.

Eyelids: Edema; lag; retraction; fat prolapse.

Lacrimal Gland: Enlargement; infiltration; prolapse.

Optic Nerve: Apical optic nerve compression; atrophy; disc edema; disc hemorrhage.

Orbit: Axial proptosis; resistance to retrodisplacement of globe.

Other: Chorioretinal folds; increased intraocular pressure with eccentric gaze; retinal nerve fiber layer dropout; visual field defect; visual loss.

Precautions

The first signs of orbital Graves' disease may not develop until active hyperthyroidism has been treated and the patient rendered euthyroid or even hypothyroid. Thus, the ophthalmologist should closely monitor patients with orbital Graves' disease before and after therapy for hyperthyroidism. The response of the orbital condition to the treatment of hyperthyroidism is unpredictable; the orbital changes may improve, remain stable, or worsen.

Any patient with orbital Graves' disease who develops ptosis or fluctuating diplopia should be suspected of having coexistent myasthenia gravis.

The side effects and complications of corticosteroid therapy are well known. Chronic steroid therapy should be managed with the assistance of an internist or endocrinologist.

Orbital radiation should be performed by a radiation specialist who is experienced with irradiation of the orbit. The retrobulbar area is treated while the globe itself is shielded. Every patient should be informed of the risk, albeit very slight, of radiation-induced cataract or retinopathy.

Complications of orbital decompression include inadequate effect, loss of vision, motility disturbance, cerebrospinal fluid leaks, lacrimal outflow obstruction, sinus mucocele, sinus hematoma, oral-antral fistula, infraorbital anesthesia, and eyelid malpositions.

Complications of surgery for lid retraction include ptosis (usually more prominent nasally), persistent retraction (usually more prominent temporally), contour abnormalities, ocular irritation or lid thickening induced by spacers (e.g., sclera), and damage to the lacrimal gland and its ducts.

Eye muscle surgery for restrictive myopathy has the same risks as standard strabismus surgery. However, exposure is usually more difficult because of the tethering effect of the muscles. Adhesions and scarring are more of a problem because of the orbital inflammation, especially in reoperations.

Comments

CT scanning is of great value in the diagnosis of orbital Graves' disease. It is also virtually mandatory before orbital decompression is undertaken. A CT scan should be obtained with a high-resolution scanner. Thick sections through the orbit are almost useless; slice thickness should be 5 mm or thinner and must include both axial and coronal projections to permit a full display of muscle enlargement and optic nerve compression. MRI scans give good detail of intraorbital structures, but they suffer from poor delineation of the bony orbit. Orbital ultrasonography is also of great value. The best orbital assessment comes from imaging with a combination of CT scanning and orbital ultrasound.

References

Burde RM: The orbit. *In* Lessell S, van Dalen JTW (eds): Neuro-ophthalmology, 1982. Amsterdam, Excerpta Medica, 1982, vol 2, pp 272–279.

Kennerdell JS, Maroon JC, Buerger GF: Comprehensive surgical management of proptosis in dysthyroid orbitopathy. Orbit 6:153–179, 1987.

McCord CD Jr: Current trends in orbital decompression. Ophthalmology 92:21–33, 1985.

Putterman AM: Surgical treatment of thyroid-related upper eyelid retraction. Ophthalmology 88:507–512, 1981.

Rootman J: Graves' Orbitopathy. *In*: Rootman J:

Diseases of the Orbit. Philadelphia, JB Lippincott, 1988, pp 241–280.

Schorr N, Seiff SR: The four stages of surgical rehabilitation of the patient with dysthyroid ophthalmopathy. Ophthalmology 93:476–483, 1986.

Sergott RC, et al: The clinical immunology of Graves' ophthalmopathy. Ophthalmology 88: 484–487, 1981.

ORBITAL HEMORRHAGES 376.32

KLAUS D. TEICHMANN, M.D., F.R.C.S(C), F.R.A.C.O.

Riyadh, Kingdom of Saudi Arabia

Orbital hematoma may develop spontaneously, particularly in patients with local vascular diseases (venous anomalies, advanced atherosclerosis, aneurysms of the ophthalmic artery, arteriovenous malformations, carotid cavernous fistula, hemangioma, lymphangioma) or be associated with systemic disorders (anemia, leukemia, hemophilia and other clotting disorders, uremia, scurvy, sickle cell disease, malaria, hypertension) or with increased venous pressure (straining, labor, Valsalva maneuver, head-down position). Most frequently, however, it occurs with trauma. Hemorrhage after retrobulbar injection is common (up to 3 per cent), but can be avoided with proper technique. Although usually benign, central retinal artery occlusion (CRAO) or ischemic optic nerve damage may ensue, particularly with intraneural sheath hemorrhage. More dangerous is bleeding after orbital or lid surgery where the orbital septum was opened and fat was removed. The incidence of blindness after blepharoplasty is reported to be less than 1 in 1000. Prevention is very important in these cases and consists of appropriate pre-, intra-, and postoperative measures.

THERAPY

Supportive. Most orbital hemorrhages require no treatment, only observation. One should check for pain, loss of vision, proptosis, ecchymosis, raised intraocular pressure (IOP), afferent pupillary defect, optic disc swelling or pallor, and complete or partial CRAO.

Analgesics may be used generously for ocular and orbital pain while preparing for surgery; however, aspirin should be avoided. If vomiting and nausea are present, antiemetics may be given.

Systemic. Control of blood pressure is important because hypertension can lead to uncontrollable hemorrhage, whereas hypotension may further reduce the already compromised circulation of retina and optic nerve. Bleeding diathesis should be ruled out and treated as required. Intravenous acetazolamide or hyperosmotic agents cannot decompress the orbit effectively.

Surgical. When vision is seriously threatened, surgical intervention is mandatory. As the survival time of vital structures during ischemia is limited (maximum 100 minutes in complete CRAO), time is precious and orbital decompression should be performed promptly. Immediate, although often short-lived, relief is obtained by canthotomy or cantholysis, or both. These procedures are much safer and more effective than anterior chamber paracentesis, which may convert a hard globe with a formed anterior chamber into a hard globe with an absent anterior chamber and the additional problem of angle-closure glaucoma. Imaging techniques (CT scan, MRI, ultrasound) are useful in guiding the surgeon, as the hematoma may be intraconal, extraconal, or more rarely subperiosteal or within the optic nerve sheath, but they often require too much time. Evacuation of a pocket of blood by needle aspiration or transseptal incision may sometimes gain time for more definitive treatment. Exploration of an operating site may indentify the source of the bleeding and permit the meticulous cautery of bleeding points, drainage of fluid blood, and removal of blood clots. Where necessary, the intraconal space should be entered by insertion of a fine hemostat through the intermuscular septum. The most likely source of acute bleeding is the ophthalmic artery or its branches, including the anterior and posterior ethmoidal arteries. These latter arteries can be approached, for clamping and cautery, via a semicircular incision medially to the nasal canthus followed by wide opening of the periorbita and removal of ethmoidal cells including the lamina papyracea. In diffuse oozing, the local application of hemostatics (topical thrombin, absorbable gelatin sponge, microfibrillar collagen) and compression can be used to achieve hemostasis. The increased volume of orbital tissues in cases of diffuse bleeding may require bony decompression, with removal of the orbital floor and the medial orbital wall. If the optic nerve compression is localized in the orbital apex, the posterior ethmoids must be removed. Decompression of the optic nerve sheath is mandatory when central retinal artery circulation is compromised by intraneural sheath hemorrhage. The pupillary response to light, visual acuity, or flash visual-evoked potentials can serve as guides for success. The wound should only be closed after all bleeding has ceased. It is advisable to insert a drain.

Ocular or Periocular Manifestations

Conjunctiva: Chemosis; hyperemia; subconjunctival hemorrhage.

Eyelids: Swelling; ecchymosis; edema; tightness; ptosis; rarely lid retraction.

Other: Ocular and periorbital pain; loss of vision; proptosis; immobility of the globe; sensory and motor abnormalities of the pupil; marked elevation of IOP; cloudy cornea; disc pallor or disc edema; pulsating or collapsed retinal arteries; rarely cherry red spot, cloudy swelling of the retina, or choroidal folds.

PRECAUTIONS

Special attention should be paid preoperatively to determine the existence of hypertension, renal disease, Graves' disease, cardiovascular disease, glaucoma, and the use of such drugs as aspirin, heparin, dicumarol, or warfarin. If a patient is suspected of having a bleeding disorder, the prothrombin time (PT), partial thromboplastin time (PTT), platelet count, bleeding time, and clotting time should be determined before surgery. During surgery, meticulous hemostasis by cautery, ligatures, hemostats, and simple compression should be observed. Orbital fat should never be pulled forward. Prolapsing fat should be clamped, cut, and cauterized. The distal stump of fat should be examined for bleeding before releasing it into the orbit. Moist gelfoam segments, soaked in thrombin solution and applied to the sites where fat was excised, may help promote hemostasis. The excessive use of epinephrine in local anesthesia is dangerous; it may provoke a marked rise in blood pressure or cause a deceptively bloodless field during surgery, with diffuse oozing setting in after vasoconstriction has subsided. A rubber drain (Penrose) or a suction drain (Hemovac) is advisable for deep orbital surgery. Tight bandages, if used at all, should not be left on for longer than 30 to 60 minutes; if pain is reported they should be removed immediately. Gauze pads soaked in iced saline may decrease postoperative swelling and abort hemorrhage. The patient's head should be elevated 30 to 40° after lid and orbital surgery. Close postoperative observation is mandatory. The patient should be asked to report the onset of severe or sudden pain. In case of doubt one should look for proptosis, the pupils should be checked, vision tested, and the fundus examined to rule out vascular occlusion or a compromised circulation.

Orbital decompression is not free of complications. Diplopia and enophthalmos are frequent sequelae that may require additional therapy at a later date. Blindness may follow any type of orbital surgery. A conservative approach should therefore be used whenever feasible, particularly in spontaneous orbital hemorrhage and in hematomas that follow retrobulbar injections, both of which tend to have a good prognosis.

COMMENTS

In any orbital surgery, the wound should not be closed until bleeding has stopped completely.

Visual damage is caused by CRAO, posterior ciliary artery occlusion, or optic nerve compression with disturbance of its blood supply. Optic nerve circulation seems to be more easily compromised than retinal circulation. Because of this fact and their short-lived effect and possible complications, anterior chamber paracentesis or posterior sclerotomy is not recommended. Direct compression applied to the orbit may help stop the bleeding, but at the same time it reduces the perfusion of important tissues. The same is true for compression of a carotid artery.

Despite the fact that early (immediate) orbital decompression is indicated in severe cases, occasionally even delayed intervention (up to several days) has proved beneficial. Further complications of orbital hemorrhage include delayed wound healing, infection and abscess formation, and discoloration of the skin. Fibrosis may develop later and cause motility problems, lid retraction, and ectropion.

References

Anderson RL, Edwards JJ: Bilateral visual loss after blepharoplasty. Ann Plast Surg 5:288–292, 1980.

Brooks AMV, Finkelstein E: Spontaneous orbital haemorrhage. Br J Ophthalmol 68:838–840, 1984.

Callahan MA: Prevention of blindness after blepharoplasty. Ophthalmology 90:1047–1051, 1983.

Feibel RM: Current concepts in retrobulbar anesthesia. Surv Ophthalmol 30:102–110, 1985.

Goldberg RA, Marmor MF, Shorr N, Christenbury JD: Blindness following blepharoplasty: Two case reports, and a discussion of management. Ophthalmic Surg 21:85–89, 1990.

Kelly PW, May DR: Central retinal artery occlusion following cosmetic blepharoplasty. Br J Ophthalmol 64:918–922, 1980.

Kersten RC, Rice CD: Subperiosteal orbital haematoma: Visual recovery following delayed drainage. Ophthalmic Surg 18:423–427, 1987.

Kraushar MF, Seelenfreud MH, Freilich DB: Central retinal artery closure during orbital hemorrhage from retrobulbar injection. Trans Am Acad Ophthalmol Otolaryngol 78:65–69, 1974.

Krohel GB, Wright JE: Orbital hemorrhage. Am J Ophthalmol 88:254–258, 1979.

McCartney DL, Char DH: Return of vision following orbital decompression after 36 hours of postoperative blindness. Am J Ophthalmol 100:602–604, 1980.

Putterman AM: Temporary blindness after cosmetic blepharoplasty. Am J Ophthalmol 80:1081–1083, 1975.

Sullivan KL, Brown GC, Forman AR, Sergott RC, Flanagan JC: Retrobulbar anesthesia and retinal vascular obstruction. Ophthalmology 90:373–377, 1983.

Uthoff D: Preoperative preparation for cataract surgery with intraocular lens implantation. Klin Mbl Augenheilkd 188:160–162, 1986.

Waller RR: Is blindness a realistic complication in blepharoplasty procedures? Ophthalmology 85:730–735, 1978.

REFRACTIVE DISORDERS

ANISOMETROPIA 367.31
(Asymmetropia)

MELVIN L. RUBIN, M.D.

Gainesville, Florida

In anisometropia, the refractive errors of the two eyes are unequal. The two eyes may be myopic or hypermetropic in unequal degrees; one eye may be emmetropic and the other eye ametropic, or one eye may be hypermetropic and the other myopic, a condition termed antimetropia. Except for the uncommon instances of uniocular disease or injury, anisometropia is usually genetically determined by factors related to the axial length of the eye.

Anisometropia may be of varying degrees; clinically, an anisometropia of greater than 2 diopters is considered to be of high degree. However, differences up to 3 diopters are not uncommon, and disparities up to 34 diopters have been recorded. In anisometropia of significant degree, the vision may be binocular, alternating, or uniocular. Binocular vision is the rule in the lesser degrees of defect; however, since the uncorrected image of one eye is always blurred, attempts at fusion frequently bring on symptoms of accommodative asthenopia. In greater degrees of error, fusion is usually impossible, and vision is either alternating or uniocular. Alternating vision can actually be advantageous if one eye is myopic and the patient is a presbyope. The myopic eye is used for near, the other for distance. This condition is called monovision. In a hyperopic youngster, uniocular vision may cause the more hyperopic eye to become amblyopic or to deviate. These risks must be considered when deciding on an optical correction.

THERAPY

Ocular. In dealing with small degrees of anisometropia, full optical correction of both eyes is desirable. In higher degrees, however, full correction presents problems, owing to the differences in size of the images in each corrected eye and irregularities of peripheral distortion. Whenever the eyes move from the primary position, an artificial heterophoria is created with full spectacle correction in highly anisometropic eyes. Therefore, each patient must be considered a separate case, with attention given to the amount of discomfort and disability the patient is suffering without correction and the amount likely to be experienced with correction.

Full correction is especially desirable for children under the age of 12 years. If binocular vision is weak or muscular imbalance is marked, orthoptic exercises should be undertaken, and proper treatment for a squint should be given. In some young patients, temporary occlusion of the better eye may be indicated.

In adults with small degrees of anisometropia and some degree of binocular vision, an attempt should be made to use full correction spectacles. Adults who use either eye alternately for near or far work may be best left untreated, unless symptoms of eyestrain are definitely present.

Whenever possible, contact lenses should be prescribed in preference to spectacles, since contact lenses usually minimize inequality of images by bringing the lens as close as possible to the principal planes. Thus, the artificial heterophoria caused by dissimilar spectacle lenses is largely eliminated and the aniseikonia is likely to be reduced.

PRECAUTIONS

With full correction in highly anisometropic eyes, prismatic imbalances may result that interfere with single binocular vision. This is particularly true for vertical imbalances that are induced when the eyes look down to read. The lines of sight pass through points on the lens that are several millimeters below the optical center, and the vertical displacement of the reading matter is greater for one eye than the other. This creates an artificial heterophoria.

Full correction spectacles, even with small degrees of anisometropia, are uncomfortable at first. However, if the spectacles are used constantly, difficulties often disappear in a few weeks' time. Every attempt should be made to see that the spectacles are worn constantly, especially in children.

COMMENTS

Although it is difficult to assess the degree to which ametropia may be axial or refractive, it is a good assumption to consider differences in the corneal powers of the two eyes as measured by a keratometer to be indicative of refractive ametropia. Unilateral aphakia results in refractive ametropia and the formation of unequal images. This can be corrected with either a contact lens or an intraocular implant. Axial ametropia may be measured by ultrasonography.

References

Duke-Elder S (ed): System of Ophthalmology. St. Louis, CV Mosby, 1970, Vol V, pp 505–511.

Katz M: The human eye as an optical system. *In* Duane TD (ed): Clinical Ophthalmology. Hagerstown, MD, Harper & Row, 1982, Vol I, pp 33: 1–52.

Milder B, Rubin ML: The Fine Art of Prescribing Glasses without Making a Spectacle of Yourself. 2nd ed. Gainesville, Triad Scientific, 1991, pp 217–253.

Rubin ML: Optics for Clinicians, 2nd ed. Gainesville, Triad Scientific, 1974, pp 141–188.

ASTIGMATISM 367.20

SOREN S. BARNER, M.D., M.D.O.S.

Copenhagen, Denmark

Astigmatism is an optical condition in which the refractive power of the eye varies along different meridians. The resulting blurring of the image is caused by the presence of toroidal rather than spherical curvatures of the refracting surfaces. The term "astigmatism" is derived from the Greek words meaning "without a point." In *simple* astigmatism, one principal meridian is emmetropic. Both principal meridians are either myopic or hyperopic in *compound* astigmatism. In *mixed* astigmatism, one meridian is myopic, and the other is hyperopic. If the principal meridians are at right angles to each other, the astigmatism is termed *regular* and can be corrected by cylindrical lenses. In the majority of cases, the steepest meridian is vertical or "with the rule," creating *direct* astigmatism. If the horizontal curvature is steeper, the astigmatism is termed *inverse* or "against the rule." Irregular astigmatism is caused by corneal pathology (scars, keratoconus), lenticular disease (cataract), or uneven corneal pressure caused by lid tumors (chalazion). Aspherical curvature of the anterior surface of the cornea is the most common cause of astigmatism, but also curvature variations of the surfaces of the lens, cataract formation, or an improperly implanted intraocular lens may contribute to the total astigmatism. The influence of heredity in regular astigmatism is difficult to assess. Dominant inheritance with incomplete penetrance is generally accepted to be the more important means of transmission. Usually, astigmatic errors are associated with axial refractive errors. Induced meridional changes after surgery may be pronounced, especially after penetrating keratoplasty, complicated cataract extraction, and plastic surgery of the eyelids. Small degrees of direct astigmatism (<0.5 diopters) are physiologic and rarely cause any symptoms. Larger degrees, astigmatism "against the rule," or errors with an oblique axis may account for decreased visual acuity, asthenopia, frontal headaches, and tilting of the head. Estimation of the degree and axis of the toricity is carried out by keratometry, retinoscopy, and refraction.

THERAPY

Ocular. Since the purpose of refraction is to make the patients comfortable rather than to achieve theoretic optical perfection, small astigmatic errors do not require correction if they produce no symptoms. However, insufficient visual acuity or asthenopic complaints caused by astigmatism should be corrected fully by spectacles. The optical correction of astigmatism is usually achieved by a combination of spherical and cylindrical lenses, as an axial error is often present. The corrective cylinder may either be concave or convex, but it is advisable to use minus cylinders as much as possible. An initial estimation of the degree and axis is usually carried out by keratometry. After a careful refraction, the final prescription may be found to differ significantly from the keratometric measurements because of lenticular errors. It is important to assess the binocular comfort during the refraction and to measure the cylindrical error for near before prescribing glasses.

Instead of spectacles, contact lenses may be used to correct astigmatism. Mild to moderate degrees of corneal toricity are best corrected with spherical contact lenses. An ultrathin lens can be used to correct errors of 1.0 diopter or less. A conventional spherical lens may be used to correct less than 2.0 diopters if the radius of curvature of the lens is halfway between that of the steeper and flatter corneal meridian. If the astigmatism is around 3.0 diopters, a large diameter hard spherical lens may provide stability on the toric cornea. High degrees of astigmatic errors are best corrected with toric contact lenses. To provide stability and avoid rotation of the cylinder axis, a prism ballast may be incorporated into the lens. Truncation is another method to keep the cylinder axis and the astigmatic axis aligned. A small segment of the circular arc of the lower portion of the lens is cut off, and rotation will be stopped by the lower eyelid. Smaller degrees of meridional errors can be corrected by soft lenses. For high degrees of astigmatism, it is advisable to use hard contact lenses.

Surgical. Surgical procedures to control or eliminate excessive degrees of corneal astigmatism have been introduced, and the term "refractive keratoplasty" is used to define controlled surgical alteration of corneal curvatures or thickness in order to induce a physiologic optical correction of the refractive status. The operations have been advocated in pronounced astigmatic anisometropia and persistent high astigmatic errors postoperatively after keratoplasty, cataract extraction, or other surgical interventions involving corneal incisions. Relaxing incisions are aimed at flattening the steeper meridian in contrast to the wedge-resection technique, which is a steepening procedure. Modified radial incisions of the anterior corneal surface—radial keratotomy—and nonintersecting transverse incisions were until recently the most widely used surgical methods to correct corneal astigmatism. A reduction of 10 diopters of astigmatism has been obtained by these operations. Thermokeratoplasty is a different method employed to correct corneal asymmetry. The induced change in corneal curvature is caused by shrinkage of collagen fibers in contact with a hot thermoprobe. With the introduction of the excimer laser for photorefractive keratectomy (PRK), a whole new dimension has been added to refractive surgery. The excimer laser interacts with tissue mainly by photochemical rather than thermal means. The laser releases short pulses in the extreme UV spectrum, virtually vaporizing and ablating the chemical bonds holding the tissue together. The result is an ultra smooth surface ready to heal quickly with a reduced risk of scar formation. Two to four parallel transverse excisions are usually employed for moderate degrees of astigmatism. Refractive keratoplasty or keratorefraction is at present considered a rather controversial method of correcting astigmatism. Various surgical keratometers have therefore been devised to prevent postoperative astigmatism by controlled suture adjustment during the operation.

Ocular or Periocular Manifestations

Cornea: Toric or irregular curvature.
Lens: Cataract; toric or irregular curvature.
Other: Amblyopia; asthenopia; decreased visual acuity; strabismus.

PRECAUTIONS

Patients with moderate or high degrees of astigmatism usually have no other ocular symptoms than insufficient visual acuity. More often, small degrees of hypermetropic or mixed astigmatism give rise to eyestrain and headache, owing to the constant accommodative effort needed to obtain a clear retinal image. It is therefore advisable to correct fully the error in order not to induce an accommodative effort. By prescribing toric spectacles, a meridional aniseikonic error and a declination error are introduced, and the patient must be warned of initial distortion of binocular single vision as compared to the accustomed uncorrected vision. As a rule, however, children adapt quickly to the new visual situation. A change in the dioptric power of the cylinder usually produces less transient symptoms than a change in the axis. If there are no ocular or visual complaints, it is unwise to change either the power of the axis or the cylinder on a routine examination, even if an improvement in visual acuity is found with a different lens. Presbyopes who do not wear spectacles for distance usually need no cylindrical correction for near. As in anisometropia of other etiology, unilateral astigmatism may be responsible for strabismus and amblyopia in childhood. In pathologic degrees of monocular corneal toricity, refractive surgery may be considered to prevent amblyopia. A transient change in astigmatism is frequently associated with uncontrolled diabetes mellitus, and metabolic regulation is necessary before a new prescription is given.

COMMENTS

Provided that there are no ocular or visual complaints, small astigmatic errors do not require correction. Far too many spectacles incorporate an unnecessary cylindrical correction as a result of a theoretic rather than a biologic refraction. It is to be remembered that 95 per cent of individuals of any population are clinically detectable as astigmatic in some degree and that the lenticular astigmatism tends to neutralize the corneal error. A small degree of astigmatism "with the rule" is the usual condition in the first few years of life. During the school years, the astigmatism changes little. From early adult life onward, there is a tendency for the direct astigmatism to decrease or even to be converted into astigmatism "against the rule." The persistent physiologic 0.5 diopter of astigmatism "with the rule" is best ignored.

References

Barner SS: Surgical treatment of corneal astigmatism. Ophthalmic Surg 7:43–48, 1976.

Barner SS: Surgical control of excessive corneal astigmatism. Experimental and clinical results. J Br Contact Lens Assoc 8:37–38, 1979.

Duke-Elder S (ed): System of Ophthalmology. St. Louis, CV Mosby, 1970, Vol V, pp 274–295.

Ellis W: Radial Keratotomy and Astigmatism Surgery, 2nd ed. Berkeley, Kugler & Ghedini, 1986.

Sloane AE, Garcia GE: Manual of Refraction, 3rd ed. Boston, Little, Brown, 1979.

Stein HA, Slatt BJ: Fitting Guide for Hard and Soft Contact Lenses. A Practical Approach, 2nd ed. St. Louis, CV Mosby, 1983, pp 222–226.

Troutman RC: Corneal Astigmatism. Etiology, Prevention and Management. St. Louis, CV Mosby, 1992.

Waring GO: Refractive Keratotomy for Myopia and Astigmatism. St. Louis, CV Mosby, 1991.

HYPEROPIA 367.0
(Far-Sightedness, Hypermetropia)
GEORGE W. WEINSTEIN, M.D.

Morgantown, West Virginia

Hyperopia is a refractive error of the eye in which parallel rays of light focus behind the photoreceptor layer of the retina when the eye is at rest, resulting in a blurred image. Various optical components of this condition include flattening of the cornea or lens, a shallow anterior chamber, a low effective refractivity of the lens, and a small axial length of the eye. Classically, the hyperopic eye is smaller than normal, not only in its anteroposterior diameter but also in all its meridians. The cornea of the classical hypermetrope is small, the lens is large, and the anterior chamber is shallow. Often, the retina has a peculiar sheen (shot-silk retina), which is often associated with accentuated reflexes on the vessels. The vessels may show congenital abnormalities, such as tortuosity and abnormal branching. Symptoms vary with the amount of optical error present, but are usually absent, especially in the young with low degrees of error. In higher degrees of hyperopia, visual blurring is marked, and the patient often holds an object at a distance in order to see it more clearly. Alternatively, the patient may hold a book very close to the eye in an attempt to employ maximum accommodation. Symptoms of eyestrain frequently occur, owing to excessive accommodation and the forced disassociation between it and convergence. Headaches may be a real problem, and the patient may show an apparent divergent squint. The degree of simple hyperopia occurring without malformations of the globe or other pathologic evidences varies considerably; in the vast majority of cases, it is under 3 diopters, although very high values over 20 diopters may occur. The various ocular components that may cause hyperopia seem to be inherited as a dominant trait.

THERAPY

Ocular. As a rule, it is best to undercorrect hyperopia as long as there is some active accommodation. This is true for most young and middle-aged individuals. Since these patients unconsciously utilize accommodation, full correction would result in overcorrection. For this reason there is little need to prescribe spectacles of 1 diopter or less for young hyperopes. The asthenopic symptoms that bring these patients to the office can usually be managed more effectively in other ways. Many of these individuals are in the midst of stressful periods, such as examination times, and tire themselves by reading for long hours into the night. This eyestrain is a manifestation of their overall fatigue, and glasses are not likely to be helpful.

For older individuals who show increasing amounts of manifest hyperopia, the spectacle correction should begin to approach the full amount obtained with refraction. Even so, one should not attempt to correct any of the hyperopia "uncovered" by cycloplegics, but should rely on the "manifest refraction" for this purpose.

In hyperopia, a corrective contact lens is closer to the far point behind the eye than is a corrective spectacle lens. Therefore, the contact lens needs a higher plus power than does the spectacle lens. As the vertex distance is shifted from the usual spectacle plane (10 to 15 mm) to zero for the contact lens, negligible or small power changes are produced for low degrees of hyperopia. For larger amounts of hyperopia in aphakia, the power change is usually quite significant, and calculations or tables based on calculations must be used to determine it.

Ocular or Periocular Manifestations

Anterior Chamber: Shallow.
Ciliary Body: Failure of ciliary muscles; spasm of ciliary muscles.
Cornea: Flat; small.
Lens: Flat; large.
Retina: Macula farther than normal from optic disc; shot-silk retina; vascular tortuosity.
Other: Accommodative asthenopia; convergent squint; divergent squint; eyestrain; overaccommodation; pseudopapillitis.

PRECAUTIONS

The typical hyperopic eye, with its relatively large lens and shallow anterior chamber, is of the type that is predisposed to closed-angle glaucoma. Therefore, mydriatics must be used with care in hyperopes.

COMMENTS

Hyperopia is the normal optical condition in infants and apparently persists throughout life in some 50 per cent of the population in most areas of the world. The 2 to 3 diopters of hyperopia present in infants usually decrease steadily in the early years of life, although they may increase in some hyperopes between the ages of 5 and 14 years. Any residual hyperopia tends to remain stationary until middle age, at which time it tends to increase owing to lenticular changes.

References

Duke-Elder S (ed): System of Ophthalmology. St. Louis, CV Mosby, 1968, Vol IV, pp 257–267.
Weinstein GW: Correction of ametropia with spectacle lenses. *In* Duane TD (ed): Clinical Ophthalmology. Hagerstown, MD, Harper & Row, 1982, Vol 1, pp 36:1–6.

MYOPIA 367.1

ROBERT H. BEDROSSIAN, M.D., M.Sc.,

Vancouver, Washington

and RICHARD ELANDER, M.D.

Santa Monica, California

The word "myopia" is derived from the Greek word *myops*, which means "to half close the eye." This describes the action of "squinting," which many nearsighted people do to improve their distance vision. The optical condition of the eye is such that the posterior focal point lies anterior to the retina. It is the result of an imbalance in the relationship between the refracting components (cornea and lens) and the axial length of the eye. The term "physiologic myopia" is used when these three components lie within the normal distribution curve and/or no pathologic process contributes to the nearsightedness. *Physiologic myopia* usually begins during the rapid growth phase of the body, starting as early as 5 years of age. Myopia generally increases until the normal growth of the individual is completed. In females, it is usually completed between the ages of 13 and 15, and between 15 to 17 years of age in males. However, the onset of myopia may be unrelated to physical growth and not become evident until the late teens or early twenties. It is more likely to occur in those who use their eyes extensively for near work. Recent studies from Denmark have indicated that there is an increase in axial length and vitreous chamber depth. The corneal curvature, anterior chamber depth, and lens thickness are almost constant.

Pathologic myopia occurs when there is excessive expansion of the posterior segment of the eye from the ora serrata to the posterior pole. This is a serious condition that may lead to loss of vision because of the structural changes that occur. It may be congenital and associated with maternal toxemia, rubella, prematurity, and congenital glaucoma. In pathologic myopia, gradual degenerative changes in the fundus occur as the sclera, choroid, and retina become thinner. These changes may occur even with a stable refraction. The earliest fundus change is a large crescent adjacent to the disc, which is followed by localized pale or tessellated patches. With continued thinning of the posterior pole, cracks appear in the retina as the posterior staphyloma enlarges. Black spots surrounded by a pale area, known as Fuchs' spots, may appear centrally. These spots are the result of subretinal neovascularization and leakage. Sudden and permanent loss of central vision may occur with these changes. Punched-out areas of atrophy finally appear. They may coalesce and leave areas of "bare" sclera. The peripheral retina also shows areas of "white without pressure" and increasing lattice degeneration. Paving-stone degeneration, as well as pigmentary degeneration, may also

occur. These changes usually correlate with axial elongation that can be seen by A- and B-scan ultrasonography. Because retinal tears and retinal detachments occur more frequently in the myopic eye compared to the hyperopic or ametropic eye, the peripheral retina should be evaluated carefully. The anterior segment is not immune from changes. Anterior insertion of the iris and remnants of mesoderm in the angle may be seen. Also associated is an increased incidence of ocular hypertension and glaucoma. Indentation tonometry is frequently inaccurate because of low scleral rigidity. These eyes may also be damaged from pressure that would be considered normal. Nuclear cataracts are a common complication of high myopia. It may be difficult to distinguish between the increasing nearsightedness associated with nuclear sclerosis and that with active progression of pathologic myopia. Cataract surgery in the highly myopic individual has an increased incidence of retinal detachment. Topical corticosteroids should be prescribed with caution, as many high myopes respond with increased pressure. The most common course of pathologic myopia is progression and additional degenerative changes. Intraocular pressures should be kept well below normal limits, if possible, to prevent increased enlargement of the scleral shell. Visual fields are also difficult to evaluate because the field defects from myopia are similar to or overlap glaucomatous changes. Fortunately, pathologic myopia is not common, but must be treated with great care when present.

Night myopia is an entity that results in increased nearsightedness when the light level is reduced. The amount is variable between individuals and has been reported to be up to 6 diopters.

THERAPY

Ocular. Spectacles and contact lenses are standard forms of correction for the visual impairment from nearsightedness. To make them more acceptable, new spectacle frame and lens designs, as well as new contact lens materials, are constantly being introduced into the marketplace.

Most studies on the prevention of myopia or on the alteration of the optical properties of the eye have been directed toward environmental factors that may aggravate increasing myopia. The amount of accommodation, nutrition, and posterior segment pressure are factors that are considered most frequently. A great majority of the studies are reported in the optometric literature.

Data from such studies are frequently questioned because of the difficulty in obtaining adequately controlled human studies. There is evidence, however, that continued accommodation and close work aggravate the progression of myopia. Most medical therapy aims at relaxing accommodation, which alleviates the long sustained accommodation that some authorities believe increases the pressure in the posterior segment of the eye. This increased pressure in turn stretches the sclera.

Some studies have suggested that bifocals are of help in myopia. The proponents of this form of treatment argue that the reason why bifocals are unsuccessful is that most are not high enough for children to use them. The top of the bifocal must be at least at the lower edge of the pupil, and the glasses must be fitted so that they stay in position. Prisms to neutralize convergence have also been suggested. Relaxation of accommodation by periodic gaze into the distance while doing close work is advocated by the Japanese. Biofeedback to control accommodation has also been reported in some studies to be effective.

The use of contact lenses and orthokeratology as a method of stabilizing or decreasing myopia still has some enthusiasts. Most patients are fitted with contact lenses about the time that their nearsightedness would normally stop progressing. In many instances, it may be more a coincidence rather than a result of contact lenses that the myopia does not progress. Although some individuals seem to have a permanent decrease in their myopia after orthokeratology, the results are very unpredictable. Retainer lenses are needed in most instances after the myopia has decreased. Corneal warpage with increased astigmatism, central corneal scarring, and keratoconus have been reported from the continued use of contact lenses. Polymegathism of the corneal endothelium may represent the first stages of permanent damage to the cornea from the long continued use of contact lenses. Although these conditions may be less of a problem with the rapidly increasing use of either soft lenses or gas-permeable semirigid lenses, they may still be of concern.

The use of 1 per cent atropine solution in the eye at night on a daily basis is effective in retarding or stopping the increase in myopia in most individuals. If atropine is used in both eyes, bifocals are also necessary. In very low myopes, the atropine can be used in one eye for several months and then in the other eye. This regimen eliminates the need for bifocals, but does not stop the progression of myopia in the untreated eye. In some individuals who have used atropine for a long time, there may be an increase or progression of the myopia. In these individuals, the pupil usually reacts, and they have partial accommodation. Occasionally, sensitivity to atropine occurs, and the eye becomes red and irritated. If this occurs, 0.25 per cent scopolamine may be used. Photochromic or tinted lenses are helpful in those individuals who have light sensitivity when their pupils are dilated. On rare occasions, psychologic disturbances may occur. The long continued use of drops may make this form of therapy psychologically unacceptable for the parents and the child. Lowering the intraocular pressure with timolol may reduce the further development of myopia in a small number of patients with pathologic myopia.

Systemic. Decreased scleral rigidity and elasticity may result from poor nutrition. Therefore, proper nutrition should be encouraged. The elimination of raw sugar, soda pop, candy, jelly sandwiches, and "junk foods" from the diet and the use of vitamin supplements, particularly vitamin A and vitamin C, have been reported as stabilizing the myopia. A recent study has reported that zinc supplements stop progressive myopia. The onset of juvenile diabetes may also be associated with progressive myopia and should be ruled out.

Surgical. Surgically altering the cornea is becoming a more accepted option for the correction of myopia in selected individuals. Radial keratotomy continues to be, by far, the most common surgical procedure. Since most of the effect of radial keratotomy is obtained with the first four incisions, it is increasingly common to use this number in the initial surgery in lower degrees of myopia. Eight incisions may be reserved for higher degrees of myopia in the initial surgery. Additional incisions may be added at a future time if needed. The amount of surgical correction depends primarily on the patient's age, the size of the optical zone, and the number and depth of the incisions. A central optical zone of less than 3 mm is not advisable. Cutting from the limbus toward the optical zone seems to produce more effect than cutting the optical zone outward. Corrections up to 7 and 8 diopters may be reached in older patients (40 or 50 years of age). Various computer programs and charts may be used to assist in determining the effects of the surgery. Late effects (2 to 3 years after surgery) can occur, which has made most surgeons more conservative in their approach. Transverse incisions to correct astigmatism are now made either during the initial surgical procedure or at a later date. They are single or in pairs, 2 to 3 mm in length, and with an optical zone greater than 5 mm. Although still unpredictable, they can be quite effective.

The number of keratomileusis procedures seems to have leveled off. It may well be the most effective treatment of high myopia, but because of its complexity, it remains a procedure done in only a few centers. The unpredictability and late regression of epikeratophakia have limited its use in recent times. Its usefulness is continuing to be researched. Another development is the use of a "nonfreeze" technique to obtain cornea lenticules.

The excimer laser is coming into increasing use, and it looks promising. It works by photoablating some of the corneal structure. It may be used not only as a way to perform radial keratotomy as a primary procedure, but also as a source of resculpting the anterior cornea in eyes that have had radial keratotomy. Other forms of laser energy, such as the Holmium laser, are being studied. Many laboratories are evaluating various instruments and computer programs.

Other avenues of approach include the intrastromal use of hydrogel lenses and materials of a higher index of refraction. These include polysulfone and polycarbonate. The routine use of these materials seems several years away. Which of these procedures will become the dominant one in the future is difficult to predict. Perhaps a combination will be the end result.

More controversial is the recent interest in anterior chamber lenses in phakic eyes and clear lens extraction with or without an intraocular lens. These procedures are being used in increasing numbers in Europe. It seems that their possible side effects (including the loss of accommodation) may be too great for their widespread introduction for the correction of myopia. Nevertheless, much activity is taking place in this field and may show promise for the future.

Thinned areas of scleral ectasia in the posterior pole may be reinforced with scleral grafts. Fascia lata, lyophilized dura, and synthetic materials have also been used. Powdered collagen injections have been used in over 3000 patients in Russia for pathologic myopia and degeneration. They report stability in over 50 per cent of patients with a 3-year or longer follow-up.

PRECAUTIONS

Patients on long-term use of cycloplegics should be followed closely. They should be seen every 4 to 6 months with periodic fundus and tension examinations. If a patient has any family history of retinal disease or cone degeneration, cycloplegics on a continued basis should be used with extreme caution. Psychologic problems may also develop with the use of cycloplegics and bifocals. Fellow students may comment about the bifocals or dilated pupils.

Corneal warpage is much less of a problem now than when nonpermeable hard lenses were common. If it does occur, the patient should be fitted with gas-permeable or soft lenses with the warning that the lenses may need to be changed as stability of the cornea is achieved. An ideal fit with contact lenses should eliminate or minimize spectacle blur.

Surgical therapy of myopia should be considered only after honest and fully informed consent is obtained. Patients have to be aware of the unpredictability of the procedure, as well as the side effects, such as glare and variable vision. Infections can occur, but are fortunately quite rare. Concerns over long-term corneal decompensation now seem to be less important. The main advantage of epikeratophakia is its reversibility, but keratomileusis seems to give a more stable result. Irregular astigmatism is a major potential problem with both of these procedures, as is late epithelial healing. Obviously, clear lens extraction with or without an intraocular lens has all the potential complications of cataract extraction with the added risks of operating on a highly myopic eye. Patients who are considered for this procedure should have a careful examination of the retinal periphery before any surgery. All retinal weaknesses and defects should be considered for treatment by a retinal specialist. Frequent postoperative evaluations of the retinal periphery should also be made to determine any potential hazards. In addition, cystoid macular edema, corneal dystrophy, iritis, choroidal hemorrhage, and endophthalmitis are possible complications of lens extraction with intraocular lens insertion.

COMMENTS

Spectacle glasses to correct myopia should be fitted as close to the eye as possible so that the lens strength and thickness of the glasses, changes in image size, and prismatic displacement may be reduced. Newer techniques of designing spectacle lenses have decreased their weight and made them much more cosmetically acceptable. Contact lenses may be a great help in patients with anisometropia. Despite the evidence that myopia may be aggravated by close work, the prohibition of all reading and close work in children with progressive myopia is unwarranted. Participation in normal day-to-day activities and exercise, as well as good nutrition, should be encouraged. If there are fluctuations in vision, systemic factors should be considered. Minimal diabetes without a spillover of glucose in the urine may cause a fluctuation in the refraction or an increase in myopia. A nonfasting blood sugar should be taken in situations of this nature. Early nuclear cataracts and the use of certain antihypertensive drugs, tranquilizers, and steroids must be ruled out as possible causes. Pseudomyopia and ciliary spasm can occur in individuals who are in jobs where they use their eyes to a great extent. The use of mild cycloplegics at night may eliminate some of the ciliary spasm and permit satisfactory distance vision without glasses.

The economic impact of myopia is a serious consideration. In the United States 40 to 50 per cent of all individuals have myopia. In certain countries, such as Taiwan, the incidence may be as high as 75 per cent. Anything that can be done to prevent severe myopia should be considered beneficial to the patient in the long run and may decrease the cost of medical eye care. Decreased distance visual acuity and dependence upon glasses may prevent some individuals from obtaining certain jobs because of safety factors. These individuals may be candidates for refractive surgery.

References

Bedrossian RH: The effect of atropine on myopia. Ophthalmology 86:717, 1979.

Salz JJ, Maguen E, et al: One year results of excimer laser photorefractive keratectomy for myopia. Refract Corneal Surg 8:269–273, 1992.

Thornton SP: Astigmatic keratotomy. A review of basic concepts with case report. J Cataract Refract Surg 16:430–435, 1990.

Waring GO, Lynn MJ, et al: Stability of refraction during 4 years after radial keratotomy in the PERK study. Am J Ophthalmol 111:133–144, 1991.

Weintraub J (ed): Fourth International Conference on Myopia, Myopia International Research Foundation, 1991.

SECTION 33

RETINA

ABETALIPOPROTEINEMIA
272.5
(Bassen-Kornzweig Syndrome)

and HOMOZYGOUS FAMILIAL HYPOBETALIPO-PROTEINEMIA

RICHARD G. WELEBER, M.D.,
and D. ROGER ILLINGWORTH, M.D., Ph.D.

Portland, Oregon

Phenotypic abetalipoproteinemia may occur on the basis of two genotypically distinct disorders in which affected patients are homozygotes. In the classic form of abetalipoproteinemia, the disorder is transmitted as an autosomal recessive trait, and obligate heterozygote parents have normal concentrations of plasma cholesterol. In contrast, the heterozygous parents of patients with homozygous hypobetalipoproteinemia display reduced levels of plasma cholesterol (70 to 120 mg/dl), and this disorder is transmitted by an autosomal dominant mode of inheritance.

The biochemical and clinical features of abetalipoproteinemia and homozygous hypobetalipoproteinemia are similar; both disorders are characterized by hypocholesterolemia (plasma cholesterol, 25 to 30 mg/dl), the presence of abnormal spiculated red cells (acanthocytes), and fat malabsorption with steatorrhea. These features are present from birth; progressive neurologic symptoms (areflexia, proprioceptive deficits, dysmetria, and ataxia) and pigmentary retinal degeneration develop insidiously in untreated patients and first become clinically evident in childhood (4 to 10 years of age). Other clinical findings that may occur in older patients include myocardial fibrosis, kyphoscoliosis, pes cavus, ophthalmoplegia, ptosis, strabismus, cataracts, and nystagmus.

The biochemical defects present in patients with abetalipoproteinemia and homozygous hypobetalipoproteinemia seem to differ, but both result in the virtual absence of lipoproteins containing apoprotein B48 and B100 from plasma. Recent studies have demonstrated that apoprotein B100 is present in increased amounts in the liver of patients with the autosomal recessive form of abetalipopro-

teinemia and that messenger RNA levels are increased. These data have been interpreted to indicate that this disorder is caused by an as-yet undefined abnormality in the secretion of apoprotein B containing lipoproteins from the liver and intestine. In contrast, immunologically detectable apoprotein B and messenger RNA concentrations of apoprotein B are markedly reduced in the liver of patients with homozygous hypobetalipoproteinemia, inferring that this disorder results from defects in the apoprotein B gene. No gross deletions in the apoprotein B gene have been observed in any of the patients with abetalipoproteinemia studied to date. In contrast, truncated species of apoprotein B have been reported in patients with hypobetalipoproteinemia. Apoprotein B48 is necessary for the assembly and secretion of chylomicrons by the intestinal mucosa, whereas apoprotein B100 is an essential component of very low (VLDL) and low-density lipoproteins (LDL) that are secreted by the liver. High-density lipoproteins do not contain apoprotein B and are the only lipoproteins present in the plasma of patients with phenotypic abetalipoproteinemia. Impaired chylomicron formation in the intestinal mucosa results in malabsorption of dietary fats and the fat-soluble vitamins (particularly A, E, and K), whereas the inability to form hepatic VLDL and LDL results in hypocholesterolemia from the liver. Hepatic transport of vitamin A on retinol-binding protein is normal, but the transport of vitamin E, which is normally carried on LDL, is impaired. This dual impediment in both the absorption and transport of vitamin E results in undetectably low levels of vitamin E in the plasma of untreated patients. Studies have shown a striking similarity between the neurologic lesions that develop in vitamin E-deficient rhesus monkeys and those that occur in untreated patients with abetalipoproteinemia. These observations, together with the documented lack of progression in neurologic or retinal pigmentary changes observed in patients with phenotypic abetalipoproteinemia who were treated for several years with high doses of vitamins E and A, support the view that these acquired degenerative changes are attributable to vitamin E deficiency.

Abetalipoproteinemia and homozygous hypobetalipoproteinemia are both rare. At present, less than 10 cases of homozygous hypobetalipoproteinemia and 60 to 80 cases of abetalipoproteinemia have been reported in the world literature. Despite similar biochemical features, clinical findings in the reported adult patients with homozygous hypobetalipoproteinemia have suggested that this disorder may be associated with less severe neuro-ophthalmologic changes than are seen in the autosomal recessive form of abetalipoproteinemia. Although the validity of these observations in a larger number of patients remains to be established, therapeutic management of both disorders is similar. Patients with heterozygous hypobetalipoproteinemia do not seem to develop any of the neurologic or retinal abnormalities seen in the homozygous state and require no specific therapy. Indeed, because of their inherently low levels of LDL cholesterol, these patients seem to have a lower than normal incidence of coronary heart disease.

THERAPY

Systemic. Supplemental high daily doses of oral water-miscible vitamin A (10,000 to 25,000 IU) have been shown to return the serum levels for this vitamin to normal and to improve dark adaptation thresholds and the electroretinogram (ERG). Although long-term vitamin A supplementation apparently has not prevented the development of retinal pigmentary degeneration in some patients, this may have been related to the lack of supplemental vitamin E. Supplemental vitamin E (200 to 300 IU/kg daily) is of great importance in the prevention of neuromuscular manifestations and retinal degeneration. Plasma concentrations of vitamin E remain low in patients on supplemental therapy, but the recommended dosages have been shown to result in normal concentrations of vitamin E in adipose tissue and liver. Dietary restriction of triglycerides containing long-chain fatty acids is important to control the steatorrhea and gastrointestinal symptoms. Restriction of dietary fat to 10 to 15 per cent of calories is recommended, but this amount may be increased in older patients. Supplemental vitamin K (5 mg weekly) should be given and will correct the prolonged prothrombin time. Serum vitamin A, serum vitamin E, prothrombin time, ERG, dark adaptometry and detailed nerve conduction studies should be performed on a yearly basis to monitor the adequacy of therapy.

Medium-chain triglycerides are contraindicated in patients with phenotypic abetalipoproteinemia and may exacerbate hepatic steatosis and the development of cirrhosis. Although the lack of LDL cholesterol results in subnormal rates of production of steroid hormones by the maximally stimulated adrenal cortex or ovary, patients with phenotypic abetalipoproteinemia do not seem to be at risk for adrenal insufficiency, and coverage with exogenous corticosteroids during periods of major stress is not necessary.

Supportive. Abetalipoproteinemia is an autosomal recessive disorder. Consanguinity has been reported in up to 50 per cent of reported cases and attests to the rarity of the gene in the normal population. Parents and obligate heterozygotes are clinically and biochemically normal. Siblings may be affected, and the risk for homozygosity for each subsequent child to parents with one affected is 25 per cent. Similarly, the risk of a homozygous child in a family where both parents have heterozygous hypobetalipoproteinemia, an autosomal dominant trait, is also 25 per cent. Methods for the prenatal diagnosis of affected siblings have not been established.

Ocular or Periocular Manifestations

Choroid: Atrophy; choroiditis.
Eyelids: Epicanthal folds; ptosis.
Lens: Cataracts.
Optic Nerve: Pallor.
Retina: Abnormal dark adaptation; abnormal electrooculogram; hypopigmentation; macular degeneration; pigmentary degeneration; subnormal or undetectable electroretinogram; vascular attenuation.
Other: Cloudy vitreous; constriction of visual fields; decreased visual acuity; dyschromatopsia; nystagmus; paralysis of extraocular muscles; strabismus.

PRECAUTIONS

The serum from untreated patients with abetalipoproteinemia is low in vitamins A, E, and K. Vitamin D formation in the skin is normal, so supplementation of vitamin D is not necessary.

COMMENTS

The prognosis for patients with abetalipoproteinemia who are untreated or in whom the diagnosis is not made in childhood is poor; progressive retinal degeneration and neurologic dysfunction result. Treatment should be started early in the disease and continued on an indefinite basis. In newly diagnosed cases, the ERG may improve or even return to normal with the rise of serum vitamin A levels, and ataxia may markedly diminish with replacement vitamin E therapy. Although some patients have continued to slowly deteriorate both neurologically and ophthalmologically even while given supplemental vitamin E and A, the doses given may have been inadequate. Since careful monitoring of diet, fat-soluble vitamin levels, and clinical status is imperative in the management of these patients, they should be referred to tertiary medical care centers for evaluation and therapy.

In many cases where the diagnosis has been established in childhood and the patients treated with vitamins E and A, progressive neuro-ophthalmologic dysfunction has been averted. The prognosis for such patients seems good. Phenotypic abetalipoproteinemia must be regarded as one of the potentially treatable hereditary disorders associated with retinitis pigmentosa and spinocerebellar degeneration.

References

Biemer JJ, McCammon RE: The genetic relationship to abetalipoproteinemia and hypobetalipoproteinemia: A report of the occurrence of both diseases within the same family. J Lab Clin Med 85: 556–565, 1975.

Bieri JG, et al: Vitamin A and vitamin E replacement in abetalipoproteinemia. Ann Intern Med 100:238–239, 1984.

Carr RE: Abetalipoproteinemia and the eye. Birth Defects 12:385–399, 1976.

Hardman DA, et al: Molecular and metabolic basis for the metabolic disorder normotriglyceridemic abetalipoproteinemia. J Clin Invest 88:1722–1729, 1991.

Hegele RA, Angel A: Arrest of neuropathy and myopathy in abetalipoproteinemia with high dose vitamin E therapy. Can Med Assoc J 132: 40–45, 1985.

Illingworth DR, Connor WE, Miller RG: Abetalipoproteinemia: Report of two cases and review of therapy. Arch Neurol 37:659–662, 1980.

Kane JP, Havel RJ: Disorders of the biogenesis and secretion of lipoproteins containing the B apolipoproteins. *In* Scriver CR, Beaudet AL, Sly WS, Valle D (eds): The Metabolic Basis of Inherited Disease, 6th ed. New York, McGraw-Hill, 1989, Vol 1, pp 1139–1164.

Kayden HJ, Hatam LG, Traber MG: The measurement of nanograms of tocopherol from needle aspiration biopsies of adipose tissue, normal and abetalipoproteinemic subjects. J Lipid Res 24: 652–656, 1983.

Lowry MJ, et al: Electrophysiological studies in five cases of abetalipoproteinemia. Can J Neurol Sci 11:60–63, 1984.

Miller RG, et al: The neuropathy of abetalipoproteinemia. Neurology 30:1286–1291, 1980.

Nelson JS, et al: Progressive neuropathologic lesions in vitamin E–deficient rhesus monkeys. J Neuropath Exp Neurol 40:166–186, 1981.

Robison WG Jr, Kuwabara T, Bieri JG: Vitamin E deficiency and the retina: Photoreceptor and pigment epithelial changes. Invest Ophthalmol Vis Sci 18:683–690, 1979.

Ross RS, et al: Homozygous hypobetalipoproteinemia: A disease distinct from abetalipoproteinemia at the molecular level. J Clin Invest 81: 590–595, 1988.

Traber MG, et al: Lack of tocopherol in peripheral nerves of vitamin E deficient patients with peripheral neuropathy. N Engl J Med 317:262–265, 1987.

von Sallmann L, Gelderman AH, Laster L: Ocular histopathologic changes in a case of a-beta-lipoproteinemia (Bassen-Kornzweig syndrome). Doc Ophthalmol 26:451–460, 1969.

Wichman A, et al: Peripheral neuropathy in abetalipoproteinemia. Neurology 35:1279–1289, 1985.

Wolff OH, Lloyd JK, Tonks EL: A-B-lipoproteinaemia with special reference to the visual defect. Exp Eye Res 3:439–442, 1964.

Yee RD, Cogan DG, Zee DS: Ophthalmoplegia and dissociated nystagmus in abetalipoproteinemia. Arch Ophthalmol 94:571–575, 1976.

Yee RD, et al: Atypical retinitis pigmentosa in familial hypobetalipoproteinemia. Am J Ophthalmol 82:64–71, 1976.

ACUTE RETINAL NECROSIS 362.84

MARK S. BLUMENKRANZ, M.D.

Menlo Park, California

The acute retinal necrosis syndrome is comprised of the triad of confluent peripheral necrotizing retinitis, arteritis, and vitreitis. The disease is most commonly seen in young and middle-aged adults in the third through fifth decades of life and generally involves one eye, although bilateral disease may occur in up to one-third of patients at the time of presentation. Males are affected slightly more often than are females, and most patients are thought to be in good health with the exception of this problem. Infrequently, a patient may give a history of preceding herpes simplex or zoster mucocutaneous infection at a remote site. In addition to the triad of retinitis, arteritis, and vitreitis, most patients first come to the attention of the ophthalmologist with complaints of a red painful eye caused by granulomatous anterior uveitis, episcleritis, and often ocular hypertension. Additionally, optic nerve dysfunction may be present to a variable degree, ranging from no observable deficit to bare or no light perception, presumably on a vasculitic basis. The most serious and visually significant late complication of the disease is complex retinal detachment, which occurs in between 75 and 85 per cent of patients with this syndrome generally 45 to 60 days after the onset of the disease.

The disease has now been definitively linked to ocular infection by members of the herpes hominis group. It is likely that most cases of "typical" acute retinal necrosis are probably caused by herpes varicella zoster virus, although it is thought that retinal infection with either herpes simplex virus I and II may also produce this clinical picture. Rarely, cytomegalovirus has been implicated in the causation of this disease, although it is generally held that it affects only immunocompromised hosts, whereas most patients with acute retinal necrosis are found to be healthy on general physical and serologic examination and have no evidence of other opportunistic infections.

Recently, several variants of typical acute retinal necrosis have been described. A mild form has been described in adults after primary varicella infection (chicken pox). Acute retinal necrosis after varicella generally occurs in adults over the age of 21, although varicella itself is much more common in children. This variant is thought to involve fewer quadrants, have less associated vitreitis, and infrequently leads to retinal detachment.

A more severe, frequently fulminant form of acute retinal necrosis has been described in immunocompromised patients. This syndrome, termed "rapidly progressive outer retinal necrosis," is characterized by primary involvement of the outer retina, with sparing of the inner retina and retinal vasculature until later in the disease. The disease has been almost exclusively associated with AIDS, and it usually leads to total retinal involvement, severe optic atrophy, retinal detachment, and loss of light perception in most individuals despite antiviral therapy with acyclovir.

THERAPY

Ocular. The anterior granulomatous uveitis is treated by a combination of cycloplegics and steroids. Generally, prednisolone is administered every 2 to 6 hours, depending on the severity of the anterior inflammation, and a long-acting cycloplegic, such as 1 per cent atropine, is given two to four times daily. In those patients with associated ocular hypertension, a topical oculohypotensive agent, generally a beta blocker, such as 0.5 per cent timolol or 0.5 per cent betaxolol, is administered. The ocular hypertension is generally not severe enough to warrant the use of an oral carbonic anhydrase inhibitor, although one may be required occasionally in rare instances. The cycloplegic-steroid combination can be tapered proportionally to the improvement in the anterior uveitis.

Systemic. The opaque confluent retinal lesions, which are known to be associated with active viral infection, respond promptly to treatment with systemic acyclovir. The drug is generally administered at a dosage of 1.5 gm/square meter[§] daily in three equally divided doses, for a minimum of 7 days. Although lower dosages than this have been employed for the successful treatment of other systemic herpetic infections (generally simplex), the higher dosage is recommended because of the well-documented frequency of herpes zoster varicella virus in this condition and its relatively greater resistance to acyclovir (ED-50 3 to 4 μM) compared with herpes simplex (ED-50 0.1 to 1.6 μM). The acute retinal lesions of viral origin are first noted to regress on average 4 days after the initiation of therapy, but require approximately 1 month for complete resolution. For that reason, as well as documented cases of persistence of active virus after only 1 week of intravenous therapy, supplemental therapy with oral acyclovir at a dosage of 15 to 30 mg/kg daily (usually 200 mg five times daily) is generally recommended as well. Retrospective analysis of patients treated both before the era of acyclovir therapy and subsequently suggests that acyclovir reduces the incidence of acute retinal necrosis in the fellow eye from approximately 85 to 25 per cent after 2 years.

Because of the invariable presence of retinal arteritis, frequent optic disc swelling, and vasculitis, treatment with aspirin[‡] at a dosage of 650 mg daily is also recommended for 1 to 2 months after the initiation of the disease. There is some evidence to suggest that this regimen may favorably affect abnormal platelet function that has been reported in this syndrome.

Lastly, because of the severity of vitreitis and potential optic nerve dysfunction, oral steroid therapy is also recommended. Generally it is begun 24 to 48 hours after the initiation of acyclovir therapy because of the potential risk of enhanced viral replication with steroids. Prednisone[‡] at a dosage of 40 to 80 mg daily in conjunction with an antacid should be given, depending on the severity of the vitreitis and papillitis, for at least 1 week with gradual tapering depending on the response to therapy. In general, oral steroids are required for a minimum of 3 to 4 weeks. Despite specific antiviral therapy with acyclovir, many patients actually demonstrate a worsening of the vitreitis during the early phase of the disease under treatment, which can be partially ameliorated by the oral steroids. In cases where there is profound loss of vision that is presumably related to optic nerve dysfunction and in cases of recent onset, some consideration can be given to very high-dose intravenous therapy with methylprednisolone,[‡] although the benefit of this treatment remains unproven.

Surgical. Despite successful regression of the peripheral retinal lesions of viral origin, as many as 85 per cent of patients treated with acyclovir, steroids, and aspirin may still go on to develop retinal detachment, frequently associated with proliferative vitreoretinopathy (PVR). There is some evidence to suggest that, if the peripheral retinal lesions of viral etiology are surrounded by prophylactic photocoagulation (media permitting), the frequency of the incidence of retinal detachment can be reduced by approximately 50 per cent. Often, however, there is severe enough vitreous inflammation and opacification to preclude successful photocoagulation. It is recommended that, in all patients in whom the media permit, at least a triple row of argon or krypton photocoagulation be applied to the posterior extent of existing lesions as well. Prophylactic vitrectomy with photocoagulation, with or without scleral buckling, has been recommended as one means of reducing the likelihood of subsequent retinal detachment. The benefit of this form of therapy remains unproven and controversial, although it may be employed in selected cases depending on the clinical circumstances.

When prophylactic treatment is unsuccessful or cannot be employed, complicated retinal detachment frequently occurs (in up to 85 per cent of cases). This condition seems to be caused by the combination of severe vitreoretinal traction forces resulting from the vitreitis and the development of large tractional tears in postnecrotic retina. It has been established that these detachments respond poorly to conventional scleral buckling techniques and require use of a vitrectomy and long-acting vitreous substitutes for successful long-term reattachment. There is evidence to suggest that employing the additional step of scleral buckling in conjunction with vitrectomy, endophotocoagulation, and long-acting gas tamponade may actually increase the need for reoperation and the frequency of postoperative complications (choroidal detachment, ocular hypertension, fibrin syndrome).

Ocular or Periocular Manifestations

Conjunctiva: Conjunctival hyperemia without a follicular response (acute phase of disease); mild lid swelling; orbital vascular engorgement.
Cornea: Granulomatous keratic precipitates (early phases of disease).
Iris: Vascular engorgement that may be confused with rubeosis.
Optic Nerve: Hyperemia; pale.
Retina: Circular or nummular opacities that appear to involve the outer retina and choroid (early phase of disease); dentate or saw-toothed, yellow-gray, flat, confluent infiltrates in the far periphery with their apices directed toward the optic nerve.
Sclera: Episcleritis.
Vitreous: Inflammatory cells; progressive cicatrization.
Other: Moderate to severe pain.

PRECAUTIONS

The major causes of permanent visual dysfunction in this syndrome are related to the sequela of retinal detachment, which still occurs at a distressingly high rate. In addition to the prompt initiation of therapy with acyclovir, oral steroids, and aspirin, photocoagulation should be administered promptly, if the ocular media permit, to reduce the likelihood of retinal detachment. Although most patients show a relatively prompt resolution of the retinal lesions on acyclovir therapy, in some instances, the lesions may actually persist or increase despite antiviral therapy. In such instances, the dosages should be carefully checked with the pharmacy to ascertain that a full complement of 1.5 gm square meter is being administered daily. It is likely that drug resistance will occur with the increased availability and treatment with various antivirals, although this response has not been well documented in the case of acute retinal necrosis. There is no evidence to suggest that

treatment with topical antiviral agents, such as trifluridine or idoxuridine, is beneficial. Although other antiviral agents have been shown to be effective systemically for other herpetic infections (vidarabine and ganciclovir[+] (DHPG)), concerns regarding potential toxicity with these agents weigh against their routine use.

Because acyclovir is only converted to its active form, acycloguanosine triphosphate, in cells infected with herpes simplex or zoster varicella virus because they contain a unique thymidine kinase, the drug is remarkably nontoxic against normal human and ocular cells. Nonetheless, toxicity may occur at the highest drug levels and is generally associated with crystallization in the urinary tract. For this reason, adequate oral fluid intake is recommended with acyclovir therapy, as well as an appropriate reduction in dosage in the presence of existing renal failure or other significant medical problems.

COMMENTS

The emergence of increasing numbers of patients with this syndrome over the past 10 years is somewhat puzzling and suggests that either the prevalence of herpes simplex and zoster infection is increasing, with the consequent increased incidence of ocular complications, or a mutant strain (e.g., herpes viruses with a predilection for retinal involvement) has evolved. Why this should result in such a high rate of retinal detachment relative to other known ocular infections, such as cytomegalovirus, toxoplasmosis, or toxocariasis, remains unknown, but the availability of specific antiviral therapy, as well as other prophylactic measures, including photocoagulation, has improved the visual prognosis of this syndrome considerably in recent years.

References

Blumenkranz MS, et al: Treatment of the acute retinal necrosis syndrome with intravenous acyclovir. Ophthalmology 93:296–300, 1986.
Blumenkranz MS, et al: Vitrectomy for retinal detachment associated with acute retinal necrosis. Am J Ophthalmol 106:426–429, 1988.
Carney MD, et al: Acute retinal necrosis. Retina 6:85, 1986.
Culbertson WW, et al: Varicella zoster virus as a cause of the acute retinal necrosis syndrome. Ophthalmology 93:559–569, 1986.
Forster DJ, Dugel PU, Frangieh GT, et al: Rapidly progressive outer retinal necrosis in acquired immunodeficiency syndrome. Am J Ophthalmol 110:341–348, 1990.
Han DP, et al: Laser photocoagulation in the acute retinal necrosis syndrome. Arch Ophthalmol 105:1051, 1987.
Palay DA, Sternberg P, Davis J, et al: Decrease in the risk of bilateral ARN by acyclovir therapy. Am J Ophthalmol 112:250–255, 1991.
Young NJA, Bird AC: Bilateral acute retinal necrosis. Br J Ophthalmol 62:581, 1978.

BRANCH RETINAL VEIN OCCLUSION 362.36

FRONCIE A. GUTMAN, M.D.,
and ROBERT E. FOSTER, M.D.

Cleveland, Ohio

Occlusion of one of the tributaries of the central retinal vein is a relatively common retinal vascular abnormality that is second only to diabetic retinopathy. Branch retinal vein occlusion produces a classic ophthalmoscopic picture that usually is recognized easily. The site of venous obstruction is at an arteriovenous crossing where the retinal vessels share a common adventitial sheath. In almost all cases of branch retinal vein occlusion, the artery is found anterior (toward the vitreous cavity) to the vein. Most branch vein obstructions occur in the temporal retina, particularly the superotemporal quadrant. Superficial hemorrhages and retinal edema are invariably present in the area of the retina drained by the obstructed vein. Hemorrhage is usually moderate or heavy with a flame-shaped appearance. Cotton-wool spots usually reflect the degree of local ischemia and are transient. Branch retinal vein occlusion is usually a unilateral finding, although approximately 3 to 10 per cent of patients eventually have bilateral involvement.

Risk factors for branch retinal vein occlusion include a history of hypertension, as well as a hyperopic refractive error. Since 85 per cent of patients suffering a branch retinal vein occlusion have systemic hypertension or other signs of systemic vascular disease, a general medical evaluation is necessary to identify coincident systemic disease. Increased intraocular pressure is not a substantial risk factor for branch retinal vein occlusion, unlike central retinal vein occlusion.

Visual acuity may be reduced by several conditions, including macular edema, intraretinal or vitreous hemorrhage, or foveal ischemia. The two complications of temporal retinal branch vein occlusion usually associated with a poor visual prognosis are macular edema and preretinal neovascularization. Untreated macular edema complicating temporal retinal branch vein occlusion has an unpredictable course and frequently a poor visual prognosis. Photocoagulation with laser paramacular grid therapy improves the visual prognosis for eyes with chronic macular edema that have a visual acuity of 20/40 or worse. Preretinal neovascularization develops in a significant number (19 to 41 per cent) of untreated eyes with temporal retinal branch vein occlusion, and approximately 60 per cent of these eyes will develop vitreous hemorrhages. The preretinal neovascularization develops at the disc and within areas of peripheral retina drained by the obstructed vein. Only rarely does it develop in noninvolved retina. Similarly, anterior segment neovascularization rarely develops after branch retinal vein occlusion.

THERAPY

Surgical. All patients whose eyes develop any form of preretinal neovascularization or macular edema associated with decreased visual acuity should be considered candidates for photocoagulation. Photocoagulation can be used to reverse macular edema and to induce atrophy of preretinal neovascularization. Since macular edema and preretinal neovascularization are such disparate clinical manifestations of the same disease, the indications for and the techniques of photocoagulation in these two complications must be considered separately.

Patients with macular edema are considered candidates for photocoagulation if the macular edema has been present for a minimum of 3 months and if the distance visual acuity is 20/40 or worse. Evaluation of these patients should include a careful refraction to determine both the best corrected distance and near visual acuities, as well as visual fields to evaluate the density of central or paracentral scotomas. Fluorescein angiography is helpful in identifying the leaking intraretinal microvascular abnormalities and assessing the degree of foveal ischemia. The photocoagulation technique consists of argon laser therapy to the sites of leakage associated with the paramacular intraretinal microvascular abnormalities. Sites of leakage and areas of capillary nonperfusion are identified readily on the fluorescein angiogram. Care should be taken to avoid sites of retinal hemorrhage, the capillary-free zone, and shunt vessels crossing the midline raphe. Treatment inside of the capillary-free zone causes a direct insult to the foveal cones. Treatment to the shunt vessels crossing the horizontal midline raphe may destroy collateral vessels and exacerbate stasis within the area of retina drained by the obstructed vein. One hundred-micron spot sizes are used to create a moderate-intensity burn at the sites of intraretinal leakage as determined by fluorescein angiography. If there are paramacular patches of concentrated diffuse intraretinal microangiopathic abnormalities, these areas may be treated by applying 100-μm spot burns spaced one width burn apart in a grid-like pattern. Confluent burns should be avoided to minimize the size and density of the scotoma created by destruction of the photoreceptor cells in the macula. Eyes with visual loss from intraretinal hemorrhage in the fovea or from foveal capillary nonperfusion are thought to have a poor visual prognosis with or without laser therapy.

Treatment efficacy may be assessed with a post treatment fluorescein angiographic study 2 to 4 months after the initial photocoagulation treatment. If there is persistent intraretinal leakage and the visual acuity has not improved significantly, additional treatment may be considered.

Once preretinal neovascularization has been identified, photocoagulation should be considered because of the significant risk of vitreous hemorrhage. Preretinal neovascularization may develop at the disc or may present as a focal frond within the peripheral retina drained by the obstructed vein. The recommended technique for photocoagulation is argon laser therapy, utilizing large (200 to 500 µM) photocoagulation burns of moderate intensity. If a peripheral focal frond is present, it can be treated directly. For preretinal neovascularization on the disc, a pattern of scattered treatment to the peripheral retina drained by the obstructed vein is recommended. Photocoagulation burns are spaced one burn width apart and are applied to all areas of the retina drained by the obstructed vein. Contiguous burns may be applied to areas of capillary nonperfusion. If a patient has both preretinal neovascularization of the disc and peripheral preretinal neovascularization, the two techniques are combined.

After treatment, clinical examination and fluorescein angiography will document the changes in the preretinal neovascularization. Involution or atrophy of preretinal neovascularization is clinically recognized by the loss of vascularity in the preretinal frond and is confirmed by an absence of fluorescein leakage and staining. A skeleton of preretinal fibrous tissue may remain.

If initial treatment has not totally destroyed the preretinal neovascularization, an additional fluorescein angiographic study should be performed to identify ischemic areas of the retina. Additional treatment should be applied to these ischemic areas and to previously untreated portions of the retina drained by the obstructed vein.

PRECAUTIONS

Although a thrombus within the affected vein is a consistent histopathologic finding in branch retinal vein occlusion, there is no contemporary controlled prospective study that evaluates the benefits of anticoagulant and fibrinolytic therapy. This may be partially explained by two observations. First, patients with branch retinal vein occlusion are frequently not seen for several weeks or months after the onset of symptoms. In addition, thrombus organization in the form of recanalization and endothelial cell proliferation may occur quite early (within 10 to 14 days). If thrombus organization has already commenced at the time of initial evaluation, the potential benefits of anticoagulant or fibrinolytic therapy would seem quite limited.

The complications seen after photocoagulation for preretinal neovascularization include vitreous hemorrhage, rhegmatogenous retinal detachment, traction retinal detachment, and macular epiretinal membrane formation. However, since all of these complications may develop in the natural course of branch retinal venous occlusive disease, their relationship to photocoagulation treatment remains uncertain.

COMMENTS

The ultimate goal in the treatment of macular edema is to improve the functional quality of central vision. For this reason, patients being considered as candidates for photocoagulation should have their distance and near visual acuities separately and carefully assessed. If a patient has only one eye with functional vision and has some level of useful reading vision, observation may be considered with deferral of photocoagulation.

The visual prognosis for eyes with macular edema is favorably influenced by laser photocoagulation. In the Branch Vein Occlusion Study, 60 per cent of treated eyes achieved a visual acuity of 20/40 or better compared to 34 per cent of untreated eyes. Remission of the macular edema and improvement in visual acuity are very gradual processes, occurring over a 6- to 12-week interval. As long as there is an improvement in visual acuity and fluorescein angiographic evidence of decreased leakage, retreatment should be deferred. If there are no signs of a remission, at least 6 weeks of observation are recommended before considering additional laser treatment. Patients with pretreatment findings, such as a visual acuity of 20/200 or worse, a dense sector scotoma, intraretinal foveal hemorrhage, and significant foveal capillary nonperfusion, may have a poor visual prognosis with or without photocoagulation.

The goal of treatment of eyes with neovascularization is to decrease the risk of vitreous hemorrhage. Twenty-two per cent of all branch retinal vein occlusions develop preretinal neovascularization, as compared to 12 per cent of eyes treated with scatter argon photocoagulation. However, the risk of neovascularization is increased in eyes with large areas of ischemia, which was defined as 5 or more disc diameters of capillary nonperfusion in the Branch Vein Occlusion Study. For this reason, eyes with extensive areas of capillary nonperfusion should be frequently and prospectively watched for early signs of preretinal neovascularization. Eyes with complete posterior vitreous detachments are at less risk for neovascularization and subsequent vitreous hemorrhage than eyes with no or partial posterior vitreous detachments.

In eyes with preretinal neovascularization, peripheral scattered laser photocoagulation promotes destruction of the neovascular fronds and reduces the incidence of vitreous hemorrhage by 50 per cent. Atrophy of neovascular fronds is usually evident within 2 to 8 weeks after photocoagulation therapy. If a vitreous hemorrhage occurs shortly after the initial treatment, it may clear without recurrence. However, if vitreous hemorrhage recurs at a later time and neovascular fronds are still present, additional peripheral laser treatment may be indicated.

Inferior temporal retinal branch vein occlusions with associated vitreous hemorrhage are more difficult to treat because the vitreous hemorrhage gravitates over that portion of the retina affected by the obstruction and limits the evaluation by fluorescein angiography and visualization for photocoagulation. If vitreous hemorrhage obscures the retina, laser therapy utilizing red wavelengths may be more effective than argon in producing photocoagulation burns and also may minimize thermal effects to the vitreous. Another alternative when vitreous hemorrhage obscures the involved retina is transconjunctival cryosurgery. For cases of chronic, severe, vitreous hemorrhage, vitrectomy facilitates clearing of the vitreous media and may be combined with endophotocoagulation treatment of the involved retina. Infrequently, eyes with neovascularization may develop tractional or rhegmatogenous retinal detachments, which may be repaired with vitreoretinal surgery.

References

Appiah AP, Trempe CL: Differences in contributory factors among hemicentral, central, and branch retinal vein occlusions. Ophthalmology 96:364–366, 1989.

Birchall CH, et al: Visual field changes in branch retinal "vein" occlusion. Arch Ophthalmol 94: 747–754, 1976.

Branch Vein Occlusion Study Group: Argon laser photocoagulation for macular edema in branch vein occlusion. Am J Ophthalmol 98:271–282, 1984.

Branch Vein Occlusion Study Group: Argon laser scatter photocoagulation for prevention of neovascularization and vitreous hemorrhage in branch vein occlusion. Arch Ophthalmol 104:34–41, 1986.

Cox MS, Whitmore PV, Gutow RF: Treatment of intravitreal and prepapillary neovascularization following branch retinal vein occlusion. Trans Am Acad Ophthalmol Otolaryngol 79:387–393, 1975.

Feist RM, et al: Branch retinal vein occlusion and quadratic variation in arteriovenous crossings. Am J Ophthalmol 113:664–668, 1990.

Finkelstein D: Retinal branch vein occlusion. In Ryan SF (ed): Retina. St. Louis, CV Mosby, 1989, Vol 2, pp 427–432.

Frangieh GT, et al: Histopathologic study of nine branch retinal vein occlusions. Arch Ophthalmol 100:1132–1140, 1982.

Gutman FA: Macular edema in branch retinal vein occlusion: Prognosis and management. Trans Am Acad Ophthalmol Otolaryngol 83:488–492, 1977.

Gutman FA, Zegarra H: The natural course of temporal retinal branch vein occlusion. Trans Am Acad Ophthalmol Otolaryngol 78:178–192, 1974.

Gutman FA, et al: Photocoagulation in retinal branch vein occlusion. Ann Ophthalmol 13:1359–1363, 1981.

Johnson RL, et al: Risk factors of branch retinal vein occlusion. Arch Ophthalmol 103:1831–1832, 1985.

Kado M, Trempe CL: Role of vitreous in branch retinal vein occlusion. Am J Ophthalmol 105:20–24, 1988.

Michels RG, Gass JDM: The natural course of retinal vein obstruction. Trans Am Acad Ophthalmol Otolaryngol 78:166–177, 1974.

Miller SD: Argon laser photocoagulation for macular edema in branch vein occlusion. Am J Ophthalmol 99:218–219, 1985.

Pollack A, et al: The fellow eye in retinal vein occlusive disease. Ophthalmology 96:842–845, 1989.

Russell SR, et al: Vitrectomy for complicated retinal detachments secondary to branch retinal vein occlusions. Am J Ophthalmol 108:6–9, 1989.

Weinberg D, et al: Anatomy of arteriovenous crossings in branch retinal vein occlusions. Am J Ophthalmol 109:298–302, 1990.

CENTRAL OR BRANCH RETINAL ARTERY OCCLUSION 362.31
(BRAO, CRAO)

MICHAEL H. GOLDBAUM, M.D., and LEONARD S. KIRSCH, M.D., F.R.C.S.(C)

San Diego, California

The significance of managing patients with retinal artery occlusion goes beyond attempts to restore vision. Approximately 90 per cent of patients with central retinal artery occlusion have an associated underlying disease, the identification and treatment of which may reduce morbidity or increase longevity for the patient. Of all retinal arterial occlusions, 60 per cent involve the central retinal artery, 35 per cent are in a branch retinal artery, and 5 per cent affect a cilioretinal artery. The average age of patients with central retinal artery occlusion is 60 years. Males predominate in a ratio of 2:1, and obstructions occur bilaterally in 1 to 2 per cent of patients.

The causes of occlusion of the retinal arteries may be classified into broad groups: emboli arising spontaneously from upstream vessels or the heart, iatrogenic emboli, focal inflammation or degeneration of the retinal artery as it enters the eye, disorders of the blood or clotting mechanism, pressure to the eye or the central retinal artery in the optic nerve, carotid insufficiency, spasm of the central retinal or ophthalmic artery, hypovolemic shock, injury to the ophthalmic or retinal artery, and anomalies or kinks in the retinal artery.

Most occlusions are caused by emboli, and the remainder are probably due to locally induced thrombosis. The clinical presentation is a function of the size of the embolus and where it lodges in the circulation. Any embolus, if small enough to enter the ophthalmic artery and large enough to obstruct the central retinal artery, may produce infarction of the retina. Platelet-fibrin clots are barely visible, grayish, nonrefractile plugs that may originate from an ulcerated atheroma in the carotid artery, from mural thrombi secondary to myocardial infarction or atrial fibrillation, or from mitral valve prolapse. Bright yellow, refractile cholesterol crystals (Hollenhorst plaques) often arise from carotid ulcerations. Calcific emboli are large, white, oval, moderately refractile bodies at or near the optic disc that usually develop secondary to diseased aortic or mitral valves. Atrial myxoma, a benign cardiac neoplasm, may be the source of multiple, spontaneous retinal emboli in a young patient. Other sources of emboli include fat from long bone fractures, and talc or cornstarch in intravenous drug abusers. Facial or orbital injection may inadvertently force substances upstream into the carotid system that then go downstream to reach the eye as iatrogenic emboli. Carotid angiography may liberate embolic material. Awareness of these potential procedural complications may aid in their prevention.

Thrombosis of the retinal arteries may occur secondary to hemorrhage into an ulcerative arteriosclerotic plaque, inflammation, or degeneration of the arterial wall. Turbulent blood flow from irregularities of plaques encroaching on the vessel lumen can induce thrombus formation that completes the obstruction. Temporal arteritis, systemic lupus erythematosus, and other connective tissue disorders may cause an obstructive arteritis. Furthermore, thrombus formation can occur from such blood dyscrasias as Waldenstrom's macroglobulinemia, multiple myeloma, sickle hemoglobinopathies, or disseminated intravascular coagulation.

Prolonged elevation of intraocular pressure above systolic pressure can result from scleral buckles, improper calibration of machines that control the infusion of fluids or gases during vitreoretinal surgery, or unrecognized pressure on the eye during general anesthesia for orthopedic or neurosurgical procedures. Occlusive pressure in the central retinal or ophthalmic artery may develop from intraorbital implants, tumors, edema, hemorrhage, or emphysema. Elevated intrasheath pressure from hemorrhage or injection into the optic nerve subarachnoid space can close the central retinal artery within the optic nerve.

Acute obstruction of the central retinal artery may be brief with recovery of visual function in minutes, may be transient or partial with recuperation of some or all visual function in hours, or may be complete and of sufficient duration to produce permanent visual loss. The gradient of the partial pressure of oxygen from the patent choroidal circulation to the retina after central retinal artery occlusion is adequate for prolonged survival, but not enough for sustained viability of the inner two-thirds of the retina. Experimental complete occlusion of the central retinal artery in rhesus monkeys for less than 100 minutes allowed full recovery of retinal function; progressively longer occlusion time resulted in successively less recovery of visual function. The recovery of partial or complete vision in patients with central retinal artery occlusion may occur after several hours or days if the occlusion is not complete.

Brief slowing of the retinal blood flow or lowering of the retinal blood pressure may cause a fleeting (generally less than 10 minutes) blindness (amaurosis fugax) in the affected eye. This symptom occurs frequently in the course of stenotic carotid arterial atherosclerosis and is observed occasionally in valvular heart disease and systemic arteritides. Often, amaurosis fugax is caused by emboli, and its occurrence should prompt a search for carotid occlusive disease. Residuals of such an event may persist in the retina as cholesterol emboli and cotton-wool spots. The presence of retinal emboli is evidence that the carotid artery is not occluded completely.

The main symptom of central retinal artery occlusion is a sudden, painless loss of vision to the level of counting fingers or hand movements in the affected eye. If the vision is no light perception, an occlusion of the ophthalmic artery should be considered as a possible cause. Occasionally, amaurosis fugax occurs hours or days before the prolonged visual loss. In approximately 25 per cent of eyes with central retinal artery occlusion, a cilioretinal artery spares part or all of the macula, and there remains a corresponding island of visual field. Conversely, obstruction of a cilioretinal artery alone causes a coinciding scotoma.

Upon ocular examination, a relative afferent pupillary defect is almost invariably present if the event is unilateral or bilaterally asymmetric. Retinal ischemic edema becomes visible as a pale grayish-white discoloration within 5 to 10 minutes after onset of the occlusion. At this time, the affected arteries may be thin and empty or have pulsatile or stationary blood segments appearing as "boxcarring." The veins are darker than normal. After 70 minutes of deprivation of blood flow through the central retinal artery, the retina reaches maximal whiteness. The fovea has a characteristic cherry red or brown color because it still receives adequate nutrition from the choroid.

Approximately one-third of patients have incomplete occlusion of the central retinal artery; the presenting visual acuity in these patients may range from 20/30 to hand motion. Restoration of the circulation may be heralded by slow flow or intermittent spurts of blood. When the occlusion is incomplete, the final vision correlates positively with the presenting vision and negatively with the duration of visual impairment.

The electroretinogram (ERG) can serve to

determine if the retinal artery obstruction is accompanied by choroidal occlusion. In a pure central retinal artery occlusion, the B-wave is lost as a result of inner retinal ischemia, but the A-wave remains since the photoreceptors still function. With ophthalmic artery occlusion or infarction of both the retinal and choroidal circulation from extraocular pressure, both the A- and B-waves of the ERG are lost. Fluorescein angiography may have normal arm-to-retinal circulation time or may reveal insufficiency of the preocular circulation by delayed arm-to-retinal circulation time. There is slowing or cessation of retinal arterial filling, increased arteriovenous transit time, and attenuation of the vasculature. With reperfusion, the fluorescein angiogram may appear normal despite persistently decreased vision.

THERAPY

Whatever treatment is used, prompt action improves the chance for success. Complete occlusion for more than 6 hours probably produces irreversible retinal damage.

Preventive. The iatrogenic causes can be anticipated, and surgical procedures should be altered to reduce the risk of occlusion. For example, after a scleral buckle is placed, the patency of the central retinal artery can be verified by indirect ophthalmoscopy. The probability of retrobulbar injection into the optic nerve or its sheath may be reduced by having the eye gaze in primary position, rather than superonasally.

Systemic. Underlying causes of retinal artery occlusion are treated directly. For instance, the effect of sickle hemoglobinopathies can be reduced with exchange transfusions. For central retinal artery occlusion due to such arteritides as temporal arteritis, high-dose corticosteroids may prevent visual loss in a fellow eye or rarely improve visual function in an affected eye. Prednisone, 1.5 to 2.0 mg/kg orally per day, is instituted with tapering over 6 to 18 months while following symptoms and the erythrocyte sedimentation rate. Hemodynamically significant atherosclerotic carotid disease amenable to surgery is treated most effectively by endarterectomy.

Ocular. The rationale for treatment of central retinal artery occlusion is to restore blood flow and prevent irreversible cell death. No treatments have yet been devised that are wholly satisfactory, in part because of the delayed presentation of many patients. Attempts to treat arterial occlusions are directed toward dislodging the embolus downstream and providing increased oxygenation of the retina. Methods to displace the embolus include trying to dilate the involved artery, increasing the pressure gradient across the blockage, and jarring the embolus. Although inhaled 5 per cent carbon dioxide gas is a potent vasodilator, it has not been found to dilate the central retinal artery in normal subjects. Retinal oxygenation may be improved by diffusion from the choroid with 95 per cent inhaled oxygen, but this has the treatment disadvantage of autoregulatory constriction of the normal central retinal artery. Carbogen, a mixture of 95 per cent oxygen and 5 per cent carbon dioxide, may be administered by face mask for up to 36 hours both to induce vasodilation and increase oxygenation; however, this treatment is probably not efficacious in most cases. The tissue effects of the 95 per cent oxygen may be offset by reduced ocular perfusion from generalized vascular dilation induced by the carbon dioxide. Retrobulbar injection of vasodilators or smooth muscle relaxants has not been demonstrated to dilate the retinal arteries or to improve retinal blood flow. Intravenous administration of 0.5 to 1.0 gm acetazolamide lowers intraocular pressure relatively rapidly, thereby increasing the intravascular pressure gradient across the embolus. Carbonic anhydrase inhibitors, it should be noted, are contraindicated in patients with sickle cell hemoglobinopathies. Anterior chamber paracentesis or digital ocular massage to enhance aqueous humor outflow, followed by the abrupt release of pressure, increases the pressure gradient across the obstruction; in addition, ocular massage has the potential benefit of mechanically dislodging the embolus.

The goal of treatment of the thrombus in a retinal artery is lysis of the clot. If the occlusion is incomplete, the body's natural fibrinolysis may occur in time for preservation of retinal function. Thrombolytic agents have been demonstrated to be effective in the treatment of acute myocardial infarction. The logical extension of this concept is the intracarotid injection of urokinase[‡] or tissue plasminogen activator.[‡] A recent report indicates that urokinase injected into the proximal portion of the ophthalmic artery may dramatically improve the visual outcome in some selected patients with central retinal artery occlusion if given within 6 hours; however, a well-controlled trial with an adequate number of patients will be necessary to evaluate fully the efficacy of fibrinolytic agents. Fibrinolytic therapy or systemic anticoagulation should be performed by physicians experienced in the use of these agents.

Surgical. When hemorrhage or edema causes the intraorbital pressure to exceed the systolic pressure of the ophthalmic or central retinal artery, decompression can be accomplished by orbital paracentesis or canthotomy. Optic nerve decompression reduces the pressure from traumatic intrasheath hemorrhage around the orbital optic nerve.

PRECAUTIONS

Patients with central retinal artery occlusion should also be followed for 3 months after the occlusion for the development of rubeosis iridis. Approximately 18 per cent of all patients with central retinal artery occlusion develop neovascularization of the iris, which is a much higher incidence than previously believed. Furthermore, roughly 15 per cent of all patients progress to neovascular glaucoma.

COMMENTS

The prognosis for visual recovery varies with the site of the obstruction. Ophthalmic artery occlusion generally has a grim prognosis. In central retinal artery occlusion, 70 per cent of eyes have a final vision of 20/400 or worse. By contrast, 90 per cent of eyes with branch retinal artery obstruction retain vision of 20/40 or better. Therefore, while patients with central retinal artery occlusions are treated vigorously to try to avert a poor outcome, patients with branch arterial occlusions are usually not given local therapy to dislodge the embolus. However, it must be emphasized that the search for an associated systemic disease is crucial regardless of the ocular presentation. For example, an erythrocyte sedimentation rate (preferably Westergren) and temporal artery biopsy must be performed in patients over 55 years of age suspected of having temporal arteritis. Noninvasive B-scan ultrasonography and Doppler tests of the carotid may reveal ulcerative plaques or significant carotid occlusion. A physician experienced in the management of cerebrovascular or cardiovascular disease may be helpful in the evaluation of the patient for carotid stenosis, cardiac valvular disorders, mural thrombosis, atrial myxomas, or temporal arteritis. In one study, the expected survival in patients with central retinal artery obstruction was 5.5 years compared to 15.4 years for an age-matched control population. In another report, patients with retinal arterial emboli had a 56 per cent mortality rate over 9 years compared to a 27 per cent rate for age-matched controls without emboli. Identification and treatment of underlying disorders may decrease the risk of morbidity or reduced longevity.

References

Augsburger JJ, Magargal LE: Visual prognosis following treatment of acute central retinal artery obstruction. Br J Ophthalmol 64:913–917, 1980.

Brown GC, Magargal LE: Central retinal artery obstruction and visual acuity. Ophthalmology 89:14–19, 1982.

Brown GC, Shields JA: Cilioretinal arteries and retinal arterial occlusion. Arch Ophthalmol 97:84–92, 1979.

Bull DA, et al: Correlation of ophthalmic findings with carotid artery stenosis. J. Cardiovasc Surg (Torino) 33:401–406, 1992.

Chawluk JB, et al: Atherosclerotic carotid artery disease in patients with retinal ischemic syndromes. Neurology 38:858–863, 1988.

Deutsch TA, et al: Effects of oxygen carbon dioxide on the retinal vasculature in humans. Arch Ophthalmol 101:1278–1280, 1983.

Duker JS, Sivalingam A, Brown GC, Reber R: A prospective study of acute central artery obstruction. The incidence of secondary ocular neovascularization. Arch Ophthalmol 109:339–342, 1991.

Ffytche TJ: A rationalization of treatment of central retinal artery occlusion. Trans Ophthalmol Soc UK 94:468–479, 1974.

Hayreh SS, Weingeist TA: Experimental occlusion of the central artery of the retina. I. Ophthalmoscopic and fluorescein angiographic studies. Br J Ophthalmol 64:896–912, 1980.

Hayreh SS, Weingeist TA: Experimental occlusion of the central artery of the retina. IV. Retinal tolerance time to acute ischaemia. Br J Ophthalmol 64:818–825, 1980.

Hirayama Y, et al: Bifemelane in the treatment of central retinal artery or vein obstruction. Clin Ther 12:230–235, 1990.

Jampol LM, et al: Ischemia of ciliary arterial circulation from ocular compression. Arch Ophthalmol 93:1311–1317, 1975.

Lorentzen SE: Occlusion of the central retinal artery: A follow-up. Acta Ophthalmol 47:690–703, 1969.

Perkins SA, et al: The idling retina: Reversible visual loss in central retinal artery obstruction. Ann Ophthalmol 19:3–6, 1987.

Ros MA, Magargal LE, Uram M: Branch retinal-artery obstruction: A review of 201 eyes. Ann Ophthalmol 21:103–107, 1989.

Rossman H: Treatment of retinal arterial occlusion. Ophthalmologica 180:68–74, 1980.

Savino PJ, Glaser JS, Cassady J: Retinal stroke: Is the patient at risk? Arch Ophthalmol 95:1185–1189, 1977.

Schmidt D, Schumacher M, Wakhloo AK: Microcatheter urokinase infusion in central retinal artery occlusion. Am J Ophthalmol 113:429–434, 1992.

Wise GN, Dollery CT, Henkind P: The Retinal Circulation. New York, Harper & Row, 1971.

CENTRAL SEROUS CHORIORETINOPATHY 362.41
(Central Serous Retinopathy)

JAMES C. FOLK, M.D.,
and CHRISTINE E.P.- BARTOS, M.D.

Iowa City, Iowa

Central serous chorioretinopathy (CSC) is a disease in which a serous detachment of the neurosensory retina is caused by leakage from the retinal pigment epithelium (RPE). The disease affects patients 20 to 55 years of age, with males outnumbering females by 10 to 1. Patients notice decreased vision, metamorphopsia, micropsia, and a positive central scotoma. The cause of this disease is unknown, but it typically occurs in males who are hard driving and have "type A" personalities. Often, the patient relates the onset of the disease to a time of unusual stress or anxiety, and some researchers believe the disease may be caused by higher-than-normal levels of circulating serum epinephrine.

THERAPY

Supportive. There is no proven medical treatment for central serous chorioretinopathy. Patients who present with their first episode can be reassured that they have at least a 90 per cent chance of retinal reattachment with an improvement of vision to 20/30 or better without treatment. Studies have shown that laser treatment directed to the site of RPE leakage hastens the resolution of the subretinal fluid and decreases the risk of recurrence, but does not improve the ultimate visual acuity even over a prolonged follow-up period. These studies contained relatively few patients and used Snellen visual acuity as an end point, which may be a relatively insensitive test of dysfunction in these patients. Although nearly all patients with a resolved episode of central serous chorioretinopathy have 20/30 or better acuity, many are persistently bothered by blurred vision, a relative scotoma, metamorphopsia, or poor color vision in the affected eye. It remains unknown whether the risk or severity of these symptoms would be decreased by a more rapid resolution of the subretinal fluid induced by laser treatment.

Surgical. A reasonable approach to patients with a first episode of central serous chorioretinopathy is to perform an initial fluorescein angiogram to rule out other causes of subretinal fluid and then to see the patient again 2 months later. If the fluid has not resolved after 2 months, treatment should be considered, especially if the leak is 300 μM or more from the foveal center. The angiogram should be repeated to locate the area(s) of RPE leakage. An appropriate frame of the angiogram should then be magnified on a viewer, and the area of RPE corresponding to the leakage found by examining the patient with a contact lens at the slit-lamp should be measured. A retrobulbar anesthetic* is usually unnecessary, but the patient should fixate on some target with the opposite eye and should be told not to move suddenly. Digital pressure on the fundus contact lens or the use of the larger "Yanuzzi" contact lens also helps minimize inadvertent movement of the eye being treated. Either argon green or krypton red laser can be used at a 100- to 200-μM spot size and a 0.1-second duration. The power should be set very low and increased gradually until a gray or light white burn is achieved that is sufficient. Often, only three or four gentle burns are required to treat the area of leakage.

No patching or drops are needed after treatment. The patient should return in 4 weeks or any time that either vision or metamorphopsia worsens. The fluorescein angiogram should be repeated if there is a suspicion of choroidal neovascularization or 2 months after treatment if the subretinal fluid has not resolved.

Ocular or Periocular Manifestations

Retina: Loss of foveal reflex; multiple yellow precipitates on the posterior surface of detached retina; retinal pigment epithelial detachment, atrophy, and pigmentation; serous neurosensory detachment.

Other: Central scotoma; decreased color vision; decreased vision; induced hyperopia; metamorphopsia; micropsia.

PRECAUTIONS

Before making a diagnosis of central serous chorioretinopathy, other cases of a macular neurosensory retinal detachment must be ruled out. These other causes include an optic pit, a choroidal tumor, a peripheral or posterior retinal break, and a choroidal neovascular membrane. Subtle choroidal neovascularization can be missed easily in these patients. Both the fundus and the fluorescein angiogram must be studied carefully for signs of choroidal neovascularization, such as hemorrhage, a grayish color to the retinal pigment epithelium, or a vascular-like structure that fills with fluorescein dye. The risk of choroidal neovascularization increases greatly in older patients with drusen and in patients with histoplasmosis scars, angioid streaks, or high myopia. Patients with choroidal neovascular membranes have a much poorer prognosis than those with central serous retinopathy. Usually, these membranes must be treated thoroughly and promptly to decrease the risk of visual loss.

Patients with central serous chorioretinopathy must also be warned that they may have persistent symptoms of blurred vision or a scotoma even after successful treatment, that there is a small risk of developing choroidal neovascularization, and that the subretinal fluid can recur later. There is also a small (perhaps 5 per cent) risk of choroidal neovascularization developing later at the site of laser treatment. This risk may increase over time.

COMMENTS

Patients with an acute episode of central serous chorioretinopathy can be followed safely, but laser treatment should be considered if the fluid does not resolve in 2 months. Laser treatment should be considered sooner, perhaps within a month, in patients with recurrent episodes because their risk of visual loss is greater and treatment seems to decrease the rate of recurrence. Recent studies with prolonged follow-up of central serous patients revealed that many continue to lose vision slowly. Included in this group of patients who lose vision are those who have chronic central serous retinopathy with multiple episodes of serous fluid. The serous detachment in these patients is often very shallow and difficult to detect over the atrophic RPE. These patients should have fluorescein angiography to determine whether there is a RPE leak. The leak may be minimal and subtle, but usually can be differentiated from the other areas of RPE atrophy or window defects, especially late in the angiogram. The leaks in these patients are usually treated in order to eliminate the subretinal fluid, but whether this treatment ultimately preserves vision remains unknown.

References

Dellaporta A: Central serous retinopathy. Trans Am Ophthalmol Soc 74:144–153, 1976.

Folk JC, et al: Visual function abnormalities in central serous retinopathy. Arch Ophthalmol 102:1299–1302, 1984.

Ficker L, et al: Long-term follow-up of a prospective trial of argon laser photocoagulation in the treatment of central serous retinopathy. Br J Ophthalmol 72:829–834, 1988.

Frederick AR Jr: Multifocal and recurrent (serous) choriodopathy (MARC) syndrome: A new variety of idiopathic central serous choroidopathy. Doc Ophthalmol 56:203–235, 1984.

Jalkh AE, et al: Retinal pigment epithelium decompensation. I. Clinical features and natural course. Ophthalmology 91:1544–1548, 1984.

Jalkh AE, et al: Retinal pigment epithelium decompensation. II. Laser treatment. Ophthalmology 91:1549–1553, 1984.

Klein ML, et al: Experience with nontreatment of central serous choroidopathy. Arch Ophthalmol 91:247–250, 1974.

Levine R, et al: Long-term follow-up of idiopathic central serous chorioretinopathy by fluorescein angiography. Ophthalmology 96:854–859, 1989.

Novak MA, et al: Krypton and argon laser photocoagulation for central serous chorioretinopathy. Retina 7:162–169, 1987.

Robertson DM, et al: Direct, indirect, and sham laser photocoagulation in the management of central serous retinopathy. Am J Ophthalmol 95:457–466, 1983.

Schatz H, et al: Subretinal neovascularization following argon laser photocoagulation treatment for central serous chorioretinopathy: Complication or misdiagnosis. Trans Am Acad Ophthalmol Otolaryngol 83:893–906, 1977.

Watzke RC, et al: Ruby laser photocoagulation therapy of central serous retinopathy. Part I: A controlled clinical study. Part II: Factors affecting prognosis. Trans Am Acad Ophthalmol Otolaryngol 78:205–211, 1974.

Watzke RC, et al: Direct and indirect laser photocoagulation of central serous choroidopathy. Am J Ophthalmol 88:914–918, 1979.

Yamuzzi LA: Type-A behavior and central serous chorioretinopathy. Retina 7:111–130, 1987.

COATS' DISEASE 362.15
(Massive Exudative Retinitis, Retinal Telangiectasia)

WILLIAM TASMAN, M.D.

Philadelphia, Pennsylvania

Coats' disease is a nonhereditary abnormality of the retinal vasculature that was first described by Coats in 1908. Associated with the abnormal retinal vasculature is subretinal exudation that may involve the macula. Peripheral retinal telangiectasis is common, and fluorescein angiography frequently reveals retinal ischemia in the areas of telangiectasis. In some cases, microaneurysmal-type changes can occur in the posterior pole. Exudation in the periphery and posterior pole is another hallmark of the disorder. Histologically, cholesterol crystals are seen in the retina. Although the vitreous is usually clear, in advanced cases vitreous hemorrhage and/or detachment of the sensory retina may occur. Occasionally proliferative vitreoretinopathy can ensue. In the end stages of unsuccessfully treated Coats' disease, neovascular glaucoma may develop. When the diagnosis is equivocal, CT scanning is a valuable test because of its ability to delineate intraocular morphology, calcified subretinal densities, and, through the use of contrast enhancement, vascularities in the subretinal space.

Coats' disease is much more common in males than females, but does affect both sexes. It is unilateral in 90 per cent of cases and is diagnosed most often between the ages of 2 and 10 years.

THERAPY

Surgical. Treatment is directed at elimination of the abnormal vessels. Both laser photocoagulation and cryotherapy are useful in eliminating the retinal telangiectasis, but when the exudation is marked, cryotherapy may be more effective than laser. Usually two to three treatment sessions are necessary at 4- to 6-week intervals to destroy the abnormal vasculature. Those patients with two or fewer quadrants have the best prognosis. The outlook becomes more guarded when three or more quadrants are involved.

Patients with advanced Coats' disease may develop serous retinal detachment. Although scleral buckling with drainage of subretinal fluid followed by cryotherapy to the abnormal vessels can lead to retinal reattachment, many such eyes are now better managed by pars plana vitrectomy, internal drainage of subretinal fluid and cholesterol crystals, and endolaser therapy.

With the elimination of the telangiectasis, exudation will begin to clear. This is a slow process, and it may take as much as 1 year until all of the exudate has absorbed. When the macula is involved, an organized fibrotic scar may remain permanently in the fovea.

Ocular or Periocular Manifestations

Retina: Cholesterol crystals; exudates; telangiectasis; microaneurysms; nonrhegmatogenous retinal detachment.
Vitreous: Hemorrhage; proliferative vitreoretinopathy.
Other: Neovascular glaucoma.

PRECAUTIONS

Even in patients who have been treated successfully, recurrences have been noted as much as 5 years later. It is therefore recommended that patients be followed at 6-month intervals so that if further treatment becomes necessary it can be done before the process becomes too extensive.

COMMENTS

Cryotherapy and photocoagulation have proved effective in salvaging many eyes with Coats' disease. Sometimes, however, macular vision does not return if the exudation has been present in the foveal area. It is important to consider the following conditions in the differential diagnosis of Coats' disease: angiomatosis retina, retinoblastoma, familial exudative vitreoretinopathy, retinopathy of prematurity, nematode infestation, and X-linked retinoschisis.

References

Coats G: Forms of retinal disease with massive exudation. Roy Lond Ophthalmol Hosp Rep 18: 440–525, 1907–1908.
Egerer I, Tasman W, Tomer TL: Coats' disease. Arch Ophthalmol 92:109–112, 1974.
Fox KR: Coats' disease. Metabol Pediatr Ophthalmol 4:121–124, 1980.
Haik BG: Advanced Coats' disease. Trans Am Ophthalmol Soc 89:371–476, 1991.
Harris GS: Coats' disease, diagnosis and treatment. Can J Ophthalmol 5:311–320, 1970.
Ridley M, et al: Coats' disease: Evaluation of management. Ophthalmology 89:1381–1387, 1982.

DIFFUSE UNILATERAL SUBACUTE NEURORETINITIS 363.05
(DUSN)

JOSEPH E. ROBERTSON, JR., M.D.
Portland, Oregon

Diffuse unilateral subacute neuroretinitis is a clinical syndrome characterized by visual loss, vitreitis, papillitis, and recurrent crops of gray white retinal lesions. Progressive visual loss, optic atrophy, retinal vessel narrowing, and diffuse pigment epithelial degeneration may also develop in time. Ocular larvae migrans of nematode origin have been associated with diffuse unilateral subacute neuroretinitis. Initially, *Toxocara canis* was speculated as the nematode causing diffuse unilateral subacute neuroretinitis, but more recently, *Baylisascaris* larvae, especially *B. procyonis* from raccoons, are suspected as the probable cause of diffuse unilateral subacute neuroretinitis. When visualized, the intraocular nematodes are usually detected initially in the macular area during biomicroscopy. They range in size from 400 to 2,000 μM long, are white, often with a glistening sheen, smooth, and gently tapered at both ends. The largest diameter of the nematode is approximately 0.05 times its length. Endemic areas of the United States for this disease seem to be the Southeast and Midwest. The nematode may persist in the fundus for up to 3 years; the various sizes of worm reported are probably due to variations in its age. The nematode is actually identified in only a minority of cases, and it is the other clinical signs that usually lead to the diagnosis. Other clinical presentations include coarse clumping of subretinal pigment that is occasionally arranged in a pattern suggesting tracks and scattered focal chorioretinal atrophic scars. Progressive changes in the structure and function of the eye continue as long as the worm remains viable. There is a reduction in amplitude of both the electroretinogram and electro-oculogram that is proportional to the degree of intraocular damage. In advanced cases, both may be severely reduced or nearly extinguished. The end stage of this process may appear ophthalmoscopically similar to advanced retinitis pigmentosa. However, it is generally quite readily differentiated from retinitis pigmentosa by its unilateral presentation.

THERAPY

Surgical. The traditional treatment for this disorder has been laser photocoagulation of the worm when it can be visualized in the subretinal space. This treatment is effective in destroying the nematode and arresting the destructive process. The toxic damage and atrophic changes that have occurred before initiation of therapy are generally irreversible, although the accompanying inflammation usually slowly subsides after laser treatment.

Systemic. Unfortunately, even extensive biomicroscopic examination may sometimes fail to localize the nematode. Previously, use of antihelmintic agents was generally considered unsuccessful. Recently there has been interest in using oral thiabendazole[‡] as a treatment for this disorder. Treatment with thiabendazole does seem to be effective, but its use is still reserved for those cases not amenable to laser therapy. The recommended dose is 22 mg/kg given two times a day for 2 to 4 days. The maximum daily dose is 3 gm.

Ocular or Periocular Manifestations

Optic Nerve: Atrophy; edema; papillitis.
Retina and Retinal Pigment Epithelium: Diffuse or focal atrophy; multifocal gray-white lesions; nematode present; vascular narrowing.
Vitreous: Vitreitis.
Other: Visual loss.

PRECAUTIONS

The pathogenesis of this condition seems to involve a local toxic tissue effect on the outer retina caused by the worm products left in the wake and a more diffuse toxic reaction affecting both inner and outer retinal tissues. Although the variability of the inflammatory signs suggests that both the local and diffuse tissue damage are governed by the immune response of the patient, corticosteroids do not seem to have any beneficial effect in preventing this damage.

COMMENTS

Any patient with late or early signs of the neuroretinitis should be investigated for nematodes and questioned for exposure to raccoons or skunks. Biomicroscopy and indirect ophthalmoscopy with a +15 diopter lens or a fundus camera are required to locate the smaller worms. Although inflammatory signs, particularly vitreous cells, are usually present in the late as well as the early stages of the disease, they may be absent, even in an extensively damaged eye containing a viable nematode.

References

Gass JDM, Braunstein RA: Further observations concerning the diffuse unilateral subacute neuroretinitis syndrome. Arch Ophthalmol *101*: 1689–1697, 1983.
Gass JDM, Scelfo R: Diffuse unilateral subacute neuroretinitis. J Roy Soc Med *71*:95–111, 1978.
Gass JDM, et al: Diffuse unilateral subacute neuroretinitis. Ophthalmology *85*:521–545, 1978.
Gass JDM, et al: Successful oral therapy in diffuse unilateral subacute neuroretinitis. Transactions Amer Ophth Soc *89*:97–112, discussion 113–116, 1991.
Gass JDM, et al: Oral therapy in diffuse unilateral subacute neuroretinitis. Arch Ophthalmol *110*: 675–680, 1992.
Kazacos KR, et al: Diffuse unilateral subacute neuroretinitis syndrome: Probable cause. Arch Ophthalmol *102*:967–968, 1984.
Oppenheim S, Rogell G, Peyser R: Diffuse unilateral subacute neuroretinitis. Ann Ophthalmol *17*: 336–338, 1985.

EALES' DISEASE 379.23
(Angiopathia Retinae Juvenilis, Inflammatory Disease of the Retinal Veins, Primary Perivasculitis of the Retina, Primary Retinal Hemorrhage in Young Men, Retinal Periphlebitis, Vasculitis Retinae, Vitreous Hemorrhage of Unknown Etiology)

MICHAEL L. KLEIN, M.D.

Portland, Oregon

Eales' disease was first described in 1880 as a condition in young men that was characterized by recurrent intraocular hemorrhages associated with enlarged and tortuous retinal veins and with concurrent findings of headache, constipation, and epistaxis. Soon thereafter, inflammation of the retinal veins was implicated in this disease entity, leading to subsequent recognition of periphlebitis as its most important feature. The most commonly proposed etiology has been allergy to tuberculoprotein. In recent years, several disease entities have been identified, each having clinical features indistinguishable from Eales' disease. Thus, the diagnosis of this disease has become less common.

Today, the term "Eales' disease" usually refers to cases of retinal phlebitis without apparent etiology. Most cases (more than 80 per cent) involve both eyes, and men are affected more frequently than women. Intraocular inflammation may be present in the early stages of the condition. Sheathing and obstruction of retinal veins (and arterioles), usually in the periphery, are typically associated with retinal hemorrhages and peripheral capillary nonperfusion. The development of neovascularization, with its sequelae of vitreous hemorrhage, fibrous proliferation, retinal detachment in the posterior segment, and neovascular glaucoma in the anterior segment, complete the full spectrum of ocular changes that may be seen in Eales' disease. The condition has been associated with a higher incidence of exposure to tuberculosis, and an increased likelihood of vestibuloauditory dysfunction has been reported.

THERAPY

Surgical. Laser photocoagulation is recommended for those cases with retinal neovascularization. Scatter treatment in the nonperfused area surrounding the new vessels and in the area peripheral to them should be applied to produce regression. It may be supplemented with local treatment to the new vessels if they are lying flat on the retina. Panretinal photocoagulation is indicated for neovascular glaucoma.

Vitrectomy should be considered for those cases in which vitreous hemorrhage has not cleared after a period of observation. During this waiting period, ultrasonography should be employed to establish that an accompanying retinal detachment is not present. If so, immediate surgical intervention may be indicated.

Ocular. No form of medical therapy has been shown to be of any benefit. Systemic corticosteroids[‡] have been used extensively, but their value has not been established.

Ocular or Periocular Manifestations

Anterior Segment: Rubeosis irides; neovascular glaucoma.
Optic Nerve: Edema.
Retina: Capillary nonperfusion; detachment; hemorrhages; macular edema, neovascularization; perivascular exudate; perivascular sheathing; vasculitis; venous obstruction.
Vitreous: Hemorrhage.

PRECAUTIONS

Photocoagulation can be associated with complications that include hemorrhage from treated neovascular fronds, choroidal hemorrhage, choroidal vitreal neovascularization, and macular pucker.

COMMENTS

Before a diagnosis of Eales' disease can be made, patients must receive a thorough workup to rule out several known conditions that produce this clinical picture. These include varieties of hemoglobinopathies, blood dyscrasias, connective tissue disorders, and inflammatory diseases. A chest x-ray should be included in such a workup to rule out sarcoidosis and tuberculosis.

References

Geiser SC, Murphy RP: Eales disease. *In* Ryan SJ (ed): Retina. St. Louis, CV Mosby, 1989, Vol 2, pp 535–539.
Renie WA, Murphy RP, Anderson KC, et al: The evaluation of patients with Eales' disease. Retina 3:243–248, 1983.
Spitznas M: Eales' disease: Clinical picture and treatment with photocoagulation. *In* L'Esperance FA Jr (ed): Current Diagnosis and Management of Chorioretinal Diseases. St. Louis, CV Mosby, 1977, pp 513–521.

GYRATE ATROPHY OF THE CHOROID AND RETINA WITH HYPERORNITHINEMIA 363.57
(Ornithine-δ-Amino Transaminase Deficiency)

RICHARD G. WELEBER, M.D.,
and NANCY G. KENNAWAY, D.Phil.

Portland, Oregon

Gyrate atrophy of the choroid and retina is a rare, autosomal recessive, progressive dystrophy that is associated with hyperornithinemia and deficient activity of ornithine-δ-amino transaminase (OAT), which is a pyridoxal phosphate-dependent enzyme required for the synthesis of proline from ornithine. The disease is characterized by circular patches of total vascular choroidal atrophy, which begin in the periphery in early childhood, enlarge and coalesce, and eventually extend toward the posterior pole. Constriction of the visual field, night blindness, cataracts, defective color vision, retinal vascular leakage, peripapillary atrophy, and macular changes develop as the disease progresses. Rarely, macular edema results. Myopia of moderate to severe degree is frequent. Legal blindness usually occurs in the fourth to fifth decade. Electroretinogram (ERG) responses and electro-oculogram (EOG) light-induced rise of the resting potential of the eye, as measured by the light to dark ratios, are consistently abnormal and eventually obliterated. Seizures or abnormal electroencephalography or both have been reported. Although the neuromuscular and electromyographic examinations are normal, eosinophilic subsarcolemmal deposits, which appear as tubular aggregates on electron microscopy, are seen on muscle biopsy. They may be secondary to inhibition of creatine synthesis by ornithine.

Parents who are carriers of this condition are normal clinically. Siblings may be affected and should be evaluated by determination of serum ornithine levels and fundus examination, as eye disease may be unrecognized.

At least two forms of gyrate atrophy with hyperornithinemia are known: a vitamin B$_6$-nonresponsive form, and a slightly milder vitamin B$_6$-responsive form. Only a few per cent of patients with gyrate atrophy are vitamin B$_6$ responsive. An even milder form of total vascular atrophy of the peripheral choroid and retina resembling gyrate atrophy exists; these patients have normal serum ornithine levels and normal OAT activity in cultured skin fibroblasts.

THERAPY

Systemic. Supplemental pyridoxine in daily doses of 15 to 20 mg can result in over 50 per cent reduction of the serum ornithine level in vitamin B_6-responsive patients; large doses (600 to 750 mg daily) have produced mild improvement in the ERG, EOG, and dark adaptometry in certain patients. However, chorioretinal atrophy has continued to progress at a slow rate despite partially reduced serum ornithine levels after vitamin B_6 administration. Because of the reported peripheral neuropathy that can occur with high-dose pyridoxine, the authors recommend only modest dietary supplementation in the range of 15 to 20 mg pyridoxine daily for those patients proven biochemically to respond to vitamin B_6 with a reduction of serum or plasma ornithine levels.

Severe dietary arginine restriction can reduce the elevated serum ornithine levels in patients who do not respond biochemically to oral pyridoxine. Some patients have had stabilization or improvements in visual acuity, ERG, visual field, color vision, and dark adaptometry after prolonged marked reduction of serum ornithine by dietary restriction of arginine. However, more recent studies have documented continual progression of atrophy of choroid and retina despite normal or near-normal plasma ornithine concentrations in children 3 to 4.5 years of age.

Oral supplementation with creatine (1.5 gm daily) has been reported to reverse the muscle abnormalities but has no effect on the retina. Supplementary proline has been suggested to possibly lessen the progression of the retinal lesions in some patients; however, this treatment has not been proven to be beneficial.

Ocular. No known topical therapy is effective. Optical correction of myopia is indicated. Occasionally, cataract extraction is warranted.

Ocular or Periocular Manifestations

Choroid: Atrophy.
Iris: Atrophy; loss of pigment.
Lens: Subcapsular cataracts.
Optic Nerve: Pallor; peripapillary atrophy.
Retina: Abnormal dark adaptometry; abnormal EOG; atrophy; macular edema; epiretinal membrane; subnormal or nonrecordable ERG; traction schisis; vascular leakage and shunt vessels; vascular sheathing and attenuation.
Vitreous: Opacity.
Other: Constriction of visual fields; de-creased visual acuity; dyschromatopsia; moderate to high myopia.

PRECAUTIONS

Only approximately 5 per cent of patients with gyrate atrophy respond clinically and biochemically to oral pyridoxine supplementation. Further studies will be necessary in these patients who do respond to determine whether the long-term course of the disease can be slowed or halted.

Vitamin B_6 is present in varying amounts in food and multiple vitamin preparations. At least one patient has been incorrectly considered a nonresponder because of failure to respond to dietary supplemental pyridoxine at a time when the patient was already receiving pyridoxine in multiple vitamin preparations sufficient to lower serum ornithine. Therefore, patients should be without any supplemental pyridoxine for several weeks before judging their biochemical responsiveness to oral vitamin B_6.

Dietary restriction of arginine requires an extremely low-protein diet that is both unpalatable and potentially dangerous. Careful monitoring of serum ammonia and nitrogen balance is essential.

Periodic documentation of retinal function over many years will be needed to determine stability or progression of the disease.

COMMENTS

Gyrate atrophy is one of the very few hereditary dystrophies of the choroid and retina that is potentially treatable. However, since treatment requires extensive clinical and biochemical evaluation and monitoring, patients should be referred to tertiary care centers, preferably those where active research on such disorders is in progress.

References

Berson EL, Schmidt SY, Shih VE: Ocular and biochemical abnormalities in gyrate atrophy of the choroid and retina. Ophthalmology 85:1018–1027, 1978.

Dalton K, Dalton MJ: Characteristics of pyridoxine overdose neuropathy syndrome. Acta Neurol Scand 76:8, 1987.

Hayasaka S, et al: Clinical trials of vitamin B_6 and proline supplementation for gyrate atrophy of the choroid and retina. Br J Ophthalmol 69:283–290, 1985.

Kaiser-Kupfer MI, Valle D: Clinical, biochemical and therapeutic aspects of gyrate atrophy. In Osbourne N, Chader J (eds): Progress in Retinal Research. Oxford, Pergamon, 1986, p 179.

Kaiser-Kupfer MI, et al: Gyrate atrophy of the choroid and retina: Improved visual function following reduction of plasma ornithine by diet. Science 210:1128–1131, 1980.

Kennaway NG, Weleber RG, Buist NRM: Gyrate atrophy of choroid and retina: Deficient activity of ornithine ketoacid aminotransferase in cultured skin fibroblasts. N Engl J Med 297:1180, 1977.

McInnes RR, et al: Hyperornithinaemia is gyrate atrophy of the retina: Improvement of vision during treatment with a low-arginine diet. Lancet 1:513–517, 1981.

Schaumburg H, Kaplan J, Windebank A, Vick N, Rasmus S, Pleasure D, Brown MJ: Sensory neuropathy from pyridoxine abuse. A new megavitamin syndrome. N Engl J Med 309:445–448, 1983.

Shih VE, et al: Ornithine ketoacid transaminase deficiency in gyrate atrophy of the choroid and retina. Am J Hum Genet 30:174–179, 1978.

Valle D, Simell O: The hyperornithinemias. In Scriver CR, Beaudet AL, Sly WS, Valle D (eds): The Metabolic Basis of Inherited Disease, 6th ed. New York, McGraw-Hill, 1989, Vol 1, pp 599–627.

Vannas-Sulonen K, Simell O, Sipilä I: Gyrate atrophy of the choroid and retina: The ocular disease progresses despite normal or near normal plasma ornithine concentration. Ophthalmology 94:1428–1433, 1987.

Vannas-Sulonen K, et al: Gyrate atrophy of the choroid and retina: A five-year follow-up of creatine supplementation. Ophthalmology 92:1719–1727, 1985.

Weleber RG, Kennaway NG: Clinical trial of vitamin B_6 for gyrate atrophy of the choroid and retina. Ophthalmology 88:316–324, 1981.

Weleber RG, Kennaway NG: Gyrate atrophy of the choroid and retina. In Heckenlively JR (ed): Retinitis Pigmentosa. Philadelphia, JB Lippincott, 1988, pp 198–220.

Weleber RG, Kennaway NG, Buist NRM: Gyrate atrophy of the choroid and retina: Approaches to therapy. Int Ophthalmol 4:23–32, 1981.

Weleber RG, Wirtz MK, Kennaway NG: Gyrate atrophy of the choroid and retina: Clinical and biochemical heterogeneity and response to vitamin B_6. Birth Defects 18:219–230, 1982.

PERIPHERAL RETINAL BREAKS AND DEGENERATION 362.60

JULIAN J. NUSSBAUM, M.D.,

Detroit, Michigan

and H. MACKENZIE FREEMAN, M.D.

Boston, Massachusetts

The most common degenerative processes affecting the peripheral retina include retinal breaks, cystoid degeneration, acquired retinoschisis, paving-stone degeneration, lattice degeneration, peripheral tapetoretinal degeneration, and snowflake degeneration.

Peripheral retinal breaks may be classified into three types. The most common retinal break to cause retinal detachment is a retinal tear, which occurs as a result of increasing vitreous traction on a vitreoretinal adhesion. Tears are usually U- or V-shaped, with the base located anteriorly and the flap pointing posteriorly. Occasionally, the flap may be completely avulsed and appears as an operculum floating freely in the vitreous cavity. Histologic studies reveal that a retinal tear shows smooth, rounded edges and a vitreoretinal adhesion. The photoreceptor layer of the retinal flap may demonstrate various stages of degeneration, depending on the age of the tear, and subretinal fluid may occasionally be seen along its margins.

Rhegmatogenous detachments caused by dialyses, a disinsertion of the retina from the ora serrata, usually occur more slowly than those caused by other retinal breaks. There are three types of retinal dialyses. Dialysis of the retina may occur in utero, leading to subsequent retinal detachment at birth or even in later years. A second type of dialysis accompanies blunt ocular trauma, is the most common cause of traumatic retinal detachment, and is usually found superonasally. A third type of dialysis occurs spontaneously in individuals most often under 20 years and nearly always under 40 years of age. This type of dialysis affects the lower temporal quadrants, is frequently bilateral, and is occasionally familial. On pathologic examination, the dialysis is seen as a separation of the retina from the nonpigmented ciliary epithelium at the ora serrata. With trauma, an associated avulsion of the vitreous base and detachment of the ciliary epithelium may be seen as a ribbon-like structure in the vitreous.

Retinal holes are the least common retinal breaks that cause retinal detachment. They are round or oval shaped and may be seen alone or in areas of retinal degeneration. When studied pathologically, retinal holes have smooth borders without an operculum or flap and are usually found within the area of the vitreous base.

Cystoid degeneration may appear as small, closely packed, parallel reddish cysts that run in a meridional direction around the peripheral retina and sometimes involve the teeth of the ora serrata. There is a greater predilection for the temporal retina. In "typical" cystoid degeneration, microcysts are located in the outer plexiform and outer nuclear layers, whereas in "reticular" cystoid degeneration, these cysts lie primarily in the nerve fiber layer. This is a benign condition seen in most eyes of patients older than 8 years of age and requires no treatment.

Acquired retinoschisis may initially appear as an exaggeration of cystoid degeneration of the peripheral retina. It is most often located in the inferotemporal quadrant. This degenerative process may progress nasally and, in rare cases, posteriorly, sometimes forming a large cyst-like elevation. The thin inner layer appears transparent, with the exception of the retinal vessels and small snowflake-like deposits that help identify it. The outer layer may appear as a faint gray haze over the red choroidal pattern. When retinal holes occur in acquired retinoschisis, they are usually small and numerous in the inner layer, but tend to be large in the outer layer. Histologic examination shows that the splitting occurs in the outer plexiform layer, with the schisis cavity bridged by the remnants of neural processes and Müller's cells. Retinal detachment is rare in acquired retinoschisis, but may occasionally be seen when breaks are present in both layers of the schisis cavity.

Scalloped, sharply demarcated, yellow-white areas of chorioretinal atrophy characterize the lesions seen in paving-stone degeneration. Histologically, there is loss of pigment epithelium and underlying choriocapillaris, leaving an atrophic retina opposed to Bruch's membrane. Because of this loss, the retina may remain attached in these areas, even when the remainder of the retina is detached. Tears may sometimes occur along the margins of paving-stone degeneration.

Lattice degeneration is a circumferentially oriented lesion of retinal thinning that is usually located at or anterior to the equator. Pigment clumping is common. Its name is derived from the interlacing branching pattern of sclerotic vessels bridging the lesion. Although less than 1 per cent of patients with lattice degeneration subsequently develop a retinal detachment, approximately one-fourth to one-third of retinal detachments are attributable to retinal breaks associated with lattice degeneration. These breaks are usually atrophic, round holes within lattice or retinal tears along the margins where the strong vitreoretinal adhesion exists. Studied microscopically, it is an area of inner retinal atrophy with overlying vitreous liquefaction and persistent strong vitreous adhesion to its margins.

Peripheral tapetoretinal degeneration appears clinically as diffuse chorioretinal atrophy and granular pigment clumping. It is essentially an exaggeration of the periphery changes seen in the normally aging eye. Histopathologically, it consists of retinal pigment epithelial and choriocapillaris atrophy with secondary photoreceptor loss. It is a benign process requiring no treatment.

Snowflake degeneration is characterized clinically by a myriad of yellow-white dots resembling snowflakes that are primarily located in the peripheral retina. It is a hereditary progressive process associated with vitreous degeneration and devascularization of the affected retinal areas. The lesions become pigmented in later stages. Patients with snowflake degeneration have a higher incidence of retinal breaks and detachment, as well as presenile cataract formation.

THERAPY

Supportive. It is important to have an understanding of which retinal breaks should be treated and which can be observed. The incidence of retinal breaks without retinal detach-

ment is approximately 7.8 per cent affecting about 16 million persons in the United States. Since the annual incidence of retinal detachment is about 1 in 9000 persons, it is obvious that the majority of retinal breaks do not result in retinal detachment and therefore do not require treatment. Therefore, when a retinal break is found, consideration should be given not only to the characteristics of the break itself but also to other ocular findings, including conditions in the other eye and the patient's age, occupation, activity level, and family history of retinal detachment.

The characteristics of the retinal break are important factors in deciding whether treatment is indicated. All symptomatic or asymptomatic retinal tears and retinal dialyses should be treated. The larger and the greater the number of retinal breaks, the stronger and more urgent are the indications for treatment. Retinal detachment from breaks located superiorly, temporally, and posteriorly poses a greater threat to the macula than those located nasally, anteriorly, and inferiorly. For this reason, prophylactic treatment of retinal breaks with the above-mentioned characteristics is recommended.

Retinal breaks found in eyes with high myopia, retinopathy of prematurity, vitreous hemorrhage, and chronic uveitis have a greater predisposition toward retinal detachment. Treatment is indicated when breaks occur in eyes with a developing cataract because the ability to visualize an early detachment decreases as the lens becomes more cataractous. In addition, it is important to study the fellow eye for retinal breaks, and a history of retinal detachment in the fellow eye is a strong indication for treatment.

Retinal breaks found in patients with Marfan's syndrome, Wagner-Stickler syndrome, Ehlers-Danlos syndrome, and atopic dermatitis should be treated because of the poorer prognoses associated with these connective tissue diseases.

Surgical. The treatment of retinal breaks without detachment involves one or a combination of three modalities: photocoagulation, cryopexy, or scleral buckling with or without an encircling band. Photocoagulation is a valuable tool for the nonsurgical treatment of retinal breaks. It is often the treatment of choice for round holes in areas of chorioretinal degeneration without evidence of vitreous traction or hemorrhage. Photocoagulation may also be used in retinal tears and in the treatment of outer layer breaks in retinoschisis. With the advent of indirect ophthalmoscopic laser delivery systems, retinal breaks are easily treated when located both posteriorly as well as anterior to the equator. Using this modality, treatment of retinal breaks is performed in an outpatient setting with the patient either in the seated or supine position and without the need for a contact lens. The pupil is dilated as widely as possible; only topical anesthetics are used. After the area of the retinal break or breaks is visualized with the indirect ophthalmoscope, three to five rows of laser burns are placed around the posterior, lateral, and, where applicable, anterior margins of the lesions. Lesions are of moderate intensity. Average settings vary according to the type of laser used; the presence of corneal, lenticular, or vitreous opacities; and the degree of pigment epithelial and choroidal pigmentation.

Cryotherapy is ideally suited for anteriorly located retinal breaks in the presence of significant media opacities, such as vitreous hemorrhage or cataract. It is carried out in an outpatient setting with topical and subconjunctival anesthesia. Subconjunctival anesthesia is preferred over retrobulbar anesthesia when treatment is not extensive. It is a safer procedure because the needle tip is always visualized under the conjunctiva. In highly myopic eyes, retrobulbar anesthesia may be hazardous because the needle could penetrate a large posterior staphyloma. After the globe has been anesthetized, the bulbar conjunctiva is gently grasped with smooth forceps over the quadrant where treatment is to be performed. Two per cent lidocaine is then injected subconjunctivally, utilizing a tuberculin syringe and a short 30-gauge needle. When extensive treatment is indicated or when the patient is very young, or very old, or debilitated, the procedure may be done in the operating room with cardiac monitoring. Treatment is carried out under direct visualization, using indirect ophthalmoscopy and scleral depression with the tip of the cryoprobe. Pressure should be firm, and the probe tip should not be moved once freezing has commenced. Two rows of overlapping cryo lesions are placed along the posterior, lateral, and, when possible, the anterior margins of the lesion, as well as freezing the break itself.

After photocoagulation or cryotherapy is completed, topical antibiotics are administered, and the eye is temporarily patched for 24 hours (if not monocular). The patient is re-examined 2 weeks later, at which time pigmentation should be seen in the treated areas. If adequate treatment is noted, the patient is re-examined at 2 months and then every 6 to 12 months, depending on the nature of the underlying pathology (high myopia with lattice degeneration, history of giant tear in the fellow eye, etc.).

Scleral buckling reduces vitreous traction, and it may be beneficial in treating patients with large horseshoe tears and vitreous hemorrhage or in patients with multiple or recurrent retinal breaks. The use of an encircling element provides permanent indentation and reduces the incidence of buckle extrusion. When treating a retinal break with scleral buckling procedures, it is important to provide adequate treatment margins with cryopexy or laser photocoagulation.

PRECAUTIONS

Treatment must provide an adequate margin of chorioretinal adhesion along all borders of the retinal break. However, excessive photocoagulation or cryotherapy should be avoided because it may cause complications, including retinal or choroidal hemorrhage, exudative choroidal and retinal detachment, and preretinal membrane formation or contracture. When performing indirect ophthalmoscopic laser photocoagulation, corneal drying must be avoided to reduce the possibility of corneal burns.

COMMENTS

It must be remembered that the great majority of peripheral retinal degeneration and breaks do not result in retinal detachment and warrant no intervention. No form of prophylactic therapy is free from the risk of complications. Therefore, when a retinal break is found, the decision "to treat or not to treat" should be made on a patient-by-patient basis.

References

Benson WE, Morse PH: The prognosis of retinal detachment due to lattice degeneration. Ann Ophthalmol 10:1197–1200, 1978.

Byer NE: Lattice degeneration of the retina. Surv Ophthalmol 23:213–248, 1979.

Foos RY: Retinal holes. Am J Ophthalmol 86:354–358, 1978.

Freeman HM: Fellow eyes of giant retinal breaks. Trans Am Ophthalmol Soc 76:343–382, 1978.

Friberg TR: Principles of photocoagulation using binocular indirect ophthalmoscope laser delivery systems. Int Ophthalmol Clin 30:89–94, 1990.

Hagler WS, Jarrett WH II, Chang M: Rhegmatogenous retinal detachment following chorioretinal inflammatory disease. Am J Ophthalmol 86:373–379, 1978.

Hirose T, Wolf E, Schepens CL: Retinal functions in snowflake degeneration. Ann Ophthalmol 12:1135–1146, 1980.

Hirose T, et al: Acquired retinoschiasis: Observations and treatment. In Pruett RC, Regan CDJ (eds): Retina Congress. New York, Appleton-Century-Crofts, 1974, pp 489–504.

McPherson A, O'Malley R, Beltangady SS: Management of the fellow eyes of patients with rhegmatogenous retinal detachment. Ophthalmology 88:922–934, 1981.

Pollak A, Oliver M: Argon laser photocoagulation of symptomatic flap tears and retinal breaks of fellow eyes. Br J Ophthalmol 65:469–472, 1981.

Sigelman J: Vitreous base classification of retinal tears: Clinical application. Surv Ophthalmol 25:59–74, 1980.

Smiddy WE, Flynn HW Jr, Nicholson DH, Clarkson JG, et al: Results and complications in treated retinal breaks. Am J Ophthalmol 113:603–604, 1991.

Takahashi M, et al: Biomicroscopic evaluation and photography of liquefied vitreous in some vitreoretinal disorders. Arch Ophthalmol 99:1555–1559, 1981.

Tolentino FI, Schepens CL, Freeman HM: Vitreoretinal Disorders: Diagnosis and Management. Philadelphia, WB Saunders, 1976.

Verdaguer J, Vaisman M: Treatment of symptomatic retinal breaks. Am J Ophthalmol 87:783–788, 1979.

REFSUM'S DISEASE 356.3
(Heredopathia Atactica Polyneuritiformis, Phytanic Acid Oxidase Deficiency)

RICHARD G. WELEBER, M.D.

Portland, Oregon

Refsum's disease is a rare autosomal recessive syndrome characterized by chronic polyneuropathy, cerebellar ataxia, atypical retinitis pigmentosa, and ichthyosiform skin lesions. Raised tissue and blood levels of phytanic acid, an abnormality related to deficient phytanic acid oxidation, are present. The age of onset varies from the first to the fifth decade of life. Although phytanic acid is stored in fatty tissues, symptoms of the disease are related to the concentration of phytanic acid in the blood, rather than total body stores. The earliest symptom is almost invariably night blindness, which usually occurs before age 20. Electroretinogram responses are profoundly abnormal or nondetectable. The disturbance in retinal pigmentation, which early in the disease is often limited to the periphery, may be granular, rather than "bone-spicule." Weakness in the extremities, unsteadiness of gait, and a history of chronic exacerbations and remission are common. Complete external ophthalmoplegia has been reported. Often, the diagnosis of Friedreich's ataxia is entertained. However, tendon reflexes that are initially undetectable may return weeks or months later. Invariably, cerebrospinal fluid shows an elevation of protein content without pleocytosis. Hearing may become defective, and cataracts may occur. Orthopedic deformities of the foot and epiphyseal dysplasia have been reported. Ichthyosiform skin lesions may wax and wane with the rising and falling of the serum phytanic acid level. Impairment of renal function has also been reported. Impaired atrial-ventricular conduction, bundle-branch blocks, and cardiac arrhythmia may have contributed to the occasional occurrence of sudden death. When untreated, the life expectancy is shortened.

THERAPY

Systemic. Since phytanic acid is not metabolized in patients with Refsum's disease and the only source of phytanic acid in humans is dietary, restriction of oral intake of phytanic acid and, to a lesser extent, phytol, which can be converted into phytanic acid, has been advised and found beneficial. Specifically, dietary intake of dairy products and ruminant fats, both of which contain phytanic acid must be markedly curtailed. Caution should be observed to avoid starvation diets, as they can cause rapid mobilization of body stores of phytanic acid with a marked increase in the elevation of serum phytanic levels, acute toxicity, cardiac arrhythmias, and possible cardiac arrest. Plasma exchange seems to be a very useful treatment to lower plasma phytanic acid concentrations rapidly and has a very definite role in the treatment of acute toxic states.

Supportive. Refsum's disease is an autosomal recessive genetic trait. Carriers with dietary loading may show elevated phytanic acid levels. However, carrier detection is best determined by assay of phytanic acid alpha-oxidase activity in cultured skin fibroblasts. Since cultured amniocentesis cells show the enzyme activity, antenatal diagnosis of the affected or carrier state is theoretically possible.

Ocular or Periocular Manifestations

Optic Nerve: Partial demyelination.
Retina: Lipid deposits in pigment epithelium with degeneration of overlying photoreceptors.
Sclera: Lipid deposits.
Other: Lipid deposits in trabecular meshwork.

PRECAUTIONS

If started early, dietary restriction may possibly prevent the development of neuromuscular and retinal changes. However, no conclusive evidence of improvement in retinal function has been reported with dietary or plasma exchange therapy. This may reflect the extent of irreversible damage to the retina. Early recognition and prompt treatment may forestall the development of these irreversible visual changes, although no improvement in the vision of patients with well-advanced disease should be expected. Since careful monitoring of diet and serum phytanic levels is required, these patients should be referred to tertiary medical centers for medical evaluation and therapy.

COMMENTS

Definite clinical and biochemical improvement has been reported with reduction of dietary phytanic acid and plasma exchange. Muscle strength, tendon reflexes, sensory and motor nerve conduction, and certain objective tests of coordination have improved with treatment. The ichthyosiform rash and cardiac arrhythmias also clear as the serum phytanic acid decreases. One 39-year-old patient treated with dietary restriction over the past 13 years has shown only minimal progression of the visual findings during this period of time.

References

Gibberd FB, et al: Heredopathia atactica polyneuritiformis (Refsum's disease) treated by diet and plasma-exchange. Lancet 1:575–578, 1979.

Hansen E, Bachen NI, Flage T: Refsum's disease. Eye manifestations in a patient treated with low phytol low phytanic acid diet. Acta Ophthalmol 57:899–913, 1979.

Kahlke W: Refsum-Syndrome. Lipoidchemische Untersuchungen bei 9 Fällen. Klin Wochenschr 42:1011–1016, 1964.

Masters-Thomas A, et al: Heredopathia atactica polyneuritiformis (Refsum's disease): 1. Clinical features and dietary management. J Hum Nutr 34:245–250, 1980.

Masters-Thomas A, et al: Heredopathia atactica polyneuritiformis (Refsum's disease): 2. Estimation of phytanic acid in foods. J Hum Nutr 34:251–254, 1980.

Penovich PE, et al: Note on plasma exchange therapy in Refsum's disease. Adv Neurol 21:151–153, 1978.

Refsum S: Heredopathia atactica polyneuritiformis; familial syndrome not hitherto described; contribution to clinical study of hereditary diseases of nervous system. Acta Psychiatr Neurol 38(Suppl):1–303, 1946.

Refsum S: Heredopathia atactica polyneuritiformis phytanic acid storage disease (Refsum's disease) with particular reference to ophthalmological disturbances. Metabol Ophthalmol 1:73–79, 1977.

Steinberg D: Refsum disease. In Scriver CR, Beaudet AL, Sly WS, Valle D (eds): The Metabolic Basis of Inherited Disease, 6th ed. New York, McGraw-Hill, 1989, Vol 2, pp 1533–1550.

Steinberg D, et al: Conversion of U-C^{14}-phytol to phytanic acid and its oxidation in heredopathia atactica polyneuritiformis. Biochem Biophys Res Commun 19:783–789, 1965.

Steinberg D, et al: Refsum's disease—a recently characterized lipoidosis involving the nervous system. Ann Intern Med 66:365–395, 1967.

Steinberg D, et al: Phytanic acid in patients with Refsum's syndrome and response to dietary treatment. Arch Intern Med 125:75–87, 1970.

RETINAL DETACHMENT 361.9

HARVEY LINCOFF, M.D.,

New York, New York

and INGRID KREISSIG, M.D.

Duebington, Germany

Retinal detachment is a separation of the sensory retina from the pigment epithelium. There are three mechanisms of detachment: rhegmatogenous or break-induced, tractional, and exudative. It is necessary to distinguish which mechanism is operative in the patient because the management for each is different.

Rhegmatogenous retinal detachment is by far the most frequent type, although its incidence is only 1 in 20,000 individuals. The retina separates because a break (tear, hole) occurs in the sensory retina and allows fluid from the vitreous to seep between the retina and the pigment epithelium. Tearing of the retina is an acute symptomatic episode characterized by flashes as nerve fibers part and by spots as retinal blood vessels are ruptured and bleed.

The detachment of the retina proceeds in a predictable manner from the retinal break that has caused it. After first separating the retina around the break, subretinal fluid dissects to the ora serrata. If the break is in the superior retina, once a significant bulla has formed, the effects of gravity and motion cause a rapid progression dependently and toward the disc. The patient perceives the advance as a dense curtain with a convex edge encroaching on the visual field. Detachments that originate from a break in the inferior retina move upward toward the disc, but more slowly.

Rhegmatogenous detachments have convex edges and convex surfaces. If the detachment is of any duration, it will extend from ora to disc. The retina loses its transparency because it is out of contact with the pigment epithelial pump that clears it. Finding the retinal break confirms its rhegmatogenous nature.

Tractional retinal detachment occurs in eyes with diabetic retinopathy or perforating injury or as a complication of retinal detachment surgery. All of these disorders can provoke an abnormal bonding of the cortical vitreous to the internal surface of the retina. In the diabetic patient, vascular leakage incites proliferation of glial cells and fibroblasts on the surface of the retina. Actin filaments that have been demonstrated in the proliferating cells contract and create the tractional forces that detach the retina. The retina in patients with perforating injuries detach because cortical vitreous, which is attached to the retina, prolapses through the wound and pulls upon the retina.

Tractional detachments progress slowly and not infrequently arrests. Rarely, a taut vitreous membrane pulls free from the surface of the retina without causing a retinal tear and the retina reattaches. Tractional detachment in the periphery may be without symptoms, unless hemorrhage or a retinal tear intervenes. The cellular structure and physiology of retinal traction—periretinal vitreoretinopathy—are under intense investigation. Cell growth inhibitors, such as fluorouracil, have been injected into vulnerable eyes to inhibit periretinal vitreoretinopathy.

The topography of the tractional retinal detachment is diagnostic of its nature. All of its surfaces and some of its borders are concave. It can occur centrally or peripherally, but has a limited extent. In the diabetic patient, it tends to begin centrally around the disc and along the major vessels. The detachment rarely progresses beyond the equator, and peripheral vision can be maintained for years. If a retinal break occurs, peripheral vision is lost within hours because the detachment rapidly extends to the ora serrata. The change in surface contour from concave to convex confirms the rhegmatogenous conversion.

Exudative retinal detachment arises from choroidal tumors (melanoma and metastatic tumors), retinal tumors (retinoblastoma and angioma), and some poorly understood inflammatory disorders, such as Coats' disease and Harada's disease. The detachment becomes symptomatic only after it invades the macula and interferes with central vision. Like rhegmatogenous detachments, exudative detachments have convex surfaces and convex borders. Unlike rhegmatogenous detachments, exudative detachments characteristically shift to that portion of the eye that is dependent. When the patient is upright, the subretinal fluid distributes symmetrically around 6 o'clock; when the patient is on his or her side, fluid runs up the dependent side. In the supine position, fluid collects centrally, and small amounts may be overlooked. Patients with small amounts of fluid report that they have poor vision upon awakening in the morning and that their vision improves as the day progresses. Maximum exudative detachments may elevate the retina in all four quadrants and detach the ciliary epithelium. In this circumstance, the retina bulges anteriorly behind the lens and is perceptible with a pen light.

THERAPY

Surgical.
RHEGMATOGENOUS DETACHMENT. Most operations for rhegmatogenous detachment can be completed in less than 2 hours and can be done under retrobulbar anesthesia. A lid block is unnecessary. An adequate scleral field is made available if the conjunctival incision extends 90° to either side of the breaks. The breaks are localized by directing a scleral depressor or a cryo probe to them while the retina is being observed with the indirect ophthalmoscope. The position of the break is marked on the sclera with ink or catheter. The edges of the break are treated with transscleral cryopexy.

The break is closed by compressing an elastic silicone sponge over it, with a mattress suture tied under tension. One mattress suture with long intrascleral limbs (6 mm) is preferable to multiple sutures with short intrascleral passages because short sutures tend to tear out of the sclera. Compression of the sponge causes an abrupt rise in the intraocular pressure, and it is necessary to monitor the central retinal artery to ascertain that it has not closed. Momentary closure or a pulsating artery is not infrequent. The artery reopens in minutes unless the patient has glaucoma. Reopening can be accelerated by digital mas-

sage. As the eye decompresses over the ensuing hours, the sponge expands beneath the break, creating a buckle (intrusion) high enough to close it. With the pathway between the vitreous and subretinal space closed by the buckle, the fluid beneath the retina is absorbed by the pigment epithelium and the retina reattaches, usually within 24 hours. Whenever posssible, the scleral sponge is oriented with its long axis in a radial direction. This direction is chosen because the retina, fixed at the disc and ora serrata, tends to form radial folds when detached. Circumferentially oriented buckles augment this tendency. When a fold falls into alignment with the retinal tear that is stretched across the circumferential buckle, the tear opens like a fish's mouth (called fish mouthing), and vitreous fluid continues to leak into the subretinal space, sustaining the detachment. Radial buckles fill the folds that make for fish mouthing and prevent this complication.

Most retinal breaks are smaller than 3 mm and can be closed by a radial sponge 5 mm in diameter that is sewn in place with an 8-mm mattress suture; 8 mm is the half-circumference of the sponge and the width of the buckle. Breaks as large as 6 mm can be closed by a 7.5-mm oval sponge, which is held in place with a 10-mm mattress suture. Breaks as large as 8 mm can be closed with two 7.5-mm overlapping sponges that are tied in place with a single mattress suture with intrascleral limbs 14 mm apart. The 8-mm break and two sponges side by side mark the limit of the radial sponge operation. Three or more sponges under a mattress suture wider than 14 mm have little compression potential and make a poor buckle.

Radial buckling without drainage of subretinal fluid can be used for breaks larger than 8 mm (40° at the equator) and up to 14 mm (70°) by resorting to a scleral pouch operation. The pouch is made from a Dacron-reinforced silicone sheet cut to a radial shape and sewn over the retinal break. The elastic buckling effect is obtained by stuffing the pouch that is created with silicone sponge pellets. The pouch operation is time consuming, but has a reattachment rate of 95 per cent, which is as good as that of the other sponge operations.

Tears longer than 70° are fortunately infrequent. When encountered they can only be buckled circumferentially; the posterior edge of a radial pouch larger than 70° would intrude upon the posterior pole. Because circumferential buckling of long tears is especially prone to cause "fish mouthing," these tears are treated instead with intravitreal tamponades of air, gas, or silicone oil with and without vitrectomy.

The perfluorocarbon gases, which expand the injected volume by two to five times, have simplified and diminished the morbidity of intraocular gas tamponades by eliminating the need to drain subretinal fluid or vitrectomy to make space for an adequate gas bubble. Because of the success of the expanding gases in treating large tears (60 to 70 per cent), the gas technique has been proposed as a primary outpatient procedure for less formidable retinal detachments. The procedure is called pneumatoretinopexy. However, intraocular gas augments and may even provoke periretinal vitreoretinopathy (PVR) and is not appropriate for detachments that might be treated with an external buckle, a procedure with less morbidity and a better rate of reattachment.

Ninety per cent of retinal detachments are suitable for treatment without drainage of subretinal fluid. Four per cent of these will fail to reattach completely because of another break that was undetected. Providing that the break that was buckled was the superior one, the upper border of the detachment will fall close to the level of the secondary break and help detect it. Three per cent will fail because the buckle was inadequate because it was either too small or was poorly placed. Three per cent will fail because of periretinal vitreoretinopathy. Patients in the first two categories will respond to a second buckling operation without drainage of subretinal fluid. Patients who fail because of PVR may require additional buckling or a vitrectomy.

One per cent of patients will have delayed absorption because their pigment epithelium and choriocapillaris function inadequately; these patients are usually elderly or myopic with an atrophic pigment epithelium and choriocapillaris. They probably should have been drained initially, particularly if the break is in the inferior retina. If the break is superior it is likely to become secure on the buckle. The patient may then be left to absorb residual fluid over weeks or months. He or she is cautioned to sleep with the head elevated to prevent pooling of the fluid in the macula during sleep.

Less than 10 per cent of patients are selected for drainage in the primary procedure. The indications are (1) the retinal break is on the posterior slope of a bulla, and localization may be uncertain because of parallax; (2) glaucoma; (3) the sclera is staphylomatous and will not tolerate an increase in intraocular pressure; and (4) there is advanced periretinal vitreoretinopathy, and the break is posterior and caught up in a traction configuration.

TRACTION DETACHMENT. Posterior traction detachments are a late complication of diabetic retinopathy. They were refractory to treatment until the advent of vitrectomy, an operation that strips or severs the proliferative membranes on the surface of the retina. The operation has a significant morbidity, and recurrence is frequent. Vitrectomy is usually deferred until the macula becomes detached.

Peripheral traction detachments occur in eyes with retinopathy of prematurity, peripheral choroiditis, perforating injuries, or peripheral vasculopathies, such as sickle cell disease. The loss of vision in the periphery may not be noticed by the patient. An examination of the peripheral retina reveals a concave elevation of the retina. The elevation may extend to the ora serrata, but rarely progresses posteriorly beyond the equator. Unless a break occurs and the detachment becomes rhegmatogenous, treatment is best deferred. Prophylactic scleral buckling has little value because the buckle cannot be made high enough to relieve traction without causing anterior chamber ischemia. Vitrectomy seems a correct approach, but is technically difficult to perform in the periphery. On the other hand, after an anterior perforating injury, a vitrectomy that removes or at least severs the intravitreal track of the prolapsed cortical vitreous reduces the incidence of traction detachment in this group of patients. A recent trial indicated that cryopexy or laser coagulation to the avascular periphery of premature infants with retinopathy of prematurity reduces the incidence of traction detachment in the developing child.

EXUDATIVE DETACHMENT. The therapy of exudative retinal detachments is directed at obliterating the exudating lesion. The detachment that might accompany a melanoma will flatten within weeks after the tumor is treated with a radioactive plaque containing iodine 125. The detachment that might result from a metastatic tumor to the choroid will regress after moderate doses of beam radiation. The detachment associated with retinoblastoma will regress after plaque or beam radiation to the tumors. Reattachment of the exudative detachment that occurs with angiomatosis of the retina will occur if the lesion is destroyed with light or cryocoagulation. Large retinal angiomas are difficult to manage because they tend to exudate as an acute response to laser or cryocoagulation. Preliminary coagulation around the angioma will not contain the exudative response. The exudative detachment that accompanies Coats' disease will regress if the vascular lesions can be obliterated with photocoagulation. The detachment that accompanies uveitis and Harada's disease may respond to steroid therapy.

One should not attempt to drain subretinal fluid in an exudative detachment because the drainage site must be elevated for access. This elevation causes the subretinal fluid to shift away from the drainage site and makes perforation of the retina or incarceration a likely consequence.

A retinal detachment secondary to cytomegalovirus infestation of the retina occurs in immunosuppressed patients and 20 per cent of patients afflicted with AIDS. The retina rapidly become necrotic over large areas and may detach because of one or more retinal holes. Multiple holes and retinal necrosis make the detachment unsuitable for a buckle operation. A vitrectomy and replacement of the vitreous with silicone oil can reattach the retina and restore useful vision in these eyes. The oil operation is complicated by the subsequent development of cataract and glaucoma. However, the limited life expectancy of the AIDS patient who demonstrates cytomegalovirus retinitis is likely to preclude the development of these complications.

PRECAUTIONS

The drainage of subretinal fluid is the most traumatic part of a retinal detachment procedure and has a significant intraocular morbidity; it can cause hemorrhage, retinal incarceration, choroidal effusion, and uveitis. The occurrence of hemorrhage may be minimized by transilluminating the choroid at the drainage site before perforating. Transillumination reveals the choroidal vessels and enables the surgeon to avoid them. Incarceration of the retina into the drainage site can be avoided by keeping the retina under ophthalmic observation while the subretinal fluid is draining. The drainage site should be closed when the retina approaches the wall of the eye. Choroidal effusion and uveitis may result from the temporary hypotony that occurs after drainage. Both are usually benign, and the eye recovers spontaneously or with steroid therapy.

The extraocular complications of scleral buckling are infection of the buckle and diplopia. With the use of closed-cell silicone sponges and prophylactic subtenon gentamicin at the conclusion of the operation, the incidence of infection has fallen to less than 0.5 per cent. The manifestations of an infected explant depend upon the infecting organism. Infections caused by *Proteus* or *Staphylococcus aureus* become evident in the first to third postoperative week because a draining fistula presents anterior to the explant in the line of the conjunctival incision. Antibiotics will not cure the condition. The complaint of pain signals uveal irritation by the organism or its toxin and indicates the need to remove the implant without delay. Most postoperative infections are, however, caused by *S. epidermidis* and are more benign. They manifest as a chronic red, sticky eye that persists for months after the operation. An examination of the conjunctival wound anterior to the buckle reveals a flat, fleshy granuloma emanating from it. Excision of the granuloma and the applications of antibiotics ameliorate the symptoms, but they will recur. A permanent cure can only be effected by removing the explant. The incidence of redetachment after removing a buckle is 10 per cent. The orbit is sterile 5 days after the explant is removed and will accept rebuckling if the retina detaches.

Diplopia occurs when a sponge is fixed beneath a rectus muscle, especially when it is fixed anteriorly to the equator. If the sponge is radially oriented, the incidence of diplopia can be reduced if the muscle is transplanted adjacent to the explant. The temporary balloon buckle eliminates this complication. The balloon causes diplopia when it is beneath a rectus muscle, but within hours after it is deflated and removed, the muscle functions normally again.

COMMENTS

Reattachment of the retina is obtained by an operation directed solely at closing the retinal breaks. The breaks are found preoperatively by examination techniques that include indirect ophthalmoscopy with scleral depression and slit-lamp biomicroscopy through a three-mirror contact lens or a wide-angle indirect contact lens with scleral depression. Finding the breaks can be a laborious task if they are small. The task can be made easier by first defining the shape of the detachment, because the shape indicates the location of the primary break (the superior break that alone could produce the detachment).

Retinal detachments occur in one of three patterns: (1) detachments that extend into the superior temporal or nasal quadrants; (2) superior detachments that cross the 12 o'clock radian and proceed down both sides of the eye to become total, and (3) inferior detachments. The analysis of a large series of retinal detachments indicated that in superior nasal or temporal detachments the primary break lies within $1^1/_2$ clock hours of the superior border of the detachment 98 per cent of the time; in superior detachments that cross the 12 o'clock radian, the break lies within a triangle whose apex is at 12 o'clock and whose sides intersect the equator 1 hour to either side of 12 o'clock 93 per cent of the time; in inferior detachments, the higher border of the detachment indicates that side of the 6 o'clock radian on which the break will be found 95 per cent of the time. More than one break is present in about 60 per cent of retinal detachments. The secondary breaks tend to be located, in order of frequency, adjacent to the primary break or remote from the primary break but in the same latitude.

Immobilization of the eye preoperatively by binocular occlusion and bedrest are useful adjuncts to therapy. Immobilization can curtail progression of the retinal detachment and may effect some regression. In a few patients (about 10 per cent), it will effect complete reattachment of the retina and enable the repair to be accomplished solely by applying laser or cryopexy to the edge of the break. The earliest sign of settling of the retina is a crinkling effect on the posterior edges of the bullae. If the crinkling sign appears after overnight occlusion, it is worth delaying an operation in the expectation of additional settling and possibly complete reattachment.

References

Algvere P, Rosengren B: Immobilization of the eye. Evaluation of a new method in retinal detachment surgery. Acta Ophthalmol 55:303–316, 1977.

Blumenkranz MS, et al: Fluorouracil for the treatment of massive periretinal proliferation. Am J Ophthalmol 94:458–467, 1982.

Coleman DJ: Early vitrectomy in the management of the severely traumatized eye. Am J Ophthalmol 93:543–551, 1982.

Cryotherapy for Retinopathy of Prematurity Cooperative Group: Multicenter trial of cryotherapy for retinopathy of prematurity: Preliminary study. Arch Ophthalmol 106:471–479, 1988.

Kreissig I, et al: The treatment of difficult retinal detachments with an expanding gas bubble without vitrectomy. Graefes Arch Clin Exp Ophthalmol 224:51–54, 1986.

Lincoff H: The rationale for radial buckling. Mod Probl Ophthalmol 12:484–491, 1974.

Lincoff H, Kreissig I: Patterns of non-rhegmatogenous elevations of the retina. Br J Ophthalmol 58:899–906, 1974.

Lincoff H, Kreissig I: Results with a temporary balloon buckle for the repair of retinal detachment. Am J Ophthalmol 92:245–251, 1981.

Lincoff H, Kreissig I, Hahn YS: An elastic pouch operation for large retinal tears. Arch Ophthalmol 97:708–710, 1979.

Machemer R: Vitrectomy in diabetic retinopathy. Removal of preretinal proliferations. Trans Am Acad Ophthalmol Otolaryngol 79:394–395, 1975.

Tasman W, et al: Cryotherapy for active retinopathy of prematurity. Ophthalmology 93:580–585, 1986.

RETINAL EMBOLI 362.33

DAVID J. WILSON, M.D.

Portland, Oregon

An embolism is the sudden partial or complete obstruction of a vessel by a clot or foreign material brought to its place of lodgement by the blood current. Retinal emboli are of particular interest because the accessibility of the retinal circulation to examination permits documentation of suspected emboli.

A great variety of materials have been reported as retinal emboli, including platelets and fibrin, cholesterol, calcific material from diseased heart valves, fat following long-bone fracture, air after chest compression injuries, atrial myxoma, metastatic tumor, amniotic fluid, septic emboli in bacterial endocarditis, leukocyte aggregates, talc and corn starch in intravenous drug abusers, corticosteroids after intranasal or retrobulbar steroid injections, and cloth material from prosthetic heart valves. By far, the most common source of retinal emboli is ulcerated atheromatous plaques in the carotid artery. These emboli may occur spontaneously or after manipulation of the carotid arteries during arteriography or surgery.

From a therapeutic viewpoint, retinal emboli are important because of their ocular sequelae and because they indicate the potential for emboli to the brain. Emboli are probably the most common cause of branch retinal artery occlusion and are a major cause of central retinal artery occlusion. However, other causes of arterial occlusion that should be considered in the differential diagnosis include atheromatous disease of the central retinal artery and arteritis of the retinal vessels. For additional information, see the article on central or branch retinal artery occlusion.

THERAPY

Ocular. The goals of treatment are improvement in vision and movement of the emboli to a more distal location in the retinal circulation. Treatment should be administered without delay. It has been demonstrated in monkeys that occlusion of the central retinal artery longer than approximately 100 minutes results in irreversible retinal damage. The patient should be placed in the supine position with the legs elevated. If this is not successful, brisk tapping and massaging of the eye are performed to try and move the emboli downstream. An anterior chamber paracentesis may be done to improve the arterial perfusion pressure, and intravenous acetazolamide (0.5 to 1.0 gm) may be given to prolong ocular hypotony. If these measures are not successful, treatment with Carbogen (95 per cent oxygen and 5 per cent carbon dioxide) by mask should be tried. This therapy should be continued for 50 minutes of every hour for 24 to 36 hours if any sign of improvement is observed.

Recently, tissue plasminogen activators have been used in the treatment of occluded coronary arteries. Animal experiments have suggested that these agents may be of benefit in platelet fibrin emboli of the retinal circulation. A single report on the use of urokinase and tissue plasminogen activator administered via a catheter in the proximal ophthalmic artery has been published. This study reported encouraging results in patients treated within the first 6 hours after occlusion. However, this markedly invasive form of therapy should be employed only under carefully defined clinical guidelines because of the risk for cerebrovascular accident.

Systemic. In addition to treating the ocular consequences of retinal emboli, treatment of the source of the emboli should be attempted to prevent additional retinal emboli or emboli to the brain. Consultation with an internist, neurologist, or cardiologist may be beneficial in evaluating the carotid arteries for evidence of atherosclerosis, the heart for valvular disease (including mitral valve prolapse) and atrial myxoma, and the hematologic status for evidence of a hypercoagulable state (particularly the lupus anticoagulant). Before recommending carotid endarterectomy for carotid artery disease, it is important to weigh the risks and benefits for each particular patient.

Ocular or Periocular Manifestations

Optic Nerve: Anterior ischemic optic neuropathy.

Retina: Central or branch retinal artery occlusion; retinal emboli.

Other: Cerebrovascular accident; signs of cardiac valvular disease; transient ischemic attacks.

PRECAUTIONS

Approximately 5 per cent of cases of central retinal artery occlusion are caused by giant cell arteritis. These cases should be differentiated from cases of embolic central retinal artery occlusion by history, erythrocyte sedimentation rate, and temporal artery biopsy.

COMMENTS

The treatment of retinal artery occlusion as a result of emboli is usually unsatisfactory. Few patients regain lost vision. However, in the setting of an acute embolic occlusion, the above measures should be employed to minimize the amount of visual loss. A systemic evaluation to determine the source of the emboli is important to prevent subsequent emboli.

References

Hayreh SS, Weingeist TA: Experimental occlusion of the central retinal artery of the retina. IV: Retinal tolerance time to acute ischemia. Br J Ophthalmol 64:818–825, 1980.

Levine SR, et al: Visual symptoms associated with the presence of a lupus anticoagulant. Ophthalmology 95:686–692, 1988.

Mayberg MR, Wilson SE, Yatsu F, et al: Carotid endarterectomy and prevention of cerebral ischemia in symptomatic carotid stenosis. JAMA 266: 3289–3294, 1991.

Rossmann H: Treatment of retinal arterial occlusion. Ophthalmologica 180:68–74, 1980.

Schmidt D, Schumacher M, Wakhloo AK: Microcatheter urokinase infusion in central retinal artery occlusion. Am J Ophthalmol 113:429–434, 1992.

Trobe JD: Carotid endarterectomy: Who needs it? Ophthalmology 94:725–730, 1987.

Vine AK, et al: Recombinant tissue plasminogen activator to lyse experimentally induced retinal arterial thrombi. Am J Ophthalmol 105:266–270, 1988.

Young BR, Rosenbaum TJ: Treatment of acute central retinal artery occlusion. Mayo Clin Proc 53: 408–410, 1978.

RETINAL VEIN OBSTRUCTION 362.30

LARRY E. MAGARGAL, M.D., F.A.C.S.

Philadelphia, Pennsylvania

Patients with retinal vein obstruction typically present with painless visual loss. The fundus is characterized by venous dilation and tortuosity, retinal hemorrhages and nerve fiber layer infarction, and retinal edema distal to the site of obstruction. Retinal vein obstructions are divided into macular, peripheral, temporal, hemispheric, and central according to the drainage area affected and are classified as hyperpermeable ("nonischemic"), indeterminate ("mixed"), or ischemic according to the angiographic pattern. Hyperpermeable venous occlusive disease is characterized by a perfused, but leaking capillary system, whereas ischemic occlusions show widespread zones of capillary nonperfusion on fluorescein angiography. A clinically useful fluorescein angiogram may be difficult to obtain because of patient refusal or dye allergies, lens changes, small pupil, or extensive retinal hemorrhages. Even with a high-quality fluorescein angiogram, there can be disagreement among experienced observers concerning the amount of capillary nonperfusion, and progressive ischemia occurs in at least 20 per cent of eyes over time, necessitating reclassification. Consideration of other parameters, such as visual acuity, presence of an afferent pupillary defect, number of cotton-wool spots, extent of retinal hemorrhages, and visual field defects can be useful in classifying the vein occlusion clinically. Electroretinography may also prove useful for determination of significant ischemia in some cases. Clinically, acute ischemic venous obstruction exhibits nerve fiber layer infarcts and more extensive retinal hemorrhages than hyperpermeable patterns.

Venous obstruction may be the result of impaired venous outflow, impaired arterial inflow (hypoperfusion), or hyperviscosity syndromes caused by intravascular or platelet coagulation pathway abnormalities. Impaired venous outflow is caused most often by progression of external compression of the vein by its diseased companion retinal artery at an arteriovenous crossing. For example, since the central retinal artery and vein share a common adventitial sheath as they pass through the lamina cribosa, atherosclerosis, optic disc drusen, optic disc edema, or other changes in the optic nerve head architecture, such as glaucomatous disc cupping, may promote central retinal vein occlusion. Impaired arterial inflow is usually related to high-grade ipsilateral internal carotid artery stenosis, which produces chronic ophthalmic artery insufficiency that can manifest initially as venous stasis retinopathy or can culminate in the ocular ischemic syndrome in those cases progressing to severe carotid stenosis. Stagnation thrombosis may be caused by an increase in the cellular components of the bloodstream, as in polycythemia or leukemia, or by an increase in the noncellular components of the bloodstream, as in the hyperglobulinemic conditions; the thrombosis may also be related to abnormalities in the size, shape, or aggregability of red blood cells and/or platelets. Uncommonly, when inflammation is associated with an acute vein obstruction, a marked cellular reaction is present in the vitreous (vitritis), definite foci of inflammation are in the retina (retinitis), and/or there may be perivascular infiltration (phlebitis). "Occult" inflammation has been suggested as a cause of central retinal vein occlusion in young people, but remains unproven. Central retinal vein occlusion is bilateral in about 5 per cent of cases, and bilaterality is more common when there is an underlying hyperviscosity condition.

The risk of developing complications is directly related to the type of venous obstruction and the degree and duration of retinal ischemia. In hyperpermeable patterns, the extent and duration of macular edema are the main therapeutic concerns, whereas in ischemic patterns, neovascularization and its sequelae are prominent. The principal complications of central retinal vein obstruction are iris neovascularization and secondary neovascular glaucoma, which occur in 20 per cent of cases overall (1 per cent of hyperpermeable cases and 60 per cent of ischemic ones). Retinal neovascularization, seen in 2 to 3 per cent of cases, and optic disc neovascularization, present in 25 per cent of cases, may lead to vitreous hemorrhage and traction retinal detachment. Some degree of macular edema is universal. Ischemic central retinal vein obstructions tend to progress from early stages of iris neovascularization to complete angle closure and absolute glaucoma within weeks. Patients at greatest risk of developing neovascular glaucoma tend to be older and have a higher incidence of pre-existent open-angle glaucoma and atherosclerotic vascular disease.

Branch retinal vein obstruction causes visual loss by associated macular edema or vitreous hemorrhage from retinal or disc neovascularization. After proliferative diabetic retinopathy, branch vein occlusion is the second leading retinal vascular cause of spontaneous vitreous hemorrhage. Neovascular glaucoma occurs in less than 1 per cent of patients with ischemic temporal branch retinal vein obstructions. Macular vein occlusion (17 per cent of all branch vein occlusions) is universally associated with macular edema, but neovascular complications do not occur, presumably because of the small area of retina involved. Ischemic hemispheric vein occlusions have a 20 per cent risk of developing optic disc or retinal neovascularization and a 15 per cent risk of neovascular glaucoma. Peripheral retinal vein occlusions are usually asymptomatic unless there are associated retinal neovascularization and vitreous hemorrhage. Disc neovascularization and neovascular glaucoma are exceedingly rare in patients with peripheral vein occlusions.

THERAPY

Systemic. Therapy with steroids or anticoagulants (heparin or warfarin) has been unsuccessful in achieving significant visual improvement or lessening the incidence of neovascular complications. No medical therapy has proven to be of value in improving visual function in patients with venous occlusive disease associated with impaired venous outflow. In cases where a high-grade, hemodynamically significant carotid stenosis is associated with venous stasis retinopathy, carotid surgery may be of benefit. If hematologic abnormalities can be identified, comprehensive management of the venous occlusive disease should include treatment of the underlying condition. For instance, aspirin, sulfinpyrazone, or antiplatelet agents may be useful in the management of patients with increased platelet aggregability, or plasmapheresis may be indicated in certain hyperviscosity conditions. The safety and efficacy of an intravenous fibrinolytic agent (tissue plasminogen activator) are currently being prospectively evaluated, but it seems to be of value only within a few hours after the obstruction, a time when very few patients are first seen.

Surgical. Prophylactic panretinal photocoagulation has been shown to virtually eliminate the risk of developing neovascular glaucoma in these otherwise high-risk ischemic eyes. Although panretinal photocoagulation can cause regression of iris and angle neovascularization, the intraocular pressure will remain elevated if the anterior chamber angle has been substantially obliterated by peripheral anterior synechiae. To achieve a comfortable, cosmetically acceptable eye, consideration may be given to cyclodestructive and/or shunt-type glaucoma surgery. The inherent difficulties in following high-risk patients clinically and angiographically at frequent intervals over extended periods of time, the tendency for the rapid progression of early iris neovascularization to neovascular glaucoma, and the relatively poor results following treatment in advanced cases make essential the early recognition of high-risk eyes capable of developing neovascular glaucoma and the initiation of prophylactic panretinal photocoagulation the treatment of choice in this disorder. Hyperpermeable cases, which have only a 1 per cent risk of developing neovascular glaucoma, can be followed and treated if they convert to an ischemic pattern. Treatment with macular grid laser photocoagulation to manage chronic macular edema is currently being studied prospectively.

The Branch Vein Occlusion Study has offered some guidelines for the management of macular edema and neovascularization associated with branch vein occlusion. Patients at least 3 months after vein occlusion with persistent macular edema and with decreased vision to the 20/40 range or worse are eligible for a grid laser photocoagulation treatment to the edematous retina outside the foveal avascular zone. Treatment benefit was noted after 3 years of follow-up, with the average visual acuity in the treatment group of 20/40 to 20/50 versus 20/70 in the untreated eyes.

The incidence of disc and retinal neovascularization at 3 years in eyes with at least 5 disc diameters of retinal ischemia was reduced from 22 to 12 per cent by sector photocoagulation to the involved extrafoveal area. After 3-year follow-up of eyes with posterior segment neovascularization, vitreous hemorrhage was reduced from 61 to 29 per cent in cases treated with sector laser photocoagulation. Despite evidence that prophylactic laser reduces the incidence of neovascularization, there was no conclusive evidence that long-term visual acuity was improved compared to eyes receiving laser after neovascularization developed. Clinical judgment is very important in individualizing the treatment of each case so as to achieve the best result for the patient. Some experts recommend that patients with attached or incomplete vitreous detachment and significant nonperfusion must be followed more closely.

Ocular or Periocular Manifestations

Anterior Chamber: Posterior synechiae; angle vessels; angle closure; cells and flare (with neovascular glaucoma).

Iris: Neovascularization; peripheral anterior synechiae.

Optic Nerve: Collateral vessels; edema; glaucomatous cupping (often best seen contralaterally); hemorrhage; neovascularization; optic atrophy.

Retina: Attenuated arteries; breaks; collateral vessels; cotton-wool spots; cystic degeneration; edema; exudate; hemorrhage; microaneurysm; neovascularization; preretinal membranes; traction retinal detachment (late); venous dilation.

Vitreous: Hemorrhage; neovascularization; inflammatory cells (rare).

Other: Afferent pupillary defect; glaucoma; ophthalmic artery disease.

PRECAUTIONS

Retinal vein obstruction occurs with increased frequency in patients over 50 years of age with systemic hypertension and generalized vascular disease. Diabetes mellitus is also more common in patients with vein occlusions than in the general population. Pre-existing increased intraocular pressure is a risk factor in central retinal vein occlusion, with one-third of patients demonstrating contralateral pressure elevation and disc cupping, but is found much less often (about 10 per cent) in branch vein, macular vein, and hemispheric vein occlusions. Other systemic conditions, such as hematologic abnormalities, coagulation disorders, collagen diseases, hyperproteinemias, and hyperlipidemias, are less commonly associated with retinal vein occlusions. In young patients with vein occlusions, abnormal platelet function is detected in about 50 per cent, particularly in patients with migraine syndromes, mitral valve prolapse, and those on certain hormonal therapies. Because of the diversity of associated conditions, it is recommended that the ophthalmologist obtain appropriate consultations to help detect these associated conditions.

COMMENTS

Patients with an ischemic central retinal vein occlusion and a visual acuity of 20/400 or worse should be offered prompt panretinal photocoagulation treatment to reduce the risk of developing painful neovascular glaucoma and possible loss of the eye. Hyperpermeable vein occlusions with good acuity should be followed and grid laser photocoagulation of persistent macular edema undertaken as indicated. There is no proof that any medication, including antiplatelet agents (such as low-dose aspirin), prevents hyperpermeable patterns from progressing to ischemic ones, but there are compelling systemic benefits of using antiplatelet agents for underlying disease.

Branch vein occlusion with persistent macular edema should be treated with laser photocoagulation to improve visual acuity in appropriate cases. Scatter laser photocoagulation in eyes with neovascularization and branch vein occlusion reduces the risk of subsequent vitreous hemorrhage. In cases not receiving laser treatment, close follow-up is important to detect progressive ischemia, which occurs in about 20 per cent of cases and places the eye at increased risk of neovascularization and its consequences.

References

Augsburger JJ, Magargal LE: Visual prognosis following treatment of acute central retinal artery obstruction. Br J Ophthalmol 64:913–917, 1980.

Brown GC, Magargal LE: Central retinal artery obstruction and visual acuity. Ophthalmology 89:14–19, 1982.

Brown GC, Shields JA: Cilioretinal arteries and retinal arterial occlusion. Arch Ophthalmol 97:84–92, 1979.

Bull DA, et al: Correlation of ophthalmic findings with carotid artery stenosis. J Cardiovasc Surg (Torino) 33:401–406, 1992.

Chawluk JB, et al: Atherosclerotic carotid artery disease in patients with retinal ischemic syndromes. Neurology 38:858–863, 1988.

Deutsch TA, et al: Effects of oxygen carbon dioxide on the retinal vasculature in humans. Arch Ophthalmol 101:1278–1280, 1983.

Duker JS, Sivalingam A, Brown GC, Reber R: A prospective study of acute central artery obstruction. The incidence of secondary ocular neovascularization. Arch Ophthalmol 109:339–342, 1991.

Ffytche TJ: A rationalization of treatment of central retinal artery occlusion. Trans Ophthalmol Soc UK 94:468–479, 1974.

Hayreh SS, Weingeist TA: Experimental occlusion of the central artery of the retina. IV. Retinal tolerance time to acute ischaemia. Br J Ophthalmol 64:818–825, 1980.

Hayreh SS, Weingeist TA: Experimental occlusion of the central artery of the retina. I. Ophthalmoscopic and fluorescein angiographic studies. Br J Ophthalmol 64:896–912, 1980.

Hirayama Y, et al: Bifemelane in the treatment of central retinal artery or vein obstruction. Clin Ther 12:230–235, 1990.

Jampol LM, et al: Ischemia of ciliary arterial circulation from ocular compression. Arch Ophthalmol 93:1311–1317, 1975.

Magargal LE, et al: Neovascular glaucoma following branch retinal vein obstruction. Glaucoma 3:333–335, 1981.

Magargal LE, et al: Neovascular glaucoma following central retinal vein obstruction. Ophthalmology 88:1095–1101, 1981.

Magargal LE, et al: Efficacy of panretinal photocoagulation in preventing neovascular glaucoma following ischemic central retinal vein obstruction. Ophthalmology 89:780–784, 1982.

Magargal LE, et al: Retinal ischemia and risk of neovascularization following central retinal vein obstruction. Ophthalmology 89:1241–1245, 1982.

Magargal LE, et al: Temporal branch retinal vein obstruction: A review. Ophthalmic Surg 17:240–246, 1986.

Sanborn GE, Magargal LE: Characteristics of the hemispheric retinal vein occlusion. Ophthalmology 91:1616–1624, 1984.

RETINITIS PIGMENTOSA 362.74

SAUL MERIN, M.D.

Jerusalem, Israel

Retinitis pigmentosa is an inherited progressive disease of the retina that is characterized by early and diffuse functional retinal abnormalities, a subnormal or "extinct" (nonrecordable) electroretinogram, early involvement of the retinal pigment epithelium and visual receptors, and an outcome of severely impaired vision or blindness. The symptoms of retinitis pigmentosa usually become apparent during the second decade of life, but are sometimes present in early childhood. Night blindness is usually the earliest symptom, followed by progressive loss of peripheral visual fields. Sometimes, central vision is involved early due to macular edema or atrophic maculopathy. Before the involvement of central vision, the patient may be aware of the deterioration of color vision. Progression of morphologic changes of the fundus depends upon the genetic entity and varies in different types of retinitis pigmentosa.

THERAPY

Ocular. A flush-fitting, opaque scleral contact lens to produce monocular complete light deprivation has been used to slow down the degenerative changes that may occur when the eye is exposed to light, but a follow-up of two such patients for 5 years did not reveal any significant difference in the natural course of the disease. The possibility that partial and selective light restriction may be of benefit is being investigated. Until the final results of these studies become known, recommendations based on theoretical and clinical considerations suggest that patients with retinitis pigmentosa wear dark sunglasses for outdoor use, especially in bright sunlight. Side shields added to the dark sunglasses are helpful to restrict further the amount of sunlight reaching the eye. Special sunglasses that reduce considerably (more than 75 per cent) the total transmission of light and cut out the lower wavelengths of light and the ultraviolet rays are produced by several manufacturers and are commercially available. Almost all patients fitted by such glasses report subjective visual improvement, mainly through enhanced contrasts. However, objective measurements confirmed such an improvement in only a proportion of cases.

Correction of associated refractive errors and the use of low-vision aids may help improve central vision. Optical devices may be used to widen the visual fields in patients with good central vision and narrow visual fields. An image intensifier may be used to improve vision in the darkness. Early clinical trials have been encouraging. A wide-field-high-intensity lantern has also been found useful and practical for night mobility.

Acetazolamide (Diamox), in amounts of 125 mg or 250 mg twice a day, was used successfully to improve central vision in patients with macular edema associated with retinitis pigmentosa. It was also reported that, with prolonged use of this medication, a progressive increase in extrafoveal retinal sensitivity was noted.

Surgical. Patients with advanced retinitis pigmentosa often suffer from a posterior cortical cataract. Even when the electroretinogram is very low or extinct, such patients may benefit from cataract extraction if their macular function is still preserved. In such cases, the best preoperative test is the visual evoked potential; its presence indicates good macular function. Studies indicate increased patient satisfaction when an intraocular lens is implanted. An ultraviolet-shielded intraocular lens is advisable.

Some patients with retinitis pigmentosa develop telangiectatic capillaries in the retina, followed by extensive intraretinal and subretinal leakage of the Coats'-like variety and neovascularization on the disc and elsewhere. Panretinal photocoagulation by laser was found to be effective in reducing the complications from this condition, especially recurrent intravitreal hemorrhage.

Grid laser therapy has been used to reduce visual loss associated with cystoid macular edema, which is frequently found in retinitis pigmentosa patients. Its beneficial effect has not yet been confirmed.

Supportive. Genetic counseling should be provided. The probability of an affected person having affected children depends on the mode of inheritance if the genetic type can be accurately diagnosed. In isolated cases, the risk of affected children depends on the severity of the disease in the affected parent, the gender, and the prevalence of the various types of retinitis pigmentosa in the family population. The discovery of the gene encoding rhodopsin on chromosome 3 led to the identification of many (at least 13) point mutations of this gene associated with autosomal dominant retinitis pigmentosa. Identification of the mutation in a specific family is helpful for counseling and prognosis.

Ocular or Periocular Manifestations

Choroid: Disappearance of choriocapillaries; loss of larger choroidal vessels (late).
Optic Nerve: Pallor.
Retina: Attenuated arteries; depigmentation of pigmentary epithelium; edematous (tapetal) reflex of pigmentary epithelium; fine pigmentary stippling; thinning; vascular pigmentary sheathing.
Other: Dyschromatopsia; midperipheral ring scotoma; night blindness; progressive constriction of peripheral visual fields; visual loss.

PRECAUTIONS

Many drugs, operations, and bizarre procedures for the treatment of retinitis pigmentosa have been suggested. These include anticoagulants,[‡] xanthinol niacinate[‡] and other vasodilators, RNA, retrobulbar injections* of hyaluronidase and acid phosphates, and even subconjunctival injection* of peat distillate. Transplantation of human placenta, practiced for many years, continues to be used by some. Surgical transplantation of strips of extraocular muscles has been suggested to improve choroidal blood flow. It has been reported that patients responded favorably to exposure to ultrasonics and acupuncture. However, reliable evidence of the success of any of the treatments mentioned above is not available.

ENCAD is a hydrolysate of yeast RNA, used extensively in the former Soviet Union for treatment of hereditary retinal degenera-

tions including retinitis pigmentosa. However, several other studies did not show any benefit from this treatment.

Vitamin A[‡] has been used for the treatment of retinitis pigmentosa, but there is no evidence of a beneficial effect from this vitamin or its derivatives; it is possible that such treatment even has a deleterious effect. Vitamin E[‡] has also been employed in the treatment of this disease; it too probably has no demonstrable benefit in the isolated form of retinitis pigmentosa.

Intramuscular injections of a ganglioside, use of cyclosporine A, and the administration of docosahexaenoic acid are three other more recently attempted therapies for retinitis pigmentosa and allied diseases. Their value has not been confirmed.

COMMENTS

Retinitis pigmentosa is associated with a variety of disease entities, including lipid disorders, mucopolysaccharidosis, spinocerebellar degenerations, and other seemingly unrelated conditions. Their association with retinitis pigmentosa is still not understood, but it is conceivable that in some of these diseases, such as Refsum's syndrome, dietary control may prove useful in avoiding or retarding some of the retinal changes observed. Combined vitamin A and E therapy seems to be efficient in arresting the visual deterioration of retinitis pigmentosa associated with abetalipoproteinemia. Transplantation of RPE cells and photoreceptors is being attempted on an investigational basis in animals. This new approach carries hope for a more efficient therapy of retinitis pigmentosa in the future.

References

Berson EL: Light deprivation and retinitis pigmentosa. Vision Res 20:1179–1184, 1980.
Birch DG, Anderson JL, Fish GE: Longitudinal measures in children receiving ENCAD for hereditary retinal degeneration. Doc Ophthalmol 77:185–192, 1991.
Bishara S, et al: Combined vitamin A and E therapy prevents retinal electrophysiological deterioration in abetalipoproteinemia. Br J Ophthalmol 66:767–770, 1982.
Chen JC, Fitzke FW, Bird AC: Long-term effect of acetazolamide in a patient with retinitis pigmentosa. Invest Ophthalmol Vis Sci 31:1914–1918, 1990.
Cox SN, Hay E, Bird AC: Treatment of chronic macular edema with acetazolamide. Arch Ophthalmol 106:1190–1195, 1988.
Dryja TP, McGee TL, Hahn LB, et al: Mutations within the rhodopsin gene in patients with autosomal dominant retinitis pigmentosa. N Engl J Med 323:1302–1307, 1990.
Fishman GA, Gilbert LD, Fiscella RG, et al: Acetazolamide for treatment of chronic macular edema in retinitis pigmentosa. Am J Ophthalmol 107:1445–1452, 1989.
Jacobson SG, Kemp CM, Sung C-H, Nathans J: Ret-

inal function and rhodopsin levels in autosomal dominant retinitis pigmentosa with rhodopsin mutations. Am J Ophthalmol 112:256–271, 1991.

Katznelson LA, Khoroshilova-Maslova IP, Eliseyeva RF: A new method of treatment of retinitis pigmentosa/pigment abiotrophy. Ann Ophthalmol 22:167–172, 1990.

Le Gargasson JF, Rigaudière F, Grall Y, et al: Retinal protection using glasses filtering short wavelengths in patients with hereditary degenerative diseases. First electrophysiologic results. Ophthalmology 3:65–66, 1989.

Lenk W: Nutritional and metabolic aspects of heredopathia atactica polyneuritiformis (Refsum's syndrome). Nutr Metab 16:366–374, 1974.

Merin S, Auerbach E: Retinitis pigmentosa. Surv Ophthalmol 20:303–346, 1976.

Merin S: Inherited Eye Diseases. Diagnosis and Clinical Management. New York, Marcel Dekker, 1991, pp 219–279.

Muller DPR, Lloyd JK, Bird AC: Long-term management of abetalipoproteinaemia. Possible role for vitamin E. Arch Dis Child 52:209–214, 1977.

Newsome DA, Blacharski PA: Grid photocoagulation for macular edema in patients with retinitis pigmentosa. Am J Ophthalmol 103:161–166, 1987.

Runge P, et al: Oral vitamin E supplements can prevent the retinopathy of abetalipoproteinemia. Br J Ophthalmol 70:166–173, 1986.

Steinberg D, et al: Phytanic acid in patients with Refsum's syndrome and response to dietary treatment. Arch Intern Med 125:75–87, 1970.

Uliss AE, Gregor ZJ, Bird AC: Retinitis pigmentosa and retinal neovascularization. Ophthalmology 93:1599–1603, 1986.

Van den Berg TJ: Red glasses and visual function in retinitis pigmentosa. Doc Ophthalmol 73:255–274, 1989.

RETINOPATHY OF PREMATURITY 362.21
(Retrolental Fibroplasia, RLF, ROP)

ROBERT E. KALINA, M.D.

Seattle, Washington

Retinopathy of prematurity (ROP) is a disorder of immature retinal blood vessels occurring in premature infants. The incidence is related inversely to birth weight. Oxygen in excess of need is thought to play a role by causing vaso-obliteration in the immature peripheral retina, but other factors likely also play a causative role. Presumably in response to peripheral retinal ischemia, neovascularization later develops just posterior to the junction of vascularized and nonvascularized retina. Such neovascularization most reliably is detected 6 or more weeks after birth and usually regresses spontaneously. However, in some cases, fibrous proliferation, vitreous hemorrhage, and retinal detachment supervene, and the proliferative phase leads to irreversible cicatricial changes. Cicatricial changes may range from mild dragging of the retina compatible with good visual acuity to a complete retrolental mass and phthisis bulbi. Cicatricial changes are usually completed by 15 months of age or earlier.

THERAPY

Supportive. The best therapy for ROP is prevention. The recognition of the causal relationship of oxygen in excess of need to ROP produced a dramatic decline in its incidence, but new cases continue to occur, despite the sophisticated neonatal intensive care techniques and oxygen monitoring that are available today. In general, modern-day cases seem to be less severe than those occurring in the past. However, the most severe cases now occur in very low birth weight infants (<1000 gm), a group more likely to survive with modern neonatal techniques. Since prematurity has become the most important cause of ROP, prevention ultimately rests with public health measures designed to reduce the incidence of premature birth.

Premature infants weighing less than 1251 to 1500 gm at birth should be examined for ROP at approximately 6 weeks of age. Infants showing ROP or those in whom vascularization of the peripheral retina is incomplete should be examined again at intervals of 1 to 4 weeks, depending upon the severity of the disease process. The binocular indirect ophthalmoscope should be used, together with an eyelid speculum, after dilation of the pupils with 2.5 per cent phenylephrine combined with either 0.5 per cent cyclopentolate or 0.5 per cent tropicamide. Children with cicatricial changes should be followed throughout life, particularly in the childhood and adolescent years, to prevent further visual loss because of amblyopia, retinal detachment, or angle-closure glaucoma.

Ocular. No topical ophthalmic preparation is known to be effective in preventing or treating ROP. However, severe proliferative ROP is associated with marked ocular inflammation, and instillation of a small amount of 0.5 per cent atropine ointment once daily may reduce posterior synechiae formation or at least allow them to form in a dilated position to permit fundus evaluation.

Surgical. In a prospective controlled clinical trial, cryotherapy has been shown to decrease the risk of severe visual loss by about 50 per cent when applied to the peripheral avascular zone of eyes with "threshold" ROP (Stage 3 "plus"; 5-8 clock hours). Subsequently, reports of indirect laser photocoagulation have claimed equivalent results with greater ease of application, particularly in Zone 1 disease. Since the proliferative changes of ROP have such a remarkable propensity for regression and because treatment may be associated with severe early or delayed complications, extending treatment to "pre-threshold" ROP should be approached with caution.

In eyes in which retinal detachment has developed, cryotherapy or laser is no longer appropriate. Scleral buckling is reasonable for rhegmatogenous retinal detachment, but definite retinal breaks rarely are confirmed in retinal detachments caused by acute ROP.

In eyes with chronic tractional/exudative retinal detachment, microsurgical techniques of lensectomy and vitrectomy with or without scleral buckling, usually applied between 3 and 12 months of age, have been successful in reattaching the retina in some cases. Even among eyes with initial anatomic success, however, visual results usually are disappointing.

Systemic. Vitamin E,[‡] an antioxidant, has been found to modify favorably the proliferative retinal vascular changes found in the kitten after oxygen exposure. Preliminary clinical reports have suggested that vitamin E may be efficacious in humans, but a committee of the Institute of Medicine determined that present evidence did not support the use of vitamin E as prophylaxis for ROP. Most institutions are withholding vitamin E supplementation in excess of the amount that is normally part of neonatal intensive care for other indications.

Ocular or Periocular Manifestations

Iris: Anterior or posterior synechiae; neovascularization.
Optic Nerve: Pallor.
Retina: Attenuated vessels; detachment; dilated vessels; "dragged" appearance; folds; hemorrhage; neovascularization; pigmentary changes; retrolental mass; vascular tortuosity.
Vitreous: Haze; hemorrhage; traction.
Other: Amblyopia; anisometropia; cataract; glaucoma; leukokoria; myopia; pseudostrabismus; shallow anterior chamber.

PRECAUTIONS

Because topical medications may cause adverse side effects in premature infants, 10 per cent phenylephrine and 1 per cent cyclopentolate should not be used. If atropine is to be used, the concentration of 0.5 per cent is recommended, preferably in an ointment form. Since absorption and systemic toxic effects of ocular medications occur mainly through the nasal mucosa, the amount applied should be minimized (never more than one drop at a time), and excess solution should be wiped away promptly. It may also be helpful to apply pressure on the closed eyelid over the area of the lacrimal sac for a few seconds after instillation of a drop.

Ophthalmoscopic examinations may be traumatic and potentially hazardous to the critically ill infant. Since ROP does not progress to "threshold" for treatment until an average of 37 weeks gestational age, examination should be delayed until the infant has stabilized and the risk from topical medications and eye examination can be minimized.

COMMENTS

In addition to recommending treatment for "threshold" ROP, the ophthalmologist may provide a valuable service to premature infants and their families. Families deserve to learn of ROP and its potential complications from the neonatal staff, rather than to discover their infant's visual disability at home. Identification of affected infants may lead to early diagnosis and treatment of complications that threaten further visual loss.

The continuing occurrence of ROP today, despite the sophisticated medical care available, deserves emphasis. Prematurity has superseded oxygen as the prime etiologic factor. Arterial oxygen monitoring has reached a high degree of accuracy, but is limited by intermittent sampling, particularly in infants requiring chronic oxygen therapy and thus at greatest risk for ROP. Transcutaneous oxygen monitoring is helpful in neonatal care, but has not been shown to reduce the incidence of ROP.

Not all cases of proliferative vascular retinopathy in infancy and childhood are ROP. Other etiologic factors should be sought, particularly in other than very low birth weight infants.

References

Cryotherapy for Retinopathy of Prematurity Cooperative Group: Multicentered trial of cryotherapy for retinopathy of prematurity. Arch Ophthalmol 106:471–479, 1988.
Flynn JT, et al: A randomized, prospective trial of transcutaneous oxygen monitoring. Ophthalmology 94:630–638, 1987.
Institute of Medicine: Vitamin E and Retinopathy of Prematurity. Report of a Study by a Committee of the Institute of Medicine, Division of Health Sciences Policy. Washington, DC, National Academy Press, 1986, pp 1–24.
McNamara JA, et al: Laser photocoagulation for stage 3+ retinopathy of prematurity. Ophthalmology 98:576–580, 1991.
Quinn GE, et al: Visual acuity in infants after vitrectomy for severe retinopathy of prematurity. Ophthalmology 98:5–13, 1991.

RETINOSCHISIS 361.10

LOUIS DAILY, M.D., Ph.D.(Ophth.)

Houston, Texas

Retinoschisis is a condition in which the sensory retina splits at any level between the inner and outer nuclear layers. This split usually occurs bilaterally at the outer plexiform layer, with the accumulation of a mucopolysaccharide-rich viscous fluid within the intervening space. As the schisis progresses, the neural elements of the retina are first stretched and finally lysed, producing absolute visual loss in the affected areas. The bulging internal wall of the cavity is thin and immobile and often has a "beaten metal" appearance. A band of prominent cystoid degeneration separating the cavity from the ora serrata is a common feature. Pigmentary lines usually are a demarcation of a secondary retinal detachment or outer layer breaks in acquired retinoschisis.

Retinoschisis can be degenerative (senile acquired), inherited (juvenile idiopathic), or tractional in etiology. Senile retinoschisis occurs as a result of a degenerative change at the periphery of the retina, affects about 3 per cent of the population, and increases in frequency from the second decade onward. Retinoschisis can be a slowly progressive, self-limited disease, or it can lead to holes in both the inner and outer walls and subsequent rhegmatogenous detachment. In the rarer idiopathic or juvenile retinoschisis, a widespread vitreoretinal degeneration occurs that is characterized by onset in the first decade, a hereditary pattern (usually sex-linked and recessive), common macular involvement, and a much poorer prognosis (visual loss 9 per cent, vitreous hemorrhage 5 per cent, retinal detachment 11 per cent). Juvenile retinoschisis has been associated with other vitreoretinal anomalies, including Goldmann-Favre syndrome and skeletal anomalies. Tractional retinoschisis may complicate tractional retinal detachment in advanced proliferative diabetic retinopathy. Tractional retinoschisis in diabetic retinopathy must be differentiated from tractional retinal detachment, which requires different surgical maneuvers. Because of coexisting vitreous hemorrhage and/or cataract, visualization may be imperfect. Additional clues to the presence of tractional retinoschisis are the absence of a pigmented line demarcating the edge of a retinal detachment, the persistence of a concave contour of the inner layer in the presence of holes, and whitening of the outer layer by photocoagulation. Unusual and anecdotal causes of clinically observed retinoschisis have been intraretinal hemorrhage in battered babies, retinoschisis secondary to retinal telangiectasia, and tractional retinoschisis in retinopathy of prematurity. The retinal elevation that communicates with optic nerve pits may be a schisis-like separation of the internal layers of the retina.

THERAPY

Supportive. The diseased gene in X-linked retinoschisis (RS) has been assigned to the short arm of the X chromosome (Xp22.2-p21.2 region) by linkage studies. Heterozygote carriers also frequently express the disease. Carrier detection and prenatal diagnosis may justify genetic counseling.

Ocular. Retinoschisis associated with Goldmann-Favre vitreoretinal degeneration has been treated with cyclosporine and bromocriptine in two patients with regression of macular edema and flattening of the retinoschisis.

Surgical. Because of the high incidence of serious complications, prophylactic treatment by photocoagulation or preferably by cryotherapy for senile retinoschisis without holes in the outer layer is contraindicated unless the schisis extends to no less than 20 degrees from the macula (a rare occurrence) and does not appear progressive. Cryotherapy performed in two stages—the anterior two thirds first and the remainder several weeks later—probably results in fewer complications, such as macular puckering or massive vitreous or preretinal membrane contraction. The inner layer of the schisis need not be collapsed completely to prevent progression. If the macula is threatened or retinal detachment has developed in the affected eye or is attributed to retinoschisis in the fellow eye, treatment should be done. A retinal detachment associated with retinoschisis should be treated first and has been managed successfully without scleral buckling and with or without vitrectomy by simultaneous external or internal subretinal fluid drainage and intraocular gas injection; this treatment resulted in spontaneous collapse of the retinoschisis. When residual schisis is great, the cyst-like fluid should be evacuated during retinal detachment surgery, but the inner layer need not be collapsed completely to prevent schisis progression. Giant outer layer breaks are managed by a variety of surgical techniques, including scleral buckling, cryotherapy or laser, or intraocular gas and postoperative positioning.

Photocoagulation can be performed with either the zenon arc coagulator or an argon (all wave or green) laser and can delimit posterior progression. If used directly on the schisis, photocoagulation must be heavy enough to include the external plexiform layer in the final limiting scar. Settings for either type of laser should be determined by the visible whitening effect of coagulation on the external layer. If part of the schisis is 3 disc diameters or closer to the macula's edge, the coagulation settings of the argon laser for the schisis itself should be 500 to 1000 nm beam diameters for 0.1- to 0.2-second exposure at 500 to 1200 mW power. Cryotherapy, preferably done under direct observation with an indirect ophthalmoscope, should result in whitening of the outer retinal layers and overlapping of the frozen areas.

Because X-linked juvenile retinoschisis is slowly progressive and surgery produces a high incidence of serious complications, prophylactic surgery to halt its progression is rarely indicated. Photocoagulation may be indicated for recurrent vitreous hemorrhage. The only other indication for surgical treatment of this form of retinoschisis is a rhegmatogenous retinal detachment; vitreous traction on the inner wall of the raised schisis cavity can require vitrectomy, gas fluid exchange, and endolaser.

Ocular or Periocular Manifestations

Optic Nerve: Atrophy.

Retina: Atrophy; "beaten metal" appearance; cysts; deposits; detachment; holes; macular degeneration; peripheral cystoid degeneration; vitreoretinal traction; subretinal fibrosis; thinning; perivascular sheathing.

Vitreous: Traction.

Other: Decreased visual acuity; scotoma; visual field defects.

PRECAUTIONS

Retinoschisis can be confused with rhegmatogenous retinal detachment. Clinical differentiation can nearly always be made by slit-lamp examination through the three-mirror Goldmann contact lens. The inner layer of the schisis, as identified by its blood vessels, can be seen by retroillumination or direct, diffuse, or focal illumination in wide or narrow optical sections. The origin of the schisis can be found with the focal beam. In optical section, the inner layer is thinner and more translucent than a detached retina. It is usually immobile, not exhibiting the undulations seen in recent retinal detachments. With the indirect ophthalmoscope it exhibits the "beaten metal" appearance. Using these examinations, as well as transillumination, fluorescein angiography, and ultrasonography, one should easily be able to differentiate schisis from retinal detachment. The lesions' progress should be watched carefully. If it has extended posterior to the equator, the visual field should be charted for damage, which does not arise until the central area is threatened.

COMMENTS

The prognosis for the most commonly observed form of retinoschisis, senile (acquired) retinoschisis, is generally good, for it can remain stationary indefinitely or progress very slowly, and even "schisis-detachment" can remain asymptomatic and nonprogressive. Treatment for asymptomatic retinoschisis would seem to be justified very infrequently.

References

Alitalo T, et al: Genetic mapping of 12 marker loci in the Xp22.3-p21 region. Hum Genet *86*:599–603, 1991.

Ambler JS, et al: The management of retinal detachment complicating degenerative retinoschisis. Am J Ophthalmol *107*:171–176, 1989.

Byer N: Long-term natural history study of senile retinoschisis with implications for management. Ophthalmology *93*:1127–1137, 1986.

Dobbie JG: Should retinoschisis be treated? *In* Brockhurst RJ (ed): Controversy in Ophthalmology. Philadelphia, WB Saunders, 1977, pp 551–561.

Garweg J, et al: Die Behandlung des Goldmann-Favre Syndroms mit Cyclosporin A und Bromocriptin. Klin Mbl Augenheilk *199*:199–205, 1991.

Greenwald MJ, et al: Traumatic retinoschisis in battered babies. Ophthalmology *93*:618–625, 1986.

Jabbour NM, et al: Stage 5 retinopathy of prematurity: Prognostic value of morphologic findings. Ophthalmology *94*:1640–1645, 1987.

Kaplan J, et al: Contribution to carrier detection and genetic counseling in X-linked retinoschisis. J Med Genet *28*:383–388, 1991.

Kellner U, et al: X-chromosomale kongenitale Retinoschisis. Fortschr Ophthalmol *87*:264–268, 1990.

Lang GE, et al: Autosomal dominante vitreoretinale Dystrophie mit Skelettdysplasie in einer Generation. Klin Mbl Augenheilk *198*:207–214, 1991.

Lincoff H, et al: Retinoschisis associated with optic nerve pits. Arch Ophthalmol *106*:61–67, 1988.

Lincoff H, et al: Tractional elevations of the retina in patients with diabetes. Am J Ophthalmol *113*:235–242, 1992.

Michel-Awad A, et al: Diagnostic antenatal de certaines maladies hereditaires cecitantes. Ophthalmologie *4*:237–239, 1990.

Scott R, et al: Pars plana vitrectomy in the management of retinal detachments associated with degenerative retinoschisis. Ophthalmology *97*:470–474, 1990.

SUBRETINAL NEOVASCULAR MEMBRANES 362.16

HUNTER L. LITTLE, M.D., F.A.C.S.

Menlo Park, California

Subretinal neovascular membranes (SRNM) are proliferative blood vessels arising from the choriocapillaris and extending through breaks in Bruch's membrane into the tissue plane between Bruch's membrane and the retinal pigment epithelium (RPE). When present in the posterior pole of the eye, they pose a significant threat of loss of central vision. Subretinal neovascular membranes cause serous and hemorrhagic detachments of the retinal pigment epithelium and of the sensory retina in the macula in both senile macular degeneration and the presumed ocular histoplasmosis syndrome, leading to macular destruction and loss of central vision in both diseases. Furthermore, subretinal neovascularization is a frequent sequela in the natural course of soft drusen and serous detachment of the retinal pigment epithelium in elderly patients. Senile macular degeneration is the leading cause of blindness in the United

States for people over 60 years of age and in ocular histoplasmic choroidopathy, which ranks second only to diabetes as the leading cause of legal blindness for people under 50 years who live within endemic areas of histoplasmosis in the central and eastern United States.

The clinical findings are best seen with the fundus contact lens. They include subretinal fluid hemorrhage beneath the sensory retina or beneath the retinal pigment epithelium, subretinal exudate, retinal striae, and a notched contour to an RPE detachment. Angiographic findings for subretinal neovascular membranes include reticular vascular pattern, bicycle wheel pattern, serpiginous margin, bright irregular fluorescein spots, and adjacent blocked fluorescence from hemorrhage. In addition to clinical and angiographic findings, one frequently sees a grayish discoloration at the level of the RPE that corresponds to the subretinal neovascular membrane. If the overlying RPE is atrophic, one can even see the membrane. Subretinal neovascular membranes can be multiple in origin. Occult SRNM commonly occur in age-related (senile macular) degeneration and present with only blurred, poorly outlined areas of fluorescence on angiography, usually with subretinal fluid. One should always suspect SRNM in a patient over 50 years of age presenting with subretinal fluid in the macula.

Age-related macular degeneration and the ocular histoplasmosis syndrome are the most frequent causes of subretinal neovascular membranes; however, SRNM may also occur in the following conditions: angioid streaks, traumatic ruptures of Bruch's membrane, choroidal scars (rarely with toxoplasmosis or photocoagulation scars), myopic degeneration, overlying choroidal nevi (rarely), end-stage Best's vitelliform macular degeneration, serpiginous or geographic choroiditis, acute multifocal posterior plaquoid posterior epitheliopathy, hamartoma of the retinal pigment epithelium, and optic nerve drusen.

THERAPY

Surgical. The indications for photocoagulation are threatened loss of vision, the presence of serous or hemorrhagic detachment of the sensory retina or the RPE or both within the macula, and evidence of the location of a subretinal neovascular membrane. Photocoagulation is performed rarely in the presence of foveal involvement by the SRNM; it is done only for moderately small SRNM (1 disc diameter or less) in eyes with vision of 20/200 or less.

Laser photocoagulation of subretinal neovascular membranes requires intense confluent photocoagulation burns covering the entire subretinal neovascular membrane and extending, when possible, approximately 200 μM beyond the peripheral margin of the membrane. Typical treatment parameters include a 200-μM diameter burn, 0.2-second exposure time, and 400 to 500 mW of power. These settings are typical for the green argon laser photocoagulator. The power levels for krypton laser photocoagulation are usually lower and the exposure times longer in order to minimize the risk of choroidal hemorrhage. Typical settings for the krypton laser include a 200-μM diameter burn and 0.5- to 1.0-second exposure times with 100 to 200 mW of power. With red wavelength lasers, the SRNM is first covered with minimal to moderate reaction using 0.2- to 0.5-second exposures; the power is increased gradually with repeated additional layers of photocoagulation over the entire SRNM until the lesion is gray to moderately white. Pressure may be applied to the contact lens to immobilize the eye and to minimize hemorrhage during the course of treatment. The rhodamine dye laser, using 577 to 630 nm, is used with settings ranging from those with argon green to those with krypton red. Since argon blue is absorbed by xanthophyll pigment, green, yellow, orange, and red are preferable wavelengths. Yellow to red (577 to 647 nm) wavelengths are preferable as they are totally transmitted by xanthophyll. Repeat fluorescein angiograms are done within 2 weeks, and subsequent treatment is performed if residual leakage is detected. Inadequate treatment results in hemorrhage and recurrence of the subretinal neovascular membrane.

PRECAUTIONS

Photocoagulation vasculitis must be distinguished from recurrent subretinal neovascular membrane. The retinal vessels overlying subretinal neovascular membranes are damaged by argon laser photocoagulation. These retinal vessels will show fluorescence because of increased permeability during the first 3 to 4 weeks after photocoagulation. Such fluorescence from photocoagulation vasculitis must be distinguished from recurrent subretinal neovascularization.

Special mention is made of the progressive enlargement of photocoagulation scars that is noted 1 to 4 years after photocoagulation. This enlargement is evident by comparing the width of the scar shortly after photocoagulation when it corresponds to the zone of the fresh photocoagulation burns with the width of the scar after several years. This phenomenon explains the progressive visual loss after the successful eradication of juxtafoveal subretinal neovascular membranes. The probable cause of circumferential retinal pigment epithelial atrophy is subliminal coagulation by heat transfer from the adjacent photocoagulation burns.

COMMENTS

The Macular Photocoagulation Study reported in a randomized control fashion that laser photocoagulation of subretinal neovascular membranes associated with senile macular degeneration reduced the loss of vision as compared with the natural course of the untreated eyes. The incidence of severe visual loss for treated eyes was 24 versus 45 per cent for untreated eyes. Successful management of subretinal neovascular membranes requires early diagnosis; proper case selection for treatment; intense, confluent photocoagulation of the entire membrane and repeat treatment until subretinal neovascular membrane is destroyed; avoidance of the fovea and preretinal blood; early and prolonged follow-up with fluorescein angiography, repeat photocoagulation (when indicated), daily Amsler grid checks, and discontinuation of aspirin and other medications that alter coagulation.

Recurrent subretinal neovascular membranes occur in 30 to 40 per cent of eyes. For this reason, retreatment is frequently indicated within the first 2 to 3 months of follow-up. Recurrences are more frequent when treating lesions within 300 μM of the fovea, presumably because one is restricted in the extent that one can treat around such membranes.

Studies are in progress to evaluate the indocyanine green angiography and diode laser photocoagulation in the management of SRNM. In contrast to fluorescein, which leaks from the SRNM into the surrounding subretinal pigment epithelial or subretinal spaces, indocyanine green remains bound to the SRNM, thus making it more effective for the detection of SRNM in the presence of a large retinal pigment epithelial detachment or turbid hemorrhagic subretinal fluid. Furthermore, the diode laser with its 800 nm wavelength may prove to be more useful in photocoagulation of juxtafoveal or subfoveal SRNM, since it seems to produce less retinal damage than do argon, krypton, and rhodamine dye lasers.

In conclusion, early detection and treatment with close follow-up are essential. Therefore, patients with macular drusen are urged to monitor their vision daily for distortion or blurring of the Amsler grid, straight line, and reading material; for altered color vision (television, or road signs); and for central or paracentral scotoma. Should any changes occur, patients are urged to report to their ophthalmologist within 24 to 48 hours for evaluation.

References

Bird AC: Treatment of senile disciform macular degeneration. Trans Ophthalmol Soc NZ 29:21–25, 1977.

Bressler, et al: Natural course of choroidal neovascular membranes within foveal avascular zone in senile macular degeneration. Am J Ophthalmol 93:157–163, 1982.

Fine SL: Macular photocoagulation study. Arch Ophthalmol 93:832, 1980.

Gutman FA: The natural course of active choroidal lesions in the presumed ocular histoplasmosis syndrome. Trans Am Ophthalmol Soc 77:515–541, 1979.

Little HL, Jack RL, Vassiliadis A: Argon laser photocoagulation of subretinal neovascular membranes. Trans Am Ophthalmol Soc 78:167–189, 1980.

Macular Photocoagulation Study Group: Argon laser photocoagulation for senile macular degeneration: Results of a randomized clinical trial. Arch Ophthalmol 100:912–918, 1982.

Macular Photocoagulation Study Group: Recurrent choroidal neovascularization after argon laser photocoagulation for neovascular maculopathy. Arch Ophthalmol 104:503–512, 1986.

Macular Photocoagulation Study Group: Argon laser photocoagulation for neovascular maculopathy: Three-year results from randomized clinical trial. Arch Ophthalmol 104:694–701, 1986.

Puliafito CA, Destro M, To K, Dobi E: Dye enhanced photocoagulation of choroidal neovascularization. Invest Ophthalmol Vis Sci 29(Suppl):414, 1988.

Ryan SJ: The development of an experimental model of subretinal neovascularization in disciform macular degeneration. Trans Am Ophthalmol Soc 77:707–745, 1979.

Sabates FN, Lee KY, Ziemianski MC: A comparative study of argon and krypton laser photocoagulation in the treatment of presumed ocular histoplasmosis syndrome. Ophthalmology 89:729–734, 1982.

Sarks SH: New vessel formation beneath the retinal pigment epithelium in senile eyes. Br J Ophthalmol 57:951–965, 1973.

Teeters VW, Bird AC: The development of neovascularization of senile disciform macular degeneration. Am J Ophthalmol 76:1–18, 1973.

Trempe CL, et al: Macular photocoagulation. Optimal wavelength selection. Ophthalmology 89:721–728, 1982.

Yanuzzi L, Slakter J, Sorenson J, Guyer D, Orlock D: Digital indocyanine green videoangiography and choroidal neovascularization. Retina 12:191–223, 1992.

THE WHITE DOT SYNDROMES 363.15

(Acute Posterior Multifocal Placoid Pigment Epitheliopathy, Birdshot Chorioretinopathy, Diffuse Unilateral Subacute Neuroretinitis, Multifocal Choroiditis and Panuveitis, Multiple Evanescent White Dot Syndrome, Presumed Ocular Histoplasmosis, Punctate Inner Choroidopathy, Punctate Outer Retinal Toxoplasmosis, Retinal Pigment Epitheliitis, Serpiginous Choroiditis, Subretinal Fibrosis and Uveitis, Vitiliginous Chorioretinopathy)

JON D. WALKER, M.D.,
and JAMES C. FOLK, M.D.

Iowa City, Iowa

The term "white dot syndrome" refers to several acquired diseases that cause inflammation and multifocal lesions at the level of the outer retina, retinal pigment epithelium, and inner choroid. Eleven separate diseases are generally included in this category. These diseases are all different, and the descriptive use of the term "white dot syndrome" does not at all imply a common appearance, etiology, or prognosis. Furthermore, there are numerous other causes of "white dots" in the fundus, but the usually acute, multifocal inflammatory nature of these eleven entities distinguish them from, for instance, vascular problems, such as cotton-wool spots, or hereditary or degenerative changes, such as Stargardt's disease, drusen, or cobblestone degeneration.

The entities included in this article are retinal pigment epitheliitis (RPE-itis), multiple evanescent white dot syndrome (MEWDS), acute posterior multifocal placoid pigment epitheliopathy (AMPPE), serpiginous choroiditis, presumed ocular histoplasmosis (POHS), punctate inner choroidopathy (PIC), multifocal choroiditis and panuveitis (MCP), subretinal fibrosis and uveitis (SFU), birdshot or vitiliginous chorioretinopathy, punctate outer retinal toxoplasmosis (PORT), and diffuse unilateral subacute neuroretinitis (DUSN).

Because there are many differences between the entities, any classification becomes somewhat arbitrary. However, one classification scheme follows:

- Primarily involving the retinal pigment epithelium, with mild effects: RPE-itis, MEWDS
- Primarily involving the inner choroid and RPE, with more marked effects: AMPPE and serpiginous
- The multifocal choroidopathies: POHS, PIC, MCP, and SFU
- Primarily involving the outer choroid: birdshot (vitiliginous) chorioretinopathy
- The two infectious etiologies: PORT, DUSN

RETINAL PIGMENT EPITHELIITIS. This is a very rare entity occurring primarily in young patients in the third decade. It is thought to involve focal inflammation at the level of the RPE with surrounding RPE edema. A viral precipitant has been postulated, but none has been identified. It usually involves a unilateral mild decrease in vision. There are usually two to four clusters of dark grayish spots surrounded by a hypopigmented halo. Fluorescein angiography may be normal, or the halo may become more hyperfluorescent with time. Symptoms usually resolve within 6 to 12 weeks. There is some question whether this condition may be related to central serous retinopathy or RPE degeneration syndromes. There has also been one case report of a choroidal neovascular membrane (CNVM).

MULTIPLE EVANESCENT WHITE DOT SYNDROME (MEWDS). This disease also occurs in younger patients with a female preponderance. It is thought to possibly involve post-

viral RPE inflammation with secondary retinal and photoreceptor changes. Vision is usually moderately decreased in the 20/40 to 20/200 range. The patients complain of photopsias, a scotoma, or decreased vision. There are multiple soft, gray-white spots in the posterior pole and midperiphery. The dots can be very faint and are seen best in the midperiphery. Initially it was thought to be primarily unilateral; however, a few spots are often seen in the fellow eye on close examination. There is usually a small amount of posterior vitreous cell as well. The white dots themselves usually last about 3 weeks and then fade. The patient may have an enlarged blind spot on perimetry that lasts longer. The fovea of the involved eye demonstrates a peculiar and almost pathognomonic orangish granular appearance. Often this may be the only physical finding to explain the patient's symptoms, particularly if the white spots have faded acutely. The fluorescein angiogram shows early hyperfluorescence of the dots with late staining. Each spot appears to be a cluster of smaller dots arranged in a wreath-like pattern. The ERG shows a decreased A-wave and early receptor potential. The prognosis is excellent, and most patients recover. However, usually some subjective decrease in visual function persists, and the enlarged blind spot may take months to resolve. Recurrences are unusual; the development of a CNVM has been reported, but is rare. The authors often make a presumptive diagnosis of this entity in patients presenting with a big blind spot syndrome, a small amount of posterior vitreous cell, and an orangish granularity of the fovea even if the acute white lesions are no longer present.

ACUTE POSTERIOR MULTIFOCAL PLACOID PIGMENT EPITHELIOPATHY (AMPPE). This disease has a predilection for patients in the third decade of life. There is no known sexual predisposition. Approximately one-third of patients have a prior viral syndrome, and this condition may represent some sort of postviral hypersensitivity process. There is some controversy as to whether it is a primary inflammation of the retinal pigment epithelium or choroidal vasculitis with choroidal lobule closure and secondary RPE changes. Patients usually present with a fairly rapid decrease in vision, the severity of which depends on whether lesions are present directly under the fovea. It is usually bilateral, with the second eye being involved in days to weeks. Classically there are large yellow-white creamy infiltrates at the level of the RPE and inner choroid. This disease is remarkable for the rate at which pigment changes develop. They usually begin in 1 to 2 weeks, and variations in pigment reaction can occur almost on a day-to-day basis. The infiltrates may form one large central lesion. Several associated ocular findings have been noted, including papillitis, serous retinal detachment (although some authorities feel this symptom implies the Vogt-

Koyanagi-Harada syndrome), retinal vasculitis, macular edema, superficial retinal hemorrhages, and episcleritis. There is usually no anterior chamber or vitreous cells, although they may be present. The geographic lesions on fluorescein angiography have a classic early hypofluorescence and late hyperfluorescence with leakage appearance. The symptoms usually resolve in 1 to 2 months. Of note, this syndrome is the only white dot syndrome that has been associated with mortality. There have been two case reports of death from associated cerebrovasculitis. Other systemic associations include red blood cell casts in the urine, thyroiditis, hearing changes, erythema nodosum, headache, and CSF pleocytosis. Most patients do not have these systemic associations. However, if a patient complains of a particularly severe headache or neurologic symptoms, referral should be considered. The prognosis is generally good, with most patients returning to 20/30 vision or better, but there are usually persistent scotomas or metamorphopsia. Recurrences and secondary choroidal neovascular membranes (CNVM) are rare.

SERPIGINOUS CHOROIDITIS. This disease has a tendency to strike older patients compared to the other white dot syndromes. The average age is in the fifth decade, but younger patients can also develop the disease. There is no clear racial or sexual predisposition, no known systemic association. Patients present with blurred vision and/or floaters. The pathology shows aggregates of lymphocytes in the choroid, presumably causing focal choriocapillaris and RPE damage. The active areas are gray-white and usually occur at the edge of previous atrophy. The active edge may remain active for months, gradually resolving to RPE mottling and atrophy. The disease usually starts at the disc and spreads centripetally in a serpiginous fashion with pseudopod-like projections. Twenty per cent of patients, however, have isolated macular lesions as the initial site of involvement. Multifocal noncontiguous recurrences can also occur. Focal phlebitis and retinal neovascularization have been rarely described. A fluorescein angiogram is characteristic, with the atrophic areas showing staining along the edge where functional choriocapillaris exists. The acute lesions are similar to AMPPE lesions with early hypofluorescence and late hyperfluorescence. Electrophysiologic testing is usually abnormal in proportion to the amount of retinal destruction. The course is characterized by recurrences occurring at times ranging from weeks to years. Progression may be asymptomatic if the macula is not involved and may explain why these patients present in an older age range. Choroidal neovascular membranes occur in up to 25 per cent of patients. Early serpiginous choroiditis may be difficult to differentiate from other focal inflammations, such as toxoplasmosis or AMPPE. Usually, the diagnosis becomes clear as the patient is

followed and recurrences occur. In general, the prognosis is fair, with at least one eye preserving useful vision. However, the prognosis can be very poor if foveal involvement or a CNVM develops.

PRESUMED OCULAR HISTOPLASMOSIS SYNDROME (POHS). Histoplasmosis capsulotum is found in river valleys, such as the Mississippi and Ohio, between 45° north and 45° south latitude. In these areas about 90 per cent of the people are skin test positive, yet only 1.6 to 2.6 per cent will have the discrete chorioretinal scars known as histo spots. The disease can present in any decade, but is more common in the fourth decade. It seems to be rare in African-Americans. The primary histoplasmosis infection is usually benign and often consists of flu symptoms or cough lasting 2 days to 2 weeks. The organism invades the lungs and then disseminates, especially to the reticuloendothelial system, leaving multiple focal calcified granulomas. A multifocal choroiditis also occurs. Presumably the organism is killed, but leaves behind residual nests of stimulated, immunoreactive cells. Either there is a chronic low level of smoldering inflammation, or some precipitate causes a nest of cells to flare up, resulting in local exudation (an active histo spot). This flare-up may cause further scarring or stimulate neovascularization with subsequent disciform scar formation. The initial multifocal inflammation that occurs with disease dissemination is asymptomatic, which is why one never sees acute multifocal active histo (unless the patient has fulminant disseminated disease, often seen in the immunosuppressed patient). It may be that because primary infections are usually acquired in childhood, the acute inflammation is less likely to be noticed.

In any event, the patient becomes symptomatic, not from the peripheral scars, but from scars present in the posterior pole. Two possibilities can occur, although it may be difficult to separate the two. The most common problem is that a CNVM develops in the area of the prior histo scar. It can cause disciform scarring and loss of central vision if not treated with laser photocoagulation. The technique for treating these neovascular membranes is covered elsewhere. Another possibility is that the scar becomes more active from an inflammatory standpoint. It can generate a small amount of subretinal fluid secondary to the inflammation. The patient can then become symptomatic without the presence of a full-blown neovascular membrane. This type of inflammatory reaction may respond quite well to systemic steroids or resolve over time without treatment. It is very important to monitor the patient closely for the development of a CNVM. Any symptomatic histoplasmosis patient must be assumed to have a neovascular membrane until proven otherwise. The Macula Photocoagulation Study has clearly demonstrated the benefit of laser treatment to CNVMs not involving the fovea in POHS patients.

PUNCTATE INNER CHOROIDOPATHY. Almost all the patients with this entity are myopic females with an average age of 27. The patients usually present with symptoms of decreased vision, scotomas, and photopsias. The symptoms are usually unilateral, but the findings are generally bilateral, albeit asymmetric. The patients have small gray-yellow spots, 0.1 to 0.2 disc diameters, in the posterior pole and periphery. Serous elevations can develop over the spots. As in POHS, the eyes are quiet with little or no anterior chamber or vitreous cells.

Symptoms usually decrease after about 1 month, although patients can have blurred vision and photopsias for a longer time. The spots evolve to atrophic scars very similar to those seen in the POHS. Skin and serologic tests for histoplasmosis have generally been negative in these patients, however.

The prognosis is usually excellent, with almost all patients returning to 20/20 unless there is a subfoveal lesion. However, 40 per cent of these patients develop a CNVM from the parafoveal scars in approximately 3 to 12 months or sometimes later. These CNVMs respond well to laser, but can also resolve without treatment. Subfoveal CNVMs have a guarded prognosis. The initial disease itself does not recur. Some patients have photopsias for years, but do not develop new lesions or further visual loss.

MULTIFOCAL CHOROIDITIS AND PANUVEITIS (MCP). Unlike POHS and PIC, this entity has a tendency to have more vitreous inflammation, more leakage from spots, and more recurrences. It is also known as the pseudo-histoplasmosis syndrome because of the similar appearance of the multifocal scars in the two diseases. There is a female preponderance with an average age of about 33. Patients usually complain of floaters and blurred vision, but may also note photopsias and visual field defects. The initial vision loss ranges from mild to severe, depending on the amount of cystoid macular edema or the presence of a CNVM. Most patients have at least a mild anterior chamber reaction; 90 to 100 per cent of patients have a significant number of inflammatory cells in the vitreous, which distinguishes this entity from POHS and PIC. Approximately one-third of patients may have peripapillary pigment changes. There are often many more lesions than are present in POHS or PIC. More lesions are often seen in the nasal fundus.

Acute lesions are grayish-yellow infiltrates at the level of the RPE and inner choroid. They tend to be smaller than the scars seen in POHS. It is not uncommon for patients to have both acute, symptomatic spots and old, quiet scars. The size of the scars is also often variable. Fluorescein angiography of only very acute lesions shows early hypofluorescence. Both acute and semiacute lesions show late staining. Old punched-out scars may act as window defects. Disc staining and cystoid macular edema may also be present. Approximately one-third of these patients may develop a CNVM. Of note, this disease can be recurrent with either new spots developing or simply recurrent inflammation in the eye without any change in the number of spots. Some authorities feel it is important to check Epstein-Barr titers in this entity, viral capsid antigen (IGG and IGM), Epstein-Barr nuclear antigen, and Epstein-Barr early antigen. Others have shown that sarcoidosis can create this clinical picture and recommend a blind conjunctival biopsy for granulomas. The prognosis is fair if inflammation can be controlled. The development of a CNVM results in a more guarded prognosis.

PROGRESSIVE SUBRETINAL FIBROSIS AND UVEITIS. This entity is the most severe of the multifocal choroidopathies. As with MCP, it can be recurrent and progressive. Unfortunately, these patients have a tendency to develop extensive subretinal fibrosis that results in marked visual loss. It is not clear whether this tendency to form fibrosis is a function of the host's immune response or the inciting agent. All the patients so far have been females, usually in their twenties. No etiologic agent has been identified.

The patients present with a fairly acute decrease in vision that progresses. The disease is bilateral, but often asymmetric. It is common for one eye to be involved first and the second eye to follow months later. It starts as a posterior to midperipheral multifocal choroiditis with 0.1 to 0.5 disc diameter whitish lesions in the RPE and inner choroid. Often, many small lesions are clustered in the posterior pole between the temporal vascular arcades. A small amount of yellowish subretinal fluid may be seen overlying the spots; this seems to indicate a poor prognosis. Approximately one-third of patients have an anterior chamber reaction and one-half to two-thirds have mild vitreous cells. With follow-up, some of the initial dots disappear, but others develop progressive fibrotic extensions that coalesce and spread under the posterior pole. The fibrosis often begins in the area of yellow subretinal fluid. These fibrotic bands are usually nonpigmented. CME can be superimposed on the process. A CNVM may also develop, but the appearance is not classic and they seem to be only a small part of the overall fibrotic response.

The prognosis is poor. The vision often drops to count fingers or hand motions over months to years. Recurrent episodes of the multifocal choroiditis stage may occur. The fibrosis stage usually progresses to a certain point and then stops. In its end stage this entity needs to be distinguished from other causes of subretinal fibrosis, such as a CNVM, retinal detachment, or old inflammatory scarring.

BIRDSHOT CHORIORETINOPATHY. Whereas the previous entities involve the RPE and inner choroid, birdshot chorioretinopathy seems to involve the outer choroid. It is a disease of older patients, with an average age of 52. There is a small female preponderance. It is rare in non-Caucasians. This disease has a marked association with HLA 29, which implies some sort of defect in immunoregulation.

Clinically, the patients present with floaters and blurred vision. They may develop problems with nyctalopia and decreased color vision in later stages. The vision is usually mildly decreased. The disease is almost always bilateral, but can be asymmetric. The external eye is usually quiet. Around 10 per cent of patients have an anterior chamber reaction, and at least 80 per cent have vitreous cells and opacities. The lesions are usually oval, from one-quarter to 1 disc diameter. They may be very subtle, particularly in blond fundi. The lesions are most often found around the disc and nasal periphery. They appear to swirl or radiate outward from around the disc into the periphery. The macula itself is usually not involved with the lesions. Unlike the other entities, the lesions usually do not develop pigmentation. The lesions themselves are usually less visible on fluorescein angiography than on color photographs, due to their deep level in the choroid and minimal interference with the RPE and choriocapillaris. Rarely, neovascularization of the retina can occur.

Most patients with this entity do fairly well. A large study suggested that approximately 50 per cent would have vision better than 20/60 in 5 years. Most of the vision loss is related to cystoid macular edema. The disease may stabilize and become quiet, although this process may take years. There does seem to be a subset of patients who develop progressively worsening vision, pale discs, and constricted visual field and have a much poorer prognosis.

PUNCTATE OUTER RETINAL TOXOPLASMOSIS (PORT). This disease seems to be a variant of toxoplasmosis with smaller, often multifocal outer retinal lesions. The epidemiology seems to be the same as regular toxoplasmosis, although this variant may have a tendency to be seen in younger patients. PORT probably represents a very early form of toxoplasmosis that is picked up sooner because the patients are more rapidly symptomatic. The disease is usually unilateral, although the patient may have old toxo scars in the other eye. The lesions are whitish, involve the outer retina, and are usually smaller than the usual toxoplasmic retinitis, ranging from 1/10 to 1/2 disc diameter. Usually the lesions are around an older toxo scar, which makes the differentiation of this entity fairly straightforward. Unlike typical toxoplasmosis, this disease has a tendency to have much less anterior chamber and vitreous reaction, probably because the inflammation has not broken through the full thickness of the retina. The disease usually resolves into a typical toxo-type scar, but can resolve into multifocal tiny white dots (25 to 75 μm) that may represent actual toxoplasmosis cysts.

DIFFUSE UNILATERAL SUBACUTE NEURORETINITIS (DUSN). This entity was formerly known as the "unilateral wipe-out syndrome." It is also a disease of younger patients, with most patients being in their second decade. It seems to be more common in the Southeast and Northern Midwest. It is caused by two unidentified nematodes, a smaller one in the Southwest and a larger one in the upper Midwest. The worm moves around in the subretinal space, and the pathophysiology seems to involve a focal toxic and/or inflammatory response to the presence of the worm and its local byproducts. There is also a diffuse toxic effect on the whole retina, which seems to be the main cause of the decreased vision. Clinically, patients present with early loss of vision associated with vitritis, papillitis, and retinal vasculitis. Patients can have an anterior uveitis, although it is usually mild. There is usually an afferent pupillary defect. The disease is almost always unilateral. The patients have recurrent crops of evanescent gray-white outer retinal dots ranging from one-quarter to one disc diameter. The dots usually fade in a few days; they may leave no changes or can resolve into histoplasmosis-like scars. The worm is usually located near the spots. Fluorescein angiography demonstrates disc and vascular leakage. Acute dots are hypofluorescent early and stain late. Of note, the ERG is usually decreased in all stages of the disease and is very helpful early on if the diagnosis is being considered. If the disease is suspected, it is important to look very carefully for the presence of the worm. Systemic evaluations for helminths are negative. With time the patients develop diffuse RPE mottling and optic atrophy. This entity should be kept in mind in patients who have extensive scarring in one eye with a normal fellow eye. It is possible that many cases of "unilateral retinitis pigmentosa" are in fact old cases of DUSN.

DIFFERENTIAL DIAGNOSIS. When entertaining the diagnosis of one of the white dot syndromes, it is of paramount importance to be sure that the patient does not have a disseminated infection of which a multifocal choroiditis is the primary manifestation. In general, white dot patients are very healthy, perhaps with an antecedent viral infection. Patients who are sick, debilitated, or immunosuppressed should raise one's suspicion for another etiology. This is especially true of AIDS patients, in whom an infectious etiology must be assumed. These patients are usually referred to their internists for an evaluation of a possible metastatic infection. A careful review of systems looking for evidence of systemic disease is mandatory in these patients. Multifocal infections, such as bacterial sepsis, mycobacteria, syphilis, Lyme disease, fungal infections and *Pneumocystis*, need to be considered depending on the clinical situation.

Viral infections in the eye, such as cytomegalovirus and especially slower variants of the acute retinal necrosis syndrome, may present with a multifocal picture. In most cases, however, the presentation is usually characteristic or becomes obvious in a short period of time. In general, the authors feel it is important to evaluate the patient for syphilis and Lyme disease. Both entities have been reported to create manifestations similar to some of the white dot syndromes. Often the patient's sexual history or associated systemic symptoms raise one's suspicion for one of these entities. Fungal infections can create a multifocal choroiditis or chorioretinitis as well. Usually the lesions are fluffier than any of the white dot syndromes, and again the patient's systemic status or recent medical history almost always provides an etiologic clue.

Certain autoimmune diseases need to be considered as well. Sarcoidosis can often present with diffuse intraocular inflammation and a multifocal picture. The authors usually obtain a chest x-ray and angiotensin-converting enzyme (ACE) level on patients with multifocal lesions. A high normal ACE level can also be a clue, and it is not unreasonable to consider a blind conjunctival biopsy as a further investigation in these patients. There does seem to be a subset of older white females who present with an MCP-type picture who in fact have sarcoidosis. These older patients usually have numerous small lesions in the inferior retinal periphery, but a few can have large granulomas in the posterior pole. Most of the other systemic autoimmune diseases that can affect the posterior part of the eye, such as lupus, Behçet's disease, or systemic vasculitis, do not present as multifocal choroidopathies. Instead, these entities usually present with diffuse intraocular inflammation or retinal vasculitis. As a result, unless the patient has a very suggestive history, laboratory tests to evaluate for these entities are not done. A patient's CBC and chemistry profile are often checked, not so much as a diagnostic maneuver but rather to assess their general medical status, particularly if immunosuppressive therapy is required. A PPD is included, more to define the patient's TB status before immunosuppression than to look for a TB-associated multifocal choroiditis, which would be unusual in an otherwise healthy patient. If the patient seems to have MCP, Epstein-Barr titers can be done. If the diagnosis of birdshot choroidopathy is entertained, testing for HLA A29 can be done to strengthen the diagnosis.

Finally, one must always keep in mind that masquerade processes, such as ocular lymphoma, metastatic disease, and choroidal leukemia, may present as a multifocal choroidal process. They often, but not always, have larger, more mass-like lesions or sub-RPE yellow deposits that differ from the smaller scars of the white dot syndromes. Usually, ultrasound examination, the systemic diagnosis, or lack of a response to treatment will suggest this type of process.

The work-up can be calibrated to the level of severity of the specific process. For instance, given the mild visual loss and characteristic changes in retinal pigment epitheliitis or MEWDS, no workup is necessary. With the more severe MCP or SFU, a full work-up is usually done. If the diagnosis of PORT is suspected, a toxoplasmosis titer is done.

Once the clinician is satisfied that the patient has one of the white dot syndromes, rather than a systemic disease, differentiation is usually fairly simple. It depends largely on the clinical appearance and degree of severity. Sometimes a period of observation is required in order for all the clinical manifestations of the disease to become apparent. For instance, both PIC and MCP can present initially as a multifocal process. However, MCP usually has more intraocular inflammation and often proves to be recurrent and to require immunosuppression. Serpiginous choroiditis may also be problematic initially, particularly if it starts in one localized area and the characteristic pattern of scarring is not present. Again, the diagnosis usually becomes apparent with follow-up.

THERAPY

The overall approach to the white dot syndromes is very straightforward. In general, if there is little inflammation and the vision is not markedly decreased, no treatment is required. If there is more inflammation, or more significant visual loss, immunosuppression may be necessary, usually with depot or oral corticosteroids. Those entities, such as POHS, PIC, and MCP, that have a high risk of a CNVM require continuous monitoring with the Amsler grid and laser treatment if necessary. Retinal pigment epitheliitis requires no treatment.

Systemic. More specific guidelines for therapy include the use of topical steroids and cycloplegics if there is significant anterior chamber reaction. If the decision to use systemic corticosteroids has been made, one should usually start the patient on a dose of 1 to 1.5 mg/kg (60 to 80 mg) a day of prednisone. The patient should be seen in 1 to 2 weeks. The steroids can be gradually tapered depending on the clinical response. Although it is difficult to generalize, patients can often be tapered over a 4- to 6-week course. Depending on severity, flare-ups may require returning to the initial dose or simply going back to the lowest dose at which inflammation was controlled. If the patient is not a steroid responder, posterior subtenon injections of Kenalog,* 20 to 40 mg, may control inflammation with minimal systemic risk. More specific treatment guidelines for each white dot entity follow:

MULTIPLE EVANESCENT WHITE DOT SYNDROME. No treatment is required for this entity. Patients should understand that, even with complete recovery, their vision may not be perfect. They should also be made aware that if they have a big blind spot, it may persist but is rarely permanent. CNVM from MEWDS is rare.

AMPPE. Because of the multifocal creamy appearance of these lesions, these patients generally merit more of a systemic work-up than MEWDS or retinal pigment epitheliitis. However, AMPPE usually resolves on its own without the need for treatment. Some authorities feel that severe vision loss or significant vitreous cells merit the use of corticosteroids. Others routinely treat patients with corticosteroids and feel that this therapy provides more rapid regression. There are no controlled studies to support any of these approaches.

SERPIGINOUS. Because this entity has a tendency to be recurrent and destructive, many authorities are more aggressive in treating it. However, the recurrent nature and slow resolution of the lesions make the assessment of treatment difficult. The disease may respond to the regimen of corticosteroids described above or to subtenon injections of 20 to 40 mg of Kenalog.* Many patients prove refractory. Isolated reports have suggested that these patients may respond to triple-agent immunosuppression (prednisone, imuran, and cyclosporine) similar to that used in renal transplantation. Others feel that very high-dose intravenous steroids may be useful. Such patients generally have vision-threatening disease and require referral to a tertiary care center.

POHS. Once the diagnosis of POHS has been made on clinical grounds, the patient should have continuous Amsler grid monitoring at home. If a CNVM develops, laser treatment should be performed if the membrane does not involve the center of the fovea. If the patient seems to be having an inflammatory exacerbation of a histo spot, the corticosteroid regimen discussed above usually proves very effective in controlling the flare-up. Subtenon steroids are also useful. This type of patient needs to be monitored closely for the development of a CNVM.

PIC. This entity is usually self-limited and does not require treatment. As with the other multifocal choroidopathies, there is a danger of a CNVM occurring later. As a result, these patients require continuous monitoring with the Amsler grid. Some patients have chronic photopsias, but retain excellent vision.

MCP. Because this entity tends to be recurrent and more severe, these patients may be more likely to require systemic corticosteroids. Perhaps 30 per cent of patients will not respond well to steroids and may require more aggressive immunosuppression, such as cyclosporine A. They also require continuous Amsler grid monitoring for the development

of a CNVM. Although controversial, some authorities feel there is an association with Epstein-Barr virus. If Epstein-Barr viral titers are suggestive of a chronic infection, some feel that acyclovir therapy may help control inflammation. Visual field testing should be part of the management of these patients, as they may occasionally have diffuse visual dysfunction without an obvious change in the number or activity of spots. Steroids may improve acute exacerbations of visual field loss. Most authorities attempt laser photocoagulation if the CNVM is in an extrafoveal location. Corticosteroids should also be tried in patients with CNVM to treat any inflammatory component.

SFU. This entity has a very poor prognosis. Some investigators have been able to prevent severe visual loss with the aggressive use of corticosteroids to decrease scarring. Preliminary reports also suggest that the aggressive use of other systemic immunosuppressive agents, before the fibrosis becomes fully developed, may prevent visual loss. This usually involves the use of a second-line immunosuppressive, such as cyclosporine. Many patients have severe visual loss in both eyes despite aggressive treatment. Again, referral to a tertiary care center is suggested.

BIRDSHOT. Because this entity has a tendency to be chronic, it is generally felt that treatment should be reserved for flare-ups that significantly decrease vision. In general, these patients can be treated if the vision falls below 20/40 or if they become significantly symptomatic from vitreous opacities. The usual treatment involves subtenon Kenalog* or systemic corticosteroids. Some patients with severe disease have been tried on second-line immunosuppressive agents with some success. Rarely, patients may have retinal neovascularization, which often responds to drugs that control the inflammation, but angiography should be used to evaluate nonperfusion. Significant ischemia may require scatter photocoagulation. Visual fields should also be followed to watch for slowly progressive field loss that may respond to low-dose steroids.

PORT. This entity responds to the usual therapy for toxoplasmosis and is covered in the article on toxoplasmosis.

DUSN. The primary treatment in this entity is to identify the worm and to kill it with photocoagulation. There does not seem to be a significant inflammatory response when this treatment is undertaken. The search for the worm should be directed to the areas of the white inflammatory lesions. If the worm cannot be identified but the diagnosis is fairly certain, there has been some success using antihelmintic drugs in combination with corticosteroids. The dose that has been used is 22 mg/kg of thiabendazole twice a day for 3 to 4 days. Generally, the vision does not improve with treatment, but only stabilizes. A vigorous attempt to find the worm early should be done, however, to try to avoid severe visual loss.

COMMENTS

A few important points need to be kept in mind when treating patients with the white dot syndromes. It is very important to use both the clinical history and physical examination to eliminate a systemic infectious cause for a multifocal choroiditis. Only then can the clinician be assured that immunosuppressive treatment can be performed safely. Any multifocal process that progresses in spite of presumably appropriate treatment requires re-evaluation for an infectious etiology. A lymphoproliferative process must also be considered, particularly if there appear to be masses or deposits in the subretinal or sub-RPE space.

The clinician must monitor the patient for the development of signs that could suggest the subretinal fibrosis and uveitis syndrome: multiple spots in the posterior pole, an accumulation of a yellowish subretinal fluid, or noticeable subretinal fibrosis. It is important to recognize this entity because of the poor prognosis and because of the possible role of early multiple drug immunosuppression.

One must constantly reassess the risks and benefits of the therapy in these entities. Steroids may be required intermittently, but usually long-term immunosuppression is not necessary. If continuous treatment is found to be required, internal medicine or rheumatologic consultation should be obtained to assist in the prevention and management of potential corticosteroid or immunosuppressive complications. Finally, the patient must be warned about the late development of a neovascular membrane, particularly if the patient has one of the multifocal choroidopathies (POHS, PIC, MCP, SFU) or serpiginous choroidopathy.

References

Cantrill HL, Folk JC: Multifocal choroiditis associated with progressive subretinal fibrosis. Am J Ophthalmol 101:170–180, 1986.

Doft BH, Gass JDM: Punctate outer retinal toxoplasmosis. Arch Ophthalmol 103:1332–1336, 1985.

Dreyer RF, Gass JDM: Multifocal choroiditis and panuveitis. Arch Ophthalmol 102:1776–1784, 1984.

Folk JC, Pulido JS, Wolf MD: White dot chorioretinal inflammatory syndromes. Focal Points, December 1990, American Academy of Ophthalmology.

Gass JDM: Stereoscopic Atlas of Macular Diseases. St. Louis, CV Mosby, 1987.

Gass JDM, Callanan DG, Bowman B: Oral therapy in diffuse unilateral subacute neuroretinitis. Arch Ophthalmol 110:675–680, 1992.

Hooper PL, Kaplan HJ: Triple-agent immunosuppression in serpiginous choroiditis. Ophthalmology 98:944–952, 1991.

Krill AE, Deutman AF: Acute retinal pigment epitheliitis. Am J Ophthalmol 74:193–205, 1972.

Mamalis N, Daily MJ: Multiple evanescent white dot syndrome. Ophthalmology 94:1209–1212, 1987.

Priem HA, Oosterhuis JA: Birdshot chorioretinopathy: Clinical characteristics and evolution. Br J Ophthalmol 72:646–659, 1988.

Watzke RC, Packer AJ, Folk JC, Benson WE, Burgess D, Ober RR: Punctate inner choroidopathy. Am J Ophthalmol 98:572–584, 1984.

Wolf MD, Alward WLM, Folk JC: Long-term visual function in acute posterior multifocal placoid pigment epitheliopathy. Arch Ophthalmol 109:800–803, 1991.

SECTION 34

SCLERA

EPISCLERITIS 379.00

PETER G. WATSON, M.D., F.R.C.S., F.R.C.Ophth.

Cambridge, England

Episcleritis is an inflammation of the fascial coats of the eye, which lie between the conjunctiva and the sclera. It is usually a mild, self-limiting, recurrent disease that is sometimes caused by exogenous inflammatory stimuli. Episcleritis is twice as common in females as in males and has its peak incidence in the fourth decade. There are two clinical types, simple and nodular. The most common is simple episcleritis, in which there are intermittent bouts of moderate or severe inflammation at 1- to 3-month intervals. These episodes usually last 7 to 10 days and occur more commonly in the spring or fall than in summer or winter. Only rarely can the precipitating factor be found, but attacks are often precipitated by stress. Patients with nodular episcleritis give no history of periodicity, but rather of prolonged mild attacks of inflammation. Almost all the patients with this condition have some intercurrent systemic disease.

THERAPY

Supportive. Since the disease is self-limiting with little to no permanent damage to the eye, episcleritis does not generally require any treatment. However, some patients demand treatment, and a few need help because of the severity and duration of the attack. Occasionally, a clear history of an exogenous sensitization can be obtained, and removal of this agent will prevent recurrent attacks. Desensitization is not indicated in the prevention of recurrent attacks and has even precipitated attacks.

Ocular. Although simple episcleritis requires no treatment, nodular episcleritis is more indolent and may require local corticosteroid drops or anti-inflammatory agents for its control. Topical ophthalmic application of 0.5 per cent prednisolone, 0.1 per cent dexamethasone, and 0.1 per cent betamethasone* daily may be used.

Systemic. In rare instances when nodular episcleritis is unresponsive, systemic anti-inflammatory agents may need to be given. Flurbiprofen,[‡] 100 mg three times daily, is usually effective until inflammation is sup-

pressed. If there is no response to flurbiprofen, indomethacin[‡] should be used. It is usually administered as 100 mg daily and decreased to 75 mg when there is a response. Many patients who do not respond to one nonsteroidal anti-inflammatory agent may well respond to another.

Ocular or Periocular Manifestations

Conjunctiva: Chemosis; hyperemia.
Cornea: Diffuse stromal haze adjacent to limbus (limited to repeated episcleritis attacks in the same position); hypesthesia; vascularization.
Other: Lacrimation; ocular pain; photophobia.

PRECAUTIONS

Up to 11 per cent of patients with episcleritis may have hyperuricemia. When clinical gout gets out of control, symptoms of episcleritis may occur in some patients. Long-term continuous therapy with steroid preparations should not be permitted because of the damage of inducing cataract and glaucoma.

COMMENTS

Episcleritis is fairly common and seems to occur spontaneously without any known cause. It may recur in the same spot or alternate to the fellow eye or the other side of the same eye. Although nodular episcleritis is managed in the same way as simple episcleritis, it has a more protracted course. The majority of attacks last 5 to 10 days; however, there is no definite pattern. Over half of the patients have intermittent attacks that usually last 3 to 6 years, although some have been known to last up to 30 years. Episcleritis starting before puberty usually ceases at puberty; episcleritis starting before menopause usually ceases with the menopause. A hormonal factor has, however, never been demonstrated.

References

Fraunfelder FT, Watson PG: Evaluation of eyes enucleated for scleritis. Br J Ophthalmol 60:227–230, 1976.

Watson PG, Hayreh SS: Scleritis and episcleritis. Br J Ophthalmol 60:163–191, 1976.

Watson PG, Hazleman BL: The Sclera and Systemic Disorders. Philadelphia, WB Saunders, 1976.

SCLERAL STAPHYLOMA AND DEHISCENCES 379.11

BISHARA M. FARIS, M.D., F.A.C.S.,

Worcester, Massachusetts

and H. MACKENZIE FREEMAN, M.D.

Boston, Massachusetts

Localized weakening of the sclera may lead to an oval or elliptical thin area through which the choroid is visible. When flat and meridionally oriented, such areas are termed *scleral dehiscences*; they are referred to as *staphylomas* when bulging.

Staphylomas are classified as anterior or posterior, depending on their relationship to the equator of the eye. Posterior staphylomas are found in myopes over −8 diopters, as well as in patients with the connective tissue disorders of Ehlers-Danlos and Marfan's syndromes. Anterior staphylomas are frequent operative findings in the nontraumatic rhegmatogenous retinal detachment population, with a reported incidence of 14 per cent. Less commonly, they occur in eyes with increased intraocular pressure and recurrent necrotizing scleritis and after deep scleral resection for episcleral malignancies. Anterior staphylomas have also been reported after subconjunctival injections of corticosteroids.

THERAPY

Supportive. Since a sustained elevation of intraocular pressure, especially in the pediatric age group, may result in anterior scleral dehiscences and staphyloma formation, the lowering of such pressure by carbonic anhydrase inhibitors, adrenergics, beta-adrenergic blocking agents, and miotics is in order. Forceful rubbing of the eyeballs produces a marked elevation in pressure and should be avoided.

Surgical. When dehiscences and staphylomas are discovered in the area to be buckled during retinal detachment surgery, certain operative precautions should be taken to prevent accidental rupture of the globe. When localizing the retinal breaks, the indentation should be produced by a cotton-tipped applicator, rather than a metal electrode. Dissection of the flaps in thin sclera is hazardous; therefore, the surgeon may elect to dissect small scleral flaps anterior and posterior to the dehiscence or staphyloma in order to cover the hard silicone implant and to buckle the areas of retinal breaks sufficiently. The blunt edges of the implant should extend over thin scleral zones and the end of healthy sclera. In cases where the thinning is extensive, it may be safer to omit undermining scleral flaps and to use an episcleral silicone sponge.

Diathermy increases scleral rigidity, thereby elevating intraocular pressure. Thus, it is mandatory that chorioretinal adhesion be produced by cryoapplications, rather than by diathermy. The cryoprobe tip should be applied gently and should not be removed until it has completely thawed. Premature probe movements may rupture the sclera.

The assistant surgeon has an important role to play during surgery. Gentle exposure of the globe prevents sudden increases in intraocular pressure and subsequent rupture of the globe. It is always safer to disinsert more recti muscles to obtain good exposure of the surgical field than to resort to forceful exposure.

The use of intravenous acetazolamide and mannitol is advised in all cases, unless there is a medical contraindication. Paracentesis, as a means to lower intraocular pressure, may be used as a last resort.

When uveal tissue does bulge through dehiscences or staphylomas despite all measures taken, such areas should be covered immediately by a silicone rubber patch that is glued with cyanoacrylate adhesive.

During surgery for episcleral malignancies, scleral resection is done whenever there is evidence of scleral involvement. Deep resections involving two-thirds or more of the scleral thickness may predispose to the formation of dehiscences and staphylomas. In such cases, it is wise to cover the resected zones by a preserved scleral graft or an autogenous pretibial periosteal patch graft.

Ocular or Periocular Manifestations

Sclera: Blue coloration; rupture; thinning.
Other: Glaucoma; myopia; retinal detachment.

PRECAUTIONS

A history of staphylomas in one eye should alert the surgeon to the possibility of their occurrence in the fellow eye. The presence or extent of a staphyloma in the fellow eye may be determined by placing a hand-held transilluminator on the cornea and observing the light transmitted through the thinned sclera.

COMMENTS

Anterior scleral staphylomas are most often located in the superior temporal quadrants. Hence, these quadrants should be avoided when subconjunctival injections of antibiotics and corticosteroids are indicated. Staphylomas may be associated with glaucoma and nontraumatic retinal detachment. When encountered during retinal detachment surgery, they can be the site of rupture of the globe unless specific operative measures are taken.

References

Edelstein AJ, Ashrafzadeh MT, Schneider J: Patch grafts for staphylomas of the anterior segment of the eye. Ophthalmic Surg 1:38–42, 1970.

Faris B, Freeman HM, Schepens CL: Scleral dehiscences, anterior staphyloma and retinal detachments—Part 1: Incidence and pathogenesis. Trans Am Acad Ophthalmol Otolaryngol 79:851–853, 1975.

Freeman HM, Schepens CL, Faris B: Scleral dehiscences, anterior staphyloma, and retinal detachment—Part 2: Surgical management. Trans Am Acad Ophthalmol Otolaryngol 79:854–857, 1975.

Koenig SB, Sanitato JJ, Kaufman HE: Long-term follow-up study of scleroplasty using autogenous periosteum. Cornea 9:139–143, 1990.

Phillips CI, Dobbie JG: Posterior staphyloma and retinal detachment. Am J Ophthalmol 55:332–335, 1963.

Stewart RH, Garcia CA: Staphyloma following cyclocryotherapy. Ophthalmic Surg 5:28–29, 1974.

Watzke RC: Scleral staphylomas and retinal detachment. Arch Ophthalmol 70:796–804, 1963.

SCLERITIS 379.00

PETER G. WATSON, M.D., F.R.C.S., F.R.C.Ophth.

Cambridge, England

Scleritis is a severe inflammatory process that involves the opaque collagenous outer coat of the eye. The inflammatory stimuli are almost always of endogenous origin and result in granuloma formation and a vasculitis that involves both the superficial and deeper scleral vasculature. Scleritis is often a manifestation of a chronic systemic inflammation, such as rheumatoid arthritis, systemic vasculitis, Wegener's granulomatosis, or other connective tissue disease. It always has a protracted course if untreated; even when well treated, recurrence is the rule. Complications are largely preventable, but if they occur, scleritis becomes one of the gravest eye diseases. Scleral inflammation usually occurs anterior to the equator, but posterior scleritis is not uncommon and often remains undiagnosed. The anterior variety is divided into diffuse, nodular, or necrotizing types. Necrotizing scleritis is further subdivided into that with inflammation and that without (scleromalacia perforans). Necrotizing scleritis has a very poor prognosis unless vigorously treated, and it usually indicates the presence of some systemic disease. B-scan ultrasonography should always be performed to exclude posterior scleritis.

THERAPY

Systemic. Bacterial infections and other conditions for which there is a specific therapy should be treated. If no such condition is detected or the scleritis is associated with a connective tissue disease, anti-inflammatory or immunosuppressive agents should be administered. Flurbiprofen[+] or indomethacin[‡] controls most attacks of diffuse or nodular scleritis. The usual daily dosage of flurbiprofen is 300 mg daily until inflammation is suppressed and pain subsides. It is a characteristic finding in all patients with scleritis that the pain is relieved as soon as the inflammatory reaction is suppressed, even though the external appearance of the eye remains the same. The presence or absence of pain may even be used to titrate the dosage of the drug in some patients. If there is no response to flurbiprofen, indomethacin can be used. It is usually administered as 100 mg daily and decreased to 75 mg when there is a response. Many patients respond to indomethacin when they do not respond to flurbiprofen, and vice versa. Therefore, both drugs may need to be tried. If there is no response to the above anti-inflammatory medications within 1 or 2 weeks or if any avascular areas appear in the sclera or episclera, systemic corticosteroids are indicated. Initially, 80 mg of prednisolone is given daily. The dosage is then decreased according to the clinical response as rapidly as possible to a maintenance level of 15 mg a day in divided doses. At this point, an additional anti-inflammatory agent is added, and corticosteroids are further decreased in 2.5-mg steps. If inflammation recurs, increased corticosteroid dosages are required.

Immunosuppressive therapy may need to be added in patients with severe necrotizing scleritis that is not controlled by high doses of corticosteroids or in those who are developing complications with large maintenance doses of steroids. Cyclophosphamide[‡] is the drug of choice and is started at 100 mg daily, increasing the dose to 150 to 200 mg over the next 2 weeks. Side effects are frequent and severe when this drug is used for immunosuppression in this disease, and it should therefore only be used in desperate situations. It is mandatory to monitor the lymphocyte count during therapy.

In the occasional patient who has destructive scleral disease caused by a venulitis as diagnosed on fluorescein angiography, it may be necessary to give pulse intravenous therapy. Scleromalacia perforans (necrotizing scleritis without accompanying inflammation) is caused by arteriolar obstruction and is not treatable unless caught before sequestration of tissue occurs. The cause of the necrotizing disease should be investigated. If there is evidence of a systemic vasculitis or an immune complex disorder in the presence of severe, destructive disease, a pulse dose of 500 mg of methylprednisolone should be given intravenously over 1 to 2 hours together with 500 mg of cyclophosphamide given intravenously over a period of several hours and washed through by intravenous infusion over the next

24 hours to minimize the chances of developing a hemorrhagic cystitis. This regime may be repeated at intervals dependent on the response. Oral daily therapy of 100 mg of cyclophosphamide or less may be sufficient to control the systemic manifestations if given with low maintenance doses of 15 mg of prednisolone. Pulse intravenous therapy is potentially hazardous and should only be resorted to under desperate circumstances and under the control of an internist experienced in its use. It has, however, proved to be vision saving.

Ocular. Although not usually necessary, systemic anti-inflammatory drugs may be used in conjunction with topical ophthalmic corticosteroid solution or ointment or 10 per cent oxyphenbutazone* ointment. This regimen gives subjective relief and comfort to some patients. Once the disease has been suppressed, certain patients can stop the systemic therapy and keep the inflammation under control by using topical ophthalmic medication infrequently.

Occasionally, intraorbital injection of corticosteroids* can be given in patients who cannot tolerate systemic corticosteroids. The effects are transient and require frequent reinjections, often at weekly intervals. Patients tolerate this form of therapy poorly, and it is seldom satisfactory for routine use. *Subconjunctival corticosteroids should never be given, as scleral lysis may result.*

Surgical. Biopsy should only be performed if it is absolutely essential to establish an obscure diagnosis. Scleral nodules often contain pultaceous material; if punctured, an area of bare sclera that will not heal will result. Surgery is reserved for patients who are resistant to medical treatment, who have a perforated globe, or whose disease is so extensive when first seen that the scleral defect could not possibly be closed by the normal reparative processes. The surgery, which varies from conjunctival excision to full anterior segment replacement, is always difficult and full of unrecognized hazards because of the softness of the inflamed tissues and the limited power of healing. If an autoimmune process is involved in the local lesion, corneoscleral grafting can be used to remove the source of antigen. *Surgery should never be performed until a complete immunosuppressive regimen has been established.*

Ocular or Periocular Manifestations

Choroid or Retina: Annular choroidal detachments; exudative retinal detachments; macular edema; subretinal mass; disc edema.
Conjunctiva: Chemosis; hyperemia.

Cornea: Epithelial or sclerosing keratitis; hypesthesia; limbal guttering; lipid deposits; nummular opacity.
Eyelids: Edema; lower lid retraction.
Sclera: Episcleral salmon-pink coloration; thinning and perforation; vascular engorgement.
Other: Cataract; increased intraocular pressure; lacrimation; miosis; myopia; papilledema; paresis of extraocular muscles; photophobia; proptosis; uveitis; visual field defects.

PRECAUTIONS

Unfortunately, the drugs that achieve effective suppression of intercurrent systemic disease are often ineffective in controlling the eye complications. The drugs used to control scleritis have numerous side effects and require long-term administration. It is essential to withdraw the corticosteroids as rapidly as possible. Subconjunctival injections of corticosteroids are contraindicated.

COMMENTS

Scleritis is often the first sign of underlying systemic connective tissue disease. Therefore, it is vital that the disease be recognized early and treated in conjunction with a rheumatologist or internist. Investigations to eliminate serious diseases can be kept to a minimum in episcleritis but need to be more extensive in patients with diffuse and nodular scleritis and should be exhaustive in patients with necrotizing scleral disease. In one series, 27 per cent of patients with necrotizing scleritis were dead within 5 years because of underlying systemic disease.

Local corticosteroid therapy is ineffective in suppressing the inflammation of scleritis, but may increase the patient's comfort. Systemic treatment is required. Treatment only suppresses the inflammation sufficiently to allow normal repair of tissues to occur and must be continued while the disease follows its natural course, which, although usually between 6 months and 6 years, occasionally lasts a lifetime.

References

Fraunfelder FT, Watson PG: Evaluation of eyes enucleated for scleritis. Br J Ophthalmol 60:227–230, 1976.

Watson PG: The nature and the treatment of scleral inflammation. Trans Ophthalmol Soc UK 102:257–281, 1982.

Watson PG, Hayreh SS: Scleritis and episcleritis. Br J Ophthalmol 60:163–191, 1976.

Watson PG, Hazleman BL: The Sclera and Systemic Disorders. Philadelphia, WB Saunders, 1976.

SCLEROMALACIA PERFORANS 379.04

JAMES V. AQUAVELLA, M.D.

Rochester, New York

The term "scleromalacia perforans" was coined by van der Hoeve in 1934 to describe a rare ocular condition that occurs mainly in postmenopausal females suffering from long-standing polyarticular rheumatoid arthritis. The condition also occurs as a sequelae to ocular carcinoma in AIDS and in predisposed patients subsequent to ocular surgery after a latent period of several months.

The principal feature is the formation of multiple areas of deep scleral ulceration, which coalesce to reveal the underlying uveal tissue. The condition is of insidious onset and is often asymptomatic. Yellowish necrotic lesions appear in the anterior sclera between the limbus and the equator with no evidence of active inflammation. Tissue loss apparently follows occlusion of smaller episcleral capillaries. The underlying pathology has been characterized as immune-complex-mediated vasculitis. There may be involvement of larger branches of the anterior and posterior ciliary vessels. With sequestration of necrotic tissue, the choroid is exposed. Although the overlying conjunctiva may be thinned, only rarely do these cases progress to frank perforation or anterior staphyloma. Such complications are associated with secondary glaucoma.

Although the number of lesions varies, they can coalesce into large areas of scleral necrosis. Complications include uveitis, secondary glaucoma, cataract, and perforation. All of the lesions share the same pathologic features. The presence of rheumatoid nodules in other parts of the body is common in this patient population.

THERAPY

Ocular. Treatment is indicated only if the patient is symptomatic or if complications exist. Topical glucocorticoids in the form of 1 per cent prednisolone four to six times daily along with cycloplegics may be used to control uveitis. Topical antiglaucoma medication is often required on a long-term basis.

On occasion, 100 to 250 mg of oral prednisolone daily may be necessary. Nonsteroidal anti-inflammatory drugs have not proven to be of value. Once the inflammatory process has been stabilized, steroids should be slowly tapered over a period of several weeks. Oral prednisolone, in combination with other anti-inflammatory agents, such as phenylbutazone,[‡] or cytotoxic agents[‡] (cyclophosphamide) may be helpful. Low-dose cyclosporine (5 mg/kg per day) has been reported to be effective in conjunction with a minimum controlling systemic steroid dosage. Intensive anti-inflammatory therapy seems to produce rapid resolution and may prevent progression of lesions. Since these patients often suffer from rheumatoid arthritis, a comprehensive medical approach is indicated.

Surgical. Surgical techniques use free or rotational autografts to reinforce the sclera and to avoid uveal exposure. Autologous sclera, fascia lata, aorta, and, more recently, periosteum and tarsus have also been used for grafting. The surgeon should be careful not to rupture the choroid during the placement of the graft. It is important for the grafts to be covered totally by sliding conjunctiva or by utilizing donor conjunctiva from other sites in the same or the fellow eye. When no conjunctiva is available, the mucous membrane has been used.

Ocular or Periocular Manifestations

Cornea: Aseptic necrosis; pannus; ulceration.

Extraocular Muscles: Limitation of motion; tendonitis.

Sclera: Episcleritis; scleritis.

Other: Cataract; retinal vasculitis; secondary glaucoma; uveitis.

PRECAUTIONS

Careful observation after the initiation of systemic immunosuppressive therapy is important in view of the known deleterious effects of these drugs. Periocular injections of corticosteroids are absolutely contraindicated. When surgical therapy is undertaken, one should be aware of the potential for recurrence. It is important to differentiate true scleromalacia perforans from other forms of scleral necrosis secondary to inflammatory conditions in which patients are more symptomatic.

COMMENTS

Scleromalacia perforans, although uncommon, poses a major management problem. If the patient is asymptomatic in the absence of complications, no therapy may be necessary. Once a decision to intervene has been made, comprehensive medical therapy with both topical and systemic corticosteroids, often accompanied by immunosuppressive drugs, must be instituted. If these measures fail, surgical modalities using overlying grafts with various materials may have to be considered. Homologous sclera and autologous periosteum are readily available.

References

Bick MW: Surgical treatment of scleromalacia perforans. Arch Ophthalmol 61:907–917, 1959.

Breslin CW, Katz JI, Kaufman HE: Surgical management of necrotizing scleritis. Arch Ophthalmol *95*:2038–2040, 1977.

de la Maza MS, Tauber J, Foster CS: Scleral grafting for necrotizing scleritis. Ophthalmology *96*:306–310, 1989.

Hakin KN, Ham J, Lightman SL: Use of cyclosporin in the management of steroid-dependent non-necrotizing scleritis. Br J Ophthalmol *75*:340–341, 1991.

Kaufman HE, Thomas EL: Prevention and treatment of symblepharon. Am J Ophthalmol *88*: 419–423, 1979.

Kaufman LM, Folk ER, Miller MT, Tessler HH: Necrotizing scleritis following strabismus surgery for thyroid ophthalmopathy. J Pediatr Ophthalmol Strabismus *26*:236–238, 1989.

Kim RY, Seiff SR, Howes, Jr. EL, O'Donnell JJ: Necrotizing scleritis secondary to conjunctival squamous cell carcinoma in acquired immunodeficiency syndrome. Am J Ophthalmol *109*:231–233, 1990.

Rootman DS, Insler MS, Kaufman HE: Rotational tarsal conjunctival flap in the treatment of scleral necrosis. Ophthalmic Surg *19*:808–810, 1988.

Taffet S, Carter GZ: Scleromalacia perforans: A useful surgical modification in fascia lata or scleral grafting. Arch Ophthalmol *69*:287–289, 1963.

Watson PG: The nature and the treatment of scleral inflammation. Trans Ophthalmol Soc UK *102*: 257–281, 1982.

Watson PG: Immunosuppressive therapy. Ocular Inflammation Ther *1*:51–54, 1983.

Watson PG, Bovey E: Anterior segment fluorescein angiography in the diagnosis of scleral inflammation. Ophthalmology *92*:1–11, 1985.

Watson PG, Hazleman BL: The Sclera and Systemic Disorders. Philadelphia, WB Saunders, 1976.

SECTION 35

VITREOUS

FAMILIAL EXUDATIVE VITREORETINOPATHY
743.51
(Autosomal Dominant Exudative Vitreoretinopathy, Criswick-Schepens Syndrome, FEVR)

JOSEPH E. ROBERTSON, JR., M.D.

Portland, Oregon

Familial exudative vitreoretinopathy (FEVR) is a hereditary abnormality of the peripheral retina that simulates retinopathy of prematurity in its cicatricial stage. This disorder is inherited predominantly as an autosomal dominant trait, with a high degree of penetrance and variable expressivity.

A pedigree in which this condition is transmitted in an X-linked recessive manner has now been described. A careful family history must be elicited to ensure an accurate diagnosis and provide proper genetic counseling. Available data now strongly suggest that the locus for dominant exudative vitreoretinopathy maps on 11q. However, only a limited number of patients have been studied, and this finding will require confirmation in other pedigrees. To date, no chromosomal mapping studies for the X-linked recessive form of this disorder have been published.

The early stages of the disease indicate that it is likely a disease of small retinal vessels, rather than a true vitreoretinopathy. The developmental disorder probably affects the peripheral retinal vessels during the last few months of intrauterine life. A wide variety of retinal vascular abnormalities have been observed in the extreme fundus periphery, particularly in the temporal retinal sector. They include the presence of an avascular zone in the extreme periphery, vasodilation and arteriovenous anastomosis in the peripheral vascular zone, a V-shaped avascular zone along the temporal meridian, and neovascularization. Vitreoretinal adhesion invariably occurs along or peripheral to the equator and is often located along the peripheral margin of the vascularized retina. Other retinal abnormalities include ectopia of the macula, cystoid degeneration, falciform retinal folds, and retinoschisis. The condition is thought to be particularly stable once the patient reaches 20 years of age.

THERAPY

Supportive. Although the expression of familial exudative vitreoretinopathy may range from the extremely mild stages of the disease to the more advanced stage with visual loss, genetic counseling is indicated for patients even with the sole clinical finding of isolated intraretinal deposits. In afflicted patients, the risk of the condition developing to some degree with each pregnancy is 50 per cent. Although most patients who become blind from this disorder do so by the end of the second decade, all individuals with this disease have an ongoing increased risk of retinal detachment and deserve ongoing follow-up.

Surgical. Scleral buckling without vitreous surgery is indicated in retinal detachment without posterior tearing of fixed retinal folds. Cryopexy or laser photocoagulation of the breaks should be initiated when symptomatic tears are experienced or when new tears with persistent vitreous traction are noted. Vitreous surgery is used when it is anticipated that (1) scleral buckling alone cannot compensate for vitreous traction sufficiently to reattach the retina, (2) dense hemorrhage accompanies the detachment, or (3) posterior breaks are involved.

Ocular or Periocular Manifestations

Cornea: Band keratopathy.
Iris: Atrophy; rubeosis.
Lens: Cataracts.
Macula: Cystoid degeneration; ectopia.
Retina: Detachment; exudate; hemorrhage; holes; neovascularization.
Vitreous: Hemorrhage; organization; traction.
Other: Neovascular glaucoma; phthisis bulbi; posterior synechiae; visual loss.

PRECAUTIONS

Retinopathy of prematurity and FEVR may be inseparable entities when morphologic characteristics are considered solely. Differentiation of these two disorders is most reliably achieved by a clinical history outlining the familial tendency and the absence of prematurity or supplemental oxygen administration. FEVR may rank among the major causes of retinal detachment, particularly in juvenile patients.

COMMENTS

Since the disease may be transmitted by autosomal dominant inheritance, family members of the patient should be examined ophthalmoscopically. The major threats to vision are posed by retinal hemorrhages, edema, and detachment. Progression of the disease is usually limited to the early years of life. Recent evidence suggests that pathologic progression of FEVR, regardless of disease stage, is not inevitable.

References

Bergen RL, Glassman R: Familial exudative vitreoretinopathy. Ann Ophthalmol 15:275–276, 1983.
Boldrey EE, et al: The histopathology of familial exudative vitreoretinopathy. A report of two cases. Arch Ophthalmol 103:238–241, 1985.
Criswick VG, Schepens CL: Familial exudative vitreoretinopathy. Am J Ophthalmol 68:578, 1969.
Feldman EL, Norris JL, Cleasby GW: Autosomal dominant exudative vitreoretinopathy. Arch Ophthalmol 101:1532–1535, 1983.
Friedrich CA, Francis KA, Kim HC: Familial exudative vitreoretinopathy (FEVR) and platelet dysfunction (Letter). Br J Ophthalmol 73:477–478, 1989.
Gole GA, Goodall K, James MJ: Familial exudative vitreoretinopathy. Br J Ophthalmol 69:76, 1985.
Laqua H: Familial exudative vitreoretinopathy. Graefes Arch Clin Exp Ophthalmol 213:121, 1980.
Li Y, Fuhrmann C, Schwinger E, Gal A, Laqua H: The gene for autosomal dominant familial exudative vitreoretinopathy (Criswick-Schepens) on the long arm of chromosome 11 (Letter). Am J Ophthalmol 113:712–713, 1992.
Miyakubo H, Inohara N, Hashimoto K: Retinal involvement in familial exudative vitreoretinopathy. Ophthalmologica 185:125–135, 1982.
Nicholson DH, Galvis V: Criswick-Schepens syndrome (familial exudative vitreoretinopathy). A study of a Colombian kindred. Arch Ophthalmol 102:1519–1522, 1984.
Ohkubo H, Tanino T: Electrophysiological findings in familial exudative vitreoretinopathy. Doc Ophthalmol 65:461–469, 1987.
Plager DA, Orgel IK, Ellis FD, Hartzer M, et al: X-linked recessive familial exudative vitreoretinopathy. Am J Ophthalmol 114:145–148, 1992.
Swanson D, Rush P, Bird AC: Visual loss from retinal oedema in autosomal dominant exudative vitreoretinopathy. Br J Ophthalmol 66:627–629, 1982.
Van Nouhuys CE: Dominant exudative vitreoretinopathy and other vascular developmental disorders of the peripheral retina. Doc Ophthalmol 54:1–415, 1982.

PERSISTENT HYPERPLASTIC PRIMARY VITREOUS 743.51
(PHPV)

RONALD C. PRUETT, M.D.

Boston, Massachusetts

Persistent hyperplastic primary vitreous (PHPV) is a congenital, usually nonhereditary syndrome caused by anomalous development of the primary vitreous-hyaloid artery complex. Two clinical forms are recognized: anterior (formerly called persistent tunica vasculosa lentis) and posterior (previously known as ablatio falciformis congenita or congenital retinal fold). Intermediate forms also occur. Most commonly, the condition is unilateral and presents in an otherwise normal child, the product of an uncomplicated full-term pregnancy with no history of perinatal oxygen administration. Leukokoria, strabismus, and poor vision are frequent initial complaints. When found bilaterally, PHPV is more likely to be of the posterior variety.

The most common findings in anterior PHPV are microphthalmos, a shallow anterior chamber with an embryonic filtration angle, and abnormally large iris blood vessels. The lens may be small and clear initially, but a posterior capsular defect may be seen with fibrovascular invasion, hemorrhage, and cataract formation. The cataract may absorb spontaneously or swell, causing secondary angle-closure glaucoma or rarely a phacoanaphylactoid reaction. A persistent hyaloid artery with retrolental fibrovascular membrane that contracts and draws the ciliary processes centrally may also be present. The retina may be clinically normal, but can show histologic abnormalities and detachment in some eyes.

Posterior PHPV is characterized by relative microcornea and a deep anterior chamber, although the filtration angle may appear immature. The lens is usually clear and of normal size; in rare cases, the lens may be colobomatous, cataractous, or subluxated. Peripheral equatorially oriented vitreous membranes fanning out from a radially oriented vitreous stalk that emanates from the disc and contains hyaloid vascular remnants may also be present. In addition, a radial retinal fold in any meridian associated with a vitreous stalk, hypoplastic disc, attenuated and sometimes sheathed retinal vessels, pigmentation and dragging of macula, and retinal detachment are frequent signs. Histologically, the neurosensory retina is abnormal, but the retinal pigment epithelium is uninvolved.

THERAPY

Surgical. There are three objectives in the management of PHPV: avoidance of unnecessary enucleation because of incorrect diagnosis, management of complications, and improvement of visual function and ocular cosmesis.

If one is aware of the polymorphism of the syndrome and utilizes appropriate methods available for investigation, misdiagnosis in potentially useful eyes will be infrequent. Eyes with anterior PHPV and relatively clear lenses or a cataract that is undergoing spontaneous reabsorption can be followed conservatively. Those with lens swelling and actual or threatened angle closure are best managed surgically, using a closed system for fragmentation and aspiration of the cataract and fibrovascular membrane. Similar techniques are indicated for those eyes with grossly normal macula that have lens or vitreous opacities thought sufficient to threaten amblyopia. Vitreous hemorrhage, with or without suspected retinal detachment, requires careful ultrasonic evaluation, followed by closed vitrectomy and scleral buckling in selected cases. In those with posterior PHPV, progressive retinal detachment is the principal indication for surgical intervention. It may be caused by increasing vitreoretinal traction by contracting membranes associated with the persistent hyaloid vascular complex. A localized traction detachment may respond to surgery using vitreous scissors or to closed vitrectomy in more extensively involved eyes. Scleral buckling can provide further relief of vitreoretinal traction and is definitely indicated for those with rhegmatogenous detachment.

Strabismus surgery, refraction, contact lens fitting, and selective occlusion therapy can be useful in PHPV, depending upon the individual problem encountered. Although the cosmetic appearance of an eye can often be improved, the prognosis for visual function must always be guarded. Severely malformed eyes do not achieve better than 20/200 acuity. Less involved eyes can achieve more useful vision, and those with minor anomalies may have essentially normal acuity and require only long-term follow-up examinations.

Precautions

When the manifestations of PHPV are primarily anterior, the consideration of possible monocular retinoblastoma accounts for the majority of these children's eyes that are enucleated. Findings that would tend to rule out that diagnosis include microphthalmos, absence of true neovascularization of the iris, ciliary processes drawn into the pupillary aperture, and other signs of anomalous development, such as an embryonic angle configuration. Further supportive evidence for PHPV would be no family history of retinoblastoma, failure to demonstrate intraocular tumefaction by B-scan ultrasonography, and absence of tumor calcification on ocular x-ray examination. CT scan and magnetic resonance studies and cytopathologic examination of vitreous biopsy materials also can be helpful.

Electroretinography, a visually evoked response, and an electrically evoked response may provide additional clues to the correct diagnosis and give some estimate of potential function.

Posterior PHPV may be confused with other conditions that produce a radial retinal fold, such as retinopathy of prematurity, chronic posterior uveitis, nematode infestation, and occult intraocular foreign body. PHPV is usually unilateral, whereas retinopathy of prematurity is bilateral. Individuals with the latter condition most often have a history of premature birth with oxygen administration. Their eyes tend to be myopic with retinal folds that are symmetric and directed temporally. Microcornea, immature angle structure, hyaloid artery remnants, and other signs of maldevelopment are lacking. These signs are also absent in eyes with other types of acquired retinal fold. A history of chronic uveitis, which may be bilateral, recent acquisition of a dog or cat, ocular trauma, or prior good vision in the involved eye would suggest noncongenital disease. Ancillary studies that can be helpful include serum antibody titers, x-rays of the eye and skull, an eosinophil count, and examination of pet stool for parasites.

Comments

PHPV is an unusual syndrome, and its fundamental cause is still unknown. Although the majority of cases present sporadically, rare familial cases have been seen, and the anomaly occurs as a heritable disorder in Doberman and Staffordshire Bull Terrior dogs. Careful examination of immediate family members is worthwhile to search for subclinical manifestations of maldevelopment. In the absence of evidence of a hereditary factor, there is no reason at present to advise the parents of such children not to bear additional offspring. Nor would the patients be expected to produce children similarly affected.

References

Caudill JW, Streeten BW, Tso MOM: Phacoanaphylactoid reaction in persistent hyperplastic primary vitreous. Ophthalmology 92:1153–1158, 1985.

Federman JL, et al: The surgical and nonsurgical management of persistent hyperplastic primary vitreous. Ophthalmology 89:20–24, 1982.

Goldberg MF, Peyman GA: Pars plicata surgery in the child for papillary membranes, persistent hyperplastic primary vitreous, and infantile cataract. In Transactions of the New Orleans Academy of Ophthalmology. St. Louis, CV Mosby, 1983, pp 228–262.

Green WR: Diagnostic cytopathology of ocular fluid specimens. Ophthalmology 91:726–749, 1984.

Haddad R, Font RL, Reeser F: Persistent hyperplastic primary vitreous. A clinicopathologic study of 62 cases and review of the literature. Surv Ophthalmol 23:123–134, 1978.

Karr DJ, Scott WE: Visual acuity results following treatment of persistent hyperplastic primary vitreous. Arch Ophthalmol 104:662–667, 1986.

Lin AE, Biglan AW, Garver KL: Persistent hyperplastic primary vitreous with vertical transmission. In Ophthalmic Paediatrics and Genetics. Amsterdam, Aeolus Press, 1990, Vol 2, No 2, pp 121–122.

Mafee MF, Goldberg MF: Persistent hyperplastic primary vitreous (PHPV): Role of computed tomography and magnetic resonance. Radiol Clin North Am 25:683–692, 1987.

Nankin SJ, Scott WE: Persistent hyperplastic primary vitreous: Roto-extraction and other surgical experience. Arch Ophthalmol 95:240–243, 1977.

Peyman GA, Sanders DR, Nagpal KC: Management of persistent hyperplastic primary vitreous by pars plana vitrectomy. Br J Ophthalmol 60: 756–758, 1976.

Pollard ZF: Treatment of persistent hyperplastic primary vitreous. J Pediatr Ophthalmol Strabismus 22:180–183, 1985.

Scott WE, et al: Management and visual acuity results of monocular congenital cataracts and persistent hyperplastic primary vitreous. Aust NZ J Ophthalmol 17:143–152, 1989.

Stades FC, et al: The incidence of PHTVL/PHPV in Doberman and the results of breeding rules. Veterinary Q 13:24–29, 1991.

Stark WJ, et al: Persistent hyperplastic primary vitreous. Surgical treatment. Ophthalmology 90: 452–457, 1983.

Wells RG, Miro P, Brummond R: Color-flow Doppler sonography of persistent hyperplastic primary vitreous. J Ultrasound Med 10:405–407, 1991.

PROLIFERATIVE VITREORETINOPATHY 379.29

(Massive Periretinal Proliferation, Massive Preretinal Gliosis, Massive Preretinal Organization, Massive Vitreous Retraction, Vitreoretinal Membrane Shrinkage)

STEVE CHARLES, M.D.

Memphis, Tennessee

Proliferative vitreoretinopathy is a reparative process initiated by a full- or partial-thickness retinal break or retinopexy. Loss of contact inhibition causes the surrounding glial or retinal pigment epithelial cells to migrate to both surfaces of the retina and proliferate. These cells migrate further and cover the posterior surface of the detached posterior hyaloid face. Fibronectin-lined, coated pits serve as attachments of the retinal pigment epithelium or glial cells to collagen fiber or other components of the extracellular matrix. The migration/contraction mechanism causes tangential force on the retina and multiple starfolds. Similarly, the vitreous contracts

largely because of this hypocellular gel contraction.

THERAPY

Surgical. The surgical objective is to allow retinal conformation to the retinal pigment epithelium. In cases of moderate starfolds, *scleral buckling* without vitreous surgery is indicated. Minimal retinopexy to the breaks should be used to avoid inflammation and further proliferation. Retreatment of retinal pigment epithelium with overlapping rows of retinopexy should be avoided to reduce proliferative vitreoretinopathy. Postreattachment retinopexy helps reduce retinal pigment epithelium proliferation and overtreatment. Laser and diathermy cause less proliferative vitreoretinopathy than cryotherapy, but are more difficult to apply.

A broad, relatively high 360° encircling buckle with a smooth contour should be utilized. This is best achieved with a silicone exoplant and two or three mattress sutures per quadrant. The posterior scleral bites should be single, long, and circumferential and as posterior as possible without damage to the vortex veins. The anterior bites should be limbus parallel, and placed in the scleral condensations at the muscle ring, representing the external landmark of the ora. Elastic 5-0 monofilament sutures are preferable, with the ends cut on the knot. The broad buckle extends back to the thicker, stronger untreated retina and to the ora to prevent anterior leakage. Extensive drainage of subretinal fluid, preferably a needle drainage method, is required to achieve instant reattachment and create space for the large buckle. Anterior vitrectomy to allow paracentesis in aphakic eyes or anterior chamber paracentesis in phakic or pseudophakic eyes may be necessary to achieve volume requirements. Air (gas) injection seals the retinal breaks via a surface tension effect and allows restoration of a pressure gradient and better drainage. Because of lateral displacement of the retina, transcleral drainage of subretinal fluid should be performed very posteriorly after air injection to avoid retinal incarceration in the drainage site.

Vitreous surgery is done when it is anticipated that scleral buckling alone cannot compensate for vitreous traction and periretinal membrane contraction sufficiently to reattach the retina. In most instances, the lens should be removed with trans pars plana lensectomy to permit better removal of the anterior loop traction, decompartmentation, and proliferative vitreoretinopathy reduction. Trans pars plana lensectomy with the aspirating phacofragmenter and linear suction is the method of choice. The anterior and posterior hyaloid vitreous cortex surfaces are usually in contact in a frontal plane configuration. This frontal plane component should be removed first, preferably with a divided 20-gauge system vitreous cutter and linear suction control using minimal suction force. The anterior loop traction then should be resected with the suction cutter if sufficient distance exists between the anterior attachment at the pars plana and the posterior attachment of this former peripheral cortical vitreous to the retina at the equator. Right-angle 20-gauge scissors should be used in most instances to resect this anterior loop component 360°.

Epiretinal membrane can then be peeled free of the retina in instances when it is minimally adherent. End-opening diamond-coated forceps are used for inside-out peeling of epiretinal membranes; needles and side-opening forceps cause more trauma to the internal limiting lamina. In cases of stronger adherence, it is better to use segmentation and delamination with a 20-gauge right-angle scissor with blades parallel to the retina (Charles modification of the Sutherland scissors). Segmentation of the epiretinal membrane in the center of a starfold and between each fold releases the tangential traction. If the membrane is dense and well developed, it can be delaminated from the retinal surface using both scissor blades between the retina and membrane. The goal is to release sufficient tangential traction to allow retinal conformation to the retinal pigment epithelium without necessarily removing all membranes.

Subretinal membranes can be segmented or removed with duckbill forceps if they are creating sufficient contour change in the retina to prevent reattachment. This can be accomplished through a pre-existing retinal break, or a retinotomy can be created for this purpose, using the scissors.

Incremental retinectomy after fluid/air exchange and internal drainage of subretinal fluid can be effective tools to release tangential forces on the retina when the retina is incarcerated in a wound or previous drain site or when dense membranes are strongly adherent over broad areas of atrophic retina.

Air (gas) tamponade should be used in all cases requiring vitrectomy because the tamponade effect of the posterior hyaloid face has been removed. Internal fluid gas exchange allows creation of a total fill of the vitreous space without hypotony or multiple small bubbles. A 20 per cent gaseous mixture of sulfur hexafluoride[‡] or a 15 per cent concentration of C_3F_8 may be used to prolong the absorption of the bubble. Concentrations greater than 20 per cent are not used because the expansion characteristics would cause elevation of intraocular pressure with a total fill. The gas is injected through the infusion cannula, preferably using a power gas injector. Fluid egress is accomplished through a tapered, bent 20-gauge cannula held near the optic nerve and controlled by a foot-controlled linear suction system.

Internal drainage of subretinal fluid with the same tapered bent cannula placed through a convenient retinal break and held near the retinal pigment epithelium allows hydraulic reattachment. A brief, high transretinal pressure gradient forces the still foreshortened retina against the retinal pigment epithelium. The appearance of subretinal air indicates the failure to release all tangential forces on the retina and the need for further segmentation, delamination, retinectomy, scleral buckling, resection, or it may indicate inoperability. Minimal transcleral diathermy or preferably laser endophotocoagulation is then placed around each retinal break, using the operating microscope for visualization.

Scleral buckling as described earlier, using a 9- to 10-mm wide 360° silicone exoplant imbricated flush with the surface of the globe and sewed end-to-end, is utilized. It is a mistake to think of proliferative vitreoretinopathy as a localized disease and to buckle only the abnormal-appearing areas. An encircling band is not required. Care should be taken to avoid muscle removal or damage to the vortex veins if buckle revision is thought to be indicated.

Ocular or Periocular Manifestations

Retina: Epiretinal membranes; fixed folds; starfolds; subretinal placoid or dendritic proliferation.
Vitreous: Condensation; contraction; pigmentation; posterior vitreous detachment.
Other: Visual loss.

PRECAUTIONS

Vitreous (periretinal membrane) surgery should be done immediately when it is apparent that conventional scleral buckling alone will not be effective. Vitreous surgery is a proven modality for this problem that no longer should be considered experimental. Care should be taken to minimize trauma to the internal limiting lamina by the use of scissor segmentation delamination, rather than peeling. Hydraulic reattachment is preferable to the injection of an expansile sulfur hexafluoride bubble and partial drainage of subretinal fluid because it permits intraoperative recognition of the need for further mechanical release of tangential traction.

Minimal retinopexy and the liberal use of subconjunctival corticosteroids* decrease the release of fibrin and reduce proliferation along this matrix.

COMMENTS

The above techniques have a 95 per cent intraoperative anatomic success, with 65 per cent long-term anatomic success and 50 per cent long-term visual success with acuities better than 5/200. With the possibility of bilateral visual loss, it is mandatory to consider this procedure with its greater success rate and 2- to 3-hour operating time to retain an ambulatory vision eye.

Silicone oil[‡] is increasingly widespread for long-term surface tension management. A combined multicenter trial has shown equal efficacy to C_3F_8 gas. More difficult cases with retinal defects that cannot conform to the RPE must be managed with lifetime silicone surface tension management.

Its purpose is rhegmatogenous defined and treated. No antiproliferative drugs have yet proven to be effective.

References

Charles S: Vitrectomy for retinal detachment. Trans Ophthalmol Soc UK 100:542–549, 1980.

Charles S: Vitreous Microsurgery. Baltimore, Williams & Wilkins, 1981.

Machemer R, van Horn D, Aaberg TM: Pigment epithelial proliferation in human retinal detachment with massive periretinal proliferation. Am J Ophthalmol 85:181–191, 1978.

van Horn DL, et al: Glial cell proliferation in human retinal detachment with massive periretinal proliferation. Am J Ophthalmol 84:383–393, 1977.

VITREOUS HEMORRHAGE 379.23

RICHARD L. WINSLOW, M.D.,
and BRUCE C. TAYLOR, M.D.

Dallas, Texas

Vitreous hemorrhage, whether associated with trauma or occurring spontaneously, is a secondary diagnosis. Successful treatment depends on identifying the specific cause of the hemorrhage. In traumatic cases, one must determine if the hemorrhage has resulted from a ruptured retinal vessel, a retinal tear, or a perforating injury. The most common causes of spontaneous hemorrhage are proliferative diabetic retinopathy, posterior vitreous detachment, retinal tear without detachment, proliferative vein occlusion, retinal detachment, intraocular lens, and proliferative sickle retinopathy. Miscellaneous causes must be considered if the more common causes are absent. Occasionally, the source of the vitreous hemorrhage can never be identified. However, every attempt must be made to identify the specific cause of the vitreous hemorrhage so that specific therapy may be instituted.

THERAPY

Supportive. The patient should avoid heavy lifting, stooping, and vigorous physical activity, all of which might produce further vitreous hemorrhage. If there is no view of the retina, diagnostic ultrasonography is required to rule out a retinal detachment. Bedrest for several days with the head elevated and both eyes patched is also helpful to allow settling of the vitreous hemorrhage inferiorly so that the superior retina may be visualized. This is often diagnostic because over 80 per cent of retinal tears associated with vitreous hemorrhage occur in the superior quadrants.

Surgical. Traumatic vitreous hemorrhage may require no therapy if there is merely a ruptured retinal vessel. If a retinal tear or dialysis is noted, cryotherapy or photocoagulation should be applied to surround the retinal break. Vitrectomy and scleral buckling procedures may be required if retinal detachment occurs.

The causes of spontaneous vitreous hemorrhage may be grouped into proliferative, rhegmatogenous, and miscellaneous. The major proliferative causes include diabetic retinopathy, vein occlusion, and sickle retinopathy, which can all be treated with photocoagulation. In proliferative diabetic retinopathy, panretinal photocoagulation is extremely helpful in preventing further vitreous hemorrhage. Either xenon or argon laser photocoagulation may be used, but argon treatment is probably preferable. Laser panretinal photocoagulation is performed using a three-mirror Goldmann lens or a Rodenstock panfunduscopic lens to visualize the retina. The laser settings include a spot size of 400 to 500 µM for 0.2 seconds and a power setting adequate to produce moderate whitening of the retina. Burns are spread from 0.5 to 1 burn width apart throughout the peripheral retina, extending posteriorly no closer than 2 disc diameters from the fovea and 1 disc diameter from the disc. The total number of burns averages between 1200 to 1600, which are usually done in three to four sessions, using only topical anesthesia. Retrobulbar anesthesia may be used, but is rarely necessary. If further vitreous hemorrhage or vascular proliferation occurs, additional photocoagulation may be applied to areas between the original burns.

Argon laser photocoagulation may be used in a similar technique to prevent further vitreous hemorrhage from a proliferative branch vein occlusion. Burns are made only in the affected sector. In central retinal vein occlusion, panretinal photocoagulation is useful in preventing both recurrent vitreous hemorrhage and rubeosis iridis.

Proliferative sickle retinopathy can be treated with a scatter technique of photocoagulation applied to the peripheral areas of capillary dropout, which are present anterior to the peripheral "sea fans." The capillary dropout may be localized more specifically with fluorescein angiography.

Scatter cryotherapy may be used for proliferative diabetic retinopathy if the vitreous hemorrhage fails to clear adequately to permit photocoagulation. If the conjunctiva is not opened, two rows of three to four cryo applications are made in each quadrant 12 to 16 mm posterior to the limbus. The freeze is monitored with indirect ophthalmoscopy to produce moderate whitening of the retina. In areas where vitreous hemorrhage obscures the view, the cryo application is timed similarly to those areas that could be visualized.

Cryotherapy may also be used to treat peripheral "sea fans" in proliferative sickle retinopathy if vitreous hemorrhage prevents photocoagulation. The best technique is to use a single freeze-thaw, allowing the ice ball to extend into the vitreous until it totally engulfs the "sea fan."

In the rhegmatogenous group, no therapy is required for a posterior vitreous detachment associated with vitreous hemorrhage. Superficial retinal hemorrhages may be seen at the disc margin or equatorial region. This is a diagnosis of exclusion and can be made only after periodic examinations, performed while the vitreous hemorrhage is clearing, demonstrate a vitreous detachment but fail to show a retinal tear.

If a retinal break is present, it should be surrounded by cryotherapy so that the freezes extend into healthy retina and are contiguous. The retina should just be made to whiten. Extensive, prolonged, or repeated cryo applications are to be avoided, since they may result in excessive retinal thinning or necrosis, as well as the release of viable retinal pigment epithelial (RPE) cells that migrate through the retinal tear into the vitreous cavity. Later proliferation of these RPE cells may result in macular pucker or proliferative vitreoretinopathy. Posterior retinal breaks may be surrounded by photocoagulation if they cannot be reached with the cryoprobe. The laser indirect ophthalmoscope may also be used in conjunction with scleral indentation to treat peripheral retinal tears.

In approximately 7 per cent of retinal tears, a retinal vessel bridges the tear and is not torn completely. It may be the source of recurrent vitreous hemorrhage and can usually be managed simply with cryotherapy or laser to surround the tear, since the recurrent hemorrhage is commonly self-limiting. Laser therapy may occasionally be used to occlude the bridging vessel by applying 0.5- to 1-second burns of 400 to 500 μM in size to the vessel in an area where the vessel is in flat retina. This technique may require repeated attempts at approximately 1-week intervals to occlude the vessel. Fluorescein angiography may be helpful in demonstrating the complete interruption of blood flow in the bridging vessel. Only rarely is a localized scleral buckle required to relieve the vitreous traction on the vessel and to prevent further vitreous hemorrhage.

When a retinal detachment is detected, a routine scleral buckle is performed if the retinal breaks can be visualized adequately. Customarily, an encircling solid or sponge explant is sutured over the retinal break after it has been surrounded by cryotherapy and the subretinal fluid has been drained. If the retinal breaks cannot be visualized adequately, a vitrectomy must first be performed, followed by a scleral buckling procedure.

In the modern era of ophthalmology, vitreous hemorrhage associated with the use of intraocular lenses has also been seen. The hemorrhage usually originates in the anterior segment, but migrates into the vitreous. The source of the hemorrhage has been the angle in angle-supported lenses, the pupillary margin in iris-supported lenses (particularly those with metal loops that can erode the pupillary margin), and the ciliary body or posterior surface of the iris in posterior chamber lenses. Usually, this hemorrhage is self-limited, but occasionally the lens must be removed. In some cases involving posterior chamber lens chafe of the iris, the contact between lens and iris may be moved by using mydriatic or miotic drops, thereby preventing further hemorrhage. In addition, laser applied to the area of chafe may cauterize the bleeding iris or cause photomydriasis, thereby reducing the lens-iris chafe.

Ocular or Periocular Manifestations

Iris: Rubeosis iridis (with proliferative diabetic retinopathy and central retinal vein occlusion).
Lens: Posterior subcapsular cataract.
Retina: Macular pucker; traction retinal detachment.
Other: Hemolytic glaucoma (particularly in the aphakic patient).

PRECAUTIONS

Patients with proliferative diabetic retinopathy are prone to develop rubeosis iridis, particularly if the lens is removed. Patients with central retinal vein occlusion are candidates for rubeosis iridis, particularly in the first 6 months after the occlusion. In the early stages, rubeosis iridis can often be controlled with panretinal photocoagulation. Patients with sickle cell hemoglobinopathy are prone to develop anterior segment necrosis after scleral buckling. Exchange transfusion before surgery and avoidance of muscle disinsertion may be helpful in preventing this complication.

COMMENTS

Proliferative diabetic retinopathy is by far the most common cause of spontaneous vitreous hemorrhage, accounting for 32 to 54 per cent of all cases. This diagnosis can usually be made by a history of diabetes or examination of the fellow eye. Once diabetes is excluded, the most common etiology is a retinal tear with or without retinal detachment, which accounts for 33 to 64 per cent of the spontaneous vitreous hemorrhages in nondiabetic patients. The presence of a retinal tear must be ruled out by careful, repeated funduscopic examination, using indirect ophthalmoscopy and scleral indentation.

References

Blankenship GW, Okun E: Retinal tributary vein occlusion: History and management by photocoagulation. Arch Ophthalmol 89:363–368, 1973.

Branch Vein Occlusion Study Group: Argon laser scatter photocoagulation for prevention of neovascularization and vitreous hemorrhage in branch vein occlusion. Arch Ophthalmol 104:34–41, 1986.

Cox MS, Whitmore PV, Gutow RF: Treatment of intravitreal and prepapillary neovascularization following branch retinal vein occlusion. Trans Am Acad Ophthalmol Otolaryngol 79:387–393, 1975.

Davis MD: Natural history of retinal breaks without detachment. Arch Ophthalmol 92:183–194, 1974.

Diabetic Retinopathy Study Research Group: Preliminary report on effects of photocoagulation therapy. Am J Ophthalmol 81:383–396, 1976.

Diabetic Retinopathy Vitrectomy Study Research Group: Early vitrectomy for severe hemorrhage in diabetic retinopathy. Arch Ophthalmol 103:1644–1652, 1985.

Diabetic Retinopathy Vitrectomy Study Research Group: Two-year course of visual acuity in severe proliferative diabetic retinopathy with conventional management. Ophthalmology 92:494–502, 1985.

Diabetic Retinopathy Vitrectomy Study Research Group: Early vitrectomy for severe proliferative diabetic retinopathy in eyes with useful vision. Ophthalmology 95:1307–1320, 1988.

Goldbaum MH, et al: Cryotherapy of proliferative sickle retinopathy. II: Triple freeze-thaw cycle. Br J Ophthalmol 63:97–101, 1979.

Hanscom TA: Indirect treatment of peripheral retinal neovascularization. Am J Ophthalmol 93:88–91, 1982.

Jaffe NS: Complications of acute posterior vitreous detachment. Arch Ophthalmol 79:568–571, 1968.

Ross WH, Gottner MJ: Peripheral retinal cryopexy for subtotal vitreous hemorrhage. Am J Ophthalmol 105:377–382, 1988.

Schimek RA, Spencer R: Cryopexy treatment of proliferative diabetic retinopathy. Retinal cryoablation in patients with severe vitreous hemorrhage. Arch Ophthalmol 97:1276–1280, 1979.

Winslow RL, Taylor BC: Spontaneous vitreous hemorrhage: Etiology and management. South Med J 73:1450–1452, 1980.

VITREOUS WICK SYNDROME 379.26

RICHARD S. RUIZ, M.D.

Houston, Texas

The vitreous wick syndrome consists of microscopic wound breakdown with subsequent vitreous prolapse, which creates a tiny vitreous wick from the external surface to the inner eye. Severe intraocular inflammation secondary to bacterial endophthalmitis may develop. Infection seems to gain entrance into the eye by way of the vitreous wick, and the fistula fails to heal because of the external vitreous. When inflammation is present, the patient presents with sudden pain, a peaked pupil, and a rupture of the anterior hyaloid membrane. This syndrome usually occurs 2 weeks or more after uncomplicated cataract surgery.

THERAPY

Surgical. Surgical repair should be carried out without delay. At the time of surgery, an anterior chamber tap for culture and sensitivity studies is taken through the fistulous opening. Using an operating microscope, the fistulous tract is carefully examined, and the vitreous wick is identified, stretched with forceps, and excised flush with the surface of the corneoscleral wound. The wound defect is then converted to a linear incision with the razor blade knife and closed tightly with several sutures. A large air bubble is instilled in the anterior chamber to push the vitreous away from the wound. In the case of mild inflammation or no inflammation, nothing further is done. When there is severe intraocular inflammation with heavy opacification of the vitreous and hypopyon formation, an anterior vitrectomy using a suitable vitrectomy instrument should be considered. The fistulous opening is then enlarged suitably, and the vitrectomy instrument with infusion and aspiration ports is introduced into the anterior chamber. All opacified vitreous, hypopyon exudate, and other inflammatory debris are removed carefully. The instrument is then directed into the posterior segment, where an anterior vitrectomy is carried out. All aspirated material is collected and concentrated for culture and sensitivity studies. The vitrectomy instrument is then withdrawn, and depending upon the severity of the inflammation, one may consider the introduction of intraocular antibiotics. The fistulous opening, which has been enlarged, is now tightly sutured and the tone of the globe re-established with balanced salt solution.

Ocular. When intraocular inflammation is present, large doses of topical antibiotics are indicated for several weeks until the inflammation subsides.

Systemic. Large doses of systemic antibiotics and corticosteroids are used in exactly the same manner as in bacterial endophthalmitis from other causes. As soon as sensitivity and culture reports are available, antibiotics may be suitably adjusted for specific organisms.

Ocular or Periocular Manifestations

Anterior Chamber: Cells and flare; hypopyon; leak.
Pupil: Peaked.
Vitreous: Exudates; prolapse; rupture of anterior hyaloid membrane; strands.
Other: Decreased visual acuity; inflammation; ocular pain; visual loss.

PRECAUTIONS

To prevent the vitreous wick syndrome, limbus-based conjunctival flaps should be used to cover the corneoscleral sutures. These sutures should be completely buried beneath the flap. Corneoscleral sutures should not be tied tightly as they cut through the tissue, causing a fistulous opening.

If fornix-based conjunctival flaps are used, it is important to realize that careful and repeated observations are necessary for at least 1 month after routine uncomplicated cataract extraction. If peaking of the pupil is observed in the postoperative period, careful slit-lamp evaluation of the vitreous face and corneoscleral wound is indicated. If vitreous adherence without wick formation is seen, the external surface of the wound should be carefully examined at close intervals in the event that vitreous prolapse develops. If a vitreous wick should develop, surgical repair should be carried out without delay.

COMMENTS

It seems reasonable that wound leakage may be largely responsible for vitreous adherence to the posterior wound after cataract surgery, particularly where definite, taut strands are noted. It is the aqueous leak that causes the vitreous to move anteriorly and become incarcerated in the fistulous opening. Often this will stop the leak, much like an iris adhesion; however, in some cases, the process progresses to frank vitreous prolapse through the wound. It seems possible that wound leak might also be responsible for anterior hyaloid rupture with or without vitreous adherence or prolapse.

Vitreous prolapsing through the fistula has the appearance of a glob of mucus on the external surface of the globe. The clinical diagnosis can be confirmed by gently stroking the externalized vitreous, which results in movement of vitreous gel in the anterior chamber and subsequent pupillary movement. A Seidel test is usually positive when gentle pressure is applied to the globe.

References

Rice TA, Michels RG: Current surgical management of the vitreous wick syndrome. Am J Ophthalmol 85:656–661, 1978.

Ruiz RS, Teeters VW: The vitreous wick syndrome. A late complication following cataract extraction. Am J Ophthalmol 70:483–490, 1970.

DRUG ROSTER

ABBREVIATIONS USED IN THE DRUG ROSTER

Arg.—Argentina
Austral.—Australia
Aust.—Austria
Belg.—Belgium
Braz.—Brazil
Canad.—Canada
Cz.—Czechoslovakia
Denm.—Denmark
Fin.—Finland
Fr.—France
G.B.—Great Britain
Germ.—Germany
Gr.—Greece
Hung.—Hungary
Ind.—India
Ire.—Ireland
Isr.—Israel

Ital.—Italy
Jap.—Japan
Mex.—Mexico
Mon.—Monaco
Neth.—Netherlands
Nig.—Nigeria
Norw.—Norway
N.Z.—New Zealand
Pol.—Poland
Port.—Portugal
S. Afr.—South Africa
Scand.—Scandinavia
Span.—Spain
Swed.—Sweden
Switz.—Switzerland
USA—United States
U.S.S.R—Union of Soviet
Socialist Republics

ACETAMINOPHEN

Proprietary Names: Aceta, Alba-Temp, Alvedon (Swed.), Anapap, Anelix, Anuphen, Apamide, Apap, Atasol (Canad.), Ben-u-ron (Germ.), Calpol (G.B.), Campain (Canad.), Capital, Ceetamol (Austral.), Cen-Apap, Cetamol (Ire.), Chemcetaphen (Canad.), Datril, Dapa, Dimindol, Dolamin (Austral.), Dolanex, Doliprane (Fr.), Dymadon (Austral.), Febridol, Febrigesic, Febrogesic, G-1, Janupap, Korum, Lestemp, Liquiprin, Lyteca, Med-Apap, Napamol (S. Afr.), Nebs, Neopap, Nevrol (Austral.), Nilprin, Pacemol (N.Z.), Pamol (G.B.), Panado, (S. Afr.), Panadol (G.B.), Panodil (Swed.), Paracet (Austral.), Paracetamol (G.B.), Parasin (Austral.), Parmol (Austral.), Parten, Pediaphen (Canad.), Phenaphen, Phendex, Placemol (Austral.), Pirin, Proval, Pyrapap, Restin (S. Afr.), Rounox (Canad.), Salzone (G.B.), SK-Apap, Sub-Due, Taper, Temetan, Temlo, Tempra, Tenlap, Termidor (Swed.), Ticelgesic (G.B.), Tylenol, Valadol, Valorin.

Preparations

Oral: Capsules, 300 and 500 mg; drops, 60 mg/0.6 ml; elixir or syrup, 120 and 150 mg/ 5 ml; tablets, 300 and 325 mg; tablets (chewable), 120 mg.

Rectal: Suppositories, 120, 300, 600, and 900 mg.

Usual Dosages

Oral, Rectal: Adults, 300 to 600 mg at 4-hour intervals if necessary; total daily dose should not exceed 2.4 gm. Children 6 to 12 years of age, 150 to 300 mg; 1 to 6 years, 60 to 120 mg; under 1 year, 60 mg. These amounts are given as single doses every 4 to 6 hours, but the total dose should not exceed 1.2 gm.

ACETAMINOPHEN/CODEINE COMBINATION

Proprietary Names: Aceta with Codeine, Apap with Codeine, Empracet with Codeine, Phenaphen 2, 3, 4, Tylenol with Codeine 1, 2, 3, 4.

Preparations

Oral: Capsules, 300 mg acetaminophen with 30 to 60 mg codeine; elixir, 120 mg acetaminophen with 12 mg codeine/5 ml; tablets, 300 or 325 mg acetaminophen with 7.5, 15, 30, or 60 mg codeine.

Usual Dosages

Oral: The usual adult dose is one or two tablets or capsules every 4 hours as required.

---

* Route of administration not approved by FDA.
† Drug not approved by FDA for any indication.
‡ Drug not approved by FDA for this particular indication.
§ Indicated dosage above the manufacturer's recommendation.

ACETAZOLAMIDE

Proprietary Names: Defiltran (Fr.), Diamox, Diazol (S. Afr.), Didoc (Jap.), Diuramid (Pol.), Glaucomide (Austral.), Glaupax (Swed.), Hydrazol.

Preparations

Injection: Powder, 500-mg vial.
Oral: Capsules (timed-release), 500 mg; tablets, 125 and 250 mg.

Usual Dosages

Intramuscular, Intravenous: 500 mg may be administered parenterally and may be repeated in 2 to 4 hours.
Oral: Adults, 250 mg every 6 hours. Children, 10 to 15 mg/kg daily in divided doses. The timed-release preparation can be given every 12 hours, but may not be as effective as regular tablets. For epilepsy, the suggested total daily dose is 8 to 30 mg/kg in divided doses.

ACETOHEXAMIDE

Proprietary Names: Dimelor (G.B.), Dymelor, Ordimel (Swed.).

Preparations

Oral: Tablets, 250 and 500 mg.

Usual Dosages

Oral: Dosage should be individualized. Usual range, 0.25 to 1.5 gm daily.

ACETYLCHOLINE

Proprietary Names: Acecoline (Canad., Fr.), Covochol (S. Afr.), Miochol.

Preparations

Injection: Two-compartment vial containing 20 mg of acetylcholine chloride and 100 mg of mannitol in the lower compartment and 2 ml of sterile water in the upper compartment.

Usual Dosages

Intracameral: 0.5 to 2 ml of a freshly prepared 1:100 solution instilled in the anterior chamber.
Retrobulbar: 25 mg in 1 ml initially, 50 to 75 mg (2 to 3 ml) per injection, depending upon the response.

ACETYLCYSTEINE

Proprietary Names: Airbron (G.B., Canad.), Fluimucil (Germ., Ital., Neth., Span., Switz.), Inspir (Swed.), Lysomucil (Belg.), Mucofilm Sol (Jpn.), Mucolyticum (Germ.), Mucomist (Ital.), Mucomyst, Nac (Canad.), Parvolex (G.B.).

Preparations

Topical Ophthalmic: Eyedrops containing 2, 5, 10, or 20 per cent acetylcysteine are prepared by dilution of 20 per cent solution with hydroxypropyl methylcellulose. This preparation should be adjusted to pH 9 with 4 per cent sodium hydroxide solution and prepared aseptically.

Usual Dosages

Topical Ophthalmic: Preparation may be applied up to four times daily.

ACETYLSALICYLIC ACID

See Aspirin.

ACICLOVIR

See Acyclovir.

ACTH

See Corticotropin.

ACYCLOGUANOSINE

See Acyclovir.

ACYCLOVIR (ACICLOVIR, ACYCLOGUANOSINE)

Proprietary Names: Acicloftal (Ital.), Acyvir (Ital.), Clovix (Ital.), Cusiviral (Span.), Cycloviran (Ital.), Maynar (Span.), Milavir (Span.), Sifiviral (Ital.), Viclovir (Span.), Vipral (Span.), Virherpes (Span.), Virmen (Span.), Zovirax (Austral., Canad., Fr., G.B., Ger., Ire., Ital., Neth., S. Afr., Span., Swed., Switz., USA).

Preparations

Injection: Powder.
Oral: Capsules, 200 mg.
Topical: Ointment, 5 per cent.
Topical Ophthalmic: No ophthalmic preparation is commercially available, but a 3 per cent ointment in petrolatum base may be prepared.

Usual Dosages

Intravenous (Slow): 5 mg/kg (250 mg/square meter) may be infused at a constant rate over 1 hour every 8 hours (15 mg/kg, daily dose).
Oral: Usual dosage is 200 mg two to five times daily.
Topical: A sufficient quantity of ointment may be used to adequately cover all lesions every 3 hours or up to six times per day for 7 days.
Topical Ophthalmic: Approximately one-half inch of ointment is administered into the lower conjunctival sac five times daily at 3-hour intervals.

ADRENOCORTICOTROPIC HORMONE

See Corticotropin.

ALLOPURINOL

Proprietary Names: Bloxanth (Canad.), Epidropal (Germ.), Foligan (Germ.), Lopurin, Urosin (Germ.), Zyloprim, Zyloric (G.B.).

Preparations

Oral: Tablets, 100 and 300 mg.

Usual Dosages

Oral: Dose range, 100 to 800 mg daily.

ALPHA-TOCOPHEROL

See Vitamin E.

ALPRAZOLAM

Proprietary Names: Tafil (Ger.), Trankimazin (Span.), Valeans (Ital.), Xanax (Austral.,

Canad., Fr., G.B., Ire., Ital., Switz., USA), Xanor (S. Afr.).

Preparations

Oral: Tablets, 0.25, 0.5, 1, and 2 mg.

Usual Dosages

Oral: Used in the treatment of anxiety disorders in doses of 0.25 to 0.5 mg three times daily, increased where necessary up to a total daily dose of 3 to 4 mg. Doses of up to 10 mg daily have been used in the treatment of panic attacks and depression.

ALTEPLASE

Proprietary Name: Activase.

Preparations

Injection: Lyophilized powder, 20 mg (11.6 million IU) and 50 mg (29 million IU).

Usual Dosages

Intravenous: The usual recommended dose for coronary artery thrombus is 100 mg given as 60 mg in the first hour (of which 6 to 10 mg is given as a bolus over the first 1 to 2 minutes), 20 mg over the second hour, and 20 mg over the third hour.

ALUMINUM ACETATE

Proprietary Names: Acid Mantle, Alsol (Germ.), Domeboro, Eddikesur (Denm.), Euceta (Neth., Switz.).

Preparations

Topical: Solution, 5 per cent.

Usual Dosages

Topical: Solution may be diluted 1:10 to 1:40 and appplied three to four times daily.

ALUMINUM HYDROXIDE

Proprietary Names: Adagel (Austral.), Aldrox (Arg., Belg.), Allulose (Norw.), Alterna GEL, Alu-Cap, Alugelibys (Span.), Alumag (S. Afr.), Aluminox (Neth.), Alusorb (Austral.), Alu-Tab, Amphojel, Amphotabs (Austral.), Basaljel (Austral., Canad.), Dialume, Gammagel (Ital.), Gastracol (Switz.), Gelox (Austral.),

Minajel (Austral.), Palliacol (Germ.), Pepsamar (Span.), Uldecan (Span.).

Preparations

Oral: Suspension (gel), 320 mg/5 ml; tablets (dried gel), 300 and 600 mg.

Usual Dosages

Oral: In conjunction with dietary phosphate restriction in the management of hyperphosphatemia, 30 to 40 ml is administered three to four times daily.

AMANTADINE

Proprietary Names: Contenton (Germ.), Mantadix (Fr.), PK-Merz (Germ.), Symmetrel, Virofral (Swed.).

Preparations

Oral: Capsules, 100 mg; syrup, 500 mg/5 ml.

Usual Dosages

Oral: Range, 100 to 500 mg daily in divided doses.

AMIKACIN

Proprietary Names: Amikin, Amiklin (Fr.), Amukin (Belg., Neth.), BB-K8 (Ital., Mex.), Biclin (Span.), Biklin (Arg., Denm., Germ., Jap., Swed.), Pierami (Ital.).

Preparations

Injection: Solution, 50 to 250 mg/ml.

Usual Dosages

Intramuscular, Intravenous: Adults, children and older infants, 15 mg/kg daily in two or three equally divided doses. The total dose should not exceed 1.5 gm. Neonates, a loading dose of 10 mg/kg is given, followed by 7.5 mg every 12 hours. Dosage should be reduced when given to patients with impaired renal function.

---

* Route of administration not approved by FDA.
† Drug not approved by FDA for any indication.
‡ Drug not approved by FDA for this particular indication.
§ Indicated dosage above the manufacturer's recommendation.

AMINOBENZOIC ACID

See Para-Aminobenzoic Acid.

AMINOCAPROIC ACID

Proprietary Names: Amicar, Capracid (Ital.), Capralense (Fr.), Caprolisin (Ital.), Capramol (Belg., Fr., Ital., Switz.), Caproamin Fides (Span.), Ekaprol (Austral.), Epsamon (Switz.), Epsikapron (G.B., S. Afr., Swed., Switz.), Hemocaprol (Fr., Span., Switz.), Ipsilon (Arg.).

Preparations

Injection: Solution, 250 mg/ml.
Oral: Syrup, 1.25 gm/5 ml; tablets, 500 mg.

Usual Dosages

Intravenous, Oral: For acute bleeding syndromes caused by elevated fibrinolytic activity, 4 to 5 gm should be administered during the first hour, followed by 1 gm/hour for 8 hours or until the hemorrhagic condition is under control. When the bleeding tendency is chronic in nautre, daily dosage of 5 to 30 gm administered in divided doses at 3- to 6-hour intervals has been recommended.

AMITRIPTYLINE

Proprietary Names: Amitid, Amizol (G.B.), Annolytin (Jap.), Deprex (Canad.), Domical (G.B.), Elatrol (Canad.), Elavil, Endep, Larozyl (Swed.), Lentizol (G.B.), Levate (Canad.), Mareline (Canad.), Novotriptyn (Canad.), Saroten (G.B.), SK-Amitriptyline, Tryptanol (Austral., S. Afr.), Tryptizol (G.B.).

Preparations

Injection: Solution, 10 mg/ml.
Oral: Tablets, 10, 25, 50, 75, and 100 mg; capsules, 25 and 50 mg.

Usual Dosages

Intramuscular: Adults, initially 80 to 120 mg daily in four divided doses. The oral route should be substituted as soon as possible.
Oral: Adults, initially 75 mg daily in divided doses. A few hospitalized patients may require as much as 300 mg daily. Elderly patients and adolescents, 10 mg three times daily and 20 mg at bedtime.

AMMONIATED MERCURY

Proprietary Name: Ammoniated Mercury.

Preparations

Topical Ophthalmic: Ointment, 3 per cent.

Usual Dosages

Topical Ophthalmic: A small amount one or two times daily.

AMOBARBITAL

Proprietary Names: Amal (Austral.), Amsal (Austral.), Amylbarb (Austral.), Amylobarbitone (G.B.), Amylobeta (Austral.), Amylosol (Austral.), Amytal, Eunoctal (Fr.), Isomyl (Swed.), Isonal (Canad.), Mylodorm (Austral.), Mylosed (Austral.), Neur-Amyl (Austral.), Novamobarb (Canad.), Restal (Austral.), Schiwanox (Germ.), Sedal (Austral.), Sednotic (Austral.), Stadadorm (Germ.).

Preparations

Injection: Powder, 125, 250, and 500 mg.
Oral: Elixir, 22 and 44 mg/5 ml; tablets 15, 30, 50, and 100 mg; capsules, 65 and 200 mg.

Usual Dosages

Intramuscular: Adults, 65 to 500 mg. No more than 5 ml should be injected at any one site.
Oral: As a hypnotic, 100 to 200 mg. As a sedative, up to 600 mg daily in divided doses. Children up to 1 year, 15 to 50 mg; 1 to 5 years, 50 to 60 mg; 6 to 12 years, 60 to 120 mg.

AMOXICILLIN

Proprietary Names: Amoxil, Amoxycillin (G.B.), Clamoxyl (Germ., (Jap.), Imacillin (Swed.), Larotid, Polymox, Pasetocin (Jap.), Robamox, Sawacillin (Jap.), Sumox, Trimox, Ulymox, Utimox.

Preparations

Oral: Capsules, 250 and 500 mg; drops for suspension (pediatric), 50 mg/ml; powder for suspension, 125 and 250 mg/5 ml; suspension, 3 gm.

Usual Dosages

Oral: Adults and children over 20 kg, 250 to 500 mg daily. Children less than 20 mg, 20 to 40 mg/kg daily. These amounts are administered in divided doses at 8-hour intervals. Larger doses may be required for persistent or severe infections. For gonorrheal or urethral infections caused by *N. gonorrhoeae*, 3 gm as a single oral dose are recommended.

AMOXICILLIN/CLAVULANATE POTASSIUM COMBINATION

Proprietary Name: Augmentin.

Preparations

Oral: Powder for suspension, 125 or 250 mg amoxicillin and 31.25 or 62.5 mg clavulanate potassium/5 ml; tablets, 250 or 500 mg amoxicillin and 125 mg clavulanate potassium; tablets (chewable), 125 or 250 mg amoxicillin and 31.25 or 62.5 mg clavulanate potassium.

Usual Dosages

Oral: For adults and children over 40 kg, usual dose is 250 mg of amoxicillin and 125 mg of clavulanate potassium every 8 hours. For more severe infections, 500 mg of amoxicillin and 125 mg of clavulanate potassium every 8 hours. In children under 40 kg, usual dose is 20 mg/kg daily in divided doses every 8 hours. For more severe infections, 40 mg/kg daily may be given in divided doses every 8 hours.

AMPHETAMINE

Proprietary Names: Badrin (Austral.), Benzedrine.

Preparations

Oral: Tablets, 5 and 10 mg.

Usual Dosages

Oral: The usual daily dose is 5 to 60 mg in divided doses. Amphetamine should be administered at the lowest effective dosage and adjusted individually.

---

*Route of administration not approved by FDA.
† Drug not approved by FDA for any indication.
‡ Drug not approved by FDA for this particular indication.
§ Indicated dosage above the manufacturer's recommendation.

AMPHOTERICIN B

Proprietary Names: Ampho-Moronal (Germ.), Fungilin (G.B.), Fungizone.

Preparations

Injection: Powder, 50 mg.
Topical Ophthalmic: No ophthalmic form is available, but aqueous suspension containing 0.1 to 5 mg/ml may be prepared from powder marked for intravenous use. Saline solution should *not* be used with amphotericin B, since saline solution will precipitate amphotericin B.

Usual Dosages

Intracameral: 20 to 30 µg in 0.1 to 0.2 ml of sterile 5 per cent dextrose in water.
Intrathecal: A total of 50 mg is diluted with at least 150 ml of 5 per cent dextrose injection (for intraventricular injection) or 10 per cent dextrose without preservative (for hyperbaric translumbar injection) to a final concentration of about 0.25 mg/ml. Therapy is initiated with 0.1 ml, and the dose is gradually increased until the patient can tolerate 0.5 mg, the usual maximum dose, without excessive discomfort. The minimal tolerated dose is given at 48- to 72-hour intervals.
Intravenous (Slow): Dosage must be adjusted individually according to severity of the disease and tolerance of patient. Therapy is usually instituted with a daily dose of 0.25 mg/kg and *gradually* increased as tolerance permits. The optimal dose is unknown. Total daily dosage may range up to 1.0 mg/kg or alternate-day dosages ranging up to 1.5 mg/kg. *Under no circumstances* should a total daily dosage of 1.5 mg/kg be exceeded. Several months of therapy are usually necessary.
Intravitreal: 4 to 5 µg in 0.1 to 0.2 ml of sterile 5 per cent dextrose in water.
Subconjunctival: 0.75 to 3 mg in 0.5 ml of sterile 5 per cent dextrose in water. Doses as large as 5 mg in a 0.5 ml suspension have occasionally been administered.
Topical Ophthalmic: One drop of a suspension containing 0.1 to 5.0 mg/ml in sterile 5 per cent dextrose in water every 30 minutes.

AMPICILLIN

Proprietary Names: Acillin, A-Cillin, Alpen, Amblosin (Germ.), Amcill, Amipenix (Jap.), Ampen (Canad.), Amperil, Ampexin (Canad.), Ampicin (Canad.), Ampilean (Canad.), Ampilum (Ital.), Ampilux (Ital.), Ampipenin (Swed.), Astrapen (Austral.), Binotal (Germ.), D-Amp, D-Cillin, Deripen (Germ.), Doktacillin (Swed.), Domicillin (Jap.), Omnipen, Pen A or A/N, Pen-Bristol (Germ.), Penbriten, Penbritine (Fr.), Penbrock (Germ.), Pencline (Fr.), Pensyn, Pentrex (S. Afr.), Pentrexyl (G.B.), Pfizerpen A., Polycillin, Principen, Ro-ampen, Roampicillin, SK-Ampicillin, Supen, Suractin (Germ.), Synpenin (Jap.), Totacillin, Totapen (Fr.), Vidopen (G.B.).

Preparations

Injection: Powder for solution, 250 mg/ml in 2.5-gm containers; powder, 0.125, 0.25, 0.5, 1, 2, and 4 gm.
Oral: Capsules, 250 and 500 mg; drops (pediatric), 10 mg/ml; powder for suspension (pediatric), 100 mg/ml; powder for suspension, 125, 250, and 500 mg/5 ml; tablets (chewable), 125 mg.

Usual Dosages

Intracameral, Intravitreal: 500 µg in 0.1 to 0.2 ml of isotonic sodium chloride injection.
Intramuscular: Adults and children over 20 kg, 250 to 500 mg four times daily at 6-hour intervals; less than 20 kg, 25 to 50 mg/kg daily in divided doses at 6- or 8-hour intervals.
Intravenous: Adults and children over 20 kg, 250 to 500 mg four times daily at 6-hour intervals. Children under 20 kg, 25 to 50 mg/kg daily in divided doses every 6 hours. For severe infections, doses up to 2 gm every 6 hours may be used. Patients have been successfully treated for bacterial meningitis with doses of 8 to 14 gm daily; the drug is administered every 3 to 4 hours.
Oral: Adults and children over 20 kg, 250 to 500 mg four times daily at 6-hour intervals; children less than 20 kg, 25 to 50 mg/kg daily in divided doses every 6 to 8 hours. Higher doses up to 12 gm daily should be used for stubborn or severe infections. For urethritis caused by *N. gonorrhoeae,* 3.5 gm as a single oral dose is recommended. In stubborn infections, therapy may be required for several weeks.
Subconjunctival: 50 to 250 mg in 0.5 ml of isotonic sodium chloride injection or sterile water for injection.
Topical Ophthalmic: One drop of a solution containing 40 to 100 mg/ml is given every 1 to 4 hours. Fortified ampicillin eyedrops are prepared with ampicillin trihydrate.

AMPICILLIN/PROBENECID COMBINATION

Proprietary Names: Polycillin-PRB, Principen with Probenecid, Probampacin.

---

* Route of administration not approved by FDA.
† Drug not approved by FDA for any indication.
‡ Drug not approved by FDA for this particular indication.
§ Indicated dosage above the manufacturer's recommendation.

Preparations

Oral: Capsules, 3.5 gm ampicillin and 1 gm probenecid; powder for suspension, 3.5 mg ampicillin and 1 gm probenecid.

Usual Dosages

Oral: Usual dosage is a single dose of 3.5 gm of ampicillin and 1 gm of probenecid.

ANTIMONY MEGLUMINE

Proprietary Names: Glucantim (Ital.), Glucantime (Fr., Span.).

Preparations

Injection: Powder.

Usual Dosages

Intramuscular, Intravenous: A dose of 100 mg/kg may be administered daily for 10 to 12 days and repeated if required after an interval of 4 to 6 weeks.

APRACLONIDINE

Proprietary Name: Iopidine.

Preparations

Topical Ophthalmic: Solution, 1 per cent.

Usual Dosages

Topical Ophthalmic: One drop may be applied to the affected eye(s) once daily.

ARGENTUM NITRATE

See Silver Nitrate.

ARTIFICIAL TEARS

See Hydroxyethyl Cellulose, Hydroxypropyl Cellulose, Hydroxypropyl Methylcellulose, Methylcellulose, Polyvinyl Alcohol.

---

*Route of administration not approved by FDA.
† Drug not approved by FDA for any indication.
‡ Drug not approved by FDA for this particular indication.
§ Indicated dosage above the manufacturer's recommendation.

ASCORBIC ACID (VITAMIN C)

Proprietary Names: Ascorbef (G.B.), Ascorbicap, Cebid, Cecon, Cetane, Cevalin, Cevi-Bid, Ce-Vi-Sol, Cevita, C-Span, Dull-C, Flavorcee, Roscorbic (G.B.), Vita-C.

Preparations

Injection: Solution 100, 250, and 500 mg/ml.
Oral: Capsules (timed-release), 500 mg; crystals, 4 gm/5 ml; liquid, 35 mg/0.6 ml; powder, 4 gm/5 ml; solution, 100 mg/ml; syrup 500 mg/5 ml; tablets, 50, 100, 250, 500, and 1000 mg; tablets (chewable), 100, 250, and 500 mg; tablets (timed-release), 0.5 and 1.5 gm.

Usual Dosages

Intramuscular, Intravenous, Oral: Adults, average protective dose is 70 to 150 mg daily. For scurvy, 0.3 to 1.0 gm daily is recommended. To enhance wound healing, 300 to 500 mg daily for 7 to 10 days both preoperatively and postoperatively are adequate. For severe burns, 1.0 to 2.0 gm daily are recommended until healing has occurred or grafting operations are complete.

ASPIRIN (ACETYLSALICYLIC ACID)

Proprietary Names: Acetophen (Canad.), Acetylin (Germ.), Acetyl-Sal (Canad.), Albyl-Selters (Swed.), Ancasal (Canad.), Apernyl (Swed.), Aquaprin (S. Afr.), A.S.A., Asadrine (Canad.), Asagran (G.B.), Aspasol (S. Afr.), Aspegic (Fr.), Aspergum, Aspirisucre (Fr.), Aspirjen, Aspisol (Austral.), Babiprin (Ire.), Bamyl (Swed.), Bayer Aspirin, Bi-prin (Austral.), Breoprin (G.B.), Buffinol, Caprin (G.B.), Cetasal (Canad.), Chu-Pax (G.B.), Claragine (Fr.), Clariprin (Austral.), Codral Junior (Austral.), Colfarit (Germ.), Disprill (Swed.), Ecotrin, Elsprin (Austral.), Entericin, Entrophen (Canad.), Extren, Godamed (Germ.), Infatabs A (Austral.), Instantine (Swed.), Ivepirine (Fr.), Juvepirine (Fr.), Levius (G.B.), Measurin, Monasalyl (Canad.), Neopirine-25 (Canad.), Nova-Phase (Canad.), Novasen (Canad.), Novosprin (Austral.), Nu-seals Aspirin (G.B.), Premaspin (Swed.), Prodol (Austral.), Provoprin-500 (Austral.), Rhonal (Canad., Fr.), Sal-Adult/Infant (Canad.), Seclopyrine (Fr.), Solcetas (Austral.), Solusal (Austral.), St. Joseph Aspirin, Supasa (Canad.), Tasprin-Sol (G.B.), Triaphen-10 (Canad.), Zorprin.

Preparations

Oral: Capsules, 325 mg; tablets, 65, 81, 162, 325, 500, and 650 mg; tablets (buffered),

325 mg; tablets (chewable), 81 mg; tablets (enteric-coated), 300 and 600 mg; tablets (timed-release), 650 mg.

Usual Dosages

Oral, Rectal: Range, 300 mg to 8 gm daily in divided doses; children, 11 to 130 mg/kg daily.

ASPIRIN/CAFFEINE/BUTALBITAL COMBINATION

Proprietary Names: B-A-C, Fiorinal, Isollyl, Lanorinal, Lorprn, Marnal.

Preparations

Oral: Capsules, 325 or 650 mg aspirin, 40 or 50 mg caffeine, and 40 or 50 mg butalbital; tablets, 325 or 650 mg aspirin, 40 or 50 mg caffeine, and 40 or 50 mg butalbital.

Usual Dosages

Oral: The usual adult dose is one or two tablets or capsules every 4 hours as needed for pain. Total daily dosage should not exceed six tablets or capsules.

ASPIRIN/CODEINE COMBINATION

Proprietary Names: Ascodeen, Ascriptin with Codeine, Codasa, Codasa Forte.

Preparations

Oral: Capsules, 300 mg aspirin with 15 mg codeine, 325 mg aspirin with 15 or 30 mg codeine, 560 mg aspirin with 30 mg codeine; tablets, 325 mg aspirin with 15 or 30 mg codeine.

Usual Dosages

Oral: Two capsules or tablets every 3 to 4 hours when necessary.

ASTEMIZOLE

Proprietary Name: Hismanal (Belg.).

---

* Route of administration not approved by FDA.
† Drug not approved by FDA for any indication.
‡ Drug not approved by FDA for this particular indication.
§ Indicated dosage above the manufacturer's recommendation.

Preparations

Oral: Tablets, 10 mg.

Usual Dosages

Oral: A single daily dose of 10 mg is recommended. In patients with severe symptoms, a regimen of 30 mg daily for 1 week, followed by 10 mg daily, may be employed.

ATROPINE

Proprietary Names: Atropair, Atropinol (Germ.), Atropisol, Atropt (Austral.), Atroptol (Austral.), BufOpto Atropine, Isopto Atropine, Ocu-Tropine, Spersatropine (S. Afr.).

Preparations

Topical Ophthalmic: Ointment, 0.5 and 1 per cent; solution, 1, 2, 3, and 4 per cent.

Usual Dosages

Topical Ophthalmic: One drop of 1 or 2 per cent atropine solution (or 1 per cent ointment) may be instilled one to three times daily. A stronger concentration or more frequent administration may be necessary in very severe inflammations. As the inflammation subsides, the frequency of administration may be reduced to twice weekly.

AURANOFIN

Proprietary Name: Ridaura.

Preparations

Oral: Capsules, 3 mg.

Usual Dosages

Oral: Initially, 6 mg daily administered as a single dose or in two divided doses. Dosage may be increased up to 9 mg daily.

AUROTHIOGLUCOSE

Proprietary Names: Aureotan (Germ.), Solganal.

Preparations

Injection: Suspension, 50 mg/ml.

Usual Dosages

Intramuscular: Adults, initially single weekly injections of 10 mg the first week, 25 mg the second week, 25 or 50 mg the third week, and 50 mg each week thereafter until a total dosage of 0.8 to 1 gm has been administered.

AZATADINE

Proprietary Names: Idulamine (Arg.), Indulian (Fr.), Optimine, Zadine (Austral.).

Preparations

Oral: Tablets, 1 mg.

Usual Dosages

Oral: Adults, 1 to 2 mg twice daily.

AZATHIOPRINE

Proprietary Names: Imuran, Imurek (Germ.), Imurel (Aust., Fr., Swed.).

Preparations

Injection: Powder (lyophilized) equivalent to 100 mg of azathioprine.
Oral: Tablets, 50 mg.

Usual Dosages

Intravenous, Oral: The dose must be individualized. The used initial dosage is 3 to 5 mg/kg once daily; maintenance, 1 to 4 mg/kg once daily.

AZIDOTHYMIDINE

See Zidovudine.

AZITHROMYCIN

Proprietary Name: Zithromax.

Preparations

Oral: Capsules, 250 mg.

---

*Route of administration not approved by FDA.
† Drug not approved by FDA for any indication.
‡ Drug not approved by FDA for this particular indication.
§ Indicated dosage above the manufacturer's recommendation.

Usual Dosages

Oral: 500 mg as a single dose on the first day followed by 250 mg once daily on days 2 through 5 for a total dose of 1.5 gm. The usual dose for infections due to *Chlamydia* is the equivalent of 1 gm as a single dose.

AZT

See Zidovudine.

AZTREONAM

Proprietary Names: Azactam (Austral., Ire., Fr., G.B., Ger., Ital., Neth., Span., Swed., Switz., USA), Primbactam (Ital.), Urobactam (Span.).

Preparations

Injection: Lyophilized powder, single-dose 500 mg/vial, 1 gm/vial, 2 gm/vial, 500 mg/bottle, 1 gm/bottle, 2 gm/bottle.

Usual Dosages

Intramuscular, Intravenous: Deep intramuscular injection or intravenously by slow injection over 3 to 5 minutes or infusion over 20 to 60 minutes. Doses range from 1 to 8 gm daily administered in divided doses every 6 to 12 hours according to the severity of the infection. Single doses over 1 gm should be administered by the intravenous route.

BACITRACIN

Proprietary Name: Baciguent.

Preparations

Injection: Powder, 10,000 and 50,000 units.
Topical: Ointment, 500 units/gm.
Topical Ophthalmic: Ointment, 500 units/gm.

Usual Dosages

Intramuscular: For infants under 2.5 kg, 900 units/kg in two to three divided doses. For infants over 2.5 kg, 1000 units/kg daily in two to three divided doses.
Topical: Ointment may be applied two to three times daily.
Topical Ophthalmic: Ointment is instilled in affected eye one to three times daily or more frequently. In severe infections, one drop of solution containing 10,000 units/ml is instilled every hour until improvement oc-

curs; the frequency of administration is then reduced.

Subconjunctival: 10,000 units in 0.5 ml of isotonic sodium chloride injection once or twice daily.

BACITRACIN/POLYMYXIN B COMBINATION

Proprietary Names: Ak-Poly-Bac Ocumycin.

Preparations

Topical Ophthalmic: Ointment, 500 units bacitracin and 10,000 units polymyxin B/gm.

Usual Dosages

Topical Ophthalmic: A small amount every 3 or 4 hours may be applied, depending on the severity of the infection.

BACLOFEN

Proprietary Name: Lioresal.

Preparations

Oral: Tablets, 10 mg, 20 mg.

Usual Dosages

Oral: Initially, 5 mg three times daily, increased by 15 mg daily every fourth day to 20 mg three times daily. The total daily dose should not exceed a maximum of 80 mg daily.

BALANCED SALT SOLUTION

Proprietary Name: BSS.

Preparations

Intraocular: Ophthalmic irrigation solution, 15, 30, 250, and 500 ml bottles.

Usual Dosages

Intraocular: An adequate amount is used to irrigate the ocular tissues.

---

* Route of administration not approved by FDA.
† Drug not approved by FDA for any indication.
‡ Drug not approved by FDA for this particular indication.
§ Indicated dosage above the manufacturer's recommendation.

BCG VACCINE

Proprietary Name: BCG Vaccine.

Preparations

Injection: Lyophilized vaccine reconstituted with 1 ml of sterile water for injection.

Usual Dosages

Intradermal: A dose of 0.1 ml is administered.

BCNU

See Carmustine.

BELLADONNA

Proprietary Names: Belladonna Extract, Leaf, or Tincture, Bellafolin (Germ.), Bellafoline (Fr.).

Preparations

Oral: Tablets, 15 mg.

Usual Dosages

Oral: 15 mg three times daily.

BENOXINATE

Proprietary Names: Cebesine (Fr.), Conjuncain (Germ.), Dorsacaine, Novesin (Switz.), Novesina (Ital.), Novesine (Austral., Belg., Fr., Germ., Neth.), Oftalmocaina (Arg.), Oxybuprocaine (G.B.), Poen Caina (Arg.).

Preparations

Topical Ophthalmic: Solution, 0.4 per cent.

Usual Dosages

Topical Ophthalmic: One drop of solution may be instilled and may be repeated for three doses if necessary.

BENZATHINE PENICILLIN G

Proprietary Names: Ben-P (Canad.), Bicillin, Dibencil, Duapen (Canad.), Dulpecen-G (Austral.), Extencilline (Fr.), LPG (Austral.), Neolin (G.B.), Penidural (G.B.), Penilente-LA (S. Afr.), Permapen, Tardocillin (Germ.).

Preparations

Injection: Powder; suspension, 300,000 and 600,000 units/ml.

Usual Dosages

Intramuscular: Adults, 1.2 million units in a single dose; older children, a single injection of 900,000 units; infants and children under 27.3 kg, a single dose of 300,000 to 600,000 units. For venereal infections in adults, 2.4 million units followed by one or two doses of 2.4 million units at 7-day intervals. For congenital syphilis in children under 2 years of age, 50,000 units/kg.

BENZYLPENICILLIN POTASSIUM

See Potassium Penicillin G.

BETA CAROTENE

Proprietary Name: Solatene.

Preparations

Oral: Capsules, 30 mg.

Usual Dosages

Oral: The usual adult dosage is 30 to 300 mg administered either as a single daily dose or in divided doses, preferably with meals.

BETAINE

Proprietary Names: Acidol-Pepsin, Somatyl (Fr., Ital.), Stea-16 (Belg.).

Preparations

Oral: Tablets, 388 mg betaine and 97 mg pepsin.

Usual Dosages

Oral: One to three tablets dissolved in a glass of water three times daily, preferably after meals.

---

*Route of administration not approved by FDA.
† Drug not approved by FDA for any indication.
‡ Drug not approved by FDA for this particular indication.
§ Indicated dosage above the manufacturer's recommendation.

BETAMETHASONE

Proprietary Names: Bentelan (Ital.), Betapred (Swed.), Betnelan (Austral.), Betnesol (G.B.), Celestan (Germ.), Celestene (Fr.), Celestona (Swed.), Celestone.

Preparations

Injection: Solution, 3 mg/ml.
Oral: Tablets, 0.6 mg; syrup, 0.6 mg/5 ml.
Topical: Cream, 0.01, 0.2, and 0.25 per cent.
Topical Ophthalmic: No preparation is commercially available. A 0.1 per cent solution may be prepared.

Usual Dosages

Intralesional: 1.5 to 6.0 mg, depending on the size of the affected area.
Oral: Maintenance dose, 0.5 to 1.2 mg daily; dose range, 0.6 to 8.4 mg daily.
Subconjunctival: 3 to 6 mg administered in 0.5 to 1 ml.
Topical: Formulations are applied sparingly in very thin films one to four times daily.
Topical Ophthalmic: One drop of a 0.1 per cent solution every 1 to 2 hours until a response is attained.

BETANIDINE

See Bethanidine.

BETAXOLOL

Proprietary Name: Betoptic.

Preparations

Topical Ophthalmic: Solution, 0.5 per cent.

Usual Dosages

Topical Ophthalmic: The usual dose is one drop in the affected eye(s) twice daily.

BETHANECHOL

Proprietary Names: Besacolin (Jap.), Duvoid, Iricoline (Fr.), Mechothane (G.B.), Mictrol, Myotonachol, Myotonine (G.B.), Urecholine, Uro-Carb (Austral.), Urolax, Vesicholine.

Preparations

Oral: Tablets, 5, 10, 25, and 50 mg.

Usual Dosages

Oral: Adult, 5 to 50 mg three or four times daily to maximum dosage of 120 mg.

BETHANIDINE (BETANIDINE)

Proprietary Names: Batel (Span.), Benzoxine (Jap.), Betaling (Jap.), Esbaloid (Canad.), Esbatal (Arg., Austral., Belg., G.B., Ital., Neth., S. Afr., Scand.), Eusmanid (Aust.), Hypersin (Jap.), Regulin (Scand.).

Preparations

Topical Ophthalmic: No ophthalmic preparation is commercially available in the United States.

Usual Dosages

Topical Ophthalmic: One drop of a 5 to 10 per cent solution twice daily.

BLEOMYCIN

Proprietary Names: Blenoxane, Bleo-S (Jap.), Oil Bleo (Jap.).

Preparations

Injection: Powder, 15 units.

Usual Dosages

Intramuscular, Intravenous, Subcutaneous: Because of the possibility of an anaphylactoid reaction, lymphoma patients should be treated with 2 units or less for the first two doses. If no reaction occurs, then 0.25 to 0.50 units/kg (10 to 20 units/square meter) may be given weekly or twice weekly.

BORIC ACID

Proprietary Name: Irigate.

Preparations

Topical Ophthalmic: Crystals; granules; ointment, 5 and 10 per cent; powder; solution, 2 and 5 per cent.

---

* Route of administration not approved by FDA.
† Drug not approved by FDA for any indication
‡ Drug not approved by FDA for this particular indication.
§ Indicated dosage above the manufacturer's recommendation.

Usual Dosages

Topical Ophthalmic: Solution or ointment is applied as required.

BOTULINUM A TOXIN

Proprietary Name: Oculinum.

Preparations

Injection: Powder (lyophilized), in 50-ng vials.

Usual Dosages

Intramuscular, Subcutaneous: Botulinim A toxin is diluted in normal saline without preservatives immediately before injection. To prevent breakdown of the toxin, the vial is turned gently, but should not be shaken. The usual dosage is a volume of 0.1 ml containing 0.025 to 5 units (1 unit = 1×10^{-5} μg) injected at six to ten separate sites per eye, or for a total volume of 2 ml or 20 injections per treatment. The total dose may vary in different individuals, but is usually between 12.5 and 75 units per eye.

BOTULISM ANTITOXIN

Proprietary Names: Botulinum Antiserum, Botulinus Antitoxin, Botulism Antitoxin Bivalent Type E, Trivalent Botulinus Antitoria.

Preparations

Injection: Solution containing 10,000 units of each type container (Antitoxin Bivalent Types A and B).

Usual Dosages

Intramuscular, Intravenous: Adults, 10,000 units of type A, B, and E antitoxin every 4 hours until the toxic condition has been alleviated. The antitoxin is diluted 1 : 10 with 10 per cent dextrose for injection before use. The first 10 ml is injected slowly over a 5-minute period; the remainder can be given more rapidly after 15 minutes.

BROMHEXINE

Proprietary Names: Aletor (Span.), Bisolvon (G.B.), Bromcilate (Span.), Brocokin (Ital.), Dakroy Biciron (Germ.), Ophtosol (Germ.).

Preparations

Oral: Elixir, 4 mg/5 ml; tablets, 8 mg.

Usual Dosages

Oral: The usual adult dose is 8 to 16 mg three or four times daily.

BROMOCRIPTINE

Proprietary Names: Parlodel, Pravidel (Germ., Swed.).

Preparations

Oral: Tablets, 2.5 mg.

Usual Dosages

Oral: Initially, 2.5 mg three or four times daily. The dose is increased weekly by increments of 2.5 mg over a period of 3 to 8 weeks until beneficial effects or intolerable adverse effects are noted. A total daily dose of 30 mg is generally considered minimal with a maximum daily amount of 150 mg.

BROMPHENIRAMINE

Proprietary Names: Dimegan (Fr.), Dimetane, Dimotane (G.B.), Ebalin (Germ.), Ilvin (Germ., Swed.), Rolabromophen, Symptom 3, Veltane.

Preparations

Oral: Solution, 2 mg/5 ml; tablets, 4 mg; tablets (extended-release), 8 and 12 mg.

Usual Dosages

Oral: The usual adult dosage is 4 to 8 mg three or four times daily. Alternatively, an extended-release formulation containing 8 or 12 mg may be administered every 8 to 12 hours.

BUPIVACAINE

Proprietary Names: Carbostesin (Germ.), Marcain (G.B.), Marcaine.

---

*Route of administration not approved by FDA.
† Drug not approved by FDA for any indication.
‡ Drug not approved by FDA for this particular indication.
§ Indicated dosage above the manufacturer's recommendation.

Preparations

Injection: Solution, 0.25, 0.5, and 0.75 per cent.

Usual Dosages

Injection: For retrobulbar block, 1.5 to 2 ml of a 0.5 or 0.75 per cent solution is injected inside the muscle cone behind the globe. Light pressure may be applied intermittently for 3 to 5 minutes after the injection.

BUPRENORPHINE

Proprietary Names: Buprenex, Temgesic (G.B., Norw.).

Preparations

Injection: Solution, 0.3 mg/ml in ampules of 1 and 2 ml.
Sublingual: Tablets, 200 µg.

Usual Dosages

Intramuscular, Intravenous: Adults, usual dosage is 0.3 mg given at intervals of up to every 6 hours.
Sublingual: The usual adult dosage is 200 µg.

BUPROPION

Proprietary Name: Wellbutrin.

Preparations

Oral: Tablets, 75 mg and 100 mg.

Usual Dosages

Oral: Initial dose of 100 mg twice daily by mouth. If necessary, this dose may be increased after at least 3 days to 100 mg three times daily. In severe cases, if no improvement has been observed after several weeks of therapy, the dose may be increased further to a maximum of 150 mg three times daily.

BUROW'S SOLUTION

See Aluminum Acetate.

CALAMINE

Proprietary Name: Calamine.

Preparations

Topical: Lotion.

Usual Dosages

Topical: A sufficient amount of lotion to cover the affected area is applied twice daily.

CALCIFEDIOL

Proprietary Names: Calderol, Dédrogyl (Fr.), Hidroferol (Span.).

Preparations

Oral: Capsules, 20 and 50 μg.

Usual Dosages

Oral: Usual doses are 50 to 125 μg daily.

CALCITONIN

Proprietary Names: Calcimar, Calcitar (Fr., Ital., Jap.), Calcitare (G.B.), Cacitonina (Ital.), Calsyn (Fr.), Calsynar (G.B.), Cibacalcin (Neth., N.Z.), Miacalcic (Austral., G.B., Norw., N.Z., Swed.), Salcatonin (G.B.), Staporox (Fr.).

Preparations

Injection: Lyophilized powder, 400 MRC units/vial with 4 ml of gelatin as diluent. The final volume should be approximately 0.5 to 1.0 ml.

Usual Dosages

Intramuscular: For hypercalcemia, 100 to 400 MRC units once or twice daily.
Intramuscular, Subcutaneous: For Paget's disease, adults, initially 50 to 100 MRC units daily or three times a week until a satisfactory clinical or biochemical response is obtained. For maintenance, 50 MRC units three times a week. In patients who relapse, larger doses should be tried, but do not consistently improve the clinical response.

CALCITRIOL (1α,25 DIHYDROXYVITAMIN D₃)

Proprietary Name: Rocaltrol.

---

* Route of administration not approved by FDA.
† Drug not approved by FDA for any indication.
‡ Drug not approved by FDA for this particular indication.
§ Indicated dosage above the manufacturer's recommendation.

Preparations

Oral: Capsules, 0.25 μg.

Usual Dosages

Oral: The recommended initial dose is 0.25 μg daily. If a satisfactory response is not observed, dosage may be increased by 0.25 μg daily at 2- to 4-week intervals.

CALCIUM CARBONATE

Proprietary Names: Alka-2, Alka-Mints, Amitone, Calcilac, Calcileve (Fr.), Calglycine, Cal-tab (Austral.), Chooz, Dicarbosil, El-Da-Mint, Equilet, Mallamint, Os-Cal 500, Spar-Cal (Austral.), Spentacid, Titracid, Titralac, Trialka, Tums.

Preparations

Oral: Powder, tablets, 0.65 and 1.25 gm; tablets (chewable), 330, 350, 420, 500, 750, and 850 mg.

Usual Dosages

Oral: Adults, 1 to 2 gm three times daily with meals. The powdered preparation is mixed with water or sprinkled on food.

CALCIUM CHLORIDE

Proprietary Name: Chloro-Calcion (Fr.).

Preparations

Injection: Solution 5 and 10 per cent.
Oral: Powder.

Usual Dosages

Intravenous (Slow): Adults, 10 to 30 ml of a 5 per cent solution.
Oral: Adults, 4 to 8 gm daily in four divided doses, given with demulcent. Children, 300 mg/kg of a 2 per cent solution given daily in four divided doses.

CALCIUM CITRATE

Proprietary Name: Citracal.

Preparations

Oral: Tablets, 950 mg.

Usual Dosages

Oral: The usual dosage is 0.95 to 1.9 gm three to four times daily.

CALCIUM EDETATE

See Edetate Calcium Disodium.

CALCIUM GLUBIONATE

Proprietary Name: Neo-Calglucon.

Preparations

Oral: Solution, 1.8 gm/5 ml.

Usual Dosages

Oral: Adults, 20 gm daily in divided doses.

CALCIUM GLUCONATE

Proprietary Names: Sandocal (G.B.), Vical (Ital.), Weifa-Kalk (Norw.).

Preparations

Injection: Powder; solution, 10 per cent.
Oral: Tablets, 325, 500, 650 mg, and 1 gm.

Usual Dosages

Intravenous: Adults, initially, 20 ml of a 10 per cent solution injected slowly, followed by a slow infusion of a 0.3 to 0.8 per cent solution over a period of 3 to 12 hours. Children, 500 mg/kg daily in divided doses.
Oral: Adults, 15 gm daily in divided doses. Children, 500 mg/kg daily in divided doses.

CALCIUM LACTATE

Proprietary Name: Calcium Lactate.

Preparations

Oral: Powder; tablets, 325 and 650 mg.

---

*Route of administration not approved by FDA.
† Drug not approved by FDA for any indication.
‡ Drug not approved by FDA for this particular indication.
§ Indicated dosage above the manufacturer's recommendation.

Usual Dosages

Oral: Adults, 1.5 to 3 gm three times daily with meals. Children, 500 mg/kg daily in divided doses.

CAPSAICIN

Proprietary Names: Axsain, Zostrix.

Preparations

Topical: Cream, .025 and .075 per cent.

Usual Dosages

Topical: Cream may be applied to affected area three to four times daily.

CARBACHOL

Proprietary Names: Carbacel, Isopto Carbachol, Isopto-Karbakolin (Swed.), Miostat, Mistura, PV Carbachol (Canad.).

Preparations

Topical Ophthalmic: Solution, 0.75, 1.5, 2.25, and 3 per cent.

Usual Dosages

Topical Ophthalmic: The frequency and concentration of instillation depend upon the patient's response to therapy.

CARBAMAZEPINE

Proprietary Names: Tegretal (Germ.), Tegretol.

Preparations

Oral: Tablets, 200 mg.

Usual Dosages

Oral: Adults and adolescents; initial 400 mg in two divided doses on first day, increased by 200 mg daily with the total dose divided into three or four equal portions. Doses up to 1.6 gm daily have been used in adults in rare instances. Children under 6 years, 100 mg daily initially; 6 to 12 years, 100 mg twice daily initially.

CARBENICILLIN

Proprietary Names: Anabactyl (Germ.), Carbapen (Austral.), Fugacillin (Swed.), Geocillin, Geopen, Microcillin (Germ.), Pyopen.

Preparations

Injection: Powder, 1, 2, 5, and 10 gm.
Oral: Tablets equivalent to 382 mg.

Usual Dosages

Intramuscular: Adults, 1 to 2 gm every 6 hours. Children, 50 to 200 mg/kg daily in divided doses every 4 to 6 hours.
Intravenous: For septicemia and severe systemic, respiratory, or soft tissue infections, adults, 300 to 500 mg/kg daily; children, 400 to 500 mg/kg daily. The drug can be administered in divided doses every 4 to 6 hours or by continuous or intermittent infusion. The recommended maximum intravenous dose is 40 gm per day.
Subconjunctival: 100 to 250 mg in 0.5 ml of isotonic sodium chloride injection or sterile water for injection.

CARBIDOPA/LEVODOPA COMBINATIONS

Proprietary Name: Sinemet.

Preparations

Oral: Tablets 10 or 25 mg carbidopa and 100 or 250 mg levodopa.

Usual Dosages

Oral: The suggested initial dosage is one tablet of Sinemet-10/100 three times daily. The amount may be increased gradually by one tablet every day or every other day up to six tablets daily. If a larger dose is needed, one table to Sinemet-25/250 three times daily may be administered.

CARBONIC ANHYDRASE INHIBITORS

See Acetazolamide, Dichlorphenamide, Ethoxzolamide, Methazolamide.

---

* Route of administration not approved by FDA.
† Drug not approved by FDA for any indication.
‡ Drug not approved by FDA for this particular indication.
§ Indicated dosage above the manufacturer's recommendation.

CARBOXYMETHYLCELLULOSE

Proprietary Name: Celluvisc.

Preparations

Topical Ophthalmic: Solution, 1 per cent.

Usual Dosages

Topical Ophthalmic: One to two drops as needed.

CARMUSTINE (BCNU)

Proprietary Name: BiCNU.

Preparations

Injection: Powder, 100 mg and 3 ml diluent.

Usual Dosages

Intravenous: The recommended dose as a single agent in previously untreated patients is 200 mg/square meter every 6 weeks. This may be given as a single dose or divided into daily injections, such as 100 mg/square meter on 2 successive days. When used in combination with other myelosuppressive drugs, dosage should be adjusted accordingly.

CARTEOLOL

Proprietary Names: Arteolol (Span.), Arteoptic (Ger., Switz.), Carteol (Fr., Ital.), Cartrol, Endak (Ger.), Mikelan (Fr., Jap., S. Afr., Span.), Ocupress, Teoptic (G.B.).

Preparations

Topical Ophthalmic: Solution 1 and 2 per cent.

Usual Dosages

Topical Ophthalmic: One drop of solution may be applied to each eye twice daily.

CEFACLOR

Proprietary Names: Ceclor, Distaclor (G.B.), Panoral (Germ.).

Preparations

Oral: Capsules, 250 and 500 mg; powder (for suspension), 125 and 250 mg/5 ml.

Usual Dosages

Oral: Adults, 250 mg every 8 hours; for severe infections, this amount may be increased to a maximum of 4 gm daily. Children, 20 to 40 mg/kg daily in equally divided doses every 8 hours.

CEFAZOLIN

Proprietary Names: Ancef, Celmetin (Swed.), Kefzol.

Preparations

Injection: Powder, 0.25, 0.5, and 1.0 gm and bulk (5 and 10 gm).
Topical Ophthalmic: No commercial preparations are available. Fortified cefazolin eyedrops can be prepared from the powder.

Usual Dosages

Intramuscular, Intravenous: Adults, 250 and 500 mg every 8 hours; in severe infections, 0.5 to 1.5 gm may be given every 6 hours. Children and infants over 1 month of age, 25 to 100 mg/kg daily in three of four divided doses. Doses of 0.5 to 1.0 gm every 12 hours may be given for pneumococcal pneumonia or acute uncomplicated urinary tract infections in either adults or children. Patients with impaired renal function should receive reduced dosages.
Intravitreal: 1.0 to 2.25 mg in 0.1 to 0.2 ml suspension.
Retrobulbar: 0.5 to 1.0 ml of a suspension containing 100 mg/ml.
Subconjunctival: 50 to 100 mg in 0.5 ml of isotonic sodium chloride injection or sterile water for injection.
Topical Ophthalmic: One drop of a solution containing 40 to 50 mg/ml every hour until improvement occurs; then reduce frequency.

CEFOTAXIME

Proprietary Name: Claforan.

---

*Route of administration not approved by FDA.
† Drug not approved by FDA for any indication.
‡ Drug not approved by FDA for this particular indication.
§ Indicated dosage above the manufacturer's recommendation.

Preparations

Injection: Powder, 1, 2, and 10 gm/vial.

Usual Dosages

Intramuscular, Intravenous: Adults, 2 to 12 gm daily in equally divided doses every 4 to 6 hours. The usual dosage for moderate to severe infections is 1 to 2 gm every 8 hours. The maximum daily dosage should not exceed 12 gm.

CEFOXITIN

Proprietary Names: Mefoxin, Mefoxitin (Denm., Germ., Swed., Switz.).

Preparations

Injection: Powder (equivalent to base), 1 and 2 gm.

Usual Dosages

Intramuscular, Intravenous: The usual adult dosage range is 1 to 2 gm every 6 to 8 hours. For life-threatening infections, 2 gm every 4 hours or 3 gm every 6 hours.

CEFTAZIDIME

Proprietary Names: Fortaz, Tazicef, Tazidime.

Preparations

Injection: Powder, 0.5, 1.0, and 2.0 gm/vial.

Usual Dosages

Intramuscular, Intravenous: The usual recommended dose is 1 gm every 8 to 12 hours.

CEFTIZOXIME

Proprietary Name: Cefizox.

Preparations

Injection: Powder, 1 or 2 gm in 28-, 50-, and 100-ml vials.

Usual Dosages

Intramuscular, Intravenous: Adults, 2 to 12 gm daily in equally divided doses every 8 to

12 hours. Children (6 months or older), 150 to 200 mg/kg daily in equally divided doses every 6 to 8 hours.

CEFTRIAXONE

Proprietary Name: Rocephin.

Preparations

Injection: Powder, 0.25, 0.5, 1, 2, and 10 gm.

Usual Dosages

Intramuscular, Intravenous: Adults, usual dose is 1 to 2 gm once daily (or in equally divided doses every 12 hours). The total daily dose should not exceed 4 gm. For uncomplicated gonococcal infections, 250 mg intramuscularly as a single dose may be administered.

CEFUROXIME

Proprietary Names: Curoxim (Ital.), Itorex (Ital.), Kefurox, Ultroxim (Ital.), Zinacef.

Preparations

Injection: Powder, 0.75, 1.5, and 7.5 gm/ vial.
Oral: Tablets, 125, 250, and 500 mg.

Usual Dosages

Intramuscular, Intravenous: Adults, 2.25 to 9.0 gm daily in equally divided doses every 8 hours. Infants and children over 3 months, 50 to 100 mg/kg daily in equally divided doses every 6 to 8 hours.
Oral: Adults and children 12 years of age and over, 250 mg every 12 hours. For severe infections or infections caused by less susceptible organisms, 500 mg every 12 hours may be used.

CELLULOSE, OXIDIZED

See Oxidized Cellulose.

CEPHALEXIN

Proprietary Names: Ceporex (G.B.), Ceporexine (Fr., Swed.), Keflex, Oracef (Germ.).

---

* Route of administration not approved by FDA.
† Drug not approved by FDA for any indication.
‡ Drug not approved by FDA for this particular indication.
§ Indicated dosage above the manufacturer's recommendation.

Preparations

Oral: Capsules, 250 and 500 mg; drops (pediatric), 100 mg/ml (after reconstitution); suspension, 125 and 250 mg/5 ml (after reconstitution).

Usual Dosages

Oral: The daily dose should not exceed 4 gm because of possible renal damage. In adults, 250 mg every 6 hours is recommended; children, 25 to 50 mg/kg in four divided doses. For severe infections, this dose may be doubled. If more than 4 gm is needed, a parenteral cephalosporin preparation should be substituted.

CEPHALORIDINE

Proprietary Names: Ceporan (Austral., Canad., S. Afr., Swed.), Ceporin (G.B.), Keflodin (Fr.), Kefspor (Germ., Swed.), Loridine.

Preparations

Injection: Powder, 0.5 and 1 gm.

Usual Dosages

Intracameral, Intravitreal: 250 μg in 0.1 to 0.2 ml of isotonic sodium chloride injection.
Intramuscular, Intravenous: The daily dose should not exceed 4 gm because of possible renal damage. Adults, 0.5 to 1.0 gm three or four times a day at equally spaced intervals. Children, 30 to 50 mg/kg daily, preferably intramuscular, in three divided doses at equally spaced intervals. These routes should not be used in premature or full-term infants less than 1 month old. Since large doses may produce tubular necrosis, appropriate reduction in dosage should be made in patients with impaired renal function. Mixing with solutions containing other antibiotics is not recommended.
Subconjunctival: 50 to 100 mg in 0.5 ml of isotonic sodium chloride injection or sterile water for injection.
Topical Ophthalmic: One drop of solution containing 50 to 100 mg/ml is instilled every hour until improvement occurs. The frequency of administration is then reduced.

CEPHALOTHIN

Proprietary Names: Cefalotine (Fr.), Cepovenin (Germ.), Keflin.

Preparations

Injection: Powder, 0.25, 0.5, 1, 2, and 4 gm.
Topical Ophthalmic: No ophthalmic form is

available, but a solution for topical use can be made from the powder.

Usual Dosages

Intramuscular, Intravenous: Adults, 1 to 2 gm every 4 to 6 hours; children, 200 mg/kg daily in four divided doses; premature and full-term newborn infants, 100 mg/kg daily in four divided doses.

Subconjunctival: 50 to 100 mg in 0.5 ml of isotonic sodium chloride injection or sterile water for injection.

Topical Ophthalmic: One drop of solution containing 50 to 100 mg/ml every hour until improvement occurs; then frequency is reduced.

CEPHAPIRIN

Proprietary Names: Ambrocef (Ital.), Ambrotina (Ital.), Brisfirina (Span.), Brisporin (Ital.), Bristocef (Germ.), Cefadyl, Cefaloject (Fr.), Cefatrexil (Arg.), Cefatrexyl (Austral., Belg., Jap., N.Z., Switz.).

Preparations

Injection: Powder, 1, 2, 4, and 20 gm.

Usual Dosages

Intramuscular, Intravenous: Adults, 0.5 to 1.0 gm every 4 to 6 hours; in severe infections, up to 12 gm daily in divided doses. Children, 40 to 80 mg/kg in four equally divided doses.

CEPHRADINE

Proprietary Names: Anspor, Cefril (S. Afr.), Eskacef (G.B.), Sefril (Germ.), Velosef.

Preparations

Injection: Powder, 0.025, 0.250, 0.5, 1, 2, and 4 gm.

Oral: Capsules, 250 and 500 mg; suspension, 125 and 250 mg/5 ml.

Usual Dosages

Intramuscular, Intravenous: Adults, 2 to 4 gm daily in equally divided doses every 6

---

*Route of administration not approved by FDA.

† Drug not approved by FDA for any indication.

‡ Drug not approved by FDA for this particular indication.

§ Indicated dosage above the manufacturer's recommendation.

hours. In severe infections, the dose may be increased to a maximum of 8 gm. Infants and children, 50 to 100 mg/kg daily in equally divided doses every 6 hours.

Oral: Adults, 250 to 500 mg every 6 hours or 0.5 to 1.0 gm every 12 hours. Severe infections may require large doses. Infants over 9 months and children, 25 to 50 mg/kg daily in four divided doses. The maximum daily dose should not exceed 4 gm.

CHLORAL HYDRATE

Proprietary Names: Aquachoral, Chloradorm (Austral.), Chloralate (Austral.), Chloraldurat (Germ.), Chloralex (Canad.), Chloralix (Austral.), Chloralixir (Canad.), Chloralvan (Canad.), Chloratol (Canad.), Cohidrate, Dormel (Austral.), Eudorm (Austral.), Felsules, H.S. Need, Kessodrate, Lanchloral (Austral.), Maso-Chloral, Nigracap (Canad.), Noctec, Novochlorhydrate (Canad.), Oradrate, Rectules, SK-Chloral Hydrate.

Preparations

Oral: Capsules, 225, 250, 450, and 500 mg, elixir; syrup, 250 and 500 mg/5 ml.

Rectal: Suppositories, 60, 120, 300, 460, 500, 600, and 900 mg.

Usual Dosages

Oral, Rectal: As sedative, adults, 250 mg three times daily after meals. As hypnotic, adults, 0.5 to 1.0 gm 15 to 30 minutes before bedtime. The daily dosage for adults should not exceed 2 gm.

CHLORAMBUCIL

Proprietary Names: Chloraminophene (Fr.), Leukeran.

Preparations

Oral: Tablets, 2 and 5 mg.

Usual Dosages

Oral: The usual dosage is 0.1 to 0.2 mg/kg daily for 3 to 6 weeks as required.

CHLORAMPHENICOL

Proprietary Names: Ak-Chlor, Amphicol, Antibiopto, Aquamycetin (Germ.), Bipimycetin (Ind.), Catilan (Germ.), Chlomin (Austral.), Chloramex (S. Afr.), Chloramol (Austral.), Chloramphycin (Ind.), Chloramsaar (Germ.),

Chlorcetin, Chlorcol (S. Afr.), Chlornicol (S. Afr.), Chlorofair, Chloromycetin, Clorfen (S. Afr.), Cloroptic, Cylphenicol, Econochlor, Enicol (Canad.), Fenicol (Canad.), Gotimycin (Germ.), Jatcetin (S. Afr.), Kamaver (Germ.), Kemicetin (G.B.), Kemicetine, Lennacol (S. Afr.), Leukomycin (Germ.), Mychel, Mycinol (Canad.), Nevimycin (Germ.), Novochlorocap (Canad.), Ocu-Chlor, Oleomycetin (Germ.), Opclor (Austral.), Ophthochlor, Pantovernil (Germ.), Paraxin, Pentamycetin (Canad.), Sintomicetine (Fr.), Solnicol (Fr.), Tifomycine (Fr.), Troymycetin (S. Afr.).

Preparations

Oral: Capsules, 50, 100, and 250 mg.
Topical Ophthalmic: Ointment, 1 per cent; solution, 0.5 per cent.

Usual Dosages

Intracameral, Intravitreal: 1 to 2 mg in 0.2 to 0.5 ml of isotonic sodium chloride injection.
Intravenous: Adults, 50 mg/kg daily in divided doses every 6 to 8 hours. Oral therapy should replace intravenous administration as soon as possible. This drug should not be used parenterally in children except to initiate therapy for meningitis or severe sepsis, when 100 mg/kg daily can be given.
Oral: Adults, children, and infants over 2 weeks of age, 50 mg/kg daily in divided doses every 6 to 8 hours. In patients in whom the half-life of the drug may be increased (e.g., those with impaired liver function), the interval between doses may have to be increased. Premature infants, 25 mg/kg daily in divided doses every 4 to 6 hours. For all infants, it is advisable to monitor chloramphenicol blood levels frequently and, ideally, to maintain the blood level of drug between 10 and 20 μg/100 ml.
Subconjunctival: 1.25 to 2 mg in 0.5 ml of isotonic sodium chloride injection.
Topical Ophthalmic: For severe conjunctivitis or corneal ulcers, one drop of a 0.5 per cent aqueous solution every 30 minutes. For mild conjunctivitis, one drop of a 0.5 per cent aqueous solution is applied at 1- to 2-hour intervals or ointment is instilled three to four times daily.

CHLORDIAZEPOXIDE

Proprietary Names: A-Poxide, Brigen-G, Calmoden (G.B.), Chemdipoxide (Canad.),

---

* Route of administration not approved by FDA.
† Drug not approved by FDA for any indication.
‡ Drug not approved by FDA for this particular indication.
§ Indicated dosage above the manufacturer's recommendation.

Chlordiazachel, Corax (Canad.), C-Tran (Canad.), Diapax (Canad.), Elenium (Pol.), Libritabs, Librium, Lo Tense, Medilium (Canad.), Menrium, Murcil, Nack (Canad.), Novopoxide (Canad.), Protensin (Canad.), Relaxil (Canad.), Risolid (Swed.), Screen, SK-Lygen, Solium (Canad.), Tenex, Trilium (Canad.), Tropium (G.B.), Via-Quil (Canad.), Zetran.

Preparations

Injection: Powder, 100 mg in 5 ml in dry-filled containers.
Oral: Capsules, 5, 10, and 25 mg; tablets, 5, 10, and 25 mg.

Usual Dosages

Intramuscular, Intravenous: 50 to 100 mg, repeated in 2 to 4 hours or given three to four times daily, if necessary.
Oral: 10 to 100 mg daily in three of four divided doses.

CHLOROQUINE

Proprietary Names: Aralen, Arechin (Pol.), Avoclor (G.B.), Chlorocon, Chlorquin (Austral.), Malaquin (Austral.), Malarex (Denm.), Malarivon (G.B.), Nivaquine (G.B.), Resochin (G.B.), Roquine, Siragan (Aust.), Tresochin (Swed.).

Preparations

Injection: Solution, 50 mg/ml (equivalent to 40 mg of base).
Oral: Tablets, 500 mg (equivalent to 300 mg of base).

Usual Dosages

Intramuscular, Oral: 150 to 900 mg of chloroquine base daily in divided doses.

CHLOROTHIAZIDE

Proprietary Names: Diuril, Diurilix (Fr.), Flumen (Ital.), Minzil (Ital.), Salisan (Denm.), Saluren (Ital.), Saluric (G.B.), SK-Chlorothiazide, Yadalan (Span.).

Preparations

Oral: Suspension, 250 mg/5 ml; tablets, 250 and 500 mg.

Usual Dosages

Oral: Adults, intially, 500 mg twice daily. Children, 20 mg/kg daily in two divided doses.

CHLORPHENIRAMINE

Proprietary Names: Alermine, Allerbid, Allergex (Austral., S. Afr.), Allergisan (Swed.), Allerhist (S. Afr.), Allertab, Al-R, Antagonate, Ardehist, Barachlor, Chestamine, Chlo-Amine, Chlor-4/100, Chloraman, Chloramate, Chloramin (Austral.), Chloren, Chlormene, Chlorohist, Chlorophen, Chloroton, Chlorpen, Chlor-Span, Chlortab, Chlor-Trimeton, Chlor-Tripolon (Canad.), Chlortrone (Canad.), Cosea, Drize, Haynon (G.B.), Histacon, Histadur, Histaids (Austral.), Histalon (Canad.), Histaspan, Histex, Histol, H-Stadur, Lorphen, Malachlor, Nasahist, Niratron, Panahist, Phenetron, Piranex (Austral.), Piriton (G.B.), Pyranistan, Rhinihist, Teldrin, Trymegen.

Preparations

Oral: Capsules (extended-release), 6 and 12 mg; solution, 2 mg/5 ml; tablets, 4 mg; tablets (timed-release), 8 and 12 mg.

Usual Dosages

Oral: Adults, 2 to 4 mg three or four times daily (tablets, syrup), or 8 to 12 mg one to three times daily (timed-release form).

CHLORPROMAZINE

Proprietary Names: Chloractil, Chlor-Promanyl (Canad.), Chlorprom-Ez-Ets (Canad.), Chlorzine, Elmarine (Canad.), Hibernal (Swed.), Klorazin (S. Afr.), Klorazine, Klorpromex (Swed.), Komazine, Largactil, Megaphen (Germ.), Onazine (Canad.), Plegomazine (Austral.), Procalm (Austral.), Promachel, Promachlor, Promacid (Austral.), Promapar, Promaz, Promosol (Canad.), Psychozine, Serazone (Austral.), Sonazine, Terpium, Thoradex, Thorazine.

Preparations

Injection: Solution, 25 mg/ml.
Oral: Capsules (sustained-release), 30, 75, 150, 200, and 300 mg; concentrate, 30 and 100

---

*Route of administration not approved by FDA.

† Drug not approved by FDA for any indication.

‡ Drug not approved by FDA for this particular indication.

§ Indicated dosage above the manufacturer's recommendation.

mg/ml; syrup, 10 mg/5 ml; tablets, 10, 25, 50, 100, and 200 mg.
Rectal: Suppositories, 25 and 100 mg.

Usual Dosages

Intramuscular: For emesis in adults, 25 mg initially, which may be increased to 50 mg and repeated every 3 to 4 hours if necessary; children, 0.5 mg/kg every 4 to 6 hours. For acute psychosis in hospitalized adults, 25 to 100 mg initially, repeated in 1 to 4 hours as necessary.
Oral: For emesis in adults, 10 to 25 mg every 4 to 6 hours; children, 0.5 mg/kg every 4 to 6 hours. For severe psychosis in adults, a daily dosage of 200 to 600 mg initially in divided doses may be administered and increased if necessary (maximum 2 gm daily); children, 0.5 mg/kg every 4 to 6 hours.
Rectal: For emesis, adults, 50 to 100 mg every 6 to 8 hours; children, 1 mg/kg every 6 to 8 hours. For psychosis in children, 1 mg/kg every 6 to 8 hours.

CHLORPROPAMIDE

Proprietary Names: Chloromide (Canad.), Chloronase (Canad., Germ.), Diabetal (Swed.), Diabetoral (Germ.), Diabett, Diabines (Swed.), Diabinese, Melitase (G.B.), Novopropamide (Canad.), Stabinol (Canad.).

Preparations

Oral: Tablets, 100 and 250 mg.
Rectal: Suppositories, 25 and 100 mg.

Usual Dosages

Oral: Dosage must be individualized. The usual range is 100 to 500 mg daily (maximum, 750 mg).
Rectal: Adults, 50 to 100 mg every 6 to 8 hours; children, 1 mg/kg every 6 to 8 hours.

CHLORTETRACYCLINE

Proprietary Names: Aureomycin, Aureomycine (Fr.), Chlortet (Austral.), CTC, Topmycin (S. Afr.).

Preparations

Injection: Powder, 500 mg buffered with sodium glycinate.
Oral: Capsules, 50, 100, and 250 mg.
Topical Ophthalmic: Ointment, 1 per cent.

Usual Dosages

Intravenous: Adults, 500 mg every 6 to 12 hours, restricted to total daily dose of 2 gm for initiation of treatment or for very severe infections; children 10 to 20 mg/kg daily divided into two doses.

Oral: Adults, 250 to 500 mg every 6 hours (loading dose of 1 gm may be used); children, 25 to 50 mg/kg daily in four doses.

Topical Ophthalmic: Ointment applied three or four times daily.

CHLORTHALIDONE

Proprietary Names: Hygroton, Igroton (Ital.), Uridon (Canad.).

Preparations

Oral: Tablets, 50 and 100 mg.

Usual Dosages

Oral: Adults, initially 50 to 100 mg daily or 100 mg on alternate days or three times weekly; some patients may require a dose of 200 mg.

CHOLECALCIFEROL (VITAMIN D₃)

Proprietary Names: D-Muslin (Germ.), Provitina D₃ (Germ.), Ultar "D", Vigorsan D₃ (Germ.).

Preparations

Oral: Capsules, 0.25 and 1 μg.

Usual Dosages

Oral: Dosage must be individualized, but the following daily intakes are recommended: infants under 1 year, 7.5 μg; children 1 to 4 years, 10 μg; in pregnancy and lactation, 10 μg.

CHOLESTYRAMINE RESIN

Proprietary Names: Cuemid (Austral., Germ., Scand.), Quantalan (Aust., Germ., Port., Switz.), Questran.

Preparations

Oral: Powder or 9-gm packets containing 4 gm of cholestyramine resin.

---

* Route of administration not approved by FDA.

† Drug not approved by FDA for any indication.

‡ Drug not approved by FDA for this particular indication.

§ Indicated dosage above the manufacturer's recommendation.

Usual Dosages

Oral: Adults, 10 to 16 gm of resin daily in divided doses.

CHOLINE

Proprietary Name: Neurotropan (Germ.).

Preparations

Oral: Powder; tablets, 250 mg.

Usual Dosages

Oral: Adults, initially 1 gm four times daily, with the amount gradually increased over a 3- to 8-week period to a maximum of 4 to 5 gm four times daily.

CHYMOTRYPSIN

Proprietary Names: Alpha Chymar, Alphacutanee (Fr.), Aphlozyme (Fr.), Catarase, Chymar (G.B.), Chymar-Zon (G.B.), Enzeon, Kimopsin (Austral., Jap.), Quimotrase (Canad.), Zolyse, Zonulyn (Canad.), Zonulysin (G.B.).

Preparations

Injection: Powder (lyophilized), 750 units (1 mg) with 5 ml of diluent; two-compartment vial containing lyophilized powder, 300 units in lower compartment and sodium chloride injection 2 ml in upper compartment.

Topical Ophthalmic: No preparation is commercially available. A solution of 750 units dissolved in 5 ml of solvent may be prepared.

Usual Dosages

Intracameral: For enzymatic zonulolysis in intracapsular lens extraction, 0.2 to 0.5 ml of a freshly prepared 1 : 5000 or 1 : 10,000 solution is injected slowly behind the iris into the posterior chamber. One to two minutes after injection of the enzyme, the anterior chamber should be irrigated with 2 ml of the diluent, sodium chloride injection, or a balanced salt solution.

Topical Ophthalmic: Solution may be applied three to four times daily.

CIMETIDINE

Proprietary Name: Tagamet.

Preparations

Oral: Tablets, 200, 300, 400, and 800 mg.

Usual Dosages

Oral: The usual dosage is 300 to 400 mg two to four times daily, usually given with or immediately after meals and at bedtime for 3 to 6 weeks.

CIPROFLOXACIN

Proprietary Names: Baycip (Span.), Cetraxal (Span., Ital.), Ciflox (Fr., Ital.), Ciloxan, Cipro, Ciprobay (Ger., S. Afr.), Ciproxin (Austral., G.B., Ire., Ital., Neth., Swed.), Ciproxine (Switz.), Cunesin (Span.), Flociprin (Ital.), Rigoran (Span.), Septocipro (Span.), Velmonit (Span.).

Preparations

Injection: 200 and 400 mg.
Oral: Tablets, 250, 500, and 750 mg.
Topical Ophthalmic: Solution, 0.3 per cent.

Usual Dosages

Intravenous: 100 to 400 mg twice daily
Oral: 250 to 750 mg twice daily.
Topical Ophthalmic: For corneal ulcer, two drops into affected eye every 15 minutes for the first 6 hours and then two drops into the affected eye every 30 minutes for the remainder of the first day. On second day, instill two drops in the affected eye hourly. On the third through fourteenth day, place two drops in the affected eye every 4 hours. For bacterial conjunctivitis, one to two drops into conjunctival sac every 2 hours while awake for 2 days and one to two drops every 4 hours while awake for the next 5 days.

CISPLATIN

Proprietary Names: Cisplatyl (Fr.), Neoplatin (G.B.), Platinex (Germ.), Platinol.

Preparations

Injection: Powder (lyophilized), 10 mg/vial.

---

*Route of administration not approved by FDA.
† Drug not approved by FDA for any indication.
‡ Drug not approved by FDA for this particular indication.
§ Indicated dosage above the manufacturer's recommendation.

Usual Dosages

Intravenous: When given as a single agent, 100 mg/square meter once every 4 weeks.

CLINDAMYCIN

Proprietary Names: Cleocin, Dalacin C (G.B.), Sobelin (Germ.).

Preparations

Injection: Solution, 150 mg/ml.
Oral: Capsules, 75 and 150 mg; granules for suspensions, 75 mg/5 ml.
Topical Ophthalmic: No ophthalmic preparation is commercially available. Fortified clindamycin eyedrops may be prepared in a concentration of 50 mg/ml.

Usual Dosages

Intramuscular: Adults, 0.6 to 2.7 gm daily in two, three, or four equally divided doses; children over 1 month of age, 15 to 40 mg/kg in three or four equally divided doses.
Intravenous: Adults, 0.6 to 2.7 gm daily in two, three, or four equally divided doses; children over 1 month of age, 15 to 25 mg/kg in three or four equally divided doses.
Intravitreal: 0.1 to 1.0 mg in 0.1 to 0.2 ml of sterile solution for injection.
Oral: Adults, 150 to 450 mg every 6 hours (capsules) or 8 to 25 mg/kg daily in three or four divided doses (granules). For children 10 kg or less, 37.5 mg three times daily is minimum dose.
Subconjunctival: 15 to 40 mg in a 0.5 ml aqueous solution.
Topical Ophthalmic: One drop of a solution containing 50 mg/ml clindamycin may be given every 1 to 4 hours.

CLOBETASOL

Proprietary Names: Butavat (Gr.), Clobesol (Ital.), Dermadex (Arg.), Dermatovate (Mex.), Dermoval (Fr.), Dermovat (Scand.), Dermovate (G.B.), Dermoxin (Germ.), Dermoxinate (Germ.), Psorex (Nig.), Temovate.

Preparations

Topical: Cream, 0.05 per cent; ointment, 0.05 per cent.

Usual Dosages

Topical: Cream or ointment is applied to affected area twice daily.

CLOBETASONE

Proprietary Names: Emovat (Denm.), En-ovate (Neth.), Eumovate (G.B.).

Preparations

Topical Ophthalmic: Solution, 0.1 per cent.

Usual Dosages

Topical Ophthalmic: One to two drops are applied to affected eye(s) two or three times daily.

CLOFAZIMINE

Proprietary Name: Lamprene.

Preparations

Oral: Capsules, 100 mg.

Usual Dosages

Oral: 100 to 300 mg daily, up to 1.2 gm daily has been given when required.

CLOFIBRATE

Proprietary Names: Aterosol (Swed.), Atheromide (Jap.), Atheropront (Germ.), Atromidin (Swed.), Atromid-S, Claresan (rR.), Lipavlon (Fr.), Liprinal (G.B.), Recolip (Swed.), Regelan (Germ.), Skleromexe (Germ.).

Preparations

Oral: Capsules, 500 mg.

Usual Dosages

Oral: Adults, 500 mg two to four times daily.

CLONAZEPAM

Proprietary Names: Clonopin, Iktorivil (Swed.), Rivotril (G.B.).

---

* Route of administration not approved by FDA.
† Drug not approved by FDA for any indication.
‡ Drug not approved by FDA for this particular indication.
§ Indicated dosage above the manufacturer's recommendation.

Preparations

Oral: Tablets, 0.5, 1, and 2 mg.

Usual Dosages

Oral: Adults, initially 1.5 mg daily in three divided doses. Dosage then may be increased by increments of 0.5 to 1 mg every third day until seizures are adequately controlled or adverse effects intervene (maximum, 20 mg daily).

CLORAZEPATE

Proprietary Names: Clorazecaps, Clora-zetabs, Gen-Xene, Nansius (Span.), Novoclo-pate (Canad.), Transene (Ital.), Tranxene (Austral., Canad., Fr., G.B., Neth., S. Afr., U.S.A.), Tranxilen (Swed.), Tranxilium (Ger., Span., Switz.).

Preparations

Oral: Tablets, 3.75, 7.5, 15, 22.5, and 11.25 mg.

Usual Dosages

Oral: Usual daily dose is 30 mg, adjusted gradually within the range of 15 to 60 mg. May be administered as a single dose of 15 mg at bedtime. Maximum daily dosage is 90 mg.

CLOTRIMAZOLE

Proprietary Names: Canastene (Belg.), Canesten (G.B.), Empecid (Arg., Jap.), Eparol (Germ.), Lotrimin, Mycelex, Panmicol (Arg.), Trimysten (Fr.).

Preparations

Oral: Powder.
Topical: Cream, 1 per cent; solution, 1 per cent.
Topical Ophthalmic: No ophthalmic preparation is commercially available. A 1 per cent solution in arachnis oil may be prepared by dissolving in chloroform, mixing with arachnis oil, and driving off the chloroform by heat. A 1 per cent suspension may also be obtained by mixing 10 mg of powder with 1 ml of artificial tears to form a suspension that must be shaken before each instillation to re-suspend the drug.

Usual Dosages

Oral: Up to 54 mg/kg daily.
Topical: Sufficient amount of cream or so-

lution to cover infected and surrounding area is applied twice daily.

Topical Ophthalmic: Drops may be instilled every 4 hours.

CLOXACILLIN

Proprietary Names: Austrastaph (Austral.), Clocillin (Jap.), Cloxapen, Cloxypen (Fr.), Ekvacillin (Swed.), Orbenin, Orbenine (Fr.), Prostaphlin-A (S. Afr.), Staphobristol (Germ.), Staphybiotic (Fr.), Tegophen.

Preparations

Oral: Capsules, 250 and 500 mg; powder for solution, 125 mg/5 ml.

Usual Dosages

Oral: Adults and children weighing 20 kg or more, 0.25 to 1.0 gm every 4 to 6 hours.

COAL TAR

Proprietary Name: Coal Tar.

Preparations

Topical: Ointment, 1, 4, and 5 per cent.

Usual Dosages

Topical: A 1 to 5 per cent concentration of coal tar in zinc oxide paste, petrolatum, or a washable base is applied two or three times daily.

COCAINE

Proprietary Name: Cocaine.

Preparations

Topical: No pharmaceutical dosage form is available; compounding by pharmacist is necessary.

Topical Ophthalmic: Solution, 4 and 10 per cent.

---

*Route of administration not approved by FDA.

† Drug not approved by FDA for any indication.

‡ Drug not approved by FDA for this particular indication.

§ Indicated dosage above the manufacturer's recommendation.

Usual Dosages

Topical: For temporary paralysis, a 10 per cent solution is placed on small cotton pledgets and applied to the nasal or punctal mucosa. No more than 200 mg should be used in a 70-kg patient over a 30-minute period.

Topical Ophthalmic: One or two drops of solution may be instilled and repeated. Care must be taken to remove excess in the fornices to prevent nasal absorption.

CODEINE

Proprietary Names: Codicept (Germ.), Codlin (Austral.), Paveral (Canad.), Tricodein (Germ.).

Preparations

Injection: Tablets (hypodermic), 15, 30, and 60 mg.

Oral: Tablets (triturates), 15, 30, and 60 mg.

Usual Dosages

Intramuscular, Oral, Subcutaneous: Adults, 30 to 60 mg four to six times daily as necessary. Children, 0.5 mg/kg four to six times daily.

COLCHICINE

Proprietary Names: Aqua-Colchin (Austral.), Colcin (Austral.), Colchineos (Fr., S. Afr.), Colgout (Austral.), Coluric (Austral.).

Preparations

Injection: Solution, 0.5 mg/ml.

Oral: Granules, 0.5 mg; tablets, 0.5 and 0.6 mg.

Usual Dosages

Intravenous: Acute attacks, 1 or 2 mg initially, followed by 0.5 mg every 3 to 6 hours as necessary (single treatment not to exceed 4 mg).

Oral: Adults, 1 or 1.2 mg initially, followed by 0.5 or 0.6 mg every 2 hours (maximum daily dose of 7 or 8 mg).

COLESTIPOL

Proprietary Name: Colestid.

Preparations

Oral: Powder in 5-gm packets and 500-gm bottles with scoop providing 5 gm/scoop.

Usual Dosages

Oral: Adults, 15 to 30 gm daily given with meals in two to four divided doses.

COLISTIMETHATE

Proprietary Names: Colimycine (Fr.), Colistinat (Swed.), Colistin Sulphomethate (G.B.), Coly-Mycin (Austral.), Colomycin Injection (G.B.), Coly-Mycin M.

Preparations

Injection: Powder equivalent to 150 mg colistin base.
Topical Ophthalmic: No ophthalmic form is available, but solution for topical use (1.5 to 3 mg/ml) can be made from powder.

Usual Dosages

Intramuscular, Intravenous: Adults, 2.5 to 5 mg/kg daily in two to four divided doses. Children, 5 mg/kg daily maximum, 300 mg in four divided doses. Premature and full-term newborn infants, 2.5 mg/kg daily in four divided doses.
Subconjunctival: 15 to 20 mg in 0.5 mg of isotonic sodium chloride injection or sterile water for injection. Doses as large as 37.5 mg have been used occasionally.
Topical Ophthalmic: One drop of a solution containing 1.5 to 3 mg/ml is instilled every 10 minutes for severe infections and every 1 to 4 hours for mild infections.

COLISTIN

Proprietary Names: Colimycine (Fr.), Colomycin (G.B.), Coly-Mycin (Austral.), Coly-Mycin S.

Preparations

Oral: Powder, 300 mg providing the equivalent of 25 mg of colistin base/5 ml when suspended in 37 ml of distilled water.
Topical Ophthalmic: Lyophilized powder

---

* Route of administration not approved by FDA.
† Drug not approved by FDA for any indication.
‡ Drug not approved by FDA for this particular indication.
§ Indicated dosage above the manufacturer's recommendation.

for solution equivalent to 5 to 10 mg colistin base dissolved in 1 ml.

Usual Dosages

Oral: Infants and children, 3 to 5 mg/kg daily in three divided doses.
Topical Ophthalmic: One to two drops every 1 to 2 hours, day and night. The frequency of administration can be reduced as the infection clears.

COLLAGEN, HEMOSTATIC

See Hemostatic Collagen.

CORTICOTROPIN (ACTH)

Proprietary Names: Acortan (Germ.), Acthar, Acthelea (Arg.), Acton (Swed.), Actonar (Arg.), Cortrophin, Depot-Acethropan (Germ.), Durackin (Canad.), Reacthin (Swed.).

Preparations

Injection: Gel (repository), 40 and 80 units/ml; powder (lyophilized), 25 and 40 units; solution, 20 units/ml.

Usual Dosages

Intramuscular, Subcutaneous: For therapeutic use, 40 units of aqueous solution daily in four divided doses (10 units every 6 hours), or 40 units of gel (repository) or aqueous suspension with zinc hydroxide (repository) every 12 to 24 hours.
Intravenous: A continuous 48-hour infusion (40 units every 12 hours) may be given.

CORTISONE

Proprietary Names: Adricort, Cortal (Swed.), Cortate (Austral.), Cortelan (G.B.), Cortemel (S. Afr.), Cortilen (Ital.), Cortistab (G.B.), Cortistan, Cortisyl (G.B.), Cortogen (S. Afr.), Cortone, Pantisone.

Preparations

Injection: Suspension, 25 and 50 mg/ml.
Oral: Tablets, 5, 10, and 25 mg.
Topical Ophthalmic: Ointment, 1.5 per cent; suspension, 2.5 and 5.0 per cent.

Usual Dosages

Intramuscular: For anti-inflammatory effects, 75 to 300 mg daily for serious disease.

Oral: For anti-inflammatory effects, 25 to 50 mg daily for mild chronic diseases. In acute, life-threatening disease, 125 to 300 mg daily in at least four divided doses.

Subconjunctival: 0.5 ml of a 2.5 per cent suspension.

Topical Ophthalmic: One drop of a 0.5 per cent suspension every 1 to 2 hours until a response is obtained; the frequency then is reduced. For severe conditions, a 1.5 or 2.5 per cent suspension may be used. The ointment preparation is applied three or four times daily or as a nighttime medication when the suspension is used during the day.

COUMARIN DERIVATIVES

See Dicumarol, Warfarin.

CREDE'S SOLUTION

See Silver Nitrate.

CROMOLYN SODIUM

Proprietary Names: Opticrom, Opticron (Fr.).

Preparations

Oral: Capsules, 100 mg.
Topical Ophthalmic: Solution, 2 and 4 per cent.

Usual Dosages

Oral: The usual dosage is 400 to 800 mg equally divided in four doses.
Topical Ophthalmic: One or two drops in each eye four to six times daily at regular intervals.

CRYSTALLINE PENICILLIN

See Potassium Penicillin G, Sodium Penicillin G.

CYCLIZINE

Proprietary Names: Marezine, Marzine (G.B.), Valoid (G.B.).

Preparations

Injection: Solution, 50 mg/ml.
Oral: Tablets, 50 mg.

Usual Dosages

Intramuscular: Adults, 50 mg every 4 to 6 hours.
Oral: Adults, 50 mg repeated every 4 to 6 hours up to 200 mg daily. Children 6 to 12 years of age, 25 mg up to three times daily.

CYCLOGUANIL PAMOATE

Proprietary Name: Camolar (G.B.).

Preparations

Injection: Oily injection containing equivalent of 140 mg of cycloguanil base in each ml.

Usual Dosages

Intramuscular: Adults, equivalent of 350 mg or 5 to 6 mg/kg cycloguanil base every 3 or 4 months; children up to 4 years, 140 mg; children 5 to 10, 280 mg.

CYCLOPENTOLATE

Proprietary Names: Ak-Pentolate, Ciclolux (Ital.), Cyclogyl, Cyclopen (Austral.), Cyplegin (Jap.), Mydplegic (Canad.), Mydrilate (G.B.), Ocu-Pentolate, Pentolair, Zyklolat (Germ.).

Preparations

Topical Ophthalmic: Solution, 0.5, 1.0, and 2.0 per cent.

Usual Dosages

Topical Ophthalmic: One drop of 0.5 or 1.0 per cent solution will sustain mydriasis/cycloplegia for approximately 24 hours. In patients with darkly pigmented irides, 2 per cent solution may be necessary.

CYCLOPHOSPHAMIDE

Proprietary Names: Cytoxan, Endoxan (Austral., Fr., Germ., S. Afr.), Endoxana (G.B.), Enduxan (Braz.), Genoxal (Span.), Procytox (Canad.), Sendoxan (Norw., Swed.).

Preparations

Injection: Powder, 100, 200, and 500 mg.
Oral: Tablets, 25 and 50 mg.

Usual Dosages

Intravenous, Oral: The initial loading dose is 40 to 50 mg/kg intravenously or 1 to 5 mg/kg orally. Maintenance dosage may be started as soon as the leukocyte count returns to 3000 to 4000 cells/cubic meter. One to 5 mg/kg orally daily, 10 to 15 mg/kg intravenously every 7 to 10 days, or 3 to 5 mg/kg intravenously twice weekly may be used.

CYCLOSPORINE (CYCLOSPORIN A)

Proprietary Name: Sandimmune.

Preparations

Injection: Solution, 50 mg/ml cyclosporine with 650 mg of polyoxyethylated castor oil and 32.9 per cent alcohol.
Oral: Solution, 100 mg/ml of cyclosporine with 12.5 per cent alcohol.

Usual Dosages

Intravenous: Initially, 5 to 6 mg/kg daily.
Oral: Initially, 15 mg/kg daily, tapered to maintenance level of 5 to 10 mg/kg daily.

CYPROHEPTADINE

Proprietary Names: Antegan (Austral.), Nuran (Germ.), Periactin, Periactinol (Germ.), Vimicon (Canad.).

Preparations

Oral: Syrup, 2 mg/5 ml; tablets, 4 mg.

Usual Dosages

Oral: Adults, 4 to 20 mg daily in divided doses. Dosage must be individualized and should not exceed 0.5 mg/kg daily.

---

* Route of administration not approved by FDA.
† Drug not approved by FDA for any indication.
‡ Drug not approved by FDA for this particular indication.
§ Indicated dosage above the manufacturer's recommendation.

CYPROTERONE ACETATE

Proprietary Name: Androcur (Denm., G.B., Germ., Ital., Neth., Norw., Span., Swed., Switz.).

Preparations

Oral: Tablets, 50 mg.

Usual Dosages

Oral: The usual dose is 50 mg twice daily, increased if necessary after 4 weeks to 200 or 300 mg daily in divided doses until a response is achieved.

CYSTEINE

Proprietary Name: Cysteine.

Preparations

Topical Ophthalmic: Eyedrops containing 1.5 per cent cysteine are prepared by adding 1.5 gm cysteine and 10 mg benzalkonium chloride in iso-osmotic solution to 100 ml.

Usual Dosages

Topical Ophthalmic: Preparation may be applied up to four times daily.

CYTARABINE

Proprietary Names: Alexan (Belg., Germ.), Aracytine (Fr.), Cytosar.

Preparations

Injection: Powder (lyophilized), 100 and 500 mg with diluent.

Usual Dosages

Intramuscular, Subcutaneous: For maintenance of remissions, 1 mg/kg weekly.
Intravenous Infusion: 0.5 to 1 mg/kg daily infused for any desired period (1, 4, 12, or 24 hours) for 10 days, increased to 2 mg/kg until remission or hematologic toxicity.
Intravenous Injection (Rapid): 2 mg/kg daily for 10 days, increased to 4 mg/kg daily if no hematologic depression; continue until remission or hematologic toxicity.

DACARBAZINE

Proprietary Name: DTIC-Dome.

Preparations

Injection: Powder, 100 and 200 mg.

Usual Dosages

Intravenous: 2 to 4.5 mg/kg daily for 10 days every 28 days or 250 mg/square meter daily for 5 days every 3 weeks.

DACTINOMYCIN

Proprietary Name: Cosmegen.

Preparatopms

Injection: Powder, 0.5 mg with 20 mg of mannitol per vial.

Usual Dosages

Intravenous: Adults, 0.5 mg daily for a maximum of 5 days; single weekly doses of 2 mg for 3 weeks have been tolerated; children, 0.015 mg/kg daily for 5 days (maximum dose, 0.5 mg). Alternatively, a total dose of 2.4 mg/square meter may be given over a 1-week period to adults or children at monthly intervals.

DANAZOL

Proprietary Names: Cylomen (Canad.), Danatrol (Belg., Fr., Switz.), Danocrine, Danokrin (Aust.), Danol (G.B.), Ladogar (S. Afr.), Winobanin (Germ.).

Preparations

Oral: Capsules, 200 mg.

Usual Dosages

Oral: 300 to 600 mg daily with a break of 5 to 7 days every 7 days for treatment of hereditary angioedema.

DANTROLENE

Proprietary Name: Dantrium.

---

*Route of administration not approved by FDA.
† Drug not approved by FDA for any indication.
‡ Drug not approved by FDA for this particular indication.
§ Indicated dosage above the manufacturer's recommendation.

Preparations

Oral: Capsules, 25, 50, 75, and 100 mg.

Usual Dosages

Oral: Initial 25 mg twice daily, increased to three to four times daily and then to 100 mg or, rarely, 200 mg four times daily. Children, similar approach with 1 mg/kg once or twice daily; maximum dose is 100 mg four times daily.

DAPSONE

Proprietary Name: Avlosulfon.

Preparations

Oral: Tablets, 25 and 100 mg.

Usual Dosages

Oral: Adults, first and second weeks, 25 mg twice weekly; third and fourth weeks, 50 mg twice weekly; thereafter, 50 mg daily. A maintenance dosage of 100 to 200 mg daily also has been used. Children, 0.35 mg/kg administered in the same schedule as adults.

DAUNORUBICIN

Proprietary Names: Cerubidin (G.B.), Cerubidine, Daunoblastin (Germ.), Daunoblastina (Ital.), Ondena (Germ.).

Preparations

Injection: Powder for solutions, in vials containing the equivalent of 20 mg of daunorubicin.

Usual Dosages

Intravenous: 1 mg/kg at intervals of 1 to 4 days or 2 mg/kg at intervals of 4 to 7 days, depending on type of neoplasm.

DEFEROXAMINE

Proprietary Names: Desferal, Desferrioxamine (G.B.).

Preparations

Injection: Powder (lyophilized), 500 mg.
Topical Ophthalmic: No ophthalmic preparation is commercially available. Eyedrops

may be prepared by dissolving 500 mg in a sterile vehicle containing 0.5 per cent methylcellulose, 1 per cent benzyl alcohol, and water for injection to 5 ml. A 5 per cent ophthalmic ointment may be prepared in a base of cetyl alcohol, wool fat, white soft paraffin, and liquid paraffin.

Usual Dosages

Intramuscular, Intravenous: An initial dose of 1 gm should be administered at a rate not to exceed 15 mg/kg/hour. This may be followed by 0.5 gm every 4 hours for two doses; subsequent doses of 0.5 gm may be necessary every 4 to 12 hours. Total amount administered should not exceed 6 gm in a 24-hour period.

Subconjunctival: For iron deposits in the deeper layers of the cornea and in the iris and lens, 0.5 ml of a 10 per cent solution is injected twice a week for 8 to 10 weeks.

Topical Ophthalmic: For treatment of superficial iron deposits in the cornea, a 10 per cent solution of deferoxamine in 1 per cent methylcellulose is used four times daily for several weeks. Alternatively, the drug may be applied in a 5 per cent concentration in any ointment base.

DEMECARIUM

Proprietary Names: Humorsol, Tosmilen (G.B.).

Preparations

Topical Ophthalmic: Solution, 0.125 and 0.25 per cent.

Usual Dosages

Topical Ophthalmic: The frequency and concentration of instillation depend upon the patient's response to therapy.

DESMOPRESSIN

Proprietary Names: Dav Ritter (Switz.), DDAVP, Minirin (Austral., Germ., Ital., Norw., Swed.), Minurin (Denm.).

Preparations

Intranasal: Solution, 0.1 mg/ml.

Usual Dosages

Intranasal: The usual dosage range in adults is 0.1 to 0.4 ml daily, either as a single dose or divided into two or three doses.

DESONIDE

Proprietary Names: Apolar (Norw., Swed.), Locapred (Fr.), PR 100 (Ital.), Prenacid (Ital.), Reticus (Ital.), Sine-Fluor (Span.), Steroderm (Ital.), Tridesilon, Tridesonit (Fr.).

Preparations

Topical: Cream, 0.05 per cent; ointment, 0.05 per cent.

Usual Dosages

Topical: Preparation is applied two or three times daily or is used under occlusive dressings.

DEXAMETHASONE

Proprietary Names: Acidocort (Fr.), Ak-Dex, Auxiloson (Germ.), Auxison (Aust., Fr.), Carulon (Jap.), Cebedex (Fr.), Corson (Jap.), Cortisumman (Germ.), Dalaron, Decacort (Swed.), Decadron, Decaesadril (Ital.), Decaject, Decameth, Decasone (Austral.), Decasterolone (Ital.), Decofluor (Ital.), Dectan (Jap.), Dectancyl (Fr.), Deksone, Delladec, Deronil, Desacort (Ital.), Desacortone (Ital.), Desalark (Ital.), Desameton (Ital.), Deseronil (Ital.), Dethamedin (Jap.), Dexacen, Dexacortal (Swed.), DexaCortisyl (Austral., G.B.), Dexair, Dexamed (Germ.), Dexamethadrone (Canad.), Dexaport, Dexa-Scheroson (Germ.), Dexa-Sine (Germ.), Dexasone, Dexinolon (Germ.), Dexmethsone (Austral.), Dexon, Dexone, Dezone, Egocort (Austral.), Fluormone (Ital.), Fluorocort (Ital.), Fortecortin (Germ.), Hexadrol, Isopto-Maxidex (Swed.), Luxazone (Ital.), Maxidex, Metasolon (Jap.), Millicorten (Germ.), Miral, Moco (Jap.), Ocu-Dex, Oradexon (Austral, G.B.), Orgadrone (Jap.), Penthasone (Canad.), Predni-F (Germ.), Savacort-D, Sawasone (Jap.), SK-Dexamethasone, Soludecadron (Fr.), Solurex, Spersadex (Germ., S. Afr.), Tendron.

Preparations

Injection: Solution, 24 mg/ml.
Injection (Subconjunctival): Solution, 0.1 per cent.
Oral: Elixir, 0.5 mg/5 ml; tablets, 0.25, 0.5, 0.75, and 1.5 mg.
Topical Ophthalmic: Ointment, 0.05 per cent; suspension, 0.1 per cent.

Usual Dosages

Intravenous, Oral: The initial dosage varies from 0.5 to 9 mg daily. Doses higher than 9 mg may be required in severe diseases.
Retrobulbar: 0.5 to 1.0 ml of a solution containing 4 mg/ml.
Subconjunctival: 0.5 ml of a 0.1 per cent solution.
Topical Ophthalmic: One drop of a 0.1 per cent suspension every 1 to 2 hours until a response is obtained. Alternatively, the ointment may be instilled three or four times daily initially and once or twice daily for maintenance.

DEXTRAN (LOW MOLECULAR WEIGHT)

Proprietary Names: Dextraven (G.B.), Gentran, Hyskon, LMD, LMWD, Lomodex (G.B.), Macrodex, Perfadex (Swed.), Rheomacrodex, Rheotran.

Preparations

Injection: Solution, 10 per cent.

Usual Dosages

Intravenous: 10 to 20 ml/kg should be administered; the first 500 ml rapidly infused with the remainer given more slowly. Total daily dose should not exceed 20 ml/kg. If therapy is longer than 24 hours, daily dose should not exceed 10 ml/kg.

DEXTROTHYROXINE

Proprietary Names: Biotirmone (Fr.), Choloxin, Debetrol (Fr.), Dethyron (Denm.), Dynothel (Germ.), Nadrothyron (Germ.).

Preparations

Oral: Tablets, 1, 2, 4, and 6 mg.

Usual Dosages

Oral: Adults, initial daily dose should be 1 to 2 mg, increased in 1- to 2-mg increments at intervals of not less than 1 month to a maximum level of 4 to 8 mg daily.

*Route of administration not approved by FDA.
† Drug not approved by FDA for any indication.
‡ Drug not approved by FDA for this particular indication.
§ Indicated dosage above the manufacturer's recommendation.

DFP

See Isoflurophate.

DHPG

See Ganciclovir.

DHT

See Dihydrotachysterol.

DIAZEPAM

Proprietary Names: Aliseum (Ital.), Alupram (G.B.), Ansiolin (Ital.), Antenex (Austral.), Anxicalm (Ire.), Apozepam (Swed.), Atensine (G.B., Ire.), Benzopin (S. Afr.), Betapam (S. Afr.), Calmigen (Ire.), Diaceplex (Span.), Dialar (G.B.), Diaquel (S. Afr.), Diazemuls (Austral., Canad., G.B., Ger., Ire., Neth.), Doval (S. Afr.), Drenian (Span.), Ducene (Austral.), Eridan (Ital.), Ethipam (S. Afr.), Evacalm (G.B.), Lamra (Ger.), Mandro-Zep (Ger.), Meval (Canad.), Neurolytril (Ger.), Noan (Ital.), Novazam (Fr.), Novodipam (Canad.), Paceum (Switz.), Pax (S. Afr.), Pro-Pam (Austral.), Psychopax (Switz.), Rimapam (G.B.), Scriptopam (S. Afr.), Sico Relax (Span.), Solis (G.B.), Stesolid (G.B., Neth., Span., Swed., Switz.), Tensium (G.B.), Tranquirit (Ital.), Tranquo (Ger.), Valaxona (Ger.), Valiquid (Ger.), Valitran (Ital.), Valium (Austral., Canad., Fr., G.B., Ger., Ire., Ital., Neth., S. Afr., Span., Swed., Switz., USA), Valrelease, Vatran (Ital.), Vivol (Canad.).

Preparations

Injection: Solution, 5 mg/ml.
Oral: Tablets, 2, 5, and 10 mg.

Usual Dosages

Intramuscular, Intravenous: Adults, 5 to 10 mg initially; this dose may be repeated in 2 to 4 hours if necessary, up to a maximum of 30 mg in 8 hours. Children, 0.05 to 0.2 mg/kg initially, repeated in 3 to 4 hours if necessary. The dose should not exceed 0.5 mg/kg in an 8-hour period.
Oral: Adults, 4 to 40 mg in divided doses or single dose of 2.5 to 10 mg at bedtime. Children over 12 years of age, 0.12 to 0.8 mg/kg daily, divided into three or four doses.

DIBROMOPROPAMIDINE

Proprietary Names: Brolene (Austral., G.B., S. Afr.).

Preparations

Topical Ophthalmic: Ointment, 0.15 per cent.

Usual Dosages

Topical Ophthalmic: A small quantity is applied to the affected eye(s) one to two times daily.

DICHLORPHENAMIDE

Proprietary Names: Daranide, Oralcon (Swed.), Oratrol.

Preparations

Oral: Tablets, 50 mg.

Usual Dosages

Oral: The usual initial adult dose is 100 to 200 mg, followed by 100 mg every 12 hours until the desired response is obtained. Maintenance dosage in adults is usually 25 to 50 mg one to three times daily.

DICLOFENAC

Proprietary Names: Aflamin (Ital.), Blesin (Jap.), Dichronic (Jap.), Neriodin (Jap.), Prophenatin (Jap.), Seecoren (Jap.), Sofarin (Jap.), Tsudohmin (Jap.), Voltaren (Arg., Belg., Denm., Germ., Ital., Jap., Neth., Span., Switz.), Voltarene (Fr.), Voltarol (G.B.).

Preparations

Oral: Tablets, 25 and 50 mg.
Topical Ophthalmic: 0.1 per cent solution, 2.5 and 5 ml.

Usual Dosages

Oral: 25 to 50 mg three times daily.
Topical Ophthalmic: 24 hours after surgery, four times daily for 2 weeks.

DICLOXACILLIN

Proprietary Names: Constaphyl (Germ.), Dichlor-Stapenor (Germ.), Diclocil (Fr., S.

---

* Route of administration not approved by FDA
† Drug not approved by FDA for any indication.
‡ Drug not approved by FDA for this particular indication.
§ Indicated dosage above the manufacturer's recommendation.

Afr.), Diclocila (Swed.), Dycill, Dynapen, Pathocil, Stafopenin (Swed.), Veracillin.

Preparations

Injection: Vials, 250 mg.
Oral: Capsules, 125, 250, and 500 mg; suspension 62.5 mg/5 ml.

Usual Dosages

Intramuscular: Adults and children weighing 40 kg or more, 125 to 250 mg every 6 hours; less than 40 kg, 12.5 to 25 mg/kg daily in four equal doses.
Oral: Adults and children weighing 40 kg or more, 125 to 250 mg every 6 hours; less than 40 kg, 12.5 to 25 mg/kg daily in four equal doses.

DICUMAROL (DICOUMAROL)

Proprietary Names: AP (Swed.), Dufalone (Canad.).

Preparations

Oral: Capsules, 25, 50, and 100 mg; tablets, 25, 50 and 100 mg.

Usual Dosages

Oral: Adults, 200 to 300 mg on the first day, followed by 25 to 200 mg daily, using prothrombin time determinations as a guide.

DIDANOSINE

Proprietary Name: Videx.

Preparations

Oral: Chewable buffered tablets, 25, 50, 100, and 150 mg.
Injection: Powder, 100, 167, 250, and 375 mg.

Usual Dosages

Oral, Injection: Recommended starting dose is 125 mg to 300 mg dependent on weight, with a dosing interval of 12 hours.

DIETHYLCARBAMAZINE

Proprietary Names: Banocide, Carbilazine (Austral.), Ethodryl (G.B.), Franocide, Hetrazan, Notezine (Fr.).

Preparations

Oral: Tablets, 50 mg.

Usual Dosages

Oral: 2 to 4 mg/kg three times daily for 1 to 4 weeks.

DIGITALIS

Proprietary Names: Digifortis, Digiglusin, Digiplex (Fr.), Digitalysat (Germ.), Pil-Digis.

Preparations

Oral: Capsules, 100 mg; tablets, 100 mg; tincture, 100 mg/ml.

Usual Dosages

Oral: Adults, initially, 1.2 to 1.5 mg over a period of 24 to 48 hours; maintenance dose, 100 mg daily.

DIHYDROTACHYSTEROL (DHT, VITAMIN D₁)

Proprietary Names: AT-10 (G.B.), Atecen (Swed.), Calcamine (Fr.), Dihydral (Belg., Neth., Span.), Dygratyl (Denm., Swed.), Hytakerol.

Preparations

Oral: Capsules, 0.125 mg; solution (in oil), 0.25 mg/ml; tablets, 0.125, 0.2, and 0.4 mg.

Usual Dosages

Oral: Adults, initially 0.75 to 2.5 mg daily; specific dosage is determined by frequent estimations of serum calcium levels. For maintenance, 0.25 to 1.75 mg weekly has been given. Larger doses may be required for some patients.

DIHYDROXYACETONE

Proprietary Names: Chromelin, Dy-O-Derm, Vitadye.

---

*Route of administration not approved by FDA.
† Drug not approved by FDA for any indication.
‡ Drug not approved by FDA for this particular indication.
§ Indicated dosage above the manufacturer's recommendation.

Preparations

Topical: Solution, 5 per cent; suspension, 5 per cent.

Usual Dosages

Topical: Solution or suspension is applied to depigmented patches of skin. This may give rise to patchy appearance, which is rectified by repeated application.

1α,25 DIHYDROXYVITAMIN D₃

See Calcitriol.

DIIODOHYDROXYQUIN (DIIODOHYDROXYQUINOLINE)

Proprietary Names: Diodoquin, Direxiode (Austral., Fr.), Embequin (G.B.), Floraquin, Florequin (Swed.), Ioquin (Fr.), Moebiquin, Panaquin, Vaam-DHQ (Austral.), Yodoxin.

Preparations

Oral: Powder; tablets, 210 and 650 mg.

Usual Dosages

Oral: The usual adult dosage is 630 to 650 mg three times daily; a daily dose of 2 gm should not be exceeded.

DIMENHYDRINATE

Proprietary Names: Amosyt (Swed.), Andrumin (Austral.), Aviomarine (Pol.), Dramamine, Dramavol (Canad.), Dymenol (Canad.), Epharetard (Germ.), Gravol (G.B.), Neo-Metic (Canad.), Novodimenate (Canad.), Novomina (Germ.), Prevenause (Canad.), Travamine (Canad.), Vomex A (Germ.), Vomital (Canad.).

Preparations

Injection: Solution, 50 mg/ml.
Oral: Liquid, 12.5 mg/4 ml; tablets, 50 mg.
Rectal: Suppositories, 100 mg.

Usual Dosages

Intramuscular: Adults, 50 mg as needed; children 5 mg/kg divided into four doses during a 24-hour period (maximum, 300 mg/day).
Intravenous: Adults, 50 mg diluted in 10

ml of sodium chloride injection and injected over a period of 2 minutes.

Oral: Adults, 50 to 100 mg every 4 hours; children, 25 to 50 mg three times daily.

Rectal: Adults, 100 mg once or twice daily.

DIMETHYL SULFOXIDE (DMSO)

Proprietary Names: Domoso, Rimso-50.

Preparations

Injection: Solution, 50 per cent.

Usual Dosages

Intravesical: 50 ml of a 50 per cent solution may be instilled slowly by catheter directly into the bladder.

DINITROCHLOROBENZENE

Proprietary Name: Dinitrochlorobenzene.

Preparations

Topical: No topical preparations are commercially available.

Usual Dosages

Topical: Initially, 2 mg may be applied to the skin to induce a systemic hypersensitivity reaction. Later, much smaller quantities are applied to the tumor to induce local reaction and necrosis.

DIPHENHYDRAMINE

Proprietary Names: Alericap (Austral.), Allerdryl, Baramine, Bax, Benachior, Benadryl, Benahist, Ben-Allergin, Bendylate, Benhydramil (Canad.), Bentrac, Benylin, Bonyl, Bidramine (Austral.), Dabylen (Germ.), Desentol (Swed.), Dihydral (S. Afr.), Diphen-Ex, Dhydramine (S. Afr.), Eldadryl, Fenylhist, Histergan (G.B.), Histine, Hyrexin, Lensen, Nordryl, Notose, Phen-Amin 50, Phenamine, Rodryl, Rohydra, SK-Diphenhydramine, Span-Lanin, Tusstat.

---

* Route of administration not approved by FDA.
† Drug not approved by FDA for any indication.
‡ Drug not approved by FDA for this particular indication.
§ Indicated dosage above the manufacturer's recommendation.

Preparations

Injection: Solution, 10 and 50 mg/ml.
Oral: Capsules, 25 and 50 mg; elixir, 12.5 mg/5 ml.

Usual Dosages

Intramuscular: Children, 5 mg/kg divided into four doses during a 24-hour period (maximum, 300 mg/day).

Intramuscular, Intravenous: Adults, 10 mg initially. The subsequent dose may be increased to 20 to 50 mg every 2 to 3 hours (maximum, 400 mg/day).

Oral: For motion sickness, adults, 50 mg one-half hour before departure and 50 mg before each meal. Children, 5 mg/kg divided into four doses during a 24-hour period (maximum, 300 mg/day). For sedative effect, 25 to 50 mg three or four times daily.

DIPHTHERIA AND TETANUS TOXOIDS AND PERTUSSIS (DPT) VACCINE

Proprietary Names: Di-Te-Tuss (Germ.), DT Coq Adsorbe (Fr.), DT Perthydral (Fr.), Tri-Immunol, Triogen, Triple Antigen, Tri-Solgen, Trivax (G.B.), Vaccin Ipad DTC (Fr.).

Preparations

Injection: 6.7, 7.5, or 12.5 Lf units diptheria toxoid, 5 Lf units tetanus toxoid, and 4 protective units pertussis vaccine/0.5 ml.

Usual Dosages

Intramuscular: Infants 2 months of age, initially 0.5 ml followed by two more doses at 4- to 8-week intervals. A reinforcing fourth dose is given 7 to 12 months after the third, and a booster dose is given when the child is 5 to 6 years old.

DIPHTHERIA ANTITOXIN

Proprietary Name: Diphtheria Antitoxin.

Preparations

Injection: Vials of 1000, 5000, 10,000, 20,000, and 40,000 units.

Usual Dosages

Intramuscular, Intravenous: Adults and children, for prophylaxis, 1000 to 10,000 units. Adults and children, for treatment, 20,000 to 120,000 units, depending upon duration of illness, degree of toxicity, and site of membrane. The dose may be repeated as indicated.

DIPIVEFRIN (DPE)

Proprietary Name: Propine.

Preparations

Topical Ophthalmic: Solution, 0.1 per cent.

Usual Dosages

Topical Ophthalmic: The usual dosage is one drop in the eye(s) every 12 hours.

DIPYRIDAMOLE

Proprietary Names: Anginal (Jap.), Coribon (Ital.), Coronarine (Fr.), Corosan (Ital.), Coroxin (Ital.), Dipyrida (Germ.), Functiocardon (Germ.), Natyl (Fr.), Novodil (Ital.), Peridamol (Fr.), Persantin (Arg., Austral., Denm., G.B., Germ., Ital., Neth., Norw., S. Afr., Span., Switz.), Persantine, Prandiol (Fr.), Stenocardil (Ital.), Stenocor (Ital.), Stimolcardio (Ital.), Trancocard (Ital.), Viscor (Ital.).

Preparations

Oral: Tablets, 25 and 100 mg.

Usual Dosages

Oral: The recommended dosage is 50 mg three times a day, taken at least 1 hour before meals.

DMSO

See Dimethyl Sulfoxide.

DOXEPIN

Proprietary Names: Adapin, Aponal (Germ.), Quitaxon (Austral., Fr., S. Afr.), Sinequan, Sinquan (Germ.).

Preparations

Oral: Capsules, 10, 25, 50, 75, 100, and 150 mg; solution, 10 mg/ml.

---

*Route of administration not approved by FDA.
† Drug not approved by FDA for any indication.
‡ Drug not approved by FDA for this particular indication.
§ Indicated dosage above the manufacturer's recommendation.

Usual Dosages

Oral: Adults, initially 75 to 150 mg daily in divided doses. For maintenance, 25 to 150 mg daily (maximum, 300 mg daily).

DOXORUBICIN

Proprietary Names: Adriamycin, Adriblastin (Germ.), Adriblastina (Ital.), Adriblastine (Fr., Switz.), Farmiblastina (Span.), Rubex (Ire.).

Preparations

Injection: Powder (lyophilized), 10, 20, and 50 mg with 5, 10, and 25 ml, respectively, of sodium chloride injection to give a final concentration of 2 mg/ml.

Usual Dosages

Intravenous: Adults, 60 to 75 mg/square meter, administered as a single dose at 21-day intervals. Alternatively, 20 to 30 mg/square meter may be given daily for 3 days at 3- or 4-week intervals. Total dosage with either regimen should not exceed 550 mg/square meter.

DOXYCYCLINE

Proprietary Names: Doxin (Austral.), Doxy-II, Doxychel, Idocyklin (Swed.), Vibramycin, Vibramycine (Fr.), Vibra-Tabs, Vibraveineuse (Fr.), Vibravenös (Germ.).

Preparations

Injection: Powder equivalent to 100 to 200 mg of doxycycline.
Oral: Capsules, 50 and 100 mg; powder for suspension, 25 mg/5 ml after reconstitution.

Usual Dosages

Intravenous: Adults and children weighing at least 45 kg, initially, 200 mg daily given in one or two infusions, followed by 100 to 200 mg daily (depending upon the severity of infection) given in one or two infusions; children under 45 kg, 2 mg/kg daily in one or two infusions, followed by 1 or 2 mg/kg given in one or two infusions.
Oral: The usual adult dose is 100 mg at 12-hour intervals for two doses, followed by 100 mg once a day. In the management of more severe infections, up to 300 mg daily may be administered.

DPE

See Dipivefrin.

DROPERIDOL

Proprietary Names: Dridol (Swed.), Droleptan (G.B.), Inapsin (S. Afr.), Inapsine.

Preparations

Injection: Solution, 2.5 mg/ml.

Usual Dosages

Intramuscular, Intravenous: The usual dosage is 2.5 to 10 mg.

ECHOTHIOPHATE

Proprietary Names: Echodide, Echothiopate (G.B.), Phospholine.

Preparations

Topical Ophthalmic: Lyophilized sterile powder, 1.5, 3, 6.25, and 12.5 mg to make 0.03, 0.06, 0.125, and 0.25 per cent solutions, respectively.

Usual Dosages

Topical Ophthalmic: The frequency and concentration of instillation depend upon the patient's response to therapy.

ECONAZOLE

Proprietary Names: Ecostatin (G.B.), Epi-Pevaryl (Germ.), Mycopevaryl (Swed.), Pevaryl (G.B.), Skilar (Ital.), Spectazole.

Preparations

Topical: Cream, 1 per cent; lotion, 1 per cent; pessaries, 150 mg; powder, 1 per cent.
Topical Ophthalmic: No ophthalmic preparation is commercially available.

---

* Route of administration not approved by FDA.
† Drug not approved by FDA for any indication.
‡ Drug not approved by FDA for this particular indication.
§ Indicated dosage above the manufacturer's recommendation.

Usual Dosages

Topical Ophthalmic: A 1 per cent solution may be applied to the affected and surrounding areas twice a day for up to 8 to 12 weeks.

EDETATE CALCIUM DISODIUM

Proprietary Names: Calcium Disodium Versenate, Disodium Calcium Edetate (G.B.), Sodium Calciumedetate (G.B.).

Preparations

Topical Ophthalmic: No ophthalmic preparation is commercially available. A 4 per cent solution may be prepared with 4.1 gm of edetate calcium disodium, 10 mg of chlorhexidine acetate, and sterile water for injection to 100 ml.

Usual Dosages

Topical Ophthalmic: For the inactivation of epithelial collagenase, the eye is irrigated with 4 per cent solution.

EDETATE DISODIUM (EDTA, ETHYLENEDIAMINE TETRAACETIC ACID)

Proprietary Names: Chealamide, Disotate, Endrate, Sodium Versenate.

Preparations

Injection: Solution, 150 mg/ml in 20-ml vials.
Topical Ophthalmic: No ophthalmic preparation is commercially available. The intravenous solution must be diluted to the desired concentration with isotonic sodium chloride solution used for injection.

Usual Dosages

Intravenous (Slow): 15 to 50 mg/kg.
Topical Ophthalmic: The eye is irrigated with 0.35 to 1.85 per cent solution.

ENDROPHONIUM

Proprietary Name: Tensilon.

Preparations

Injection: Solution, 10 mg/ml.

Usual Dosages

Intravenous: For diagnosis, adults, 3 to 4 mg injected within 15 to 30 seconds; if no response occurs within 45 seconds, additional increments up to 10 mg; children, 0.2 mg/kg, 20 per cent of total dose given within 1 minute, remainder if tolerated.

EDTA

See Edetate Disodium.

EHDP

See Etidronate Disodium.

ELEDOISIN

Proprietary Name: Eledosin.

Preparations

Topical Ophthalmic: Solution, 400 µg/ml.

Usual Dosages

Topical Ophthalmic: One to two drops are applied to each affected eye three times daily.

EPHEDRINE

Proprietary Names: Bofedrol, Ectasule Minus, Efedrinetter (Swed.), Ephedroides (Fr.), Isofedrol, Nefrytol-Junior (S. Afr.), Slo-Fedrin, Spaneph (G.B.).

Preparations

Oral: Capsules, 25 and 50 mg; syrup, 10 and 20 mg/5 ml.

Usual Dosages

Oral: Range, 25 to 400 mg daily.

EPINEPHRINE

Proprietary Names: Adremad (Fr.), Adrenalin, Adrenaline (G.B.), Adrenatrate,

Asmatane, Asmolin, Asthma Meter, Bronkaid, Dysne-Inhal (Canad.), Dyspne (Austral.). E1/2, E2, Epifrin, Epinal, Epitrate, Eppy, Glaucon, Glauconin (Swed.), Glaufrin (Swed.), Glin-Epin (Austral.), Glycirenan (Germ.), Intranefrin (Canad.), Liadren (Ital.), Lyophrin (G.B.), Medihaler-Epi, Micronefrin, Mistura E, Mytrate, Primatene, Simplene (G.B.), Suprarenin, Sus-Phrine, Vaponefrin.

Preparations

Injection: Solution, 1 : 1000 (1 mg/ml).
Topical Ophthalmic: Solution, 0.1, 0.25, 0.5 1.0, and 2.0 per cent.

Usual Dosages

Intramuscular, Intravenous, Subcutaneous: Adults, initially 0.5 ml of a 1 : 1000 solution injected intramuscularly or subcutaneously, followed by 0.25 to 0.5 ml of a 1 : 10,000 solution given intravenously every 5 to 15 minutes.
Topical Ophthalmic: In primary open-angle glaucoma and other chronic glaucomas, one drop of 1 or 2 per cent solution in each eye, once or twice daily.

ERGOCALCIFEROL (VITAMIN D$_2$)

Proprietary Names: Calciferol, Deltalin, Deltavit (Ital.), Drisdol, Ostelin (Austral.), Ostoforte (Canad.), Radiostol (Canad.), Savitol (Germ.), Sterogyl (G.B.).

Preparations

Oral: Capsules, 25,000 IU (0.625 mg) and 50,000 IU (1.25 mg); tablets, 50,000 IU (1.25 mg).
Injection: Solution in oil, 500,000 IU (12.5 mg)/ml.

Usual Dosages

Intramuscular, Oral: 50,000 to 400,000 IU daily; dosage must be adjusted to the needs of the patient.

ERGOTAMINE

Proprietary Names: Ergate (S. Afr.), Ergomar, Ergostat, Ergotart (Austral.), Etin (Austral.), Exmigra (Neth.), Exmigrex (Fin.), Femergin (G.B.), Gynergen, Lingraine (G.B.), Lingran (Swed.), Lengrene (Norw.), Medihaler-Ergotamine.

---

*Route of administration not approved by FDA.
† Drug not approved by FDA for any indication.
‡ Drug not approved by FDA for this particular indication.
§ Indicated dosage above the manufacturer's recommendation.

Preparations

Inhalation: Solution, 9 mg/ml.
Injection: Solution, 0.5 mg/ml.
Oral: Tablets, 1 mg.
Sublingual: Tablets, 2 mg.

Usual Dosages

Inhalation: Adults, single inhalation (0.36 mg) at onset of attack, repeated if necessary at intervals of no less than 5 minutes to a total of six inhalations in 24 hours (maximum, 12 mg in 1 week).
Intramuscular, Subcutaneous: Adults, 0.25 to 0.5 mg at onset of attack, repeated in 40 minutes if necessary; maximum of 1 mg in 1 week.
Oral: Adults, 1 to 2 mg at onset, repeated every 30 minutes; maximum of 6 mg in 24 hours and 12 mg in 1 week.
Sublingual: Adults, 2 mg at onset, repeated every 30 minutes if necessary. Dosage must not exceed 6 mg in 24 hours or 10 mg in 1 week.

ERGOTAMINE/BELLADONNA/ CAFFEINE/PENTOBARBITAL COMBINATION

Proprietary Name: Cafergot P-B.

Preparations

Oral: Tablets, 1 mg ergotamine, 0.125 mg belladonna, 100 mg caffeine, and 30 mg pentobarbital.
Rectal: Suppositories, 2 mg ergotamine, 0.25 mg belladonna, 100 mg caffeine, and 60 mg pentobarbital.

Usual Dosages

Oral: Adults, two tablets at the onset of attack. An additional tablet may be taken every 30 minutes, if needed, but the amount generally should be limited to a total of six tablets per attack or no more than ten tablets per week.
Rectal: Adults, one-half to one suppository at the onset of an attack. Another suppository may be used in 1 hour if needed; the total amount should not exceed two suppositories per attack or no more than five suppositories per week.

---

* Route of administration not approved by FDA.
† Drug not approved by FDA for any indication.
‡ Drug not approved by FDA for this particular indication.
§ Indicated dosage above the manufacturer's recommendation.

ERGOTAMINE/BELLADONNA/ PHENOBARBITAL COMBINATION

Proprietary Name: Bellergal.

Preparations

Oral: Tablets, 0.3 mg ergotamine, 0.1 mg belladonna, and 20 mg phenobarbital; tablets (timed-release), 0.6 mg ergotamine, 0.2 mg belladonna, and 40 mg phenobarbital.

Usual Dosages

Oral: Adults, two tablets at the onset of an attack. An additional tablet may be taken every 30 minutes, if needed, but the amount generally should be limited to a total of six tablets per attack or no more than ten tablets per week.

ERGOTAMINE/CAFFEINE COMBINATION

Proprietary Name: Cafergot.

Preparations

Oral: Tablets, 1 mg ergotamine and 100 mg caffeine.
Rectal: Suppositories, 2 mg ergotamine and 100 mg caffeine.

Usual Dosages

Oral: Adults, two tablets at the onset of an attack. An additional tablet may be taken every 30 minutes, if needed, but the amount generally should be limited to a total of six tablets per attack or no more than ten tablets per week.
Rectal: Adults, one-half to one suppository at the onset of an attack. Another suppository may be used in 1 hour if needed; the total amount should not exceed two suppositories per attack or no more than five suppositories per week.

ERYTHROMYCIN

Proprietary Names: Abboject (S. Afr.), Abboticin (Swed.), Abboticine (Fr.), Bristamycin, Chemthromycin (Canad.), E-Biotic, E.E.S., Emcinka (Canad.), EMU-V (Austral., S. Afr.), E-Mycin Eratrex (Austral.), Eromel (S. Afr.), Eromycin (Austral.), Erostin (Austral.), Erycen (G.B.), Erycinum (Germ.), Erypar, Erythrocin, Erythromid (G.B.), Erythromycetine (Canad.), Erythroped (G.B.), Erythro-ST (Jap.), Ethril, Ethryn (Austral.), Ilosone Ilotycin, Kesso-Mycin, Neo-Erycinum (Germ.), Novorythro (Canad.), Paediathrocin (Germ.), Pedia-mycin, Pfizer-E, Propiocine (Fr.), Retcin (G.B.), Robimycin, RP-Mycin, Rythrocaps (S. Afr.), SK-Erythromycin, Wyamycin.

Preparations

Injection: Powder, 0.5 and 1 gm; solution, 50 mg/ml.
Oral: Tablets (enteric-coated), 250 mg.
Rectal: Suppositories, 125 mg.
Topical: Ointment, 1 per cent.
Topical Ophthalmic: Ointment, 0.5 per cent.

Usual Dosages

Intramuscular (Deep): Adults, 100 mg initially, repeated at 4- to 8-hour intervals (total daily dose, 5 to 8 mg/kg). The recommended dose for children weighing over 13.6 kg is 50 mg every 4 to 6 hours, or a total of 12 mg/kg daily.
Intravenous: Adults, 1 to 4 gm daily in divided doses. Children, 50 mg/kg daily in four divided doses. Premature and full-term newborn infants, 10 mg/kg dailly in four divided doses. For severe infections, 15 to 20 mg/kg may be given.
Oral: Adults, initially 500 mg followed by 250 mg every 6 hours. For severe infections, 4 gm or more daily in divided doses. Children, 30 to 50 mg/kg daily in divided doses. For severe infections, the dose may be doubled.
Subconjunctival: Up to 100 mg in 0.5 ml of isotonic sodium chloride injection.
Topical: Preparation may be applied to the affected area three or four times daily.
Topical Ophthalmic: Ointment preparation is applied one or more times daily.

ETHACRYNIC ACID (ETACRYNIC ACID)

Proprietary Names: Crinuryl (Isr.), Edecril (Austral., Jap.), Edecrin, Hydromedrin (Germ.).

Preparations

Injection: Powder, 50 mg/vial.
Oral: Tablets, 25 and 50 mg.

---

*Route of administration not approved by FDA.
† Drug not approved by FDA for any indication.
‡ Drug not approved by FDA for this particular indication.
§ Indicated dosage above the manufacturer's recommendation.

Usual Dosages

Intravenous: For adults, the usual dose is 50 mg or 0.5 to 1.0 mg/kg. In children, initially, 1 mg/kg. These doses may be increased if necessary.
Oral: Adults, initially, 50 to 100 mg daily. If an adequate response is not obtained, the daily dosage may be increased, usually in increments of 25 or 50 mg. For maintenance, the dose and frequency of administration must be determined individually. Children, initially, 25 mg daily. Dosage may be increased gradually by increments of 25 mg.

ETHAMBUTOL

Proprietary Names: Dexambutol (Fr.), Etibi (Canad.), Miambutol (Ital.), Myambutol.

Preparations

Oral: Tablets, 100 and 400 mg.

Usual Dosages

Oral: Adults, for initial treatment, 25 mg/kg daily as a single dose for 10 to 12 days, followed by 15 mg/kg daily as a single dose. For treatment, 25 mg/kg daily as a single dose. After 60 days of treatment, the dose may be reduced to 15 mg/kg daily. Therapy should be continued until bacteriologic conversion occurs or until maximal clinical improvement is noted. Information is inadequate to establish dosage for children under 13 years of age.

ETHINYL ESTRADIOL

Proprietary Names: Duramen (Switz.), Edrol (Austral.), Estigyn (Austral.), Estinyl, Eticyclin Forte (Switz.), Etifollin (Norw.), Etivex (Swed.), Farmacyrol Forte (Germ.), Feminone, Gynolett (Germ.), Linoral (Swed.), Lynoral (Austral., Belg., G.B., Germ., Neth., Switz.), Primogyn (Austral.), Progynon C or M (Austral., Germ., Span., Switz.).

Preparations

Oral: Powder, 1 gm; tablets, 0.02, 0.05, and 0.5 mg.

Usual Dosages

Oral: For hypogonadism, 0.05 mg one to three times daily for the first 2 weeks of an arbitrary cycle, with the addition of a progestin for the last 2 weeks.

ETHOXZOLAMIDE

Proprietary Names: Cardrase, Ethamide.

Preparations

Oral: Tablets, 125 mg.

Usual Dosages

Oral: In the adjunctive treatment of glaucoma in adults, 62.5 to 250 mg may be administered two to four times daily.

ETHYLENEDIAMINE TETRAACETIC ACID

See Edetate Disodium.

ETIDRONATE DISODIUM (EHDP)

Proprietary Names: Calcimux (Arg.), Didronel, Etidron (Ital.).

Preparations

Oral: Tablets, 200 mg.

Usual Dosages

Oral: For Paget's disease, a single daily dose should be given 2 hours before a meal. Initially, 5 mg/kg is given daily for a period not to exceed 6 months. Larger doses should be reserved for use when there is a need for rapid suppression of increased bone turnover or prompt reduction of elevated cardiac output. When doses greater than 10 mg/kg daily are given, the treatment period should not exceed 3 months; the daily dosage should not exceed 20 mg/kg.

ETOPOSIDE

Proprietary Name: Vepesid.

Preparations

Injection: Solution, 100 mg/5 ml.
Oral: Capsules, 50 mg.

---

* Route of administration not approved by FDA.
† Drug not approved by FDA for any indication.
‡ Drug not approved by FDA for this particular indication.
§ Indicated dosage above the manufacturer's recommendation.

Usual Dosages

Intravenous: 35 to 100 mg/square meter.
Oral: 100 to 200 mg/square meter.

ETRETINATE

Proprietary Names: Tegason (G.B.), Tegison.

Preparations

Oral: Capsules, 10 and 25 mg.

Usual Dosages

Oral: Initially, 0.75 to 1.0 mg/kg daily taken in divided doses. A maximum dose of 1.5 mg/kg should not be exceeded. Maintenance doses are 0.5 to 0.75 mg/kg daily.

FENOPROFEN

Proprietary Names: Fenopron (G.B.), Fepron (Belg., Ital., Neth.), Feprona (Germ.), Nalfon, Nalgesic (Fr.), Progesic.

Preparations

Oral: Pulvules, 300 mg; tablets, 200, 300, and 600 mg.

Usual Dosages

Oral: For osteoarthritis, the recommended initial dose is 300 to 600 mg four times daily.

FIBRINOLYSIN

Proprietary Names: Lyovac, Thrombolysin.

Preparations

Injection: Vial, 50,000 units.

Usual Dosages

Intravenous: The dosage of 50,000 to 100,000 units per hour for 1 to 6 hours each day is recommended. Dosage may be repeated for 3 or 4 consecutive days, depending on patient response. A single dose of 100,000 units may be adequate in the treatment of uncomplicated thrombophlebitis, but extensive or organized venous thrombi may require a total of 250,000 to 400,000 units.

FLUCONAZOLE

Proprietary Names: Biozolene (Ital.), Diflucan (G.B., Ger., Ital., Neth., S. Afr., Swed., Switz., USA), Elazor (Ital.), Fungata (Ger.), Triflucan (Fr.).

Preparations

Injection: Solution, 2 mg/ml.
Oral: Tablets, 50, 100, and 200 mg.

Usual Dosages

Injection, Oral: 100 to 400 mg per day, depending on patient's response to therapy.

FLUCYTOSINE

Proprietary Names: Alcobon (G.B.), Ancobon, Ancotil (Arg., Austral., Canad., Denm., Fr., Germ., Jap., Norw., Swed., Switz.).

Preparations

Oral: Capsules, 250 and 500 mg.
Topical Ophthalmic: Solution, 1 and 1.5 per cent.

Usual Dosages

Oral: Adults and children, 50 to 150 mg/kg daily in divided doses at 6-hour intervals.
Topical Ophthalmic: One or two drops of solution may be given hourly.

FLUMETHASONE

Proprietary Name: Locorten.

Preparations

Topical: Cream, 0.03 per cent.

Usual Dosages

Topical: Preparation is applied to affected area three or four times daily or is used under occlusive dressings.

---

*Route of administration not approved by FDA.
† Drug not approved by FDA for any indication.
‡ Drug not approved by FDA for this particular indication.
§ Indicated dosage above the manufacturer's recommendation.

FLUOCINOLONE

Proprietary Names: Flucort (Jap.), Fluonid, Jellin (Germ.), Loaclyn (Ital.), Synalar, Synamol (Canad.), Synemol.

Preparations

Topical: Cream, 0.01, 0.025, and 0.2 per cent; ointment, 0.025 per cent; solution, 0.01 per cent.

Usual Dosages

Topical: Preparation is applied three to four times daily as needed or used under occlusive dressings.

FLUOCINONIDE

Proprietary Names: Lidex, Topsyn.

Preparations

Topical: Cream, 0.05 per cent; gel, 0.05 per cent; ointment, 0.05 per cent.

Usual Dosages

Topical: Preparation is applied three or four times daily as needed.

FLUORESCEIN

Proprietary Names: Ak-Fluor, Fluor-Amps (G.B.), Fluorescite, Fluoreseptic, Fluorets (G.B.), Fluor-I-Strip, Fluoro-I-Strip (G.B.), Ful-Glo, Funduscein.

Preparations

Injection: Solution, 5 and 10 per cent.
Topical Ophthalmic: Applicators impregnated with 0.6, 1.0, and 9.0 mg/strip; solution, 2 per cent.

Usual Dosages

Intravenous: Adults, 500 mg (10 ml of a 5 per cent solution or 5 ml of a 10 per cent solution) is injected rapidly into an arm vein. The dye should appear in the central retinal artery in 9 to 15 seconds.
Topical Ophthalmic: For detection of epithelial defects, a fluorescein strip moistened with ophthalmic irrigating solution is used to touch the conjunctiva, or one drop of solution is placed in the conjunctival sac.

FLUORINATED CORTICOSTEROIDS

See Betamethasone, Dexamethasone, Flumethasone, Fluocinolone, Fluocinonide, Flurandrenolide, Halcinonide, Triamcinolone.

FLUOROMETHOLONE

Proprietary Names: FML Liquifilm, Oxylone.

Preparations

Topical Ophthalmic: Suspension, 0.1 per cent.

Usual Dosages

Topical Ophthalmic: One drop every 1 or 2 hours until response; then frequency is reduced.

FLUOROURACIL

Proprietary Names: Adrucil, Efudex, Fluoroplex, 5 FU.

Preparations

Injection: Solution, 50 mg/ml.
Topical: Cream, 5 per cent; solution, 1, 2, and 5 per cent.

Usual Dosages

Intravenous: Daily dosage is based on 12 mg/kg, but should not exceed 800 mg regardless of the patient's weight.
Subconjunctival: 0.1 ml of a solution containing 50 mg/ml.
Topical: Preparation is applied twice daily.

FLUOXETINE

Proprietary Names: Adofen (Span.), Fluctin (Ger.), Fluctine (Switz.), Fluoxeren (Ital.), Prozac (Canad., G.B., Ital., Neth., S. Afr., Span., USA), Reneuron (Span.).

Preparations

Oral: Capsules, 20 mg; liquid suspension, 20 mg/5 ml.

---

* Route of administration not approved by FDA.
' Drug not approved by FDA for any indication.
‡ Drug not approved by FDA for this particular indication.
§ Indicated dosage above the manufacturer's recommendation.

Usual Dosages

Oral: Initial dose 20 mg/day; doses up to 80 mg daily in divided doses may be employed if necessary.

FLURANDRENOLIDE

Proprietary Names: Cordran, Drenison (G.B.), Drocort (Swed.), Haelen (G.B.), Sermaba (Germ.).

Preparations

Topical: Cream and ointment, 0.025 and 0.05 per cent; lotion, 0.05 per cent; tape 4 µg/square centimeter.

Usual Dosages

Topical: Preparation is applied two or three times daily or is used under occlusive dressings. The tape is applied once every 12 hours.

FLURBIPROFEN

Proprietary Names: Ansaid, Cebutid (Fr.), Froben (G.B., S. Afr., Switz.), Ocufen.

Preparations

Oral: Tablets, 50 and 100 mg.
Topical Ophthalmic: Solution, 0.03 per cent.

Usual Dosages

Oral: 100 to 400 mg daily.
Topical Ophthalmic: A total of four drops should be administered, with instillation of one drop approximately every 30 minutes beginning 2 hours before surgery.

FOLIC ACID

Proprietary Names: Acfol (Span.), Folacid (Neth.), Folacin (Norw., Swed.), Folaemin (Neth.), Folasic (Austral.), Foldine (Fr.), Folettes (Austral.), Folico (Ital.), Folina (Ital.), Folsan (Germ.), Folvite, Nifolin Denm.), Novofolacid (Canad.).

Preparations

Injection: Solution, 5 mg/ml.
Oral: Tablets, 0.1, 0.25, 0.4, 0.8, and 1 mg.

Usual Dosages

Intramuscular, Intravenous, Oral, Subcutaneous (Deep): Up to 1 mg daily. Oral dosage of 0.1 mg daily is considered sufficient as a nutritional supplement. To prevent megaloblastic anemia of pregnancy and fetal damage, up to 1 mg daily throughout pregnancy has been suggested.

FOSCARNET

Proprietary Name: Foscavir.

Preparations

Injection: Solution, 24 mg/ml.

Usual Dosages

Intravenous: The usual initial dose is 60 mg/kg given at a constant rate over a minimum of 1 hour every 8 hours for 2 to 3 weeks. The recommended maintenance dose is 90 mg/kg/day given as an intravenous infusion over 2 hours.

F₃T

See Trifluridine.

FUROSEMIDE

Proprietary Names: Arasemide (Jap.), Dryptal (G.B.), Franyl (Jap.), Frusemide (G.B.), Frusid (G.B.), Furantral (Pol.), Impugan (Swed.), Lasilix (Fr.), Lasix, Seguril (Span.).

Preparations

Injection: Solution, 10 mg/ml.
Oral: Solution, 10 mg/ml; tablets, 20, 40, and 80 mg.

Usual Dosages

Intravenous: Adults, 80 to 100 mg every 1 to 2 hours until an adequate response is obtained and other therapeutic modalities can be instituted. Children, 25 to 50 mg every 4 hours.
Oral: Adults, 20 to 80 mg as a single dose

---

*Route of administration not approved by FDA.
† Drug not approved by FDA for any indication.
‡ Drug not approved by FDA for this particular indication.
§ Indicated dosage above the manufacturer's recommendation.

initially. Children, 1 to 2 mg/kg once or twice daily initially.

GAMMA BENZENE HEXACHLORIDE

See Lindane.

GANCICLOVIR (DHPG)

Proprietary Names: Cymevan (Fr.), Cymeven (Ger.), Cymevene (G.B., Neth., Span., Swed., Switz.), Cytovene.

Preparations

Injection: Powder.

Usual Dosages

Intravenous: Initially, the usual daily adult dosage is 7.5 to 10 mg/kg given in divided doses at 8- to 12-hour intervals. Maintenance therapy is 5 to 6 mg/kg daily.
Intravitreal: 200 μg in 0.1 ml of aqueous solution.

GAS-GANGRENE ANTITOXIN

Proprietary Name: Gas-Gangrene Antitoxin.

Preparations

Injection: Solution, 2500 units/ml.

Usual Dosages

Intramuscular, Intravenous: The usual prophylactic dose is 25,000 units, which may be doubled or repeated if necessary. The therapeutic dose is at least 75,000 units and may be repeated every 4 to 6 hours, according to the response of the patient.

GELATIN SPONGE (ABSORBABLE)

Proprietary Name: Gelfoam.

Preparations

Topical: Sponges, sizes 12, 50, 100, and 200.

Usual Dosages

Topical: The sponges may be applied dry or saturated with sodium chloride solution for injection to the bleeding area.

GEMFIBROZIL

Proprietary Name: Lopid.

Preparations

Oral: Capsules, 300 mg.

Usual Dosages

Oral: The usual dose is 0.9 to 1.5 gm daily in divided doses.

GENTAMICIN

Proprietary Names: Cidomycin (G.B.), Garamycin, Garamycina (Swed.), Genoptic, Gentalline (Fr.), Genticin (G.B.), Geomycine (Belg.), Refobacin (Germ.), Sulmycin (Germ.), U-Gencin.

Preparations

Injection: Solution, 10 and 40 mg/ml.
Topical Ophthalmic: Ointment, 3 mg/ml; solution, 3 mg/ml.

Usual Dosages

Intramuscular, Intravenous: Adults and children (with normal renal function), 3 mg/kg daily administered in three equally divided doses. The usual dosage is 80 mg three times daily for patients weighing more than 60 kg, and 60 mg three times daily for patients weighing 60 kg or less. In serious and life-threatening infections, up to 5 mg/kg daily administered in three or four equally divided doses may be required.
Intravitreal: 100 to 400 µg in 0.1 to 0.2 ml of isotonic sodium chloride injection.
Retrobulbar: 0.5 to 1.0 ml of a solution containing 40 mg/ml.
Subconjunctival: 1.25 to 30 mg in a 0.5 ml aqueous solution. The pediatric solution for injection without preservatives is preferred for subconjunctival injections.
Topical Ophthalmic: One drop of a solution 3 to 15 mg/ml is given every 1 to 4 hours, or the ointment preparation is applied two or three times daily. Fortified gentamicin eye-drops are prepared by adding 2 ml of the parenteral preparation containing 40 mg/ml to the 5-ml dropper bottle of the gentamicin

---

* Route of administration not approved by FDA.
† Drug not approved by FDA for any indication.
‡ Drug not approved by FDA for this particular indication.
§ Indicated dosage above the manufacturer's recommendation.

ophthalmic solution to produce a concentration of 13.6 mg/ml.

GENTIAN VIOLET

Proprietary Names: Crystal Violet (G.B.), Genapax.

Preparations

Topical: Solution, 0.5, 1.0, and 2.0 per cent.

Usual Dosages

Topical: Solution should be applied to lesions with cotton two to three times daily.

GLYCERIN (GLYCEROL)

Proprietary Names: Glyrol, Luxoral (Ital.), Ophthalgan, Osmoglyn.

Preparations

Oral: Solution, 50 (0.6 gm/ml) and 75 (0.94 gm/ml) per cent.
Topical Ophthalmic: Solution, 0.5 per cent.

Usual Dosages

Oral: One to 1.5 gm/kg usually given as a 50 or 75 per cent solution.
Topical Ophthalmic: One drop of solution may be instilled into the eye every 3 or 4 hours for reduction of corneal edema.

GOLD SALTS

See Auranofin, Aurothioglucose, Gold Sodium Thiomalate.

GOLD SODIUM THIOMALATE (SODIUM AUROTHIOMALATE)

Proprietary Names: Myochrysine, Myocrisin (G.B.), Tauredon (Germ.).

Preparations

Injection: Solution, 10, 25, 50, and 100 mg/ml.

Usual Dosages

Intramuscular: Adults, initially, single weekly injections of 10 mg the first week, 25 mg the second week, 25 or 50 mg the third week, and 50 mg each week thereafter until a total dosage of 0.8 to 1 gm has been administered.

GRISEOFULVIN

Proprietary Names: Fulcin (G.B.), Fulvicin-P/G, Fulvicin-U/F, Grifulvin V, Grisactin, Grisefuline (Fr.), Grisovin (G.B.), Grisowen, Gris-PEG, Lamoryl (Swed.), Likuden M (Germ.).

Preparations

Oral: Capsules, 125 and 250 mg; suspension, 125 mg/5 ml; tablets, 125, 250, and 500 mg.

Usual Dosages

Oral: Adults, 0.5 to 1 gm daily in divided doses. Children, approximately 5 to 10 mg/kg in single or divided doses.

GUANETHIDINE

Proprietary Name: Ismelin.

Preparations

Oral: Tablets, 10 and 25 mg.
Topical Ophthalmic: Preparation is not commerically available in the United States.

Usual Dosages

Oral: Adults, for ambulatory patients, initially, 10 mg daily. The dosage may be increased by increments of 10 mg every 5 to 7 days. In hospitalized patients, initial dose is 25 to 50 mg daily, increased by 25 to 50 mg daily or every other day as indicated. Because of the drug's long half-life, the maximal effect may not be observed for 7 to 14 days and it may be necessary to reduce the dose slightly after an initial antihypertensive effect has been obtained. Children, initially, 0.2 mg/kg daily, increased by the same amount every 7 to 10 days if required.
Topical Ophthalmic: One drop of a 5 to 10 per cent solution twice daily.

---

*Route of administration not approved by FDA.
† Drug not approved by FDA for any indication.
‡ Drug not approved by FDA for this particular indication.
§ Indicated dosage above the manufacturer's recommendation.

GUANIDINE

Proprietary Name: Guanidine.

Preparations

Oral: Tablets, 125 mg.

Usual Dosages

Oral: An initial daily test dose of 10 mg/kg is given. The total dose is arrived at by daily increments. A dosage of 10 to 58 mg/kg daily is administered in three to four divided doses.

HALCINONIDE

Proprietary Name: Halog.

Preparations

Topical: Cream, 0.1 per cent; ointment, 0.025 and 0.1 per cent; solution, 0.1 per cent.

Usual Dosages

Topical: Preparation is applied three or four times daily as needed.

HALOPERIDOL

Proprietary Names: Haldol, Serenace (G.B.).

Preparations

Injection: Solution, 5 mg/ml.
Oral: Solution, 2 mg/ml; tablets, 0.5, 1, 2, 5, and 10 mg.

Usual Dosages

Intramuscular: 1 to 5 mg given every 12 hours as needed.
Oral: 1 to 5 mg twice daily.

HALOPROGIN

Proprietary Names: Halotex, Mycanden (Arg., Germ., S. Afr.), Mycilan (Belg., Fr.), Polik (Jap.).

Preparations

Topical: Cream, 1 per cent; solution, 1 per cent.

Usual Dosages

Topical: The preparation is applied liberally to the affected area twice daily for 2 to 3 weeks.

HEMOSTATIC COLLAGEN (ABSORBABLE)

Proprietary Names: Avitene, Instat.

Preparations

Topical: Fiber squares, 70 mm × 35 or 70 mm × 1 mm.

Usual Dosages

Topical: Small squares or fibrous form may be applied directly to the source of bleeding.

HEPARIN

Proprietary Names: Calciparin (Germ.), Calciparine (Austral., Fr.), Cutheparine (Fr.), Depo-Heparin, Disebrin (Ital.), Hamocura (Germ.), Hepacarin (Jap.), Hepalean (Canad.), Hepathrom, Hep-Lock, Heprinar, Lipo-Hepin, Liquaemin, Liquemin (Germ.), Liquemine (Fr.), Norheparin (Germ.), Panheprin, Thrombophob (Germ.), Thrombo-Vetren (Germ.), Vetren (Germ.).

Preparations

Injection: Gel (for repository injection), 20,000 units/ml; solution, 200, 1000, 5000, 7500, 10,000, 15,000, 20,000, and 40,000 units/ml.

Usual Dosages

Intravenous: 10,000 USP units initially, then 5000 to 10,000 units four to six times daily. By intravenous infusion, 20,000 to 40,000 units/L at a rate of 15 to 30 units per minute.
Subcutaneous: 10,000 to 20,000 units initially, then 8000 to 10,000 units three times daily, according to prothrombin time response.

---

* Route of administration not approved by FDA.
† Drug not approved by FDA for any indication.
‡ Drug not approved by FDA for this particular indication.
§ Indicated dosage above the manufacturer's recommendation.

HOMATROPINE

Proprietary Names: Homatrocel, Isopto Homatropine, SMP Homatropine (G.B.).

Preparations

Topical Ophthalmic: Solution, 2 and 5 per cent.

Usual Dosages

Topical Ophthalmic: One drop instilled two to four times daily.

HYALURONIDASE

Proprietary Names: Alidase, Hyalas (Swed.), Hyalase (G.B.), Hyason (Belg.), Jalovis (Ital.), Jaluran (Ital.), Kinetin (Germ.), Permease (Aust.), Seravase (S. Afr.), Wydase.

Preparations

Injection: Powder (lyophilized), 150 and 1500 units; solution, 150 units/ml.
Topical Ophthalmic: No preparation is commercially available. A solution of 750 units dissolved in 1 ml physiologic saline may be prepared.

Usual Dosages

Infiltration: For local anesthesia of the eye, 150 units are dissolved in 1 ml of a 2 per cent procaine and 0.4 per cent potassium sulfate solution. For nerve block, 0.4 ml of this mixture is diluted to 10 ml, and two drops (0.12 ml) of epinephrine are added before injection.
Topical Ophthalmic: Solution may be applied three to four times daily.

HYDROCHLOROTHIAZIDE

Proprietary Names: Aquarius (Canad.), Chemhydrazide (Canad.), Chlorzide, Delco-Retic, Direma (G.B.), Diucen-H, Diuchlor H (Canad.), Diu-Scrip, Esidrex (G.B.), Esidrix, Hydrazide (Canad.), Hydrid (Canad.), Hydro-Aquil (Canad.), Hydrodiuretex (Canad.), Hydro-Diuril, Hydromal, Hydrosaluret (Canad.), HydroSaluric (G.B.), Hydrozide, Hyeloril, Hyperetic, Kenazide, Lexxor, Loqua, Mictrin, Neo-Codema (Canad.), Neoflumen (Austral.), Novohydrazide (Canad.), Oretic, Ro-Hydrazide, SK-Hydrochlorothiazide, Thiuretic, Urozide (Canad.), Zide.

Preparations

Oral: Tablets, 25, 50, and 100 mg.

Usual Dosages

Oral: Adults, initially 25 to 50 mg twice daily. Children, 2 mg/kg daily in two divided doses.

HYDROCORTISONE

Proprietary Names: Actocortin (Germ., Swed.), A-Hydrocort, Anusol-HC, Barriere-HC (Canad.), Bio-Cort (Canad.), Bio-Cortex, Biosone, Cetacort, Corlan (G.B.), Corphos, Cortamed (Canad.), Cortef, Cortenema, Cortiment (Canad., Swed.), Cortomister (Fr.), Efcortelan (G.B.), Efcortesol (G.B.), Eldecort, Emo-Cort (Canad.), Ficortril (Germ., Swed.), Flebocortid (Austral., Ital.), Heb-Cort, Hycor (Austral.), Hycorace, Hydrocort, Hydrocortal (Swed.), Hydrocortemel (S. Afr.), Hydrocortistab (G.B.), Hydrocortisone, Hydrosone, Hynax (Austral.), Hysone-A (Austral.), Idrocortisone (Ital.), Intracort (Austral.), Komed HC, Manticor (Canad.), Microcort (Canad.), Nordicort (Austral.), Novohydrocort (Canad.), Nutracort, Pabracort (G.B.), Panhydrosone, Phiacort (Austral.), Polycort (S. Afr.), Scheroson (Austral.), Scheroson F (Germ.), Sigmacort (Austral.), Siguent Hycor (Austral.), Solu-Cortef, Solu-Glyc (Swed.), Span-Ster, Squibb-HC (Austral.), Sterocort (Canad.), Tega-cort, Unicort (Canad.), Venocort (Austral.), Venocortin (S. Afri.), Wincort (Canad.).

Preparations

Injection (Ophthalmic): Suspension, 2.5 per cent.
Topical: Cream, 0.125, 0.2, 0.25, 0.5, and 1.0 per cent; lotion, 0.125, 0.25, 0.5, and 1 per cent; ointment, 1 and 2.5 per cent.
Topical Ophthalmic: Ointment, 0.5, 1.5, and 2.5 per cent; solution, 0.2 per cent; suspension, 0.5 and 2.5 per cent.

Usual Dosages

Intramuscular: For emergency situations when the intravenous route is not feasible, 100 to 250 mg initially, repeated until an adequate response is discernible. Maximum daily dose is 1 gm.
Intravenous: For conditions other than shock, 100 to 500 mg initially, repeated if necessary. Dosage may be reduced for infants and children.
Subconjunctival: 0.5 ml of a 2.5 per cent suspension.

---

*Route of administration not approved by FDA.
† Drug not approved by FDA for any indication.
‡ Drug not approved by FDA for this particular indication.
§ Indicated dosage above the manufacturer's recommendation.

Topical: Preparation is applied three or four times daily as required.
Topical Ophthalmic: One or two drops of a 0.2 per cent solution or 0.5 per cent suspension every 1 or 2 hours until a response is obtained; the frequency then is reduced. For severe conditions, a 2.5 per cent suspension may be used. The ointment preparation is applied three or four times daily or as a nighttime medication when the suspension is used during the day.

HYDROGEN PEROXIDE

Proprietary Name: Hydrogen Peroxide.

Preparations

Topical: Solution, 3 per cent.

Usual Dosages

Topical: Application to wounds and mucous membranes helps in debridement by loosening masses of infected detritus in wounds.

HYDROXOCOBALAMIN

Proprietary Names: Acimexan (Switz.), Acuo-Godabion B12 (Span.), Alpha Redisol, Alpha-Ruvite, Aquo-Cytobion (Germ.), Aquodavur (Span.), Axlon (Germ.), Behepan (Swed.), Berubilong (Germ.), Biocobal VCA (Ital.), Bradirubra (Ital.), Cobalidrina (Ital.), Cobalin-H (G.B.), Cobalvit (Ital.), Depogamma (Germ.), Docevita (Span.), Docivit Depo (Germ.), Dodecavit (Fr.), Dosixbe (Arg.), Droxodoce (Arg.) Droxofor (Arg.), Forta-B12 (Belg.), Fravit B_{12} (Ital.), Hidroxuber (Span.), Hydrocobamine (Neth.), Hydroxo B_{12}, Idrozima (Ital.), Liodozal (Switz.), Longicobal (Ital.), Macrabin H (Ind.), Mega-B12 (Belg.), Megamilbedoce (Span.), Milbedoce Depot (Span.), Natur B_{12} (Ital.), Neo-Betalin 12, Neo-Cytamen (Arg., Austral., G.B., Ital., S. Afr.), Novidroxin (Germ.), Novobedouze (Belg., Fr., Switz.), Red 1000 (Ital.), Rossobivit (Ital.), Rubesol-LA, Rubitard B_{12} (Ital.), Sytobex-H, Vibeden (Denm.), Vitarubin Depot (Switz.).

Preparations

Injection: Solution, 100, 250, and 1000 µg/ml.

Usual Dosages

Intramuscular: For patients with demonstrable neurologic damage, 1 mg may be given once weekly for several months, then once or twice monthly for another year. Neurologic damage that cannot be reversed within 12 to 18 months must be considered irreversible.

HYDROXYCHLOROQUINE

Proprietary Names: Ercoquin (Norw., Swed.), Plaquenil, Plaquinol (Port.), Quensyl (Germ.).

Preparations

Oral: Tablets, 200 mg (equivalent to 155 mg of base).

Usual Dosages

Oral: The average adult dosage is 200 mg once or twice daily.

HYDROXYETHYL CELLULOSE

Proprietary Names: Adsorbotear, Ciba Vision Lens Drops, Comfort Tears, Gonioscopic Prism Solution, Lens Fresh Lubricating and Rewetting Drops, Neo-Tears, Optocrymal (Canad.), TearGard.

Preparations

Topical Ophthalmic: Solution.

Usual Dosages

Topical Ophthalmic: One or two drops in the eyes(s) instilled three times daily or as needed.

HYDROXYPROPYL CELLULOSE

Proprietary Name: Lacrisert.

Preparations

Topical Ophthalmic: Ophthalmic insert, 5 mg.

Usual Dosages

Topical Ophthalmic: One ophthalmic insert may be instilled in each eye one to two times daily.

---

* Route of administration not approved by FDA.
† Drug not approved by FDA for any indication.
‡ Drug not approved by FDA for this particular indication.
§ Indicated dosage above the manufacturer's recommendation.

HYDROXYPROPYL METHYLCELLULOSE

Proprietary Names: Celacol HPM, Contactisol (Canad.), Goniosol, Hypromellose, Isopto Alkaline, Isopt-Fluid (Germ.), Isopto Plain, Isopto Tears, Lacril, Methocel HG, Methopt (Austral.), Tearisol.

Preparations

Topical Ophthalmic: Solution, 0.5, 0.8, 1.0, and 2.5 per cent.

Usual Dosages

Topical Ophthalmic: One drop in the eye several times a day.

HYDROXYSTILBAMIDINE

Proprietary Name: Hydroxystilbamidine.

Preparations

Injection: Powder, 225 mg.

Usual Dosages

Intravenous (Slow Infusion): The daily dose range for adults is 225 mg in 200 ml of 5 per cent dextrose injection or sodium chloride injection, up to a total of 5 to 25 gm. In most cases, a maximum of 8 gm is recommended.

HYDROXYUREA

Proprietary Names: Hydrea, Litalir (Germ.).

Preparations

Oral: Capsules, 500 mg.

Usual Dosages

Oral: 80 mg/kg as a single dose every 3 days or 20 to 30 mg/kg daily.

HYDROXYZINE

Proprietary Names: Atarax, Atazina (Ital.), Aterax (S. Afr.), Masmoran (Germ.), Neocalma (Ital.), Neurozina (Ital.), Paxistil (Belg.), Sedaril, Vistaril.

Preparations

Injection: Solution, 25, 50, and 100 mg/ml.
Oral: Capsules, 25, 50, and 100 mg; suspension, 25 mg/ml; syrup, 10 mg/5 ml; tablets, 10, 25, 50, and 100 mg.

Usual Dosages

Intramuscular: Adults, for serious psychiatric conditions, 50 to 100 mg initially and every 4 to 6 hours as needed.
Oral: For anxiety, adults, 225 to 400 mg daily divided in three or four doses. For pruritus in adults, 25 mg three to four times daily; children over 6 years, 50 to 100 mg daily in divided doses; children under 6 years, 50 mg daily in divided doses.

HYOSCINE

See Scopolamine.

HYPEROSMOTIC AGENTS

See Glycerin, Isosorbide, Mannitol, Urea.

IBUPROFEN

Proprietary Names: Brufen (G.B.), Motrin.

Preparations

Oral: Tablets, 300 and 400 mg.

Usual Dosages

Oral: 300 or 400 mg three or four times daily may be administered.

IDOXURIDINE (IDU)

Proprietary Names: Dendrid, Herpid (G.B.), Herpidu (S. Afr.), Herplex, Iduridine (Germ., Swed.), Iduviran (Fr.), Kerecid (G.B.), Ophthalmadine (G.B.), Stoxil, Synmiol (Germ.), Virunguent (Germ.).

Preparations

Topical Ophthalmic: Ointment, 0.5 per cent; solution, 0.1 per cent.

---

*Route of administration not approved by FDA.
† Drug not approved by FDA for any indication.
‡ Drug not approved by FDA for this particular indication.
§ Indicated dosage above the manufacturer's recommendation.

Usual Dosages

Topical Ophthalmic: One drop of the solution instilled every hour during the day and every 2 hours at night. The ointment is applied four or five times daily or as nighttime medication when the solution is used during the day. Treatment should be continued for at least 2 weeks.

IFOSFAMIDE

Proprietary Names: Cyfos, Holoxan (Fr., Germ., Neth.), Ifex, Mitoxana, Naxamide.

Preparations

Injection: Powder in vials of 0.5, 1.0 and 2.0 gm.

Usual Dosages

Intravenous: A total dose for each course is 8 to 10 gm/square meter administered as a single daily dose over 3 to 10 days.

IMIPENEM/CILASTATIN COMBINATION

Proprietary Name: Primaxin.

Preparations

Injection: Powder (equivalent to base), 250 mg of imipenem and 250 mg of cilastatin.

Usual Dosages

Intravenous: The daily dosage should not exceed 50 mg/kg or 4 gm, whichever is lower. The usual adult dosage is 500 mg every 6 hours.

IMIPRAMINE

Proprietary Names: Berkomine (G.B.), Censtim (Austral.), Chemipramine (Canad.), Co-Caps Imipramine (G.B.), Dimipressin (G.B.), Imavate, Imiprin (Austral.), Impranil (Canad.), Impril (Canad.), Iramil (Austral.), Janimine, Melipramine (Austral.), Norpramine (G.B.), Novopramine (Canad.), Oppanyl (G.B.), Panpramine S. Afr.), Praminil (G.B.), Presamine, Prodepress (Austral.), SK-Pramine, Somipra (Austral.), Thymopramine (S. Afr.), Tofranil, W.D.D.

Preparations

Injection: Solution, 12.5 mg/ml.
Oral: Capsules, 75, 100, 125, and 150 mg; tablets, 10, 25, and 50 mg.

Usual Dosages

Intramuscular: Adults, initially up to 100 mg daily in divided doses. The oral route should be substituted as soon as possible.

Oral: Adults (hospitalized), initially, 100 mg daily in divided doses, increased gradually to 200 mg daily; 250 to 300 mg daily may be given if there is no response after 2 weeks. Adults (outpatients), initially, 75 mg increased to 150 mg daily in divided doses; for maintenance, 50 to 150 mg daily at bedtime (maximum, 300 mg daily). Adolescents and elderly patients, initially, 30 to 40 mg daily (maximum, 100 mg daily).

INDOMETHACIN (INDOMETACIN)

Proprietary Names: Amuno (Germ.), Confortid (Swed.), Imbrilon (G.B.), Inacid (Span.), Indacin (Jap.), Indocid (G.B.), Indocin, Indomee (Swed.), Infrocin (Canad.), Metindol (Pol.), Mezolin (Jap.).

Preparations

Oral: Capsules, 25 and 50 mg.
Topical Ophthalmic: No commercial preparations are available. A 1 per cent solution may be prepared by dissolving 10 mg of indomethacin in 1 ml of sesame oil or water.

Usual Dosages

Oral: 50 to 200 mg daily in divided doses.
Topical Ophthalmic: Solution may be administered three or four times daily.

INFLUENZA VIRUS VACCINE

Proprietary Names: Fluax, Fluogen, Fluvirin (G.B.), Fluzone, Influvac (G.B.), MFV-Ject (Fr., G.B.).

Preparations

Injection: Suspension, 100 µg/ml.

Usual Dosages

Intramuscular: For adults and children older than 12 years of age, the usual dosage is 0.5 ml administered as a single dose.

---

* Route of administration not approved by FDA.
† Drug not approved by FDA for any indication.
‡ Drug not approved by FDA for this particular indication.
§ Indicated dosage above the manufacturer's recommendation.

INSULIN

Proprietary Names: Actrapid, Deposulin (Germ.), Endopancrine (Fr.), Insulatard NPH, Lentard, Lente (Iletin or Insulin), Mixtard, Monotard, NPH Iletin, Protamine (Zinc and Iletin), Regular (Iletin or Insulin), Semilente (Iletin or Insulin), Semitard, Ultralente (Iletin or Insulin), Ultratard, Velosulin.

Preparations

Injection: Solution and suspension, 40, 80, 100, and 500 units/ml.

Usual Dosages

Intramuscular, Intravenous, Subcutaneous: The number and size of daily doses are dependent upon patient's need.

INTERFERON-ALPHA

Proprietary Names: Alferon, Intron A, Roferon-A, Wellferon.

Preparations

Injection: Powder, 18 million units/vial; solution, 3 or 6 million units/ml.
Topical Ophthalmic: No ophthalmic preparation is commercially available. A solution containing 30 million units/ml may be prepared by using parenteral preparations.

Usual Dosages

Intramuscular, Subcutaneous: Initially, the usual dose is 3 million units daily. The recommended maintenance dose is 3 million units 3 times weekly. Doses higher than 3 million units are not recommended.
Topical Ophthalmic: Two drops may be applied to the eye(s) daily.

INTERFERON GAMMA

Proprietary Name: Interferon Gamma.

Preparations

Injection: Lyophilized powder for reconstitution with sterile water. One mg is equivalent to 20 million units.

Usual Dosages

Intramuscular, Subcutaneous: The usual daily dose is 1 to 10 million units (0.125 to 0.5

mg)/square meter. Depending on the severity, the duration of administration may last several months.

INTERLEUKIN-2

Proprietary Name: Cetus.

Preparations

Infection: Solution.

Usual Dosages

Intravenous: Initially, the usual dose is 30,000 to 100,000 units/kg every 8 hours.

ISOFLUROPHATE (DFP)

Proprietary Names: Diflupyl (Fr.), Dyflos (G.B.), Floropryl.

Preparations

Topical Ophthalmic: Ointment, 0.025 per cent; solution, 0.1 per cent.

Usual Dosages

Topical Ophthalmic: One drop daily or 1/4-inch strip of ointment every 12 to 72 hours.

ISOMETHEPTENE/ DICHLORALPHENAZONE COMBINATION

Proprietary Name: Midrin.

Preparations

Oral: Capsules, 65 mg isometheptene and 100 mg dichloralphenazone.

Usual Dosages

Oral: At first sign of a migraine attack, two capsules should be taken, followed by one capsule every hour until migraine is relieved. Maximum dose is five capsules in a 12-hour period.

---

*Route of administration not approved by FDA.
† Drug not approved by FDA for any indication.
‡ Drug not approved by FDA for this particular indication.
§ Indicated dosage above the manufacturer's recommendation.

ISONIAZID

Proprietary Names: Cedin (Germ.), Cotinazin, Dinacrin, Dow-Isoniazid, Hydronsan (Jap., S. Afr.), Hyzyd, INH, Isobicina (Ital.), Isotamine (Canad.), Isotinyl (Austral.), Isozid (Germ.), Laniazid, Neoteben (Germ.), Niconyl, Nidaton, Nydrazid, Panazid, Rimifon (G.B.), Rolazid, Tb-Phlogin (Germ.), Teebaconin, Tibinide (Swed.), Triniad, Uniad.

Preparations

Injection: Solution, 100 mg/ml.
Oral: Syrup, 50 mg/5 ml; tablets, 100 and 300 mg.

Usual Dosages

Intramuscular, Oral: Adults, 5 mg/kg daily in a single dose (maximum, 300 mg daily). Children inactivate this drug faster than adults and may be given 30 mg/kg daily in a single dose (maximum, 300 mg daily). The larger doses should be used for atypical infection. For prophylactic use, adults, 300 mg daily in a single dose; children, 10 mg/kg daily in a single dose (maximum, 300 mg daily).

ISOPROTERENOL

Proprietary Names: Aerolone, Isoprenaline (G.B.), Isuprel, Norisodrine, Vapo-Iso.

Preparations

Inhalation: Aerosol, 0.2 and 0.25 per cent; solution for nebulization, 0.031, 0.062, 0.25, 0.5, and 1.0 per cent.
Injection: Solution, 0.02 and 0.2 mg/ml.
Sublingual: Tablets, 10 and 15 mg.

Usual Dosages

Inhalation: For treatment of bronchospasm during mild acute asthmatic attacks, the usual dose is 120 to 262 μg (one or two inhalations of a 0.25 per cent solution) administered via a metered aerosol.
Intramuscular, Intravenous, Subcutaneous: The usual adult bolus dose is 0.02 to 0.06 mg, with subsequent doses ranging from 0.01 to 0.2 mg.
Sublingual: Adults, usual dose is 10 to 20 mg. Daily dosage should not exceed 60 mg. Children, usual dose is 5 to 10 mg. Daily dosage should not exceed 30 mg.

ISOSORBIDE

Proprietary Name: Isosorbide.

Preparations

Oral: Solution, 45 per cent.

Usual Dosages

Oral: Adults, initially, 1.5 gm/kg may be given up to four times daily. The usual dose range is 1 to 3 gm/kg two to four times a day as needed.

IVERMECTIN

Proprietary Names: Cardomec, Eqvalan, Heartgard-30, Ivomec (G.B.), Zimecterin.

Preparations

Oral: Tablets.

Usual Dosages

Oral: A single oral dose of 12 mg annually.

KANAMYCIN

Proprietary Names: Kamycine (Fr.), Kanabristol (Germ.), Kanasig (Austral.), Kanmy (S. Afr.), Kannasyn (G.B.), Kantrex, Kantrox (Swed.), Klebcil.

Preparations

Injection: Solution, 37.5, 250, and 333 mg/ml.

Usual Dosages

Intramuscular: To achieve continuously high blood levels, 15 mg/kg daily in divided doses every 6 to 8 hours. Otherwise, a dose of 7.5 mg/kg every 12 hours should not be exceeded.
Intravenous: This route is used only if intramuscular route is not possible. The dose should not exceed 15 mg/kg daily and must be administered slowly.

KETOCONAZOLE

Proprietary Name: Nizoral.

---

* Route of administration not approved by FDA.
† Drug not approved by FDA for any indication.
‡ Drug not approved by FDA for this particular indication.
§ Indicated dosage above the manufacturer's recommendation.

Preparations

Oral: Suspension, 100 mg/5 ml; tablets, 200 mg.
Topical: Cream, 2 per cent.
Topical Ophthalmic: No ophthalmic preparation is commercially available.

Usual Dosages

Oral: The recommended starting dose is 200 mg in a single daily dose. In very serious infections, the dose may be increased up to 1.2 gm daily.
Topical Ophthalmic: A 1 to 2 per cent solution may be applied to the affected and surrounding areas twice a day for up to 8 to 12 weeks.

KETOROLAC

Proprietary Name: Toradol.

Preparations

Injection: Solution, 15 and 30 mg/ml.
Oral: Tablets, 10 mg.

Usual Dosages

Intramuscular Injection: Initial dose of 30 or 60 mg as a loading dose, followed by half of the loading dose. Maximum recommended daily dose is 150 mg for the first day and 120 mg/day thereafter.
Oral: 10 mg as needed every 4 to 6 hours with a maximum dosage of 40 mg daily; prolonged treatment is not recommended.

KETOTIFEN

Proprietary Names: Zaditen (Belg., G.B., Germ., Lux., Neth., Switz.).

Preparations

Oral: Capsules, 1 mg; elixir, 1 mg/5 ml; tablets, 1 mg.

Usual Dosages

Oral: The usual daily dose is 1 mg twice daily.

LEUCOVORIN

Proprietary Names: Lederfoline (Fr.), Ledervorin (Neth.), Ledervorin Calcium (Belg.).

Preparations

Injection: Powder, 50 mg; solution, 3 mg/ml.

Usual Dosages

Intramuscular, Intravenous, Oral, Subcutaneous (Deep): Up to 1 mg daily; maintenance dose of 0.1 to 0.25 mg daily.

LEVAMISOLE

Proprietary Names: Decaris (Denm., Hung.), Ergamisol (Belg., Ital., S. Afr.), Ketrax (G.B.), Meglum (Arg.), Solaskil (Fr.), Stimamizol (Arg.).

Preparations

Oral: Syrup, 40 mg/5 ml; tablets, 40 mg.

Usual Dosages

Oral: An initial daily dose of 40 mg is recommended, increasing the amount by 40 mg every 2 weeks to a maximum of 150 mg.

LEVOBUNOLOL

Proprietary Name: Betagan.

Preparations

Topical Ophthalmic: Solution, 0.5 per cent.

Usual Dosages

Topical Ophthalmic: The usual dose is one drop in the affected eye(s) one to two times daily.

LEVODOPA

Proprietary Names: Bendopa, Berkdopa (G.B.), Bio Dopa, Brocadopa (G.B.), Dopar, Dopastral (Swed.), Emeldopa (S. Afr.), Helfodopa (Germ.), Larodopa, Ledopa (Fr.), Levopa (G.B.), Parda, Parkidopa (Swed.), Rio-Dopa, Sobiodopa (Fr.), Speciadopa (Fr.), Syndopa (Austral.), Veldopa (G.B.).

---

*Route of administration not approved by FDA.
† Drug not approved by FDA for any indication.
‡ Drug not approved by FDA for this particular indication.
§ Indicated dosage above the manufacturer's recommendation.

Preparations

Oral: Capsules 100, 250, and 500 mg; tablets, 100, 250, and 500 mg.

Usual Dosages

Oral: The usual initial dosage is 0.5 to 1.0 gm daily, divided into two or more doses. The usual optimal therapeutic dosage should not exceed 8 gm daily.

LEVOTHYROXINE

Proprietary Names: Cytolen, Eltroxin (G.B.), Euthyrox (Germ.), Letter, Levaxin (Swed.), Levoid, Levothroid, Noroxine, Oroxine (Austral.), Percutacrine, Thyroxinique (Fr.), Synthroid, Thyratabs (Swed.), Thyrine (Austral.), Thyroxevan (Austral.), Thyroxinal (Austral.), Thyroxine (G.B.).

Preparations

Oral: Tablets, 0.025, 0.05, 0.1, 0.15, 0.175, 0.2, and 0.3 mg.

Usual Dosages

Oral: Initially, 0.05 to 0.1 mg daily, increased by increments of 0.05 to 0.1 mg at 2- to 2-week intervals until the desired response is maintained. Most patients can be maintained in a full clinical euthyroid state with doses of 0.1 to 0.2 mg daily.

LIDOCAINE

Proprietary Names: Anaesthol (Germ.), Anestacon, Ardecaine, Canocaine, Dolicaine, Indolor (S. Afr.), L-Caine, Leostesin (S. Afr.), Lida-Mantle, Lidocaton (G.B.), Lidothesin (G.B.), Lignane (S. Afr.), Lignocaine (G.B.), Lignostab (G.B.), Nervocaine, Norocaine, Nurocain (Austral.), Rocaine, Sarnacaine (Austral.), Stanacaine, Ultracaine, Xylestesin (Germ.), Xylocaine, Xylocard (G.B.), Xylotox (G.B.).

Preparations

Injection: Solution, 0.5, 1.0, 1.5, 2.0, 4.0, and 5.0 per cent.
Topical: Jelly, 2 per cent; ointment, 2.5 and 5.0 per cent; solution, 2 and 4 per cent.

Usual Dosages

Infiltration: Without epinephrine, for extensive procedures, 25 to 60 ml of a 0.5 per cent solution or 10 to 30 ml of a 1 per cent solution; for minor surgery and relief of pain, 2 to 50 ml of a 0.5 per cent solution. With epinephrine 1:200,000, up to 50 ml of a 1 per cent solution.

Topical: The 2 per cent solution is generally recommended for topical anesthesia. The 4 per cent solution should be used only when the lower concentration does not provide adequate anesthesia. The maximum dose is 10 ml of the 2 per cent or 5 ml of the 4 per cent concentration.

LINCOMYCIN

Proprietary Names: Albiotic (Germ.), Cillimycin (Germ.), Lincocin, Mycivin (G.B.).

Preparations

Injection: Solution, 300 mg/ml.
Oral: Capsules, 250 and 500 mg.

Usual Dosages

Intramuscular: Adults, 0.6 to 1.2 gm daily. Children and infants over 1 month, 10 to 20 mg/kg daily.
Intravenous: Adults, 0.6 to 1.0 gm every 8 to 12 hours. Maximum daily dose should not exceed 8 gm. Children and infants over 1 month, 10 to 20 mg/kg daily in two or three divided doses.
Oral: Adults, 500 mg three or four times daily. Children and infants over 1 month, 30 to 60 mg/kg in three or four divided doses.
Subconjunctival: 150 mg in a 0.5 ml aqueous solution.

LINDANE (GAMMA BENZENE HEXACHLORIDE)

Proprietary Names: Aphtris (Fr.), Elentol (Fr.), Gamene, Jacutin (Germ.), Lorexane (G.B.), Kevellada (Canad.), Kwell.

Preparations

Topical: Cream, lotion, and shampoo, 1 per cent.

Usual Dosages

Topical: Cream or lotion is applied with soft brush and washed off thoroughly after 24

---

* Route of administration not approved by FDA.
† Drug not approved by FDA for any indication.
‡ Drug not approved by FDA for this particular indication.
§ Indicated dosage above the manufacturer's recommendation.

hours using a soft brush. For head lice, shampoo is applied, lathered, and rinsed thoroughly after 5 minutes; this may be repeated in 1 week if indicated. For pubic lice, shampoo applied as above, or after a scrub bath as outlined previously, thin layer of lotion is applied to affected area and washed off 24 hours later.

LIOTHYRONINE

Proprietary Names: Cynomel (Fr.), Cytomel, Tertroxin (G.B.), Triiodothyronine (G.B.), Trithyrone (Fr.).

Preparations

Oral: Tablets, 5, 25, and 50 μg.

Usual Dosages

Oral: Intially, 25 μg daily, increased by increments of 12.5 to 25 μg at intervals of 1 to 2 weeks until the desired response is maintained. The usual maintenance dose is up to 75 to 100 μg daily.

LITHIUM

Proprietary Names: Camcolit (G.B.), Carbolith (Canad.), Eskalith, Hypnorex (Germ.), Lithane, Lithicarb (Austral.), Lithionit (Swed.), Lithium Duriles (Germ.), Lithium Oligosol (Fr.), Lithobid, Litho-Carb (Canad.), Lithonate, Lithotabs, Maniprex (Belg.), Neurolithium (Fr.), Pfi-Lith, Phasal (G.B.), Priadel (G.B.), Quilonum (Germ., S. Afr.).

Preparations

Oral: Capsules, 300 mg, syrup, 8 mEq/5 ml; tablets, 300 mg.

Usual Dosages

Oral: Dosage should be individualized on the basis of serum levels and response.

LORAZEPAM

Proprietary Names: Almazine (G.B.), Ativan (Austral., Canad., G.B., Ire., S. Afr., USA), Control (Ital., Switz.), Donix (Span.), Duralozam (Ger.), Idalprem (Span.), Laubeel (Ger.), Lorans (Ital.), Loraz, Novolorazem (Canad.), Orfidal (Span.), Pro Dorm (Ger.), Punktyl (Ger.), Sedizepan (Span.), Somagerol (Ger.), Tavor (Ger., Ital.), Temesta (Fr., Neth., Swed., Switz.), Tolid (Ger.), Tran-Qil (S. Afr.), Tranqipam (S. Afr.).

Preparations

Injection: 2 and 4 mg/ml.
Oral: Tablets, 0.5, 1, and 2 mg.

Usual Dosages

Intramuscular: 0.05 mg/kg up to a maximum of 4 mg.
Intravenous: 2 mg total or 0.02 mg/lb, whichever is smaller.
Oral: 1 to 4 mg daily in two to three divided doses with the largest dose taken at night; up to 10 mg daily.

LOVASTATIN (MEVINOLIN)

Proprietary Name: Mevacor.

Preparations

Oral: Tablets, 20 mg.

Usual Dosages

Oral: The dose range is 20 to 80 mg daily in single or divided doses.

LUBRICANTS

See Petroleum, Artificial Tears.

MALATHION

Proprietary Names: Derbac (G.B.), Noury Hoofdlotion (Neth.), Prioderm.

Preparations

Topical: Liquid, 0.05 per cent; lotion, 0.05 per cent; shampoo, 1 per cent.

Usual Dosages

Topical: The recommended treatment for head lice is two applications 1 week apart.

MANNITOL

Proprietary Names: Manicol (Fr.), Osmitrol, Osmosol (Austral.), Resectisol.

---

* Route of administration not approved by FDA.
† Drug not approved by FDA for any indication.
‡ Drug not approved by FDA for this particular indication.
§ Indicated dosage above the manufacturer's recommendation.

Preparations

Injection: Solution, 5, 10, 15, and 20 per cent.

Usual Dosages

Intravenous: 0.5 to 2 gm/kg given as a 20 per cent solution is infused slowly over a period of 30 to 60 minutes.

MEASLES, MUMPS, AND RUBELLA VIRUS VACCINE LIVE

Proprietary Name: M-M-R.

Preparations

Injection: 1000 $TCID_{50}$ measles virus vaccine live, 5000 $TCID_{50}$ mumps virus vaccine live, and 1000 $TCID_{50}$ rubella virus vaccine live/0.5 ml.

Usual Dosages

Subcutaneous: The usual dose is 0.5 ml administered as a single dose.

MEBENDAZOLE

Proprietary Names: Mebendacin (Span.), Mebutar (Arg.), Nemasole (Arg.), Vermox.

Preparations

Oral: Tablets (chewable), 100 mg.

Usual Dosages

Oral: Adults and children, 100 mg given morning and evening for 3 consecutive days for most infections. Enterobiasis can usually be treated with a single 100-mg dose; if a cure is not achieved with initial therapy, a second course 3 weeks later may be beneficial.

MECHLORETHAMINE

Proprietary Names: Caryolysine (Fr.), Cloramin (Ital.), Erasol (Denm.), Mustargen, Mustine (G.B.).

Preparations

Injection: Powder, 10 mg.
Topical: No topical preparations are commercially available, but a 0.02 to 0.1 per cent solution can be prepared.

Usual Dosages

Intravenous: The usual dosage is 0.4 mg/kg per course of therapy, given in a single dose or on 2 separate days. The interval between courses of therapy is usually 3 to 6 weeks.

Topical: Solution may be applied daily for 4 weeks in treatment of mycosis fungoides.

MECLIZINE (MECLOZINE)

Proprietary Names: Antivert, Antrizine, Bonamine (Canad., Germ.), Bonine, Calmonal (Germ.), Dizmiss, Eldezine, Lamine, Mecazine (Canad.), Motion Cure, Navicalm (S. Afr.), Postafen (Germ., Swed.), Roclizine, Ru-Vert-M, Veritab, Vertizine, Vertrol, Wehvert.

Preparations

Oral: Tablets, 12.5, 25, and 50 mg; tablets (chewable), 25 mg.

Usual Dosages

Oral: The daily dose is 25 to 50 mg in single or divided doses.

MEDRYSONE

Proprietary Name: HMS Liquifilm.

Preparations

Topical Ophthalmic: Suspension, 1 per cent.

Usual Dosages

Topical Ophthalmic: One drop of suspension every 1 or 2 hours until response is obtained; frequency is then reduced.

MELPHALAN

Proprietary Name: Alkeran.

Preparations

Oral: Tablets, 2 mg.

---

* Route of administration not approved by FDA.
† Drug not approved by FDA for any indication.
‡ Drug not approved by FDA for this particular indication.
§ Indicated dosage above the manufacturer's recommendation.

Usual Dosages

Oral: The usual dosage is 6 mg daily.

MENADIOL

Proprietary Names: Kappadione, Synkayvite.

Preparations

Injection: Solution, 5, 10, and 37.5 mg/ml.
Oral: Tablets, 5 mg.

Usual Dosages

Intramuscular, Intravenous, Oral, Subcutaneous: The usual adult therapeutic dose is 5 to 15 mg.

MENADIONE

Proprietary Name: Menadione.

Preparations

Oral: Powder; tablets, 5 mg.

Usual Dosages

Oral: The usual adult therapeutic dose is 2 to 10 mg.

MEPACRINE

See Quinacrine.

MEPERIDINE (PETHIDINE)

Proprietary Names: Demerol, Dolantin (Germ.), Dolosal (Fr.), Pethoid (Austral.), Phytadon (Canad.), Suppolosal (Fr.).

Preparations

Injection: Solution, 50, 75, and 100 mg/ml.
Injection: Elixir, 50 mg/5 ml; tablets, 50 and 10 mg.

Usual Dosages

Intramuscular, Intravenous (Slow), Oral, Subcutaneous: Adults, 50 to 150 mg every 3 to 4 hours as necessary. Children, 1 to 1.5 mg/kg (maximum dose, 100 mg) administered orally, subcutaneously, or intramuscularly. The dose may be repeated at intervals of 3 to 4 hours if necessary.

MERCAPTAMINE

Proprietary Names: Cysteamine (G.B.), Lambratene (Ital.).

Preparations

Injection, Oral: Powder.
Topical Ophthalmic: No ophthalmic preparation is commercially available.

Usual Dosages

Oral: A 5 per cent solution may be given in an initial daily dose of 30 mg/kg, divided into four equal parts. This may be increased to 60 mg/kg after 4 weeks, to 90 mg/kg after a further 4 weeks, and then maintained at this dose.
Topical Ophthalmic: A solution containing 0.1 per cent mercaptamine may be prepared with the powder for injection.

METHACHOLINE

Proprietary Name: Methacholine.

Preparations

Injection: Ampule, 1 and 10 gm.

Usual Dosages

Subcutaneous: 10 to 25 mg.

METHAZOLAMIDE

Proprietary Name: Neptazane.

Preparations

Oral: Tablets, 50 mg.

Usual Dosages

Oral: The usual adult dosage is 50 to 100 mg two or three times daily.

---

*Route of administration not approved by FDA.
† Drug not approved by FDA for any indication.
‡ Drug not approved by FDA for this particular indication.
§ Indicated dosage above the manufacturer's recommendation.

METHICILLIN

Proprietary Names: Azapen, Belfacillin (Swed.), Celbenin, Cinopenil (Germ.), Flabelline (Fr.), Lucopenin (Denm.), Metin (Austral.), Penistaph (Fr.), Staphcillin, Synticillin (Denm.).

Preparations

Injection: Powder (buffered), 1, 4, and 6 gm (900 mg methicillin base/gm).

Usual Dosages

Intracameral: 1 mg in 0.2 to 0.5 ml of isotonic sodium chloride injection.
Intramuscular: Adults, 1 gm every 6 hours. Infants and children, 25 mg/kg every 6 hours.
Intravenous: Adults, 1 gm every 6 hours. Higher doses may be required in the treatment of severe infections, and intramuscular doses of up to 8 gm a day and intravenous doses of 8 to 24 gm a day have been used.
Subconjunctival: 50 to 150 mg in 0.5 ml of isotonic sodium chloride injection or sterile water for injection.

METHIMAZOLE

Proprietary Name: Tapazole.

Preparations

Oral: Tablets, 5 and 10 mg.

Usual Dosages

Oral: Adults, 15 to 60 mg daily for initial treatment of hyperthyroidism and 5 to 15 mg daily for maintenance.

METHOCARBAMOL

Proprietary Names: Delaxin, Lumirelax (Fr.), Metho-500, Methocabal (Jap.), Parabaxin, Robaxin, Romethocarb, SK-Methocarbamal, Tresortil (Denm.).

Preparations

Injection: Solution, 100 mg/ml.
Oral: Tablets, 500 and 750 mg.

Usual Dosages

Intravenous: Adults, 1 to 3 gm daily at a rate not exceeding 3 ml/min.
Oral: Adults, initially, 1.5 to 2 gm four

times daily for 48 to 72 hours; for maintenance, 1 gm four times daily.

METHOTREXATE

Proprietary Names: Ledertrexate (Fr.),
Mexate.

Preparations

Injection: Solution, 2.5, 20, 25, 50, 100, and
250 mg/ml.
Oral: Tablets, 2.5 mg.

Usual Dosages

Intramuscular: In the management of rheumatoid arthritis, parenteral dosage regimen
often consists of 7.5 to 15 mg given intramuscularly once weekly.
Oral: For psoriasis chemotherapy, divided
dose schedule recommends 2.5 mg at 12-hour
intervals for three doses or at 8-hour intervals
for four doses each week. When remission is
achieved and supportive care in antineoplastic chemotherapy has produced general clinical improvement, maintenance therapy of 30
mg/square meter is administered two times
weekly either by mouth or intramuscularly. In
the management of rheumatoid arthritis, oral
dosage regimen often consists of 2.5 mg administered at 12-hour intervals for three doses
each week.

METHOXSALEN

Proprietary Names: Oxsoralen, Oxsoralen
Ultra, Soloxsalen (Canad.).

Preparations

Oral: Capsules, 10 mg.
Topical: Lotion, 1 per cent.

Usual Dosages

Oral: 20 to 70 mg followed by UV
irradiation.
Topical: Application followed by UV
irradiation.

METHYLCELLULOSE

Proprietary Names: BFL (Canad.), Cellu-
lone (Austral.), Cologel, Hydrolose, Isopto-

---

* Route of administration not approved by FDA.
† Drug not approved by FDA for any indication.
‡ Drug not approved by FDA for this particular
indication.
§ Indicated dosage above the manufacturer's
recommendation.

Plain, Lacril (Canad.), Methocel A, Methulose,
Tearisol, Viscosae (Denm.), Visulose.

Preparations

Topical Ophthalmic: Solution, 0.25, 0.5, and
1 per cent.

Usual Dosages

Topical Ophthalmic: One drop as needed.

METHYLENE BLUE (METHYLTHIONINE)

Proprietary Names: Desmoidpillen
(Germ.), M-B Tabs, Urolene Blue, Wright's
Stain.

Preparations

Injection: Solution, 1 to 5 per cent.

Usual Dosages

Injection: In the form of a 2 per cent sterile
stolution, it is used to outline various body
cavities.

METHYLPREDNISOLONE

Proprietary Names: A-Methapred, Depo-
Medrate (Germ.), Depo-Medrol, Depo-Med-
rone (G.B.), Depo-Pred, Dura-Meth, Medra-
lone, Medrate (Germ.), Medrol, Medules,
Mepred, Rep-Pred, Solu-Medrol, Solu-Med-
rone (G.B.), Urbason (Germ., Swed.).

Preparations

Injection: Aqueous suspension, 20, 40 and
80 mg/ml; powder, 40, 125, 500 mg, and 1
gm. The aqueous suspension for injection
may be used for subconjunctival injection.
Oral: Capsules, 2 and 4 mg; tablets, 2, 4,
8, 16, 24, and 32 mg.

Usual Dosages

Intravenous: Initially, 10 to 40 mg. For high
dose therapy, 30 mg/kg infused over 10 to 20
minutes.
Oral: The initial dosage may vary from 4
to 48 mg daily depending on the specific disease entity being treated. It should be empha
sized that dosage requirements are variable
and must be individualized on the basis of the
disease under treatment and the response of
the patient.

Subconjunctival: 0.5 ml of a suspension containing 20, 40, or 80 mg/ml. This dose may be repeated every 3 to 5 weeks.

METHYLTESTOSTERONE

Proprietary Names: Android, Glosso-Sterandryl (Fr.), Mesteron (Pol.), Metandren, Neohombreol M, Oreton Methyl, Testin (Norw.), Testomet (Austral.), Testred, Virilon.

Preparations

Oral: Tablets, 5 and 10 mg.

Usual Dosages

Buccal: 10 mg sublingually may reduce the frequency and severity of angioedema attacks.

METHYLTHIONINE

See Methylene Blue.

METHYSERGIDE

Proprietary Names: Desril (G.B.), Desernil (Fr.), Sansert.

Preparations

Oral: Tablets, 2 mg.

Usual Dosages

Oral: Adults, 2 to 8 mg daily in divided doses.

METRONIDAZOLE

Proprietary Names: Clont (Germ.), Debetrol (Arg.), Deflamon (Ital.), Elyzol (Scand.), Entizol (Pol.), Flagyl, Fossyol (Germ.), Gineflavir (Ital.), Kreucosan (Germ.), Meronidal (Jap.), Metrolag (Switz.), Nalox (Arg.), Neo-Tric (Canad.), Nida (Jap.), Novonidazol (Canad.), Rathimed N (Germ.), Salandol (Jap.), Sanatrichom (Germ.), Tranoxa (Arg.), Trichocide (Jap.), Tricho-Gynaedron (Germ.), Trichos Cordes (Germ.), Trichomal (Denm.), Trichozole (Austral.), Tricocet (Ital.), Tricofin

(Arg.), Tricowas (Span.), Trikacide (Canad.), Trivazol (Ital.), Vagilen (Ital.), Vaginyl (G.B.).

Preparations

Oral: Tablets, 200 and 250 mg.

Usual Dosages

Oral: Adults, 250 mg three times daily for 7 days; course may be repeated if needed after interval of 4 to 6 weeks.

METIPRANOLOL

Proprietary Names: Betanol (Mon.), Beta-Ophtiole (Neth., S. Afr.), Disorate (Ger.), Glauline (G.B.), Optipranolol.

Preparations

Topical Ophthalmic: 0.1 and 0.3 per cent solution.

Usual Dosages

Topical Ophthalmic: One drop of solution may be applied to affected eye(s) twice daily.

MEVINOLIN

See Lovastatin.

MICONAZOLE

Proprietary Names: Albistat (Belg., Neth.), Andergin (Ital.), Daktar (Germ., Norw., Swed.), Daktarin (G.B.), Deralbine (Arg.), Dermonistat (G.B.), Epi-Monistat (Germ.), Fungisidin (Span.), Micatin, Micotef (Ital.).

Preparations

Injection: Solution, 10 mg/ml in 20-ml ampules.
Oral: Available from Centers for Disease Control.
Topical: Cream, 2 per cent.
Topical Ophthalmic: No ophthalmic preparation is commercially available. A 1 per cent solution in arachnis oil may be prepared by dissolving in chloroform, mixing with arachnis oil, and driving off chloroform by heat. A 2 per cent ointment form may also be prepared. A 1 per cent solution may also be obtained by using the intravenous preparation containing 10 mg/ml.

---

*Route of administration not approved by FDA.
† Drug not approved by FDA for any indication.
‡ Drug not approved by FDA for this particular indication.
§ Indicated dosage above the manufacturer's recommendation.

Usual Dosages

Intravenous: A daily dosage of 25 to 30 mg/kg in two or three equally divided doses at 8- or 12-hour intervals.
Intravitreal: 40 µg in 0.1 to 0.2 ml of sterile aqueous solution.
Subconjunctival: 5 to 10 mg in a 0.5 ml aqueous solution.
Topical: A sufficient amount of cream to cover the affected area is applied twice daily.
Topical Ophthalmic: Preparation is applied to affected and surrounding areas twice a day. Ophthalmic form is applied up to 8 to 12 weeks.

MINOCYCLINE

Proprietary Names: Klinomycin (Germ.), Minocin, Minomycin (Austral., S. Afr.), Mynocine (Fr.), Ultramycin (Canad.), Vectrin.

Preparations

Injection: Powder, 100 mg (of base).
Oral: Capsules, 50 and 100 mg (of base); syrup, 50 mg (of base)/5 ml.

Usual Dosages

Intravenous: Adults, 200 mg followed by 100 mg every 12 hours (maximum, 400 mg daily). Children 8 to 12 years of age, 4 mg/kg initially followed by 2 mg/kg every 12 hours.
Oral: Adults and children over 12 years of age, 200 mg initially, followed by 100 mg every 12 hours. Children 8 to 12 years of age, 4 mg/kg daily in divided doses every 12 hours.

MITHRAMYCIN

See Plicamycin.

MITOMYCIN

Proprietary Names: Ametycine (Fr.), Mutamycin (Canad., Neth., Swed., Switz., USA).

Preparations

Injection: Solution, 5, 20, and 40 mg.
Topical Ophthalmic: No ophthalmic prepa-

---

* Route of administration not approved by FDA.
† Drug not approved by FDA for any indication.
‡ Drug not approved by FDA for this particular indication.
§ Indicated dosage above the manufacturer's recommendation.

ration is commercially available; however, a 0.02 to 0.04 per cent solution can be prepared.

Usual Dosages

Injection: The usual initial dose is 10 to 20 mg/square meter body surface given as a single dose through an infusion, repeated every 6 to 8 weeks. It may be given intravenously in divided doses of 20 mg/square meter daily for 5 days and repeated after 2 days.
Topical Ophthalmic: One drop may be applied twice daily for 5 to 14 days in the affected eye.

MONOBENZONE

Proprietary Names: Aloquin (Austral.), Benoquin, Depigman (Germ., Neth., Switz.), Dermochinona (Ital.), Leucodinine (Belg.).

Preparations

Topical: Cream, 20 per cent; ointment, 20 per cent.

Usual Dosages

Topical: Preparation is applied to the affected area two or three times daily.

MOXISYLYTE

Proprietary Names: THY (G.B.), Thymoxamine (G.B.).

Preparations

Topical Ophthalmic: Solution, 0.1, 0.2, and 0.5 per cent.

Usual Dosages

Topical Ophthalmic: The frequency and concentration of instillation depend upon the patient's response to therapy.

MUMPS VIRUS VACCINE LIVE

Proprietary Name: Mumpsvax.

Preparations

Injection: 5000 TCID$_{50}$/0.5 ml.

Usual Dosages

Subcutaneous: The usual dosage is 0.5 ml administered as a single dose.

MUPIROCIN

Proprietary Name: Bactroban.

Preparations

Topical: Ointment, 2 per cent.

Usual Dosages

Topical: A small amount of ointment is applied to the affected area three times daily.

NAFCILLIN

Proprietary Name: Nafcil, Unipen.

Preparations

Injection: Powder, 0.5, 1, and 2 gm.
Oral: Capsules, 250 mg; powder for solution, 250 mg/5 ml; tablets, 500 mg.

Usual Dosages

Intramuscular: Adults, 500 mg every 4 to 6 hours; children, 25 mg/kg twice daily; newborn infants, 10 mg/kg twice daily.
Intravenous: Adults, 0.5 to 1.0 gm in 15 to 30 ml of water for injection or sodium chloride injection infused over a 10-minute period for 4 hours or dissolved in 150 ml of sodium chloride injection and given by slow intravenous drip. Up to 8 gm daily can be given for serious infections. Older infants and children, 50 mg/kg daily in six divided doses.
Oral: Adults, 0.25 to 1.0 gm every 4 to 6 hours, preferably 2 hours before meals. Children, 25 to 50 mg/kg daily in four divided doses. Newborn infants, 10 mg/kg twice daily.

NALOXONE

Proprietary Name: Narcan.

---

*Route of administration not approved by FDA.
† Drug not approved by FDA for any indication.
‡ Drug not approved by FDA for this particular indication.
§ Indicated dosage above the manufacturer's recommendation.

Preparations

Injection: Solution, 0.02, 0.4, and 1.0 mg/ml.

Usual Dosages

Intramuscular, Intravenous, Subcutaneous: For narcotic overdose in adults, the initial dose is 0.4 to 2.0 mg intravenously, which may be repeated at 2- to 3-minute intervals up to 10 mg. For pruritus an intravenous infusion of 2.0 to 6.4 mg may be administered over a 4-hour period.

NAPHAZOLINE

Proprietary Names: Ak-Con, Albalon, Allerest, Clear Eyes, Degest, Naphcon, Opticon, Vasoclear.

Preparations

Topical Ophthalmic: Solution, 0.012 and 0.1 per cent.

Usual Dosages

Topical Ophthalmic: One drop is instilled every 2 to 3 hours or as needed until symptoms subside.

NAPROXEN

Proprietary Names: Anaprox, Naprosyn, Naxen (Mex.), Proxen (Aust., Germ., Switz.).

Preparations

Oral: Tablets, 250 mg.

Usual Dosages

Oral: Adults, 500 to 750 mg daily in divided doses.

NATAMYCIN

Proprietary Names: Myprozine, Natacyn.

Preparations

Topical Ophthalmic: Suspension, 5 per cent.

Usual Dosages

Topical Ophthalmic: One drop of a 5 per cent suspension every 1 to 2 hours. The effect may be enhanced by concomitant treatment with 1 per cent potassium iodide solution, also applied topically.

NEOARSPHENAMINE

Proprietary Name: Collunovar (Fr.).

Preparations

Injection: Powder.

Usual Dosages

Intravenous: Usual dosage is 150 to 600 mg.

NEOMYCIN

Proprietary Names: Bykomycin (Germ.), Emelmycin (S. Afr.), Herisan Antibiotic (Canad.), Myacyne (Germ.), Mycifradin, Myciguent, Neobiotic, Neobram (Austral.), Neocin (Canad.), Neomate (Austral.), Neomin (G.B.), Neo Morrhuol (Austral.), Neopan (S. Afr.), Neopt (Austral.), Nivemycin (G.B.).

Preparations

Injection: Powder, 500 mg.
Oral: Solution, 125 mg/5 ml; tablets, 500 mg.
Topical: Cream, 5 mg/gm; ointment, 5 mg/gm.
Topical Ophthalmic: Ointment, 3.5 and 5.0 mg/ml.

Usual Dosages

Oral: For diarrhea caused by enteropathogenic *E. coli*, adults, 50 mg/kg daily in four divided doses; newborn and premature infants, 10 to 50 mg/kg daily in four divided doses; older infants and children, 50 to 100 mg/kg daily in four divided doses.
Topical: Preparation may be applied two to three times daily.
Topical Ophthalmic: Ointment is applied one to three times daily.

NEOMYCIN/HYDROCORTISONE COMBINATION

Proprietary Names: Ak-Neo-Cort, Neo-Cortef.

---

* Route of administration not approved by FDA.
† Drug not approved by FDA for any indication.
‡ Drug not approved by FDA for this particular indication.
§ Indicated dosage above the manufacturer's recommendation.

Preparations

Topical Ophthalmic: Ointment, 0.5 per cent neomycin and 1.5 per cent hydrocortisone; solution, 0.5 per cent neomycin and 1.5 per cent hydrocortisone.

Usual Dosages

Topical Ophthalmic: Preparation is applied two to three times daily.

NEOMYCIN/POLYMYXIN B COMBINATION

Proprietary Names: Polyspectin Liquifilm, Statrol.

Preparations

Topical Ophthalmic: Ointment, 5 mg neomycin and 6000 units/gm polymyxin B; solution, 5 gm neomycin and 5000 units/ml polymyxin B.

Usual Dosages

Topical Ophthalmic: One drop of solution in lower conjunctival sac(s) several times daily as required. A 0.5-inch ribbon of ointment is instilled in conjunctival sac(s) at night when used adjunctively with the solution.

NEOMYCIN/POLYMYXIN B/BACITRACIN COMBINATION

Proprietary Names: Mycitracin, Neo-Polycin, Neosporin, Polyspectrin S.O.P., Pyocidin.

Preparations

Topical Ophthalmic: Ointment, 5000 units/gm polymyxin B, 400 units/gm bactracin, and 5 mg/gm neomycin.

Usual Dosages

Topical Ophthalmic: A small amount of ointment may be applied to the conjunctival sac several times daily or as required until a favorable response is observed. The number of daily applications may then be reduced until the disorder is under control.

NEOMYCIN/POLYMYXIN B/GRAMICIDIN COMBINATION

Proprietary Name: Neosporin.

Preparations

Topical Ophthalmic: Solution, 1.75 mg neomycin, 10,000 units polymyxin B, and 0.025 mg gramicidin/ml.

Usual Dosages

One or two drops of solution in the affected eye(s) are instilled two to four times daily, or more frequently as required, for 7 to 10 days. In acute infections, drops may be applied every 15 to 30 minutes.

NEOSTIGMINE

Proprietary Name: Prostigmin.

Preparations

Injection: Solution, 0.25, 0.50, and 1 mg/ml.
Topical Ophthalmic: Solution, 5 per cent.

Usual Dosages

Intramuscular: Adults, 15 mg/kg daily in divided doses every 6 hours. The total daily dose should not exceed 1 gm.
Subcutaneous: 0.5 to 2 mg.
Topical Ophthalmic: A dosage of one to two drops may be applied two to six times daily.

NIACIN (NICOTINIC ACID)

Proprietary Names: Acidemel (S. Afr.), Diacin, Efacin, Niac, Nicangin (Swed.), Nico-400, Nicobid, Nicocap, Nicolar, Niconacid (Germ.), Ni Cord, Nico-Span, Nicotinex, Nicyl (Fr.), Ni-Span, SK-Niacin, Span Niacin, Vasotherm, Wampocap.

Preparations

Oral: Tablets, 500 mg.

Usual Dosages

Oral: Adults, initially, 100 mg three times daily, increased to 1.5 to 6.0 gm divided into three doses given with or after meals.

---

*Route of administration not approved by FDA.
† Drug not approved by FDA for any indication.
‡ Drug not approved by FDA for this particular indication.
§ Indicated dosage above the manufacturer's recommendation.

NIFEDIPINE

Proprietary Names: Adalat, Adalate (Fr.), Nifelate (Arg.), Procardia.

Preparations

Oral: Capsules, 10 and 20 mg.

Usual Dosages

Oral: The usual dosage range is 10 to 20 mg three times daily. The maximum daily dose is 180 mg.

NIRIDAZOLE

Proprietary Name: Ambilhar.

Preparations

Oral: Tablets, 500 mg.

Usual Dosages

Oral: Adults and children, 25 mg/kg daily in two divided doses for 5 to 7 days in schistosomiasis and 7 to 10 days in dracunculiasis.

NITROGEN MUSTARD

See Mechlorethamine.

NITROGLYCERIN

Proprietary Names: Anginine (Austral.), Angised (S. Afr.), Ang-O-Span, Cardabid, Corobid, Gilucor Nitro (Germ.), Glyceryl Trinitrate (G.B.), Glynite (Canad.), Gly-Trate, Klavi Kordal, Lenitral (Fr.), Niglycon, Niong, Nitora, Nitrangin (Germ.), Nitrine, Nitro-Bid, Nitrocap, Nitrocels, Nitrocontin (G.B.), Nitro-Dial, Ni-trodyl, Nitroglyn, Nitrol, Nitrolar, Nitrolex TD, Nitrolingual (Germ.), Nitro-Lyn, Nitro Mack Retard (Germ.), Nitronet, Nitrong, Nitroprn, Nitrorectal (Germ.), Nitroretard (Swed.), Nitro-SA, Nitrospan, Nitrostabilin (Canad.), Nitrostat, Nitro-TD, Nitrotym, Nitrozell Retard (Germ.), Sustac (G.B.), Trates, Triagin (Austral.), Vasitrin (Austral.), Vasoglyn.

Preparations

Oral: Capsules (extended-release), 2.5, 6.5, and 9 mg; tablets (extended-release), 1.3, 2.6, and 6.5 mg.
Sublingual: Tablets, 0.15, 0.3, 0.4, and 0.6 mg.

Usual Dosages

Oral: 1.3 to 9 mg of extended-release formulation may be administered every 8 to 12 hours.

Sublingual: 0.15 to 0.6 mg repeated in 5 minutes if necessary, but no more than 1.8 mg should be used within a 15-minute period.

NYSTATIN

Proprietary Names: Adiclair (Ger.), Bio-fanal (Ger.), Canida-Lokalicid (Ger.), Candio-Hermal (Ger., Switz.), Canstat (S. Afr.), Cordes Nystatin Soft (Ger.), Moronal (Ger.), Mycostatin (Austral., Canad., Ire., Ital., S. Afr., Span., Swed., USA), Mycostatine (Fr., Switz.), Mykundex (Ger.), Mykundex Mono (Ger.), Nadostine (Canad.), Nilstat (Austral., Canad., USA), Nyaderm (Canad.), Nyspes (G.B.), Nystan (G.B.), Nystatin-Dome (G.B.), Nysta-vescent (G.B.), Nystex.

Preparations

Oral: Pastilles, 200,000 units each, Suspension, 50 million, 150 million, 1 billion, 2 billion, and 5 billion units.

Topical: Cream, 15- and 30-gm tubes; ointment, 15 gm; topical powder, 15 gm.

Topical Ophthalmic: No ophthalmic preparation is commercially available.

Usual Dosages

Oral: Pastilles, one to two four or five times daily for up to 14 days; suspension, 1/8 tsp. (approx. 500,000 units) in 1/2 cup of water.

Topical: Cream, ointment, powder: Apply liberally to affected area twice daily.

Topical Ophthalmic: One drop of suspension of 20,000 units/ml applied four times daily.

OFLOXACIN

Proprietary Names: Flobacin (Ital.), Floxin, Oflocet (Fr., Ital.), Oflocin (Ital.), Tarivid (G.B., Ger., Ire., Jap., Neth., S. Afr., Swed., Switz.).

Preparations

Injection: Solution, 20 and 40 mg/ml.
Oral: Tablets, 200, 300 and 400 mg.

---

* Route of administration not approved by FDA.
† Drug not approved by FDA for any indication.
‡ Drug not approved by FDA for this particular indication.
§ Indicated dosage above the manufacturer's recommendation.

Usual Dosages

Injection: The usual dose is 200 to 400 mg administered by slow infusion over 60 minutes every 12 hours.

Oral: The usual dose is 200 to 400 mg every 12 hours.

ORAZEPAM

Proprietary Names: Adumbran (Ger., Ital., Span.), Alepam (Austral.), Alopam (Swed.), Anxiolit (Switz.), Aplakil (Span.), Azutranquil (Ger.), Benzotran (Austral.), Constantonin (Ger.), Durazepam (Ger.), Limbial (Ital.), Murelax (Austral.), Noctazepam (Ger.), Norkotral N (Ger.), Novoxapam (Canad.), Oxaline (S. Afr.), Oxanid (G.B.), Oxa-Puren (Ger.), Praxiten (Ger.), Psiquiwas (Span.), Purata (S. Afr.), Quilibrex (Ital.), Seresta (Fr., Neth., Swtiz.), Serax, Serepax (Austral., S. Afr., Swed.), Seresta (Fr., Neth., Switz.), Serpax (Ital.), Sigacalm (Ger.), Sobile (Span.), Sobril (Swed.), Uskan (Ger., Switz.), Zapex (Canad.), Zaxopam.

Preparations

Oral: Capsules, 10, 15, and 30 mg; tablets, 15 mg.

Usual Dosages

Oral: 15 to 30 mg three to four times daily. Because of the drug's flexibility and the range of emotional disturbances responsive to it, dosage should be individualized for maximum beneficial effects.

OSMOTIC AGENTS

See Glycerin, Isosorbide, Mannitol, Urea.

OXACILLIN

Proprietary Names: Bactocill, Bristopen (G.B., Fr.), Cryptocillin (Germ.), Prostaphlin, Staphenor (Germ.).

Preparations

Injection: Powder, 0.25, 0.5, 1, 2, and 4 gm.

Usual Dosages

Intramuscular: Adults and children weighing more than 40 kg, 0.25 to 1.0 gm every 4 to 6 hours (up to 8 gm daily may be given for severe infections). Children weighing less than 40 kg, 50 to 100 mg/kg daily (or more in severe infections) in equal doses every 4 to 6 hours. Newborns and premature infants, 25 mg/kg daily.

Intravenous: When administered by direct infusion, the dose should be well diluted and given over a period of approximately 10 to 15 minutes. Doses should be comparable to those administered intramuscularly; for severe infections, 1 gm or more may be given intravenously every 3 to 4 hours.

OXAMNIQUINE

Proprietary Names: Mansil (Braz.), Vansil (S. Afr.).

Preparations

Oral: Powder.

Usual Dosages

Oral: Adults, 15 mg/kg as a single dose; children, 20 mg/kg in two equally divided doses 2 to 8 hours apart.

OXIDIZED CELLULOSE

Proprietary Names: Hemo-Pak, Oxycel, Surgicel.

Preparations

Topical: Pads, 3″ × 3″; pledgets, 2″ × 1″ × 1″; strips, 5″ or 36″ × 0.5″, 3″, 14″, or 18″ × 2″, and 4″ × 8″.

Usual Dosages

Topical: Minimal amounts of an appropriate size are laid on the bleeding site.

OXYMETHOLONE

Proprietary Names: Adroyd, Anadrol-50, Anadroyd (Belg.), Anapolon (G.B.), Anasteron (Denm., Norw., Swed.), Anasteronal (Span.), Nastenon (Fr.), Oxitosono-50 (Span.), Pardroyd (Germ.), Plenastril (Germ., Switz.), Synasteron (Belg.), Zenalosyn (Neth.).

---

*Route of administration not approved by FDA.
† Drug not approved by FDA for any indication.
‡ Drug not approved by FDA for this particular indication.
§ Indicated dosage above the manufacturer's recommendation.

Preparations

Oral: Tablets, 5, 10, and 50 mg.

Usual Dosages

Oral: The usual adult dose is 5 to 10 mg daily.

OXYPHENBUTAZONE

Proprietary Names: Butapirone (Ital.), Iridil (Ital.), Oxalid, Phlogase (Germ.), Rheumapax (Swed.), Tandacote (G.B.), Tandearil, Tanderil (G.B.).

Preparations

Oral: Tablets, 100 mg.
Topical Ophthalmic: No ophthalmic preparation is available commercially. A 5 per cent solution or 10 per cent ointment may be prepared by the pharmacist.

Usual Dosages

Oral: Range, 100 to 600 mg.
Topical Ophthalmic: Preparation is applied three to four times daily.

OXYTETRACYCLINE

Proprietary Names: Abbocin (G.B.), Berkmycen (G.B.), Biotet (S. Afr.), Bobbamycin (Austral.), Chemocycline (G.B.), Clinimycin (G.B.), Dalimycin, Galenomycin (G.B.), Imperacin (G.B.), Lenocycline (S. Afr.), Macocyn (Germ.), 0-4-cycline (S. Afr.), Oppamycin (G.B.), Otetryn, Oxamycen (Jap.), Oxlopar, Oxycycline (Austral.), Oxydon (G.B.), Oxy-Dumocyclin (Swed.), Oxyject, Oxy-Kesso-Tetra, Oxymycin (G.B.), Oxytetral (Swed.), Roxy (S. Afr.), Stecsolin (G.B.), Terramycin, Terravenös (Germ.), Tetlong (S. Afr.), Tetramel (S. Afr.), Tetramine, Tetra-Tablinen (Germ.), Unimycin (G.B.), Uri-Tet, Vendarcin (Austral., Germ., Neth., S. Afr.).

Preparations

Oral: Tablets, 250 mg.
Topical Ophthalmic: Ointment, 0.5 per cent.

Usual Dosages

Oral: Adults, 1 gm daily in divided doses; a total of 2 to 4 gm may be given to severely ill patients. Children, 25 to 50 mg/kg daily in four divided doses.

Topical Ophthalmic: Ointment preparation may be applied two to three times daily.

PAPAVERINE

Proprietary Names: Artegodan (Germ.), Cerebid, Cerespan, Dilaspan, Dipav, Dylate, Kavrin, Myobid, P-200, Pameion (Ital.), Panergon (Germ., Switz.), Papaverlumin Fuerte (Span.), Pavabid, Pava-2 Caps, Pavacap, Pavacen, Pavakey, Pavased, Pavatran, Pava-Wol, Paverine, Paveron (Germ.), Pavine TD, Qua-Bid, Sustaverine, Therapav, Vasal, Vasocap, Vaso-Pav, Vasospan.

Preparations

Oral: Capsules (timed-release), 150 mg; tablets, 30, 60, 100, and 200 mg.

Usual Dosages

Oral: The usual dosage range for adults is 60 to 300 mg one to five times daily. Timed-release capsules may be given every 8 to 12 hours.

PARA-AMINOBENZOIC ACID

Proprietary Names: PABA, pabaGel, Pabanol, Pre Sun, Sunbrella.

Preparations

Topical: Jelly, 5 per cent; solution, 5 per cent; suspension, 5 per cent.

Usual Dosages

Topical: Preparation should be applied uniformly and generously to all exposed skin surfaces before exposure to UVB light.

PAROMOMYCIN

Proprietary Names: Aminoxidin (Ital.), Gabbromicina (Arg.), Gabbromycin (Germ.), Gabbroral (Arg., Belg., Ital.), Gabromicina (Span.), Gaboral (Span.), Humagel (Fr.), Humatin, Paramicina (Ital.), Sinosid (Ital.).

---

* Route of administration not approved by FDA.
† Drug not approved by FDA for any indication.
‡ Drug not approved by FDA for this particular indication.
§ Indicated dosage above the manufacturer's recommendation.

Preparations

Oral: Capsules, 250 mg.
Topical Ophthalmic: No ophthalmic preparation is commercially available.

Usual Dosages

Oral: For intestinal amebiasis, 25 to 35 mg/kg daily in three divided doses for 5 to 10 days.
Topical Ophthalmic: A 0.1 per cent solution may be applied to affected eye(s) twice daily.

PENICILLAMINE

Proprietary Names: Cuprenil (Pol.), Cuprimine, Depamine (G.B.), Depen, Distamine (G.B.), D-Penamine (Austral.), Metalcaptase (Germ.), Trolovol (Germ.).

Preparations

Oral: Capsules, 250 mg.

Usual Dosages

Oral: Adults, for cystinuria, 2 gm daily, with a range of 1 to 4 gm daily in divided doses. For rheumatoid arthritis, 125 to 250 mg initially as a single daily dose; the amount may be increased by increments of 250 mg/day at 2- to 3-month intervals with the average daily maintenance dose at 500 to 750 mg. The maximum daily dosage is usually 1 gm, but up to 1.5 gm may be required in some patients.

PENICILLIN G

See Benzathine Penicillin G, Potassium Penicillin G, Procaine Penicillin G, Sodium Penicillin G.

PENICILLIN V

Proprietary Names: Acipen-V (Neth.), Biotic, Fenospen (Ital.), Oracilline (Belg., Fr.), Penbec-V (Canad.), Pengrocill (Switz.), Penoral (S. Afr.), Tripapenicillina (Ital.), V-Cillin, Veekay (S. Afr.), V-Pen, Widocillin (Switz.).

Preparations

Oral: Capsules, 250 mg; suspension, 125 to 250 mg/5 ml; tablets, 125, 250, and 500 mg.

Usual Dosages

Oral: Adults, for mild to moderate infections, 125 to 250 mg three times daily; for severe infections, 500 mg three times daily or 250 mg every 4 hours. Children, for mild to moderate infections, 125 to 250 mg three times daily; for severe infections, 250 mg four times daily. Infants, 12.5 to 50 mg/kg daily in three to six divided doses.

PENTAMIDINE

Proprietary Names: Lomidine (Fr., Germ.), Pentam.

Preparations

Injection: Powder, 200 and 300 mg/vial.
Topical Ophthalmic: No ophthalmic preparation is commercially available. A 1 per cent solution may be prepared with 10 mg pentamidine powder mixed with 1 ml artificial tears.

Usual Dosages

Intramuscular, Intravenous: The usual dosage is 300 mg daily or an alternate days until 12 to 15 doses are given; a second course can be administered 1 or 2 weeks later.
Topical Ophthalmic: One or two drops of 1 per cent solution may be instilled in the affected eye(s) one to four times daily.

PENTAZOCINE

Proprietary Names: Fortal (Belg., Fr), Fortalgesic (Swed., Switz.), Fortral (G.B.), Fortralin (Scand.), Talwin.

Preparations

Injection: Solution, 30 mg/ml.
Oral: Tablets, 50 mg.

Usual Dosages

Intramuscular, Intravenous, Subcutaneous: Adults, 30 mg every 3 to 4 hours as necessary; single doses in excess of 30 mg intravenously or 60 mg intramuscularly or subcutaneously are not advisable. The total daily dose should not exceed 360 mg. Children under 12 years of age, dosage is not established.
Oral: Adults, 50 mg every 3 to 4 hours as necessary. This may be increased to 100 mg if necessary. The daily dose should not exceed

---

*Route of administration not approved by FDA.
† Drug not approved by FDA for any indication.
‡ Drug not approved by FDA for this particular indication.
§ Indicated dosage above the manufacturer's recommendation.

600 mg. Children under 12 years of age, dosage is not established.

PERGOLIDE

Proprietary Names: Celance (G.B.), Permax.

Preparations

Oral: Tablets, 0.05, 0.25, and 1 mg.

Usual Dosages

Oral: Initial recommended dosage is 0.05 mg for the first 2 days. This dose should then be gradually increased by 0.1 or 0.15 mg/day every third day over the next 12 days of therapy. The dosage may then be increased by 0.25 mg daily every third day until optimal dosage is achieved. Usually administered in divided doses three times daily.

PERMETHRIN

Proprietary Name: Nix.

Preparations

Topical: Liquid, 1 per cent.

Usual Dosages

Topical: A sufficient volume to saturate the hair and scalp should be applied and allowed to remain on the hair for 10 minutes before rinsing off with water.

PETHIDINE

See Meperidine.

PETROLATUM (WHITE PETROLATUM)

Proprietary Names: Duolube, Duratears, Lacri-Lube, Moroline, Refresh PM.

Preparations

Topical: Ointment.
Topical Ophthalmic: Ointment.

Usual Dosages

Topical: Small amount of ointment may be applied as needed.
Topical Ophthalmic: Small amount of ointment may be applied as needed.

PHENOXYMETHYLPENICILLIN POTASSIUM

See Potassium Penicillin V.

PHENYLBUTAZONE

Proprietary Names: Butagesic (Canad.), Butalan (Austral.), Butalgin (Austral.), Butaphen (Austral.), Butapirazol (Pol.), Butarex (Austral.), Butazolidin, Butazone (G.B.), Butina (S. Afr.), Butoroid (Austral.), Butoz (Austral.), Butozone (S. Afr.), Butrex (S. Afr.), Buzon (Austral.), Chembutazone (Canad.), Diossidone (Ital.), Ecobutazone (Canad.), Elmedal (Germ.), Eributazone (Canad.), Ethibute (G.B.), Flexazone (G.B.), Intrabutazone (Canad.), Kadol (Ital.), Malgesic (Canad.), Merizone (Canad.), Nadozone (Canad.), Neo-Zoline (Canad.), Novophenyl (Canad.), Oppazone (G.B.), Panazone (S. Afr.), Phenbutazol (Canad.), Phenybute (Austral.), Phenylbetazone (Canad.), Praecirheumin (Germ.), Tazone (Canad.), Tetnor (G.B.), Ticinil (Ital.), Wescozone (Canad.).

Preparations

Oral: Tablets, 100 mg.

Usual Dosages

Oral: Initially, 300 to 600 mg daily in divided doses. A 1-week trial period is considered adequate to determine response. If symptoms can be controlled with a maintenance dose of 100 to 200 mg daily, the drug may be given for longer periods under careful supervision.

PHENYLEPHRINE

Proprietary Names: Ak-Dilate, Ak-Nefrin, Alcon-Efrin, Degest (Austral., Canad.), Dilatair, Efricel, I-Care (Austral.), Isopto Frin, Isopto Phenylephrine (Austral.), Mistura D, Mydfrin, Neo-Synephrine, Ocu-Phrin, Ocugestrin, Prefrin, Tear-Efrin.

Preparations

Topical Ophthalmic: Solution, 0.12, 0.125, 0.2, 2.5, and 10 per cent.

---

* Route of administration not approved by FDA.
† Drug not approved by FDA for any indication.
‡ Drug not approved by FDA for this particular indication.
§ Indicated dosage above the manufacturer's recommendation.

Usual Dosages

Topical Ophthalmic: Solution may be applied one to three times daily.

PHENYTOIN

Proprietary Names: Dantoin (Canad.), Difhydan (Swed.), Dihycon, Di-Hydan (Fr.), Dilabid, Dilantin, Di-Phen, Diphentyn (Canad.), Diphenyl, Diphenylan, Ditoin (Austral.), Divulsan (Canad.), Ekko, Epanutin (G.B.), Fenantoin (Swed.), Kessodanten, Novodiphenyl (Canad.), Phenhydan (Germ.), Phentoin (Austral.), Pyoredol (Fr.), Solantyl (Fr.), Toin, Zentropil (Germ.).

Preparations

Injection: Powder for solution containing approximately 50 mg/ml when diluted with special solvent provided.
Oral: Capsules, 30 to 100 mg; suspension, 30 mg/5ml (pediatric) and 125 mg/5ml; tablets (pediatric), 50 mg.

Usual Dosages

Intramuscular, Intravenous: Adults, 150 to 250 mg followed if necessary by 100 to 150 mg 30 minutes later. The rate of administration should not exceed 50 mg/minute. Higher doses may be required to control seizures.
Oral: Dosage must be individualized. Adults, initially, 300 mg daily. The maintenance dose is usually 100 mg three to four times daily.

PHOSPHATE SALTS

Proprietary Names: K-Phos, Neutra-Phos.

Preparations

Oral: Capsules, 250 mg phosphorus, 7.125 or 14.25 mEq potassium, and 0 or 7.125 mEq sodium; solution, 250 mg phosphorus, 7.125 or 14.25 mEq potassium, and 0 or 7.125 mEq sodium/75 ml; tablets, 114, 126, or 250 mg phosphorus, 45, 90, or 144 mg potassium, and 0, 67, 134, or 298 mg sodium.

Usual Dosages

Oral: Adults, 2 to 4 gm of phosphorus daily in divided doses.

PHYSOSTIGMINE

Proprietary Name: Isopto Eserine.

Preparations

Topical Ophthalmic: Ointment, 0.25 per cent; solution, 0.1, 0.25, and 0.5 per cent.

Usual Dosages

Topical Ophthalmic: In primary open-angle and other chronic glaucomas, one drop of 0.25 or 0.5 per cent solution in each eye every 4 to 6 hours; ointment is used at night.

PHYTONADIONE (VITAMIN K₁)

Proprietary Names: AquaMEPHYTON, Konakion, MEPHYTON.

Preparations

Injection: Solution, 2 and 10 mg/ml.
Oral: Tablets, 5 mg.

Usual Dosages

Intramuscular, Intravenous, Oral, Subcutaneous: In the treatment of hypoprothrombinemia resulting from malabsorption syndromes, 2 to 25 mg may be administered to adults initially and repeated if necessary, depending on the severity of the deficiency and the response to the drug.

PILOCARPINE

Proprietary Names: Adsorbocarpine, Akarpine, Almocarpine, Isopto Carpine, Isopto-Pilocarpine (Fr.), Licarpin (Swed.), Marticarpine (Fr.), Mio-Carpine-SMP (S. Afr.), Mistura P, Nova-Carpine (Canad.), Ocu-Carpine, Ocusert, Pilocar, Pilocarpina Lux (Ital.), Pilocel, Pilokair, Pilomiotin, Pilopine, Pilopt (Austral.), Piloptic, PV Carpine, Spersacarpine (S. Afr., Swed.).

Preparations

Topical Ophthalmic: Gel, 4 per cent; Ocusert, 20 to 40 μg of pilocarpine released each hour for 1 week; solution, 0.25, 0.5, 1.0, 2.0, 3.0, 4.0, 5.0, 6.0, 8.0, and 10 per cent.

---

*Route of administration not approved by FDA.
† Drug not approved by FDA for any indication.
‡ Drug not approved by FDA for this particular indication.
§ Indicated dosage above the manufacturer's recommendation.

Usual Dosages

Topical Ophthalmic: The frequency and concentration of instillation depend upon the patient's response to therapy.

PIPERACILLIN

Proprietary Names: Pentcillin (Jap.), Pipracil, Pipril (G.B., Germ.).

Preparations

Injection: Powder, 2, 3, 4, and 40 gm.

Usual Dosages

Intramuscular, Intravenous: For serious infections, the usual dosage is 3 to 4 gm administered every 4 to 6 hours as a 20- to 30-minute infusion. The maximum dose is 24 gm, although higher doses have been used. Intramuscular injections should be limited to 2 gm/site.

PIPERAZINE

Proprietary Names: Adipalit (Ital.), Ancazine (Canad.), Antelmina (Fr.), Antepar, Antivermine (Pol.), Ascalix (G.B.), Bryrel, Citrazine (Austral.), Dietelmin (Fr.), Divermex (Austral.), Entacyl (G.B.), Eraverm (Germ.), Helmezine (G.B.), Lumbrioxyl (Fr.), Multifuge, Oxucide, Oxypel (Canad.), Paravermin (Germ.), Perin, Pinsirup, Pin-Tega, Pipenin (Jap.), Piperasol (Pol.), Piperol (Fr.), Piperzinal (Canad.), Pipril, Piprosan (Austral.), Razine, Stavermol (Germ.), Tasnon (Germ.), Ta-Verm, Uvilon (Germ.), Vermago, Vermicompren (Germ.), Vermolina (Austral.).

Preparations

Oral: Syrup, 500 mg/5 ml; tablets, 500 mg (in terms of hexahydrate salt).

Usual Dosages

Oral: For roundworms, adults, 3.5 gm once daily for 2 consecutive days; children, 75 mg/kg (maximum, 3.5 gm) once daily for 2 consecutive days. For pinworms, adults and children, 65 mg/kg (maximum, 2.5 gm) once daily for 7 consecutive days. In severe infections, the above doses may be repeated at a 1-week interval.

PIROXICAM

Proprietary Name: Feldene.

Preparations

Oral: Capsules, 10 and 20 mg.

Usual Dosages

Oral: The usual daily dosage is 20 mg administered as a single or divided dose.

PLICAMYCIN (MITHRAMYCIN)

Proprietary Name: Mithracin.

Preparations

Injection: Powder (for solution) in vials containing 2500 µg plicamycin, 100 mg mannitol, and sufficient disodium phosphate to adjust pH to 7.

Usual Dosages

Intravenous: 25 µg/kg as a single dose by direct injection or added to 5 per cent dextrose in water and infused gradually over a 4- to 8-hour period.

PNEUMOCOCCAL VACCINE

Proprietary Names: Pneumovax, Pnu-Imune.

Preparations

Injection: 25 µg/0.5 ml.

Usual Dosages

Intramuscular, Subcutaneous: A single dose of 0.5 ml is injected.

POLYMYXIN B

Proprietary Names: Aerosporin, Polmix (Austral.).

Preparations

Injection: Powder, 500,000 units (equivalent to polymyxin standard 50 mg).

---

* Route of administration not approved by FDA.
† Drug not approved by FDA for any indication.
‡ Drug not approved by FDA for this particular indication.
§ Indicated dosage above the manufacturer's recommendation.

Topical Ophthalmic: For ophthalmic administration, the sterile powder is reconstituted by adding 20 to 50 ml of sterile water for injection or 0.9 per cent sodium chloride injection to a vial labeled as containing 500,000 units of polymyxin B. This provides solutions containing approximately 10,000 to 25,000 units/ml (10,000 units = 1 mg).

Usual Dosages

Intravenous: 15,000 to 25,000 units/kg daily. Infants may tolerate up to 40,000 units/kg daily if needed.
Subconjunctival: Up to 10,000 units daily.
Topical Ophthalmic: One drop of solution every hour as frequently as needed. The interval between doses may be increased if a favorable therapeutic response occurs.

POLYVINYL ALCOHOL

Proprietary Names: AKWA Tears, Barnes-Hind Wetting Solution, Contique Artificial Tears, Hypotears, Liquifilm Forte, Liquifilm Tears, Pre-Sert, Total.

Preparations

Topical Ophthalmic: Solution, 1.4, 2, and 3 per cent.

Usual Dosages

Topical Ophthalmic: Solution may be used as a subsititute for tears, and one or two drops may be applied to the eyes as needed.

POTASSIUM IODIDE

Proprietary Names: Jodetten (Germ.), KI-N, Pherajod (Germ.), Pima, Solvejod (Swed.), SSKI.

Preparations

Oral: Solution, 300 mg/0.3 ml and 1 gm/ml.
Topical Ophthalmic: No ophthalmic preparation is commercially available. A 10 per cent solution can be prepared by dilution.

Usual Dosages

Oral: For use as an antifungal agent, 0.6 to 1 ml of a saturated solution (100 per cent) three times daily; amount is increased by 0.06 ml at each dose until the maximum tolerated dose is reached. Maximum daily dose is 12 to 15 ml.

Topical Ophthalmic: For fungal ulcers, 1 to 10 per cent solutions may be instilled in the conjunctival sac four to six times daily.

POTASSIUM PENICILLIN G (BENZYLPENICILLIN POTASSIUM)

Proprietary Names: Abbocillin (Canad.), Abbocillin-G (Austral.), Arcocillin, Biotic-T, Burcillin-G, Cilloral, Cryspen, Crystapen (G.B.), Deltapen, Dymocillin (Canad.), Eskacillin 100 (G.B.), Falapen (G.B.), Fivepen (Canad.), Forpen (Canad.), G-Recillin-T, Hyasorb, Hylenta (Canad.), Ka-Pen (Canad.), K-Cillin, Kesso-Pen, K-Pen, Lanacillin, Lemicillin, Liquapen, Nece-Pen (Fr.), Neo-Pens (Canad.), Novopen (Canad., S. Afr.), P-50 (Canad.), Paclin G, Palocillin, Parcillin, Penalev, Pencitabs (Canad.), Penevan (Austral.), Penioral (Canad.), Peniset (Austral.), Pensol (Austral.), Pensorb, Pentids, Pfizerpen G, Pharmacillin (Germ.), Purapen G (G.B.), SK-Penicillin G, Solupen (G.B.), Specilline G (Fr.), Sugracillin, Tabillin (G.B.), Therapen-K (Canad.), Tu Cillin, Wescopen (Canad.).

Preparations

Injection: Powder; suspension for injection.

Usual Dosages

Intramuscular, Intravenous: Adults, 300,000 to 1.2 million units daily. Doses as large as 60 million units daily have been infused for certain serious infections. Children, 300,000 to 1.2 million units daily. Doses as large as 10 million units daily may be necessary (by intravenous infusion). Premature or full-term newborn infants, 600,000 units daily in two divided doses.
Oral: Adults and children, 600,000 to 3 million units daily.

POTASSIUM PENICILLIN V (PHENOXYMETHYLPENICILLIN POTASSIUM)

Proprietary Names: Abbocillin VK (Austral.), Acocillin (Swed.), Apopen (Swed.), Apsin VK (G.B.) Arcasin (Germ.), Beromycin (Germ.), Betapen-VK, Biotic-V, Bopen V-K, Bramcillin (Austral.), Calciopen (Swed.), Calcipen (Austral., Norw.), Caps-Pen V (Austral.), Cilicaine-V or VK (Austral.), Cillaphen (Austral.), Co-Caps Penicillin V-K (G.B.), Co-

cillin V-K, Compocillin-VK, Corcillin V (S. Afr.), Crystapen V (G.B.), Crystapen-VK (Austral.), CVK (G.B.), CVL (Austral.), Darocillin (S. Afr.), Deltacillin (S. Afr.), Diacipen-VK (S. Afr.), Distaquaine V or V-K (G.B.), Dowpen VK, Econocil-VK (G.B.), Econopen V (G.B.), Falcopen V or VK (Austral.), Fenoxicillin (Denm.), Fenoxypen (Germ., S. Afr., Swed.), GPV (G.B.), Hi-Pen (Canad.), Ia-pen (G.B.), Icipen (G.B.), Isocillin (Germ.), Ispenoral (Germ.), Jatcillin (S. Afr.), Kabipenin (Germ.), Kavepenin (Swed.), Kesso-Pen-VK, Lanacillin VK, Ledercillin VK, LPV (Austral.), LV, Meropenin (Swed.), Nadopen-V (Canad.), Norcilin (G.B.), Novopen-V (Canad.), Nutracillin (S. Afr.), Oracilline (Fr.), Orapen (S. Afr.), Oratren (Germ.), Orvepen (Neth.), Ospen (Fr., Germ.), Ospeneff (G.B.), Paclin VK, Pancillen (Austral.), Penaper VK, Pencompren (Germ.), Pengen-VK, Penicals (G.B.), Penicillin V-K (Austral.), Peni-Vee (K) (Austral.), Penoxyl VK (G.B.), Pen-Vee (Canad.), Pen-Vee K, Pfipen V (Austral.), Pfizerpen VK, Phenethicillin, P-Mega-Tablinen (Germ.), Propen-VK (Austral.), PVF K (Canad.), PVK (Austral.), PVO (Austral.), QIDpen VK, Repen-VK, Robicillin VK, Rocilin (Austral., Norw.), Ro-Cillin VK, Roscopenin (Swed.), Saropen-VK, SK-Penicillin VK, Stabillin V-K (G.B.), Suspen V (Austral.), Ticillin V-K (G.B.), Tikacillin (Swed.), Uticillin VK, V-Cil-K (G.B.), V-Cillin K, VC-K (Canad.), Veecillin (Austral.), Veekay (S. Afr.), Veetids, Vepen (Swed.), Viacillin (Swed.), Vicin (Austral.), Vikacillin (S. Afr.), Viraxacillin-V (Austral.), V-Pen, VPV (Austral.), Weifapenin (Scand.), Win-V-K (Canad.).

Preparations

Oral: Granules for solution, 125 and 250 mg/5 ml; powder for drops, 125 mg/2.5 ml; powder for solution, 125 and 250 mg/5 ml; tablets, 125, 250, and 500 mg.

Usual Dosages

Oral: Adults and children over 12 years of age, 125 to 500 mg (200,000 to 800,000 units) every 6 to 8 hours for 10 days. Infants and small children, 25,000 to 100,000 units/kg daily in three to six divided doses.

POVIDONE-IODINE

Proprietary Names: ACU-dyne, Betadine, Betaisodona (Germ.), Betiadine (Arg.), Biodine, Bridine (Canad.), Disadine (G.B.), Efodine, Final Step, Frepp, Frepp/Sepp, Iodex, Iso-Betadine (Belg.), Isobetadine (Denm.), Isodine, Jodocur (Ital.), Mallisol, Neojodin (Jap.), Nutradine (S. Afr.), Operand, Pervinox (Arg.), Pevidine (G.B.), Pharmadine Polydine, Povadyne, Proviodine (Canad.), PV-I (G.B.),

---

*Route of administration not approved by FDA.
† Drug not approved by FDA for any indication.
‡ Drug not approved by FDA for this particular indication.
§ Indicated dosage above the manufacturer's recommendation.

Savlon Dry (Austral.), Surgi-Sep, Topionic (Span.), Videne (G.B.).

Preparations

Topical: Ointment, 1 per cent; solution, 1, 7.5, and 10 per cent.

Usual Dosages

Topical: Preparation is applied directly to the affected area(s) as needed.

PRAZIQUANTEL

Proprietary Names: Cesol (Germ.), Biltricide (Germ.).

Preparations

Oral: Powder.

Usual Dosages

Oral: 40 to 60 mg/kg administered as a single or multiple dose.

PRAZOSIN

Proprietary Names: Hypovase (G.B.), Minipres (Arg.), Minipress, Peripress (Scand.).

Preparations

Oral: Capsules, 1, 2, and 5 mg.

Usual Dosages

Oral: Initially, 1 mg two or three times daily. The usual maintenance dosage is 6 to 15 mg daily in divided doses.

PREDNISOLONE

Proprietary Names: Adnisolone (Austral.), Ak-Pred, Ak-Tate, Alto-Pred (G.B.), Bio-Pred, Codelcortone (G.B.), Codelsol (G.B.), Cordrol, Dacortin H (Span.), Decortin-H (Germ.), Delcort-E, Delcortol (Denm.), Delta-Cortef, Deltacortenolo (Ital.), Delta-cortilen

(Ital.), Deltacortril (G.B.), Deltalone (G.B.), Delta Phoricol (G.B.), Deltasolone (Austral.), Deltastab (G.B.), Deltidrosol (Ital.), Di-Adreson-F (G.B.), Di-Pred, Donisolone (Jap.), Dua-Pred, Duo-Cort, Durapred, Econopred, Encortolone (Pol.), Endoprenovis (Ital.), Erbacort (Fr.), Fernisolone-P, Hostacortin-H (Germ.), Hydeltra, Hydeltrasol, Hydrocortancyl (Fr.), Hydrosol, Inflamase, Jectasone, Keteocort H (Germ.), Key-Pred, Lenisolone (S. Afr.), Marsolone (G.B.), Mecortolon (Pol.), Meticortelone, Metreton, Nisolone, Nor-Pred, Nova-Pred (Canad.), Ocu-Pred, Ocu-Pred-A, Ocu-Pred Forte, Optocort (Austral.), Panacort, Panafcortelone (Austral.), Panisolone, Paracortol (Austral.), Phortisolone (Fr.), Poly-Pred (S. Afr.), Precortalon (Swed.), Pre-Cortisyl (G.B.), Predair, Predair-A, Predair Forte, Predalone, Pred-Cylsma (Swed.), Predeltilone (S. Afr.), Predenema (G.B.), Pred Forte, Predicort, Pred Mild, Prednelan (N.Z.), Prednesol (G.B.), PredniCoelin (Germ.), Predni-H (Germ.), Predniretard (Fr.), Prednisol (Ital.), Predonine (Jap.), Predoxine, Predsol (G.B.), Predulose, Prelone (Austral.), PSP-IV, Rolesone (Fr.), Ropredlone, Savacort-50/100, Scherisolon (Austral., Germ.), Sigpred, Sintisone (G.B.), Sodasone, Solone (Austral.), Sol-Pred, Solucort (Fr.), Solu-Dacortin (Aust., Austral, Swed.), Solu-Decortin-H (Germ.), Solu-Pred, Solu Predalone, Ster-5, Steraject-50, Sterane, Sterofrin (Austral.), Ulacort, Ultracorten-H (Germ.), Ultracortenol (Austral., Germ.).

Preparations

Injection: Powder, 66.9 mg equivalent to 50 mg prednisolone; solution equivalent to 20 mg/ml prednisolone; suspension, 20, 25, 50, and 100 mg/ml.
Oral: Tablets, 5 mg.
Topical Ophthalmic: Ointment, 0.25 per cent; solution, 0.125, 0.5, and 1.0 per cent; suspension, 0.12, 0.125, and 1.0 per cent.

Usual Dosages

Intramuscular, Intravenous: 4 to 60 mg daily.
Oral: The initial dosage may vary from 5 to 60 mg daily, depending on the specific disease entity being treated. Higher initial dosage may be required in selected patients. It should be emphasized that dosage requirements are variable and must be individualized on the basis of the disease under treatment and the response of the patient.
Retrobulbar: 0.5 to 1.0 ml of solution containing 25 mg/ml.
Topical Ophthalmic: One drop of 0.12 to 1 per cent suspension every 2 to 4 hours until a response is obtained. The frequency is then reduced. The ointment preparation is applied three to four times daily or as a nighttime

---

medication when the solution is used during the day.

PREDNISONE

Proprietary Names: Adasone (Austral.), Ancortone (Ital.), Colisone (Canad.), Cortancyl (Fr.), Dabroson (Germ.), Dacortin (Span.), Decortin (Germ.), DeCortisyl (G.B.), Delcortin (Denm.), Deltacortene (Ital.), Deltacortone (G.B.), Delta Prenovis (Ital.), Deltasone, Deltison (Swed.), Di-Adreson (G.B.), Encorton (Pol.), Erftopred (Germ.), Hostacortin (Germ.), Inocortyl (Fr.), Keteocort (Germ.), Keysone, Lisacort, Marsone (G.B.), Maso-Pred, Meticorten, Nisone (Span.), Orasone, Panafcort (Austral., S. Afr.), Pan-Sone, Paracort (Canad.), Parmenison (Aust.), Pred-5, Predeltin (S. Afr.), Prednicen-M, Prednilong (S. Afr.), Prednilonga (Germ.), Predniment (Germ.), Predni-Tablinen (Germ.), Prednital (Ital.), Presone (Austral.), Propred (Austral.), Rectodelt (Germ.), Ropred, Sarogesic Servisone, SK-Prednison, Sone (Austral.), Sterapred, Ultracorten (Germ.), Urtilone (Fr.), Wescopred (Canad.), Winpred (Canad.).

Preparations

Oral: Tablets 1, 2.5, 5, 10, 20, 25, and 50 mg.

Usual Dosages

Oral: The initial dosage may vary from 5 to 60 mg daily, depending upon the specific disease entity being treated. Higher initial dosages may be required in selected patients. It should be emphasized that dosage requirements are variable and must be individualized on the basis of the disease under treatment and the response of the patient.

PRIMAQUINE

Proprietary Name: Primaquine.

Preparations

Oral: Tablets, 26.3 mg (equivalent to 15 mg of base).

Usual Dosages

Oral: (Doses expressed in terms of the base.) To prevent relapses, adults, 15 mg; chil-

---

*Route of administration not approved by FDA.
† Drug not approved by FDA for any indication.
‡ Drug not approved by FDA for this particular indication.
§ Indicated dosage above the manufacturer's recommendation.

---

dren, 1.75 mg/4.5 kg. The dose is given daily for 14 days, concomitantly with other antimalarial drugs given on the first 3 days of an acute attack.

PROBENECID

Proprietary Names: Benacen, Benemid, Benemide (Fr.), Benn, Benuryl (Canad.), Panuric (S. Afr.), Probalan, Probecid (Norw., Swed.), Probemid (Span.), Proben (S. Afr.), Prebenid (Belg.), Procid (Austral.), Robenecid, SK-Probenecid, Solpurin (Ital.), Uroben (Ital.), Urocid (Ital.).

Preparations

Oral: Tablets, 500 mg.

Usual Dosages

Oral: Adults, for treatment of gout, 250 mg twice daily for 1 week, followed by 500 mg twice daily thereafter. When used in combination with penicillin therapy, the recommended dosage is 2 gm daily in divided doses.

PROBUCOL

Proprietary Name: Lorelco.

Preparations

Oral: Tablets, 250 mg.

Usual Dosages

Oral: Adults, 500 mg twice daily taken with meals.

PROCAINE

Proprietary Names: Anucaine, Durathesia, Neocaine, Novocain, P45 (Austral.), Planocaine (S. Afr.), Rectocaine, Unicaine, Westocaine (Canad.).

Preparations

Injection: Solution, 1, 2, and 10 per cent.

Usual Dosages

Nerve Block: With or without epinephrine 1 : 200,000, up to 50 ml of the 1 per cent or 25 ml of the 2 per cent solution.

PROCAINE PENICILLIN G (AQUEOUS)

Proprietary Names: Almopen (S. Afr.), Aquacaine G (Austral.), Aquacillin (Austral.), Ayercillin (Canad.), Cilicaine (Austral.), Crysticillin AS, Depocillin, Depocillin (S. Afr.), Duracillin AS, Eskacillin (G.B.), Evacilin (Austral.), Flo-Cillin, Flocilline (Fr.), Francacilline (Canad.), Hostacillin (Austral.), Hydracillin (Swed.), Ibacillin (Canad.), Megapen (Austral.), Novocillin (S. Afr.), Parencillin, Penlator, Pentids-P, Pfizerpan-AS, Procillin (Austral., S. Afr.), Pro-Stabillin AS (G.B.), Suspenin (Swed.), Therapen (Canad.), Viraxacillin (Austral.), Wycillin.

Preparations

Injection: Powder; suspension for injection.

Usual Dosages

Intramuscular: Adults and children, 600,000 to 1 million units daily in one or two doses, depending upon the condition being treated. Doses as large as 4.8 million units divided into at least two doses have been injected at different sites at one visit for certain serious infections. Ten days to 2 weeks of therapy are usually sufficient.

PROCARBAZINE

Proprietary Names: Matulane, Natulan (G.B.), Natulanar (Swed.).

Preparations

Oral: Capsules, 50 mg.

Usual Dosages

Oral: Single or divided doses of 2 to 4 mg/kg daily are recommended for the first week. Daily doses should then be maintained at 4 to 6 mg/kg daily until the white blood count falls below 4000/cubic millimeter or the platelets fall below 100,000/cubic millimeter.

PROCHLORPERAZINE

Proprietary Names: Anit-Naus (Austral.), Compazine, Stemetil (G.B.), Tementil (Fr.), Vertigon (G.B.).

---

*Route of administration not approved by FDA.
† Drug not approved by FDA for any indication.
‡ Drug not approved by FDA for this particular indication.
§ Indicated dosage above the manufacturer's recommendation.

Preparations

Injection: Solution, 5 mg/ml.
Oral: Capsules (sustained-release), 10, 15, and 30 mg; syrup, 5 mg/5 ml; tablets, 5, 10, and 25 mg.
Rectal: Suppositories, 2.5, 5.0, and 25.0 mg.

Usual Dosages

Intramuscular: Adults, 5 to 10 mg every 3 to 4 hours (maximum, 40 mg daily).
Oral: Adults, 5 to 10 mg three to four times daily.
Rectal: Adults, 25 mg twice daily.

PROMETHAZINE

Proprietary Names: Atosil (Germ.), Avomine (G.B.), Fellozine, Ganphen, Histantil (Canad.), K-Phen, Lemprometh, Lenazine (S. Afr.), Lergigan (Swed.), Methazine, Meth-Zine (Austral.), Pentazine, Phenergen, Phenerhist, Phenerject, Progan (Austral.), Promethapar, Prorex, Prothazine (Austral.), Provigan, Quadnite, Remsed, Rolamethazine, Sigazine, ZiPan.

Preparations

Injection: Solution, 25 and 50 mg/ml.
Oral: Syrup, 6.25 and 25 mg/5 ml; tablets, 12.5, 25, and 50 mg.
Rectal: Suppositories, 25 and 50 mg.

Usual Dosages

Intramuscular, Intravenous, Rectal: Adults, 25 mg repeated in 2 hours if necessary.
Intramuscular, Oral: Children, 0.5 mg/kg at bedtime or 0.13 mg/kg in the morning or when necessary.
Oral: Adults, 25 mg at bedtime or 12.5 mg four times daily.

PROPAMIDINE

Proprietary Name: Brolene (Austral., G.B.).

Preparations

Topical Ophthalmic: Solution, 0.1 per cent.

Usual Dosages

Topical Ophthalmic: One or two drops of solution in the affected eye(s) are instilled two to four times daily, or more frequently as required, for 7 to 10 days. In acute infections, drops may be applied every 15 to 30 minutes. Treatment should not be prolonged for longer than 1 week.

PROPARACAINE (PROXYMETACAINE)

Proprietary Names: Ak-Taine, Alcaine, Kainair, Keracaine (Fr.), Ocu-Caine, Ophthaine, Ophthetic.

Preparations

Tropical Ophthalmic: Solution, 0.5 per cent.

Usual Dosages

Topical Ophthalmic: For minor procedures, one drop of solution is instilled before the procedure. For deeper anesthesia, more frequent instillation is required.

PROPOXYPHENE

Proprietary Names: Algaphan (Austral.), Antalvic (Fr.), Darvon, Depronal SA (G.B.), Develin (Germ.), Dextropropoxyphene (G.B.), Dolene, Dolocap, Dolotard (Swed.), Doloxene, Erantin (Germ.), Harmar, Mardon, Pro-65 (Canad.), Propox 65, Propoxychel, Proxagesic, Ropoxy, Scrip-Dyne, SK-65, S-Pain-65.

Preparations

Oral: Capsules, 32 and 65 mg; suspension, 50 mg/5 ml; tablets, 100 mg.

Usual Dosages

Oral: 65 (hydrochloride salt) or 100 mg (napsylate salt) three or four times daily.

PROPRANOLOL

Proprietary Names: Docitron (Germ.), Herzul (Jap.), Inderal, Kemi (Jap.).

Preparations

Injection: Solution, 1 mg/ml.
Oral: Tablets, 10, 40, 80, and 160 mg.

---

*Route of administration not approved by FDA.
† Drug not approved by FDA for any indication.
‡ Drug not approved by FDA for this particular indication.
§ Indicated dosage above the manufacturer's recommendation.

Usual Dosages

Intravenous (Slow): 1 to 10 mg.
Oral: 20 mg to 2 gm daily in divided doses; the initial dose should not exceed 40 mg.

PROPYLTHIOURACIL

Proprietary Names: Propacil, Propycil (Germ.), Propyl-Thyracil (Canad.), Thyreostat II (Germ.), Tiotil (Swed.).

Preparations

Oral: Tablets, 50 mg.

Usual Dosages

Oral: For management of hyperthyroidism, adults, initially 300 to 400 mg daily in divided doses every 8 hours. Some patients may require as much as 900 mg daily for initial control. For maintenance, 100 to 300 mg is given daily in three divided doses.

PSORALENS

See Methoxsalen, Trioxsalen.

PYRANTEL

Proprietary Names: Antiminth, Aut (Arg.), Cobantril (Switz.), Combantrin (Arg., Austral., Belg., Canad., Fr., Ital., Neth., S. Afr.), Helmex (Germ.), Lombriareu (Span.), Trilombrin (Span.).

Preparations

Oral: Suspension, 250 mg/5 ml.

Usual Dosages

Oral: Adults and children, for roundworms and pinworms, 11 mg/kg (maximum, 1 gm); for hookworms, this dose is given for 3 consecutive days. Repeated in 1 month if indicated.

PYRAZINAMIDE

Proprietary Names: Piraldina (Ital.), Pyrafat (Germ.), Pyrazide (S. Afr.), Tebrazid (Belg., Canad.), Zinamide (Austral., G.B.).

Preparations

Oral: Tablets, 500 mg.

Usual Dosages

Oral: Adults, 20 to 35 mg/kg daily in one or more doses (maximum, 3 gm daily).

PYRETHRINS

Proprietary Names: A-200 Pyrinate, Barc, Blue, Licetrol, Pyrinyl, R&C, RID, Tisit, Tisit Blue, Triple X.

Preparations

Topical: Gel, 0.18, 0.3, or 0.33 per cent pyrethrins, 2.2, 3.0, or 4.0 per cent piperonyl butoxide, and 1, 2, or 4.8 per cent petrolatum; liquid, 0.18, 0.2, or 0.3 per cent pyrethrins, 2.0, 2.2, or 3.0 per cent piperonyl butoxide, 0.8, 1.2, or 5.5 per cent petrolatum, and 2.4 per cent benzyl alcohol, 0.2 per cent pyrethrins, 20 per cent piperonyl butoxide, and 0.8 per cent kerosene, 0.3 per cent pyrethrins and 2 per cent piperonyl butoxide; shampoo, 0.17 or 0.3 per cent pyrethrins, 2 or 3 per cent piperonyl butoxide, 1.2 per cent petrolatum, and 2.4 per cent benzyl alcohol.

Usual Dosages

Topical: Preparation is applied undiluted to infected areas, allowed to remain no longer than 10 minutes, and rinsed thoroughly with warm water and soap or shampoo; no more than two consecutive applications within 24 hours.

PYRIDOSTIGMINE

Proprietary Names: Mestinon, Regonol.

Preparations

Oral: Syrup, 60 mg/5 ml; tablets, 60 mg; tablets (timed-release), 180 mg.

Usual Dosages

Oral: Range, 0.06 mg to 1.5 gm daily.

PYRIDOXINE (VITAMIN B₆)

Proprietary Names: B₆-Vicotrat (Germ.), Becilan (Fr.), Bedoxine (Belg.), Beesix, Bena-

---

don (G.B.), Bivit-6 (Ital.), Comploment (G.B.), Dermo 6 (Fr.), Dextamina B6 (Span.), Farmobion B₆ (Ital.), Gonabion B6 (Span.), Gravidox, Hexa-Betalin, Hexapyral (Swed.), Hexavibex, Hexobion (Germ., Span.), Lactosec 200 (S. Afr.), Pan B-6, Pydox (Austral.), Pyricamphre (Fr.), Pyroxin (Austral.), Rodex, Seibion (Ital.), Sibevit B6 (Span.), Vitanoxi B6 (Span.), Xanturenasi (Ital.).

Preparations

Injection: Solution, 50 and 100 mg/ml.
Oral: Tablets, 10, 25, 50, and 100 mg.

Usual Dosages

Intramuscular, Intravenous, Oral: In cases of dietary deficiency, 10 to 20 mg daily for 3 weeks. For drug-induced deficiency, 100 mg daily for 3 weeks followed by a 30-mg maintenance dose daily. For inborn errors of metabolism, as much as 600 mg a day and a daily intake of 30 mg for life.

PYRIMETHAMINE

Proprietary Names: Daraprim, Erbaprelina (Ital.), Tindurin (Hung.).

Preparations

Oral: Tablets, 25 mg.

Usual Dosages

Oral: For treatment of chloroquine-resistant *P. falciparum* malaria, adults 25 mg twice daily for the first 3 days of treatment with quinine and sulfadiazine. For ocular toxoplasmosis, adults, initially 100 to 150 mg. Then 25 mg is administered twice daily for 8 weeks, followed by 25 mg once daily for an additional 8 weeks. Finally, 25 mg is given every other day until a total of 6 months of therapy have been completed. Sulfadiazine should be given concomitantly.

QUINACRINE

Proprietary Name: Atabrine.

Preparations

Oral: 100-mg tablets.

Usual Dosages

Oral: 100 mg twice daily.

---

* Route of administration not approved by FDA.
† Drug not approved by FDA for any indication.
‡ Drug not approved by FDA for this particular indication.
§ Indicated dosage above the manufacturer's recommendation.

QUININE

Proprietary Names: Bi-quinate (Austral.), Coco-Quinine, Dentojel (Canad.), Quinamm, Quinate (Austral.), Quinbisan (Austral.), Quine, Quinsan (Austral.).

Preparations

Injection: Powder.
Oral: Capsules, 130, 200, and 325 mg; tablets, 325 mg.

Usual Dosages

Intravenous: Adults, 600 mg every 8 hours until a clinical response is obtained (usually at least 3 days).
Oral: For treatment of chloroquine-resistant *P. falciparum* malaria, adults, 650 mg every 8 hours for 14 days in combination with pyrimethamine and sulfadiazine.

RABIES IMMUNE GLOBULIN (RIG)

Proprietary Name: Hyperab.

Preparations

Injection: Vial, 2 ml (300 IU) and 10 ml (1500 IU).

Usual Dosages

Intramuscular: 20 IU/kg; half of materials should be infiltrated around the wound if possible. Used in conjunction with 14 or 21 doses of rabies vaccine; when this serum is used for immediate delivery of preformed antibody, a total of 21 doses of rabies vaccine is preferred, either as 21 daily doses or 14 doses in the first 7 days followed by 7 daily doses; three booster doses of vaccine follow: one 10 days after completion of the series, the second 20 days later, and the third 90 days later.

RABIES VACCINE

Proprietary Name: Rabies Vaccine.

Preparations

Injection: Powder.

---

*Route of administration not approved by FDA.
† Drug not approved by FDA for any indication.
‡ Drug not approved by FDA for this particular indication.
§ Indicated dosage above the manufacturer's recommendation.

Usual Dosages

Subcutaneous: Adults and child for pre-exposure immunoprophylaxis, two 1-ml doses administered in outer aspect of the upper arm at approximately 1-month intervals, followed by booster dose after 6 or 7 months; booster doses repeated until antibody response detectable; persons in high-risk occupations should be given booster dose at least every 2 years; if bitten by rabid animal, five daily doses of vaccine, followed by booster dose 20 days after last injection. For postexposure immunoprophylaxis, when given without rabies immune globulin or antiserum, 14 daily injections should be administered, using doses recommended by manufacturer; when given with rabies immune globulin or antiserum, 21 doses are administered; these may be given as 21 daily doses or 14 doses during the first 7 days and then 7 daily doses; three supplemental doses of vaccine should be given 10, 20, and 90 days after completion of 14- or 21-day course.

RANITIDINE

Proprietary Names: Azantac (Fr.), Coralen (Span.), Mauran (Ital.), Nodol (Ital.), Novoranidine (Canad.), Quantor (Span.), Ran H2 (Span.), Raniben (Ital.), Ranibloc (Ital.), Ranidil (Ital.), Ranidin (Span.), Ranilonga (Span.), Raniplex (Fr.), Ranix (Span.), Ranuber (Span.), Sostril (Ger.), Tanidina (Span.), Terposen (Span.), Toriol (Span.), Trigger (Ital.), Ulcex (Ital.), Ulkobrin (Ital.), Zantac (Austral., Canad., G.B., Ire., Ital., Neth., S. Afr., Span., Swed., USA), Zantic (Ger., Switz.).

Preparations

Injection: Solution, 25 mg/ml.
Oral: Syrup, tablets, 150 and 300 mg.

Usual Dosages

Injection, Intramuscular or Intravenous: 50 mg every 6 to 8 hours.
Oral: 150 mg or 10 ml (2 tsp equivalent to 150 mg) twice daily; tablets, 300 mg once daily or 150 mg twice daily.

RETINOL

See Vitamin A.

RIFAMPIN (RIFAMPICIN)

Proprietary Names: Rifa (Germ.), Rimactane, Rifadin.

Preparations

Oral: Capsules, 300 mg.
Topical Ophthalmic: Ointment, 1 per cent.

Usual Dosages

Oral: Adults, 600 mg in a single daily administration. In serious infections, a maximum daily dose of 1.2 gm may be given. Children, 10 to 20 mg/kg (not to exceed 600 mg) daily.
Topical Ophthalmic: Ointment preparation may be applied two to three times daily.

SALICYLATES

See Aspirin, Sodium Salicylate.

SCOPOLAMINE (HYOSCINE)

Proprietary Names: Isopto Hyoscine, Scopolamina Lux (Ital.), Scopos (Fr.).

Preparations

Injection: Solution, 0.3, 0.4, 0.5, 0.6, and 1 mg/ml.
Oral: Tablets, 0.4 and 0.6 mg.
Topical Ophthalmic: Ointment, 0.2 per cent; solution, 0.2, 0.25, 0.3, 0.5, and 1.0 per cent.

Usual Dosages

Intramuscular: Adults, 0.4 mg; infants 4 to 7 months, 0.1 mg; 7 months to 3 years, 0.15 mg; 3 to 8 years, 0.2 mg; 8 to 12 years, 0.3 mg.
Oral, Subcutaneous: Adults, 0.6 to 1 mg; children, 0.006 mg/kg.
Topical Ophthalmic: One drop applied in the eyes three to four times daily or more frequently if required.

SELEGILINE

Proprietary Names: Eldeprine (Fr.), Eldepryl (G.B., Neth., S. Afr., Swed., USA), Jumex (Ital.), Jumexal (Switz.), Movergan (Ger.), Plurimen (Span.).

Preparations

Oral: Tablets, 5 mg.

Usual Dosages

Oral: The recommended dosage is 10 mg daily administered as divided doses of 5 mg each taken at breakfast and lunch.

SELENIUM

Proprietary Names: Selenitrace, Selepen.

Preparations

Injection: 40 and 50 µg/ml in 10- and 30-ml vials.

Usual Dosages

Intravenous: Adults, recommended daily intake is 20 to 50 µg. In deficiency states, 100 µg daily for 1 month reverses the deficiency symptoms without toxicity.

SILVER NITRATE (ARGENTUM NITRATE, CREDE'S SOLUTION)

Proprietary Name: Mova Nitrat (Germ.).

Preparations

Topical Ophthalmic: Solution, 0.5, 0.67 and 1 per cent.

Usual Dosages

Topical Ophthalmic: One drop may be applied to each eye.

SITOSTEROLS

Proprietary Name: Cytellin.

Preparations

Oral: Suspension, 3 gm/15 ml.

Usual Dosages

Oral: Adults, 12 to 24 gm daily, given in divided doses immediately before meals.

SODIUM ASCORBATE

Proprietary Names: Cenolate, Cevita.

Preparations

Injection: Solution, 250 and 562.5 mg/ml.
Oral: Crystals, 1020 mg/1.25 ml; powder, 1020 mg/1.25 ml; tablets, 585 mg.

Usual Dosages

Intramuscular, Intravenous, Oral: Adults, the average protective dose is 70 to 150 mg daily. For scurvy, 0.3 to 1.0 gm daily is recommended. To enhance wound healing, 300 to 500 mg daily for 7 to 10 days both preoperatively and postoperatively are adequate. For severe burns, 1.0 to 2.0 gm daily is recommended until healing has occurred or grafting operations are complete.

SODIUM AUROTHIOMALATE

See Gold Sodium Thiomalate.

SODIUM CHLORIDE

Proprietary Names: Adsorbonac, Hyperopto, Hypersal, Muro-128, Ocean, Ocurins.

Preparations

Injection: Solution 0.45, 0.9, 3, and 5 per cent.
Topical Ophthalmic: Ointment, 5 per cent; solution, 2 and 5 per cent.

Usual Dosages

Intravenous: Adults and children, as required to correct dehydration and increase calcium excretion.
Topical Ophthalmic: One drop in eye(s) every 3 or 4 hours. Ointment may be applied as necessary as directed by the physican.

SODIUM CITRATE/CITRIC ACID COMBINATION

Proprietary Name: Bicitra.

Preparations

Oral: Liquid, 500 mg sodium citrate and 334 mg citric acid/5 ml.

---

*Route of administration not approved by FDA.
† Drug not approved by FDA for any indication.
‡ Drug not approved by FDA for this particular indication.
§ Indicated dosage above the manufacturer's recommendation.

Usual Dosages

Oral: Adults, 10 to 30 ml diluted in 30 to 90 ml water after meals and at bedtime.

SODIUM HYALURONATE

Proprietary Names: Connettivina (Germ., Ital.), Healon.

Preparations

Injection: Syringes, 10 mg/ml.
Topical Ophthalmic: No ophthalmic preparation is commercially available. The preparation intended for injection may be used to obtain the desired concentration.

Usual Dosages

Incracameral: A sufficient amount is slowly and carefully introduced.
Topical Ophthalmic: For treatment of keratoconjunctivitis sicca, 0.1 to 0.2 per cent may be applied two to four times daily or more frequently if needed.

SODIUM IODIDE[131]

Proprietary Names: Iodotope I-131, Oriodide-131, Theriodide-131.

Preparations

Oral: Capsules, 1, 3, 5, 6, 7, 8, 9, and 10 millicuries; solution, 1 to 200 millicuries.

Usual Dosages

Oral: For treatment of suitable patients with Graves' disease and hyperthyroidism, the usual dose is 4 to 10 millicuries. If the first treatment is not successful, retreatment after an interval of 3 or 4 months is usually recommended. Larger doses are required for suitable patients with toxic nodular goiter.

SODIUM PENICILLIN G

Proprietary Names: Gonopen (N.Z.), Novopen (S. Afr.), Specilline (Fr.).

Preparations

Injection: Powder (for solution), 1 and 5 million units.
Topical Ophthalmic: Ointment, 1000 units/gm.

Usual Dosages

Intracameral: 1000 to 4000 units in 0.2 to 0.5 ml of isotonic sodium chloride injection.

Intravenous: Adults, 8 to 20 million units daily; children, 200,000 to 400,000 units/kg daily in four divided doses; premature and full-term newborn infants, 40,000 to 80,000 units/kg daily in four divided doses.

Subconjunctival: 500,000 to 1 million units in 0.5 ml of isotonic sodium chloride injection or sterile water for injection.

Topical Ophthalmic: Ointment may be used several times daily. Fortified sodium penicillin G eyedrops are prepared by adding 15 to 600 mg (25,000 to 1 million units) with 50 mg of sodium citrate and 0.002 per cent phenylmercuric nitrate to 10 ml sterile water for injection.

SODIUM SALICYLATE

Proprietary Names: Alysine, Ancosal (Austral.), Ensalate (Austral.), Enterosalicyl (Fr., Swed.), Enterosalyl (G.B.), Idocyl (Swed.), Klev (Canad.), Rhumax (Austral.), Uracel.

Preparations

Oral: Tablets, 300 and 600 mg.

Usual Dosages

Oral: 600 mg every 4 to 6 hours as necessary (range, 300 mg to 4 gm daily).

SODIUM STIBOGLUCONATE

See Stibogluconate Sodium.

SPECTINOMYCIN

Proprietary Names: Actinospectacin, Trobicin.

Preparations

Injection: Powder, 2 and 4 gm (supplied with 3.5 and 6.5 ml of diluent, respectively).

Usual Dosages

Intramuscular: Adults, 2 to 4 gm. The larger doses are indicated for retreatment af-

ter other antibiotic therapy has failed or for patients living in areas where resistance to penicillin is known to be prevalent. The larger dose should be divided between two gluteal injection sites.

SPIRAMYCIN

Proprietary Names: Rovamycin (G.B.), Selectomycin (Germ.).

Preparations

Oral: Syrup, 125 mg/5 ml; tablets, 250 mg.

Usual Dosages

Oral: 2 to 4 gm daily in divided doses.

SPIRONOLACTONE

Proprietary Name: Aldactone.

Preparations

Oral: Tablets, 25 mg.

Usual Dosages

Oral: Adults, 50 to 100 mg daily; children, 3.3 mg/kg daily in divided doses.

STIBOCAPTATE

Proprietary Name: Astiban (G.B.).

Preparations

Injection: Powder, 0.5 and 10 gm.

Usual Dosages

Intramuscular: A 10 per cent solution is prepared in water for injection and should be used in 24 hours if unrefrigerated; refrigerated solution may be used if colorless and clear. The total dose is divided into five equal amounts and given once or twice a week or, in hospitalized patients, as often as every day, depending upon tolerance of patient. Adults, 40 mg/kg in five divided doses; children 6 years and older, 50 mg/kg in five divided doses.

STIBOGLUCONATE SODIUM

Proprietary Name: Pentostam.

' Route of administration not approved by FDA.
[†] Drug not approved by FDA for any indication.
[‡] Drug not approved by FDA for this particular indication.
[§] Indicated dosage above the manufacturer's recommendation.

Preparations

Injection: Solution, 330 mg/ml.

Usual Dosages

Intramuscular, Intravenous (Slow): A course of treatment consists of six to ten daily injections, each of 6 ml, repeated if necessary on two occasions after 10-day intervals.

STREPTOKINASE

Proprietary Names: Kabikinase, Streptase.

Preparations

Injection: Powder, 100,000, 250,000, 600,000 and 750,000 IU.

Usual Dosages

Intravenous: A loading dose of 250,000 IU is administered over a 30-minute period. After the loading dose, a maintenance infusion is given for 24 to 72 hours.

STREPTOMYCIN

Proprietary Names: Darostrep (S. Afr.), Isoject-Streptomycin Injection, Novostrep (S. Afr.), Orastrep (G.B.), Strepolin (Austral., S. Afr.), Streptevan (Austral.), Strept-evanules (Austral.), Streptosol (Canad., S. Afr.), Strycin.

Preparations

Injection: Powder (for solution), 1 and 5 gm; solution, 200, 400, and 500 mg/ml.

Usual Dosages

Intramuscular: Adults, 0.5 to 2 gm daily in two divided doses for 7 to 10 days and 1 gm daily thereafter for no longer than 3 weeks. Children, 20 to 30 mg/kg daily in divided doses. In severe infections, 2 to 4 gm daily (adults) or 20 to 40 mg/kg (children) in divided doses every 6 to 12 hours.

---

*Route of administration not approved by FDA.
† Drug not approved by FDA for any indication.
‡ Drug not approved by FDA for this particular indication.
§ Indicated dosage above the manufacturer's recommendation.

SUCCINYLCHOLINE (SUXAMETHONIUM)

Proprietary Names: Anectine, Brevidil E/M (G.B.), Celocurin-Klorid (Swed.), Lysthenon (Germ.), Pantolax (Germ.), Quelicin, Scoline (Austral., Canad., S. Afr.), Succinyl (Germ.), Sucostrin, Sux-Cert.

Preparations

Injection: Powder, 0.5 and 1.0 gm; solution, 20 mg/ml.

Usual Dosages

Intramuscular: The usual dosage is 2.5 mg/kg, but single doses should not exceed 150 mg.
Intravenous: For short procedures, 10 to 30 mg given over 10 to 30 seconds. Up to 80 mg may be required by some patients.

SULFACETAMIDE

Proprietary Names: Acetopt (Austral.), Ak-Sulf, Albucid (G.B.), Bleph-10, Cetamide, Isopto Cetamide, Ocu-Sul-10/15/30, Op-Sulfa, Optamide (Austral.), Optiole S (Canad.), Sulamyd, Sulf-10, Sulfacel, Sulfair, Sulphacalyre (G.B.), Sulphacetamide (G.B.), Sulten-10, Vasosulf (G.B.).

Preparations

Topical Ophthalmic: Ointment, 10 and 30 per cent; solution, 10, 15, and 30 per cent.

Usual Dosages

Topical Ophthalmic: For acute cases, frequent administration of 10 or 15 per cent solution every 10 to 30 minutes. For chronic cases, 10 per cent ointment applied three or four times daily or 30 per cent solution three or four times daily in combination with 10 per cent ointment used at bedtime.

SULFADIAZINE

Proprietary Names: Adiazine (Fr.), Coco-Diazine, Diazyl (Austral.), Microsulfon, Solu-Diazine (Canad.), Sulfadets (Canad.), Sulphadiazine (G.B.).

Preparations

Oral: Suspension, 500 mg/5 ml; tablets, 500 mg; tablets (chewable), 300 mg.

Usual Dosages

Oral: The usual loading dose in adults is 2 to 4 gm, with a maintenance dose of 2 to 4 gm daily in three to six divided doses. For treatment of chloroquine-resistant *P. falciparum* malaria, adults, 2 gm daily for the first 6 days of therapy with pyrimethamine and quinine. For ocular toxoplasmosis, adults, 4 gm daily in four divided doses for 1 to 3 weeks, then 2 gm daily in four divided doses until a total of 6 weeks of therapy has been completed.

SULFAFURAZOLE

See Sulfisoxazole.

SULFALENE

Proprietary Names: Kelfizina (Arg., Belg., Ital., Neth.), Kelfizine (G.B.), Longum (Arg., Belg., Germ., Neth.), Policydal (Jap.).

Preparations

Oral: Suspension, 100 mg/ml in 10- and 20-ml bottles; tablets for suspension, 2 gm.

Usual Dosages

Oral: In adults, 2 gm once a week in a single dose. For children, the dose is 30 mg/kg once a week.

SULFAMETHOXAZOLE

Proprietary Name: Gantanol.

Preparations

Oral: Suspension, 500 mg/5 ml; tablets, 500 mg.

Usual Dosages

Oral: Adults, 2 gm initially, then 1 gm two or three times daily. Children over 2 months of age, initially 60 mg/kg (maximum, 2 gm), then half of this amount every 12 hours.

Route of administration not approved by FDA.
† Drug not approved by FDA for any indication.
‡ Drug not approved by FDA for this particular indication.
§ Indicated dosage above the manufacturer's recommendation.

SULFAMETHOXAZOLE/ TRIMETHOPRIM COMBINATION

See Trimethoprim/Sulfamethoxazole Combination.

SULFASALAZINE

Proprietary Names: Azulfidine, Salazopyrin, Salazopyrine (Fr.), Salicylazosulfapyridine, S.A.S.-500, S.A.S.P., Sulcolon, Sulphasalazine (G.B.).

Preparations

Oral: Tablets, 500 mg.

Usual Dosages

Oral: Initially, adults, 1 to 4 gm daily in four to eight divided doses; for maintenance, up to 2 gm daily in four divided doses. To prevent attacks of chronic ulcerative colitis, 3 gm may be necessary daily in divided doses.

SULFINPYRAZONE

Proprietary Names: Anturan (Agr., Austral., Belg., Canad., Denm., G.B., S. Afr., Span., Switz.), Anturane, Anturano (Germ.), Enturen (Ital., Neth.), Zynol (Canad.).

Preparations

Oral: Capsules, 200 mg; tablets, 100 mg.

Usual Dosages

Oral: Dose range, 200 to 800 mg daily.

SULFISOXAZOLE (SULFAFURAZOLE)

Proprietary Names: Gantrisin, Gantrisine (Fr.), Lipo Gantrisin, Novosoxazole (Canad.), SK-Soxazole, Sosol, Soxomide, Sulfagen (Canad.), Sulfalar, Sulfizin, Sulfizole (Canad.), Sulphafurazole (G.B.), US-67 (Canad.).

Preparations

Oral: Liquid (timed-release), 1 gm/5 ml; suspension (pediatric), 500 mg/5 ml; syrup, 500 mg/5 ml; tablets, 500 mg.
Topical Ophthalmic: Ointment, 4 per cent; solution, 4 per cent.

Usual Dosages

Oral: Adults, 2 to 4 gm initially, then 1 to 2 gm every 4 to 6 hours.
Topical Ophthalmic: Ointment is applied three or four times daily.

SULINDAC

Proprietary Names: Arthrocine (Fr.), Artribid (Port.), Citireuma (Ital.), Clinoril, Imbaral (Germ.).

Preparations

Oral: Tablets, 150 and 200 mg.

Usual Dosages

Oral: The usual maximum dosage is 400 mg/day.

SUPROFEN

Proprietary Name: Surfrex (Belg.).

Preparations

Topical Ophthalmic: No commercial preparation is available, but a 0.5 per cent solution may be prepared.

Usual Dosages

Topical Ophthalmic: Solution may be administered three to four times daily.

SUXAMETHONIUM

See Succinylcholine.

TERBUTALINE

Proprietary Names: Brethine, Bricanyl (G.B.), Bristurin (Jap.), Feevone (Austral.), Filair (G.B.), Terbasmin (Ital., Span.).

Preparations

Injection: Solution, 1 mg/ml.
Oral: Tablets, 2.5 and 5 mg.

Usual Dosages

Oral: Adults, initially, 2.5 mg three times daily at approximately 8-hour intervals, increased gradually over a period of 2 to 4 weeks to 5 mg three times daily. Children 12 years and under, 1.25 to 2.5 mg three times daily at approximately 6- to 8-hour intervals, increasing the dose, if needed and tolerated, to a maximum of 5 mg daily.
Subcutaneous: Adults, 0.25 mg repeated in 15 to 30 minutes if necessary; no more than 0.5 mg should be administered in any 4-hour period. Children, 0.01 mg/kg (maximum total dose, 0.25 mg). The dose may be repeated once in 30 minutes if necessary, but usually is effective for 4 hours.

TERFENADINE

Proprietary Name: Seldane.

Preparations

Oral: Tablets, 60 mg.

Usual Dosages

Oral: Adults, 60 mg twice daily.

TETANUS AND DIPHTHERIA TOXOIDS (TD) ADSORBED

Proprietary Names: Tetanus and Diphtheria Toxoid.

Preparations

Injection: 5 Lf units tetanus toxoid and 1.4, 1.5, or 2 Lf units diphtheria toxoid/0.5 ml or 10 Lf units tetanus toxoid and 2 Lf units diphtheria toxoid/0.5 ml.

Usual Dosages

Intramuscular: Adults and children, 7 years and older, two injections of 0.5 ml with an interval of at least 4 weeks between injections. A reinforcing dose to complete basic immunization is given 6 to 12 months later and every 10 years thereafter.

TETANUS ANTITOXIN (EQUINE OR BOVINE)

Proprietary Name: Tetanus Antitoxin.

Preparations

Injection: Ampules of 1500, 10,000, 15,000, and 50,000 units.

Usual Dosages

Intramuscular: Adults and children, for prophylaxis 5000 to 10,000 units within 24 hours after injury. If 48 hours have elapsed between the time of injury and treatment, a dose of 10,000 to 20,000 units is recommended.

Intravenous: Adults and children, for treatment, 40,000 to 100,000 units or more.

TETANUS IMMUNE GLOBULIN (TIG)

Proprietary Names: Homo-Tet, Hyper-Tet, Tet-Conn-G.

Preparations

Injection: Syringe, 250 unit; vial, 250 unit.

Usual Dosages

Intramuscular: For prophylaxis, adults and children, 250 units as a single dose. For treatment, the optimal therapeutic dose has not been established; 3000 to 6000 units are usually cited, but doses as large as 10,000 units have been used.

TETANUS TOXOID

Proprietary Names: Tetanol (Germ.), Tetatoxoid (Germ.), Tetavax (Fr.), T-Immun (Germ.).

Preparations

Injection: Ampules, 0.5 ml; vials, 5 ml.

Usual Dosages

Intramuscular: Adults and children, 0.5 ml for three injections; second injection given 4 to 6 weeks after first, and third given 6 months to 1 year after second. A booster dose is given every 10 years.

TETRACYCLINE

Proprietary Names: Achromycin, Ambramycin-P (S. Afr.), Amer-Tet, Amtet, Austramycin (Austral.), Bicycline, Bristacycline, Bristrex, Capcycline (S. Afr.), Cefracycline (Canad.), Centet, Chemcycline (Canad.), Co-

---

* Route of administration not approved by FDA.
† Drug not approved by FDA for any indication.
‡ Drug not approved by FDA for this particular indication.
§ Indicated dosage above the manufacturer's recommendation.

Caps, Tetracycline (G.B.), Cycline, Cyclopar, Decabiotic (Canad.), Decycline (Canad.), Dema, Desamycin, Dumocyclin (Swed.), Economycin (G.B.), Fed-Mycin, Fermentmycin (S. Afr.), Florocycline (Fr.), Gene-Cycline (Canad.), G-Mycin, GT250/500 (Canad.), GT-Liquid (Canad.), Hexacycline (Fr.), Hostacyclin (Germ.), Hostacycline (Austral., S. Afr.), Hydracycline (Austral.), Kesso-Tetra, Lemtrex, Lexacycline, Maso-Cycline, Maytrex, Mericycline, Miriamycine (Fr.), Muracine (Canad.), Neo-tetrine (Canad.), Nor-Tet, Novotetra (Canad.), Oppacyn (G.B.), Paltet, Panmycin, Partrex, Pexobiotic (Canad.), Phosmycine (S. Afr.), Piracaps, Polycycline, QIDtet, Quadcin (N.Z.), Quadracycline-V (Austral.), Quatrax (Austral.), Retet, Rexamycin, Robitet, Ro-Cycline, Sanclomycine (Fr.), Sarocycline, Scotrex, Sifacycline (Fr.), SK-Teteracycline, Steclin, Sumycin, Supramycin N (Germ.), Sustamycin (G.B.), Svedocyklin (Swed.), T-125/250, T-Caps, Tet-Cy, Tetrabiotic (Canad.), Tetra-C, Tetracap (Austral., Canad.), Tetrachel, Tetracitro S (Germ.), Tetraclor, Tetra-Co, Tetracrine (Canad.), Tetracyn, Tetracyne (Fr.), Tetradecin Novum (Swed.), Tetral (Canad.), Tetralan, Tetralean (Canad.), Tetralution (Germ.), Tetram, Tetramax, Tetramykoin (Austral.), Tetrex, Tetrosol (Canad.), T-Liquid (Canad.), Totomycin (G.B.), Trexin, Triacycline (Canad.), T-Tabs (Canad.), U-Tet, Wintracin (Canad.).

Preparations

Injection: Solution 100, 250, and 500 mg.
Oral: Capsules, 100, 125, 250, and 500 mg; syrup, 125 mg/5 ml; tablets, 50, 100, 125, and 250 mg.
Topical: Powder with diluent to make solution, 2.2 mg/ml.
Topical Ophthalmic: Ointment, 1 and 3 per cent; suspension in oil, 1 per cent.

Usual Dosages

Intramuscular: Children, 25 mg/kg daily in four divided doses (intravenous route preferred). This route should not be used in newborn infants.
Intravenous: Children, 15 mg/kg daily in four divided doses. This route should not be used in newborn infants.
Oral: Adults, 1 to 4 gm daily divided into three to four doses.
Subconjunctival: 2.5 to 5.0 mg in 0.5 ml of isotonic sodium chloride injection.
Topical: 0.5 to 1.0 ml of the prepared solution is applied twice daily.
Topical Ophthalmic: One drop of a 0.5 per cent solution is instilled every 30 minutes to 2 hours. Solutions should be freshly prepared every 24 to 48 hours and kept refrigerated. Ointment may be applied directly to the affected area every 2 hours or more often, as the severity of the infection and the degree of

response indicate. Severe or stubborn ocular infections may require treatment for many days.

TETRAHYDROZOLINE

Proprietary Names: Murine Plus, Soothe, Tetracon, Visine.

Preparations

Topical Ophthalmic: Solution, 0.05 per cent.

Usual Dosages

Topical Ophthalmic: One or two drops are instilled every 2 to 3 hours or as needed until symptoms subside.

THIABENDAZOLE

Proprietary Names: Mintezol, Minzolum (Germ.).

Preparations

Oral: Suspension, 500 mg/5 ml; tablets (chewable), 500 mg.
Topical Ophthalmic: No ophthalmic preparation is commercially available. A 1 to 4 per cent solution in a cremophore base or in arachnis oil may be prepared.

Usual Dosages

Oral: 25 to 100 mg/kg, up to a maximum of 3 gm, in two divided doses daily, for 2 to 7 days.
Topical Ophthalmic: Solution is applied to affected and surrounding areas twice a day.

THIAMINE (VITAMIN B₁)

Proprietary Names: B-1, Betalin S, Bewon.

Preparations

Oral: Tablets, 100, 250, and 500 mg.

---

*Route of administration not approved by FDA.
† Drug not approved by FDA for any indication.
‡ Drug not approved by FDA for this particular indication.
§ Indicated dosage above the manufacturer's recommendation.

Usual Dosages

Oral: For thiamine deficiency syndromes, 5 to 10 mg three times daily.

THIOTEPA

Proprietary Names: Thio-Tepa (G.B.), Tifosyl (Swed.).

Preparations

Injection: Vial, 15 mg.

Usual Dosages

Topical Ophthalmic: For the treatment of pterygium, a solution of 0.05 per cent may be administered to the eye every 3 hours during the waking period for 6 to 8 weeks.

THROMBIN

Proprietary Names: Thrombinar, Thrombostat.

Preparations

Topical: Powder, 1000, 5000, 10,000, and 20,000 units.

Usual Dosages

Topical: For general use, concentrations of 1000 units/10 ml are used on the bleeding site. When bleeding is profuse, concentrations as high as 1000 to 2000 units/ml may be required.

THYROGLOBULIN

Proprietary Names: Proloid, Thyractin.

Preparations

Oral: Tablets, 16, 32, 65, 100, 130, 200, and 325 mg (1 gr = 65 mg).

Usual Dosages

Oral: Dosage should be started in small amounts and increased gradually with increments at intervals of 1 to 2 weeks. Usual maintenance dose is 0.5 to 3.0 gr (32 to 200 mg) daily.

TICARCILLIN

Proprietary Names: Aerugipen (Germ.), Tarcil (Austral.), Ticar, Ticarpen (Neth., Switz.).

Preparations

Injection: Powder, 1, 3, and 6 gm (equivalent to base).

Usual Dosages

Intramuscular, Intravenous: The usual adult dose in the treatment of severe gram-negative infections is the equivalent of 15 to 25 gm daily in divided doses every 4 to 8 hours, although 3 gm may be given every 3 hours in very severe infection. Children may be given 200 to 300 mg/kg daily in divided doses. In the treatment of uncomplicated urinary tract infections, the usual dosage is equivalent to 3 to 4 gm in divided doses daily intramuscularly or by slow intravenous infusion.

TIMOLOL

Proprietary Names: Timoptic, Timoptol (Austral., Fr., G.B., Neth., N.Z., S. Afr.).

Preparations

Topical Ophthalmic: Solution, 0.25 and 0.5 per cent.

Usual Dosages

Topical Ophthalmic: One drop of solution may be applied to each eye twice daily. If systemic side effects occur, punctal occlusion should be done.

TISSUE PLASMINOGEN ACTIVATOR

See Alterplase, Streptokinase, Urokinase.

TITANIUM DIOXIDE

Proprietary Names: Titanium Dioxide.

Preparations

Topical: Ointment, 20 per cent; paste, 20 per cent.

---

* Route of administration not approved by FDA.
† Drug not approved by FDA for any indication.
‡ Drug not approved by FDA for this particular indication.
§ Indicated dosage above the manufacturer's recommendation.

Usual Dosages

Topical: Preparation may be applied two or three times daily as needed.

TOBRAMYCIN

Proprietary Names: Brulamycin (Hung.), Gernebcin (Germ.), Nebcina (Denm. Norw., Swed.), Nebcin, Nebcine (Fr.), Nebicina (Ital.), Obracin (Belg., Neth., Switz.), Tobra (Arg.), Tobracin (Jap.), Tobradistin (Span.), Tobrex.

Preparations

Injection: Solution, 10 to 40 mg/ml.
Topical Ophthalmic: Ointment, 0.3 per cent; solution, 0.3 per cent.

Usual Dosages

Intramuscular, Intravenous: According to the severity of infection, a total daily dose of 3 to 5 mg/kg is usually given in equally divided amounts every 8 hours. Daily dosage should not exceed 5 mg/kg unless serum levels are monitored.
Subconjunctival: 2.5 to 40 mg in 0.5 ml of isotonic sodium chloride injection or sterile water for injection.
Topical Ophthalmic: In mild to moderate disease, drug may be instilled two to three times daily. In severe infections, hourly applications may be used until improvement, after which treatment should be reduced before discontinuation. Fortified tobramycin eyedrops may be prepared to produce a concentration of 15 mg/ml.

TOLBUTAMIDE

Proprietary Names: Arcosal (Denm.), Artosin (Austral., Germ. S. Afr., Swed.), Chembutamide (Canad.), Dolipol (Fr.), Insilange-D (Jap.), Ipoglicone (Ital.), Mellitol (Canad.), Mobenol (Canad.), Neo-Dibetic (Canad.). Nigloid (Jap.), Novobutamide (Canad.), Oramide (Canad.), Oribetic, Orinase, Pramidex (G.B.), Rastinon (G.B.), SK-Tolbutamide, Tolbutol (Canad.), Tolbutone (Canad.), Wescotol (Canad.).

Preparations

Oral: Tablets, 500 mg.

Usual Dosages

Oral: Dosages should be individualized. Usual dose is 500 mg twice daily with a range of 0.25 to 3 gm daily.

TOLMETIN

Proprietary Names: Tolectin, Tolmex (Ital.).

Preparations

Oral: Capsules, 400 mg; tablets, 200 mg.

Usual Dosages

Oral: The recommended starting dose for adults is 400 mg three times daily, preferably including a dose on arising and a dose at bedtime.

TOLNAFTATE

Proprietary Names: Aftate, Focusan (Swed.), Sporiderm (Fr.), Sporiline (Fr.), Tinacidin (Austral.), Tinactin, Tonoftal (Germ.).

Preparations

Topical: Cream, 1 per cent; gel, 1 per cent; powder, 1 per cent; solution, 1 per cent.

Usual Dosages

Topical: One to two drops of solution or a small amount of cream or powder is rubbed into lesions twice daily for 2 to 3 weeks.

TRAZODONE

Proprietary Names: Deprax (Span.), Desyrel, Molipaxin (G.B., Ire., S. Afr.), Pragmarel (Fr.), Thombran (Ger.), Trazolan (Neth.), Trialodine, Trittico (Ital., Switz.).

Preparations

Oral: Tablets, 50, 100, 150, and 300 mg.

Usual Dosages

Oral: Initial dose of 150 mg daily in divided doses. May be increased by 50 mg/day every 3 to 4 days. Maximum dose should not exceed 400 mg/day in divided doses. Dosage during prolonged maintenance therapy should be kept at the lowest effective level.

---

*Route of administration not approved by FDA.

† Drug not approved by FDA for any indication.

‡ Drug not approved by FDA for this particular indication.

§ Indicated dosage above the manufacturer's recommendation.

TRANEXAMIC ACID

Proprietary Names: Amcacid (Ital.), Amchafibrin (Span.), Anvitoff (Germ., Switz.), Carxamin (Jap.), Cyclokapron (Arg., Belg.), Cyklokapron (Denm., G.B., Germ., Neth., Norw., S. Afr., Swed., Switz.), Exacyl (Fr.), Frenolyse (Fr.), Hexapromin (Jap.), Hexatron (Jap.), Tranex (Ital.), Tranexan (Jap.), Transamin (Jap.), Trasmalon (Jap.), Ugurol (Ital.).

Preparations

Injection: Solution, 100 mg/ml.
Oral: Syrup, 500 mg/5 ml; tablets, 500 mg.

Usual Dosages

Intravenous (Slow): 0.5 to 1.0 gm given two to three times daily over a period of at least 5 minutes.
Oral: 1.0 to 1.5 gm two to three times daily.

TRETINOIN

Proprietary Names: A-Acido (Arg.), Aberel, Aberela (Norw.), Acid A Vit (Belg., Neth.), Acnavit (Denm.), Acretin (Belg.), Airol (Arg., Austral, Denm., Germ., Ital., Norw., S. Afr., Switz.), A-vitaminsyre (Denm.), Avitoin (Norw.), Cordes VAS (Germ.), Dermairol (Swed.), Dermojuventus (Span.), Effederm (Fr.), Epi-Aberel (Germ.), Eudyna (Germ.), Retin-A.

Preparations

Topical: Cream, 0.05 and 0.1 per cent; gel, 0.01 and 0.025 per cent; liquid, 0.05 per cent.
Topical Ophthalmic: No ophthalmic preparation is commercially available. A preparation of 0.1 per cent tretinoin in arachnis oil may be made.

Usual Dosages

Topical: One application daily to the involved areas.
Topical Ophthalmic: One application of 0.1 per cent tretinoin in arachnis oil may be applied three times daily.

TRIAMCINOLONE

Proprietary Names: Acetospan, Adcortyl (G.B.), Amcort, Aristocort, Aristo-Pak, Aristosol, Aristospan, Cenocort, Cino-40, Delphicort (Germ.), Kenacomb (Austral.), Kenacort, Kenalog, Kenalone (Austral.), Ledercort (G.B.), Lederspan (G.B.), Rocinolone, SK-Triamcinolone, Solodelf (Germ.), Solutedarol (Fr.), Spencort, Tedarol (Fr.), Tracilon, Triamalone (Canad.), Triamcin, Triamcort (Ital.), Triam Forte, Triamolone, Tri-Kort, Vertalog, Volon (Germ.), Volonimat (Germ.).

Preparations

Injection: Suspension (aqueous), 10 and 40 mg/ml.
Topical: Cream, 0.025, 0.1, and 0.5 per cent; lotion, 0.025 and 0.1 per cent; ointment, 0.025 and 0.1 per cent; suspension, 0.007 and 0.1 per cent.

Usual Dosages

Intralesional: The size of the lesion determines the total amount of drug needed, the concentration used, and the number and pattern of injection sites. (For small lesions, 5 mg/2 ml divided over several locations.)
Retrobulbar: 10 to 40 mg/ml in 0.5 to 1.0 ml.
Topical: Preparation is applied three or four times daily.

TRICHLOROACETIC ACID

Proprietary Name: Trichloracetic Acid.

Preparations

Topical: Solution, 15 to 100 per cent.

Usual Dosages

Intralesional: After removal of the contents of an epithelial implantation cyst of the anterior chamber, the cyst may be injected with 10 to 20 per cent trichloroacetic acid. This is allowed to remain from 30 to 120 seconds before it is withdrawn.
Topical Ophthalmic: A 10 to 25 per cent aqueous solution has been used to cauterize the surface of the cornea in treatment of recurrent erosion, bullous keratopathy, and other painful corneal diseases. The corneal epithelium may first be scraped with a knife. The solution should be applied to the surface of the eye for 15 seconds and then flushed with water or saline.

---

* Route of administration not approved by FDA.
† Drug not approved by FDA for any indication.
‡ Drug not approved by FDA for this particular indication.
§ Indicated dosage above the manufacturer's recommendation.

TRIFLURIDINE (F₃T)

Proprietary Names: Bephen (Germ.), TFT (Neth.), Triherpine (Lux.), Viroptic.

Preparations

Topical Ophthalmic: Solution, 1 per cent.

Usual Dosages

Topical Ophthalmic: One drop in the eye(s) every 2 hours while awake until herpetic lesion is completely re-epithelialized, then one drop every 4 hours for 7 days.

TRIHEXYPHENIDYL

Proprietary Names: Anti-Spas (Austral.), Antitrem, Aparkane (Canad.), Artane, Benzhexol (G.B.), Hexyphen, Novohexidyl (Canad.), Pargitan (Germ., Swed.), Peragit (Dermn., Norw.), Pipanol, Tremin, Trihexy (Canad.), Trixyl (Canad.).

Preparations

Oral: Capsules (timed-release), 5 mg; elixir, 2 mg/5 ml; tablets, 2 and 5 mg.

Usual Dosages

Oral: The total daily dosage usually ranges between 5 and 15 mg and is administered in divided doses according to the patient's need.

TRIMEPRAZINE

Proprietary Names: Penectyl (Canad.), Repeltin (Germ.), Temaril, Theralen (Swed.), Theralene (Fr., Germ.), Vallergan (G.B.).

Preparations

Oral: Capsules (timed-release), 5 mg; syrup, 2.5 mg/5 ml; tablets, 2.5 mg.

Usual Dosages

Oral: Adults, 10 mg daily divided into two to four doses.

TRIMETHOPRIM/SULFAMETHOXAZOLE COMBINATION

Proprietary Names: Abacin (Ital.), Abactrim (Span.), Ampliespectrum (Span.), Bacterial (Ital.), Bacticel (Arg.), Bactifor (Span.), Bactramin (Jap.), Bactrim, Bactrimel (Neth.), Baktar (Jap.), Biosulten (Span.), Brogenit (Span.), Chemitrin (Ital.), Co-Trim (S. Afr.), Cotrim (Germ.), Cotrimox (G.B.), Co-Trimoxazole (G.B.), Dhas (Span.), Drylin (Germ.), Duratrimet (Germ.), Espectrin (Braz.), Eusaprim (Aust., Belg., Fin., Fr., Germ., Ital., Neth., Norw., Swed., Switz.), Fectrim (G.B.), Gantaprim (Ital.), Gantrim (Ital.), Helveprim (Switz.), Hulin (Span.), Isotrim (Ital.), Ixazolina (Span.), Kepinol (Germ.), Kitaprim (Span.), Lescot (Arg.), Magisprim (Ital.), Medixin (Ital.), Metroprin (Span.), Mezenol (S. Afr.), Microtrim (Germ.), Missile (Arg.), Nodilon (G.B.), Nopil (Switz.), Omsat (Germ.), Oxaprim (Ital.), Paitrin (Ital.), Purbac (S. Afr.), Septocid (Ital.), Septra, Septran (S. Afr.), Septrin, Sigaprim (Germ.), Sinerbactin (Span.), Soifasul (Span.), Sulfacet (Germ.), Sulfotrim (Denm., Neth., Switz.), Sulfotrimin (Germ.), Surpim (Ital.), System (Ital.), Tacumil (Span.), Teleprim (Ital.), Thoxaprim (S. Afr.), TMS (Germ.), Trib (Austral.), Trigonyl (Germ.), Trim (Ital.), Trimesulf (Ital.), Trimetoprim-Sulfa (Norw., Swed.), Trisazol (Span.), Trisural (Denm.), Ultrasept (S. Afr.), Uro-Septra (Braz.).

Preparations

Injection: Solution, 80 mg trimethoprim and 400 mg sulfamethoxazole/5 ml.
Oral: Suspension, 40 mg trimethoprim and 200 mg sulfamethoxazole/5 ml; tablets, 80 mg trimethoprim and 400 mg sulfamethoxazole or 160 mg trimethoprim and 800 mg sulfamethoxazole.
Topical Ophthalmic: No ophthalmic preparation is commercially available.

Usual Dosages

Intravenous: Total daily dose of 8 to 20 mg/kg (based on trimethoprim component) may be given in three or four equally divided doses over a period of 60 to 90 minutes.
Oral: Adults and children over 12 years of age, two tablets every 12 hours for 12 to 14 days for urinary tract infections. For severe infections, the daily amount may be increased by half and given in three divided doses. For patients with impaired renal function, the usual dose may be given initially and subsequent doses reduced by one-third to one-half with a 12-hour interval between doses.
Topical Ophthalmic: One drop of a solution containing 16 mg trimethoprim and 80 mg

---

*Route of administration not approved by FDA.
† Drug not approved by FDA for any indication.
‡ Drug not approved by FDA for this particular indication.
§ Indicated dosage above the manufacturer's recommendation.

sulfamethoxazole may be administered every 1 to 4 hours.

TRIMETHOPRIM SULFATE AND POLYMYXIN B SULFATE COMBINATION

Proprietary Names: Polytrim (G.B., Neth., S. Afr., USA).

Preparations

Topical Ophthalmic: Solution.

Usual Dosages

Topical Ophthalmic: One drop every 3 hours may be applied to the affected eye(s) up to six times daily for a period of 7 to 10 days.

TRIOXSALEN

Proprietary Name: Trisoralen.

Preparations

Oral: Tablets, 5 mg.

Usual Dosages

Oral: 20 to 80 mg daily followed by UV irradiation.

TRIPELENNAMINE

Proprietary Names: PBZ, Pyribenzamine, Ro-Hist.

Preparations

Oral: Tablets, 25 and 50 mg.

Usual Dosages

Oral: 25 to 600 mg daily.

TRISULFAPYRIMIDINES

Proprietary Names: Neotrizine, Quadetts, Quadramoid, Sulfonsol, Sulfose, Triple Sulfas, Terfonyl, Trisem.

Preparations

Oral: Suspension, 500 mg/5 ml; tablets, 500 mg.

Usual Dosages

Oral: Adults, 3 to 4 gm initially, then 1 gm every 6 hours. Children and infants over 2 months, 75 mg/kg initially, then 150 mg/kg daily in four to six divided doses.

TROPICAMIDE

Proprietary Names: Mydracyl, Mydriafair, Mydriaticum (Germ.), Myriaticum (S. Afr.), Ocu-Tropic, Tropicacyl.

Preparations

Topical Ophthalmic: Solution, 0.5 and 1 per cent.

Usual Dosages

Topical Ophthalmic: For ophthalmoscopy, one drop of 0.5 or 1 per cent tropicamide may be supplemented with 10 per cent phenylephrine. For refraction, one drop of 1 per cent tropicamide repeated in 5 minutes.

TYPHOID VACCINE

Proprietary Name: Typhoid Vaccine.

Preparations

Injection: Suspension, 8 units/ml in vials of 5, 10, and 20 ml.

Usual Dosages

Subcutaneous: For primary immunization of adults and children over 10 years of age, two doses of 0.5 ml may be administered at an interval of 4 or more weeks. For children under 10 years of age, two doses of 0.25 ml may be administered at an interval of 4 or more weeks.

UREA

Proprietary Names: Aquacare, Aqua Lacten, Carmol, Nutraplus, U-Lactin, Ureaphil, Urevert (G.B.).

---

* Route of administration not approved by FDA.
† Drug not approved by FDA for any indication.
‡ Drug not approved by FDA for this particular indication.
§ Indicated dosage above the manufacturer's recommendation.

Preparations

Injection: Powder (lyophilized), 40 and 90 gm.
Topical: Cream, 2, 10, and 20 per cent; lotion 2 and 10 per cent.

Usual Dosages

Intravenous: Adults, 0.5 to 2 gm/kg given as a 30 per cent solution, administered at a rate of 60 drops/minute. Children, 0.5 to 1.5 gm/kg infused over 30-minute period.
Topical: Preparation may be applied two or three times daily.

UROKINASE

Proprietary Names: Abbokinase, Breokinase, Win-Kinase.

Preparations

Injection: Powder, 250,000 IU.

Usual Dosages

Intravenous: Using a solution containing 50,000 IU/ml, the usual priming dose is 4400 IU/kg at a rate of 90 ml/hour for 10 minutes, followed by continuous infusion of 4400 IU/kg at a rate of 15 ml/hour for 12 hours.
Intervitreal: 25,000 IU in 0.3 ml of distilled water.

VACCINIA IMMUNE GLOBULIN (HUMAN)

Proprietary Name: Vacciniabulin (Germ.).

Preparations

Injection: A sterile solution of globulins derived from blood plasma of adult human donors who have been vaccinated against smallpox. Each 100 ml contains 15 to 19 gm of protein, of which not less than 90 per cent is globulin.

Usual Dosages

Intramuscular: Adults, prophylactic, 0.3 ml/kg; therapeutic, 0.6 ml/kg. Children, prophylactic, 0.3 to 0.5 ml/kg; therapeutic, 0.6 to 1 ml/kg.

VANCOMYCIN

Proprietary Names: Diatracin (Span.), Vancocin.

Preparations

Injection: Powder, 500 mg.
Oral: Powder, 10 gm.
Topical Ophthalmic: No ophthalmic preparation is commercially available.

Usual Dosages

Intravenous: Adults, 2 gm daily in two to four divided doses. Doses of 3 to 4 gm daily are used for seriously ill patients with normal renal function. Children, 40 mg/kg daily. The dose should be diluted with 100 to 200 ml of sodium chloride injection or 5 per cent dextrose injection and given slowly to lessen the possibility of thrombophlebitis.
Intravitreal: 0.1 to 1.0 mg in 0.1 ml of isotonic sodium chloride for injection.
Oral: Adults, maximum daily dose of 4 gm in aqueous solution in doses of 0.5 to 1.0 gm every 6 hours.
Subconjunctival: 25 mg in a 0.5 ml aqueous solution.
Topical Ophthalmic: One drop of a solution containing 50 mg/ml of vancomycin may be given every 1 to 4 hours.

VASOPRESSIN

Proprietary Name: Pitressin.

Preparations

Injection: Solution, 10 pressor units/0.5 ml.

Usual Dosages

Intramuscular, Subcutaneous: For the treatment of diabetes insipidus, the dosage is 5 to 10 units repeated two or three times daily as needed.

VERCURONIUM

Proprietary Name: Norcuron.

Preparations

Injection: Solution, 10 and 20 mg.

---

*Route of administration not approved by FDA.
† Drug not approved by FDA for any indication.
‡ Drug not approved by FDA for this particular indication.
§ Indicated dosage above the manufacturer's recommendation.

Usual Dosages

Intravenous: 0.08 to 0.10 mg/kg given as a bolus injection.

VERAPAMIL

Proprietary Names: Anpec (Austral.), Apo-Verap (Canad.), Azupamil (Ger.), Berkatens (Ire.), Calan, Cardiagutt (Ger.), Cardibeltin (Ger.), Coraver (Swed.), Cordilox (G.B.), Dignover (Ger.), Drosteakard (Ger.), Durasoptin (Ger.), Flamon (Switz.), Geangin (G.B., Neth.), Half Securon (G.B.), Isoptin (Canad., Ger., G.B., Ire., Ital., Neth., S. Afr., Swed., Switz., USA), Isoptine (Fr.), Manidon (Sp.), Novoveramil (Canad.), Praecicor (Ger.), Quasar (Ital.), Securon (G.B.), Univer (G.B.), Vasomil (S. Afr.), Veracim (Switz.), Veradil (Austral.), Veradurat (Ger.), Verahexal (Ger.), Veraloc (Swed.), Veramex (Ger.), Veranorm (Ger.), Verelan (Ire., USA), Veroptinstada (Ger.), Verpamil (S. Afr.).

Preparations

Injection: Solution, 5 and 10 mg/4 ml.
Oral: Tablets, 40, 80, and 120 mg; sustained release, 120, 180, and 240 mg.

Usual Dosages

Injection: 5 to 10 mg injected over a period of 2 to 3 minutes.
Oral: Dose is individualized based on titration.

VIDARABINE

Proprietary Name: Vira-A.

Preparations

Topical Ophthalmic: Ointment, 3 per cent.

Usual Dosages

Topical Ophthalmic: Approximately one-half inch of ointment is administered into the lower conjunctival sac five times daily at 3-hour intervals.

VINBLASTINE

Proprietary Names: Periblastine (S. Afr.), Velbe (Austral., Canad., Fr., G.B., Ger., Ital., Neth., Swed., Switz.), Velsar.

Preparations

Injection: Powder (lyophilized), 10 mg.

Usual Dosages

Intravenous: To initiate therapy for adults, 3.7 mg/square meter is administered. The following dosages are given at weekly intervals: 5.5, 7.4, 9.25, and 11.1 mg/square meter. The maximum adult dose should not exceed 18.5 mg/square meter. For most adult patients, the weekly dosage proves to be 5.5 to 7.4 mg/square meter.

VINCRISTINE

Proprietary Name: Oncovin.

Preparations

Injection: Powder, 1 and 5 mg with diluent.

Usual Dosages

Intravenous: A usual dose of 1.4 mg/square meter is recommended, with a pediatric dosage of 2 mg/square meter. Vincristine is usually administered as a single dose at weekly intervals.

VITAMIN A (RETINOL)

Proprietary Names: A 313 (Fr.), Acon, Alphalin, A-Mulsin (Germ.), Anatola (Canad.), Arovit (Fr., Germ., Swed.), Aquasol A, Atamin Forte (Austral.), Avibon (Fr.), A-Vicotrat (Germ.), Avita (S. Afr.), A-Vitan, Carotin (Austral.), Dispatabs, Fab-A-Vit (S. Afr.), Halivite (Fr.), Ido-A (Swed.), Ro-A-Vit (G.B.) Solatene, Solu-A, Vi-Alpha, Vogan (Germ.).

Preparations

Injection: Solution, 50,000 and 100,000 IU/ml.
Oral: Capsules, 5000, 25,000, 50,000, and 100,000 IU; solution (in oil), 50,000 IU/ml; tablets, 50,000, 75,000, and 150,000 IU.

Usual Dosages

Intramuscular: In severe vitamin A deficiency, adults and children over 8 years of age, 50,000 to 100,000 IU daily for 3 days, followed by 50,000 IU daily for 2 weeks.
Oral: In severe vitamin A deficiency, adults and children over 8 years, 100,000 IU daily for 3 days, followed by 50,000 IU daily for 2 weeks and 10,000 to 20,000 IU daily for another 2 months.

VITAMIN B₁

See Thiamine.

VITAMIN B₆

See Pyridoxine.

VITAMIN B COMPLEX

Proprietary Names: B-50/100/125, Becotin, Bejectal, Betalin, Mega-B, Orexin, Solu-B.

Preparations

Injection: Ampules; two separate vials of sterile solution, the contents of which when mixed provide 10 ml of solution; vials.
Oral: Pulvules, 10 mg B_1, 10 mg B_2, 4.1 mg B_6, 50 mg niacinamide, 25 mg pantothenic acid, and 1 μg B_{12}; softab, 10 mg B_1, 5 mg B_6, and 15 μg B_{12}; tablets, 100 mg B_1, 100 mg B_6, 100 μg B_{12}, 100 mg niacinamide, 100 μg folic acid, and 100 mg pantothenic acid.

Usual Dosages

Intramuscular, Intravenous: Before administration, 4 ml of solution No. 2 should be aseptically withdrawn and added to solution No. 1 vial if using two spearate vial preparations. Ordinarily 2 ml at each injection should be adequate, although 5 ml or even more may be given if indicated.
Oral: Usual dosage is one pulvule or tablet daily.

VITAMIN C

See Ascorbic Acid.

VITAMIN D₁

See Dihydrotachysterol.

VITAMIN D₂

See Ergocalciferol.

---

* Route of administration not approved by FDA.
† Drug not approved by FDA for any indication.
‡ Drug not approved by FDA for this particular indication.
§ Indicated dosage above the manufacturer's recommendation.

VITAMIN D₃

See Calcitriol or Cholecalciferol.

VITAMIN E (ALPHA-TOCOPHEROL)

Proprietary Names: Aquasol E, Dalfatol, Dextamina-E Fuerte (Span.), Dif-Vitamin E (Span.), E-Ferol, Egermol (Belg.), Eprolin, Epsilan-M, E Sir (Ital.), Esorb, Eta-Monovit (Ital.), E-Toplex, Everol (Span.), Evion (Span.), E-Vites, Fertilvit (Ital.), Godabion E (Span.), Ilitia (Ital.), Invite E (Austral.), Lan-E, Lethopherol, Na-To-Caps, Natopherol, Pertropin, Propan E (S. Afr.), Solucap E, Tocerol (Austral.), Tocopher, Tocopherex, Tocopherol, Tocovite (Austral.), Vascuals, Viteril (Ital.).

Preparations

Injection: Solution 100, 200, 220, and 500 units/ml.
Oral: Capsules, 30, 50, 100, 200, 400, 500, 600, 800, and 1000 units; elixir, 333 units/5 ml; solution, 50 units/ml; tablets, 100, 200, 300, and 400 units.
Topical: Cream, 30, 60, and 120 gm; liquid, 10, 15, 30, and 60 ml; oil, 15, 30, and 60 ml; ointment, 45 and 60 gm.

Usual Dosages

Intramuscular, Oral: Four to five times RDA in suspected deficiency.
Topical: A thin layer is applied over the affected area(s).

VITAMIN K

See Menadiol, Menadione, Phytonadione.

WARFARIN

Proprietary Names: Athrombin-K, Coumadin, Coumadine (Fr.), Marevan (G.B.), Panwarfin, Waran (Swed.), Warfilone (Canad.), Warnerin (Canad.).

Preparations

Injection: Powder (lyophilized), 50 mg with 2 ml of diluent and 75 mg with 3 ml of diluent.
Oral: Tablets, 2, 2.5, 5, 7.5, 10, and 25 mg.

---

*Route of administration not approved by FDA.
† Drug not approved by FDA for any indication.
‡ Drug not approved by FDA for this particular indication.
§ Indicated dosage above the manufacturer's recommendation.

Usual Dosages

Intramuscular, Intravenous, Oral: 30 to 50 mg initially; subsequent doses, 3 to 10 mg daily, according to prothrombin activity of the blood.

WHITE PETROLATUM

See Petrolatum.

YELLOW MERCURIC OXIDE

Proprietary Name: Yellow Mercuric Oxide.

Preparations

Topical Ophthalmic: Ointment, 1 and 2 per cent.

Usual Dosages

Topical Ophthalmic: A small quantity is applied one to two times daily.

ZALCITABINE

Proprietary Name: Hivid.

Preparations

Oral: Tablets, 0.375 and 0.750 mg.

Usual Dosages

Oral: Suggested dosage regimen is 0.75 mg three times daily by mouth, in association with zidovudine 200 mg three times daily.

ZIDOVUDINE (AZIDOTHYMIDINE, AZT)

Proprietary Name: Retrovir.

Preparations

Oral: Capsules, 100 mg.

Usual Dosages

Oral: The usual dose is 200 mg administered every 4 hours around the clock.

ZINC GLUCONATE

Proprietary Name: Zinc.

Preparations

Oral: Tablets, 10, 25, 50, and 100 mg.

Usual Dosages

Oral: As a dietary adjunct, two to three tablets daily.

ZINC OXIDE

Proprietary Names: Continuous Coverage, Covermark, Dermablend.

Preparations

Topical: Ointment, 20 per cent; paste, 25 per cent.

Usual Dosages

Topical: Preparation may be applied two to three times daily as needed.

ZINC SULFATE

Proprietary Names: Bufopto Zinc Sulfate, Medizinc, Op-Thal-Zin, Orazinc, Scrip-Zinc, Solvezinc (Autral.), Solvezink (Denm., Norw., Swed.), Verazinc, Zinc-200, Zincaps (Austral.), Zinc-Glenwood, Zincomed (G.B.), Zin-Cora, Zinc Sulphate (G.B.), Zinklet (Denm.).

Preparations

Oral: Capsules, 220 mg (50 mg zinc); tablets, 66 mg (15 mg zinc).
Topical Ophthalmic: Ointment, 0.5 per cent; solution, 0.1, 0.2, and 0.25 per cent.

Usual Dosages

Oral: 66 to 220 mg daily.
Topical Ophthalmic: Application of the solution or ointment is required two to four times a day.

---

* Route of administration not approved by FDA.
† Drug not approved by FDA for any indication.
‡ Drug not approved by FDA for this particular indication.
§ Indicated dosage above the manufacturer's recommendation.

INDEX

Note: Page numbers followed by t refer to tables.

Cercarian conjunctivitis, 135
Cerebral palsy, 271–273
Cerebrospinal fluid, absorption of, in intracranial
hypertension, 290–291
examination of, in leptospirosis, 30
in syphilis, 5–6, 16
Chalazion, differential diagnosis of, 352, 360
pathogenesis of, 563
therapy for, 563–564
Chalcosis, 371–373
Chandler's syndrome, 670–671
Chaulmoogra oil, 29
CHED, 479
Chemical conjunctivitis, 472
Chiasmal glioma, 329
Chickenpox, 111
Child. See also *Infant; Juvenile* entries.
aphakic contact lenses in, 706
aphakic glaucoma in, 656–658
cataract surgery in, 705–706
migraine in, 285, 287
pupillary block glaucoma in, 641
Chlamydia infection. See also *Conjunctivitis, inclusion;
Trachoma.*
in Reiter's syndrome, 420
ocular manifestations of, 457, 484
ophthalmia neonatorum and, 473–474
phlyctenulosis and, 510–511
Chloral hydrate, 841
Chlorambucil, 842
for anterior uveitis, 624
for Behçet's disease, 409
for juvenile arthritis, 228
for sarcoidosis, 422
side effects of, 228
Chloramphenicol, 842
contact dermatitis and, 203
for bacterial conjunctivitis, 457
for *Escherichia coli* infection, 21
for *Fusobacterium* infection, 22–23
for influenza, 26–27
for Koch-Weeks bacillus infection, 28
for orbital cellulitis, 749–750
for Rocky Mountain spotted fever, 82
for scrub typhus, 84
for typhoid fever, 55
for yersiniosis, 58
optic atrophy and, 727
side effect(s) of, bone marrow depression as, 58, 81
gastric, 23, 58, 81
hematologic, 23, 58, 81, 457
optic nerve atrophy as, 727
rash as, 58
Chlorazepate, 289
Chlordiazepoxide, 842
for pruritus, 219
Chloroquine, 842
for leishmaniasis, 121
for malaria, 130
for rheumatoid arthritis, 235
for sarcoidosis, 422
for systemic lupus erythematosus, 240
optic atrophy and, 727
side effects of, 131, 423, 727
Chlorothiazide, 843
Chlorpheniramine, 220
Chlorpromazine, 843
for herpes zoster infection, 97
for nystagmus, 547
Chlorpropamide, 843

Chlortetracycline, 843–844
for conjunctivitis, 420
Chlorthalidone, 844
for hypoparathyroidism, 148
side effects of, 412
Cholecalciferol, 844. See also *Calcitrol; Vitamin D.*
Cholestasis, intrahepatic, 217
Cholestyramine resin, 844
for fat malabsorption, 177
Cholinergic urticaria, 217, 223–224
Cholinesterase inhibitor(s), 133
Chondro-osteodystrophy, 173–174
Chorioretinopathy, birdshot, 801–802
clinical manifestations of, 804–805
therapy for, 807
central serous, 775–777
vitiliginous, 801
Choristoma, dermoid, 314–316
Choroid, angioid streaks in, 440
atrophy of, with hyperornithemia, 780–781
coloboma of, 532
concussion of, 385–386
detachment of, 441–444
hemorrhagic, 433
kissing, 442
effusion of, 442, 444
expulsive hemorrhage of, 448–450
folds in, 444–445
laceration of, 385–386
melanoma of, glaucoma with, 631, 633
malignant, 349, 450–453
metastasis to, 631
neovascular membrane of, 802–804
neovascularization of, 445–447, 776
rupture of, 386, 447–448
tumors of, macular edema and, 715t
retinal detachment and, 787
Choroidal tap, 443
Choroiditis, choroidal detachment in, 441
multifocal, 801–802
clinical manifestations of, 804
therapy for, 806–807
serpiginous, 801–802
clinical manifestations of, 803
therapy for, 807
Choroidopathy, punctate inner, 801–802
clinical manifestations of, 804
therapy for, 806–807
Chronic progressive external ophthalmoplegia, with
ragged red fibers, 274–276
Chvostek's sign, 145, 147
Chylomicronemia, 181
Chymotrypsin, 844
for ligneous conjunctivitis, 470–471
Cicatricial ectropion, 567, 569
Cicatricial entropion, 570–571
Cicatricial pemphigoid, 458–461
Cilia, in intradermal nevus, 589
loss of, 584–585
Ciliary body, accommodative spasm in, 665
block of, 646–648
concussion of, 387–388
epithelial tumors of, 632
laceration of, 387–388
melanoma of, glaucoma with, 631
malignant, 349, 450–453
metastasis to, 631, 633
Ciliary neuralgia, 277–278
Ciliary spasm, 680
Ciliochoroidal detachment, 441–444, 651

ISBN 0-7216-4913-0

90038

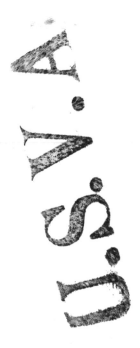